Newly Approved Medications

Naldemedine (Symproic)	An opioid antagonist for opioid-induced constipation
Naloxegol (Movantik)	Treatment of opioid induced constipation for chronic pain
Neratinib (Nerlynx)	Kinase inhibitor for extended adjuvant treatment of breast cancer
Niraparib (Zejula)	A PARP inhibitor for recurrent epithelial ovarian, fallopian tube, or primary peritoneal cancer
Ocrelizumab (Ocrevus)	A monoclonal antibody for relapsing or primary progressive forms of multiple sclerosis
Olaratumab (Lartruvo)	A PDGFR-alpha blocking antibody for soft tissue sarcoma
Plecanatide (Trulance)	A guanylate cyclase-C agonist for chronic idiopathic constipation
Ponatinib (Iclusig)	Kinase inhibitor for treatment of acute lymphoblastic and chronic myeloid leukemia
Ribociclib (Kisqali)	A kinase inhibitor for postmenopausal women with advanced breast cancer
Rucaparib (Rubraca)	An oral PARP inhibitor for certain types of advanced ovarian cancer
Safinamide (Xadago)	An MAO-B inhibitor for Parkinson's patients experiencing "off" episodes
Sarilumab (Kevzara)	Treatment of moderate to severe active rheumatoid arthritis
Sofosbuvir/velpatasvir/ voxilaprevir (Vosevi)	Fixed combination for treatment of chronic HCV genotypes 1, 2, 3, 4, 5 or 6
*Telotristat (Xermelo)	An oral tryptophan hydroxylase inhibitor for carcinoid syndrome diarrhea
Valbemazine (Ingrezza)	A selective VMATZ inhibitor for the treatment of tardive dyskinesia
Ziv-Aflibercept (Zaltrap)	Treatment of colorectal cancer, metastatic

*Featured on Evolve only

D0189700

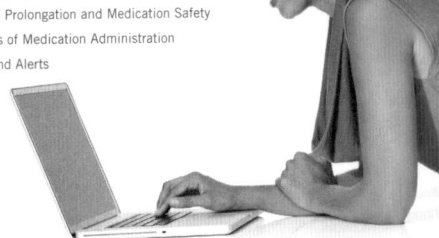

Saunders

NURSING
DRUG
HANDBOOK
2019

ROBERT J. KIZIOR, BS, RPh
Department of Pharmacy
Alexian Brothers Medical Center
Elk Grove Village, Illinois

Keith J. Hodgson, RN, BSN, CCRN
Staff Nurse, Intensive Care Unit
Former Staff Nurse, Emergency
Department
St. Joseph's Hospital
Tampa, Florida

ELSEVIER

REF
615.1
S257
2019

ELSEVIER

3251 Riverport Lane
St. Louis, Missouri 63043

SAUNDERS NURSING DRUG HANDBOOK 2019

ISBN: 978-0-323-60885-5
ISSN: 1098-8661

Notices

Practitioners and researchers must always rely on their own experience and knowledge in evaluating and using any information, methods, compounds, or experiments described herein. Because of rapid advances in the medical sciences, in particular, independent verification of diagnoses and drug dosages should be made. To the fullest extent of the law, no responsibility is assumed by Elsevier, authors, editors, or contributors for any injury and/or damage to persons or property as a matter of products liability, negligence, or otherwise, or from any use or operation of any methods, products, instructions, or ideas contained in the material herein.

ISBN: 978-0-323-60885-5

Executive Content Strategist: Sonya Seigafuse
Content Development Manager: Lisa Newton
Senior Content Development Specialist: Tina Kaemmerer, Charlene Ketchum
Publishing Services Manager: Julie Eddy
Project Manager: Mike Sheets
Design Direction: Ryan Cook

Printed in the United States of America

Last digit is the print number: 9   8   7   6   5   4   3   2   1

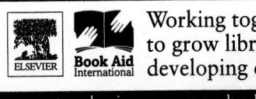

Working together
to grow libraries in
developing countries

www.elsevier.com • www.bookaid.org

CONTENTS

AUTHOR BIOGRAPHIES

Robert (Bob) J. Kizior, BS, RPh

Bob graduated from the University of Illinois School of Pharmacy and is licensed to practice in the state of Illinois. He has worked as a hospital pharmacist for more than 40 years at Alexian Brothers Medical Center in Elk Grove Village, Illinois—a suburb of Chicago. Bob is the Pharmacy Surgery Coordinator for the Department of Pharmacy, where he participates in educational programs for pharmacists, nurses, physicians, and patients. He plays a major role in coordinating pharmacy services in the OR satellite. Bob is a former adjunct faculty member at William Rainey Harper Community College in Palatine, Illinois.

An avid sports fan, Bob also has eclectic tastes in music that range from classical, big band, rock 'n' roll, and jazz to country and western. Bob spends much of his free time reviewing the professional literature to stay current on new drug information.

Keith J. Hodgson, RN, BSN, CCRN

Keith was born into a loving family in Chicago, Illinois. His mother, Barbara B. Hodgson, was an author and publisher of several medication products, and her work has been a part of his life since he was a child. By the time he was 4 years old, Keith was already helping his mother with the drug cards by stacking the draft pages that were piled up throughout their home.

Because of his mother's influence, Keith contemplated becoming a nurse in college, but his mind was fully made up after he shadowed his sister in the Emergency Department. Keith received his Associates Degree in Nursing from Hillsborough Community College and his Bachelor of Science in Nursing from the University of South Florida in Tampa, Florida. Keith started his career in the Emergency Department and now works in the Trauma/Neurological/Surgical Intensive Care Unit at St. Joseph's Hospital in Tampa, Florida.

Keith's favorite interests include music, reading, Kentucky basketball, and, if he gets the chance, watching every minute of the Olympic Games.

REVIEWERS

Janis McMillan, MSN, RN, CNE
Associate Clinical Professor
Northern Arizona University School of Nursing
Flagstaff, Arizona

Shelby Bottemiller, PharmD
Clinical Adjunct Faculty
Washington State University
Spokane, Washington

Judith L. Myers, MSN, RN
Formerly, Assistant Professor of Nursing
Grand View University
Des Moines, Iowa

CONSULTANTS*

Katherine B. Barbee, MSN, ANP, F-NP-C
Kaiser Permanente
Washington, District of Columbia

Marla J. DeJong, RN, MS, CCRN, CEN, Capt
Wilford Hall Medical Center
Lackland Air Force Base, Texas

Diane M. Ford, RN, MS, CCRN
Andrews University
Berrien Springs, Michigan

Denise D. Hopkins, PharmD
College of Pharmacy
University of Arkansas
Little Rock, Arkansas

Barbara D. Horton, RN, MS
Arnot Ogden Medical Center School of Nursing
Elmira, New York

Mary Beth Jenkins, RN, CCRN, CAPA
Elliott One Day Surgery Center
Manchester, New Hampshire

Kelly W. Jones, PharmD, BCPS
McLeod Family Medicine Center
McLeod Regional Medical Center
Florence, South Carolina

Linda Laskowski-Jones, RN, MS, CS, CCRN, CEN
Christiana Care Health System
Newark, Delaware

Jessica K. Leet, RN, BSN
Cardinal Glennon Children's Hospital
St. Louis, Missouri

Denise Macklin, BSN, RNC, CRNI
President, Professional Learning Systems, Inc.
Marietta, Georgia

Judith L. Myers, MSN, RN
Health Sciences Center
St. Louis University School of Nursing
St. Louis, Missouri

Kimberly R. Pugh, MSEd, RN, BS
Nurse Consultant
Baltimore, Maryland

Regina T. Schiavello, BSN, RNC
Wills Eye Hospital
Philadelphia, Pennsylvania

Gregory M. Susla, PharmD, FCCM
National Institutes of Health
Bethesda, Maryland

---

*The author acknowledges the work of the consultants in previous edition(s).

ACKNOWLEDGMENTS

I would like to thank my co-author Bob Kizior for his knowledge, experience, support, and friendship. We would like to give special thanks to Sonya Seigafuse, Charlene Ketchum, Julie Eddy, Mike Sheets, and the entire Elsevier team for their superior dedication, hard work, and belief in us. Without this wonderful team, none of this would be possible.

Keith J. Hodgson, RN, BSN, CCRN

DEDICATION

I dedicate my work to the practicing nurse, those aspiring to become nurses, and to all health care professionals who are dedicated to the art and science of healing.

Bob Kizior, BS, RPh

I dedicate this work to my sister, Lauren, a foundation for our family; my sister, Kathryn, for her love and support; my father, David Hodgson, the best father a son could have; my brothers-in-law, Andy and Jim, great additions to the family; the grandchildren, Paige Olivia, Logan James, Ryan James, and Dylan Boyd; to Jen Nicely for always being there; and to my band of brothers, Peter, Jamie, Miguel, Ritch, George, Jon, Domingo, Ben, Craig, Pat, and Shay.

We also make a special dedication to Barbara B. Hodgson, RN, OCN. She truly was a piece of something wonderful. Barbara often gave her love and support without needing any in return, and would do anything for a smile. Not only was she a colleague and a friend, she was also a small business owner, an artist, a dreamer, and an innovator. We hope the pride we offer in her honor comes close to what she always gave us. Her dedication and perseverance lives on.

Keith J. Hodgson, RN, BSN, CCRN

BIBLIOGRAPHY

Lexi-Comp's Drug Information Handbook, ed 26, Hudson, OH, 2017–2018, Lexi-Comp.

Medical Letter on Drugs and Therapeutics: 2016–2017, Pharmacists Letter: 2017.

Takemoto CK, Hodding JH, Kraus DM: *Lexi-Comp's Pediatric Dosage Handbook*, ed 23, Hudson, OH, 2016–2017, Lexi-Comp.

Trissel LA: *Handbook of Injectable Drugs*, ed 19, Bethesda, MD, 2016, American Society of Health-System Pharmacists.

ILLUSTRATION CREDITS

Kee JL, Hayes ER, McCuiston LE, editors: *Pharmacology: A Nursing Process Approach*, ed 7, Philadelphia, 2012, Saunders.

Mosby's GenRx, ed 12, St. Louis, 2004, Mosby.

PREFACE

Nurses are faced with the ever-challenging responsibility of ensuring safe and effective drug therapy for their patients. Not surprisingly, the greatest challenge for nurses is keeping up with the overwhelming amount of new drug information, including the latest FDA-approved drugs and changes to already approved drugs, such as new uses, dosage forms, warnings, and much more. Nurses must integrate this information into their patient care quickly and in an informed manner.

Saunders Nursing Drug Handbook 2019 is designed as an easy-to-use source of current drug information to help the busy nurse meet these challenges. What separates this book from others is that it guides the nurse through patient care to better practice and better care.

This handbook contains the following:

1. **An IV compatibility chart.** This handy chart is bound into the handbook to prevent accidental loss.
2. **The Drug Classifications section.** The action and uses for some of the most common clinical and pharmacotherapeutic classes are presented. Unique to this handbook, each class provides an at-a-glance table that compares all the generic drugs within the classification according to product availability, dosages, side effects, and other characteristics. Its half-page color tab ensures you can't miss it!
3. **An alphabetical listing of drug entries by generic name.** Red letter thumb tabs help you page through this section quickly. Information on medications that contain a Black Box Alert is an added feature of the drug entries. This alert identifies those medications for which the FDA has issued a warning that the drugs may cause serious adverse effects. Tall Man lettering, with emphasis on certain syllables to avoid confusing similar sounding/looking medications, is shown in slim red capitalized letters (e.g., *aceta**ZOLAMIDE***). High Alert drugs with a color icon 〓 are considered dangerous by The Joint Commission and the Institute for Safe Medication Practices (ISMP) because if they are administered incorrectly, they may cause life-threatening or permanent harm to the patient. The entire High Alert generic drug entry sits on a red-shaded background so that it's easy to spot! To make scanning pages easier, each new entry begins with a shaded box containing the generic name, pronunciation, trade name(s), fixed combination(s), and classification(s).
4. **A comprehensive reference section.** Appendixes include vital information on calculation of doses; controlled drugs; chronic wound care; drugs of abuse; equianalgesic dosing; herbals: common natural medicines; lifespan, cultural aspects, and pharmacogenomics of drug therapy; normal laboratory values; cytochrome P450 enzymes; antidotes or reversal agents; preventing medication errors; parenteral fluid administration; and Common Terminology Criteria for Adverse Events (CTCAE).
5. **Drugs by Disorder.** You'll find Drugs by Disorder in the front of the book for easy reference. It lists common disorders and the drugs most often used for treatment.
6. **The index.** The comprehensive index is located at the back of the book on light red pages. Undoubtedly the best tool to help you navigate the handbook, the comprehensive index is organized by showing generic drug names in **bold,** trade names in regular type, classifications in *italics,* and the page number of the main drug entry listed first and in **bold.**

A DETAILED GUIDE TO THE SAUNDERS NURSING DRUG HANDBOOK

An intensive review by consultants and reviewers helped us to revise the **Saunders Nursing Drug Handbook** so that it is most useful in both educational and clinical practice. The main objective of the handbook is to provide essential drug information in a user-friendly format. The bulk of the handbook contains an alphabetical listing of drug entries by generic name.

To maintain the portability of this handbook and meet the challenge of keeping content current, we have also included additional information for some medications on the Evolve® Internet site. Users can also choose from 100 monographs for the most commonly used medications and customize and print drug cards. Evolve® also includes drug alerts (e.g., medications removed from the market) and drug updates (e.g., new drugs, updates on existing entries). Information is periodically added, allowing the nurse to keep abreast of current drug information.

We have incorporated the IV Incompatibilities/Compatibilities ▦ heading. The drugs listed in this section are compatible or incompatible with the generic drug when administered directly by IV push, via a Y-site, or via IV piggyback. We have highlighted the intravenous drug administration and handling information with a special heading icon ▧ and have broken it down by Reconstitution, Rate of Administration, and Storage.

We present entries in an order that follows the logical thought process the nurse undergoes whenever a drug is ordered for a patient:

- What is the drug?
- How is the drug classified?
- What does the drug do?
- What is the drug used for?
- Under what conditions should you **not** use the drug?
- How do you administer the drug?
- How do you store the drug?
- What is the dose of the drug?
- What should you monitor the patient for once he or she has received the drug?
- What do you assess the patient for?
- What interventions should you perform?
- What should you teach the patient?

The following are included within the drug entries:

Generic Name, Pronunciation, Trade Names. Each entry begins with the generic name and pronunciation, followed by the U.S. and Canadian trade names. Exclusively Canadian trade names are followed by a red maple leaf ✦. Trade names that were most prescribed in the year 2016 are underlined in this section.

Black Box Alert. This feature highlights drugs that carry a significant risk of serious or life-threatening adverse effects. Black Box Alerts are ordered by the FDA.

Do Not Confuse With. Drug names that sound similar to the generic and/or trade names are listed under this heading to help you avoid potential medication errors.

Fixed-Combination Drugs. Where appropriate, fixed-combinations, or drugs made up of two or more generic medications, are listed with the generic drug.

Pharmacotherapeutic and Clinical Classification Names. Each entry includes both the pharmacotherapeutic and clinical classifications for the generic drug.

Action/Therapeutic Effect. This section describes how the drug is predicted to behave, with the expected therapeutic effect(s) under a separate heading.

Pharmacokinetics. This section includes the absorption, distribution, metabolism, excretion, and half-life of the medication. The half-life is bolded in red for easy access.

Uses/Off-Label. The listing of uses for each drug includes both the FDA uses and the off-label uses. The off-label heading is shown in bold red for emphasis.

Precautions. This heading incorporates a discussion about when the generic drug is contraindicated or should be used with caution. The cautions warn the nurse of specific situations in which a drug should be closely monitored.

Lifespan Considerations ⧗. This section includes pregnancy/lactation data and age-specific information concerning children and elderly people.

Interactions. This heading enumerates drug, food, and herbal interactions with the generic drug. As the number of medications a patient receives increases, awareness of drug interactions becomes more important. Also included is information about therapeutic and toxic blood levels in addition to the altered lab values that show what effects the drug may have on lab results.

Product Availability. Each drag monograph gives the form and availability of the drug. The icon ⬤ identifies noncrushable drug forms.

Administration/Handling. Instructions for administration are given for each route of administration (e.g., IV, IM, PO, rectal). Special handling, such as refrigeration, is also included where applicable. The routes in this section are always presented in the order IV, IM, SQ, and PO, with subsequent routes in alphabetical order (e.g., Ophthalmic, Otic, Topical. **IV administration** 🗄 is broken down by reconstitution, rate of administration (how fast the IV should be given), and storage (including how long the medication is stable once reconstituted).

IV Incompatibilities/IV Compatibilities ▦. These sections give the nurse the most comprehensive compatibility information possible when administering medications by direct IV push, via a Y-site, or via IV piggyback.

Indications/Routes/Dosage. Each entry provides specific dosing guidelines for adults, elderly, children, and patients with renal and/or hepatic impairment. Dose modification for toxicity has been added where applicable. Dosages are clearly indicated for each approved indication and route.

Side Effects. Side effects are defined as those responses that are usually predictable with the drug, are **not** life-threatening, and may or may not require discontinuation of the drug. Unique to this handbook, side effects are grouped by frequency listed from highest occurrence percentage to lowest so that the nurse can focus on patient care without wading through myriad signs and symptoms of side effects.

Adverse Effects/Toxic Reactions. Adverse effects and toxic reactions are very serious and often life-threatening undesirable responses that require prompt intervention from a health care provider.

Nursing Considerations. Nursing considerations are organized as care is organized. That is:

- What needs to be assessed or done before the first dose is administered? (Baseline Assessment)
- What interventions and evaluations are needed during drug therapy? (Intervention/Evaluation)
- What explicit teaching is needed for the patient and family? (Patient/Family Teaching)

Saunders Nursing Drug Handbook is an easy-to-use source of current drug information for nurses, students, and other health care providers. It is our hope that this handbook will help you provide quality care to your patients.

We welcome any comments you may have that would help us to improve future editions of the handbook. Please contact us via the publisher at *http://evolve.elsevier. com/SaundersNDH*.

Robert J. Kizior, BS, RPh
Keith J. Hodgson, RN, BSN, CCRN

DRUGS BY DISORDER

Note: Not all medications appropriate for a given condition are listed, nor are those not listed inappropriate.
Generic names appear first, followed by brand names in parentheses.

Alcohol dependence
Acamprosate (Campral)
Disulfiram (Antabuse)
Naltrexone (Depade, ReVia, Vivitrol)

Allergic rhinitis
Nasal Spray
Azelastine (Astelin, Astepro)
Azelastine/fluticasone (Dymista)
Beclomethasone (Beconase AQ, Qnasl)
Budesonide (Rhinocort Allergy Spray)
Ciclesonide (Omnaris, Zetonna)
Flunisolide
Fluticasone (Flonase Sensimist Allergy Relief)
Mometasone (Nasonex)
Nasal spray
Olopatadine (Patanase)
Triamcinolone (Nasacort Allergy 24 HR)
Oral Form
Cetirizine (Zyrtec Allergy)
Cetirizine/Pseudoephedrine (Zyrtec-D 12 hour)
Desloratadine (Clarinex)
Desloratadine/Pseudoephedrine (Clarinex-D 12 hour)
Fexofenadine (Allegra)
Fexofenadine/Pseudoephedrine (Allegra-D 12 hour, Allegra-D 24 hour)
Levocetirizine (Xyzal Allergy 24 hour)
Loratadine (Alavert, Claritin)
Loratadine/Pseudoephedrine (Alavert-D 12 hour, Claritin-D 12 hour, Claritin-D 24 hour)
Montelukast (Singulair)

Allergic conjunctivitis
Alcaftadine (Lastacaft)
Azelastine – generic
Bepotastine (Bepreve)

Cromolyn – generic
Emedastine (Emadine)
Epinastine (Elestat)
Ketorolac (Acular)
Ketotifen (Alaway, Zaditor)
Lodoxamide (Alomide)
Loteprednol (Alrex, Lotemax)
Nedocromil (Alocril)
Olopatadine (Pataday, Patanol, Pazeo)
Prednisone (Pred Mild)

Alzheimer's disease
Donepezil (Aricept, Aricept ODT)
Galantamine (Razadyne, Razadyne ER)
Memantine/Donepezil (Namzaric)
Memantine (Namenda, Namenda XR)
Rivastigmine (Exelon, Exelon Patch)

Angina
Amlodipine (Norvasc)
Atenolol (Tenormin)
Diltiazem (Cardizem, Dilacor)
Isosorbide (Imdur, Isordil)
Metoprolol (Lopressor)
Nadolol (Corgard)
Nicardipine (Cardene)
Nifedipine (Adalat, Procardia)
Nitroglycerin
Propranolol (Inderal)
Verapamil (Calan, Isoptin)

Anxiety
Alprazolam (Xanax)
Buspirone (BuSpar)
Diazepam (Valium)
Hydroxyzine (Atarax, Vistaril)
Lorazepam (Ativan)
Oxazepam (Serax)
Paroxetine (Paxil)
Trazodone (Desyrel)
Venlafaxine (Effexor)

Arrhythmias
Adenosine (Adenocard)
Amiodarone (Cordarone, Pacerone)
Digoxin (Lanoxin)
Diltiazem (Cardizem, Dilacor)
Disopyramide (Norpace)
Dofetilide (Tikosyn)
Dronedarone (Multaq)
Esmolol (Brevibloc)
Flecainide (Tambocor)
Ibutilide (Corvert)
Lidocaine
Metoprolol (Lopressor)
Mexiletine (Mexitil)
Propafenone (Rythmol)
Propranolol (Inderal)
Sotalol (Betapace)
Verapamil (Calan, Isoptin)

Arthritis, rheumatoid (RA)
Abatacept (Orencia)
Adalimumab (Humira)
Anakinra (Kineret)
Azathioprine (Imuran)
Certolizumab (Cimzia)
Etanercept (Enbrel)
Golimumab (Simponi)
Hydroxychloroquine (Plaquenil)
Infliximab (Remicade)
Leflunomide (Arava)
Methotrexate
Prednisone (Deltasone)
Rituximab (Rituxan)
Sarilumab (Kevzara)
Sulfasalazine (Azulfidine-EN)
Tocilizumab (Actemra)
Tofacitinib (Xeljanz)

Asthma
Albuterol (Proventil, Ventolin)
Aminophylline (Theophylline)
Arformoterol (Brovana)
Beclomethasone (Beclovent, Vanceril)
Budesonide (Pulmicort)
Ciclesonide (Alvesco)
Cromolyn (Crolom, Intal)
Epinephrine (Adrenalin)
Flunisolide (AeroBid)
Fluticasone (Flovent)
Hydrocortisone (Solu-Cortef)
Ipratropium (Atrovent)

Levalbuterol (Xopenex)
Mepolizumab (Nucala)
Metaproterenol (Alupent)
Methylprednisolone (Solu-Medrol)
Mometasone (Asmanex)
Montelukast (Singulair)
Prednisolone (Prelone)
Prednisone (Deltasone)
Reslizumab (Cinqair)
Salmeterol (Serevent)
Terbutaline (Brethine)
Theophylline (Slo-Bid)
Zafirlukast (Accolate)

Attention-deficit hyperactivity disorder (ADHD)
Amphetamine (Adzenys XR-ODT, Dyanavel XR)
Atomoxetine (Strattera)
Clonidine (Catapres, Kapvay)
Desipramine (Norpramin)
Dexmethylphenidate (Focalin, Focalin XR)
Dextroamphetamine (Dexedrine, Zenzedi)
Guanfacine (Intuniv)
Lisdexamfetamine (Vyvanse)
Methylphenidate (Concerta, Daytrana, Focalin, Methylin, Ritalin)
Mixed amphetamine (dextroamphetamine and amphetamine salts) (Adderall, Adderall XR)

Benign prostatic hypertrophy (BPH)
Alfuzosin (Uroxatral)
Doxazosin (Cardura)
Dutasteride (Avodart)
Fesoterodine (Toviaz)
Finasteride (Proscar)
Mirabegron (Myrbetriq)
Silodosin (Rapaflo)
Tadalafil (Cialis)
Tamsulosin (Flomax)
Terazosin (Hytrin)
Tolterodine (Detrol)

Bipolar disorder
Aripiprazole (Abilify)
Asenapine (Saphris)
Carbamazepine (Tegretol)
Lamotrigine (Lamictal)
Lithium (Lithobid)
Lurasidone (Latuda)

Olanzapine (Zyprexa)
Olanzapine/Fluoxetine (Symbyax)
Oxcarbazepine (Trileptal)
Paliperidone (Invega)
Quetiapine (Seroquel)
Risperidone (Risperdal)
Valproic acid (Depakene, Depakote)
Ziprasidone (Geodon)

Bladder hyperactivity
Darifenacin (Enablex)
Oxybutynin (Ditropan, Gelnique)
Solifenacin (VESIcare)
Tolterodine (Detrol)
Trospium (Sanctura)

Bronchospasm
Albuterol (Proventil, Ventolin)
Bitolterol (Tornalate)
Levalbuterol (Xopenex)
Metaproterenol (Alupent)
Salmeterol (Serevent)
Terbutaline (Brethine)

Cancer
Abarelix (Plenaxis)
Abiraterone (Zytiga)
Ado-trastuzumab (Kadcyla)
Afatinib (Gilotrif)
Aldesleukin (Proleukin)
Alemtuzumab (Campath)
Alitretinoin (Panretin)
Altretamine (Hexalen)
Anastrozole (Arimidex)
Arsenic trioxide (Trisenox)
Asparaginase (Elspar)
Atezolizumab (Tecentriq)
Avelumab (Bavencio)
Axitinib (Inlyta)
Azacitidine (Vidaza)
BCG (TheraCys, Tice BCG)
Belinostat (Beleodaq)
Bendamustine (Treanda)
Bevacizumab (Avastin)
Bexarotene (Targretin)
Bicalutamide (Casodex)
Bleomycin (Blenoxane)
Blinatumomab (Blincyto)
Bortezomib (Velcade)
Bosutinib (Bosulif)

Brentuximab (Adcetris)
Brigatinib (Alunbrig)
Busulfan (Myleran)
Cabazitaxel (Jevtana)
Cabozantinib (Cabometyx)
Capecitabine (Xeloda)
Carboplatin (Paraplatin)
Carfilzomib (Kyprolis)
Carmustine (BiCNU)
Ceritinib (Zykadia)
Cetuximab (Erbitux)
Chlorambucil (Leukeran)
Cisplatin (Platinol)
Cladribine (Leustatin)
Clofarabine (Clolar)
Cobimetinib (Cotellic)
Crizotinib (Xalkori)
Cyclophosphamide (Cytoxan)
Cytarabine (Ara-C, Cytosar)
Dabrafenib (Tafinlar)
Dacarbazine (DTIC)
Dactinomycin (Cosmegen)
Daratumumab (Darzalex)
Dasatinib (Sprycel)
Daunorubicin (Cerubidine, DaunoXome)
Degarelix (Firmagon)
Denileukin (Ontak)
Dinutuximab (Unituxin)
Docetaxel (Taxotere)
Doxorubicin (Adriamycin, Doxil)
Durvalumab (Imfinzi)
Elotuzumab (Empliciti)
Enzalutamide (Xtandi)
Epirubicin (Ellence)
Eribulin (Halaven)
Erlotinib (Tarceva)
Estramustine (Emcyt)
Etoposide (VePesid)
Everolimus (Afinitor)
Fludarabine (Fludara)
Fluorouracil
Flutamide (Eulexin)
Fulvestrant (Faslodex)
Gefitinib (Iressa)
Gemcitabine (Gemzar)
Goserelin (Zoladex)
Hydroxyurea (Hydrea)
Ibritumomab (Zevalin)
Ibrutinib (Imbruvica)
Idarubicin (Idamycin)

Idelalisib (Zydelig)
Ifosfamide (Ifex)
Imatinib (Gleevec)
Interferon alfa-2b (Intron A)
Ipilimumab (Yervoy)
Irinotecan (Camptosar)
Ixabepilone (Ixempra)
Ixazomib (Ninlaro)
Lapatinib (Tykerb)
Letrozole (Femara)
Leuprolide (Lupron)
Lenvatinib (Lenvima)
Lomustine (CeeNU)
Mechlorethamine (Mustargen)
Megestrol (Megace)
Melphalan (Alkeran)
Mercaptopurine (Purinethol)
Methotrexate
Midostaurin (Rydapt)
Mitomycin (Mutamycin)
Mitotane (Lysodren)
Mitoxantrone (Novantrone)
Necitumumab (Portrazza)
Nelarabine (Arranon)
Neratinib (Nerlynx)
Nilotinib (Tasigna)
Nilutamide (Nilandron)
Niraparib (Zejula)
Nivolumab (Opdivo)
Obinutuzumab (Gazyva)
Ofatumumab (Arzerra)
Olaparib (Lynparza)
Olaratumab (Lartruvo)
Omacetaxine (Synribo)
Osimertinib (Tagrisso)
Oxaliplatin (Eloxatin)
Paclitaxel (Taxol)
Palbociclib (Ibrance)
Panitumumab (Vectibix)
Panobinostat (Farydak)
Pazopanib (Votrient)
Pegaspargase (Oncaspar)
Pembrolizumab (Keytruda)
Pemetrexed (Alimta)
Pentostatin (Nipent)
Pertuzumab (Perjeta)
Plicamycin (Mithracin)
Pomalidomide (Pomalyst)
Ponatinib (Iclusig)
Pralatrexate (Folotyn)

Procarbazine (Matulane)
Ramucirumab (Cyramza)
Rasburicase (Elitek)
Regorafenib (Stivarga)
Ribociclib (Kisqali)
Rituximab (Rituxan)
Romidepsin (Istodax)
Rucaparib (Rubraca)
Sipuleucel-T (Provenge)
Sonidegib (Odomzo)
Sorafenib (Nexavar)
Streptozocin (Zanosar)
Sunitinib (Sutent)
Tamoxifen (Nolvadex)
Temozolomide (Temodar)
Temsirolimus (Torisel)
Teniposide (Vumon)
Thioguanine
Thiotepa (Thioplex)
Tipifarnib (Zarnestra)
Tipiracil/trifluridine (Lonsurf)
Topotecan (Hycamtin)
Toremifene (Fareston)
Tositumomab (Bexxar)
Trabectedin (Yondelis)
Trametinib (Mekinist)
Trastuzumab (Herceptin)
Tretinoin (ATRA, Vesanoid)
Valrubicin (Valstar)
Vandetanib (Caprelsa)
Vemurafenib (Zelboraf)
Venetoclax (Venclexta)
Vinblastine (Velban)
Vincristine (Oncovin)
Vinorelbine (Navelbine)
Vismodegib (Erivedge)
Vorinostat (Zolinza)
Ziv-Aflibercept (Zaltrap)

Cerebrovascular accident (CVA)
Aspirin
Clopidogrel (Plavix)
Heparin
Nimodipine (Nimotop)
Prasugrel (Effient)
Warfarin (Coumadin)

**Chronic Obstructive Pulmonary
Disease (COPD)**
Inhaled short-acting Antimuscarinic

Ipratropium (Atrovent HFA)
Inhaled short-acting Beta-2 Agonists (SABA)
Albuterol (ProAir HFA, Proventil HFA, Ventolin HFA)
Levalbuterol (Xopenex HFA)
Inhaled short-acting Beta-2 Agonist (SABA)/short-acting Antimuscarinic (SAMA)
Albuterol/Ipratropium (Combivent Respimat)
Inhaled long-acting Beta-2 Agonists (LABA)
Arformoterol (Brovana)
Indacaterol (Arcapta Neohaler)
Olodaterol (Striverdi Respimat)
Salmeterol (Serevent Diskus)
Formoterol (Perforomist)
Inhaled long-acting Antimuscarinic Agents (LAMA)
Aclidinium (Tudorza Pressair)
Glycopyrrolate (Seebri Neohaler)
Tiotropium (Spiriva Respimat)
Umeclidinium (Incruse Ellipta)
Inhaled long-acting Beta-2 Agonists (LABA)/long-acting Antimuscarinic Agents (LAMA)
Glycopyrrolate/formoterol (Bevespi)
Glycopyrrolate/indacaterol (Utibron Neohaler)
Tiotropium/olodaterol (Stiolto Respimat)
Umeclidinium/vilanterol (Anoro Ellipta)
Inhaled Corticosteroids
Beclomethasone (QVAR)
Budesonide (Pulmicort)
Ciclesonide (Alvesco)
Flunisolide (Aerospan HFA)
Fluticasone (Flovent Diskus, Flovent HFA)
Mometasone (Asmanex HFA, Asmanex Twisthaler)
Inhaled Corticosteroids/long-acting Beta-2 Agonists (LABA)
Fluticasone/salmeterol (Advair Diskus)
Fluticasone/vilanterol (Breo Ellipta)
Budesonide/formoterol (Symbicort)

Crohn's disease
Azathioprine
Adalimumab (Humira)

Certolizumab (Cimzia)
Corticosteroids
Infliximab (Inflectra, Remicade)
6-Mercaptopurine
Ustekinumab (Stelara)
Vedolizumab (Entyvio)

Constipation
Bisacodyl (Dulcolax)
Docusate (Colace)
Lactulose (Kristalose)
Lubiprostone (Amitiza)
Methylcellulose (Citrucel)
Milk of magnesia (MOM)
Polyethylene glycol (MiraLAX)
Psyllium (Metamucil)
Senna (Senokot)

Deep vein thrombosis (DVT)
Dalteparin (Fragmin)
Edoxaban (Savaysa)
Enoxaparin (Lovenox)
Heparin
Tinzaparin (Innohep)
Warfarin (Coumadin)

Depression
SSRIs
Citalopram (Celexa)
Escitalopram (Lexapro)
fluoxetine (Prozac, Prozac Weekly)
paroxetine (Paxil, Paxil CR)
sertraline (Zoloft)
SNRIs
Desvenlafaxine (Pristiq, Khedezla)
Duloxetine (Cymbalta)
Venlafaxine (Effexor XR)
Levomilnacipran (Fetzima)
TCAs
Amitriptyline (Elavil)
Nortriptyline (Pamelor)
MAOIs
Phenelzine (Nardil)
Selegiline (Emsam)
Other
Bupropion (Wellbutrin SR, Aplenzin, Forfivo XL)
Mirtazapine (Remerol, Remeron SolTab)
Trazodone (Oleptro)
Vilazodone (Viibryd)
Vortioxetine (Trintellix)

Diabetes
Biguanides
Metformin (Glucophage, Glucophage
   XR, Glumetza, Fortamet, Riomet)
Sulfonylureas
Glimepiride (Amaryl)Glipizide
   (Glucotrol, Glucotrol XL)
Glyburide (Glynase)
GLP-1 Receptor Agonists
Albiglutide (Tanzeum)
Dulaglutide (Trulicity)
Exenatide (Byetta, Bydureon)
Liraglutide (Victoza)
Lixisenatide (Adlyxin)
DDP-4 Inhibitors
Alogliptin (Nesina)
Linagliptin (Tradjenta)
Saxagliptin (Onglyza)
Sitagliptin (Januvia)
SGLT2 Inhibitors
Canagliflozin (Invokana)
Dapagliflozin (Farxiga)
Empagliflozin (Jardiance)
Meglitinides
Nataglinide (Starlix)
Repaglinide (Prandin)
Thiazolidinediones
Pioglitazone (Actos)
Rosiglitazone (Avandia)
Alpha-Glucosidase Inhibitors
Acarbose (Precose)
Miglitol (Glyset)
Other
Colesevelam (Welchol)
Bromocriptine (Cycloset)
Pramlintide (Symlin)
Insulin
Rapid-Acting
Insulin aspart (Novolog)
Insulin glulisine (Apidra)
Insulin lispro (Humalog)
Insulin inhalation powder (Afrezza)
Regular Insulin
Humulin R
Novolin R
Intermediate Insulin
NPH (Humulin N, Novolin N)
Long-Acting Insulin
Insulin detemir (Levemir)
Insulin glargine (Lantus, Toujeo,
   Basaglar)
Insulin degludec (Tresiba)

Diabetic peripheral neuropathy
Amitriptyline (Elavil)
Bupropion (Wellbutrin)
Capsaicin (Trixaicin)
Carbamazepine (Tegretol)
Citalopram (Celexa)
Desipramine (Norpramin)
Duloxetine (Cymbalta)
Gabapentin (Neurontin)
Lamotrigine (Lamictal)
Lidocaine patch (Lidoderm)
Nortriptyline (Pamelor)
Oxcarbazepine (Trileptal)
Oxycodone (OxyContin)
Paroxetine (Paxil)
Pregabalin (Lyrica)
Tramadol (Ultram)
Valproic acid (Depakote)
Venlafaxine, extended-release
   (Effexor XR)

Diarrhea
Bismuth subsalicylate (Pepto-Bismol)
Diphenoxylate and atropine (Lomotil)
Fidaxomicin (Dificid)
Kaolin-pectin (Kaopectate)
Loperamide (Imodium)
Octreotide (Sandostatin)
Rifaximin (Xifaxan)

Edema
Amiloride (Midamor)
Bumetanide (Bumex)
Chlorthalidone (Hygroton)
Ethacrynic acid (Edecrin)
Furosemide (Lasix)
Hydrochlorothiazide (HydroDIURIL)
Indapamide (Lozol)
Metolazone (Zaroxolyn)
Spironolactone (Aldactone)
Torsemide (Demadex)
Triamterene (Dyrenium)

Epilepsy
Brivaracetam (Briviact)
Carbamazepine (Tegretol)
Clobazam (Onfi)
Clonazepam (Klonopin)
Clorazepate (Tranxene)
Diazepam (Valium)
Eslicarbazepine (Aptiom)
Ethosuximide (Zarontin)

Ezogabine (Potiga)
Fosphenytoin (Cerebyx)
Gabapentin (Neurontin)
Lacosamide (Vimpat)
Lamotrigine (Lamictal, Lamictal ODT, Lamictal XR)
Levetiracetam (Keppra)
Lorazepam (Ativan)
Midazolam (Versed)
Oxcarbazepine (Trileptal)
Perampanel (Fycompa)
Phenobarbital
Phenytoin (Dilantin)
Pregabalin (Lyrica)
Primidone (Mysoline)
Rufinamide (Banzel)
Tiagabine (Gabitril)
Topiramate (Qudexy XR, Topamax Trokendi XR)
Valproic acid (Depakene, Depakote)
Vigabatrin (Sabril)
Zonisamide (Zonegran)

Esophageal reflux, esophagitis
Cimetidine (Tagamet)
Dexlansoprazole (Dexilant)
Esomeprazole (Nexium)
Famotidine (Pepcid)
Lansoprazole (Prevacid)
Nizatidine (Axid)
Omeprazole (Prilosec)
Pantoprazole (Protonix)
Rabeprazole (AcipHex)
Ranitidine (Zantac)

Fever
Acetaminophen (Tylenol)
Aspirin
Ibuprofen (Advil, Caldolor, Motrin)
Naproxen (Aleve, Anaprox, Naprosyn)

Fibromyalgia
Acetaminophen (Tylenol)
Amitriptyline (Elavil)
Carisoprodol (Soma)
Citalopram (Celexa)
Cyclobenzaprine (Flexeril)
Duloxetine (Cymbalta)
Fluoxetine (Prozac)
Gabapentin (Neurontin)
Milnacipran (Savella)

Paroxetine (Paxil)
Pregabalin (Lyrica)
Tramadol (Ultram)
Venlafaxine (Effexor)

Gastric/Duodenal Ulcer
Cimetidine (Tagamet)
Esomeprazole (Nexium)
Famotidine (Pepcid)
Lansoprazole (Prevacid)
Nizatidine (Axid)
Omeprazole (Prilosec)
Pantoprazole (Protonix)
Rabeprazole (AcipHex)
Ranitidine (Zantac)
Sucralfate (Carafate)

Gastritis
Cimetidine (Tagamet)
Famotidine (Pepcid)
Nizatidine (Axid)
Ranitidine (Zantac)

Gastroesophageal reflux disease (GERD)
Cimetidine (Tagamet)
Dexlansoprazole (Dexilant)
Esomeprazole (Nexium)
Famotidine (Pepcid)
Lansoprazole (Prevacid)
Nizatidine (Axid)
Omeprazole (Prilosec)
Pantoprazole (Protonix)
Rabeprazole (AcipHex)
Ranitidine (Zantac)

Glaucoma
Acetazolamide (Diamox)
Apraclonidine (Iopidine)
Betaxolol (Betoptic)
Bimatoprost (Lumigan)
Brimonidine (Alphagan)
Brinzolamide (Azopt)
Carbachol
Dorzolamide (Trusopt)
Echothiophate iodide (Phospholine)
Latanoprost (Xalatan)
Levobunolol (Betagan)
Pilocarpine (Isopto Carpine)
Tafluprost (Zioptan)
Timolol (Timoptic)

Travoprost (Travatan)
Unoprostone (Rescula)

Gout
Allopurinol (Zyloprim)
Colchicine (Colcrys)
Febuxostat (Uloric)
Ibuprofen (Motrin)
Indomethacin (Indocin)
Lesinurad (Zurampic)
Naproxen (Naprosyn)
Pegloticase (Krystexxa)
Piroxicam (Feldene)
Probenecid (Benemid)
Sulindac (Clinoril)

Heart failure (HF)
Bisoprolol (Zebeta)
Bumetanide (Bumex)
Candesartan (Atacand)
Captopril (Capoten)
Carvedilol (Coreg)
Digoxin (Lanoxin)
Dobutamine (Dobutrex)
Dopamine (Intropin)
Enalapril (Vasotec)
Eplerenone (Inspra)
Fosinopril (Monopril)
Furosemide (Lasix)
Hydralazine (Apresoline)
Isosorbide (Isordil)
Ivabradine (Corlanor)
Lisinopril (Prinivil, Zestril)
Losartan (Cozaar)
Metoprolol (Lopressor)
Milrinone (Primacor)
Nitroglycerin
Quinapril (Accupril)
Ramipril (Altace)
Sacubitril/valsartan (Entresto)
Spironolactone (Aldactone)
Torsemide (Demadex)
Valsartan (Diovan)

Hepatitis B
Adefovir (Hepsera)
Entecavir (Baraclude)
Lamivudine (Epivir)
Peginterferon alpha-2a (Pegasys)
Telbivudine (Tyzeka)
Tenofovir (Viread)

Hepatitis C
Daclatasvir (Daklinza)
Elbasvir/Grazoprevir (Zepatier)
Ledipasvir/Sofosbuvir (Harvoni)
Ombitasvir/paritaprevir/ritonavir
    (Technivie)
Ombitasvir/paritaprevir/ritonavir/
    dasabuvir (Viekira Pak)
Peginterferon alfa-2a (Pegasys)
Peginterferon alfa-2b (Pegintron)
Ribavirin (Copegus, Rebetol,
    Ribasphere)
Simeprevir (Olysio)
Sofosbuvir (Sovaldi)
Sofosbuvir/Velpatasvir (Epclusa)
Sofosbuvir/Velpatasvir/Voxilaprevir
    (Vosevi)

Human immunodeficiency virus (HIV)
Abacavir (Ziagen)
Atazanavir (Reyataz)
Cobicistat (Tybost)
Darunavir (Prezista)
Delavirdine (Rescriptor)
Didanosine (Videx)
Dolutegravir (Tivicay)
Efavirenz (Sustiva)
Elvitegravir (Vitekta)
Emtricitabine (Emtriva)
Enfuvirtide (Fuzeon)
Etravirine (Intelence)
Fosamprenavir (Lexiva)
Indinavir (Crixivan)
Lamivudine (Epivir)
Lopinavir/ritonavir (Kaletra)
Maraviroc (Selzentry)
Nelfinavir (Viracept)
Nevirapine (Viramune)
Raltegravir (Isentress)
Rilpivirine (Edurant)
Ritonavir (Norvir)
Saquinavir (Invirase)
Stavudine (Zerit)
Tenofovir (Viread)
Tesamorelin (Egrifta)
Tipranavir (Aptivus)
Zidovudine (AZT, Retrovir)

Hyperphosphatemia
Aluminum salts
Calcium salts

Ferric Citrate (Auryxia)
Lanthanum (Fosrenol)
Sevelamer (Renagel)

Hypertension
Thiazide Diuretics
Hydrochlorothiazide
Loop Diuretics
Bumetanide (Bumex)
Furosemide (Lasix)
Aldosterone Antagonists
Eplerenone (Inspra)
Spironolactone (Aldactone)
ACE Inhibitors
Benazepril (Lotensin)
Enalapril (Vasotec)
Lisinopril (Zestril, Prinivil)
Quinapril (Accupril)
Ramipril (Altace)
ARBs
Azilsartan (Edarbi)
Candesartan (Atacand)
Irbesartan (Avapro)
Losartan (Cozaar)
Valsartan (Diovan)
Calcium channel Blockers
Dihydropyridines
Amlodipine (Norvasc)
Nifedipine (Adalat CC, Procardia XL)
Nondihydropyridines
Diltiazem (Cardizem LA, Taztia XT)
Verapamil (Calan)
Beta Blockers
Atenolol (Tenormin)
Carvedilol (Coreg, Coreg CR)
Labetalol
Metoprolol (Lopressor, Toprol XL)
Nebivolol (Bystolic)
Central Alpha-adrenergic Agonists
Clonidine (Catapres)
Direct Vasodilators
Hydralazine (Apresoline)

Hypertriglyceridemia
Atorvastatin (Lipitor)
Colesevelam (Welchol)
Fenofibrate (Tricor)
Fluvastatin (Lescol)
Gemfibrozil (Lopid)
Icosapent (Vascepa)

Lovastatin (Mevacor)
Niacin (Niaspan)
Omega-3 acid ethyl esters (Lovaza)
Pravastatin (Pravachol)
Rosuvastatin (Crestor)
Simvastatin (Zocor)

Hyperuricemia
Allopurinol (Zyloprim)
Febuxostat (Uloric)
Pegloticase (Krystexxa)
Probenecid (Benemid)

Hypotension
Dobutamine (Dobutrex)
Dopamine (Intropin)
Ephedrine
Epinephrine
Norepinephrine (Levophed)
Phenylephrine (Neo-Synephrine)

Hypothyroidism
Levothyroxine (Levoxyl, Synthroid)
Liothyronine (Cytomel)
Thyroid

Idiopathic thrombocytopenic purpura (ITP)
Cyclophosphamide (Cytoxan)
Dexamethasone (Decadron)
Hydrocortisone (Solu-Cortef)
Immune globulin intravenous
Methylprednisolone (Solu-Medrol)
Prednisone
Rh_o(D) immune globulin (RhoGAM)
Rituximab (Rituxan)

Insomnia
Diphenhydramine (Benadryl)
Estazolam (ProSom)
Eszopiclone (Lunesta)
Flurazepam (Dalmane)
Ramelteon (Rozerem)
Suvorexant (Belsomra)
Temazepam (Restoril)
Zaleplon (Sonata)
Zolpidem (Ambien, Edluar)

Inflammatory bowel disease (Crohn's disease, ulcerative colitis)
Adalimumab (Humira)

Azathioprine (Imuran)
Balsalazide (Colazal, Giazo)
Budesonide (Entocort EC, Uceris)
Certolizumab (Cimzia)
Cyclosporine (Sandimmune)
Golimumab (Simponi)
Hydrocortisone (Colocort, Cortifoam)
Infliximab (Remicade)
Mercaptopurine (Purinethol)
Mesalamine (Apriso, Asacol HD, Delzicol, Lialda, Pentasa)
Methotrexate (Otrexup, Rasuvo)
Olsalazine (Dipentum)
Prednisone
Sulfasalazine (Azulfidine)
Tacrolimus (Prograf)
Vedolizumab (Entyvio)

Irritable Bowel Syndrome with Constipation
Chloride channel Activator
Lubiprostone (Amitiza)
Guanylate cyclase-C Receptor Agonist
Linaclotide (Linzess)

Irritable Bowel Syndrome with diarrhea
Antibiotic
Rifaximin (Xifaxan)
Mu-Opioid Receptor Agonist/ Delta-Opioid Receptor Antagonist
Eluxadoline (Viberzi)
5-HT modulators
Alosetron (Lotronex)
Ondansetron (Zofran)

Lipid disorders
Statins
Atorvastatin (Lipitor)
Fluvastatin (Lescol)
Lovastatin (Altoprev)
Pitavastatin (Livalo)
Pravastatin (Pravachol)
Rosuvastatin (Crestor)
Simvastatin (Zocor)
Cholesterol Absorption Inhibitor
Ezetimibe (Zetia)
PCSK9 Inhibitors
Alirocumab (Praluent)
Evolocumab (Repatha)

Bile Acid Sequestrants
Colesevelam (Welchol)
Colestipol (Colestid)
Cholestyramine (Questran)
Fibrates
Gemfibrozil (Lopid)
Fenofibrate (Lipofen, Lofibra, Tricor, Antara, Fibricor, Trilipix)
Fish Oil
Icosapent ethyl (Vascepa)
Omega-3 acid ethyl esters (Lovaza)

Migraine headaches
Almotriptan (Axert)
Dihydroergotamine (DHE 45, Migranal)
Eletriptan (Relpax)
Ergotamine/caffeine (Cafergot)
Frovatriptan (Frova)
Naratriptan (Amerge)
Rizatriptan (Maxalt)
Sumatriptan (Imitrex)
Zolmitriptan (Zomig, Zomig-ZMT)

Multiple sclerosis (MS)
Alemtuzumab (Lemtrada)
Daclizumab (Zinbryta)
Dalfampridine (Ampyra)
Dimethyl fumarate (Tecfidera)
Fingolimod (Gilenya)
Glatiramer (Copaxone)
Interferon beta-1a (Avonex, Rebif)
Interferon beta-1b (Betaseron, Extavia)
Ocrelizumab (Ocrevus)
Peginterferon beta-la (Plegridy)
Mitoxantrone (Novantrone)
Natalizumab (Tysabri)
Teriflunomide (Aubagio)

Myelodysplastic syndrome
Azacitidine (Vidaza)
Clofarabine (Clolar)
Decitabine (Dacogen)
Lenalidomide (Revlimid)

Myocardial infarction (MI)
Alteplase (Activase)
Aspirin
Atenolol (Tenormin)
Captopril (Capoten)
Clopidogrel (Plavix)
Dalteparin (Fragmin)
Diltiazem (Cardizem, Dilacor)

Enalapril (Vasotec)
Enoxaparin (Lovenox)
Heparin
Lidocaine
Lisinopril (Prinivil, Zestril)
Metoprolol (Lopressor)
Morphine
Nitroglycerin
Propranolol (Inderal)
Quinapril (Accupril)
Ramipril (Altace)
Reteplase (Retavase)
Warfarin (Coumadin)

Nausea
Aprepitant (Emend)
Chlorpromazine (Thorazine)
Dexamethasone (Decadron)
Dimenhydrinate (Dramamine)
Dronabinol (Marinol)
Droperidol (Inapsine)
Fosaprepitant (Emend)
Granisetron (Kytril)
Hydroxyzine (Vistaril)
Lorazepam (Ativan)
Meclizine (Antivert)
Metoclopramide (Reglan)
Nabilone (Cesamet)
Ondansetron (Zofran)
Palonosetron (Aloxi)
Prochlorperazine (Compazine)
Promethazine (Phenergan)
Rolapitant (Varubi)

Obesity
Benzphetamine (Didrex)
Bupropion (Wellbutrin)
Bupropion/naltrexone (Contrave)
Diethylpropion (Tenuate)
Exenatide (Bydureon, Byetta)
Lorcaserin (Belviq)
Methamphetamine (Desoxyn)
Orlistat (Alli, Xenical)
Phendimetrazine (Bontril)
Phentermine (Ionamin)
Phentermine and topiramate (Qsymia)

Obsessive-compulsive disorder (OCD)
Citalopram (Celexa)
Clomipramine (Anafranil)

Escitalopram (Lexapro)
Fluoxetine (Prozac)
Fluvoxamine (Luvox)
Paroxetine (Paxil)
Sertraline (Zoloft)

Organ transplant, rejection prophylaxis
Azathioprine (Imuran)
Basiliximab (Simulect)
Belatacept (Nulojix)
Cyclophosphamide (Cytoxan, Neosar)
Cyclosporine (Sandimmune)
Daclizumab (Zenapax)
Everolimus (Zortress)
Mycophenolate (CellCept)
Sirolimus (Rapamune)
Tacrolimus (Prograf)

Osteoarthritis
Acetaminophen (Tylenol)
Celecoxib (Celebrex)
Diclofenac (Cataflam, Pennsaid, oltaren)
Duloxetine (Cymbalta)
Etodolac (Lodine)
Flurbiprofen (Ansaid)
Ibuprofen (Motrin)
Ketoprofen (Orudis)
Meloxicam (Mobic)
Nabumetone (Relafen)
Naproxen (Naprosyn)
Sulindac (Clinoril)
Tramadol (Ultram)

Osteoporosis
Alendronate (Fosamax)
Calcitonin (Miacalcin)
Calcium salts
Conjugated estrogens/bazedoxifene (Duavee)
Denosumab (Prolia)
Ibandronate (Boniva)
Raloxifene (Evista)
Risedronate (Actonel)
Teriparatide (Forteo)
Vitamin D
Zoledronic acid (Reclast)

Paget's disease
Alendronate (Fosamax)
Calcitonin (Miacalcin)

Etidronate (Didronel)
Pamidronate (Aredia)
Risedronate (Actonel)
Tiludronate (Skelid)
Zoledronic acid (Reclast)

Pain, mild to moderate
Acetaminophen (Tylenol)
Aspirin
Celecoxib (Celebrex)
Codeine
Diclofenac (Cataflam, Voltaren, Zipsor)
Diflunisal (Dolobid)
Etodolac (Lodine)
Flurbiprofen (Ansaid)
Ibuprofen (Advil, Caldolor, Motrin)
Ketorolac (Toradol)
Naproxen (Anaprox, Naprosyn)
Salsalate (Disalcid)
Tramadol (Ultram)

Pain, moderate to severe
Butorphanol (Stadol)
Fentanyl (Onsolis, Sublimaze)
Hydromorphone (Dilaudid)
Methadone (Dolophine)
Morphine (MS Contin)
Morphine/naltrexone (Embeda)
Nalbuphine (Nubain)
Oxycodone (OxyFast, Roxicodone)
Oxymorphone (Opana)
Ziconotide (Prialt)

Panic attack disorder
Alprazolam (Xanax)
Clonazepam (Klonopin)
Paroxetine (Paxil)
Sertraline (Zoloft)
Venlafaxine (Effexor)

Parkinsonism
Apomorphine (Apokyn)
Carbidopa/levodopa (Sinemet, Sinemet CR)
Entacapone (Comtan)
Pimavanserin (Nuplazid)
Pramipexole (Mirapex)
Rasagiline (Azilect)
Ropinirole (Requip)
Rotigotine (Neupro)

Selegiline (Eldepryl, Zelapar)
Tolcapone (Tasmar)

Peptic ulcer disease
Cimetidine (Tagamet)
Dexlansoprazole (Dexilant)
Esomeprazole (Nexium)
Famotidine (Pepcid)
Lansoprazole (Prevacid)
Nizatidine (Axid)
Omeprazole (Prilosec)
Pantoprazole (Protonix)
Rabeprazole (AcipHex)
Ranitidine (Zantac)
Sucralfate (Carafate)

Pneumonia
Amoxicillin (Amoxil)
Amoxicillin/clavulanate (Augmentin)
Ampicillin (Polycillin)
Azithromycin (Zithromax)
Cefaclor (Ceclor)
Cefpodoxime (Vantin)
Ceftriaxone (Rocephin)
Cefuroxime (Kefurox, Zinacef)
Clarithromycin (Biaxin)
Co-trimoxazole (Bactrim, Septra)
Erythromycin
Gentamicin (Garamycin)
Levofloxacin (Levaquin)
Linezolid (Zyvox)
Moxifloxacin (Avelox)
Piperacillin/Tazobactam (Zosyn)
Tobramycin (Nebcin)
Vancomycin (Vancocin)

Pneumonia, *Pneumocystis jiroveci*
Atovaquone (Mepron)
Clindamycin (Cleocin)
Co-trimoxazole (Bactrim, Septra)
Pentamidine (Pentam)
Trimethoprim (Proloprim)

Post-traumatic stress disorder (PTSD)
Amitriptyline (Elavil)
Aripiprazole (Abilify)
Citalopram (Celexa)
Escitalopram (Lexapro)
Fluoxetine (Prozac)
Imipramine (Tofranil)
Lamotrigine (Lamictal)

Olanzapine (Zyprexa)
Paroxetine (Paxil)
Phenelzine (Nardil)
Prazosin (Minipress)
Propranolol (Inderal)
Quetiapine (Seroquel)
Risperidone (Risperdal)
Sertraline (Zoloft)
Topiramate (Topamax)
Valproic acid (Depakote)
Venlafaxine (Effexor)
Ziprasidone (Geodon)

Pruritus
Amcinonide (Cyclocort)
Cetirizine (Zyrtec)
Clemastine (Tavist)
Clobetasol (Temovate)
Cyproheptadine (Periactin)
Desloratadine (Clarinex)
Desonide (Tridesilon)
Desoximetasone (Topicort)
Diphenhydramine (Benadryl)
Fluocinolone (Synalar)
Fluocinonide (Lidex)
Halobetasol (Ultravate)
Hydrocortisone (Cort-Dome,
  Hytone)
Hydroxyzine (Atarax, Vistaril)
Prednisolone (Prelone)
Prednisone (Deltasone)
Promethazine (Phenergan)

Psychotic disorders
Aripiprazole (Abilify)
Asenapine (Saphris)
Brexpiprazole (Rexulti)
Cariprazine (Vraylar)
Chlorpromazine (Thorazine)
Clozapine (Clozaril)
Fluphenazine (Prolixin)
Haloperidol (Haldol)
Iloperidone (Fanapt)
Loxapine (Adasuve)
Lurasidone (Latuda)
Olanzapine (Zyprexa, Zyprexa Zydis)
Paliperidone (Invega)
Pimavanserin (Nuplazid)
Quetiapine (Seroquel, Seroquel XR)
Risperidone (Risperdal)
Thioridazine (Mellaril)

Thiothixene (Navane)
Ziprasidone (Geodon)

Pulmonary arterial hypertension
Ambrisentan (Letairis)
Bosentan (Tracleer)
Epoprostenol (Flolan)
Iloprost (Ventavis)
Macitentan (Opsumit)
Riociguat (Adempas)
Selexipag (Uptravi)
Sildenafil (Revatio)
Tadalafil (Adcirca)
Treprostinil (Remodulin, Tyvaso)

Respiratory distress syndrome (RDS)
Beractant (Survanta)
Calfactant (Infasurf)
Poractant alfa (Curosurf)

Restless legs syndrome
Cabergoline (Dostinex)
Carbamazepine (Tegretol)
Carbidopa/levodopa (Sinemet)
Clonazepam (Klonopin)
Gabapentin (Horizant, Neurontin)
Levodopa
Pramipexole (Mirapex)
Pregabalin (Lyrica)
Ropinirole (Requip)
Rotigotine (Neupro)

Schizophrenia
Aripiprazole (Abilify)
Asenapine (Saphris)
Brexpiprazole (Rexulti)
Cariprazine (Vraylar)
Chlorpromazine (Thorazine)
Clozapine (Clozaril)
Fluphenazine (Prolixin)
Haloperidol (Haldol)
Iloperidone (Fanapt)
Lurasidone (Latuda)
Olanzapine (Zyprexa, Zyprexa Zydis)
Paliperidone (Invega, Invega Sustenna)
Quetiapine (Seroquel, Seroquel XR)
Risperidone (Risperdal)
Thioridazine (Mellaril)
Thiothixene (Navane)
Ziprasidone (Geodon)

Smoking cessation
Bupropion (Zyban)
Nicotine (NicoDerm, Nicotrol)
Varenicline (Chantix)

Thrombosis
Apixaban (Eliquis)
Dalteparin (Fragmin)
Edoxaban (Savaysa)
Enoxaparin (Lovenox)
Fondaparinux (Arixtra)
Heparin
Tinzaparin (Innohep)
Warfarin (Coumadin)

Thyroid disorders
Levothyroxine (Levoxyl, Synthroid)
Liothyronine (Cytomel)
Thyroid

Transient ischemic attack (TIA)
Aspirin
Clopidogrel (Plavix)
Prasugrel (Effient)
Warfarin (Coumadin)

Tremor
Atenolol (Tenormin)
Chlordiazepoxide (Librium)
Diazepam (Valium)
Lorazepam (Ativan)
Metoprolol (Lopressor)
Nadolol (Corgard)
Propranolol (Inderal)

Tuberculosis (TB)
Bedaquiline (Sirturo)
Cycloserine (Seromycin)
Ethambutol (Myambutol)
Isoniazid (INH)
Pyrazinamide
Rifabutin (Mycobutin)
Rifampin (Rifadin)
Rifapentine (Priftin)

Urticaria
Cetirizine (Zyrtec)
Cimetidine (Tagamet)

Clemastine (Tavist)
Cyproheptadine (Periactin)
Diphenhydramine (Benadryl)
Hydroxyzine (Atarax, Vistaril)
Loratadine (Claritin)
Promethazine (Phenergan)
Ranitidine (Zantac)

Vertigo
Dimenhydrinate (Dramamine)
Diphenhydramine (Benadryl)
Meclizine (Antivert)
Scopolamine (Trans-Derm Scop)

Vomiting
Aprepitant (Emend)
Chlorpromazine (Thorazine)
Dexamethasone (Decadron)
Dimenhydrinate (Dramamine)
Dronabinol (Marinol)
Droperidol (Inapsine)
Fosaprepitant (Emend)
Granisetron (Kytril)
Hydroxyzine (Vistaril)
Lorazepam (Ativan)
Meclizine (Antivert)
Metoclopramide (Reglan)
Nabilone (Cesamet)
Ondansetron (Zofran)
Palonosetron (Aloxi)
Prochlorperazine (Compazine)
Promethazine (Phenergan)
Rolapitant (Varubi)
Scopolamine (Trans-Derm Scop)
Trimethobenzamide (Tigan)

Zollinger-Ellison syndrome
Aluminum salts
Cimetidine (Tagamet)
Esomeprazole (Nexium)
Famotidine (Pepcid)
Lansoprazole (Prevacid)
Omeprazole (Prilosec)
Pantoprazole (Protonix)
Rabeprazole (AcipHex)
Ranitidine (Zantac)

DRUG CLASSIFICATION CONTENTS

allergic rhinitis nasal preparations

Alzheimer's disease agents

angiotensin-converting enzyme (ACE) inhibitors

angiotensin II receptor antagonists

antianxiety agents

antiarrhythmics

antibiotics

antibiotic: aminoglycosides

antibiotic: cephalosporins

antibiotic: fluoroquinolones

antibiotic: macrolides

antibiotic: penicillins

anticoagulants/antiplatelets/ thrombolytics

anticonvulsants

antidepressants

antidiabetics

antidiarrheals

antifungals: systemic mycoses

antiglaucoma agents

antihistamines

antihyperlipidemics

antihypertensives

antimigraine (triptans)

antipsychotics

antivirals

beta-adrenergic blockers

bronchodilators

calcium channel blockers

chemotherapeutic agents

contraception

corticosteroids

corticosteroids: topical

diuretics

H_2 antagonists

hepatitis C virus

hormones

human immunodeficiency virus (HIV) infection

immunosuppressive agents

laxatives

multiple sclerosis agents

nonsteroidal anti-inflammatory drugs (NSAIDs)

nutrition: enteral

nutrition: parenteral

obesity management

osteoporosis

Parkinson's disease treatment

proton pump inhibitors

rheumatoid arthritis

sedative-hypnotics

skeletal muscle relaxants

smoking cessation agents

vitamins

Allergic Rhinitis Preparations

USES

Relieve symptoms associated with allergic rhinitis. These symptoms include rhinorrhea, nasal congestion, pruritus, sneezing, postnasal drip, nasal pain.

Allergic rhinitis or hay fever is an inflammation of the nasal airways occurring when an allergen (e.g., pollen) is inhaled. This triggers antibody production. The antibodies bind to mast cells, which contain histamine. Histamine is released, causing symptoms of allergic rhinitis.

ACTION

Intranasal corticosteroids: Depress migration of polymorphonuclear leucocytes and fibroblasts, reverse capillary permeability, and stabilize nasal membranes to prevent/control inflammation. First-line therapy for moderate to severe symptoms or where nasal congestion is the dominant complaint.

Intranasal antihistamines: Reduce histamine-mediated symptoms of allergic rhinitis, including pruritus, sneezing, rhinorrhea, watery eyes. Second-line therapy for intermittent nasal symptoms where congestion is not dominant.

Intranasal mast cell stabilizers: Inhibit the mast cell release of histamine and other inflammatory mediators.

Intranasal anticholinergics: Block acetylcholine in the nasal mucosa. Effective in treating rhinorrhea associated with allergic rhinitis.

Intranasal decongestants: Vasoconstrict the respiratory mucosa, provide short-term relief of nasal congestion. Used only as adjuvant therapy for 3–5 days.

Oral antihistamines: First line therapy for mild symptoms or where sneezing/itching is primary complaint.

Oral decongestants: For primary complaint of nasal congestion.

CORTICOSTEROIDS—INTRANASAL

Generic (Brand)	Adult Dose	Pediatric Dose	Side Effects
Beclomethasone (Beconase AQ) (Qnasl)	Beconase AQ: 1–2 sprays in each nostril 2 times/day Qnasl: 80 mcg/spray: 2 sprays in each nostril once daily	Beconase AQ: 6–11 yrs: 1–2 sprays in each nostril 2 times/day Qnasl: 4–11 yrs: 40 mcg/spray: 1 spray in each nostril once daily	Altered taste and smell, epistaxis, burning, stinging, headache, nasal septum perforation
Budesonide (Rhinocort Allergy Spray, Rhinocort Aqua)	Rhinocort Aqua: 1–4 sprays in each nostril daily Rhinocort Allergy Spray: 1–2 sprays in each nostril once daily	Rhinocort Allergy Spray, Rhinocort Aqua: 6–11 yrs: 1–2 sprays in each nostril daily	Bronchospasm, cough, epistaxis, nasal/throat irritation

	Adult Dose	Pediatric Dose	Side Effects
Ciclesonide (Omnaris, Zetonna)	Omnaris: 2 sprays in each nostril daily Zetonna: 1 spray in each nostril daily	Omnaris: 6–11 yrs: 2 sprays in each nostril daily (seasonal allergic rhinitis only)	Fever, headache, nausea, cough, epistaxis, nasal septum disorder
Flunisolide (Nasalide)	2 sprays in each nostril 2 or 3 times/day (maximum: 8 sprays in each nostril daily)	6–14 yrs: 2 sprays in each nostril 2 times/day or 1 spray in each nostril 3 times/day (maximum: 4 sprays in each nostril daily)	Nasal burning/stinging, nasal dryness/irritation
Fluticasone (Flonase Sensimist, Flonase Allergy Relief)	Flonase, Flonase Allergy Relief, Flonase Sensimist: 1–2 sprays in each nostril once daily	Flonase Sensimist: 2–11 yrs: 1 spray in each nostril daily Flonase Allergy Relief: 4–11 yrs: 1 spray in each nostril once daily	Dizziness, fever, headache, nausea, cough, epistaxis
Fluticasone/Azelastine (Dymista)	1 spray in each nostril 2 times/day	Not indicated in children younger than 6 yrs	Same as fluticasone and azelastine
Mometasone (Nasonex)	2 sprays in each nostril daily	2–11 yrs: 1 spray in each nostril daily	Headache, nasopharyngitis, sinusitis
Triamcinolone (Nasacort Allergy 24 HR, Nasacort AQ)	1–2 sprays in each nostril daily	2–5 yrs: 1 spray in each nostril once daily 6–11 yrs: 1–2 sprays in each nostril daily	Bronchitis, chest congestion, cough, epistaxis, pharyngitis, sinusitis

ANTIHISTAMINES—INTRANASAL

Generic (Brand)	Adult Dose	Pediatric Dose	Side Effects
Azelastine Astepro 0.1%, 0.15%	Azelastine: 1–2 sprays in each nostril 2 times/day Astepro 0.1%, 0.15%: 1–2 sprays in each nostril two times/day or 2 sprays each nostril once daily (for seasonal allergic rhinitis)	Azelastine: 5–11 yrs: 1 spray in each nostril 2 times/day. Astepro 0.1%: 2–5 yrs: 1 spray 2 times/day. Astepro 0.1% or 0.15%: 6–11 yrs: 1 spray 2 times/day.	Sedation, epistaxis, nasal irritation
Azelastine/Fluticasone (Dymista)	1 spray in each nostril 2 times/day	Not approved for children younger than 6 yrs	Same as azelastine and fluticasone
Olopatadine (Patanase)	2 sprays in each nostril 2 times/day	6–11 yrs: 1 spray in each nostril 2 times/day	Same as azelastine

Continued

MAST CELL STABILIZERS

Generic (Brand)	Adult Dose	Pediatric Dose	Side Effects
Cromolyn (Nasalcrom)	1 spray in each nostril 3–6 times/day	2–11 yrs: 1 spray in each nostril 3–6 times/day	Nasal irritation, unpleasant taste

ANTICHOLINERGICS

Generic (Brand)	Adult Dose	Pediatric Dose	Side Effects
Ipratropium (Atrovent) 0.03%	2 sprays in each nostril 2–3 times/day	6–12 yrs: 2 sprays in each nostril 2–3 times/day	Nasal irritation, epistaxis, dizziness, headache, blurry vision
Ipratropium (Atrovent) 0.06%	2 sprays in each nostril 3–4 times/day	5–12 yrs: 2 sprays in each nostril 3–4 times/day	Same as ipratropium 0.03%

DECONGESTANTS

Generic (Brand)	Adult Dose	Pediatric Dose	Side Effects
Oxymetazoline (Afrin, Neo-Synephrine 12 HR)	2–3 sprays 2 times/day	6–11 yrs: 2–3 sprays 2 times/day	Insomnia, tachycardia, nervousness, nausea, vomiting, transient burning, headache, rebound congestion if used longer than 72 hrs
Phenylephrine (Neo-Synephrine Cold and Sinus, Vicks Sinus)	2–3 drops/sprays q4h as needed (0.25% or 0.5%)	6–11 yrs: 2–3 drops/sprays (0.25%) q4h as needed 1–5 yrs: 2–3 drops/sprays (0.125%) q4h as needed	Restlessness, nervousness, headache, rebound nasal congestion, burning, stinging, dryness

Alzheimer's Disease

Dementia is a general term used describing a decline in mental ability that is severe enough to interfere with the function of daily living. Alzheimer's disease (AD) is the most common cause of dementia. Cognitive loss in AD is associated with depletion of acetylcholine (involved with learning and memory). AD is confirmed only at autopsy and is characterized by the presence of beta-amyloid plaques on the outer portions of neurons.

Currently, two classes of medications are used as therapies for AD, *acetylcholinesterase inhibitors (AChEIs)* and an *N-methyl-D-aspartate (NMDA) receptor antagonist.*

AChEIs increase the concentration of acetylcholine and may have beneficial effects on dementia. NMDA receptor antagonist mechanism of action is unclear, but may reduce glutamatergic overstimulation at the NMDA receptor, which may have symptomatic benefits on dementia.

ACETYLCHOLINESTERASE INHIBITORS

Name	Uses	Availability	Dose/Titration	Adverse Effects
Donepezil (Aricept, Aricept ODT)	Mild, moderate, severe AD	**T:** 5 mg, 10 mg, 23 mg **ODT:** 5 mg, 10 mg	Initially, 5 mg once/d, may increase to 10 mg once/d after 4-6 wks. After 3 months, if sub-optimal response, may increase to 23 mg once/d	Nausea, vomiting, abdominal cramping, diarrhea, bradycardia, syncope
Galantamine (Razadyne, Razadyne ER)	Mild, moderate AD	**T:** 4 mg, 8 mg, 12 mg **OS:** 4 mg/ml **ER:** 8 mg, 16 mg, 24 mg	**T, OS:** Initially, 4 mg bid; may increase to 8 mg bid after 4 wks, then to 12 mg bid after additional 4 wks **ER:** Initially, 8 mg once/d, may increase to 16 mg once/d after 4 wks, then to 24 mg once/d after additional 4 wks	Nausea, vomiting, diarrhea, weight loss, decreased appetite, syncope
Rivastigmine (Exelon, Exelon Patch)	Mild, moderate AD Patch also approved for severe AD	**C:** 1.5 mg, 3 mg, 4.5 mg, 6 mg **OS:** 2 mg/ml **PATCH:** 4.6 mg/24 hrs, 9.5 mg/24 hrs, 13.3 mg/24 hrs	**C, OS:** Initially, 1.5 mg bid, may increase in increments of 1.5 mg bid every 2 wks up to 6 mg bid	Nausea, vomiting, abdominal cramping, diarrhea, bradycardia, syncope, loss of appetite, weight loss

Continued

ACETYLCHOLINESTERASE INHIBITORS—cont'd

NMDA Receptor Antagonist

Memanatine (Namenda, Namenda XR)	Moderate, severe AD	**T:** 5 mg, 10 mg **OS:** 2 mg/ml **XR:** 7 mg, 14 mg, 21 mg, 28 mg	**T, OS:** Initially, 5 mg once/d, may increase in increments of 5 mg/wk up to 10 mg bid	Dizziness, headache, diarrhea, constipation, confusion

NMDA Receptor Antagonist/ Acetylcholinesterase Inhibitor

Memantine/done-pezil (Namzaric)	Moderate, severe AD	**ER:** 14/10 mg, 28/10 mg	**14/10 mg:** Once/d in evening in patients previously stabilized on memantine 5 mg bid or 14 mg once/d and donepezil 10 mg once/d **28/10 mg:** Once/d in evening in patients previously stabilized on memantine 10 mg bid or 28 mg once/d and donepezil 10 mg once/d	Refer to individual agents for adverse effects

C: capsule, *ER:* extended release, *OS:* oral solution, *T:* tablet, *XR:* extended release

Angiotensin-Converting Enzyme (ACE) Inhibitors

USES

Treatment of hypertension (HTN), adjunctive therapy for heart failure (HF).

ACTION

Antihypertensive: Inhibits angiotensin-converting enzyme (ACE). ACE catalyzes conversion of angiotensin I to angiotensin II, a potent vasoconstrictor that also stimulates aldosterone secretion by adrenal cortex. Beneficial effects in HTN/HF appear to be suppression of the renin-angiotensin-aldosterone system. Reduces peripheral arterial resistance.

HF: Decreases peripheral vascular resistance (afterload), pulmonary capillary wedge pressure (preload); improves cardiac output, exercise tolerance.

Frequent or Severe Side Effects

Class Effects

Cough, hypotension, rash, acute renal failure (in pts with renal artery stenosis), angioedema, hyperkalemia, mild-moderate loss of taste, hepatotoxicity, pancreatitis, blood dyscrasias, renal damage

ACE INHIBITORS

Name	Availability	Uses	Dosage Range (per day)
Benazepril (Lotensin)	**T:** 5 mg, 10 mg, 20 mg, 40 mg	HTN	**HTN:** Initially, 10 mg/day. Usual dose: 20–80 mg once/d or divided bid.
Captopril (Capoten)	**T:** 12.5 mg, 25 mg, 50 mg, 100 mg	HTN	**HTN:** Initially, 12.5–25 mg 2–3 times/day. Usual dose: 50–100 mg 2 times/day.
		HF	**HF:** Initially, 6.25 mg 3 times/day. Target: 50 mg 3 times/day.
Enalapril (Vasotec)	**T:** 2.5 mg, 5 mg, 10 mg, 20 mg **IV:** 1.25 mg/ml	HTN	**HTN:** Initially, 2.5–5 mg/day; may increase at 1–2 wk intervals. Usual dose: 5–40 mg once/d or divided bid.
		HF	**HF:** Initially, 2.5 mg 2 times/day, may increase at 1–2 wk intervals. Target: 20 mg/day in 1–2 divided doses.
Fosinopril (Monopril)	**T:** 10 mg, 20 mg, 40 mg	HTN	**HTN:** Initially, 10 mg/day. Usual dose: 10–80 mg once/d.
		HF	**HF:** Initially, 5–10 mg/day. Target: 10–40 mg/day.

Continued

ACE INHIBITORS—cont'd

Name	Availability	Uses	Dosage Range (per day)	Frequent or Severe Side Effects
Lisinopril (Prinivil, Zestril)	**T:** 2.5 mg, 5 mg, 10 mg, 20 mg, 40 mg	HTN	**HTN:** Initially, 5–10 mg/day. Usual dose: 10–40 mg/once/d.	
		HF	**HF:** Initially, 2.5–5 mg/day. Target: 20–40 mg/day.	
Moexipril (Univasc)	**T:** 7.5 mg, 15 mg	HTN	**HTN:** Initially, 3.75–7.5 mg/day. Usual dose: 7.5–30 mg/day in 1–2 divided doses.	
Perindopril (Aceon)	**T:** 2 mg, 4 mg, 6 mg	HTN	**HTN:** Initially, 4 mg/day. May increase at 1–2 wk intervals. Usual dose: 4–8 mg once/d or divided bid.	
Quinapril (Accupril)	**T:** 5 mg, 10 mg, 20 mg, 40 mg	HTN	**HTN:** Initially, 10–20 mg once daily. Usual dose: 10–40 mg once/d or divided bid.	
		HF	**HF:** Initially, 5 mg 2 times/day. Titrate to 20–40 mg/day in 2 divided doses.	
Ramipril (Altace)	**C:** 1.25 mg, 2.5 mg, 5 mg, 10 mg	HTN	**HTN:** Initially, 2.5 mg once daily. Usual dose: 2.5–20 mg once/d or divided bid.	
		HF	**HF:** Initially, 1.25–2.5 mg once daily. Target: 10 mg once daily.	
Trandolapril (Mavik)	**T:** 1 mg, 2 mg, 4 mg	HTN	**HTN:** Initially, 1–2 mg once daily. Usual dose: 2–8 mg once/d or divided bid.	
		HF	**HF:** Initially, 1 mg once daily. Target: 4 mg once daily.	

C, Capsules; *HF,* heart failure; *HTN,* hypertension; *T,* tablets.

Angiotensin II Receptor Antagonists

USES

Treatment of hypertension (HTN) alone or in combination with other antihypertensives. Treatment of heart failure (HF).

ACTION

Angiotensin II receptor antagonists (AIIRA) block vasoconstrictor and aldosterone-secreting effects on angiotensin II by selectively blocking the binding of angiotensin II to AT_1 receptors in vascular smooth muscle and the adrenal gland, causing vasodilation and a decrease in aldosterone effects.

ANGIOTENSIN II RECEPTOR ANTAGONISTS

Name	Availability	Uses	Dosage Range (per day)	Frequent or Severe Side Effects
Azilsartan (Edarbi)	**T:** 40 mg, 80 mg	HTN	40–80 mg once daily	**Class Effects** Hypotension, rash, acute renal failure (in pts with renal artery stenosis), hyperkalemia, mild-moderate loss of taste, hepatotoxicity, pancreatitis, blood dyscrasias, renal damage
Candesartan (Atacand)	**T:** 4 mg, 8 mg, 16 mg, 32 mg	HTN HF	Initially, 16 mg once daily. Usual dose: 8–32 mg in 1–2 divided doses Initially 4–8 mg once daily. Double dose at 2 wk intervals. Target: 32 mg once daily.	
Eprosartan (Teveten)	**T:** 400 mg, 600 mg	HTN	Initially, 600 mg/day. Usual dose: 600–once/d	
Irbesartan (Avapro)	**T:** 75 mg, 150 mg, 300 mg	HTN Nephropathy	150–300 mg once daily 300 mg once daily	
Losartan (Cozaar)	**T:** 25 mg, 50 mg, 100 mg	HTN Nephropathy	Initially, 50 mg once daily. Usual dose: 25–100 mg/once/d or divided bid. Initially, 50 mg/day; may increase to 100 mg/day.	
Olmesartan (Benicar)	**T:** 5 mg, 20 mg, 40 mg	HTN	Initially, 20 mg once daily. May increase to 40 mg once daily after 2 wks.	

Continued

ANGIOTENSIN II RECEPTOR ANTAGONISTS—cont'd

Name	Availability	Uses	Dosage Range (per day)	Frequent or Severe Side Effects
Telmisartan (Micardis)	**T:** 40 mg, 80 mg	HTN CV risk reduction	Initially 40 mg once daily. Usual dose: 40–80 mg once daily. 80 mg once daily	
Valsartan (Diovan)	**T:** 80 mg, 160 mg	HTN	Initially, 80 or 160 mg once daily. Usual dose: 80–320 mg once daily	
		HF	Initially 20–40 mg 2 times/day. Titrate to 80–160 mg 2 times/day.	
		Post MI	Initially, 20 mg 2 times/day. Titrate to target of 160 mg 2 times/day	

CV, Cardiovascular; *HF,* heart failure; *HTN,* hypertension; *MI,* myocardial Infarction; *T,* tablets.

Antianxiety Agents

USES

Treatment of anxiety including generalized anxiety disorder (GAD), panic disorder, obsessive-compulsive disorder (OCD), social anxiety disorder (SAD), post-traumatic stress disorder (PTSD), and acute stress disorder. In addition, some benzodiazepines are used as hypnotics, anticonvulsants to prevent delirium tremors during alcohol withdrawal, and as adjunctive therapy for relaxation of skeletal muscle spasms.

Midazolam, a short-acting benzodiazepine, is used for preop sedation and relief of anxiety for short diagnostic/endoscopic procedures (see individual monograph for midazolam).

◄**ALERT▶** Refer to individual entries of nonbenzodiazepine drugs for more information on uses and actions.

ACTION

Benzodiazepines are the largest and most frequently prescribed group of antianxiety agents. The exact mechanism is unknown, but they may increase the inhibiting effect of gamma-aminobutyric acid (GABA), which inhibits nerve impulse transmission by binding to specific benzodiazepine receptors in various areas of the central nervous system (CNS).

ANTIANXIETY AGENTS

Name	Availability	Uses	Dosage	Side Effects
Benzodiazepine				
Alprazolam (Xanax)	**T:** 0.25 mg, 0.5 mg, 1 mg, 2 mg **S:** 1 mg/ml **ER:** 0.5 mg, 1 mg, 2 mg, 3 mg **ODT:** 0.25 mg, 0.5 mg, 1 mg, 2 mg	Anxiety, panic disorder	Initially, 0.25–0.5 mg 3 times/day. May increase every 3–4 days. Maximum: 4 mg/day.	Drowsiness, weakness, fatigue, ataxia, slurred speech, confusion, lack of coordination, impaired memory, paradoxical agitation, dizziness, nausea
Chlordiazepoxide (Librium)	**C:** 5 mg, 10 mg, 25 mg **T:** 10 mg, 25 mg **I:** 100 mg	Anxiety, alcohol withdrawal	Anxiety: 5–10 mg 3–4 times/day up to 20–25 mg 3–4 times/day. Alcohol withdrawal: Initially, 50–100 mg. May increase to 300 mg/24 hrs.	Drowsiness, fatigue, ataxia, memory impairment
Clorazepate (Tranxene)	**T:** 3.75 mg, 7.5 mg, 15 mg **SD:** 11.25 mg, 22.5 mg	Anxiety, alcohol withdrawal, anticonvulsant	7.5–15 mg 2–4 times/day.	Hypotension, drowsiness, fatigue, ataxia, memory impairment, headache, nausea
Diazepam (Valium)	**T:** 2 mg, 5 mg, 10 mg **S:** 5 mg/5 ml **I:** 5 mg/ml	Anxiety, alcohol withdrawal, anticonvulsant, muscle relaxant	2–10 mg, 2–4 times/day.	Hypotension, ataxia, drowsiness, fatigue, vertigo
Lorazepam (Ativan)	**T:** 0.5 mg, 1 mg, 2 mg **S:** 2 mg/ml **I:** 2 mg/ml, 4 mg/ml	Anxiety, alcohol withdrawal	Initially, 2–3 mg/day in 2–3 divided doses. Usual dose: 2–6 mg/day in divided doses.	Sedation, respiratory depression, ataxia, dizziness, headache

Continued

ANTIANXIETY AGENTS—cont'd

Name	Availability	Uses	Dosage	Side Effects
Nonbenzodiazepine				
Buspirone (BuSpar)	**T:** 5 mg, 7.5 mg, 10 mg, 15 mg, 30 mg	Anxiety	Initially, 7.5 mg 2 times/day. May increase every 2–3 days by 2.5 mg bid. Maximum: 30 mg 2 times/day.	Dizziness, light-headedness, headaches, nausea, restlessness
Hydroxyzine (Atarax, Vistaril)	**T:** 10 mg, 25 mg, 50 mg **C:** 25 mg, 50 mg, 100 mg **S:** 10 mg/5 ml	Anxiety	50–100 mg 4 times/day	Drowsiness; dry mouth, nose, and throat
Paroxetine (Paxil)	**S:** 10 mg/5 ml **T:** 10 mg, 20 mg, 30 mg, 40 mg **T (CR):** 12.5 mg, 25 mg, 37.5 mg	Anxiety, depression, obsessive-compulsive disorder, panic disorder	Initially, 20 mg once daily. May increase by 10 mg/day at 1 wk intervals up to 50 mg/day. **CR:** Initially, 12.5 mg/day. May increase by 12.5 mg/day at 1 wk intervals up to 37.5 mg/day.	Drowsiness; dry mouth, nose, and throat; dizziness, diarrhea, diaphoresis, constipation, vomiting, tremors
Venlafaxine (Effexor)	**C (ER):** 37.5 mg, 75 mg, 150 mg **T (ER):** 37.5 mg, 75 mg, 150 mg	Anxiety, depression	Initially 37.5–75 mg once daily. May increase by 75 mg/day at least every 4 days up to 225 mg/day.	Drowsiness, nausea, headaches, dry mouth

C, Capsules; *CR,* controlled-release; *ER,* extended-release; *I,* Injection; *ODT,* orally disintegrating tablet; *S,* solution; *SD,* single dose; *T,* tablets.

Antiarrhythmics

USES

Prevention and treatment of cardiac arrhythmias, such as premature ventricular contractions, ventricular tachycardia, premature atrial contractions, paroxysmal atrial tachycardia, atrial fibrillation and flutter.

ACTION

The antiarrhythmics are divided into four classes based on their effects on certain ion channels and/or receptors located on the myocardial cell membrane. Class I is further divided into three subclasses (IA, IB, IC) based on electrophysiologic effects.

Class I: Blocks cardiac sodium channels and slows conduction velocity, prolonging refractory period and decreasing automaticity of sodium-dependent tissue.

Class IA: Blocks sodium and potassium channels.

Class IB: Shortens the repolarization phase.

Class IC: Slows conduction velocity; no effect on repolarization phase.

Class II: Slows sinus and atrioventricular (AV) nodal conduction.

Class III: Blocks cardiac potassium channels, prolonging the repolarization phase of electrical cells.

Class IV: Inhibits the influx of calcium through its channels, causing slower conduction through the sinus and AV nodes; decreases contractility.

ANTIARRHYTHMICS

Name	Availability	Uses	Dosage Range	Side Effects
Class IA				
Disopyramide (Norpace, Norpace CR)	**C:** 100 mg, 150 mg **C (ER):** 100 mg, 150 mg	AF, WPW, PSVT, PVCs, VT	**C:** 100–200 mg q6h. **ER:** 200–400 mg q12h.	Dry mouth, blurred vision, urinary retention, HF, proarrhythmia, heart block, nausea, vomiting, diarrhea, hypoglycemia, nervousness
Procainamide (Procan-SR, Pronestyl)	**I:** 100 mg/ml, 500 mg/ml	AF, WPW, VT	Loading dose: 15–18 mg/kg over 20–30 min. Maintenance dose: 1–4 mg/min as a continuous infusion.	Hypotension, fever, agranulocytosis, SLE, headaches, proarrhythmia, confusion, disorientation, GI symptoms, hypotension

Continued

ANTIARRHYTHMICS—cont'd

Name	Availability	Uses	Dosage Range	Side Effects
Quinidine (Quinaglute, Quinidex)	**T:** 200 mg, 300 mg **T (ER):** 300 mg, 324 mg **I:** 80 mg/ml	AF, WPW, PVCs, VT	**A (PO):** 400 mg q6h. **(ER):** 300–q8–12h or 648 mg q8h.	Diarrhea, hypotension, nausea, vomiting, cinchonism, fever, bitter taste, heart block, thrombocytopenia, proarrhythmia
Class IB				
Lidocaine (Xylocaine)	**I:** 300 mg for IM **IV Infusion:** 2 mg/ml, 4 mg/ml	PVCs, VT, VF	**IV:** Initially, 1–1.5 mg/kg. May repeat 0.5–0.75 mg/kg q5–10 min. Maximum cumulative dose: 3 mg/kg, then 1–4 mg/min infusion	Drowsiness, agitation, muscle twitching, seizures, paresthesia, proarrhythmia, slurred speech, tinnitus, cardiac depression, bradycardia, asystole
Mexiletine (Mexitil)	**C:** 150 mg, 200 mg, 250 mg	PVCs, VT, VF	**A:** Initially, 200 mg q8h. Adjust every 2–3 days in 50–100 mg increments. Maximum: 1,200 mg/day.	Drowsiness, agitation, muscle twitching, seizures, paresthesia, proarrhythmia, nausea, vomiting, blood dyscrasias, hepatitis, fever
Class IC				
Flecainide (Tambocor)	**T:** 50 mg, 100 mg, 150 mg	AF, PSVT, life-threatening ventricular arrhythmias	**A:** Initially, 100 mg q12h. May increase by 50 mg q12h at 4 day intervals. Maximum: 400 mg/day.	Dizziness, tremors, bradycardia, heart block, HF, GI upset, neutropenia, flushing, blurred vision, metallic taste, proarrhythmia
Propafenone (Ryth mol)	**T:** 150 mg, 225 mg, 300 mg **ER:** 225 mg, 325 mg, 425 mg	PAF, WPW, life-threatening ventricular arrhythmias	**A: T:** Initially, 150 mg q8h. May increase at 3–4 day intervals up to 300 mg q8h. **ER:** Initially, 225 mg q12h. May increase at a minimum of 5 days up to 425 mg q12h.	Dizziness, blurred vision, altered taste, nausea, exacerbation of asthma, proarrhythmia, bradycardia, heart block, HF, GI upset, bronchospasm, hepatotoxicity

Class II (Beta-Blockers)			
Acebutolol (Sectral)	C: 100 mg, 200 mg, 400mg	Ventricular arrhythmias	A: Initially, 200 mg 2 times/day. Maintenance: 600–1200 mg/day in divided doses.	Bradycardia, hypotension, depression, nightmares, fatigue, sexual dysfunction, SLE, arthritis, myalgia
Esmolol (Brevibloc)	I: 10 mg/ml	Supraventricular tachycardia	A: 50–200 mcg/kg/min	Hypotension, heart block, HF, bronchospasm
Propranolol (Inderal)	T: 10 mg, 20 mg, 40 mg	Tachyarrhythmias	A: Initially, 10–30 mg 3–4 times/day Maintenance: 10–40 mg 3–4 times/day	Bradycardia, hypotension, depression, nightmares, fatigue, sexual dysfunction, heart block, bronchospasm
Class III			
Amiodarone (Corda rone, Pacerone)	T: 100 mg, 200 mg, 400 mg I: 50 mg/ml	AF, PAF, PSVT, life-threatening ventricular arrhythmias	A (PO): 800–1,600 mg/day in divided doses for 1–3 wks, then 600–800 mg/day in divided doses (IV): 150 mg bolus, then 900 mg over 18 hrs	Blurred vision, photophobia, constipation, ataxia, proarrhythmia, pulmonary fibrosis, bradycardia, heart block, hyperthyroidism or hypothyroidism, peripheral neuropathy, GI upset, blue-gray skin, optic neuritis, hypotension
Dofetilide (Tikosyn)	C: 125 mcg, 250 mcg, 500 mcg	AF, A flutter	A: Individualized	Torsades de pointes, hypotension
Dronedarone (Multaq)	T: 400 mg	AF, A flutter	A (PO): 400 mg 2 times/day	Diarrhea, nausea, abdominal pain, vomiting, asthenia
Ibutilide (Corvert)	I: 0.1 mg/ml	AF, A flutter	A (greater than 60 kg): 1 mg over 10 min; (less than 60 kg): 0.01 mg/kg over 10 min	Torsades de pointes

Continued

ANTIARRHYTHMICS—cont'd

Name	Availability	Uses	Dosage Range	Side Effects
Sotalol (Betapace)	**T:** 80 mg, 120 mg, 160 mg	AF, PAF, PSVT, life-threatening ventricular arrhythmias	**A (IV):** Initially, 80 mg 2 times/day. May increase at 3 day intervals up to 160 mg 2 times/day.	Fatigue, dizziness, dyspnea, bradycardia, proarrhythmia, heart block, hypotension, bronchospasm
Class IV (Calcium Channel Blockers)				
Diltiazem (Cardizem)	**I:** 25 mg/ml vials **Infusion:** 1 mg/ml	AF, A flutter, PSVT	**A (IV):** 20–25 mg bolus, then infusion of 5–15 mg/hr	Hypotension, bradycardia, dizziness, headaches, heart block, asystole, HF
Verapamil (Calan, Isoptin)	**I:** 5 mg/2 ml	AF, A flutter, PSVT	**A (IV):** 5–10 mg	Hypotension, bradycardia, dizziness, headaches, constipation, heart block, HF, asystole, fatigue, edema, nausea

A, Adults; *AF,* atrial fibrillation; *A flutter,* atrial flutter; *C,* capsules; *HF,* heart failure; *ER,* extended-release; *I,* Injection; *PAF,* paroxysmal atrial fibrillation; *PSVT,* paroxysmal supraventricular tachycardia; *PVCs,* premature ventricular contractions; *SLE,* systemic lupus erythematosus; *SR,* sustained-release; *T,* tablets; *VT,* ventricular tachycardia; *WPW,* Wolff-Parkinson-White syndrome.

Antibiotics

USES

Treatment of wide range of gram-positive or gram-negative bacterial infections, suppression of intestinal flora before surgery, control of acne, prophylactically to prevent rheumatic fever, prophylactically in high-risk situations (e.g., some surgical procedures or medical conditions) to prevent bacterial infection.

ACTION

Antibiotics are natural or synthetic compounds that have the ability to kill or suppress the growth of microorganisms.

One means of classifying antibiotics is by their antimicrobial spectrum. Narrow-spectrum agents are effective against few microorganisms. Broad-spectrum agents (e.g., aminoglycosides are effective against gram-negative aerobes), whereas broad-spectrum agents are effective against a wide variety of microorganisms (e.g., fluoroquinolones are effective against gram-positive cocci and gram-negative bacilli).

Antimicrobial agents may also be classified based on their mechanism of action.

- Agents that inhibit cell wall synthesis or activate enzymes that disrupt the cell wall, causing a weakening in the cell, cell lysis, and death. Include penicillins, cephalosporins, vancomycin, imidazole antifungal agents.
- Agents that act directly on the cell wall, affecting permeability of cell membranes, causing leakage of intracellular substances. Include antifungal agents amphotericin and nystatin, polymyxin, colistin.

- Agents that bind to ribosomal subunits, altering protein synthesis and eventually causing cell death. Include aminoglycosides.
- Agents that affect bacterial ribosome function, altering protein synthesis and causing slow microbial growth. Do not cause cell death. Include chloramphenicol, clindamycin, erythromycin, tetracyclines.
- Agents that inhibit nucleic acid metabolism by binding to nucleic acid or interacting with enzymes necessary for nucleic acid synthesis. Inhibit DNA or RNA synthesis. Include rifampin, metronidazole, fluoroquinolones (e.g., ciprofloxacin).
- Agents that inhibit specific metabolic steps necessary for microbial growth, causing a decrease in essential cell components or synthesis of nonfunctional analogues of normal metabolites. Include trimethoprim, sulfonamides.
- Agents that inhibit viral DNA synthesis by binding to viral enzymes necessary for DNA synthesis, preventing viral replication. Include acyclovir, vidarabine.

SELECTION OF ANTIMICROBIAL AGENTS

The goal of therapy is to achieve antimicrobial action at the site of infection sufficient to inhibit the growth of the microorganism. The agent selected should be the most active against the most likely infecting organism, least likely to cause toxicity or allergic reaction. Factors to consider in selection of an antimicrobial agent include the following:

- Sensitivity pattern of the infecting microorganism
- Location and severity of infection (may determine route of administration)
- Pt's ability to eliminate the drug (status of renal and hepatic function)
- Pt's defense mechanisms (includes both cellular and humoral immunity)
- Pt's age, pregnancy status, genetic factors, allergies, CNS disorder, preexisting medical problems

CATEGORIZATION OF ORGANISMS BY GRAM STAINING

Gram-Positive Cocci	Gram-Negative Cocci	Gram-Positive Bacilli	Gram-Negative Bacilli
Aerobic *Staphylococcus aureus* *Staphylococcus epidermidis* *Streptococcus pneumoniae* *Streptococcus pyogenes* *Viridans streptococci* *Enterococcus faecalis* *Enterococcus faecium* **Anaerobic** *Peptostreptococcus spp.* *Peptococcus spp.*	**Aerobic** *Neisseria gonorrhoeae* *Neisseria meningitidis* *Moraxella catarrhalis*	**Aerobic** *Listeria monocytogenes* *Bacillus anthracis* *Corynebacterium diphtheriae* **Anaerobic** *Clostridium difficile* *Clostridium perfringens* *Clostridium tetani* *Actinomyces spp.*	**Aerobic** *Escherichia coli* *Klebsiella pneumoniae* *Proteus mirabilis* *Serratia marcescens* *Acinetobacter spp.* *Pseudomonas aeruginosa* *Enterobacter spp.* *Haemophilus influenzae* *Legionella pneumophila* **Anaerobic** *Bacteroides fragilis* *Fusobacterium spp.*

Antibiotic: Aminoglycosides

USES

Treatment of serious infections when other less-toxic agents are not effective, are contraindicated, or require adjunctive therapy (e.g., with penicillins or cephalosporins). Used primarily in the treatment of infections caused by gram-negative microorganisms, such as those caused by *Proteus, Klebsiella, Pseudomonas, Escherichia coli, Serratia,* and *Enterobacter.* Inactive against most gram-positive microorganisms. Not well absorbed systemically from GI tract (must be administered parenterally for systemic infections). Oral agents are given to suppress intestinal bacteria.

ACTION

Bactericidal. Transported across bacterial cell membrane; irreversibly bind to specific receptor proteins of bacterial ribosomes. Interfere with protein synthesis, preventing cell reproduction and eventually causing cell death.

ANTIBIOTIC: AMINOGLYCOSIDES

Name	Availability	Dosage Range	Side Effects
Amikacin	**I:** 50 mg/ml, 250 mg/ml	**A:** 5–7.5 mg/kg q8h or 15–20 mg/kg once daily **C:** 5–7.5 mg/kg q8h	Nephrotoxicity, neurotoxicity, ototoxicity (both auditory and vestibular), hypersensitivity (skin itching, redness, rash, swelling)
Gentamicin	**I:** 10 mg/ml, 40 mg/ml	**A:** 4–7 mg/kg once daily or 1–2.5 mg/kg q8–12h **C:** 2–2.5 mg/kg q8h	Same as amikacin
Tobramycin	**I:** 10 mg/ml, 40 mg/ml	**A:** 5–7 mg/kg once daily or 1–2.5 mg/kg q8h **C:** 2–2.5 mg/kg q8h	Same as amikacin

A, Adults; *C (dosage),* children; *I,* Injection; *T,* tablets.

Antibiotic: Cephalosporins

USES

Broad-spectrum antibiotics, which, like penicillins, may be used in a number of diseases, including respiratory diseases, skin and soft tissue infection, bone/joint infections, genitourinary infections, prophylactically in some surgical procedures.

First-generation cephalosporins have activity against gram-positive organisms (e.g., streptococci and most staphylococci) and activity against most gram-negative organisms, including *Escherichia coli, Klebsiella pneumoniae, Proteus mirabilis, Salmonella,* and *Shigella.*

Second-generation cephalosporins have same effectiveness as first-generation and increased activity against gram-negative organisms, including *Haemophilus influenzae, Neisseria, Enterobacter,* and several anaerobic organisms.

Third-generation cephalosporins are less active against gram-positive organisms but more active against the Enterobacteriaceae with some activity against *Pseudomonas aeruginosa, Serratia* spp., and *Acinetobacter* spp.

Fourth-generation cephalosporins have good activity against gram-positive organisms (e.g., *Staphylococcus*

ACTION

aureus) and gram-negative organisms (e.g., *Pseudomonas aeruginosa, E. coli, Klebsiella,* and *Proteus*).

Fifth-generation cephalosporins have good activity against gram-positive organisms (e.g., *Staphylococcus aureus, Streptococcus* spp.) and gram-negative organisms (e.g., *E. coli, Klebsiella* spp.).

Cephalosporins inhibit cell wall synthesis or activate enzymes that disrupt the cell wall, causing cell lysis and cell death. May be bacteriostatic or bactericidal. Most effective against rapidly dividing cells.

ANTIBIOTIC: CEPHALOSPORINS

Name	Availability	Dosage Range	Side Effects
First-Generation			
Cefadroxil (Duricef)	C: 500 mg T: 1 g S: 125 mg/5 ml, 250 mg/5 ml, 500 mg/5 ml	A: 500 mg–1 g C: 15 mg/kg q12h	Abdominal cramps/pain, fever, nausea, vomiting, diarrhea, headaches, oral/vaginal candidiasis
Cefazolin (Ancef)	I: 500 mg, 1 g, 2 g	A: 500 mg–2 g q6–8h C: 25–100 mg/kg/day divided q6–8h	Fever, rash, diarrhea, nausea, pain at injection site

Cephalexin (Keflex, Keftab)	C: 250 mg, 500 mg T: 250 mg, 500 mg, 1 g	A: 250 mg–1 g q6–12h C: 25–100 mg/kg/day divided q6–8h	Headache, abdominal pain, diarrhea, nausea, dyspepsia
Second-Generation			
Cefaclor (Ceclor)	C: 250 mg, 500 mg T (ER): 500 mg S: 125 mg/5 ml, 187 mg/5 ml, 250 mg/5 ml, 375 mg/5 ml	A: 250–500 mg q8h ER: 500 mg q12h C: 20–40 mg/kg/day q8–12h	Rash, diarrhea, increased transaminases May have serum sickness-like reaction
Cefotetan	I:1g, 2g	A: 500 mg–3 g q12h C: 20–40 mg/kg q12h	Diarrhea, increased AST, ALT, hypersensitivity reactions
Cefoxitin (Mefoxin)	I:1g,2g	A: 1–2 g q6–8h C: 80–160 mg/kg/day divided q6h	Diarrhea
Cefprozil (Cefzil)	T: 250 mg, 500 mg S: 125 mg/5 ml, 250 mg/5 ml	A: 500 mg q12–24h C: 7.5–15 mg/kg q12h	Dizziness, abdominal pain, diarrhea, nausea, increased AST, ALT
Cefuroxime (Ceftin, Kefurox, Zinacef)	T: 125 mg, 250 mg, 500 mg S: 125 mg/5 ml, 250 mg/5 ml I: 750 mg, 1.5 g	A (PO): 125–500 mg q12h (IM/IV): 750 mg–1.5 g q8–12h C (PO): 10–15 mg/kg q12h (IM/IV): 75–150 mg/kg/day divided q8h	Diarrhea, nausea, vomiting, thrombophlebitis, increased AST, ALT
Third-Generation			
Cefdinir (Omnicef)	C: 300 mg S: 125 mg/5 ml	A: 300 mg q12h or 600 mg once daily C: 7 mg/kg q12h or 14 mg/kg once daily	Headache, hyperglycemia, abdominal pain, diarrhea, nausea
Cefditoren (Spectracef)	T: 200 mg, 400 mg	A: 200–400 mg q12h C: (>11 yrs): 200–400 mg q12h	Diarrhea, nausea
Cefotaxime (Claforan)	I: 500 mg, 1 g, 2 g	A: 1–2 g q4–12h C: 50–300 mg/kg/day divided q4–6h	Rash, diarrhea, nausea, pain at injection site

Continued

ANTIBIOTIC: CEPHALOSPORINS—cont'd

Name	Availability	Dosage Range	Side Effects
Cefpodoxime (Vantin)	T: 100 mg, 200 mg S: 50 mg/5 ml, 100 mg/5 ml	A: 100–400 mg q12h C: 5 mg/kg q12h	Rash, diarrhea, nausea
Ceftazidime (Fortaz, Tazicef, Tazidime)	I: 500 mg, 1 g, 2 g	A: 500 mg–2 g q8—12h C: 30–50 mg/kg q8h	Diarrhea, pain at injection site
Ceftibuten (Cedax)	C: 400 mg S: 90 mg/5 ml, 180 mg/5 ml	A: 400 mg once daily C: 4.5 mg/kg bid or 9 mg/kg once daily	Headache, nausea, diarrhea
Ceftriaxone (Rocephin)	I: 250 mg, 500 mg, 1 g, 2 g	A: 1–2 g q12–24h C: 50–100 mg/kg/day divided q12–24h	Rash, diarrhea, eosinophilia, increased AST, ALT
Fourth-Generation			
Cefepime (Maxipime)	I: 1g, 2g	A: 1–2 g q8–12h C: 50 mg/kg q8–12h	Rash, diarrhea, nausea; increased AST, ALT
Fifth-Generation			
Ceftaroline (Teflaro)	I: 400 mg, 600 mg	A: 600 mg q12h	Headache, insomnia, rash, pruritus, diarrhea, nausea
Fixed-Combinations			
Ceftazidime/avibactam (Avycaz)	I: 2 g ceftazidime/0.5 g avibactam	A: 2.5 g q8h	Nausea, vomiting, constipation, anxiety
Ceftolozane/tazobactam (Zerbaxa)	I: 1 g ceftolozane/0.5 g tazobactam	A: 1.5 g q8h	Nausea, diarrhea, headache, pyrexia

A, Adults; *C,* capsules; *C (dosage),* children; *ER,* extended-release; *I,* Injection; *S,* suspension; *T,* tablets.

Antibiotic: Fluoroquinolones

USES

Fluoroquinolones act against a wide range of gram-negative and gram-positive organisms. They are used primarily in the treatment of lower respiratory infections, skin/skin structure infections, urinary tract infections, and sexually transmitted diseases.

ACTION

Bactericidal. Inhibit DNA gyrase in susceptible microorganisms, interfering with bacterial DNA replication and repair.

ANTIBIOTIC: FLUOROQUINOLONES

Name	Availability	Dosage Range	Side Effects
Ciprofloxacin (Cipro)	**T:** 100 mg, 250 mg, 500 mg, 750 mg **S:** 250 mg/5 ml, 500 mg/5 ml **I:** 200 mg, 400 mg	**A (PO):** 250–750 mg q12h; **(IV):** 200–400 mg q12h	Dizziness, headaches, anxiety, drowsiness, insomnia, abdominal pain, nausea, diarrhea, vomiting, phlebitis (parenteral)
Delafloxacin (Baxdela)	**T:** 450 mg **I:** 300 mg	**A (PO):** 450 mg q12h; **(IV):** 300 mg q12h	Nausea, diarrhea, headache, elevation of transaminases, vomiting
Gemifloxacin (Factive)	**T:** 320 mg	**A:** 320 mg once daily	Headache, dizziness, rash, diarrhea, nausea
Levofloxacin (Levaquin)	**T:** 250 mg, 500 mg, 750 mg **I:** 250 mg, 500 mg, 750 mg **OS:** 250 mg/10 ml	**A (PO/IV):** 250–750 mg/day as single dose	Headache, insomnia, dizziness, rash, nausea, diarrhea, constipation
Moxifloxacin (Avelox)	**T:** 400 mg **I:** 400 mg	**A:** 400 mg/day	Headache, dizziness, insomnia, nausea, diarrhea
Ofloxacin	**T:** 300 mg, 400 mg	**A:** 200–400 mg q12h	Dizziness, headache, insomnia, abdominal cramps, diarrhea, nausea

A, Adults; *I*, Injection; *OS*, oral solution; *PO*, oral; *S*, suspension; *T*, tablets.

Antibiotic: Macrolides

USES

Macrolides act primarily against most gram-positive microorganisms and some gram-negative cocci. Azithromycin and clarithromycin appear to be more potent than erythromycin. Macrolides are used in the treatment of pharyngitis/tonsillitis, sinusitis, chronic bronchitis, pneumonia, uncomplicated skin/skin structure infections.

ACTION

Bacteriostatic or bactericidal. Reversibly binds to the P site of the 50S ribosomal subunit of susceptible organisms, inhibiting RNA-dependent protein synthesis.

ANTIBIOTIC: MACROLIDES

Name	Availability	Dosage Range	Side Effects
Azithromycin (Zithromax)	T: 250 mg, 600 mg S: 100 mg/5 ml, 200 mg/5 ml, 1-g packet I: 500 mg	A (PO): 500 mg once, then 250 mg once daily (IV): 500 mg/day C (PO/IV): 5–10 mg/kg once daily	PO: Nausea, diarrhea, vomiting, abdominal pain IV: Pain, redness, swelling at injection site
Clarithromycin (Biaxin)	T: 250 mg, 500 mg T (XL): 500 mg S: 125 mg/5 ml	A: 250–500 mg q12h (or XL 1,000 mg once daily) C: 7.5 mg/kg q12h	Headaches, loss of taste, nausea, vomiting, diarrhea, abdominal pain/discomfort
Erythromycin (EES, Eryc, EryPed, Ery-Tab, Erythrocin, PCE)	T: 200 mg, 250 mg, 333 mg, 400 mg, 500 mg C: 250 mg S: 100 mg/2.5 ml, 125 mg/5 ml, 200 mg/5 ml, 250 mg/5 ml, 400 mg/5 ml	A (PO): 250–500 mg q6h (IV): 500 mg–1 g q6h C (PO): 7.5 mg/kg q6h (IV): 15–20 mg/kg/day in divided doses q6h	PO: Nausea, vomiting, diarrhea, abdominal pain IV: Inflammation, phlebitis at injection site

A, Adults; *C,* capsules; *C (dosage),* children; *I,* Injection; *S,* suspension; *T,* tablets; *XL,* long-acting.

Antibiotic: Penicillins

USES

Penicillins (also referred to as beta-lactam antibiotics) may be used to treat a large number of infections, including pneumonia and other respiratory diseases, urinary tract infections, septicemia, meningitis, intra-abdominal infections, gonorrhea and syphilis, bone/joint infection.

Penicillins are classified based on an antimicrobial spectrum:

Natural penicillins are very active against gram-positive cocci but ineffective against most strains of *Staphylococcus aureus* (inactivated by enzyme penicillinase).

Penicillinase-resistant penicillins are effective against penicillinase-producing *Staphylococcus aureus* but are less effective against gram-positive cocci than the natural penicillins.

Broad-spectrum penicillins are effective against gram-positive cocci and some gram-negative bacteria (e.g., *Haemophilus influenzae, Escherichia coli, Proteus mirabilis, Salmonella,* and *Shigella*).

Extended-spectrum penicillins are effective against gram-negative organisms, including *Pseudomonas aeruginosa, Enterobacter, Proteus* spp., *Klebsiella, Serratia* spp., and *Acinetobacter* spp.

ACTION

Penicillins inhibit cell wall synthesis or activate cell wall enzymes, which disrupt the bacterial cell wall, causing cell lysis and cell death. May be bacteriostatic or bactericidal. Most effective against bacteria undergoing active growth and division.

ANTIBIOTIC: PENICILLINS

Name	Availability	Dosage Range	Side Effects
Natural			
Penicillin G benzathine (Bicillin, Bicillin LA)	**I:** 600,000 units, 1.2 million units, 2.4 million units	**A:** 1.2–2.4 million units as single dose **C:** 25,000–50,000 units/kg as single dose	Mild diarrhea, nausea, vomiting, headaches, sore mouth/tongue, vaginal itching/discharge, allergic reaction (including anaphylaxis, skin rash, urticaria, pruritus)

Continued

ANTIBIOTIC: PENICILLINS—cont'd

Name	Availability	Dosage Range	Side Effects
Penicillin G potassium (Pfizerpen)	**I:** 1, 2, 3, 5 million-unit vials	**A:** 2–4 million units q4h **C:** 100,000–400,000 units/kg/ day divided q4–6h	Rash, injection site reaction, phlebitis
Penicillin V potassium (Apo-Pen-VK)	**T:** 250 mg, 500 mg **S:** 125 mg/5 ml, 250 mg/5 ml	**A:** 250–500 mg q6–8h **C:** 25–50 mg/kg/day in divided doses q6–8h	Diarrhea, nausea, vomiting
Penicillinase-Resistant			
Dicloxacillin (Dynapen, Pathocil)	**C:** 125 mg, 250 mg, 500 mg **S:** 62.5 mg/5 ml	**A:** 125–500 mg q6h **C:** 25–50 mg/kg/day divided q6h	Abdominal pain, diarrhea, nausea
Nafcillin (Unipen)	**I:**500 mg, 1 g, 2g	**A (IV):** 500 mg–2 g q4–6h **C (IV):** 50–200 mg/kg/day in divided doses q4–6h	Inflammation, pain, phlebitis Increased risk of interstitial nephritis
Oxacillin (Bactocill)	**C:** 250 mg, 500 mg **S:** 250 mg/5 ml **I:** 250 mg, 500 mg, 1 g, 2 g	**A (IV):** 1–2 g q4–6h **C (IV):** 25–50 mg/kg q6h	Diarrhea, nausea, vomiting Increased risk of hepatotoxicity, interstitial nephritis
Broad-Spectrum			
Amoxicillin (Amoxil, Trimox)	**T:** 125 mg, 250 mg, 500 mg, 875 mg **C:** 250 mg, 500 mg **S:** 200 mg/5 ml, 400 mg/5 ml, 125 mg/5 ml, 250 mg/5 ml	**A:** 250–500 mg q8h or 500–875 g q12h **C:** 20–90 mg/kg/day divided q8–12h	Diarrhea, colitis, nausea

Amoxicillin/ clavulanate (Augmentin)	**T:** 250 mg, 500 mg, 875 mg **T (chewable):** 125 mg, 200 mg, 250 mg, 400 mg **S:** 125 mg/5 ml, 200 mg/5 ml, 250 mg/5 ml, 400 mg/5 ml	**A:** 875 mg q12h or 250–500 mg q8h **C:** 25–90 mg/kg/day divided q 12h	Diarrhea, rash, nausea, vomiting
Ampicillin (Principen)	**C:** 250 mg, 500 mg **S:** 125 mg/5 ml, 250 mg/5 ml **I:** 125 mg, 250 mg, 500 mg, 1 g, 2 g	**A (PO):** 250–500 mg q6h **(IV):** 500 mg–2 g q6h **C (PO):** 12.5–50 mg/kg q6h **(IV):** 25–50 mg/kg q6h	Nausea, vomiting, diarrhea
Ampicillin/sulbactam (Unasyn)	**I:**1.5 g, 3 g	**A:** 1.5–3 g q6h **C:** 25–50 mg/kg q6h	Local pain at injection site, rash, diarrhea
Extended-Spectrum			
Piperacillin/tazobactam (Zosyn)	**I:** 2.25 g, 3.375 g, 4.5 g	**A:** 3.375 g q6h or 4.5 g q6–8h **C:** 240–300 mg/kg/day divided q8h	Diarrhea, insomnia, headache, fever, rash

A, Adults; *C*, capsules; *C (dosage)*, children; *I*, Injection; *PO*, oral; *S*, suspension; *T*, tablets.

Anticoagulants/Antiplatelets/Thrombolytics

USES	ACTION
Treatment and prevention of venous thromboembolism, acute MI, acute cerebral embolism; reduce risk of acute MI; reduction of total mortality in pts with unstable angina; prevent occlusion of saphenous grafts following open heart surgery; prevent embolism in select pts with atrial fibrillation, prosthetic heart valves, valvular heart disease, cardiomyopathy. Heparin also used for acute/chronic consumption coagulopathies (disseminated intravascular coagulation).	*Anticoagulants:* Inhibit blood coagulation by preventing the formation of new clots and extension of existing ones *but do not dissolve formed clots.* Anticoagulants are subdivided. *Heparin* (including low molecular weight heparin): Indirectly interferes with blood coagulation by blocking the conversion of prothrombin to thrombin and fibrinogen to fibrin. *Coumarin:* Acts indirectly to prevent synthesis in the liver of vitamin K–dependent clotting factors. *Direct Thrombin Inhibitors:* Inhibit thrombin from converting fibrinogen to fibrin. *Factor Xa Inhibitors:* Inhibits platelet activation and fibrin clot formation. *Antiplatelets:* Interfere with platelet aggregation. Effects are irreversible for life of platelet. Medications in this group act by different mechanisms. Aspirin irreversibly inhibits cyclo-oxygenase and formation of thromboxane A_2. Clopidogrel, dipyridamole, prasugrel, and ticlopidine have similar effects as aspirin and are known as adenosine diphosphate (ADP) inhibitors. Abciximab, eptifibatide, and tirofiban block binding of fibrinogen to the glycoprotein IIb/IIIa receptor on platelet surface (known as platelet glycoprotein IIb/IIIa receptor antagonists). *Thrombolytics:* Act directly or indirectly on fibrinolytic system to dissolve clots (converting plasminogen to plasmin, an enzyme that digests fibrin clot).

ANTICOAGULANTS/ANTIPLATELETS/THROMBOLYTICS

Name	Availability	Uses	Side Effects
Anticoagulants			
Direct Thrombin Inhibitors			
Argatroban	I: 100 mg/ml	Prevent/treat VTE in pts with HIT or at risk for HIT undergoing PCI	Bleeding, hypotension, hematuria

Bivalirudin (Angiomax)	I: 250-mg vials	Pts with unstable angina undergoing PTCA	Bleeding, hypotension, pain, headache, nausea, back pain
Dabigatran (Pradaxa)	C: 75 mg, 110 mg, 150 mg	Reduce risk for stroke/embolism with nonvalvular atrial fibrillation, prevent/treat DVT/PE, postoperative prophylaxis of DVT/PE following hip replacement	Bleeding, gastritis, dyspepsia
Desirudin (Iprivask)	I: 15 mg	Prophylaxis of DVT following hip surgery	Bleeding
Heparin, Low Molecular Weight Heparins			
Dalteparin (Fragmin)	I: 2,500 units, 5,000 units, 7,500 units, 10,000 units	Prevent DVT following hip surgery, abdominal surgery, unstable angina or non–Q-wave MI	Bleeding, hematoma, increased ALT, AST, pain at injection site, bruising
Enoxaparin (Lovenox)	I: 30 mg, 40 mg, 60 mg, 80 mg, 100 mg, 120 mg, 150 mg	Prevent DVT following hip surgery, knee surgery, abdominal surgery, unstable angina or non–Q-wave MI, acute illness	Bleeding, thrombocytopenia, hematoma, increased ALT, AST, nausea, bruising
Heparin	I: 1,000 units/ml, 2,500 units/ml, 5,000 units/ml, 7,500 units/ml, 10,000 units/ml, 20,000 units/ml	Prevent/treat VTE	Bleeding, thrombocytopenia, skin rash, itching, burning
Tinzaparin (Innohep)	I: 10,000 units/ml, 20,000 units/ml vials	Treat DVT/PE, prevent VTE following surgery	Bleeding, thrombocytopenia, increased ALT, injection site hematoma
Factor Xa Inhibitor			
Apixaban (Eliquis)	T: 2.5 mg, 5 mg	Reduce risk of stroke/embolism in nonvalvular atrial fibrillation Prevent VTE post hip/knee replacement surgery, prevent/treat recurrence	Bleeding, nausea, anemia

Continued

ANTICOAGULANTS/ANTIPLATELETS/THROMBOLYTICS—cont'd

Name	Availability	Uses	Side Effects
Betrixaban (Bevyxxa)	C: 40 mg, 80 mg	Prophylaxis of VTE in adults with acute medical illness at risk for thromboembolic complications due to restricted mobility, other VTE risk factors	Bleeding
Edoxaban(Savaysa)	T: 15 mg, 30 mg, 60 mg	Prevent thromboembolism in nonvalvular atrial fibrillation, treat DVT/PT	Bleeding, anemia, rash, abnormal liver function tests
Fondaparinux (Arixtra)	I: 2.5 mg, 5 mg, 7.5 mg, 10 mg	Prophylaxis of DVT following hip fracture, abdominal surgery, hip surgery, knee surgery, treat DVT/PE	Bleeding, thrombocytopenia, hematoma, fever, nausea, anemia
Rivaroxaban (Xarelto)	T: 10 mg	Prevent DVT post knee, hip replacement. Prevent thromboembolism in atrial fibrillation. Prevent/treat DVT/PE	Bleeding
Coumarin			
Warfarin (Coumadin)	PO: 1 mg, 2 mg, 2.5 mg, 3 mg, 4 mg, 5 mg, 6 mg, 7.5 mg, 10 mg. I: 5 mg	Prevent/treat VTE in pts; prevent systemic embolism in pts with heart valve replacement, valve heart disease, MI, atrial fibrillation	Bleeding, skin necrosis, anorexia, nausea, vomiting, diarrhea, rash, abdominal cramps, purple toe syndrome, drug interactions (see individual monograph)
Antiplatelets			
Abciximab (ReoPro)	I: 2 mg/ml	Adjunct to PCI to prevent acute cardiac ischemic complications (with heparin and aspirin)	Bleeding, hypotension, nausea, vomiting, back pain, allergic reactions, thrombocytopenia
Aspirin	PO: 81 mg, 165 mg, 325 mg, 500 mg, 650 mg	TIA acute MI, chronic stable/unstable angina, revascularization procedures Prevent reinfarction and thromboembolism post MI	Tinnitus, dizziness, hypersensitivity, dyspepsia, minor bleeding, GI ulceration

Clopidogrel (Plavix)	PO: 75 mg	Reduce risk of stroke, MI, or vascular death in pts with recent MI, noncardioembolic stroke, peripheral artery disease. Reduce CV death, MI, stroke, reinfarction in pts with non-STEMI/STEMI	Bleeding, rash, pruritus, bruising, epistaxis
Cangrelor (Kengreal)	I: 50 mg	Adjunct to PCI to reduce risk of MI, repeat coronary revascularization, stent thrombosis	Bleeding
Eptifibatide (Integrilin)	I: 0.75 mg/ml, 2 mg/ml	Treat acute coronary syndrome	Bleeding, hypotension
Prasugrel (Effient)	PO: 5 mg, 10 mg	Reduce thrombotic cardiovascular events in pts with ACS to be managed with PCI (including stenting)	Bleeding, hypotension
Ticagrelor (Brilinta)	PO: 60 mg, 90 mg	Reduce thrombotic cardiovascular events in pts with ACS	Bleeding, dyspnea
Tirofiban (Aggrastat)	I: 50 mcg/ml, 250 mcg/ml	Treat acute coronary syndrome	Bleeding, thrombocytopenia, brady-cardia, pelvic pain
Vorapaxar (Zontivity)	T: 2.08 mg	Reduce thrombotic cardiovascular events (e.g., MI, stroke) in pts with history of MI or peripheral arterial disease	Bleeding
Thrombolytics			
Alteplase (Activase)	I: 50 mg, 100 mg	Acute MI, acute ischemic stroke, pulmonary embolism	Bleeding, epistaxis
Tenecteplase (TNKase)	I: 50 mg	Acute MI	Bleeding, hematuria

ACS, Acute coronary syndrome; *DTV,* deep vein thrombosis; *HIT,* heparin-induced thrombocytopenia; *I,* injection; *MI,* myocardial infarction; *PCI,* percutaneous coronary intervention; *PO,* oral; *PTCA,* percutaneous transluminal coronary angioplasty; *STEMI,* ST segment elevation MI; *T,* tablet; *TIA,* transient ischemic attack; *VTE,* venous thromboembolism.

Anticonvulsants

USES

Anticonvulsants are used to treat seizures. Seizures can be divided into two broad categories: partial seizures and generalized seizures. *Partial seizures* begin locally in the cerebral cortex, undergoing limited spread. Simple partial seizures do not involve loss of consciousness but may evolve secondarily into generalized seizures. Complex partial seizures involve impairment of consciousness.

Generalized seizures may be convulsive or nonconvulsive and usually produce immediate loss of consciousness.

ACTION

Anticonvulsants can prevent or reduce excessive discharge of neurons with seizure foci or decrease the spread of excitation from seizure foci to normal neurons. The exact mechanism is unknown but may be due to (1) suppressing sodium influx, (2) suppressing calcium influx, or (3) increasing the action of gamma-aminobutyric acid (GABA), which inhibits neurotransmitters throughout the brain

ANTICONVULSANTS

Name	Availability	Uses	Dosage Range	Side Effects
Brivaracetam (Briviact)	I: 10 mg/ml S: 10 mg/ml T: 10 mg, 25 mg, 50 mg, 75 mg, 100 mg	Partial-onset seizure	A: Initially, 50 mg bid. (May decrease to 25 mg bid or increase to 100 mg bid)	Nausea, vomiting, dizziness, fatigue, angioedema, psychiatric symptoms
Carbamazepine (Carbatrol, Carnexiv, Epitol, Tegretol, Tegretol XR)	S: 100 mg/5 ml T (chewable): 100 mg T: 200 m g T (ER): 100 mg, 200 mg, 400 mg C (ER): 100 mg, 200 mg, 300 mg I:10 mg/ml	Complex partial, tonic-clonic, mixed seizures; trigeminal neuralgia	**Note:** Refer to monograph for IV dosage A: Initially, 400 mg/day in 2 divided doses. May increase up to 200 mg/day at weekly intervals up to 800–1,600 mg/day in 2–3 doses. C: Initially, 200 mg/day in 2 divided doses. May increase by 100 mg/day at weekly intervals up to 400–800 mg/day in 3–4 doses.	Dizziness, diplopia, leukopenia, drowsiness, blurred vision, headache, ataxia, nausea, vomiting, hyponatremia, rash, pruritus

Clonazepam (Klonopin)	**T:** 0.5 mg, 1 mg, 2 mg	Petit mal, akinetic, myoclonic, absence seizures	**A:** Initially, not to exceed 1.5 mg in 3 divided doses. May increase q3days up to 2–8 mg/day in 1–2 divided doses.	CNS depression, sedation, ataxia, confusion, depression, behavior disorders, respiratory depression
Ezogabine (Potiga)	**T:** 50 mg, 200 mg, 300 mg, 400 mg	Partial onset seizures	**A:** Initially, 100 mg 3 times/day. May increase at weekly intervals up to 150 mg/day. Usual dose: 200–400 mg 3 times/day.	Dizziness, somnolence, fatigue, confusion, vertigo, tremor, balance disorder, urinary retention
Fosphenytoin (Cerebyx)	**I:** 50 mg PE/ml	Status epilepticus, seizures occurring during neurosurgery	**A:** 15–20 mg PE/kg bolus, then 4–6 mg PE/kg/day maintenance.	Burning, itching, paresthesia, nystagmus, ataxia
Gabapentin (Neurontin)	**C:** 100 mg, 300 mg, 400 mg **S:** 250 mg/5 ml	Partial and generalized seizures	**A:** 300 mg 3 times/day. Usual dose: 900–1,800 mg/day in 3 doses.	CNS depression, fatigue, drowsiness, dizziness, ataxia, nystagmus, blurred vision, confusion; may cause weight gain
Lacosamide (Vimpat)	**T:** 50 mg, 100 mg, 150 mg, 200 mg **S:** 10 mg/ml **I:** 10 mg/ml	Adjunctive therapy, partial seizures	**A:** Monotherapy: Initially, 100 mg 2 times/day. May increase at weekly intervals by 50 mg 2 times/day. Maintenance: 150–200 mg 2 times/day. Adjunctive: Initially, 50 mg 2 times/day. May increase by 50 mg 2 times/day. Maintenance: 100–200 mg 2 times/day.	Diplopia, headache, dizziness, nausea

Continued

ANTICONVULSANTS—cont'd

Name	Availability	Uses	Dosage Range	Side Effects
Lamotrigine (Lamictal)	T: 25 mg, 100 mg, 150 mg, 200 mg. T (ER): 25 mg, 50 mg, 100 mg, 200 mg, 250 mg, 300 mg T (ODT): 25 mg, 50 mg, 100 mg, 200 mg T (Chew): 5 mg, 25 mg	Partial seizures, primary generalized tonic-clonic seizures, generalized seizures of Lennox-Gastaut syndrome	A: Refer to individual monograph.	Dizziness, ataxia, drowsiness, diplopia, nausea, rash, headache, vomiting, insomnia, incoordination
Levetiracetam (Keppra)	T: 250 mg, 500 mg, 750 mg, 1,000 mg S: 100 mg/ml T(ER): 500 mg, 750 mg	Adjunctive therapy, partial seizures, primary tonic-clonic seizures, myoclonic seizures	A: T: Initially, 500 mg 2 times/day. May increase q2wks by 500mg/dose. Usual dose: 1,500 mg 2 times/day. ER: Initially, 1,000 mg once daily. May increase q2wks by 1,000 mg/day up to 3,000 mg once daily.	Dizziness, drowsiness, weakness, irritability, hallucinations, psychosis
Oxcarbazepine (Trileptal)	T: 150 mg, 300 mg, 600 mg T(ER): 150 mg, 300 mg, 600 mg	Partial seizures	A: T: 600 mg/day in 2 divided doses. May increase by 600 mg/day at weekly intervals up to 1,200 mg/day in 2 divided doses. ER: 600 mg once daily. May increase by 600 mg/day at weekly intervals up to 1,200–2,400 mg/day.	Drowsiness, dizziness, headaches, diplopia, ataxia, nausea, vomiting, hyponatremia, skin reactions
Perampanel (Fycompa)	S: 0.5 mg/ml T: 2 mg, 4 mg, 6 mg, 8 mg, 10 mg, 12 mg	Partial onset seizure, primary generalized tonic clonic seizure	A, C (12 yrs or older): Initially, 2 mg daily at hs. May increase by 2 mg/d at weekly intervals. Usual dose: 8–12 mg qhs	Weight gain, abnormal gait, dizziness, headache, somnolence, serious psychiatric reactions.
Phenobarbital	T: 30 mg, 60 mg, 100 mg I: 65 mg, 130 mg	Tonic-clonic, partial seizures; status epilepticus	A(PO): 100–300 mg/day; (IM/IV): 200–600 mg. C (PO): 3–5 mg/kg/day; (IM/IV): 100–400 mg.	CNS depression, sedation, paradoxical excitement and hyperactivity, rash, hypotension

Phenytoin (Dilantin)	C: 30 mg, 100 mg T (chewable): 50 mg S: 125 mg/5 ml I: 50 mg/ml	Tonic-clonic, psychomotor seizures	**A:** Initially, 100 mg 3 times/day. May increase at 7–10 days intervals. Usual dose: 400 mg /day. **C:** Initially, 5 mg/kg/day in 2–3 divided doses. May increase at 7–10 day intervals. Usual dose: 4–8 mg/kg/day in 1–3 doses.	Nystagmus, ataxia, hypertrichosis, gingival hyperplasia, rash, osteomalacia, lymphadenopathy
Pregabalin (Lyrica)	C: 25 mg, 50 mg, 75 mg, 100 mg, 150 mg, 200 mg, 225 mg, 300 mg	Adjunctive therapy, partial seizures	**A:** Initially 150 mg/day (75 mg 2 times/day or 50 mg 3 times/day) up to 600 mg/day in 2 or 3 doses.	Confusion, drowsiness, dizziness, ataxia, weight gain, dry mouth, blurred vision, peripheral edema, myopathy, angioedema, decreased platelet count
Primidone (Mysoline)	T: 50 mg, 250 mg	Complex partial, akinetic, tonic-clonic seizures	**A:** 750–1250 mg/day in 3–4 doses **C:** 10–25 mg/kg/day	CNS depression, sedation, paradoxical excitement and hyperactivity, rash, dizziness, ataxia
Rufinamide (Banzel)	S: 40 mg/ml T: 200 mg, 400 mg	Lennox-Gastaut syndrome (adjunct)	**A:** Initially, 400–800 mg/day in 2 divided doses. May increase by 400–800 mg/day every other day **C:** Initially, 10 mg/kg/day in 2 divided doses. May increase by 10 mg/kg/day every other day up to 45 mg/kg/day. **Maximum:** 3,200 mg/day.	Fatigue, dizziness, headache, nausea, drowsiness
Tiagabine (Gabitril)	T: 4 mg, 12 mg, 16 mg, 20 mg	Partial seizures	**A:** Initially, 4 mg up to 56 mg/day in 2–4 doses. May increase by 4–8 mg/day at weekly intervals **C:** Initially, 4 mg up to 32 mg/day in 2–4 doses. May increase by 4–8 mg/day at weekly intervals.	Dizziness, asthenia, nervousness, anxiety, tremors, abdominal pain

Continued

ANTICONVULSANTS—cont'd

Name	Availability	Uses	Dosage Range	Side Effects
Topiramate (Topamax)	**T:** 25 mg, 100 mg, 200 mg, **C (Sprinkle):** 15 mg, 25 mg, **C (ER 24HR Sprinkle) (Qudexy XR):** 25 mg, 50 mg, 100 mg, 150 mg, **C XR (Trokendi XR):** 25 mg, 50 mg, 100 mg, 200 mg	Partial seizures, Lennox-Gastaut syndrome	See individual monograph.	Drowsiness, dizziness, headache, ataxia, confusion, weight loss, diplopia
Valproic acid (Depakene, Depakote)	**C:** 250 mg, **S:** 250 mg/5 ml, **Sprinkles:** 125 mg, **T:** 125 mg, 250 mg, 500 mg, **T (ER):** 500 mg, **I:** 100 mg/ml	Complex partial, absence seizures	**A, C:** Initially, 15 mg/kg/day. May increase by 5–10 mg/kg/day at weekly intervals up to 60 mg/kg/day.	Nausea, vomiting, tremors, thrombocytopenia, hair loss, hepatic dysfunction, weight gain, decreased platelet function
Vigabatrin (Sabril)	**T:** 500 mg, **PS:** 500 mg	Infantile spasms, refractory complex partial seizures	**A:** Initially, 500 mg 2 times/day. May increase by 500 mg increments at weekly intervals up to 1,500 mg 2 times/day. **C:** Initially, 250 mg 2 times/day. May increase by 500 mg/day at weekly intervals up to 1,000 mg 2 times/day.	Vision changes, eye pain, abdominal pain, agitation, confusion, mood/mental changes, abnormal coordination, weight gain
Zonisamide (Zonegran)	**C:** 100 mg	Partial seizures	**A:** Initially, 100 mg/day. May increase to 200 mg/day after 2 wks, then 300 mg/day up to 400 mg/day at 2 wk intervals.	Drowsiness, dizziness, anorexia, diarrhea, weight loss, agitation, irritability, rash, nausea, cognitive side effects, kidney stones

A, Adults; *C,* capsules; *C (dosage),* children; *ER,* extended-release; *I,* Injection; *ODT,* orally disintegrating tablets; *PE,* phenytoin equivalent; *PO,* oral; *PS,* powder sachet; *S,* suspension; *T,* tablets.

Antidepressants

USES

Used primarily for the treatment of depression. Depression can be a chronic or recurrent mental disorder presenting with symptoms such as depressed mood, loss of interest or pleasure, guilt feelings, disturbed sleep/appetite, low energy, and difficulty in thinking. Depression can also lead to suicide.

ACTION

Antidepressants include tricyclics, monoamine oxidase inhibitors (MAOIs), selective serotonin reuptake inhibitors (SSRIs), serotonin-norepinephrine reuptake inhibitors (SNRIs), and other antidepressants. Depression may be due to reduced functioning of monoamine neurotransmitters (e.g., norepinephrine, serotonin [5-HT], dopamine) in the CNS (decreased amount and/or decreased effects at the receptor sites). Antidepressants block metabolism, increase amount/effects of monoamine neurotransmitters, and act at receptor sites (change responsiveness/ sensitivities of both presynaptic and postsynaptic receptor sites).

ANTIDEPRESSANTS

Name	Availability	Uses	Dosage Range (per day)	Side Effects
Tricyclics				
Amitriptyline (Elavil)	**T:** 10 mg, 25 mg, 50 mg, 75 mg, 100 mg, 150 mg	Depression, neuropathic pain	Initially, 25–100 mg at bedtime or in divided doses. Usual dose: 100–300 mg/day.	Drowsiness, blurred vision, constipation, confusion, postural hypotension, cardiac conduction defects, weight gain, seizures, dry mouth
Desipramine (Norpramin)	**T:** 10 mg, 25 mg, 50 mg, 75 mg, 100 mg, 150 mg	Depression, neuropathic pain	Initially, 25–100 mg at bedtime or in divided doses. Usual dose: 100–300 mg/day.	Dizziness, drowsiness, fatigue, headache, anorexia, diarrhea, nausea

Continued

ANTIDEPRESSANTS—cont'd

Name	Availability	Uses	Dosage Range (per day)	Side Effects
Imipramine (Tofranil)	**T:** 10 mg, 25 mg, 50 mg, **C:** 75 mg, 100 mg, 125 mg, 150 mg	Depression, enuresis, neuro-pathic pain, panic disorder, ADHD	Initially, 25–100 mg at bedtime or in divided doses. Usual dose: 100–300 mg/day.	Dizziness, fatigue, headache, vomiting, xerostomia
Nortriptyline (Aventyl, Pamelor)	**C:** 10 mg, 25 mg, 50 mg, 75 mg **S:** 10 mg/5 ml	Depression, neuropathic pain, smoking cessation	Initially, 50–100 mg once daily. Usual dose: 50–150 mg once daily.	Dizziness, fatigue, headache, anorexia, xerostomia
Selective Serotonin Reuptake Inhibitors				
Citalopram (Celexa)	**T:** 10 mg, 20 mg, 40 mg **ODT:** 40 mg **S:** 10 mg/5 ml	Depression, OCD, panic disorder	20–40 mg	Insomnia or sedation, nausea, agitation, headaches
Escitalopram (Lexapro)	**T:** 5 mg, 10 mg, 20 mg **S:** 5 mg/5 ml	Depression, GAD	10–20 mg	Insomnia or sedation, nausea, agitation, headaches
Fluoxetine (Prozac)	**C:** 10 mg, 20 mg, 40 mg **C (DR):** 90 mg **T:** 10 mg, 20 mg **S:** 20 mg/5 ml	Depression, OCD, bulimia, panic disorder, anorexia, bipolar disorder, premenstrual syndrome	Initially, 10–20 mg once daily. Usual dose: 20 mg once daily. **DR:** 90 mg once weekly.	Akathisia, sexual dysfunction, skin rash, urticaria, pruritus, decreased appetite, asthenia, diarrhea, drowsiness, headaches, diaphoresis, insomnia, nausea, tremors
Paroxetine (Paxil)	**T:** 10 mg, 20 mg, 30 mg, 40 mg **S:** 10 mg/5 ml **ER:** 12.5 mg, 25 mg, 37.5 mg	Depression, OCD, panic attack, SAD	Initially/usual dose: 20 mg once daily. **ER:** Initially, 12.5–25 mg once daily. Usual dose: 25 mg once daily.	Asthenia, constipation, diarrhea, diaphoresis, insomnia, nausea, sexual dysfunction, tremors, vomiting, urinary frequency or retention

Drug	Forms	Indications	Dosage	Side Effects
Sertraline (Zoloft)	T: 25 mg, 50 mg, 100 mg, S: 20 mg/ml	Depression, OCD, panic attack	50–200 mg	Sexual dysfunction, dizziness, drowsiness, anorexia, diarrhea, nausea, dry mouth, abdominal cramps, decreased weight, headaches, increased diaphoresis, tremors, insomnia
Vortioxetine (Trintellix)	T: 5 mg, 10 mg, 15 mg, 20 mg	Depression	Initially, 10 mg once daily. Usual dose: 10–20 mg once daily.	Nausea, constipation
Serotonin-Norepinephrine Reuptake Inhibitors				
Desvenlafaxine (Pristiq)	T: 25 mg, 50 mg, 100 mg	Depression	50–100 mg	Nausea, dizziness, insomnia, hyperhidrosis, constipation, drowsiness, decreased appetite, anxiety, male sexual function disorders
Duloxetine (Cymbalta)	C: 20 mg, 30 mg, 60 mg	Depression, fibromyalgia, neuropathic pain	Initially, 30–60 mg once daily. Usual dose: 60 mg once daily or 2 divided doses.	Nausea, dry mouth, constipation, decreased appetite, fatigue, diaphoresis, hyperglycemia
Venlafaxine (Effexor)	T: 25 mg, 37.5 mg, 50 mg, 75 mg, 100 mg, 150 mg, 225 mg T(ER): 37.5 mg, 75 mg, 150 mg	Depression, anxiety	Initially, 25 mg 3 times or (ER): 37.5 mg once daily. Usual dose: 75 mg 3 times/day or (ER) 75–225 mg once daily.	Increased blood pressure, agitation, sedation, insomnia, nausea
Other				
Brexpiprazole (Rexulti)	T: 0.25 mg, 0.5 mg, 1 mg, 2 mg, 3 mg, 4 mg	Depression	Initially, 0.5–1 mg/day. May increase at weekly interval to 1 mg/day. **Maximum:** 3 mg/day.	Weight gain, akathisia
Bupropion (Wellbutrin)	T: 75 mg, 100 mg SR: 100 mg, 150 mg, 200 mg	Depression, smoking cessation, ADHD, bipolar disorder	Initially, 100 mg 2 times/day. Usual dose: 100 mg 3 times/day. SR: Initially, 150 mg once daily. Usual dose: 150 mg 2 times/day.	Insomnia, irritability, seizures

Continued

ANTIDEPRESSANTS—cont'd

Name	Availability	Uses	Dosage Range (per day)	Side Effects
Mirtazapine (Remeron)	**T:** 7.5 mg, 15 mg, 30 mg, 45 mg	Depression	Initially, 15 mg once at bedtime. Usual dose: 30–45 mg once daily.	Sedation, dry mouth, weight gain, agranulocytosis, hepatic toxicity
Trazodone (Desyrel)	**T:** 50 mg, 100 mg, 150 mg, 300 mg **ER:** 150 mg, 300 mg	Depression	Initially, 75 mg 2 times/day or **(ER):** 150 mg once daily. Usual dose: 150 mg bid or **(ER):** 150–375 mg once daily.	Sedation, orthostatic hypotension, priapism
Vilazodone (Viibryd)	**T:** 10 mg, 20 mg, 40 mg	Depression	Initially, 10 mg once daily. Usual dose: 40 mg once daily.	Diarrhea, nausea, dizziness, dry mouth, insomnia, vomiting, decreased libido

ADHD, Attention-deficit hyperactivity disorder; *C,* capsules; *DR,* delayed-release; *ER,* extended-release; *GAD,* generalized anxiety disorder; *OC,* oral concentrate; *OCD,* obsessive-compulsive disorder; *ODT,* orally disintegrating tablets; *S,* suspension; *SAD,* social anxiety disorder; *SR,* sustained-release; *T,* tablets.

Antidiabetics

USES

Insulin: Treatment of insulin-dependent diabetes (type 1) and non–insulin-dependent diabetes (type 2). Also used in acute situations such as ketoacidosis, severe infections, major surgery in otherwise non–insulin-dependent diabetics. Administered to pts receiving parenteral nutrition. Drug of choice during pregnancy. All insulins, including long-acting insulins, can cause hypoglycemia and weight gain.

Alpha-glucosidase inhibitors: Adjunct to diet and exercise for management of type 2 diabetes mellitus.

Biguanides: Adjunct to diet and exercise for management of type 2 diabetes mellitus.

ACTION

Dipeptidyl peptidase 4 inhibitors (DPP-4): Adjunct to diet and exercise for management of type 2 diabetes mellitus.

Meglitinide: Adjunct to diet and exercise for management of type 2 diabetes mellitus.

Sulfonylureas: Adjunct to diet and exercise for management of type 2 diabetes mellitus.

Thiazolidinediones: Adjunct to diet and exercise for management of type 2 diabetes mellitus.

Sodium-glucose co-transporter 2 (SGLT2): Adjunct to diet and exercise for management of type 2 diabetes mellitus.

Insulin: A hormone synthesized and secreted by beta cells of Langerhans' islet in the pancreas. Controls storage and utilization of glucose, amino acids, and fatty acids by activated transport systems/enzymes. Inhibits breakdown of glycogen, fat, protein. Insulin lowers blood glucose by inhibiting glycogenolysis and gluconeogenesis in liver; stimulates glucose uptake by muscle, adipose tissue. Activity of insulin is initiated by binding to cell surface receptors.

Alpha-glucosidase inhibitors: Work locally in small intestine, slowing carbohydrate breakdown and glucose absorption.

Biguanides: Inhibit hepatic gluconeogenesis, glycogenolysis; enhance insulin sensitivity in muscle and fat.

DPP-4: Inhibit degradation of endogenous incretins, which increases insulin secretion, decreases glucagon secretion.

Meglitinide: Stimulates pancreatic insulin secretion.

Sulfonylureas: Stimulate release of insulin from beta cells of the pancreas.

Thiazolidinediones: Enhance insulin sensitivity in muscle and fat.

SGLT2: Blocks glucose reabsorption in proximal tubule in the kidney, increases urinary glucose excretion.

ANTIDIABETICS

INSULIN

Type	Onset	Peak	Duration	Comments
Rapid-Acting				
Apidra, glulisine	10–15 min	1–1.5 hrs	3–5 hrs	Stable at room temp for 28 days Can mix with NPH
Humalog, lispro	15–30 min	0.5–2.5 hrs	6–8 hrs	Stable at room temp for 28 days Can mix with NPH

Continued

ANTIDIABETICS—cont'd

Type	Onset	Peak	Duration	Comments
Novolog, aspart	10–20 min	1–3 hrs	3–5 hrs	Stable at room temp for 28 days Can mix with NPH
Short-Acting				
Humulin R, Novolin R, regular	30–60 min	1–5 hrs	6–10 hrs	Stable at room temp for 28 days Can mix with NPH
Intermediate-Acting				
Humulin N, Novolin N, NPH	1–2 hrs	6–14 hrs	16–24 hrs	Stable at room temp for 28 days Can mix with aspart, lispro, glulisine
Long-Acting				
Basaglar, glargine	1–4 hrs	No significant peak	24 hrs	Do NOT mix with other insulins Stable at room temp for 28 days
Lantus, glargine	1–4 hrs	No significant peak	24 hrs	Do NOT mix with other insulins Stable at room temp for 28 days
Levemir, detemir	0.8–2 hrs	No significant peak	12–24 hrs (dose dependent)	Do NOT mix with other insulins Stable at room temp for 42 days
Toujeo, glargine	1–6 hrs	No significant peak	Longer than 24 hrs	Do NOT mix with other insulins Stable at room temp for 28 days
Tresiba, degludec	0.5–1.5 hrs	12 hrs	42 hrs	Do NOT mix with other insulins Stable at room temp for 56 days

ORAL AGENTS

Name	Availability	Dosage Range	Side Effects
Sulfonylureas			
Glimepiride (Amaryl)	**T:** 1 mg, 2 mg, 4 mg	Initially, 1–2 mg/day. May increase by 1–2 mg q1–2 weeks. **Maximum:** 8 mg/day	Hypoglycemia, dizziness, headache, nausea, flu-like syndrome
Glipizide (Glucotrol)	**T:** 5 mg, 10 mg **T (XL):** 5 mg	**T:** Initially, 5 mg/day. May increase by 2.5–5 mg q3–4 days. **(XL):** Initially, 5 mg/day. **Maximum:** 20 mg/day	Dizziness, nervousness, anxiety, diarrhea, tremor
Glyburide (DiaBeta, Micronase)	**T:** 1.25 mg, 2.5 mg, 5 mg **PT:** 1.5 mg, 3 mg	**T:** Initially, 2.5–5 mg/day. May increase by 2.5 mg/day at weekly intervals up to 20 mg/day **PT:** Initially, 1.5–3 mg/day. May increase by 1.5 mg at weekly intervals up to 12 mg/day	Dizziness, headache, nausea
Alpha-Glucosidase Inhibitors			
Acarbose (Precose)	**T:** 25 mg, 50 mg, 100 mg	Initially, 25 mg 3 times/day. May increase at 4–8 wk intervals. Usual dose: 50–100 mg 3 times/day	Flatulence, diarrhea, abdominal pain, increased risk of hypoglycemia when used with insulin or sulfonylureas
Miglitol (Glyset)	**T:** 25 mg, 50 mg, 100 mg	Initially, 25 mg 3 times/day. May increase at 4–8 wk intervals to 50 mg 3 times/day, then 100 mg 3 times/day	Flatulence, diarrhea, abdominal pain, rash
Dipeptidyl Peptidase Inhibitors			
Alogliptin (Nesina)	**T:** 6.25 mg, 12.5 mg, 25 mg	6.25–25 mg/day	Nasopharyngitis, cough, headache, upper respiratory tract infections
Linagliptin (Tradjenta)	**T:** 5 mg	5 mg/day	Arthralgia, back pain, headache
Saxagliptin (Onglyza)	**T:** 2.5 mg, 5 mg	2.5–5 mg/day	Upper respiratory tract infection, urinary tract infection, headache

Continued

ANTIDIABETICS—cont'd

Name	Availability	Dosage Range	Side Effects
Sitagliptin (Januvia)	**T:** 25 mg, 50 mg, 100 mg	25–100 mg/day	Nasopharyngitis, upper respiratory infection, headaches, modest weight gain, increased incidence of hypoglycemia when added to a sulfonylurea
Biguanides			
Metformin (Glucophage)	**T:** 500 mg, 850 mg, 1,000 mg **XR:** 500 mg, 750 mg, 1,000 mg	**T:** Initially, 500 mg 2 times/day or 850 mg once daily. May increase by 500 mg/day at weekly intervals up to 2,550 mg/day **(XR):** Initially, 500–1,000 mg/day. May increase by 500 mg/day at weekly intervals up to 2,500 mg/day	Nausea, vomiting, diarrhea, loss of appetite, metallic taste, lactic acidosis (rare but potentially fatal complication)
Glucagon-Like Peptide-1 (GLP-1)			
Albiglutide (Tanzeum)	**I:** 30 mg, 50 mg	30–50 mg once weekly	Diarrhea, nausea, upper respiratory tract infection, injection site reaction
Exenatide (Byetta)	**I:** 5 mcg, 10 mcg	5–10 mcg 2 times/day	Diarrhea, dizziness, dyspnea, headaches, nausea, vomiting
Exenatide extended-release (Bydureon)	**I:** 2 mg	2 mg once weekly	Diarrhea, nausea, headache
Liraglutide (Victoza)	**I:** 0.6 mg, 1.2 mg, 1.8 mg (6 mg/ml)	Initially, 0.6 mg/day. May increase at weekly intervals up to 1.2 mg/day, then 1.8 mg/day	Headache, nausea, diarrhea
Lixisenatide (Adlyxin)	**I:** 50 mcg/ml, 100 mcg/ml	20 mcg SC once/d	Nausea, vomiting, headache, dizziness

Meglitinides			
Nateglinide (Starlix)	T: 60 mg, 120 mg	60–120 mg 3 times/day	Hypoglycemia, upper respiratory infection, dizziness, back pain, flu-like syndrome
Repaglinide (Prandin)	T: 0.5 mg, 1 mg, 2 mg	0.5–1 mg with each meal. Usual dose: 0.5–4 mg/day (**Maximum:** 16 mg/day)	Headache, hypoglycemia, upper respiratory infection
SGLT2			
Canagliflozin (Invokana)	T: 100 mg, 300 mg	100–300 mg/day before first meal of day	Genital mycotic infections, recurrent urinary tract infections, increased urinary frequency, hypotension, increased serum creatinine, LDL, Hgb, Hct. Hyperkalemia, hypermagnesemia, hyperphosphatemia, fractures
Dapagliflozin (Farxiga)	T: 5 mg, 10 mg	5–10 mg/day in morning	Genital mycotic infections, recurrent urinary tract infections, increased urinary frequency, hypotension, increased serum creatinine, LDL, Hgb, Hct. Hyperphosphatemia, fractures
Empagliflozin (Jardiance)	T: 10 mg, 25 mg	10–25 mg/day in morning	Genital mycotic infections, recurrent urinary tract infections, increased urinary frequency, hypotension, increased serum creatinine, LDL, Hgb, Hct

Continued

ANTIDIABETICS—cont'd

Name	Availability	Dosage Range	Side Effects
Thiazolidinediones			
Pioglitazone (Actos)	**T:** 15 mg, 30 mg, 45 mg	15–30 mg/day	Mild to moderate peripheral edema, weight gain, increased risk of HF, associated with reduced bone mineral density and increased incidence of fractures
Rosiglitazone (Avandia)	**T:** 2 mg, 4 mg, 8 mg	Initially, 4 mg/day. May increase at 8–12 weeks to 8 mg/day as a single or 2 divided doses	Increased cholesterol, weight gain, back pain, upper respiratory tract infection
Miscellaneous			
Bromocriptine (Cycloset)	**T:** 0.8 mg	1.6–4.8 mg/day	Nausea, fatigue, dizziness, vomiting
Colesevelam (Welchol)	**T:** 625 mg **S:** 1.875 g, 3.75 g packet	3.75 g/day	Constipation, dyspepsia, nausea
Pramlintide (Symlin)	**I:** 1,500 mcg/1.5 ml, 2,700 mcg/2.7 ml	Type 1: 15–60 mcg immediately prior to meals Type 2: 60–120 mcg immediately prior to meals	Abdominal pain, anorexia, head-aches, nausea, vomiting, severe hypoglycemia may occur when used in combination with insulin (reduction in dosages of short-acting, including premixed, insulins recommended)

HF, Heart failure; *I,* Injection; *PT,* prestab; *S,* suspension; *T,* tablets; *XL,* extended-release; *XR,* extended-release.

Antidiarrheals

USES

Acute diarrhea, chronic diarrhea of inflammatory bowel disease, reduction of fluid from ileostomies.

ACTION

Systemic agents: Act as smooth muscle receptors (enteric) disrupting peristaltic movements, decreasing GI motility, increasing transit time of intestinal contents.

Local agents: Adsorb toxic substances and fluids to large surface areas of particles in the preparation. Some of these agents coat and protect irritated intestinal walls. May have local anti-inflammatory action.

ANTIDIARRHEALS

Name	Availability	Type	Dosage Range
Bismuth (Pepto-Bismol)	**T:** 262 mg **C:** 262 mg **L:** 130 mg/15 ml, 262 mg/15ml, 524 mg/15 ml	Local	**A:** 2 T or 30 ml **C (9–12 yrs):** 1 T or 15 ml **C (6–8 yrs):** 2/3 T or 10 ml **C (3–5 yrs):** 1/3 T or 5 ml
Diphenoxylate with atropine (Lomotil)	**T:** 2.5 mg **L:** 2.5 mg/5 ml	Systemic	**A:** 5 mg 4 times/day **C:** 0.3–0.4 mg/kg/day in 4 divided doses (L)
Loperamide (Imodium)	**C:** 2 mg **T:** 2mg **L:** 1 mg/5 ml, 1 mg/ml	Systemic	**A:** Initially, 4 mg **(Maximum:** 16 mg/day) **C (9–12 yrs):** 2 mg 3 times/day **C (6–8 yrs):** 2 mg 2 times/day **C (2–5 yrs):** 1 mg 3 times/day **(L)**

A, Adults; *C*, capsules; *C (dosage)*, children; *L*, liquid; *S*, suspension; *T*, tablets.

Antifungals: Systemic Mycoses

Systemic mycoses are subdivided into opportunistic infections (candidiasis, aspergillosis, cryptococcosis, and mucormycosis) that are seen primarily in debilitated or immunocompromised hosts and nonopportunistic infections (blastomycosis, histoplasmosis, and coccidioidomycosis) that occur in any host. Treatment can be difficult because these infections often resist treatment and may require prolonged therapy.

ANTIFUNGALS: SYSTEMIC MYCOSES

Name	Indications	Side Effects
Amphotericin B	Potentially life-threatening fungal infections, including aspergillosis, blastomycosis, coccidioidomycosis, cryptococcosis, histoplasmosis, systemic candidiasis	Fever, chills, headache, nausea, vomiting, nephrotoxicity, hypokalemia, hypomagnesemia, hypotension, dyspnea, arrhythmias, abdominal pain, diarrhea, increased hepatic function tests
Amphotericin B lipid complex (Abelcet)	Invasive fungal infections	Chills, fever, hypotension, headache, nausea, vomiting
Amphotericin B liposomal (AmBisome)	Empiric therapy for presumed fungal infections in febrile neutropenic pts, treatment of cryptococcal meningitis in HIV-infected pts, treatment of *Aspergillus, Candida, Cryptococcus* infections, treatment of visceral leishmaniasis	Peripheral edema, tachycardia, hypotension, chills, insomnia, headache
Amphotericin colloidal dispersion (Amphotec)	Invasive *Aspergillus*	Hypotension, tachycardia, chills, fever, vomiting
Anidulafungin (Eraxis)	Candidemia, esophageal candidiasis	Diarrhea, hypokalemia, increased hepatic function tests, headache

Drug	Uses	Side Effects
Caspofungin (Cancidas)	Candidemia, invasive aspergillosis, empiric therapy for presumed fungal infections in febrile neutropenic pts	Headache, nausea, vomiting, diarrhea, increased hepatic function tests
Fluconazole (Diflucan)	Treatment of vaginal candidiasis; oropharyngeal, esophageal candidiasis; and cryptococcal meningitis. Prophylaxis to decrease incidence of candidiasis in pts undergoing bone marrow transplant receiving cytotoxic chemotherapy and/or radiation	Nausea, vomiting, abdominal pain, diarrhea, dysgeusia, increased hepatic function tests, liver necrosis, hepatitis, cholestasis, headache, rash, pruritus, eosinophilia, alopecia
Isavuconazonium (Cresemba)	Treatment of invasive aspergillosis, invasive mucormycosis	Nausea, vomiting, diarrhea, increased hepatic enzymes, hypokalemia, constipation, dyspnea, cough, peripheral edema, back pain
Itraconazole (Sporanox)	Blastomycosis, histoplasmosis, aspergillosis, onychomycosis, empiric therapy of febrile neutropenic pts with suspected fungal infections, treatment of oropharyngeal and esophageal candidiasis	Congestive heart failure, peripheral edema, nausea, vomiting, abdominal pain, diarrhea, increased hepatic function tests, liver necrosis, hepatitis, cholestasis, headache, rash, pruritus, eosinophilia
Ketoconazole (Nizoral)	Candidiasis, chronic mucocutaneous candidiasis, oral thrush, candiduria, blastomycosis, coccidioidomycosis	Nausea, vomiting, abdominal pain, diarrhea, gynecomastia, increased LFT, liver necrosis, hepatitis, cholestasis, headache, rash, pruritus, eosinophilia
Micafungin (Mycamine)	Esophageal candidiasis, Candida infections, prophylaxis in pts undergoing hematopoietin stem cell transplantation	Fever, chills, hypokalemia, hypomagnesemia, hypocalcemia, myelosuppression, thrombocytopenia, nausea, vomiting, abdominal pain, diarrhea, increased LFT, dizziness, headache, rash, pruritus, pain or inflammation at injection site, fever
Posaconazole (Noxafil)	Prevent invasive aspergillosis and Candida infections in pts 13 yrs and older who are immunocompromised, treatment of oropharyngeal candidiasis	Fever, headaches, nausea, vomiting, diarrhea, abdominal pain, hypokalemia, cough, dyspnea
Voriconazole (Vfend)	Invasive aspergillosis, candidemia, esophageal candidiasis, serious fungal infections	Visual disturbances, nausea, vomiting, abdominal pain, diarrhea, increased LFT, liver necrosis, hepatitis, cholestasis, headache, rash, pruritus, eosinophilia

Antiglaucoma Agents

USES

Reduction of elevated intraocular pressure (IOP) in pts with open-angle glaucoma and ocular hypertension.

ACTION

Medications decrease IOP by two primary mechanisms: decreasing aqueous humor (AH) production or increasing AH outflow.

- *Miotics (direct acting and indirect acting):* Constrict pupils, opening channels in the trabecular meshwork, reducing resistance to outflow of AH.
- *Alpha₂ agonists:* Activate receptors in ciliary body, inhibiting aqueous secretion and increasing uveoscleral aqueous outflow.
- *Beta blockers:* Reduce production of aqueous humor.
- *Carbonic anhydrase inhibitors:* Decrease production of AH by inhibiting enzyme carbonic anhydrase.
- *Prostaglandins:* Increase outflow of aqueous fluid through uveoscleral route.

ANTIGLAUCOMA AGENTS

Name	Availability	Dosage Range	Side Effects
Miotics			
Carbachol (Isopto-Carbachol)	**S:** 1.5%, 3%	1 drop qid	Brow ache, corneal toxicity, conjunctival inflammation, transient myopia, blurred vision, retinal detachment
Pilocarpine (Isopto Carpine Pilopine HS [Gel])	**G:** 4% **S:** 1%, 2%, 4%	**S:** 1 drop qid **G:** 1 drop HS	Same as carbachol

Alpha₂ Agonists

Apraclonidine (Iopidine)	S: 0.5%, 1%	1 drop tid	Fatigue, somnolence, local allergic reaction, dry eyes, stinging
Brimonidine (Alphagan HP)	S: 0.1%, 0.15%, 0.2%	1 drop tid	Same as apraclonidine

Prostaglandins

Bimatoprost (Lumigan)	S: 0.01%	1 drop daily in evening	Conjunctival hyperemia; darkening of iris, eyelids; increase in length, thickness, and number of eyelashes; local irritation; itching; dryness; blurred vision
Latanoprost (Xalatan)	S: 0.005%	1 drop daily in evening	See bimatoprost
Tafluprost (Zioptan)	S: 0.0015%	1 drop daily in evening	See bimatoprost
Travoprost (Travatan)	S: 0.004%	1 drop daily in evening	See bimatoprost

Beta Blockers

Betaxolol (Betoptic, Betoptic-S)	Suspension (Betoptic-S): 0.25% S (Betoptic): 0.5%	Betoptic-S: 1 drop 2 times/day Betoptic: 1–2 drops 2 times/day	Fatigue, dizziness, bradycardia, respiratory depression, mask symptoms of hypoglycemia, block effects of beta agonists in treatment of asthma
Carteolol (Ocupress)	S: 1%	1 drop 2 times/day	Same as betaxolol
Levobunolol (Betagan)	S: 0.25%, 0.5%	1 drop 1–2 times/day	Same as betaxolol
Metipranolol (OptiPranolol)	S: 0.3%	1 drop 2 times/day	Same as betaxolol
Timolol (Betimol, Istalol, Timoptic, Timoptic XE)	S: 0.25%, 0.5% G, Timoptic XE: 0.25%, 0.5%	S: 1 drop 2 times/day (Istalol): 1 drop daily G: 1 drop daily	Same as betaxolol

Continued

ANTIGLAUCOMA AGENTS—cont'd

Carbonic Anhydrase Inhibitors

Brinzolamide (Azopt)	Suspension: 1%	1 drop 3 times/day	Bitter taste, stinging, redness, burning, conjunctivitis, dry eyes, blurred vision
Dorzolamide (Trusopt)	S: 2%	1 drop 3 times/day	Same as brinzolamide
Combinations			
Brimonidine/timolol (Combigan)	0.2%/0.5%	1 drop bid	See individual agents
Brinzolamide/Brimonidine (Simbrinza)	1%/0.2%	1 drop tid	See individual agents
Timolol/dorzolamide (Cosopt)	0.5%/2%	1 drop bid	See individual agents

C, Capsules; *G,* gel; *O,* ointment; *S,* solution; *T,* tablets.

Antihistamines

USES

Symptomatic relief of upper respiratory allergic disorders. Allergic reactions associated with other drugs respond to antihistamines, as do blood transfusion reactions. Used as a second-choice drug in treatment of angioneurotic edema. Effective in treatment of acute urticaria and other dermatologic conditions. May also be used for preop sedation, Parkinson's disease, and motion sickness.

ACTION

Antihistamines (H_1 antagonists) inhibit vasoconstrictor effects and vasodilator effects on endothelial cells of histamine. They block increased capillary permeability, formation of edema/wheal caused by histamine. Many antihistamines can bind to receptors in CNS, causing primarily depression (decreased alertness, slowed reaction times, drowsiness) but also stimulation (restlessness, nervousness, inability to sleep). Some may counter motion sickness.

ANTIHISTAMINES

Name	Availability	Dosage Range	Side Effects
Cetirizine (Zyrtec)	T: 5 mg, 10 mg C: 5 mg, 10 mg T (chew): 5 mg/10 mg S: 5 mg/5 ml	A: 5–10 mg/day C (6–12 yrs): 5–10 mg/day C (2–5 yrs): 2.5–5 mg/day	Headache, somnolence, fatigue, abdominal pain, dry mouth
Desloratadine (Clarinex)	T: 5 mg ODT: 2.5 mg, 5 mg S: 0.5 mg/ml	A, C (12 yrs and older): 5 mg/day C (6–11 yrs): 2.5 mg/day C (1–5 yrs): 1.25 mg/day C (6–11 mos): 1 mg/day	Dizziness, fatigue, headache, nausea
Dimenhydrinate (Dramamine)	T: 50 mg T (chew): 25 mg, 50 mg	A: 50–100 mg q4–6h C: 12.5–50 mg q6–8h	Dizziness, drowsiness, headache, nausea
Diphenhydramine (Benadryl)	T: 25 mg, 50 mg C: 25 mg, 50 mg L: 12.5 mg/5 ml	A: 25–50 mg q6–8h C (6–11 yrs): 12.5–25 mg q4–6h C (2–5 yrs): 6.25 mg q4–6h	Chills, confusion, dizziness, fatigue, headache, sedation, nausea
Fexofenadine (Allegra)	T: 30 mg, 60 mg, 180 mg ODT: 30 mg S: 30 mg/5 ml	A: 60 mg q12h or 180 mg/day C (2–11 yrs): 30 mg q12h, (6–23 mos): 15 mg bid	Headache, vomiting, fatigue, diarrhea
Hydroxyzine (Atarax)	T: 10 mg, 25 mg, 50 mg C: 25 mg, 50 mg, 100 mg S: 10 mg/5 ml	A: 25 mg q6–8h C: 2 mg/kg/day in divided doses q6–8h	Dizziness, drowsiness, fatigue, headache
Levocetirizine (Xyzal)	T: 5 mg S: 2.5 mg/ml	A, C (12 yrs and older): 5 mg once daily in evening C (6–11 yrs): 2.5 mg once daily in evening (6 mos–5 yrs): 1.25 mg once daily	Fatigue, fever, somnolence, vomiting

Continued

ANTIHISTAMINES—cont'd

Name	Availability	Dosage Range	Side Effects
Loratadine (Claritin)	**ODT:** 10 mg **T(chew):** 5 mg **T:** 10 mg **S:** 1 mg/ml	**A:** 10 mg/day **C (6–12 yrs):** 10 mg/day (2–5 yrs): 5 mg/day	Fatigue, headache, malaise, somnolence, abdominal pain
Promethazine (Phenergan)	**T:** 12.5 mg, 25 mg, 50 mg **S:** 6.25 mg/5 ml	**A:** 25 mg at bedtime or 12.5 mg q8h **C:** 0.5 mg/kg at bedtime or 0.1 mg/kg q6-8h	Confusion, dizziness, drowsiness, fatigue, constipation, nausea, vomiting

A, Adults; *C,* capsules; *C (dosage),* children; *L* liquid; *ODT,* orally disintegrating tablet; *S,* syrup; *SR,* sustained-release; *T,* tablets.

Antihyperlipidemics

USES	ACTION
Cholesterol management.	*Bile acid sequestrants:* Bind bile acids in the intestine; prevent active transport and reabsorption and enhance bile acid excretion. Depletion of hepatic bile acid results in the increased conversion of cholesterol to bile acids. *HMG-CoA reductase inhibitors (statins):* Inhibit HMG-CoA reductase, the last regulated step in the synthesis of cholesterol. Cholesterol synthesis in the liver is reduced. *Niacin (nicotinic acid):* Reduces hepatic synthesis of triglycerides and secretion of very low density lipoprotein (VLDL) by inhibiting the mobilization of free fatty acids from peripheral tissues. *Fibric acid:* Increases the oxidation of fatty acids in the liver, resulting in reduced secretion of triglyceride-rich lipoproteins, and increases lipoprotein lipase activity and fatty acid uptake. *Cholesterol absorption inhibitor:* Acts in the gut wall to prevent cholesterol absorption through the intestinal villi. *Omega fatty acids:* Exact mechanism unknown. Mechanisms may include inhibition of acyl-CoA, decreased lipo-genesis in liver, increased lipoprotein lipase activity. *PCSK9 inhibitors:* Binds with high-affinity and specificity to LDL cholesterol receptors, promoting their degradation.

ANTIHYPERLIPIDEMICS

Name	Primary Effect	Dosage	Comments/Side Effects
Bile Acid Sequestrants			
Cholestyramine (Prevalite, Questran)	Decreases LDL Increases HDL, TG	4 g 1–2 times/day May increase over 1 hr interval. Usual dose: 8–16 g/day in 2 divided doses	May bind drugs given concurrently. Take at least 1 hr before or 4–6 hrs after cholestyramine. **Side Effects:** Constipation, heartburn, nausea, vomiting, stomach pain
Colesevelam (Welchol)	Decreases LDL Increases HDL, TG	3.75 g once daily or 1.875 g 2 times/day	Take with food. **Side Effects:** Constipation, dyspepsia, weakness, myalgia, pharyngitis
Colestipol (Colestid)	Decreases LDL Increases TG	**G:** Initially, 5 g once or twice daily. May increase by 5 g/day q1–2 mos. Maintenance: 5–30 g/day. **T:** Initially, 2 g once or twice daily. May increase by 2 g 2 times/day at 1–2 mo intervals. Maintenance: 2–16 g/day	Do not crush tablets. May bind drugs given concurrently. Take at least 1 hr before or 4–6 hrs after colestipol. **Side Effects:** Constipation, headache, dizziness, anxiety, vertigo, drowsiness, nausea, vomiting, diarrhea, flatulence
Cholesterol Absorption Inhibitor			
Ezetimibe (Zetia)	Decreases LDL Increases HDL Decreases TG	10 mg once daily	Administer at least 2 hrs before or 4 hrs after bile acid sequestrants. **Side Effects:** Dizziness, headache, fatigue, diarrhea, abdominal pain, arthralgia, sinusitis, pharyngitis
Fibrio Acid			
Fenofibrate (Antara, Lofibra, Tricor, Triglide)	Decreases TG Decreases LDL Increases HDL	**Antara:** 43–130 mg/day **Lofibra:** 67–200 mg/day **Tricor:** 48–145 mg/day **Triglide:** 50–160 mg/day **Fenoglide:** 40–120 mg/day **Lipofen:** 50–150 mg/day	May increase levels of ezetimibe. Concomitant use of statins may increase rhabdomyolysis, elevate CPK levels, and cause myoglobinuria. **Side Effects:** Abdominal pain, constipation, diarrhea, respiratory complaints, headache, fever, flu-like syndrome, asthenia

Continued

ANTIHYPERLIPIDEMICS—cont'd

Name	Primary Effect	Dosage	Comments/Side Effects
Fenofibric acid (Fibricor, Trilipix)	Decreases TG, LDL Increases HDL	**Trilipix:** 45–135 mg/day **Fibricor:** 35–105 mg/day	May give without regard to meals. Concomitant use of statins may increase rhabdomyolysis. **Side Effects:** Headache, upper respiratory tract infection, pain, nausea, dizziness, nasopharyngitis
Gemfibrozil (Lopid)	Decreases TG Increases HDL	600 mg 2 times/day	Give 30 min before breakfast and dinner. Concomitant use of statins may increase rhabdomyolysis, elevate CPK levels, and cause myoglobinuria. **Side Effects:** Fatigue, vertigo, headache, rash, eczema, diarrhea, abdominal pain, nausea, vomiting, constipation
Niacin			
Niacin, nicotinic acid (Niacor, Niaspan)	Decreases LDL,TG Increases HDL	**Regular-release (Niacor):** 1 g tid **Extended-release (Niaspan):** 1 g at bedtime	Diabetics may experience a dose-related elevation in glucose. **Side Effects:** Increased LFT, hyperglycemia, dyspepsia, itching, flushing, dizziness, insomnia
Statins			
Atorvastatin (Lipitor)	Decreases LDL,TG Increases HDL	Initially, 10–20 mg/day. Range: 10–80 mg/day	May interact with CYP3A4 inhibitors (e.g., amiodarone, diltiazem, cyclosporine, grapefruit juice) increasing risk of myopathy. **Side Effects:** Myalgia, myopathy, rhabdomyolysis, headache, chest pain, peripheral edema, dizziness, rash, abdominal pain, constipation, diarrhea, dyspepsia, nausea, flatulence, increased LFT, back pain, sinusitis
Fluvastatin (Lescol)	Decreases LDL,TG Increases HDL	40–80 mg/day	Primarily metabolized by CYP2C9 enzyme system. May increase levels of phenytoin, rifampin. May lower fluvastatin levels. **Side Effects:** Headache, fatigue, dyspepsia, diarrhea, nausea, abdominal pain, myalgia, myopathy, rhabdomyolysis

Lovastatin (Mevacor)	Decreases LDL, TG Increases HDL	Initially, 20 mg/day. Adjust at 4 wk intervals. **Maximum:** 80 mg/day	May interact with CYP3A4 inhibitors (e.g., amiodarone, diltiazem, cyclosporine, grapefruit products) increasing risk of myopathy. **Side Effects:** Increased CPK levels, headache, dizziness, rash, constipation, diarrhea, abdominal pain, dyspepsia, nausea, flatulence, myalgia, myopathy, rhabdomyolysis
Pitavastatin (Livalo)	Decreases LDL, TG Increases HDL	Initially, 2 mg/day. May increase at 4 wk intervals to 4 mg/day	Erythromycin, rifampin may increase concentration. **Side Effects:** Myalgia, back pain, diarrhea, constipation, pain in extremities
Pravastatin (Pravachol)	Decreases LDL, TG Increases HDL	Initially, 40 mg/day. Titrate to response. Range: 10–80 mg/day	May be less likely to be involved in drug interactions. Cyclosporine may increase pravastatin levels. **Side Effects:** Chest pain, headache, dizziness, rash, nausea, vomiting, diarrhea, increased LFTs, cough, flu-like symptoms, myalgia, myopathy, rhabdomyolysis
Rosuvastatin (Crestor)	Decreases LDL, TG Increases HDL	Initially, 10–20 mg/day. Titrate to response. Range: 5–40 mg/day	May be less likely to be involved in drug interactions. Cyclosporine may increase rosuvastatin levels. **Side Effects:** Chest pain, peripheral edema, headache, rash, dizziness, vertigo, pharyngitis, diarrhea, nausea, constipation, abdominal pain, dyspepsia, sinusitis, flu-like symptoms, myalgia, myopathy, rhabdomyolysis

Continued

ANTIHYPERLIPIDEMICS—cont'd

Name	Primary Effect	Dosage	Comments/Side Effects
Simvastatin (Zocor)	Decreases LDL, TG Increases HDL	5–40 mg/day	May interact with CYP3A4 inhibitors (e.g., amiodarone, diltiazem, cyclosporine, grapefruit products) increasing risk of myopathy. **Side Effects:** Constipation, flatulence, dyspepsia, increased LFTs, increased CPK, upper respiratory tract infection
Omega Fatty Acids			
Icosapent (Vascepa)	Decreases TG	2 g 2 times/day	**Side Effects:** Arthralgia
Lovaza	Decreases TG Increases LDL, HDL	2 g 2 times/day or 4 g once daily	Use with caution with fish or shellfish allergy. **Side Effects:** Eructation, dyspepsia, taste perversion
PCSK9 Inhibitors			
Alirocumab (Praluent)	Decreases LDL	**SQ:** 75 mg q2wks	**Side Effects:** Hypersensitivity reactions (e.g., rash), nasopharyngitis, injection site reactions, influenza
Evolcumab (Repatha)	Decreases LDL	**SQ:** 140 mg q2wks or 420 mg qmo	**Side Effects:** Nasopharyngitis, upper respiratory tract infection, influenza, back pain, injection site reactions

CPK, Creatine Phosphokinase; *G,* granules; *HDL,* high-density lipoprotein; *LDL,* low-density lipoprotein; *SQ,* subcutaneous; *T,* tablets; *TG,* triglycerides.

Antihypertensives

USES

Treatment of mild to severe hypertension.

ACTION

Many groups of medications are used in the treatment of hypertension.

ACE inhibitors: Decrease conversion of angiotensin I to angiotensin II, a potent vasoconstrictor, reducing peripheral vascular resistance and B/P.

Alpha agonists (central action): Stimulate alpha$_2$-adrenergic receptors in the cardiovascular centers of the CNS, reducing sympathetic outflow and producing an antihypertensive effect.

Alpha antagonists (peripheral action): Block alpha$_1$ adrenergic receptors in arterioles and veins, inhibiting vasoconstriction and decreasing peripheral vascular resistance, causing a fall in B/P.

Angiotensin receptor blockers: Block vasoconstrictor effects of angiotensin II by blocking the binding of angiotensin II to AT1 receptors in vascular smooth muscle, helping blood vessels to relax and reduce B/P.

Beta blockers: Decrease B/P by inhibiting beta, adrenergic receptors, which lowers heart rate, heart workload, and the heart's output of blood.

Calcium channel blockers: Reduce B/P by inhibiting flow of extracellular calcium across cell membranes of vascular tissue, relaxing arterial smooth muscle.

Diuretics: Inhibit sodium (Na) reabsorption, increasing excretion of Na and water. Reduce plasma, extracellular fluid volume, and peripheral vascular resistance.

Renin inhibitors: Directly inhibit renin, decreasing plasma renin activity (PRA), inhibiting conversion of angiotensinogen to angiotensin, producing antihypertensive effect.

Vasodilators: Directly relax arteriolar smooth muscle, decreasing vascular resistance. Exact mechanism unknown.

ANTIHYPERTENSIVES

Name	Availability	Dosage Range	Side Effects
(ACE) Inhibitors			
Benazepril (Lotensin)	**T:** 5 mg, 10 mg, 20 mg, 40 mg	20–80 mg/day as single or 2 divided doses	Postural dizziness, headache, cough
Captopril	**T:** 12.5 mg, 25 mg, 50 mg, 100 mg	50–100 mg 2 times/day	Rash, cough, hyperkalemia
Enalapril (Vasotec)	**T:** 2.5 mg, 5 mg, 10 mg, 20 mg	5–40 mg/day in 1–2 divided doses	Hypotension, chest pain, syncope, headache, dizziness, fatigue
Fosinopril	**T:** 10 mg, 20 mg,40 mg	10–80 mg once/d or divided bid	Dizziness, cough, hyperkalemia
Lisinopril (Prinivil, Zestril)	**T:** 2.5 mg, 5 mg, 10 mg, 20 mg, 30 mg, 40 mg	10–40 mg once/d	Hypotension, headache, fatigue, dizziness, hyperkalemia, cough
Quinapril	**T:** 5 mg, 10 mg, 20 mg, 40 mg	10–80 mg once/d or divided bid	Hypotension, dizziness, fatigue, headache, myalgia, hyperkalemia
Ramipril (Altace)	**T or C:** 1.25 mg, 2.5 mg, 5 mg, 10 mg	2.5–20 mg once/d or divided bid	Cough, hypotension, angina, headache, dizziness, hyperkalemia
Alpha Agonists: Central Action			
Clonidine (Catapres)	**T:** 0.1 mg, 0.2 mg,0.3 mg **P:** 0.1 mg/hr, 0.2 mg/hr, 0.3 mg/hr	**PO:** 0.1–0.8 mg divided bid or tid **Topical:** 0.1–0.6 mg/wk	Sedation, dry mouth, heart block, rebound hypertension, contact dermatitis with patch, bradycardia, drowsiness
Alpha Agonists: Peripheral Action			
Doxazosin (Cardura)	**T:** 1 mg, 2 mg, 4 mg, 8 mg	**PO:** 2–16 mg/day	Dizziness, vertigo, headaches
Prazosin (Minipress)	**C:** 1 mg, 2 mg, 5 mg	**PO:** 6–20 mg/day	Dizziness, light-headedness, headaches, drowsiness, palpitations, fluid retention
Terazosin (Hytrin)	**C:** 1 mg, 2 mg, 5 mg, 10 mg	**PO:** 1–20 mg/day	Dizziness, headaches, asthenia (loss of strength, energy)

Angiotensin Receptor Blockers

Azilsartan (Edarbi)	**T:** 40 mg, 80 mg	40–80 mg once/d	Diarrhea, hypotension, nausea, cough
Candesartan (Atacand)	**T:** 4 mg, 8 mg, 16 mg, 32 mg	8–32 mg once/d or divided bid	Hypotension, dizziness, headache, hyperkalemia
Eprosartan (Teveten)	**T:** 400 mg, 600 mg	600 mg once/d	Headache, cough, dizziness
Irbesartan (Avapro)	**T:** 75 mg, 150 mg, 300 mg	150–300 mg once/d	Fatigue, diarrhea, cough
Losartan (Cozaar)	**T:** 25 mg, 50 mg, 100 mg	25–100 mg once/d or divided bid	Chest pain, fatigue, hypoglycemia, weakness, cough, hypotension
Olmesartan (Benicar)	**T:** 5 mg, 20 mg, 40 mg	20–40 mg once/d	Dizziness, headache, diarrhea, flu-like symptoms
Valsartan (Diovan)	**T:** 80 mg, 160 mg, 320 mg	80–320 mg once/d	Dizziness, fatigue, increased BUN

Beta Blockers

Atenolol (Tenormin)	**T:** 25 mg, 50 mg, 100 mg	50–100 mg once/d	Fatigue, bradycardia, reduced exercise tolerance, increased triglycerides, bronchospasm, sexual dysfunction, masked hypoglycemia
Bisoprolol (Zebeta)	**T:** 5 mg, 10 mg	5–20 mg once/d	Fatigue, insomnia, diarrhea, arthralgia, upper respiratory infections
Carvedilol (Coreg, Coreg CR)	**T:** 3.125 mg, 6.25 mg, 12.5 mg, 25 mg; **CR:** 10 mg, 20 mg, 40 mg, 80 mg	**T:** 12.5–50 mg divided bid; **CR:** 20–80 mg once/d	Orthostatic hypotension, fatigue, dizziness
Metoprolol (Lopressor)	**T:** 25 mg, 37.5 mg, 50 mg, 75 mg, 100 mg	100–450 mg bid or tid	Hypotension, bradycardia, fatigue, 1st degree heart block, dizziness
Metoprolol XL (Toprol XL)	**T:** 25 mg, 50 mg, 100 mg, 200 mg	25–400 mg once/d	Same as metoprolol
nebivolol (Bystolic)	**T:** 2.5 mg, 5 mg, 10 mg, 20 mg	5–40 mg once/d	Upper respiratory tract infection, dizziness, fatigue

Continued

ANTIHYPERTENSIVES—cont'd

Name	Availability	Dosage Range	Side Effects
Calcium Channel Blockers			
Amlodipine (Norvasc)	**T:** 2.5 mg, 5 mg, 10 mg	2.5–10 mg once/d	Headache, fatigue, peripheral edema, flushing, worsening heart failure, rash, gingival hyperplasia, tachycardia
Diltiazem CD (Cardizem CD)	**C:** 120 mg, 180 mg, 240 mg, 300 mg	240–360 mg once/d	Dizziness, headache, bradycardia, heart block, worsening heart failure, edema, constipation
Felodipine (Plendil)	**T:** 2.5 mg, 5 mg, 10 mg	2.5–10 mg once/d	Headache, flushing, peripheral edema, rash, gingival hyperplasia, tachycardia
Nifedipine XL (Adalat CC, Procardia XL)	**T:** 30 mg, 60 mg, 90 mg	30–90 mg once/d	Flushing, peripheral edema, headache, dizziness, nausea
Verapamil SR (Calan SR)	**T:** 120 mg, 180 mg, 240 mg **T (Sustained-Release):** 120 mg, 180 mg	**T (Immediate-Release):** 80–160 mg tid **T (Sustained-Release):** 240–480 mg once/d or divided bid	Headache, gingival hyperplasia, constipation
Diuretics			
Chlorthalidone (Hygroton)	**T:** 25 mg, 50 mg	12.5–25 mg/day	Same as hydrochlorothiazide
Hydrochlorothiazide (Hydrodiuril)	**T:** 25 mg, 50 mg	12.5–50 mg/day	Hypokalemia, hyperuricemia, hypomagnesemia, hyperglycemia Pancreatitis, rash, photosensitivity, hyponatremia, hypercalcemia, hypercholesterolemia, hypertriglyceridemia

Renin Inhibitor		
Aliskiren (Tekturna)	**T:** 150 mg, 300 mg	**PO:** 150–300 mg/day	Diarrhea, dyspepsia, headache, dizziness, fatigue, upper respiratory tract infection

Vasodilators		
Hydralazine (Apresoline)	**T:** 10 mg, 25 mg, 50 mg, 100 mg	**PO:** 40–300 mg/day	Headaches, palpitations aggravation of angina, dizziness, fluid retention, nasal congestion
Minoxidii (Loniten)	**T:** 2.5 mg, 10 mg	**PO:** 10–40 mg/day	Rapid/irregular heartbeat, hypertrichosis, peripheral edema aggravation of angina, fluid retention

C, Capsules; *P,* patch; *T,* tablets.

Antimigraine (Triptans)

USES

Treatment of migraine headaches with or without aura in adults 18 yrs and older.

ACTION

Triptans are selective agonists of the serotonin (5-HT) receptor in cranial arteries, which cause vasoconstriction and reduce inflammation associated with antidromic neuronal transmission correlating with relief of migraine headache.

TRIPTANS

Name	Availability	Dosage Range	Contraindications	Common Side Effects
Almotriptan (Axert)	**T:** 6.25 mg, 12.5 mg	6.25–12.5 mg; may repeat after 2 hrs (**Maximum:** 25 mg/day)	Ischemic heart disease, angina pectoris, arrhythmias, previous MI, uncontrolled hypertension, hemiplegic or basilar migraine, peripheral vascular disease	Drowsiness, dizziness, paresthesia, nausea, vomiting, headache, xerostomia
Eletriptan (Relpax)	**T:** 20 mg, 40 mg	**A:** 20–40 mg; may repeat after **2** hrs (**Maximum: 2** hrs (**Maximum:** 80 mg/day)	Same as almotriptan	Chest pain, dizziness, drowsiness, headache, paresthesia, nausea, xerostomia, weakness
Frovatriptan (Frova)	**T:** 2.5 mg	2.5 mg; may repeat after 2 hrs; no more than 3 **T**/day (**Maximum:** 7.5 mg/day)	Same as almotriptan	Hot/cold sensations, dizziness, fatigue, headaches, skeletal pain, dyspepsia, flushing, paresthesia, drowsiness, xerostomia, nausea
Naratriptan (Amerge)	**T:** 1 mg, 2.5 mg	1–2.5 mg; may repeat once after 4 hrs (**Maximum:** 5 mg/day)	Same as almotriptan plus severe renal/hepatic disease	Neck pain, pain, nausea, fatigue
Rizatriptan (Maxalt, Maxalt-MLT)	**T:** 5 mg, 10 mg **DT:** 5 mg, 10 mg	5 or 10 mg; may repeat after 2 hrs (**Maximum:** 30 mg/day)	Same as almotriptan	Chest pain, drowsiness, xerostomia, weakness, paresthesia, nausea, dizziness, drowsiness, fatigue

Sumatriptan (Imitrex, Sumavel DosePro, Onzetra, Xsail, Zecuity)	**T:** 25 mg, 50 mg, 100 mg, **NS:** 5 mg, 10 mg, 20 mg, **I:** 4 mg, 6 mg, **NP:** 8 pouches of 2 nose pieces each 11 mg/ piece	**PO:** 25–100 mg; may repeat after 2 hrs (**Maximum:** 200 mg/day), **NS:** 5–20 mg; may repeat after 2 hrs (**Maximum:** 40 mg/day), **Subcutaneous:** 3–6 mg; may repeat after 1 hr (**Maximum:** 12 mg/day), **NP:** 22 mg; may repeat after 2 hrs (**Maximum:** 44 mg/day)	Same as almotriptan plus severe hepatic dysfunction	*Oral:* Hot/cold flashes, paresthesia, malaise, fatigue *Injection:* Atypical sensations, flushing, chest pain/discomfort, injection site reaction, dizziness, vertigo, paresthesia, dizziness; bleeding, bruising, swelling, erythema at injection site *Nasal:* Discomfort, nausea, vomiting, altered taste *Transdermal:* Localized pain, skin discoloration, allergic contact dermatitis, pruritus, local irritation
Zolmitriptan (Zomig, Zomig-ZMT)	**T:** 2.5 mg, 5 mg, **DT:** 2.5 mg, 5 mg, **NS:** 2.5 mg/0.1 ml, 5 mg/0.1 ml	**PO:** 2.5–5 mg; may repeat after 2 hrs (**Maximum:** 10 mg/day), **NS:** 1 spray (2.5 or 5 mg) at onset of migraine headache; may repeat after 2 hrs (**Maximum:** 10 mg/day)	Same as almotriptan plus symptomatic Wolff-Parkinson-White syndrome	Atypical sensations, pain, nausea, dizziness, asthenia, drowsiness

A, Adults; *DT,* disintegrating tablets; *I,* Injection; *NP,* nasal powder; *NS,* nasal spray; *T,* tablets.

Antipsychotics

USES	ACTION	SIDE EFFECTS (Please refer to individual monographs)
Antipsychotics are primarily used in managing schizophrenia. They may also be used in treatment of bipolar disorder, schizoaffective disorder, and irritability associated with autism. The goals in treating schizophrenia include targeting symptoms, preventing relapse, and increasing adaptive functioning. Use of antipsychotic medications is the mainstay of schizophrenia management.	The precise mechanism of action of antipsychotic medications is unknown, but they have been categorized into two groups: *Typical (traditional):* Associated with high dopamine antagonism and low serotonin antagonism. *Atypical:* Those having moderate to high dopamine antagonism and high serotonin antagonism and those having low dopamine antagonism and high serotonin antagonism.	*Typical versus atypical:* Typical antipsychotics are associated with a greater risk of extrapyramidal side effects, and atypicals are associated with a greater risk of weight gain. *Endocrine:* Hyperprolactinemia, weight gain, increased risk of diabetes. *Cardiovascular:* Orthostatic hypotension, electrocardiographic changes. *Lipids:* Increased triglycerides, cholesterol. *Central nervous system:* Dystonic reactions, akathisia, pseudo-parkinsonism, tardive dyskinesia, sedation, risk of seizures.

TYPICAL ANTIPSYCHOTICS

Name	Uses	Dosage (Oral)
Fluphenazine	Adult psychosis	1–5 mg/day
Haloperidol (Haldol)	Adult and child psychosis	1–15 mg/day
Thioridazine	Adult, adolescent, child schizophrenia and psychosis	200–800 mg/day
Thiothixene (Navane)	Adult and adolescent schizophrenia	Moderate: 15 mg/day Severe: 20–30 mg/day

ATYPICAL ANTIPSYCHOTICS

Name	Uses	Dosage
Aripiprazole (Abilify)	Adult and adolescent schizophrenia; adult and child bipolar 1 disorder; adult major depressive disorder; irritability with adolescent autism	10–15 mg/day
Brexipiprazole (Rexulti)	Adult schizophrenia; adult major depressive disorder	2–4 mg/day
Cariprazine (Vraylar)	Adult schizophrenia, bipolar I disorder (manic or mixed episodes)	1.5–6 mg/day
Clozapine (Clozaril)	Schizophrenia; suicidal behavior in adult schizophrenia and schizoaffective disorder	300–450 mg/day
Iloperidone (Fanapt)	Adult schizophrenia	12–24 mg/day
Lurasidone (Latuda)	Adult schizophrenia, bipolar I disorder (manic or mixed episodes)	40–160 mg/day
Olanzapine (Zyprexa)	Adult, adolescent, and child schizophrenia; adult, adolescent mania in bipolar I disorder	10–20 mg/day
Paliperidone (Invega)	Adult and adolescent schizophrenia; adult schizoaffective disorder	3–12 mg/day
Quetiapine (Seroquel)	Adult and adolescent schizophrenia; adult, adolescent, and child bipolar I disorder	400–800 mg/day
Risperidone (Risperdal)	Adult and adolescent schizophrenia; adult, adolescent, and child bipolar I disorder; irritability with adolescent and child autism	4–8 mg/day
Ziprasidone (Geodon)	Adult schizophrenia; manic or mixed episodes associated with adult bipolar I disorder	40–160 mg/day

Antivirals

USES

Treatment of HIV infection. Treatment of cytomegalovirus (CMV) retinitis in pts with AIDS, acute herpes zoster (shingles), genital herpes (recurrent), mucosal and cutaneous herpes simplex virus (HSV), chickenpox, and influenza A viral illness.

ACTION

Effective antivirals must inhibit virus-specific nucleic acid/ protein synthesis. Possible mechanisms of action of antivirals used for non-HIV infection may include inference with viral DNA synthesis and viral replication, inactivation of viral DNA polymerases, incorporation and termination of the growing viral DNA chain, prevention of release of viral nucleic acid into the host cell, or interference with viral penetration into cells.

ANTIVIRALS

Name	Availability	Uses	Side Effects
Abacavir (Ziagen)	**T:** 300 mg **OS:** 20 mg/ml	HIV infection	Nausea, vomiting, loss of appetite, diarrhea, headaches, fatigue, hypersensitivity reactions
Acyclovir (Zovirax)	**T:** 400 mg, 800 mg **C:** 200 mg **I:** 50 mg/ml	Mucosal/cutaneous HSV-1 and HSV-2, varicella-zoster (shingles), genital herpes, herpes simplex, encephalitis, chickenpox	Malaise, anorexia, nausea, vomiting, light-headedness
Adefovir (Hepsera)	**T:** 10 mg	Chronic hepatitis B	Asthenia, headaches, abdominal pain, nausea, diarrhea, flatulence, dyspepsia
Amantadine (Symmetrel)	**T:** 100 mg **C:** 100 mg **S:** 50 mg/5 ml	Influenza A	Anxiety, dizziness, headaches, nausea, loss of appetite
Cidofovir (Vistide)	**I:** 75 mg/ml	CMV retinitis	Decreased urination, fever, chills, diarrhea, nausea, vomiting, headaches, loss of appetite

Darunavir (Prezista)	T: 75 mg, 150 mg, 400 mg, 600 mg, 800 mg	HIV infection	Diarrhea, nausea, vomiting, headaches, skin rash, constipation
Delavirdine (Rescriptor)	T: 100 mg, 200 mg	HIV infection	Diarrhea, fatigue, rash, headaches, nausea
Didanosine(Videx)	C: 125 mg, 200 mg, 250 mg, 400 mg **Powder for suspension: 2 g, 4 g**	HIV infection	Peripheral neuropathy, anxiety, headaches, rash, nausea, diarrhea, dry mouth
Efavirenz (Sustiva)	C: 50 mg, 200 mg T: 600 mg	HIV infection	Diarrhea, dizziness, headaches, insomnia, nausea, vomiting, drowsiness
Etravirine (Intelence)	T: 25 mg, 100 mg, 200 mg	HIV infection	Rash, nausea, abdominal pain, vomiting
Famciclovir (Famvir)	T: 125 mg, 250 mg, 500 mg	Herpes zoster, genital herpes, herpes labialis, mucosal/cutaneous herpes simplex	Headaches, nausea
Foscarnet (Foscavir)	I: 24 mg/ml	CMV retinitis, HSV infections	Decreased urination, abdominal pain, nausea, vomiting, dizziness, fatigue, headaches
Ganciclovir (Cytovene)	I: 500 mg	CMV retinitis, CMV disease	Sore throat, fever, unusual bleeding/bruising
Indinavir (Crixivan)	C: 200 mg, 400 mg	HIV infection	Blood in urine, weakness, nausea, vomiting, diarrhea, headaches, insomnia, altered taste
Lamivudine (Epivir)	T: 100 mg, 150 mg, 300 mg OS: 5 mg/ml, 10 mg/ml	HIV infection, chronic hepatitis B	Nausea, vomiting, abdominal pain, paresthesia
Lopinavir/ritonavir (Kaletra)	T: 100 mg/25 mg, 200 mg/50 mg OS: 80 mg/20 mg per ml	HIV infection	Diarrhea, nausea

Continued

ANTIVIRALS—cont'd

Name	Availability	Uses	Side Effects
Maraviroc (Selzentry)	**T:** 150 mg, 300 mg	HIV infection	Cough, pyrexia, upper respiratory tract infection, rash, musculoskeletal symptoms, abdominal pain, dizziness
Nelfinavir (Viracept)	**T:** 250 mg, 625 mg	HIV infection	Diarrhea
Oseltamivir (Tamiflu)	**C:** 30 mg, 45 mg, 75 mg **S:** 6 mg/ml	Influenza A or B	Diarrhea, nausea, vomiting
Raltegravir (Isentress)	**T:** 400 mg **T (chew):** 25 mg, 100 mg	HIV infection	Nausea, headache, diarrhea, pyrexia
Ribavirin (Virazole)	**Aerosol:** 6 g **OS:** 40 mg/ml **T:** 200 mg, 400 mg, 600 mg	Lowers respiratory infections in infants, children due to respiratory syncytial virus (RSV), chronic hepatitis C	Anemia
Ritonavir (Norvir)	**C:** 100 mg **T:** 100 mg **OS:** 80 mg/ml	HIV infection	Weakness, diarrhea, nausea, decreased appetite, vomiting, altered taste
Saquinavir (Invirase)	**C:** 200 mg **T:** 500 mg	HIV infection	Weakness, diarrhea, nausea, oral ulcers, abdominal pain
Stavudine (Zerit)	**C:** 15 mg, 20 mg, 30 mg, 40 mg **OS:** 1 mg/ml	HIV infection	Paresthesia, decreased appetite, chills, fever, rash

Tenofovir (Viread)	**T:** 150 mg, 200 mg, 250 mg, 300 mg **Powder (oral):** 40 mg/g	HIV infection	Diarrhea, nausea, pharyngitis, headaches
Valacyclovir (Valtrex)	**T:** 500 mg, 1 g	Herpes zoster, genital herpes, herpes labialis, chickenpox	Headaches, nausea
Valganciclovir (Valcyte)	**T:** 450 mg **OS:** 50 mg/ml	CMV retinitis	Anemia, abdominal pain, diarrhea, headaches, nausea, vomiting, paresthesia
Zanamivir (Relenza)	**Inhalation:** 5 mg	Influenza A and B	Cough, diarrhea, dizziness, headaches, nausea, vomiting
Zidovudine (Retrovir)	**C:** 100 mg **S:** 50 mg/5 ml **I:** 10 mg/ml	HIV infection	Fatigue, fever, chills, headaches, nausea, muscle pain

C, Capsules; *I*, Injection; *OS*, oral solution; *S*, syrup; *T*, tablets.

Beta-Adrenergic Blockers

USES

Management of hypertension, angina pectoris, arrhythmias, hypertrophic subaortic stenosis, migraine headaches, MI (prevention), glaucoma.

ACTION

Beta-adrenergic blockers competitively block adrenergic receptors, located primarily in myocardium, and beta$_2$-adrenergic receptor's, located primarily in bronchial and vascular smooth muscle. By occupying beta-receptor sites, these agents prevent naturally occurring or administered epinephrine/norepinephrine from exerting their effects. The results are basically opposite to those of sympathetic stimulation.

Effects of beta, blockade include slowing heart rate, decreasing cardiac output and contractility; effects of beta$_2$ blockade include bronchoconstriction, increased airway resistance in pts with asthma or COPD. Beta blockers can affect cardiac rhythm/automaticity (decrease sinus rate, SA/AV conduction; increase refractory period in AV node); decrease systolic and diastolic B/P; exact mechanism unknown but may block peripheral receptors, decrease sympathetic outflow from CNS, or decrease renin release from kidney. All beta blockers mask tachycardia that occurs with hypoglycemia. When applied to the eye, reduce intraocular pressure and aqueous production.

BETA-ADRENERGIC BLOCKERS

Name	Availability	Indication	Dosage Range	Frequent or Severe Side Effects
Acebutolol (Sectral)	C: 200 mg, 400 mg	HTN, ventricular arrhythmia	**HTN:** Initially, 400 mg once daily or 2 divided doses. Usual dose: 200–1200 mg once/d or divided bid **Arrhythmia:** Initially, 200 mg 2 times/day. Gradually increase to 300–600 mg 2 times/day	**CLASS:** Fatigue, depression, bradycardia, decreased exercise tolerance, erectile dysfunction, heart failure, may aggravate hypoglycemia, increase incidence of diabetes, insomnia, increase triglycerides, decrease cholesterol. Sudden withdrawal may exacerbate angina and myocardial infarction.

Atenolol (Tenormin)	**T:** 25 mg, 50 mg, 100 mg	HTN, angina, MI	**Angina:** Initially, 50 mg once daily. May increase to 100 mg once daily after one wk **HTN:** Initially, 50 mg once daily. May increase to 100 mg once daily after 2 wks **MI:** 50 mg bid or 100 mg once daily
Bisoprolol (Zebeta)	**T:** 5 mg, 10 mg	HTN	Initially, 5 mg once daily. May increase to 10 mg/day, then 20 mg/day. Usual dose: 5-10 mg/day
Carvedilol (Coreg)	**T:** 3.125 mg, 6.25 mg, 12.5 mg, 25 mg **C (SR):** 10 mg, 20 mg, 40 mg, 80 mg	HF, LVD after MI, HTN	**Immediate-Release HF:** Initially, 3.25 mg 2 times/day. May increase at 2 wk intervals to 6.25 mg 2 times/day, then 12.5 mg 2 times/day, then 25 mg 2 times/day **LVD after MI:** Initially, 6.25 mg 2 times/day. May increase q3—10 days to 12.5 mg 2 times/day, then 25 mg 2 times/day **HTN:** Initially, 6.25 mg 2 times/day. May increase q7—14 days to 12.5 mg 2 times/day, then 25 mg 2 times/day **Extended-Release HF:** 10—80 mg once daily **LVD after MI:** 10-80 mg once daily **HTN:** 20-80 mg once daily
Labetalol (Trandate)	**T:** 100 mg, 200 mg, 300 mg	HTN	Initially, 100 mg 2 times/day. May increase q2-3 days in 100 mg 2 times/day increments. Usual dose: 200—1200 mg 2 times/day

Continued

BETA-ADRENERGIC BLOCKERS—cont'd

Name	Availability	Indication	Dosage Range	Frequent or Severe Side Effects
Metoprolol (Lopressor [IR], Toprol XL [SR])	**T (IR):** 50 mg, 100 mg **T (SR):** 25 mg, 50 mg	HTN, angina, HF, MI	**IR:** **Angina:** Initially, 50 mg 2 times/day. May increase up to 400 mg/day **HTN:** Initially, 100 mg once daily. May increase at weekly intervals up to 450 mg/day divided bid or tid **Post-MI:** 100 mg bid **SR:** **Angina:** 100–400 mg once daily **HF:** 12.5–200 mg once daily **HTN:** 25–400 mg once daily	
Nadolol (Corgard)	**T:** 20 mg, 40 mg, 80 mg	HTN, angina	**Angina, HTN:** Initially, 40 mg once/day. Usual dose: 40–320 mg once daily	
Nebivolol (Bystolic)	**T:** 2.5 mg, 5 mg, 10 mg, 20 mg	HTN	Initially, 5 mg once daily. May increase at 2 wk intervals up to 40 mg/once/d	
Pindolol (Visken)	**T:** 5 mg, 10 mg	HTN	Initially, 5 mg 2 times/day. May increase to 10–40 mg/day. **Maximum:** 60 mg/day divided bid	

| Propranolol (Inderal) | T (IR): 10 mg, 20 mg, 40 mg, 60 mg, 80 mg
C (SR): 60 mg, 80 mg, 120 mg, 160 mg
S: 4 mg/ml, 8 mg/ml
I: 1 mg/ml | HTN, angina, MI, arrhythmias, migraine, essential tremor, hypertrophic subaortic stenosis | **IR:**
Angina: 80–320 mg/day in 2–4 divided doses
Arrhythmias: 10–30 mg 3–4 times/day
HTN: 40 mg bid up to 240 mg/day in 2–3 divided doses
Hypertrophic subaortic stenosis: 20–40 mg 3–4 times/day
Post-MI: 180-240 mg/day in 2–4 divided doses
Migraine: Initially, 80 mg/day. May increase gradually up to 240 mg/day in divided doses
Tremor: Initially, 40 mg 2 times/day. Usual dose: 120–320 mg/day
SR:
Angina: Initially, 80 mg once daily. May increase q3-7days up to 320 mg/day
HTN: 80–120 mg once daily at bedtime
Migraine: Initially, 80 mg once daily. Gradually increase up to 240 mg once daily
Hypertrophic subaortic stenosis: 80–160 mg once daily |

C, Capsules; *HF,* heart failure; *HTN,* hypertension; *I,* Injection; *LVD,* left ventricular dysfunction; *S,* solution; *SR,* sustained-release; *T,* tablets.

Bronchodilators

USES

Relief of bronchospasm occurring during anesthesia and in bronchial asthma, bronchitis, emphysema.

ACTION

Inhaled corticosteroids: Exact mechanism unknown. May act as anti-inflammatories, decrease mucus secretion.

Beta₂-adrenergic agonists: Stimulate beta receptors in lung, relax bronchial smooth muscle, increase vital capacity, decrease airway resistance.

Anticholinergics: Inhibit cholinergic receptors on bronchial smooth muscle (block acetylcholine action).

Leukotriene modifiers: Decrease effect of leukotrienes, which increase migration of eosinophils, producing mucus/edema of airway wall, causing bronchoconstriction.

Methylxanthines: Directly relax smooth muscle of bronchial airway, pulmonary blood vessels (relieve bronchospasm, increase vital capacity). Increase cyclic 3,5-adenosine monophosphate.

BRONCHODILATORS

Name	Availability	Dosage Range	Side Effects
Anticholinergics			
Aclidinium (Tudorza)	Inhalation powder: 400 mcg/actuation	A: 400 mcg 2 times/day	Headache, nasopharyngitis, cough
Glycopyrrolate (Seebri Neohaler)	**Inhalation Capsule:** 15.6 mcg/cap	A: One inhalation 2 times/day	Fatigue, diarrhea, nausea, arthralgia, nasopharyngitis, upper respiratory tract infection, wheezing
Ipratropium (Atrovent)	**NEB:** 0.02% (500 mcg) **MDI:** 17 mcg/actuation	A **(NEB):** 500 mcg q6-8h A **(MDI):** 2 puffs 4 times/day	Upper respiratory tract infection, bronchitis, sinusitis, headache, dyspnea

Tiotropium (Spiriva, Spiriva Respimat)	Inhalation powder: 18 mcg/ capsule Aerosol Solution: 1.25 mcg/ inhalation	A: Once/day (inhaled twice) Aerosol Solution: 2 inhalations once daily	Xerostomia, upper respiratory tract infection, sinusitis, pharyngitis
Umeclidinium (Incruse Ellipta)	Inhalation powder: 62.5 mcg/blister	A: One inhalation once daily	Nasopharyngitis, upper respiratory tract infection, cough, arthralgia
Bronchodilators			
Arformoterol (Brovanna)	NEB: 15 mcg/2 ml	Neb: 15 mcg 2 times/day	Pain, diarrhea, sinusitis, leg cramps, dyspnea, rash, flu syndrome, peripheral edema
Albuterol (ProAir HFA, ProAir Respiclick Proventil HFA, Ventolin HFA)	DPI: 90 mcg/actuation MDI: 90 mcg/actuation NEB: 2.5 mg/3 ml, 2.5 mg/0.5 ml, 0.63-1.25 mg/3 ml	DPI: 1-2 inhalations q4–6h as needed MDI: 2 inhalations q4–6h as needed NEB: 1.25–5 mg q4–6h as needed	Tachycardia, skeletal muscle tremors, muscle cramping, palpitations, insomnia, hypokalemia, increased serum glucose
Albuterol/ipratropium (Combivent Respimat, DuoNeb)	MDI: 90 mcg albuterol/ 18 mcg ipratropium/actuation NEB: 2.5 mg albuterol/ 0.5 mg ipratropium/3 ml	MDI: 1 inhalation 4 times/day as needed NEB: 2.5 mg/0.5 mg 4 times/day as needed	Same as individual listing for albuterol and ipratropium
Formoterol (Foradil, Perforomist)	NEB: 20 mcg/2 ml	NEB: 20 mcg q12h	Diarrhea, nausea, asthma exacerbation, bronchitis, infection
Formoterol/budesonide (Symbicort)	MDI: 80,160 mcg/ 4.5 mcg/ inhalation	MDI: 2 inhalations 2 times/day	Same as individual listing for formoterol and budesonide
Formoterol/mometasone (Dulera)	MDI: 5 mcg/100 mcg, 5 mcg/200 mcg	MDI: 2 inhalations 2 times/day	Same as individual listing for formoterol and beclomethasone

Continued

BRONCHODILATORS—cont'd

Name	Availability	Dosage Range	Side Effects
Indacaterol (Arcapta)	**DPI:** 75 mcg/capsule	**DPI:** 75 mcg once daily	Cough, oropharyngeal pain, nasopharyngitis, headache, nausea
Levalbuterol (Xopenex)	**MDI:** 45 mcg/actuation **NEB:** 0.31, 0.63, 1.25 mg/ 3 ml, 1.25 mg/0.5 ml	**MDI:** 2 inhalations q4–6h as needed **NEB:** 0.31–1.25 mg q6–8h	Tremor, rhinitis, viral infection, headache, nervousness, asthma, pharyngitis, rash
Olodaterol (Striverdi Respimat)	**MDI:** 2.5 mcg/actuation	**MDI:** 2 inhalations once daily	Nasopharyngitis, rash, dizziness, cough, bronchitis, upper respiratory tract infections
Olodaterol/tiotropium (Stiolto Respimat)	**MDI:** 2.5 mcg/2.5 mcg	**MDI:** 2 inhalations once daily	Nasopharyngitis, cough, back pain
Salmeterol (Serevent Diskus)	**DPI:** 50 mcg/blister	**DPI:** 50 mcg q12h	Headache, pain, throat irritation, nasal congestion, bronchitis, pharyngitis
Salmeterol/fluticasone (Advair Diskus, Advair HFA)	**DPI:** 100, 250, 500 mcg/ 50 mcg/blister **MDI:** 45, 115, 230 mcg/21 mcg/inhalation	**DPI:** 1 inhalation 2 times/day **MDI:** 2 inhalations 2 times/day	Same as individual listing for salmeterol and fluticasone
Vilanterol/umeclidinium (Anoro Ellipta)	**DPI:** 25 mcg/62.5 mcg	**DPI:** Once daily	Pharyngitis, sinusitis, lower respiratory tract infections, constipation, diarrhea, muscle spasms, neck/chest pain
Inhaled Corticosteroids			
Beclomethasone (Qvar)	**MDI:** 40, 80 mcg/inhalation	**MDI:** 40-320 mcg 2 times/day	Cough, hoarseness, headache, pharyngitis

Budesonide (Pulmicort Flexhaler, Pulmicort Respules)	**DPI: (Flexhaler):** 90,180 mcg/inhalation **DPI: (Turbuhaler):** 200 mcg/inhalation **NEB: (Respules):** 0.25, 0.5 mg/2 ml	**DPI: (Flexhaler):** 180–720 mcg 2 times/day **DPI: (Turbuhaler):** 400–2,400 mcg/day in 2–4 divided doses **NEB: (Respules):** 250–500 mcg 1–2 times/day or 1 mg once daily	Headache, nausea, respiratory infection, rhinitis
Ciclesonide (Alvesco HFA)	HFA: 80, 160 mcg/inhalation	HFA: 80–320 mcg 2 times/day	Headache, nasopharyngitis, upper respiratory infection, epistaxis, nasal congestion, sinusitis
Fluticasone (Arnuity Ellipta, Flovent Diskus, Flovent HFA)	**DPI: (Flovent Diskus):** 50, 100, 250 mcg/blister **(Arnuity Ellipta):** 100 mcg, 200 mcg/activation **MDI: (Flovent HFA):** 44, 110, 220 mcg/inhalation	**DPI: (Flovent Diskus):** 100–1,000 mcg 2 times/day **(Arnuity Ellipta):** 100–200 mcg once daily **MDI: (Flovent HFA):** 88–880 mcg 2 times/day	Headache, nasal congestion, pharyngitis, sinusitis, respiratory infections
Formoterol/budesonide (Symbicort)	MDI: 80,160 mcg/4.5 mcg/inhalation	MDI: 2 inhalations 2 times/day	Same as individual listing for formoterol and budesonide
Mometasone (Asmanex Twisthaler)	DPI: 110–220 mcg/inhalation	DPI: 220–880 mcg once daily in evening or 220 mcg bid	Same as beclomethasone
Salmeterol/fluticasone (Advair Diskus, Advair HFA)	**DPI:** 100, 250, 500 mcg/blister **MDI:** 45,115, 230 mcg/21 mcg/inhalation	**DPI:** 1 inhalation 2 times/day **MDI:** 2 inhalations 2 times/day	Same as individual listing for salmeterol and fluticasone
Vilanterol/fluticasone (Breo Ellipta)	**DPI:** 25 mcg/100 mcg; 25 mcg/200 mcg	**DPI:** 1 inhalation once daily	Nasopharyngitis, upper respiratory infection, headache, oral candidiasis

Continued

BRONCHODILATORS—cont'd

Name	Availability	Dosage Range	Side Effects
Leukotriene Modifiers			
Montelukast (Singulair)	**T:** 4 mg, 5 mg, 10 mg	**A:** 10 mg/day **C (6–14 yrs):** 5 mg/day **C (2–5 yrs):** 4 mg/day	Dyspepsia, increased LFT, cough, nasal congestion, headache, dizziness, fatigue
Zafirlukast (Accolate)	**T:** 10 mg, 20 mg	**A, C (12 yrs and older):** 20 mg 2 times/day **C (5–11 yrs):** 10 mg 2 times/day	Headache, nausea, diarrhea, infection
PDE-4 Inhibitor			
Roflumilast (Daliresp)	**T:** 500 mcg	**A:** 500 mcg once daily	Headache, dizziness, insomnia

A, Adults; *C (dosage),* children; *DPI,* dry powder inhaler; *HFA,* hydrofluoroalkane; *MDI,* metered dose inhaler; *NEB,* nebulization; *T,* tablets.

Calcium Channel Blockers

USES

Treatment of essential hypertension, treatment of and prophylaxis of angina pectoris (including vasospastic, chronic stable, unstable), prevention/control of supraventricular tachyarrhythmias, prevention of neurologic damage due to subarachnoid hemorrhage.

ACTION

Calcium channel blockers inhibit the flow of extracellular Ca^{2+} ions across cell membranes of cardiac cells, vascular tissue. They relax arterial smooth muscle, depress the rate of sinus node pacemaker, slow AV conduction, decrease heart rate, produce negative inotropic effect (rarely seen clinically due to reflex response). Calcium channel blockers decrease coronary vascular resistance, increase coronary blood flow, reduce myocardial oxygen demand. Degree of action varies with individual agent.

CALCIUM CHANNEL BLOCKERS

Name	Availability	Indications	Dosage Range	Side Effects
Amlodipine (Norvasc)	T: 2.5 mg, 5 mg, 10 mg	HTN, angina	**HTN:** Initially, 2.5–5 mg once daily. May titrate q7–14 days up to 10 mg/day **Angina:** 5–10 mg once daily	Headache, peripheral edema, dizziness, flushing, rash, gingival hyperplasia, tachycardia
Diltiazem (Cardizem)	T: 30 mg, 60 mg, 90 mg, 120 mg **(ER):** 120 mg, 180 mg, 240 mg, 300 mg, 360 mg, 420 mg C **(SR-12HR):** 60 mg, 90 mg, 120 mg, **(ER-24HR):** 120 mg, 180 mg, 240 mg, 300 mg, 360 mg, 420 mg **I:** 5 mg/ml	**PO:** HTN, angina **IV:** Arrhythmias	**See monograph** **HTN:** 120–540 mg/day **Angina:** 120–480 mg/day **I:** 20–25 mg IV bolus, then 5–15 mg/hr infusion	Constipation, flushing, hypotension, dizziness, AV block, bradycardia, headache, edema, HF
Felodipine (Plendil)	T: 2.5 mg, 5 mg, 10 mg	HTN	Initially, 5 mg/day. May increase q2wks. Usual dose: 5–10 mg/day	Headache, peripheral edema, dizziness, flushing, rash, gingival hyperplasia, tachycardia

Continued

CALCIUM CHANNEL BLOCKERS—cont'd

Name	Availability	Indications	Dosage Range	Side Effects
Isradipine	**C:** 2.5 mg, 5 mg	HTN	Initially, 2.5 mg 2 times/day. May increase at 2–4 wk intervals at 2.5–5 mg increments. Usual dose: 5–10 mg 2 times/day	Headache, peripheral edema, dizziness, flushing, rash, gingival hyperplasia, tachycardia
Nicardipine (Cardene)	**C (IR):** 20 mg, 30 mg **C (ER):** 30 mg, 45 mg,60 mg **I:** 2.5 mg/ml	HTN, angina	**Angina/HTN:** Initially, 20–30 mg 3 times/day. May increase q3days. Usual dose: 20–40 mg 3 times/day	Headache, peripheral edema, dizziness, flushing, rash, gingival hyperplasia, tachycardia
Nifedipine (Adalat, Procardia)	**C (IR):** 10 mg, 20 mg **T (ER):** 30 mg, 60 mg, 90 mg	HTN, angina	**HTN (ER):** Initially, 30–60 mg once daily. Usual dose: 90–120 mg once daily **Angina (IR):** 10–20 mg tid or **(ER):** Initially, 30–60 mg once daily. Titrate up to 90 mg daily. **Maximum:** 120 mg	Headache, peripheral edema, dizziness, flushing, rash, gingival hyperplasia, tachycardia
Nimodipine (Nimotop, Nymalize)	**C:** 30 mg **S:** 60 mg/20 ml	Prevent neurologic damage following subarachnoid hemorrhage	60 mg q4h for 21 days	Nausea, reduced B/P, headache, rash, diarrhea
Verapamil (Calan, Isoptin)	**T (IR):** 40 mg, 80 mg, 120 mg **T (SR):** 120 mg, 180 mg, 240 mg	HTN, angina	**Angina (IR):** Initially, 40–120 mg 3 times/day. Usual dose: 80–160 mg tid or **(SR):** Initially, 180 mg at HS. May increase at weekly intervals up to 480 mg/day **HTN (IR):** Initially, 80 mg 3 times/day. Usual dose: 240–480 mg/day in divided doses **(SR):** Initially, 120–180 mg/day. May increase at weekly intervals to 240 mg/day, then 180 mg 2 times/day. **Maximum:** 240 mg 2 times/day	Constipation, dizziness, tachycardia, AV block, bradycardia, headache, edema, HF

C, Capsules; *CR,* controlled-release; *ER,* extended-release; *HTN,* hypertension; *I,* injection; *S,* solution; *SR,* sustained-release; *T,* tablets.

Chemotherapeutic Agents

USES

Treatment of a variety of cancers; may be palliative or curative. Treatment of choice in hematologic cancers. Often used as adjunctive therapy (e.g., with surgery or irradiation); most effective when tumor mass has been removed or reduced by radiation. Often used in combinations to increase therapeutic results, decrease toxic effects. Certain agents may be used in nonmalignant conditions: polycythemia vera, psoriasis, rheumatoid arthritis, or immunosuppression in organ transplantation (used only in select cases that are severe and unresponsive to other forms of therapy). Refer to individual monographs.

ACTION

Most antineoplastics can be divided into alkylating agents, antimetabolites, anthracyclines, plant alkaloids, and topoisomerase inhibitors. These agents affect cell division or DNA synthesis. Newer agents (monoclonal antibodies and tyrosine kinase inhibitors) directly target a molecular abnormality in certain types of cancer. Hormones modulate tumor cell behavior without directly attacking those cells. Some agents are classified as miscellaneous.

CHEMOTHERAPEUTIC AGENTS

Name	Uses	Category	Side Effects
Abiraterone (Zytiga)	Prostate Cancer	Antiandrogen	Joint swelling, hypokalemia, edema, muscle discomfort, hot flashes, diarrhea, UTI, cough, hypertension, arrhythmia, dyspepsia, upper respiratory tract infection
Aldesleukin (Proleukin)	Melanoma (metastatic), Renal Cell (metastatic)	Biologic response modifier	Hypotension, sinus tachycardia, nausea, vomiting, diarrhea, renal impairment, anemia, rash, fatigue, agitation, pulmonary congestion, dyspnea, fever, chills, oliguria, weight gain, dizziness

Continued

CHEMOTHERAPEUTIC AGENTS—cont'd

Name	Uses	Category	Side Effects
Alectinib (Alecensa)	Non-small cell lung cancer (NSCLC), metastatic	Kinase inhibitor	Constipation, fatigue, edema, myalgia
Anastrozole (Arimidex)	Breast cancer	Aromatase inhibitor	Peripheral edema, chest pain, nausea, vomiting, diarrhea, constipation, abdominal pain, anorexia, pharyngitis, vaginal hemorrhage, anemia, leukopenia, rash, weight gain, diaphoresis, increased appetite, pain, headaches, dizziness, depression, paresthesia, hot flashes, increased cough, dry mouth, asthenia, dyspnea, phlebitis
Arsenic trioxide (Trisenox)	Acute promyelocytic leukemia (APL)	Miscellaneous	AV block, GI hemorrhage, hypertension, hypoglycemia, hypokalemia, hypomagnesemia, neutropenia, oliguria, prolonged QT interval, seizures, sepsis, thrombocytopenia
Asparaginase (Elspar)	Acute lymphoblastic leukemia (ALL)	Miscellaneous	Anorexia, nausea, vomiting, hepatic toxicity, pancreatitis, nephrotoxicity, clotting factor abnormalities, malaise, confusion, lethargy, EEG changes, respiratory distress, fever, hyperglycemia, depression, stomatitis, allergic reactions, drowsiness
Atezolizumab (Tecentriq)	NSCLC, metastatic, urothelial carcinoma, locally advanced or metastatic	Miscellaneous	Fatigue, decreased appetite, nausea, urinary tract infections, constipation, pyrexia
Avelumab (Bavencio)	Merkel cell carcinoma	PD-L1 blocking antibody	Fatigue, musculoskeletal pain, diarrhea, nausea, infusion-related reactions, rash, decreased appetite, peripheral edema
Axitinib (Inlyta)	Renal cell carcinoma, advanced	Kinase inhibitor	Diarrhea, hypertension, fatigue, decreased appetite, nausea, dysphoria, vomiting, asthenia, constipation
Azacitidine (Vidaza)	Myelodysplastic (MDS) syndrome	DNA methylation inhibitor	Edema, hypokalemia, weight loss, myalgia, cough, dyspnea, upper respiratory tract infection, back pain, pyrexia, weakness

Drug	Uses	Classification	Side effects/adverse reactions
BCG (TheraCys, Tice BCG)	Bladder cancer	Biologic response modulator	Nausea, vomiting, anorexia, diarrhea, dysuria, hematuria, cystitis, urinary urgency, anemia, malaise, fever, chills
Belinostat (Beleodaq)	Peripheral T-cell lymphoma	Miscellaneous	Nausea, fatigue, pyrexia, anemia, vomiting
Bendamustine (Treanda)	Chronic lymphocytic leukemia (CLL), Non-Hodgkin lymphoma (NHL)	Alkylating agent	Neutropenia, pyrexia, thrombocytopenia, nausea, anemia, leukopenia, vomiting
Bevacizumab (Avastin)	Cervical cancer, persistent/recurrent/metastatic, colorectal cancer, metastatic, glioblastoma, NSCLC, nonsquamous	Monoclonal antibody	Increased B/P, fatigue, blood clots, diarrhea, decreased WBCs, headaches, decreased appetite, stomatitis
Bexarotene (Targretin)	Cutaneous T-cell lymphoma	Miscellaneous	Anemia, dermatitis, fever, hypercholesterolemia, infection, leukopenia, peripheral edema
Bicalutamide (Casodex)	Prostate cancer, metastatic	Antiandrogen	Gynecomastia, hot flashes, breast pain, nausea, diarrhea, constipation, nocturia, impotence, pain, muscle pain, asthenia, abdominal pain
Bleomycin (Blenoxane)	Head/neck cancers, Hodgkin lymphoma, malignant pleural effusion, testicular cancer	Antibiotic	Nausea, vomiting, anorexia, stomatitis, hyperpigmentation, alopecia, pruritus, hyperkeratosis, urticaria, pneumonitis progression to fibrosis, weight loss, rash
Blinatumomab (Blincyto)	Acute lymphoblastic leukemia (ALL)	Miscellaneous	Pyrexia, headache, peripheral edema, febrile neutropenia, nausea, hypokalemia, tremor, rash, constipation
Bortezomib (Velcade)	Mantle cell lymphoma, multiple myeloma	Proteasome inhibitor	Anxiety, dizziness, headaches, insomnia, peripheral neuropathy, pruritus, rash, abdominal pain, decreased appetite, constipation, diarrhea, dyspepsia, nausea, vomiting, arthralgia, dyspnea, asthenia, edema, pain
Bosutinib (Bosulif)	Chronic myelogenous leukemia (CML)	Kinase inhibitor	Nausea, diarrhea, thrombocytopenia, vomiting, abdominal pain, anemia, fever, fatigue

Continued

CHEMOTHERAPEUTIC AGENTS—cont'd

Name	Uses	Category	Side Effects
Brentuximab (Adcetris)	Anaplastic large cell lymphoma, Hodgkin lymphoma (relapsed, refractory, post-autologous hematopoietic stem cell transplant)	Miscellaneous	Neutropenia, peripheral sensory neuropathy, fatigue, nausea, anemia, upper respiratory tract infection, diarrhea, pyrexia, thrombocytopenia, cough, vomiting
Brigatinib (Alunbrig)	NSCLC, metastatic	Kinase inhibitor	Nausea, diarrhea, fatigue, cough, headache
Busulfan (Myleran)	Chronic myeloid leukemia (CML)	Alkylating agent	Nausea, vomiting, hyperuricemia, myelosuppression, skin hyperpigmentation, alopecia, anorexia, weight loss, diarrhea, stomatitis
Cabazitaxel (Jevtana)	Prostate cancer, metastatic	Microtubule inhibitor	Neutropenia, anemia, leukopenia, thrombocytopenia, diarrhea, fatigue, nausea, vomiting, constipation, asthenia, abdominal pain, hematuria, anorexia, peripheral neuropathy, dyspnea, alopecia
Capecitabine (Xeloda)	Breast cancer, metastatic, colorectal cancer	Antimetabolite	Nausea, vomiting diarrhea, stomatitis, myelosuppression, palmar-plantar erythrodysesthesia syndrome, dermatitis, fatigue, anorexia
Carboplatin (Paraplatin)	Ovarian cancer, advanced	Alkylating agent	Nausea, vomiting, nephrotoxicity, myelosuppression, alopecia, peripheral neuropathy, hypersensitivity, ototoxicity, asthenia, diarrhea, constipation
Carfilzomib (Kyprolis)	Multiple myeloma, relapsed/refractory	Proteasome inhibitor	Anemia, fatigue, nausea, thrombocytopenia, dyspnea, diarrhea, pyrexia
Carmustine (BiCNU)	Brain tumors, multiple myeloma, Hodgkin lymphoma, relapsed/refractory, NHL, relapsed/refractory	Alkylating agent	Anorexia, nausea, vomiting, myelosuppression, pulmonary fibrosis, pain at injection site, diarrhea, skin discoloration
Ceritinib (Zykadia)	NSCLC, metastatic	Kinase inhibitor	Diarrhea, nausea, increased LFTs, vomiting, abdominal pain, fatigue, decreased appetite, constipation

Drug	Uses	Classification	Side Effects/Adverse Reactions
Cetuximab (Erbitux)	Colorectal cancer, metastatic, head/neck cancer, squamous cell	Monoclonal antibody	Dyspnea, hypotension, acne-like rash, dry skin, weakness, fatigue, fever, constipation, abdominal pain
Chlorambucil (Leukeran)	Lymphomas, chronic lymphocytic leukemia (CLL)	Alkylating agent	Myelosuppression, dermatitis, nausea, vomiting, hepatic toxicity, anorexia, diarrhea, abdominal discomfort, rash
Cisplatin (Platinol-AQ)	Bladder cancer, advanced, ovarian cancer, metastatic, testicular cancer, metastatic	Alkylating agent	Nausea, vomiting, nephrotoxicity, myelosuppression, neuropathies, ototoxicity, anaphylactic-like reactions, hyperuricemia, hypomagnesemia, hypophosphatemia, hypokalemia, hypocalcemia, pain at injection site
Cladribine (Leustatin)	Hairy cell leukemia	Antimetabolite	Nausea, vomiting, diarrhea, myelosuppression, chills, fatigue, rash, fever, headaches, anorexia, diaphoresis
Cobimetinib (Cotellic)	Melanoma, unresectable or metastatic	Kinase inhibitor	Diarrhea, photosensitivity reaction, nausea, vomiting, pyrexia, increased ALT, AST, alkaline phosphatase
Crizotinib (Xalkori)	NSCLC, metastatic	Tyrosine kinase inhibitor	Vision disorders, nausea, vomiting, diarrhea, edema, constipation
Cyclophosphamide (Cytoxan)	ALL, AML, breast cancer, CML, Hodgkin lymphoma, multiple myeloma, NHL, ovarian carcinoma	Alkylating agent	Nausea, vomiting, hemorrhagic cystitis, myelosuppression, alopecia, interstitial pulmonary fibrosis, amenorrhea, azoospermia, diarrhea, darkening skin/fingernails, headaches, diaphoresis
Cytarabine (Ara-C, Cytosar)	AML, ALL, CML, meningeal leukemia	Antimetabolite	Anorexia, nausea, vomiting, stomatitis, esophagitis, diarrhea, myelosuppression, alopecia, rash, fever, neuropathies, abdominal pain
Dabrafenib (Tafinlar)	Melanoma, metastatic or unresectable	Kinase inhibitor	Hyperkeratosis, headache, pyrexia, arthralgia, constipation, alopecia, rash, cough, palmer-plantar erythrodysesthesia syndrome, papilloma
Dacarbazine (DTIC)	Hodgkin lymphoma, metastatic malignant melanoma	Alkylating agent	Nausea, vomiting, anorexia, hepatic necrosis, myelosuppression, alopecia, rash, facial flushing, photosensitivity, flu-like symptoms, confusion, blurred vision

Continued

CHEMOTHERAPEUTIC AGENTS—cont'd

Name	Uses	Category	Side Effects
Daratumumab (Darzalex)	Multiple myeloma, relapsed/refractory	Monoclonal antibody	Fatigue, nausea, infusion reactions, back pain, pyrexia, nausea, upper respiratory tract infections
Dasatinib (Sprycel)	ALL, CML	Tyrosine kinase inhibitor	Pyrexia, pleural effusion, febrile neutropenia, GI bleeding, pneumonia, thrombocytopenia, dyspnea, anemia, cardiac failure, diarrhea
Daunorubicin (Cerubidine)	ALL, AML	Anthracycline	HF, nausea, vomiting, stomatitis, mucositis, diarrhea, hematuria, myelosuppression, alopecia, fever, chills, abdominal pain
Daunorubicin liposomal (DaunoXome)	Kaposi sarcoma	Anthracycline	Nausea, diarrhea, abdominal pain, anorexia, vomiting, stomatitis, myelosuppression, rigors, back pain, headaches, neuropathy, depression, dyspnea, fatigue, fever, cough, allergic reactions, diaphoresis
Dinutuximab (Unituxin)	Neuroblastoma	Monoclonal antibody	Pain, arthralgia, myalgia, neuralgia, pyrexia, hypotension, vomiting, diarrhea, urticaria, hypoxia
Docetaxel (Taxotere)	Breast cancer, NSCLC, prostate, gastric, head/neck cancers	Antimicrotubular	Hypotension, nausea, vomiting, diarrhea, mucositis, myelosuppression, rash, paresthesia, hypersensitivity, fluid retention, alopecia, asthenia, stomatitis, fever
Doxorubicin (Adriamycin)	Breast cancer, metastatic cancers	Anthracycline	Cardiotoxicity, including HF, arrhythmias, nausea, vomiting, stomatitis, esophagitis, GI ulceration, diarrhea, anorexia, hematuria, myelosuppression, alopecia, hyperpigmentation of nail beds and skin, local inflammation at injection site, rash, fever, chills, urticaria, lacrimation, conjunctivitis
Doxorubicin liposomal (Doxil)	AIDS-related Kaposi sarcoma, multiple myeloma, ovarian cancer, advanced	Anthracycline	Neutropenia, palmar-plantar erythrodysesthesia syndrome, cardiomyopathy, HF
Durvalumab (Imfinzi)	Urothelial carcinoma, advanced and metastatic	PD-L1 blocking antibody	Fatigue, musculoskeletal pain, constipation, decreased appetite, nausea, peripheral edema, UTI
Elotuzumab (Empliciti)	Multiple myeloma, relapsed/refractory	Immunostimulatory antibody	Fatigue, diarrhea, pyrexia, constipation, cough, peripheral neuropathy, nasopharyngitis, decreased appetite, upper respiratory tract infections, pneumonia

Drug	Uses	Classification	Side Effects
Enasidenib (Idhifa)	AML, refractory	Isocitrate dehydrogenase-2 inhibitor	Nausea, vomiting, diarrhea, elevated bilirubin, decreased appetite
Enzalutamide (Xtandi)	Prostate cancer, metastatic	Antiandrogen	Fatigue, weakness, back pain, diarrhea, tissue swelling, musculoskeletal pain, headache, upper respiratory tract infections, blood in urine, spinal cord compression
Epirubicin (Ellence)	Breast cancer, adjuvant	Anthracycline	Anemia, leukopenia, neutropenia, infection, mucositis
Erlotinib (Tarceva)	NSCLC, pancreatic cancer	Tyrosine kinase inhibitor	Diarrhea, rash, nausea, vomiting
Etoposide (VePesid)	Small cell lung cancer, testicular cancer	Podophyllotoxin derivative	Nausea, vomiting, anorexia, myelosuppression, alopecia, diarrhea, drowsiness, peripheral neuropathies
Everolimus (Afinitor)	Breast cancer, advanced, neuroendocrine tumors, renal cell carcinoma, advanced, subependymal giant cell astrocytoma	mTOR kinase inhibitor	Stomatitis, infections, asthenia, fatigue, cough, diarrhea
Exemestane (Aromasin)	Breast cancer	Aromatase inactivator	Dyspnea, edema, hypertension, mental depression
Fludarabine (Fludara)	CLL	Antimetabolite	Nausea, diarrhea, stomatitis, bleeding, anemia, myelosuppression, skin rash, weakness, confusion, visual disturbances, peripheral neuropathy, coma, pneumonia, peripheral edema, anorexia
Fluorouracil (Adrucil, Efudex)	Breast, colon, gastric, pancreatic, rectal cancers, basal cell carcinoma	Antimetabolite	Nausea, vomiting, stomatitis, GI ulceration, diarrhea, anorexia, myelosuppression, alopecia, skin hyperpigmentation, nail changes, headaches, drowsiness, blurred vision, fever

Continued

CHEMOTHERAPEUTIC AGENTS—cont'd

Name	Uses	Category	Side Effects
Flutamide (Eulexin)	Prostate cancer	Antiandrogen	Hot flashes, nausea, vomiting, diarrhea, hepatitis, impotence, decreased libido, rash, anorexia
Fulvestrant (Faslodex)	Breast cancer, metastatic or advanced	Estrogen receptor antagonist	Asthenia, pain, headaches, injection site pain, flu-like symptoms, fever, nausea, vomiting, constipation, anorexia, diarrhea, peripheral edema, dizziness, depression, anxiety, rash, increased cough, UTI
Gefitinib (Iressa)	NSCLC	Tyrosine kinase inhibitor	Diarrhea, rash, acne, nausea, dry skin, vomiting, pruritus, anorexia
Gemcitabine (Gemzar)	Breast, NSCLC, ovarian, pancreatic cancers	Antimetabolite	Increased LFT, nausea, vomiting, diarrhea, stomatitis, hematuria, myelosuppression, rash, mild paresthesia, dyspnea, fever, edema, flu-like symptoms, constipation
Goserelin (Zoladex)	Breast cancer, prostate cancer	Hormone agonist	Hot flashes, sexual dysfunction, erectile dysfunction, gynecomastia, lethargy, pain, lower urinary tract symptoms, headaches, nausea, depression, diaphoresis
Hydroxyurea (Hydrea)	CML, head/neck cancers	Antimetabolite	Anorexia, nausea, vomiting, stomatitis, diarrhea, constipation, myelosuppression, fever, chills, malaise
Ibrutinib (Imbruvica)	CLL, small lymphocytic lymphoma, mantle cell lymphoma, Waldenstrom macroglobulinemia	Kinase inhibitor	Neutropenia, thrombocytopenia, diarrhea, anemia, musculoskeletal pain, rash, nausea, bruising, fatigue, hemorrhage, pyrexia
Idarubicin (Idamycin PFS)	Acute myeloid leukemia (AML)	Anthracycline	HF, arrhythmias, nausea, vomiting, stomatitis, myelosuppression, alopecia, rash, urticaria, hyperuricemia, abdominal pain, diarrhea, esophagitis, anorexia
Idelalisib (Zydelig)	CLL, follicular B-cell non-Hodgkin lymphoma, small lymphocytic lymphoma	Kinase inhibitor	Diarrhea, pyrexia, fatigue, nausea, cough, abdominal pain, pneumonia, increased ALT/AST

Ifosfamide (Ifex)	Testicular cancer	Alkylating agent	Nausea, vomiting, hemorrhagic cystitis, myelosuppression, alopecia, lethargy, drowsiness, confusion, hallucinations, hematuria
Imatinib (Gleevec)	ALL, CML, dermatofibro-sarcoma protuberans, GIST, chronic eosinophilic leukemias, myelodysplastic/myelo-proliferative disease	Tyrosine kinase inhibitor	Nausea, fluid retention, hemorrhage, musculoskeletal pain, arthralgia, weight gain, pyrexia, abdominal pain, dyspnea, pneumonia
Interferon alfa-2b (Intron-A)	AIDS-related Kaposi sar-coma, follicular lym-phoma, hairy cell leuke-mia, malignant melanoma	Miscellaneous	Mild hypotension, hypertension, tachycardia with high fever, nausea, diarrhea, al-tered taste, weight loss, thrombocytopenia, myelosuppression, rash, pruritus, my-algia, arthralgia associated with flu-like symptoms
Ipilimumab (Yervoy)	Melanoma, unresectable or metastatic, melanoma, adjuvant	Miscellaneous	Fatigue, diarrhea, pruritus, rash, colitis
Irinotecan (Camptosar)	Colorectal cancer, metastatic, pancreatic adenocarcinoma, metastatic	Camptothecin	Diarrhea, nausea, vomiting, abdominal cramps, anorexia, stomatitis, increased AST, severe myelosuppression, alopecia, diaphoresis, rash, weight loss, dehydra-tion, increased serum alkaline phosphatase, headaches, insomnia, dizziness, dys-pnea, cough, asthenia, rhinitis, fever, back pain, chills
Ixabepilone (Ixempra)	Breast cancer	Antimicrotubular	Peripheral sensory neuropathy, fatigue, myalgia, alopecia, nausea, vomiting, stomatitis, diarrhea, anorexia, abdominal pain
Ixazomib (Ninlaro)	Multiple myeloma	Proteasome inhibitor	Diarrhea, constipation, thrombocytopenia, peripheral neuropathy, nausea, peripheral edema, back pain, vomiting
Lapatinib (Tykerb)	Breast cancer	Tyrosine kinase inhibitor	Diarrhea, palmar-plantar erythrodysesthesia, nausea, rash, vomiting, fatigue

Continued

CHEMOTHERAPEUTIC AGENTS—cont'd

Name	Uses	Category	Side Effects
lenalidomide (Revlimid)	Mantle cell lymphoma, multiple myeloma, myelodysplastic syndromes	Immunomodulator	Diarrhea, pruritus, rash, fatigue, DVT, pulmonary embolism, thrombocytopenia, neutropenia, upper respiratory tract infection, cellulitis, hypertension, peripheral neuropathy
Lenvatinib (Lenvima)	Renal cell carcinoma, advanced, thyroid cancer, differentiated	Kinase inhibitor	Hypertension, fatigue, diarrhea, arthralgia, decreased weight, nausea, stomatitis, headache, vomiting, proteinuria, abdominal pain
Letrozole (Femara)	Breast cancer in postmenopausal women	Aromatase inhibitor	Hypertension, nausea, vomiting, constipation, diarrhea, abdominal pain, anorexia, rash, pruritus, musculoskeletal pain, arthralgia, fatigue, headaches, dyspnea, coughing, hot flashes
Leuprolide (Lupron)	Prostate cancer, advanced	Hormone agonist	Hot flashes, gynecomastia, nausea, vomiting, constipation, anorexia, dizziness, headaches, insomnia, paresthesia, bone pain
Lomustine (CeeNU)	Brain tumors, Hodgkin lymphoma	Alkylating agent	Anorexia, nausea, vomiting, stomatitis, hepatotoxicity, nephrotoxicity, myelosuppression, alopecia, confusion, slurred speech
Megestrol (Megace)	Breast cancer, endometrial cancer	Hormone	Deep vein thrombosis, Cushing-like syndrome, alopecia, carpal tunnel syndrome, weight gain, nausea
Melphalan (Alkeran)	Multiple myeloma, ovarian cancer	Alkylating agent	Anorexia, nausea, vomiting, myelosuppression, diarrhea, stomatitis
Mercaptopurine (Purinethol)	ALL	Antimetabolite	Anorexia, nausea, vomiting, stomatitis, hepatic toxicity, myelosuppression, hyperuricemia, diarrhea, rash
Methotrexate (Rheumatrex)	ALL, trophoblastic neoplasms, breast cancer, head and neck cancer, cutaneous T-cell lymphoma, lung cancer, advanced NHL, osteosarcoma	Antimetabolite	Nausea, vomiting, stomatitis, GI ulceration, diarrhea, hepatic toxicity, renal failure, cystitis, myelosuppression, alopecia, urticaria, acne, photosensitivity, interstitial pneumonitis, fever, malaise, chills, anorexia

Midostaurin (Rhydapt)	AML, aggressive systemic mastocytosis (ASM)	Kinase inhibitor	Febrile neutropenia, nausea, mucositis, vomiting, headache, petechiae, musculoskeletal pain, epistaxis, hyperglycemia, upper respiratory tract infections
Mitomycin (Mutamycin)	Gastric cancer, pancreatic cancer	Antibiotic	Anorexia, nausea, vomiting, stomatitis, diarrhea, renal toxicity, myelosuppression, alopecia, pruritus, fever, hemolytic uremic syndrome, weakness
Mitotane (Lysodren)	Adrenocortical carcinoma	Miscellaneous	Anorexia, nausea, vomiting, diarrhea, skin rashes, depression, lethargy, drowsiness, dizziness, adrenal insufficiency, blurred vision, impaired hearing
Mitoxantrone (Novantrone)	Acute nonlymphocytic leukemias, prostate cancer, advanced hormone refractory	Anthracenedione	HF, tachycardia, EKG changes, chest pain, nausea, vomiting, stomatitis, mucositis, myelosuppression, rash, alopecia, urine discoloration (bluish green), phlebitis, diarrhea, cough, headaches, fever
Necitumumab (Portrazza)	NSCLC (squamous) metastatic	Epidermal growth factor receptor (EGFR) antagonist	Rash, hypomagnesemia
Nelarabine (Arranon)	T-cell acute lymphoblastic leukemia/lymphoma	Antimetabolite	Anemia, neutropenia, thrombocytopenia, nausea, vomiting, diarrhea, fatigue, fever, dyspnea, severe neurologic events (convulsions, peripheral neuropathy)
Neratinib (Nerlynx)	Breast cancer	Kinase inhibitor	Diarrhea, nausea, abdominal pain, fatigue, vomiting, stomatitis, muscle spasms increase AST/ALT UTI
Nilotinib (Tasigna)	CML	Tyrosine kinase inhibitor	Rash, pruritus, nausea, fatigue, headache, constipation, diarrhea, vomiting, thrombocytopenia, neutropenia
Nilutamide (Nilandron)	Prostate cancer, metastatic	Antiandrogen	Hypertension, angina, hot flashes, nausea, anorexia, increased hepatic enzymes, dizziness, dyspnea, visual disturbances, impaired adaptation to dark, constipation, decreased libido
Niraparib (Zejula)	Epithelial carcinoma, fallopian tube or peritoneal cancer	PARP inhibitor	Thrombocytopenia, anemia, neutropenia, leukopenia, palpitations, nausea, vomiting, stomatitis, UTI, elevated AST/ALT, dyspnea, hypertension

Continued

CHEMOTHERAPEUTIC AGENTS—cont'd

Name	Uses	Category	Side Effects
Nivolumab (Opdivo)	Melanoma, unresectable or metastatic, head and neck cancer, squamous cell (recurrent or metastatic), Hodgkin lymphoma, NSCLC, metastatic, renal cell cancer, advanced	Miscellaneous	Fatigue, dyspnea, musculoskeletal pain, decreased appetite, cough, nausea, constipation
Obinutuzumab (Gazyva)	CLL, follicular lymphoma	Monoclonal antibody	Infusion reactions, thrombocytopenia, febrile neutropenia, lymphopenia, bone marrow failure, tumor lysis syndrome
Ofatumumab (Arzerra)	CLL	Monoclonal antibody	Fever, cough, diarrhea, fatigue, rash, infections, septic shock, neutropenia, thrombocytopenia, infusion reactions
Olaparib (Lynparza)	Ovarian cancer, advanced	Miscellaneous	Anemia, fatigue, nausea, vomiting, diarrhea, dysgeusia, dyspepsia, headache, decreased appetite
Olaratumab (Lartruvo)	Soft tissue sarcoma	PDGFR-alpha blocking antibody	Nausea, fatigue, musculoskeletal pain, mucositis, alopecia, vomiting, neuropathy, headache
Omacetaxine (Synribo)	CML	Protein synthesis inhibitor	Diarrhea, nausea, fatigue, pyrexia, asthenia, vomiting, anorexia, headache, thrombocytopenia, neutropenia, leukopenia, lymphopenia
Osimertinib (Tagrisso)	NSCLC, metastatic	Kinase inhibitor	Diarrhea, rash, dry skin, nail toxicity
Oxaliplatin (Eloxatin)	Colon cancer	Alkylating agent	Fatigue, neuropathy, abdominal pain, dyspnea, diarrhea, nausea, vomiting, anorexia, fever, edema, chest pain, anemia, thrombocytopenia, thromboembolism, altered hepatic function tests

Drug	Use	Classification	Side Effects
Paclitaxel (Taxol)	Breast cancer, Kaposi sarcoma, NSCLC, ovarian cancer	Antimicrotubular	Hypertension, bradycardia, EKG changes, nausea, vomiting, diarrhea, mucositis, myelosuppression, alopecia, peripheral neuropathies, hypersensitivity reaction, arthralgia, myalgia
Palbociclib (Ibrance)	Breast cancer, advanced	Kinase inhibitor	Neutropenia, leukopenia, fatigue, anemia, upper respiratory tract infection, nausea, stomatitis, alopecia, diarrhea, thrombocytopenia, decreased appetite, vomiting, asthenia, peripheral neuropathy, epistaxis
Panitumumab (Vectibix)	Colorectal cancer metastatic	Monoclonal antibody	Pulmonary fibrosis, severe dermatologic toxicity, infusion reactions, abdominal pain, nausea, vomiting, constipation, skin rash, fatigue
Panobinostat (Farydak)	Multiple myeloma	Miscellaneous	Diarrhea, fatigue, nausea, peripheral edema, decreased appetite, pyrexia, vomiting
Pazopanib (Votrient)	Renal cell carcinoma, soft tissue sarcoma	Kinase inhibitor	Diarrhea, hypertension, nausea, fatigue, vomiting, hepatotoxicity, hemorrhagic events
Pegaspargase (Oncaspar)	ALL	Miscellaneous	Hypotension, anorexia, nausea, vomiting, hepatotoxicity, pancreatitis, depression of clotting factors, malaise, confusion, lethargy, EEG changes, respiratory distress, hypersensitivity reaction, fever, hyperglycemia, stomatitis
Pemetrexed (Alimta)	NSCLC, nonsquamous, mesothelioma	Antimetabolite	Anorexia, constipation, diarrhea, neuropathy, anemia, chest pain, dyspnea, rash, fatigue
Pentostatin (Nipent)	Hairy cell leukemia	Antibiotic	Nausea, vomiting, hepatic disorders, elevated hepatic function tests, leukopenia, anemia, thrombocytopenia, rash, fever, upper respiratory infection, fatigue, hematuria, headaches, myalgia, arthralgia, diarrhea, anorexia
Pertuzumab (Perjeta)	Breast cancer, metastatic	HER2/neu receptor antagonist	Alopecia, diarrhea, nausea, neutropenia, rash, fatigue, peripheral neuropathy
Pomalidomide (Pomalyst)	Multiple myeloma, relapsed/refractory	Immunomodulator	Dyspnea, fatigue, peripheral edema, anorexia, rash, hypertension, pyrexia, myelosuppression, thrombocytopenia
Ponatinib (Iclusig)	ALL, CML	Kinase inhibitor	Abdominal pain, rash, fatigue, hypertension, pyrexia, myelosuppression, leukopenia, arthralgia, vomiting

Continued

CHEMOTHERAPEUTIC AGENTS—cont'd

Name	Uses	Category	Side Effects
Procarbazine (Matulane)	Hodgkin lymphoma, non-Hodgkin lymphomas, CNS tumors	Alkylating agent	Nausea, vomiting, stomatitis, diarrhea, constipation, myelosuppression, pruritus, hyperpigmentation, alopecia, myalgia, paresthesia, confusion, lethargy, mental depression, fever, hepatic toxicity, arthralgia, respiratory disorders
Ramucirumab (Cyramza)	Colorectal cancer, metastatic, gastric cancer, advanced or metastatic, NSCLC, metastatic	Miscellaneous	Diarrhea, hypertension
Regorafenib (Stivarga)	Colorectal cancer, GIST	VEGF inhibitor	Asthenia, fatigue, mucositis, weight loss, fever, GI perforation, hemorrhage, infections, PPES
Ribociclib (Kisqali)	Breast cancer, metastatic or advanced	Kinase inhibitor	Neutropenia, nausea, fatigue, diarrhea, leukopenia, alopecia, vomiting, headache
Rituximab (Rituxan)	CLL, non-Hodgkin lymphoma	Monoclonal antibody	Hypotension, arrhythmias, peripheral edema, nausea, vomiting, abdominal pain, leukopenia, thrombocytopenia, neutropenia, rash, pruritus, urticaria, angioedema, myalgia, headaches, dizziness, throat irritation, rhinitis, bronchosnasm, hypersensitivity reaction
Rucaparib (Rubraca)	Ovarian cancer, advanced	PARP inhibitor	Nausea, fatigue, vomiting, anemia, decreased appetite, diarrhea, thrombocytopenia, dyspnea, increased AST/ALT, decreased Hgb, platelets, ANC
Sipuleucel-T (Provenge)	Prostate cancer, metastatic	Miscellaneous	Chills, fatigue, fever, back pain, nausea, headache, joint ache
Sonidegib (Odomzo)	Basal cell carcinoma, locally advanced	Hedgehog pathway inhibitor	Muscle spasms, alopecia, dysgeusia, fatigue, nausea, diarrhea, decreased weight, musculoskeletal pain, myalgia, headache, abdominal pain, vomiting, pruritus
Sorafenib (Nexavar)	Hepatocellular cancer, renal cell cancer, advanced, thyroid cancer	Tyrosine kinase inhibitor	Fatigue, alopecia, nausea, vomiting, anorexia, constipation, diarrhea, neuropathy, dyspnea, cough, asthenia, pain

Sunitinib (Sutent)	GIST, pancreatic neuroendocrine tumors, advanced, renal cell carcinoma, advanced	Tyrosine kinase inhibitor	Hypotension, edema, fatigue, headache, fever, dizziness, rash, hyperpigmentation, diarrhea, nausea, dyspepsia, altered taste, vomiting, neutropenia, thrombocytopenia, increased ALT/AST
Tamoxifen (Nolvadex-D)	Breast cancer	Estrogen receptor antagonist	Skin rash, nausea, vomiting, anorexia, menstrual irregularities, hot flashes, pruritus, vaginal discharge or bleeding, myelosuppression, headaches, tumor or bone pain, ophthalmic changes, weight gain, confusion
Temozolomide (Temodar)	Anaplastic astrocytoma, glioblastoma multiforme	Alkylating agent	Amnesia, fever, infection, leukopenia, neutropenia, peripheral edema, seizures, thrombocytopenia
Temsirolimus (Torisel)	Renal cell carcinoma, advanced	mTOR kinase inhibitor	Rash, asthenia, mucositis, nausea, edema, anorexia, thrombocytopenia, leukopenia
Thioguanine (Tabloid)	AML	Antimetabolite	Anorexia, stomatitis, myelosuppression, hyperuricemia, nausea, vomiting, diarrhea
Thiotepa (Thioplex)	Bladder cancer, papillary, breast cancer	Alkylating agent	Anorexia, nausea, vomiting, mucositis, myelosuppression, amenorrhea, reduced spermatogenesis, fever, hypersensitivity reactions, pain at injection site, headaches, dizziness, alopecia
Tipiracil/trifluridine (Lonsurf)	Colorectal cancer, metastatic	Miscellaneous	Asthenia, fatigue, nausea, diarrhea, vomiting, decreased appetite, pyrexia, abdominal pain
Topotecan (Hycamtin)	Cervical cancer, recurrent or resistant, ovarian cancer, metastatic, SCLC, relapsed	Camptothecin	Nausea, vomiting, diarrhea, constipation, abdominal pain, stomatitis, anorexia, neutropenia, leukopenia, thrombocytopenia, anemia, alopecia, headaches, dyspnea, paresthesia
Toremifene (Fareston)	Breast cancer	Estrogen receptor antagonist	Elevated hepatic function tests, nausea, vomiting, constipation, skin discoloration, dermatitis, dizziness, hot flashes, diaphoresis, vaginal discharge or bleeding, ocular changes, cataracts, anxiety

Continued

CHEMOTHERAPEUTIC AGENTS—cont'd

Name	Uses	Category	Side Effects
Trabectedin (Yondelis)	Soft tissue sarcoma	Alkylating agent	Nausea, vomiting, fatigue, diarrhea, decreased appetite, peripheral edema, dyspnea, headache; increased ALT, AST, alkaline phosphatase; neutropenia, thrombocytopenia, anemia
Trametinib (Mekinist)	Melanoma, metastatic or unresectable	MEK inhibitor	Rash, peripheral edema, pyrexia, malignancies, fatigue, hemorrhagic events, HF
Trastuzumab (Herceptin)	Gastric cancer, metastatic, breast cancer, metastatic	Monoclonal antibody	HF, heart murmur (S_3 gallop), nausea, vomiting, diarrhea, abdominal pain, anorexia, rash, peripheral edema, back or bone pain, asthenia (loss of strength, energy), headaches, insomnia, dizziness, cough, dyspnea, rhinitis, pharyngitis
Tretinoin (Vesanoid)	Acute promyelocytic leukemia	Miscellaneous	Flushing, nausea, vomiting, diarrhea, constipation, dyspepsia, mucositis, leukocytosis, dry skin/mucous membranes, rash, pruritus, alopecia, dizziness, anxiety, insomnia, headaches, depression, confusion, intracranial hypertension, agitation, dyspnea, shivering, fever, visual changes, earaches, hearing loss, bone pain, myalgia, arthralgia
Valrubicin (Valstar)	Bladder cancer	Anthracycline	Dysuria, hematuria, urinary frequency/incontinence/urgency
Vandetanib (Caprelsa)	Thyroid cancer, medullary	Tyrosine kinase inhibitor	Diarrhea, rash, acne, nausea, hypertension, headache, fatigue, decreased appetite, abdominal pain
Vemurafenib (Zelboraf)	Melanoma, metastatic or unresectable	Kinase inhibitor	Arthralgia, alopecia, fatigue, malignancies, dermatological reactions
Venetoclax (Venclexta)	CLL	BCL-2 inhibitor	Diarrhea, neutropenia, anemia, nausea, upper respiratory tract infections, thrombocytopenia, fatigue
Vinblastine (Velban)	Mycosis fungoides, Hodgkin lymphoma, lymphocytic lymphoma, testicular cancer, Kaposi sarcoma	Vinca alkaloid	Nausea, vomiting, stomatitis, constipation, myelosuppression, alopecia, peripheral neuropathy, loss of deep tendon reflexes, paresthesia, diarrhea

Drug	Classification	Uses	Adverse Effects
Vincristine (Oncovin)	Vinca alkaloid	ALL, Hodgkin lymphoma, non-Hodgkin lymphomas, Wilm's tumor, neuroblastoma, rhabdomyosarcoma	Nausea, vomiting, stomatitis, constipation, pharyngitis, polyuria, myelosuppression, alopecia, numbness, paresthesia, peripheral neuropathy, loss of deep tendon reflexes, headaches, abdominal pain
Vincristine liposomal (Marqibo)	Vinca alkaloid	ALL	Constipation, nausea, pyrexia, fatigue, peripheral neuropathy, febrile neutropenia, diarrhea, anemia, reduced appetite, insomnia
Vinorelbine (Navelbine)	Vinca alkaloid	NSCLC	Elevated LFT, nausea, vomiting, constipation, ileus, anorexia, stomatitis, myelosuppression, alopecia, vein discoloration, venous pain, phlebitis, interstitial pulmonary changes, asthenia, fatigue, diarrhea, peripheral neuropathy, loss of deep tendon reflexes
Vismodegib (Erivedge)	Hedgehog pathway inhibitor	Basal cell carcinoma, metastatic or locally advanced	Alopecia, muscle spasms, dysgenesia, weight loss, fatigue, nausea, diarrhea, reduced appetite, vomiting, arthralgia
Vorinostat (Zolinza)	Histone deacetylase inhibitor	Cutaneous T-cell lymphoma	Diarrhea, fatigue, nausea, thrombocytopenia, anorexia, dysgeusia
ziv-aflibercept (Zaltrap)	Miscellaneous	Colorectal cancer, metastatic	Leukopenia, neutropenia, diarrhea, proteinuria, increased ALT/AST, stomatitis, thrombocytopenia, hypertension, epistaxis, headache, abdominal pain

AV, Atrioventricular; *C,* capsules; *EEG,* electroencephalogram; *EKG,* electrocardiogram; *HF,* heart failure; *I,* Injection; *LFT,* liver function test; *T,* tablets; *UTI,* urinary tract Infection.

Contraception

ACTION	CLASSIFICATION
Combination oral contraceptives decrease fertility primarily by inhibition of ovulation. In addition, they can promote thickening of the cervical mucus, thereby creating a physical barrier for the passage of sperm. Also, they can modify the endometrium, making it less favorable for nidation.	Oral contraceptives either contain both an estrogen and a progestin (combination oral contraceptives) or contain only a progestin (progestin-only oral contraceptives). The combination oral contraceptives have three subgroups: *Monophasic:* Daily estrogen and progestin dosage remains constant.	*Biphasic:* Estrogen remains constant, but the progestin dosage increases during the second half of the cycle. *Triphasic:* Progestin changes for each phase of the cycle. *Four-phasic:* Contains four progestin/estrogen combinations during the 20-day cycle.

Over the past several years, options have expanded to include a combined hormonal patch (Ortho Evra), vaginal ring (NuvaRing), and extended cycle contraceptives (e.g., Loestrin-24 FE, Seasonale, Seasonique, Yaz). The latest oral contraceptive, Natazia, is a four-phase dosing regimen (estradiol steps down and dienogest, a progestin, steps up during the cycle to help avoid breakthrough bleeding).

COMMON COMPLAINTS WITH ORAL CONTRACEPTIVES

Too much estrogen	Nausea, bloating, breast tenderness, increased B/P, melasma, headache
Too little estrogen	Early or midcycle breakthrough bleeding, increased spotting, hypomenorrhea
Too much progestin	Breast tenderness, headache, fatigue, changes in mood
Too little progestin	Late breakthrough bleeding
Too much androgen	Increased appetite, weight gain, acne, oily skin, hirsutism, decreased libido, increased breast size, breast tenderness, increased LDL cholesterol, decreased HDL cholesterol

B/P, Blood pressure; *HDL,* high-density lipoprotein; *LDL,* low-density lipoprotein.

CONTRACEPTIVES

Name	Estrogen Content	Progestin Content
Low-Dose Monophasic Pills		
Aubra Aviane Falmina Lessina Lutera Orsythia Sronyx	EE 20 mcg	Levonorgestrel 0.1 mg
Gildess 1/20 Junel 1/20 Junel Fe 1/20 Loestrin Fe 1/20 Microgestin Fe 1/20 Tarina Fe 1/20	EE 20 mcg	Norethindrone 1 mg
Altavera Levora Marlissa Portia-28	EE 30 mcg	Levonorgestrel 0.15 mg
Cryselle-28 Lo/Ovral-28 Low-Ogestrel, -28	EE 30 mcg	Norgestrel 0.3 mg
Gildess 1.5/30 Junel 1.5/30 Junel Fe 1.5/30 Larin 1.5/30 Loestrin Fe 1.5/30 Microgestin 1.5/30 Microgestin Fe 1.5/30	EE 30 mcg	Norethindrone acetate 1.5 mg

Continued

CONTRACEPTIVES—cont'd

Name	Estrogen Content	Progestin Content
Apri Desogen Ortho-Cept Reclipsen	EE 30 mcg	Desogestrel 0.15 mg
Yasmin Ocella Syeda	EE 30 mcg	Drospirenone 3 mg
Kelnor 1/35 Zovia 1/35	EE 35 mcg	Ethynodiol diacetate 1 mg
Ortho-Cyclen Mononessa Previfem Sprintec	EE 35 mcg	Norgestimate 0.25 mg
Necon 1/50 Norinyl 1+50	Mestranol 50 mcg	Norethindrone 1 mg
Balziva Femcon Fe Gildagia Zenchent	EE 35 mcg	Norethindrone 0.4 mg
Brevicon-28 Modicon Necon 0.5/35 Nortrel 0.5/35	EE 35 mcg	Norethindrone 0.5 mg (total of 10.5 mg/cycle)
Necon 1/35–28 Norinyl 1+35 Nortrel 1/35 Ortho-Novum 1/35–28	EE 35 mcg	Norethindrone 1 mg (total of 21 mg/cycle)

High-Dose Monophasic Pills

Name	EE	Progestin
Zovia 1/50–28	EE 50 mcg	Ethynodiol diacetate 1 mg
Ogestrel 0.5/50–28	EE 50 mcg	Norgestrel 0.5 mg

Biphasic Pills

Name	EE	Progestin
Azurette / Kariva / Mircette	EE 20 mcg × 21 days, placebo × 2 days, 10 mcg × 5 days	Desogestrel 0.15 mg × 21 days
Necon 10/11	EE 35 mcg	Norethindrone 0.5 mg × 10 days, 1 mg × 11 days

Triphasic Pills

Name	EE	Progestin
Tilia / Tri-Legest Fe	EE 20 mcg × 5 days, 30 mcg × 7 days, 35 mcg × 9 days	Norethindrone 1 mg × 21 days
Ortho Tri-Cyclen Lo	EE 25 mcg × 21 days	Norgestimate 0.18 mg × 7 days, 0.215 mg × 7 days, 0.25 mg × 7 days
Caziant / Cyclessa / Velivet	EE 25 mcg × 21 days	Desogestrel 0.1 mg × 7 days, 0.125 mg × 7 days, 0.15 mg × 7 days
Enpresse / Trivora	EE 30 mcg × 6 days, 40 mcg × 5 days, 30 mcg × 10 days	Levonorgestrel 0.05 mg × 6 days, 0.075 mg × 5 days, 0.125 mg × 10 days
Ortho Tri-Cyclen / Trinessa / Tri-Previfem / Tri-Sprintec	EE 35 mcg × 21 days	Norgestimate 0.18 mg × 7 days, 0.215 mg × 7 days, 0.25 mg × 7 days
Aranelle / Leena / Tri-Norinyl	EE 35 mcg × 21 days	Norethindrone 0.5 mg × 7 days, 1 mg × 9 days, 0.5 mg × 5 days
Ortho-Novum 7/7/7 / Nortrel 7/7/7 / Necon 7/7/7	EE 35 mcg × 21 days	Norethindrone 0.5 mg × 7 days, 0.75 mg × 7 days, 1 mg × 7 days

Continued

CONTRACEPTIVES—cont'd

Name	Estrogen Content	Progestin Content
Four Phasic		
Natazia	Estradiol 3 mg × 2 days, then 2 mg × 22 days, then 1 mg × 2 days, then 2-day pill-free interval	Dienogest none × 2 days, then 2 mg × 5 days, then 3 mg × 17 days, then none for 4 days
Extended-Cycle Pills		
Loestrin FE	EE 20 mcg × 24 days	Norethindrone 1 mg × 24 days
Jolessa	EE 30 mcg × 84 days	Levonorgestrel 0.15 mg × 84 days
Quartette Quasense	EE 20 mcg × 42 days, 25 mcg × 21 days, 30 mcg × 21 days, then 10 mcg × 7 days	Levonorgestrel 0.15 mg × 84 days
Seasonique	EE 30 mcg × 84 days, 10 mcg × 7 days	Levonorgestrel 0.15 mg × 84 days
Yaz Gianvi	EE 20 mcg × 24 days	Drospirenone 3 mg × 24 days
Continuous Cycle Pill		
Amethyst	EE 20 mcg	Levonorgestrel 90 mcg
Progestin-Only Pills		
Camilla Errin Jolivette Nor-QD Nora-BE	N/A	Norethindrone 0.35 mg
Emergency Contraception		
Plan B Next Choice	N/A	Levonorgestrel 0.75-mg tablets taken 12 hrs apart
Ella	N/A	Ulipristal 30 mg one time within 5 days after unprotected intercourse

Hormonal Alternative to Oral Contraception

Depo-Provera CI Medroxyprogesterone Acetate	None
	Medroxyprogesterone 150 mg
Depo-SubQ Provera 104	None
	Medroxyprogesterone 104 mg
Implanon	None
	Etonogestrel (release rate varies overtime)
Kyleena	None
	19.5 mg for 5 yrs
Liletta	None
	52 mg for 3 yrs
Mirena	None
	Levonorgestrel 20 mcg/day for 5 yrs
NuvaRing	Ethinyl estradiol 15 mcg/day
	Etonogestrel 0.12 mg/day
Ortho Evra	Ethinyl estradiol 20 mcg/day
	Norelgestromin 200 mcg/day
Skyla	None
	13.5 mg for 3 yrs

Corticosteroids

USES

Replacement therapy in adrenal insufficiency, including Addison's disease. Symptomatic treatment of multiorgan disease/conditions. Rheumatoid arthritis (RA), osteoarthritis, severe psoriasis, ulcerative colitis, lupus erythematosus, anaphylactic shock, acute exacerbation of asthma, status asthmaticus, organ transplant.

ACTION

Suppress migration of polymorphonuclear leukocytes (PML) and reverse increased capillary permeability by their anti-inflammatory effect. Suppress immune system by decreasing activity of lymphatic system.

CORTICOSTEROIDS

Name	Availability	Route of Administration	Side Effects
Beclomethasone (Beconase, Qnasl, QVAR)	**Aerosol (oral inhalation), QVAR:** 40 mcg/inhalation, 80 mcg/inhalation **Aerosol (spray, intranasal), Qnasl:** 80 mcg/inhalation, **Beconase:** 42 mcg/inhalation **Suspension (intranasal), Beconase:** 42 mcg/inhalation	Inhalation, intranasal	**I:** Cough, dry mouth/throat, headaches, throat irritation, increased blood glucose **Nasal:** Headaches, sore throat, intranasal ulceration, increased blood glucose
Betamethasone (Celestone)	**I:** 6 mg/ml	IV, intralesional, intra-articular	Nausea, vomiting, increased appetite, weight gain, insomnia, increased blood glucose
Budesonide (Pulmicort, Rhinocort)	**Nasal:** 32 mcg/spray **Suspension for nebulization:** 250 mcg, 500 mcg	Intranasal	Headaches, sore throat, intranasal ulceration, increased blood glucose
Cortisone (Cortone)	**T:** 5 mg, 10 mg, 25 mg	PO	Insomnia, nervousness, increased appetite, indigestion, increased blood glucose
Dexamethasone (Decadron)	**T:** 0.5 mg, 1 mg, 4 mg, 6 mg **OS:** 0.5 mg/5 ml **I:** 4 mg/ml, 10 mg/ml	PO, parenteral	Insomnia, weight gain, increased appetite, increased blood glucose
Fludrocortisone (Florinef)	**T:** 0.1 mg	PO	Edema, headache, peptic ulcer, increased blood glucose
Flunisolide (Nasalide)	**Nasal:** 25 mcg/spray	Inhalation, intranasal	Headache, nasal congestion, pharyngitis, upper respiratory infections, altered taste/ smell, increased blood glucose
Fluticasone (Flonase, Flovent)	**Inhalation:** 44 mcg, 110 mcg, 220 mcg **Nasal:** 50 mcg, 100 mcg	Inhalation, intranasal	Headache, burning/stinging, nasal congestion, upper respiratory infections, increased blood glucose
Hydrocortisone (Solu-Cortef)	**T:** 5 mg, 10 mg, 25 mg **I:** 100 mg, 250 mg, 500 mg, 1 g	PO, parenteral	Insomnia, headache, nausea, vomiting, increased blood glucose
Methylprednisolone (Solu-Medrol)	**T:** 4 mg **I:** 40 mg, 125 mg, 500 mg, 1 g, 2 g	PO, parenteral	Headache, insomnia, nervousness, increased appetite, nausea, vomiting, increased blood glucose

Prednisolone (Prelone)	**T:** 5 mg **OS:** 5 mg/5 ml, 15 mg/5 ml	PO	Headache, insomnia, weight gain, nausea, vomiting, increased blood glucose
Prednisone	**T:** 1 mg, 2.5 mg, 5 mg, 10 mg, 20 mg, 50 mg	PO	Headache, insomnia, weight gain, nausea, vomiting, increased blood glucose
Triamcinolone (Kenalog, Nasacort AQ)	**Injection, suspension:** 10 mg/ml, 40 mg/ml **Intranasal, suspension:** 55 mcg/inhalation	IM, inhalation (nasal)	**PO:** Insomnia, increased appetite, nausea, vomiting, increased blood glucose **I:** Cough, dry mouth/throat, headaches, throat irritation, increased blood glucose

I, Injection; *OS,* oral suspension; *T,* tablets.

Corticosteroids: Topical

USES

Provide relief of inflammation/pruritus associated with corticosteroid-responsive disorders (e.g., contact dermatitis, eczema, insect bite reactions, first- and second- degree localized burns/sunburn).

ACTION

Diffuse across cell membranes, form complexes with cytoplasm. Complexes stimulate protein synthesis of inhibitory enzymes responsible for anti-inflammatory effects (e.g., inhibit edema, erythema, pruritus, capillary dilation, phagocytic activity).

Topical corticosteroids can be classified based on potency:

May use for facial and intertriginous application for only limited time.

High potency: For more severe inflammatory conditions (e.g., lichen simplex chronicus, psoriasis). May use for facial and intertriginous application for short time only. Used in areas of thickened skin due to chronic conditions.

Low potency: Modest anti-inflammatory effect, safest for chronic application, facial and intertriginous application, with occlusion, for infants/young children.

Medium potency: For moderate inflammatory conditions (e.g., chronic eczematous dermatoses).

Very high potency: Alternative to systemic therapy for local effect (e.g., chronic lesions caused by psoriasis). Increased risk of skin atrophy. Used for short periods on small areas. Avoid occlusive dressings.

CORTICOSTEROIDS: TOPICAL

Name	Availability	Potency	Side Effects
Alclometasone (Aclovate)	**C**, **O**: 0.05%	Low	Skin atrophy, contact dermatitis, stretch marks on skin, enlarged blood vessels in the skin, hair loss, pigment changes, secondary infections
Amcinonide (Cyclocort)	**C**, **O**, **L**: 0.1%	High	Same as alclometasone
Betamethasone dipropionate	**C**, **O**, **G**, **L**: 0.05%	High	Same as alclometasone
Betamethasone valerate	**C**: 0.01%, 0.05%, 0.1% **O**: 0.1% **L**: 0.1%	High	Same as alclometasone
Clobetasol (Temovate)	**C**, **O**: 0.05%	High	Same as alclometasone
Desonide (Tridesilon)	**C**, **O**, **L**: 0.05%	Low	Same as alclometasone
Desoximetasone (Topicort)	**C**: 0.25%, 0.5% **O**: 0.25% **G**: 0.05%	High	Same as alclometasone
Fluocinolone (Synalar)	**C**: 0.01%, 0.025%, 0.2% **O**: 0.025%	High	Same as alclometasone
Fluocinonide (Lidex)	**C**, **O**, **G**: 0.05%	High	Same as alclometasone
Flurandrenolide (Cordran)	**C**, **O**, **L**: 0.025%, 0.05%	Medium	Same as alclometasone
Fluticasone (Cutivate)	**C**: 0.05% **O**: 0.005%	Medium	Same as alclometasone
Halobetasol (Ultravate)	**C**, **O**: 0.05%	High	Same as alclometasone
Hydrocortisone (Hytone)	**C**, **O**: 0.5%, 1%, 2.5%	Medium	Same as alclometasone
Mometasone (Elocon)	**C**, **O**, **L**: 0.1%	Medium	Same as alclometasone
Prednicarbate (Dermatop)	**C**: 0.1%	Medium	Same as alclometasone
Triamcinolone (Aristocort, Kenalog)	**C**, **O**, **L**: 0.025%, 0.1%, 0.5%	Medium	Same as alclometasone

C, Cream; *G*, gel; *L*, lotion; *O*, ointment.

Diuretics

USES	ACTION
Thiazides: Management of edema resulting from a number of causes (e.g., HF, hepatic cirrhosis); hypertension either alone or in combination with other antihypertensives.	Increase the excretion of water/sodium and other electrolytes via the kidneys. Exact mechanism of antihypertensive effect unknown; may be due to reduced plasma volume or decreased peripheral vascular resistance. Subclassifications of diuretics are based on their mechanism and site of action.
Loop: Management of edema associated with HF, cirrhosis of the liver, and renal disease. Furosemide used in treatment of hypertension alone or in combination with other antihypertensives.	*Thiazides:* Act at cortical diluting segment of nephron, block reabsorption of Na, Cl, and water; promote excretion of Na, Cl, K, and water. *Loop:* Act primarily at the thick ascending limb of Henle's loop to inhibit Na, Cl, and water absorption.
Potassium-sparing: Adjunctive treatment with thiazides, loop diuretics in treatment of HF and hypertension.	*Potassium-sparing:* Spironolactone blocks aldosterone action on distal nephron (causes K retention, Na excretion). Triamterene, amiloride act on distal nephron, decreasing Na reuptake, reducing K secretion.

DIURETICS

Name	Availability	Dosage Range	Side Effects
Thiazide, Thiazide-related			
Chlorothiazide (Diuril)	**T:** 250 mg, 500 mg **S:** 250 mg/5 ml **I:** 500 mg	**Edema:** 500–1,000 mg 1–2 times/day **HTN:** 500–2,000 mg/day in 1–2 divided doses	**CLASS** Hyperuricemia, hypokalemia, hypomagnesemia, hyperglycemia, hyponatremia, hypercalcemia, hypercholesterolemia, hypertriglyceridemia, pancreatitis, rash, photosensitivity
Chlorthalidone	**Hygroton:** 25 mg, 50 mg, 100 mg	**Edema:** Initially, 50–100 mg once daily or 100 mg every other day. **Maximum:** 200 mg/day	
Hydrochlorothiazide	**T:** 12.5 mg, 25 mg, 50 mg **C:** 12.5 mg	**Edema:** 25–100 mg/day in 1–2 divided doses **HTN:** Initially, 12.5–25 mg once daily. May increase up to 50 mg/day in 1 or 2 divided doses	
Indapamide (Lozol)	**T:** 1.25 mg, 2.5 mg	**Edema:** Initially, 2.5 mg/day. May increase after 1 wk to 5 mg/day **HTN:** Initially, 2.5 mg/day. May increase q4wks to 2.5 mg, then to 5 mg/day	
Metolazone (Zaroxolyn)	**T:** 2.5 mg, 5 mg, 10 mg	**Edema:** 2.5–20 mg once daily **HTN:** 2.5–5 mg once daily	
Loop			
Bumetanide (Bumex)	**T:** 0.5 mg, 1 mg, 2 mg **I:** 0.25 mg/ml	**Edema:** Initially, 0.5–2 mg/dose 1–2 times/day. **Maximum:** 10 mg/day	**CLASS** Dehydration, hypokalemia, hyponatremia, hypomagnesemia, hyperglycemia, metabolic alkalosis, hyperuricemia, blood dyscrasias, rash, hypercholesterolemia, hypertriglyceredemia
Furosemide (Lasix)	**T:** 20 mg, 40 mg, 80 mg **OS:** 10 mg/ml, 40 mg/5 ml **I:** 10 mg/ml	**HTN:** 20–80 mg/day in 2 divided doses **Edema: PO:** 20–80 mg/dose. May increase by 20–40 mg/dose up to 600 mg/day. **IV:** 20–40 mg/dose. May increase by 20 mg/dose. **Maximum:** 200 mg/dose	
Torsemide (Demadex)	**T:** 5 mg, 10 mg, 20 mg, 100 mg **I:** 10 mg/ml	**Edema:** 10–200 mg/day **HTN:** Initially, 5 mg/day. May increase after 4–6 wks to 10 mg/day	

Potassium-sparing

Amiloride (Midamor)	**T:** 5 mg	**HF/Edema:** Initially, 5 mg/day. May increase to 10 mg/day	Hyperkalemia, nausea, abdominal pain, diarrhea, rash, headache
Eplerenone (Inspra)	**T:** 25 mg, 50 mg	**HF:** Initially, 25 mg/day, titrate to 50 mg once daily. **HTN:** Initially, 50 mg/day. May increase to 50 mg 2 times/day	Hyperkalemia, hyponatremia
Spironolactone (Aldactone)	**T:** 25 mg, 50 mg, 100 mg	**Edema:** 25–200 mg/day in 1 or 2 divided doses. **HTN:** 50–100 mg/day in 1 or2 divided doses. **Hypokalemia:** 25–100 mg/day. **HF:** Initially, 12.5–25 mg once daily. **Maximum:** 50 mg/day	Hyperkalemia, nausea, vomiting, abdominal cramps, diarrhea, hyponatremia, gynecomastia, menstrual abnormalities, rash
Triamterene (Dyrenium)	**C:** 50 mg, 100 mg	**Edema, HTN:** 100–300 mg/day in 1–2 divided doses	Hyperkalemia, nausea, abdominal pain, nephrolithiasis

C, Capsules; *HF,* heart failure; *HTN,* hypertension; *I,* Injection; *OS,* oral solution; *S,* suspension; *T,* tablets.

H₂ Antagonists

USES

Short-term treatment of duodenal ulcer (DU), active benign gastric ulcer (GU), maintenance therapy of DU, pathologic hypersecretory conditions (e.g., Zollinger-Ellison syndrome), gastroesophageal reflux disease (GERD), and prevention of upper GI bleeding in critically ill pts.

ACTION

Inhibit gastric acid secretion by interfering with histamine at the histamine H₂ receptors in parietal cells. Also inhibit acid secretion caused by gastrin. Inhibition occurs with basal (fasting), nocturnal, food-stimulated, or fundic distention secretion. H₂ antagonists decrease both the volume and H₂ concentration of gastric juices.

H₂ ANTAGONISTS

Name	Availability	Dosage Range	Side Effects
Cimetidine (Tagamet)	T: 200 mg, 300 mg, 400 mg, 800 mg L: 300 mg/5 ml	**Treatment of DU:** 800 mg at bedtime, 400 mg 2 times/day or 300 mg 4 times/day **Maintenance of DU:** 400 mg at bedtime **Treatment of GU:** 800 mg at bedtime or 300 mg 4 times/day **GERD:** 400 mg 4 times/day or 800 mg 2 times/day **Hypersecretory:** 300 mg 4 times/day. **Maximum:** 2,400 mg/day	Headaches, fatigue, dizziness, confusion, diarrhea, gynecomastia
Famotidine (Pepcid)	T: 10 mg, 20 mg, 40 mg OS: 40 mg/5 ml I: 10 mg/ml	**Treatment of DU:** 40 mg/day in 1 or 2 divided doses **Maintenance of DU:** 20 mg/day **Treatment of GU:** 40 mg/day at bedtime **GERD:** 20 mg 2 times/day for 6 wks **Hypersecretory:** Initially, 20 mg q6h. May increase up to 160 mg q6h	Headaches, dizziness, diarrhea, constipation, abdominal pain, tinnitus

Name	Forms	Indications/Dosage	Side Effects
Nizatidine (Axid)	**OS:** 15 mg/ml **C:** 75 mg, 150 mg, 300 mg	**Treatment of GU:** 300 mg at hs or 150 mg 2 times/day **GERD:** 150 mg 2 times/day **Treatment of DU:** 300 mg at hs or 150 mg 2 times/day **Maintenance of DU:** 150 mg/day at bedtime	Fatigue, urticaria, abdominal pain, constipation, nausea
Ranitidine (Zantac)	**T:** 75 mg, 150 mg, 300 mg **C:** 150 mg, 300 mg **Syrup:** 15 mg/ml **I:** 25 mg/ml	**Treatment of DU:** 300 mg at hs or 150 mg 2 times/day **Maintenance of DU:** 150 mg/day at bedtime **Treatment of GU:** 150 mg 2 times/day **GERD:** 150 mg 2 times/day **Hypersecretory:** 150 mg 2 times/day. **Maximum:** 6 g/day **Erosive Esophagitis:** Treatment: 150 mg 4 times/day. Maintenance: 150 mg 2 times/day	Blurred vision, constipation, nausea, abdominal pain

C, Capsules; *DT,* disintegrating tablets; *DU,* duodenal ulcer; *GERD,* gastroesophageal reflux disease; *GU,* gastric ulcer; *I,* Injection; *L,* liquid; *OS,* oral suspension; *T,* tablets.

Hepatitis C Virus

Hepatitis C virus (HCV) is the leading blood borne infection in the US. HCV is transmitted by exposure to infected blood products. Risk factors for acquiring HCV include injection drug use, receiving contaminated blood products, needle sticks, and vertical transmission. If untreated, HCV may progress to chronic HCV and long-term sequelae including cirrhosis and hepatocellular carcinoma. There are seven known genotypes of HCV (genotypes 1–7) which impact the selection of initial therapy and treatment response. Genotype 1 is the most common and is further subtyped into genotypes 1a and 1b.

Currently, there are two indirect-acting antivirals and seven direct-acting antivirals approved for the treatment of chronic HCV

ACTION

Indirect Acting Antivirals (IAA)

Alpha Interferons (peg-interferons): Induces immune response against HCV, inhibiting viral replication

Ribavirin: Exact mechanism unknown but has activity against several RNA and DNA viruses

Direct Acting Antivirals (DAA)

NS3/4A Protease Inhibitors (PIs): Targets the serine protease NS3/NS4 that is responsible for processing HCV polyprotein and producing new viruses.

Nonstructural Protein 5A (NS5A) Inhibitors: Suppress the NS5A protein, that is essential for viral assembly and replication.

Nonstructural Protein 5B (NS5B) Inhibitors: Suppress the NS5B RNA-dependent RNA polymerase that is responsible for HCV replication.

ANTI-HEPATITIS C VIRUS PREPARATIONS

Name	Type	Genotype	Dosage	Side Effects
Elbasvir, grazoprevir (Zepatier)	DAA NS5A/NS3/4A protease inhibitor	1, 4	**Genotype 1a:** One tablet daily for 12 wks (16 wks with baseline NS5A polymorphins) **Genotype 1b:** One tablet daily for 12 wks **Genotype 4:** One tablet daily for 12 wks (16 wks peginterferon/ribavirin experienced)	Fatigue, headache, nausea
Glecaprivir, pibrentasvir (Mavyret)	DAA NS5A/NS3/4A protease inhibitor	1, 2, 3, 4, 5, 6	**Genotypes 1, 2, 3, 4, 5, 6:** Three tablets once daily. Treatment duration 8-16 wks based on patients that are mono-infected, and coinfected with compensated liver disease (with or without cirrhosis) and with or without renal impairment	Headache, fatigue
Simeprevir (Olysio)	DAA (NS3/4A-PI)	1, 4	150 mg once daily plus peginterferon and ribavirin for 12 wks, then additional 12–36 wks of peginterferon and ribavirin 150 mg once daily plus sofosbuvir for 12 wks without cirrhosis or 24 wks with cirrhosis	(With peginterferon, ribavirin): rash, itching, nausea, photosensitivity (With sofosbuvir): fatigue, headache, nausea, insomnia, pruritus, rash, dizziness, diarrhea
Sofosbuvir (Sovaldi)	DAA (NS5B)	1, 2, 3, 4	**Genotypes 1, 4:** 400 mg once daily plus peginterferon and ribavirin for 12 wks 400 mg once daily plus simeprevir for 12 wks without cirrhosis or 24 wks with cirrhosis **Genotypes 2, 3:** 400 mg once daily plus ribavirin for 12 wks for genotype 2 or 24 wks for genotype 3	(With peginterferon, ribavirin): Fatigue, headache, nausea, insomnia, anemia (With simeprevir): fatigue, headache, nausea, insomnia, pruritus, rash, dizziness, diarrhea
Ledipasvir, Sofosbuvir (Harvoni)	DAA (NS5A/NS5B)	1, 4, 5, 6	**Genotype 1:** One tablet (90 mg/400 mg) for 12 wks in treatment-naïve pt with or without cirrhosis and treatment-experienced pt without cirrhosis; for 24 wks for treatment-experienced pts with cirrhosis **Genotypes 4, 5, 6:** One tablet daily for 12 wks	Fatigue, headache, nausea, diarrhea, insomnia; elevations in bilirubin, lipase, and creatinine kinase

Continued

ANTI-HEPATITIS C VIRUS PREPARATIONS—cont'd

Name	Type	Genotype	Dosage	Side Effects
Ombitasvir, Paritaprevir, Ritonavir, Dasabuvir (Viekira Pak)	DAA (NS5A/protease inhibitor/CYP3A inhibitor/polymerase inhibitor)	1	Two ombitasvir, paritaprevir, ritonavir tablets (12.5 mg, 75 mg, 50 mg) once daily in the morning plus one dasabuvir 250 mg tablet 2 times/day Patients with **genotype 1a or 1b with cirrhosis** will also receive ribavirin for 12 wks (genotype 1 a with cirrhosis: 12–24 wks based on treatment history; liver transplant pts: 24 wks)	(With ribavirin): fatigue, nausea, itching, insomnia (Without ribavirin): nausea, itching, insomnia
Peginterferon alfa 2a (Pegasys)	IAA (Interferon)	1, 2, 3, 4	180 mcg SQ wkly for 12–48 wks based on antiviral regimen, pt history, response	(With ribavirin): fatigue, weakness, fever, myalgia, headache
Peginterferon alfa 2b (PegIntron)	IAA (Interferon)	1, 2, 3, 4	1.5 mcg/kg SQ wkly for 12–48 wks based on antiviral regimen, pt history, response	(With ribavirin): injection site reaction, fatigue, weakness, headache, rigors, fever, nausea, myalgia, insomnia, mood instability, hair loss
Ribavirin (Copegus, Ribasphere)	IAA (Nucleoside analogue)	1, 2, 3, 4	**Genotypes 2, 3** 400 mg 2 times/day (with peginterferon) **Genotypes 1, 4** < 75 kg: 400 mg qam and 600 mg qpm 75kg or greater: 600 mg 2 times/day	(With peginterferon): fatigue, weakness, headache, rigors, fever, nausea, myalgia, insomnia, mood instability, hair loss
Daclatasvir (Daklinza)	DAA (NS5A)	3	60 mg once daily with sofosbuvir for 12 wks	Headache, fatigue
Ombitasvir, paritaprevir, ritonavir (Technivie)	DAA (NS5A/protease Inhibitor/CYP3A inhibitor)	4	Two tablets once daily with ribavirin for 12 wks	Asthenia, fatigue, nausea, insomnia
Sofosbuvir/velpatasvir (Epclusa)	DAA (NS5B/NS5A)	1, 2, 3, 4, 5, 6	One tablet daily for 12 wks	Insomnia, anemia, headache, fatigue, nausea, diarrhea
Sofosbuvir/velpatasvir/voxilaprevir (VOSEVI)	DAA (NS5B/ NS5A/protease inhibitor)	1, 2, 3, 4, 5, 6	One tablet daily for 12 wks	Headache, fatigue, diarrhea, nausea

Hormones

USES

Functions of the body are regulated by two major control systems: the nervous system and the endocrine (hormone) system. Together they maintain homeostasis and control different metabolic functions in the body.

Hormones are concerned with control of different metabolic functions in the body (e.g., rates of chemical reactions in cells, transporting substances through cell membranes, cellular metabolism [growth/secretions]). By definition, a hormone is a chemical substance secreted into body fluids by cells and has control over other cells in the body.

Hormones can be local or general:

- Local hormones have specific local effects (e.g., acetylcholine, which is secreted at parasympathetic and skeletal nerve endings).

- *General hormones* are mostly secreted by specific endocrine glands (e.g., epinephrine/norepinephrine are secreted by the adrenal medulla in response to sympathetic stimulation), transported in the blood to all parts of the body, causing many different reactions.

Some general hormones affect all or almost all cells of the body (e.g., thyroid hormone from the thyroid gland increases the rate of most chemical reactions in almost all cells of the body); other general hormones affect only specific tissue (e.g., ovarian hormones are specific to female sex organs and secondary sexual characteristics of the female).

ACTION

Endocrine hormones almost never directly act intracellularly affecting chemical reactions. They first combine with hormone receptors either on the cell surface or inside the cell (cell cytoplasm or nucleus). The combination of hormone and receptors alters the function of the receptor, and the receptor is the direct cause of the hormone effects. Altered receptor function may include the following:

Altered cell permeability, which causes a change in protein structure of the receptor, usually opening or closing a channel for one or more ions. The movement of these ions causes the effect of the hormone.

Activation of intracellular enzymes immediately inside the cell (e.g., hormone combines with receptor that then becomes the activated enzyme adenyl cyclase, which causes formation of cAMP).

◀**ALERT▶** cAMP has effects inside the cell. It is not the hormone but cAMP that causes these effects.

Regulation of hormone secretion is controlled by an internal control system, the negative feedback system:

- Endocrine gland oversecretes.
- Hormone exerts more and more of its effect.

Continued

Hormones—cont'd

ACTION—cont'd

- Target organ performs its function.
- Too much function in turn feeds back to endocrine gland to decrease secretory rate.

The endocrine system contains many glands and hormones. A summary of the important glands and their hormones secreted are as follows:

The pituitary gland (hypophysis) is a small gland found in the sella turcica at the base of the brain. The pituitary is divided into two portions physiologically: the anterior pituitary (adenohypophysis) and the posterior pituitary (neurohypophysis). Six important hormones are secreted from the anterior pituitary and two from the posterior pituitary.

Anterior pituitary hormones:
- Growth hormone (GH)
- Adrenocorticotropin (corticotropin)
- Thyroid-stimulating hormone (thyrotropin) (TSH)
- Follicle-stimulating hormone (FSH)
- Luteinizing hormone (LH)
- Prolactin

Posterior pituitary hormones:
- Antidiuretic hormone (vasopressin)
- Oxytocin

Almost all secretions of the pituitary hormones are controlled by hormonal or nervous signals from the hypothalamus. The hypothalamus is a center of information concerned with the well-being of the body, which in turn is used to control secretions of the important pituitary hormones just listed. Secretions from the posterior pituitary are controlled by nerve signals originating in the hypothalamus; anterior pituitary hormones are controlled by hormones secreted within the hypothalamus. These hormones are as follows:

- Thyrotropin-releasing hormone (TRH) releasing thyroid-stimulating hormone
- Corticotropin-releasing hormone (CRH) releasing adrenocorticotropin
- Growth hormone-releasing hormone (GHRH) releasing growth hormone and growth hormone inhibitory hormone (GHIH) (same as somatostatin)
- Gonadotropin-releasing hormone (GnRH) releasing the two gonadotropic hormones LH and FSH
- Prolactin inhibitory factor (PIF) causing inhibition of prolactin and prolactin-releasing factor

ANTERIOR PITUITARY HORMONES

All anterior pituitary hormones (except growth hormone) have as their principal effect stimulating target glands.

GROWTH HORMONE (GH)

Growth hormone affects almost all tissues of the body. GH (somatotropin) causes growth in almost all tissues of the body (increases cell size, increases mitosis with increased number of cells, and differentiates certain types of cells). Metabolic effects include increased rate of protein synthesis, mobilization of fatty acids from adipose tissue, decreased rate of glucose utilization.

THYROID-STIMULATING HORMONE (TSH)

Thyroid-stimulating hormone controls secretion of the thyroid hormones. The thyroid gland is located immediately below the larynx on either side of and anterior to the trachea and secretes two significant hormones, thyroxine (T_4) and triiodothyroxine (T_3), which have a profound effect on increasing the metabolic rate of the body. The thyroid gland also secretes calcitonin, an important hormone for calcium metabolism. Calcitonin promotes deposition of calcium in the bones, which decreases calcium concentration in the extracellular fluid.

ADRENOCORTICOTROPIN

Adrenocorticotropin causes the adrenal cortex to secrete adrenocortical hormones. The adrenal glands lie at the superior poles of the two kidneys. Each gland is composed of two distinct parts: the adrenal medulla and the cortex. The adrenal medulla, related to the sympathetic nervous system, secretes the hormones epinephrine and norepinephrine. When stimulated, they cause constriction of blood vessels, increased activity of the heart inhibitory effects on the GI tract, and dilation of the pupils. The adrenal cortex secretes corticosteroids, of which there are two major types: mineralocorticoids and glucocorticoids. Aldosterone, the principal mineralocorticoid, primarily affects electrolytes of the extracellular fluids. Cortisol, the principal glucocorticoid, affects glucose, protein, and fat metabolism.

LUTEINIZING HORMONE (LH)

Luteinizing hormone plays an important role in ovulation and causes secretion of female sex hormones by the ovaries and testosterone by the testes.

FOLLICLE-STIMULATING HORMONE (FSH)

Follicle-stimulating hormone causes growth of follicles in the ovaries before ovulation and promotes formation of sperm in the testes.

Ovarian sex hormones are estrogens and progestins. Estradiol is the most important estrogen; progesterone is the most important progestin.

Estrogens mainly promote proliferation and growth of specific cells in the body and are responsible for development of most of the secondary sex characteristics. Primarily cause cellular proliferation and growth of tissues of sex organs/other tissue related to reproduction. Ovaries, fallopian tubes, uterus, vagina increase in size. Estrogen initiates growth of breast and milk-producing apparatus, external appearance.

Progesterone stimulates secretion of the uterine endometrium during the latter half of the female sexual cycle, preparing the uterus for implantation of the fertilized ovum. Decreases the frequency of uterine contractions (helps prevent expulsion of the implanted ovum). Progesterone promotes development of breasts, causing alveolar cells to proliferate, enlarge, and become secretory in nature.

Testosterone is secreted by the testes and formed by the interstitial cells of Leydig. Testosterone production increases under the stimulus of the anterior pituitary gonadotropic hormones. It is responsible for distinguishing characteristics of the masculine body (stimulates the growth of male sex organs and promotes the development of male secondary sex characteristics,

e.g., distribution of body hair; effect on voice, protein formation, and muscular development).

PROLACTIN

Prolactin promotes the development of breasts and secretion of milk

POSTERIOR PITUITARY HORMONES

ANTIDIURETIC HORMONE (ADH) (VASOPRESSIN)

ADH can cause antidiuresis (decreased excretion of water by the kidneys). In the presence of ADH, the permeability of the renal-collecting ducts and tubules to water increases, which allows water to be absorbed, conserving water in the body. ADH in higher concentrations is a very potent vasoconstrictor, constricting arterioles everywhere in the body, increasing B/P.

OXYTOCIN

Oxytocin contracts the uterus during the birthing process, esp. toward the end of the pregnancy, helping expel the baby. Oxytocin also contracts myoepithelial cells in the breasts, causing milk to be expressed from the alveoli into the ducts so that the baby can obtain it by suckling.

Continued

Hormones—cont'd

ACTION—cont'd

PANCREAS

The pancreas is composed of two tissue types: *acini* (secrete digestive juices in the duodenum) and islets of *Langerhans* (secrete insulin/glucagons directly into the blood). The islets of Langerhans contain three cells: alpha, beta, and delta. Alpha cells secrete glucagon, beta cells secrete insulin, and delta cells secrete somatostatin.

Insulin promotes glucose entry into most cells, thus controlling the rate of metabolism of most carbohydrates. Insulin also affects fat metabolism.

Glucagon effects are opposite those of insulin, the most important of which is increasing blood glucose concentration by releasing it from the liver into the circulating body fluids.

Somatostatin (same chemical as secreted by the hypothalamus) has multiple inhibitory effects: depresses secretion of insulin and glucagon, decreases GI motility decreases secretions/absorption of the GI tract.

Human Immunodeficiency Virus (HIV) Infection

USES	ACTION
Antiretroviral agents are used in the treatment of HIV infection.	*Nucleoside reverse transcriptase inhibitors (NRTIs)* compete with natural substrates for formation of proviral DNA by reverse transcriptase inhibiting viral replication.
	Nucleotide reverse transcriptase inhibitors (NRTIs) inhibit reverse transcriptase by competing with the natural substrate deoxyadenosine triphosphate and by DNA chain termination.
	Non-nucleoside reverse transcriptase inhibitors (NNRTIs) directly bind to reverse transcriptase and block RNA-dependent and DNA-dependent DNA polymerase activities by disrupting the enzyme's catalytic site.
	Protease inhibitors (PIs) bind to the active site of HIV-1 protease and prevent the processing of viral gag and gag-pol polyprotein precursors resulting in immature, noninfectious mal particles.
	Fusion inhibitors interfere with the entry of HIV-1 into cells by inhibiting fusion of viral and cellular membranes. *CCR5 co-receptor antagonist* selectively binds to human chemokine receptor CCR5 present on cell membrane preventing HIV-1 from entering cells.
	Integrase inhibitor inhibits catalytic activity of HIV-1 integrase, an HIV-1 encoded enzyme required for viral replication.

ANTIRETROVIRAL AGENTS FOR TREATMENT OF HIV INFECTION

Name	Availability	Dosage Range	Side Effects
Nucleoside Analogues			
Abacavir (Ziagen)	**T:** 300 mg **OS:** 20 mg/ml	**A:** 300 mg 2 times/day or 600 mg once daily	Nausea, vomiting, malaise, rash, fever, headaches, asthenia, fatigue, hyper-sensitivity reactions
Didanosine (Videx EC)	**DR:** 125 mg, 200 mg, 250 mg, 400 mg **OS:** 2 g/bottle, 4 g/bottle	**DR (weighing 60 kg or more):** 400 mg once daily; **(weighing 25-59 kg):** 250 mg once daily; **(weighing 20-24 kg):** 200 mg once daily **OS (weighing more than 60 kg):** 200 mg q12h or 400 mg once daily; **(weighing less than 60 kg):** 125 mg q12h or 250 mg once daily	Peripheral neuropathy, pancreatitis, diarrhea, nausea, vomiting, headaches, insomnia, rash, hepatitis, seizures
Emtricitabine (Emtriva)	**C:** 200 mg **OS:** 10 mg/ml	**A:** 200 mg/day **(C)** 240 mg/day **(OS)**	Headaches, insomnia, depression, diarrhea, nausea, vomiting, rhinitis, asthenia, rash
Lamivudine (Epivir)	**T:** 100 mg, 150 mg, 300 mg **OS:** 5 mg/ml, 10 mg/ml	**A:** 150 mg 2 times/day or 300 mg once daily **C:** 4 mg/kg 2 times/day	Diarrhea, malaise, fatigue, headaches, nausea, vomiting, abdominal pain, peripheral neuropathy, arthralgia, myalgia, skin rash
Stavudine (Zerit)	**C:** 15 mg, 20 mg, 30 mg, 40 mg **OS:** 1 mg/ml	**A (weighing more than 60 kg):** 40 mg 2 times/day (20 mg 2 times/day if peripheral neuropathy occurs); **(weighing 60 kg or less):** 30 mg 2 times/day (15 mg 2 times/day if peripheral neuropathy occurs)	Peripheral neuropathy, anemia, leukopenia, neutropenia
Zidovudine (Retrovir)	**C:** 100 mg **T:** 300 mg **Syrup:** 50 mg/5 ml, 10 mg/ml	**A:** 300 mg 2 times/day	Anemia, granulocytopenia, myopathy, nausea, malaise, fatigue, insomnia

Continued

ANTIRETROVIRAL AGENTS FOR TREATMENT OF HIV INFECTION—cont'd

Name	Availability	Dosage Range	Side Effects
Nucleotide Analogues			
Tenofovir TAF (Vemlidy)	**T:** 25 mg	**A:** 25 mg once daily	Headache, abdominal pain, fatigue, cough, nausea, back pain
Tenofovir TDF (Viread)	**T:** 300 mg	**A:** 300 mg once daily	Nausea, vomiting, diarrhea, headache, fatigue
Non-nucleoside Analogues			
Delavirdine (Rescriptor)	**T:** 100 mg, 200 mg	**A:** 200 mg 3 times/day for 14 days, then 400 mg 3 times/day	Rash, nausea, headaches, elevated hepatic function tests
Efavirenz (Sustiva)	**C:** 50 mg, 200 mg **T:** 600 mg	**A:** 600 mg/day **C:** 200-600 mg/day based on weight	Headaches, dizziness, insomnia, fatigue, rash, nightmares
Etravirine (Intelence)	**T:** 100 mg, 200 mg	**A:** 200 mg 2 times/day	Skin reactions (e.g., Stevens-Johnson syndrome, erythema multiforme), nausea, abdominal pain, vomiting
Nevirapine (Viramune, Viramune XR)	**T:** 200 mg **T (ER):** 400 mg **S:** 50 mg/ml	**A:** 200 mg/day for 14 days, then (if no rash) 200 mg 2 times/day	Rash, nausea, fatigue, fever, headaches, abnormal hepatic function tests
Rilpivirine (Edurant)	**T:** 25 mg	**A:** 25 mg once daily with a meal	Depression, insomnia, headache, rash
Protease Inhibitors			
Atazanavir (Reyataz)	**C:** 100 mg, 150 mg, 200 mg, 300 mg	**A:** 400 mg/day or 300 mg (with 100 mg ritonavir) once daily	Headaches, diarrhea, abdominal pain, nausea, rash
Darunavir (Prezista)	**T:** 400 mg, 600 mg	**A:** 600 mg 2 times/day (with ritonavir 100 mg) or 800 mg once daily with ritonavir 100 mg	Diarrhea, nausea, vomiting, headaches, skin rash, constipation
Fosamprenavir (Lexiva)	**T:** 700 mg **OS:** 50 mg/ml	**A:** 1,400-2,800 mg/day with 100 mg ritonavir	Headaches, fatigue, rash, nausea, diarrhea, vomiting, abdominal pain

Indinavir (Crixivan)	**C:** 200 mg, 400 mg	**A:** 800 mg q8h or 800 mg 2 times/day with ritonavir 100 mg	Nephrolithiasis, hyperbilirubinemia, abdominal pain, asthenia, fatigue, flank pain, nausea, vomiting, diarrhea, headaches, insomnia, dizziness, altered taste
Lopinavir/ritonavir (Kaletra)	**C:** 133/33 mg **OS:** 80/20 mg	**A:** 400 mg/100 mg 2 times/day or 800 mg/200 mg once daily **C (4-12 yrs):** 10-13 mg/kg 2 times/day	Diarrhea, nausea, vomiting, abdominal pain, headaches, rash
Nelfinavir (Viracept)	**T:** 250 mg **Oral Powder:** 50 mg/g	**A:** 750 mg q8h or 1,250 mg 2times/day **C:** 20-25 mg/kg q8h	Diarrhea, fatigue, asthenia, headaches, hypertension, impaired concentration
Ritonavir (Norvir)	**C:** 100 mg **OS:** 80 mg/ml	**A:** Titrate up to 800 mg/day based on protease inhibitor	Nausea, vomiting, diarrhea, altered taste, fatigue, elevated LFT and triglyceride levels
Saquinavir (Invirase)	**C:** 200 mg **T:** 500 mg	**A:** 1,000 mg 2 times/day with ritonavir 100 mg	Diarrhea, elevated LFTs, hypertriglycerides, cholesterol, abnormal fat accumulation, hyperglycemia
Tipranavir (Aptivus)	**C:** 250 mg **OS:** 100 mg/ml	**A:** 500 mg (with 200 mg ritonavir) 2 times/day	Diarrhea, nausea, fatigue, headaches, vomiting
Fusion Inhibitors			
Enfuvirtide (Fuzeon)	**I:** 108 mg (90 mg when reconstituted)	**Subcutaneous:** 90 mg 2 times/day	Insomnia, depression, peripheral neuropathy, decreased appetite, constipation, asthenia, cough
CCR5 Antagonists			
Maraviroc (Selzentry)	**T:** 150 mg, 300 mg	**A:** 300 mg 2 times/day **CYP3A4 inducers:** 600 mg 2 times/day **CYP3A4 inhibitors:** 150 mg 2 times/day	Cough, pyrexia, upper respiratory tract infections, rash, musculoskeletal symptoms, abdominal pain, dizziness

Continued

ANTIRETROVIRAL AGENTS FOR TREATMENT OF HIV INFECTION—cont'd

Name	Availability	Dosage Range	Side Effects
Integrase Inhibitor			
Raltegravir (Isentress)	**T:** 400 mg	**A:** 400 mg 2 times/day	Nausea, headache, diarrhea, pyrexia
Dolutegravir (Tivicay)	**T:** 50 mg	**A:** 50 mg once daily or 50 mg bid (with CYP3A inducers or resistance)	Insomnia, headache

A, Adults; *C,* capsules; *C* (dosage), children; *DR,* delayed-release; *ER,* extended-release; *I,* Injection; *OS,* oral solution; *S,* suspension; *T,* tablets; *TAF,* tenofovir alafenamide; *TDF,* tenofovir disoproxil fumarate.

FIXED-COMBINATION THERAPIES

Brand Name	Generic Name	Dosage
Atripla	Efavirenz 600 mg Emtricitabine 200 mg Tenofovir (TDF) 300 mg	1 tablet once daily
Combivir	Lamivudine 150 mg Zidovudine 300 mg	1 tablet twice daily
Complera	Emtricitabine 200 mg Rilpivirine 27.5 mg Tenofovir (TDF) 300 mg	1 tablet once daily
Descovy	Emtricitabine 200 mg Tenofovir (TAF) 25 mg	1 tablet once daily
Epzicom	Abacavir 600 mg Lamivudine 300 mg	1 tablet once daily
Evotaz	Atazanavir 300 mg Cobicistat 150 mg	1 tablet once daily

Name	Composition	Dosage
Genvoya	Cobicistat 150 mg Elvitegravir 150 mg Emtricitabine 200 mg Tenofovir (TAF) 10 mg	1 tablet once daily
Odefsey	Emtricitabine 200 mg Rilpivirine 25 mg Tenofovir (TAF) 25 mg	1 tablet once daily
Prezcobix	Cobicistat 150 mg Darunavir 800 mg	1 tablet once daily
Stribild	Cobicistat 150 mg Elvitegravir 150 mg Emtricitabine 200 mg Tenofovir (TDF) 300 mg	1 tablet once daily
Triumeq	Abacavir 600 mg Dolutegravir 50 mg Lamivudine 300 mg	1 tablet once daily
Trizivir	Abacavir 300 mg Lamivudine 150 mg Zidovudine 300 mg	1 tablet twice daily
Truvada	Emtricitabine 200 mg Tenofovir (TDF) 300 mg	1 tablet once daily

TAF, tenofovir alafenamide; *TDF,* tenofovir disoproxil fumarate.

Immunosuppressive Agents

USES

Improvement of both short- and long-term allograft survivals

ACTION

Basiliximab: An interleukin-2 (IL-2) receptor antagonist inhibiting IL-2 binding. This prevents activation of lymphocytes, and the response of the immune system to antigens is impaired.

Cyclosporine: Inhibits production and release of IL-2.

Daclizumab: An IL-2 receptor antagonist inhibiting IL-2 binding.

Mycophenolate: A prodrug that reversibly binds and inhibits inosine monophosphate dehydrogenase (IMPD), resulting in inhibition of purine nucleotide synthesis; inhibiting DNA and RNA synthesis and subsequent synthesis of T and B cells.

Sirolimus: Inhibits IL-2–stimulated T-lymphocyte activation and proliferation, which may occur through formation of a complex.

Tacrolimus: Inhibits IL-2–stimulated T-lymphocyte activation and proliferation, which may occur through formation of a complex.

IMMUNOSUPPRESSIVE AGENTS

Name	Availability	Dosage	Side Effects
Basiliximab (Simulect)	**I:** 10 mg, 20 mg	20 mg for 2 doses (on day of transplant, then 4 days after transplantation)	Abdominal pain, asthenia, cough, dizziness, dyspnea, dysuria, edema, hypertension, infection, tremors
Cyclosporine (Neoral, Sandimmune)	**C:** 25 mg, 50 mg, 100 mg **S:** 100 mg/ml **I:** 50 mg/ml	Dose dependent on type of transplant and formulation	Hypertension, hyperkalemia, nephrotoxicity, coarsening of facial features, hirsutism, gingival hyperplasia, nausea, vomiting, diarrhea, hepatotoxicity, hyperuricemia, hypertriglyceridemia, hypercholesterolemia, tremors, paresthesia, seizures, risk of infection/malignancy
Mycophenolate (CellCept, Myfortic)	**Cellcept:** **C:** 250 mg **I:** 500 mg **S:** 200 mg/ml **T:** 500 mg **Myfortic:** **T(DR):** 180 mg, 320 mg	**Cellcept:** 1–1.5 g 2 times/day based on type of transplant **Myfortic:** **Renal:** 720 mg 2 times/day	Diarrhea, vomiting, leukopenia, neutropenia, infections
Sirolimus (Rapamune)	**S:** 1 mg/ml **T:** 0.5 mg, 1 mg, 2 mg	2–6 mg/day	Dyspnea, leukopenia, thrombocytopenia, hyperlipidemia, abdominal pain, acne, arthralgia, fever, diarrhea, constipation, headaches, vomiting, weight gain
Tacrolimus (Prograf)	**C:** 0.5 mg, 1 mg, 5 mg **I:** 5 mg/ml **C(ER):** 0.5 mg,1 mg, 5 mg **T(ER):** 0.75 mg, 1 mg, 4 mg	**Heart:** 0.075 mg/kg/day in 2 divided doses q12h **Kidney:** 0.1–0.2 mg/kg/day in 2 divided doses q12h **Liver:** 0.1–0.15 mg/kg/day in 2 divided doses q12h	Nephrotoxicity, neurotoxicity, hyperglycemia, nausea, vomiting, photophobia, infections, hypertension, hyperlipidemia

C, Capsules; *DR,* Delayed release; *ER,* extended release; *I,* Injection; *S,* oral solution or suspension; *T,* tablets.

Laxatives

USES

Short-term treatment of constipation; colon evacuation before rectal/bowel examination; prevention of straining (e.g., after anorectal surgery, MI); to reduce painful elimination (e.g., episiotomy, hemorrhoids, anorectal lesions); modification of effluent from ileostomy, colostomy; prevention of fecal impaction; removal of ingested poisons.

ACTION

Laxatives ease or stimulate defecation. Mechanisms by which this is accomplished include (1) attracting, retaining fluid in colonic contents due to hydrophilic or osmotic properties; (2) acting directly or indirectly on mucosa to decrease absorption of water and NaCl; or (3) increasing intestinal motility, decreasing absorption of water and NaCl by virtue of decreased transit time.

Bulk-forming: Act primarily in small/large intestine. Retain water in stool, may bind water, ions in colonic lumen (soften feces, increase bulk); may increase colonic bacteria growth (increases fecal mass). Produce soft stool in 1–3 days.

Osmotic agents: Act in colon. Similar to saline laxatives. Osmotic action may be enhanced in distal ileum/colon by bacterial metabolism to lactate, other organic acids. This decrease in pH increases motility, secretion. Produce soft stool in 1–3 days.

Saline: Acts in small/large intestine, colon (sodium phosphate). Poorly, slowly absorbed; causes hormone cholecystokinin release from duodenum (stimulates fluid secretion, motility); possesses osmotic properties; produces watery stool in 2–6 hrs (small doses produce semifluid stool in 6–12 hrs).

Stimulant: Acts in colon. Enhances accumulation of water/electrolytes in colonic lumen, enhances intestinal motility. May act directly on intestinal mucosa. Produces semifluid stool in 6–12 hrs.

◄ALERT► Bisacodyl suppository acts in 15–60 min.

Stool softener: Acts in small/large intestine. Hydrates and softens stools by its surfactant action, facilitating penetration of fat and water into stool. Produces soft stool in 1–3 days.

LAXATIVES

Name	Onset of Action	Uses	Side Effects/Precautions
Bulk-forming			
Methylcellulose (Citrucel)	12–24 hrs up to 3 days	Treatment of constipation for postpartum women, elderly, pts with diverticulosis, irritable bowel syndrome, hemorrhoids	Gas, bloating, esophageal obstruction, colonic obstruction, calcium and iron malabsorption
Psyllium (Metamucil)	Same as methylcellulose	Treatment of chronic constipation and constipation associated with rectal disorders; management of irritable bowel syndrome	Diarrhea, constipation, abdominal cramps, esophageal/colon obstruction, bronchospasm
Stool Softener			
Docusate (Colace, Surfak)	1–3 days	Treatment of constipation due to hard stools, in painful anorectal conditions, and for those who need to avoid straining during bowel movements	Stomachache, mild nausea, cramping, diarrhea, irritated throat (with liquid and syrup dose forms)
Saline			
Magnesium citrate (Citrate of Magnesia, Citro-Mag)	30 min–3 hrs	Bowel evacuation prior to certain surgical and diagnostic procedures	Hypotension, abdominal cramping, diarrhea, gas formation, electrolyte abnormalities
Magnesium hydroxide	30 min–3 hrs	Short-term treatment of occasional constipation	Electrolyte abnormalities can occur; use caution in pts with renal or cardiac impairment; diarrhea, abdominal cramps, hypotension
Sodium phosphate (Fleet Phospho-Soda)	2–15 min	Relief of occasional constipation; bowel evacuation prior to certain surgical and diagnostic procedures	Electrolyte abnormalities; do not use for pts with HF, severe renal impairment, ascites, GI obstruction, active inflammatory bowel disease

Continued

LAXATIVES—cont'd

Name	Onset of Action	Uses	Side Effects/Precautions
Osmotic			
Lactulose (Kristalose)	24–48 hrs	Short-term relief of constipation	Nausea, vomiting, diarrhea, abdominal cramping, bloating, gas
Polyethylene glycol (MiraLax)	24–48 hrs	Short-term relief of constipation	Bitter taste, diarrhea
Stimulant			
Bisacodyl (Dulcolax)	**PO:** 6–12 hrs **Rectal:** 15–60 min	Short-term relief of constipation	Electrolyte imbalance, abdominal discomfort, gas, potential for overuse/abuse
Senna (Senokot)	6–12 hrs	Short-term relief of constipation	Abdominal discomfort, cramps

GI, Gastrointestinal; *HF,* heart failure.

Multiple Sclerosis

Multiple sclerosis (MS) is the most common autoimmune disorder affecting central nervous system. MS is a demyelinating disease where insulating covers of nerve cells in the brain and spinal cord are damaged which disrupts the ability of parts of the nervous system to communicate. Symptoms may include double vision, blindness in one eye, muscle weakness, trouble with sensation or coordination.

Presently, there is no cure for MS. Treatment attempts to improve function and prevent new attacks.

MEDICATIONS FOR MULTIPLE SCLEROSIS

Name	Dosage	Side Effects
Alemtuzumab (Lemtrada)	12 mg IV once/day x 5 days followed 1 year later by 12 mg IV once/day x 3 days	Rigors, tremors nausea, vomiting, rash, fatigue, hypotension, urticarial, pruritus, skeletal pain, headache, diarrhea, neutropenia, anemia, thrombocytopenia, respiratory toxicity (dyspnea, cough, pneumonitis, infections).
Daclizumab (Zinbryta)	150 mg SQ once/month	Autoimmune disorders (hepatitis, lymphadenopathy, noninfectious colitis), depression, severe hypersensitivity reactions, infections
Dimethyl fumarate (Tecfidera)	240 mg PO bid	Flushing, abdominal pain, diarrhea, nausea, vomiting, dyspepsia, lymphopenia, hepatotoxicity, PML
Fingolimod (Gilenya)	0.5 mg PO once daily	Headache, back pain, cough, infections, hypersensitivity reactions, elevated LFTs, bradycardia, AV block, macular edema, decreased pulmonary function

Continued

MEDICATIONS FOR MULTIPLE SCLEROSIS—cont'd

Name	Dosage	Side Effects
Glatiramer (Copaxone, Glatopa)	**Copaxone:** 20 mg SQ once/day or 40 mg 3 x/wk **Glatopa:** 20 mg SQ once/day	Pain, erythema, inflammation, pruritus at injection site, arthralgia, transient chest pain, post-injection reactions (chest pain, palpitations, dyspnea)
Interferon beta 1a (Avonex, Rebif)	**Avonex:** 30 mcg IM weekly **Rebif:** 44 mcg 3 times/week	Headache, flu-like symptoms, myalgia, depression with suicidal ideation, generalized pain, asthenia, chills, injection site reaction, hypersensitivity reactions, anemia, hepatotoxicity.
Interferon beta 1b (Betaseron, Extavia)	250 mcg SQ every other day	Headache, flu-like symptoms, myalgia, upper respiratory tract infection, depression with suicidal ideation, generalized pain, asthenia, chills, fever, injection site reaction, hypersensitivity reactions, anemia, hepatotoxicity, seizures.
Mitoxantrone	12 mg/m2 iv q3 months	Nausea, vomiting, diarrhea, cough, headache, stomatitis, abdominal discomfort, fever, alopecia, cardiotoxicity, myelosuppression , acute/chronic myeloid leukemia
Natalizumab (Tysabri)	300 mg IV q4 wks	Headache, fatigue, depression, arthralgia, infections, hypersensitivity reactions, hepatotoxicity, progressive multifocal leukoencephalopathy (PML)
Ocrelizumab (Ocrevus)	600 mg IV q6 months	Infusion reactions (Pruritus, rash, urticaria, erythema), respiratory tract infections, skin infections, malignancies, PML
Pegylated interferon beta 1a (Plegridy)	125 mcg SQ q2 weeks	Headache, flu-like symptoms, myalgia, depression with suicidal ideation, generalized pain, asthenia, chills, injection site reaction, hypersensitivity reactions, anemia, hepatotoxicity, elevated LFT, seizures.
Teriflunomide (Aubagio)	7 or 14 mg PO once/day	Headache, diarrhea, nausea, alopecia, paresthesia, abdominal pain, elevated LFTs, neutropenia, leukopenia, hepatic failure, acute renal failure, toxic epidermal necrolysis

Nonsteroidal Anti-Inflammatory Drugs (NSAIDs)

USES

Provide symptomatic relief from *pain/inflammation* in the treatment of musculoskeletal disorders (e.g., rheumatoid arthritis [RA], osteoarthritis, ankylosing spondylitis), *analgesic* for low to moderate pain, *reduction in fever* (many agents not suited for routine/prolonged therapy due to toxicity). By virtue of its action on platelet function, aspirin is used in treatment or prophylaxis of diseases associated with hypercoagulability (reduces risk of stroke/heart attack).

ACTION

Exact mechanism for anti-inflammatory, analgesic, antipyretic effects unknown. Inhibition of enzyme cyclooxygenase, the enzyme responsible for prostaglandin synthesis, appears to be a major mechanism of action. May inhibit other mediators of inflammation (e.g., leukotrienes). Direct action on hypothalamus heat-regulating center may contribute to antipyretic effect.

NSAIDs

Name	Availability	Dosage Range	Side Effects
Aspirin	**Caplet:** 500 mg. **Suppository:** 300 mg, 600 mg **T:** 325 mg **T (EC):** 81 mg, 325 mg **T (chew):** 81 mg	**Analgesic/antipyretic:** 325–650 mg q4–6h prn or 975 mg q6h prn or 500–1000 mg q4–6h prn	GI discomfort, dizziness, headaches, increased risk of bleeding
Celecoxib (Celebrex)	**C:** 50 mg, 100 mg, 200 mg, 400 mg	200 mg q12h (**Maximum:** 600 mg day 1, then 400 mg/day)	Diarrhea, back pain, dizziness, heartburn, headaches, nausea, abdominal pain
Diclofenac (Voltaren, Zipsor, Zorvolex)	**T:** 25 mg, 50 mg, 75 mg **C (Zipsor):** 25 mg **C (Zorvolex):** 18 mg, 35 mg	50 mg tid (**Zipsor):** 25 mg 4 times/day (**Zorvolex):** 18–35 mg 3 times/day	Indigestion, constipation, diarrhea, nausea, headaches, fluid retention, abdominal cramps

Continued

NSAIDs—cont'd

Name	Availability	Dosage Range	Side Effects
Diflunisal (Dolobid)	**T:** 500 mg	**Arthritis:** 0.5–1 g/day in 2 divided doses **Maximum:** 1.5 g/day **P:** 500 mg once, then 250 mg q8–12h	Headaches, abdominal cramps, indigestion, diarrhea, nausea
Etodolac (Lodine)	**T:** 400 mg, 500 mg **T (ER):** 400 mg, 500 mg, 600 mg **C:** 200 mg, 300 mg	**Arthritis:** 400 mg 2 times/day or 300 mg 2–3 times/day or 500 mg 2 times/day. **(ER):** 400 mg up to 1,000 mg once daily **P:** 200–400 mg q6–8h as needed	Indigestion, dizziness, headaches, bloated feeling, diarrhea, nausea, weakness, abdominal cramps
Fenoprofen (Nalfon)	**C:** 200 mg, 400 mg **T:** 600 mg	**Arthritis:** 400–600 mg 3–4 times/day **P:** 200 mg q4–6h as needed	Nausea, indigestion, anxiety, constipation, shortness of breath, heartburn
Ibuprofen (Advil, Caldolor, Motrin)	**I:** 100 mg/ml **T:** 100 mg, 200 mg, 400 mg, 600 mg, 800 mg **T (chewable):** 50 mg, 100 mg **C:** 200 mg **S:** 100 mg/5 ml	**Inflammatory disease:** 400–800 mg/ dose 3–4 times/day **P:** 200–400 mg/dose q4–6h as needed	Dizziness, abdominal cramps, abdominal pain, heartburn, nausea
Indomethacin (Indocin, Tivorbex)	**(Tivorbex):** 20 mg, 40 mg **C:** 25 mg, 50 mg **C (SR):** 75 mg **S:** 25 mg/5 ml	**Arthritis:** 25–50 mg/dose 2–3 times/day **Maximum:** 200 mg/day **P: (Tivorbex only):** 20 mg 3 times/ day or 40 mg 2–3 times/day	Fluid retention, dizziness, headaches, abdominal pain, indigestion, nausea
Ketoprofen (Orudis KT)	**C:** 25 mg, 50 mg **C (ER):** 200 mg	**Arthritis:** 50 mg 4 times/day or 75 mg 3 times/day **ER:** 200 mg once daily **P:** 25–50 mg q6–8h as needed	Headaches, anxiety, abdominal pain, bloated feeling, constipation, diarrhea, nausea
Ketorolac (Toradol)	**T:** 10 mg **I:** 15 mg/ml, 30 mg/ml	**P: (PO):** 10 mg q4–6h as needed; **(IM/IV):** 60–120 mg/day in divided doses	Fluid retention, abdominal pain, diarrhea, dizziness, headaches, nausea
Meloxicam (Mobic, Vivlodex)	**C: (Vivlodex):** 5 mg, 10 mg **T: (Mobic):** 7.5 mg, 15 mg **S:** 7.5 mg/5 ml	**Arthritis: (Mobic):** 7.5–15 mg once daily **(Vivlodex):** 5–10 mg once daily	Heartburn, indigestion, nausea, diarrhea, headaches

Name	Availability	Dosage Range	Side Effects
Nabumetone (Relafen)	**T:** 500 mg, 750 mg	**Arthritis:** 1–2 g/day in 1–2 divided doses	Fluid retention, dizziness, headaches, abdominal pain, constipation, diarrhea, nausea
Naproxen (Anaprox, Naprosyn)	**T:** 250 mg, 375 mg, 500 mg **T (CR):** 375 mg, 500 mg **S:** 125 mg/5 ml	**Arthritis:** 500–1,000 mg/day in 2 divided doses **Maximum:** 1,500 mg/day **P:** 500 mg once, then 500 mg q12h or 250 mg q6–8h as needed	Tinnitus, fluid retention, shortness of breath, dizziness, drowsiness, headaches, abdominal pain, constipation, heartburn, nausea
Oxaprozin (Daypro)	**C:** 600 mg **T:** 600 mg	**Arthritis:** 600–1,200 mg once daily	Constipation, diarrhea, nausea, indigestion
Piroxicam (Feldene)	**C:** 10 mg, 20 mg	**Arthritis:** 10–20 mg/day in 1–2 divided doses	Abdominal pain, stomach pain, nausea
Sulindac (Clinoril)	**T:** 150 mg, 200 mg	**Arthritis:** 150 mg bid	Dizziness, abdominal pain, constipation, diarrhea, nausea

A, Adults; *C,* capsules; *CR,* controlled-release; *ER,* extended-release; *GI,* gastrointestinal; *I,* Injection; *P,* pain; *S,* suspension; *SR,* sustained-release; *T,* tablets.

Nutrition: Enteral

	INDICATIONS	ROUTES OF ENTERAL NUTRITION DELIVERY
Enteral nutrition (EN), also known as *tube feedings*, provides food/nutrients via the GI tract using special formulas, delivery techniques, and equipment. All routes of EN consist of a tube through which liquid formula is infused.	Tube feedings are used in pts with major trauma, burns; those undergoing radiation and/or chemotherapy; pts with hepatic failure, severe renal impairment, physical or neurologic impairment; preop and postop to promote anabolism; prevention of cachexia, malnutrition; dysphagia; pts requiring mechanical ventilation.	**NASOGASTRIC (NG):** **INDICATIONS:** Most common for short-term feeding in pts unable or unwilling to consume adequate nutrition by mouth. Requires at least a partially functioning GI tract. **ADVANTAGES:** Does not require surgical intervention and is fairly easily inserted. Allows full use of digestive tract. Decreases abdominal distention, nausea, vomiting that may be caused by hyperosmolar solutions. **DISADVANTAGES:** Temporary. May be easily pulled out during routine nursing care. Has potential for pulmonary aspiration of gastric contents, risk of reflux esophagitis, regurgitation. **NASODUODENAL (ND), NASOJEJUNAL (NJ):** **INDICATIONS:** Pts unable or unwilling to consume adequate nutrition by mouth. Requires at least a partially functioning GI tract. **ADVANTAGES:** Does not require surgical intervention and is fairly easily inserted. Preferred for pts at risk for aspiration. Valuable for pts with gastroparesis.

	INITIATING ENTERAL NUTRITION
DISADVANTAGES: Temporary. May be pulled out during routine nursing care. May be dislodged by coughing, vomiting. Small lumen size increases risk of clogging when medication is administered via tube, more susceptible to rupturing when using infusion device. Must be radiographed for placement, frequently extubated. **GASTROSTOMY:** **INDICATIONS:** Pts with esophageal obstruction or impaired swallowing; pts in whom NG, ND, or NJ not feasible; when long-term feeding indicated. **ADVANTAGES:** Permanent feeding access. Tubing has larger bore, allowing noncontinuous (bolus) feeding (300–400 ml over 30–60 min q3–6h). May be inserted endoscopically using local anesthetic (procedure called *percutaneous endoscopic gastrostomy* [PEG]).	**DISADVANTAGES:** Requires surgery; may be inserted in conjunction with other surgery or endoscopically (see **ADVANTAGES**). Stoma care required. Tube may be inadvertently dislodged. Risk of aspiration, peritonitis, cellulitis, leakage of gastric contents. **JEJUNOSTOMY:** **INDICATIONS:** Pts with stomach or duodenal obstruction, impaired gastric motility; pts in whom NG, ND, or NJ not feasible; when long-term feeding indicated. **ADVANTAGES:** Allows early postop feeding (small bowel function is least affected by surgery). Risk of aspiration reduced. Rarely pulled out inadvertently. **DISADVANTAGES:** Requires surgery (laparotomy). Stoma care required. Risk of intraperitoneal leakage. Can be dislodged easily.	With continuous feeding, initiation of isotonic (about 300 mOsm/L) or moderately hypertonic feeding (up to 495 mOsm/L) can be given full strength, usually at a slow rate (30–50 ml/hr) and gradually increased (25 ml/ hr q6–24h). Formulas with osmolality greater than 500 mOsm/L are generally started at half strength and gradually increased in rate, then concentration. Tolerance is increased if the rate and concentration are not increased simultaneously.

Continued

Nutrition: Enteral—cont'd

SELECTION OF FORMULAS

Protein: Has many important physiologic roles and is the primary source of nitrogen in the body. Protein provides 4 kcal/g protein. Sources of protein in enteral feedings: sodium caseinate, calcium caseinate, soy protein, dipeptides.

Carbohydrate (CHO): Provides energy for the body and heat to maintain body temperature. Provides 3.4 kcal/g carbohydrate. Sources of CHO in enteral feedings: corn syrup, cornstarch, maltodextrin, lactose, sucrose, glucose.

Fat: Provides concentrated source of energy. Referred to as *kilocalorie dense* or *protein sparing.* Provides 9 kcal/g fat. Sources of fat in enteral feedings: corn oil, safflower oil, medium-chain triglycerides.

Electrolytes, vitamins, trace elements: Contained in formulas (not found in specialized products for renal/hepatic insufficiency).

All products containing protein, fat, carbohydrate, vitamin, electrolytes, trace elements are nutritionally complete and designed to be used by pts for long periods.

COMPLICATIONS

MECHANICAL: Usually associated with some aspect of the feeding tube.

Aspiration pneumonia: Caused by delayed gastric emptying, gastroparesis, gastroesophageal reflux, or decreased gag reflex. May be prevented or treated by reducing infusion rate, using lower-fat formula, feeding beyond pylorus, checking residuals, using small-bore feeding tubes, elevating head of bed 30–45 degrees during and for 30–60 min after intermittent feeding, and regularly checking tube placement.

Esophageal, mucosal, pharyngeal irritation, otitis: Caused by using large-bore NG tube. Prevented by use of small bore whenever possible.

Irritation, leakage at ostomy site: Caused by drainage of digestive juices from site. Prevented by close attention to skin/stoma care.

Tube, lumen obstruction: Caused by thickened formula residue, formation of formula-medication complexes. Prevented by frequently irrigating tube with clear water (also before and after giving formulas/medication), avoiding instilling medication if possible.

GASTROINTESTINAL: Usually associated with formula, rate of delivery, unsanitary handling of solutions or delivery system.

Diarrhea: Caused by low-residue formulas, rapid delivery, use of hyperosmolar formula, hypoalbuminemia, malabsorption, microbial contamination, or rapid GI transit time. Prevented by using fiber supplemented formulas, decreasing rate of delivery, using dilute formula, and gradually increasing strength.

Cramps, gas, abdominal distention: Caused by nutrient malabsorption, rapid delivery of refrigerated formula. Prevented by delivering formula by continuous methods, giving formulas at room temperature, decreasing rate of delivery.

Nausea, vomiting: Caused by rapid delivery of formula, gastric retention. Prevented by reducing rate of delivery, using dilute formulas, selecting low-fat formulas.

Constipation: Caused by inadequate fluid intake, reduced bulk, inactivity. Prevented by supplementing fluid intake, using fiber-supplemented formula, encouraging ambulation.

METABOLIC: Fluid/serum electrolyte status should be monitored. Refer to monitoring section. In addition, the very young and very old are at greater risk of developing complications such as dehydration or overhydration.

MONITORING

Daily: Estimate nutrient intake, fluid intake/output, weight of pt, clinical observations.

Weekly: Serum electrolytes (potassium, sodium, magnesium, calcium, phosphorus), blood glucose, BUN, creatinine, hepatic function tests (e.g., AST, ALT, alkaline phosphatase), 24-hr urea and creatinine excretion, total iron-binding capacity (TIBC) or serum transferrin, triglycerides, cholesterol.

Monthly: Serum albumin.

Other: Urine glucose, acetone (when blood glucose is greater than 250), vital signs (temperature, respirations, pulse, B/P) q8h.

DRUG THERAPY: DOSAGE FOR SELECTION/ ADMINISTRATION:

Drug therapy should not have to be compromised in pts receiving enteral nutrition:

* Temporarily discontinue medications not immediately necessary.
* Consider an alternate route for administering medications (e.g., transdermal, rectal, intravenous).
* Consider alternate medications when current medication is not available in alternate dosage forms.

ENTERAL ADMINISTRATION OF MEDICATIONS:

Medications may be given via feeding tube with several considerations:

* Tube type
* Tube location in the GI tract
* Site of drug action
* Site of drug absorption
* Effects of food on drug absorption
* Use of liquid dosage forms is preferred whenever possible; many tablets may be crushed; contents of many capsules may be emptied and given through large-bore feeding tubes.
* Many oral products should not be crushed (e.g., sustained-release, enteric coated, capsule granules).
* Some medications should not be given with enteral formulas because they form precipitates that may clog the feeding tube and reduce drug absorption.
* Feeding tube should be flushed with water before and after administration of medications to clear any residual medication.

Continued

Nutrition: Parenteral

Parenteral nutrition (PN), also known as *total parenteral nutrition* (TPN) or *hyperalimentation* (HAL), provides required nutrients to pts by IV route of administration. The goal of PN is to maintain or restore nutritional status caused by disease, injury, or inability to consume nutrients by other means.

INDICATIONS

Conditions when pt is unable to use alimentary tract via oral, gastrostomy, or jejunostomy route. Impaired absorption of protein caused by obstruction, inflammation, or antineoplastic therapy. Bowel rest necessary because of GI surgery or ileus, fistulas, or anastomotic leaks. Conditions with increased metabolic requirements (e.g., burns, infection, trauma). Preserve tissue reserves (e.g., acute renal failure). Inadequate nutrition from tube feeding methods.

COMPONENTS OF PN

To meet IV nutritional requirements, six essential categories in PN are needed for tissue synthesis and energy balance.

Protein: In the form of crystalline amino acids (CAA), primarily used for protein synthesis. Several products are designed to meet specific needs for pts with renal failure (e.g., NephrAmine), hepatic disease (e.g., Hepat Amine), stress/trauma (e.g., Aminosyn HBC), use in neonates and pediatrics (e.g., Aminosyn PF; TrophAmine). Calories: 4 kcal/g protein.

Energy: In the form of dextrose, available in concentrations of 5%–70%. Dextrose less than 10% may be given peripherally; concentrations greater than 10% must be given centrally. Calories: 3.4 kcal/g dextrose.

IV fat emulsion: Available in 10% and 20% concentrations. Provides a concentrated source of energy/calories (9 kcal/g fat) and is a source of essential fatty acids. May be administered peripherally or centrally.

Electrolytes: Major electrolytes (calcium, magnesium, potassium, sodium; also acetate, chloride, phosphate). Doses of electrolytes are individualized, based on many factors (e.g., renal/hepatic function, fluid status).

Vitamins: Essential components in maintaining metabolism and cellular function; widely used in PN.

Trace elements: Necessary in long-term PN administration. Trace elements include zinc, copper, chromium, manganese, selenium, molybdenum, iodine.

Miscellaneous: Additives include insulin, albumin, heparin, and H2 blockers (e.g., cimetidine, ranitidine, famotidine). Other medication may be included, but compatibility for admixture should be checked on an individual basis.

ROUTE OF ADMINISTRATION

PN is administered via either peripheral or central vein.

Peripheral: Usually involves 2–3 L/day of 5%–10% dextrose with 3%–5% amino acid solution along with IV fat emulsion. Electrolytes, vitamins, trace elements are added according to pt needs. Peripheral solutions provide about 2,000 kcal/day and 60–90 g protein/day.

ADVANTAGES: Lower risks vs. central mode of administration.

DISADVANTAGES: Peripheral veins may not be suitable (esp. in pts with illness of long duration); more susceptible to phlebitis (due to osmolalities greater than 600 mOsm/L); veins may be viable only 1–2 wks; large volumes of fluid are needed to meet nutritional requirements, which may be contraindicated in many pts.

Central: Usually utilizes hypertonic dextrose (concentration range of 15%–35%) and amino acid

solution of 3%–7% with IV fat emulsion. Electrolytes, vitamins, trace elements are added according to pt needs. Central solutions provide 2,000–4,000 kcal/day. Must be given through large central vein with high blood flow, allowing rapid dilution, avoiding phlebitis/thrombosis (usually through percutaneous insertion of catheter into subclavian vein, then advancement of catheter to superior vena cava).

ADVANTAGES: Allows more alternatives/flexibility in establishing regimens; allows ability to provide full nutritional requirements without need of daily fat emulsion; useful in pts who are fluid restricted (increased concentration), those needing large nutritional requirements (e.g., trauma, malignancy), or those for whom PN indicated more than 7–10 days.

DISADVANTAGES: Risk with insertion, use, maintenance of central line; increased risk of infection, catheter-induced trauma, and metabolic changes.

Continued

Nutrition: Parenteral—cont'd

MONITORING

May vary slightly from institution to institution.

Baseline: CBC, platelet count, prothrombin time (PT), weight, body length/head circumference (in infants), serum electrolytes, glucose, BUN, creatinine, uric acid, total protein, cholesterol, triglycerides, bilirubin, alkaline phosphatase, lactate dehydrogenase (LDH), AST, albumin, prealbumin, other tests as needed.

Daily: Weight, vital signs (temperature, pulse, respirations [TPR]), nutritional intake (kcal, protein, fat), serum electrolytes (potassium, sodium chloride), glucose (serum, urine), acetone, BUN, osmolarity, other tests as needed.

2–3 times/wk: CBC, coagulation studies (PT, partial thromboplastin time [PTT]), serum creatinine, calcium, magnesium, phosphorus, acid-base status, other tests as needed.

Weekly: Nitrogen balance, total protein, albumin, prealbumin, transferrin, hepatic function tests (AST, ALT), serum alkaline phosphatase, LDH, bilirubin, Hgb, uric acid, cholesterol, triglycerides, other tests as needed.

COMPLICATIONS

Mechanical: Malfunction in system for IV delivery (e.g., pump failure; problems with lines, tubing, administration sets, catheter). Pneumothorax, catheter misdirection, arterial puncture, bleeding, hematoma formation may occur with catheter placement.

Infectious: Infections (pts often more susceptible to infections), catheter sepsis (e.g., fever, shaking, chills, glucose intolerance where no other site of infection is identified).

Metabolic: Includes hyperglycemia, elevated serum cholesterol and triglycerides, abnormal serum hepatic function tests.

Fluid, electrolyte, acid-base disturbances: May alter serum potassium, sodium, phosphate, magnesium levels.

Nutritional: Clinical effects seen may be due to lack of adequate vitamins, trace elements, essential fatty acids.

DRUG THERAPY/ADMINISTRATION METHODS: Compatibility of other intravenous medications pts may be administered while receiving parenteral nutrition is an important concern.

Intravenous medications usually are given as a separate admixture via piggyback to the parenteral nutrition line, but in some instances may be added directly to the parenteral nutrition solution. Because of the possibility of incompatibility when adding medication directly to the parenteral nutrition solution, specific criteria should be considered:

- Stability of the medication in the parenteral nutrition solution
- Properties of the medication, including pharmacokinetics that determine if the medication is appropriate for continuous infusion
- Documented chemical and physical compatibility with the parenteral nutrition solution

In addition, when medication is given via piggyback using the parenteral nutrition line, important criteria should include the following:

- Stability of the medication in the parenteral nutrition solution
- Documented chemical and physical compatibility with the parenteral nutrition solution

Obesity Management

USES

Adjunct to diet and physical activity in the treatment of chronic, relapsing obesity.

ACTIONS

Two categories of medications are used for weight control. *Appetite suppressants:* Block neuronal uptake of norepinephrine, serotonin, dopamine, causing a feeling of fullness or satiety. *Digestion inhibitors:* Reversible lipase inhibitors that block the breakdown and absorption of fats, decreasing appetite and reducing calorie intake.

ANOREXIANTS

Name	Availability	Dosage	Side Effects
Diethylpropion (Tenuate, Tenuate Dospan)	T: 25 mg, T (CR): 75 mg	25 mg 3-4 times/day or 75 mg once daily in midmorning	Headaches, euphoria, palpitations, hypertension, pulmonary hypertension, valvular heart disease, seizures, bone marrow depression, dependence, withdrawal psychosis
Liraglutide (Victoza)	I: 18 mg/3 ml	SQ: Initially, 0.6 mg/day. May increase by 0.6 mg/day weekly up to 3 mg/day	Diarrhea, constipation, dyspepsia, fatigue, vomiting, increased heart rate, renal impairment
Lorcaserin (BelViq, Belviq XR)	C: 10 mg, T: 20 mg	(Belviq) 10 mg 2 times/day (Belviq XR): 20 mg once daily	Nausea, headache, dizziness, fatigue, dry mouth, diarrhea, constipation, hypoglycemia, hallucinations, decreased white/red blood cells, euphoria, cognitive impairment
Naltrexone/bupropion (Contrave)	T: 8 mg/90 mg	Titrate weekly up to 2 tablets 2 times/day (1 tablet once daily, then 1 tablet 2 times/day, then 2 tablets in AM and 1 in PM, then 2 tablets 2 times/day)	Suicidal ideation, mood changes, seizures, increased HR with or without B/P, allergic reactions, hepatic toxicity, nausea, vomiting, headache, dizziness, dry mouth, angle closure glaucoma

Continued

ANOREXIANTS—cont'd

Name	Availability	Dosage	Side Effects
Orlistat (Alii, Xenical)	**C:** 60 mg, 120 mg	**Alii:** 60 mg up to tid with meals **Xenical:** 120 mg tid with each meal containing fat	Flatulence, rectal incontinence, oily stools, cholelithiasis, abdominal/rectal pain, hepatitis, pancreatitis, nausea
Phentermine (Apidex-P, Suprenza)	**C:** 15 mg, 30 mg, 37.5 mg **T:** 37.5 mg **T (ODT):** 15 mg, 30 mg, 37.5 mg	15-37.5 mg/day in 1 or 2 divided doses **ODT:** 15-37.5 mg once daily in morning	Headaches, euphoria, palpitations, hypertension, pulmonary hypertension, valvular heart disease, tremor, dependence, withdrawal psychosis, CNS stimulation, GI complaints
Phentermine/topiramate (Qsymia)	**C:** 13.75 mg/23 mg	3.75 mg/23 mg to 15 mg/92 mg once daily in the morning	Paresthesia, dizziness, insomnia, depression, tachycardia, cognitive impairment, angle-closure glaucoma, hypokalemia, metabolic acidosis, constipation, dry mouth, suicidal ideation, kidney stones

AS, Appetite suppressant; *B/P,* blood pressure; *C,* capsules; *CNS,* central nervous system; *CR,* controlled-release; *DI,* digestion Inhibitor; *GI,* gastrointestinal; *HR,* heart rate; *I,* Injection; *ODT,* orally disintegrating tablets; *SQ,* subcutaneously; *T,* tablets.

Osteoporosis

HISTORY

Osteoporosis is a bone disease that can lead to fractures. Bone mineral density (BMD) is reduced, bone microarchitecture is disrupted, and the amount and variety of proteins in bone are altered. Osteoporosis primarily affects women after menopause (postmenopausal osteoporosis) but may develop in men, in anyone in the presence of particular hormonal disorders (e.g., parathyroid glands), after overconsumption of dietary proteins, or as a result of medications (e.g., glucocorticoids). Several pharmacologic options, along with lifestyle changes, that can be used to prevent and/or treat osteoporotic fractures include bisphosphonates, selective estrogen receptor modulator (SERM), parathyroid hormone (PTH), calcitonin, and monoclonal antibodies.

ACTION

Bisphosphonates: Inhibit bone resorption via actions on osteoclasts or osteoclast precursors, decrease rate of bone resorption, leading to an indirect increase in BMD.

Selective estrogen receptor modulator (SERM): Decreases bone resorption, increasing BMD and decreasing the incidence of fractures.

Parathyroid hormone: Stimulates osteoblast function, increasing gastrointestinal calcium absorption and increasing renal tubular reabsorption of calcium. This increases BMD, bone mass, and strength, resulting in a decrease in osteoporosis-related fractures.

Calcitonin: Inhibitor of bone resorption. Efficacy not observed in early postmenopausal women and is used only in women with osteoporosis who are at least 5 yrs beyond menopause.

Monoclonal antibody: Inhibits the RANK ligand (RANKL), a cytokine member of the tumor necrosis factor family. This inhibits osteoclast formation, function, and survival, which decreases bone resorption and increases bone mass and strength in cortical and trabecular bone.

BISPHOSPHONATES

Name	Availability	Dosage	Side Effects
Alendronate (Binosto, Fosamax)	**T:** 5 mg, 10 mg, 35 mg. 40 mg, 70 mg **S:** 70 mg/75ml	**Prevention:** 5 mg/day or 35 mg/wk **Treatment:** 10 mg/day or 70 mg/wk	Transient, mild hypocalcemia, hypophosphatemia, dysphagia, esophagitis, esophageal and gastric ulcer, abdominal pain, diarrhea, musculoskeletal pain. May cause jaw osteonecrosis (up to 0.04%)
Ibandronate (Boniva)	**T:** 150 mg **I:** 1 mg/ml	**Prevention and treatment:** 150 mg/mo **IV Injection: Treatment:** 3 mg/3 mos	Dyspepsia, back pain, dysphagia, esophagitis, esophageal and gastric ulcer, abdominal pain, diarrhea, musculoskeletal pain. May cause jaw osteonecrosis (up to 0.04%)
Risedronate (Actonel)	**T:** 5 mg, 30 mg, 35 mg, 150 mg **T (DR):** 35 mg	**Prevention and treatment:** 5 mg/day, 35 mg/wk, or 150 mg/mo	Hypertension, headache, rash, dysphagia, esophagitis, esophageal and gastric ulcer, abdominal pain, diarrhea, musculoskeletal pain. May cause jaw osteonecrosis (up to 0.04%)
Zoledronic acid (Reclast)	**I:** 5 mg	**Prevention: IV:** 5 mg every 2 yrs **Treatment: IV:** 5 mg every yr	Hypertension, pain, fever, headache, chills, fatigue, nausea, musculoskeletal pain

SERM

Name	Availability	Dosage	Side Effects
Raloxifene (Evista)	**T:** 60 mg	**Prevention and treatment:** 60 mg/day	Peripheral edema, arthralgia, leg cramps, muscle spasms, flu syndrome, infection. Avoid use in patients with hot flashes, history of VTE, where hip fracture is primary concern

PARATHYROID HORMONE

Name	Availability	Dosage	Side Effects
Abaloparatide (Tymos)	**I:** 2000 mcg/ml prefilled pen delivers 80 mcg/dose	**Treatment:** 80 mcg subcutaneously once daily	Hypercalciuria, dizziness, nausea, headache, fatigue, palpitations, vertigo, abdominal pain. Avoid use with pre-existing hypercalcemia
Teriparatide (Forteo)	**I:** 250 mcg/ml syringe delivers 20 mcg/dose	**Treatment:** 20 mcg subcutaneously once daily	Hypercalcemia, muscle cramps, nausea, dizziness, headache. Avoid use with metabolic bone disease, Paget's disease, previous skeletal irradiation, elevated alkaline phosphatase, severe renal impairment

CALCITONIN

Name	Availability	Dosage	Side Effects
Calcitonin (Fortical, Miacalcin)	**I (Miacalcin):** 200 units/ml **Nasal (Fortical, Miacalcin):** 200 units/activation	**Treatment: IM/Subcutaneous (Miacalcin):** 100 units every other day **Nasal:** 200 units in 1 nostril daily	Rhinitis, local nasal irritation. **Injection:** nausea, local inflammation, flushing of face, hands

MONOCLONAL ANTIBODY RANKL INHIBITOR

Name	Availability	Dosage	Side Effects
Denosumab (Prolia)	**I:** 60 mg/ml	**Subcutaneous:** 60 mg once every 6 mos	Back pain, pain in extremity, hypercholesterolemia, musculoskeletal pain, fatigue, headache, peripheral edema, dermatitis. May cause jaw osteonecrosis (up to 1.7%). Avoid use in patient with hypocalcemia, stage 5 kidney disease, dialysis

DR, Delayed-release; *I,* injection; *S,* solution (oral); *T,* tablet.

Parkinson's Disease Treatment

USES	ACTION
To slow or stop clinical progression of Parkinson's disease and to improve function and quality of life in pts with Parkinson's disease, a progressive neurodegenerative disorder.	Normal motor function is dependent on the synthesis and release of dopamine by neurons projecting from the substantia nigra to the corpus striatum. In Parkinson's disease, disruption of this pathway results in diminished levels of the neurotransmitter dopamine. Medication is aimed at providing improved function using the lowest effective dose.

TYPES OF MEDICATIONS FOR PARKINSON'S DISEASE DOPAMINE PRECURSOR

Levodopa/carbidopa:

Levodopa: Dopamine precursor supplementation to enhance dopaminergic neurotransmission. A small amount of levodopa crosses the blood-brain barrier and is decarboxylated to dopamine, which is then available to stimulate dopaminergic receptors.

Carbidopa: Inhibits peripheral decarboxylation of levodopa, decreasing its conversion to dopamine in peripheral tissues, which results in an increased availability of levodopa for transport across the blood-brain barrier.

COMT INHIBITORS

Entacapone, tolcapone: Reversible inhibitor of catechol-*O*-methyltransferase (COMT). COMT is responsible for catalyzing levodopa. In the presence of a decarboxylase inhibitor (carbidopa), COMT becomes the major metabolizing enzyme for levodopa in the brain and periphery. By inhibiting COMT, higher plasma levels of levodopa are attained, resulting in more dopaminergic stimulation in the brain and lessening the symptoms of Parkinson's disease.

DOPAMINE RECEPTOR AGONISTS

Bromocriptine: Stimulates postsynaptic dopamine type 2 receptors in the neostriatum of the CNS.

Pramipexole: Stimulates dopamine receptors in the striatum of the CNS.

Ropinirole: Stimulates postsynaptic dopamine D2 type receptors within the caudate putamen in the brain.

MONOAMINE OXIDASE B INHIBITORS

Rasagiline, Safinamide, Selegiline: Increase dopaminergic activity due to inhibition of monoamine oxidase type B (MAO B). MAO B is involved in the oxidative deamination of dopamine in the brain.

MEDICATIONS FOR TREATMENT OF PARKINSON'S DISEASE

Name	Type	Availability	Dosage	Side Effects
Amantadine	Dopamine agonist	**C:** 100 mg **Syrup:** 10 mg/ml **T:** 100 mg	100 mg 2 times/day. May increase up to 400 mg/day in divided doses	Cognitive impairment, confusion, insomnia, hallucinations, livido reticularis
Carbidopa/ levodopa (Rytary, Sinemet, Sinemet CR)	Dopamine precursor	**OD:** 10/100 mg, 25/100 mg, 25/250 mg **Immediate-release (Sinemet):** 10/100 mg, 25/100 mg, 25/250 mg **Extended-release (Sinemet CR):** 25/100 mg, 50/200 mg **(Rytary):** 23.75 mg/95 mg, 36.25 mg/145 mg, 48.75 mg/195 mg, 61.25 mg/245 mg	300–1,500 mg levodopa in divided doses **Sinemet:** 300–1,500 mg levodopa in divided doses **Sinemet CR:** Initially, 400 mg/day in 2 divided doses. May increase up to 1,600 mg levodopa in divided doses **Rytary:** Initially, 23.75 mg/95 mg 3 times/day. May increase up to 612.5 mg/2,450 mg per day in divided doses	Anorexia, nausea, orthostatic hypotension initially; hallucinations, confusion, sleep disturbances with chronic use, constipation, dry mouth, headache, dyskinesia
Entacapone (Comtan)	COMT inhibitor	**T:** 200 mg	200 mg 3–4 times/day up to maximum of 8 times/day (1,600 mg)	Dyskinesias, nausea, diarrhea, urine discoloration
Pramipexole (Mirapex, Mirapex ER)	Dopamine agonist	**T:** 0.125 mg, 0.25 mg, 0.5 mg, 0.75 mg, 1 mg, 1.5 mg **ER:** 0.375 mg, 0.75 mg, 1.5 mg, 2.25 mg, 3 mg, 3.75 mg, 4.5 mg	**T:** Initially, 0.125 mg 3 times/day. May increase q5–7 days. Usual dose: 0.5–1.5 mg 3 times/day **ER:** Initially, 0.375 mg once daily. May increase q5–7 days by 0.75 mg/dose up to 4.5 mg once daily	Side effects similar to carbidopa/ levodopa. Lower risk of dyskinesias, higher risk of hallucinations, sleepiness, edema. May cause excessive daytime sleepiness, impair impulse control (e.g., gambling)

Continued

MEDICATIONS FOR TREATMENT OF PARKINSON'S DISEASE—cont'd

Name	Type	Availability	Dosage	Side Effects
Rasagiline (Azilect)	MAO B inhibitor	**T:** 0.5 mg, 1 mg	0.5–1 mg once daily	Nausea, orthostatic hypotension, hallucinations, insomnia, dry mouth, constipation, vivid dreams. Many potential drug interactions.
Ropinirole (Requip, Requip XL)	Dopamine agonist	**T:** 0.25 mg, 0.5 mg, 1 mg, 2 mg, 3 mg, 4 mg, 5 mg **XL:** 2 mg, 4 mg, 6 mg, 8 mg, 12 mg	**T:** Initially, 0.25 mg 3 times/day. May increase at weekly intervals to 0.5 mg 3 times/day, then 0.75 mg 3 times/day, then 1 mg 3 times/day. May then increase by 1.5 mg/day up to 9 mg/day, then by 3 mg/day up to total dose of 24 mg/day in divided doses **XL:** Initially, 2 mg/day for 1–2 wks, then increase by 2 mg/day at weekly intervals	Side effects similar to carbidopa/levodopa. Lower risk of dyskinesias, higher risk of hallucinations, sleepiness, edema. May cause excessive daytime sleepiness, impair impulse control (e.g., gambling)
Rotigotine (Neupro)	Dopamine agonist	**Transdermal patch:** 1 mg/24 hrs, 2 mg/24 hrs, 3 mg/24 hrs, 4 mg/24 hrs, 6 mg/24 hrs, 8 mg/24 hrs	Early stage: Initially, 2 mg/24 hrs up to 6 mg/24 hrs Advanced stage: Initially, 4 mg/24 hrs up to 8 mg/24 hrs	Side effects similar to carbidopa/levodopa. Lower risk of dyskinesias, higher risk of hallucinations, sleepiness, edema. May cause excessive daytime sleepiness, impair impulse control (e.g. gambling)
Safinamide (Xadago)	MAO B inhibitor	**T:** 50 mg, 100 mg	Initially, 50 mg once daily. May increase after two wks to 100 mg once daily	Dyskinesia, falls, hallucinations, nausea, insomnia. Many potential drug interactions
Selegiline (Eldepryl, Zelapar)	MAO B inhibitor	**C (Eldepryl):** 5 mg **OD (Zelapar):** 1.25 mg	**C:** 5 mg with breakfast and lunch **OD:** 1.25–2.5 mg daily in the morning	Nausea, orthostatic hypotension, hallucinations, insomnia, dry mouth, constipation, vivid dreams. Many potential drug interactions.
Tolcapone (Tasmar)	COMT inhibitor	**T:** 100 mg	Initially, 100 mg 3 times/day. May increase to 200 mg 3 times/day	Dyskinesias, nausea, diarrhea, urine discoloration

C, Capsules; *COMT,* catechol-*O*-methyltransferase; *ER,* extended-release; *I,* Injection; *MAO B,* monoamine oxidase B; *OD,* orally disintegrating; *T,* tablets; *XL,* extended-release.

Proton Pump Inhibitors

USES

Treatment of various gastric disorders, including gastric and duodenal ulcers, gastroesophageal reflux disease (GERD), pathologic hypersecretory conditions.

ACTION

Suppresses gastric acid secretion by specific inhibition of the hydrogen-potassium-adenosine triphosphatase (H^+/K^+ ATPase) enzyme system, which transports the acid at the gastric parietal cells. These agents do not have anticholinergic or histamine receptor antagonistic properties.

PROTON PUMP INHIBITORS

Name	Availability	Indications	Usual Dosage	Side Effects
Dexlansoprazole (Dexilant)	**C:** 30 mg, 60 mg	Erosive esophagitis, heartburn associated with nonerosive GERD	30–60 mg/day	Diarrhea, abdominal pain, nausea, upper respiratory tract infection, vomiting, flatulence
Esomeprazole (Nexium)	**C:** 20 mg, 40 mg **I:** 20 mg, 40 mg	*Helicobacter pylori* eradication, GERD, erosive esophagitis	20–40 mg/day	Headaches, diarrhea, abdominal pain, nausea
Lansoprazole (Prevacid)	**C:** 15 mg, 30 mg **T (ODT):** 15 mg, 30 mg	Duodenal ulcer, gastric ulcer, NSAID-associated gastric ulcer, hypersecretory conditions, *H. pylori* eradication, GERD, erosive esophagitis	15–30 mg/day	Diarrhea, skin rash, pruritus, headaches
Omeprazole (Prilosec)	**C:** 10 mg, 20 mg, 40 mg	Duodenal ulcer, gastric ulcer, hypersecretory conditions, *H. pylori* eradication, GERD, erosive esophagitis	20–40 mg/day	Headaches, diarrhea, abdominal pain, nausea
Omeprazole and Sodium Bicarbonate (Zegerid)	**P:** 20 mg, 40 mg	Duodenal ulcer, benign gastric ulcer, GERD, erosive esophagitis	20–40 mg/day	Headaches, abdominal pain, diarrhea, nausea
Pantoprazole (Protonix)	**T:** 20 mg, 40 mg **I:** 40 mg	Erosive esophagitis, hypersecretory conditions	40 mg/day	Diarrhea, headaches
Rabeprazole (Aciphex)	**T:** 20 mg **S:** 5 mg, 10 mg	Duodenal ulcer, hypersecretory conditions, *H. pylori* eradication, GERD, erosive esophagitis	20 mg/day	Headaches

C, Capsules; *GERD,* gastroesophageal reflux disease; *I,* Injection; *NSAID,* nonsteroidal anti-Inflammatory drug; *ODT,* orally disintegrating tablets; *P,* powder for suspension; *S,* sprinkles; *T,* tablets.

Rheumatoid Arthritis

Rheumatoid arthritis (RA) is an autoimmune disease associated with progressive disability, systemic complications, early death, and socioeconomic costs. RA affects most joints and their surrounding tissues. RA is characterized by synovial inflammation and hyperplasia, autoantibody production (e.g., rheumatoid factor), cartilage and bone destruction, and systemic features (e.g., cardiovascular, pulmonary, psychological, skeletal disorders). The clinical hallmark of RA is polyarticular synovial inflammation of peripheral joints (typically in the hands, resulting in pain, stiffness, and some degree of irreversible joint damage; deformity; and disability).

Medications used in RA include disease-modifying antirheumatic drugs (DMARDS) and biologic agents, including tumor necrosis factor (TNT) inhibitors.

DMARDS

Name	Dosage	Side Effects/Comments
Hydroxychloroquine (Plaquenil)	Induction: 400–600 mg/day for 4–12 wks Maintenance: 200–400 mg/day	**Side Effects:** nausea, epigastric pain, hemolysis may occur in pts with G6PD deficiency, retinal toxicity with long-term use
Leflunomide (Arava)	Induction: 100 mg/day X 3 days Maintenance: 10–20 mg/day	**Side Effects:** diarrhea, respiratory tract infection, hypertension, headache, reversible alopecia, rash, myelosuppression, and/or elevated hepatic enzymes **Comments:** contraindicated for use during pregnancy
Methotrexate (oral) (Rheumatrex, Trexall) Methotrexate (injectable) Otrexup, Rasuvo)	Induction: 7.5–10 mg PO once/wk Maintenance: 7.5–25 mg PO once wkly Induction: 7.5 PO once wkly Maintenance: 10–25 mg IM or SQ once wkly	**Side Effects:** stomatitis, anorexia, nausea, vomiting, diarrhea, abdominal cramps, hepatic enzyme elevations, thrombocytopenia **Comments:** not recommended in pts with CrCl <30 ml/min; should not be prescribed for women who are or may become pregnant
Sulfasalazine (Azulfidine)	Induction: 3–4 g/day in divided doses Maintenance: 2 g/day in divided doses	**Side Effects:** headache, nausea, anorexia, rash, hemolysis may occur in pts with G6PD deficiency

BIOLOGIC AGENTS

TNF INHIBITORS

Name	Dosage	Side Effects/Comments
Adalimumab (Humira)	40 mg SQ once wkly or q2wks	**Side Effects:** headache, skin rash, positive ANA titer, antibody development, injection site reaction (erythema, itching, pain, swelling), upper respiratory tract infection **Comments:** increased risk for serious infections (e.g., tuberculosis, invasive fungal infections), avoid use in pts with recent history of malignancy or pre-existing demyelinating disorders
Certolizumab (Cinzia)	Induction: 400 mg SQ at 0, 2,4 wks Maintenance: 200 mg SQ every other week or 400 mg q4wks	**Side Effects:** nausea, infection, upper respiratory tract infection, skin rash **Comments:** see adalimumab
Etanercept (Enbrel)	25 mg SQ 2 times/wk or 50 mg SQ once/wk	**Side Effects:** headache, skin rash, diarrhea, injection site reactions (e.g., erythema, swelling), upper respiratory tract infection, rhinitis **Comments:** see adalimumab
Golimumab (Simponi, Simponi Aria)	Simponi: 50 mg SQ once monthly Simponi Aria: Induction: 2 mg/kg IV at 0 and 4 wks Maintenance: 2 mg/kg IV q8wks	**Side Effects:** positive ANA titer, upper respiratory tract infection (e.g., nasopharyngitis, rhinitis) **Comments:** see adalimumab
Infliximab (Remicade)	Induction: 3 mg/kg IV at 0, 2, and 6 wks Maintenance: 3 mg/kg IV q8wks	**Side Effects:** nausea, diarrhea, abdominal pain, increased ANA titer, upper respiratory tract infection, sinusitis, cough, pharyngitis **Comments:** see adalimumab

OTHER BIOLOGIC AGENTS

Name	Dosage	Side Effects/Comments
Abatacept (Orencia)	**IV:** 500 mg, 750 mg, or 1,000 mg IV at 0,2, and 4 wks, then q4wks **SQ:** 125 mg SQ once/wk	**Side Effects:** nausea, UTIs, acute exacerbation of COPD, hypertension, headache, dizziness **Comments:** may increase risk of serious infections (e.g., pneumonia, pyelonephritis, cellulitis, diverticulitis)
Rituximab (Rituxan)	1,000 mg IV twice, 2 wks apart	**Side Effects:** hypotension, peripheral edema, abdominal pair anemia, arthralgia, infusion site reactions **Comments:** Pts at high risk for hepatitis B virus infection should be screened before beginning therapy
Sarilumab (Kevzara)	**SQ:** 200 mg q2wks	**Side Effects:** neutropenia, increased ALT, injection site reactions (e.g., erythema), upper respiratory tract infections, UTI **Comments:** screening for tuberculosis recommended
Tocilizumab (Actemra)	**IV:** Induction: 4 mg/kg IV q4wks Maintenance: 8 mg/kg q4 wks **SQ:** Induction: 162 mg SQ every other week Maintenance: 162 mg once wkly	**Side Effects:** hypertension, upper abdominal pain, increased ALT/ AST, injection site reactions, neutropenia, dyslipidemia **Comments:** severe complications including GI perforation and hypersensitivity with anaphylaxis have been reported
Tofacitinib (Xeljanz)	5 mg PO bid	**Side Effects:** diarrhea, nasopharyngitis, upper respiratory infections, headache hypertension, increased LFT, dyslipidemia, cytopenias have been reported **Comments:** screening for tuberculosis recommended, increased incidence of solid cancers detected

ANA, Antinuclear antibodies; *CNS*, central nervous system; *COPD*, chronic obstructive pulmonary disease; *GI*, gastrointestinal; *UTI*, urinary tract Infection.

Sedative-Hypnotics

USES

Treatment of insomnia (i.e., difficulty falling asleep initially, frequent awakening, awakening too early).

ACTION

Benzodiazepines are the most widely used agents and largely replace barbiturates due to greater safety, lower incidence of drug dependence. Benzodiazepines nonselective bind to at least three receptor subtypes accounting for sedative, anxiolytic, relaxant, and anticonvulsant properties. Benzodiazepines enhance the effect of the inhibitory neurotransmitter gamma-aminobutyric acid (GABA), which inhibits impulse transmission in the CNS reticular formation in brain. Benzodiazepines decrease sleep latency, number of nocturnal awakenings, and time spent in awake stage of sleep; increase total sleep time. The *nonbenzodiazepines* zaleplon and Zolpidem preferentially bind with one receptor subtype, reducing sleep latency and nocturnal awakenings and increasing total sleep time. Ramelteon is a selective agonist of melatonin receptors (responsible for determining circadian rhythms and synchronizing sleep-wake cycles).

SEDATIVE-HYPNOTICS

Name	Availability	Dosage Range	Side Effects
Benzodiazepines			
Estazolam	**T:** 1 mg, 2 mg	**A:** 1–2 mg **E:** 0.5–1 mg	Daytime sedation, memory and psychomotor impairment, tolerance, withdrawal reactions, rebound insomnia, dependence
Flurazepam	**C:** 15 mg, 30 mg	**A/E:** 15–30 mg **E:** 15 mg	Headaches, unpleasant taste, dry mouth, dizziness, anxiety, nausea
Temazepam (Restoril)	**C:** 7.5 mg, 15 mg, 30 mg	**A:** 15–30 mg **E:** 7.5–15 mg	Same as flurazepam

Continued

SEDATIVE-HYPNOTICS—cont'd

Name	Availability	Dosage Range	Side Effects
Nonbenzodiazepines			
Doxepin (Silenor)	**T:** 3 mg, 6 mg	**A, E:** 3–6 mg	Somnolence, dizziness, nausea, upper respiratory tract infections, nasopharyngitis, hypertension, headache
Eszopiclone (Lunesta)	**T:** 1 mg, 2 mg, 3 mg	**A:** 1–3 mg **E:** 1–2 mg	Headaches, unpleasant taste, dry mouth, dizziness, anxiety, nausea
Ramelteon (Rozerem)	**T:** 8 mg	**A, E:** 8 mg	Headaches, dizziness, fatigue, nausea
Suvorexant (Belsomra)	**T:** 5 mg, 10 mg, 15 mg, 20 mg	**A, E:** 10–20 mg	Next day somnolence, leg weakness
Zaleplon (Sonata)	**C:** 5 mg, 10 mg	**A:** 10–20 mg **E:** 5 mg	Headaches, dizziness, myalgia, drowsiness, asthenia, abdominal pain
Zolpidem (Ambien, Ambien CR, Edluar, Intermezzo, Zolpimist)	**T:** 5 mg, 10 mg **CR:** 6.25 mg, 12.5 mg **SL (Edluar):** 5 mg, 10 mg **(Intermezzo):** 1.75 mg, 3.5 mg **OS:** 5 mg/actuation	**OS, T, SL (Edluar):** 5 mg (females, elderly); 5–10 mg (males) (Intermezzo): 1.75 mg (females, elderly); 3.5 mg (males) **CR:** 6.25 mg (females, elderly); 6.25–12.5 mg (males)	Dizziness, daytime drowsiness, headaches, confusion, depression, hangover, asthenia

A, Adults; *C,* capsules; *CR,* controlled-release; *E,* elderly; *OS,* oral solution; *SL,* sublingual; *T,* tablets.

Skeletal Muscle Relaxants

USES

Central acting muscle relaxants: Adjunct to rest, physical therapy for relief of discomfort associated with acute, painful musculoskeletal disorders (i.e., local spasms from muscle injury).

Baclofen, dantrolene, diazepam: Treatment of spasticity characterized by heightened muscle tone, spasm, loss of dexterity caused by multiple sclerosis, cerebral palsy, spinal cord lesions, CVA.

ACTION

Central acting muscle relaxants: Exact mechanism unknown. May act in CNS at various levels to depress polysynaptic reflexes; sedative effect may be responsible for relaxation of muscle spasm.

Baclofen, diazepam: May mimic actions of gamma-aminobutyric acid on spinal neurons; do not directly affect skeletal muscles.

Dantrolene: Acts directly on skeletal muscle, relieving spasticity.

SKELETAL MUSCLE RELAXANTS

Name	Indication	Dosage Range	Side Effects/Comments
Baclofen (Lioresal)	Spasticity associated with multiple sclerosis, spinal cord injury	Initially 5 mg 3 times/day Increase by 5 mg 3 times/day q3days **Maximum:** 20 mg 4 times/day	Drowsiness, dizziness, GI effects Caution with renal impairment, seizure disorders Withdrawal syndrome (e.g., hallucinations, psychosis, seizures)
Carisoprodol (Rela)	Discomfort due to acute, painful, musculoskeletal conditions	250–350 mg 4 times/day	Drowsiness, dizziness, GI effects Hypomania at higher than recommended doses Withdrawal syndrome Hypersensitivity reaction (skin reaction, bronchospasm, weakness, burning eyes, fever) or idiosyncratic reaction (weakness, visual or motor disturbances, confusion) usually occurring within first 4 doses

Continued

SKELETAL MUSCLE RELAXANTS—cont'd

Name	Indication	Dosage Range	Side Effects/Comments
Chlorzoxazone (Lorzone)	Discomfort due to acute, painful, musculoskeletal conditions	Initially 250–500 mg 3–4 times/day **Maximum:** 750 mg 3–4 times/day	Drowsiness, dizziness, GI effects, rare hepatotoxicity Hypersensitivity reaction (urticaria, itching) Urine discoloration to orange, red, or purple
Cyclobenzaprine (Flexeril)	Muscle spasm, pain, tenderness, restricted movement due to acute, painful, musculoskeletal conditions	Initially 5–10 mg 3 times/day	Drowsiness, dizziness, GI effects Anticholinergic effects (dry mouth, urinary retention) Quinidine-like effects on heart (QT prolongation) Long half-life
Dantrolene (Dantrium)	Spasticity associated with multiple sclerosis, cerebral palsy, spinal cord injury	Initially 25 mg/day for 1 wk, then 25 mg 3 times/day for 1 wk, then 50 mg 3 times/day for 1 wk, then 100 mg 3 times/day **Maximum:** 100 mg 4 times/day	Drowsiness, dizziness, GI effects Contraindicated with hepatic disease Dose-dependent hepatotoxicity Diarrhea that is dose dependent and may be severe, requiring discontinuation
Diazepam (Valium)	Spasticity associated with cerebral palsy, spinal cord injury; reflex spasm due to muscle, joint trauma or inflammation	2–10 mg 3–4 times/day	Drowsiness, dizziness, GI effects Abuse potential
Metaxalone (Skelaxin)	Discomfort due to acute, painful, musculoskeletal conditions	800 mg 3–4 times/day	Drowsiness (low risk), dizziness, GI effects Paradoxical muscle cramps Mild withdrawal syndrome Contraindicated in serious hepatic or renal disease
Methocarbamol (Robaxin)	Discomfort due to acute, painful, musculoskeletal conditions	Initially 1,500 mg 4 times/day **Maintenance:** 1,000 mg 4 times/day	Drowsiness, dizziness, GI effects Urine discoloration to brown, brown-black, or green

Orphenadrine (Norflex)	Discomfort due to acute, painful, musculoskeletal conditions	100 mg 2 times/day	Drowsiness, dizziness, GI effects Long half-life Anticholinergic effects (dry mouth, urinary retention) Rare aplastic anemia Some products may contain sulfites
Tizanidine (Zanaflex)	Spasticity	Initially 4 mg q6–8h (**maximum** 3 times/day), may increase by 2–4 mg as needed/tolerated **Maximum:** 36 mg (limited information on doses greater than 24 mg)	Drowsiness, dizziness, GI effects Hypotension (20% decrease in B/P) Hepatotoxicity (usually reversible) Withdrawal syndrome (hypertension, tachycardia, hypertonia) Effect is short lived (3–6 hrs) Dose cautiously with creatinine clearance less than 25 ml/min

B/P, Blood pressure; *GI,* gastrointestinal.

Smoking Cessation Agents

Tobacco smoking is associated with the development of lung cancer and chronic obstructive pulmonary disease. Smoking is harmful not just to the smoker but also to family members, coworkers, and others breathing cigarette smoke.

Quitting smoking decreases the risk of developing lung cancer, other cancers, heart disease, stroke, and respiratory illnesses. Several medications have proved useful as smoking cessation aids. Nausea and light-headedness are possible signs of overdose of nicotine warranting a reduction in dosage.

SMOKING CESSATION AGENTS

Name	Availability	Dose Duration	Cautions/Side Effects	Comments
Bupropion (Zyban)	**T:** 150 mg	150 mg every morning for 3 days, then 150 mg 2 times/day Start 1–2 wks before quit date **Duration:** 7–12 wks up to 6 mos for maintenance	History of seizure, eating disorder, use of MAOI within previous 14 days, bipolar disorder **Side Effects:** Insomnia, dry mouth, tremor, rash	Stop smoking during second wk of treatment and use counseling support services along with medication
Clonidine (Catapres, Catapres-TTS)	**T:** 0.1 mg, 0.2 mg **Patch:** 0.1 mg/24 hrs, 0.2 mg/24 hrs, 0.3 mg/24 hrs	**Oral:** 0.15–0.75 mg/day **Patch:** 0.1–0.2 mg daily **Duration:** 3–10 wks	Rebound hypertension. **Side Effects:** Dry mouth, drowsiness, dizziness, sedation, constipation	Abrupt discontinuation can result in anxiety, agitation, headaches, tremors accompanied or followed by rapid rise in B/P

Nicotine gum (Nicorette)	Squares: 2 mg, 4 mg	1 gum q1–2h for 6 wks, then q2–4h for 3 wks then q4–8h for 3 wks **Maximum:** 24 pieces/day **Duration:** up to 12 wks	Recent MI (within 2 wks), serious arrhythmias, serious or worsening angina pectoris **Side Effects:** Dyspepsia, mouth soreness, hiccups	2 mg recommended for pts smoking less than 25 cigarettes/day, 4 mg for pts smoking 25 or more cigarettes/day Chew until a peppery or minty taste emerges and then "park" between cheek and gums to facilitate nicotine absorption through oral mucosa Chew slowly and intermittently to avoid jaw ache and achieve maximum benefit Only water should be taken 15 min before and during chewing
Nicotine inhaler (Nicotrol)	Cartridge: 10 mg (delivers 4 mg nicotine)	4–16 cartridges daily; taper frequency of use over the last 6–12 mos **Duration:** up to 6 mos	Recent MI (within 2 wks), serious arrhythmias, serious or worsening angina pectoris **Side Effects:** Local irritation of mouth and throat, coughing, rhinitis	Use at or above room temperature (cold temperatures decrease amount of nicotine inhaled)
Nicotine lozenge (Nicorette Lozenges)	Lozenges: 2 mg, 4 mg	One lozenge q 1–2h for 6 wks, then q2–4h for 3 wks, then q4–8h for 3 wks **Maximum:** 5 lozenges in 6 hrs; 20 lozenges in 1 day	Recent MI (within 2 wks), serious arrhythmias, serious or worsening angina pectoris **Side Effects:** Local skin reaction, insomnia, nausea, sore throat	First cigarette smoked within 30 min of waking, use 4 mg; after 30 min of waking, use 2 mg Use at least 9 lozenges/day first 6 wks Only 1 lozenge at a time, 5 per 6 hrs and 20 per 24 hrs Do not chew or swallow
Nicotine nasal spray (Nicotrol NS)	10 mg/ml (delivers 0.5 mg/spray)	8–40 doses/day A dose consists of one 0.5 mg delivery to each nostril; initial dose is 1–2 sprays/hr, increasing as needed **Duration:** 3–6 mos	Recent MI (within 2 wks), serious arrhythmias, serious or worsening angina pectoris **Side Effects:** Nasal irritation	Do not sniff, swallow, or inhale through nose while administering nicotine doses (may increase irritation) Tilt head back slightly for best results

Continued

SMOKING CESSATION AGENTS—cont'd

Name	Availability	Dose Duration	Cautions/Side Effects	Comments
Nicotine patch (NicoDerm CQ)	**Nicoderm CQ:** 7 mg/24 hrs, 14 mg/24 hrs, 21 mg/24 hrs **Nicotrol:** 5 mg/16 hrs, 10 mg/16 hrs, 15 mg/16 hrs	Apply upon waking on quit date: **Nicoderm CQ (greater than 10 cigarettes/day):** 21 mg/24 hrs for 4 wks, then 14 mg/24 hrs for 2 wks, then 7 mg/24 hrs for 2 wks **(10 or fewer cigarettes/day):** 14 mg/24 hrs for 6 wks, then 7 mg/24 hrs for 2 wks	Recent MI (within 2 wks), serious arrhythmias, serious or worsening angina pectoris **Side Effects:** Local skin reaction, insomnia	The 16- and 24-hr patches are of comparable efficacy Begin with a lower-dose patch in pts smoking 10 or fewer cigarettes/day Place new patch on relatively hair-free location, usually between neck and waist, in the morning If insomnia occurs, remove the 24-hr patch prior to bedtime or use the 16-hr patch Rotate patch site to diminish skin irritation
Nortriptyline (Pamelor)	**T:** 25 mg, 50 mg, 75 mg, 100 mg	Initially 25 mg/day, increasing gradually to target dose of 75–100 mg/day 10–28 days prior to selected "quit" date, continue for 12 wks or more after "quit" day **Duration:** up to 12 wks	Risk of arrhythmias **Side Effects:** Sedation, dry mouth, blurred vision, urinary retention, light-headedness, shaky hands	Initiate therapy 10–28 days before the quit date to allow steady state of nortriptyline at target dose
Varenicline (Chantix)	**T:** 0.5 mg, 1 mg	**Days 1–3:** 0.5 mg daily; **days 4–7:** 0.5 mg 2 times/day; **day 8 to end of treatment:** 1 mg 2 times/day **Duration:** begin 1 wk before set quit date, continue for 12 wks. May use additional 12 wks if failed to quit after first 12 wks	**Side Effects:** Nausea; sleep disturbances; headaches; may impair ability to drive, operate machinery; depressed mood; altered behavior; suicidal ideation reported	Use lower dosage if not able to tolerate nausea and vomiting Use counseling support services along with medication

B/P, Blood pressure; *MAOI,* monoamine oxidase inhibitor; *MI,* myocardial infarction; *T,* tablets.

Vitamins

INTRODUCTION

Vitamins are organic substances required for growth, reproduction, and maintenance of health and are obtained from food or supplementation in small quantities (vitamins cannot be synthesized by the body or the rate of synthesis is too slow/inadequate to meet metabolic needs). Vitamins are essential for energy transformation and regulation of metabolic processes. They are catalysts for all reactions using proteins, fats, carbohydrates for energy, growth, and cell maintenance.

WATER SOLUBLE

Water-soluble vitamins include vitamin C (ascorbic acid), B_1 (thiamine), B_2 (riboflavin), B_3 (niacin), B_5 (pantothenic acid), B_6 (pyridoxine), folic acid, B_{12} (cyanocobalamin). Water-soluble vitamins act as coenzymes for almost every cellular reaction in the body. B-complex vitamins differ from one another in both structure and function but are grouped together because they first were isolated from the same source (yeast and liver).

FAT SOLUBLE

Fat-soluble vitamins include vitamins A, D, E, and K. They are soluble in lipids and are usually absorbed into the lymphatic system of the small intestine and then into the general circulation. Absorption is facilitated by bile. These vitamins are stored in the body tissue when excessive quantities are consumed. May be toxic when taken in large doses (see sections on individual vitamins).

VITAMINS

Name	Uses	Deficiency	Side Effects
Vitamin A (Aquasol A)	Required for normal growth, bone development, vision, reproduction, maintenance of epithelial tissue	Dry skin, poor tooth development, night blindness	**High dosages:** Hepatotoxicity, cheilitis, facial dermatitis, photosensitivity, mucosal dryness
Vitamin B₁ (thiamine)	Important in red blood cell formation, carbohydrate metabolism, neurologic function, myocardial contractility, growth, energy production	Fatigue, anorexia, growth retardation	**Large parenteral doses:** May cause pain on injection
Vitamin B₂ (riboflavin)	Necessary for function of coenzymes in oxidation-reduction reactions, essential for normal cellular growth, assists in absorption of iron and pyridoxine	Numbness in extremities, blurred vision, photophobia, cheilosis	Orange-yellow discoloration in urine

Continued

VITAMINS—cont'd

Name	Uses	Deficiency	Side Effects
Vitamin B₃ (niacin)	Coenzyme for many oxidation-reduction reactions	Pellagra, headache, anorexia, memory loss, insomnia	**High dosages (more than 500 mg):** Nausea, vomiting, diarrhea, gastritis, hepatotoxicity, skin rash, facial flushing, headaches
Vitamin B₅ (pantothenic acid)	Precursor to coenzyme A, important in synthesis of cholesterol, hormones, fatty acids	Natural deficiency unknown	Occasional GI disturbances (e.g. diarrhea)
Vitamin B₆ (pyridoxine)	Enzyme cofactor for amino acid metabolism, essential for erythrocyte production, Hgb synthesis	Neuritis, anemia, lymphopenia	**High dosages:** May cause sensory neuropathy
Vitamin B₁₂ (cyanocobalamin)	Coenzyme in cells, including bone marrow, CNS, and GI tract, necessary for lipid metabolism, formation of myelin	Gastrointestinal disorders, anemias, poor growth	Skin rash, diarrhea, pain at injection site
Vitamin C (ascorbic acid)	Cofactor in various physiologic reactions, necessary for collagen formation, acts as antioxidant	Poor wound healing, bleeding gums, scurvy	**High dosages:** May cause calcium oxalate crystalluria, esophagitis, diarrhea
Vitamin D (Calciferol)	Necessary for proper formation of bone, calcium, mineral homeostasis, regulation of parathyroid hormone, calcitonin, phosphate	Rickets, osteomalacia	Hypercalcemia, kidney stones, renal failure, hypertension, psychosis, diarrhea, nausea, vomiting, anorexia, fatigue, headaches, altered mental status
Vitamin E (Aquasol E)	Antioxidant, promotes formation, functioning of red blood cells, muscle, other tissues	Red blood cell breakdown	**High dosages:** GI disturbances, malaise, headaches

CNS, Central nervous system; *F,* females; *GI,* gastrointestinal; *M,* males.

abacavir

a-**bak**-a-veer
(Ziagen)

■ **BLACK BOX ALERT** ■ Serious, sometimes fatal hypersensitivity reactions, lactic acidosis, severe hepatomegaly with steatosis (fatty liver) have occurred.

FIXED-COMBINATION(S)

Epzicom: abacavir/lamiVUDine (antiretroviral): 600 mg/300 mg. **Triumeq:** abacavir/dolutegravir (integrase inhibitor)/lamiVUDine (antiretroviral): 600 mg/50 mg/300 mg. **Trizivir:** abacavir/lamiVUDine (antiretroviral)/zidovudine (antiretroviral): 300 mg/150 mg/300 mg.

◆CLASSIFICATION

PHARMACOTHERAPEUTIC: Antiretroviral agent. **CLINICAL:** Antiviral.

USES

Treatment of HIV-1 infection, in combination with at least two other antiretroviral agents.

PRECAUTIONS

Contraindications: Hypersensitivity to abacavir (do **not** rechallenge). Pts testing positive for the HLA-B *5701 allele are at increased risk for hypersensitivity reaction. Moderate or severe hepatic impairment. **Cautions:** Mild hepatic disease. Pts at risk for coronary heart disease (e.g., hypertension, hyperlipidemia, diabetes, smoking). Pts at risk for hepatotoxicity (e.g., female gender, obesity), pts with plasma HIV RNA levels greater than 100,000 copies/mL.

ACTION

Interferes with HIV viral RNA-dependent DNA polymerase. **Therapeutic Effect:** Inhibits/prevents HIV replication in infected cells.

PHARMACOKINETICS

Rapidly absorbed after PO administration. Widely distributed, including to cerebrospinal fluid (CSF) and erythrocytes. Metabolized in liver. Protein binding: 50%. Primarily excreted in urine. Unknown if removed by hemodialysis. **Half-life:** 1.5 hrs.

⧗ LIFESPAN CONSIDERATIONS

Pregnancy/Lactation: Unknown if excreted in breast milk. Breastfeeding not recommended (may increase potential for HIV transmission, adverse effects). **Children:** Safety and efficacy not established in pts less than 3 mos of age. **Elderly:** No age-related precautions noted.

INTERACTIONS

DRUG: Alcohol may increase concentration, risk of toxicity. **HERBAL:** None significant. **FOOD:** None known. **LAB VALUES:** May increase serum amylase, ALT, AST, CPK, GGT, blood glucose, triglycerides. May decrease Hgb, leukocytes, lymphocytes.

AVAILABILITY (Rx)

Solution, Oral: 20 mg/mL. **Tablets:** 300 mg.

ADMINISTRATION/HANDLING

PO
• May give without regard to food. • Oral solution may be refrigerated. Do not freeze.

INDICATIONS/ROUTES/DOSAGE

HIV Infection (in Combination with Other Antiretrovirals)
PO: ADULTS, ELDERLY: 300 mg twice daily or 600 mg once daily. **CHILDREN 3 MOS–16 YRS:** Oral solution (weight-based dosing): 8 mg/kg twice daily or 16 mg/kg once daily. **Maximum:** 300 mg twice daily. (Alternative dosing) **CHILDREN 14 KG OR GREATER:** Tablets, oral solution (weight-based dosing): **14–19 kg:** 150 mg (½ tab) twice daily or 300 mg once daily. **20–24 kg:** 150 mg (½ tab) in AM, 300 mg (1 tab) in PM or 450 mg once daily. **25 kg or greater:** 300 mg (1 tab) twice daily or 600 mg once daily.

Dosage in Renal Impairment
No dose adjustment.

 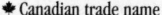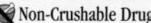

Dosage in Hepatic Impairment
Mild Impairment: 200 mg twice daily (oral solution recommended). **Moderate to Severe Impairment:** Not recommended (contraindicated by manufacturer).

SIDE EFFECTS

ADULT: Frequent   (47%–11%): Nausea, nausea with vomiting, diarrhea, decreased appetite. **Occasional (39%–11%):** Insomnia. **CHILDREN: Frequent:** Nausea with vomiting, fever, headache, diarrhea, rash. **Occasional (9%):** Decreased appetite.

ADVERSE EFFECTS/ TOXIC REACTIONS

Hypersensitivity reaction may be life-threatening. Signs and symptoms include fever, rash, fatigue, intractable nausea/vomiting, severe diarrhea, abdominal pain, cough, pharyngitis, dyspnea. Life-threatening hypotension may occur. Lactic acidosis, severe hepatomegaly with steatosis may occur.

NURSING CONSIDERATIONS

BASELINE ASSESSMENT

Obtain CBC, LFT before beginning therapy and at periodic intervals during therapy. Question history of hypersensitivity reaction. Question for possibility of pregnancy. Increased risk of sensitivity (cutaneous, GI, pulmonary) in those with positive HLA-B*5701 genotype status. Offer emotional support.

INTERVENTION/EVALUATION

Stop abacavir if 3 or more of the following occur: rash, fever, GI disturbances (diarrhea, nausea, vomiting), flu-like symptoms, respiratory difficulty. Assess for nausea, vomiting. Monitor daily pattern of bowel activity, stool consistency. Assess dietary pattern; monitor for weight loss. Monitor lab values, hepatic function.

PATIENT/FAMILY TEACHING

• Immediately report allergic reactions of any kind. • Do not take any medications, including OTC drugs, without consulting physician. • Avoid alcohol.

• Small, frequent meals may offset anorexia, nausea. • Abacavir is not a cure for HIV infection, nor does it reduce risk of transmission to others. • Pt must continue practices to prevent HIV transmission.

abaloparatide

a-**bal**-oh-**par**-a-tide
(Tymlos)

■ **BLACK BOX ALERT** ■ May cause a dose-dependent increase in the incidence of osteosarcoma. It is unknown whether abaloparatide will cause osteosarcoma in humans. Avoid use in pts at risk for osteosarcoma (e.g., pts with Paget's disease of bone or unexplained elevations of alkaline phosphatase, pediatric and young adults with open epiphyses, pts with bone metastasis or skeletal malignancies, hereditary disorders predisposing to osteosarcoma, or prior history of external beam or implant radiation involving the skeleton. Cumulative use of parathyroid analogs (e.g., teriparatide) for more than 2 yrs during a pt's lifetime is not recommended.
Do not confuse abaloparatide with teriparatide.

◆CLASSIFICATION

PHARMACOTHERAPEUTIC: Parathyroid hormone receptor agonist. **CLINICAL:** Osteoporosis agent.

USES

Treatment of postmenopausal women with osteoporosis at high risk for fracture, defined as history of osteoporotic fracture, multiple risk factors for fracture, or pts who have failed or are intolerant to other osteoporosis therapy.

PRECAUTIONS

Contraindications: Hypersensitivity to abaloparatide. **Cautions:** Pts at risk for hypercalcemia (e.g., hyperparathyroidism, renal impairment, severe dehydration; history of hypercalciuria, urolithiasis). Avoid use in pts at increased risk for osteosarcoma (e.g., pts with Paget's disease of bone or unexplained elevations of alkaline phosphatase, open epiphyses, bone or skeletal malignancies, hereditary disorders predisposing to osteosarcoma, prior radiation therapy involving the skeleton). Not recommended in pts with cumulative use of parathyroid analogs greater than 2 yrs during lifetime.

ACTION

Bone formation predominates at low dose. **Therapeutic Effect:** Increases bone mineral density and bone formation markers, decreasing risk of vertebral and nonvertebral fractures.

PHARMACOKINETICS

Widely distributed. Metabolism not specified. Degraded into small peptides via proteolytic enzymes. Protein binding: 70%. Peak plasma concentration: 0.51 hrs. Excreted primarily in urine. Not expected to be removed by dialysis. **Half-life:** 1.7 hrs.

⏳ LIFESPAN CONSIDERATIONS

Pregnancy/Lactation: Not indicated in females of reproductive potential. Unknown if distributed in breast milk or crosses the placenta. **Children:** Safety and efficacy not established. **Elderly:** No age-related precautions noted.

INTERACTIONS

DRUG: None known. **HERBAL:** None significant. **FOOD:** None known. **LAB VALUES:** May increase serum calcium, uric acid; urine calcium.

AVAILABILITY (Rx)

Prefilled Injector Pens: 3120 mcg/1.56 mL (2000 mcg/mL). Delivers 30 doses of 80 mcg.

ADMINISTRATION/HANDLING

Subcutaneous
• Visually inspect for particulate matter or discoloration. Solution should appear clear, colorless. • Do not use if solution is cloudy, discolored, or if visible particles are observed. • Insert needle subcutaneously into the periumbilical region of the abdomen (avoid a 2-inch area around the navel) and inject solution. • Do not inject into areas of active skin disease or injury such as sunburns, skin rashes, inflammation, skin infections, or active psoriasis. • Do not administer IV or intramuscularly. • Rotate injection sites.
Storage • Refrigerate unused injector pens. • After first use, store at room temperature for up to 30 days. • Do not freeze or expose to heating sources.

INDICATIONS/ROUTES/DOSAGE

Postmenopausal Osteoporosis
SQ: ADULTS, ELDERLY: 80 mcg once daily. Give with supplemental calcium and vitamin D if dietary intake is inadequate.
Dosage in Renal Impairment
No dose adjustment.
Dosage in Hepatic Impairment
Not specified; use caution.

SIDE EFFECTS

Frequent (58%): Injection site reactions (edema, pain, redness). **Occasional (10%–5%):** Dizziness, nausea, headache, palpitations. **Rare (3%–2%):** Fatigue, upper abdominal pain, vertigo.

ADVERSE EFFECTS/TOXIC REACTIONS

May increase risk of osteosarcoma. Hypercalcemia reported in 3% of pts. Tachycardia occurred in 2% of pts (usually within 15 min after injection). Orthostatic hypotension reported in 4% of pts (usually within 4 hrs after injection). Hypercalciuria and urolithiasis reported in 20% and 2% of pts, respectively. Immunogenicity (auto-abaloparatide antibodies) occurred in 49% of pts.

NURSING CONSIDERATIONS

BASELINE ASSESSMENT
Obtain baseline parathyroid hormone level. Screen for risk of osteosarcoma,

hypercalcemia (as listed in Precautions); prior use of parathyroid analogs. Assess pt's willingness to self-inject medication.

INTERVENTION/EVALUATION

Monitor bone mineral density, parathyroid hormone level; serum calcium. Monitor urinary calcium levels, esp. in pts with pre-existing hypercalciuria or active urolithiasis. Due to risk of orthostatic hypotension, administer the first several doses with the pt in the lying or sitting position. Monitor for orthostatic hypotension (dizziness, palpitations, tachycardia, nausea, syncope). If orthostatic hypotension occurs, place pt in supine position. Assess need for calcium, vitamin D supplementation.

PATIENT/FAMILY TEACHING

• Receive the first several injections while lying or sitting down. Slowly go from lying to standing to avoid an unusual drop in blood pressure. Immediately sit or lie down if dizziness, near-fainting, palpitations occur. • Report symptoms of high calcium levels (e.g., constipation, lethargy, nausea, vomiting, weakness); severe bone pain. • An increased heart rate may occur after injection and will usually subside within 6 hrs. • A health care provider will show you how to properly prepare and inject your medication. You must demonstrate correct preparation and injection techniques before using medication at home. • Vitamin D and calcium supplementation may be required if dietary intake is inadequate.

---

abatacept

a-**bay**-ta-sept
(Orencia)
Do not confuse Orencia with Oracea.

◆ CLASSIFICATION

PHARMACOTHERAPEUTIC: Selective T-cell costimulation modulator. **CLINICAL:** Rheumatoid arthritis agent.

USES

Reduction of signs and symptoms, progression of structural damage in adults with moderate to severe rheumatoid arthritis (RA) alone or in combination with other disease-modifying antirheumatic medications. Treatment of active adult psoriatic arthritis. Treatment of moderate to severe active polyarticular juvenile idiopathic arthritis in pts 2 yrs and older. May use alone or in combination with methotrexate. Note: Do not use with anakinra or tumor necrosis factor [TNF] antagonists.

PRECAUTIONS

Contraindications: Hypersensitivity to abatacept. **Cautions:** Chronic, latent, or localized infection; conditions predisposing to infections (diabetes, indwelling catheters, renal failure, open wounds); COPD (higher incidence of adverse effects); elderly, hx recurrent infections.

ACTION

Inhibits T-lymphocyte activation, necessary in the inflammatory cascade leading to joint inflammation and destruction. Blocks production of inflammatory mediators. **Therapeutic Effect:** Induces positive clinical response in adult pts with moderate to severely active RA or juvenile idiopathic arthritis.

PHARMACOKINETICS

Higher clearance with increasing body weight. Age, gender do not affect clearance. **Half-life:** 8–25 days.

⌛ LIFESPAN CONSIDERATIONS

Pregnancy/Lactation: Crosses placenta; unknown if distributed in breast milk. **Children:** Safety and efficacy not established in pts younger than 6 yrs. **Elderly:** Cautious use due to increased risk of serious infection and malignancy.

INTERACTIONS

DRUG: May increase risk of infection, decrease efficacy of immune response associated with **live vaccines** (do not give concurrently or within 2 mos of stopping abatacept). **Tumor necrosis factor (TNF) antagonists (adalimumab, etanercept, inFLIXimab)** may increase risk of infection. **HERBAL:** Echinacea may decrease concentration/effects. **FOOD:** None known. **LAB VALUES:** None significant.

AVAILABILITY (Rx)

IV Injection, Powder for Reconstitution: 250 mg. **Subcutaneous Injection, Solution:** 50 mg/0.4 mL, 87.5 mg/0.7 mL, 125 mg/mL single-dose prefilled syringe.

ADMINISTRATION/HANDLING

 IV

Reconstitution • Reconstitute each vial with 10 mL Sterile Water for Injection using the silicone-free syringe provided with each vial and an 18- to 21-gauge needle. • Rotate solution gently to prevent foaming until powder is completely dissolved. • From a 100-mL 0.9% NaCl infusion bag, withdraw and discard an amount equal to the volume of the reconstituted vials (for 2 vials remove 20 mL, for 3 vials remove 30 mL, for 4 vials remove 40 mL), resulting in final volume of 100 mL. • Slowly add the reconstituted solution from each vial into the infusion bag using the same syringe provided with each vial. • Concentration in the infusion bag will be 10 mg/mL or less abatacept.
Rate of Administration • Infuse over 30 min using a 0.2 to 1.2 micron low protein-binding filter.
Storage • Store vials, prefilled syringes in refrigerator. • Any reconstitution that has been prepared by using siliconized syringes will develop translucent particles and must be discarded. • Solution should appear clear and colorless to pale yellow. Discard if solution is discolored or contains precipitate. • Solution is stable for up to 24 hrs after reconstitution.

• Reconstituted solution may be stored at room temperature or refrigerated.

Subcutaneous
• Allow syringe to warm to room temperature (30–60 min). • Inject in front of thigh, outer areas of upper arms, or abdomen. • Avoid areas that are tender, bruised, red, scaly, or hard. • Do not rub injection site. • Rotate injection sites.

▨ IV INCOMPATIBILITY

Do not infuse concurrently in same IV line as other agents.

INDICATIONS/ROUTES/DOSAGE

Note: Discontinue in pts developing serious infection.

Rheumatoid Arthritis (RA), Psoriatic Arthritis
IV: BODY WEIGHT 101 KG OR MORE: 1 g (4 vials) given as a 30-min infusion. Following initial therapy, give at 2 wks and 4 wks after first infusion, then q4wks thereafter. **BODY WEIGHT 60–100 KG:** 750 mg (3 vials) given as a 30-min infusion. Following initial therapy, give at 2 wks and 4 wks after first infusion, then q4wks thereafter. **BODY WEIGHT 59 KG OR LESS:** 500 mg (2 vials) given as a 30-min infusion. Following initial therapy, give at 2 wks and 4 wks after first infusion, then q4wks thereafter.
Subcutaneous: Following a single IV infusion, 125 mg given within 24 hrs of infusion, then 125 mg once a week (subcutaneous administration may be initiated without an IV loading dose). **Transitioning from IV to SQ:** Give 1st SQ dose instead of next scheduled IV dose.

Juvenile Idiopathic Arthritis
Note: Dose based on body weight at each administration. **IV: CHILDREN 6 YRS AND OLDER, WEIGHING LESS THAN 75 KG:** 10 mg/kg. **CHILDREN WEIGHING 75–100 KG:** 750 mg. **GREATER THAN 100 KG:** 1,000 mg. Following initial therapy, give 2 wks and 4 wks after first infusion, then q4wks thereafter.

Dosage Adjustment for Toxicity
Discontinue in pts developing a serious infection.

Dosage in Renal/Hepatic Impairment
No dose adjustment.

SIDE EFFECTS

Frequent (18%): Headache. **Occasional (9%–6%):** Dizziness, cough, back pain, hypertension, nausea.

ADVERSE EFFECTS/TOXIC REACTIONS

Upper respiratory tract infection, nasopharyngitis, sinusitis, UTI, influenza, bronchitis occur in 5% of pts. Serious infections, including pneumonia, cellulitis, diverticulitis, acute pyelonephritis, occur in 3% of pts. Hypersensitivity reaction (rash, urticaria, hypotension, dyspnea) occurs rarely. May increase risk of malignancies.

NURSING CONSIDERATIONS

BASELINE ASSESSMENT

Assess onset, type, location, duration of pain/inflammation. Inspect appearance of affected joint for immobility, deformities, skin condition. Screen for latent TB infection prior to initiating therapy.

INTERVENTION/EVALUATION

Assess for therapeutic response: relief of pain, stiffness, swelling; increased joint mobility; reduced joint tenderness; improved grip strength. Monitor for hypersensitivity reaction. Diligently screen for infection.

PATIENT/FAMILY TEACHING

• Notify physician if infection, hypersensitivity reaction, infusion-related reaction occurs. • Do not receive live vaccines during treatment or within 3 mos of its discontinuation. • COPD pts must report worsening of respiratory symptoms.

abciximab

ab-**sik**-si-mab
(ReoPro)

◆CLASSIFICATION

PHARMACOTHERAPEUTIC: Glycoprotein IIb/IIIa receptor inhibitor. **CLINICAL:** Antiplatelet; antithrombotic.

USES

Adjunct to aspirin and heparin therapy to prevent cardiac ischemic complications in pts undergoing percutaneous coronary intervention (PCI) and those with unstable angina not responding to conventional medical therapy when PCI is planned within 24 hrs. **OFF-LABEL:** Support PCI during ST-segment elevation myocardial infarction (STEMI).

PRECAUTIONS

Contraindications: Hypersensitivity to abciximab. Active internal bleeding, arteriovenous malformation or aneurysm, CVA with residual neurologic deficit, history of CVA (within the past 2 yrs) or oral anticoagulant use within the past 7 days unless PT is less than 1.2 times control, history of vasculitis, hypersensitivity to murine proteins, intracranial neoplasm, prior IV dextran use before or during percutaneous transluminal coronary angioplasty (PTCA), recent surgery or trauma (within the past 6 wks), recent GI or GU bleeding (within the past 6 wks), thrombocytopenia (less than 100,000/mm^3), and severe uncontrolled hypertension. Concomitant use of another glycoprotein IIb/IIIa inhibitor. **Cautions:** Increased risk of bleeding in pts who weigh less than 75 kg; pts older than 65 yrs; pts with history of GI disease; pts receiving thrombolytics; PTCA in less than 12 hrs of onset of symptoms for acute MI; prolonged PTCA (longer than 70 min); failed PTCA.

ACTION

Binds to GP IIb/IIIa receptor sites on platelets. **Therapeutic Effect:** Inhibits platelet aggregation.

PHARMACOKINETICS

Rapidly cleared from plasma. Initial-phase half-life is less than 10 min; second-phase half-life is 30 min.

⧗ LIFESPAN CONSIDERATIONS

Pregnancy/Lactation: Unknown if distributed in breast milk. **Children:** Safety and efficacy not established. **Elderly:** Increased risk of major bleeding.

INTERACTIONS

DRUG: Alteplase, **apixaban, argatroban,** aspirin, **clopidogrel,** dipyridamole, **ibuprofen, naproxen, rivaroxaban, warfarin** may increase risk of bleeding. **HERBAL:** Glucosamine, herbals with anticoagulant/antiplatelet activity (e.g., ginseng, ginkgo) may increase risk of bleeding. **FOOD:** None known. **LAB VALUES:** Increases activated clotting time (ACT), prothrombin time (PT), activated partial thromboplastin time (aPTT); decreases platelet count.

AVAILABILITY (Rx)

Injection Solution: 2 mg/mL (5-mL vial).

ADMINISTRATION/HANDLING
🖉 IV

Reconstitution • Bolus dose: Withdraw bolus dose into syringe using a 0.2 or 0.5 micron low protein-binding filter. • **Continuous infusion:** Withdraw dose through a 0.2 or 0.5 micron low protein-binding filter and further dilute into 250 mL D₅W or 0.9% NaCl.

Rate of Administration • Bolus given over 1 min.
Administration Precautions • Give in separate IV line; do not add any other medication to infusion. • For bolus injection and continuous infusion, use sterile, nonpyrogenic, low protein-binding 0.2 or 0.22 micron filter.

Storage • Store vials in refrigerator. • Solution appears clear, colorless. • Do not shake. • Prepared solution is stable for 12 hrs. Discard any unused portion left in vial or if preparation contains opaque particles.

▣ IV INCOMPATIBILITY

Administer in separate line; no other medication should be added to infusion solution.

▣ IV COMPATIBILITIES

Adenosine (Adenocard), argatroban, atropine sulfate, bivalirudin (Angiomax), diphenhydrAMINE (Benadryl), fentaNYL (Sublimaze), metoprolol (Lopressor), midazolam (Versed).

INDICATIONS/ROUTES/DOSAGE

Percutaneous Coronary Intervention (PCI)
IV Bolus: ADULTS: 0.25 mg/kg 10–60 min before PCI, then 12-hr IV infusion of 0.125 mcg/kg/min. **Maximum:** 10 mcg/min.

PCI (Unstable Angina)
IV Bolus: ADULTS: 0.25 mg/kg, followed by 18- to 24-hr infusion of 10 mcg/min, ending 1 hr after procedure.

Dosage in Renal/Hepatic Impairment
No dose adjustment.

SIDE EFFECTS

Frequent (16%–12%): Nausea, hypotension. **Occasional (9%):** Vomiting. **Rare (3%):** Bradycardia, confusion, dizziness, pain, peripheral edema, UTI.

ADVERSE EFFECTS/TOXIC REACTIONS

Major bleeding complications may occur. Hypersensitivity reaction may occur. Atrial fibrillation or flutter, pulmonary edema, complete AV block occur occasionally.

NURSING CONSIDERATIONS

BASELINE ASSESSMENT

Concomitant heparin gtt should be discontinued 4 hrs before arterial sheath removal (or per facility protocol). Maintain pt on bed rest for 6–8 hrs following sheath removal or drug discontinuation, whichever is later. Check platelet count, PT, aPTT, PFA before infusion (assess for preexisting blood abnormalities), 2–4 hrs following treatment, and at 24 hrs or before discharge, whichever is first. Check insertion site, distal pulse of affected limb while femoral artery sheath is in place, and then routinely for 6 hrs following femoral artery sheath removal. Minimize need for injections, blood draws, catheters, other invasive procedures.

INTERVENTION/EVALUATION

Monitor ACT, PT, aPTT, platelet count, Hgb, Hct. Stop abciximab and/or heparin infusion if serious bleeding occurs that is uncontrolled by pressure. Observe for mental status changes, headache, stroke-like symptoms, evidence of intracranial hemorrhage. Assess skin for ecchymosis, petechiae, particularly at femoral arterial access, also at catheter insertion, arterial and venous puncture, cutdown, needle sites. Handle pt carefully and as infrequently as possible to prevent bleeding. Do not obtain B/P in lower extremities (possible deep vein thrombi). Assess for decrease in B/P, increase in pulse rate, complaint of abdominal or back pain, evidence of GI hemorrhage. Question for increase in discharge during menses. Assess urinary output for hematuria. Monitor for hematoma. Use care in removing any dressing, tape.

PATIENT/FAMILY TEACHING

• Assess skin for bruising up to 3 days after infusion. • Report signs of bleeding such as bloody stool or urine, nosebleeds. Immediately report symptoms of bleeding into the brain such as confusion, difficulty speaking, headache, one-sided weakness, seizures, vision loss. • Do not take herbal supplements unless approved by physician who originally started therapy.

---

abiraterone

a-bir-a-ter-one
(Zytiga)
Do not confuse Zytiga with Zetia or ZyrTEC.

◆CLASSIFICATION

PHARMACOTHERAPEUTIC: Androgen biosynthesis inhibitor. **CLINICAL:** Antineoplastic.

USES

Treatment of metastatic castration-resistant prostate cancer in combination with predniSONE.

PRECAUTIONS

Contraindications: Hypersensitivity to abiraterone. Use in women who are pregnant or may become pregnant. **Cautions:** History of cardiovascular disease (especially HF, recent MI, or ventricular arrhythmia) due to potential for hypertension, hypokalemia, fluid retention; moderate hepatic impairment; adrenal insufficiency. Avoid use with strong CYP3A4 inducers.

ACTION

Inhibits androgen production in adrenal gland, testes, and prostate tumors. Inhibits formation of testosterone precursors. **Therapeutic Effect:** Lowers serum testosterone to castrate levels.

PHARMACOKINETICS

Protein binding: 99%. Primarily excreted in feces. **Peak plasma concentration:** 2 hrs. **Half-life:** 12 hrs (up to 19 hrs with hepatic impairment).

⧖ LIFESPAN CONSIDERATIONS

Pregnancy/Lactation: Contraindicated in women who are or may become pregnant. **Children:** Safety and efficacy not established. **Elderly:** No age-related precautions noted.

INTERACTIONS

DRUG: May increase concentration/toxicity of **silodosin, tamoxifen, thioridazine, topotecan.** May decrease effect of **clopidogrel, traMADol.** **CYP3A4 inhibitors (e.g., clarithromycin, ketoconazole)** may increase concentration. **CYP3A4 inducers (e.g., carBAMazepine)** may decrease concentration. **HERBAL:** St. John's wort may decrease levels/effects. **FOOD:** Do not give with **food** (no **food** should be consumed for at least 2 hrs before or 1 hr after dose). **LAB VALUES:** May increase serum ALT, AST, bilirubin, triglycerides. May decrease serum potassium, phosphate.

AVAILABILITY (Rx)

🔖 Tablets: 250 mg, 500 mg.

ADMINISTRATION/HANDLING
PO
• Give on empty stomach only (at least 1 hr before or 2 hrs after food). • Give with water. • Administer whole. Do not break, crush, dissolve, or divide tablets. Women who are or may become pregnant should wear gloves if handling the tablets.

INDICATIONS/ROUTES/DOSAGE
◀ **ALERT** ▶ Consider increased dosage of predniSONE during unusual stress or infection. Interrupting predniSONE therapy may induce adrenocorticoid insufficiency.

Metastatic Castration-Resistant Prostate Cancer
PO: ADULTS, ELDERLY: 1,000 mg once daily (with predniSONE 5 mg 2 times/day).

Dosage Modification

Hepatic enzymes greater than upper limit of normal (ULN) (during treatment)

Lab Values	Recommendation
ALT, AST elevations greater than 5 × ULN or bilirubin greater than 3 × ULN with 1,000 mg	Interrupt treatment and restart at 750 mg once ALT, AST less than 2.5 × ULN or bilirubin less than 1.5 × ULN.
ALT, AST elevations greater than 5 × ULN or bilirubin greater than 3 × ULN with 750 mg	Interrupt treatment and restart at 500 mg once ALT, AST less than 2.5 × ULN or bilirubin less than 1.5 × ULN.

If hepatotoxicity occurs at reduced dose of 500 mg daily, discontinue treatment.

Dosage Adjustment for Concomitant Strong CYP3A4 Inducers
Increase abiraterone dose to 1,000 mg twice daily.

Dosage in Renal Impairment
No dose adjustment.

Dosage in Hepatic Impairment
Mild Impairment: No dosage adjustment necessary. **Moderate Impairment:** Reduce dose to 250 mg daily. Discontinue if serum ALT, AST greater than 5 times ULN or serum bilirubin greater than 3 times ULN. **Severe Impairment:** Avoid use.

SIDE EFFECTS

Frequent (30%–26%): Joint swelling/discomfort, peripheral edema, muscle spasm, musculoskeletal pain, hypokalemia. **Occasional (19%–6%):** Hot flashes, diarrhea, UTI, cough, hypertension, urinary frequency, nocturia. **Rare (less than 6%):** Heartburn, upper respiratory tract infection.

ADVERSE EFFECTS/ TOXIC REACTIONS

Mineralocorticoid excess (severe fluid retention, hypokalemia, hypertension) may compromise pts with prior cardiovascular history. Safety not established in pts with left ventricular ejection fraction

 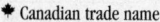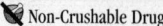

less than 50%. Tachycardia, atrial fibrillation, supraventricular tachycardia, atrial flutter, complete AV block, bradyarrhythmia reported in 7% of pts. Chest pain, unstable angina, HF reported in less than 4% of pts. Stress, infection, or interruption of daily steroids may cause adrenocortical insufficiency. Hepatotoxicity (serum ALT, AST greater than 5 times ULN) reported in 2% of pts. Pts with hepatic impairment are more likely to develop hepatotoxicity.

NURSING CONSIDERATIONS

BASELINE ASSESSMENT

Obtain baseline BMP, LFT. Evaluate history of HF, myocardial infarction, arrhythmias, angina pectoris, peripheral edema, hepatic impairment, adrenal or pituitary abnormalities, left ventricular ejection fraction (if applicable). Question possibility of pregnancy before treatment. Question history of corticosteroid intolerance if applicable.

INTERVENTION/EVALUATION

Assess for peripheral edema behind medial malleolus (sacral area in bedridden patients). Monitor BMP, LFT. Monitor for mineralocorticoid excess (hypokalemia, hypertension, fluid retention) at least once monthly. Assess for cardiac arrhythmia if hypokalemia occurs. Obtain EKG for palpitations, dyspnea, dizziness. Monitor for signs and symptoms of adrenocortical insufficiency during predniSONE interruption, periods of stress, infection. Measure serum ALT, AST, alkaline phosphatase, bilirubin every 2 wks for 3 mos, then monthly. If hepatotoxicity occurs, dosage modification will be necessary. Pts with moderate hepatic impairment must have LFT every wk for first month, then every 2 wks for 2 mos, then monthly. If serum ALT, AST above 5 times ULN or serum bilirubin above 3 times ULN, treatment should be discontinued.

PATIENT/FAMILY TEACHING

• Must be taken on empty stomach (no food 2 hrs before and 1 hr after dose). • If taken with food, toxic levels may result. • Sexually active men must wear condoms during treatment and for 1 wk after treatment. • Women who are pregnant or are planning pregnancy may not touch medication without gloves. • Dizziness, palpitations, headache, confusion, muscle weakness, leg swelling/discomfort may become more apparent during periods of unusual stress, infection, or interruption of predniSONE therapy. • Blood tests will be performed routinely. • Report signs of liver problems (yellowing of skin, bruising, light-colored stool, right upper quadrant pain), chest pain, palpitations. • An increase in urinary frequency or nocturia is expected as treatment becomes therapeutic. • Do not chew, crush, dissolve, or divide tablets.

acetaminophen
TOP 100

a-**seet**-a-**min**-oh-fen
(Abenol ✤, Acephen, Apo-Acetaminophen ✤, Atasol ✤, Feverall, Mapap, Ofirmev, Tempra ✤, Tylenol, Tylenol Arthritis Pain, Tylenol Children's Meltaways, Tylenol Junior Meltaways, Tylenol Extra Strength)

■ **BLACK BOX ALERT** ■ Potential for severe liver injury. Acetaminophen injection associated with acute liver failure.
Do not confuse Acephen with Aciphex, Feverall with Fiberall, Fioricet with Fiorinal, Percocet with Percodan, Tylenol with atenolol, timolol, Tylenol PM, or Tylox, or Vicodin with Hycodan.

FIXED-COMBINATION(S)

Capital with Codeine, Tylenol with Codeine: acetaminophen/codeine: 120 mg/12 mg per 5 mL. **Endocet:** acetaminophen/oxyCODONE: 325 mg/5

mg, 325 mg/7.5 mg, 325 mg/10 mg.
Fioricet: acetaminophen/caffeine/
butalbital: 325 mg/40 mg/50 mg. **Hycet:** acetaminophen/HYDROcodone:
325 mg/7.5 mg per 15 mL. **Norco:**
acetaminophen/HYDROcodone: 325
mg/5 mg, 325 mg/7.5 mg, 325 mg/10
mg. **Percocet:** acetaminophen/oxy-
CODONE: 325 mg/5 mg. **Tylenol with
Codeine:** acetaminophen/codeine:
300 mg/15 mg, 300 mg/30 mg, 300
mg/60 mg. **Ultracet:** acetaminophen/
traMADol: 325 mg/37.5 mg. **Vicodin:** acetaminophen/HYDROcodone:
300 mg/5 mg. **Vicodin ES:**
acetaminophen/HYDROcodone:
300 mg/7.5 mg. **Vicodin HP:**
acetaminophen/HYDROcodone: 300
mg/10 mg. **Xartemis XR:** acetamino-
phen/oxyCODONE: 325 mg/7.5 mg.
Xodol: acetaminophen/HYDROcodone:
300 mg/5 mg, 300 mg/7.5 mg, 300
mg/10 mg.

◆CLASSIFICATION

PHARMACOTHERAPEUTIC: Central
analgesic. **CLINICAL:** Non-narcotic
analgesic, antipyretic.

USES

PO, Rectal: Temporary relief of mild to
moderate pain, headache, fever.
IV: (Additional) Management of moderate to severe pain when combined with
opioid analgesia.

PRECAUTIONS

Contraindications: Hypersensitivity to acetaminophen. (Ofirmev): severe hepatic impairment or severe active liver disease. **Cautions:** Sensitivity to acetaminophen; severe
renal impairment; alcohol dependency, hepatic impairment, or active hepatic disease;
chronic malnutrition and hypovolemia
(Ofirmev); G6PD deficiency (hemolysis
may occur). Limit dose to less than 4 g/day.

ACTION

Appears to inhibit prostaglandin synthesis in the CNS and, to a lesser extent,
block pain impulses through peripheral
action. Acts centrally on hypothalamic
heat-regulating center, producing peripheral vasodilation (heat loss, skin
erythema, diaphoresis). **Therapeutic
Effect:** Results in antipyresis. Produces
analgesic effect.

PHARMACOKINETICS

Route	Onset	Peak	Duration
PO	Less than 60 min	1–3 hrs	4–6 hrs

Rapidly, completely absorbed from GI
tract; rectal absorption variable. Protein
binding: 20%–50%. Widely distributed to
most body tissues. Metabolized in liver.
Excreted in urine. Removed by hemodialysis. **Half-life:** 1–4 hrs (increased
in pts with hepatic disease, elderly, neonates; decreased in children).

⧗ LIFESPAN CONSIDERATIONS

Pregnancy/Lactation: Crosses placenta; distributed in breast milk. Routinely used in all stages of pregnancy; appears safe for short-term use. **Children/
Elderly:** No age-related precautions
noted.

INTERACTIONS

DRUG: Alcohol (chronic use), **hepatotoxic medications (e.g., phenytoin),
hepatic enzyme inducers (e.g., phenytoin, rifAMPin)** may increase risk of
hepatotoxicity with prolonged high dose
or single toxic dose. May increase risk
of bleeding with **warfarin** with chronic,
high-dose use. **HERBAL: St. John's wort**
may decrease blood levels. **FOOD: Food**
may decrease rate of absorption. **LAB
VALUES:** May increase serum ALT, AST,
bilirubin; prothrombin levels (may indicate hepatotoxicity).

AVAILABILITY (OTC)

Caplets: 325 mg, 500 mg, 650 mg.
Elixir: 160 mg/5 mL. **Injection, Solution
(Ofirmev):** 1,000 mg/100 mL glass vial.
Liquid (Oral): 160 mg/5 mL, 500 mg/5 mL,

---

500 mg/15 mL. **Solution (Oral Drops):** 80 mg/0.8 mL. **Suppository:** 80 mg, 120 mg, 325 mg, 650 mg. **Suspension:** 160 mg/5 mL. **Tablets:** 325 mg, 500 mg. **Tablets (Chewable):** 80 mg. **Tablets (Orally Disintegrating):** 80 mg, 160 mg.

 Caplets: (Extended-Release [Tylenol Arthritis Pain]): 650 mg.

ADMINISTRATION/HANDLING

IV

Reconstitution • Does not require further dilution. • Store at room temperature. • Withdraw doses less than 1,000 mg. • Place in separate empty, sterile container.
Rate of Administration • Infuse over 15 min.
Stability • Once opened or transferred, stable for 6 hrs at room temperature.

PO

• Give without regard to meals. • Tablets may be crushed. • Do not crush extended-release caplets. • Suspension: Shake well before use. • Take with full glass of water.

Rectal

• Moisten suppository with cold water before inserting well up into rectum. • Do not freeze suppositories.

INDICATIONS/ROUTES/DOSAGE

Note: Over-the-counter (OTC) use of acetaminophen should be limited to 3,000 mg/day.

Analgesia and Antipyresis
IV: ADULTS, ADOLESCENTS WEIGHING 50 KG OR MORE: 1,000 mg q6h or 650 mg q4h. **Maximum single dose:** 1,000 mg; **maximum total daily dose:** 4,000 mg. **ADULTS, ADOLESCENTS WEIGHING LESS THAN 50 KG:** 15 mg/kg q6h or 12.5 mg/kg q4h. **Maximum single dose:** 750 mg; **maximum total daily dose:** 75 mg/kg/day (3,750 mg). **CHILDREN 2–12 YRS:** 15 mg/ kg q6h or 12.5 mg/kg q4h. **Maximum single dose:** 750 mg. **Maximum:** 75

mg/kg/day, not to exceed 3,750 mg/ day. **INFANTS AND CHILDREN LESS THAN 2 YRS:** 7.5–15 mg/kg q6h. **Maximum:** 60 mg/kg/day. **NEONATES:** (Limited data available) Loading dose: 20 mg/kg. **PMA 37 or greater than 37 wks:** 10 mg/ kg/dose q6h. **Maximum:** 40 mg/kg/ day. **PMA 33–36 wks:** 10 mg/kg/dose q8h. **Maximum:** 40 mg/kg/day. **PMA 28–32 wks:** 10 mg/kg/dose q12h. **Maximum:** 22.5 mg/kg/day.
PO: ADULTS, ELDERLY, CHILDREN 13 YRS AND OLDER: (Regular Strength) 325–650 mg q4–6h. **Maximum:** 3,250 mg/day unless directed by health care provider. (Extra Strength) 1000 mg q6h. **Maximum:** 3,000 mg/day unless directed by health care provider. **CHILDREN 12 YRS AND YOUNGER:** (Weight dosing preferred; if not available, use age. Doses may be repeated q4h. **Maximum:** 5 doses/day.)

Age	Weight (Kg)	Dose
11–12 yrs	32.7–43.2	480 mg
9–10 yrs	27.3–32.6	400 mg
6–8 yrs	21.8–27.2	320 mg
4–5 yrs	16.4–21.7	240 mg
2–3 yrs	10.9–16.3	160 mg
1–<2 yrs	8.2–10.8	120 mg
4–11 mos	5.4–8.1	80 mg
0–3 mos	2.7–5.3	40 mg

NEONATES: Term: 10–15 mg/kg/ dose q4–6h. **Maximum:** 75 mg/kg/day. **GA 33–37 wks or term less than 10 days:** 10–15 mg/kg/dose q6h. **Maximum:** 60 mg/kg/day. **GA: 28–32 wks:** 10–12 mg/kg/dose q6–8h. **Maximum:** 40 mg/kg/day.
Rectal: ADULTS: 325–650 mg q4–6h. **Maximum:** 4 g/24 hrs. **CHILDREN:** 10–20 mg/kg/dose q4–6h as needed. **Maximum:** 5 doses/24 hrs. **NEONATES: Term:** Initially, 30 mg/ kg/once, then 20 mg/kg/dose q6–8h. **Maximum:** 90 mg/kg/day. **GA 33–37 wks or term less than 10 days:** Initially, 30 mg/kg once, then 15 mg/kg/ dose q8h. **Maximum:** 60 mg/kg/day. **GA: 28–32 wks:** 20 mg/kg/dose q12h. **Maximum:** 40 mg/kg/day.

Dosage in Renal Impairment

Creatinine Clearance	Frequency
Oral	
10–50 mL/min	q6h
Less than 10 mL/min	q8h
Continuous renal replacement therapy	q6h
IV	
30 mL/min or less (use caution, decrease daily dose, extend dosing interval)	

Dosage in Hepatic Impairment

Use with caution. IV contraindicated with severe impairment.

SIDE EFFECTS

💚 **Rare:** Hypersensitivity reaction.

ADVERSE EFFECTS/TOXIC REACTIONS

Early Signs of Acetaminophen Toxicity: Anorexia, nausea, diaphoresis, fatigue within first 12–24 hrs. **Later Signs of Toxicity:** Vomiting, right upper quadrant tenderness, elevated LFTs within 48–72 hrs after ingestion. **Antidote:** Acetylcysteine (see Appendix J for dosage).

NURSING CONSIDERATIONS

BASELINE ASSESSMENT

If given for analgesia, assess onset, type, location, duration of pain. Effect of medication is reduced if full pain response recurs prior to next dose. Assess for fever. Assess LFT in pts with chronic usage or history of hepatic impairment, alcohol abuse.

INTERVENTION/EVALUATION

Assess for clinical improvement and relief of pain, fever. **Therapeutic serum level:** 10–30 mcg/mL; **toxic serum level:** greater than 200 mcg/mL. Do not exceed maximum daily recommended dose: 4 g/day.

PATIENT/FAMILY TEACHING

• Consult physician for use in children younger than 2 yrs, oral use longer than 5 days (children) or longer than 10 days (adults), or fever lasting longer than 3 days. • Severe/recurrent pain or high/continuous fever may indicate serious illness. • Do not take more than 4 g/day (3 g/day if using OTC [over-the-counter]). Actual OTC dosing recommendations may vary by product and/or manufacturer. Many nonprescription combination products contain acetaminophen. Avoid alcohol.

acetylcysteine

a-**seet**-il-**sis**-teen
(Acetadote, Cetylev, Mucomyst ♣, Parvolex ♣)
Do not confuse acetylcysteine with acetylcholine, or Mucomyst with Mucinex.

◆CLASSIFICATION

PHARMACOTHERAPEUTIC: Respiratory inhalant, intratracheal. **CLINICAL:** Mucolytic, antidote.

USES

Inhalation: Adjunctive treatment for abnormally viscid mucous secretions present in acute and chronic bronchopulmonary disease and in pulmonary complications of cystic fibrosis and surgery, diagnostic bronchial studies. **Injection, PO:** Antidote in acute acetaminophen toxicity.

PRECAUTIONS

Contraindications: Hypersensitivity to acetylcysteine. **Cautions:** Pts with bronchial asthma; debilitated pts with severe respiratory insufficiency (increases risk of anaphylactoid reaction).

ACTION

Mucolytic splits linkage of mucoproteins, reducing viscosity of pulmonary secretions. Acetaminophen toxicity: Hepatoprotective by restoring hepatic glutathione and enhancing nontoxic conjugation of acetaminophen. **Therapeutic Effect:** Facilitates removal of pulmonary secretions by coughing, postural drainage, mechanical means. Protects against acetaminophen overdose-induced hepatotoxicity.

⧖ LIFESPAN CONSIDERATIONS

Pregnancy/Lactation: Unknown if distributed in breast milk. **Children/Elderly:** No age-related precautions noted.

INTERACTIONS

DRUG: None significant. **HERBAL:** None significant. **FOOD:** None known. **LAB VALUES:** None significant.

AVAILABILITY (Rx)

Inhalation Solution (Mucomyst): 10% (100 mg/mL), 20% (200 mg/mL). **Injection Solution (Acetadote):** 20% (200 mg/mL). **Tablets, Effervescent:** 500 mg, 2.5 g.

ADMINISTRATION/HANDLING

 IV

The total dose is 300 mg/kg administered over 21 hrs. Dose preparation is based on pt weight. Total volume administered should be adjusted for pts less than 40 kg and for pts requiring fluid restriction. Store unopened vials at room temperature. Following dilution in D₅W, solution is stable for 24 hrs at room temperature. Color change of opened vials may occur (does not affect potency).

Three-Bag Method (as Antidote): Loading, Second, and Third Doses, Pts Greater Than or Equal to 40 kg:
Loading dose: 150 mg/kg in 200 mL of diluent administered over 60 min.
Second dose: 50 mg/kg in 500 mL of diluent administered over 4 hrs.
Third dose: 100 mg/kg in 1,000 mL of diluent administered over 16 hrs.

Pts Greater Than 20 kg but Less Than 40 kg:
Loading dose: 150 mg/kg in 100 mL of diluent administered over 60 min.

Second dose: 50 mg/kg in 250 mL of diluent administered over 4 hrs.
Third dose: 100 mg/kg in 500 mL of diluent administered over 16 hrs.

Pts Less Than or Equal to 20 kg:
Loading dose: 150 mg/kg in 3 mL/kg of body weight of diluent administered over 60 min.
Second dose: 50 mg/kg in 7 mL/kg of body weight of diluent administered over 4 hrs.
Third dose: 100 mg/kg in 14 mL/kg of body weight of diluent administered over 16 hrs.

PO
• For treatment of acetaminophen overdose. • Give as 5% solution. • Dilute 20% solution 1:3 with cola, orange juice, other soft drink. • Give within 1 hr of preparation.

Inhalation, Nebulization
• 20% solution may be diluted with 0.9% NaCl or sterile water; 10% solution may be used undiluted.

▦ IV COMPATIBILITIES

Cefepime (Maxipime), cefTAZidime (Fortaz).

INDICATIONS/ROUTES/DOSAGE

Bronchopulmonary Disease
Inhalation, Nebulization
◀**ALERT**▶ Bronchodilators should be given 10–15 min before acetylcysteine. **ADULTS, ELDERLY, CHILDREN:** 3–5 mL (20% solution) 3–4 times/day or 6–10 mL (10% solution) 3–4 times/day. Range: 1–10 mL (20% solution) q2–6h or 2–20 mL (10% solution) q2–6h. **INFANTS:** 1–2 mL (20%) or 2–4 mL (10%) 3–4 times/day.
Intratracheal: ADULTS, CHILDREN: 1–2 mL of 10% or 20% solution instilled into tracheostomy q1–4h.

Acetaminophen Overdose
◀**ALERT**▶ It is essential to initiate treatment as soon as possible after over-

dose and, in any case, within 24 hrs of ingestion.

PO *(Effervescent Tablets, Oral Solution 5%):* **ADULTS, ELDERLY, CHILDREN:** Loading dose of 140 mg/kg, followed in 4 hrs by maintenance dose of 70 mg/kg q4h for 17 additional doses (or until acetaminophen assay reveals nontoxic level). Repeat dose if emesis occurs within 1 hr of administration.

IV: ADULTS, ELDERLY, CHILDREN: (Consists of 3 doses. Total Dose: 300 mg/kg.) 150 mg/kg infused over 60 min, then 50 mg/kg infused over 4 hrs, then 100 mg/kg infused over 16 hrs (see Administration/Handling for dilution). **GREATER THAN 100 KG:** (Consists of 3 doses. Total Dose: 30 g.) 15 g over 60 min; 5 g over 4 hrs; 10 g over 16 hrs. Duration of administration may vary depending on acetaminophen levels and LFTs obtained during treatment. Pts who still have detectable levels of acetaminophen or elevated LFT results continue to benefit from additional acetylcysteine administration beyond 24 hrs.

Diagnostic Bronchial Studies
Inhalation, Nebulization: ADULTS: 1–2 mL of 20% solution or 2–4 mL of 10% solution 2–3 times before the procedure.

SIDE EFFECTS

IV: (10%): Nausea, vomiting. **(7%–6%):** Acute flushing, erythema. **(4%):** Pruritus. **Frequent: Inhalation:** Stickiness on face, transient unpleasant odor. **Occasional: Inhalation:** Increased bronchial secretions, throat irritation, nausea, vomiting, rhinorrhea. **Rare: Inhalation:** Rash. **PO:** Facial edema, bronchospasm, wheezing, nausea, vomiting.

ADVERSE EFFECTS/ TOXIC REACTIONS

Large doses may produce severe nausea/vomiting. **(Less than 2%):** Serious anaphylactoid reactions including cough, wheezing, stridor, respiratory distress, bronchospasm, hypotension, and death

have been known to occur with IV administration.

NURSING CONSIDERATIONS

BASELINE ASSESSMENT

Mucolytic: Assess pretreatment respirations for rate, depth, rhythm. **IV antidote:** Obtain baseline LFT, PT/INR and drug screen. For use as antidote, obtain acetaminophen level to determine need for treatment with acetylcysteine.

INTERVENTION/EVALUATION

If bronchospasm occurs, discontinue treatment, notify physician; bronchodilator may be added to therapy. Monitor rate, depth, rhythm, type of respiration (abdominal, thoracic). Observe sputum for color, consistency, amount. **IV antidote:** Administer within 8 hrs of acetaminophen ingestion for maximal hepatic protection; ideally, within 4 hrs after immediate-release and 2 hrs after liquid acetaminophen formulations.

PATIENT/FAMILY TEACHING

• Slight, disagreeable sulfuric odor from solution may be noticed during initial administration but disappears quickly. • Adequate hydration is important part of therapy. • Follow guidelines for proper coughing and deep breathing techniques. • Auscultate lung sounds.

acyclovir

a-**sye**-klo-veer
(Apo-Acyclovir ✦, Zovirax)
Do not confuse acyclovir with ganciclovir, Retrovir, or valACYclovir, or Zovirax with Doribax, Valtrex, Zithromax, Zostrix, Zyloprim, or Zyvox.

FIXED-COMBINATION(S)

Lipsovir: acyclovir/hydrocortisone (a steroid): 5%/1%.

 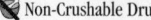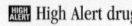

◆CLASSIFICATION

PHARMACOTHERAPEUTIC: Synthetic nucleoside. **CLINICAL:** Antiviral.

USES

Parenteral
Treatment of initial and prophylaxis of recurrent mucosal and cutaneous herpes simplex virus (HSV-1 and HSV-2) in immunocompromised pts. Treatment of severe initial episodes of herpes genitalis in immunocompetent pts. Treatment of herpes simplex encephalitis including neonatal herpes simplex virus. Treatment of herpes zoster (shingles) in immunocompromised pts.

Oral
Treatment of initial episodes and prophylaxis of recurrent herpes simplex (HSV-2 genital herpes). Treatment of chickenpox (varicella). Acute treatment of herpes zoster (shingles). **OFF-LABEL:** (Parenteral/Oral): Prevention of HSV reactivation in HIV-positive pts; hematopoietic stem cell transplant (HSCT); during periods of neutropenia in pts with cancer; prevention of VZV reactivation in allogenic HSCT; treatment of disseminated HSC or VZV in immunocompromised pts with cancer; empiric treatment of suspected encephalitis in immunocompromised pts with cancer; treatment of initial and prophylaxis of recurrent mucosal and cutaneous herpes simplex infections in immunocompromised pts.

Topical
Cream: Treatment of recurrent herpes labialis (cold sores) in immunocompetent pts. **Ointment:** Management of initial genital herpes. Treatment of mucocutaneous HSV in immunocompromised pts.

PRECAUTIONS

Contraindications: Use in neonates when acyclovir is reconstituted with Bacteriostatic Water for Injection containing benzyl alcohol. Hypersensitivity to acyclovir, valACYclovir. **Cautions:** Immunocompromised pts (thrombocytopenic purpura/hemolytic uremic syndrome reported); elderly, renal impairment, use of other nephrotoxic medications. IV Use: Pts with underlying neurologic abnormalities, serious hepatic/electrolyte abnormalities, substantial hypoxia.

ACTION

Converts to acyclovir triphosphate, which competes for viral DNA polymerase, becoming part of DNA chain. **Therapeutic Effect:** Interferes with DNA synthesis and viral replication. Virustatic.

PHARMACOKINETICS

15%–30% absorbed from GI tract. Bioavailability: 10%–20%; minimal absorption following topical application. Protein binding: 9%–36%. Widely distributed. Partially metabolized in liver. Excreted primarily in urine. Removed by hemodialysis. **Half-life:** 2.5 hrs (increased in renal impairment).

⧗ LIFESPAN CONSIDERATIONS

Pregnancy/Lactation: Crosses placenta; distributed in breast milk. **Children:** Safety and efficacy not established in pts younger than 2 yrs (younger than 1 yr for IV use). **Elderly:** Age-related renal impairment may require decreased dosage. May experience more neurologic effects (e.g., agitation, confusion, hallucinations).

INTERACTIONS

DRUG: Nephrotoxic medications may increase risk of nephrotoxicity. **HERBAL:** None significant. **FOOD:** None known. **LAB VALUES:** May increase serum ALT, AST, BUN, creatinine.

AVAILABILITY (Rx)

Cream: 5%. **Injection, Powder for Reconstitution:** 500 mg. **Injection, Solution:** 50 mg/mL. **Ointment:** 5%. **Suspension, Oral:** 200 mg/5 mL. **Tablets:** 400 mg, 800 mg. **Tablet (buccal):** 50 mg.

🐾 **Capsules:** 200 mg.

ADMINISTRATION/HANDLING

 IV

Reconstitution • Add 10 mL Sterile Water for Injection to each 500-mg vial (50 mg/mL). Do not use Bacteriostatic Water for Injection containing benzyl alcohol or parabens (will cause precipitate). • Shake well until solution is clear. • Further dilute with at least 100 mL D₅W or 0.9 NaCl. Final concentration should be 7 mg/mL or less. (Concentrations greater than 10 mg/mL increase risk of phlebitis.)

Rate of Administration • Infuse over at least 1 hr (nephrotoxicity due to crystalluria and renal tubular damage may occur with too-rapid rate). • Maintain adequate hydration during infusion and for 2 hrs following IV administration.

Storage • Store vials at room temperature. • Solutions of 50 mg/mL stable for 12 hrs at room temperature; may form precipitate if refrigerated. • IV infusion (piggyback) stable for 24 hrs at room temperature.

PO
• May give without regard to food. • Do not crush/break capsules. • Store capsules at room temperature.

Topical
(Ointment): • Avoid contact with eye. • Use finger cot/rubber glove to prevent autoinoculation.
(Cream): • Apply to cover only cold sores or area with symptoms. • Rub until it disappears.

▦ IV INCOMPATIBILITIES

Aztreonam (Azactam), diltiaZEM (Cardizem), DOBUTamine (Dobutrex), DOPamine (Intropin), levoFLOXacin (Levaquin), meropenem (Merrem IV), ondansetron (Zofran), piperacillin and tazobactam (Zosyn).

▦ IV COMPATIBILITIES

Allopurinol (Alloprim), amikacin (Amikin), ampicillin, ceFAZolin (Ancef), cefotaxime (Claforan), cefTAZidime (Fortaz), cefTRIAXone (Rocephin), cimetidine (Tagamet), clindamycin (Cleocin), diphenhydrAMINE (Benadryl), famotidine (Pepcid), fluconazole (Diflucan), gentamicin, heparin, HYDROmorphone (Dilaudid), imipenem (Primaxin), LORazepam (Ativan), magnesium sulfate, methylPREDNISolone (SOLU), metoclopramide (Reglan), metroNIDAZOLE (Flagyl), morphine, multivitamins, potassium chloride, propofol (Diprivan), raNITIdine (Zantac), vancomycin.

INDICATIONS/ROUTES/DOSAGE

Genital Herpes (Initial Episode)
IV: ADULTS, ELDERLY: 5–10 mg/kg q8h for 2–7 days. Followed with oral therapy to complete at least 10 days of therapy.
PO: ADULTS, ELDERLY, CHILDREN 12 YRS AND OLDER: 200 mg q4h 5 times/day for 10 days or 400 mg 3 times/day for 7–10 days. **CHILDREN YOUNGER THAN 12 YRS:** 40–80 mg/kg/day in 3–4 divided doses for 5–10 days. **Maximum:** 1,200 mg/day.
Topical: ADULTS: (Ointment) ½ inch for 4-inch square surface q3h (6 times/day) for 7 days.

Genital Herpes (Recurrent)
Intermittent Therapy
PO: ADULTS, ELDERLY, CHILDREN 12 YRS AND OLDER: 200 mg q4h 5 times/day for 5 days or 400 mg 3 times/day for 5–10 days or 800 mg 2 times/day for 5 days or 800 mg 3 times/day for 2 days. **CHILDREN YOUNGER THAN 12 YRS:** 20 mg/kg 3 times/day for 5 days. **Maximum:** 400 mg/dose.
Chronic Suppressive Therapy
PO: ADULTS, ELDERLY, CHILDREN 12 YRS AND OLDER: 400 mg 2 times/day for up to 12 mos. **CHILDREN YOUNGER THAN 12 YRS:** 20 mg/kg twice daily. **Maximum:** 400 mg/dose.

Herpes Simplex Mucocutaneous
PO: ADULTS, ELDERLY: 400 mg 5 times/day for 5–10 days. **CHILDREN:** 20 mg/kg 4 times/day for 5–7 days. **Maximum:** 800 mg/dose.

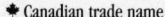 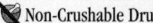

IV: ADULTS, ELDERLY, CHILDREN: 5–10 mg/kg/dose q8h for 7 days.
Topical: ADULTS: (Ointment) ½ inch for 4-inch square surface q3h (6 times/day) for 7 days.

Herpes Simplex Encephalitis
IV: ADULTS, ELDERLY, CHILDREN 12 YRS AND OLDER: 10 mg/kg q8h for 14–21 days. **CHILDREN 3 MOS–YOUNGER THAN 12 YRS:** 15–20 mg/kg q8h for 14–21 days.

Herpes Zoster (Shingles)
IV: ADULTS, CHILDREN 12 YRS AND OLDER: (immunocompromised) 10 mg/kg/dose q8h for 7–10 days. **CHILDREN YOUNGER THAN 12 YRS:** (immunocompromised) 10 mg/kg/dose q8h for 7–10 days.
PO: ADULTS, ELDERLY, CHILDREN 12 YRS AND OLDER: 800 mg q4h 5 times/day for 7–10 days.

Herpes Labialis (Cold Sores)
Topical: ADULTS, ELDERLY, CHILDREN 12 YRS AND OLDER: Apply to affected area 5 times/day for 4 days. **Buccal Tablet:** 50 mg as a single dose to upper gum region.

Varicella-Zoster (Chickenpox)
◀**ALERT**▶ Begin treatment within 24 hrs of onset of rash.
PO: ADULTS, ELDERLY, CHILDREN OLDER THAN 12 YRS AND CHILDREN 2–12 YRS, WEIGHING 40 KG OR MORE: 800 mg 4 times/day for 5 days. **CHILDREN 2–12 YRS, WEIGHING LESS THAN 40 KG:** 20 mg/kg 4 times/day for 5 days. **Maximum:** 800 mg/dose.

Usual Neonatal Dosage
HSV (treatment) (IV): 20 mg/kg/dose q8–12h for 14–21 days.
HSV (chronic suppression) (PO): 300 mg/m²/dose q8h following IV therapy for 6 mos.
Varicella-Zoster (IV): 10 mg/kg/dose q8h for 5–10 days.

Dosage in Renal Impairment
Dosage and frequency are modified based on severity of infection and degree of renal impairment.
PO: Normal dose 200 mg q4h, 200 mg q8h, or 400 mg q12h.
Creatinine clearance 10 mL/min and less: 200 mg q12h.
PO: Normal dose 800 mg q4h.
Creatinine clearance greater than 25 mL/min: Give usual dose and at normal interval, 800 mg q4h. **Creatinine clearance 10–25 mL/min:** 800 mg q8h. **Creatinine clearance less than 10 mL/min:** 800 mg q12h.
IV:

Creatinine Clearance	Dosage
Greater than 50 mL/min	100% of normal q8h
25–50 mL/min	100% of normal q12h
10–24 mL/min	100% of normal q24h
Less than 10 mL/min	50% of normal q24h
Hemodialysis (HD)	2.5–5 mg/kg q24h (give after HD)
Peritoneal dialysis (PD)	50% normal dose q24h
Continuous renal replacement therapy (CRRT)	5–10 mg/kg q12–24h (q12h for viral meningo-encephalitis/VZV infection)

Dosage in Hepatic Impairment
Mild to Moderate Impairment: No dose adjustment. **Severe Impairment:** Use caution.

SIDE EFFECTS
Frequent: Parenteral (9%–7%): Phlebitis or inflammation at IV site, nausea, vomiting. **Topical (28%):** Burning, stinging. **Occasional: Parenteral (3%):** Pruritus, rash, urticaria. **PO (12%–6%):** Malaise, nausea. **Topical (4%):** Pruritus. **Rare: PO (3%–1%):** Vomiting, rash, diarrhea, headache. **Parenteral (2%–1%):** Confusion, hallucinations, seizures, tremors. **Topical (less than 1%):** Rash.

ADVERSE EFFECTS/ TOXIC REACTIONS

Rapid parenteral administration, excessively high doses, or fluid and electrolyte imbalance may produce renal failure. Toxicity not reported with oral or topical use.

NURSING CONSIDERATIONS

BASELINE ASSESSMENT

Question for history of allergies, esp. to acyclovir. Assess herpes simplex lesions before treatment to compare baseline with treatment effect.

INTERVENTION/EVALUATION

Assess IV site for phlebitis (heat, pain, red streaking over vein). Evaluate cutaneous lesions. Ensure adequate ventilation. Manage chickenpox and disseminated herpes zoster with strict isolation. Encourage fluid intake.

PATIENT/FAMILY TEACHING

• Drink adequate fluids. • Do not touch lesions with bare fingers to prevent spreading infection to new site. • Continue therapy for full length of treatment. • Space doses evenly. • Use finger cot/rubber glove to apply topical ointment. • Avoid sexual intercourse during duration of lesions to prevent infecting partner. • Acyclovir does not cure herpes infections. • Pap smear should be done at least annually due to increased risk of cervical cancer in women with genital herpes.

---

adalimumab

a-da-**lim**-ue-mab
(Cyltezo, <u>Humira</u>)

■ **BLACK BOX ALERT** ■ Increased risk for serious infections. Tuberculosis, invasive fungal infections, bacterial and viral opportunistic infections have occurred. Test for tuberculosis prior to and during treatment. Lymphoma, other malignancies reported in children/ adolescents. Hepatosplenic T-cell lymphoma reported primarily in pts with Crohn's disease or ulcerative colitis and concomitant azaTHIO-prine or mercaptopurine.
Do not confuse Humira with HumaLOG or HumuLIN, or adalimumab with belimumab or ipilimumab.

◆CLASSIFICATION

PHARMACOTHERAPEUTIC: Monoclonal antibody. **CLINICAL:** Rheumatoid arthritis agent.

USES

Reduces signs/symptoms, progression of structural damage and improves physical function in adults with moderate to severe RA. May be used alone or in combination with other disease-modifying antirheumatic drugs. First-line treatment of moderate to severe RA, treatment of psoriatic arthritis, treatment of ankylosing spondylitis, to induce/maintain remission of moderate to severe active Crohn's disease, moderate to severe plaque psoriasis in pts 6 yrs of age and older. Reduces signs and symptoms of moderate to severe active polyarticular juvenile rheumatoid arthritis in pts 2 yrs and older. Treatment of active ulcerative colitis in pts unresponsive to immunosuppressants. Treatment of moderate to severe hidradenitis suppurativa. Treatment of uveitis (non-infectious intermediate, posterior and panuveitis) in adults.

PRECAUTIONS

Contraindications: Hypersensitivity to adalimumab. Severe infections (e.g., sepsis, TB). **Cautions:** Pts with chronic infections or pts at risk for infections (e.g., diabetes, indwelling catheters, renal failure, open wounds), elderly, decreased left ventricular function, HF, demyelinating disorders, invasive fungal infections, history of malignancies.

  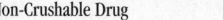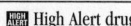

ACTION

Binds specifically to tumor necrosis factor (TNF) alpha cell, blocking its interaction with cell surface TNF receptors. **Therapeutic Effect:** Decreases signs/symptoms of RA, psoriatic arthritis, ankylosing spondylitis, Crohn's disease, ulcerative colitis. Inhibits progression of rheumatoid and psoriatic arthritis. Reduces epidermal thickness, inflammation of plaque psoriasis.

PHARMACOKINETICS

Metabolism not specified. Elimination not specified. **Half-life:** 10–20 days.

⧗ LIFESPAN CONSIDERATIONS

Pregnancy/Lactation: Unknown if distributed in breast milk. **Children:** Safety and efficacy not established. **Elderly:** Cautious use due to increased risk of serious infection and malignancy.

INTERACTIONS

DRUG: Abatacept, anakinra, immunosuppressive therapy may increase risk of infections. May decrease efficacy of immune response with **live vaccines** (should not give concurrently). **HERBAL: Echinacea** may decrease effects. **FOOD:** None known. **LAB VALUES:** May increase serum cholesterol, other lipids, alkaline phosphatase.

AVAILABILITY (Rx)

Injection Solution: 10 mg/0.2 mL, 20 mg/0.4 mL, 40 mg/0.8 mL in prefilled syringes.

ADMINISTRATION/HANDLING

Subcutaneous
• Refrigerate; do not freeze. • Discard unused portion. • Rotate injection sites. Give new injection at least 1 inch from an old site and never into area where skin is tender, bruised, red, or hard. • Give in thigh or lower abdomen. • Avoid areas within 2 inches of navel.

INDICATIONS/ROUTES/DOSAGE

Rheumatoid Arthritis (RA)
Subcutaneous: ADULTS, ELDERLY: 40 mg every other wk. Dose may be increased to 40 mg/wk in pts not taking methotrexate.

Ankylosing Spondylitis, Psoriatic Arthritis
Subcutaneous: ADULTS, ELDERLY: 40 mg every other wk.

Crohn's Disease
Subcutaneous: ADULTS, ELDERLY, CHILDREN 6 YRS AND OLDER WEIGHING 40 KG OR MORE: Initially, 160 mg given as 4 injections on day 1 or 2 injections/day over 2 days, then 80 mg 2 wks later (day 15). **Maintenance:** 40 mg every other wk beginning at day 29. **CHILDREN 6 YRS AND OLDER WEIGHING 17–39 KG:** 80 mg (2 40-mg injections on day 1), then 40 mg 2 wks later. **Maintenance:** 20 mg every other wk beginning at day 29.

Plaque Psoriasis, Uveitis
Subcutaneous: ADULTS, ELDERLY: Initially, 80 mg as a single dose, then 40 mg every other wk starting 1 wk after initial dose.

Juvenile Rheumatoid Arthritis
Subcutaneous: CHILDREN 2 YRS AND OLDER, WEIGHING 10–14 KG: 10 mg every other wk. **WEIGHING 15–29 KG:** 20 mg every other wk. **WEIGHING 30 KG OR MORE:** 40 mg every other wk.

Ulcerative Colitis
Subcutaneous: ADULTS, ELDERLY: Initially, 160 mg (4 injections in 1 day or 2 injections over 2 days) then 80 mg 2 wks later (day 15), then 40 mg every other wk beginning on day 29.

Hidradenitis Suppurativa
Subcutaneous: ADULTS, ELDERLY: Initially, 160 mg (4 injections day 1) or 80 mg (2 injections on days 1 and 2), then 80 mg 2 wks later (day 15), then 40 mg weekly beginning day 29.

Dosage in Renal/Hepatic Impairment
No dose adjustment.

SIDE EFFECTS

Frequent (20%): Injection site erythema, pruritus, pain, swelling. **Occasional (12%–9%):** Headache, rash, sinusitis, nausea. **Rare (7%–5%):** Abdominal or back pain, hypertension.

ADVERSE EFFECTS/ TOXIC REACTIONS

Hypersensitivity reactions (rash, urticaria, hypotension, dyspnea), infections (primarily upper respiratory tract, bronchitis, urinary tract) occur rarely. May increase risk of serious infections (pneumonia, tuberculosis, cellulitis, pyelonephritis, septic arthritis). May increase risk of reactivation of hepatitis B virus in pts who are chronic carriers. May cause new–onset or exacerbation of central nervous demyelinating disease; worsening and new–onset HF. May increase risk of malignancies. Immunogenicity (anti-adalimumab autoantibodies) occured in 12% of pts.

NURSING CONSIDERATIONS

BASELINE ASSESSMENT

Assess onset, type, location, duration of pain or inflammation. Inspect appearance of affected joints for immobility, deformities, skin condition. Review immunization status/screening for TB. If pt is to self-administer, instruct on subcutaneous injection technique, including areas of the body acceptable for injection sites.

INTERVENTION/EVALUATION

Monitor lab values, particularly CBC. Assess for therapeutic response: relief of pain, stiffness, swelling; increased joint mobility; reduced joint tenderness; improved grip strength.

PATIENT/FAMILY TEACHING

• Injection site reaction generally occurs in first month of treatment and decreases in frequency during continued therapy. • Do not receive live vaccines during treatment. • Report rash, nausea. • A health care provider will show you how to properly prepare and inject your medication. You must demonstrate correct preparation and injection techniques before using medication.

adefovir

a-**def**-o-veer
(Hepsera)

■ **BLACK BOX ALERT** ■ May cause HIV resistance in unrecognized or untreated HIV infection. Lactic acidosis, severe hepatomegaly with steatosis (fatty liver), acute exacerbation of hepatitis have occurred. Use with caution in pts with renal dysfunction or in pts at risk for renal toxicity.

◆CLASSIFICATION

PHARMACOTHERAPEUTIC: Antiviral. **CLINICAL:** Hepatitis B agent.

USES

Treatment of chronic hepatitis B virus infection in adults with evidence of active viral replication based on persistent elevations of serum ALT or AST or histologic evidence.

PRECAUTIONS

Contraindications: Hypersensitivity to adefovir. **Cautions:** Pts with known risk factors for hepatic disease (female gender, obesity, prolonged treatment), renal impairment, elderly. Concurrent administration with tenofovir-containing products.

ACTION

Interferes with hepatitis B viral RNA-dependent DNA polymerase, an enzyme, causing DNA chain termination after its incorporation into viral DNA. **Therapeutic Effect:** Prevents viral cell replication.

PHARMACOKINETICS

Rapidly converted to adefovir in intestine. Binds to proteins after PO administration. Protein binding: less than 4%. Excreted

---

 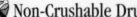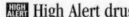

in urine. **Half-life:** 7 hrs (increased in renal impairment).

⧗ LIFESPAN CONSIDERATIONS

Pregnancy/Lactation: Unknown if drug crosses placenta or is distributed in breast milk. **Children:** Safety and efficacy not established. **Elderly:** Age-related renal impairment, decreased cardiac function require cautious use.

INTERACTIONS

DRUG: Nephrotoxic agents (e.g., **IV contrast dye, cyclosporine, gentamicin, vancomycin), NSAIDs** may increase risk of renal toxicity. May alter effects of **tenofovir** (avoid concomitant use). **HERBAL:** None significant. **FOOD: Alcohol** may increase risk of hepatotoxicity. **LAB VALUES:** May increase serum ALT, AST, amylase.

AVAILABILITY (Rx)

Tablets: 10 mg.

ADMINISTRATION/HANDLING

PO
• Give without regard to food.

INDICATIONS/ROUTES/DOSAGE

Note: Continue for 6 months or longer after HBeAg seroconversion.

Chronic Hepatitis B (Normal Renal Function)
PO: **ADULTS, ELDERLY, CHILDREN 12 YRS AND OLDER:** 10 mg once daily.

Chronic Hepatitis B (Impaired Renal Function)
PO: **ADULTS, ELDERLY WITH CREATININE CLEARANCE 20–49 ML/MIN:** 10 mg q48h. **ADULTS, ELDERLY WITH CREATININE CLEARANCE 10–19 ML/MIN:** 10 mg q72h. **ADULTS, ELDERLY ON HEMODIALYSIS:** 10 mg every 7 days following dialysis.

Dosage in Hepatic Impairment
No adjustment needed.

SIDE EFFECTS

Frequent (13%): Asthenia. **Occasional (9%–4%):** Headache, abdominal pain, nausea, flatulence. **Rare (3%):** Diarrhea, dyspepsia.

ADVERSE EFFECTS/ TOXIC REACTIONS

Nephrotoxicity, characterized by increased serum creatinine and decreased glomerular filtration rate (GFR), is treatment-limiting toxicity of adefovir therapy. Lactic acidosis, severe hepatomegaly occur rarely, particularly in female pts.

NURSING CONSIDERATIONS

BASELINE ASSESSMENT

Obtain baseline renal function lab values before therapy begins and routinely thereafter. Pts with renal insufficiency, preexisting or during treatment, may require dose adjustment. HIV antibody testing should be performed before therapy begins (unrecognized or untreated HIV infection may result in emergence of HIV resistance).

INTERVENTION/EVALUATION

Monitor I&O. Closely monitor for adverse reactions in those taking other medications that are excreted renally or with other drugs known to affect renal function.

PATIENT/FAMILY TEACHING

• Report nausea, vomiting, abdominal pain. • Avoid alcohol. • Do not take over-the-counter anti-inflammatory drugs. • Report decreased urinary output, dark-colored urine.

---

adenosine

ah-**den**-oh-seen
(Adenocard, Adenoscan)

◆CLASSIFICATION

PHARMACOTHERAPEUTIC: Cardiac agent, diagnostic aid. **CLINICAL:** Antiarrhythmic.

USES

Adenocard: Treatment of paroxysmal supraventricular tachycardia (PSVT), including pts associated with accessory bypass tracts (Wolff-Parkinson-White syndrome). **Adenoscan:** Adjunct in diagnosis in myocardial perfusion imaging or stress echocardiography. **OFF-LABEL:** Acute vasodilator testing in pulmonary artery hypertension.

PRECAUTIONS

Contraindications: Hypersensitivity to adenosine. Second- or third-degree AV block, symptomatic bradycardia, sick sinus syndrome (except in pts with functioning pacemaker). Bronchoconstrictive or bronchospastic lung disease, asthma. **Cautions:** Pts with first-degree AV block, bundle branch block; concurrent use of drugs that slow AV conduction (e.g., digoxin, verapamil); autonomic dysfunction, pericarditis, pleural effusion, carotid stenosis, uncorrected hypovolemia; elderly, pts with bronchoconstriction.

ACTION

Slows impulse formation in SA node and conduction time through AV node. Acts as a diagnostic aid in myocardial perfusion imaging or stress echocardiography by causing coronary vasodilation and increased blood flow. **Therapeutic Effect:** Restores normal sinus rhythm.

PHARMACOKINETICS

Rapidly cleared from circulation via cellular uptake. Metabolized via phosphorylation or deamination. **Half-life:** Less than 10 secs.

⌛ LIFESPAN CONSIDERATIONS

Pregnancy/Lactation: Unknown if distributed in breast milk. Do not breastfeed until approved by physician. **Children/Elderly:** No age-related precautions noted.

INTERACTIONS

DRUG: Methylxanthines (e.g., theophylline) may decrease effect. **Dipyridamole, nicotine** may increase effect.

CarBAMazepine may increase degree of heart block caused by adenosine. **HERBAL:** None significant. **FOOD:** Avoid **caffeine** (may decrease effect). **LAB VALUES:** None significant.

AVAILABILITY (Rx)

Injection Solution (Adenocard): 3 mg/mL in 2-mL, 4-mL vials. **Injection Solution (Adenoscan):** 3 mg/mL in 20-mL, 30-mL vials.

ADMINISTRATION/HANDLING

 IV

Rate of Administration • Administer very rapidly (over 1–2 sec) undiluted directly into vein, or if using IV line, use closest port to insertion site. If IV line is infusing any fluid other than 0.9% NaCl, flush line first. • After rapid bolus injection, follow with 0.9% NaCl rapid flush, B/P. **Storage** • Store at room temperature. Solution appears clear. • Crystallization occurs if refrigerated; if crystallization occurs, dissolve crystals by warming to room temperature. • Discard unused portion.

⊞ IV INCOMPATIBILITIES

Any drug or solution other than 0.9% NaCl, D_5W, Ringer's lactate, or abciximab.

INDICATIONS/ROUTES/DOSAGE

Paroxysmal Supraventricular Tachycardia (PSVT) (Adenocard)
Rapid IV Bolus: ADULTS, ELDERLY, CHILDREN WEIGHING 50 KG OR MORE: Initially, 6 mg given over 1–2 sec. If first dose does not convert within 1–2 min, give 12 mg; may repeat 12-mg dose in 1–2 min if no response has occurred. Follow each dose with 20 mL 0.9% NaCl by rapid IV push. **CHILDREN WEIGHING LESS THAN 50 KG:** Initially 0.05–0.1 mg/kg. (**Maximum:** 6 mg). If first dose does not convert within 1–2 min, may increase dose by 0.05–0.1 mg/kg. May repeat until sinus rhythm is established or up to a maximum single dose of 0.3 mg/kg or 12 mg. Follow each dose with 5–10 mL 0.9% NaCl by rapid IV push.

  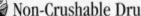

Diagnostic Testing (Adenoscan)
IV Infusion: ADULTS: 140 mcg/kg/min for 6 min using syringe or infusion pump. Total dose: 840 mcg/kg. Thallium is injected at midpoint (3 min) of infusion.

Dosage in Renal/Hepatic Impairment
No dose adjustment.

SIDE EFFECTS

Frequent (18%–12%): Facial flushing, dyspnea. **Occasional (7%–2%):** Headache, nausea, light-headedness, chest pressure. **Rare (1% or less):** Paresthesia, dizziness, diaphoresis, hypotension, palpitations; chest, jaw, or neck pain.

ADVERSE EFFECTS/ TOXIC REACTIONS

Frequently produces transient, short-lasting heart block.

NURSING CONSIDERATIONS

BASELINE ASSESSMENT

Identify arrhythmia per cardiac monitor, 12-lead EKG, and assess apical pulse, B/P.

INTERVENTION/EVALUATION

Assess cardiac performance per continuous EKG. Monitor B/P, apical pulse (rate, rhythm, quality). Monitor respiratory rate. Monitor serum electrolytes.

PATIENT/FAMILY TEACHING

• May induce feelings of impending doom, which resolves quickly. • Flushing/headache may occur temporarily following administration. • Report continued chest pain, light-headedness, head or neck pain, difficulty breathing.

ado-trastuzumab emtansine

ado-tras-**tooz**-oo-mab
(Kadcyla)
■ **BLACK BOX ALERT** ■ Do not substitute ado-trastuzumab for trastuzumab. Hepatotoxicity,

hepatic failure may lead to death. Monitor hepatic function prior to each dose. May decrease left ventricular ejection fraction (LVEF). Embryo-fetal toxicity may result in birth defects and/or fetal demise.
Do not confuse ado-trastuzumab with trastuzumab.

◆CLASSIFICATION

PHARMACOTHERAPEUTIC: HER2-targeted antibody and microtubule inhibitor conjugate. **CLINICAL:** Antineoplastic.

USES

Treatment of HER2-positive, metastatic breast cancer in pts who have previously received trastuzumab and a taxane agent separately or in combination, or pts who have developed recurrence within 6 mos of completing adjuvant therapy.

PRECAUTIONS

Contraindications: Hypersensitivity to trastuzumab. **Cautions:** History of cardiomyopathy, HF, MI, arrhythmias, hepatic disease, thrombocytopenia, pulmonary disease, peripheral neuropathy, pregnancy.

ACTION

Inhibits proliferation of tumor cells that overexpress human epidermal growth factor receptor 2 (HER2). Promotes cellular death (apoptosis) by mediating release of cytotoxic catabolytes. Disrupts cellular microtubule networks. **Therapeutic Effect:** Inhibits tumor cell survival in HER2-positive breast cancer.

PHARMACOKINETICS

Metabolized in liver. Protein binding: 93%. Peak plasma concentration: 30–90 min. **Half-life:** 4 days.

⌛ LIFESPAN CONSIDERATIONS

Pregnancy/Lactation: May cause fetal harm. Use contraception during treatment and up to 6 mos after discontinuation. Unknown if distributed in breast milk. Do not breastfeed. **Children:** Safety and efficacy not established. **Elderly:** No age-related precautions noted.

INTERACTIONS

DRUG: CYP3A4 inhibitors (e.g., ketoconazole, ritonavir) may increase concentration/effect. **HERBAL:** None significant. **FOOD:** None known. **LAB VALUES:** May increase serum ALT, AST, bilirubin. May decrease platelets, serum potassium.

AVAILABILITY (Rx)

Lyophilized Powder for Injection: 100-mg vial, 160-mg vial.

ADMINISTRATION/HANDLING

◀ALERT▶ Use 0.22-micron in-line filter. Do not administer IV push or bolus.

 IV

Reconstitution • Use proper chemotherapy precautions. • Slowly inject 5 mL of Sterile Water for Injection into 100-mg vial or 8 mL Sterile Water for Injection for 160-mg vial. • Final concentration: 20 mg/mL. • Gently swirl until completely dissolved. • Do not shake. • Inspect for particulate matter/discoloration. • Calculate dose from 20 mg/mL vial. • Further dilute in 250 mL of 0.9% NaCl only. • Invert bag to mix (do not shake).

Rate of Administration • Infuse using 0.22-micron in-line filter. • Infuse initial dose over 90 min. • Infuse subsequent doses over 30 min. • Slow or interrupt infusion rate if hypersensitivity reaction occurs.

Storage • Refrigerate unused vials. • Reconstituted vials, diluted solutions should be used immediately (may be refrigerated for up to 24 hrs).

▦ IV INCOMPATIBILITIES

Do not use dextrose-containing solutions.

INDICATIONS/ROUTES/DOSAGE

Note: Do not substitute with conventional trastuzumab (Herceptin).

Metastatic Breast Cancer
IV Infusion: ADULTS/ELDERLY: 3.6 mg/kg every 3 wks until disease progression or unacceptable toxicity.

Dose Modification
Reduction Schedule for Adverse Effects:
Initial dose: 3.6 mg/kg. First reduction: 3 mg/kg. Second reduction: 2.4 mg/kg. **Elevated Serum ALT, AST:** If less than 5 times upper limit of normal (ULN), continue same dose. If 5–20 times ULN, hold until less than 5 times ULN and reduce by one dose level. If greater than 20 times ULN, discontinue. **Elevated Serum Bilirubin:** Hold until less than 1.5 times ULN, then continue same dose. If 3–10 times ULN, hold until less than 1.5 times ULN, then reduce by one dose level. If greater than 10 times ULN, discontinue. **Left Ventricular Dysfunction:** If LVEF greater than 45%, continue same dose. If LVEF 40%–45% with a decrease less than 10% from baseline, continue dose (or reduce) and repeat LVEF in 3 wks. If LVEF 40%–45% with decrease greater than 10% from baseline, hold and repeat assessment in 3 wks. Discontinue therapy if no recovery within 10% of baseline, LVEF less than 40%, or symptomatic HF. **Thrombocytopenia:** If platelet count is 25,000–50,000 cells/mm³, hold until level greater than 75,000 cells/mm³ and then continue same dose. If platelet count is less than 25,000 cells/mm³, hold until level greater than 75,000 cells/mm³ and reduce one dose level.

Dosage in Renal/Hepatic Impairment
No dose adjustment.

SIDE EFFECTS

Frequent (40%–21%): Nausea, fatigue, musculoskeletal pain, headache, constipation, diarrhea. **Occasional (19%–7%):** Abdominal pain, vomiting, pyrexia, arthralgia, asthenia, cough, dry mouth, stomatitis, myalgia, insomnia, rash, dizziness, dyspepsia, chills, dysgeusia, peripheral edema. **Rare (6%–3%):** Pruritus, blurry vision, dry eye, conjunctivitis, lacrimation.

ADVERSE EFFECTS/ TOXIC REACTIONS

Hepatotoxicity may include elevated transaminase, nodular regenerative hyperplasia, portal hypertension. Left ventricular dysfunction reported in 1.8% of pts. Interstitial lung disease (ILD), including pneumonitis, may lead to ARDS. Hypersensitivity reactions reported in 1.4% of pts. Thrombocytopenia (34% of pts) may increase risk of bleeding. Peripheral neuropathy observed rarely. Approx. 5.3% of pts tested positive for anti–ado-trastuzumab antibodies (immunogenicity).

NURSING CONSIDERATIONS

BASELINE ASSESSMENT

Obtain baseline CBC, BMP; PT/INR if on anticoagulants. Confirm HER2-positive titer. Screen for baseline HF, hepatic impairment, peripheral edema, pulmonary disease, thrombocytopenia. Obtain negative pregnancy test before initiating treatment. Question current breastfeeding status. Obtain baseline echocardiogram for LVEF status.

INTERVENTION/EVALUATION

Observe for hypersensitivity reactions during infusion. Monitor LFT, potassium levels before and during treatment. Obtain LVEF q3mos or with any dose reduction regarding LVEF status. Assess for bruising, jaundice, right upper quadrant (RUQ) abdominal pain. Obtain anti–ado-trastuzumab antibody titer if immunogenicity suspected. Obtain stat EKG for palpitations or irregular pulse, chest X-ray for difficulty breathing, cough, fever. Monitor for neurotoxicity (peripheral neuropathy).

PATIENT/FAMILY TEACHING

• Blood levels will be monitored routinely. • Avoid pregnancy. • Contraception should be used during treatment and up to 6 mos after discontinuation. • Report black/tarry stools, RUQ abdominal pain, nausea, bruising, yellowing of skin or eyes, difficulty breathing, palpitations, bleeding. • Avoid alcohol. • Treatment may reduce the heart's ability to pump; expect routine echocardiograms. • Report bleeding of any kind or extremity numbness, tingling, weakness, pain.

afatinib

a-**fa**-ti-nib
(Gilotrif)
Do not confuse afatinib with ibrutinib, dasatinib, gefitinib, or SUNItinib.

◆CLASSIFICATION

PHARMACOTHERAPEUTIC: Kinase inhibitor. **CLINICAL:** Antineoplastic.

USES

First-line treatment of metastatic non–small cell lung cancer (NSCLC) in pts with epidermal growth factor (EDGF) exon 19 deletions or exon 21 (L858R) substitution mutations. Treatment of metastatic, squamous NSCLC progressing after platinum-based chemotherapy.

PRECAUTIONS

Contraindications: Hypersensitivity to afatinib. **Cautions:** Hepatic impairment; severe renal impairment; pts with hx of keratitis, severe dry eye, ulcerative keratitis, or use of contact lenses; hypovolemia; pulmonary disease; ulcerative lesions. Patients with GI disorders associated with diarrhea (e.g., Crohn's disease), cardiac risk factors, and/or decreased left ventricular ejection fraction.

ACTION

Highly selective blocker of ErbB family (e.g., HER2); irreversibly binds to intracellular tyrosine kinase domain.

Therapeutic Effect: Inhibits tumor growth, causes tumor regression.

PHARMACOKINETICS

Readily absorbed following PO administration. Enzymatic metabolism is minimal. Protein binding: 95%. Peak plasma concentration: 2–5 hrs. Excreted in feces (85%), urine (4%). **Half-life:** 37 hrs.

⏳ LIFESPAN CONSIDERATIONS

Pregnancy/Lactation: May cause fetal harm. Unknown if distributed in breast milk. Must either discontinue drug or discontinue breastfeeding. Contraception recommended during treatment and up to 2 wks after discontinuation. **Children:** Safety and efficacy not established. **Elderly:** No age-related precautions noted.

INTERACTIONS

DRUG: P-glycoprotein inhibitors (e.g., amiodarone, cycloSPORINE, ketoconazole) may increase concentration/effect. **P-glycoprotein inducers (e.g., carBAMazepine, rifAMPin)** may decrease concentration/effect. **HERBAL:** None significant. **FOOD: High-fat meals** may decrease absorption. **LAB VALUES:** May increase serum ALT, AST. May decrease serum potassium.

AVAILABILITY (Rx)

Tablets: 20 mg, 30 mg, 40 mg.

ADMINISTRATION/HANDLING

PO
• Give at least 1 hr before or 2 hrs after meal. Do not take missed dose within 12 hrs of next dose.

INDICATIONS/ROUTES/DOSAGE

Non–Small Cell Lung Cancer
PO: ADULTS/ELDERLY: Initially, 40 mg once daily until disease progression or no longer tolerated. Do not take missed dose within 12 hrs of next dose.

Dose Modification
Chronic Use of P-glycoprotein (P-gp) Inhibitors: Reduce daily dose by 10 mg if tolerated. Resume previous dose after discontinuation of inhibitor if tolerated. **Chronic Use of P-glycoprotein Inducers:** Increase daily dose by 10 mg if tolerated. May resume initial dose 2–3 days after discontinuation of P-gp inducer. **Moderate to Severe Diarrhea (more than 48 hrs):** Withhold dose until resolution to mild diarrhea. **Moderate Cutaneous Skin Reaction (more than 7 days):** Withhold dose until reaction resolves, then reduce dose appropriately. **Suspected Keratitis:** Withhold until appropriately ruled out. If keratitis confirmed, continue only if benefits outweigh risks.

Permanent Discontinuation
Discontinue if persistent severe diarrhea, respiratory distress, severe dry eye, or life-threatening bullous, blistering, exfoliating lesions, persistent ulcerative keratitis, interstitial lung disease, symptomatic left ventricular dysfunction occurs.

Dosage in Renal/Hepatic Impairment
eGFR 15–29 mL/min: Decrease dose to 30 mg. **Severe Impairment:** Avoid use.

SIDE EFFECTS

Frequent (96%–58%): Diarrhea, rash, dermatitis, stomatitis, paronychia (nail infection). **Occasional (31%–11%):** Dry skin, decreased appetite, pruritus, epistaxis, weight loss, cystitis, pyrexia, cheilitis (lip inflammation), rhinorrhea, conjunctivitis.

ADVERSE EFFECTS/TOXIC REACTIONS

Diarrhea may lead to severe, sometimes fatal, dehydration or renal impairment. Bullous and exfoliative skin lesions occur rarely. Rash, erythema, acneiform lesions occur in 90% of pts. Palmar-plantar erythrodysesthesia syndrome (PPES), a chemotherapy-induced skin condition that presents with redness, swelling, numbness, skin sloughing of the hands and feet, has been reported. Interstitial lung disease (ILD), including pulmonary infiltration, pneumonitis, ARDS, allergic alveolitis, reported in 2% of pts. Hepatotoxicity reported in 10% of pts. Keratitis symptoms, such as eye inflammation, lacrimation, light sensitivity, blurred vision, red eye, occurred in 1% of pts.

NURSING CONSIDERATIONS

BASELINE ASSESSMENT

Obtain baseline CBC, BMP, visual acuity. Obtain negative pregnancy test before initiating therapy. Question current breastfeeding status. Screen for history/co-morbidities, contact lens use. Receive full medication history, including herbal products. Assess skin for lesions, ulcers, open wounds.

INTERVENTION/EVALUATION

Monitor renal/hepatic function tests, urine output. Encourage PO intake. Assess for hydration status. Offer antidiarrheal medication for loose stool. Report oliguria, dark or concentrated urine. Immediately report skin lesions, vision changes, dry eye, severe diarrhea. Obtain chest X-ray if ILD suspected.

PATIENT/FAMILY TEACHING

• Most pts experience diarrhea, and severe cases may lead to dehydration or kidney failure; maintain adequate hydration. • Avoid pregnancy; contraception should be used during treatment and up to 2 wks after discontinuation. • Report any yellowing of skin or eyes, abdominal pain, bruising, black/tarry stools, dark urine, decreased urine output. • Minimize exposure to sunlight. • Immediately report eye problems (pain, swelling, blurred vision, vision changes) or skin blistering/redness. • Do not eat 1 hr before or 2 hrs after dose. • Do not wear contact lenses (may increase risk of keratitis).

albiglutide

al-bi-**gloo**-tide
(Tanzeum)

■ **BLACK BOX ALERT** ■ Thyroid C-cell tumors have occurred in animal studies with glucagon-like peptide-1 (GLP-1) receptor agonists; unknown if relevant in humans.
Do not confuse albiglutide with exenatide, dulaglutide, or liraglutide.

◆CLASSIFICATION

PHARMACOTHERAPEUTIC: Glucagon-like peptide-1 (GLP-1) receptor agonist. **CLINICAL:** Antidiabetic.

USES

Adjunct to diet and exercise to improve glycemic control in pts with type 2 diabetes mellitus.

PRECAUTIONS

Contraindications: Personal/family history of medullary thyroid carcinoma (MTC). Pts with multiple endocrine neoplasia syndrome type 2 (MEN2). Hypersensitivity to albiglutide. **Cautions:** Pts with hx pancreatitis, renal impairment. Not recommended in pts with preexisting severe GI disease, diabetic ketoacidosis; type 1 diabetes mellitus; pancreatitis; or as a first-line treatment regimen.

ACTION

Agonist of human glucagon-like peptide-1 (GLP-1). Increases glucose-dependent insulin secretion, decreases inappropriate glucagon secretion. Slows gastric emptying. **Therapeutic Effect:** Augments glucose-dependent insulin secretion.

PHARMACOKINETICS

Metabolized by protein degradation into small peptides, amino acids by proteolytic enzymes. Protein binding: Not specified. Peak plasma concentration: 3–5 days. Steady state reached in 4–5 wks. **Half-life:** 5 days.

⚕ LIFESPAN CONSIDERATIONS

Pregnancy/Lactation: Likely distributed in breast milk; drug is albumin-based protein therapeutic. Must either discontinue drug or discontinue breast-feeding. Due to extended clearance period, recommend discontinuation of therapy at least 1 mo before planned pregnancy. **Children:** Safety and efficacy not established in pts younger than 18 yrs. **Elderly:** No age-related precautions noted.

INTERACTIONS

DRUG: Insulin, metFORMIN, sulfonylureas may increase hypoglycemic effect. May decrease effect of **PO drugs requiring rapid onset** due to delayed gastric emptying. **HERBAL: Fenugreek, flaxseed, ginseng, gotu kola** may increase risk of hypoglycemia. **FOOD:** None known. **LAB VALUES:** Expected to decrease serum glucose, Hgb A1c. May increase serum ALT, GGT.

AVAILABILITY (Rx)

Prefilled Injector Pens: 30 mg, 50 mg.

ADMINISTRATION/HANDLING

Subcutaneous • Administer any time of day, without regard to meals, on same day each week. May change administration day if last dose was given more than 4 days ago. If dose is missed, administer within 3 days of missed dose. If more than 3 days pass after missed dose, wait until next regularly scheduled dose. • If refrigerated, allow pen to sit at room temperature for 15 min before using.
Reconstitution • See manufacturer guidelines.
Administration • Subcutaneously insert needle into abdomen, thigh, or upper arm region. • Press injection button until "click" is heard, then hold button for additional 5 sec to deliver full dose. • Do not reuse needle. • Rotate injection sites.
Storage • Mixed solution should appear yellow, free of all particles. • Use within 8 hrs of reconstitution. • Once needle is attached, use immediately; product can clog needle if allowed to dry after priming. • Refrigerate unused pens; do not freeze. • Once dispensed, may store pen at room temperature up to 4 wks.

INDICATIONS/ROUTES/DOSAGE

Type 2 Diabetes Mellitus
Subcutaneous: ADULTS/ELDERLY: 30 mg once weekly into abdomen, thigh, or upper arm region. May increase to 50 mg once weekly if glycemic response inadequate. **Missed Dose:** Administer within 3 days after missed dose, then resume on usual day of administration. If longer than 3 days, skip missed dose and resume administration on next regular weekly dose.
Dose Modification
Concomitant Use with Insulin Secretagogue (e.g., Sulfonylurea) or Insulin: Consider reduced dose based on glycemic goal.

Dosage in Renal/Hepatic Impairment
No dose adjustment.

SIDE EFFECTS

Occasional (14%–5%): Upper respiratory tract infection, diarrhea, nausea, injection site reactions (hematoma, erythema, rash), cough, back pain, arthralgia, sinusitis, influenza. **Rare (3%–2%):** Dyspepsia, vomiting, gastric reflux.

ADVERSE EFFECTS/TOXIC REACTIONS

May increase risk of acute renal failure or worsening of chronic renal impairment (esp. with dehydration), severe gastroparesis, thyroid C-cell tumors. May increase risk of hypoglycemia when used with other hypoglycemic agents or insulin. Dyspnea, pruritus, rash may indicate hypersensitivity reaction. Other adverse events include appendicitis (0.3% of pts), atrial fibrillation/flutter (1% of pts), pancreatitis (0.3% of pts), pneumonia (1.8% of pts). Immunogenicity (anti-alglutide antibody formation) reported

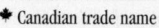 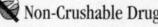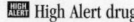

in 5.5% of pts. Some pts with antibody formation also tested positive for antibodies to GLP-1 and human albumin. May cause increased risk of hepatic injury.

NURSING CONSIDERATIONS

BASELINE ASSESSMENT

Obtain baseline fasting glucose level, Hgb A1c; BMP, LFT if applicable. Question history of medullary thyroid carcinoma, multiple neoplasia syndrome type 2, pancreatitis. Receive full medication history, including herbal products. Screen for use of other hypoglycemic agents or insulin. Assess pt's understanding of diabetes management, routine home glucose monitoring. Assess hydration status.

INTERVENTION/EVALUATION

Monitor capillary blood glucose levels, Hgb A1c; hepatic/renal function in pts with renal impairment reporting severe gastrointestinal reactions including gastroparesis, vomiting, diarrhea. Screen for thyroid tumors (dysphagia, dyspnea, persistent hoarseness, neck mass). If tumor is suspected, consider endocrinologist consultation. Clinical significance of serum calcitonin level or thyroid ultrasound with GLP-1-associated thyroid tumors is debated/unknown. Assess for hypoglycemia, hyperglycemia, hypersensitivity/allergic reaction. Screen for glucose-altering conditions: fever, stress, surgical procedures, trauma. Obtain dietary consult for nutritional education. Encourage PO intake.

PATIENT/FAMILY TEACHING

• A health care provider will show you how to properly prepare and inject your medication. You must demonstrate correct preparation and injection techniques before using medication. • Diabetes mellitus requires lifelong control. Diet and exercise are principal parts of treatment; do not skip or delay meals. Test blood sugar regularly. • When taking additional medications to lower blood sugar or when glucose demands are altered (fever, infection, stress, trauma), have low blood sugar treatment available (glucagon, oral dextrose). • Monitor daily calorie intake. • Report suspected pregnancy or plans of breastfeeding. • Therapy may increase risk of thyroid cancer; report lumps or swelling of the neck, hoarseness, trouble swallowing, shortness of breath. • Persistent, severe abdominal pain that radiates to the back (with or without vomiting) may indicate acute pancreatitis. • Rash, itching, hives may indicate allergic reaction.

albumin

al-**bue**-min
(Albuked-5, Albuked-25, <u>Albuminar-5</u>, <u>Albuminar-25</u>, AlbuRx, Albutein, <u>Buminate</u>, Flexbumin, Plasbumin-5, Plasbumin-25)
Do not confuse albumin with albuterol, or Buminate with bumetanide.

◆CLASSIFICATION

PHARMACOTHERAPEUTIC: Plasma protein fraction. **CLINICAL:** Blood derivative.

USES

Hypovolemia plasma volume expansion, maintenance of cardiac output in treatment of shock or impending shock. May be useful in treatment of ovarian hyperstimulation syndrome, acute/severe nephrosis, cirrhotic ascites, adult respiratory distress syndrome (ARDS), cardiopulmonary bypass, hemodialysis. **OFF-LABEL:** Large-volume paracentesis. In cirrhotics, with diuretics to help facilitate diuresis.

PRECAUTIONS

Contraindications: Hypersensitivity to albumin. Pts at risk for volume overload (e.g., severe anemia, HF, renal insufficiency). Dilution with Sterile Water for

Injection may cause hemolysis or acute renal failure. **Cautions:** Pts for whom sodium restriction is necessary, hepatic/renal failure (added protein load). Avoid 25% concentration in preterm infants (risk of intraventricular hemorrhage).

ACTION

Blood volume expander. **Therapeutic Effect:** Provides increase in intravascular oncotic pressure, mobilizes fluids into intravascular space.

PHARMACOKINETICS

Route	Onset	Peak	Duration
IV	15 min (in well-hydrated pt)	N/A	Dependent on initial blood volume

Distributed throughout extracellular fluid. **Half-life:** 15–20 days.

⌛ LIFESPAN CONSIDERATIONS

Pregnancy/Lactation: Unknown if drug crosses placenta or is distributed in breast milk. **Children/Elderly:** No age-related precautions noted.

INTERACTIONS

DRUG: None significant. **HERBAL:** None significant. **FOOD:** None known. **LAB VALUES:** May increase serum alkaline phosphatase.

AVAILABILITY (Rx)

Injection Solution: (5%): 50 mL, 250 mL, 500 mL. **(25%):** 20 mL, 50 mL, 100 mL.

ADMINISTRATION/HANDLING

📁 IV

Reconstitution • A 5% solution may be made from 25% solution by adding 1 volume 25% to 4 volumes 0.9% NaCl (NaCl preferred). Do not use Sterile Water for Injection (life-threatening hemolysis, acute renal failure can result).
Rate of Administration • Give by IV infusion. Rate is variable, depending on use, blood volume, concentration of sol-

ute. 5%: Do not exceed 2–4 mL/min in pts with normal plasma volume, 5–10 mL/min in pts with hypoproteinemia. 25%: Do not exceed 1 mL/min in pts with normal plasma volume, 2–3 mL/min in pts with hypoproteinemia. 5% is administered undiluted; 25% may be administered undiluted or diluted in 0.9% NaCl. • May give without regard to pt blood group or Rh factor.
Storage • Store at room temperature. Appears as clear brownish, odorless, moderately viscous fluid. • Do not use if solution has been frozen, appears turbid, contains sediment, or if not used within 4 hrs of opening vial.

🔲 IV INCOMPATIBILITIES

Lipids, micafungin (Mycamine), midazolam (Versed), vancomycin (Vancocin), verapamil (Isoptin).

🔲 IV COMPATIBILITIES

DiltiaZEM (Cardizem), LORazepam (Ativan).

INDICATIONS/ROUTES/DOSAGE

◄**ALERT**► 5% should be used in hypovolemic or intravascularly depleted pts. 25% should be used in pts in whom fluid and sodium intake must be minimized.

Usual Dosage
IV: ADULTS, ELDERLY: Initially, 25 g; may repeat in 15–30 min.

Hypovolemia
IV: ADULTS, ELDERLY, ADOLESCENTS: 5% albumin: 12.5–25 g (250–500 mL), repeat after 15–30 min, as needed. **CHILDREN:** 0.5–1 g/kg/dose (10–20 mL/kg/dose of 5% albumin). Repeat in 30-min intervals as needed.

Hemodialysis
IV: ADULTS, ELDERLY: 50–100 mL (12.5–25 g) of 25% albumin as needed.

Dosage in Renal/Hepatic Impairment
No dose adjustment.

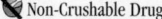

SIDE EFFECTS

Occasional: Hypotension. **Rare:** High dose in repeated therapy: altered vital signs, chills, fever, increased salivation, nausea, vomiting, urticaria, tachycardia.

ADVERSE EFFECTS/ TOXIC REACTIONS

Fluid overload may occur, marked by increased B/P, distended neck veins. Pulmonary edema may occur, evidenced by labored respirations, dyspnea, rales, wheezing, coughing. Neurologic changes, including headache, weakness, blurred vision, behavioral changes, incoordination, isolated muscle twitching, may occur.

NURSING CONSIDERATIONS

BASELINE ASSESSMENT

Obtain B/P, pulse, respirations immediately before administration. Adequate hydration required before albumin is administered.

INTERVENTION/EVALUATION

Monitor B/P for hypotension/hypertension. Assess frequently for evidence of fluid overload, pulmonary edema (see **Adverse Effects/Toxic Reactions**). Check skin for flushing, urticaria. Monitor I&O ratio (watch for decreased output). Assess for therapeutic response (increased B/P, decreased edema).

---

albuterol

TOP 100

al-**bue**-ter-ol
(Airomir ✦, Apo-Salvent ✦, PMS-Salbutamol ✦, ProAir HFA, ProAir RespiClick, Proventil HFA, Ventolin HFA, VoSpire ER)
Do not confuse albuterol with albumin or atenolol, Proventil with Bentyl, PriLOSEC, or Prinivil, or Ventolin with Benylin or Vantin.

FIXED-COMBINATION(S)

Combivent Respimat: albuterol/ ipratropium (a bronchodilator): 100 mcg/20 mcg per actuation. **DuoNeb:** albuterol/ipratropium 3 mg/0.5 mg.

◆CLASSIFICATION

PHARMACOTHERAPEUTIC: Sympathomimetic (adrenergic agonist). **CLINICAL:** Bronchodilator.

USES

Treatment or prevention of bronchospasm due to reversible obstructive airway disease, prevention of exercise-induced bronchospasm.

PRECAUTIONS

Contraindications: Hypersensitivity to albuterol. Severe hypersensitivity to milk protein (powder for inhalation). **Cautions:** Hypertension, cardiovascular disease, hyperthyroidism, diabetes, HF, convulsive disorders, glaucoma, hypokalemia, arrhythmias.

ACTION

Stimulates $beta_2$-adrenergic receptors in lungs, resulting in relaxation of bronchial smooth muscle. **Therapeutic Effect:** Relieves bronchospasm and reduces airway resistance.

PHARMACOKINETICS

Route	Onset	Peak	Duration
PO	15–30 min	2–3 hrs	4–6 hrs
PO (extended-release)	30 min	2–4 hrs	12 hrs
Inhalation	5–15 min	0.5–2 hrs	2–5 hrs

Rapidly, well absorbed from GI tract; rapidly absorbed from bronchi after inhalation. Metabolized in liver. Primarily excreted in urine. **Half-life:** 3.8–6 hrs.

☒ LIFESPAN CONSIDERATIONS

Pregnancy/Lactation: Appears to cross placenta; unknown if distributed in breast milk. May inhibit uterine contractility. **Children:** Safety and efficacy not established in pts younger than 2 yrs (syrup) or younger than 6 yrs (tablets). **Elderly:** May be more sensitive to

---

tremor or tachycardia due to age-related increased sympathetic sensitivity.

INTERACTIONS

DRUG: Beta-blockers (e.g., carvedilol, labetalol, metoprolol) antagonize effects. May produce bronchospasm. **Atomoxetine, MAOIs, tricyclic antidepressants (e.g., amitriptyline, doxepin)** may potentiate cardiovascular effects. May increase effects of **loop diuretics (e.g., furosemide)** (produce hypokalemia), **sympathomimetics** (increase CNS stimulation). **HERBAL: St. John's wort** may decrease level/effects. **Ephedra, yohimbe** may cause CNS stimulation. **FOOD:** None known. **LAB VALUES:** May increase blood glucose level. May decrease serum potassium level.

AVAILABILITY (Rx)

Aerosol, Powder Breath Activated Inhalation (ProAir RespiClick): 90 mcg/actuation. **Aerosol Solution, Inhalation (ProAir HFA, Proventil HFA, Ventolin HFA):** 90 mcg/spray. **Solution for Nebulization:** 0.63 mg/3 mL (0.021%), 1.25 mg/3 mL (0.042%), 2.5 mg/3 mL (0.084%), 5 mg/mL (0.5%). **Syrup:** 2 mg/5 mL. **Tablets:** 2 mg, 4 mg.

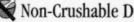 **Tablets (Extended-Release [VoSpire ER]):** 4 mg, 8 mg.

ADMINISTRATION/HANDLING

PO

• Do not break, crush, dissolve, or divide extended-release tablets. • Administer with food.

Inhalation Aerosol

• Shake container well before inhalation. • Prime prior to first use. A spacer is recommended for use with MDI. • Wait 2 min before inhaling second dose (allows for deeper bronchial penetration). • Rinse mouth with water immediately after inhalation (prevents mouth/throat dryness).

Inhalation Powder

• Device is breath activated. • Do not use with spacer. • Do not wash or put any part of inhaler to water.

Nebulization

• Administer over 5–15 min.

INDICATIONS/ROUTES/DOSAGE

Acute Bronchospasm, Exacerbation of Asthma

Inhalation: ADULTS, ELDERLY, CHILDREN OLDER THAN 12 YRS: (Acute, Severe): 4–8 puffs q20min up to 4 hrs, then q1–4h as needed. **CHILDREN 12 YRS AND YOUNGER:**(Acute,Severe): 4–8 puffs q20min for 3 doses, then q1–4h as needed. **Nebulization: ADULTS, ELDERLY, CHILDREN OLDER THAN 12 YRS:** (Acute, Severe): 2.5–5 mg q20min for 3 doses, then 2.5–10 mg q1–4h or 10–15 mg/hr continuously. **CHILDREN 12 YRS AND YOUNGER:** 0.15 mg/kg q20min for 3 doses (minimum: 2.5 mg), then 0.15–0.3 mg/kg q1–4h as needed. **Maximum:** 10 mg q1–4h as needed or 0.5 mg/kg/hr by continuous inhalation.

Chronic Bronchospasm

PO: ADULTS, CHILDREN OLDER THAN 12 YRS: 2–4 mg 3–4 times/day. **Maximum:** 8 mg 4 times/day. **ELDERLY:** 2 mg 3–4 times/day. **Maximum:** 8 mg 4 times/day. **CHILDREN 6–12 YRS:** 2 mg 3–4 times/day. **Maximum:** 24 mg/day. **CHILDREN 2–5 YRS:** 0.1–0.2 mg/kg/dose 3 times/day. **Maximum:** 4 mg 3 times/day. **PO: (Extended-Release): ADULTS, CHILDREN OLDER THAN 12 YRS:** 4–8 mg q12h. **Maximum:** 32 mg/day. **CHILDREN 6–12 YRS:** 4 mg q12h. **Maximum:** 24 mg/day. **Nebulization: ADULTS, ELDERLY, CHILDREN 12 YRS AND OLDER:** 2.5 mg 3–4 times/day as needed. Children 2–11 yrs: 0.63–1.25 mg 3–4 times/day as needed. **Inhalation: ADULTS, ELDERLY, CHILDREN:** 2 puffs q4–6h as needed.

Exercise-Induced Bronchospasm

Inhalation: ADULTS, ELDERLY, CHILDREN 5 YRS AND OLDER: 2 puffs 5 min before exercise. **CHILDREN 4 YRS AND YOUNGER:** 1–2 puffs 5 min before exercise.

Dosage in Renal/Hepatic Impairment

No dose adjustment.

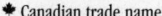 ✦ Canadian trade name   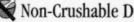 Non-Crushable Drug   ⚠ High Alert drug

SIDE EFFECTS

Frequent (27%–4%): Headache, restlessness, nervousness, tremors, nausea, dizziness, throat dryness and irritation, pharyngitis, B/P changes including hypertension, heartburn, transient wheezing. **Occasional (3%–2%):** Insomnia, asthenia, altered taste. **Inhalation:** Dry, irritated mouth or throat; cough, bronchial irritation. **Rare:** Drowsiness, diarrhea, dry mouth, flushing, diaphoresis, anorexia.

ADVERSE EFFECTS/TOXIC REACTIONS

Excessive sympathomimetic stimulation may produce palpitations, ectopy, tachycardia, chest pain, slight increase in B/P followed by substantial decrease, chills, diaphoresis, blanching of skin. Too-frequent or excessive use may lead to decreased bronchodilating effectiveness and severe, paradoxical broncho-constriction.

NURSING CONSIDERATIONS

BASELINE ASSESSMENT

Assess lung sounds, pulse, B/P, color, characteristics of sputum noted. Offer emotional support (high incidence of anxiety due to difficulty in breathing and sympathomimetic response to drug).

INTERVENTION/EVALUATION

Monitor rate, depth, rhythm, type of respiration; quality and rate of pulse; EKG; serum potassium, glucose; ABG determinations. Assess lung sounds for wheezing (bronchoconstriction), rales.

PATIENT/FAMILY TEACHING

• Follow guidelines for proper use of inhaler. • A health care provider will show you know to properly prepare and use your medication. You must demonstrate correct preparation and injection techniques before using medication. • Increase fluid intake (decreases lung secretion viscosity). • Do not take more than 2 inhalations at any one time (excessive use may produce paradoxical bronchoconstriction or decreased bronchodilating effect). • Rinsing mouth with water immediately after inhalation may prevent mouth/throat dryness. • Avoid excessive use of caffeine derivatives (chocolate, coffee, tea, cola, cocoa).

alectinib

al-**ek**-ti-nib
(Alecensa)
Do not confuse alectinib with afatinib, ibrutinib, imatinib, or gefitinib.

◆CLASSIFICATION

PHARMACOTHERAPEUTIC: Kinase inhibitor. **CLINICAL:** Antineoplastic.

USES

First line treatment of pts with anaplastic lymphoma kinase (ALK)–positive metastatic non–small cell lung cancer (NSCLC).

PRECAUTIONS

Contraindications: Hypersensitivity to alectinib. **Cautions:** Baseline anemia, leukopenia; bradycardia, bradyarrhythmias, chronic edema, diabetes, dehydration, electrolyte imbalance, hepatic/renal impairment, HF, ocular disease, pulmonary disease, history of thromboembolism.

ACTION

Inhibits tyrosine kinase activity and tumor cell proliferation. Inhibits autophosphorylation of ALK and ALK-dependent signaling proteins. **Therapeutic Effect:** Inhibits lung cancer growth and metastasis.

PHARMACOKINETICS

Metabolized in liver. Protein binding: Greater than 99%. Peak plasma concentration: 4 hrs. Steady state reached in 7 days. Excreted in feces (98%), urine (less than 0.5%). **Half-life:** 33 hrs.

⏳ LIFESPAN CONSIDERATIONS

Pregnancy/Lactation: Avoid pregnancy; may cause fetal harm. Females of reproductive potential should use effective contraception during treatment and for at least 1 wk after discontinuation. Unknown if distributed in breast milk. Breastfeeding not recommended during treatment and for at least 1 wk after discontinuation. Males with female partners of reproductive potential must use barrier methods during treatment and up to 3 mos after discontinuation. **Children:** Safety and efficacy not established. **Elderly:** Safety and efficacy not established.

INTERACTIONS

DRUG: None significant. **HERBAL:** None significant. **FOOD:** High-fat, high-calorie meals increase absorption/exposure. **LAB VALUES:** May increase serum alkaline phosphatase, ALT, AST, bilirubin, CPK, creatinine, glucose. May decrease serum calcium, potassium, phosphate, sodium; Hgb, Hct, lymphocytes, RBCs.

AVAILABILITY (Rx)

🜲 Capsules: 150 mg.

ADMINISTRATION/HANDLING
PO
• Give with food. • Administer whole; do not break, crush, cut, or open capsules. • If a dose is missed or vomiting occurs during administration, give next dose at regularly scheduled time.

INDICATIONS/ROUTES/DOSAGE

Non–Small Cell Lung Cancer
PO: ADULTS, ELDERLY: 600 mg twice daily until disease progression or unacceptable toxicity.

Dose Reduction Schedule
First dose reduction: 450 mg twice daily. **Second dose reduction:** 300 mg twice daily. Permanently discontinue if unable to tolerate 300 mg twice daily.

Dose Modification
Bradycardia
Symptomatic bradycardia: Withhold treatment until recovery to asymptomatic bradycardia or to a heart rate of 60 bpm or greater, then resume at reduced dose level (if pt not taking concomitant medications known to cause bradycardia). **Symptomatic bradycardia in pts taking concomitant medications known to cause bradycardia:** Withhold treatment until recovery to asymptomatic bradycardia or heart rate of 60 bpm or greater. If concomitant medication can be adjusted or discontinued, then resume at same dose. If concomitant medication cannot be adjusted or discontinued, then resume at reduced dose level. **Life-threatening bradycardia in pts who are not taking concomitant medications known to cause bradycardia:** Permanently discontinue. **Life-threatening bradycardia in pts who are taking concomitant medications known to cause bradycardia:** Withhold treatment until recovery to asymptomatic bradycardia or heart rate of 60 bpm or greater. If concomitant medication can be adjusted or discontinued, then resume at reduced dose level with frequent monitoring. Permanently discontinue if bradycardia recurs despite dose reduction.

CPK Elevation
CPK elevation greater than 5 times upper limit of normal (ULN): Withhold treatment until recovery to baseline or less than or equal to 2.5 times ULN, then resume at same dose. **CPK elevation greater than 10 times ULN or second occurrence of CPK elevation greater than 5 times ULN:** Withhold treatment until recovery to baseline or less than or equal to 2.5 times ULN, then resume at reduced dose level.

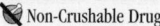

Hepatotoxicity

Serum ALT or AST elevation greater than 5 times ULN with total bilirubin less than or equal to 2 times ULN: Withhold treatment until serum ALT or AST recovers to baseline or less than or equal to 3 times ULN, then resume at reduced dose level. **Serum ALT or AST elevation greater than 3 times ULN with total serum bilirubin greater than 2 times ULN in the absence of cholestasis or hemolysis:** Permanently discontinue. **Total bilirubin elevation greater than 3 times ULN:** Withhold treatment until recovery to baseline or less than or equal to 1.5 times ULN, then resume at reduced dose level.

Pulmonary

Any grade treatment-related interstitial lung disease/pneumonitis: Permanently discontinue.

Dosage in Renal Impairment

Mild to moderate impairment: No dose adjustment. **Severe impairment:** Not specified; use caution.

Dosage in Hepatic Impairment

Mild impairment: No dose adjustment. **Moderate to severe impairment:** Not specified; use caution.

SIDE EFFECTS

Frequent (41%–19%): Fatigue, asthenia, constipation, edema (peripheral, generalized, eyelid, periorbital), myalgia, musculoskeletal pain, cough, generalized rash, papular rash, pruritus, macular rash, maculopapular rash, acneiform dermatitis, erythema, nausea. **Occasional (18%–10%):** Headache, diarrhea, dyspnea, back pain, vomiting, increased weight, blurred vision, vitreous floaters, visual impairment, reduced visual acuity, asthenopia, diplopia, photosensitivity.

ADVERSE EFFECTS/TOXIC REACTIONS

Approx. 23% of pts required at least one dose reduction. Median time to first dose reduction was 48 days. Decreased Hgb levels were reported in 56% of pts. Drug-induced hepatotoxicity with elevations of serum ALT/AST greater than 5 times ULN reported in 4%–5% of pts. Most reported cases of hepatotoxicity occurred during first 2 mos of therapy. Grade 3 interstitial lung disease occurred in less than 1% of pts. Symptomatic bradycardia reported in 7.5% of pts. Severe myalgia, musculoskeletal pain occurred in 29% of pts. CPK elevation occurred in 43% of pts. Other serious adverse effects may include endocarditis, hemorrhage (unspecified), intestinal perforation, pulmonary embolism.

NURSING CONSIDERATIONS

BASELINE ASSESSMENT

Obtain baseline CBC, CPK, BMP, LFT; serum ionized calcium, phosphate; capillary blood glucose, urine pregnancy, vital signs. Obtain baseline EKG in pts with history of arrhythmias, HF, concurrent use of medications known to bradycardia. Question possibility of pregnancy or plans of breastfeeding. Question history of hepatic/renal impairment, pulmonary embolism, diabetes, cardiac/pulmonary disease. Screen for medication known to cause bradycardia. Assess visual acuity. Verify ALK-positive NSCLC test prior to initiation.

INTERVENTION/EVALUATION

Monitor CBC routinely; LFTs q2wks during first 2 mos of treatment, then periodically thereafter (or more frequently in pts with hepatic impairment). Obtain BMP, serum ionized calcium, magnesium if arrhythmia or severe dehydration occurs. Monitor vital signs (esp. heart rate). Obtain EKG for bradycardia, chest pain, dyspnea. Worsening cough, fever, dyspnea may indicate interstitial lung disease/pneumonitis. Monitor for hepatotoxicity, hyperglycemia, vision changes, myalgia, musculoskeletal pain.

PATIENT/FAMILY TEACHING

• Blood levels, EKGs will be monitored routinely. • Report history of heart problems including extremity swelling, HF, slow heart rate. Therapy may decrease your heart rate; report dizziness, chest pain, palpitations, or fainting. • Worsening cough, fever, or shortness of breath may indicate severe lung inflammation. • Avoid pregnancy; contraception recommended during treatment and for up to 7 days after final dose. Do not breastfeed. Males with female partners of reproductive potential should use condoms during sexual activity during treatment and up to 3 mos after final dose. • Blurry vision, confusion, frequent urination, increased thirst, fruity breath may indicate high blood sugar levels. • Report any yellowing of skin or eyes, upper abdominal pain, bruising, black/tarry stools, dark urine. • Do not take newly prescribed medication unless approved by doctor who originally started treatment. • Avoid prolonged sun exposure/ tanning beds. Use high SPF sunscreen and lip balm to protect against sunburn. • Take with food. • Avoid alcohol.

alendronate

a-**len**-dro-nate
(Apo-Alendronate ✣, Binosto, Fosamax)
Do not confuse alendronate with risedronate, or Fosamax with Flomax.

FIXED-COMBINATION(S)

Fosamax Plus D: alendronate/cho-lecalciferol (vitamin D analogue): 70 mg/2,800 international units, 70 mg/5,600 international units.

◆CLASSIFICATION

PHARMACOTHERAPEUTIC: Bisphos-phonate. **CLINICAL:** Bone resorption inhibitor, calcium regulator.

USES

Fosamax: Treatment of osteoporosis in men. Treatment of glucocorticoid-in-duced osteoporosis in men and women with low bone mineral density who are receiving at least 7.5 mg predniSONE (or equivalent). Treatment and pre-vention of osteoporosis in males and postmenopausal women. Treatment of Paget's disease of the bone in pts who are symptomatic, at risk for future com-plications, or with alkaline phosphatase equal to or greater than 2 times ULN. **Binosto:** Treatment of osteoporosis in males and postmenopausal women.

PRECAUTIONS

Contraindications: Hypocalcemia, ab-normalities of the esophagus, inability to stand or sit upright for at least 30 min, sensitivity to alendronate or other bisphosphonates; oral solution or effer-vescent tablet should not be used in pts at risk for aspiration. **Cautions:** Renal im-pairment, dysphagia, esophageal disease, gastritis, ulcers, or duodenitis.

ACTION

Inhibits bone resorption via actions on osteoclasts or osteoclast precursors. **Therapeutic Effect:** Leads to increased bone mineral density. **Paget's disease:** Decreases bone formation, but bone has a more normal architecture.

PHARMACOKINETICS

Poorly absorbed after PO administration. Protein binding: 78%. After PO admin-istration, rapidly taken into bone, with uptake greatest at sites of active bone turnover. Excreted in urine, feces (as unabsorbed drug). **Terminal half-life:** Greater than 10 yrs (reflects release from skeleton as bone is resorbed).

⧖ LIFESPAN CONSIDERATIONS

Pregnancy/Lactation: Possible incom-plete fetal ossification, decreased maternal weight gain, delay in delivery. Unknown if distributed in breast milk. Breastfeeding not recommended. **Children:** Safety and efficacy not established. **Elderly:** No age-related precautions noted.

INTERACTIONS

DRUG: Calcium, antacids may de-crease absorption. **Aspirin, NSAIDs**

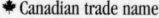 ✣ Canadian trade name　　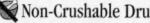 Non-Crushable Drug　　██ High Alert drug

may increase risk of ulcers, upper GI adverse effects. **HERBAL:** None significant. **FOOD:** Concurrent **beverages, dietary supplements, food** may interfere with absorption. **Caffeine** may reduce efficacy. **LAB VALUES:** Reduces serum calcium, phosphate. Significant decrease in serum alkaline phosphatase noted in pts with Paget's disease.

AVAILABILITY (Rx)

Solution, Oral: 70 mg/75 mL. **Tablets:** 5 mg, 10 mg, 35 mg, 40 mg, 70 mg. **Tablets, Effervescent: (Binosto):** 70 mg.

ADMINISTRATION/HANDLING

PO
• Give at least 30 min before first food, beverage, or medication of the day. • **Tablets, Effervescent:** Dissolve in 4 oz water. Wait at least 5 min after effervescence stops. Stir for 10 sec and drink. **Oral Solution:** Follow with at least 2 oz of water.

INDICATIONS/ROUTES/DOSAGE

Note: Consider discontinuing after 3–5 yrs for osteoporosis in pts at low risk for fractures.

Osteoporosis (in Men)
PO: ADULTS, ELDERLY: 10 mg once daily in the morning or 70 mg weekly.

Glucocorticoid-Induced Osteoporosis
PO: ADULTS, ELDERLY: 5 mg once daily in the morning. **POSTMENOPAUSAL WOMEN NOT RECEIVING ESTROGEN:** 10 mg once daily in the morning.

Postmenopausal Osteoporosis
PO: *(Treatment):* **ADULTS, ELDERLY:** 10 mg once daily in the morning or 70 mg weekly.
PO: *(Prevention):* **ADULTS, ELDERLY:** 5 mg once daily in the morning or 35 mg weekly.

Paget's Disease
PO: ADULTS, ELDERLY: 40 mg once daily in the morning for 6 mos.

Dosage in Renal Impairment
Not recommended in pts with creatinine clearance less than 35 mL/min.

Dosage in Hepatic Impairment
No dose adjustment.

SIDE EFFECTS

Frequent (8%–7%): Back pain, abdominal pain. **Occasional (3%–2%):** Nausea, abdominal distention, constipation, diarrhea, flatulence. **Rare (less than 2%):** Rash; severe bone, joint, muscle pain.

ADVERSE EFFECTS/TOXIC REACTIONS

Overdose produces hypocalcemia, hypophosphatemia, significant GI disturbances. Esophageal irritation occurs if not given with 6–8 oz of plain water or if pt lies down within 30 min of administration. May increase risk of osteonecrosis of the jaw.

NURSING CONSIDERATIONS

BASELINE ASSESSMENT
Obtain baseline serum calcium, phosphate, alkaline phosphatase. Hypocalcemia, vitamin D deficiency must be corrected before beginning therapy. Assess pt's ability to remain upright for at least 30 minutes.

INTERVENTION/EVALUATION
Monitor chemistries (esp. serum calcium, phosphorus, alkaline phosphatase levels).

PATIENT/FAMILY TEACHING
• Expected benefits occur only when medication is taken with full glass (6–8 oz) of plain water, first thing in the morning and at least 30 min before first food, beverage, or medication of the day is taken. Any other beverage (mineral water, orange juice, coffee) significantly reduces absorption of medication. • Do not lie down for at least 30 min after taking medication (potentiates delivery to stomach, reducing risk of

esophageal irritation). • Report new swallowing difficulties, pain when swallowing, chest pain, new/worsening heartburn. • Consider weight-bearing exercises, modify behavioral factors (e.g., cigarette smoking, alcohol consumption). • Supplemental calcium and vitamin D should be taken if dietary intake inadequate.

alfuzosin

al-fue-**zoe**-sin
(Apo-Alfuzosin 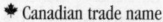, Uroxatral, Xatral 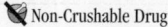)

◆CLASSIFICATION

PHARMACOTHERAPEUTIC: Alpha$_1$-adrenergic blocker. **CLINICAL:** Benign prostatic hyperplasia agent.

USES

Treatment of signs and symptoms of benign prostatic hyperplasia (BPH). **OFF-LABEL:** Facilitates expulsion of ureteral stones.

PRECAUTIONS

Contraindications: Hypersensitivity to alfuzosin. Moderate to severe hepatic impairment; concurrent use of strong CYP3A4 inhibitors (e.g., ketoconazole) or other alpha-adrenergic blockers. **Cautions:** Pts with known QT interval prolongation (congenital or acquired). Severe renal or mild hepatic impairment.

ACTION

Blocks adrenoreceptors of lower urinary tract (e.g., prostate, bladder neck). **Therapeutic Effect:** Relaxes smooth muscle; improves urinary flow, symptoms of prostatic hyperplasia.

PHARMACOKINETICS

Readily absorbed (decreased under fasting conditions). Protein binding: 90%. Metabolized in liver. Primarily excreted in urine. **Half-life:** 10 hrs.

⧗ LIFESPAN CONSIDERATIONS

Pregnancy/Lactation: Not indicated for use in this pt population. **Children:** Not indicated for use in this pt population. **Elderly:** No age-related precautions noted.

INTERACTIONS

DRUG: Other alpha-blocking agents (e.g., doxazosin, prazosin, tamsulosin, terazosin) may have additive effect. **CYP3A4 inhibitors (e.g., ritonavir, ketoconazole), PDE5 inhibitors (e.g., sildenafil)** may increase level/effects. **HERBAL: St. John's wort** may decrease level/effects. **FOOD: Food** increases absorption. **LAB VALUES:** None significant.

AVAILABILITY (Rx)

Tablets (Extended-Release): 10 mg.

ADMINISTRATION/HANDLING

PO
• Give immediately after the same meal each day. • Swallow whole; do not break, crush, dissolve, or divide extended-release tablets.

INDICATIONS/ROUTES/DOSAGE

Benign Prostatic Hyperplasia
PO: ADULTS: 10 mg once daily, after same meal each day.

Dosage in Renal/Hepatic Impairment
See Precautions.

SIDE EFFECTS

Frequent (7%–6%): Dizziness, headache, malaise. **Occasional (4%):** Dry mouth. **Rare (3%–2%):** Nausea, dyspepsia (heartburn, epigastric discomfort), diarrhea, orthostatic hypotension, tachycardia, drowsiness.

ADVERSE EFFECTS/TOXIC REACTIONS

Ischemia-related chest pain reported in 2% of pts. Priapism has been reported.

NURSING CONSIDERATIONS

BASELINE ASSESSMENT
Question for sensitivity to alfuzosin, use of other alpha-blocking agents (doxazosin, prazosin, tamsulosin, terazosin). Obtain B/P.

INTERVENTION/EVALUATION
Assist with ambulation if dizziness occurs. Report headache. Monitor for hypotension. Question for improvement in urine flow, hesitancy.

PATIENT/FAMILY TEACHING
• Take after the same meal each day. • Avoid tasks that require alertness, motor skills until response to drug is established. • Do not chew, crush, dissolve, or divide extended-release tablets.

---

alirocumab

al-i-**rok**-ue-mab
(Praluent)
Do not confuse alirocumab with adalimumab or raxibacumab.

◆CLASSIFICATION
PHARMACOTHERAPEUTIC: Proprotein convertase subtilisin kexin 9 (PCSK9) inhibitor, monoclonal antibody. **CLINICAL:** Antihyperlipidemic.

USES
Treatment of hyperlipidemia. Adjunct to diet and maximally tolerated statin therapy for the treatment of adults with heterozygous familial hypercholesterolemia or clinical atherosclerotic cardiovascular disease who require additional lowering of low-density lipoprotein cholesterol (LDL-C).

PRECAUTIONS
Contraindications: Severe hypersensitivity to alirocumab. **Cautions:** Hepatic impairment.

ACTION
Prevents binding of PCSK9 to LDL receptors on hepatocytes. Increases hepatic uptake of LDL. **Therapeutic Effect:** Decreases serum cholesterol levels.

PHARMACOKINETICS
Distributed primarily in circulatory system. Metabolized by protein degradation into small peptides, amino acids. Peak plasma concentration: 3–7 days. Steady state reached by 2–3 doses. **Half-life:** 17–20 days.

⧗ LIFESPAN CONSIDERATIONS
Pregnancy/Lactation: May cross placental barrier, esp. during second and third trimesters. Unknown if distributed in breast milk. Human immunoglobulin G is present in breast milk. **Children:** Safety and efficacy not established. **Elderly:** No age-related precautions noted.

INTERACTIONS
DRUG: None known. **HERBAL:** None significant. **FOOD:** None known. **LAB VALUES:** Expected to decrease serum LDL-C levels. May increase serum ALT, AST.

AVAILABILITY (Rx)
Injection Solution: 75 mg/mL, 150 mg/mL in single-dose, prefilled syringe or pen.

ADMINISTRATION/HANDLING
Subcutaneous
• Visually inspect for particulate matter or discoloration. Solution should appear clear, colorless to pale yellow. • Allow pen/syringe to warm to room temperature for 30–40 min prior to use. • Subcutaneously insert needle into abdomen, thigh, or upper arm region and inject solution. It may take up to 20 sec to fully inject dose. • Do not inject into areas of active skin disease or injury such as sunburns, skin rashes, inflammation, or skin infections. • Rotate injection sites.

Storage
• Refrigerate unused pens/syringes in outer carton. • Do not freeze. • Discard

---

if pen/syringe has been at room temperature more than 24 hrs or longer. • Protect from light.

INDICATIONS/ROUTES/DOSAGE

Hyperlipidemia

SQ: ADULTS, ELDERLY: 75 mg once every 2 wks. May increase to maximum dose of 150 mg once every 2 wks if response inadequate. If a dose is missed, administer within 7 days of scheduled dose, then resume normal schedule. If missed dose is not within 7 days, wait until next scheduled dose. Less frequent dosing: 300 mg q4wks.

Dosage in Renal Impairment
No dose adjustment.

Dosage in Hepatic Impairment
Mild to Moderate Impairment: No dose adjustment. **Severe Impairment:** Use caution.

SIDE EFFECTS

Occasional (11%–7%): Nasopharyngitis, injection site reactions (e.g., erythema, itching, swelling, pain/tenderness, bruising/contusion). **Rare (5%–2%):** Diarrhea, bronchitis, myalgia, muscle spasm, sinusitis, cough, musculoskeletal pain.

ADVERSE EFFECTS/TOXIC REACTIONS

Serious hypersensitivity reactions (e.g., pruritus, rash, urticaria), including some serious events (e.g., hypersensitivity vasculitis, hypersensitivity reactions requiring hospitalization), have been reported. Infections such as UTI (5% of pts) and influenza (6% of pts) have occurred. Neurologic events such as confusion, memory impairment reported in less than 1% of pts. Immunogenicity (anti-alirocumab antibodies) reported in 5% of pts. Pts who developed neutralizing antibodies had a higher incidence of injection site reactions.

NURSING CONSIDERATIONS

BASELINE ASSESSMENT
Obtain baseline LDL-C level, LFT. Question history of hypersensitivity reaction, hepatic impairment. Assess skin for sunburns, skin rashes, inflammation, or skin infections.

INTERVENTION/EVALUATION
Obtain LDL-C level within 4–8 wks after treatment initiation or with any dose titration. Monitor for hypersensitivity reactions. If hypersensitivity reaction occurs, discontinue therapy and treat symptoms accordingly; monitor until symptoms resolve. Monitor for infections including UTI, influenza.

PATIENT/FAMILY TEACHING
• A health care provider will show you how to properly prepare and inject your medication. You must demonstrate correct preparation and injection techniques before using medication. • Treatment may cause serious allergic reactions such as itching, hives, rash, or more serious reactions requiring hospitalization. If allergic reaction occurs, immediately seek medical attention. • Do not reuse prefilled pens/syringes.

---

aliskiren   HIGH ALERT

a-lis-**kye**-ren
(Rasilez ✤, Tekturna)
■ **BLACK BOX ALERT** ■ May cause fetal injury, mortality. Discontinue as soon as possible once pregnancy detected.
Do not confuse Tekturna with Valturna.

FIXED-COMBINATION(S)

Amturnide: aliskiren/amLODIPine (a calcium channel blocker)/hydroCHLOROthiazide (a diuretic): 150 mg/5 mg/12.5 mg, 300 mg/5 mg/12.5 mg, 300 mg/5 mg/25 mg, 300 mg/10 mg/12.5 mg, 300 mg/10 mg/25 mg.

Tekamlo: aliskiren/amLODIPine (a calcium channel blocker): 150 mg/5 mg, 150 mg/10 mg, 300 mg/5 mg, 300 mg/10 mg. **Tekturna HCT:** aliskiren/hydroCHLOROthiazide (a diuretic): 150 mg/12.5 mg, 150 mg/25 mg, 300 mg/12.5 mg, 300 mg/25 mg. **Valturna:** aliskiren/valsartan (an angiotensin II receptor antagonist): 150 mg/160 mg, 300 mg/320 mg.

◆CLASSIFICATION

PHARMACOTHERAPEUTIC: Renin-inhibitor. **CLINICAL:** Antihypertensive.

USES

Treatment of hypertension (not recommended as initial treatment). May be used alone or in combination with other antihypertensives.

PRECAUTIONS

Contraindications: Hypersensitivity to aliskiren. Concurrent use with ACE inhibitor or Angiotensin II Receptor Blockers in pts with diabetes. **Cautions:** Severe renal impairment. History of angioedema, dialysis, nephrotic syndrome, renovascular hypertension. Concurrent use with P-glycoprotein inhibitors (e.g., cycloSPORINE).

ACTION

Direct renin inhibitor. Decreases plasma renin activity (PRA), inhibiting the conversion of angiotensinogen to angiotensin I, decreasing the formation of angiotensin II. **Therapeutic Effect:** Reduces B/P.

PHARMACOKINETICS

Peak plasma concentration reached within 1–3 hrs. Protein binding: 49%. Metabolized in liver. Minimally excreted in urine. Peak plasma steady-state levels reached in 7–8 days. **Half-life:** 24 hrs.

⊠ LIFESPAN CONSIDERATIONS

Pregnancy/Lactation: Carcinogenic potential to fetus. May cause fetal/neonatal morbidity, mortality. Unknown if distributed in breast milk. **Children:** Safety and efficacy not established. **Elderly:** No age-related precautions noted.

INTERACTIONS

DRUG: **CycloSPORINE, itraconazole** may increase concentration/effect. **HERBAL:** **Ephedra, ginseng, yohimbe** may worsen hypertension. **Garlic, black cohosh** may increase antihypertensive effect. **FOOD:** **High-fat meals** substantially decrease absorption. **Grapefruit products** may reduce antihypertensive effects. Separate by 4 hrs. **LAB VALUES:** May increase serum BUN, creatinine, uric acid, creatinine kinase, potassium. May decrease Hgb, Hct.

AVAILABILITY (Rx)

Tablets, Film-Coated: 150 mg, 300 mg.

ADMINISTRATION/HANDLING

PO

• High-fat meals substantially decrease absorption. • Consistent administration with regard to meals is recommended. • Do not break, crush, dissolve, or divide film-coated tablets.

INDICATIONS/ROUTES/DOSAGE

Hypertension
PO: ADULTS, ELDERLY: Initially, 150 mg/day. May increase to 300 mg/day.

Dosage in Renal Impairment
Mild to moderate impairment: No dose adjustment. **Severe impairment:** Use caution.

Dosage in Hepatic Impairment
No dose adjustment.

SIDE EFFECTS

Rare (2%–1%): Diarrhea, particularly in women, elderly (older than 65 yrs), gastroesophageal reflux, cough, rash.

ADVERSE EFFECTS/TOXIC REACTIONS

Angioedema, periorbital edema, edema of hands, generalized edema have been reported.

NURSING CONSIDERATIONS

BASELINE ASSESSMENT

Correct hypovolemia in pts on concurrent diuretic therapy. Obtain B/P and apical pulse immediately before each dose, in addition to regular monitoring (be alert to fluctuations). If excessive reduction in B/P occurs, place pt in supine position, feet slightly elevated.

INTERVENTION/EVALUATION

Assess for edema. Monitor I&O; weigh daily. Monitor B/P, renal function tests, potassium, Hgb, Hct.

PATIENT/FAMILY TEACHING

• Pregnant pts should avoid second- and third-trimester exposure to aliskiren. • Report swelling of face/lips/tongue, difficulty breathing. • Avoid strenuous exercise during hot weather (risk of dehydration, hypotension). • Do not chew, crush, dissolve, or divide film-coated tablets.

---

allopurinol

al-oh-**pure**-i-nol
(Aloprim, Apo-Allopurinol ✹,
Zyloprim)
**Do not confuse allopurinol
with Apresoline or haloperidol,
or Zyloprim with Zorprin or
Zovirax.**

FIXED-COMBINATION(S)

Duzallo: allopurinol/leinurad (uric acid transporter-1 inhibitor): 200 mg/200 mg, 300 mg/200 mg.

◆CLASSIFICATION

PHARMACOTHERAPEUTIC: Xanthine oxidase inhibitor. **CLINICAL:** anti-gout

USES

PO: Management of primary or secondary gout (e.g., acute attack, nephropathy). Treatment of secondary hyperuricemia that may occur during cancer treatment. Management of recurrent uric acid and calcium oxalate calculi. **Injection:** Management of elevated uric acid in cancer treatment for leukemia, lymphoma, or solid tumor malignancies.

PRECAUTIONS

Contraindications: Severe hypersensitivity to allopurinol. **Cautions:** Renal/hepatic impairment; pts taking diuretics, mercaptopurine or azaTHIOprine, other drugs causing myelosuppression. Do not use in asymptomatic hyperuricemia.

ACTION

Decreases uric acid production by inhibiting xanthine oxidase, an enzyme responsible for converting xanthine to uric acid. **Therapeutic Effect:** Reduces uric acid concentrations in serum and urine.

PHARMACOKINETICS

Route	Onset	Peak	Duration
PO, IV	2–3 days	1–3 wks	1–2 wks

Well absorbed from GI tract. Widely distributed. Protein binding: less than 1%. Metabolized in liver. Excreted primarily in urine. Removed by hemodialysis. **Half-life:** 1–3 hrs; metabolite, 12–30 hrs.

⧗ LIFESPAN CONSIDERATIONS

Pregnancy/Lactation: Unknown if drug crosses placenta or is distributed in breast milk. **Children/Elderly:** No age-related precautions noted.

INTERACTIONS

DRUG: Loop or thiazide diuretics (e.g., furosemide, hydroCHLOROthiazide) may increase level/effect. May increase effect of **oral anticoagulants (e.g., warfarin).** May increase concentration, toxicity of **azaTHIOprine, mercaptopurine. Amoxicillin, ampicillin** may increase incidence of rash. **HERBAL:** None significant. **FOOD:** None known. **LAB VALUES:** May increase serum BUN, alkaline phosphatase, ALT, AST, creatinine.

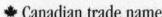 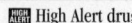

AVAILABILITY (Rx)

Injection, Powder for Reconstitution (Aloprim): 500 mg. **Tablets (Zyloprim):** 100 mg, 300 mg.

ADMINISTRATION/HANDLING

 IV

Reconstitution • Reconstitute 500-mg vial with 25 mL Sterile Water for Injection (concentration of 20 mg/mL). • Further dilute with 0.9% NaCl or D_5W (50–100 mL) to a concentration of 6 mg/mL or less.
Rate of Administration • Infuse over 15–60 min. Daily doses can be given as a single infusion or in equally divided doses at 6-, 8-, or 12-hr intervals.
Storage • Solution should appear clear and colorless. • Store unreconstituted vials at room temperature. • Do not refrigerate reconstituted and/or diluted solution. Must administer within 10 hrs of preparation. • Do not use if precipitate forms or solution is discolored.

PO
• Give after meals with plenty of fluid. • Fluid intake should yield slightly alkaline urine and output of approximately 2 L in adults. • Dosages greater than 300 mg/day to be administered in divided doses.

▓ IV INCOMPATIBILITIES

Amikacin (Amikin), carmustine (BiCNU), cefotaxime (Claforan), clindamycin (Cleocin), cytarabine (Ara-C), dacarbazine (DTIC), diphenhydrAMINE (Benadryl), DOXOrubicin (Adriamycin), doxycycline (Vibramycin), gentamicin, haloperidol (Haldol), hydrOXYzine (Vistaril), IDArubicin (Idamycin), imipenem-cilastatin (Primaxin), methylPREDNISolone (SOLU-Medrol), metoclopramide (Reglan), ondansetron (Zofran), streptozocin (Zanosar), tobramycin, vinorelbine (Navelbine).

▓ IV COMPATIBILITIES

Bumetanide (Bumex), calcium gluconate, furosemide (Lasix), heparin, HYDROmorphone (Dilaudid), LORazepam (Ativan), morphine, potassium chloride.

INDICATIONS/ROUTES/DOSAGE

◀**ALERT**▶ Doses greater than 300 mg should be given in divided doses.

Gout
PO: ADULTS, CHILDREN OLDER THAN 10 YRS: Initially, 100 mg/day. Increase at weekly intervals needed to achieve desired serum uric acid level. **(Mild):** 200–300 mg/day. **(Moderate to Severe):** 400–600 mg/day in 2–3 divided doses. **Maximum:** 800 mg/day.

Secondary Hyperuricemia Associated with Chemotherapy
PO: ADULTS, CHILDREN OLDER THAN 10 YRS: 600–800 mg/day in 2–3 divided doses for 2–3 days starting 1–2 days before chemotherapy. **CHILDREN 6–10 YRS:** 300 mg/day in 2–3 divided doses. **CHILDREN YOUNGER THAN 6 YRS:** 150 mg/day in 3 divided doses.
◀**ALERT**▶ **IV:** Daily dose can be given as single infusion or at 6-, 8-, or 12-hr intervals.
IV: ADULTS, ELDERLY, CHILDREN 10 YRS OR OLDER: 200–400 mg/m²/day beginning 24–48 hrs before initiation of chemotherapy. **CHILDREN YOUNGER THAN 10 YRS:** 200 mg/m²/day beginning 24–48 hrs before initiation of chemotherapy. **Maximum:** 600 mg/day.

Recurrent Uric Acid Calcium Oxalate Calculi
PO: ADULTS: 200–300 mg/day in single or divided doses.

Dosage in Renal Impairment
Dosage is modified based on creatinine clearance. **PO:** Removed by hemodialysis. Administer dose following hemodialysis or administer 50% supplemental dose.

IV/PO

Creatinine

Clearance	Dosage
10–20 mL/min	200 mg/day
3–9 mL/min	100 mg/day
Less than 3 mL/min	100 mg at extended intervals
HD	100 mg q48h (increase cautiously to 300 mg)

Dosage in Hepatic Impairment
No dose adjustment.

SIDE EFFECTS

Occasional: PO: Drowsiness, unusual hair loss. **IV:** Rash, nausea, vomiting. **Rare:** Diarrhea, headache.

ADVERSE EFFECTS/ TOXIC REACTIONS

Pruritic maculopapular rash, possibly accompanied by malaise, fever, chills, joint pain, nausea, vomiting should be considered a toxic reaction. Severe hypersensitivity reaction may follow appearance of rash. Bone marrow depression, hepatotoxicity, peripheral neuritis, acute renal failure occur rarely.

NURSING CONSIDERATIONS

BASELINE ASSESSMENT

Obtain baseline BMP, LFT. Instruct pt to drink minimum of 2,500–3,000 mL of fluid daily while taking medication.

INTERVENTION/EVALUATION

Discontinue medication immediately if rash or other evidence of allergic reaction occurs. Monitor I&O (output should be at least 2,000 mL/day). Assess serum chemistries, uric acid, hepatic function. Assess urine for cloudiness, unusual color, odor. **Gout:** Assess for therapeutic response: relief of pain, stiffness, swelling; increased joint mobility; reduced joint tenderness; improved grip strength.

PATIENT/FAMILY TEACHING

• May take 1 wk or longer for full therapeutic effect. • Maintain adequate hydration; drink 2,500–3,000 mL of fluid daily while taking medication. • Avoid tasks that require alertness, motor skills until response to drug is established. • Avoid alcohol (may increase uric acid).

almotriptan

al-moe-**trip**-tan
(Axert)
Do not confuse almotriptan with alvimopan, or Axert with Antivert.

◆CLASSIFICATION

PHARMACOTHERAPEUTIC: Serotonin receptor agonist (5-HT$_{1B}$). **CLINICAL:** Antimigraine.

USES

Acute treatment of migraine headache with or without aura in adults. Acute treatment of migraine headache in adolescents 12–17 yrs with history of migraine with or without aura and having attacks usually lasting 4 or more hrs when left untreated.

PRECAUTIONS

Contraindications: Hypersensitivity to almotriptan. Cerebrovascular disease (e.g., recent stroke, transient ischemic attacks), peripheral vascular disease (e.g., ischemic bowel disease), hemiplegic or basilar migraine, ischemic heart disease (including angina pectoris, history of MI, silent ischemia, and Prinzmetal's angina), uncontrolled hypertension, use within 24 hrs of ergotamine-containing preparations or another 5-HT$_{1B}$ agonist. **Cautions:** Mild to moderate renal or hepatic impairment, pt profile suggesting cardiovascular risks, controlled hypertension; history of CVA, sulfonamide allergy.

ACTION

Binds selectively to serotonin receptors in cranial arteries producing a

---

 ✣ Canadian trade name   🦺 Non-Crushable Drug   🔲 High Alert drug

vasoconstrictive effect. Decreases inflammation associated with relief of migraine. **Therapeutic Effect:** Produces relief of migraine headache.

PHARMACOKINETICS

Well absorbed after PO administration. Protein binding: 35%. Metabolized by liver. Primarily excreted in urine. **Half-life:** 3–4 hrs.

⌛ LIFESPAN CONSIDERATIONS

Pregnancy/Lactation: Unknown if distributed in breast milk. **Children:** Safety and efficacy not established in pts younger than 12 yrs. **Elderly:** No age-related precautions noted.

INTERACTIONS

DRUG: Ergotamine-containing drugs may produce vasospastic reaction. **MAOIs** may increase concentration. Combined use of **SSRIs** or **SNRIs (e.g., FLUoxetine, fluvoxaMINE, PARoxetine, sertraline)** may produce weakness, hyperreflexia, incoordination. **CYP3A4 inhibitors (e.g., erythromycin, itraconazole, ketoconazole, ritonavir)** may increase plasma concentration/effect. **HERBAL:** None significant. **FOOD:** None known. **LAB VALUES:** None significant.

AVAILABILITY (Rx)

🖌 **Tablets:** 6.5 mg, 12.5 mg.

ADMINISTRATION/HANDLING

PO
• Swallow whole; do not break, crush, dissolve, or divide tablets. • Take with full glass of water. • May give without regard to food.

INDICATIONS/ROUTES/DOSAGE

Migraine Headache
PO: ADULTS, ELDERLY, ADOLESCENTS 12–17 YRS: Initially, 6.25–12.5 mg as a single dose. If headache returns, dose may be repeated after 2 hrs. **Maximum:** 2 doses/24 hrs (25 mg).

Concurrent Use of CYP3A4 Inhibitors
ADULTS, ELDERLY: Recommended initial dose is 6.25 mg, maximum daily dose is 12.5 mg. Avoid use in pts with renal or hepatic impairment AND use of CYP3A4 inhibitors.

Dosage in Renal Impairment
CrCl 30 mL/min or less: Initially, 6.25 mg in a single dose. **Maximum:** 12.5 mg/day.

Dosage in Hepatic Impairment
Initially, 6.25 mg in a single dose. **Maximum:** 12.5 mg/day.

SIDE EFFECTS

Rare (2%–1%): Nausea, dry mouth, headache, dizziness, somnolence, paresthesia, flushing.

ADVERSE EFFECTS/ TOXIC REACTIONS

Excessive dosage may produce tremor, redness of extremities, decreased respirations, cyanosis, seizures, chest pain. Serious arrhythmias occur rarely but particularly in pts with hypertension, diabetes, obesity, smokers, and those with strong family history of coronary artery disease.

NURSING CONSIDERATIONS

BASELINE ASSESSMENT

Question for history of peripheral vascular disease, cardiac conduction disorders, CVA. Question pt regarding onset, location, duration of migraine, and possible precipitating factors.

INTERVENTION/EVALUATION

Evaluate for relief of migraine headache and associated photophobia, phonophobia (sound sensitivity), nausea, vomiting.

PATIENT/FAMILY TEACHING

• Take a single dose as soon as symptoms of an actual migraine attack appear. • Medication is intended to relieve migraine, not to prevent or reduce number of attacks. • Lie down in quiet, dark room for additional benefit after taking medication. • Avoid tasks that require alertness, motor skills until response to drug is established. • Report immediately if palpitations, pain or tightness in chest or throat, or pain or weakness of extremities occurs. • Swallow whole; do not chew, crush, dissolve, or divide tablets.

ALPRAZolam

al-**praz**-oh-lam
(ALPRAZolam Intensol, ALPRAZolam XR, Apo-Alpraz ✢, Niravam, Xanax, Xanax XR)
Do not confuse ALPRAZolam with LORazepam, or Xanax with Tenex, Tylox, Xopenex, Zantac, or ZyrTEC.

◆CLASSIFICATION

PHARMACOTHERAPEUTIC: Benzodiazepine (Schedule IV). **CLINICAL:** Antianxiety.

USES

Management of generalized anxiety disorders (GAD). Short-term relief of symptoms of anxiety, panic disorder, with or without agoraphobia. Anxiety associated with depression. **OFF-LABEL:** Anxiety in children. Preoperative anxiety.

PRECAUTIONS

Contraindications: Hypersensitivity to ALPRAZolam. Acute narrow angle-closure glaucoma, concurrent use with ketoconazole or itraconazole or other potent CYP3A4 inhibitors. **Cautions:** Renal/hepatic impairment, predisposition to urate nephropathy, obese pts. Concurrent use of CYP3A4 inhibitors/inducers and major CYP3A4 substrates; debilitated pts, respiratory disease, depression (esp. suicidal risk), elderly (increased risk of severe toxicity). History of substance abuse.

ACTION

Enhances the inhibitory effects of the neurotransmitter gamma-aminobutyric acid in the brain. **Therapeutic Effect:** Produces anxiolytic effect due to CNS depressant action.

PHARMACOKINETICS

Well absorbed from GI tract. Protein binding: 80%. Metabolized in liver. Primarily excreted in urine. Minimal removal by hemodialysis. **Half-life:** 6–27 hrs.

⌛ LIFESPAN CONSIDERATIONS

Pregnancy/Lactation: Crosses placenta; distributed in breast milk. Chronic ingestion during pregnancy may produce withdrawal symptoms, CNS depression in neonates. **Children:** Safety and efficacy not established. **Elderly:** Use small initial doses with gradual increase to avoid ataxia (muscular incoordination) or excessive sedation. May have increased risk of falls, delirium.

INTERACTIONS

DRUG: Potentiated effects when used with **other CNS depressants (including alcohol). CYP3A4 inhibitors (e.g., antifungal agents [azole], OLANZapine, protease inhibitors, SSRIs)** may increase CNS effect. **CYP3A4 inducers (e.g., carBAMazepine, rifAMPin)** may decrease effect. **HERBAL: Gotu kola, kava kava, St. John's wort, valerian** may increase CNS depressant effect. **St. John's wort, yohimbe** may decrease effectiveness. **FOOD: Grapefruit products** may increase level, effects. **LAB VALUES:** None significant.

AVAILABILITY (Rx)

Solution, Oral (ALPRAZolam Intensol): 1 mg/mL. **Tablets (Orally Disintegrating [Niravam]):** 0.25 mg, 0.5 mg, 1 mg, 2 mg. **Tablets (Immediate-Release [Xanax]):** 0.25 mg, 0.5 mg, 1 mg, 2 mg.
🔲 **Tablets (Extended-Release [Xanax XR]):** 0.5 mg, 1 mg, 2 mg, 3 mg.

 ✢ Canadian trade name   🔲 Non-Crushable Drug   🟥 High Alert drug

ADMINISTRATION/HANDLING

PO, Immediate-Release
• May give without regard to meals. • Tablets may be crushed. • If oral intake is not possible, may be given sublingually.

PO, Extended-Release
• Administer once daily. • Do not break, crush, dissolve, or divide extended-release tablets. Swallow whole.

PO, Orally Disintegrating
• Place tablet on tongue, allow to dissolve. • Swallow with saliva. • Administration with water not necessary. • If using ½ tab, discard remaining ½ tab.

INDICATIONS/ROUTES/DOSAGE

Anxiety Disorders
PO: *(Immediate-Release, Oral Concentrate, ODT)* : **ADULTS:** Initially, 0.25–0.5 mg 3 times/day. May titrate q3–4days. **Maximum:** 4 mg/day in divided doses. **CHILDREN, YOUNGER THAN 18 YRS:** 0.125 mg 3 times/day. May increase by 0.125–0.25 mg/dose. **Maximum:** 0.06 mg/kg/day or 0.02 mg/kg/dose. Range: 0.375–3 mg/day. **ELDERLY, DEBILITATED PTS, PTS WITH HEPATIC DISEASE OR LOW SERUM ALBUMIN:** Initially, 0.25 mg 2–3 times/day. Gradually increase to optimum therapeutic response.

Anxiety with Depression
PO: ADULTS: (average dose required) 2.5–3 mg/day in divided doses.

Panic Disorder
PO *(Immediate-Release, Oral Concentrate, ODT)*: **ADULTS:** Initially, 0.5 mg 3 times/day. May increase at 3- to 4-day intervals in increments of 1 mg or less a day. Range: 5–6 mg/day. **Maximum:** 10 mg/day. **ELDERLY:** Initially, 0.125–0.25 mg twice daily. May increase in 0.125-mg increments until desired effect attained.
PO: *(Extended-Release)*:
◄**ALERT►** To switch from immediate-release to extended-release form, give total daily dose (immediate-release) as a single daily dose of extended-release form.
ADULTS: Initially, 0.5–1 mg once daily. May titrate at 3- to 4-day intervals. Range: 3–6 mg/day. **ELDERLY:** Initially, 0.5 mg once daily.

Dosage in Renal Impairment
No dose adjustment.

Dosage in Hepatic Impairment
Severe Disease: Immediate-Release: 0.25 mg 2–3 mg times/day. **Extended-Release:** 0.5 mg once daily.

SIDE EFFECTS

Frequent (41%–20%): Ataxia, light-headedness, drowsiness, slurred speech (particularly in elderly or debilitated pts). **Occasional (15%–5%):** Confusion, depression, blurred vision, constipation, diarrhea, dry mouth, headache, nausea. **Rare (4% or less):** Behavioral problems such as anger, impaired memory; paradoxical reactions (insomnia, nervousness, irritability).

ADVERSE EFFECTS/ TOXIC REACTIONS

Abrupt or too-rapid withdrawal may result in restlessness, irritability, insomnia, hand tremors, abdominal/muscle cramps, diaphoresis, vomiting, seizures. Overdose results in drowsiness, confusion, diminished reflexes, coma. Blood dyscrasias noted rarely. **Antidote:** Flumazenil (see Appendix J for dosage).

NURSING CONSIDERATIONS

BASELINE ASSESSMENT
Assess degree of anxiety; assess for drowsiness, dizziness, light-headedness. Assess motor responses (agitation, trembling, tension), autonomic responses (cold/clammy hands, diaphoresis). Initiate fall precautions.

INTERVENTION/EVALUATION
For pts on long-term therapy, perform hepatic/renal function tests, CBC periodically. Assess for paradoxical reaction, particularly during early therapy.

Evaluate for therapeutic response: calm facial expression, decreased restlessness, insomnia. Monitor respiratory and cardiovascular status.

PATIENT/FAMILY TEACHING

• Drowsiness usually disappears during continued therapy. • If dizziness occurs, change positions slowly from recumbent to sitting position before standing. • Avoid tasks that require alertness, motor skills until response to drug is established. • Smoking reduces drug effectiveness. • Sour hard candy, gum, sips of water may relieve dry mouth. • Do not abruptly withdraw medication after long-term therapy. • Avoid alcohol. • Do not take other medications without consulting physician.

---

alteplase HIGH ALERT

al-te-plase
(Activase, Cathflo Activase)
Do not confuse alteplase or Activase with Altace, or Activase with Cathflo Activase.

◆CLASSIFICATION

PHARMACOTHERAPEUTIC: Tissue plasminogen activator (tPA). **CLINICAL:** Thrombolytic.

USES

Treatment of ST-elevation MI for lysis of thrombi in coronary arteries, acute ischemic stroke, acute massive pulmonary embolism. Treatment of occluded central venous catheters. **OFF-LABEL:** Acute peripheral occlusive disease, prosthetic valve thrombosis. Acute ischemic stroke presenting 3–4½ hrs after onset of symptoms.

PRECAUTIONS

Contraindications: Hypersensitivity to alteplase. Active internal bleeding, AV malformation or aneurysm, bleeding diathesis CVA, intracranial neoplasm, intracranial or intraspinal surgery or trauma, recent (within past 2 mos), severe uncontrolled hypertension, suspected aortic dissection. **Cautions:** Recent (within 10 days) major surgery or GI bleeding, OB delivery, organ biopsy, recent trauma or CPR, left heart thrombus, endocarditis, severe hepatic disease, pregnancy, elderly, cerebrovascular disease, diabetic retinopathy, thrombophlebitis, occluded AV cannula at infected site.

ACTION

Binds to fibrin in a thrombus and converts entrapped plasminogen to plasmin, initiating fibrinolysis. **Therapeutic Effect:** Degrades fibrin clots, fibrinogen, other plasma proteins.

PHARMACOKINETICS

Rapidly metabolized in liver. Primarily excreted in urine. **Half-life:** 35 min.

⧖ LIFESPAN CONSIDERATIONS

Pregnancy/Lactation: Use only when benefit outweighs potential risk to fetus. Unknown if drug crosses placenta or is distributed in breast milk. **Children:** Safety and efficacy not established. **Elderly:** May have increased risk of bleeding; monitor closely.

INTERACTIONS

DRUG: Heparin, low molecular weight heparins, medications altering platelet function (e.g., clopidogrel, NSAIDs, thrombolytics), oral anticoagulants (e.g., warfarin) increase risk of hemorrhage. **HERBAL:** Cat's claw, dong quai, evening primrose, feverfew, garlic, ginkgo, ginseng, green tea, horse chestnut, red clover may increase risk of bleeding due to antiplatelet activity. **FOOD:** None known. **LAB VALUES:** Decreases plasminogen, fibrinogen levels during infusion, decreases clotting time (confirms the presence of lysis). May decrease Hgb, Hct.

AVAILABILITY (Rx)

Injection, Powder for Reconstitution: 2 mg (Cathflo Activase), 50 mg (Activase), 100 mg (Activase).

ADMINISTRATION/HANDLING
IV

Reconstitution • Activase: Reconstitute immediately before use with Sterile Water for Injection. • Reconstitute 100-mg vial with 100 mL Sterile Water for Injection (50-mg vial with 50 mL sterile water) without preservative to provide a concentration of 1 mg/mL. • **Activase Cathflo:** Add 2.2 mL Sterile Water for Injection to provide concentration of 1 mg/mL. • Avoid excessive agitation; gently swirl or slowly invert vial to reconstitute.

Rate of Administration • Activase: Give by IV infusion via infusion pump (see Indications/Routes/Dosage). • If minor bleeding occurs at puncture sites, apply pressure for 30 sec; if unrelieved, apply pressure dressing. • If uncontrolled hemorrhage occurs, discontinue infusion immediately (slowing rate of infusion may produce worsening hemorrhage). • Avoid undue pressure when drug is injected into catheter (can rupture catheter or expel clot into circulation). • Instill dose into occluded catheter. • After 30 min, assess catheter function by attempting to aspirate blood. • If still occluded, let dose dwell an additional 90 min. • If function not restored, a second dose may be instilled.

Storage • Activase: Store vials at room temperature. • After reconstitution, solution appears colorless to pale yellow. • Solution is stable for 8 hrs after reconstitution. Discard unused portions.

IV INCOMPATIBILITIES

DOBUTamine (Dobutrex), DOPamine (Intropin), heparin.

IV COMPATIBILITIES

Lidocaine, metoprolol (Lopressor), morphine, nitroglycerin, propranolol (Inderal).

INDICATIONS/ROUTES/DOSAGE

Acute MI
IV Infusion: ADULTS WEIGHING MORE THAN 67 KG: Total dose: 100 mg over 90 min, starting with 15-mg bolus over 1–2 min, then 50 mg over 30 min, then 35 mg over 60 min. **ADULTS WEIGHING 67 KG OR LESS: Total dose:** Start with 15-mg bolus over 1–2 min, then 0.75 mg/kg over 30 min (**maximum:** 50 mg), then 0.5 mg/kg over 60 min (**maximum:** 35 mg). **Maximum total dose:** 100 mg.

Acute Pulmonary Emboli
IV Infusion: ADULTS: 100 mg over 2 hrs. May give as a 10-mg bolus followed by 90 mg over 2 hrs. Institute or reinstitute heparin near end or immediately after infusion when activated partial thromboplastin time (aPTT) or thrombin time (TT) returns to twice normal or less.

Acute Ischemic Stroke
◀**ALERT**▶ Dose should be given within the first 3 hrs of the onset of symptoms. Recommended total dose: 0.9 mg/kg. **Maximum:** 90 mg.
IV Infusion: ADULTS WEIGHING 100 KG OR LESS: 0.09 mg/kg as IV bolus over 1 min, then 0.81 mg/kg as continuous infusion over 60 min. **WEIGHING GREATER THAN 100 KG:** 9 mg bolus over 1 min, then 81 mg as continuous infusion over 60 min.

Central Venous Catheter Clearance
IV: ADULTS, ELDERLY: Up to 2 mg; may repeat after 2 hrs. If catheter functional, withdraw 4–5 mL blood to remove drug and residual clot.

Usual Neonatal Dosage
Occluded IV Catheter: Use 1 mg/mL conc (**maximum:** 2 mg/2 mL) leave in lumen up to 2 hrs, then aspirate.

Systemic Thrombosis: 0.1–0.6 mg/kg/hr for 6 hrs.

Dosage in Renal/Hepatic Impairment
No dose adjustment.

SIDE EFFECTS

Frequent: Superficial bleeding at puncture sites, decreased B/P. **Occasional:** Allergic reaction (rash, wheezing, bruising).

ADVERSE EFFECTS/TOXIC REACTIONS

Severe internal hemorrhage, intracranial hemorrhage may occur. Lysis of coronary thrombi may produce atrial or ventricular arrhythmias or stroke.

NURSING CONSIDERATIONS

BASELINE ASSESSMENT

Assess for contraindications to therapy. Obtain baseline B/P, apical pulse. Record weight. Evaluate 12-lead EKG, cardiac enzymes, electrolytes. Assess Hct, platelet count, thrombin time (TT), prothrombin time (PT), activated partial thromboplastin time (aPTT), fibrinogen level before therapy is instituted. Type and screen blood.

INTERVENTION/EVALUATION

Perform continuous cardiac monitoring for arrhythmias. Check B/P, pulse, respirations q15min until stable, then hourly. Check peripheral pulses, heart and lung sounds. Monitor for chest pain relief and notify physician of continuation or recurrence (note location, type, intensity). Assess for bleeding: overt blood, occult blood in any body substance. Monitor aPTT per protocol. Maintain B/P; avoid any trauma that might increase risk of bleeding (e.g., injections, shaving). Assess neurologic status frequently.

amikacin

am-i-**kay**-sin
(Amikin)

■ **BLACK BOX ALERT** ■ May cause neurotoxicity, nephrotoxicity, and/or neuromuscular blockade and respiratory paralysis. Ototoxicity usually is irreversible; nephrotoxicity usually is reversible.
Do not confuse amikacin or Amikin with Amicar, or amikacin with anakinra.

◆CLASSIFICATION

PHARMACOTHERAPEUTIC: Aminoglycoside. **CLINICAL:** Antibiotic.

USES

Treatment of serious infections due to *Pseudomonas,* other gram-negative organisms (*Proteus, Serratia,* other gram-negative bacilli), including biliary tract, bone and joint, CNS, intra-abdominal, skin and soft tissue, urinary tract. Treatment of bacterial pneumonia, septicemia. **OFF-LABEL:** *Mycobacterium avium* complex (MAC).

PRECAUTIONS

Contraindications: Hypersensitivity to amikacin, other aminoglycosides. **Cautions:** Preexisting renal impairment, auditory or vestibular impairment, hypocalcemia, elderly, pts with neuromuscular disorder, dehydration, concomitant use of neurotoxic or nephrotoxic medications.

ACTION

Inhibits protein synthesis in susceptible bacteria by binding to 30S ribosomal unit. **Therapeutic Effect:** Interferes with protein synthesis of susceptible microorganisms.

PHARMACOKINETICS

Rapid, complete absorption after IM administration. Protein binding: 0%–10%. Widely distributed (penetrates

 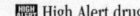

blood-brain barrier when meninges are inflamed). Excreted unchanged in urine. Removed by hemodialysis. **Half-life:** 2–4 hrs (increased in renal impairment, neonates; decreased in cystic fibrosis, burn pts, febrile pts).

⧗ LIFESPAN CONSIDERATIONS

Pregnancy/Lactation: Readily crosses placenta; small amounts distributed in breast milk. May produce fetal nephrotoxicity. **Children:** Neonates, premature infants may be more susceptible to toxicity due to immature renal function. **Elderly:** Higher risk of toxicity due to age-related renal impairment, increased risk of hearing loss.

INTERACTIONS

DRUG: Nephrotoxic (e.g., **cyclosporine, gentamicin, IV contrast dye, NSAIDS**) and ototoxic medications (e.g., **aspirin, gentamicin, furosemide, quinine**) may increase toxicity. May increase effects of **cycloSPORINE, neuromuscular blocking agents.** **HERBAL:** None significant. **FOOD:** None known. **LAB VALUES:** May increase serum creatinine, BUN, ALT, AST, bilirubin, LDH. May decrease serum calcium, magnesium, potassium, sodium. **Therapeutic levels:** Peak: life-threatening infections: 25–40 mcg/mL; serious infections: 20–25 mcg/mL; urinary tract infections: 15–20 mcg/mL. **Trough:** Less than 8 mcg/mL. **Toxic levels:** Peak: greater than 40 mcg/mL; **trough:** greater than 10 mcg/mL.

AVAILABILITY (Rx)

Injection Solution: 250 mg/mL.

ADMINISTRATION/HANDLING

 IV

Reconstitution • Dilute to concentration of 0.25–5 mg/mL in 0.9% NaCl or D₅W.
Rate of Administration • Infuse over 30–60 min.

Storage • Store vials at room temperature. • Solution appears clear but may become pale yellow (does not affect potency). • Intermittent IV infusion (piggyback) is stable for 24 hrs at room temperature, 2 days if refrigerated. • Discard if precipitate forms or dark discoloration occurs.

IM
• To minimize discomfort, give deep IM slowly. • Less painful if injected into gluteus maximus rather than in lateral aspect of thigh.

▦ IV INCOMPATIBILITIES

Amphotericin, azithromycin (Zithromax), propofol (Diprivan).

▦ IV COMPATIBILITIES

Amiodarone (Cordarone), aztreonam (Azactam), calcium gluconate, cefepime (Maxipime), cimetidine (Tagamet), ciprofloxacin (Cipro), clindamycin (Cleocin), dexmedetomidine (Precedex), diltiaZEM (Cardizem), diphenhydrAMINE (Benadryl), enalapril (Vasotec), esmolol (BreviBloc), fluconazole (Diflucan), furosemide (Lasix), levoFLOXacin (Levaquin), LORazepam (Ativan), magnesium sulfate, midazolam (Versed), morphine, ondansetron (Zofran), potassium chloride, raNITIdine (Zantac), vancomycin.

INDICATIONS/ROUTES/DOSAGE

Usual Parenteral Dosage
IV, IM: ADULTS, ELDERLY, CHILDREN, INFANTS: 5–7.5 mg/kg/dose q8h. **NEONATES:** 15 mg/kg/dose q12–48h (based on wgt).

Dosage in Renal Impairment
Dosage and frequency are modified based on degree of renal impairment and serum drug concentration. After a loading dose of 5–7.5 mg/kg, maintenance dose and frequency are based on serum creatinine levels and creatinine clearance.

Creatinine Clearance	Dosing Interval
50 mL/min or greater	q8h
30–49 mL/min	q12–18h
10–29 mL/min	q18–24h
Less than 10 mL/min	q48–72h
Hemodialysis	q48–72h (give after HD on dialysis days)
Continuous renal replacement therapy (CRRT)	Initially, 10 mg/kg, then 7.5 mg/kg q24–48h

Dosage in Hepatic Impairment
No dose adjustment.

SIDE EFFECTS

Frequent: Phlebitis, thrombophlebitis. **Occasional:** Rash, fever, urticaria, pruritus. **Rare:** Neuromuscular blockade (difficulty breathing, drowsiness, weakness).

ADVERSE EFFECTS/TOXIC REACTIONS

Serious reactions include nephrotoxicity (increased thirst, decreased appetite, nausea, vomiting, increased BUN and serum creatinine levels, decreased creatinine clearance); neurotoxicity (muscle twitching, visual disturbances, seizures, paresthesia); ototoxicity (tinnitus, dizziness, loss of hearing).

NURSING CONSIDERATIONS

BASELINE ASSESSMENT

Obtain BUN, serum creatinine. Dehydration must be treated prior to aminoglycoside therapy. Establish baseline hearing acuity before beginning therapy. Question for history of allergies, esp. to aminoglycosides and sulfite. Obtain specimen for culture, sensitivity before giving first dose (therapy may begin before results are known).

INTERVENTION/EVALUATION

Monitor I&O (maintain hydration), urinalysis. Monitor results of serum peak/trough levels. Be alert to ototoxic, neurotoxic, nephrotoxic symptoms (see Adverse Effects/Toxic Reactions). Check IM injection site for pain, induration. Evaluate IV site for phlebitis. Assess skin rash, diarrhea, superinfection (particularly genital/anal pruritus), changes of oral mucosa. When treating pts with neuromuscular disorders, assess respiratory response carefully. **Therapeutic levels:** Peak: life-threatening infections: 25–40 mcg/mL; serious infections: 20–25 mcg/mL; urinary tract infections: 15–20 mcg/mL. **Trough:** Less than 8 mcg/mL. **Toxic levels:** Peak: greater than 40 mcg/mL; **trough:** greater than 10 mcg/mL.

PATIENT/FAMILY TEACHING

• Continue antibiotic for full length of treatment. • Space doses evenly. • IM injection may cause discomfort. • Report any hearing, visual, balance, urinary problems, even after therapy is completed. • Do not take other medications without consulting physician.

---

amiodarone

a-mi-**oh**-da-rone
(Apo-Amiodarone ✦, Nexterone, Pacerone)

■ **BLACK BOX ALERT** ■ Pts should be hospitalized when amiodarone is initiated. Alternative therapies should be tried first before using amiodarone. Only indicated for pts with life-threatening arrhythmias due to risk of toxicity. Pulmonary toxicity may occur without symptoms. Hepatotoxicity is common, usually mild (rarely possible). Can exacerbate arrhythmias.

Do not confuse amiodarone with aMILoride, dronedarone, or Cordarone with Cardura.

◆CLASSIFICATION

PHARMACOTHERAPEUTIC: Cardiac agent. **CLINICAL:** Antiarrhythmic.

✦ Canadian trade name   🔰 Non-Crushable Drug   HIGH ALERT High Alert drug

USES

Management of life-threatening recurrent ventricular fibrillation, hemodynamically unstable ventricular tachycardia (VT) unresponsive to other therapy. **OFF-LABEL:** Treatment of atrial fibrillation, paroxysmal supraventricular tachycardia (SVT); ventricular tachyarrhythmias.

PRECAUTIONS

Contraindications: Hypersensitivity to amiodarone, iodine. Bradycardia-induced syncope (except in the presence of a pacemaker), second- and third-degree AV block (except in presence of a pacemaker); severe sinus node dysfunction, causing marked sinus bradycardia; cardiogenic shock. **Cautions:** May prolong QT interval. Thyroid disease, electrolyte imbalance, hepatic disease, hypotension, left ventricular dysfunction, pulmonary disease. Pts taking warfarin, surgical pts.

ACTION

Prolongs duration of myocardial cell action potential and refractory period by acting directly on all cardiac tissue. Decreases AV and sinus node function. **Therapeutic Effect:** Suppresses arrhythmias.

PHARMACOKINETICS

Route	Onset	Peak	Duration
PO	3 days–3 wks	1 wk–5 mos	7–50 days after discontinuation

Slowly, variably absorbed from GI tract. Protein binding: 96%. Extensively metabolized in liver. Excreted via bile; not removed by hemodialysis. **Half-life:** 26–107 days; metabolite: 61 days.

LIFESPAN CONSIDERATIONS

Pregnancy/Lactation: Crosses placenta; distributed in breast milk. May adversely affect fetal development. **Children:** Safety and efficacy not established. **Elderly:** May be more sensitive to effects on thyroid function. May experience increased incidence of ataxia, other neurotoxic effects.

INTERACTIONS

DRUG: Sofosbuvir may cause severe bradycardia. May increase **thioridazine** concentration and produce additive prolongation of QT interval. May increase cardiac effects with **other antiarrhythmics.** May increase effect of **beta blockers (e.g., carvedilol, labetalol, metoprolol), oral anticoagulants (e.g., warfarin).** May increase concentration, toxicity of ARIPiprazole, **colchicine, digoxin, phenytoin.** May increase risk of **simvastatin** toxicity, myopathy, rhabdomyolysis. **HERBAL: St. John's wort** may decrease effect. **Ephedra** may worsen arrhythmia. Herbals with hypotensive properties may increase levels/effects of amiodarone. **FOOD: Grapefruit products** may alter effect. Avoid use during therapy. **LAB VALUES:** May increase serum ALT, AST, alkaline phosphatase, ANA titer. May cause changes in EKG, thyroid function test results. **Therapeutic serum level:** 0.5–2.5 mcg/mL; toxic serum level not established.

AVAILABILITY (Rx)

Infusion (Pre-Mix): Nexterone: 150 mg/100 mL; 360 mg/200 mL. **Injection, Solution (Cordarone IV):** 50 mg/mL, 3 mL, 9 mL, 18 mL. **Tablets:** 100 mg (Pacerone), 200 mg (Cordarone, Pacerone), 400 mg (Pacerone).

ADMINISTRATION/HANDLING

 IV

Reconstitution • Infusions longer than 2 hrs must be administered/diluted in glass or polyolefin bottles. • Dilute loading dose (150 mg) in 100 mL D_5W (1.5 mg/mL). • Dilute maintenance dose (900 mg) in 500 mL D_5W (1.8 mg/mL). Concentrations greater than 3 mg/mL cause peripheral vein phlebitis.

Rate of Administration • Does not need protection from light during administration. • Administer through central venous catheter (CVC) if possible, using in-line filter. • Bolus over 10 min (15 mg/min) not to exceed 30 mg/min; then

1 mg/min over 6 hrs; then 0.5 mg/min over 18 hrs. • Infusions longer than 1 hr, concentration not to exceed 2 mg/mL unless CVC used.

Storage • Store at room temperature. • Stable for 24 hrs when diluted in glass or polyolefin containers; stable for 2 hrs when diluted in PVC containers.

PO

• Give consistently with regard to meals to reduce GI distress. • Tablets may be crushed. • Do not give with grapefruit products.

🔳 IV INCOMPATIBILITIES

CeFAZolin (Ancef), heparin, sodium bicarbonate.

🔳 IV COMPATIBILITIES

Dexmedetomidine (Precedex), DOBUTamine (Dobutrex), DOPamine (Intropin), furosemide (Lasix), insulin (regular), labetalol (Normodyne), lidocaine, LORazepam (Ativan), midazolam (Versed), morphine, nitroglycerin, norepinephrine (Levophed), phenylephrine (Neo-Synephrine), potassium chloride, vancomycin.

INDICATIONS/ROUTES/DOSAGE

Ventricular Arrhythmias
PO: ADULTS, ELDERLY: Initially, 800–1,600 mg/day in 1–2 divided doses for 1–3 wks. After arrhythmia is controlled or side effects occur, reduce to 600–800 mg/day for 4 wks. **Maintenance:** 400 mg/day.
IV Infusion: ADULTS, ELDERLY: Initially, 1,050 mg over 24 hrs; 150 mg over 10 min, then 360 mg over 6 hrs; then 540 mg over 18 hrs. May continue at 0.5 mg/min. After first 24 hrs, infuse 720 mg/24 hrs (0.5 mg/min) with a concentration of 1–6 mg/mL.

Dosage in Renal Impairment
No dose adjustment.

Dosage in Hepatic Impairment
Use caution.

SIDE EFFECTS

Expected: Corneal microdeposits noted in almost all pts treated for more than 6 mos (can lead to blurry vision). **Occasional (greater than 3%): PO:** Constipation, headache, decreased appetite, nausea, vomiting, paresthesia, photosensitivity, muscular incoordination. **Parenteral:** Hypotension, nausea, fever, bradycardia. **Rare (less than 3%): PO:** Bitter or metallic taste, decreased libido, dizziness, facial flushing, blue-gray coloring of skin (face, arms, and neck), blurred vision, bradycardia, asymptomatic corneal deposits, rash, visual disturbances, halo vision.

ADVERSE EFFECTS/ TOXIC REACTIONS

Serious, potentially fatal pulmonary toxicity (alveolitis, pulmonary fibrosis, pneumonitis, acute respiratory distress syndrome) may begin with progressive dyspnea and cough with crackles, decreased breath sounds, pleurisy, HF, or hepatotoxicity. May worsen existing arrhythmias or produce new arrhythmias.

NURSING CONSIDERATIONS

BASELINE ASSESSMENT

Obtain baseline serum ALT, AST, alkaline phosphatase, EKG; pulmonary function tests, CXR in pts with pulmonary disease. Assess B/P, apical pulse immediately before drug is administered (if pulse is 60/min or less or systolic B/P is less than 90 mm Hg, withhold medication, contact physician).

INTERVENTION/EVALUATION

Monitor for symptoms of pulmonary toxicity (progressively worsening dyspnea, cough). Dosage should be discontinued or reduced if toxicity occurs. Assess pulse for quality, rhythm, bradycardia. Monitor EKG for cardiac changes (e.g., widening of QRS, prolongation of PR and QT intervals). Notify physician of any significant interval changes. Assess for nausea, fatigue, paresthesia, tremor. Monitor for signs of hypothyroidism (periorbital

 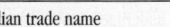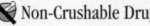

edema, lethargy, pudgy hands/feet, cool/ pale skin, vertigo, night cramps) and hyperthyroidism (hot/dry skin, bulging eyes [exophthalmos], frequent urination, eyelid edema, weight loss, difficulty breathing). Monitor serum ALT, AST, alkaline phosphatase for evidence of hepatic toxicity. Assess skin, cornea for bluish discoloration in pts who have been on drug therapy longer than 2 mos. Monitor thyroid function test results. If elevated hepatic enzymes occur, dosage reduction or discontinuation is necessary. Monitor for therapeutic serum level (0.5–2.5 mcg/ mL). Toxic serum level not established.

PATIENT/FAMILY TEACHING

• Protect against photosensitivity reaction on skin exposed to sunlight. • Bluish skin discoloration gradually disappears when drug is discontinued. • Report shortness of breath, cough. • Outpatients should monitor pulse before taking medication. • Do not abruptly discontinue medication. • Compliance with therapy regimen is essential to control arrhythmias. • Restrict salt, alcohol intake. • Avoid grapefruit products. • Recommend ophthalmic exams q6mos. • Report any vision changes, signs/symptoms of cardiac arrhythmias.

amitriptyline

a-mi-**trip**-ti-leen
(Apo-Amitriptyline ✤, Levate ✤, Novo-Tryptyn ✤, Elavil)

■ **BLACK BOX ALERT** ■ Increased risk of suicidal thinking and behavior in children, adolescents, young adults 18–24 yrs with major depressive disorder, other psychiatric disorders.
Do not confuse amitriptyline with aminophylline, imipramine, or nortriptyline, or Elavil with Eldepryl, enalapril, Equanil, or Mellaril.

FIXED-COMBINATION(S)

Limbitrol: amitriptyline/chlordiazePOXIDE (an antianxiety): 12.5 mg/5 mg, 25 mg/10 mg.

◆CLASSIFICATION

PHARMACOTHERAPEUTIC: Tricyclic. **CLINICAL:** Antidepressant, antineuralgic, antibulimic.

USES

Treatment of depression. **OFF-LABEL:** Neuropathic pain, related to diabetic neuropathy or postherpetic neuralgia; treatment of migraine. Treatment of depression in children, post-traumatic stress disorder (PTSD).

PRECAUTIONS

Contraindications: Hypersensitivity to amitriptyline. Acute recovery period after MI, co-administered with or within 14 days of MAOIs. **Cautions:** Prostatic hypertrophy, history of urinary retention or obstruction, narrow-angle glaucoma, diabetes, seizures, hyperthyroidism, cardiac/hepatic/renal disease, schizophrenia, xerostomia, visual problems, constipation or bowel obstruction, elderly, increased intraocular pressure (IOP), hiatal hernia, suicidal ideation.

ACTION

Blocks reuptake of neurotransmitters (norepinephrine, serotonin) at presynaptic membranes, increasing availability at postsynaptic receptor sites. Strong anticholinergic activity. **Therapeutic Effect:** Antidepressant effect.

PHARMACOKINETICS

Rapidly and well absorbed from GI tract. Protein binding: 90%. Metabolized in liver. Primarily excreted in urine. Minimal removal by hemodialysis. **Half-life:** 10–26 hrs.

⧗ LIFESPAN CONSIDERATIONS

Pregnancy/Lactation: Crosses placenta; minimally distributed in breast milk. **Children:** More sensitive to increased dosage, toxicity, increased risk of suicidal ideation, worsening of depression. **Elderly:** Increased risk of toxicity. Increased sensitivity to anticholinergic effects. Caution in pts with cardiovascular disease.

INTERACTIONS

DRUG: CNS depressants (e.g., alcohol, anticonvulsants, barbiturates, phenothiazines, sedative-hypnotics) may increase sedation, respiratory depression, hypotensive effect. May increase concentrations of **dronedarone, thioridazine, toremifine, ziprasidone.** QUEtiapine may increase level/effect. May increase risk of hypertensive crisis, hyperpyresis, seizures with **MAOIs. HERBAL:** St. John's wort may decrease levels. **Gotu kola, kava kava, St. John's wort, valerian** may increase CNS depression. **FOOD:** None known. **LAB VALUES:** May alter EKG readings (flattened T wave), serum glucose (increase or decrease). **Therapeutic serum level:** Peak: 120–250 ng/mL; **toxic serum level:** greater than 500 ng/mL.

AVAILABILITY (Rx)

Tablets: 10 mg, 25 mg, 50 mg, 75 mg, 100 mg, 150 mg.

ADMINISTRATION/HANDLING

PO
• Give with food or milk if GI distress occurs.

INDICATIONS/ROUTES/DOSAGE

Depression
PO: ADULTS: Initially, 25–50 mg/day as a single dose at bedtime, or in divided doses. May gradually increase up to 100–300 mg/day. Titrate to lowest effective dosage. **ELDERLY:** 10 mg 3 times/day and 20 mg at bedtime. **ADOLESCENTS:** 10 mg 3 times/day and 20 mg at bedtime.

Pain Management
PO: ADULTS, ELDERLY: 25–50 mg at bedtime. May increase to 150 mg/day. **CHILDREN:** Initially, 0.1 mg/kg. May increase over 2 wks to 0.5–2 mg/kg at bedtime.

Dosage in Renal/Hepatic Impairment
Use with caution.

SIDE EFFECTS

Frequent: Dizziness, drowsiness, dry mouth, orthostatic hypotension, headache, increased appetite, weight gain, nausea, unusual fatigue, unpleasant taste. **Occasional:** Blurred vision, confusion, constipation, hallucinations, delayed micturition, eye pain, arrhythmias, fine muscle tremors, parkinsonian syndrome, anxiety, diarrhea, diaphoresis, heartburn, insomnia. **Rare:** Hypersensitivity, alopecia, tinnitus, breast enlargement, photosensitivity.

ADVERSE EFFECTS/TOXIC REACTIONS

Overdose may produce confusion, seizures, severe drowsiness, changes in cardiac conduction, fever, hallucinations, agitation, dyspnea, vomiting, unusual fatigue, weakness. Abrupt withdrawal after prolonged therapy may produce headache, malaise, nausea, vomiting, vivid dreams. Blood dyscrasias, cholestatic jaundice occur rarely.

NURSING CONSIDERATIONS

BASELINE ASSESSMENT

Observe and record behavior. Assess psychological status, thought content, suicidal ideation, sleep patterns, appearance, interest in environment. For pts on long-term therapy, hepatic/renal function tests, blood counts should be performed periodically.

INTERVENTION/EVALUATION

Supervise suicidal-risk pt closely during early therapy (as depression lessens, energy level improves, increasing suicide potential). Assess appearance, behavior, speech pattern, level of interest, mood. Monitor B/P for hypotension, pulse, arrhythmias. **Therapeutic**

✦ Canadian trade name   🐴 Non-Crushable Drug   🔲 High Alert drug

serum level: Peak: 120–250 ng/mL; **toxic serum level:** greater than 500 ng/mL.

PATIENT/FAMILY TEACHING

• Go slowly from lying to standing. • Tolerance to postural hypotension, sedative and anticholinergic effects usually develops during early therapy. • Maximum therapeutic effect may be noted in 2–4 wks. • Sensitivity to sun may occur. • Report visual disturbances. • Do not abruptly discontinue medication. • Avoid tasks that require alertness, motor skills until response to drug is established. • Avoid alcohol. • Sips of water may relieve dry mouth.

---

amLODIPine   [TOP 100]

am-**loe**-di-peen
(Apo-amLODIPine ✲, Norvasc)
Do not confuse amLODIPine with aMILoride, or Norvasc with Navane or Vascor.

FIXED-COMBINATION(S)

Anturnide: amLODIPine/aliskiren (a renin inhibitor)/hydroCHLOROthiazide (a diuretic): 5 mg/150 mg/12.5 mg, 5 mg/300 mg/12.5 mg, 5 mg/300 mg/25 mg, 10 mg/300 mg/12.5 mg, 10 mg/300 mg/25 mg. **Azor:** amLODIPine/olmesartan (an angiotensin II receptor antagonist): 5 mg/20 mg, 10 mg/20 mg, 5 mg/40 mg, 10 mg/40 mg. **Caduet:** amLODIPine/atorvastatin (hydroxymethylglutaryl-CoA [HMG-CoA] reductase inhibitor): 2.5 mg/10 mg, 2.5 mg/20 mg, 2.5 mg/40 mg, 5 mg/10 mg, 10 mg/10 mg, 5 mg/20 mg, 10 mg/20 mg, 5 mg/40 mg, 10 mg/40 mg, 5 mg/80 mg, 10 mg/80 mg. **Exforge:** amLODIPine/valsartan (an angiotensin II receptor antagonist): 5 mg/160 mg, 10 mg/160 mg, 5 mg/320 mg, 10 mg/320 mg. **Exforge HCT:** amLODIPine/valsartan/hydroCHLOROthiazide (a diuretic): 5 mg/160 mg/12.5 mg, 5 mg/160 mg/25 mg, 10 mg/160 mg/12.5 mg, 10 mg/160 mg/25 mg, 10 mg/320 mg/25 mg. **Lotrel:** amLODIPine/benazepril (an angiotensin-converting enzyme [ACE] inhibitor): 2.5 mg/10 mg, 5 mg/10 mg, 5 mg/20 mg, 5 mg/40 mg, 10 mg/20 mg, 10 mg/40 mg. **Prestalia:** amLODIPine/perindopril (an ACE inhibitor): 2.5 mg/3.5 mg; 5 mg/7 mg; 10 mg/14 mg. **Tekamlo:** amLODIPine/aliskiren (a renin inhibitor): 5 mg/150 mg, 5 mg/300 mg, 10 mg/150 mg, 10 mg/300 mg. **Tribenzor:** amLODIPine/olmesartan/hydroCHLOROthiazide: 5 mg/20 mg/12.5 mg, 5 mg/40 mg/12.5 mg, 5 mg/40 mg/25 mg, 10 mg/40 mg/12.5 mg, 10 mg/40 mg/25 mg. **Twynsta:** amLODIPine/telmisartan (an angiotensin II receptor antagonist): 5 mg/40 mg, 5 mg/80 mg, 10 mg/40 mg, 10 mg/80 mg.

◆CLASSIFICATION

PHARMACOTHERAPEUTIC: Calcium channel blocker. **CLINICAL:** Antihypertensive, antianginal.

USES

Management of hypertension, coronary artery disease (chronic stable angina, vasospastic [Prinzmetal's or variant] angina).

PRECAUTIONS

Contraindications: Hypersensitivity to amLODIPine. **Cautions:** Hepatic impairment, severe aortic stenosis, hypertrophic cardiomyopathy with outflow tract obstruction.

ACTION

Inhibits calcium movement across cardiac and vascular smooth muscle cell membranes. **Therapeutic Effect:** Dilates coronary arteries, peripheral arteries/arterioles. Decreases total peripheral vascular resistance and B/P by vasodilation.

PHARMACOKINETICS

Route	Onset	Peak	Duration
PO	0.5–1 hr	N/A	24 hrs

Slowly absorbed from GI tract. Protein binding: 95%–98%. Metabolized in liver. Excreted primarily in urine. Not removed by hemodialysis. **Half-life:** 30–50 hrs (increased in elderly, pts with hepatic cirrhosis).

⧖ LIFESPAN CONSIDERATIONS

Pregnancy/Lactation: Unknown if drug crosses placenta or is distributed in breast milk. **Children:** Safety and efficacy not established. **Elderly:** Half-life may be increased, more sensitive to hypotensive effects.

INTERACTIONS

DRUG: May increase level of **simvastatin. Azole antifungals, cycloSPORINE, protease inhibitors (e.g., darunavir, ritonavir)** may increase concentration. **CarBAMazepine, rifAMPin** may decrease level/effect. **HERBAL: St. John's wort** may decrease concentration. **Ephedra, yohimbe** may worsen hypertension. **Garlic** may increase antihypertensive effect. **FOOD: Grapefruit products** may increase concentration, hypotensive effects. **LAB VALUES:** May increase hepatic enzyme levels.

AVAILABILITY (Rx)

Tablets: 2.5 mg, 5 mg, 10 mg.

ADMINISTRATION/HANDLING

PO

• May give without regard to food.

INDICATIONS/ROUTES/DOSAGE

Hypertension

PO: ADULTS: Initially, 5 mg/day as a single dose. May titrate every 7–14 days. **Maximum:** 10 mg/day. **SMALL-FRAME, FRAGILE, ELDERLY:** 2.5 mg/day as a single dose. May titrate q7–14 days. **Maximum:** 10 mg/day. **CHILDREN 6–17 YRS:** 2.5–5 mg/day.

CAD

PO: ADULTS: 5–10 mg/day as a single dose. **ELDERLY, PTS WITH HEPATIC INSUFFICIENCY:** 5 mg/day as a single dose.

Dosage in Renal Impairment

No dose adjustment.

Dosage in Hepatic Impairment

ADULTS, ELDERLY: (Hypertension) Initially, 2.5 mg/day. (Angina) Initially, 5 mg/day. Titrate slowly in pts with severe impairment.

SIDE EFFECTS

Frequent (greater than 5%): Peripheral edema, headache, flushing. **Occasional (5%–1%):** Dizziness, palpitations, nausea, unusual fatigue or weakness (asthenia). **Rare (less than 1%):** Chest pain, bradycardia, orthostatic hypotension.

ADVERSE EFFECTS/ TOXIC REACTIONS

Overdose may produce excessive peripheral vasodilation, marked hypotension with reflex tachycardia, syncopy.

NURSING CONSIDERATIONS

BASELINE ASSESSMENT

Assess baseline renal/hepatic function tests, B/P, apical pulse.

INTERVENTION/EVALUATION

Assess B/P (if systolic B/P is less than 90 mm Hg, withhold medication, contact physician). Assess for peripheral edema behind medial malleolus (sacral area in bedridden pts). Assess skin for flushing. Question for headache, asthenia.

PATIENT/FAMILY TEACHING

• Do not abruptly discontinue medication. • Compliance with therapy regimen is essential to control hypertension. • Avoid tasks that require alertness, motor skills until response to drug is established. • Do not ingest grapefruit products.

---

amoxicillin

a-**mox**-i-sil-in
(Apo-Amoxi ✦, Moxatag,
Novamoxin ✦)
**Do not confuse amoxicillin with
amoxapine or Atarax.**

◆CLASSIFICATION

PHARMACOTHERAPEUTIC: Penicillin.
CLINICAL: Antibiotic.

USES

Treatment of susceptible infections due to
streptococci, *E. coli, E. faecalis, P. mirabilis, H. influenzae, N. gonorrhoeae,*
including ear, nose, and throat; lower
respiratory tract; skin and skin structure;
UTIs; acute uncomplicated gonorrhea;
H. pylori. **OFF-LABEL:** Treatment of Lyme
disease and typhoid fever. Postexposure
prophylaxis for anthrax exposure.

PRECAUTIONS

Contraindications: Hypersensitivity to
amoxicillin, other beta-lactams. **Cautions:** History of allergies (esp. cephalosporins), infectious mononucleosis,
renal impairment, asthma.

ACTION

Inhibits bacterial cell wall synthesis.
Therapeutic Effect: Bactericidal in
susceptible microorganisms.

PHARMACOKINETICS

Well absorbed from GI tract. Protein
binding: 20%. Partially metabolized
in liver. Primarily excreted in urine.
Removed by hemodialysis. **Half-
life:** 1–1.3 hrs (increased in renal
impairment).

☒ LIFESPAN CONSIDERATIONS

Pregnancy/Lactation: Crosses placenta, appears in cord blood, amniotic
fluid. Distributed in breast milk in low
concentrations. May lead to allergic sensitization, diarrhea, candidiasis, skin rash in
infant. **Children:** Immature renal function
in neonate/young infant may delay renal
excretion. **Elderly:** Age-related renal impairment may require dosage adjustment.

INTERACTIONS

DRUG: Allopurinol may increase
incidence of rash. **Probenecid** may
increase concentration, toxicity risk.
May decrease effect of **oral contraceptives. HERBAL:** None significant.
FOOD: None known. **LAB VALUES:** May
increase serum ALT, AST, bilirubin,
BUN, creatinine, LDH. May cause positive Coombs' test.

AVAILABILITY (Rx)

Capsules: 250 mg, 500 mg. **Powder
for Oral Suspension:** 125 mg/5 mL,
200 mg/5 mL, 250 mg/5 mL, 400 mg/5
mL. **Tablets:** 500 mg, 875 mg. **Tablets
(Chewable):** 125 mg, 250 mg. **Tablets,
Extended-Release (Moxatag):** 775 mg.

ADMINISTRATION/HANDLING

PO
• Give without regard to meals. • Instruct pt to chew/crush chewable tablets
thoroughly before swallowing. • Oral
suspension dose may be mixed with
formula, milk, fruit juice, water,
cold drink. • Give immediately after
mixing. • After reconstitution, oral
suspension is stable for 14 days at either room temperature or refrigerated.

INDICATIONS/ROUTES/DOSAGE

Susceptible Infections
PO: ADULTS, ELDERLY: 250–500 mg q8h
or 500–875 mg q12h or 775 mg (Moxatag) once daily. **CHILDREN OLDER THAN 3
MOS:** 25–50 mg/kg/day in divided doses
q8h. Maximum single dose: 500 mg.
CHILDREN 3 MOS AND YOUNGER: 25–50
mg/kg/day in divided doses q8h. **NEO-
NATE:** 20–30 mg/kg/day in divided doses
q12h.

H. Pylori Infection
PO: ADULTS, ELDERLY: 1 g twice daily in
combination with at least 1 other antibiotic

and an acid-suppressing agent (proton pump inhibitor or H₂ antagonist).

Otitis Media
PO: CHILDREN: 80–90 mg/kg/day in 2 divided doses. **NEONATES:** 30–40 mg/kg/day in divided doses q8h.

Dosage in Renal Impairment
◀ALERT▶ Immediate-release 875-mg tablet or 775-mg extended-release tablet should not be used in pts with creatinine clearance less than 30 mL/min. Dosage interval is modified based on creatinine clearance. **Creatinine clearance 10–30 mL/min:** 250–500 mg q12h. **Creatinine clearance less than 10 mL/min:** 250–500 mg q24h.

Dosage in Hepatic Impairment
No dose adjustment.

SIDE EFFECTS
Frequent: GI disturbances (mild diarrhea, nausea, vomiting), headache, oral/vaginal candidiasis. **Occasional:** Generalized rash, urticaria.

ADVERSE EFFECTS/TOXIC REACTIONS
Antibiotic-associated colitis, other superinfections (abdominal cramps, severe watery diarrhea, fever) may result from altered bacterial balance in GI tract. Severe hypersensitivity reactions, including anaphylaxis, acute interstitial nephritis, occur rarely.

NURSING CONSIDERATIONS
BASELINE ASSESSMENT
Question for history of allergies (esp. penicillins, cephalosporins), renal impairment.

INTERVENTION/EVALUATION
Promptly report rash, diarrhea (fever, abdominal pain, mucus and blood in stool may indicate antibiotic-associated colitis). Be alert for superinfection: fever, vomiting, diarrhea, anal/genital pruritus, black "hairy" tongue, oral mucosal

changes (ulceration, pain, erythema). Monitor renal/hepatic function tests.

PATIENT/FAMILY TEACHING
• Continue antibiotic for full length of treatment. • Space doses evenly. • Take with meals if GI upset occurs. • Thoroughly crush or chew the chewable tablets before swallowing. • Report rash, diarrhea, other new symptoms.

---

amoxicillin/clavulanate

a-**mox**-i-sil-in/**klav**-yoo-la-nate
(Apo-Amoxi-Clav ✦, <u>Augmentin</u>, Augmentin ES 600, <u>Augmentin XR</u>, Clavulin ✦, Novo-Clavamoxin ✦)
Do not confuse Augmentin with amoxicillin or Azulfidine.

◆CLASSIFICATION
PHARMACOTHERAPEUTIC: Penicillin. **CLINICAL:** Antibiotic.

USES
Treatment of susceptible infections due to *streptococci, E. coli, E. faecalis, P. mirabilis,* beta-lactamase producing *H. influenzae, Klebsiella* spp., *M. catarrhalis,* and *S. aureus* (not methicillin-resistant *Staphylococcus aureus* [MRSA]), including lower respiratory, skin and skin structure, UTIs, otitis media, sinusitis. **OFF-LABEL:** Chronic antimicrobial suppression of prosthetic joint infection.

PRECAUTIONS
Contraindications: Hypersensitivity to amoxicillin, clavulanate, any penicillins; history of cholestatic jaundice or hepatic impairment with amoxicillin/clavulanate therapy. Augmentin XR (additional): Severe renal impairment (CrCl less than 30 mL/min), hemodialysis pt. **Cautions:** History of allergies, esp. cephalosporins; renal impairment, infectious mononucleosis.

✦ Canadian trade name   🗎 Non-Crushable Drug   🔲 High Alert drug

ACTION

Amoxicillin inhibits bacterial cell wall synthesis. Clavulanate inhibits bacterial beta-lactamase. **Therapeutic Effect:** Amoxicillin is bactericidal in susceptible microorganisms. Clavulanate protects amoxicillin from enzymatic degradation.

PHARMACOKINETICS

Well absorbed from GI tract. Protein binding: 20%. Partially metabolized in liver. Primarily excreted in urine. Removed by hemodialysis. **Half-life:** 1–1.3 hrs (increased in renal impairment).

⧗ LIFESPAN CONSIDERATIONS

Pregnancy/Lactation: Crosses placenta, appears in cord blood, amniotic fluid. Distributed in breast milk in low concentrations. May lead to allergic sensitization, diarrhea, candidiasis, skin rash in infant. **Children:** Immature renal function in neonate/young infant may delay renal excretion. **Elderly:** Age-related renal impairment may require dosage adjustment.

INTERACTIONS

DRUG: Allopurinol may increase incidence of rash. **Probenecid** may increase concentration, toxicity risk. May decrease effect of **oral contraceptives. HERBAL:** None significant. **FOOD:** None known. **LAB VALUES:** May increase serum ALT, AST. May cause positive Coombs' test.

AVAILABILITY (Rx)

Powder for Oral Suspension (Amoclan, Augmentin): 125 mg–31.25 mg/5 mL, 200 mg–28.5 mg/5 mL, 250 mg–62.5 mg/5 mL, 400 mg–57 mg/5 mL, 600 mg–42.9 mg/5 mL. **Tablets (Augmentin):** 250 mg–125 mg, 500 mg–125 mg, 875 mg–125 mg. **Tablets (Chewable [Augmentin]):** 200 mg–28.5 mg, 400 mg–57 mg.

Tablets (Extended-Release [Augmentin XR]): 1,000 mg–62.5 mg.

ADMINISTRATION/HANDLING

PO

• Store tablets at room temperature. • After reconstitution, oral suspension is stable for 10 days but should be refrigerated. • May mix dose of suspension with milk, formula, or juice and give immediately. • Give without regard to meals. • Give with food to increase absorption, decrease stomach upset. • Instruct pt to chew/crush chewable tablets thoroughly before swallowing. • Do not break, crush, dissolve, or divide extended-release tablets.

INDICATIONS/ROUTES/DOSAGE

Note: Dosage based on amoxicillin component.

Usual Adult Dosage

PO: ADULTS, ELDERLY: 250 mg q8h or 500 mg q8–12h or 875 mg q12h or 2,000 mg q12h.

Usual Pediatric Dosage

PO: CHILDREN OLDER THAN 3 MOS, WEIGHING 40 KG OR MORE: (Mild-Moderate): 500 mg q12h or 250 mg q8h. **(Severe):** 875 mg q12h or 500 mg q8h. **(Extended-Release):** 2,000 mg q12h. **WEIGHING LESS THAN 40 KG: (Mild-Moderate):** 25 mg/kg/day in 2 divided doses or 20 mg/kg/day in 3 divided doses. **(Severe):** 45 mg/kg/day in 2 divided doses or 40 mg/kg/day in 3 divided doses. **Maximum Single Dose:** 500 mg. **LESS THAN 3 MOS:** Amoxicillin 30 mg/kg/day divided q12h using 125 mg/5mL suspension only.

Usual Neonate Dosage

PO: NEONATES, CHILDREN YOUNGER THAN 3 MOS: 30 mg/kg/day (125 mg/5 mL suspension) in divided doses q12h.

Dosage in Renal Impairment

◀ **ALERT** ▶ Do not use 875-mg tablet or extended-release tablets for creatinine clearance less than 30 mL/min. Dosage and frequency are modified based on creatinine clearance. **Creatinine clearance 10–30 mL/min:** 250–500 mg q12h. **Creatinine clearance less than 10 mL/min:** 250–500 mg q24h. **HD:** 250–500 mg q24h, give dose during and after dialysis. **PD:** 250 mg q12h.

Dosage in Hepatic Impairment

No dose adjustment (see Contraindications).

SIDE EFFECTS

Occasional (9%–4%): Diarrhea, loose stools, nausea, skin rashes, urticaria. **Rare (less than 3%):** Vomiting, vaginitis, abdominal discomfort, flatulence, headache.

ADVERSE EFFECTS/ TOXIC REACTIONS

Antibiotic-associated colitis, other superinfections (abdominal cramps, severe watery diarrhea, fever) may result from altered bacterial balance in GI tract. Severe hypersensitivity reactions, including anaphylaxis, acute interstitial nephritis, occur rarely.

NURSING CONSIDERATIONS

BASELINE ASSESSMENT

Question for history of allergies, esp. penicillins, cephalosporins, renal impairment.

INTERVENTION/EVALUATION

Promptly report rash, diarrhea (fever, abdominal pain, mucus and blood in stool may indicate antibiotic-associated colitis). Be alert for signs of superinfection, including fever, vomiting, diarrhea, black "hairy" tongue, ulceration or changes of oral mucosa, anal/genital pruritus. Monitor renal/hepatic tests with prolonged therapy.

PATIENT/FAMILY TEACHING

• Continue antibiotic for full length of treatment. • Space doses evenly. • Take with meals if GI upset occurs. • Thoroughly crush or chew the chewable tablets before swallowing. • Notify physician if rash, diarrhea, other new symptoms occur.

amphotericin B ▪️HIGH ALERT▪️

am-foe-**ter**-i-sin
(<u>Abelcet</u>, <u>AmBisome</u>, Amphotec, Fungizone ✦)

■ **BLACK BOX ALERT** ■ (Nonliposomal) To be used primarily for pts with progressive, potentially fatal fungal infection. Not to be used for noninvasive forms of fungal disease (oral thrush, vaginal candidiasis).

◆CLASSIFICATION

PHARMACOTHERAPEUTIC: Polyene antifungal. **CLINICAL:** Antifungal, antiprotozoal.

USES

Abelcet: Treatment of aspergillosis or any type of invasive fungal infections refractory or intolerant to Fungizone. **AmBisome:** Empiric treatment of fungal infection in febrile neutropenic pts. *Aspergillus, Candida* species, *Cryptococcus* infections refractory to Fungizone or pt with renal impairment or toxicity with Fungizone. Treatment of cryptococcal meningitis in HIV-infected pts. Treatment of visceral leishmaniasis. **Amphotec:** Treatment of invasive aspergillosis in pts with renal impairment or toxicity or prior treatment failure with Fungizone. **Fungizone:** Treatment of life-threatening fungal infections caused by susceptible fungi, including *Candida* spp., *Histoplasma, Cryptococcus, Aspergillus, Blastomyces.* **OFF-LABEL:** Abelcet, Amphotec: Serious *Candida* infections. **AmBisome:** Treatment of systemic histoplasmosis infection.

PRECAUTIONS

Contraindications: Hypersensitivity to amphotericin B. **Cautions:** Concomitant use with other nephrotoxic drugs; renal impairment.

ACTION

Generally fungistatic but may become fungicidal with high dosages or very susceptible microorganisms. Binds to sterols in fungal cell membrane. **Therapeutic Effect:** Alters fungal cell membrane permeability, allowing loss of potassium, other cellular components, resulting in cell death.

PHARMACOKINETICS

Protein binding: 90%. Widely distributed. Metabolism not specified. Cleared by nonrenal pathways. Minimal removal by hemodialysis. Amphotec and Abelcet are not dialyzable. **Half-life:** Fungizone, 24 hrs (increased in neonates and children); Abelcet, 7.2 days; AmBisome, 100–153 hrs; Amphotec, 26–28 hrs.

⏳ LIFESPAN CONSIDERATIONS

Pregnancy/Lactation: Crosses placenta; unknown if distributed in breast milk. **Children:** Safety and efficacy not established, but use the least amount for therapeutic regimen. **Elderly:** No age-related precautions noted.

INTERACTIONS

DRUG: Antineoplastic agents may increase potential for bronchospasm, renal toxicity, hypotension. **Corticosteroids (e.g., hydrocortisone, prednisone, dexamethasone), corticotropin** may cause severe hypokalemia, cardiac dysfunction. **Nephrotoxic medications (e.g., cycloSPORINE, IV contrast dye, vancomycin)** may increase nephrotoxicity. **HERBAL:** None significant. **FOOD:** None known. **LAB VALUES:** May increase serum ALT, AST, alkaline phosphatase, BUN, creatinine. May decrease serum calcium, magnesium, potassium.

AVAILABILITY (Rx)

Injection, Powder for Reconstitution: 50 mg (AmBisome, Amphotec, Fungizone), 100 mg (Amphotec). **Injection, Suspension (Abelcet):** 5 mg/mL.

ADMINISTRATION/HANDLING
📋 IV

• Use strict aseptic technique; no bacteriostatic agent or preservative is present in diluent.

Reconstitution
ABELCET
• Shake 20-mL (100-mg) vial gently until contents are dissolved. Withdraw required dose using 5-micron filter needle (supplied by manufacturer). • Dilute with D_5W to 1–2 mg/mL.
AMBISOME
• Reconstitute each 50-mg vial with 12 mL Sterile Water for Injection to provide concentration of 4 mg/mL. • Shake vial vigorously for 30 sec. Withdraw required dose and inject syringe contents through a 5-micron filter into an infusion of D_5W to provide final concentration of 1–2 mg/mL (0.2–0.5 mg/mL for infants and small children).
AMPHOTEC
• Add 10 mL Sterile Water for Injection to each 50-mg vial to provide concentration of 5 mg/mL. Shake gently. • Further dilute **only** with D_5W to a concentration of 0.1–2 mg/mL.
FUNGIZONE
• Add 10 mL Sterile Water for Injection to each 50-mg vial. • Further dilute with 250–500 mL D_5W. • Final concentration should not exceed 0.1 mg/mL (0.25 mg/mL for central infusion).
Rate of Administration • Give by slow IV infusion. Infuse conventional amphotericin over 4–6 hrs; Abelcet over 2 hrs (shake contents if infusion longer than 2 hrs); Amphotec over minimum of 2 hrs (avoid rate faster than 1 mg/kg/hr); AmBisome over 1–2 hrs.
Storage
ABELCET
• Refrigerate unreconstituted solution. Reconstituted solution is stable for 48 hrs if refrigerated, 6 hrs at room temperature.
AMBISOME
• Refrigerate unreconstituted solution. Reconstituted vials are stable for 24 hrs when refrigerated. Concentration of 1–2 mg/mL is stable for 6 hrs.
AMPHOTEC
• Refrigerate unused vials. • Reconstituted solution is stable for 24 hrs if refrigerated.

FUNGIZONE

• Refrigerate unused vials. • Once reconstituted, vials stable for 24 hrs at room temperature, 7 days if refrigerated. • Diluted solutions stable for 24 hrs at room temperature, 2 days if refrigerated.

IV INCOMPATIBILITIES

Note: Abelcet, AmBisome, Amphotec: Do not mix with any other drug, diluent, or solution. Fungizone: Allopurinol (Aloprim), aztreonam (Azactam), calcium gluconate, cefepime (Maxipime), cimetidine (Tagamet), ciprofloxacin (Cipro), dexmedetomidine (Precedex), diphenhydrAMINE (Benadryl), DOPamine (Intropin), enalapril (Vasotec), filgrastim (Neupogen), fluconazole (Diflucan), foscarnet (Foscavir), magnesium sulfate, meropenem (Merrem IV), ondansetron (Zofran), piperacillin and tazobactam (Zosyn), potassium chloride, propofol (Diprivan).

IV COMPATIBILITY

LORazepam (Ativan).

INDICATIONS/ROUTES/DOSAGE

Usual Abelcet Dose
IV Infusion *(Abelcet)*: ADULTS, CHILDREN: 3–5 mg/kg/day at rate of 2.5 mg/kg/hr.

Usual AmBisome Dose
IV Infusion *(Ambisome)*: ADULTS, CHILDREN: 3–6 mg/kg/day over 2 hrs.

Usual Amphotec Dose
IV Infusion *(Amphotec)*: ADULTS, CHILDREN: 3–4 mg/kg/day at rate no faster than 1 mg/kg/hr. **Maximum:** 6 mg/kg/day.

Fungizone, Usual Dose
IV Infusion: ADULTS, ELDERLY: Dosage based on pt tolerance and severity of infection. Initially, 1-mg test dose is given over 20–30 min. If tolerated, usual dose is 0.3–1.5 mg/kg/day or 1–1.5 mg/kg q48h. **Maximum:** 1.5 mg/kg/day. **CHILDREN:** Test dose of 0.1 mg/kg/dose (**maximum:** 1 mg) is infused over 30–60 min. If test dose is tolerated, usual

dose is 0.25–1 mg/kg/day or 1–1.5 mg/kg q48h. **NEONATES:** Initially, 0.5 mg/kg/dose once daily. May gradually increase by 0.25–0.5 mg/kg each day to maximum of 1.5 mg/kg/day. **Maintenance dose:** 0.25–1 mg/kg/day or 1–1.5 mg/kg/dose every other day.

Dosage in Renal/Hepatic Impairment
No dose adjustment.

SIDE EFFECTS

Frequent (greater than 10%): Abelcet: Chills, fever, increased serum creatinine, multiple organ failure. **AmBisome:** Hypokalemia, hypomagnesemia, hyperglycemia, hypocalcemia, edema, abdominal pain, back pain, chills, chest pain, hypotension, diarrhea, nausea, vomiting, headache, fever, rigors, insomnia, dyspnea, epistaxis, increased hepatic/renal function test results. **Amphotec:** Chills, fever, hypotension, tachycardia, increased serum creatinine, hypokalemia, bilirubinemia. **Amphocin:** Fever, chills, headache, anemia, hypokalemia, hypomagnesemia, anorexia, malaise, generalized pain, nephrotoxicity.

ADVERSE EFFECTS/ TOXIC REACTIONS

Cardiovascular toxicity (hypotension, ventricular fibrillation), anaphylaxis occur rarely. Altered vision/hearing, seizures, hepatic failure, coagulation defects, multiple organ failure, sepsis may occur. Each alternative formulation is less nephrotoxic than conventional amphotericin (Amphocin).

NURSING CONSIDERATIONS

BASELINE ASSESSMENT

Obtain baseline BMP, LFT, serum magnesium, ionized calcium. Question for history of allergies, esp. to amphotericin B, sulfite. Avoid, if possible, other nephrotoxic medications. Obtain premedication orders (antipyretics, antihistamines, antiemetics, corticosteroids) to reduce adverse reactions during IV therapy.

INTERVENTION/EVALUATION

Monitor B/P, temperature, pulse, respirations; assess for adverse reactions (fever, tremors, chills, anorexia, nausea, vomiting, abdominal pain) q15min twice, then q30min for 4 hrs of initial infusion. If symptoms occur, slow infusion, administer medication for symptomatic relief. For severe reaction, stop infusion and notify physician. Evaluate IV site for phlebitis. Monitor I&O, renal function tests for nephrotoxicity. Monitor CBC, BMP (esp. potassium), LFT, serum magnesium.

PATIENT/FAMILY TEACHING

• Prolonged therapy (wks or mos) is usually necessary. • Fever reaction may decrease with continued therapy. • Muscle weakness may be noted during therapy (due to hypokalemia).

---

ampicillin

am-pi-**sil**-in
(Apo-Ampi ✦, Novo-Ampicillin ✦, Nu-Ampi ✦)
Do not confuse ampicillin with aminophylline.

◆CLASSIFICATION

PHARMACOTHERAPEUTIC: Penicillin.
CLINICAL: Antibiotic.

USES

Treatment of susceptible infections due to streptococci, *S. pneumoniae,* staphylococci (non–penicillinase-producing), meningococci, *Listeria,* some *Klebsiella, E. coli, H. influenzae, Salmonella, Shigella,* including GI, GU, respiratory infections, meningitis, endocarditis prophylaxis. **OFF-LABEL:** Surgical prophylaxis for liver transplantation.

PRECAUTIONS

Contraindications: Hypersensitivity to ampicillin or any penicillin. Infections caused by penicillinase-producing organisms. **Cautions:** History of allergies, esp. cephalosporins, renal impairment, asthmatic pts, infectious mononucleosis.

ACTION

Inhibits cell wall synthesis in susceptible microorganisms. **Therapeutic Effect:** Bactericidal in susceptible microorganisms.

PHARMACOKINETICS

Moderately absorbed from GI tract. Protein binding: 15%–25%. Widely distributed. Partially metabolized in liver. Primarily excreted in urine. Removed by hemodialysis. **Half-life:** 1–1.5 hrs (increased in renal impairment).

⧖ LIFESPAN CONSIDERATIONS

Pregnancy/Lactation: Crosses placenta; appears in cord blood, amniotic fluid. Distributed in breast milk in low concentrations. May lead to allergic sensitization, diarrhea, candidiasis, skin rash in infant. **Children:** Immature renal function in neonates/young infants may delay renal excretion. **Elderly:** Age-related renal impairment may require dosage adjustment.

INTERACTIONS

DRUG: Allopurinol may increase incidence of rash. **Probenecid** may increase concentration, toxicity risk. May decrease effects of **oral contraceptives.** May increase level/effect of **methotrexate. HERBAL:** None significant. **FOOD:** None known. **LAB VALUES:** May increase serum ALT, AST. May cause positive Coombs' test.

AVAILABILITY (Rx)

Capsules: 250 mg, 500 mg. **Injection, Powder for Reconstitution:** 125 mg, 250 mg, 500 mg, 1 g, 2 g. **Powder for Oral Suspension:** 125 mg/5 mL, 250 mg/5 mL.

ADMINISTRATION/HANDLING

 IV

Reconstitution • For IV injection, dilute each vial with 5 mL Sterile Water for Injection or 0.9% NaCl (10 mL for 1- and 2-g vials). **Maximum concentration:** 100 mg/mL for IV push. • For intermittent IV infusion (piggyback), further dilute with 50–100 mL 0.9% NaCl. **Maximum concentration:** 30 mg/mL.
Rate of Administration • For IV injection, give over 3–5 min (125–500 mg) or over 10–15 min (1–2 g). For intermittent IV infusion (piggyback), infuse over 15–30 min. • Due to potential for hypersensitivity/anaphylaxis, start initial dose at few drops per min, increase slowly to ordered rate; stay with pt first 10–15 min, then check q10min.
Storage • IV solution, diluted with 0.9% NaCl, is stable for 8 hrs at room temperature or 2 days if refrigerated. • If diluted with D_5W, is stable for 2 hrs at room temperature or 3 hrs if refrigerated. • Discard if precipitate forms.

IM
• Reconstitute each vial with Sterile Water for Injection or Bacteriostatic Water for Injection (consult individual vial for specific volume of diluent). • Stable for 1 hr. • Give deeply in large muscle mass.

PO
• Oral suspension, after reconstitution, is stable for 7 days at room temperature, 14 days if refrigerated. • Shake oral suspension well before using. • Give orally 1–2 hrs before meals for maximum absorption.

▦ IV INCOMPATIBILITIES

DiltiaZEM (Cardizem), midazolam (Versed), ondansetron (Zofran).

▦ IV COMPATIBILITIES

Calcium gluconate, cefepime (Maxipime), dexmedetomidine (Precedex), DOPamine (Intropin), famotidine (Pepcid), furosemide (Lasix), heparin, HYDROmorphone (Dilaudid), insulin (regular), levoFLOXacin (Levaquin), lipids, magnesium sulfate, morphine, multivitamins, potassium chloride, propofol (Diprivan).

INDICATIONS/ROUTES/DOSAGE

Usual Dosage
PO: ADULTS, ELDERLY: 250–500 mg q6h. **CHILDREN:** 50–100 mg/kg/day in divided doses q6h. **Maximum:** 2–4 g/day. **IV, IM: ADULTS, ELDERLY:** 1–2 g q4–6h or 50–250 mg/kg/day in divided doses. **Maximum:** 12 g/day. **CHILDREN:** 25–200 mg/kg/day in divided doses q6h. **Maximum:** 12 g/day. **NEONATES:** 50 mg/kg/dose q6–12h.

Dosage in Renal Impairment

Creatinine Clearance	Dosage
10–50 mL/min	Administer q6–12h
Less than 10 mL/min	Administer q12–24h
Hemodialysis	1–2 g q12–24h
Peritoneal dialysis	250 mg q12h
Continuous renal replacement therapy (CRRT)	2g, then 1–2 g q6–8h

Dosage in Hepatic Impairment
No dose adjustment.

SIDE EFFECTS

Frequent: Pain at IM injection site, GI disturbances (mild diarrhea, nausea, vomiting), oral or vaginal candidiasis. **Occasional:** Generalized rash, urticaria, phlebitis, thrombophlebitis (with IV administration), headache. **Rare:** Dizziness, seizures (esp. with IV therapy).

ADVERSE EFFECTS/TOXIC REACTIONS

Antibiotic-associated colitis, other superinfections (abdominal cramps, severe watery diarrhea, fever) may result from altered bacterial balance in GI tract. Severe hypersensitivity reactions, including anaphylaxis, acute interstitial nephritis, occur rarely.

NURSING CONSIDERATIONS

BASELINE ASSESSMENT

Question for history of allergies, esp. penicillins, cephalosporins; renal impairment.

INTERVENTION/EVALUATION

Promptly report rash (although common with ampicillin, may indicate hypersensitivity) or diarrhea (fever, abdominal pain, mucus and blood in stool may indicate antibiotic-associated colitis). Evaluate IV site for phlebitis. Check IM injection site for pain, induration. Monitor I&O, urinalysis, renal function tests. Be alert for superinfection: fever, vomiting, diarrhea, anal/genital pruritus, oral mucosal changes (ulceration, pain, erythema).

PATIENT/FAMILY TEACHING

• Continue antibiotic for full length of treatment. • Space doses evenly. • More effective if taken 1 hr before or 2 hrs after food/beverages. • Discomfort may occur with IM injection. • Report rash, diarrhea, or other new symptoms.

ampicillin/ sulbactam

amp-i-**sil**-in/sul-**bak**-tam
(<u>Unasyn</u>)

◆CLASSIFICATION

PHARMACOTHERAPEUTIC: Penicillin. **CLINICAL:** Antibiotic.

USES

Treatment of susceptible infections, including intra-abdominal, skin/skin structure, gynecologic infections, due to beta-lactamase–producing organisms, including *H. influenzae, E. coli, Klebsiella, Acinetobacter, Enterobacter, S. aureus,* and *Bacteroides* spp. OFF-

LABEL: Endocarditis, community-acquired pneumonia, surgical prophylaxis, pelvic inflammatory disease.

PRECAUTIONS

Contraindications: Hypersensitivity to ampicillin, any penicillins, or sulbactam. Hx of cholestatic jaundice, hepatic impairment associated with ampicillin/sulbactam. **Cautions:** History of allergies, esp. cephalosporins; renal impairment; infectious mononucleosis; asthmatic pts.

ACTION

Ampicillin inhibits bacterial cell wall synthesis. Sulbactam inhibits bacterial beta-lactamase. **Therapeutic Effect:** Ampicillin is bactericidal in susceptible microorganisms. Sulbactam protects ampicillin from enzymatic degradation.

PHARMACOKINETICS

Protein binding: 28%–38%. Widely distributed. Partially metabolized in liver. Primarily excreted in urine. Removed by hemodialysis. **Half-life:** 1–1.3 hrs (increased in renal impairment).

⧗ LIFESPAN CONSIDERATIONS

Pregnancy/Lactation: Crosses placenta; appears in cord blood, amniotic fluid. Distributed in breast milk in low concentrations. May lead to allergic sensitization, diarrhea, candidiasis, skin rash in infant. **Children:** Safety and efficacy not established in pts younger than 1 yr. **Elderly:** Age-related renal impairment may require dosage adjustment.

INTERACTIONS

DRUG: Allopurinol may increase incidence of rash. **Probenecid** may increase concentration, toxicity risk. May decrease effect of **oral contraceptives.** May increase level/effect of **methotrexate. HERBAL:** None significant. **FOOD:** None known. **LAB VALUES:** May increase serum ALT, AST, alkaline phosphatase, LDH, creatinine. May cause positive Coombs' test.

AVAILABILITY (Rx)

Injection, Powder for Reconstitution: 1.5 g (ampicillin 1 g/sulbactam 0.5 g), 3 g (ampicillin 2 g/sulbactam 1 g).

ADMINISTRATION/HANDLING

 IV

Reconstitution • For IV injection, dilute with Sterile Water for Injection to provide concentration of 375 mg/mL. • For intermittent IV infusion (piggyback), further dilute with 50–100 mL 0.9% NaCl.
Rate of Administration • For IV injection, give slowly over minimum of 10–15 min. • For intermittent IV infusion (piggyback), infuse over 15–30 min. • Due to potential for hypersensitivity/anaphylaxis, start initial dose at few drops per min, increase slowly to ordered rate; stay with pt first 10–15 min, then check q10min.
Storage • IV solution, diluted with 0.9% NaCl, is stable for up to 72 hrs if refrigerated (4 hrs if diluted with D₅W). • Discard if precipitate forms.

IM
• Reconstitute each 1.5-g vial with 3.2 mL Sterile Water for Injection or lidocaine to provide concentration of 250 mg ampicillin/125 mg sulbactam/mL. • Give deeply into large muscle mass within 1 hr after preparation.

🔲 IV INCOMPATIBILITIES

Amiodarone (Cordarone), diltiaZEM (Cardizem), IDArubicin (Idamycin), ondansetron (Zofran).

🔲 IV COMPATIBILITIES

Famotidine (Pepcid), heparin, insulin (regular), morphine.

INDICATIONS/ROUTES/DOSAGE

Usual Dosage Range
IV, IM: ADULTS, ELDERLY, CHILDREN 13 YRS AND OLDER: 1.5–3 g q6h. **Maximum:** 12 g/day. **IV: CHILDREN 12 YRS AND YOUNGER:** 100–200 mg ampicillin/kg/

day in divided doses q6h. **Maximum:** 12 g/day (Unasyn). 8 g/day (ampicillin). **NEONATES:** 100 mg (ampicillin)/kg/day in divided doses q8–12h.

Dosage in Renal Impairment
Dosage and frequency are modified based on creatinine clearance and severity of infection.

Creatinine Clearance	Dosage
Greater than 30 mL/min	No dose adjustment
15–30 mL/min	1.5–3 g q12h
5–14 mL/min	1.5–3 g q24h
Hemodialysis	1.5–3 g q12–24h (after HD on dialysis days)
Peritoneal dialysis	1.5–3 g q12–24h
Continuous renal replacement therapy (CRRT)	3 g, then 1.5–3 g q6–12h

Dosage in Hepatic Impairment
No dose adjustment.

SIDE EFFECTS

Frequent: Diarrhea, rash (most common), urticaria, pain at IM injection site, thrombophlebitis with IV administration, oral or vaginal candidiasis. **Occasional:** Nausea, vomiting, headache, malaise, urinary retention.

ADVERSE EFFECTS/TOXIC REACTIONS

Antibiotic-associated colitis, other superinfections (abdominal cramps; severe, watery diarrhea; fever) may result from altered bacterial balance in GI tract. Severe hypersensitivity reactions, including anaphylaxis, acute interstitial nephritis, blood dyscrasias may occur. High dosage may produce seizures.

NURSING CONSIDERATIONS

BASELINE ASSESSMENT

Question for history of allergies, esp. penicillins, cephalosporins; renal impairment.

 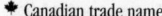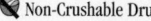 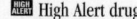

INTERVENTION/EVALUATION

Promptly report rash (although common with ampicillin, may indicate hypersensitivity) or diarrhea (fever, abdominal pain, mucus and blood in stool may indicate antibiotic-associated colitis). Evaluate IV site for phlebitis. Check IM injection site for pain, induration. Monitor I&O, urinalysis, renal function tests. Be alert for superinfection: fever, vomiting, diarrhea, anal/genital pruritus, oral mucosal changes (ulceration, pain, erythema).

PATIENT/FAMILY TEACHING

• Take antibiotic for full length of treatment. • Space doses evenly. • Discomfort may occur with IM injection. • Report rash, diarrhea, or other new symptoms.

---

anastrozole

HIGH ALERT

an-**as**-troe-zole
(Apo-Anastrozole ✦, Arimidex)
Do not confuse anastrozole with letrozole, or Arimidex with Imitrex.

◆CLASSIFICATION

PHARMACOTHERAPEUTIC: Aromatase inhibitor. **CLINICAL:** Antineoplastic hormone.

USES

Treatment of advanced breast cancer in postmenopausal women who have developed progressive disease while receiving tamoxifen therapy. First-line therapy in advanced or metastatic breast cancer in postmenopausal women. Adjuvant treatment in early hormone receptor–positive breast cancer in postmenopausal women. **OFF-LABEL:** Treatment of recurrent or metastatic endometrial or uterine cancers; treatment of ovarian cancer.

PRECAUTIONS

Contraindications: Hypersensitivity to anastrozole. Pregnancy, women who may become pregnant. **Cautions:** Preexisting ischemic cardiac disease, osteopenia (higher risk of developing osteoporosis), hyperlipidemia. May increase fall risk with fractures during therapy in pts with history of osteoporosis.

ACTION

Decreases circulating estrogen level by inhibiting aromatase, the enzyme that catalyzes the final step in estrogen production. **Therapeutic Effect:** Inhibits growth of breast cancers that are stimulated by estrogens by lowering serum estradiol concentration.

PHARMACOKINETICS

Well absorbed into systemic circulation (absorption not affected by food). Protein binding: 40%. Metabolized in liver. Eliminated by biliary system and, to a lesser extent, kidneys. **Mean half-life:** 50 hrs in postmenopausal women. Steady-state plasma levels reached in approximately 7 days.

⌧ LIFESPAN CONSIDERATIONS

Pregnancy/Lactation: Crosses placenta; may cause fetal harm. Unknown if distributed in breast milk. **Children:** Safety and efficacy not established. **Elderly:** No age-related precautions noted.

INTERACTIONS

DRUG: Estrogen therapies may reduce concentration/effects. **Tamoxifen** may reduce plasma concentration. **HERBAL:** Avoid **black cohosh, dong quai, licorice, red clover. FOOD:** None known. **LAB VALUES:** May elevate serum GGT level in pts with liver metastases. May increase serum ALT, AST, alkaline phosphatase, total cholesterol, LDL.

AVAILABILITY (Rx)

Tablets: 1 mg.

ADMINISTRATION/HANDLING

PO
- Give without regard to food.

INDICATIONS/ROUTES/DOSAGE

Breast Cancer (Advanced)
PO: ADULTS, ELDERLY: 1 mg once daily (continue until tumor progresses).

Breast Cancer (Early, Adjuvant)
PO: ADULTS, ELDERLY: 1 mg once daily.

Dosage in Renal/Hepatic Impairment
No dose adjustment.

SIDE EFFECTS

Frequent (16%–8%): Asthenia, nausea, headache, hot flashes, back pain, vomiting, cough, diarrhea. **Occasional (6%–4%):** Constipation, abdominal pain, anorexia, bone pain, pharyngitis, dizziness, rash, dry mouth, peripheral edema, pelvic pain, depression, chest pain, paresthesia. **Rare (2%–1%):** Weight gain, diaphoresis.

ADVERSE EFFECTS/TOXIC REACTIONS

Thrombophlebitis, anemia, leukopenia occur rarely. Vaginal hemorrhage occurs rarely (2%).

NURSING CONSIDERATIONS

BASELINE ASSESSMENT

Obtain baseline bone mineral density, total cholesterol, LDL, mammogram, clinical breast exam.

INTERVENTION/EVALUATION

Monitor for asthenia, dizziness; assist with ambulation if needed. Assess for headache, pain. Offer antiemetic for nausea, vomiting. Monitor for onset of diarrhea; offer antidiarrheal medication.

PATIENT/FAMILY TEACHING

- Notify physician if nausea, asthenia, hot flashes become unmanageable.

anidulafungin

a-**nid**-ue-la-**fun**-jin
(Eraxis)

◆CLASSIFICATION

PHARMACOTHERAPEUTIC: Echinocandin. **CLINICAL:** Antifungal.

USES

Treatment of candidemia, other forms of *Candida* infections (e.g., intra-abdominal abscess, peritonitis), esophageal candidiasis.

PRECAUTIONS

Contraindications: Hypersensitivity to anidulafungin, other echinocandins. **Cautions:** Hepatic impairment.

ACTION

Inhibits synthesis of the enzyme glucan (vital component of fungal cell formation), preventing fungal cell wall formation. **Therapeutic Effect:** Fungistatic.

PHARMACOKINETICS

Distributed in tissue. Moderately bound to albumin. Protein binding: 84%–99%. Slow chemical degradation; 30% excreted in feces over 9 days. Not removed by hemodialysis. **Half-life:** 40–50 hrs.

⧗ LIFESPAN CONSIDERATIONS

Pregnancy/Lactation: May be embryotoxic. Crosses placental barrier. Unknown if distributed in breast milk. **Children:** Safety and efficacy not established. **Elderly:** No age-related precautions noted.

INTERACTIONS

DRUG: None significant. **HERBAL:** None significant. **FOOD:** None known. **LAB VALUES:** May increase serum alkaline phosphatase, amylase, ALT, AST, bilirubin, calcium, creatinine, CPK, LDH, lipase. May decrease serum albumin, bicarbonate, magnesium, protein, potassium; Hgb, Hct, WBCs, neutrophils,

---

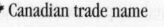 ♣ Canadian trade name   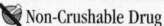 Non-Crushable Drug   **HIGH ALERT** High Alert drug

platelet count. May prolong prothrombin time (PT).

AVAILABILITY (Rx)

Injection, Powder for Reconstitution: 50-mg vial, 100-mg vial.

ADMINISTRATION/HANDLING

 IV

Reconstitution • Reconstitute each 50-mg vial with 15 mL Sterile Water for Injection (100 mg with 30 mL). Swirl, do not shake. • Further dilute 50 mg with 50 mL D_5W or 0.9% NaCl (100 mg with 100 mL, 200 mg with 200 mL).
Rate of Administration • Do not exceed infusion rate of 1.1 mg/min. Not for IV bolus injection.
Storage • Refrigerate unreconstituted vials. Reconstituted vials are stable for 24 hrs at room temperature. Infusion solution is stable for 48 hrs at room temperature.

IV INCOMPATIBILITIES

Amphotericin B (Abelcet, AmBisome), ertapenem (INVanz), sodium bicarbonate.

IV COMPATIBILITIES

Dexamethasone (Decadron), famotidine (Pepcid), furosemide (Lasix), HYDROmorphone (Dilaudid), LORazepam (Ativan), methylPREDNISolone (SOLU), morphine. Refer to IV Compatibility Chart in front of book.

INDICATIONS/ROUTES/DOSAGE

◄**ALERT**► Duration of treatment based on pt's clinical response. In general, treatment is continued for at least 14 days after last positive culture.

Candidemia, Other Candida Infections
IV: ADULTS, ELDERLY: Give single 200-mg loading dose on day 1, followed by 100 mg/day thereafter for at least 14 days after last positive culture.

Esophageal Candidiasis
IV: ADULTS, ELDERLY: Give single 100-mg loading dose on day 1, followed by 50 mg/day thereafter for a minimum of 14 days and for at least 7 days following resolution of symptoms.

Dosage in Renal/Hepatic Impairment
No dose adjustment.

SIDE EFFECTS

Rare (3%–1%): Diarrhea, nausea, headache, rigors, peripheral edema.

ADVERSE EFFECTS/ TOXIC REACTIONS

Hypokalemia occurs in 4% of pts. Hypersensitivity reaction characterized by facial flushing, hypotension, pruritus, urticaria, rash occurs rarely. Hepatitis, elevated LFT, hepatic failure was reported.

NURSING CONSIDERATIONS

BASELINE ASSESSMENT

Obtain baseline CBC, BMP, LFT. Obtain specimens for fungal culture prior to therapy. Treatment may be instituted before results are known.

INTERVENTION/EVALUATION

Monitor for evidence of hepatic dysfunction, hypokalemia. Monitor daily pattern of bowel activity, stool consistency. Assess for rash, urticaria.

PATIENT/FAMILY TEACHING

• For esophageal candidiasis, maintain diligent oral hygiene.

---

antihemophilic factor (factor VIII, AHF)

an-tee-hee-moe-**fil**-ik **fak**-tor
(**Antihemophilic Factor/von Willebrand Factor Complex:** Alphanate, Humate-P, Wilate. Human: Hemofil M, Koate-DVI, Monoclate-P. **Recombinant:** Advate, Eloctate, Kogenate FS, Recombinate, Xyntha)

◆CLASSIFICATION

PHARMACOTHERAPEUTIC: Antihemophilic agent. **CLINICAL:** Hemostatic.

USES

Human: Prevention/treatment of hemorrhagic episodes, perioperative management of hemophilia A. **Alphanate, Humate-P, Wilate:** Prevention/treatment of hemorrhagic episodes in pts with hemophilia A. Prophylaxis with surgical/invasive procedures, treatment of bleeding in pts with von Willebrand disease (vWD) when desmopressin is known or suspected to be inadequate. **Recombinant:** Management of hemophilia A, prevention and control of bleeding episodes, perioperative management of hemophilia A, prophylaxis of joint bleeding and reduce risk of joint damage in children with hemophilia A.

PRECAUTIONS

Contraindications: Hypersensitivity to any component of product. **Cautions:** Hepatic disease, pts with blood types A, B, AB (progressive anemia, intravascular hemolysis may occur).

ACTION

Assists in conversion of prothrombin to thrombin, essential for blood coagulation. Replaces missing clotting factor VIII. **Therapeutic Effect:** Produces hemostasis; corrects or prevents bleeding episodes.

PHARMACOKINETICS

Half-life: 8–27 hrs.

⏳ LIFESPAN CONSIDERATIONS

Pregnancy/Lactation: Unknown if drug crosses placenta or is distributed in breast milk. **Children:** Safety and efficacy not established. **Elderly:** No age-related precautions noted.

INTERACTIONS

DRUG: None significant. **HERBAL:** None significant. **FOOD:** None known. **LAB VALUES:** None significant.

AVAILABILITY (Rx)

Human: Injection, Powder for Reconstitution (Hemofil M, Koate-DVI, Monoclate-P): Actual number of units listed on each vial. **Alphanate:** 250 units, 500 units, 1,000 units, 1,500 units. **Elocate:** 250 units, 500 units, 750 units, 1,000 units, 1,500 units, 2,000 units, 3,000 units. **Humate-P:** 250 units, 500 units, 1,000 units. **Recombinant: Injection, Powder for Reconstitution: Advate:** 250 units, 500 units, 1,000 units, 1,500 units, 2,000 units, 3,000 units. **Kogenate, Recombinate:** 250 units, 500 units, 1,000 units. **Xyntha:** 250 units, 500 units, 1,000 units, 2,000 units.

ADMINISTRATION/HANDLING

💉 IV

Reconstitution • Warm concentrate and diluent to room temperature. • Using needle supplied by the manufacturer, add diluent to powder to dissolve, gently agitate or rotate. Do not shake vigorously. Complete dissolution may take 5–10 min. • Use second filtered needle supplied by the manufacturer, and add to infusion bag.

Rate of Administration • Advate: Over 5 min or less. **Maximum:** 10 mL/min. • **Hexilate FS, Kogenate FS:** Over 1–15 min based on pt tolerance. • **Xyntha:** Over several min. • **Hemofil M, Koate-DVI:** Over 5–10 min. **Maximum:** 10 mL/min. • **Monoclate-P:** Infuse at 2 mL/min. • **Alphanate:** 10 mL/min. • **Humate-P:** 4 mL/min.

Administration Precautions • Check pulse rate prior to and following administration. If pulse rate increases, reduce or stop administration. • After administration, apply prolonged pressure on venipuncture site. • Monitor IV site for oozing q5–15min for 1–2 hrs following administration.

Storage • May refrigerate or store at room temperature. • See individual products for specific storage durations.

⬛ IV INCOMPATIBILITIES

Do not mix with other IV solutions or medications.

INDICATIONS/ROUTES/DOSAGE

Hemophilia A, Von Willebrand Disease
IV: ADULTS, ELDERLY, CHILDREN: Dosage is highly individualized and is based on pt's weight, severity of bleeding, coagulation studies.

Dosage in Renal/Hepatic Impairment
No dose adjustment.

SIDE EFFECTS

Occasional: Allergic reaction, including fever, chills, urticaria, wheezing, hypotension, nausea, feeling of chest tightness, stinging at injection site, dizziness, dry mouth, headache, altered taste.

ADVERSE EFFECTS/TOXIC REACTIONS

Risk of transmitting viral hepatitis. Intravascular hemolysis may occur if large or frequent doses are used with blood group A, B, or AB.

NURSING CONSIDERATIONS

BASELINE ASSESSMENT

Question history of hepatic disease, prior hypersensitivity reaction. When monitoring B/P, avoid overinflation of cuff to prevent trauma, bleeding. Remove adhesive tape from any pressure dressing carefully and slowly.

INTERVENTION/EVALUATION

Following IV administration, apply prolonged pressure on venipuncture site. Monitor IV site for oozing q5–15 min for 1–2 hrs following administration. Assess for allergic reaction. Immediately report any evidence of hematuria or change in vital signs. Assess for decreases in B/P, increased pulse rate, complaint of abdominal or back pain, severe headache (may be evidence of hemorrhage). Question for increased discharge during menses. Assess skin for bruises, petechiae. Check

for excessive bleeding from minor cuts, scratches. Assess gums for erythema, gingival bleeding. Assess urine for hematuria. Evaluate for therapeutic relief of pain, reduction of swelling, restricted joint movement.

PATIENT/FAMILY TEACHING

• Report any sign of bleeding, including red or dark urine, black/red stool, coffee-ground vomitus, blood-tinged mucus from cough. • Wear identification indicating a hemolytic condition. • Bring adequate supply of agent when traveling.

---

apixaban

a-**pix**-a-ban
(Eliquis)
⬛ **BLACK BOX ALERT** ⬛ Discontinuation in absence of alternative anticoagulation increases risk for thrombotic events. Spinal or epidural hematoma resulting in paralysis may occur with neuraxial anesthesia or spinal/epidural puncture.
Do not confuse apixaban with rivaroxaban, argatroban, or dabigatran.

◆CLASSIFICATION

PHARMACOTHERAPEUTIC: Factor Xa inhibitor. **CLINICAL:** Anticoagulant.

USES

Reduces risk for stroke, systemic embolism in pts with nonvalvular atrial fibrillation. Prophylaxis of DVT following hip or knee replacement surgery. Treatment of DVT and PE. Reduces risk of recurrent DVT/PE following initial therapy.

PRECAUTIONS

Contraindications: Severe hypersensitivity to apixaban. Active pathologic bleeding. **Cautions:** Mild to moderate hepatic impairment, severe renal impairment (may increase bleeding risk). Avoid use in pts with severe hepatic impairment, prosthetic heart valve, significant rheumatic heart disease.

ACTION

Selectively blocks active site of factor Xa, a key factor in the intrinsic and extrinsic pathway of blood coagulation cascade. **Therapeutic Effect:** Inhibits clot-induced platelet aggregation, fibrin clot formation.

PHARMACOKINETICS

Readily absorbed after PO administration. Peak plasma concentration: 3–4 hrs. Protein binding: 87%. Metabolized in liver. Excreted primarily in urine, feces. **Half-life:** 12 hrs.

LIFESPAN CONSIDERATIONS

Pregnancy/Lactation: Unknown if distributed in breast milk. **Children:** Safety and efficacy not established. **Elderly:** No age-related precautions noted.

INTERACTIONS

DRUG: CYP3A4 inducers (e.g., car-BAMazepine, rifAMPin) may decrease level/effect. **Aspirin, NSAIDs, warfarin, heparin, antiplatelet agents, CYP3A4 inhibitors, (e.g., ketoconazole, clarithromycin)** may increase concentration, bleeding risk. **HERBAL:** St. John's wort may decrease level/effect. Flaxseed, garlic, ginger, ginkgo biloba, ginseng, omega-3 may increase risk of bleeding. **FOOD:** Grapefruit products may increase level/adverse effects. **LAB VALUES:** May decrease platelet count, Hgb, LFT.

AVAILABILITY (Rx)

Tablets: 2.5 mg, 5 mg.

ADMINISTRATION/HANDLING

◄**ALERT**► Discontinuation in absence of alternative anticoagulation increases risk for thrombotic events.

PO
• Give without regard to meals. • If elective surgery or invasive procedures with moderate or high risk for bleeding, discontinue apixaban at least 24–48 hrs prior to procedure.

INDICATIONS/ROUTES/DOSAGE

Nonvalvular Atrial Fibrillation
PO: ADULTS, ELDERLY: 5 mg twice daily. In pts with at least 2 of the following characteristics: age 80 yrs or older, body weight 60 kg or less, serum creatinine 1.5 mg/dL or greater, concurrent use with CYP3A4, or P-gp inhibitors (e.g., ketoconazole, ritonavir), reduce dose to 2.5 mg twice daily.

DVT/PE Treatment
PO: ADULTS/ELDERLY: 10 mg twice daily for 7 days, then 5 mg twice daily.

DVT Prophylaxis (Hip/Knee Replacement)
Note: Begin 12–24 hrs postoperatively.
ADULTS, ELDERLY: 2.5 mg twice daily (35 days for hip; 12 days for knee).

DVT Prophylaxis, Reduce Risk Recurrent DVT/PE
PO: ADULTS, ELDERLY: 2.5 mg twice daily (after at least 6 mos of treatment).

Dosage in Renal Impairment
DVT/PE/Reduce Risk Recurrent DVT, Postoperative: No adjustment. **Nonvalvular A-fib, HD: SCr < 1.5:** No adjustment. **SCr 1.5 or greater, age older than 80 yrs, weight 60 kg or less:** 2.5 mg 2 times/day.

Dosage in Hepatic Impairment
Mild Impairment: No dose adjustment. **Moderate Impairment:** Use caution. **Severe Impairment:** Not recommended.

SIDE EFFECTS

Rare (3%–1%): Nausea, ecchymosis.

A

ADVERSE EFFECTS/ TOXIC REACTIONS

Increased risk for bleeding/hemorrhagic events. May cause serious, potentially fatal bleeding, accompanied by one or more of the following: a decrease in Hgb of 2 g/dL or more; a need for 2 or more units of packed RBCs; bleeding occurring at one of the following sites: intracranial, intraspinal, intraocular, pericardial, intra-articular, intramuscular with compartment syndrome, retroperitoneal. Serious reactions include jaundice, cholestasis, cytolytic hepatitis, Stevens-Johnson syndrome, hypersensitivity reaction, anaphylaxis.

NURSING CONSIDERATIONS

BASELINE ASSESSMENT

Obtain baseline CBC. Question history of bleeding disorders, recent surgery, spinal punctures, intracranial hemorrhage, bleeding ulcers, open wounds, anemia, hepatic impairment. Obtain full medication history including herbal products.

INTERVENTION/EVALUATION

Periodically monitor CBC, stool for occult blood. Be alert for complaints of abdominal/back pain, headache, confusion, weakness, vision change (may indicate hemorrhage). Question for increased menstrual bleeding/discharge. Assess for any sign of bleeding: bleeding at surgical site, hematuria, blood in stool, bleeding from gums, petechiae, ecchymosis.

PATIENT/FAMILY TEACHING

• Do not take/discontinue any medication except on advice from physician. • Avoid alcohol, aspirin, NSAIDs, herbal supplements, grapefruit products. • Consult physician before surgery, dental work. • Use electric razor, soft toothbrush to prevent bleeding. • Report blood-tinged mucus from coughing, heavy menstrual bleeding, headache, vision problems, weakness, abdominal pain, frequent bruising, bloody urine or stool, joint pain or swelling.

apremilast

a-**pre**-mi-last
(Otezla)
Do not confuse apremilast with roflumilast.

◆CLASSIFICATION

PHARMACOTHERAPEUTIC: Phosphodiesterase 4 (PDE4) inhibitor. **CLINICAL:** Antipsoriatic arthritis agent.

USES

Treatment of adult pts with active psoriatic arthritis, moderate to severe plaque psoriasis who are candidates for phototherapy or systemic therapy.

PRECAUTIONS

Contraindications: Hypersensitivity to apremilast. **Cautions:** History of depression, severe renal impairment, suicidal ideation. Pts with latent infections (e.g., TB, viral hepatitis).

ACTION

Selectively inhibits PDE4, increasing cyclic AMP (cAMP) and inflammatory mediators. **Therapeutic Effect:** Reduces psoriatic arthritis exacerbations.

PHARMACOKINETICS

Readily absorbed after PO administration. Protein binding: 68%. Peak plasma concentration: 2.5 hrs. Metabolized in liver. Excreted in urine (58%), feces (39%). **Half-life:** 6–9 hrs.

⧗ LIFESPAN CONSIDERATIONS

Pregnancy/Lactation: Unknown if distributed in breast milk. Not recommended for nursing mothers. **Children:** Safety and efficacy not established in pts younger than 18 yrs. **Elderly:** No age-related precautions noted.

INTERACTIONS

DRUG: Strong CYP450 inducers (e.g., carBAMazepine, PHENobarbital, phenytoin, rifAMPin) may decrease concentration/effect. **HERBAL:** St. John's wort may decrease concentration/effect. **FOOD:** None significant. **LAB VALUES:** None known.

AVAILABILITY (Rx)

Tablets: 10 mg, 20 mg, 30 mg.

ADMINISTRATION/HANDLING

PO
• Give without regard to meals. Administer whole; do not crush, cut, dissolve, or divide.

INDICATIONS/ROUTES/DOSAGE

Psoriatic Arthritis, Plaque Psoriasis
PO: ADULTS/ELDERLY: Initially, titrate dose from day 1–day 5. **Day 1:** 10 mg in AM only. **Day 2:** 10 mg in AM; 10 mg in PM. **Day 3:** 10 mg in AM; 20 mg in PM. **Day 4:** 20 mg in AM; 20 mg in PM. **Day 5:** 20 mg in AM; 30 mg in PM. **Day 6/Maintenance:** 30 mg twice daily.

Dosage in Renal Impairment (CrCl less than 30 mL/min)
Days 1–3: 10 mg in AM. **Days 4–5:** 20 mg in AM, using only am schedule. **Day 6/Maintenance:** 30 mg once daily.

Dosage in Hepatic Impairment
No dose adjustment.

SIDE EFFECTS

Occasional (9%–4%): Nausea, diarrhea, headache, upper respiratory tract infection. **Rare (3% or less):** Vomiting, nasopharyngitis, upper abdominal pain.

ADVERSE EFFECTS/TOXIC REACTIONS

Increased risk of depression reported in less than 1% of pts. Weight decrease of 5%–10% of body weight occurred in 10% of pts.

NURSING CONSIDERATIONS

BASELINE ASSESSMENT

Obtain baseline weight, vital signs. Question history of depression, severe renal impairment, suicidal ideations. Screen for prior allergic reactions to drug class. Receive full medication history including herbal products. Assess degree of joint pain, range of motion, mobility.

INTERVENTION/EVALUATION

Be alert for worsening depression, suicidal ideation. Monitor for weight loss. Assess for dehydration if diarrhea occurs. Assess improvement of joint pain, range of motion, mobility.

PATIENT/FAMILY TEACHING

• Report changes in mood or behavior, thoughts of suicide, self-destructive behavior. Report weight loss of any kind. • Increase fluid intake if dehydration suspected. • Immediately notify physician if pregnancy suspected. • Do not chew, crush, dissolve, or divide tablets.

aprepitant/ fosaprepitant

a-**prep**-i-tant/fos-a-**prep**-i-tant (Emend)
Do not confuse fosaprepitant with aprepitant, fosamprenavir, or fospropofol.

◆CLASSIFICATION

PHARMACOTHERAPEUTIC: Neurokinin receptor antagonist. **CLINICAL:** Antinausea, antiemetic.

USES

PO/IV: Prevention of nausea, vomiting associated with repeat courses of moderately to highly emetogenic cancer chemotherapy. **PO:** Prevention of postop nausea, vomiting.

PRECAUTIONS

Contraindications: Hypersensitivity to aprepitant or fosaprepitant. Concurrent use with pimozide. **Cautions:** Severe hepatic impairment. Concurrent use of

medications metabolized through CYP3A4 (e.g., docetaxel, etoposide, ifosfamide, imatinib, irinotecan, PACLitaxel, vinblastine, vinCRIStine, vinorelbine).

ACTION

Inhibits substance P receptor, augments antiemetic activity of 5-HT$_3$ receptor antagonists. **Therapeutic Effect:** Prevents acute and delayed phases of chemotherapy-induced emesis.

PHARMACOKINETICS

Moderately absorbed from GI tract. Crosses blood-brain barrier. Extensively metabolized in liver. Protein binding: greater than 95%. Eliminated primarily by liver metabolism (not excreted renally). **Half-life:** 9–13 hrs.

LIFESPAN CONSIDERATIONS

Pregnancy/Lactation: Unknown if drug crosses placenta or is distributed in breast milk. **Children:** Safety and efficacy not established. **Elderly:** No age-related precautions noted.

INTERACTIONS

DRUG: Strong **CYP3A4 inhibitors (e.g., ketoconazole, clarithromycin)** may increase concentration. **Strong CYP3A4 inducers (e.g., carBAMazepine, rifAMPin)** may decrease concentration. May decrease effectiveness of **hormonal contraceptives, warfarin.** **HERBAL:** St. John's wort may decrease plasma concentration. **FOOD:** Grapefruit products may increase plasma concentration. **LAB VALUES:** May increase serum ALT, AST, alkaline phosphatase, BUN, creatinine, glucose. May produce proteinuria.

AVAILABILITY (Rx)

Capsules (Emend): 40 mg, 80 mg, 125 mg. **Injection, Powder for Reconstitution (Fosaprepitant):** 150 mg.

ADMINISTRATION/HANDLING

PO
• Give without regard to food.

IV

Reconstitution • Reconstitute each vial with 5 mL 0.9% NaCl. • Add to 145 mL 0.9% NaCl to provide a final concentration of 1 mg/mL.
Rate of Administration • Infuse over 20–30 min 30 min prior to chemotherapy.
Storage • Refrigerate unreconstituted vials. • After reconstitution, solution is stable at room temperature for 24 hrs.

IV INCOMPATIBILITIES

Do not infuse with any solutions containing calcium or magnesium.

INDICATIONS/ROUTES/DOSAGE

Prevention of Chemotherapy-Induced Nausea, Vomiting
Note: Administer in combination with a 5-HT$_3$ antagonist on day 1 and dexamethasone on days 1 through 4.
PO: ADULTS, ELDERLY, CHILDREN 12 YRS OR YOUNGER WEIGHING 30 KG OR MORE: 125 mg 1 hr before chemotherapy on day 1 and 80 mg once daily in the morning on days 2 and 3.
IV: ADULTS, ELDERLY (SINGLE-DOSE REGIMEN): 150 mg over 20–30 min 30 min prior to chemotherapy.

Prevention of Postop Nausea, Vomiting
PO: ADULTS, ELDERLY: 40 mg once within 3 hrs prior to induction of anesthesia.

Dosage in Renal/Hepatic Impairment
No dose adjustment. Caution in severe hepatic impairment.

SIDE EFFECTS

Frequent (17%–10%): Fatigue, nausea, hiccups, diarrhea, constipation, anorexia. **Occasional (8%–4%):** Headache, vomiting, dizziness, dehydration, heartburn. **Rare (3% or less):** Abdominal pain, epigastric discomfort, gastritis, tinnitus, insomnia.

ADVERSE EFFECTS/ TOXIC REACTIONS

Neutropenia, mucous membrane disorders occur rarely.

NURSING CONSIDERATIONS

BASELINE ASSESSMENT

Assess for dehydration (poor skin turgor, dry mucous membranes, longitudinal furrows in tongue).

INTERVENTION/EVALUATION

Monitor hydration, nutritional status, I&O. Assess bowel sounds for peristalsis. Assist with ambulation if dizziness occurs. Provide supportive measures. Monitor daily pattern of bowel activity, stool consistency.

PATIENT/FAMILY TEACHING

• Relief from nausea/vomiting generally occurs shortly after drug administration. • Report persistent vomiting, headache. • May decrease effectiveness of oral contraceptives.

argatroban

ar-**gat**-roe-ban
Do not confuse argatroban with Aggrastat.

◆CLASSIFICATION

PHARMACOTHERAPEUTIC: Thrombin inhibitor. **CLINICAL:** Anticoagulant.

USES

Prophylaxis or treatment of thrombosis in heparin-induced thrombocytopenia (HIT) in pts with HIT or at risk of developing HIT undergoing. Pts with or at risk for HIT undergoing percutaneous coronary procedures. **OFF-LABEL:** Maintain extracorporeal circuit patency of continuous renal replacement therapy (CRRT) in pts with HIT.

PRECAUTIONS

Contraindications: Hypersensitivity to argatroban, active major bleeding. **Cautions:** Severe hypertension, immediately following lumbar puncture, spinal anesthesia, major surgery, pts with congenital or acquired bleeding disorders, gastrointestinal ulcerations, hepatic impairment, critically ill pts.

ACTION

Direct thrombin inhibitor that reversibly binds to thrombin-active sites. Inhibits thrombin-catalyzed or thrombin-induced reactions, including fibrin formation, activation of coagulant factors V, VIII, and XIII; inhibits protein C formation, platelet aggregation. **Therapeutic Effect:** Produces anticoagulation.

PHARMACOKINETICS

Distributed primarily in extracellular fluid. Protein binding: 54%. Metabolized in liver. Primarily excreted in the feces, presumably through biliary secretion. **Half-life:** 39–51 min (prolonged in hepatic failure).

LIFESPAN CONSIDERATIONS

Pregnancy/Lactation: Unknown if excreted in breast milk. **Children:** Safety and efficacy not established in pts younger than 18 yrs. **Elderly:** No age-related precautions noted.

INTERACTIONS

DRUG: Antiplatelet agents (e.g., aspirin, clopidogrel), other anticoagulants (e.g., warfarin), thrombolytics (e.g., tissue plasminogen activator [TPA]), NSAIDs may increase the risk of bleeding. **HERBAL: Dong quai, evening primrose oil, ginkgo, policosanol, willow bark** may increase risk of bleeding. **FOOD:** None known. **LAB VALUES:** Prolongs prothrombin time (PT), activated partial thromboplastin time (aPTT), international normalized ratio (INR). May decrease Hgb, Hct.

AVAILABILITY (Rx)

Infusion (Pre-Mix): 125 mg/125 mL, 250 mg/250 mL. **Injection Solution:** 250 mg/2.5 mL vial.

ADMINISTRATION/HANDLING

 IV

Reconstitution • Dilute each 250-mg vial with 250 mL 0.9% NaCl, D₅W to provide a final concentration of 1 mg/mL.
Rate of Administration • Initial rate of administration is based on body weight at 2 mcg/kg/min (e.g., 50-kg pt infuse at 6 mL/hr). Dosage should not exceed 10 mcg/kg/min.
Storage • Discard if solution appears cloudy or an insoluble precipitate is noted. • Following reconstitution, stable for 96 hrs at room temperature or refrigerated. • Avoid direct sunlight.

⊞ IV INCOMPATIBILITY

Amiodarone (Cardarone).

⊞ IV COMPATIBILITIES

DiphenhydrAMINE (Benadryl), DOBU-Tamine (Dobutrex), DOPamine (Intropin), furosemide (Lasix), midazolam (Versed), morphine, vasopressin (Pitressin). Refer to IV Compatibility Chart in front of book.

INDICATIONS/ROUTES/DOSAGE

Heparin-Induced Thrombocytopenia (HIT)
IV Infusion: ADULTS, ELDERLY: Initially, 2 mcg/kg/min administered as a continuous infusion. After initial infusion, dose may be adjusted until steady-state aPTT is 1.5–3 times initial baseline value, not to exceed 100 sec. Dosage should not exceed 10 mcg/kg/min.

Percutaneous Coronary Intervention
IV Infusion: ADULTS, ELDERLY: Initially, administer bolus of 350 mcg/kg over 3–5 min, then infuse at 25 mcg/kg/min. Check ACT (activated clotting time) 5–10 min following bolus. If ACT is less than 300 sec, give additional bolus 150 mcg/kg, increase infusion to 30 mcg/kg/min. If ACT is greater than 450 sec, decrease infusion to 15 mcg/kg/min. Once ACT of 300–450 sec achieved, continue dose through duration of procedure.

Dosage in Renal Impairment
No dose adjustment.

Dosage in Hepatic Impairment
Moderate to Severe Impairment:
ADULTS, ELDERLY: Initially, 0.5 mcg/kg/min. **CHILDREN:** Initially, 0.2 mcg/kg/min. Adjust dose in increments of 0.05 mcg/kg/min or less.

SIDE EFFECTS

Frequent (8%–3%): Dyspnea, hypotension, fever, diarrhea, nausea, pain, vomiting, infection, cough.

ADVERSE EFFECTS/TOXIC REACTIONS

Ventricular tachycardia, atrial fibrillation occur occasionally. Major bleeding, sepsis occur rarely.

NURSING CONSIDERATIONS

BASELINE ASSESSMENT

Obtain CBC, PT, aPTT. Determine initial B/P. Minimize need for multiple injection sites, blood draws, catheters.

INTERVENTION/EVALUATION

Assess for any sign of bleeding: bleeding at surgical site, hematuria, melena, bleeding from gums, petechiae, ecchymoses, bleeding from injection sites. Handle pt carefully and infrequently to prevent bleeding. Assess for decreased B/P, increased pulse rate, complaint of abdominal/back pain, severe headache (may indicate hemorrhage). Monitor ACT, PT, aPTT, platelet count, Hgb, Hct. Question for increase in discharge during menses. Assess for hematuria. Observe skin for any occurring ecchymoses, petechiae, hematoma. Use care in removing any dressing, tape.

PATIENT/FAMILY TEACHING

• Use electric razor, soft toothbrush to prevent cuts, gingival trauma. • Report any sign of bleeding, including red/dark urine, black/red stool, coffee-ground vomitus, blood-tinged mucus from cough.

ARIPiprazole   TOP 100

ar-i-**pip**-ra-zole
(Abilify, Abilify Maintena, Aristada)

■ **BLACK BOX ALERT** ■ Increased risk of mortality in elderly pts with dementia-related psychosis, mainly due to pneumonia, HF. Increased risk of suicidal thinking and behavior in children, adolescents, young adults 18–24 yrs with major depressive disorder, other psychiatric disorders.

Do not confuse Abilify with Ambien, or ARIPiprazole with esomeprazole, omeprazole, pantoprazole, or RABEprazole (proton pump inhibitors).

◆**CLASSIFICATION**

PHARMACOTHERAPEUTIC: DOPamine agonist. **CLINICAL:** Antipsychotic agent.

USES

PO: Treatment of schizophrenia. Treatment of bipolar disorder. Adjunct treatment in major depressive disorder. Treatment of irritability associated with autistic disorder in children 6–17 yrs of age. Treatment of Tourette disorder. **IM: (Immediate-Release):** Agitation associated with schizophrenia/bipolar disorder. **(Extended-Release): Abilify Maintena:** Treatment of schizophrenia in adults. Maintenance monotherapy treatment of bipolar 1 disorder in adults. **Aristada:** Treatment of schizophrenia. **OFF-LABEL:** Schizoaffective disorder, depression with psychotic features, aggression, bipolar disorder (children), conduct disorder (children), psychosis/agitation related to Alzheimer's dementia.

PRECAUTIONS

Contraindications: Hypersensitivity to ARIPiprazole. **Cautions:** Concurrent use of CNS depressants (including alcohol), disorders in which CNS depression is a feature, cardiovascular or cerebrovascular diseases (may induce hypotension), Parkinson's disease (potential for exacerbation), history of seizures or conditions that may lower seizure threshold (Alzheimer's disease), diabetes mellitus. Pts at risk for pneumonia. Elderly with dementia.

ACTION

Provides partial agonist activity at DOPamine (D2, D3) and serotonin (5-HT$_{1A}$) receptors and antagonist activity at serotonin (5-HT$_{2A}$) receptors. **Therapeutic Effect:** Improves symptoms associated with schizophrenia, bipolar disorder, autism, depression.

PHARMACOKINETICS

Well absorbed through GI tract. Protein binding: 99% (primarily albumin). Reaches steady levels in 2 wks. Metabolized in liver. Excreted in feces (55%), urine (25%). Not removed by hemodialysis. **Half-life:** 75 hrs.

⧖ LIFESPAN CONSIDERATIONS

Pregnancy/Lactation: Unknown if drug crosses placenta. May be distributed in breast milk. Breastfeeding not recommended. **Children:** Safety and efficacy not established. **Elderly:** May increase risk of mortality in pts with dementia-related psychosis.

INTERACTIONS

DRUG: Alcohol may potentiate cognitive and motor effects. **CYP3A4 inducers** (e.g., carBAMazepine, rifampin) may decrease concentration. **CYP3A4 inhibitors** (e.g., erythromycin, ketoconazole, ritonavir)

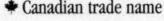 ✦ Canadian trade name   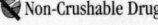 Non-Crushable Drug   ▨ **HIGH ALERT** High Alert drug

may increase concentration. **CYP2D6 inhibitors** may increase concentration/effects. **HERBAL:** St. John's wort may decrease levels. **Gotu kola, kava kava, St. John's wort, valerian** may increase CNS depression. **FOOD:** None known. **LAB VALUES:** May increase serum glucose. May decrease neutrophils, leukocytes.

AVAILABILITY (Rx)

Injection, Prefilled Syringe (Aristada): 441 mg, 662 mg, 882 mg, 1064 mg. **Injection, Solution (Abilify):** 9.75 mg/1.3 mL (7.5 mg/mL). **Solution, Oral:** 1 mg/mL. **Tablets:** 2 mg, 5 mg, 10 mg, 15 mg, 20 mg, 30 mg. **Tablets, Orally Disintegrating:** 10 mg, 15 mg. **Injection, Powder for Reconstitution (Abilify Maintena):** 300 mg, 400 mg.

ADMINISTRATION/HANDLING

IM (Abilify)
• For IM use only (inject slowly into deep muscle mass). Do not administer IV or subcutaneous.

IM (Abilify Maintena)
• Reconstitute 400-mg vial with 1.9 mL Sterile Water for Injection (300-mg vial with 1.5 mL) to provide a concentration of 100 mg/0.5 mL. Once reconstituted, administer in gluteal muscle. Do not administer via IV or subcutaneously.

PO
• Give without regard to food.

Orally Disintegrating Tablet
• Remove tablet, place entire tablet on tongue. • Do not break, split tablet. • May give without liquid.

INDICATIONS/ROUTES/DOSAGE

Note: May substitute oral solution/tablet mg per mg up to 25 mg. For 30-mg tablets, give 25 mg oral solution.
Strong CYP3A4 Inducers: ARIPiprazole dose should be doubled. **Strong CYP3A4 Inhibitors:** ARIPiprazole dose should be reduced by 50%.

Schizophrenia
PO: ADULTS, ELDERLY: Initially, 10–15 mg once daily. May increase up to 30 mg/day. Titrate dose at minimum of 2-wk intervals. **CHILDREN 13–17 YRS:** Initially, 2 mg/day for 2 days, then 5 mg/day for 2 days. May further increase to target dose of 10 mg/day. May then increase in increments of 5 mg up to maximum of 30 mg/day. **IM: ADULTS, ELDERLY: (Abilify Maintena):** Initially, 400 mg monthly (separate doses by at least 26 days). **(Aristada):** 441 mg, 662 mg or 882 mg monthly or 882 mg q6wks, or 1064 mg q2mos. IM dose based on oral dose. (In conjunction with first IM dose, administer oral aripiprazole for 21 consecutive days).

Bipolar Disorder
PO: ADULTS, ELDERLY: Monotherapy: Initially, 15 mg once daily. May increase to 30 mg/day. **Adjunct to lithium or valproic acid:** Initially, 10–15 mg. May increase to 30 mg/day based on pt tolerance. **CHILDREN 10–17 YRS:** Initially, 2 mg/day for 2 days, then 5 mg/day for 2 days. May further increase to a target of 10 mg/day. Give subsequent dose increases of 5 mg/day. **Maximum:** 30 mg/day. **IM: ADULTS, ELDERLY: (Abilify Maintena):** Initially, 400 mg monthly (separate doses by at least 26 days).

Major Depressive Disorder (Adjunct to Antidepressants)
PO: ADULTS, ELDERLY: (Abilify): Initially, 2–5 mg/day. May increase up to maximum of 15 mg/day. Titrate dose in 5-mg increments of at least 1-wk intervals.

Agitation with Schizophrenia/Bipolar Disorder
IM: ADULTS, ELDERLY (Abilify): 5.25–15 mg as a single dose. May repeat after 2 hrs. **Maximum:** 30 mg/day.

Irritability with Autistic Disorder
PO: CHILDREN 6–17 YRS: Initially, 2 mg/day for 7 days followed by increase to 5 mg/day. Subsequent increases made in 5-mg increments at intervals of at least 1 wk. **Maximum:** 15 mg/day.

Tourette Disorder
PO: CHILDREN 6–17 YRS WEIGHING 50 KG OR MORE: 2 mg/day for 2 days; then 5 mg/day for 5 days with target dose of 10 mg on day 8. **Maximum:** 20 mg/day. **LESS THAN 50 KG:** 2 mg/day for 2 days, then 5 mg/day. **Maximum:** 10 mg/day.

Dosage in Renal/Hepatic Impairment
No dose adjustment.

SIDE EFFECTS

Frequent (11%–5%): Weight gain, headache, insomnia, vomiting. **Occasional (4%–3%):** Light-headedness, nausea, akathisia, drowsiness. **Rare (2% or less):** Blurred vision, constipation, asthenia (loss of strength, energy), anxiety, fever, rash, cough, rhinitis, orthostatic hypotension.

ADVERSE EFFECTS/TOXIC REACTIONS

Extrapyramidal symptoms, neuroleptic malignant syndrome, tardive dyskinesia, hyperglycemia, ketoacidosis, hyperosmolar coma, CVA, TIA occur rarely. Prolonged QT interval occurs rarely. May cause leukopenia, neutropenia, agranulocytosis.

NURSING CONSIDERATIONS

BASELINE ASSESSMENT
Assess behavior, appearance, emotional status, response to environment, speech pattern, thought content. Correct dehydration, hypovolemia. Assess for suicidal tendencies. Question history (or family history) of diabetes. Obtain serum blood glucose level.

INTERVENTION/EVALUATION
Periodically monitor weight. Monitor for extrapyramidal symptoms (abnormal movement), tardive dyskinesia (protrusion of tongue, puffing of cheeks, chewing/puckering of the mouth). Periodically monitor B/P, pulse (particularly in pts with preexisting cardiovascular disease). Monitor serum blood glucose levels during therapy. Assess for therapeutic response (greater interest in surroundings, improved self-care, increased ability to concentrate, relaxed facial expression).

PATIENT/FAMILY TEACHING
• Avoid alcohol. • Avoid tasks that require alertness, motor skills until response to drug is established. • Report worsening depression, suicidal ideation, unusual changes in behavior, extrapyramidal effects.

---

armodafinil **HIGH ALERT**

ar-moe-**daf**-i-nil
(Nuvigil)
Do not confuse armodafinil with modafinil.

◆CLASSIFICATION

PHARMACOTHERAPEUTIC: Alpha$_1$ agonist. **CLINICAL:** CNS stimulant.

USES

Treatment of excessive daytime sleepiness associated with obstructive sleep apnea–hypopnea syndrome, narcolepsy, shift-work sleep disorder.

PRECAUTIONS

Contraindications: History of sensitivity to armodafinil or modafinil. **Cautions:** History of mitral valve prolapse, left ventricular hypertrophy, hepatic impairment, recent history of MI, unstable angina, cardiac ischemia, drug abuse, psychosis, depression, mania, renal impairment, elderly.

ACTION

Exact mechanism unknown. May bind to DOPamine reuptake carrier sites in the brain, increasing alpha activity, decreasing delta, theta, and beta activity. **Therapeutic Effect:** Improves wakefulness.

PHARMACOKINETICS

Well absorbed. Widely distributed. Mainly eliminated by hepatic metabolism

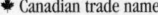

with less than 10% excreted by kidneys. Unknown if removed by hemodialysis. **Half-life:** 15 hrs.

⌛ LIFESPAN CONSIDERATIONS

Pregnancy/Lactation: Unknown if distributed in breast milk. Use caution in pregnant women. **Children:** Safety and efficacy not established in pts younger than 17 yrs. **Elderly:** Age-related renal/hepatic impairment may require decreased dosage.

INTERACTIONS

DRUG: Carbamazepine, erythromycin, ketoconazole, PHENobarbital, rifAMPin may alter concentration/effect. May reduce effects of **cycloSPORINE, oral contraceptives.** May increase concentrations of **diazePAM, omeprazole, phenytoin, propanolol, tricyclic antidepressants, warfarin. HERBAL:** None significant. **FOOD: Food** slows peak concentration by 2–4 hrs; may affect time of onset, length of drug action. **LAB VALUES:** May increase alkaline phosphatase, GGT. May decrease serum uric acid.

AVAILABILITY (Rx)

Tablets: 50 mg, 150 mg, 200 mg, 250 mg.

ADMINISTRATION/HANDLING

PO
• May give without regard to food.

INDICATIONS/ROUTES/DOSAGE

Narcolepsy, Obstructive Sleep Apnea–Hypopnea Syndrome
PO: ADULTS, ELDERLY: 150 or 250 mg/day given as a single dose in the morning.

Shift-Work Sleep Disorder
PO: ADULTS, ELDERLY: 150 mg given daily approximately 1 hr prior to the start of work shift.

Dosage in Renal/Hepatic Impairment
No dose adjustment. **Severe Hepatic Impairment:** May decrease dose.

SIDE EFFECTS

Frequent (17%–7%): Headache, nausea. **Occasional (5%–4%):** Dizziness, insomnia, dry mouth, diarrhea, anxiety. **Rare (2%):** Depression, fatigue, palpitations, dyspepsia, rash, upper abdominal pain.

ADVERSE EFFECTS/ TOXIC REACTIONS

Small risk of serious rash, including Stevens-Johnson syndrome.

NURSING CONSIDERATIONS

BASELINE ASSESSMENT

Obtain baseline evidence of narcolepsy or other sleep disorders, including pattern, environmental situations, lengths of time of sleep episodes. Question for sudden loss of muscle tone (cataplexy) precipitated by strong emotional responses before sleep episode. Assess frequency/severity of sleep episodes prior to drug therapy.

INTERVENTION/EVALUATION

Monitor sleep pattern, evidence of restlessness during sleep, length of insomnia episodes at night. Assess for dizziness, anxiety. Initiate fall precautions.

PATIENT/FAMILY TEACHING

• Avoid or limit alcohol. • Use alternative contraceptives during therapy and 1 mo after discontinuing drug (reduces effectiveness of oral contraceptives). • Report rash, depression, diarrhea, insomnia. • Sips of water may relieve dry mouth.

---

aspirin

as-pir-in
(Asaphen E.C. ♣, Ascriptin, Bayer, Bufferin, Durlaza, Ecotrin, Entrophen ♣, Novasen ♣)
Do not confuse aspirin or Ascriptin with Afrin, Aricept, or Ecotrin with Epogen.

FIXED-COMBINATION(S)

Aggrenox: aspirin/dipyridamole (an antiplatelet agent): 25 mg/200 mg. **Fiorinal:** aspirin/butalbital/caffeine (a barbiturate): 325 mg/50 mg/40 mg. **Lortab/ASA:** aspirin/HYDROcodone (an analgesic): 325 mg/5 mg. **Percodan:** aspirin/oxyCODONE (an analgesic): 325 mg/2.25 mg, 325 mg/4.5 mg. **Pravigard:** aspirin/pravastatin (a cholesterol-lowering agent): 81 mg/20 mg, 81 mg/40 mg, 81 mg/80 mg, 325 mg/20 mg, 325 mg/40 mg, 325 mg/80 mg. **Yosprala:** aspirin/omeprazole (a proton pump inhibitor [PPI]) 325 mg/40 mg, 81 mg/40 mg.

◆CLASSIFICATION

PHARMACOTHERAPEUTIC: Nonsteroidal salicylate. **CLINICAL:** Antiinflammatory, antipyretic, anticoagulant.

USES

Treatment of mild to moderate pain, fever. Reduces inflammation related to rheumatoid arthritis (RA), juvenile arthritis, osteoarthritis, rheumatic fever. Used as platelet aggregation inhibitor in the prevention of transient ischemic attacks (TIAs), cerebral thromboembolism, MI or reinfarction. **Durlaza:** Reduce risk of MI in pts with CAD or stroke in pts who have had TIA or ischemic stroke. **OFF-LABEL:** Prevention of preeclampsia; alternative therapy for preventing thromboembolism associated with atrial fibrillation when warfarin cannot be used; pericarditis associated with MI; prosthetic valve thromboprophylaxis. Adjunctive treatment of Kawasaki's disease. Complications associated with autoimmune disorders, colorectal cancer.

PRECAUTIONS

Contraindications: Hypersensitivity to salicylates, NSAIDs. Aspirin triad (asthma, rhinitis [with or without nasal polyps], aspirin intolerance). Asthma, rhinitis, nasal polyps; inherited or acquired bleeding disorders; use in children (younger than 16 yrs) for viral infections. Do not use for at least 7 days after tonsillectomy or oral surgery. **Cautions:** Platelet/bleeding disorders, severe renal/hepatic impairment, dehydration, erosive gastritis, peptic ulcer disease, sensitivity to tartrazine dyes, elderly (chronic use of doses 325 mg or greater). Avoid use in pregnancy, especially third trimester.

ACTION

Inhibits cyclo-oxygenase enzyme via acetylation. Inhibits formation of prostaglandin derivative thromboxane A. **Therapeutic Effect:** Reduces inflammatory response, intensity of pain; decreases fever; inhibits platelet aggregation.

PHARMACOKINETICS

Route	Onset	Peak	Duration
PO	1 hr	2–4 hrs	4–6 hrs

Rapidly and completely absorbed from GI tract; enteric-coated absorption delayed; rectal absorption delayed and incomplete. Protein binding: High. Widely distributed. Rapidly hydrolyzed to salicylate. **Half-life:** 15–20 min (aspirin); 2–3 hrs (salicylate at low dose); more than 20 hrs (salicylate at high dose).

⧗ LIFESPAN CONSIDERATIONS

Pregnancy/Lactation: Readily crosses placenta; distributed in breast milk. May prolong gestation and labor, decrease fetal birth weight, increase incidence of stillbirths, neonatal mortality, hemorrhage. Avoid use during last trimester (may adversely affect fetal cardiovascular system: premature closure of ductus arteriosus). **Children:** Caution in pts with acute febrile illness (Reye's syndrome). **Elderly:** May be more susceptible to toxicity; lower dosages recommended.

INTERACTIONS

DRUG: Alcohol, NSAIDs may increase risk of GI effects (e.g., ulceration).

Antacids, urinary alkalinizers increase excretion. **Anticoagulants, (e.g. enoxaparin, warfarin), heparin, thrombolytics, rivaroxaban, ticagrelor** increase risk of bleeding. **HERBAL:** Avoid **cat's claw, dong quai, evening primrose, feverfew, garlic, ginger, ginkgo, ginseng, green tea, horse chestnut, red clover** (possess antiplatelet activity). **FOOD:** None known. **LAB VALUES:** May alter serum ALT, AST, alkaline phosphatase, uric acid; prolongs prothrombin time (PT) platelet function assay. May decrease serum cholesterol, potassium, T_3, T_4.

AVAILABILITY (OTC)

Caplets: 325 mg, 500 mg. **Suppositories:** 300 mg, 600 mg. **Tablets:** 325 mg. **Tablets (Chewable):** 81 mg.

🔖 **Capsule, Extended-Release: (Durlaza)** 162.5 mg. **Tablets (Enteric-Coated):** 81 mg, 325 mg, 500 mg, 650 mg.

ADMINISTRATION/HANDLING

PO

• Do not break, crush, dissolve, or divide enteric-coated tablets or extended-release capsule. • May give with water, milk, meals if GI distress occurs.

Rectal

• Refrigerate suppositories; do not freeze. • If suppository is too soft, chill for 30 min in refrigerator or run cold water over foil wrapper. • Moisten suppository with cold water before inserting well into rectum.

INDICATIONS/ROUTES/DOSAGE

Analgesia, Fever

PO: ADULTS, ELDERLY, CHILDREN 12 YRS AND OLDER AND 50 KG OR MORE: 325–650 mg q4–6h or 975 mg q6h prn or 500–1,000 mg q4–6h prn. **Maximum:** 4 g/day. **RECTAL:** 300–600 mg q4h prn. **INFANTS, CHILDREN LESS THAN 50 KG:** 10–15 mg/kg/dose q4–6h. **Maximum:** 4 g/day or 90 mg/kg/day.

Revascularization
PO: ADULTS, ELDERLY: 80–325 mg/day.

Kawasaki's Disease
PO: CHILDREN: 80–100 mg/kg/day in divided doses q6h up to 14 days (until fever resolves for at least 48 hrs). After fever resolves, 1–5 mg/kg once daily for at least 6–8 wks.

MI, Stroke (Risk Reduction)
PO: ADULTS, ELDERLY: *Durlaza:* 162.5 mg once daily.

Dosage in Renal/Hepatic Impairment
Avoid use in severe impairment.

SIDE EFFECTS

Occasional: GI distress (including abdominal distention, cramping, heartburn, mild nausea); allergic reaction (including bronchospasm, pruritus, urticaria).

ADVERSE EFFECTS/ TOXIC REACTIONS

High doses of aspirin may produce GI bleeding and/or gastric mucosal lesions. Dehydrated, febrile children may experience aspirin toxicity quickly. Reye's syndrome, characterized by persistent vomiting, signs of brain dysfunction, may occur in children taking aspirin with recent viral infection (chickenpox, common cold, or flu). Low-grade aspirin toxicity characterized by tinnitus, generalized pruritus (may be severe), headache, dizziness, flushing, tachycardia, hyperventilation, diaphoresis, thirst. Marked toxicity characterized by hyperthermia, restlessness, seizures, abnormal breathing patterns, respiratory failure, coma.

NURSING CONSIDERATIONS

BASELINE ASSESSMENT

Do not give to children or teenagers who have or have recently had viral infections (increases risk of Reye's syndrome). Do not use if vinegar-like odor is noted (indicates chemical breakdown). Assess history of GI bleed, peptic ulcer disease, OTC use of products that may contain aspirin. Assess type, location, duration of pain, inflammation. Inspect appearance of affected joints for immobility, deformities, skin condition. **Therapeutic serum level for antiarthritic effect:** 20–30 mg/dL (toxicity occurs if level is greater than 30 mg/dL).

INTERVENTION/EVALUATION

Monitor urinary pH (sudden acidification, pH from 6.5 to 5.5, may result in toxicity). Assess skin for evidence of ecchymosis. If given as antipyretic, assess temperature directly before and 1 hr after giving medication. Evaluate for therapeutic response: relief of pain, stiffness, swelling; increased joint mobility; reduced joint tenderness; improved grip strength.

PATIENT/FAMILY TEACHING

• Do not, chew, crush, dissolve, or divide enteric-coated tablets. • Avoid alcohol, OTC pain/cold products that may contain aspirin. • Report ringing of the ears or persistent abdominal GI pain, bleeding. • Therapeutic anti-inflammatory effect noted in 1–3 wks. • Behavioral changes, persistent vomiting may be early signs of Reye's syndrome; contact physician.

---

atazanavir

TOP
100

a-ta-**zan**-a-veer
(Reyataz)
Do not confuse Reyataz with Retavase.

FIXED-COMBINATION(S)

Evotaz: atazanavir/cobicistat (antiretroviral booster): 300 mg/150 mg.

◆CLASSIFICATION

PHARMACOTHERAPEUTIC: Antiretroviral. **CLINICAL:** Protease inhibitor.

USES

Treatment of HIV-1 infection in combination with at least two other antiretroviral agents in pts 3 mos and older, weighing 5 kg or more.

PRECAUTIONS

Contraindications: Hypersensitivity to atazanavir. Concurrent use with alfuzosin, ergot derivatives, indinavir, irinotecan, lovastatin, lurasidone (when atazanavir given with ritonavir), midazolam (oral), nevirapine, pimozide, rifAMPin, sildenafil (for pulmonary arterial hypertension), St. John's wort, simvastatin, triazolam. **Cautions:** Preexisting conduction system defects (first-, second-, or third-degree AV block), diabetes, elderly, renal impairment (not recommended in end-stage renal disease or pts on hemodialysis), hemophilia A or B, hepatitis B or C virus infection. Do not use in pts younger than 3 mos (potential for kernicterus). Pts with increased transaminase levels prior to use or underlying hepatic disease.

ACTION

Binds to HIV-1 protease, inhibiting cleavage of viral precursors into functional proteins. **Therapeutic Effect:** Prevents formation of mature HIV viral cells.

PHARMACOKINETICS

Rapidly absorbed after PO administration. Protein binding: 86%. Extensively metabolized in liver. Excreted in feces (79%), urine (13%). **Half-life:** 5–8 hrs.

⧗ LIFESPAN CONSIDERATIONS

Pregnancy/Lactation: Unknown if drug crosses placenta or is distributed in breast milk. Lactic acidosis syndrome, hyperbilirubinemia, kernicterus have been reported. **Children:** Safety and efficacy not established in pts younger than 3 mos. **Elderly:** Age-related hepatic impairment may require dose reduction.

INTERACTIONS

DRUG: May increase concentration, toxicity of **amiodarone, atorvastatin, bepridil, clarithromycin, cyclo-**SPORINE**, diltiaZEM, felodipine, lidocaine, lovastatin, niCARdipine, NIFEdipine, rosuvastatin, sildenafil, simvastatin, sirolimus, tacrolimus, tadalafil, tricyclic antidepressants, vardenafil, verapamil, warfarin.** H_2-**receptor antagonists, proton pump inhibitors, rifAMPin** may decrease concentration/effects. **Ritonavir, voriconazole** may increase concentration. **HERBAL: St. John's wort** may decrease concentration/effects. **FOOD: High-fat meals** may decrease absorption. **LAB VALUES:** May increase serum bilirubin, ALT, AST, amylase, lipase. May decrease Hgb, neutrophil count, platelets. May alter LDL, triglycerides.

AVAILABILITY (Rx)

Capsules: 150 mg, 200 mg, 300 mg.
Packet, Oral: 50 mg.

ADMINISTRATION/HANDLING

PO
• Give with food. • Swallow whole; do not break or open capsules. • Administer at least 2 hrs before or 10 hrs after H

INDICATIONS/ROUTES/DOSAGE

Note: Dosage adjustment may be necessary with colchicine, bosentan, H_2 antagonists, proton pump inhibitors, PDE5 inhibitors.

HIV-1 Infection
PO: ADULTS, ELDERLY (ANTIRETROVIRAL-NAIVE): 300 mg and ritonavir 100 mg, or cobicistat 150 mg, once daily, or 400 mg (2 capsules) once daily with food in pts unable to tolerate ritonavir. **CHILDREN 6–17 YRS (NAIVE OR EXPERIENCED) WEIGHING 40 KG OR MORE: Capsules:** 300 mg once daily (with ritonavir 100 mg). **WEIGHING 20–39 KG:** 200 mg once daily (with ritonavir 100 mg). **WEIGHING 15–19 KG:** 150 mg once daily (with ritonavir 100 mg). **ADULTS,**
ELDERLY (ANTIRETROVIRAL-EXPERIENCED), PREGNANT PTS, CHILDREN WEIGHING 40 KG OR MORE: (Capsule): 300 mg and ritonavir 100 mg or cobicistat 150 mg once daily. **WEIGHING 20–39 KG:** 200 mg and ritonavir 100 mg once daily. **WEIGHING 15–19 KG:** 150 mg and ritonavir 100 mg once daily.

Powder (Naive and Experienced)
CHILDREN WEIGHING 25 KG OR MORE: 300 mg (6 packets) plus ritonavir 100 mg once daily. **WEIGHING 15–24 KG:** 250 mg (5 packets) plus ritonavir 80 mg once daily. **WEIGHING 5–14 KG:** 200 mg (4 packets) plus ritonavir 80 mg once daily.

HIV-1 Infection (Concurrent Therapy with Efavirenz)
PO: ADULTS, ELDERLY: 400 mg atazanavir, 100 mg ritonavir (as a single dose given with food), and 600 mg efavirenz as a single daily dose on an empty stomach (preferably at bedtime).

HIV-1 Infection (Concurrent Therapy with Didanosine)
PO: ADULTS, ELDERLY: Give atazanavir with food 2 hrs before or 1 hr after didanosine.

HIV-1 Infection (Concurrent Therapy with Tenofovir)
PO: ADULTS, ELDERLY: 300 mg atazanavir, 100 mg ritonavir, and 300 mg tenofovir given as a single daily dose with food. **FOR TREATMENT-EXPERIENCED PREGNANT WOMEN DURING SECOND OR THIRD TRIMESTER:** 400 mg and ritonavir 100 mg once daily.

HIV-1 Infection in Pts with Mild to Moderate Hepatic Impairment
◀ **ALERT** ▶ Avoid use in pts with severe hepatic impairment.
PO: ADULTS, ELDERLY: 300 mg once daily with food.

Dosage in Renal Impairment
HD (Naive): 300 mg with ritonavir. (Experienced): Not recommended.

SIDE EFFECTS

Frequent (16%–14%): Nausea, headache. **Occasional (9%–4%):** Rash, vomiting, depression, diarrhea, abdominal pain, fever. **Rare (3% or less):** Dizziness, insomnia, cough, fatigue, back pain.

ADVERSE EFFECTS/ TOXIC REACTIONS

Severe hypersensitivity reaction (angioedema, chest pain), jaundice may occur.

NURSING CONSIDERATIONS

BASELINE ASSESSMENT

Obtain baseline CBC, BMP, LFT, viral load before beginning therapy and at periodic intervals during therapy. Offer emotional support.

INTERVENTION/EVALUATION

Monitor lab results. Assess for nausea, vomiting; assess eating pattern. Monitor daily pattern of bowel activity, stool consistency. Assess skin for rash. Question for evidence of headache. Assess mood for evidence of depression.

PATIENT/FAMILY TEACHING

• Take with food. • Small, frequent meals may offset nausea, vomiting. • Swallow whole; do not break or open capsules. • Pt must continue practices to prevent HIV transmission. • Atazanavir is not a cure for HIV infection, nor does it reduce risk of transmission to others. • Report dizziness, light-headedness, yellowing of skin or whites of eyes, flank pain or when urinating, blood in urine, skin rash.

---

atenolol HIGH ALERT

a-**ten**-oh-lol
(Apo-Atenol ✦, Tenormin)
■ **BLACK BOX ALERT** ■ Do not abruptly discontinue; taper gradually to avoid acute tachycardia, hypertension, ischemia.

Do not confuse atenolol with albuterol, timolol, or Tylenol, or Tenormin with Imuran, Norpramin, or thiamine.

◆CLASSIFICATION

PHARMACOTHERAPEUTIC: Beta$_1$-adrenergic blocker. **CLINICAL:** Antihypertensive, antianginal, antiarrhythmic.

USES

Treatment of hypertension, alone or in combination with other agents; management of angina pectoris; management of pts with definite/suspected MI to reduce CV mortality. **OFF-LABEL:** Arrhythmia (esp. supraventricular and ventricular tachycardia), thyrotoxicosis.

PRECAUTIONS

Contraindications: Hypersensitivity to atenolol. Cardiogenic shock, uncompensated HF, second- or third-degree heart block (except with functioning pacemaker), sinus bradycardia, sinus node dysfunction, pulmonary edema, pregnancy. **Cautions:** Elderly, renal impairment, peripheral vascular disease, diabetes, thyroid disease, bronchospastic disease, compensated HF, myasthenia gravis, psychiatric disease, history of anaphylaxis to allergens, concurrent use with digoxin, verapamil, or diltiaZEM.

ACTION

Blocks beta$_1$-adrenergic receptors in cardiac tissue. **Therapeutic Effect:** Slows sinus node heart rate, decreasing cardiac output, B/P. Decreases myocardial oxygen demand.

PHARMACOKINETICS

Route	Onset	Peak	Duration
PO	1 hr	2–4 hrs	24 hrs

Incompletely absorbed from GI tract. Protein binding: 6%–16%. Minimal liver metabolism. Primarily excreted unchanged in urine. Removed by hemodialysis.

Half-life: 6–9 hrs (increased in renal impairment).

⧖ LIFESPAN CONSIDERATIONS

Pregnancy/Lactation: Readily crosses placenta; distributed in breast milk. Avoid use during first trimester. May produce bradycardia, apnea, hypoglycemia, hypothermia during delivery; low birthweight infants. **Children:** No age-related precautions noted. **Elderly:** Age-related peripheral vascular disease, renal impairment require caution.

INTERACTIONS

DRUG: Diuretics (e.g., furosemide, HCTZ), other antihypertensives (e.g., amlodipine, lisinopril, valsartan) may increase hypotensive effect. **Sympathomimetics, xanthines** may mutually inhibit effects. May mask symptoms of hypoglycemia, prolong hypoglycemic effect of **insulin, oral antidiabetic medications (e.g., glyburide). NSAIDs** may decrease antihypertensive effect. **HERBAL: Ephedra, ginseng, yohimbe** may worsen hypertension. **Garlic** may increase antihypertensive effect. **FOOD:** None known. **LAB VALUES:** May increase serum ANA titer, serum BUN, creatinine, potassium, uric acid, lipoprotein, triglycerides.

AVAILABILITY (Rx)

Tablets: 25 mg, 50 mg, 100 mg.

ADMINISTRATION/HANDLING

PO
• Give without regard to food. • Tablets may be crushed.

INDICATIONS/ROUTES/DOSAGE

Hypertension
PO: ADULTS: Initially, 25–50 mg once daily. After 1–2 wks, may increase dose up to 100 mg once daily. **ELDERLY:** Usual initial dose, 25 mg/day. **CHILDREN:** Initially, 0.5–1 mg/kg/dose given once daily. Range: 0.5–1.5 mg/kg/day. **Maximum:** 2 mg/kg/day up to 100 mg/day.

Angina Pectoris
PO: ADULTS: Initially, 50 mg once daily. May increase dose up to 200 mg once daily. **ELDERLY:** Usual initial dose, 25 mg/day.

Post-MI
PO: ADULTS: 100 mg once daily or 50 mg twice daily for 6–9 days post-MI.

Dosage in Renal Impairment
Dosage interval is modified based on creatinine clearance.

Creatinine Clearance	Maximum Dosage
15–35 mL/min	50 mg/day
Less than 15 mL/min	25 mg/day
Hemodialysis (HD)	Give dose post-HD or give 25–50 mg supplemental dose

Dosage in Hepatic Impairment
No dose adjustment.

SIDE EFFECTS

Atenolol is generally well tolerated, with mild and transient side effects. **Frequent:** Hypotension manifested as cold extremities, constipation or diarrhea, diaphoresis, dizziness, fatigue, headache, nausea. **Occasional:** Insomnia, flatulence, urinary frequency, impotence or decreased libido, depression. **Rare:** Rash, arthralgia, myalgia, confusion (esp. in the elderly), altered taste.

ADVERSE EFFECTS/ TOXIC REACTIONS

Overdose may produce profound bradycardia, hypotension. Abrupt withdrawal may result in diaphoresis, palpitations, headache, tremors. May precipitate HF, MI in pts with cardiac disease; thyroid storm in pts with thyrotoxicosis; peripheral ischemia in pts with existing peripheral vascular disease. Hypoglycemia may occur in previously controlled diabetes. Thrombocytopenia (unusual bruising, bleeding) occurs rarely. **Antidote:** Glucagon (see Appendix J for dosage).

NURSING CONSIDERATIONS

BASELINE ASSESSMENT

Assess B/P, apical pulse immediately before drug is administered (if pulse is 60/min or less, or systolic B/P is less than 90 mm Hg, withhold medication, contact physician). **Antianginal:** Record onset, quality (sharp, dull, squeezing), radiation, location, intensity, duration of anginal pain, precipitating factors (exertion, emotional stress). Assess baseline renal/hepatic function tests.

INTERVENTION/EVALUATION

Monitor B/P for hypotension, pulse for bradycardia, respiration for difficulty in breathing, EKG. Monitor daily pattern of bowel activity, stool consistency. Assess for evidence of HF: dyspnea (particularly on exertion or lying down), nocturnal cough, peripheral edema, distended neck veins. Monitor I&O (increased weight, decreased urinary output may indicate HF). Assess extremities for pulse quality, changes in temperature (may indicate worsening peripheral vascular disease). Assist with ambulation if dizziness occurs.

PATIENT/FAMILY TEACHING

• Do not abruptly discontinue medication. • Compliance with therapy essential to control hypertension, angina. • To reduce hypotensive effect, go from lying to standing slowly. • Avoid tasks that require alertness, motor skills until response to drug is established. • Advise diabetic pts to monitor blood glucose carefully (may mask signs of hypoglycemia). • Report dizziness, depression, confusion, rash, unusual bruising/bleeding. • Outpatients should monitor B/P, pulse before taking medication, following correct technique. • Restrict salt, alcohol intake. • Therapeutic antihypertensive effect noted in 1–2 wks.

atezolizumab

a-te-zoe-**liz**-ue-mab
(Tecentriq)
Do not confuse atezolizumab with daclizumab, certolizumab, eculizumab, omalizumab, or tocilizumab.

◆CLASSIFICATION

PHARMACOTHERAPEUTIC: Programmed death-ligand 1 (PD-L1) blocking antibody. Monoclonal antibody. **CLINICAL:** Antineoplastic.

USES

Treatment of pts with locally advanced or metastatic urothelial carcinoma who have disease progression during or following platinum-containing chemotherapy or have disease progression within 12 mos of neoadjuvant or adjuvant treatment with platinum-containing chemotherapy. Treatment of metastatic NSCLC in pts with disease progression during or following platinum-containing chemotherapy.

PRECAUTIONS

Contraindications: Hypersensitivity to atezolizumab. **Cautions:** Active infection; baseline anemia, lymphopenia; diabetes; pts at risk for dehydration, electrolyte imbalance; hepatic impairment, peripheral or generalized edema, neuropathy, optic disorders, interstitial lung disease; history of venous thromboembolism, intestinal obstruction, pancreatitis.

ACTION

Binds to PD-L1 and blocks interaction with both PD-L1 and B7.1 receptors. Releases the PD-1/PD-L1 pathway-mediated inhibition of the immune response (including antitumor immune response). **Therapeutic Effect:** Inhibits T-cell proliferation and cytokine production. Inhibits tumor cell growth and metastasis.

PHARMACOKINETICS

Metabolism not specified. Steady state reached in 6–9 wks. Elimination not specified. **Half-life:** 27 days.

⏳ LIFESPAN CONSIDERATIONS

Pregnancy/Lactation: Avoid pregnancy; may cause fetal harm. Unknown if distributed in breast milk; however, human immunoglobulin G is present in breast milk. Breastfeeding not recommended during treatment and for at least 5 mos after discontinuation. Females of reproductive potential should use effective contraception during treatment and up to 5 mos after discontinuation. May impair fertility in females. **Children:** Safety and efficacy not established. **Elderly:** No age-related precautions noted.

INTERACTIONS

DRUG: None known. **HERBAL:** None significant. **FOOD:** None known. **LAB VALUES:** May increase serum alkaline phosphatase, ALT, AST, creatinine, glucose. May decrease serum albumin, sodium; lymphocytes, Hgb, Hct, RBCs.

AVAILABILITY (Rx)

Injection Solution: 1,200 mg/20 mL (60 mg/60 mL).

ADMINISTRATION/HANDLING

 IV

Reconstitution • Visually inspect solution for particulate matter or discoloration. Solution should appear clear to slightly yellow. Discard if solution is cloudy or discolored or if visible particles are present. • Do not shake vial. • Withdraw 20 mL of solution from vial and dilute into a 250-mL polyvinyl chloride, polyethylene, or polyolefin infusion bag containing 0.9% NaCl. Dilute with 0.9% NaCl only. • Mix by gentle inversion. • Do not shake. • Discard partially used or empty vials.
Rate of Administration • Infuse over 60 min using sterile, nonpyrogenic, low protein-binding, 0.2- to 0.22-micron in-line filter. • If first infusion is tolerated, all subsequent infusions may be delivered over 30 mins. • Do not administer as IV bolus.

Storage • Refrigerate diluted solution up to 24 hrs or store at room temperature for no more than 6 hrs (includes time of preparation and infusion). • Do not freeze. • Do not shake.

▦ IV INCOMPATIBILITIES

Do not administer with other medications. Infuse via dedicated line.

INDICATIONS/ROUTES/DOSAGE

NSCLC, Urothelial Carcinoma

IV: ADULTS, ELDERLY: 1,200 mg q3wks until disease progression or unacceptable toxicity. No dose reductions are recommended.

Dose Modification

Based on Common Terminology Criteria for Adverse Events (CTCAE). **Withhold treatment for any of the following toxic reactions:** Grade 2 or 3 diarrhea or colitis; grade 2 pneumonitis; serum AST or ALT elevation 3–5 times upper limit of normal (ULN) or serum bilirubin elevation 1.5–3 times ULN; symptomatic hypophysitis, adrenal insufficiency, hypothyroidism, hyperthyroidism; grade 3 or 4 hyperglycemia; grade 3 rash; grade 2 ocular inflammatory toxicity, grade 2 or 3 pancreatitis; grade 3 or 4 infection, grade 2 infusion-related reactions. **Restarting treatment after interruption of therapy:** Resume treatment when adverse effects return to grade 0 or 1. **Permanently discontinue for any of the following toxic reactions:** Grade 3 or 4 diarrhea or colitis; grade 3 or 4 pneumonitis; serum AST or ALT elevation greater than 5 times ULN or serum bilirubin elevation 3 times ULN; grade 4 hypophysitis; grade 4 rash; grade 3 or 4 ocular inflammatory toxicity; grade 4 or any grade recurrent pancreatitis; grade 3 or 4 infusion-related reactions; any occurrence of encephalitis, Guillain-Barré, meningitis, meningoencephalitis, myasthenic syndrome/myasthenia gravis.

Dosage in Renal Impairment
No dose adjustment.

Dosage in Hepatic Impairment
Mild impairment: No dose adjustment.
Moderate to severe impairment: Not specified; use caution.

SIDE EFFECTS

Frequent (52%–18%): Fatigue, decreased appetite, nausea, pyrexia, constipation, diarrhea, peripheral edema. **Occasional (17%–13%):** Abdominal pain, vomiting, dyspnea, back/neck pain, rash, arthralgia, cough, pruritus.

ADVERSE EFFECTS/TOXIC REACTIONS

May cause severe immune-mediated events including adrenal insufficiency (0.4% of pts), interstitial lung disease or pneumonitis (3% of pts), colitis or diarrhea (20% of pts), hepatitis (2%–3% of pts), hypophysitis (0.2% of pts), hyperthyroidism (1% of pts), hypothyroidism (4% of pts), rash (up to 37% of pts), new-onset diabetes with ketoacidosis (0.2% of pts), pancreatitis (0.1% of pts); meningoencephalitis, myasthenic syndrome/myasthenia gravis, Guillain-Barré, ocular inflammatory toxicity (less than 1% of pts). Severe, sometimes fatal infections, including sepsis, herpes encephalitis, mycobacterial infection, occurred in 38% of pts. Urinary tract infections were the most common cause of grade 3 or higher infection, occurring in 7% of pts. Severe infusion-related reactions reported in less than 1% of pts. Other adverse events, including acute kidney injury, dehydration, dyspnea, encephalitis, hematuria, intestinal obstruction, meningitis, neuropathy, pneumonia, urinary obstruction, venous thromboembolism, were reported. Immunogenicity (auto-atezolizumab antibodies) occurred in 42% of pts.

NURSING CONSIDERATIONS

BASELINE ASSESSMENT
Obtain baseline CBC, BMP, LFT, thyroid panel, urine pregnancy, urinalysis; vital signs. Screen for history of pituitary/pulmonary/thyroid disease, autoimmune disorders, diabetes, hepatic impairment, venous thromboembolism. Conduct full dermatologic/neurologic/ophthalmologic exam. Verify use of effective contraception in females of reproductive potential. Screen for active infection. Assess hydration status.

INTERVENTION/EVALUATION
Monitor CBC, BMP, LFT, thyroid panel, vital signs. Diligently monitor for immune-mediated adverse events as listed in Adverse Effects/Toxic Reactions. Notify physician if any CTCAE toxicities occur, and initiate proper treatment. Obtain chest X-ray if interstitial lung disease, pneumonitis suspected. Due to high risk for dehydration/diarrhea, strictly monitor I&O. Encourage PO intake. If corticosteroid therapy is initiated for immune-mediated events, monitor capillary blood glucose and screen for corticosteroid side effects. Report any changes in neurologic status, including nuchal rigidity with fever, positive Kernig's sign, positive Brudzinski's sign, altered mental status, seizures. Diligently monitor for infection.

PATIENT/FAMILY TEACHING
• Blood levels will be routinely monitored. • Avoid pregnancy; treatment may cause birth defects. Do not breastfeed. Females of childbearing potential should use effective contraception during treatment and for at least 5 mos after final dose. • Treatment may cause serious or life-threatening inflammatory reactions. Report signs and symptoms of treatment-related inflammatory events in the following body systems: colon (severe abdominal pain or diarrhea); eye (blurry vision, double vision, unequal pupil size, sensitivity to light, eyelid drooping); lung (chest pain, cough,

shortness of breath); liver (bruising easily, amber-colored urine, clay-colored/tarry stools, yellowing of skin or eyes); pituitary (persistent or unusual headache, dizziness, extreme weakness, fainting, vision changes); thyroid (trouble sleeping, high blood pressure, fast heart rate [overactive thyroid]), (fatigue, goiter, weight gain [underactive thyroid]), neurologic (confusion, headache, seizures, neck rigidity with fever, severe nerve pain or loss of motor function). • Immediately report allergic reactions, bleeding of any kind, signs of infection. • Treatment may cause severe diarrhea. Drink plenty of fluids.

---

atoMOXetine

at-oh-**mox**-e-teen
(Apo-Atomoxetine ✦, <u>Strattera</u>)
■ **BLACK BOX ALERT** ■ Increased risk of suicidal thinking and behavior in children and adolescents with attention-deficit hyperactivity disorder (ADHD).
Do not confuse atomoxetine with atorvastatin.

◆CLASSIFICATION

PHARMACOTHERAPEUTIC: Norepinephrine reuptake inhibitor. **CLINICAL:** Psychotherapeutic agent.

USES

Treatment of ADHD.

PRECAUTIONS

Contraindications: Hypersensitivity to atomoxetine. Narrow-angle glaucoma, use with or within 14 days of MAOIs. Pheochromocytoma or history of pheochromocytoma. Severe cardiovascular disease. **Cautions:** Hypertension, tachycardia, cardiovascular disease (e.g., structural abnormalities, cardiomyopathy), urinary retention, moderate or severe hepatic impairment, suicidal ideation, emergent psychotic or manic symptoms, comorbid bipolar disorder, renal impairment, poor metabolizers of CYP2D6 metabolized drugs (e.g., FLUoxetine, PARoxetine). Pts predisposed to hypotension.

ACTION

Inhibits reuptake of norepinephrine. **Therapeutic Effect:** Improves symptoms of ADHD.

PHARMACOKINETICS

Rapidly absorbed after PO administration. Protein binding: 98% (primarily to albumin). Excreted in urine (80%), feces (17%). Not removed by hemodialysis. **Half-life:** 4–5 hrs (increased in moderate to severe hepatic insufficiency).

⧖ LIFESPAN CONSIDERATIONS

Pregnancy/Lactation: Unknown if distributed in breast milk. **Children:** Safety and efficacy not established in pts younger than 6 yrs. May produce suicidal thoughts in children and adolescents. **Elderly:** Age-related hepatic/renal impairment, cardiovascular or cerebrovascular disease may increase risk of adverse effects.

INTERACTIONS

DRUG: MAOIs may increase concentration/effect. **FLUoxetine, PARoxetine** may increase concentration/effect. Avoid concurrent use of **medications that can increase heart rate or B/P.** **HERBAL:** None significant. **FOOD:** None known. **LAB VALUES:** May increase hepatic enzymes, serum bilirubin.

AVAILABILITY (Rx)

Capsules: 10 mg, 18 mg, 25 mg, 40 mg, 60 mg, 80 mg, 100 mg.

ADMINISTRATION/HANDLING
PO

• Give without regard to food. • Swallow capsules whole, do not break or open (powder in capsule is ocular irritant). Give as single daily dose in the morning or 2 evenly divided doses in morning and late afternoon/early evening.

INDICATIONS/ROUTES/DOSAGE

Note: May discontinue without tapering dose.

Attention-Deficit Hyperactivity Disorder (ADHD)
PO: ADULTS, CHILDREN 6 YRS AND OLDER WEIGHING 70 KG OR MORE: Initially, 40 mg once daily. May increase after at least 3 days to 80 mg daily. **Maximum:** 100 mg. **CHILDREN 6 YRS AND OLDER WEIGHING LESS THAN 70 KG:** Initially, 0.5 mg/kg/day. May increase after at least 3 days to 1.2 mg/kg/day. **Maximum:** 1.4 mg/kg/day or 100 mg, whichever is less.

Dosage in Hepatic Impairment
Expect to administer 50% of normal atomoxetine dosage to pts with moderate hepatic impairment and 25% of normal dosage to pts with severe hepatic impairment.

Dosage in Renal Impairment
No dose adjustment.

Dosage with Strong CYP2D6 Inhibitors
ADULTS: Initially, 40 mg/day. May increase to 80 mg/day after minimum of 4 wks. **CHILDREN:** Initially, 0.5 mg/kg/day. May increase to 1.2 mg/kg/day only after minimum 4-wk interval.

SIDE EFFECTS

Frequent: Headache, dyspepsia, nausea, vomiting, fatigue, decreased appetite, dizziness, altered mood. **Occasional:** Tachycardia, hypertension, weight loss, delayed growth in children, irritability. **Rare:** Insomnia, sexual dysfunction in adults, fever.

ADVERSE EFFECTS/TOXIC REACTIONS

Urinary retention, urinary hesitancy may occur. In overdose, gastric lavage, activated charcoal may prevent systemic absorption. Severe hepatic injury occurs rarely.

NURSING CONSIDERATIONS

BASELINE ASSESSMENT
Assess pulse, B/P before therapy, following dose increases, and periodically during therapy. Assess attention span, interactions with others.

INTERVENTION/EVALUATION
Monitor urinary output; complaints of urinary retention/hesitancy may be a related adverse reaction. Monitor B/P, pulse periodically and following dose increases. Monitor for growth, attention span, hyperactivity, unusual changes in behavior, suicidal ideation. Assist with ambulation if dizziness occurs. Be alert to mood changes. Monitor fluid and electrolyte status in pts with significant vomiting.

PATIENT/FAMILY TEACHING
• Take last dose early in evening to avoid insomnia. • Report palpitations, fever, vomiting, irritability. • Monitor growth rate, weight. • Report changes in behavior, suicidal ideation, chest pain, palpitations, dyspnea.

---

atorvaSTATin   TOP 100

a-**tor**-va-sta-tin
(Apo-Atorvastatin ✦, Lipitor, Novo-Atorvastatin ✦)
Do not confuse atorvastatin with atomoxetine, lovastatin, nystatin, pitavastatin, pravastatin, or simvastatin, or Lipitor with Levatol, lisinopril, or Zocor.

FIXED-COMBINATION(S)

Caduet: atorvastatin/amLODIPine (calcium channel blocker): 10 mg/2.5 mg, 10 mg/5 mg, 10 mg/10 mg, 20 mg/2.5 mg, 20 mg/5 mg, 20 mg/10 mg, 40 mg/2.5 mg, 40 mg/5 mg, 40 mg/10 mg, 80 mg/5 mg, 80 mg/10 mg.

◆CLASSIFICATION

PHARMACOTHERAPEUTIC: Hydroxymethylglutaryl CoA (HMG-CoA) reductase inhibitor. **CLINICAL:** Antihyperlipidemic.

USES

Primary prevention of cardiovascular disease in high-risk pts. Reduces risk of stroke and heart attack in pts with type 2 diabetes with or without evidence of heart disease. Reduces risk of stroke in pts with or without evidence of heart disease with multiple risk factors other than diabetes. Adjunct to diet therapy in management of hyperlipidemias (reduces elevations in total cholesterol, LDL-C, apolipoprotein B, triglycerides in pts with primary hypercholesterolemia, homozygous familial hypercholesterolemia, heterozygous familial hypercholesterolemia in pts 10–17 yrs of age, females more than 1 yr postmenarche. **OFF-LABEL:** Secondary prevention in pts who have experienced a noncardioembolic stroke/TIA or following an acute coronary syndrome (ACS) event.

PRECAUTIONS

Contraindications: Hypersensitivity to atorvastatin. Active hepatic disease, breastfeeding, pregnancy, unexplained elevated LFT results. **Cautions:** Anticoagulant therapy; history of hepatic disease; substantial alcohol consumption; pts with prior stroke/TIA; concomitant use of potent CYP3A4 inhibitors; elderly (predisposed to myopathy).

ACTION

Inhibits HMG-CoA reductase, the enzyme that catalyzes the early step in cholesterol synthesis. **Therapeutic Effect:** Decreases LDL and VLDL, plasma triglyceride levels; increases HDL concentration.

PHARMACOKINETICS

Poorly absorbed from GI tract. Protein binding: greater than 98%. Metabolized in liver. Primarily excreted in feces (biliary). **Half-life:** 14 hrs.

⌛ LIFESPAN CONSIDERATIONS

Pregnancy/Lactation: Distributed in breast milk. Contraindicated during pregnancy. May produce fetal skeletal malformation. **Children:** Safety and efficacy not established. **Elderly:** No age-related precautions noted.

INTERACTIONS

DRUG: Strong CYP3A4 inhibitors (e.g., clarithromycin, protease inhibitors, itraconazole) may increase concentration, risk of rhabdomyolysis. **CycloSPORINE** may increase concentration. **Gemfibrozil, fibrates, niacin, colchicine** may increase risk of myopathy, rhabdomyolysis. **Strong CYP3A4 inducers (e.g., rifAMPin, efavirenz)** may decrease concentration. **HERBAL: St. John's wort** may decrease level. **FOOD: Grapefruit products** may increase serum concentrations. **Red yeast rice** may increase serum levels (2.4 mg lovastatin per 600 mg rice). **LAB VALUES:** May increase serum transaminase, creatinine kinase concentrations.

AVAILABILITY (Rx)

Tablets: 10 mg, 20 mg, 40 mg, 80 mg.

ADMINISTRATION/HANDLING

PO

• Give without regard to food or time of day. • Do not break, crush, dissolve, or divide film-coated tablets.

INDICATIONS/ROUTES/DOSAGE

Do not use in pts with active hepatic disease.
Note: Individualize dosage based on baseline LDL/cholesterol, goal of therapy, pt response. **Maximum dose with strong CYP3A4 inhibitors:** 20 mg/day.

Dyslipidemias
PO: ADULTS, ELDERLY: Initially, 10–20 mg/day (40 mg in pts requiring greater than 45% reduction in LDL-C). Range: 10–80 mg/day.

Heterozygous Hypercholesterolemia
PO: CHILDREN 10–17 YRS: Initially, 10 mg/day. **Maximum:** 20 mg/day.

Dosage in Renal Impairment
No dose adjustment.

Dosage in Hepatic Impairment
See contraindications.

SIDE EFFECTS

Common: Atorvastatin is generally well tolerated. Side effects are usually mild and transient. **Frequent (16%):** Headache. **Occasional (5%–2%):** Myalgia, rash, pruritus, allergy. **Rare (less than 2%–1%):** Flatulence, dyspepsia, depression.

ADVERSE EFFECTS/TOXIC REACTIONS

Potential for cataracts, photosensitivity, myalgia, rhabdomyolysis.

NURSING CONSIDERATIONS

BASELINE ASSESSMENT

Obtain baseline cholesterol, triglycerides, LFT. Question for possibility of pregnancy before initiating therapy. Obtain dietary history.

INTERVENTION/EVALUATION

Monitor for headache. Assess for rash, pruritus, malaise. Monitor cholesterol, triglyceride lab values for therapeutic response. Monitor LFTs, CPK.

PATIENT/FAMILY TEACHING

• Follow special diet (important part of treatment). • Periodic lab tests are essential part of therapy. • Do not take other medications without consulting physician. • Do not chew, crush, dissolve, or divide tablets. • Report dark urine, muscle fatigue, bone pain. • Avoid excessive alcohol intake, large quantities of grapefruit products.

atropine

at-roe-peen
(Lomotil: atropine/diphenoxylate [peristaltic inhibitor]: 0.025 mg/2.5 mg.)

◆CLASSIFICATION

PHARMACOTHERAPEUTIC: Acetylcholine antagonist. **CLINICAL:** Antiarrhythmic, antispasmodic, antidote, cycloplegic, antisecretory, anticholinergic.

USES

Injection: Preop to inhibit salivation/secretions; treatment of symptomatic sinus bradycardia; AV block; ventricular asystole; antidote for organophosphate pesticide poisoning. Adjuvant to decrease side effects during reversal of neuromuscular blockage.

PRECAUTIONS

Contraindications: Hypersensitivity to atropine. Narrow-angle glaucoma, pyloric stenosis, prostatic hypertrophy. **Cautions:** Autonomic neuropathy, paralytic ileus, intestinal atony, severe ulcerative colitis, toxic megacolon, renal/hepatic impairment, myocardial ischemia, hyperthyroidism, hypertension, tachyarrhythmias, HF, coronary artery disease, esophageal reflux or hiatal hernia associated with reflux esophagitis; infants, children with spastic paralysis or brain damage; elderly; biliary tract disease, chronic pulmonary disease.

ACTION

Competes with acetylcholine for common binding sites on muscarinic receptors located on exocrine glands, cardiac and smooth muscle ganglia, intramural neurons. **Therapeutic Effect:** Decreases GI motility, secretory activity, GU muscle tone (ureter, bladder); abolishes various types of reflex vagal cardiac slowing or asystole.

PHARMACOKINETICS

Rapidly and well absorbed after IM administration. Widely distributed. Metabolized in liver. Excreted in urine (30%–50% as unchanged drug). **Half-life:** 2–3 hrs.

⌛ LIFESPAN CONSIDERATIONS

Pregnancy/Lactation: Crosses placenta; distributed in breast milk. **Children/Elderly:** Increased susceptibility to atropine effects.

INTERACTIONS

DRUG: Anticholinergics (e.g., glycopyrrolate, scopolamine) may increase effects. **HERBAL:** None significant. **FOOD:** None known. **LAB VALUES:** None significant.

AVAILABILITY (Rx)

Injection (AtroPen): 0.25 mg/0.3 mL, 0.5 mg/0.7 mL, 1 mg/0.7 mL, 2 mg/0.7 mL. **Injection, Solution:** 0.4 mg/mL, 1 mg/mL.

ADMINISTRATION/HANDLING

 IV

• Must be given rapidly (prevents paradoxical slowing of heart rate).

IM

• May be given subcutaneously or IM.

▒ IV INCOMPATIBILITIES

None known.

▒ IV COMPATIBILITIES

DiphenhydrAMINE (Benadryl), droperidol (Inapsine), fentaNYL (Sublimaze), glycopyrrolate (Robinul), heparin, HYDROmorphone (Dilaudid), midazolam (Versed), morphine, potassium chloride, propofol (Diprivan).

INDICATIONS/ROUTES/DOSAGE

Preanesthetic
IV, IM, Subcutaneous: ADULTS, ELDERLY: 0.4–0.6 mg 30–60 min preop.

CHILDREN WEIGHING 5 KG OR MORE: 0.01–0.02 mg/kg/dose to maximum of 0.4 mg/dose. Minimum dose: 0.1 mg. **CHILDREN WEIGHING LESS THAN 5 KG:** 0.02 mg/kg/dose 30–60 min preop.

Bradycardia
IV: ADULTS, ELDERLY: 0.5–1 mg q5min, not to exceed total of 3 mg or 0.04 mg/kg. **CHILDREN:** 0.02 mg/kg with a minimum of 0.1 mg to a maximum of 0.5 mg as a single dose. May repeat in 5 min. **Maximum total dose:** 1 mg.

Dosage in Renal/Hepatic Impairment
No dose adjustment.

SIDE EFFECTS

Frequent: Dry mouth, nose, throat (may be severe); decreased sweating; constipation; irritation at subcutaneous or IM injection site. **Occasional:** Dysphagia, blurred vision, bloated feeling, impotence, urinary hesitancy. **Ophthalmic:** Mydriasis, blurred vision, photophobia, decreased visual acuity, tearing, dry eyes or dry conjunctiva, eye irritation, crusting of eyelid. **Rare:** Allergic reaction, including rash, urticaria; mental confusion or excitement, particularly in children; fatigue.

ADVERSE EFFECTS/TOXIC REACTIONS

Overdose may produce tachycardia, palpitations, hot/dry/flushed skin, absence of bowel sounds, increased respiratory rate, nausea, vomiting, confusion, drowsiness, slurred speech, dizziness, CNS stimulation. Overdose may also produce psychosis as evidenced by agitation, restlessness, rambling speech, visual hallucinations, paranoid behavior, delusions, followed by depression. Ophthalmic form may rarely produce increased IOP.

NURSING CONSIDERATIONS

BASELINE ASSESSMENT

Determine if pt is sensitive to atropine, homatropine, scopolamine.

INTERVENTION/EVALUATION

Monitor changes in B/P, pulse, temperature. Observe for tachycardia if pt has cardiac abnormalities. Assess skin turgor, mucous membranes to evaluate hydration status (encourage adequate fluid intake unless NPO for surgery), bowel sounds for peristalsis. Be alert for fever (increased risk of hyperthermia). Monitor I&O, palpate bladder for urinary retention. Monitor daily pattern of bowel activity, stool consistency.

PATIENT/ FAMILY TEACHING

• For preop use, explain that warm flushing feeling may occur.

---

avelumab

a-**vel**-ue-mab
(Bavencio)
Do not confuse avelumab with durvalumab, nivolumab or olaratumab.

◆CLASSIFICATION

PHARMACOTHERAPEUTIC: Programmed death ligand-1 (PD-L1) blocking antibody. Monoclonal antibody. **CLINICAL:** Antineoplastic.

USES

Treatment of adults and pediatric pts 12 yrs and older with metastatic Merkel cell carcinoma. Treatment of pts with locally advanced or metastatic urothelial carcinoma who have disease progression during or following platinum-containing chemotherapy or have disease progression within 12 mos of neoadjuvant or adjuvant treatment with platinum-containing chemotherapy.

PRECAUTIONS

Contraindications: Hypersensitivity to avelumab. **Cautions:** Acute infection, conditions predisposing to infection (e.g., diabetes, immunocompromised pts,

renal failure, open wounds); corticosteroid intolerance, hematologic cytopenias, hepatic impairment, interstitial lung disease, renal insufficiency; history of autoimmune disorders (Crohn's disease, demyelinating polyneuropathy, Guillain-Barré syndrome, Hashimoto's thyroiditis, hyperthyroidism, myasthenia gravis, rheumatoid arthritis, Type I diabetes, vasculitis); CVA, diabetes, intestinal obstruction, pancreatitis.

ACTION

Binds to PD-L1 and blocks interaction with both PD-L1 and B7.1 receptors while still allowing interaction between PD-L2 and PD-L1. PD-L1 is an immune check point protein expressed on tumor cells, down regulating anti-tumor T-Cell function. **Therapeutic Effect:** Restores immune responses, including T-cell anti-tumor function.

PHARMACOKINETICS

Widely distributed. Degraded into small peptides and amino acids via proteolytic enzymes. Steady state reached in 4–6 wks. Excretion not specified. **Half-life:** 6.1 days.

⌛ LIFESPAN CONSIDERATIONS

Pregnancy/Lactation: Avoid pregnancy; may cause fetal harm. Females of reproductive potential should use effective contraception during treatment and for at least 1 mo after discontinuation. Unknown if distributed in breast milk. However, human immunoglobulin G (IgG) is present in breastmilk and is known to cross the placenta. Breastfeeding not recommended during treatment and for at least 1 mo after discontinuation. **Children:** Safety and efficacy not established in pts younger than 12 yrs. **Elderly:** No age-related precautions noted.

INTERACTIONS

DRUG: May enhance adverse effects/toxicity of **belimumab. HERBAL:** None significant. **FOOD:** None known. **LAB VALUES:** May decrease Hgb, Hct, lymphocytes, neutrophils, platelets, RBCs. May increase

---

serum alkaline phosphatase, ALT, AST, amylase, bilirubin, glucose, GGT, lipase.

AVAILABILITY (Rx)

Injection: 200 mg/10 mL (20 mg/mL).

ADMINISTRATION/HANDLING

 IV

Preparation • Visually inspect for particulate matter or discoloration. Solution should appear clear and colorless to slightly yellow in color. • Do not use if solution is cloudy, discolored, or if visible particles are observed. • Withdraw proper volume from vial and inject into a 250-mL bag of 0.9% NaCl or 0.45% NaCl. • Gently invert to mix; avoid foaming. • Do not shake. • Diluted solution should be clear, colorless, and free of particles.

Rate of Administration • Infuse over 60 min via dedicated IV line using a sterile, non-pyrogenic, low protein-binding in-line filter.

Storage • Refrigerate unused vials. • May refrigerate diluted solution for no more than 24 hrs or store at room temperature for no more than 4 hrs. If refrigerated, allow diluted solution to warm to room temperature before infusing. • Do not freeze or shake. • Protect from light.

▨ IV INCOMPATIBILITIES

Do not mix or infuse with other medications.

INDICATIONS/ROUTES/DOSAGE

NOTE: Premedicate with acetaminophen and an antihistamine prior to the first 4 infusions. Consider premedication for subsequent infusions based on prior infusion reactions.

Urothelial Carcinoma, Merkel Cell Carcinoma

IV: ADULTS, ELDERLY, CHILDREN: 10 mg/kg every 2 wks. Continue until disease progression or unacceptable toxicity.

Dose Modification

Infusion-related reactions

CTCAE grade 1 or 2: Interrupt or decrease rate of infusion. **CTCAE grade 3 or 4:** Permanently discontinue.

Endocrinopathies (e.g., adrenal insufficiency, hyperglycemia, hyperthyroidism, hypothyroidism) (treatment-induced)

CTCAE grade 3 or 4 endocrinopathies: Withhold treatment until resolved to grade 1 or 0, then resume therapy after corticosteroid taper. Consider hormone replacement therapy if hypothyroidism occurs.

Colitis (treatment-induced)

CTCAE grade 2 or 3 diarrhea or colitis: Withhold treatment until resolved to grade 1 or 0, then resume therapy after corticosteroid taper. **CTCAE grade 4 diarrhea or colitis; recurrent grade 3 diarrhea or colitis:** Permanently discontinue.

Hepatitis (treatment-induced)

Serum ALT/AST greater than 3 and up to 5 times upper limit normal (ULN) or serum bilirubin greater than 1.5 and up to 3 times ULN: Withhold treatment until resolved to grade 1 or 0, then resume therapy. **Serum ALT/AST greater than 5 times upper limit normal (ULN) or serum bilirubin greater than 3 times ULN):** Permanently discontinue.

Nephritis and Renal Dysfunction (treatment-induced)

Serum creatinine greater than 1.5 and up to 6 times ULN: Withhold treatment until resolved to grade 1 or 0, then resume therapy after corticosteroid taper. **Serum creatinine greater than 6 times ULN:** Permanently discontinue.

Other moderate or severe symptoms of treatment-induced reactions (e.g., arthritis, bullous dermatitis, encephalitis, erythema multiform, exfoliative dermatitis, demyelination, Guillain-Barré syndrome, hemolytic anemia, histiocytic necrotizing lymphadenitis, hypophysitis, hypopituitarism, iritis, myasthenia gravis, myocarditis, myosotis, pancreatitis, pemphigoid,

psoriasis, Stevens Johnson Syndrome/toxic epidermal necrolysis, rhabdomyolysis, uveitis, vasculitis): Withhold treatment until resolved to grade 1 or 0, then resume therapy after corticosteroid taper. **Life-threatening adverse effects, recurrent severe immune-mediated reactions; requirement of predniSONE 10 mg/day or greater (or equivalent) for more than 2 wks; persistent grade 2 or 3 immune-mediated reaction lasting 12 wks or longer:** Permanently discontinue.

Pneumonitis (treatment induced)

CTCAE grade 2 pneumonitis: Withhold treatment until resolved to grade 1 or 0, then resume therapy after corticosteroid taper. **CTCAE grade 3 or 4 or recurrent grade 2 pneumonitis:** Permanently discontinue.

Dosage in Renal Impairment
Not specified; use caution.

Dosage in Hepatic Impairment
Not specified; use caution.

SIDE EFFECTS

Note: Percentage of side effects may vary depending on indication of treatment. **Frequent (50%–18%):** Fatigue, musculoskeletal pain, diarrhea, rash, infusion reactions (back pain, chills, pyrexia, hypotension), nausea, decreased appetite, peripheral edema, cough. **Occasional (17%–10%):** Constipation, arthralgia, abdominal pain, decreased weight, dizziness, vomiting, hypertension, dyspnea, pruritus, headache.

ADVERSE EFFECTS/TOXIC REACTIONS

Anemia, neutropenia, thrombocytopenia is an expected response to therapy. May cause severe, sometimes fatal cases of immune-mediated reactions such as pneumonitis (1% of pts), hepatitis (1% of pts), colitis (2% of pts), adrenal insufficiency (1% of pts), hypothyroidism, hyperthyroidism (6% of pts), type 1 diabetes mellitus including ketoacidosis (less than 1% of pts), nephritis (less than 1% of pts), other immune-mediated

effects (less than 1%). Cellulitis, CVA, dyspnea, ileus, pericardial effusion, small bowel/intestinal obstruction, renal failure, respiratory failure, septic shock, transaminitis, urosepsis may occur. Immunogenicity (auto-avelumab antibodies) reported in 4% of pts.

NURSING CONSIDERATIONS

BASELINE ASSESSMENT

Obtain ANC, CBC, BMP (esp. serum creatinine, creatinine clearance; BUN), TSH, vital signs; urine pregnancy. Question current breastfeeding status. Verify use of contraception in female pts of reproductive potential. Question history of prior hypersensitivity reaction, infusion-related reactions, allergy to corticosteroids/prednisone. Screen for history of autoimmune disorders, diabetes, pituitary/pulmonary/thyroid disease, renal insufficiency. Obtain nutrition consult. Offer emotional support.

INTERVENTION/EVALUATION

Monitor ANC, CBC, BMP, creatinine clearance, thyroid panel (if applicable); vital signs. Diligently monitor for infusion-related reactions, treatment-related toxicities, esp. during initial infusions. If immune-mediated reactions occur, consider referral to specialist; pt may require treatment with corticosteroids. Screen for allergic reactions, acute infections (cellulitis, sepsis, UTI), hepatitis, pulmonary events (dyspnea, pneumonitis, pneumonia). Monitor strict I&O, hydration status, stool frequency and consistency. Encourage proper calorie intake and nutrition. Assess skin for rash, lesions, dermal toxicities.

PATIENT/FAMILY TEACHING

• Treatment may depress your immune system and reduce your ability to fight infection. Report symptoms of infection such as body aches, burning with urination, chills, cough, fatigue, fever. Avoid those with active infection. • Avoid pregnancy; treatment may cause birth defects. Do not breastfeed. Females of childbearing potential should use effective contraception during treatment and for at least 1 mo after discontinuation. • Serious adverse reactions may affect lungs, liver, intestines, kidneys, hormonal glands, nervous system, which may require anti-inflammatory medication. • Immediately report any serious or life-threatening inflammatory symptoms in the following body systems: colon (severe abdominal pain/ swelling, diarrhea); kidneys (decreased or dark-colored urine, flank pain); lung (chest pain, severe cough, shortness of breath); liver (bruising, dark-colored urine, clay-colored/tarry stools, nausea, yellowing of the skin or eyes); nervous system (paralysis, weakness); pituitary (persistent or unusual headaches, dizziness, extreme weakness, fainting, vision changes); skin (blisters, bubbling, inflammation, rash); thyroid (trouble sleeping, high blood pressure, fast heart rate [overactive thyroid]; fatigue, goiter, weight gain [underactive thyroid]); vascular (low blood pressure, vein/artery pain or irritation). • Do not take any over-the-counter anti-inflammatory medications unless approved by your doctor.

axitinib

ax-i-ti-nib
(Inlyta)
Do not confuse axitinib with afatinib, ibrutinib, or imatinib.

◆CLASSIFICATION

PHARMACOTHERAPEUTIC: Tyrosine kinase inhibitor. **CLINICAL:** Antineoplastic.

USES

Treatment of advanced renal cell carcinoma after failure of one prior systemic chemotherapy.

PRECAUTIONS

Contraindications: Hypersensitivity to axitinib. **Cautions:** Pts with increased risk or history of thrombotic events (CVA, MI), GI perforation or fistula formation, renal/hepatic impairment, hypertension, HF. Do not use in pts with untreated brain metastasis or recent active GI bleeding.

ACTION

Inhibits vascular endothelial growth factor receptors. **Therapeutic Effect:** Blocks tumor growth, inhibits angiogenesis.

PHARMACOKINETICS

Metabolized in liver. Protein binding: greater than 99%. Excreted primarily in feces a lesser amount excreted in urine. **Half-life:** 2.5–6 hrs.

⧗ LIFESPAN CONSIDERATIONS

Pregnancy/Lactation: May cause fetal harm. Unknown whether distributed in breast milk. **Children:** Safety and efficacy not established in pts younger than 18 yrs. **Elderly:** No age-related precautions noted.

INTERACTIONS

DRUG: Strong CYP3A4/5 inhibitors (e.g., erythromycin, ketoconazole, ritonavir) may significantly increase concentration; do not use concurrently. If used, reduce dose by 50%. Coadministration with **strong CYP3A4/5 inducers (e.g., rifAMPin, phenytoin, carBAMazepine, PHENobarbital)** may significantly decrease concentration; do not use concurrently. **HERBAL: St. John's wort** may decrease concentration. **FOOD: Grapefruit products** may increase concentration. **LAB VALUES:** May decrease Hgb, WBC count, platelets, lymphocytes; serum calcium, alkaline phosphatase, albumin, sodium, phosphate, bicarbonate. May increase serum ALT, AST, bilirubin, BUN, creatinine, serum potassium, lipase, amylase; urine protein. May alter serum glucose.

AVAILABILITY (Rx)

Tablets, film-coated: 1 mg, 5 mg.

ADMINISTRATION/HANDLING

PO
• Give without regard to food. • Swallow tablets whole with full glass of water.

INDICATIONS/ROUTES/DOSAGE

Renal Cell Carcinoma
PO: ADULTS, ELDERLY: Initially, 5 mg twice daily, given approximately 12 hrs apart. If tolerated (no adverse events above grade 2, BP normal and no antihypertension use for at least 2 consecutive wks), may increase to 7 mg twice daily, then 10 mg twice daily. For adverse effects, may decrease to 3 mg twice daily, then 2 mg twice daily if adverse effects persist.

Dose Modification
Dosage with concomitant strong CYP3A4 inhibitors: Reduce dose by 50%. (Avoid concomitant use if possible.)

Dosage in Renal Impairment
No dose adjustment. Use caution in ESRD.

Dosage in Hepatic Impairment
Mild impairment: No dose adjustment.
Moderate Impairment: Reduce initial dose by 50%. **Severe Impairment:** Not recommended.

SIDE EFFECTS

Frequent (55%–20%): Diarrhea, hypertension, fatigue, decreased appetite, nausea, dysphonia, palmar-plantar erythrodysesthesia (hand-foot) syndrome, weight loss, vomiting, asthenia, constipation. **Occasional (19%–11%):** Hypothyroidism, cough, stomatitis, arthralgia, dyspnea, abdominal pain, headache, peripheral pain, rash, proteinuria, dysgeusia. **Rare (10%–2%):** Dry skin, dyspepsia, dizziness, myalgia, pruritus, epistaxis, alopecia, hemorrhoids, tinnitus, erythema.

ADVERSE EFFECTS/TOXIC REACTIONS

Arterial and venous thrombotic events (MI, CVA), GI perforation, fistula, hemorrhagic events (including cerebral hemorrhage, hematuria, hemoptysis, GI bleeding), hypertensive crisis, cardiac failure have been observed and can be fatal. Hypothyroidism requiring thyroid hormone replacement has been noted. Reversible posterior leukoencephalopathy syndrome (RPLS) has been observed.

NURSING CONSIDERATIONS

BASELINE ASSESSMENT
Obtain baseline BMP, LFT, renal function test, urine protein, serum amylase, lipase, phosphate before initiation of, and periodically throughout, treatment. Offer emotional support. Assess medical history, esp. hepatic function abnormalities. B/P should be well controlled prior to initiating treatment. Stop medication at least 24 hrs prior to scheduled surgery. Monitor thyroid function before and periodically throughout treatment.

INTERVENTION/EVALUATION
Monitor CBC, BMP, LFT, renal function test, urine protein, serum amylase, lipase, phosphate, thyroid tests. Monitor daily pattern of bowel activity, stool consistency. Assess for evidence of bleeding or hemorrhage. Assess for hypertension. For persistent hypertension despite use of antihypertensive medications, dose should be reduced. Permanently discontinue if signs or symptoms of RPLS occur (extreme lethargy, increased B/P from pt baseline, pyuria). Contact physician if changes in voice, redness of skin, or rash is noted.

PATIENT/FAMILY TEACHING
• Avoid crowds, those with known infection. • Avoid contact with anyone who recently received live virus vaccine; do not receive vaccinations. • Swallow tablet whole; do not chew, crush, dissolve, or divide. • Avoid grapefruit

products. • Report persistent diarrhea, extreme fatigue, abdominal pain, yellowing of skin or eyes, bruising easily; bleeding of any kind, esp. bloody stool or urine; confusion, seizure activity, vision loss, trouble speaking, chest pain; difficulty breathing, leg pain or swelling.

azaTHIOprine

a-za-thy-o-preen
(Apo-AzaTHIOprine ✤, Azasan, Imuran)
■ BLACK BOX ALERT ■ Chronic immunosuppression increases risk of developing malignancy.
Do not confuse azaTHIOprine with Azulfidine, azaCITIDine, or azithromycin, or Imuran with Elmiron, Imdur, or Inderal.

◆ CLASSIFICATION

PHARMACOTHERAPEUTIC: Immunologic agent. CLINICAL: Immunosuppressant.

USES

Adjunct in prevention of rejection in kidney transplantation. Treatment of rheumatoid arthritis (RA) in pts unresponsive to conventional therapy. OFF-LABEL: Treatment of dermatomyositis, polymyositis. Maintenance, remission, or reduction of steroid use in Crohn's disease, lupus nephritis, chronic refractory immune thrombocytopenic purpura.

PRECAUTIONS

Contraindications: Hypersensitivity to azaTHIOprine. Pregnant women with RA, pts previously treated for RA with alkylating agents (cyclophosphamide, chlorambucil, melphalan) may have a prohibitive risk of malignancy with azathioprine. Cautions: Immunosuppressed pts, pts with hepatic/renal impairment, active infection. Testing for genetic deficiency of thiopurine methyltransferase should be obtained. (Absence or

reduced levels increase risk of myelosuppression.)

PHARMACOKINETICS

Well absorbed from GI tract. Peak levels: 1–2 hrs. Protein binding: 30%. Metabolized in liver. Primarily excreted in urine. Half-life: 2 hrs.

ACTION

Antagonizes purine metabolism, inhibits DNA, protein, and RNA synthesis. Therapeutic Effect: Suppresses cell-mediated hypersensitivities; alters antibody production, immune response in transplant recipients. Reduces symptoms of arthritis severity.

⌛ LIFESPAN CONSIDERATIONS

Pregnancy/Lactation: May depress spermatogenesis, reduce sperm viability, count. May cause fetal harm. Do not breastfeed. Children: Safety and efficacy not established. Elderly: No age-related precautions noted.

INTERACTIONS

DRUG: Allopurinol, sulfamethoxazole/trimethoprim may increase activity, toxicity. Bone marrow depressants may increase myelosuppression. Other immunosuppressants may increase risk of infection or development of neoplasms. May increase effects of live virus vaccines. HERBAL: Avoid cat's claw, echinacea (immunostimulant properties). FOOD: None known. LAB VALUES: May decrease Hgb, serum albumin, uric acid, leukocytes, platelet count. May increase serum ALT, AST, alkaline phosphatase, amylase, bilirubin.

AVAILABILITY (Rx)

Tablets: 50 mg (Imuran), 75 mg (Azasan), 100 mg (Azasan).

ADMINISTRATION/HANDLING

PO
• Give with food or in divided doses to reduce potential for GI disturbances.
• Store oral form at room temperature.

INDICATIONS/ROUTES/DOSAGE

◀ **ALERT** ▶ Reduce dose to 1/3 or 1/4 usual dose when used with allopurinol or in low/absent thiopurine methyltransferase genetic deficiency.

Prevention of Renal Allograft Rejection

PO: ADULTS, ELDERLY, CHILDREN: 3–5 mg/kg/day on day of transplant (or 1–3 days prior to transplant), then 1–3 mg/kg/day as maintenance dose.

Rheumatoid Arthritis (RA)

PO: ADULTS, ELDERLY: Initially, 1 mg/kg/day (50–100 mg) as a single dose or in 2 divided doses for 6–8 wks. May increase by 0.5 mg/kg/day after 6–8 wks at 4-wk intervals. **Maximum:** 2.5 mg/kg/day. **Maintenance:** Lowest effective dosage. May decrease dose by 0.5 mg/kg or 25 mg/day q4wks (while other therapies, such as rest, physiotherapy, and salicylates, are maintained). May discontinue abruptly.

Dosage in Renal Impairment

Dosage is modified based on creatinine clearance.

Creatinine Clearance	Dosage
10–50 mL/min	75% of normal
Less than 10 mL/min	50% of normal
Hemodialysis	50% of normal (Adults: additional 0.25 mg/kg)
Continuous renal replacement therapy (CRRT)	75% of normal

Dosage in Hepatic Impairment

No dose adjustment.

SIDE EFFECTS

Frequent: Nausea, vomiting, anorexia (particularly during early treatment and with large doses). **Occasional:** Rash. **Rare:** Severe nausea/vomiting with diarrhea, abdominal pain, hypersensitivity reaction.

ADVERSE EFFECTS/ TOXIC REACTIONS

Increases risk of neoplasia (new abnormal-growth tumors). Significant leukopenia and thrombocytopenia may occur, particularly in pts undergoing renal transplant rejection. Hepatotoxicity occurs rarely.

NURSING CONSIDERATIONS

BASELINE ASSESSMENT

Arthritis: Assess onset, type, location, and duration of pain, fever, inflammation. Inspect appearance of affected joints for immobility, deformities, skin condition.

INTERVENTION/EVALUATION

CBC, LFT should be performed weekly during first mo of therapy, twice monthly during second and third mos of treatment, then monthly thereafter. If WBC falls rapidly, dosage should be reduced or discontinued. Assess particularly for delayed myelosuppression. Routinely watch for any change from baseline. **Arthritis:** Assess for therapeutic response: relief of pain, stiffness, swelling; increased joint mobility; reduced joint tenderness; improved grip strength.

PATIENT/FAMILY TEACHING

• Contact physician if unusual bleeding/ bruising, sore throat, mouth sores, abdominal pain, fever occurs. • Therapeutic response in rheumatoid arthritis may take up to 12 wks. • Women of childbearing age must avoid pregnancy.

azilsartan

a-zil-**sar**-tan
(Edarbi)

■ **BLACK BOX ALERT** ■ May cause fetal injury, mortality. Discontinue as soon as possible once pregnancy is detected.
Do not confuse azilsartan with losartan, irbesartan, or valsartan.

FIXED-COMBINATION(S)

Edarbyclor: azilsartan/chlorthalidone, a diuretic: 40 mg/12.5 mg, 40 mg/25 mg.

◆CLASSIFICATION

PHARMACOTHERAPEUTIC: Angiotensin II receptor blocker (ARB). **CLINICAL:** Antihypertensive.

USES

Treatment of hypertension alone or in combination with other antihypertensives.

PRECAUTIONS

Contraindications: Hypersensitivity to azilsartan. Concomitant use with aliskiren in pts with diabetes. **Cautions:** Renal/hepatic impairment, unstented renal artery stenosis, significant aortic/mitral stenosis, severe HF, volume depletion/salt-depleted pts, history of angioedema.

ACTION

Inhibits vasoconstriction, aldosterone-secreting effects of angiotension II, blocking the binding of angiotension II to AT_1 receptors. **Therapeutic Effect:** Produces vasodilation, decreases peripheral resistance, decreases B/P.

PHARMACOKINETICS

Hydrolyzed to active metabolite in GI tract. Moderately absorbed (60%). Peak plasma concentration: 1.5–3 hrs. Metabolized in liver. Protein binding: greater than 99%. Excreted in feces (55%), urine (42%). **Half-life:** 11 hrs.

⌛ LIFESPAN CONSIDERATIONS

Pregnancy/Lactation: May cause fetal harm when administered during third trimester. Unknown if distributed in breast milk. Breastfeeding not recommended. **Children:** Safety and efficacy not established. **Elderly:** Elevated creatinine levels may occur in pts older than 75 yrs.

INTERACTIONS

DRUG: ACE inhibitors (e.g., enalapril, lisinopril), potassium-sparing diuretics (e.g., spironolactone, triamterene), potassium supplements may increase risk of hyperkalemia. **NSAIDs, COX-2 inhibitors (e.g., celecoxib)** may decrease effect. **Hypotensive agents** may increase hypotensive effects. **HERBAL: Yohimbe, ephedra, licorice, ginseng** may increase B/P. **Garlic** may enhance antihypertensive effect. **FOOD:** None known. **LAB VALUES:** May increase serum creatinine. May decrease Hgb, Hct.

AVAILABILITY (Rx)

Tablets: 40 mg, 80 mg.

ADMINISTRATION/HANDLING

PO
• May give without regard to food.

INDICATIONS/ROUTES/DOSAGE

Hypertension
PO: ADULTS, ELDERLY: 80 mg once daily. Reduce to 40 mg once daily if giving high-dose diuretic concurrently.

Dosage in Renal/Hepatic Impairment
No dose adjustment.

SIDE EFFECTS

Occasional (2%–0.4%): Diarrhea, orthostatic hypotension. **Rare (0.3%):** Nausea, fatigue, muscle spasm, cough.

ADVERSE EFFECTS/TOXIC REACTIONS

Oliguria, acute renal failure may occur in pts with history of renal artery stenosis, severe HF, volume depletion.

NURSING CONSIDERATIONS

BASELINE ASSESSMENT

Obtain baseline Hgb, Hct, BMP, LFT. Obtain B/P, apical pulse immediately before each dose, in addition to regular monitoring (be alert to fluctuations). Question for possibility of pregnancy. Assess medication history (esp. diuretics). Question history of hepatic/renal impairment, renal artery stenosis, severe HF.

INTERVENTION/EVALUATION

Maintain hydration (offer fluids frequently). Monitor serum electrolytes, B/P, pulse, hepatic/renal function. Observe for symptoms of hypotension. If excessive reduction in B/P occurs, place pt in supine position, feet slightly elevated. Correct volume or salt depletion prior to treatment.

PATIENT/FAMILY TEACHING

• Take measures to avoid pregnancy. If pregnancy occurs, inform physician immediately. • Low blood pressure is more likely to occur if pt takes diuretics or other medications to control hypertension, consumes low-salt diet, experiences vomiting or diarrhea, or becomes dehydrated. • Change positions slowly, particularly from lying to standing position. • Report light-headedness or dizziness; lie down immediately. • Report swollen extremities or decreased urine output despite fluid intake.

azithromycin

a-**zith**-roe-**mye**-sin
(Apo-Azithromycin ✦, AzaSite, Novo-Azithromycin ✦, Zithromax, Zithromax TRI-PAK, Zithromax Z-PAK, Zmax)
Do not confuse azithromycin with azaTHIOprine or erythromycin, or Zithromax with Fosamax or Zovirax.

◆CLASSIFICATION

PHARMACOTHERAPEUTIC: Macrolide. **CLINICAL:** Antibiotic.

USES

IV/PO: Treatment of susceptible infections due to *Chlamydia pneumoniae, C. trachomatis, H. influenzae, Legionella, M. catarrhalis, Mycoplasma pneumoniae, N. gonorrhoeae, S. aureus., S. pneumoniae, S. pyogenes,* including mild to moderate infections of upper respiratory tract (pharyngitis, tonsillitis), lower respiratory tract (acute bacterial exacerbations, COPD, pneumonia), uncomplicated skin and skin-structure infections, sexually transmitted diseases (nongonococcal urethritis, cervicitis due to *C. trachomatis*), chancroid. Prevents disseminated *Mycobacterium avium* complex (MAC). Treatment of mycoplasma pneumonia, community-acquired pneumonia, pelvic inflammatory disease (PID). Prevention/treatment of MAC in pts with advanced HIV infection. **OFF-LABEL:** Prophylaxis of endocarditis. Prevention of pulmonary exacerbations in pts with cystic fibrosis. **Ophthalmic:** Treatment of bacterial conjunctivitis caused by susceptible infections due to *H. influenzae, S. aureus, S. mitis, S. pneumoniae.* Prevention of pulmonary exacerbations in pts with cystic fibrosis.

PRECAUTIONS

Contraindications: Hypersensitivity to azithromycin or other macrolide antibiotics. History of cholestatic jaundice/hepatic impairment associated with prior azithromycin therapy. **Cautions:** Hepatic/renal impairment, myasthenia gravis, hepatocellular and/or cholestatic hepatitis (with or without jaundice), hepatic necrosis. May prolong QT interval.

ACTION

Binds to ribosomal receptor sites of susceptible organisms, inhibiting RNA-dependent protein synthesis. **Therapeutic Effect:** Bacteriostatic or bactericidal, depending on drug dosage.

PHARMACOKINETICS

Rapidly absorbed from GI tract. Protein binding: 7%–50%. Widely distributed. Metabolized in liver. Excreted primarily by biliary excretion. **Half-life:** 68 hrs.

⌛ LIFESPAN CONSIDERATIONS

Pregnancy/Lactation: Unknown if distributed in breast milk. **Children:** Safety and efficacy not established

---

✦ Canadian trade name   🐦 Non-Crushable Drug   🔳 High Alert drug

in pts younger than 16 yrs for IV use and younger than 6 mos for oral use. **Elderly:** No age-related precautions in those with normal renal function.

INTERACTIONS

DRUG: Aluminum/magnesium-containing antacids may decrease concentration (give 1 hr before or 2 hrs after antacid). May increase levels of **amiodarone, cycloSPORINE, dronedarone, QT-prolonging medications, thioridazine, toremifene, ziprasidone. QUEtiapine** may increase concentration. **HERBAL:** None significant. **FOOD:** None known. **LAB VALUES:** May increase serum creatine phosphokinase (CPK), ALT, AST, bilirubin, LDH, potassium.

AVAILABILITY (Rx)

Injection, Powder for Reconstitution (Zithromax): 500 mg. **Ophthalmic Solution (AzaSite):** 1%. **Suspension, Oral (Zithromax):** 100 mg/5 mL, 200 mg/5 mL. **Suspension, Oral (Extended-Release [Zmax]):** 2-g single-dose packet. **Tablets:** 250 mg, 500 mg, 600 mg.

ADMINISTRATION/HANDLING

IV

Reconstitution • Reconstitute each 500-mg vial with 4.8 mL Sterile Water for Injection to provide concentration of 100 mg/mL. • Shake well to ensure dissolution. • Further dilute with 250 or 500 mL 0.9% NaCl or D$_5$W to provide final concentration of 2 mg/mL with 250 mL diluent or 1 mg/mL with 500 mL diluent. **Rate of Administration** • Infuse over 60 min (2 mg/mL). Infuse over 3 hrs (1 mg/mL). **Storage** • Store vials at room temperature. • Following reconstitution, diluted solution is stable for 24 hrs at room temperature or 7 days if refrigerated.

PO (Immediate-Release Suspension)
• Give tablets without regard to food. • May store suspension at room temperature. Stable for 10 days after reconstitution.

PO (Extended-Release Suspension)
• Do not administer oral suspension with food. Give at least 1 hr before or 2 hrs after meals. • Give Zmax within 12 hrs of reconstitution. • Give tablets with food to decrease GI effects.

PO
• Tablets: May give with food to decrease GI effects.

Ophthalmic
• Place gloved finger on lower eyelid and pull out until a pocket is formed between eye and lower lid. • Place prescribed number of drops into pocket. • Instruct pt to close eye gently for 1 to 2 min (so that medication will not be squeezed out of sac) and to apply digital pressure to lacrimal sac at inner canthus for 1 min to minimize systemic absorption.

▧ IV INCOMPATIBILITIES

CefTRIAXone (Rocephin), ciprofloxacin (Cipro), famotidine (Pepcid), furosemide (Lasix), ketorolac (Toradol), levoFLOXacin (Levaquin), morphine, piperacillin/tazobactam (Zosyn), potassium chloride.

▧ IV COMPATIBILITIES

Ceftaroline (Teflaro), doripenem (Doribax), ondansetron (Zofran), tigecycline (Tygacil), diphenhydrAMINE (Benadryl).

INDICATIONS/ROUTES/DOSAGE

Usual Dosage Range
PO: ADULTS, ELDERLY: 250–600 mg once daily or 1–2 g as single dose. *(Zmax):* 2 g as a single dose. **CHILDREN 6 MOS AND OLDER:** 5–12 mg/kg (**maximum:** 500 mg) once daily or 30 mg/kg (**maximum:** 1,500 mg) as single dose. *(Zmax):* 60 mg/kg as a single dose. **NEONATES:** 10–20 mg/kg once daily.
IV: ADULTS, ELDERLY: 250–500 mg once daily **CHILDREN, NEONATES:** 10 mg/kg once daily.

Mild to Moderate Respiratory Tract, Skin, Soft Tissue Infections
PO: **ADULTS, ELDERLY:** 500 mg day 1, then 250 mg days 2–5.

MAC Prevention
PO: **ADULTS, ELDERLY:** 1,200 mg once weekly. **CHILDREN:** 20 mg/kg once weekly. **Maximum:** 1,200 mg/dose.

MAC Treatment
PO: **ADULTS, ELDERLY:** 600 mg/day with ethambutol. **CHILDREN:** 10–12 mg/kg/day (**maximum:** 500 mg) with ethambutol.

Otitis Media
PO: **CHILDREN 6 MOS AND OLDER:** 30 mg/kg as single dose (**maximum:** 1,500 mg) or 10 mg/kg/day for 3 days (**maximum:** 500 mg) or 10 mg/kg on day 1 (**maximum:** 500 mg), then 5 mg/kg on days 2–5 (**maximum:** 250 mg).

Pharyngitis, Tonsillitis
PO: **ADULTS, ELDERLY, CHILDREN:** 12 mg/kg (**maximum:** 500 mg) on day 1, then 6 mg/kg (**maximum:** 250 mg) on days 2–5.

Pneumonia, Community-Acquired
PO *(Zmax):* **ADULTS, ELDERLY:** 2 g as single dose.
PO: **ADULTS, ELDERLY, CHILDREN 16 YRS AND OLDER:** 500 mg on day 1, then 250 mg on days 2–5 or 500 mg/day IV for 2 days, then 500 mg/day PO to complete course of therapy. **CHILDREN 6 MOS–15 YRS:** 10 mg/kg on day 1 (**maximum:** 500 mg), then 5 mg/kg (**maximum:** 250 mg) on days 2–5.

Dosage in Renal/Hepatic Impairment
Use caution.

Bacterial Conjunctivitis
Ophthalmic: **ADULTS, ELDERLY:** 1 drop in affected eye twice daily for 2 days, then 1 drop once daily for 5 days.

SIDE EFFECTS

Occasional: Systemic: Nausea, vomiting, diarrhea, abdominal pain. **Ophthalmic:** Eye irritation. **Rare: Systemic:** Headache, dizziness, allergic reaction.

ADVERSE EFFECTS/TOXIC REACTIONS

Antibiotic-associated colitis, other superinfections may result from altered bacterial balance in GI tract. Acute interstitial nephritis, hepatotoxicity occur rarely.

NURSING CONSIDERATIONS

BASELINE ASSESSMENT

Question for history of hepatitis, allergies to azithromycin, erythromycins. Assess for infection (WBC count, appearance of wound, evidence of fever).

INTERVENTION/EVALUATION

Check for GI discomfort, nausea, vomiting. Monitor daily pattern of bowel activity and stool consistency. Monitor LFT, CBC. Assess for hepatotoxicity: malaise, fever, abdominal pain, GI disturbances. Be alert for superinfection: fever, vomiting, diarrhea, anal/genital pruritus, oral mucosal changes (ulceration, pain, erythema).

PATIENT/FAMILY TEACHING

• Continue therapy for full length of treatment. • Avoid concurrent administration of aluminum- or magnesium-containing antacids. • Bacterial conjunctivitis: Do not wear contact lenses.

---

aztreonam

az-**tree**-o-nam
(Azactam, Cayston)

◆**CLASSIFICATION**
PHARMACOTHERAPEUTIC: Monobactam. **CLINICAL:** Antibiotic.

USES

Injection: Treatment of infections caused by susceptible gram-negative microorganisms *P. aeruginosa, E. coli, S. marcescens, K. pneumoniae, P. mirabilis, H. influenzae, Enterobacter, Citrobacter* spp., including lower respiratory tract, skin/skin structure, intraabdominal, gynecologic, complicated/uncomplicated UTIs; septicemia; cystic fibrosis. **Cayston:** Improve respiratory symptoms in cystic fibrosis pts with *P. aeruginosa.* **OFF-LABEL:** Surgical prophylaxis.

PRECAUTIONS

Contraindications: Hypersensitivity to aztreonam. **Cautions:** History of allergy, esp. cephalosporins, penicillins; renal impairment; bone marrow transplant pts with risk factors for toxic epidermal necrolysis (TEN).

ACTION

Binds to penicillin-binding proteins, which inhibits bacterial cell wall synthesis. **Therapeutic Effect:** Bactericidal.

PHARMACOKINETICS

Completely absorbed after IM administration. Protein binding: 56%–60%. Partially metabolized by hydrolysis. Primarily excreted unchanged in urine. Removed by hemodialysis. **Half-life:** 1.4–2.2 hrs (increased in renal/hepatic impairment).

⧗ LIFESPAN CONSIDERATIONS

Pregnancy/Lactation: Crosses placenta, distributed in amniotic fluid; low concentration in breast milk. **Children:** Safety and efficacy not established in pts younger than 9 mos. **Elderly:** Age-related renal impairment may require dosage adjustment.

INTERACTIONS

DRUG: None significant. **HERBAL:** None significant. **FOOD:** None known. **LAB VALUES:** May increase serum alkaline phosphatase, creatinine, LDH, ALT, AST levels. Produces a positive Coombs' test.

May prolong partial thromboplastin time (PTT), prothrombin time (PT).

AVAILABILITY (Rx)

Injection, Infusion Solution (Azactam): Premix 1 g/50 mL, 2 g/50 mL. **Injection, Powder for Reconstitution (Azactam):** 1 g, 2 g. **Oral Inhalation, Powder for Reconstitution (Cayston):** 75 mg.

ADMINISTRATION/HANDLING

 IV

Reconstitution • For IV push, dilute each gram with 6–10 mL Sterile Water for Injection. • For intermittent IV infusion, further dilute with 50–100 mL D$_5$W or 0.9% NaCl. Final concentration not to exceed 20 mg/mL.
Rate of Administration • For IV push, give over 3–5 min. • For IV infusion, administer over 20–60 min.
Storage • Store vials at room temperature. • Solution appears colorless to light yellow. • Following reconstitution, solution is stable for 48 hrs at room temperature or 7 days if refrigerated. • Discard if precipitate forms. Discard unused portions.

IM
• Reconstitute with at least 3 mL diluent per gram of aztreonam. • Shake immediately, vigorously after adding diluent. • Inject deeply into large muscle mass. • Following reconstitution, solution is stable for 48 hrs at room temperature or 7 days if refrigerated.

Inhalation
• Administer only with an Altera nebulizer system. • Nebulize over 2–3 min. • Give bronchodilator 15 min–4 hrs (short-acting) or 30 min–12 hrs (long-acting) before administration. • Reconstituted solution must be used immediately.

▨ IV INCOMPATIBILITIES

Acyclovir (Zovirax), amphotericin (Fungizone), LORazepam (Ativan), metroNIDAZOLE (Flagyl), vancomycin (Vancocin).

🏵 IV COMPATIBILITIES

Bumetanide (Bumex), calcium gluconate, cimetidine (Tagamet), diltiaZEM (Cardizem), diphenhydrAMINE (Benadryl), DOBUTamine (Dobutrex), DOPamine (Intropin), famotidine (Pepcid), furosemide (Lasix), heparin, HYDROmorphone (Dilaudid), insulin (regular), magnesium sulfate, morphine, potassium chloride, propofol (Diprivan).

INDICATIONS/ROUTES/DOSAGE

Severe Infections
IV: ADULTS, ELDERLY: 2 g q6–8h. **Maximum:** 8 g/day. **CHILDREN:** 30 mg/kg q6–8h. **Maximum:** 8 g/day (120 mg/kg/day).

Mild to Moderate Infections
IV: ADULTS, ELDERLY: 1–2 g q8–12h. **Maximum:** 8 g/day. **CHILDREN:** 30 mg/kg q8h. **Maximum:** 8 g/day.

Usual Neonatal Dosage
IV: 30 mg/kg/dose q6–12h.

Cystic Fibrosis
NOTE: Pretreatment with a bronchodilator is recommended.
IV: CHILDREN: 50 mg/kg/dose q6–8h up to 200 mg/kg/day. **Maximum:** 8 g/day.
Inhalation (Nebulizer): ADULTS, CHILDREN 7 YRS OR OLDER: 75 mg 3 times/day (at least 4 hrs apart) for 28 days, then off for 28-day cycle.

Dosage in Renal Impairment
Dosage and frequency are modified based on creatinine clearance and severity of infection:

Creatinine Clearance	Dosage
10–30 mL/min	50% usual dose at usual intervals
Less than 10 mL/min	25% usual dose at usual intervals
Hemodialysis	500 mg–2 g, then 25% of initial dose at usual interval
Continuous renal replacement therapy (CRRT)	2 g, then 1 g q8–12h or 2g q12h

Dosage in Hepatic Impairment
Use with caution.

SIDE EFFECTS

Frequent (greater than 5%): Cayston: Cough, nasal congestion, wheezing, pharyngolaryngeal pain, pyrexia, chest discomfort, abdominal pain, vomiting. **Occasional (less than 3%):** Discomfort and swelling at IM injection site, nausea, vomiting, diarrhea, rash. **Rare (less than 1%):** Phlebitis or thrombophlebitis at IV injection site, abdominal cramps, headache, hypotension.

ADVERSE EFFECTS/TOXIC REACTIONS

Antibiotic-associated colitis, other superinfections may result from altered bacterial balance in GI tract. Severe hypersensitivity reactions, including anaphylaxis, occur rarely.

NURSING CONSIDERATIONS

BASELINE ASSESSMENT
Question for history of allergies, esp. to aztreonam, other antibiotics.

INTERVENTION/EVALUATION
Evaluate for phlebitis, pain at IM injection site. Assess for GI discomfort, nausea, vomiting. Monitor daily pattern of bowel activity, stool consistency. Assess skin for rash. Be alert for superinfection: fever, vomiting, diarrhea, anal/genital pruritus, oral mucosal changes (ulceration, pain, erythema). Monitor renal/hepatic function.

PATIENT/FAMILY TEACHING
• Report nausea, vomiting, diarrhea, rash.

B

baclofen

bak-loe-fen
(Apo-Baclofen ✢, Gablofen, Lioresal, Novo-Baclofen ✢)

■ **BLACK BOX ALERT** ■ Abrupt withdrawal of intrathecal form has resulted in severe hyperpyrexia, obtundation, rebound or exaggerated spasticity, muscle rigidity, leading to organ failure, death.
Do not confuse baclofen with Bactroban or Beclovent, or Lioresal with lisinopril or Lotensin.

◆CLASSIFICATION

PHARMACOTHERAPEUTIC: Skeletal muscle relaxant. **CLINICAL:** Antispastic, analgesic in trigeminal neuralgia.

USES

Oral: Management of reversible spasticity associated with multiple sclerosis, spinal cord lesions. **Intrathecal:** Management of severe spasticity of spinal cord or cerebral origin in pts 4 yrs of age and older. **OFF-LABEL:** Treatment of bladder spasms, cerebral palsy, intractable hiccups or pain, Huntington's chorea, trigeminal neuralgia.

PRECAUTIONS

Contraindications: Hypersensitivity to baclofen. **Intrathecal:** IV, IM, SQ, or epidural administration in addition to intrathecal use. **Cautions:** Renal impairment, seizure disorder, elderly, autonomic dysreflexia, reduced GI motility, GI or urinary obstruction; respiratory, pulmonary, peptic ulcer disease.

ACTION

Inhibits transmission of reflexes at spinal cord level. **Therapeutic Effect:** Relieves muscle spasticity.

PHARMACOKINETICS

Well absorbed from GI tract. Protein binding: 30%. Partially metabolized in liver. Primarily excreted in urine. **Half-life:** 2.5–4 hrs.

⧗ LIFESPAN CONSIDERATIONS

Pregnancy/Lactation: Unknown if crosses placenta or distributed in breast milk. **Children:** Safety and efficacy not established in pts younger than 12 yrs. Limited published data in children. **Elderly:** Increased risk of CNS toxicity (hallucinations, sedation, confusion, mental depression); age-related renal impairment may require decreased dosage.

INTERACTIONS

DRUG: CNS depressants (e.g., **alcohol, ALPRAZolam, LORazepam, morphine, oxyCODONE, traMADol**) may potentiate effect. **HERBAL: Gotu kola, kava kava, St. John's wort, valerian** may increase CNS sedation. **FOOD:** None known. **LAB VALUES:** May increase serum ALT, AST, alkaline phosphatase, glucose.

AVAILABILITY (Rx)

Intrathecal Injection Solution: 50 mcg/mL, 500 mcg/mL, 1,000 mcg/mL, 2,000 mcg/mL. **Tablets:** 10 mg, 20 mg.

ADMINISTRATION/HANDLING

PO
• Give with food or milk. • Tablets may be crushed.

Intrathecal
• For screening, a 50 mcg/mL concentration should be used for injection. • For maintenance therapy, solution should be diluted for pts who require concentrations other than 500 mcg/mL or 2,000 mcg/mL.

INDICATIONS/ROUTES/DOSAGE

◄ **ALERT** ► Avoid abrupt withdrawal.

Spasticity
PO: ADULTS, CHILDREN 12 YRS AND OLDER: Initially, 5 mg 3 times daily. May increase by 15 mg/day (5 mg/dose) at 3-day intervals until optimal response achieved. Range: 40–80 mg/day. **Maximum:** 80 mg/day. **ELDERLY:** Initially, 5 mg 2–3 times daily. May gradually increase dosage.

Intrathecal Dose

ADULTS, ELDERLY, CHILDREN 4 YRS AND OLDER: Initially, 50 mcg as screening dose (25 mcg in very small pediatric pts) for 1 dose; observe pt for 4–8 hrs for positive response (decrease in muscle tone and/or frequency and/or severity of spasm). If response is inadequate, give 75 mcg 24h after 1st dose. If response is still inadequate, give 100 mcg 24h after 2nd dose. Initial pump dose: give double screening dose (unless efficacy of bolus maintained greater than 8 hrs, then screening dose). After 24h, dose may be increased/decreased only once q24h until satisfactory response.

Dosage in Renal Impairment
Use caution.

Dosage in Hepatic Impairment
No dose adjustment.

SIDE EFFECTS

Frequent (greater than 10%): Transient drowsiness, asthenia, dizziness, nausea, vomiting. **Occasional (10%–2%):** Headache, paresthesia, constipation, anorexia, hypotension, confusion, nasal congestion. **Rare (less than 1%):** Paradoxical CNS excitement or restlessness, slurred speech, tremor, dry mouth, diarrhea, nocturia, impotence.

ADVERSE EFFECTS/TOXIC REACTIONS

Abrupt discontinuation may produce hallucinations, seizures. Overdose results in blurred vision, seizures, myosis, mydriasis, severe muscle weakness, strabismus, respiratory depression, vomiting.

NURSING CONSIDERATIONS

BASELINE ASSESSMENT
Record onset, type, location, duration of muscular spasm, pain. Check for immobility, stiffness, swelling.

INTERVENTION/EVALUATION
For pts on long-term therapy, BMP, LFT, CBC should be performed periodically. Assess for paradoxical reaction. Observe for drowsiness, dizziness, ataxia. Assist with ambulation at all times. Evaluate for therapeutic response: decreased intensity of skeletal muscle spasm, pain.

PATIENT/FAMILY TEACHING
• Drowsiness usually diminishes with continued therapy. • Avoid tasks that require alertness, motor skills until response to drug is established. • Do not abruptly withdraw medication after long-term therapy (may result in muscle rigidity, rebound spasticity, high fever, altered mental status). • Avoid alcohol, CNS depressants.

basiliximab

ba-si-**lik**-si-mab
(Simulect)

■ **BLACK BOX ALERT** ■ Must be prescribed by a physician experienced in immunosuppression therapy and organ transplant management.
Do not confuse basiliximab with daclizumab or brentuximab.

◆CLASSIFICATION

PHARMACOTHERAPEUTIC: Monoclonal antibody. **CLINICAL:** Immunosuppressive.

USES

Adjunct with cycloSPORINE, corticosteroids in prevention of acute organ rejection in pts receiving renal transplant. **OFF-LABEL:** Treatment of refractory graft-vs-host disease, prevention of liver or cardiac transplant rejection.

PRECAUTIONS

Contraindications: Hypersensitivity to basiliximab. **Cautions:** Re-exposure to subsequent courses of basiliximab.

ACTION

Binds to and blocks receptor of interleukin-2, a protein that stimulates proliferation of T-lymphocytes, which play a major role in organ transplant rejection. **Therapeutic Effect:** Impairs response of immune system to antigens, prevents acute renal transplant rejection.

PHARMACOKINETICS

Half-life: 4–10 days (adults); 5–17 days (children).

⧖ LIFESPAN CONSIDERATIONS

Pregnancy/Lactation: Unknown if crosses placenta or distributed in breast milk. Breastfeeding not recommended. **Children/Elderly:** No age-related precautions noted.

INTERACTIONS

DRUG: Tacrolimus (topical), **trastuzumab** may increase concentration. **HERBAL:** Echinacea may decrease therapeutic effect. **Bilberry, garlic, ginger, ginseng** may increase hypoglycemic effect. **FOOD:** None known. **LAB VALUES:** May alter serum calcium, glucose, potassium; Hgb, Hct. May increase serum cholesterol, BUN, creatinine, uric acid. May decrease serum magnesium, phosphate; platelet count.

AVAILABILITY (Rx)

Injection, Powder for Reconstitution: 10 mg, 20 mg.

ADMINISTRATION/HANDLING
🖫 IV

**Reconstitution • ** Reconstitute 10-mg vial with 2.5 mL or 20-mg vial with 5 mL Sterile Water for Injection. • Shake gently to dissolve. • May further dilute with 25–50 mL 0.9% NaCl or D₅W to a final concentration of 0.4 mg/mL. • Gently invert to avoid foaming. • Do not shake.
**Rate of Administration • ** Give as IV bolus over 10 min. or as IV infusion over 20–30 min.
**Storage • ** Refrigerate unused vials. • After reconstitution, use within 4 hrs (24 hrs if refrigerated). • Discard if precipitate forms.

⧉ IV INCOMPATIBILITIES

Specific information not available. Do not add other medications simultaneously through same IV line.

INDICATIONS/ROUTES/DOSAGE

Prophylaxis of Organ Rejection
IV: ADULTS, ELDERLY, CHILDREN WEIGHING 35 KG OR MORE: 20 mg within 2 hrs before transplant surgery and 20 mg 4 days after transplant. **CHILDREN WEIGHING LESS THAN 35 KG:** 10 mg within 2 hrs before transplant surgery and 10 mg 4 days after transplant.

Dosage in Renal/Hepatic Impairment
No dose adjustment.

SIDE EFFECTS

Frequent (greater than 10%): GI disturbances (constipation, diarrhea, dyspepsia), CNS effects (dizziness, headache, insomnia, tremor), respiratory tract infection, dysuria, acne, leg or back pain, peripheral edema, hypertension. **Occasional (10%–3%):** Angina, neuropathy, abdominal distention, tachycardia, rash, hypotension, urinary disturbances (urinary frequency, genital edema, hematuria), arthralgia, hirsutism, myalgia.

ADVERSE EFFECTS/TOXIC REACTIONS

Severe, acute hypersensitivity reactions including anaphylaxis characterized by bronchospasm, capillary leak syndrome, cytokine release syndrome, dyspnea, HF, hypotension, pulmonary edema, pruritus, respiratory failure, tachycardia, rash, urticaria, wheezing have been reported. May increase risk of cytomegalovirus infection.

NURSING CONSIDERATIONS

BASELINE ASSESSMENT

Obtain baseline CBC, BMP, serum ionized calcium, phosphate, uric acid; vital signs, particularly B/P, pulse rate. Question current breastfeeding status.

INTERVENTION/EVALUATION

Diligently monitor CBC, electrolytes, renal function. Assess B/P for hypertension/hypotension, pulse for evidence of tachycardia. Question for GI disturbances, CNS effects, urinary changes. Monitor for presence of wound infection, signs of infection (fever, sore throat, unusual bleeding/bruising), hypersensitivity reaction.

PATIENT/FAMILY TEACHING

• Report difficulty in breathing or swallowing, palpitations, bruising/bleeding, rash, itching, swelling of lower extremities, weakness. • Female pts should take measures to avoid pregnancy; avoid breastfeeding.

---

beclomethasone

be-kloe-**meth**-a-sone
(Apo-Beclomethasone ✤, Beconase AQ, QNASL, QVAR, Rivanase AQ ✤)
Do not confuse beclomethasone with betamethasone or dexamethasone, or Beconase with baclofen.

◆CLASSIFICATION

PHARMACOTHERAPEUTIC: Adrenocorticosteroid. **CLINICAL:** Anti-inflammatory, immunosuppressant.

USES

Inhalation: Maintenance and prophylactic treatment of asthma in pts 5 yrs and older. **Intranasal: Beconase AQ:** Relief of seasonal/perennial rhinitis; prevention of nasal polyp recurrence after surgical removal; treatment of nonallergic rhinitis. **QNASL:** Treatment of seasonal and perennial allergic rhinitis in pts 4 yrs and older. **OFF-LABEL:** Prevention of seasonal rhinitis (nasal form).

PRECAUTIONS

Contraindications: Hypersensitivity to beclomethasone. **Oral inhalation:** Acute exacerbation of asthma, status asthmaticus. **Cautions:** Cardiovascular disease, cataracts, diabetes, elderly, glaucoma, hepatic/renal impairment, myasthenia gravis, risk for osteoporosis, peptic ulcer disease, seizure disorder, thyroid disease, ulcerative colitis; following acute MI. Avoid use in pts with untreated viral, fungal, or bacterial systemic infections.

ACTION

Controls or prevents inflammation by altering rate of protein synthesis; depresses migration of polymorphonuclear leukocytes, fibroblasts; reverses capillary permeability. **Therapeutic Effect: Inhalation:** Inhibits bronchoconstriction, produces smooth muscle relaxation, decreases mucus secretion. **Intranasal:** Decreases response to seasonal, perennial rhinitis.

PHARMACOKINETICS

Rapidly absorbed from pulmonary, nasal, GI tissue. Metabolized in liver. Protein binding: 87%. Excreted in feces (60%), urine (12%). **Half-life:** 2–4.5 hrs.

⧗ LIFESPAN CONSIDERATIONS

Pregnancy/Lactation: Unknown if crosses placenta or distributed in breast milk. **Children:** Prolonged treatment/high dosages may decrease short-term growth rate, cortisol secretion. **Elderly:** No age-related precautions noted.

INTERACTIONS

DRUG: None significant. **HERBAL:** Echinacea may decrease effects. **FOOD:** None known. **LAB VALUES:** None significant.

AVAILABILITY (Rx)

Inhalation, Oral (Qvar): 40 mcg/inhalation, 80 mcg/inhalation. **Nasal Inhalation (Beconase AQ):** 42 mcg/inhalation. **QNASL:** 40 mcg/actuation, 80 mcg/actuation.

ADMINISTRATION/HANDLING

Inhalation

• Shake container well. • Instruct pt to exhale completely, place mouthpiece between lips, inhale, hold breath as long as possible before exhaling. • Allow at least 1 min between inhalations. • Rinse mouth after each use (decreases dry mouth, hoarseness, thrush).

Intranasal

• Instruct pt to clear nasal passages as much as possible before use. • Tilt pt's head slightly forward. • Insert spray tip into nostril, pointing toward nasal passages, away from nasal septum. • Spray into one nostril while pt holds the other nostril closed, concurrently inhaling through nose to permit medication as high into nasal passages as possible.

INDICATIONS/ROUTES/DOSAGE

Asthma

Oral Inhalation *(QVAR)*: **ADULTS, EL-DERLY, CHILDREN 12 YRS AND OLDER:** 40–160 mcg twice daily. **Maximum:** 320 mcg twice daily. **CHILDREN 5–11 YRS:** 40 mcg twice daily. **Maximum:** 80 mcg twice daily.

Rhinitis, Prevention of Recurrence of Nasal Polyps

Nasal Inhalation *(Beconase AQ)*: **ADULTS, ELDERLY, CHILDREN 12 YRS AND OLDER:** 1–2 sprays in each nostril twice daily. **CHILDREN 6–11 YRS:** 1 spray each nostril twice daily. May increase to 2 sprays 2 times/day. Once adequate control achieved, decrease to 1 spray in each nostril twice daily.

Allergic Rhinitis

Nasal Inhalation *(QNASL)*: **ADULTS, ELDERLY, CHILDREN 12 YRS AND OLDER:** 80 mcg/spray: 2 sprays in each nostril daily. **Maximum:** 320 mcg (4 sprays/day). **CHILDREN, 4–11 YRS OF AGE:** 40 mcg/spray: 1 spray each nostril once daily. **Maximum:** 80 mcg/day.

Dosage in Renal/Hepatic Impairment

No dose adjustment.

SIDE EFFECTS

Frequent: Inhalation (14%–4%): Throat irritation, dry mouth, hoarseness, cough. **Intranasal:** Nasal burning, mucosal dryness. **Occasional: Inhalation (3%–2%):** Localized fungal infection (thrush). **Intranasal:** Nasal-crusting epistaxis, sore throat, ulceration of nasal mucosa. **Rare: Inhalation:** Transient bronchospasm, esophageal candidiasis. **Intranasal:** Nasal and pharyngeal candidiasis, eye pain.

ADVERSE EFFECTS/TOXIC REACTIONS

Acute hypersensitivity reaction (urticaria, angioedema, severe bronchospasm) occurs rarely. Change from systemic to local steroid therapy may unmask previously suppressed bronchial asthma condition.

NURSING CONSIDERATIONS

BASELINE ASSESSMENT

Establish baseline history for asthma, rhinitis. Question for hypersensitivity to corticosteroids.

INTERVENTION/EVALUATION

Monitor respiratory status. Auscultate lung sounds. Observe for signs of oral candidiasis. In pts receiving bronchodilators by inhalation concomitantly with inhaled steroid therapy, advise use of bronchodilator several minutes before corticosteroid aerosol (enhances penetration of steroid into bronchial tree).

PATIENT/FAMILY TEACHING

• Do not change dose schedule or stop taking drug; must taper off gradually under medical supervision. • **Inhalation:** Maintain diligent oral hygiene. • Rinse mouth with water immediately after inhalation (prevents mouth/throat dryness, fungal infection of mouth). • Report sore throat or mouth. • **Intranasal:** Report symptoms that do not improve; or if sneezing, nasal irritation occurs. • Clear nasal passages prior to use. • Improvement may take days to several weeks.

belatacept

bel-**at**-a-sept
(Nulojix)

■ **BLACK BOX ALERT** ■ Must be administered by personnel trained in administration/handling of immunosuppression therapy. Increased risk of malignancies, infection. Increased risk of post-transplant lymphoproliferative disorder (PTLD), mainly in central nervous system. Not recommended for hepatic transplants due to increased risk of graft loss, death.

◆CLASSIFICATION

PHARMACOTHERAPEUTIC: Selective T-cell costimulation blocker. **CLINICAL:** Immunosuppressive agent.

USES

Prevention of acute organ rejection in pts receiving kidney transplants (in combination with basiliximab induction, mycophenolate mofetil, corticosteroids). For use in Epstein-Barr virus (EBV) seropositive kidney transplant recipients.

PRECAUTIONS

Contraindications: Hypersensitivity to belatacept. Transplant pts who are Epstein-Barr virus (EBV) seronegative or unknown sero-status. **Cautions:** History of opportunistic infections: bacterial, mycobacterial, invasive fungal, viral, protozoal (e.g., histoplasmosis, aspergillosis, candidiasis, coccidioidomycosis, listeriosis, HIV, tuberculosis, pneumocystosis). Recent open wounds, ulcerations. Not recommended in liver transplants. Avoid use of live vaccines.

ACTION

Inhibits T-lymphocyte proliferation and production of a critical pathway in cellular immune response involved in allograft rejection. **Therapeutic Effect:** Prevents renal transplant rejection.

PHARMACOKINETICS

Half-life: 8–10 days.

⌛ LIFESPAN CONSIDERATIONS

Pregnancy/Lactation: Unknown if crosses placenta or distributed in breast milk. Must either discontinue breastfeeding or discontinue drug. **Children:** Safety and efficacy not established. **Elderly:** No age-related precautions noted.

INTERACTIONS

DRUG: May increase concentration/effects of **belimumab, mycophenolate. Pimecrolimus, tacrolimus (topical)** may increase concentration/effect. **Live vaccines** not recommended. **HERBAL:** **Echinacea, cat's claw** may reduce effect. **FOOD:** None known. **LAB VALUES:** May increase serum potassium, cholesterol, uric acid, glucose; urine protein. May decrease serum calcium, magnesium, phosphate, potassium; Hgb, Hct, WBC.

AVAILABILITY (Rx)

Lyophilized Powder for Injection: 250 mg per vial.

ADMINISTRATION/HANDLING

◄**ALERT**► Use only silicone-free disposable syringe provided. Using different syringe may produce translucent particles. Administer via dedicated line only.

📁 **IV**

Reconstitution • Reconstitute vial with 10.5 mL of suitable diluent (0.9% NaCl, D₅W, or Sterile Water for Injection) using provided syringe, 18- to 20-gauge needle. • Direct stream to glass wall (avoids foaming). • Swirl gently (do not shake). • Discard if opaque particles, discoloration, or foreign particles are present. • Infusion bag must match diluent (0.9% NaCl with 0.9% NaCl, D_5W with D_5W; may use Sterile Water for Injection with NaCl or D_5W). • To mix infusion bag, withdraw and discard volume equal to the volume of reconstituted solution. • Using same silicone-free disposable syringe, gently inject reconstituted solution into 100- to 250-mL bag (based on concentration). • Final concentration of infusion bag should range from 2 mg/mL to 10 mg/mL. • IV infusion stable for 24 hrs at room temperature.

Rate of Administration • Infuse over 30 min using infusion set with a 0.2- to 1.2-micron low-protein-binding filter.

Storage • Refrigerate vials. • Solution should be clear to slightly opalescent and colorless to slightly yellow. • May refrigerate solution up to 24 hrs. • Discard if reconstituted solution remains at room temperature longer than 24 hrs.

INDICATIONS/ROUTES/DOSAGE

Note: Dosage based on actual body weight at time of transplantation. Do not modify dose unless a change in body weight is greater than 10%.

Prophylaxis of Acute Kidney Transplant Rejection (in Combination with an Immunosuppressant)
IV: ADULTS, ELDERLY: Initial phase: 10 mg/kg on day 1 (day of transplantation, prior to implantation), day 5, end of wk 2, 4, 8, and 12 after transplantation. **Maintenance:** 5 mg/kg end of wk 16, then q4wks thereafter (plus or minus 3 days).

Dosage Modification
Infusion is based on actual body weight at the time of transplantation; modify dose for weight changes greater than 10% during treatment. Prescribed dose must be evenly divisible by 12.5 to match closest increment (0, 12.5, 25, 37.5, 50, 62.5, 75, 87.5, 100) in mg. For example, the actual dose for a

64-kg pt is 637.5 mg or 650 mg, not 640 mg.

Dosage in Renal/Hepatic Impairment
No dose adjustment.

SIDE EFFECTS

Frequent (45%–20%): Anemia, diarrhea, UTI, peripheral edema, constipation, hypertension, pyrexia, nausea, cough, vomiting, headache. **Occasional (19%–5%):** Abdominal pain, hypotension, arthralgia, hematuria, upper respiratory infection, insomnia, nasopharyngitis, back pain, dyspnea, influenza, dysuria, bronchitis, stomatitis, anxiety, dizziness, abdominal pain, muscle tremor, acne, alopecia, hyperhidrosis.

ADVERSE EFFECTS/TOXIC REACTIONS

Serious conditions, including malignancies (esp. skin cancer), progressive multifocal leukoencephalopathy (caused by JC virus), cytomegalovirus, polyoma virus nephropathy, viral reactivation (herpes zoster, hepatitis), may occur. Other opportunistic infections (bacterial, fungal, viral, protozoal) may cause tuberculosis, cryptococcal meningitis, Chagas' disease, West Nile encephalitis, Guillain-Barré syndrome, cerebral aspergillosis. Additional complications, including chronic allograft nephropathy, renal tubular necrosis, renal artery necrosis, atrial fibrillation, hematoma at incision site, wound dehiscence, lymphocele, arteriovenous fistula thrombosis, hydronephrosis, urinary incontinence, anti-belatacept antibody formation, were reported.

NURSING CONSIDERATIONS

BASELINE ASSESSMENT
Obtain baseline CBC, serum chemistries, renal function, glomerular filtration rate (GFR), serum magnesium, ionized calcium, phosphate, lipid panel, urinalysis. Evaluate pt for active tuberculosis or latent infection prior to initiating treatment

and periodically during therapy. Induration of 5 mm or greater with tuberculin skin test should be considered a positive result when assessing whether treatment for latent tuberculosis is necessary. Assess baseline mental status to compare any worsening cognitive symptoms. Obtain Epstein-Barr virus (EBV) serology prior to treatment (contraindicated in pts who are EBV seronegative). Note any skin discoloration, ulcers, excoriation, lesions. Question history of hypertension/hypotension, arrhythmia, diabetes, HIV. Receive full medication history. Question possibility of pregnancy.

INTERVENTION/EVALUATION

Monitor B/P, vital signs, I&O, weight. Diligently monitor CBC, renal function, serum electrolytes (hypokalemia may result in changes in muscle strength, muscle cramps, altered mental status, cardiac arrhythmias). Routinely monitor serum glucose levels for new-onset diabetes after transplantation, corticosteroid use. Monitor for fever, tenderness over transplantation site, skin lesions, changing characteristics of moles, neurologic deterioration related to PTLD or PML.

PATIENT/FAMILY TEACHING

• Therapy may increase risk of malignancies and life-threatening infections. • Treatment is given with immunosuppressive therapy with basiliximab induction, corticosteroids. • Report history of HIV, opportunistic infections, hepatitis, coughing of blood, or close relatives with active tuberculosis. • Avoid sunlight, sunlamps. • Seek immediate attention if toxic reactions occur. • Do not receive live vaccines. • Report pregnancy or plans of becoming pregnant. • Adhere to strict dosing schedule. • Report chest pain, palpitations, edema, fever, night sweats, weight loss, swollen glands, flu-like symptoms, stomach pain, vomiting, diarrhea, weakness, or urinary changes (color, frequency, odor, concentration, burning, blood).

belimumab

be-**lim**-oo-mab
(Benlysta)
Do not confuse belimumab with bevacizumab.

◆CLASSIFICATION

PHARMACOTHERAPEUTIC: Monoclonal antibody. **CLINICAL:** Immunosuppressant, anti-lupus agent.

USES

Treatment for active, autoantibody-positive, systemic lupus erythematosus, in addition to standard therapy.

PRECAUTIONS

Contraindications: Hypersensitivity (anaphylaxis) to belimumab. **Cautions:** Severe, active, chronic infections; depression, pts at risk for suicide, other mood changes. Avoid live vaccines within 30 days before or concurrently with belimumab.

ACTION

Blocks binding of human B-lymphocyte stimulator protein to receptors on B-lymphocyte. **Therapeutic Effect:** Reduces activity of B-cell–mediated immunity and autoimmune response.

PHARMACOKINETICS

Half-life: 19 days.

☒ LIFESPAN CONSIDERATIONS

Pregnancy/Lactation: Unknown if crosses placenta or distributed in breast milk. Contraception recommended during therapy and for at least 4 wks after discontinuation. **Children:** Safety and efficacy not established. **Elderly:** No age-related precautions noted.

INTERACTIONS

DRUG: Abatacept, belatacept, etanercept, pimecrolimus, tacrolimus (topical) may increase concentration/effect. **Cyclophosphamide** not recommended

---

✤ Canadian trade name   🐢 Non-Crushable Drug   🔲 High Alert drug

concomitantly. **HERBAL: Echinacea** may decrease effect. **FOOD:** None known. **LAB VALUES:** May decrease WBC.

AVAILABILITY (Rx)

Lyophilized Powder for Injection: 120 mg, 400 mg. **Single-Dose Prefilled Syringe:** 200 mg/mL.

ADMINISTRATION/HANDLING

Reconstitution • Allow vial to warm to room temperature (10–15 min). • Reconstitute 120-mg vial with 1.5 mL Sterile Water for Injection or 400-mg vial with 4.8 mL Sterile Water for Injection (both vials will equal final concentration of 80 mg/mL). • Direct stream toward glass wall to avoid foaming. • Gently swirl for 60 sec every 5 min until fully dissolved (usually 10–30 min). • If mechanical reconstitution device is used, do not swirl greater than 30 min or exceed 500 rpm. • Small air bubbles expected, acceptable. • Dilute in 250 mL 0.9% NaCl only. • From infusion bag, withdraw and discard volume equal to the volume of reconstituted solution. • Invert bag and gently inject solution to mix. • Infuse within 8 hrs of reconstitution.
Rate of Administration • Infuse over 1 hr.
Storage • Refrigerate vials/infusion bag until time of use. • Solution should be opalescent and colorless to pale yellow with no particles present. • Discard solution if particulate matter or discoloration observed. • Protect from sunlight.

▨ IV INCOMPATIBILITIES

Do not infuse with dextrose-based solution. Use dedicated line only.

INDICATIONS/ROUTES/DOSAGE

Active Systemic Lupus Erythematosus
IV: ADULTS, ELDERLY: Initially, 10 mg/kg q2 wks for 3 doses, then q4 wks thereafter.
SUBCUTANEOUS: ADULTS, ELDERLY: 200 mg once weekly.

Dosage in Renal/Hepatic Impairment
No dose adjustment.

SIDE EFFECTS

Frequent (15%–12%): Nausea, diarrhea. **Occasional (10%–5%):** Pyrexia, nasopharyngitis, bronchitis, insomnia, extremity pain, depression, migraine, pharyngitis. **Rare (less than 4%):** Cystitis, viral gastroenteritis.

ADVERSE EFFECTS/TOXIC REACTIONS

May increase risk of mortality. Antibelimumab antibody formation reported in less than 1%. Hypersensitivity reaction, including anaphylactic reaction, may include urticaria, pruritus, erythema, dyspnea, angioedema, hypotension (13% of pts). Infusion reactions such as nausea, headaches, flushing occur more frequently. Serious infections related to immunosuppression, including respiratory tract infection, pneumonia, nasopharyngitis, sinusitis, influenza, UTI, cellulitis, bronchitis, viral reactivation, may occur. Mental health issues, including psychiatric events (16%) and depression (6%), have been noted. Life-threatening psychiatric events and depression (including suicide) reported in less than 1%. Pts who experienced life-threatening episodes had prior psychiatric history.

NURSING CONSIDERATIONS

BASELINE ASSESSMENT

Obtain baseline CBC with differential, BMP, IgG level, vital signs. Assess history of recent immunizations, malignancies, open sores, ulcerations, weight loss, HIV infection, chronic infection. Assess psychiatric history, including insomnia, anxiety, depression, impulsiveness, suicidal ideations, mood changes. Question possibility of pregnancy, current breastfeeding.

INTERVENTION/EVALUATION

Monitor vital signs, CBC. If hypersensitivity reaction occurs, immediately notify physician. Premedication with antihistamines, antipyretics, and/or corticosteroids may prevent subsequent reactions. Discontinue treatment if anaphylactic reaction occurs; initiate appropriate medical treatment. Routinely inspect skin, paying close attention to areas that are discolored, irregular, or have ill-defined borders (may indicate malignancies). Obtain anti-belimumab antibody titer if immunogenicity suspected. Consider interrupting therapy if acute infection occurs.

PATIENT/FAMILY TEACHING

• Report any signs of allergic reaction (see Adverse Effects/Toxic Reactions). • If anaphylactic reaction occurs, pt may require rapid-sequence intubation. • Allergic reactions include itching, hives, dizziness, or difficulty breathing. • Notify physician if pregnant or plan on becoming pregnant. • Contraception recommended during treatment and at least 4 mos after discontinuation. • Report suicidal ideation, mood changes, or worsening depression. • Do not receive live vaccines 30 days before or during treatment. • Report any fever, cough, night sweats, flu-like symptoms, skin changes, or painful/burning urination.

belinostat

beh-lih-noh-stat
(Beleodaq)

◆CLASSIFICATION

PHARMACOTHERAPEUTIC: Histone deacetylase inhibitor. **CLINICAL:** Antineoplastic.

USES

Treatment of relapsed or refractory peripheral T-cell lymphoma (PTCL).

PRECAUTIONS

Contraindications: Hypersensitivity to belinostat. **Cautions:** Pts with high tumor burden, hx of hepatic impairment, thrombocytopenia. Avoid use in pts with active infection.

ACTION

Inhibits enzymatic activity of histone deacetylases by catalyzing removal of acetyl groups from lysine residues of histones and nonhistone proteins. **Therapeutic Effect:** Inhibits tumor cell growth and metastasis; causes tumor cellular death (apoptosis).

PHARMACOKINETICS

Limited tissue distribution. Metabolized in liver. Protein binding: 93%–95%. Excreted primarily in urine. **Half-life:** 1.1 hrs.

⧗ LIFESPAN CONSIDERATIONS

Pregnancy/Lactation: Has teratogenic effects; may cause fetal harm/demise. Not recommended in nursing mothers. Unknown if distributed in breast milk. Must either discontinue drug or discontinue breastfeeding. **Children:** Safety and efficacy not established. **Elderly:** No age-related precautions noted.

INTERACTIONS

DRUG: Strong UGT1A1 inhibitors (e.g., atazanavir, lopinavir, ritonavir) may increase concentration/effect. **HERBAL:** None known. **FOOD:** None significant. **LAB VALUES:** May decrease ANC, Hgb/Hct, lymphocytes, platelets, WBC; serum potassium. May increase blood lactic dehydrogenase, serum creatinine.

AVAILABILITY (Rx)

Lyophilized Powder for Injection: 500 mg vial.

ADMINISTRATION/HANDLING
 IV

Reconstitution • Maintain standard chemotherapy preparation and handling precautions. • Reconstitute each vial with 9 mL of Sterile Water for Injection, using suitable syringe for final concentration of 50 mg/mL. • Gently swirl contents until completely dissolved.

• Visually inspect for particulate matter. • Do not use if cloudiness or particulate matter observed. • Withdraw required dosage and mix into infusion bag containing 250 mL of 0.9% NaCl.
Rate of Administration • Infuse over 30 min using 0.22-micron in-line filter. • May extend infusion time to 45 min if infusion site pain or other infusion-related symptoms occur.
Storage • Reconstituted vial may be stored at room temperature (max 77°F/25°C) for up to 12 hrs. • Infusion bag may be stored at room temperature (max 77°F/25°C) for up to 36 hrs.

INDICATIONS/ROUTES/DOSAGE

Peripheral T-Cell Lymphoma
IV Infusion: ADULTS/ELDERLY: 1,000 mg/m² once daily on days 1–5 of a 21-day cycle. Cycles may be repeated every 21 days until disease progression or unacceptable toxicity.

Dose Modification
ANC should be greater than or equal to 1,000/mm³ and platelet count greater than or equal to 50,000/mm³ prior to start of each cycle or prior to resuming treatment following toxicity. Discontinue treatment if ANC nadir less than 500/mm³ or recurrent platelet count nadir less than 25,000/mm³ after two dose reductions. Other toxicities must be Grade 2 or less prior to resuming treatment.

Hematologic Toxicities
Platelet count greater than 25,000/mm³ or ANC greater than 500 cells/mm³: No change. **Platelet count less than 25,000/mm³ or ANC less than 500 cells/mm³:** Decrease dose by 25% (750 mg/m²).

Nonhematologic Toxicities
Any Grade 3 or 4: Decrease dose by 25% (750 mg/m²). **Recurrence of Grade 3 or 4 Adverse Reaction After**

Two Dosage Reductions: Discontinue treatment. **Nausea, Vomiting, Diarrhea:** Only modify dose if duration is greater than 7 days with supportive management. **Pts with Reduced UGT1A1 Activity:** Reduce starting dose to 750 mg/m² in pts known to be homozygous for UGT1A1*28 allele.

Dosage in Renal/Hepatic Impairment
No dose adjustment.

SIDE EFFECTS

Frequent (47%–29%): Nausea, fatigue, pyrexia, vomiting, anemia. **Occasional (23%–10%):** Constipation, diarrhea, dyspepsia, rash, peripheral edema, cough, pruritus, chills, decreased appetite, headache, infusion site pain, abdominal pain, hypotension, phlebitis, dizziness.

ADVERSE EFFECTS/TOXIC REACTIONS

Anemia, lymphopenia, neutropenia, thrombocytopenia are expected responses to therapy. Serious and sometimes fatal infections including pneumonia, sepsis have occurred. May cause hepatotoxicity, LFT abnormalities, tumor lysis syndrome. GI toxicities including severe diarrhea, nausea, vomiting may require use of antiemetic and antidiarrheal medication or result in dosage reduction. Nineteen percent of pts required treatment discontinuation related to toxic anemia, febrile neutropenia, multiorgan failure, ventricular fibrillation (rare).

NURSING CONSIDERATIONS

BASELINE ASSESSMENT
Obtain baseline ANC, CBC, BMP, LFT, vital signs; urine pregnancy in women of reproductive potential. Question history of anemia, arrhythmias, hepatic impairment, peripheral edema, or if pt homozygous for UGT1A1 allele (may require reduced starting dose). Question possibility of pregnancy, current breastfeeding

status. Receive full medication history including herbal products.

INTERVENTION/EVALUATION

Diligently monitor blood counts (esp. ANC, Hgb/Hct, WBC, platelet count) weekly; hepatic/renal function prior to start of first dose of each cycle, vital signs. Monitor for symptoms of hypokalemia. Screen for tumor lysis syndrome (electrolyte imbalance, uric acid nephropathy, acute renal failure). Obtain EKG if arrhythmia, palpitations occur. Notify physician if any CTCAE toxicities occur (see Appendix M). Offer antiemetics if nausea, vomiting occurs.

PATIENT/FAMILY TEACHING

• Blood levels will be routinely monitored. • Avoid pregnancy; treatment may cause birth defects or miscarriage. Do not breastfeed. • Report any abdominal pain, black/tarry stools, bruising, yellowing of skin or eyes, dark urine, decreased urine output. • Severe diarrhea may lead to dehydration. • Body aches, burning with urination, chills, cough, difficulty breathing, fever may indicate an acute infection.

---

benazepril

ben-**ay**-ze-pril
(Lotensin)
■ **BLACK BOX ALERT** ■ May cause fetal injury, mortality. Discontinue as soon as possible once pregnancy is detected.
Do not confuse benazepril with enalapril, lisinopril, or Benadryl, or Lotensin with Lioresal.

FIXED-COMBINATION(S)

Lotensin HCT: benazepril/hydrochlorothiazide (a diuretic): 5 mg/6.25 mg, 10 mg/12.5 mg, 20 mg/12.5 mg, 20 mg/25 mg. **Lotrel:** benazepril/amLODIPine (a calcium blocker): 2.5 mg/10 mg, 5 mg/10 mg, 5 mg/20 mg, 5 mg/40 mg, 10 mg/20 mg, 10 mg/40 mg.

◆CLASSIFICATION

PHARMACOTHERAPEUTIC: Angiotensin-converting enzyme (ACE) inhibitor. **CLINICAL:** Antihypertensive.

USES

Treatment of hypertension. Used alone or in combination with other antihypertensives.

PRECAUTIONS

Contraindications: Hypersensitivity to benazepril. History of angioedema with or without previous treatment with ACE inhibitors. Use with aliskiren in pts with diabetes. **Cautions:** Renal impairment; hypertrophic cardiomyopathy without flow tract obstruction; severe aortic stenosis; before, during, or immediately following major surgery; unstented renal artery stenosis; diabetes mellitus, pregnancy, breastfeeding. Concomitant use of potassium-sparing diuretics, potassium supplements.

ACTION

Decreases rate of conversion of angiotensin I to angiotensin II, a potent vasoconstrictor. Reduces peripheral arterial resistance. **Therapeutic Effect:** Lowers B/P.

PHARMACOKINETICS

Route	Onset	Peak	Duration
PO	1 hr	2–4 hrs	24 hrs

Partially absorbed from GI tract. Protein binding: 97%. Metabolized in liver. Primarily excreted in urine. Minimal removal by hemodialysis. **Half-life:** 35 min; metabolite, 10–11 hrs.

⌛ LIFESPAN CONSIDERATIONS

Pregnancy/Lactation: Crosses placenta. Unknown if distributed in breast milk. May cause fetal, neonatal mortality or morbidity. **Children:** Safety and efficacy not established. **Elderly:** May be more sensitive to hypotensive effects.

INTERACTIONS

DRUG: Diuretics (e.g., furosemide, HCTZ), antihypertensives (e.g., amlodipine, atenolol, valsartan) may increase effect. **NSAIDs** (e.g., ibuprofen, naproxen), **sympathomimetics** may decrease effect. **Potassium-sparing diuretics** (e.g., spironolactone), **potassium supplements** may cause hyperkalemia. May increase **cycloSPORINE, lithium** concentration/effect. **HERBAL:** Ephedra, ginseng, licorice may worsen hypertension. **Black cohosh, periwinkle** may have increased antihypertensive effect. **FOOD:** None known. **LAB VALUES:** May increase serum potassium, ALT, AST, alkaline phosphatase, bilirubin, BUN, creatinine, glucose. May decrease serum sodium; Hgb, Hct. May cause positive ANA titer.

AVAILABILITY (Rx)

Tablets: 5 mg, 10 mg, 20 mg, 40 mg.

ADMINISTRATION/HANDLING

• Give without regard to food.

INDICATIONS/ROUTES/DOSAGE

Hypertension (Monotherapy)
PO: ADULTS: Initially, 10 mg/day. **Maintenance:** 10–40 mg/day as single dose or in 2 divided doses. **Maximum:** 80 mg/day. **ELDERLY:** Initially, 5–10 mg/day. Range: 10–40 mg/day. **CHILDREN 6 YRS AND OLDER:** Initially, 0.2 mg/kg/day (up to 10 mg/day). Range: 0.1–0.6 mg/kg/day. **Maximum:** 40 mg/day.

Hypertension (Combination Therapy)
PO: ADULTS: Discontinue diuretic 2–3 days prior to initiating benazepril, then dose as noted above. If unable to discontinue diuretic, begin benazepril at 5 mg/day.

Dosage in Renal Impairment
CrCl less than 30 mL/min: ADULTS: Initially, 5 mg/day titrated up to maximum of 40 mg/day. **CHILDREN:** Not recommended. **HD, PD:** 25%–50% of usual dose; supplement dose not necessary.

Dosage in Hepatic Impairment
Use caution.

SIDE EFFECTS

Frequent (6%–3%): Cough, headache, dizziness. **Occasional (2%):** Fatigue, drowsiness, nausea. **Rare (less than 1%):** Rash, fever, myalgia, diarrhea, loss of taste.

ADVERSE EFFECTS/TOXIC REACTIONS

Excessive hypotension ("first-dose syncope") may occur in pts with HF, severe salt or volume depletion. Angioedema, hyperkalemia occur rarely. Agranulocytosis, neutropenia may be noted in pts with renal impairment, collagen vascular disease (scleroderma, systemic lupus erythematosus). Nephrotic syndrome may occur in pts with history of renal disease.

NURSING CONSIDERATIONS

BASELINE ASSESSMENT

Obtain CBC before therapy begins and q2wks for 3 mos, then periodically thereafter. Obtain B/P immediately before each dose, in addition to regular monitoring (be alert to fluctuations).

INTERVENTION/EVALUATION

Assist with ambulation if dizziness occurs. Monitor B/P, renal function, urinary protein, serum potassium. Monitor CBC with differential if pt has collagen vascular disease or renal impairment. If excessive reduction in B/P occurs, place pt in supine position with legs elevated. Monitor pt with renal impairment, autoimmune disease, or taking drugs that affect leukocytes or immune response.

PATIENT/FAMILY TEACHING

• To reduce hypotensive effect, go from lying to standing slowly. • Full therapeutic effect may take 2–4 wks. • Skipping doses or noncompliance with drug therapy may produce severe rebound hypertension. • Report dizziness, persistent cough.

bendamustine

ben-da-**mus**-teen
(Bendeka, <u>Treanda</u>)
**Do not confuse bendamustine
with carmustine or lomustine.**

◆CLASSIFICATION

PHARMACOTHERAPEUTIC: Alkylating agent. **CLINICAL:** Antineoplastic.

USES

Treatment of chronic lymphocytic leukemia (CLL). Treatment of indolent B-cell non-Hodgkin's lymphoma (NHL) that has progressed during or within 6 mos of treatment with riTUXimab or a riTUXimab-containing regimen. **OFF-LABEL:** Treatment of mantle cell lymphoma, relapsed multiple myeloma. First-line treatment for follicular lymphoma. Treatment of Waldenström's macroglobulinemia.

PRECAUTIONS

Contraindications: Hypersensitivity to bendamustine. (Bendeka only): polyethylene glycol 400, or propylene glycol mono-thioglycerol. **Cautions:** Myelosuppression (may increase risk of infection), renal/hepatic impairment, dehydration, HF.

ACTION

Alkylates and cross-links macromolecules, resulting in DNA, RNA, and protein synthesis inhibition. **Therapeutic Effect:** Inhibits tumor cell growth, causes cell death.

PHARMACOKINETICS

Metabolized via hydrolysis to metabolites. Protein binding: 64%–95%. Excreted primarily in feces. **Half-life:** 40 min.

⏳ LIFESPAN CONSIDERATIONS

Pregnancy/Lactation: May cause fetal harm. Unknown if distributed in breast milk. Impaired spermatogenesis, azoospermia have been reported in male pts. **Children:** Safety and efficacy not established. **Elderly:** No age-related precautions noted.

INTERACTIONS

DRUG: Ciprofloxacin, fluvoxaMINE may increase concentration, decrease plasma concentrations of active metabolites. **CYP1A2 inducers (e.g., omeprazole), nicotine** may decrease concentration. **HERBAL:** None significant. **FOOD:** None known. **LAB VALUES:** May increase serum AST, bilirubin, creatinine, glucose, uric acid. May decrease WBCs, neutrophils, Hgb, platelets; serum potassium, sodium, calcium.

AVAILABILITY (Rx)

Injection, Powder for Reconstitution: *(Treanda)*: 25 mg, 100 mg. **Injection, *(Bendeka)*:** 100 mg/4 mL.

ADMINISTRATION/HANDLING
 **IV**

Reconstitution • Reconstitute each 100-mg vial with 20 mL Sterile Water for Injection (25-mg vial with 5 mL) for final concentration of 5 mg/mL. • Powder should completely dissolve in 5 min. • Discard if particulate matter is observed. • Withdraw volume needed for required dose (based on 5 mg/mL concentration) and immediately transfer to 500-mL infusion bag of 0.9% NaCl for final concentration of 0.2–0.6 mg/mL. • Reconstituted solution must be transferred to infusion bag within 30 min of reconstitution. • After transferring, thoroughly mix contents of infusion bag. **Rate of Administration •** Infuse over 30 min for CLL or 60 min for NHL. **Storage •** Reconstituted solution should appear clear and colorless to pale yellow. • Final solution is stable for 24 hrs if refrigerated or 3 hrs at room temperature. • Administration must be completed within these stability time frames.

INDICATIONS/ROUTES/DOSAGE

◄**ALERT**► Antiemetics are recommended to prevent nausea and vomiting.

Chronic Lymphocytic Leukemia
IV Infusion: ADULTS/ELDERLY: 100 mg/ m^2 given over 30 min daily on days 1 and 2 of a 28-day cycle, up to 6 cycles.

Non-Hodgkin's Lymphoma
IV Infusion: ADULTS/ELDERLY: 120 mg/ m^2 on days 1 and 2 of a 21-day cycle, up to 8 cycles.

Dose Modification
Hematologic Toxicity: Grade 4 or greater: Withhold until ANC 1,000/ mm^3 or greater, platelet 75,000/mm^3 or greater. **CLL: Toxicity Grade 3 or greater:** Reduce dose to 50 mg/m^2 on days 1 and 2 of each treatment cycle. **Recurrence:** Reduce dose to 25 mg/^{2} on days 1 and 2 of each cycle. **NHL: Hematologic toxicity Grade 4 or nonhematologic toxicity Grade 3 or greater:** Reduce dose to 90 mg/m^2 on days 1 and 2 of each cycle. **Recurrence:** Reduce dose to 60 mg/ m^2 on days 1 and 2 of each treatment cycle.

Dosage in Renal Impairment
Not recommended in pts with CrCl less than 40 mL/min.

Dosage in Hepatic Impairment
Mild: Use caution. **Moderate to Severe:** Not recommended.

SIDE EFFECTS

Frequent (24%–16%): Fever, nausea, vomiting. **Occasional (9%–8%):** Diarrhea, fatigue, asthenia (loss of strength, energy), rash, decreased weight, nasopharyngitis. **Rare (6%–3%):** Chills, pruritus, cough, herpes simplex infections.

ADVERSE EFFECTS/TOXIC REACTIONS

Myelosuppression characterized as neutropenia (75% of pts), thrombocytopenia (77% of pts), anemia (89% of pts), leukopenia (61% of pts) is an expected response to therapy. Infection, including pneumonia, sepsis may occur. Tumor lysis syndrome may lead to acute renal failure. Worsening of hypertension occurs rarely.

NURSING CONSIDERATIONS

BASELINE ASSESSMENT
Obtain baseline CBC, BMP, LFT before treatment begins and routinely thereafter. Question for possibility of pregnancy. Offer emotional support.

INTERVENTION/EVALUATION
Offer antiemetics to control nausea, vomiting. Monitor daily pattern of bowel activity, stool consistency. Assess skin for evidence of rash. Monitor for signs of infection (fever, chills, cough, flu-like symptoms). Monitor for hypertension. Hematologic nadirs occur in 3rd week of therapy and may require dose delays if recovery to recommended values has not occurred by day 28.

PATIENT/FAMILY TEACHING
• Avoid crowds, those with known infection. • Avoid contact with anyone who recently received live virus vaccine. • Do not have immunizations without physician's approval (drug lowers body resistance). • Promptly report fever, chills, flu-like symptoms, sore throat, unusual bruising/bleeding from any site. • Male pts should be warned of potential risk to their reproductive capacities.

benztropine

benz-**trow**-peen
(Cogentin)
Do not confuse benztropine with bromocriptine or benzonatate.

◆CLASSIFICATION

PHARMACOTHERAPEUTIC: Anticholinergic. **CLINICAL:** Antiparkinson agent.

USES

Adjunctive therapy for all forms of Parkinson's disease, control of extrapyramidal reactions (except tardive dyskinesia) due to neuroleptic medications.

PRECAUTIONS

Contraindications: Hypersensitivity to benztropine. Children younger than 3 yrs (due to atropine-like adverse effects). **Cautions:** Children 3 yrs and older. Glaucoma, heart disease, hypertension, hypotension; pts with tachycardia, arrhythmias, prostatic hypertrophy, hepatic/renal impairment, obstructive diseases of GI/GU tract, urinary retention, elderly, myasthenia gravis, use during hot weather or during exercise.

ACTION

Possesses anticholinergic effects. **Therapeutic Effect:** Reduces incidence/severity of akinesia, rigidity, tremor.

PHARMACOKINETICS

Well absorbed following PO and IM administration. Metabolized in liver. PO onset of action: 1–2 hrs; IM onset of action: minutes. Pharmacologic effects may not be apparent until 2–3 days after initiation of therapy and may persist for up to 24 hrs after discontinuation of drug. **Half-life:** Extended (no specific determination).

⌛ LIFESPAN CONSIDERATIONS

Pregnancy/Lactation: Unknown if drug crosses placenta or is distributed in breast milk. **Children:** Safety and efficacy not established in pts younger than 3 yrs. **Elderly:** Increased risk for adverse reactions.

INTERACTIONS

DRUG: CNS depressants (e.g., alcohol, ALPRAZolam, LORazepam, morphine, oxyCODONE, traMADol) may increase sedative effects. May increase effects of **anticholinergics**. **HERBAL:** None significant. **FOOD:** None known. **LAB VALUES:** None significant.

AVAILABILITY (Rx)

Injection, Solution: 1 mg/mL. **Tablets:** 0.5 mg, 1 mg, 2 mg.

ADMINISTRATION/HANDLING

IM
• Inject slow, deep IM.

PO
• Give without regard to food. • Give with food if GI upset occurs.

INDICATIONS/ROUTES/DOSAGE

Parkinsonism
PO: ADULTS, ELDERLY: Initially, 0.5–1 mg at bedtime or in 2–4 divided doses. Titrate by 0.5 mg at 5- to 6-day intervals. Usual dose: 1–2 mg daily. Range: 0.5–6 mg daily. **Maximum:** 6 mg/day.

Drug-Induced Extrapyramidal Symptoms
PO, IM, IV: ADULTS, ELDERLY: Initially, 1–2 mg 2–3 times/day. Titrate at 0.5 mg q5–6days. **Usual dose:** 1–4 mg once or twice daily. **Maximum:** 6 mg/day. **CHILDREN OLDER THAN 3 YRS:** 0.02–0.05 mg/kg/dose once or twice daily.

Acute Dystonic Reactions
IV, IM: ADULTS: Initially, 1–2 mg as a single dose followed by 1–2 mg orally 1–2 times/day for up to 7–28 days to prevent recurrence.

Dosage in Renal/Hepatic Impairment
No dose adjustment.

SIDE EFFECTS

Frequent: Drowsiness, dry mouth, blurred vision, constipation, urinary retention, GI upset, photosensitivity. **Occasional:** Headache, memory loss, muscle cramps, anxiety, peripheral paresthesia, orthostatic hypotension, abdominal cramps. **Rare:** Rash, confusion, eye pain.

ADVERSE EFFECTS/TOXIC REACTIONS

Overdose may produce severe anticholinergic effects (drowsiness, tachycardia, paralytic ileus, malignant hyperthermia,

B

urinary retention, dyspnea, skin flushing, dryness of mouth/nose/throat. Severe paradoxical reactions (hallucinations, tremor, seizures, toxic psychosis) may occur.

NURSING CONSIDERATIONS

BASELINE ASSESSMENT

Assess mental status for confusion, disorientation, agitation, psychotic-like symptoms (medication frequently produces such side effects in pts older than 60 yrs). Note severity of baseline rigidity, tremors.

INTERVENTION/EVALUATION

Be alert to neurologic effects: headache, drowsiness, mental confusion, agitation. Assess for clinical reversal of symptoms (improvement of tremor of head and hands at rest, mask-like facial expression, shuffling gait, muscular rigidity). Monitor daily pattern of bowel activity, stool consistency, esp. constipation. Monitor I/O. Assess for urinary retention.

PATIENT/FAMILY TEACHING

• Avoid tasks that require alertness, motor skills until response to drug is established. • Dry mouth, drowsiness, dizziness may be an expected side effect. • Drowsiness tends to diminish or disappear with continued therapy. • Avoid alcohol. • Report sudden muscle weakness or stiffness. • Report trouble urinating, bladder pain, or distention.

---

betamethasone

bay-ta-**meth**-a-sone
(Betaderm ✦, Betaject ✦, Betnesol ✦, Celestone Soluspan, Diprolene, Luxiq, Sernivo)
Do not confuse betamethasone with dexamethasone or Luxiq with Lasix.

FIXED-COMBINATION(S)

Lotrisone: betamethasone/clotrimazole (an antifungal): 0.05%/1%.
Taclonex: betamethasone/calcipotriene (an antipsoriatic): 0.064%/0.005%.

◆CLASSIFICATION

PHARMACOTHERAPEUTIC: Adrenocorticosteroid. **CLINICAL:** Anti-inflammatory, immunosuppressant.

USES

Systemic: Anti-inflammatory, immunosuppressant in the treatment of diseases, including those of allergic, dermatologic, endocrine, GI, hematologic, respiratory, or rheumatoid origin. **Topical:** Relief of inflammatory and pruritic dermatoses. **Foam:** Relief of inflammation, itching associated with dermatosis of the scalp. **Sernivo:** Treatment of mild to moderate plaque psoriasis. **OFF-LABEL:** Accelerate fetal lung maturation in pts with preterm labor.

PRECAUTIONS

Contraindications: Hypersensitivity to betamethasone. IM administration in idiopathic thrombocytopenia purpura. **Cautions:** Hypothyroidism, hepatic/renal impairment, cardiovascular disease, diabetes, glaucoma, cataracts, myasthenia gravis, pts at risk for osteoporosis/seizures/GI disease, following acute MI, elderly, systemic fungal infections.

ACTION

Controls rate of protein synthesis, depresses migration of polymorphonuclear leukocytes/fibroblasts, reverses capillary permeability, prevents or controls inflammation. **Therapeutic Effect:** Decreases tissue response to inflammatory process.

PHARMACOKINETICS

Rapidly absorbed following PO administration. Protein binding: 64%. After topical application, limited absorption

---

systemically. Metabolized in liver. Excreted in urine. **Half-life:** 6.5 hrs.

⚗ LIFESPAN CONSIDERATIONS

Pregnancy/Lactation: Crosses placenta, distributed in breast milk. **Children:** Prolonged treatment, high-dose therapy may decrease short-term growth rate, cortisol secretion. **Elderly:** Increased risk for developing hypertension, osteoporosis.

INTERACTIONS

DRUG: **Amphotericin** may increase risk of hypokalemia. May decrease effects of **insulin, oral hypoglycemics (e.g., glimepiride, metFORMIN, SI-Tagliptin), potassium supplements.** May increase **digoxin** toxicity (due to hypokalemia). **Hepatic enzyme inducers (e.g., carBAMazepine, PHENobarbital, rifAMPin)** may decrease effect. **Live virus vaccines** may potentiate virus replication, increase vaccine side effects, decrease pt's antibody response to vaccine. **HERBAL:** **Cat's claw, echinacea** possess immunostimulant effects. **FOOD:** None known. **LAB VALUES:** May decrease serum calcium, potassium, thyroxine. May increase serum cholesterol, lipids, glucose, sodium, amylase.

AVAILABILITY (Rx)

Cream (Diprolene AF): 0.05%. **Foam** (Luxiq): 0.12%. **Gel:** 0.05%. **Injection, Suspension** (Celestone Soluspan): 3mg/mL. **Lotion** (Diprolene): 0.05%. **Ointment:** 0.05%, 0.1%. **Topical Spray:** 0.05%.

ADMINISTRATION/HANDLING

IM
• Inject slowly, deep IM into large muscle mass.

Topical
• Gently cleanse area before application. • Apply sparingly and rub into area thoroughly. • Do not apply to face, groin, axillae, or inguinal areas. Not for use on broken skin, areas of infection, or in diaper area. • Do not dispense foam directly into hands; use fingers to apply small amounts.

INDICATIONS/ROUTES/DOSAGE

Anti-Inflammation, Immunosuppression, Corticosteroid Replacement Therapy
IM: **ADULTS, ELDERLY:** 0.25–9 mg/day in 2 divided doses. **CHILDREN:** 0.02–0.3 mg/kg/day in 3–4 divided doses.

Relief of Inflamed and Pruritic Dermatoses
Topical: (Cream/Ointment): **ADULTS, ELDERLY:** 1–2 times daily. **Foam:** Apply twice daily (morning and night).

Plaque Psoriasis
Topical: **ADULTS, ELDERLY:** (Sernivo): Apply to affected areas 2 times/day for up to 4 wks.

Dosage in Hepatic Impairment
Use caution.

SIDE EFFECTS

Frequent: **Systemic:** Increased appetite, abdominal distention, nervousness, insomnia, false sense of well-being. **Topical:** Burning, stinging, pruritus. **Occasional:** **Systemic:** Dizziness, facial flushing, diaphoresis, decreased or blurred vision, mood swings. **Topical:** Allergic contact dermatitis, purpura or blood-containing blisters, thinning of skin with easy bruising, telangiectases, raised dark red spots on skin, angiomas.

ADVERSE EFFECTS/TOXIC REACTIONS

Overdose may cause systemic hypercorticism, adrenal suppression.

NURSING CONSIDERATIONS

BASELINE ASSESSMENT

Question for hypersensitivity to any corticosteroid, sulfite. Obtain baseline values for height, weight, B/P, serum glucose, electrolytes. Obtain baseline results of initial tests (tuberculosis [TB] skin test, X-rays, EKG).

INTERVENTION/EVALUATION

Monitor B/P, blood glucose, electrolytes. Apply topical preparation sparingly. Do not use on broken skin or in areas of infection. Do not apply to wet skin, face, inguinal areas.

PATIENT/FAMILY TEACHING

• Take with food, milk. • Take single daily dose in the morning. • Do not stop abruptly. • Apply topical preparations in a thin layer. • Do not receive smallpox vaccination during or immediately after therapy.

---

bethanechol

be-**than**-e-kole
(Duvoid ✤, Urecholine)
Do not confuse bethanechol with betaxolol.

◆CLASSIFICATION

PHARMACOTHERAPEUTIC: Parasympathomimetic choline ester. **CLINICAL:** Cholinergic.

USES

Treatment of acute postoperative and postpartum nonobstructive urinary retention, retention due to neurogenic bladder. **OFF-LABEL:** Treatment of gastroesophageal reflux.

PRECAUTIONS

Contraindications: Hypersensitivity to bethanechol. Mechanical obstruction of GI/GU tract, GI or bladder wall instability, hyperthyroidism, cardiac disease, bronchial asthma, peptic ulcer, epilepsy, pronounced bradycardia or hypotension, parkinsonism. **Cautions:** None known.

ACTION

Stimulates parasympathetic nervous system, increasing bladder muscle tone and causing contractions, which initiates urination. Also stimulates gastric motility, increasing gastric tone, and may restore peristalsis. **Therapeutic Effect:** May initiate urination, bladder emptying. Stimulates gastric, intestinal motility.

PHARMACOKINETICS

Route	Onset	Peak	Duration
PO	30–90 min	60 min	6 hrs

Poorly absorbed following PO administration. Does not cross blood-brain barrier. **Half-life:** Unknown.

⧗ LIFESPAN CONSIDERATIONS

Pregnancy/Lactation: Unknown if crosses placenta or distributed in breast milk. **Children/Elderly:** No age-related precautions noted.

INTERACTIONS

DRUG: Beta blockers (e.g., **labetalol, metoprolol), anticholinesterase inhibitors (e.g., donepezil, rivastigmine)** may increase effect/toxicity. **HERBAL:** None significant. **FOOD:** None known. **LAB VALUES:** May increase serum amylase, lipase, ALT, AST.

AVAILABILITY (Rx)

Tablets: 5 mg, 10 mg, 25 mg, 50 mg.

ADMINISTRATION/HANDLING

PO
• Administer 1 hr before or 2 hrs after meals.

INDICATIONS/ROUTES/DOSAGE

Nonobstructive Urinary Retention, Neurogenic Bladder
PO: ADULTS, ELDERLY: Usual dose: 10–50 mg 3–4 times/day. Minimum effective dose determined by giving 5–10 mg initially, repeating same amount at 1-hr intervals until desired response is achieved. **CHILDREN:** 0.3–0.6 mg/kg/day in 3–4 divided doses.

Dosage in Renal/Hepatic Impairment
No dose adjustment.

SIDE EFFECTS

Occasional: Belching, changes in vision, blurred vision, diarrhea, urinary urgency

---

or frequency. **Rare:** Dyspnea, chest tightness, bronchospasm.

ADVERSE EFFECTS/TOXIC REACTIONS

Overdose produces CNS stimulation (insomnia, anxiety, orthostatic hypotension), cholinergic stimulation (headache, increased salivation/diaphoresis, nausea, vomiting, flushed skin, abdominal pain, seizures).

NURSING CONSIDERATIONS

BASELINE ASSESSMENT

Ensure pt has emptied bladder prior to procedure.

INTERVENTION/EVALUATION

Monitor urine output. Palpate bladder for evidence of urinary retention.

PATIENT/FAMILY TEACHING

• Report nausea, vomiting, diarrhea, diaphoresis, increased salivary secretions, irregular heartbeat, muscle weakness, severe abdominal pain, difficulty breathing.

---

betrixaban

be-trix-a-ban
(Bevyxxa)

■ **BLACK BOX ALERT** ■ Epidural/spinal hematomas may occur in pts receiving neuraxial anesthesia or undergoing spinal puncture, resulting in long-term or permanent paralysis. Factors increasing risk of epidural/spinal hematoma include indwelling epidural catheters or concomitant use of medical products affecting hemostasis. Consider the risks before spinal procedures. **Do not confuse betrixaban with apixaban, edoxaban, or rivaroxaban.**

◆CLASSIFICATION

PHARMACOTHERAPEUTIC: Factor Xa inhibitor. **CLINICAL:** Anticoagulant.

USES

Prophylaxis of venous thromboembolism (VTE) in adult pts hospitalized for an acute medical illness who are at risk for thromboembolic complications due to moderate or severe restricted mobility and other risk factors for VTE.

PRECAUTIONS

Contraindications: Hypersensitivity to betrixaban. Major active bleeding. **Cautions:** Severe renal impairment, concomitant use of P-gp inhibitors, pts at risk for bleeding (e.g., active GI ulcerative disease, congenital/acquired disorders, hemophilia, menses, severe hypertension, open wounds; recent history of intracranial hemorrhage, lumbar puncture, spinal anesthesia, surgery, trauma). Not recommended in pts with hepatic impairment. Safety and efficacy not established in pts with prosthetic heart valves.

ACTION

Directly and selectrively inhibits factor Xa (FXa). FXa is part of the prothrombinase complex that catalyzes the conversion of prothrombin to thrombin. Thrombin activates platelets and catalyzes conversion of fibrinogen to fibrin. **Therapeutic Effect:** Inhibits fibrin clot formation.

PHARMACOKINETICS

Widely distributed. Protein binding: 60%. Peak plasma concentration: 3–4 hrs. Steady state reached in 6 days. Excreted in feces (85%), urine (11%). **Half-life:** 19–27 hrs.

⧖ LIFESPAN CONSIDERATIONS

Pregnancy/Lactation: Unknown if distributed in breast milk. May increase risk of bleeding during pregnancy/delivery. **Children:** Safety and efficacy not established. **Elderly:** No age-related precautions noted.

INTERACTIONS

DRUG: Anticoagulants (e.g., **apixaban, dabigatran, edoxaban, heparin, rivaroxaban, warfarin**), **vorapaxar** may increase risk of bleeding. **P-gp**

B

inhibitors (e.g., **amiodarone, azithromycin, ketoconazole, verapamil**) may increase concentration/effect; may increase risk of bleeding. **HERBAL:** Herbals with anticoagulant activity (e.g., **anise, bilberry**) may increase of bleeding. **FOOD:** None known. **LAB VALUES:** May decrease serum potassium.

AVAILABILITY (Rx)

Capsules: 40 mg, 80 mg.

ADMINISTRATION/HANDLING

PO

• Give with food. • If a dose is missed, administer as soon as possible on same day (do not double dose if a day is missed).

INDICATIONS/ROUTES/DOSAGE

Venous Thromboembolism

PO: ADULTS, ELDERLY: Initially, 160 mg as a single dose. **Maintenance:** 80 mg once daily for 35–42 days.

Dose Modification

Concomitant use of P-gp inhibitors: Initially, 80 mg as a single dose. **Maintenance:** 40 mg once daily for 35–42 days.

Dosage in Renal Impairment

Severe impairment (CrCl 15–29 mL/min): Initially, 80 mg as a single dose. **Maintenance:** 40 mg once daily for 35–42 days.

Dosage in Hepatic Impairment

Not recommended in hepatic impairment.

SIDE EFFECTS

Rare (3%–2%): Constipation, hypertension, headache, nausea, diarrhea.

ADVERSE EFFECTS/TOXIC REACTIONS

Hemorrhagic events, some of them fatal, were reported; events included intracranial hemorrhage; hemorrhagic CVA; epistaxis; and intra-articular, intraspinal, intraocular, GI, GU, pericardial, and retroperitoneal bleeding. Discontinuation in the absence of other adequate anticoagulants may increase the risk of ischemic events, stroke. May increase risk of epidural or spinal hematomas, which may lead to permanent or long-time paralysis. Protamine sulfate, vitamin K, tranexamic acid are not expected to reverse anticoagulant effect.

NURSING CONSIDERATIONS

BASELINE ASSESSMENT

Question history of bleeding disorders, recent surgery, spinal procedures, intracranial hemorrhage, bleeding ulcers, open wounds, trauma. Receive full medication history and screen for interactions (esp. P-gp inhibitors, herbals with anticoagulant properties). Question history of hepatic/renal impairment.

INTERVENTION/EVALUATION

Be alert for decrease in B/P, increase in pulse rate; complaints of abdominal/back pain, dysarthria, headache, confusion, weakness, vision change (may indicate hemorrhage). If internal hemorrhage suspected, recommend emergent radiologic imaging. Question for increased menstrual bleeding/discharge. Assess skin for ecchymosis, petechiae. Check for excessive bleeding from minor cuts, scratches. Monitor urine and stool for occult blood. Avoid IM injections.

PATIENT/FAMILY TEACHING

• Do not discontinue current blood thinning regimen or take any newly prescribed medications unless approved by the physician who originally started treatment. • Suddenly stopping therapy may increase the risk of blood clots or stroke. Promptly refill prescription so that the next scheduled dose is not missed. • Report bleeding of any kind (bloody urine, stool; nosebleeds; increased menstrual bleeding). If bleeding occurs, it may take longer to stop bleeding. • Immediately report signs of stroke (confusion, headache, numbness, one-sided weakness, trouble speaking, loss of vision). • Minor blunt force trauma to the head, chest, or abdomen can be life-threatening.

- Monitor changes in urine output.
- Do not take aspirin, herbal supplements, OTC nonsteroidal anti-inflammatories (may increase risk of bleeding). • Consult physician before any surgery or dental work. • Use electric razor, soft toothbrush to prevent bleeding.

bevacizumab

be-va-**siz**-ue-mab
(Avastin, Mvasi)

■ BLACK BOX ALERT ■ May result in development of GI perforation, presented as intra-abdominal abscess, fistula, wound dehiscence, wound healing complications. Severe, sometimes fatal, hemorrhagic events including central nervous system/GI/vaginal bleeding, epistaxis, hemoptysis, pulmonary hemorrhage has occurred. **Do not confuse Avastin with Astelin, or bevacizumab with cetuximab or riTUXimab.**

◆ CLASSIFICATION

PHARMACOTHERAPEUTIC: Monoclonal antibody. **CLINICAL:** Antineoplastic.

USES

First- or second-line combination chemotherapy with 5-fluorouracil (5-FU) for treatment of pts with colorectal cancer. Second-line treatment of colorectal cancer after progression of first-line treatment with bevacizumab. Treatment with CARBOplatin and PACLitaxel for nonsquamous, non–small-cell lung cancer (NSCLC). Treatment of renal cell carcinoma (metastatic) with interferon alfa, brain cancer (glioblastoma) that has progressed following prior therapy. Treatment of platinum-resistant recurrent epithelial ovarian, fallopian tube, or primary peritoneal cancer (in combination with PACLitaxel, DOXOrubicin [liposomal] or topotecan). Treatment of platinum-sensitive ovarian cancer. Treatment of persistent, recurrent, or metastatic cervical cancer (in combination with PACLitaxel and either CISplatin or topotecan). **OFF-LABEL:** Adjunctive therapy in malignant mesothelioma, ovarian cancer, prostate cancer, age-related macular degeneration. Treatment of metastatic breast cancer.

PRECAUTIONS

Contraindications: Hypersensitivity to bevacizumab. **Cautions:** Cardiovascular disease, acquired coagulopathy, preexisting hypertension, pts at risk of thrombocytopenia. Pts with CNS metastasis. Do not administer within 28 days of major surgery or active bleeding.

ACTION

Binds to and inhibits vascular endothelial growth factor, a protein that plays a major role in formation of new blood vessels to tumors. **Therapeutic Effect:** Inhibits metastatic disease progression.

PHARMACOKINETICS

Clearance varies by body weight, gender, tumor burden. **Half-life:** 20 days (range: 11–50 days).

⧗ LIFESPAN CONSIDERATIONS

Pregnancy/Lactation: May possess teratogenic effects. Potential for fertility impairment. May decrease maternal and fetal body weight, increase risk of skeletal fetal abnormalities. Breastfeeding not recommended. **Children:** Safety and efficacy not established. **Elderly:** Higher incidence of severe adverse reactions in pts older than 65 yrs.

INTERACTIONS

DRUG: SUNItinib may increase concentration/effect. May increase levels of **cloZAPine, SORAfenib, SUNItinib.** **HERBAL:** None significant. **FOOD:** None known. **LAB VALUES:** May decrease Hgb, Hct, platelet count, WBC; serum potassium, sodium. May increase urine protein.

AVAILABILITY (Rx)

Injection, Solution: 25-mg/mL vial (4 mL, 16 mL).

B

ADMINISTRATION/HANDLING
IV

◀**ALERT**▶ Do not give by IV push or bolus.

Reconstitution • Dilute prescribed dose in 100 mL 0.9% NaCl. • Avoid dextrose-containing solutions. • Discard any unused portion.

Rate of Administration • Usually given following other chemotherapy. Infuse initial dose over 90 min. • If first infusion is well tolerated, second infusion may be administered over 60 min. • If 60-min infusion is well tolerated, all subsequent infusions may be administered over 30 min.

Storage • Diluted solution may be stored for up to 8 hrs if refrigerated.

IV INCOMPATIBILITIES

Do not mix with dextrose solutions.

INDICATIONS/ROUTES/DOSAGE

Colorectal Cancer (with Fluorouracil-Based Chemotherapy)
IV: ADULTS, ELDERLY: 5 mg/kg q2wks (in combination with bolus-IFL) or 10 mg/kg q2wks in combination with FOLFOX4).

Colorectal Cancer Progression (Following Initial Bevacizumab/Fluorouracil-Based Chemotherapy)
IV: ADULTS, ELDERLY: 5 mg/kg q2wks or 7.5 mg/kg q3wks (in combination with fluoropyrimidine-irinotecan– or fluoropyrimidine-oxaliplatin–based regimen).

Non–Small-Cell Lung Cancer (NSCLC)
IV: ADULTS, ELDERLY: 15 mg/kg q3wks (in combination with CARBOplatin and PACLitaxel) for 6 cycles.

Metastatic Renal Cell Carcinoma
IV: ADULTS, ELDERLY: 10 mg/kg once q2wks (with interferon alfa).

Brain Cancer
IV: ADULTS, ELDERLY: 10 mg/kg q2wks (as monotherapy).

Ovarian Cancer (Platinum-Resistant)
IV: ADULTS, ELDERLY: 10 mg/kg q2wks with PACLitaxel, DOXOrubicin [liposomal], or wkly topotecan or 15 mg/kg q3wks (with topotecan q3wks).

Ovarian Cancer (Platinum-Sensitive)
IV: ADULTS, ELDERLY: 15 mg/kg q3wks with CARBOplatin/PACLitaxel for 6–8 cycles then 15 mg/kg q3wks as a single agent or 15 mg/kg with CARBOplatin/gemcitabine for 6–10 cycles, then 15 mg/kg q3wks as a single agent. Continue until disease progression or unacceptable toxicity.

Cervical Cancer
IV: ADULTS, ELDERLY: 15 mg/kg q3wks (in combination with PACLitaxel and either CISplatin or topotecan). Continue until disease progression or unacceptable toxicity.

Dose Adjustment for Toxicity
Temporary suspension: Mild to moderate proteinuria, severe hypertension not controlled with medical management. **Permanent discontinuation:** Wound dehiscence requiring intervention, GI perforation, hypertensive crises, serious bleeding, nephrotic syndrome.

Dosage in Renal/Hepatic Impairment
No dose adjustment.

SIDE EFFECTS

Frequent (73%–25%): Asthenia, vomiting, anorexia, hypertension, epistaxis, stomatitis, constipation, headache, dyspnea. **Occasional (21%–15%):** Altered taste, dry skin, exfoliative dermatitis, dizziness, flatulence, excessive lacrimation, skin discoloration, weight loss, myalgia. **Rare (8%–6%):** Nail disorder, skin ulcer, alopecia, confusion, abnormal gait, dry mouth.

ADVERSE EFFECTS/TOXIC REACTIONS

UTI, manifested as urinary frequency/urgency, proteinuria, occurs frequently. Most serious adverse effects include HF, deep vein thrombosis, GI perforation, wound dehiscence, hypertensive crisis, nephrotic syndrome, severe hemorrhage. Anemia, neutropenia, thrombocytopenia occur occasionally. Hypersensitivity reactions occur rarely. May increase risk of tracheoesophageal fistula development.

NURSING CONSIDERATIONS

BASELINE ASSESSMENT

Obtain baseline CBC, serum potassium, sodium levels and at regular intervals during therapy. Assess for proteinuria with urinalysis. For pts with 2+ or greater urine dipstick reading, a 24-hr urine collection is advised.

INTERVENTION/EVALUATION

Monitor B/P regularly for hypertension. Assess for asthenia. Assist with ambulation if asthenia occurs. Monitor for fever, chills, abdominal pain, epistaxis. Offer antiemetic if nausea, vomiting occurs. Monitor daily pattern of bowel activity, stool consistency.

PATIENT/FAMILY TEACHING

• Report abdominal pain, vomiting, constipation, headache. • Do not receive immunizations without physician's approval (lowers body's resistance). • Avoid contact with anyone who recently received a live virus vaccine. • Avoid crowds, those with infection. • Female pts should take measures to avoid pregnancy during treatment.

---

bicalutamide

bye-ka-**loo**-ta-mide
(Apo-Bicalutamide ✦, Casodex)

◆CLASSIFICATION

PHARMACOTHERAPEUTIC: Antiandrogen hormone. **CLINICAL:** Antineoplastic.

USES

Treatment of advanced metastatic prostatic carcinoma (in combination with luteinizing hormone-releasing hormone [LHRH] agonist analogues, e.g., leuprolide). Treatment with both drugs must be started at same time. **OFF-LABEL:** Monotherapy for locally advanced prostate cancer.

PRECAUTIONS

Contraindications: Hypersensitivity to bicalutamide. Women, esp. those who are or may become pregnant. **Cautions:** Moderate to severe hepatic impairment, diabetes.

ACTION

Competitively inhibits androgen action by binding to androgen receptors in target tissue. **Therapeutic Effect:** Prevents testosterone stimulation of cell growth in prostate cancer.

PHARMACOKINETICS

Well absorbed from GI tract. Protein binding: 96%. Metabolized in liver. Excreted in urine and feces. Not removed by hemodialysis. **Half-life:** 5.8–7 days.

⧖ LIFESPAN CONSIDERATIONS

Pregnancy/Lactation: May inhibit spermatogenesis in males. Not used in women. **Children:** Safety and efficacy not established. **Elderly:** No age-related precautions noted.

INTERACTIONS

DRUG: May increase effects of **ARIPiprazole, budesonide, colchicine, fentaNYL, salmeterol, SAXagliptin. HERBAL:** None significant. **FOOD:** None known. **LAB VALUES:** May increase serum ALT, AST, alkaline phosphatase, creatinine, bilirubin, BUN, glucose. May decrease WBC, Hgb.

AVAILABILITY (Rx)

Tablets: 50 mg.

ADMINISTRATION/HANDLING

PO

• Give without regard to food. • Give at same time each day.

INDICATIONS/ROUTES/DOSAGE

Prostatic Carcinoma

PO: ADULTS, ELDERLY: 50 mg once daily in morning or evening, given concurrently with an LHRH analogue or after surgical castration.

Dosage in Renal/Hepatic Impairment

No dose adjustment.

SIDE EFFECTS

Frequent (49%–10%): Hot flashes, breast pain, muscle pain, constipation, asthenia, diarrhea, nausea. **Occasional (9%–8%):** Nocturia, abdominal pain, peripheral edema. **Rare (7%–3%):** Vomiting, weight loss, dizziness, insomnia, rash, impotence, gynecomastia.

ADVERSE EFFECTS/TOXIC REACTIONS

Sepsis, HF, hypertension, iron deficiency anemia, interstitial pneumonitis, pulmonary fibrosis may occur. Severe hepatotoxicity occurs rarely within the first 3–4 mos after treatment initiation.

NURSING CONSIDERATIONS

BASELINE ASSESSMENT

Obtain baseline CBC, LFT, PSA, serum testosterone, luteinizing hormone (LH) levels.

INTERVENTION/EVALUATION

Monitor lab studies for changes from baseline. Perform periodic LFT. If ALT, AST increase over 2 times the upper limit of normal (ULN) or jaundice is noted, discontinue treatment. Monitor for diarrhea, nausea, vomiting.

PATIENT/FAMILY TEACHING

• Do not stop taking either medication (both drugs must be continued). • Take medications at same time each day. • Explain possible expectancy of frequent side effects. • Report persistent nausea, vomiting, diarrhea, or yellowing of skin or eyes.

bisacodyl

bis-**ak**-oh-dil
(Apo-Bisacodyl ✦, Dulcolax)

◆CLASSIFICATION

PHARMACOTHERAPEUTIC: GI stimulant. **CLINICAL:** Laxative.

USES

Treatment of constipation, colonic evacuation before examinations or procedures.

PRECAUTIONS

Contraindications: Hypersensitivity to bisacodyl. Abdominal pain, appendicitis, intestinal obstruction, nausea, undiagnosed rectal bleeding, vomiting, pregnancy, lactation. **Cautions:** Long-term use may lead to laxative dependence, loss of normal bowel function.

ACTION

Direct effect on colonic smooth musculature by stimulating intramural nerve plexi. **Therapeutic Effect:** Promotes fluid and electrolyte accumulation in colon, increasing peristalsis, producing laxative effect.

PHARMACOKINETICS

Route	Onset	Peak	Duration
PO	6–12 hrs	N/A	N/A
Rectal	15–60 min	N/A	N/A

Minimal absorption following PO and rectal administration. Absorbed drug is excreted in urine; remainder is eliminated in feces.

⌛ LIFESPAN CONSIDERATIONS

Pregnancy/Lactation: Unknown if drug crosses placenta or is distributed in breast milk. **Children:** Use with caution in pts younger than 6 yrs (usually unable to describe symptoms or more severe side effects). **Elderly:** Repeated use may cause weakness, orthostatic hypotension due to fluid, electrolyte imbalance.

INTERACTIONS

DRUG: Antacids may decrease effect, cause premature dissolution of enteric coating and possible gastric irritation. **HERBAL:** None significant. **FOOD: Milk** may cause rapid dissolution of bisacodyl. **LAB VALUES:** May increase serum glucose. May decrease serum potassium (due to fluid loss).

AVAILABILITY (OTC)

Suppositories (Dulcolax): 10 mg.

Tablets (Enteric-Coated [Dulcolax]): 5 mg.

ADMINISTRATION/HANDLING

PO
• Give on empty stomach (faster action). • Offer 6–8 glasses of water a day (aids stool softening). • Administer tablets whole; do not break, crush, dissolve, or divide. • Avoid giving within 1 hr of antacids, milk, other oral medication.

Rectal, Suppository
• If suppository is too soft, chill for 30 min in refrigerator or run cold water over foil wrapper. • Moisten suppository with cold water before inserting well into rectum.

Storage • Store rectal enema, suppositories at room temperature.

INDICATIONS/ROUTES/DOSAGE

Treatment of Constipation
PO: ADULTS, ELDERLY, CHILDREN OLDER THAN 12 YRS: 5–15 mg as needed. **Maximum:** 30 mg. **CHILDREN 3–12 YRS:** 5–10 mg or 0.3 mg/kg at bedtime or after breakfast.
Rectal, Suppository: ADULTS, ELDERLY, CHILDREN OLDER THAN 12 YRS: 10 mg to induce bowel movement. **CHILDREN 2–12 YRS:** 5–10 mg as a single dose. **CHILDREN YOUNGER THAN 2 YRS:** 5 mg.

Dosage in Renal/Hepatic Impairment
No dose adjustment.

SIDE EFFECTS

Frequent: Some degree of abdominal discomfort, nausea, mild cramps, faintness.

Occasional: Rectal administration: burning of rectal mucosa, mild proctitis.

ADVERSE EFFECTS/TOXIC REACTIONS

Long-term use may result in laxative dependence, chronic constipation, loss of normal bowel function. Overdose may result in electrolyte or metabolic disturbances (hypokalemia, hypocalcemia, metabolic acidosis, alkalosis), persistent diarrhea, vomiting, muscle weakness, malabsorption, weight loss.

NURSING CONSIDERATIONS

BASELINE ASSESSMENT
Observe for evidence of constipation. Assess pattern of bowel activity, stool consistency.

INTERVENTION/EVALUATION
Encourage adequate fluid intake. Assess bowel sounds for peristalsis. Monitor daily pattern of bowel activity, stool consistency; record time of evacuation. Assess for abdominal disturbances. Monitor serum electrolytes in those exposed to prolonged, frequent, or excessive use of medication.

PATIENT/FAMILY TEACHING
• Institute measures to promote defecation: increase fluid intake, exercise, high-fiber diet. • Do not take antacids, milk, or other medication within 1 hr of taking medication (decreased effectiveness). • Report unrelieved constipation, rectal bleeding, muscle pain or cramps, dizziness, weakness. • Do not chew, crush, dissolve, or divide tablets.

bisoprolol HIGH ALERT

bi-**soe**-proe-lol
(Apo-Bisoprolol ✦, Novo-Bisoprolol ✦, Zebeta)
Do not confuse Zebeta with DiaBeta or Zetia.

FIXED-COMBINATION(S)

Ziac: bisoprolol/hydroCHLOROthiazide (a diuretic): 2.5 mg/6.25 mg, 5 mg/6.25 mg, 10 mg/6.25 mg.

◆CLASSIFICATION

PHARMACOTHERAPEUTIC: Beta-adrenergic blocker. **CLINICAL:** Antihypertensive.

USES

Management of hypertension, alone or in combination with other medications. **OFF-LABEL:** Chronic stable angina pectoris, premature ventricular contractions, supraventricular arrhythmias, HF.

PRECAUTIONS

Contraindications: Hypersensitivity to bisoprolol. Cardiogenic shock, marked sinus bradycardia, overt HF, second- or third-degree heart block (except in pts with pacemaker). **Cautions:** Concurrent use of digoxin, verapamil, diltiaZEM, HF, history of severe anaphylaxis to allergens, renal/hepatic impairment, hyperthyroidism, diabetes, bronchospastic disease, myasthenia gravis, psychiatric disease, peripheral vascular disease, Raynaud's disease.

ACTION

Blocks beta$_1$-adrenergic receptors in cardiac tissue. **Therapeutic Effect:** Slows sinus heart rate, decreases B/P.

PHARMACOKINETICS

Well absorbed from GI tract. Protein binding: 26%–33%. Metabolized in liver. Primarily excreted in urine. Not removed by hemodialysis. **Half-life:** 9–12 hrs (increased in renal impairment).

⧗ LIFESPAN CONSIDERATIONS

Pregnancy/Lactation: Readily crosses placenta; distributed in breast milk. Avoid use during first trimester. May produce bradycardia, apnea, hypoglycemia, hypothermia during delivery, low-birth-weight infants. **Children:** Safety and efficacy not established. **Elderly:** Age-related peripheral vascular disease may increase risk of decreased peripheral circulation.

INTERACTIONS

DRUG: Diuretics (e.g., furosemide), **other antihypertensives (e.g., amlodipine, lisinopril, valsartan)** may increase hypotensive effect. May mask symptoms of hypoglycemia, prolong hypoglycemic effect of **insulin, oral hypoglycemics (e.g., glimepiride, met-FORMIN, SITagliptin).** NSAIDs (e.g., **diclofenac, ibuprofen, naproxen**) may decrease antihypertensive effect. **Verapamil, diltiaZEM, digoxin** may increase risk of bradycardia or heart block. **HERBAL: Ephedra, ginseng, yohimbe** may worsen hypertension. **Garlic** may have increased antihypertensive effect. **FOOD:** None known. **LAB VALUES:** May increase ANA titer, serum BUN, creatinine, potassium, uric acid, lipoproteins, triglycerides.

AVAILABILITY (Rx)

Tablets: 5 mg, 10 mg.

ADMINISTRATION/HANDLING

PO

- Give without regard to food.

INDICATIONS/ROUTES/DOSAGE

Hypertension

PO: ADULTS, ELDERLY: Initially, 2.5–5 mg once daily. May increase to 10 mg, then to 20 mg once daily. Usual dose: 5–10 mg once daily.

Dosage in Renal Impairment

ADULTS, ELDERLY: CrCl less than 40 mL/min: Initially, give 2.5 mg.

Dosage in Hepatic Impairment

Cirrhosis, Hepatitis: Initially, 2.5 mg.

SIDE EFFECTS

Frequent (11%–8%): Fatigue, headache. **Occasional (4%–2%):** Dizziness, arthralgia, peripheral edema, URI, rhinitis, pharyngitis, diarrhea, nausea, insomnia. **Rare (less than 2%):** Chest pain, asthenia, dyspnea, vomiting, bradycardia, dry mouth, diaphoresis, decreased libido, impotence.

ADVERSE EFFECTS/ TOXIC REACTIONS

Overdose may produce profound bradycardia, hypotension. Abrupt withdrawal may result in diaphoresis, palpitations, headache, tremors. May precipitate HF, MI in pts with cardiac disease, thyroid storm in pts with thyrotoxicosis, peripheral ischemia in those with existing peripheral vascular disease. Hypoglycemia may occur in previously controlled diabetes. Thrombocytopenia, unusual bruising/bleeding occur rarely.

NURSING CONSIDERATIONS

BASELINE ASSESSMENT

Assess baseline renal/hepatic function tests. Assess B/P, apical pulse immediately before drug is administered (if pulse is 60/min or less or systolic B/P is less than 90 mm Hg, withhold medication, contact physician).

INTERVENTION/EVALUATION

Monitor B/P, pulse for quality, irregular rate, bradycardia. Assist with ambulation if dizziness occurs. Assess for peripheral edema. Monitor daily pattern of bowel activity, stool consistency. Assess neurologic status.

PATIENT/FAMILY TEACHING

• Do not abruptly discontinue medication. • Compliance with therapy regimen is essential to control hypertension. • If dizziness occurs, sit or lie down immediately. • Avoid tasks that require alertness, motor skills until response to drug is established. • Take pulse properly before each dose and report excessively slow pulse rate (less than 60 beats/min). Report numbness of extremities, dizziness. • Do not use nasal decongestants, OTC cold preparations (stimulants) without physician's approval. • Restrict salt, alcohol intake.

---

bivalirudin

bye-**val**-i-rue-din
(Angiomax)

◆ CLASSIFICATION

PHARMACOTHERAPEUTIC: Thrombin inhibitor. **CLINICAL:** Anticoagulant.

USES

Anticoagulant in pts undergoing percutaneous transluminal coronary angioplasty (PTCA) in conjunction with aspirin and provisional glycoprotein IIb/IIIa inhibitor. Pts with heparin-induced thrombocytopenia (HIT) and thrombosis syndrome (HITTS) while undergoing percutaneous coronary intervention (PCI) (in conjunction with aspirin). **OFF-LABEL:** HIT; ST-segment elevation MI (STEMI) undergoing PCI.

PRECAUTIONS

Contraindications: Hypersensitivity to bivalirudin. Active major bleeding. **Cautions:** Renal impairment, conditions associated with increased risk of bleeding (e.g., bacterial endocarditis, recent major bleeding, CVA, stroke, intracerebral surgery, hemorrhagic diathesis, severe hypertension, severe renal/hepatic impairment, recent major surgery).

ACTION

Specifically and reversibly inhibits thrombin by binding to its receptor sites. **Therapeutic Effect:** Decreases acute myocardial ischemic complications in pts with unstable angina pectoris.

PHARMACOKINETICS

Route	Onset	Peak	Duration
IV	Immediate	N/A	1 hr

Primarily eliminated by kidneys. Twenty-five percent removed by hemodialysis. **Half-life:** 25 min (increased in moderate to severe renal impairment).

B

⧗ LIFESPAN CONSIDERATIONS

Pregnancy/Lactation: Unknown if drug crosses placenta or is distributed in breast milk. **Children:** Safety and efficacy not established. **Elderly:** Age-related renal impairment may require dosage adjustment.

INTERACTIONS

DRUG: Anticoagulants (e.g., **heparin, warfarin**), antiplatelets (e.g., **aspirin, clopidogrel**), NSAIDs (e.g., **diclofenac, ibuprofen, naproxen**), thrombolytic therapy (e.g., **TPA**) may increase risk of bleeding. **HERBAL:** Dong quai, fish oil (omega-3), feverfew, ginger, ginkgo, ginseng, garlic, licorice, saw palmetto, vitamin E may increase risk of bleeding. **FOOD:** None known. **LAB VALUES:** Prolongs activated partial thromboplastin time (aPTT), prothrombin time (PT).

AVAILABILITY (Rx)

Injection, Powder for Reconstitution: 250 mg.

ADMINISTRATION/HANDLING

💧 IV

Reconstitution • To each 250-mg vial add 5 mL Sterile Water for Injection. • Gently swirl until fully dissolved. • Dilute each vial in 50 mL D₅W or 0.9% NaCl bag to yield final concentration of 5 mg/mL (1 vial in 50 mL, 2 vials in 100 mL, 5 vials in 250 mL). • If low-rate infusion is used after initial infusion, reconstitute the 250-mg vial with added 5 mL Sterile Water for Injection. • Gently swirl until fully dissolved. • Dilute each vial in 500 mL D₅W or 0.9% NaCl bag to yield final concentration of 0.5 mg/mL. • Produces a clear, colorless solution (do not use if cloudy or contains a precipitate).
Rate of Administration • Adjust IV infusion based on aPTT or pt's body weight.
Storage • Store unreconstituted vials at room temperature. • Reconstituted solution may be refrigerated for up to 24 hrs. • Final dilution with a concentration of 0.5–5 mg/mL is stable at room temperature for up to 24 hrs.

▦ IV INCOMPATIBILITIES

Alteplase (Activase), amiodarone (Cordarone), amphotericin B (AmBisome, Abelcet), diazePAM (Valium), DOBUTamine (Dobutrex), reteplase (Retavase), streptokinase (Streptase), vancomycin (Vancocin).

▦ IV COMPATIBILITIES

Refer to IV compatibility chart in front of book.

INDICATIONS/ROUTES/DOSAGE

Anticoagulant in Pts with Unstable Angina, HIT, or HITTS Undergoing PTCA
IV: ADULTS, ELDERLY: 0.75 mg/kg as IV bolus, followed by IV infusion at rate of 1.75 mg/kg/hr for duration of procedure and up to 4 hrs postprocedure. IV infusion may be continued beyond initial 4 hrs at rate of 0.2 mg/kg/hr for up to 20 hrs.

Dosage in Renal Impairment

◄**ALERT**► Initial bolus dose remains unchanged.

Creatinine Clearance	Dosage
30 mL/min or greater	1.75 mg/kg/hr
10–29 mL/min	1 mg/kg/hr
Dialysis	0.25 mg/kg/hr

Dosage in Hepatic Impairment
No dosage adjustment.

SIDE EFFECTS

Frequent (42%): Back pain. **Occasional (15%–12%):** Nausea, headache, hypotension, generalized pain. **Rare (8%–4%):** Injection site pain, insomnia, hypertension, anxiety, vomiting, pelvic or abdominal pain, bradycardia, nervousness, dyspepsia, fever, urinary retention.

ADVERSE EFFECTS/TOXIC REACTIONS

Hemorrhagic events occur rarely, characterized by significant fall in B/P or Hgb/Hct.

B

NURSING CONSIDERATIONS

BASELINE ASSESSMENT

Assess CBC, PT/INR, aPTT, renal function. Determine initial B/P.

INTERVENTION/EVALUATION

Monitor aPTT, CBC, urine and stool specimen for occult blood, renal function studies. Monitor for evidence of bleeding. Assess for decrease in B/P, increase in pulse rate. Question for increase in vaginal bleeding during menses.

---

blinatumomab

blin-a-**toom**-oh-mab
(Blincyto)

■ **BLACK BOX ALERT** ■ Cytokine release syndrome (CRS) or neurologic toxicities, which may be life threatening or fatal, have occurred. Interrupt or discontinue treatment as recommended.
Do not confuse blinatumomab with ibritumomab or tositumomab.

◆CLASSIFICATION

PHARMACOTHERAPEUTIC: Bispecific CD-19-directed CD3 T-cell engager. **CLINICAL:** Antineoplastic.

USES

Treatment of Philadelphia chromosome-negative relapsed or refractory B-cell precursor acute lymphoblastic leukemia (ALL) in adults and children.

PRECAUTIONS

Contraindications: Hypersensitivity to blinatumomab. **Cautions:** Baseline anemia, leukopenia, neutropenia, thrombocytopenia; active infection or pts at increased risk of infection (diabetes, indwelling catheters), hepatic/renal impairment, electrolyte imbalance, high tumor burden, history of cognitive or seizure disorders, syncope, elderly.

ACTION

Activates endogenous T cells by connecting CD3 in the T-cell receptor complex with CD19 on benign and malignant B cells. Mediates proliferation of T cells, release of inflammatory cytokines, production of cytolytic proteins, and up-regulation of cell adhesions, resulting in lysis of tumor cells. **Therapeutic Effect:** Inhibits tumor cell growth and metastasis in ALL.

PHARMACOKINETICS

Widely distributed. Metabolism not specified; degrades into small peptides and amino acids via catabolic pathway. Protein binding: Not specified. Steady state reached within 24 hrs. Excretion not specified; negligible amounts excreted in urine. **Half-life:** 2.1 hrs.

☒ LIFESPAN CONSIDERATIONS

Pregnancy/Lactation: May cause fetal harm. Avoid pregnancy. Unknown if distributed in breast milk. Must either discontinue drug or discontinue breastfeeding. **Children:** Safety and efficacy not established. **Elderly:** May have increased risk of neurologic toxicities, including cognitive disorder, encephalopathy, confusion, seizure; serious infections, hepatic impairment.

INTERACTIONS

DRUG: May alter concentration of **medications with a narrow therapeutic index (e.g., cycloSPORINE, warfarin).** **HERBAL:** None significant. **FOOD:** None known. **LAB VALUES:** May decrease immunoglobulins, Hgb, Hct, neutrophils, leukocytes, platelets; serum albumin, magnesium, phosphate, potassium. May increase serum ALT, AST, bilirubin, GGT, glucose; body weight.

AVAILABILITY (Rx)

Injection, Lyophilized Powder for Reconstitution: 35 mcg/vial.

ADMINISTRATION/HANDLING

🖥 IV

• Hospitalization is recommended for the first 9 days of the first cycle and the first 2 days of the second cycle. For all subsequent cycle starts and reinitiation (e.g., if treatment is interrupted for 4 or more hrs), supervision by a health care professional or hospitalization is recommended. • Do not flush infusion line after administration, esp. when changing infusion bags. Flushing of infusion line can result in excess dosage and complications. • At end of infusion, any used solution in IV bag and IV lines should be disposed of in accordance with local requirements.

Premedication • Premedicate with dexamethasone 20 mg IV 1 hr prior to the first dose of each cycle, prior to step dose (such as cycle 1 on day 8), or when restarting an infusion after an interruption of 4 or more hrs.

Reconstitution • Reconstitution guidelines are highly specific. Infusion bags must be prepared by personnel trained in aseptic preparations and admixing of oncologic drugs following strict environmental specifications at a USP <797> compliant facility using ISO Class 5 laminar flow hood or better. • See manufacturer guidelines for details.

Rate of Administration • Administer as continuous IV infusion at a constant flow rate using an infusion pump. The pump should be programmable, lockable, nonelastomeric, and have an alarm. • Infusion bags should be infused over 24–48 hrs. Infuse the total 240-mL solution according to the instructions on the pharmacy label of the bag at one of the following constant rates: 10 mL/hr over 24 hrs, or 5 mL/hr over 48 hrs. • Infuse via dedicated line. • Use sterile, nonpyrogenic, low protein-binding, 0.2-micron in-line filter.

Storage • Refrigerate unused vials and IV solution stabilizer until time of use. • Protect from light. • Do not freeze. • Reconstituted vials may be stored at room temperature up to 4 hrs or refrigerated up to 24 hrs. • Prepared IV bag solutions may be stored at room temperature up to 48 hrs or refrigerated up to 8 days. • If prepared IV bag solution is not administered with the infusion time frame and temperature indicated, it must be discarded; do not refrigerate again.

INDICATIONS/ROUTES/DOSAGE

Note: See Administration/Handling.

Acute Lymphoblastic Leukemia (ALL)

IV: ADULTS, ELDERLY, CHILDREN: A treatment course consists of up to 2 cycles for induction followed by 3 additional cycles for consolidation and up to 4 additional cycles of continued therapy. Cycles 1–5 consist of 4 wks of continuous IV infusion followed by a 2-wk treatment-free interval. Cycles 6–9 consist of 4 wks of continuous IV infusion followed by an 8-wk treatment-free interval. **PTS WEIGHING 45 KG OR MORE:** (Induction cycle 1): Administer 9 mcg/day on days 1–7, then at 28 mcg/day on days 8–28 as continuous infusion. (Induction cycle 2, consolidation cycles 3–5, continued therapy cycles 6–9): Administer 28 mcg/day on days 1–28. **PTS WEIGHING LESS THAN 45 KG:** (Cycle 1): 5 mcg/m²/day (not to exceed 9 mcg/day) on days 1–7 and 15 mcg/m²/day (**Maximum:** 28 mcg/day) on days 8–28 as continuous infusion. (Induction cycle 2, consolidation cycles 3–5): Administer 15 mcg/m²/day (**Maximum:** 28 mcg/day) on days 1–28.

Dose Modification

(Based on Common Terminology Criteria for Adverse Events) **Note:** If interruption after an adverse event is no longer than 7 days, continue the same cycle to a total of 28 days of infusion inclusive of the days before and after the interruption in that cycle. If interruption due to an adverse event is longer than 7 days, start new cycle.

Cytokine Release Syndrome

CTCAE Grade 3: Withhold until resolved, then restart at 9 mcg/day. Increase dose to 28 mcg/day after 7 days if toxicity does not occur. **CTCAE Grade 4:** Permanently discontinue.

Neurological Toxicity

CTCAE Grade 3: Withhold until no more than Grade 1 for at least 3 days, then restart at 9 mcg/day. Increase dose to 28 mcg/day after 7 days if toxicity does not recur. If toxicity occurred at 9 mcg/day, or if toxicity takes more than 7 days to resolve, permanently discontinue. **CTCAE Grade 4:** Permanently discontinue.

Seizure

Permanently discontinue if more than one seizure occurs.

Other Clinically Relevant Adverse Reactions

CTCAE Grade 3: Withhold until no more than Grade 1, then restart at 9 mcg/day. Increase dose to 28 mcg/day after 7 days if toxicity does not recur. If toxicity takes more than 14 days to resolve, permanently discontinue. **CTCAE Grade 4:** Consider permanent discontinuation.

Elevated Hepatic Enzymes

Interrupt treatment if ALT/AST rise to greater than 5 times upper limit of normal (ULN) or bilirubin rises to more than 3 times ULN. Consider dose recommendation as listed in other clinically relevant adverse reactions or as ordered by prescriber.

Dosage in Renal Impairment

CrCl equal to or greater than 30 mL/min: No dose adjustment. **CrCl less than 30 mL/min or hemodialysis:** Not specified; use caution.

Dosage in Hepatic Impairment

Not specified; use caution. Hepatic toxicity during treatment: see dose modification.

SIDE EFFECTS

Frequent (62%–36%): Pyrexia, headache. **Occasional (25%–5%):** Peripheral edema, nausea, tremor, constipation, diarrhea, cough, fatigue, dyspnea, insomnia, chills, abdominal pain, dizziness, back pain, extremity pain, vomiting, bone pain, chest pain, decreased appetite, arthralgia, hypotension, hypertension, tachycardia, confusion, paresthesia. **Rare (4%–2%):** Aphasia, memory impairment.

ADVERSE EFFECTS/TOXIC REACTIONS

Myelosuppression (principally, anemia, leukopenia, neutropenia, thrombocytopenia) is an expected outcome of treatment. Cytokine release syndrome (CRS) may be life threatening or fatal. Symptoms of CRS may include asthenia, hypotension, nausea, pyrexia; elevated ALT/AST, bilirubin; disseminated intravascular coagulation (DIC), capillary leak syndrome, hemophagocytic lymphohistiocytosis/macrophage activation syndrome (HLH/MAS). Infusion reactions have occurred and may be clinically indistinguishable from CRS. Neurologic toxicities such as altered level of consciousness, balance disorders, confusion, disorientation encephalopathy, seizures, speech disorders, syncope occurred in approx. 50% of pts and may affect ability to drive or operate machinery. Median time to onset of neurologic toxicity was 7 days. CTCAE Grade 3 toxicities or higher occurred in 15% of pts. Serious infections such as opportunistic infections, bacterial/viral/fungal infections, sepsis, pneumonia, catheter-site infections occurred in 25% of pts. Other life-threatening or fatal events may include tumor lysis syndrome, neutropenia/febrile neutropenia, leukoencephalopathy. Medication preparation and administration errors have occurred, resulting in underdose or overdose. Immunogenicity (anti-blinatumomab antibodies) occurred in less than 1% of pts.

NURSING CONSIDERATIONS

BASELINE ASSESSMENT

Obtain baseline CBC, BMP, LFTs, serum magnesium, phosphate, ionized calcium, vital signs. Consider electrolyte correction before starting treatment. Screen for home medications requiring narrow therapeutic index. Screen for active infection, history of seizures, hepatic/renal impairment, cognitive disorders. Verify pregnancy status in women of childbearing

B

potential. Assess plans of breastfeeding. Conduct full neurologic assessment.

INTERVENTION/EVALUATION

Monitor CBC, LFTs, serum electrolytes (correct as indicated), vital signs. Monitor closely for cytokine release syndrome, neurologic toxicities, serious infection, tumor lysis syndrome, hepatic impairment. Keep area around IV site clean to reduce risk of infection. Do not adjust setting of infusion pump. Pump changes may result in dosing errors. Do not flush IV line after infusion completion. Initiate fall precautions. Monitor I&O.

PATIENT/FAMILY TEACHING

• Treatment may cause life-threatening side effects that must be immediately treated by medical personnel. • Report symptoms of cytokine release syndrome, such as chills, facial swelling, fever, low blood pressure, nausea, vomiting, weakness; any infusion-related reactions, such as difficulty breathing or skin rash. • Report any neurologic problems, such as confusion, difficulty speaking or slurred speech, loss of consciousness, loss of balance, or seizures. • Treatment may lower your white blood cell count and increase your risk of infection. Report any signs of infection, such as fever, cough, fatigue, or burning with urination. Keep area around IV catheter clean at all times to reduce risk of infection. • Do not change or alter settings on infusion pump, even if the pump alarm sounds. Any changes made to the infusion pump by anyone other than trained medical personnel can result in a dose that is too high or too low and may be life threatening. • Report symptoms of liver problems, such as bruising, confusion, dark or amber-colored urine, right upper abdominal pain, or yellowing of the skin or eyes. • Avoid tasks that require alertness, motor skills until response to drug is established. Do not drive or operate machinery. • Blood levels will be monitored routinely. • Hospitalization is required when starting therapy.

bortezomib

bor-**tez**-oh-mib
(<u>Velcade</u>)

◆CLASSIFICATION

PHARMACOTHERAPEUTIC: Protease inhibitor. **CLINICAL:** Antineoplastic.

USES

Treatment of relapsed or refractory mantle cell lymphoma. Treatment of multiple myeloma. **OFF-LABEL:** Treatment of Waldenström's macroglobulinemia; peripheral or cutaneous T-cell lymphoma; systemic light-chain amyloidosis.

PRECAUTIONS

Contraindications: Hypersensitivity to bortezomib, boron or mannitol; intrathecal administration. **Cautions:** Concomitant use of CYP3A4 inhibitors, history of syncope, concomitant use of antihypertensives; dehydration, diabetes, hepatic impairment, preexisting cardiac disease, neuropathy.

ACTION

Inhibits proteasomes (enzyme complexes regulating protein homeostasis within the cell). **Therapeutic Effect:** Produces cell-cycle arrest, apoptosis.

PHARMACOKINETICS

Widely distributed. Protein binding: 83%. Primarily metabolized by enzymatic action. Significant biliary excretion, with lesser amount excreted in urine. **Half-life:** 9–15 hrs.

⌛ LIFESPAN CONSIDERATIONS

Pregnancy/Lactation: May induce degenerative effects in ovary, degenerative changes in testes. May affect male/female fertility. Breastfeeding not recommended. **Children:** Safety and efficacy not established. **Elderly:** Increased incidence of Grade 3 or 4 thrombocytopenia.

INTERACTIONS

DRUG: CYP3A4 inhibitors (e.g., itraconazole, ketoconazole) may increase concentration/toxicity. **CYP3A4 inducers** (e.g., **rifAMPin**) may decrease concentration/effect (avoid use). **HERBAL: Green tea, green tea extracts** may diminish effect. **St. John's wort** may decrease level/effect. **FOOD: Grapefruit products** may increase concentration. **LAB VALUES:** May significantly decrease WBC, Hgb, Hct, platelet count, neutrophils.

AVAILABILITY (Rx)

Injection, Powder for Reconstitution: 3.5 mg.

ADMINISTRATION/HANDLING

 IV

Reconstitution • Reconstitute vial with 3.5 mL 0.9% NaCl to provide a concentration of 1 mg/mL.
Rate of Administration • Give as bolus IV injection over 3–5 sec.
Storage • Store unopened vials at room temperature. • Once reconstituted, solution may be stored at room temperature for up to 3 days or for 5 days if refrigerated.

Subcutaneous
Reconstitution • Reconstitute vial with 1.4 mL 0.9% NaCl to provide a concentration of 2.5 mg/mL.

INDICATIONS/ROUTES/DOSAGE

Mantle Cell Lymphoma (Initial Treatment)
IV: ADULTS, ELDERLY: 1.3 mg/m² days 1, 4, 8, 11 of a 21-day cycle for 6 cycles (in combination with riTUXimab, cyclophosphamide, DOXOrubicin, and predniSONE).

Mantle Cell Lymphoma (Relapsed)
IV: Subcutaneous: ADULTS, ELDERLY: Treatment cycle consists of 1.3 mg/m² twice wkly on days 1, 4, 8, and 11 for 2 wks of a 21-day treatment for 8 cycles. Therapy extending beyond 8 cycles may be given by standard schedule or given

once weekly for 4 wks followed by a 13-day rest period.

Multiple Myeloma (Initial Treatment)
IV: Subcutaneous: ADULTS, ELDERLY: (with melphalan and predniSONE) 1.3 mg/m² on days 1, 4, 8, 11, 22, 25, 29, 32 of a 42-day cycle for 4 cycles, then 1.3 mg/m² on days 1, 8, 22, 29 of a 42-day cycle for 5 cycles.

Multiple Myeloma (Relapsed)
IV, Subcutaneous: ADULTS, ELDERLY: 1.3 mg/m² twice wkly for 2 wks on days 1, 4, 8, 11 of a 21-day treatment cycle for 8 cycles. Therapy extending beyond 8 cycles may be given by standard schedule or given once weekly × 4 wks followed by a 13-day rest period.

Dosage Adjustment Guidelines
Withhold therapy at onset of CTCAE Grade 3 nonhematologic or Grade 4 hematologic toxicities, excluding neuropathy. When symptoms resolve, resume therapy at a 25% reduced dosage.

Dosage Adjustment Guidelines with Neuropathic Pain, Peripheral Sensory Neuropathy
For CTCAE Grade 1 toxicity with pain or Grade 2 (interfering with function but not activities of daily living [ADL]), 1 mg/m². For Grade 2 toxicity with pain or Grade 3 (interfering with ADL), withhold drug until toxicity is resolved, then reinitiate with 0.7 mg/m². For Grade 4 toxicity (permanent sensory loss that interferes with function), discontinue bortezomib.

Dosage in Renal Impairment
No dose adjustment.

Dosage in Hepatic Impairment
Mild impairment: No initial adjustment. **Moderate (bilirubin greater than 1.5–3 times upper limit of normal [ULN]) to severe (bilirubin greater than 3 times ULN) impairment:** Decrease initial dose to 0.7 mg/m² (based on tolerance may increase to 1 mg/m² or decrease to 0.5 mg/m²).

SIDE EFFECTS

Expected (65%–36%): Fatigue, malaise, asthenia, nausea, diarrhea, anorexia, constipation, fever, vomiting. **Frequent (28%–21%):** Headache, insomnia, arthralgia, limb pain, edema, paresthesia, dizziness, rash. **Occasional (18%–11%):** Dehydration, cough, anxiety, bone pain, muscle cramps, myalgia, back pain, abdominal pain, taste alteration, dyspepsia, pruritus, hypotension (including orthostatic hypotension), rigors, blurred vision.

ADVERSE EFFECTS/TOXIC REACTIONS

Thrombocytopenia occurs in 40% of pts. GI, intracerebral hemorrhage are associated with drug-induced thrombocytopenia. Anemia occurs in 32% of pts. New onset or worsening of existing neuropathy occurs in 37% of pts. Symptoms may improve in some pts upon drug discontinuation. Pneumonia occurs occasionally.

NURSING CONSIDERATIONS

BASELINE ASSESSMENT

Obtain baseline CBC. Ensure adequate hydration prior to initiation of therapy. Antiemetics, antidiarrheals may be effective in preventing, treating nausea, vomiting, diarrhea.

INTERVENTION/EVALUATION

Routinely assess B/P; monitor pt for orthostatic hypotension. Maintain strict I&O. Monitor CBC, esp. platelet count, throughout treatment. Monitor renal, hepatic, pulmonary function throughout therapy. Encourage adequate fluid intake to prevent dehydration. Monitor temperature and be alert to high potential for fever. Monitor for peripheral neuropathy (burning sensation, neuropathic pain, paresthesia, hyperesthesia). Avoid IM injections, rectal temperatures, other traumas that may induce bleeding.

PATIENT/FAMILY TEACHING

• Report new/worsening vomiting, bruising/bleeding, breathing difficulties.
• Discuss importance of pregnancy testing, avoidance of pregnancy, measures to prevent pregnancy. • Increase fluid intake. • Avoid tasks that require mental alertness, motor skills until response to drug is established.

bosutinib

boe-**sue**-ti-nib
(Bosulif)

◆CLASSIFICATION

PHARMACOTHERAPEUTIC: Tyrosine kinase inhibitor. **CLINICAL:** Antineoplastic.

USES

Treatment of chronic, accelerated, or blast phase Philadelphia chromosome–positive chronic myelogenous leukemia (CML) with resistance or intolerance to prior therapy.

PRECAUTIONS

Contraindications: Hypersensitivity to bosutinib. **Cautions:** Baseline anemia, thrombocytopenia, neutropenia; hepatic impairment, recent diarrhea, pulmonary edema, HF, fluid retention. Pts with history of pancreatitis, moderate to severe renal impairment. Avoid concurrent use of CYP3A4 inducers/inhibitors.

ACTION

Inhibits Bcr-Abl tyrosine kinase, a translocation-created enzyme, created by the Philadelphia chromosome abnormality noted in chronic myelogenous leukemia (CML). Inhibits Src-family kinase, including Src, Lyn, and Hck. **Therapeutic Effect:** Inhibits tumor cell growth and proliferation in chronic, accelerated, or blast phase CML.

PHARMACOKINETICS

Well absorbed following oral administration. Protein binding: 94%. Metabolized in liver. Excreted in feces (91%), urine (3%). **Half-life:** 22.5 hrs.

⌛ LIFESPAN CONSIDERATIONS

Pregnancy/Lactation: Potential for embryo/fetal toxicity. Avoid pregnancy. Must use effective contraception during treatment and for at least 30 days after treatment. Unknown if distributed in breast milk. Avoid breastfeeding. **Children:** Safety and efficacy not established in pts younger than 18 yrs. **Elderly:** No age-related precautions noted.

INTERACTIONS

DRUG: Strong **CYP3A inhibitors and/ or P-glycoprotein (P-gp) inhibitors** (e.g., clarithromycin, ketoconazole, ritonavir, miSOPROStol, nafcillin, salmeterol), moderate **CYP3A4 inhibitors** (e.g., ciprofloxacin, diltiaZEM, erythromycin, verapamil) may increase concentration/effect. Strong **CYP3A4 inducers** (e.g., rifAMPin, phenytoin, PHENobarbital) and moderate **CYP3A4 inducers** (e.g., bosentan, nafcillin, modafinil) may decrease concentration/ effect. **Proton pump inhibitors** (e.g., omeprazole, pantoprazole) may reduce absorption, concentration. **HERBAL:** St. John's wort may decrease effectiveness. **FOOD: Grapefruit products** may decrease bosutinib concentration. **LAB VALUES:** May decrease Hgb, platelets, WBCs, serum phosphorous. May increase serum ALT, AST, bilirubin, lipase.

AVAILABILITY (Rx)

🔖 **Tablets:** 100 mg, 500 mg.

ADMINISTRATION/HANDLING

PO
- Give with food. Do not break, crush, dissolve, or divide tablets.

INDICATIONS/ROUTES/DOSAGE

Chronic Myelogenous Leukemia (CML)
PO: ADULTS, ELDERLY: 500 mg once daily with food. If complete hematologic response not achieved by wk 8 or complete cytogenetic response not achieved by wk 12, in absence of grade 3 or higher adverse reactions, may increase to 600 mg once daily.

CML with Baseline Renal Impairment
CrCl less than 30 mL/min: 300 mg once daily. **CrCl 30–50 mL/min:** 400 mg once daily.

CML with Baseline Hepatic Impairment
PO: ADULTS: 200 mg once daily with food.

Dosage Modification
Hepatotoxicity: Withhold treatment until serum ALT, AST less than or equal to 2.5 times ULN. Then, resume at 400 mg once daily with food. Discontinue if recovery lasts longer than 4 wks or hepatotoxicity, including elevated serum bilirubin levels greater than 2 times ULN. **Severe diarrhea:** Withhold until recovery to low-grade diarrhea. Then, resume at 400 mg once daily with food. **Myelosuppression:** Withhold until absolute neutrophil count greater than 1000 cells/ mm³ and platelet count greater than 50,000 cells/mm³. Then, resume at same dose if recovery occurs within 2 wks. May reduce dose to 400 mg for recovery lasting greater than 2 wks.

SIDE EFFECTS

Frequent (82%–35%): Diarrhea, nausea, vomiting, abdominal pain, rash. **Occasional (26%–10%):** Pyrexia, fatigue, headache, cough, peripheral edema, arthralgia, anorexia, upper respiratory infection, asthenia, back pain, nasopharyngitis, dizziness, pruritus.

ADVERSE EFFECTS/TOXIC REACTIONS

Severe fluid retention may result in pleural effusion, pericardial effusion, pulmonary edema, ascites. Neutropenia, thrombocytopenia, anemia is an expected response of drug therapy. Severe diarrhea may result in fluid loss, electrolyte imbalance, hypotension. Hepatotoxicity occurred in 7%–9% of pts.

NURSING CONSIDERATIONS

BASELINE ASSESSMENT

Offer emotional support. Assess baseline weight, BMP, LFT. Confirm negative pregnancy test before initiating treatment. Obtain full medication history, including vitamins, herbal products. Screen for peripheral edema, signs/symptoms of HF, anemia.

INTERVENTION/EVALUATION

Weigh daily and monitor for unexpected rapid weight gain, edema. Monitor for changes in serum electrolytes, LFT during treatment. Offer antiemetics for nausea, vomiting. Monitor daily pattern of bowel activity, stool consistency. Monitor CBC for neutropenia, thrombocytopenia, anemia. Assess for bruising, hematuria, jaundice, right upper abdominal pain, weight loss, or acute infection (fever, diaphoresis, lethargy, productive cough).

PATIENT/FAMILY TEACHING

• Blood levels will be drawn routinely.
• Take with meals. • Drink plenty of fluids (diarrhea may result in dehydration).
• Swallow whole; do not break, chew, crush, dissolve, or divide tablets. • Strictly avoid pregnancy. • Use contraception during treatment and for at least 30 days after treatment. • Report urine changes, bloody or clay-colored stools, upper abdominal pain, nausea, vomiting, bruising, persistent diarrhea, fever, cough, difficulty breathing, chest pain. • Immediately report any newly prescribed medications. • Avoid alcohol, grapefruit products. • Discuss using antacids for indigestion, heartburn, upset stomach (omeprazole, lansoprazole, pantoprazole may reduce absorption, concentration of bosutinib). • Separate antacid dosing by more than 2 hrs before and after medication.

brentuximab vedotin

bren-**tux**-i-mab ve-**doe**-tin
(Adcetris)
■ **BLACK BOX ALERT** ■ JC virus infection resulting in progressive multifocal leukoencephalopathy and death can occur.

◆CLASSIFICATION

PHARMACOTHERAPEUTIC: Monoclonal antibody, antimitotic. **CLINICAL:** Antineoplastic.

USES

Treatment of relapsed or refractory Hodgkin's lymphoma after failure of autologous hematopoietic stem cell transplant (HSCT) or after failure of at least two prior multiagent chemotherapy regimens in pts who are not transplant candidates. Treatment of systemic anaplastic large-cell lymphoma (ALCL) after failure of at least one prior multiagent chemotherapy regimen.

PRECAUTIONS

Contraindications: Hypersensitivity to brentuximab. Avoid use with bleomycin (increased risk for pulmonary toxicity). **Cautions:** Renal/hepatic impairment, peripheral neuropathy, infusion reactions, neutropenia, tumor lysis syndrome, Stevens-Johnson syndrome, pregnancy.

ACTION

Binds to CD30-expressing cells, allowing the antibody to direct the drug to a target on lymphoma cells, disrupting the microtubule network within the cell. **Therapeutic Effect:** Induces cell cycle arrest, cell death.

PHARMACOKINETICS

Minimally metabolized. Protein binding: 68%–82%. Excreted primarily in feces (72%). **Half-life:** 4–6 days.

⧖ LIFESPAN CONSIDERATIONS

Pregnancy/Lactation: May cause fetal harm (embryo-fetal toxicities). Unknown if distributed in breast milk. **Children:** Safety and efficacy not established. **Elderly:** Safety and efficacy not established.

INTERACTIONS

DRUG: Strong CYP3A4 inhibitors (e.g., atazanavir, clarithromycin, ketoconazole) increase concentration/effect. **CYP3A4 inducers (e.g., rifAMPin)** may reduce concentration/effect. **FOOD:** None known. **HERBAL: Echinacea** may decrease effect. **LAB VALUES:** May decrease Hgb, Hct, WBC, RBC, platelets. May increase serum bicarbonate, lactate dehydrogenase, glucose, albumin, magnesium, sodium.

AVAILABILITY (Rx)

Injection, Powder for Reconstitution: 50-mg single-use vial.

ADMINISTRATION/HANDLING

 IV

Reconstitution • Reconstitute each 50-mg vial with 10.5 mL Sterile Water for Injection, directing the stream toward wall of vial and not at powder. • Gently swirl (do not shake). • This will yield a concentration of 5 mg/mL. • The dose for pts weighing over 100 kg should be calculated for 100 kg. • Reconstituted solution must be transferred to infusion bag with a minimum 100 mL diluent, yielding a final concentration of 0.4–1.8 mg/mL brentuximab. • Gently invert bag to mix solution. **Rate of Administration** • Infuse over 30 min.

Storage • Discard if solution contains particulate or is discolored; solution should appear clear to slightly opalescent, colorless. • May store solution at 36°–46°F. • Use within 24 hrs after reconstitution.

⧖ IV COMPATIBILITIES

0.9% NaCl, D₅W, lactated Ringer's.

INDICATIONS/ROUTES/DOSAGE

◀**ALERT**▶ Do not give by IV bolus or IV push.

Hodgkin's Lymphoma (Relapsed or Refractory)
IV Infusion: ADULTS, ELDERLY: 1.8 mg/kg (**Maximum:** 180 mg) infused over 30 min every 3 wks. Continue treatment until disease progression or unacceptable toxicity.

Hodgkin's Lymphoma (After HSCT)
IV Infusion: ADULTS/ELDERLY: 1.8 mg/kg (**Maximum:** 180 mg) infused over 30 min every 3 wks. Continue treatment until a maximum of 16 cycles, disease progression, or unacceptable toxicity occurs. Begin within 4–6 wks post HSCT or upon recovery from HSCT.

Systemic Anaplastic Large-Cell Lymphoma
IV Infusion: ADULTS/ELDERLY: 1.8 mg/kg (**Maximum:** 180 mg) infused over 30 min every 3 wks. Continue treatment until disease progression or unacceptable toxicity occurs.

Dosage in Renal Impairment
CrCl less than 30 mL/min: Avoid use.

Dosage in Hepatic Impairment
Mild impairment: Initial dose 1.2 mg/kg (**Maximum:** 120 mg) q3wks. **Moderate to Severe impairment:** Avoid use.

SIDE EFFECTS

◀**ALERT**▶ Effects present as mild, manageable.
Frequent (52%–22%): Peripheral neuropathy, fatigue, respiratory tract infection, nausea, diarrhea, fever, rash, abdominal pain, cough, vomiting. **Occasional (19%–11%):** Headache, dizziness, constipation, chills, bone/muscle pain, insomnia, peripheral edema, alopecia. **Rare (10%–5%):** Anxiety, muscle spasm, decreased appetite, dry skin.

ADVERSE EFFECTS/TOXIC REACTIONS

Myelosuppression characterized as neutropenia (54% of pts), peripheral neuropathy (52% of pts), thrombocytopenia (28% of pts), anemia (19% of pts) have occurred. Infusion reactions (including anaphylaxis), Stevens-Johnson syndrome have been reported. Tumor lysis syndrome may lead to acute renal failure. Progressive multifocal leukoencephalopathy (changes in mood, confusion, loss of memory, decreased strength or weakness on one side of body, changes in speech, walking, and vision) has been reported.

NURSING CONSIDERATIONS

BASELINE ASSESSMENT

Obtain baseline CBC before treatment begins and as needed to monitor response and toxicity but particularly prior to each dosing cycle. Question for evidence of peripheral neuropathy (hypoesthesia, hyperesthesia, paresthesia, burning sensation, neuropathic pain or weakness). Pts experiencing new or worsening neuropathy may require a delay, dose change, or discontinuation of treatment.

INTERVENTION/EVALUATION

Offer antiemetics to control nausea, vomiting. Monitor for hematologic toxicity (fever, sore throat, signs of local infection, bruising, unusual bleeding), symptoms of anemia (excessive fatigue, weakness). Assess response to medication. Monitor and report nausea, vomiting, diarrhea. Monitor daily pattern of bowel activity, stool consistency. Assess skin for evidence of rash.

PATIENT/FAMILY TEACHING

• Avoid crowds, persons with known infections. • Report signs of infection at once (fever, flu-like symptoms). • Avoid contact with those who recently received live virus vaccine. • Do not receive immunizations without physician's approval (drug lowers body resistance).

• Promptly report fever, easy bruising or unusual bleeding from any site. • Male pts should be warned of potential risk to their reproductive capacities.

---

brexpiprazole

brex-**pip**-ra-zole
(Rexulti)

■ **BLACK BOX ALERT** ■ Elderly pts with dementia-related psychosis are at increased risk of death, mainly due to HF, pneumonia. Increased risk of suicidal thoughts and behaviors in patients aged 24 yrs and younger with major depression, other psychiatric disorders. **Do not confuse brexpiprazole with ARIPiprazole, esomeprazole, omeprazole, or pantoprazole, or RABEprazole.**

◆CLASSIFICATION

PHARMACOTHERAPEUTIC: DOPamine agonist. **CLINICAL:** Antipsychotic agent.

USES

Adjunctive therapy to antidepressants for the treatment of major depressive disorder. Treatment of schizophrenia.

PRECAUTIONS

Contraindications: Hypersensitivity to brexpiprazole. **Cautions:** Concurrent use of CNS depressants (including alcohol) antihypertensives, disorders in which CNS depression is a feature, cardiovascular or cerebrovascular disease (may induce hypotension), Parkinson's disease, Parkinson's disease dementia, Lewy body dementia, history of seizures or conditions that may lower seizure threshold (Alzheimer's disease). Pts at risk for aspiration pneumonia, elderly, HF, diabetes. Pts at high risk for suicide. Preexisting low WBC/ANC, history of drug-induced leukopenia/neutropenia, dehydration.

ACTION

Exact mechanism of action unknown. Provides partial agonist activity at DOPamine and serotonin (5-HT$_1$A) receptors and antagonist activity at serotonin (5-HT$_2$A) receptors. **Therapeutic Effect:** Diminishes schizophrenic, depressive behavior.

PHARMACOKINETICS

Widely distributed. Metabolized in liver. Protein binding: greater than 99%. Peak plasma concentration: 4 hrs. Steady state reached in 10–12 days. Excreted in urine (25%), feces (46%). **Half-life:** 86–91 hrs.

⧗ LIFESPAN CONSIDERATIONS

Pregnancy/Lactation: Unknown if distributed in breast milk. May cause extrapyramidal and/or withdrawal symptoms in neonates if given in third trimester. **Children:** Safety and efficacy not established. **Elderly:** May have increased risk for adverse effects due to age-related hepatic, renal, cardiac disease. May increase risk of death in elderly pts with dementia-related psychosis.

INTERACTIONS

DRUG: Alcohol may potentiate cognitive and motor effects. **Strong CYP3A4 inducers (e.g., carBAMazepine, rifAMPin)** may decrease concentration/effect. **Strong CYP3A4 inhibitors (e.g., itraconazole, ketoconazole), strong CYP2D6 inhibitors (e.g., FLUoxetine, PARoxetine)** may increase concentration/effect. **HERBAL: St John's wort** may decrease concentration. **Gotu kola, kava kava, St John's wort, valerian** may increase CNS depression. **FOOD:** None known. **LAB VALUES:** May decrease leukocytes, neutrophils. May increase serum blood glucose, lipid levels.

AVAILABILITY (Rx)

Tablets: 0.25 mg, 0.5 mg, 1 mg, 2 mg, 3 mg, 4 mg.

ADMINISTRATION/HANDLING

PO
• Give without regard to food.

INDICATIONS/ROUTES/DOSAGE

Major Depressive Disorder (MDD)
PO: ADULTS, ELDERLY: Initially, 0.5–1 mg once daily. May increase at weekly intervals, to 1 mg once daily, then up to target dose of 2 mg once daily. **Maximum:** 3 mg once daily.

Schizophrenia
PO: ADULTS, ELDERLY: Initially, 1 mg once daily on days 1–4. May increase to 2 mg once daily on days 5–7, then to 4 mg once daily on day 8 based on clinical response and tolerability. **Maximum:** 4 mg once daily.

Dose Modification
Renal Impairment (CrCl less than 60 mL/min)
Maximum: 2 mg once daily for MDD, or 3 mg once daily for schizophrenia.
Hepatic Impairment
Maximum recommended dose: 2 mg once daily for MDD, or 3 mg once daily for schizophrenia.
CYP2D6 Poor Metabolizers or Pts Taking Strong CYP2D6 Inhibitors or Strong CYP3A4 Inhibitors
Administer half of the usual dose.
CYP2D6 Poor Metabolizers Taking Strong/Moderate CYP3A4 Inhibitors or Pts Taking Strong/Moderate CYP2D6 Inhibitors with Strong/Moderate CYP3A4 Inhibitors
Administer a quarter of the usual dose.
Pts Taking Strong CYP3A4 Inducers
Double the usual dose over 1–2 wks.

SIDE EFFECTS

Occasional (9%–4%): Headache, nasopharyngitis, dyspepsia, akathisia, somnolence, tremor. **Rare (3%–1%):** Constipation, fatigue, increased appetite, weight gain, anxiety, restlessness, dizziness, diarrhea, blurry vision, dry mouth, salivary hypersecretion, abdominal pain, flatulence, myalgia, abnormal dreams, insomnia, hyperhidrosis.

 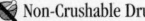

ADVERSE EFFECTS/TOXIC REACTIONS

May increase risk of death in elderly pts with dementia-related psychosis. Most deaths appeared to be cardiovascular (e.g., HF, sudden death) or infectious (e.g., pneumonia) in nature. Increased incidence of suicidal thoughts and behaviors in pts 24 yrs and younger was reported. May increase risk of neuroleptic malignant syndrome (NMS). Symptoms of NMS may include hyperpyrexia, muscle rigidity, altered mental status, autonomic instability (irregular pulse or blood pressure, tachycardia, diaphoresis, and cardiac dysrhythmia), elevated creatinine, phosphokinase, myoglobinuria (rhabdomyolysis), acute renal failure. Metabolic changes such as hyperglycemia, ketoacidosis, hyperosmolar coma, diabetes, dyslipidemia, dystonia, and weight gain may occur. Other adverse effects may include leukopenia, neutropenia, agranulocytosis, orthostatic hypotension, syncope, cerebrovascular events (e.g., CVA, transient ischemic attack), seizures, hyperthermia, dysphagia, cognitive or motor impairment, tardive dyskinesia.

NURSING CONSIDERATIONS

BASELINE ASSESSMENT

Obtain baseline BMP, capillary blood glucose, vital signs; CBC in pts with preexisting low WBC or history of leukopenia or neutropenia. Receive full medication history and screen for drug interactions. Assess behavior, appearance, emotional state, response to environment, speech pattern, thought content. Correct dehydration, hypovolemia. Assess for suicidal tendencies, history of dementia-related psychosis, HF, CVA, NMS, diabetes.

INTERVENTION/EVALUATION

Monitor weight, BMP, capillary blood glucose, vital signs. Diligently monitor for extrapyramidal symptoms, tardive dyskinesia, hypotension, syncope, cerebrovascular or cardiovascular dysfunction, NMS. Assess for therapeutic response (greater interest in surroundings, improved self-care, increased ability to concentrate, relaxed facial expression).

PATIENT/FAMILY TEACHING

• Avoid alcohol. • Avoid tasks that require alertness, motor skills until response to drug is established. • Report worsening depression, suicidal ideation, usual changes in behavior. • Treatment may cause life-threatening conditions such as involuntary, uncontrollable movements; elevated body temperature, altered mental status, high or low blood pressure, seizures. • Pts with HF or active pneumonia are at increased risk of sudden death. • Immediately report fever, cough, increased sputum production, palpitations, fainting, or signs of HF.

brigatinib

bri-**ga**-ti-nib
(Alunbrig)
Do not confuse brigatinib with axitinib, cabozantinib, ceritinib, crizotinib, erlotinib, imatinib.

◆CLASSIFICATION

PHARMACOTHERAPEUTIC: Tyrosine kinase inhibitor. **CLINICAL:** Antineoplastic.

USES

Treatment of pts with anaplastic lymphoma kinase (ALK)-positive metastatic non–small-cell lung cancer (NSCLC) who have progressed or are intolerant to crizotinib.

PRECAUTIONS

Contraindications: Hypersensitivity to brigatinib. **Cautions:** Baseline anemia, leukopenia. History of symptomatic bradycardia, bradyarrhythmias, diabetes, hepatic/renal impairment, hypertension, ocular disease, pancreatitis, pulmonary disease. Concomitant use of strong CYP3A inhibitors, beta blockers, calcium channel blockers (see Interactions).

ACTION

A broad-spectrum kinase inhibitor (activity against ALK, ROSI, IGF-1R and FLT-3). Inhibits ALK downstream signaling proteins. Has activity against cells expressing EML4-ALK. **Therapeutic Effect:** Expresses anti-tumor activity against EML-ALK; mutant forms shown in NSCLC in pts progressed with crizotinib.

PHARMACOKINETICS

Widely distributed. Metabolized in liver. Protein binding: 66%. Peak plasma concentration: 1–4 hrs. Excreted in feces (65%), urine (25%). **Half-life:** 25 hrs.

⧖ LIFESPAN CONSIDERATIONS

Pregnancy/Lactation: Avoid pregnancy; may cause fetal harm. Females of reproductive potential should use effective nonhormonal contraception during treatment and for at least 4 mos after discontinuation. Unknown if distributed in breast milk. Breastfeeding not recommended during treatment and for at least 1 wk after discontinuation. **Males:** Males with female partners of reproductive potential should use barrier methods during sexual activity during treatment for at least 3 mos after discontinuation. **Children:** Safety and efficacy not established. **Elderly:** No age-related precautions noted.

INTERACTIONS

DRUG: Strong CYP3A4 inhibitors (e.g., clarithromycin, itraconazole, ritonavir) may increase concentration/effect. **Strong CYP3A4 inducers (e.g., carbamazepine, phenytoin, rifampin)** may decrease concentration/effect. May decrease effectiveness of hormonal contraceptives. Concomitant use of **beta blockers (e.g., atenolol,** **carvedilol, metoprolol), calcium channel blockers (e.g., diltiazem, verapamil), digoxin** may increase risk of symptomatic bradycardia. **HERBAL: St. John's wort** may decrease concentration/effect. **FOOD: Grapefruit products** may increase concentration/effect. **LAB VALUES:** May increase serum alkaline phosphatase, ALT, AST, amylase, bilirubin, CPK, glucose, lipase. May decrease Hct, Hgb, lymphocytes, RBCs; serum phosphate. May prolong aPTT.

AVAILABILITY (Rx)

Tablets: 30 mg, 90 mg.

ADMINISTRATION/HANDLING

PO
• Give with or without food. • Administer tablets whole; do not break, crush, cut, or divide. • If a dose is missed or vomiting occurs after administration, do not give extra dose. Administer next dose at regularly scheduled time.

INDICATIONS/ROUTES/DOSAGE

Non–Small-Cell Lung Cancer
PO: ADULTS, ELDERLY: 90 mg once daily for 7 days. If 90-mg dose is tolerated, then increase to 180 mg once daily. Continue until disease progression or unacceptable toxicity. If treatment is interrupted for 14 days (or more) for reasons other than toxic reactions, restart at 90 mg once daily for 7 days before increasing to the dose that was previously tolerated.

Dose Reduction Schedule
First dose reduction: 90 mg once daily: Reduce to 60 mg once daily. **180 mg once daily:** Reduce to 120 mg once daily. **Second dose reduction: 90 mg once daily:** Permanently discontinue. **180 mg once daily:** Reduce to 90 mg once daily. **Third dose reduction: 90 mg once daily:** N/A. **180 mg once daily:** Reduce to 60 mg once daily. **Note:** Once dose has been reduced, do not subsequently increase dose. If pt is unable to tolerate 60-mg dose, permanently discontinue.

Dose Modification
Symptomatic Bradycardia
Withhold treatment until recovery to asymptomatic bradycardia or to a heart rate of 60 bpm or greater, then resume at reduced dose level (if pt not taking concomitant medications known to cause bradycardia). **Symptomatic bradycardia in pts taking concomitant medications known to cause bradycardia:** Withhold treatment until recovery to asymptomatic bradycardia or heart rate of 60 bpm or greater. If concomitant medication can be adjusted or discontinued, then resume at same dose. If concomitant medication cannot be adjusted or discontinued, then resume at reduced dose level. **Life-threatening bradycardia in pts who are not taking concomitant medications known to cause bradycardia:** Permanently discontinue. **Life-threatening bradycardia in pts who are taking concomitant medications known to cause bradycardia:** Withhold treatment until recovery to asymptomatic bradycardia or heart rate of 60 bpm or greater. If concomitant medication can be adjusted or discontinued, then resume at reduced dose level with frequent monitoring. Permanently discontinue if symptomatic bradycardia recurs despite dose reduction.

CPK Elevation
CTCAE grade 3 CPK elevation (greater than 5 times upper limit of normal [ULN]): Withhold treatment until recovery to baseline or less than or equal to 2.5 times ULN, then resume at same dose. **CTCAE grade 4 CPK elevation (greater than 10 times ULN) or recurrence of CTCAE grade 3 CPK elevation:** Withhold treatment until recovery to baseline or less than or equal to 2.5 times ULN, then resume at reduced dose level.

Hyperglycemia
CTCAE grade 3 serum glucose elevation (greater than 250 mg/dL or 13.9 mmol/L): If adequate medical management of hyperglycemia cannot be achieved, withhold treatment until

adequately controlled. Consider dose reduction or permanent discontinuation.

Hypertension
CTCAE grade 3 hypertension (systolic BP greater than or equal to 160 mm Hg or diastolic BP greater than or equal to 100 mm Hg); concomitant use of more than one antihypertensive drug; required medical intervention; requirement of aggressive hypertensive therapy: Withhold treatment until recovery to grade 1 or 0, then resume at reduced dose level. **CTCAE grade 4 hypertension (first occurrence) or recurrence of grade 3 hypertension:** Withhold treatment until recovery to grade 1 or 0, then either resume at reduced dose level or permanently discontinue. **Recurrence of grade 4 hypertension:** Permanently discontinue.

Lipase/Amylase Elevation
CTCAE grade 3 serum amylase or lipase elevation (greater than 2 times upper limit of normal [ULN]): Withhold treatment until recovery to grade 1 or 0 (or baseline), then resume at same dose. **CTCAE grade 4 serum amylase or lipase elevation (greater than 5 times ULN) or recurrence of grade 3 serum lipase or amylase elevation:** Withhold treatment until recovery to grade 1 or 0, then resume at reduced dose level.

Pulmonary
CTCAE grade 1 pulmonary symptoms during the first 7 days of therapy: Withhold treatment until recovery to baseline, then resume at same dose level. Do not increase dose if interstitial lung disease (ILD)/pneumonitis suspected. **CTCAE grade 1 pulmonary symptoms after the first 7 days of therapy:** Withhold treatment until recovery to baseline, then resume at same dose level. **CTCAE grade 2 pulmonary symptoms during the first 7 days of therapy:** Withhold treatment until recovery to baseline, then resume at reduced dose level. Do not increase dose if ILD/pneumonitis suspected. **CTCAE grade 2 pulmonary symptoms after**

the first 7 days of therapy: Withhold treatment until recovery to baseline, then resume at same dose level. If ILD/pneumonitis is suspected, resume at reduced dose level. With any recurrence of ILD/pneumonitis or any grade 3 or 4 pulmonary symptoms, permanently discontinue.

Visual Disturbance
CTCAE grade 2 or 3 visual disturbance: Withhold treatment until recovery to baseline, then resume at reduced dose level. **Grade 4 visual disturbance:** Permanently discontinue.

Other Toxicities
Any other CTCAE grade 3 toxicity: Withhold treatment until recovery to baseline, then resume at same dose level. **Recurrence of any other grade 3 toxicity:** Withhold treatment until recovery to baseline, then either resume at reduced dose level or permanently discontinue. **First occurrence of any other CTCAE grade 4 toxicity:** Withhold treatment until recovery to baseline, then either resume at reduced dose level or permanently discontinue. **Recurrence of any other grade 4 toxicity:** Permanently discontinue.
Concomitant use of strong CYP3A inhibitors: Reduce daily dose by 50% if strong CYP3A inhibitor cannot be discontinued. If strong CYP3A inhibitor is discontinued, then resume the dose that was previously tolerated before starting CYP3A inhibitor.

Dosage in Renal Impairment
Mild to moderate impairment: No dose adjustment. **Severe impairment:** Not specified; use caution.

Dosage in Hepatic Impairment
Mild impairment: No dose adjustment. **Moderate to severe impairment:** Not specified; use caution.

SIDE EFFECTS

Frequent (33%–19%): Nausea, fatigue, headache, dyspnea, vomiting, decreased appetite, diarrhea, constipation. **Occasional (18%–9%):** Cough, abdominal pain, rash (acneiform dermatitis, exfoliative rash, pruritic rash, pustular rash),

pyrexia, arthralgia, peripheral neuropathy, muscle spasm, extremity pain, hypertension, back pain, myalgia.

ADVERSE EFFECTS/TOXIC REACTIONS

Anemia, leukopenia are expected responses to therapy. Serious events, such as ILD/pneumonitis (3%–9% of pts), hypertension (6%–21% of pts), symptomatic bradycardia (6%–7% of pts), visual disturbance (blurred vision, diplopia, reduced visual acuity, macular edema, vitreous floaters, visual field defect, vitreous detachment, cataract [7%–10% of pts]), CPK elevation (27%–48% of pts), pancreatic enzyme elevation (27%–39%), hyperglycemia (43% of pts), may occur.

NURSING CONSIDERATIONS

BASELINE ASSESSMENT
Obtain baseline CBC, CPK, BMP, LFT; urine pregnancy, vital signs. Obtain baseline EKG in pts with history of arrhythmia, HF. Question plans for breastfeeding. Question history of hepatic/renal impairment, diabetes, cardiac/pulmonary disease, hypertension, pancreatitis. Receive full medication history and screen for interactions. Assess visual acuity. Verify ALK-positive NSCLC test prior to initiation. Obtain nutritional consult. Offer emotional support.

INTERVENTION/EVALUATION
Monitor CBC, CPK, BMP, LFT; vital signs (esp. heart rate) periodically. Obtain serum amylase, lipase in pts with severe abdominal pain, nausea, periumbilical ecchymosis (Cullen's sign), flank ecchymosis (Grey Turner's sign). Monitor for hepatotoxicity, hyperglycemia, vision changes, myalgia, musculoskeletal pain, interstitial lung disease/pneumonitis. If treatment-related toxicities occur, consider referral to specialist; pt may require treatment with corticosteroids. Screen for acute infections. Monitor I&O, hydration status, stool frequency and consistency. Encourage proper calorie intake and nutrition. Assess skin for rash, lesions.

PATIENT/FAMILY TEACHING

• Treatment may depress your immune system and reduce your ability to fight infection. Report symptoms of infection, such as body aches, burning with urination, chills, cough, fatigue, fever. Avoid those with active infection. • Therapy may decrease your heart rate, which may be life-threatening; report dizziness, chest pain, palpitations, or fainting. • Worsening cough, fever, or shortness of breath may indicate severe lung inflammation. • Avoid pregnancy. Do not breastfeed. Females of childbearing potential should use effective contraception during treatment and up to 4 mos after final dose. Males with female partners of reproductive potential should use condoms during sexual activity during treatment and for up to 3 mos after final dose. • Blurry vision, confusion, frequent urination, increased thirst, fruity breath may indicate high blood sugar levels. • Report abdominal pain, bruising around belly button or flank bruising, black/tarry stools, dark-colored urine, decreased urine output, severe muscle aches, yellowing of the skin or eyes. • Do not take newly prescribed medication unless approved by the doctor who originally started treatment. • Do not ingest grapefruit products.

---

brivaracetam

briv-a-ra-se-tam
(Briviact, Brivlera ✦)
Do not confuse brivaracetam with levETIRAcetam.

◆CLASSIFICATION

PHARMACOTHERAPEUTIC: Synaptic vesicle protein 2A ligand. **CLINICAL:** Anticonvulsant.

USES

Monotherapy or adjunctive therapy in the treatment of partial-onset seizures in pts 16 years and older with epilepsy.

PRECAUTIONS

Contraindications: Hypersensitivity to brivaracetam. **Cautions:** Baseline neutropenia, hepatic impairment; pts at high risk for suicide; history of depression, mood disorder, psychiatric disorder; history of drug abuse.

ACTION

Exact mechanism unknown. Binds to synaptic proteins that modulate neurotransmitter release in the brain. **Therapeutic Effect:** Prevents seizure activity.

PHARMACOKINETICS

Rapidly, completely absorbed following PO administration. Metabolized primarily by enzymatic hydrolysis, mediated by hepatic and extrahepatic amidase. Protein binding: less than or equal to 20%. Peak plasma concentration: 1 hr. Primarily excreted in urine (95%). **Half-life:** 9 hrs.

⧗ LIFESPAN CONSIDERATIONS

Pregnancy/Lactation: Unknown if distributed in breast milk. Must either discontinue drug or discontinue breastfeeding. **Children:** Safety and efficacy not established in pts younger than 16 yrs. **Elderly:** Not specified; use caution.

INTERACTIONS

DRUG: RifAMPin may decrease concentration/effect. May increase concentration/effect of **phenytoin, carBAMazepine. HERBAL: Ginseng, goldenseal, gotu kola, hawthorn, melatonin, valerian** may increase CNS depression. **Ginkgo** may decrease anticonvulsant effect. **FOOD:** None known. **LAB VALUES:** May decrease neutrophils, WBCs. May increase serum phenytoin (free and total) levels.

AVAILABILITY (Rx)

Tablets: 10 mg, 25 mg, 50 mg, 75 mg, 100 mg. **Oral Solution:** 10 mg/mL. **Injection Solution:** 50 mg/5 mL.

ADMINISTRATION/HANDLING

 IV

Reconstitution • Visually inspect for particulate matter or discoloration. Do not use if particulate matter or discoloration observed. • May be given without further dilution or may be mixed with 0.9% NaCl, 5% dextrose injection.

Rate of Administration • Give over 2–15 min.

Storage • Injection solution should appear clear and colorless. • Diluted solution should not be stored more than 4 hrs at room temperature. Do not freeze.

PO

• Give without regard to food. • Administer tablets whole; do not crush, cut, dissolve, or divide. • Oral solution should appear slightly viscous, clear, colorless to yellowish in color, and have a raspberry flavor. • Store oral solution at room temperature. • Discard unused oral solution remaining after 5 mos of first opening bottle. • Do not freeze oral solution. Oral solution should be delivered using calibrated measuring device (does not require dilution). May give oral solution via nasogastric tube or gastrostomy tube.

INDICATIONS/ROUTES/DOSAGE

Partial-Onset Seizures (Monotherapy or Adjunctive Therapy)
PO/IV: ADOLESCENTS, ADULTS: Initially, 50 mg twice daily. May either decrease to 25 mg twice daily or increase to 100 mg twice daily. **Maintenance:** 25–100 mg twice daily. **Maximum:** 200 mg/day. When initiating treatment, gradual dose escalation is not required. Injection solution should be administered at same dose and same frequency as tablets and oral solution. Gradually taper dose to discontinue treatment. **ELDERLY:** Consider initiating at lower end of the dosage range.

Dose Modification
Concomitant use with rifAMPin: May need to increase brivaracetam dosage by 100% (double dose).

Dosage in Renal Impairment
No dosage adjustment. Not recommended in pts with ESRD undergoing dialysis (not studied).

Dosage in Hepatic Impairment
Mild, moderate, severe impairment: Initially, 25 mg twice daily. **Maintenance:** 25–75 mg twice daily. **Maximum:** 75 mg twice daily.

SIDE EFFECTS

Occasional (16%–9%): Somnolence, sedation, dizziness, fatigue. **Rare (5%–2%):** Nausea, vomiting, ataxia, balance disorder, abnormal coordination, nystagmus, irritability, constipation.

ADVERSE EFFECTS/TOXIC REACTIONS

Sudden discontinuance may increase risk of seizure frequency and status epilepticus. May increase risk of suicidal thoughts or behavior. Psychiatric events including nonpsychotic behavior (anger, agitation, aggression, anxiety, apathy, depression, hyperactivity, irritability, mood swings, nervousness, restlessness, tearfulness) and psychotic symptoms (psychotic behavior with acute psychosis, delirium, hallucinations, paranoia) occurred in 13% of pts. Hypersensitivity reactions including bronchospasm, angioedema were reported. Clinically significant decreased WBC count (less than 3,000 cells/mm^3) and decreased neutrophil count (less than 1000 cells/mm^3) occurred in 1.8% and 0.3% of pts, respectively.

NURSING CONSIDERATIONS

BASELINE ASSESSMENT

Obtain CBC in pts with baseline neutropenia. Review history of seizure disorder (intensity, frequency, duration, LOC). Initiate seizure precautions, fall precautions. Question history of hypersensitivity reaction, hepatic impairment, psychiatric disorder; history of suicidal thoughts or behavior. Obtain urine pregnancy in female pts of reproductive potential.

INTERVENTION/EVALUATION

Periodically monitor CBC in pts with neutropenia. Monitor phenytoin levels in pts taking concomitant phenytoin (treatment may increase phenytoin levels). Observe for recurrence of seizure activity. Assess for clinical improvement (decrease in intensity/frequency of seizures). Diligently monitor for depression, changes in behavior, psychosis, suicidal ideation. Assist with ambulation if dizziness occurs.

PATIENT/FAMILY TEACHING

• Drowsiness usually diminishes with continued therapy. • Avoid tasks that require alertness, motor skills until response to drug is established. • Do not abruptly discontinue medication (may precipitate seizures). • Strict maintenance of drug therapy is essential for seizure control. • Report anxiety, anger, depression, mood swings, hostile behavior, thoughts of suicide, unusual changes in behavior. • Difficulty breathing, swelling of tongue or throat may indicate emergent allergic reaction. • Avoid alcohol.

brodalumab

broe-dal-ue-mab
(Siliq)

■ **BLACK BOX ALERT** ■ Suicidal ideation and behavior, including completed suicides, were reported with brodalumab. Screen for history of depression, suicidal ideation. Recommend mental health consultation in pts with suicidal ideation and behavior. Pts must seek immediate medical attention if new-onset suicidal ideation, anxiety, depression, mood change occurs.
Do not confuse brodalumab with avelumab, dupilumab, durvalumab, nivolumab, or sarilumab.

◆CLASSIFICATION

PHARMACOTHERAPEUTIC: Anti-interleukin 17-receptor antibody. Monoclonal antibody. **CLINICAL:** Anti-psoriasis agent.

USES

Treatment of moderate to severe plaque psoriasis in adults who are candidates for systemic therapy or phototherapy and have failed to respond or have lost response to other systemic therapies.

PRECAUTIONS

Contraindications: Hypersensitivity to brodalumab. Crohn's disease. **Cautions:** Baseline neutropenia; history of anxiety, depression, suicidal ideation and behavior, mood disorder; concomitant immunosuppressant therapy, conditions predisposing to infection (e.g., diabetes, immunocompromised pts, renal failure, open wounds), prior exposure to tuberculosis. Concomitant use of live vaccines not recommended. Not recommended in pts with active TB.

ACTION

Selectively binds to the IL-17A receptor, inhibiting the release of pro-inflammatory cytokines (involved in the pathogenesis of immune-mediated diseases, including plaque psoriasis). **Therapeutic Effect:** Blocks cytokine-induced responses.

PHARMACOKINETICS

Widely distributed. Metabolism: not specified. Degraded into small peptides and amino acids via catabolic pathway. Peak plasma concentration: 3 days. Steady state reached in 4 wks. Excretion not specified. **Half-life:** Not specified.

⧗ LIFESPAN CONSIDERATIONS

Pregnancy/Lactation: Unknown if distributed in breast milk. However, human immunoglobulin G (IgG) is present in breast milk and is known to cross the placenta. **Children:** Safety and efficacy not established. **Elderly:** No age-related precautions noted.

INTERACTIONS

DRUG: Avoid use of **live vaccines.** May decrease therapeutic effect of **BCG.** May increase adverse effects/toxicity of **belimumab, natalizumab, pimecrolimus,**

tacrolimus. **HERBAL: Echinacea** may decrease therapeutic effect. **FOOD:** None known. **LAB VALUES:** May decrease neutrophils.

AVAILABILITY (Rx)

Injection Solution: 210 mg/1.5 mL in prefilled single-dose syringe.

ADMINISTRATION/HANDLING

Subcutaneous

Preparation • Remove prefilled syringe from refrigerator and allow solution to warm to room temperature (approx. 30 min) with needle cap intact. • Visually inspect for particulate matter or discoloration. Solution should appear clear, colorless to slightly yellow in color. Do not use if solution is cloudy, discolored, or if visible particles are observed.

Administration • Insert needle subcutaneously into upper arms, outer thigh, or abdomen, and inject solution. • Do not inject into areas of active skin disease or injury, such as sunburns, skin rashes, inflammation, skin infections, or active psoriasis. • Do not administer IV or intramuscularly. • Rotate injection sites.

Storage • Refrigerate prefilled syringes in original carton until time of use. • May store at room temperature for up to 14 days. Once warmed to room temperature, do not place back into refrigerator. • Do not freeze or expose to heating sources. • Do not shake. • Protect from light.

INDICATIONS/ROUTES/DOSAGE

Plaque Psoriasis

SQ: ADULTS, ELDERLY: Initially, 210 mg once at wks 0, 1, 2. **MAINTENANCE:** 210 mg once q2wks thereafter.

Permanent Discontinuation: Consider discontinuation in pts who have not achieved an adequate response after 12–16 wks.

Dosage in Renal Impairment

Not specified; use caution.

Dosage in Hepatic Impairment

Not specified; use caution.

SIDE EFFECTS

Occasional (5%-4%): Arthralgia, headache. **Rare (3%-1%):** Fatigue, diarrhea, oropharyngeal pain, nausea, myalgia, injection site reactions (bruising, erythema, hemorrhage, pain, pruritus), conjunctivitis.

ADVERSE EFFECTS/TOXIC REACTIONS

Suicidal ideation and behavior, including completed suicides, were reported. May increase risk of tuberculosis. Infections such as bronchitis, influenza, nasopharyngitis, pharyngitis, upper respiratory tract infection, tinea infections, UTI may occur. May cause exacerbation of Crohn's disease and ulcerative colitis. Immunogenicity (auto-brodalumab antibodies) occurred in 3% of pts.

NURSING CONSIDERATIONS

BASELINE ASSESSMENT

Obtain CBC in pts with known history of neutropenia. Screen for active infection. Pts should be evaluated for active tuberculosis and tested for latent infection prior to initiating treatment and periodically during therapy. Induration of 5 mm or greater with tuberculin skin test should be considered a positive test result when assessing if treatment for latent tuberculosis is necessary. Verify pt has not received live vaccines prior to initiation. Question history of Crohn's disease, ulcerative colitis, hypersensitivity reaction; anxiety, depression, mood disorder, suicidal ideation and behavior. Conduct dermatological exam; record characteristics of psoriatic lesions. Assess pt's willingness to self-inject medication.

INTERVENTION/EVALUATION

Diligently monitor for suicidal ideation and behavior, new onset or worsening of anxiety, depression, mood disorder. Consult mental health professional if mood disorder suspected. Monitor for symptoms of tuberculosis, including those who tested negative for latent tuberculosis infection prior to initiation.

B

Interrupt or discontinue treatment if serious infection, opportunistic infection, or sepsis occurs, and initiate appropriate antimicrobial therapy. Monitor for hypersensitivity reaction, symptoms of inflammatory bowel disease. Assess skin for improvement of lesions.

PATIENT/FAMILY TEACHING

• Seek immediate medical attention if thoughts of suicide, new onset or worsening of anxiety, depression, or changes in mood occurs. • A health care provider will show you how to properly prepare and inject your medication. You must demonstrate correct preparation and injection techniques before using medication at home. • Treatment may depress your immune system response and reduce your ability to fight infection. Report symptoms of infection, such as body aches, chills, cough, fatigue, fever. Avoid those with active infection. • Do not receive live vaccines. • Expect frequent tuberculosis screening. • Report travel plans to possible endemic areas. • Treatment may cause worsening of Crohn's disease or cause inflammatory bowel disease. Report abdominal pain, diarrhea, weight loss.

---

budesonide

bue-**des**-oh-nide
(Entocort EC, Pulmicort Flexhaler, <u>Pulmicort</u>, Rhinocort Allergy, <u>Rhinocort Aqua</u>, Uceris)
Do not confuse budesonide with Budeprion.

FIXED-COMBINATION(S)

Symbicort: budesonide/formoterol (bronchodilator): 80 mcg/4.5 mcg, 160 mcg/4.5 mcg.

◆CLASSIFICATION

PHARMACOTHERAPEUTIC: Glucocorticosteroid. **CLINICAL:** Anti-inflammatory, antiallergy.

USES

Nasal: (Rx): Management of seasonal or perennial allergic rhinitis in adults and children 6 yrs and older. **(OTC):** Relief of hay fever, other upper respiratory allergies. **Nebulization, Oral Inhalation:** Maintenance or prophylaxis therapy for asthma. **PO: (Entocort EC):** Treatment of mild to moderate active Crohn's disease. Maintenance of clinical remission of mild to moderate Crohn's disease. **(Uceris):** Induction of remission in active, mild to moderate ulcerative colitis. **OFF-LABEL:** Treatment of vasomotor rhinitis.

PRECAUTIONS

Contraindications: Hypersensitivity to budesonide, primary treatment of status asthmaticus, acute episodes of asthma. Not for relief of acute bronchospasms. **Cautions:** Thyroid disease, hepatic impairment, renal impairment, cardiovascular disease, diabetes, glaucoma, cataracts, myasthenia gravis, pts at risk for osteoporosis, seizures, GI disease, post acute MI, elderly.

ACTION

Inhibits accumulation of inflammatory cells; controls rate of protein synthesis; decreases migration of polymorphonuclear leukocytes (reverses capillary permeability and lysosomal stabilization at cellular level). **Therapeutic Effect:** Relieves symptoms of allergic rhinitis, asthma, Crohn's disease.

PHARMACOKINETICS

Form	Onset	Peak	Duration
Pulmicort Respules	2–8 days	4–6 wks	—
Rhinocort Aqua	10 hrs	2 wks	—

Minimally absorbed from nasal tissue; moderately absorbed from inhalation. Protein binding: 88%. Primarily metabolized in liver. **Half-life:** 2–3 hrs.

⧗ LIFESPAN CONSIDERATIONS

Pregnancy/Lactation: Unknown if drug crosses placenta or is distributed in breast milk. **Children:** Prolonged treatment or high dosages may decrease short-term growth rate, cortisol secretion. **Elderly:** No age-related precautions noted.

INTERACTIONS

DRUG: CYP3A4 inhibitors (e.g., itraconazole, ketoconazole) may increase concentration. **HERBAL:** Echinacea may decrease effects. **FOOD:** **Grapefruit products** may increase systemic exposure. **LAB VALUES:** May decrease serum potassium.

AVAILABILITY (Rx)

Oral Inhalation Powder (Pulmicort Flexhaler): 90 mcg per inhalation; 180 mcg per inhalation. **Inhalation Suspension for Nebulization (Pulmicort):** 0.25 mg/2 mL; 0.5 mg/2 mL; 1 mg/2 mL. **Nasal Spray (Rhinocort Allergy, Rhinocort Aqua):** 32 mcg/spray.

🕭 **Capsules, Enteric-Coated (Entocort EC):** 3 mg. **Tablets, Extended-Release: (Uceris):** 9 mg.

ADMINISTRATION/HANDLING

Inhalation

• Hold inhaler in upright position to load dose. Do not shake prior to use. Prime prior to first use only. • Place mouthpiece between lips and inhale forcefully and deeply. Do not exhale through inhaler; do not use a spacer. • Rinsing mouth after each use decreases incidence of candidiasis.

Intranasal

• Instruct pt to clear nasal passages before use. • Tilt pt's head slightly forward. • Insert spray tip into nostril, pointing toward nasal passages, away from nasal septum. • Spray into one nostril while pt holds other nostril closed and concurrently inspires through nostril to allow medication as high into nasal passages as possible.

Nebulization

• Shake well before use. • Administer with mouthpiece or face mask. • Rinse mouth following treatment.

PO

• May take with or without food. Swallow whole. Do not break, crush, dissolve, or divide capsule or tablet.

INDICATIONS/ROUTES/DOSAGE

Rhinitis

Intranasal: **(Rx): ADULTS, ELDERLY, CHILDREN 6 YRS AND OLDER:** 1 spray (32 mcg) in each nostril once daily. **Maximum:** 4 sprays in each nostril once daily for adults and children 12 yrs and older; 2 sprays in each nostril once daily for children 6–11 yrs.

Intranasal: (OTC): ADULTS, ELDERLY, CHILDREN 6 YRS AND OLDER: 2 sprays in each nostril once daily. May decrease to 1 spray in each nostril once daily.

Bronchial Asthma

Nebulization: CHILDREN 12 MOS–8 YRS: *(Previous therapy with bronchodilators alone):* 0.5 mg/day as single dose or 2 divided doses. **Maximum:** 0.5 mg/day. *(Previous therapy with inhaled corticosteroids):* 0.5 mg/day as single dose or 2 divided doses. **Maximum:** 1 mg/day. *(Previous therapy of oral corticosteroids):* 1 mg/day as single dose in 2 divided doses. **Maximum:** 1 mg/day.
Oral Inhalation: *(Pulmicort Flexhaler):* **ADULTS, ELDERLY:** Initially, 360 mcg 2 times/day. **Maximum:** 720 mcg 2 times/day. **CHILDREN, 6 YRS AND OLDER:** 180 mcg 2 times/day. **Maximum:** 360 mcg 2 times/day.

Crohn's Disease

PO: ADULTS, ELDERLY: (Capsule) 9 mg once daily for up to 8 wks. Recurring episodes may be treated with a repeat 8-wk course of treatment. **Maintenance of remission:** 6 mg once daily for up to 3 mos.

Ulcerative Colitis

PO: ADULTS, ELDERLY: (Tablet) 9 mg once daily in morning for up to 8 wks.

Dosage in Renal/Hepatic Impairment
No dose adjustment.

SIDE EFFECTS

Frequent (greater than 3%): Nasal: Mild nasopharyngeal irritation, burning, stinging, dryness; headache, cough. **Inhalation:** Flu-like symptoms, headache, pharyngitis. **Occasional (3%–1%): Nasal:** Dry mouth, dyspepsia, rebound congestion, rhinorrhea, loss of taste. **Inhalation:** Back pain, vomiting, altered taste, voice changes, abdominal pain, nausea, dyspepsia.

ADVERSE EFFECTS/TOXIC REACTIONS

Acute hypersensitivity reaction (urticaria, angioedema, severe bronchospasm) occurs rarely.

NURSING CONSIDERATIONS

BASELINE ASSESSMENT

Question for hypersensitivity to any corticosteroids, components. Auscultate lung sounds.

INTERVENTION/EVALUATION

Monitor for relief of symptoms. Auscultate lung sounds. Observe proper use of medication delivery device to ensure correct technique.

PATIENT/FAMILY TEACHING

• Improvement noted in 24 hrs, but full effect may take 3–7 days. • Report if no improvement in symptoms or if sneezing, nasal irritation occurs.

---

bumetanide

bue-**met**-a-nide
(Bumex, Burinex ✦)
■ **BLACK BOX ALERT** ■ Excess dosage can lead to profound diuresis with fluid and electrolyte loss.
Do not confuse bumetanide with Buminate.

◆CLASSIFICATION

PHARMACOTHERAPEUTIC: Loop diuretic. **CLINICAL:** Diuretic.

USES

Management of edema associated with HF, renal disease, or hepatic disease.

PRECAUTIONS

Contraindications: Hypersensitivity to bumetanide. Anuria, hepatic coma, severe electrolyte depletion (until condition improves or is corrected). **Cautions:** Severe hypersensitivity to sulfonamides; hypotension.

ACTION

Enhances excretion of sodium, chloride, and, to lesser degree, potassium by direct action at ascending limb of loop of Henle and in proximal tubule. **Therapeutic Effect:** Produces diuresis.

PHARMACOKINETICS

Route	Onset	Peak	Duration
PO	30–60 min	60–120 min	4–6 hrs
IV	Rapid	15–30 min	2–3 hrs

Completely absorbed from GI tract (absorption decreased in HF, nephrotic syndrome). Protein binding: 94%–96%. Partially metabolized in liver. Primarily excreted in urine. Not removed by hemodialysis. **Half-life:** 1–1.5 hrs.

⧗ LIFESPAN CONSIDERATIONS

Pregnancy/Lactation: Unknown if drug is distributed in breast milk. **Children:** Safety and efficacy not established. **Elderly:** May be more sensitive to hypotension/electrolyte effects. Increased risk for circulatory collapse or thrombolytic episode. Age-related renal impairment may require reduced or extended dosage interval.

INTERACTIONS

DRUG: Agents inducing hypokalemia (e.g., metOLazone, hydroCHLOROthiazide) may increase risk of hypokalemia. May increase risk of **lithium** toxicity. **NSAIDs (e.g., diclofenac, naproxen)** may increase effect. **HERBAL: Ephedra, ginseng, yohimbe** may worsen hypertension. **Garlic** may have increased antihypertensive effect. **FOOD:** None known. **LAB VALUES:** May increase serum glucose, BUN, uric acid; urinary phosphate. May decrease serum calcium, chloride, magnesium, potassium, sodium.

AVAILABILITY (Rx)

Injection Solution: 0.25 mg/mL. **Tablets:** 0.5 mg, 1 mg, 2 mg.

ADMINISTRATION/HANDLING

 IV

Rate of Administration • May give undiluted but is compatible with D₅W, 0.9% NaCl, or lactated Ringer's solution. • Administer IV push over 1–2 min. • May give through Y tube or 3-way stopcock. • May give as continuous infusion.
Storage • Store at room temperature. • Stable for 24 hrs if diluted.

PO

• Give with food to avoid GI upset, preferably with breakfast (may prevent nocturia).

▨ IV INCOMPATIBILITY

Midazolam (Versed).

▨ IV COMPATIBILITIES

Aztreonam (Azactam), cefepime (Maxipime), dexmedetomidine (Precedex), diltiaZEM (Cardizem), DOBUTamine (Dobutrex), furosemide (Lasix), LORazepam (Ativan), milrinone (Primacor), morphine, piperacillin and tazobactam (Zosyn), propofol (Diprivan).

INDICATIONS/ROUTES/DOSAGE

Edema, HF
PO: ADULTS, ELDERLY: 0.5–2 mg 1–2 times/day. May repeat in 4–5 hrs for up to 2 doses. **Maximum:** 10 mg/day.
IV, IM: ADULTS, ELDERLY: 0.5–1 mg/dose; may repeat in 2–3 hrs for up to 2 doses

(**Maximum:** 10 mg/day) or 0.5–2 mg/hr by continuous IV infusion. Repeat loading dose before increasing infusion rate.

Usual Pediatric Dosage
IV, IM, PO: CHILDREN: 0.015–0.1 mg/kg/dose q6–24h. **Maximum:** 10 mg/day. **NEONATES:** 0.01–0.05 mg/kg/dose q12–48h.

Dosage in Renal/Hepatic Impairment
Use caution; contraindicated in anuria, hepatic coma.

SIDE EFFECTS

Expected: Increased urinary frequency and urine volume. **Frequent (5%):** Muscle cramps, dizziness, hypotension, headache, nausea. **Occasional (3%–1%):** Impaired hearing, pruritus, EKG changes, weakness, hives, abdominal pain, dyspepsia, musculoskeletal pain, rash, nausea, vomiting. **Rare (less than 1%):** Chest pain, ear pain, fatigue, dry mouth, premature ejaculation, impotence, nipple tenderness.

ADVERSE EFFECTS/TOXIC REACTIONS

Vigorous diuresis may lead to profound water and electrolyte depletion, resulting in hypokalemia, hyponatremia, dehydration, coma, circulatory collapse. Ototoxicity manifested as deafness, vertigo, tinnitus may occur, esp. in pts with severe renal impairment or those taking other ototoxic drugs. Blood dyscrasias, acute hypotensive episodes have been reported.

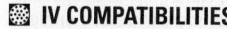

NURSING CONSIDERATIONS

BASELINE ASSESSMENT
Obtain baseline vital signs, esp. B/P for hypotension, before administration. Assess baseline electrolytes, particularly for hypokalemia, hyponatremia. Assess for edema. Observe skin turgor, mucous membranes for hydration status. Initiate I&O, obtain baseline weight.

INTERVENTION/EVALUATION

Continue to monitor B/P, vital signs, electrolytes, I&O, weight. Note extent of diuresis. Watch for changes from initial assessment (hypokalemia may result in muscle weakness, tremor, muscle cramps, altered mental status, cardiac arrhythmias; hyponatremia may result in confusion, thirst, cold/clammy skin).

PATIENT/FAMILY TEACHING

• Expect increased urinary frequency/volume. • Report auditory abnormalities (e.g., sense of fullness in ears, tinnitus). • Eat foods high in potassium such as whole grains (cereals), legumes, meat, bananas, apricots, orange juice, potatoes (white, sweet), raisins. • Rise slowly from sitting/lying position.

buprenorphine

bue-pre-**nor**-feen
(Belbuca, Buprenex, Butrans, Probuphine, Implant Kit)

■ **BLACK BOX ALERT** ■ **Transdermal:** Prolonged use during pregnancy may result in neonatal abstinence syndrome. Potential for abuse, misuse, and diversion. Do not exceed dose of one 20 mcg/hr patch due to risk of QT interval prolongation. May cause potentially life-threatening respiratory depression. **Implant:** Potential for implant migration, protrusion, expulsion, and nerve damage associated with insertion and removal.

Do not confuse Buprenex with Bumex, or buprenorphine with buPROPion.

FIXED-COMBINATION(S)

Brunavail: buprenorphine/naloxone (narcotic antagonist): 2.1 mg/0.3 mg; 4.2 mg/0.7 mg; 6.3 mg/1 mg. **Suboxone:** buprenorphine/naloxone: 2 mg/0.5 mg, 4 mg/1 mg, 8 mg/2 mg, 12 mg/3 mg. **Zubsolv:** buprenorphine/naloxone: 1.4 mg/0.36 mg; 5.7 mg/1.4 mg.

◆CLASSIFICATION

PHARMACOTHERAPEUTIC: Opioid agonist, antagonist injection (Schedule V). **CLINICAL:** Opioid dependence adjunct, analgesic.

USES

Sublingual Tablet: Treatment of opioid dependence. **Implant:** Maintenance treatment of opioid dependence in pts who achieved/sustained prolonged clinical stability on low to moderate doses of a transmucosal buprenorphine product for 3 months or longer with no need for supplemental dosing or adjustments. **Injection:** Relief of moderate to severe pain. **Transdermal, Buccal film:** Moderate to severe chronic pain requiring continuous around-the-clock opioid analgesic for extended period. **OFF-LABEL:** Injection: Heroin/opioid withdrawal in hospitalized pts.

PRECAUTIONS

Contraindications: Hypersensitivity to buprenorphine. **Transdermal patch, Buccal film:** (Additional) Significant respiratory depression, severe asthma in an unmonitored setting or in absence of resuscitation equipment, known or suspected GI obstruction, including paralytic ileus. **Cautions:** Hepatic/renal impairment, elderly, debilitated, pediatric pts, head injury/increased intracranial pressure, pts at risk for respiratory depression, hyperthyroidism, myxedema, adrenal cortical insufficiency (e.g., Addison's disease), urethral stricture, CNS depression, morbid obesity, toxic psychosis, prostatic hypertrophy, delirium tremens, kyphoscoliosis, biliary tract dysfunction, acute pancreatitis, acute abdominal conditions, acute alcoholism, pts with prolonged QT syndrome, concurrent use of antiarrhythmics, hypovolemia, cardiovascular disease, ileus, bowel obstruction, hx of seizure disorder.

ACTION

Binds to opioid receptors within CNS. **Therapeutic Effect:** Suppresses opioid withdrawal symptoms, cravings. Alters pain perception, emotional response to pain.

PHARMACOKINETICS

Route	Onset	Peak	Duration
Sublingual	15 min	1 hr	6 hrs
IV	Less than 15 min	Less than 1 hr	6 hrs
IM	15 min	1 hr	6 hrs

Excreted primarily in feces with lesser amount eliminated in urine. Protein binding: High. **Half-life: Parenteral:** 2–3 hrs; **Sublingual:** 37 hrs (increased in hepatic impairment).

⧖ LIFESPAN CONSIDERATIONS

Pregnancy/Lactation: Crosses placenta. Distributed in breast milk. Breastfeeding not recommended. Neonatal withdrawal noted in infant if mother was treated with buprenorphine during pregnancy, with onset of withdrawal symptoms generally noted on day 1, manifested as hypertonia, tremor, agitation, myoclonus. Apnea, bradycardia, seizures occur rarely. **Children:** Safety and efficacy of injection form not established in those 2–12 yrs. Safety and efficacy of tablet, fixed-combination form not established in pts 16 yrs or younger. **Elderly:** Age-related hepatic impairment may require dosage adjustment.

INTERACTIONS

DRUG: CNS depressants, MAOIs may increase CNS or respiratory depression, hypotension. **CYP3A4 inhibitors (e.g., azole antifungals, macrolide antibiotics, protease inhibitors)** may increase plasma concentration. **CYP3A4 inducers (e.g., carBAMazepine, phenytoin, rifAMPin)** may cause increased clearance of buprenorphine. May decrease effects of **other opioid analgesics. HERBAL: St. John's wort, kava kava, gotu kola, valerian** may increase CNS depression. **FOOD:** None known. **LAB VALUES:** May increase serum amylase, lipase.

AVAILABILITY (Rx)

Buccal Film: 75 mcg, 150 mcg, 300 mcg, 450 mcg, 600 mcg, 750 mcg, 900 mcg. **Implant (Probuphine):** Set of 4 implants, each containing 74.2 mg of buprenorphine (equivalent to 80 mg of buprenorphine hydrochloride). **Injection Solution (Buprenex):** 0.3 mg/1 mL. **Tablets, Sublingual:** 2 mg, 8 mg. **Transdermal Weekly Patch (Butrans):** 5 mcg/hr, 7.5 mcg/hr, 10 mcg/hr, 15 mcg/hr, 20 mcg/hr.

ADMINISTRATION/HANDLING

 IV

Reconstitution • May be diluted with lactated Ringer's solution, D₅W, 0.9% NaCl.
Rate of Administration • If given as IV push, administer over at least 2 min.

IM
• Give deep IM into large muscle mass.

Buccal Film
Moisten inside cheek. Apply with dry finger. Press and hold in place for 5 sec. Keep film in place until dissolved (approx 30 min). Do not chew, swallow, touch, or move film. Do not cut/tear. Avoid areas with open sores/lesions.

Sublingual
• Instruct pt to dissolve tablet(s) under tongue; avoid swallowing (reduces drug bioavailability). • For doses greater than 2 tablets, either place all tablets at once or 2 tablets at a time under the tongue.
Storage • Store parenteral form at room temperature. • Protect from prolonged exposure to light. • Store tablets at room temperature.

Transdermal
• Apply to clean, dry, intact, nonirritated, hairless skin of upper outer arm, upper chest, upper back, or side of chest. Hair at application site should be clipped; do not shave. • Clean site with clear water and allow to dry. Do not use soaps, alcohol, oils (may increase absorption). Press patch in place and hold for 15

seconds. • Wait minimum of 21 days before reapplying to same site. • Avoid exposing patch to external heat sources. Incidental exposure to water is acceptable. Patch may be taped in place with first-aid tape. • If patch falls off during 7-day dosing interval, apply new patch to a different skin site.

🏵 IV INCOMPATIBILITIES

DiazePAM (Valium), furosemide (Lasix), LORazepam (Ativan).

🏵 IV COMPATIBILITIES

Allopurinol (Aloprim, Zyloprim), aztreonam (Azactam), cefepime (Maxipime), diphenhydrAMINE (Benadryl), granisetron (Kytril), haloperidol (Haldol), heparin, linezolid (Zyvox), midazolam (Versed), piperacillin/tazobactam (Zosyn), promethazine (Phenergan), propofol (Diprivan).

INDICATIONS/ROUTES/DOSAGE

Opioid Dependence
Sublingual: ADULTS, CHILDREN 13 YRS AND OLDER: 8 mg on day 1, then 16 mg on day 2 and subsequent induction days. Range: 12–16 mg/day (usually over 3–4 days). **Maintenance:** Target dose 12–16 mg/day. Pts should be switched to buprenorphine/naloxone combination for maintenance and unsupervised therapy. **Implant:** Four implants inserted subdermally in upper arm for 6 mos of treatment.

Moderate to Severe Pain
IM/IV: ADULTS, CHILDREN 13 YRS AND OLDER: 0.3 mg (1 mL) q6–8h prn; may repeat once 30–60 min after initial dose. Range: 0.15–0.6 mg q4–8h prn. **ELDERLY:** 0.15 mg q6h prn. **CHILDREN 2–12 YRS:** 2–6 mcg/kg q4–6h prn.
Transdermal: ADULTS, ELDERLY: (OPIOID NAIVE): Initial dose always 5 mcg/hr once q7days. **THOSE ALREADY RECEIVING OPIOIDS:** Refer to conversion chart in package insert. Do not increase dose until pt exposed to previous dose for 72 hrs. **Buccal: ADULTS, ELDERLY: (OPIOID NAIVE):** Initially, 75 mcg once or q12h for 4 days, then 150 mcg q12h. **(OPIOID**

EXPERIENCED): Taper current opioid to no more than 30 mg oral morphine equivalent. Based on opioid dose prior to tapering: 75 mcg once daily or q12h for less than 30 mg; 150 mcg q12h for 30–89 mg; 300 mcg q12h for 90–160 mg.

Dosage in Renal Impairment
Use caution.

Dosage in Hepatic Impairment
Injection: Use caution.
Transdermal: No adjustment.

SIDE EFFECTS

Frequent (67%–10%): Sedation, dizziness, nausea. **Butrans (more than 5%):** Nausea, headache, pruritus at application site, dizziness, rash, vomiting, constipation, dry mouth. **Implant: (more than 5%):** Headache, nausea, vomiting, constipation. **Occasional (5%–1%):** Headache, hypotension, vomiting, miosis, diaphoresis. **Rare (less than 1%):** Dry mouth, pallor, visual abnormalities, injection site reaction.

ADVERSE EFFECTS/TOXIC REACTIONS

Overdosage results in cold, clammy skin, weakness, confusion, severe respiratory depression, cyanosis, pinpoint pupils, seizures, extreme drowsiness progressing to stupor, coma.

NURSING CONSIDERATIONS

BASELINE ASSESSMENT

Obtain baseline B/P, pulse rate. Assess mental status, alertness. Assess type, location, intensity of pain. Obtain history of pt's last opioid use. Assess for early signs of withdrawal symptoms before initiating therapy.

INTERVENTION/EVALUATION

Monitor for change in respirations, B/P, rate/quality of pulse, mental status. Assess lab results. Initiate deep breathing, coughing exercises, particularly in pts with pulmonary impairment. Assess for clinical improvement; record onset of relief of pain. Monitor strictly for compliance, signs of abuse or misuse.

B

PATIENT/FAMILY TEACHING

• Change positions slowly to avoid dizziness, orthostatic hypotension. • Avoid tasks that require alertness, motor skills until response to drug is established. • Avoid alcohol, sedatives, antidepressants, tranquilizers.

buPROPion

bue-**proe**-pee-on
(Aplenzin, Forfivo XL, Wellbutrin SR, Wellbutrin XL, Zyban)
■ **BLACK BOX ALERT** ■ Increased risk of suicidal thinking and behavior in children, adolescents, young adults 18–24 yrs with major depressive disorder, other psychiatric disorders. Agitation, hostility, depressed mood also reported. Use in smoking cessation may cause serious neuropsychiatric events. **Do not confuse Aplenzin with Relenza, buPROPion with busPIRone, Wellbutrin SR with Wellbutrin XL, or Zyban with Diovan or Zagam.**

◆CLASSIFICATION

PHARMACOTHERAPEUTIC: Aminoketone. **CLINICAL:** Antidepressant, smoking cessation aid.

USES

Treatment of depression, seasonal affective disorder (SAD). Zyban assists in smoking cessation. **OFF-LABEL:** Treatment of ADHD in adults, children. Depression associated with bipolar disorder.

PRECAUTIONS

Contraindications: Hypersensitivity to buPROPion. Current or prior diagnosis of anorexia nervosa or bulimia, seizure disorder, use within 14 days of MAOIs; concomitant use of other buPROPion products; pts undergoing abrupt discontinuation of alcohol or sedatives. Initiation of buPROPion in pts receiving linezolid or IV methylene blue. **Aplenzin, Forfivo XL,** **Wellbutrin XL (additional):** Conditions increasing seizure risk, severe head injury, stroke, CNS tumor/infection. **Forfivo XL (additional):** Pts receiving other dosage forms of bupropion. **Cautions:** History of seizure, cranial or head trauma, cardiovascular disease, history of hypertension or coronary artery disease, elderly, pts at high risk for suicide, renal/hepatic impairment. Concurrent use of antipsychotics, antidepressants, theophylline, steroids, stimulants, hypoglycemic agents, excessive use of alcohol, sedatives/hypnotics, opioids.

ACTION

Blocks reuptake of neurotransmitters, (DOPamine, norepinephrine) at CNS presynaptic membranes. **Therapeutic Effect:** Relieves depression. Eliminates nicotine withdrawal symptoms.

PHARMACOKINETICS

Rapidly absorbed from GI tract. Protein binding: 84%. Crosses the blood-brain barrier. Metabolized in liver. Primarily excreted in urine. **Half-life:** 14 hrs.

⧗ LIFESPAN CONSIDERATIONS

Pregnancy/Lactation: Unknown if drug crosses placenta or is distributed in breast milk. **Children:** More sensitive to increased dosage, toxicity; increased risk of suicidal ideation, worsening of depression. Safety and efficacy not established in pts younger than 18 yrs. **Elderly:** More sensitive to anticholinergic, sedative, cardiovascular effects. Age-related renal impairment may require dosage adjustment.

INTERACTIONS

DRUG: **Ritonavir, efavirenz** may reduce concentration. **CarBAMazepine, PHENobarbital, phenytoin** may decrease effectiveness. **MAOIs** may increase risk of toxicity. **Levodopa, amantadine** may increase risk of side effects. **HERBAL: Gotu kola, kava kava, St. John's wort, valerian** may increase CNS depression. **FOOD:** None known. **LAB VALUES:** May decrease WBC.

◆ Canadian trade name   🦺 Non-Crushable Drug   High Alert drug

AVAILABILITY (RX)

Tablets: 75 mg, 100 mg.

🔖 Tablets, Extended-Release (24 hr): 174 mg, 348 mg, 522 mg **(Aplenzin)**; 450 mg **(Forfivo XL)**; 150 mg, 300 mg **(Wellbutrin XL)**. Tablets, Sustained-Release (12 hr): 100 mg, 150 mg, 200 mg **(Wellbutrin SR)**, 150 mg **(Zyban)**.

ADMINISTRATION/HANDLING

PO

• Give without regard to food (give with food if GI irritation occurs). • Give at least 4-hr interval for immediate onset and 8-hr interval for sustained-release tablet to avoid seizures. • Give Aplenzin once daily in the morning. • Avoid bedtime dosage (decreases risk of insomnia). • Do not break, crush, dissolve, or divide sustained-, extended-release preparations.

INDICATIONS/ROUTES/DOSAGE

Depression

PO *(Immediate-Release)*: **ADULTS:** Initially, 100 mg twice daily. May increase to 100 mg 3 times/day no sooner than 3 days after beginning therapy. **Maximum:** 150 mg 3 times/day. **ELDERLY:** Initially, 37.5 mg 2 times/day. May increase by 37.5 q3–4days. **Maximum:** 300 mg/day in divided doses.

PO *(Sustained-Release)*: **ADULTS:** Initially, 150 mg/day as a single dose in the morning. May increase to 150 mg twice daily as early as day 4 after beginning therapy. **Maximum:** 400 mg/day in 2 divided doses. **ELDERLY:** Initially, 100 mg/day. May increase by 100 mg q3–4days. **Maximum:** 300 mg/day in divided doses.

PO *(Extended-Release)*: **ADULTS:** 150 mg once daily. May increase to 300 mg once daily as early as day 4. **Maximum:** 450 mg/day. *(Forfivo XL):* Use only after initial dose titration with other buPROPion products. *(Aplenzin)*: Initially, 174 mg once daily in morning; may increase as soon as 4 days to 348 mg/day. **Maximum:** 522 mg/day.

Smoking Cessation

PO: ADULTS, ELDERLY: (Zyban): Initially, 150 mg/day for 3 days, then 150 mg twice daily for 7–12 wks.

SAD

PO: ADULTS, ELDERLY: (Wellbutrin XL): 150 mg/day for 1 wk, then 300 mg/day. Begin in autumn (Sept–Nov). End of treatment begins in spring (Mar–Apr) by decreasing dose to 150 mg/day for 2 wks before discontinuation. **(Aplenzin):** 174 mg once daily. May increase after 1 wk to 348 mg once daily.

Dosage in Renal Impairment

Use caution.

Dosage in Hepatic Impairment

Mild to moderate impairment: Use caution, reduce dosage. **Severe impairment:** Use extreme caution. **Maximum dose:** Aplenzin: 174 mg every other day. Wellbutrin: 75 mg/day. Wellbutrin SR: 100 mg/day or 150 mg every other day. Wellbutrin XL: 150 mg every other day. Zyban: 150 mg every other day.

SIDE EFFECTS

Frequent (32%–18%): Constipation, weight gain or loss, nausea, vomiting, anorexia, dry mouth, headache, diaphoresis, tremor, sedation, insomnia, dizziness, agitation. **Occasional (10%–5%):** Diarrhea, akinesia, blurred vision, tachycardia, confusion, hostility, fatigue.

ADVERSE EFFECTS/TOXIC REACTIONS

Risk of seizures increases in pts taking more than 150 mg/dose; in pts with history of bulimia, seizure disorders, discontinuing drugs that may lower seizure threshold.

NURSING CONSIDERATIONS

BASELINE ASSESSMENT

Assess psychological status, thought content, suicidal tendencies, appearance. For pts on long-term therapy, hepatic/renal function tests should be performed periodically.

INTERVENTION/EVALUATION

Supervise suicidal-risk pt closely during early therapy and dose changes (as depression lessens, energy level improves, increasing suicide potential). Assess appearance, behavior, speech pattern, level of interest, mood changes.

PATIENT/FAMILY TEACHING

• Full therapeutic effect may be noted in 4 wks. • Avoid tasks that require alertness, motor skills until response to drug is established. • Report signs/symptoms of seizure, worsening depression, suicidal ideation, unusual behavioral changes. • Avoid alcohol. • Do not chew, crush, dissolve, or divide sustained-, extended-release tablets.

---

busPIRone

bue-**spye**-rone
(Apo-BusPIRone ◆)
Do not confuse busPIRone with buPROPion.

◆CLASSIFICATION

PHARMACOTHERAPEUTIC: Nonbarbiturate. **CLINICAL:** Antianxiety.

USES

Short-term management (up to 4 wks) of generalized anxiety disorder (GAD). **OFF-LABEL:** Augmenting medication for antidepressants.

PRECAUTIONS

Contraindications: Hypersensitivity to busPIRone. **Cautions:** Concurrent use of MAOIs, severe hepatic/renal impairment (not recommended).

ACTION

Exact mechanism of action unknown. Binds to serotonin, DOPamine at presynaptic neurotransmitter receptors in CNS. **Therapeutic Effect:** Produces anxiolytic effect.

PHARMACOKINETICS

Rapidly and completely absorbed from GI tract. Protein binding: 95%. Metabolized in liver. Primarily excreted in urine. Not removed by hemodialysis. **Half-life:** 2–3 hrs.

⧗ LIFESPAN CONSIDERATIONS

Pregnancy/Lactation: Unknown if drug crosses placenta or is distributed in breast milk. **Children:** Safety and efficacy not established. **Elderly:** No age-related precautions noted.

INTERACTIONS

DRUG: CNS depressants (e.g., **alcohol, ALPRAZolam, LORazepam, morphine, oxyCODONE, traMADol**) potentiate effect, may increase sedation. **CYP3A4 inhibitors (e.g., erythromycin, ketoconazole)** may increase concentration/effect. **CYP3A4 inducers (e.g., rifAMPin)** may decrease concentration/effect. May increase effects of MAOIs. **HERBAL: Gotu kola, kava kava, St. John's wort, valerian** may increase CNS depression. **FOOD: Grapefruit products** may increase concentration, risk of toxicity. **LAB VALUES:** May produce false-positive urine metanephrine/catecholamine assay test.

AVAILABILITY (Rx)

Tablets: 5 mg, 7.5 mg, 10 mg, 15 mg, 30 mg.

ADMINISTRATION/HANDLING

PO
• Give without regard to food. Must be consistent.

INDICATIONS/ROUTES/DOSAGE

Short-Term Management (up to 4 wks) of Anxiety Disorders
PO: ADULTS, ELDERLY: Initially, 7.5 mg twice daily. May increase every 2–3 days in increments of 2.5 mg twice daily. **Maintenance:** 10–15 mg twice daily. **Maximum:** 30 mg twice daily.

Dosage in Renal/Hepatic Impairment
Not recommended in severe impairment.

SIDE EFFECTS

Frequent (12%–6%): Dizziness, drowsiness, nausea, headache. **Occasional (5%–2%):** Nervousness, fatigue, insomnia, dry mouth, light-headedness, mood swings, blurred vision, poor concentration, diarrhea, paresthesia. **Rare:** Muscle pain/stiffness, nightmares, chest pain, involuntary movements.

ADVERSE EFFECTS/TOXIC REACTIONS

No evidence of drug tolerance, psychological or physical dependence, withdrawal syndrome. Overdose may produce severe nausea, vomiting, dizziness, drowsiness, abdominal distention, excessive pupil constriction.

NURSING CONSIDERATIONS

BASELINE ASSESSMENT

Assess degree/manifestations of anxiety. Offer emotional support. Assess motor responses (agitation, trembling, tension), autonomic responses (cold, clammy hands; diaphoresis).

INTERVENTION/EVALUATION

For pts on long-term therapy, CBC, LFT, renal function tests should be performed periodically. Assist with ambulation if drowsiness, dizziness occur. Evaluate for therapeutic response: calm facial expression, decreased restlessness, lessened insomnia, mental status.

PATIENT/FAMILY TEACHING

• Improvement may be noted in 7–10 days, but optimum therapeutic effect generally takes 3–4 wks. • Drowsiness usually disappears during continued therapy. • If dizziness occurs, slowly go from lying to standing. • Avoid tasks that require alertness, motor skills until response to drug is established. • Avoid alcohol, grapefruit products. • Be consistent in taking with regard to food.

cabazitaxel

ka-**baz**-i-**tax**-el
(Jevtana)

■ **BLACK BOX ALERT** ■ All pts should be premedicated with a corticosteroid, an antihistamine, and an H₂ serum antagonist prior to infusion. Severe hypersensitivity reactions have occurred. Immediately discontinue infusion and give appropriate treatment if hypersensitivity reaction occurs. Neutropenic deaths reported. CBC, particularly ANC, should be obtained prior to and during treatment. Do not administer with neutrophil count 1,500 cells/mm³ or less.

Do not confuse cabazitaxel with PACLitaxel or Paxil, or Jevtana with Januvia, Levitra, or Sentra.

◆CLASSIFICATION

PHARMACOTHERAPEUTIC: Microtubule inhibitor. **CLINICAL:** Antineoplastic.

USES

Used in combination with predniSONE for treatment of hormone-refractory metastatic prostate cancer previously treated with a DOCEtaxel-containing regimen.

PRECAUTIONS

Contraindications: Hypersensitivity to cabazitaxel. Severe hepatic impairment (total serum bilirubin greater than 3 times upper limit of normal [ULN]). Neutrophil count of 1,500/mm³ or less, history of hypersensitivity to polysorbate 80. **Caution:** Mild to moderate hepatic impairment (bilirubin equal to or less than 3 times ULN), elderly, pregnancy, renal impairment (CrCl less than 30 mL/min). Pts at risk for developing GI complications (e.g., GI ulceration, concomitant use of NSAIDs).

ACTION

Binds to tubulin to promote assembly into microtubules and inhibits disassembly, which inhibits microtubules depolymerization/cell division. **Therapeutic Effect:** Blocks cells in mitotic phase of cell cycle, inhibiting tumor proliferation.

PHARMACOKINETICS

Widely distributed. Metabolized in liver. Protein binding: 89%–92%. Excreted in feces (76%), urine (3.7%). **Half-life:** 95 hrs.

⌛ LIFESPAN CONSIDERATIONS

Pregnancy/Lactation: May cause fetal harm. Crosses placental barrier. Breastfeeding not recommended. **Children:** Safety and efficacy not established. **Elderly:** Pts 65 yrs and older have 5% greater risk of developing neutropenia, fatigue, dizziness, fever, urinary tract infection, dehydration.

INTERACTIONS

DRUG: Strong CYP3A4 inhibitors (e.g., atazanavir, clarithromycin, ketoconazole, ritonavir) may increase concentration/effect; avoid use. **Strong CYP3A4 inducers (e.g., carBAMazepine, PHENobarbital, phenytoin, rifAMPin)** may decrease cabazitaxel concentration effects. **Live virus vaccine** may potentiate virus replication, increase vaccine's side effects, decrease response to vaccine. **HERBAL: St. John's wort, valerian** may increase CNS depression. **St. John's wort** may decrease concentration/effect. **FOOD: Grapefruit products** may increase concentration/effects. **LAB VALUES:** May increase serum bilirubin. May decrease Hgb, Hct, neutrophils, platelets.

AVAILABILITY (Rx)

Injection: 60 mg/1.5 mL

ADMINISTRATION/HANDLING

◀**ALERT**▶ Wear gloves during preparation, handling. Two-step dilution process must be performed under aseptic conditions to prepare second (final) infusion solution. Medication undergoes two dilutions. After second dilution, administration should be initiated within 30 min.

✦ Canadian trade name   🍃 Non-Crushable Drug   🔺 High Alert drug

Reconstitution

Step 1, First Dilution: • Each vial of cabazitaxel contains 60 mg/1.5 mL; must first be mixed with entire contents of supplied diluent. • Once reconstituted, solution contains 10 mg/mL of cabazitaxel. • When transferring diluent, direct needle onto inside vial wall and inject slowly to limit foaming. • Remove syringe and needle, then gently mix initial diluted solution by repeated inversions for at least 45 sec to ensure full mixing of drug and diluent. • Do not shake. • Allow any foam to dissipate.

Step 2, Final Dilution: • Withdraw recommended dose and further dilute with 250 mL 0.9% NaCl or D_5W. • If dose greater than 65 mg is required, use larger volume of 0.9% NaCl or D_5W so that concentration of 0.26 mg/mL is not exceeded. • Concentration of final diluted solution should be between 0.10 and 0.26 mg/mL.

Rate of Administration • Infuse over 1 hr using in-line 0.22-micron filter.

Storage • Store vials at room temperature. • First dilution solution stable for 30 min. • Final diluted solution stable for 8 hrs at room temperature or 24 hrs if refrigerated.

INDICATIONS/ROUTES/DOSAGE

◄**ALERT**► Antihistamine (dexchlorpheniramine 5 mg, diphenhydrAMINE 25 mg, or equivalent antihistamine), corticosteroid (dexamethasone 8 mg or equivalent), and H_2 antagonist (raNITIdine 50 mg or equivalent H_2 antagonist) should be given at least 30 min prior to each dose to reduce risk/severity of hypersensitivity.

Hormone-Refractory Metastatic Prostate Cancer

◄**ALERT**► Monitoring of CBC is essential on wkly basis during cycle 1 and before each treatment cycle thereafter so that the dose can be adjusted.

IV Infusion: ADULTS, ELDERLY: 20–25 mg/m² given as 1-hr infusion every 3 wks in combination with 10 mg predniSONE daily throughout treatment.

Dose Modification

Grade 3 neutropenia, febrile neutropenia, grade 3 or persistent diarrhea, neuropathy: Reduce dosage to 20 mg/m² after treatment interruption.

Dosage with Strong CYP3A Inhibitors
Consider dose reduction by 25%.

Dosage in Renal Impairment
CrCl less than 15 mL/min: Use caution.

Dosage in Hepatic Impairment
Mild Impairment: 20 mg/m². **Moderate Impairment:** 15 mg/m². **Severe Impairment:** Contraindicated.

SIDE EFFECTS

Frequent (47%–16%): Diarrhea, fatigue, nausea, vomiting, constipation, esthesia, abdominal pain, anorexia, back pain. **Occasional (13%–5%):** Peripheral neuropathy, fever, dyspnea, cough, arthralgia, dysgeusia, dyspepsia, alopecia, peripheral edema, weight decrease, urinary tract infection, dizziness, headache, muscle spasm, dysuria, hematuria, mucosal inflammation, dehydration.

ADVERSE EFFECTS/TOXIC REACTIONS

Hypersensitivity reaction may include generalized rash, erythema, hypotension, bronchospasm. 94% of pts develop grade 1–4 neutropenia and associated complications including anemia, thrombocytopenia, sepsis. GI abnormalities, hypertension, arrhythmias, renal failure may occur.

NURSING CONSIDERATIONS

BASELINE ASSESSMENT

Obtain ANC, CBC, BMP, LFT, serum testosterone. Assess ANC, CBC prior to each infusion. Question history of hypersensitivity reaction; renal/hepatic impairment; intolerance to corticosteroids. Receive full medication history and screen for interactions.

INTERVENTION/EVALUATION

Monitor CBC, ANC on wkly basis during cycle 1 and before each treatment cycle thereafter; do not administer if ANC less than 1,500 cells/mm³. Monitor serum ALT, AST, renal function. Monitor for hypersensitivity reaction (rash, erythema, dyspnea). Encourage adequate fluid intake. Monitor daily pattern of bowel activity, stool consistency. Offer antiemetics if nausea, vomiting occur. Closely monitor for signs/symptoms of neutropenia.

PATIENT/FAMILY TEACHING

• Report fever, chills, persistent sore throat, unusual bruising/bleeding, pale skin, fatigue. • Avoid tasks that require alertness, motor skills until response to drug is established. • Maintain strict oral hygiene. • Do not have immunizations without physician approval (drug lowers body's resistance). • Avoid those who have received a live virus vaccine. • Avoid crowds, those with cough, sneezing. • Avoid grapefruit products. • Diarrhea may cause dehydration; drink plenty of fluids.

---

caffeine citrate

kaf-een **sit**-rate
(Cafcit)

◆CLASSIFICATION

PHARMACOTHERAPEUTIC: Citrate salt of caffeine. **CLINICAL:** Bronchial smooth muscle relaxant.

USES

Short-term treatment of apnea in premature infants from 28 wks to younger than 33 wks gestational age.

PRECAUTIONS

Contraindications: Hypersensitivity to caffeine. **Cautions:** Hepatic/renal impairment, seizure disorder. Avoid in pts with symptomatic cardiac arrhythmias, agitation, anxiety, tremors.

ACTION

Stimulates medullary respiratory center. Appears to increase sensitivity of respiratory center to stimulatory effects of CO_2. **Therapeutic Effect:** Increases alveolar ventilation, reducing severity, frequency of apneic episodes.

PHARMACOKINETICS

Rapidly distributed in the brain. Peak plasma concentration: 30–120 min (PO). **Half-life:** 3–4 days (neonates); 5 hrs (9 mos and older).

INTERACTIONS

DRUG: CNS stimulants may cause excessive CNS stimulation (e.g., nervousness, insomnia, seizures, arrhythmias). **CYP1A2 inhibitors (e.g., cimetidine, ciprofloxacin)** may increase concentration, risk of side effects. **HERBAL:** None significant. **FOOD:** None known. **LAB VALUES:** May alter serum glucose.

AVAILABILITY (Rx)

Injection Solution: 20 mg/mL. **Oral Solution:** 20 mg/mL.

ADMINISTRATION/HANDLING

PO

• May give without regard to feedings. • May administer injectable solution orally.

 IV

• Infuse loading dose over at least 30 min; maintenance dose over at least 10 min. • May give without further dilution.

▦ IV COMPATIBILITIES

Alprostadil, calcium gluconate, cefotaxime, dexamethasone, DOBUTamine, DOPamine, gentamicin, heparin, vancomycin.

▦ IV INCOMPATIBILITIES

Acyclovir (Zovirax, Sitavig), furosemide (Lasix).

INDICATIONS/ROUTES/DOSAGE

Apnea

PO, IV: Loading dose: 20 mg/kg as caffeine citrate (5–10 mg/kg as caffeine base). If theophylline given within previous 72 hrs, a modified dose (50%–75%) may be given. **Maintenance:** 5–10 mg/kg/day as caffeine citrate (2.5 mg/kg/day as caffeine base) starting 24 hrs after loading dose. Dosage adjusted based on pt response and serum caffeine concentrations.

SIDE EFFECTS

Occasional (9%–2%): Feeding intolerance, rash, gastritis, abnormal healing, dyspnea, dry skin.

ADVERSE EFFECTS/TOXIC REACTIONS

Sepsis, necrotizing enterocolitis reported in 4% of pts. Hemorrhage including GI bleeding, intracranial hemorrhage; retinopathy of prematurity, renal failure, pulmonary edema, disseminated intravascular coagulation, acidosis, accidental injury, skin breakdown reported in 2% of pts.

NURSING CONSIDERATIONS

BASELINE ASSESSMENT

Baseline serum caffeine levels should be measured in infants previously treated with theophylline (preterm infants metabolize theophylline to caffeine).

INTERVENTION/EVALUATION

Diligently monitor respirations. Assess skin for rash. Monitor heart rate, number/severity of apnea spells, serum caffeine levels. Monitor for toxic reactions.

---

calcitonin

kal-si-**toe**-nin
(Calcimar ✦, Miacalcin)
Do not confuse calcitonin with calcitriol, or Miacalcin with Micatin.

◆CLASSIFICATION

PHARMACOTHERAPEUTIC: Synthetic hormone. **CLINICAL:** Calcium regulator, bone resorption inhibitor.

USES

Parenteral: Treatment of Paget's disease of bone, hypercalcemia, postmenopausal osteoporosis in women greater than 5 yrs postmenopause. **Intranasal:** Postmenopausal osteoporosis in women more than 5 yrs postmenopause.

PRECAUTIONS

Contraindications: Hypersensitivity to calcitonin, salmon protein. **Cautions:** None known.

ACTION

Antagonizes effects of parathyroid hormone. Increases jejunal secretion of water, sodium, potassium, chloride. Inhibits osteoclast bone resorption, increases excretion of calcium, phosphate, sodium, magnesium, potassium. **Therapeutic Effect:** Regulates serum calcium concentrations.

PHARMACOKINETICS

Nasal form rapidly absorbed. Injection form rapidly metabolized primarily in kidneys. Primarily excreted in urine. **Half-life: Nasal:** 43 min; **Injection:** 70–90 min.

⧖ LIFESPAN CONSIDERATIONS

Pregnancy/Lactation: Does not cross placenta; unknown if distributed in breast milk. Safe usage during lactation not established (inhibits lactation in animals). **Children:** Safety and efficacy not established. **Elderly:** No age-related precautions noted.

INTERACTIONS

DRUG: May decrease **lithium** concentration/effects. **HERBAL:** None significant. **FOOD:** None known. **LAB VALUES:** None significant.

AVAILABILITY (Rx)

Injection Solution (Miacalcin): 200 units/mL. **Nasal Spray (Miacalcin Nasal):** 200 units/activation.

ADMINISTRATION/HANDLING

IM, Subcutaneous
• IM route preferred if injection volume greater than 2 mL. Subcutaneous injection for outpatient self-administration unless volume greater than 2 mL. • Skin test should be performed before therapy in pts suspected of sensitivity to calcitonin. • Bedtime administration may reduce nausea, flushing.

Intranasal
• Refrigerate unopened nasal spray. Store at room temperature after initial use. • Instruct pt to clear nasal passages. • Tilt head slightly forward. • Insert spray tip into nostril, pointing toward nasal passages, away from nasal septum. • Spray into one nostril while pt holds other nostril closed and concurrently inspires through nose to deliver medication as high into nasal passage as possible. Spray into one nostril daily. • Discard after 30 doses.

INDICATIONS/ROUTES/DOSAGE

Skin Testing before Treatment in Pts with Suspected Sensitivity to Calcitonin-Salmon
Note: A detailed skin testing protocol is available from the manufacturer.

Paget's Disease
IM, Subcutaneous: ADULTS, ELDERLY: 100 units/day.

Postmenopausal Osteoporosis
IM, Subcutaneous: ADULTS, ELDERLY: 100 units daily with adequate calcium and vitamin D intake.
Intranasal: ADULTS, ELDERLY: 200 units/day as a single spray in one nostril, alternating nostrils daily.

Hypercalcemia
IM, Subcutaneous: ADULTS, ELDERLY: Initially, 4 units/kg q12h; may increase to 8 units/kg q12h if no response in 2 days; may further increase to 8 units/kg q6h if no response in another 2 days.

Dosage in Renal/Hepatic Impairment
No dose adjustment.

SIDE EFFECTS

Frequent: IM, Subcutaneous (10%): Nausea (may occur soon after injection; usually diminishes with continued therapy), inflammation at injection site. **Nasal (12%–10%):** Rhinitis, nasal irritation, redness, mucosal lesions. **Occasional: IM, Subcutaneous (5%–2%):** Flushing of face, hands. **Nasal (5%–3%):** Back pain, arthralgia, epistaxis, headache. **Rare: IM, Subcutaneous:** Epigastric discomfort, dry mouth, diarrhea, flatulence. **Nasal:** Itching of earlobes, pedal edema, rash, diaphoresis.

ADVERSE EFFECTS/TOXIC REACTIONS

Pts with a protein allergy may develop a hypersensitivity reaction (rash, dyspnea, hypotension, tachycardia).

NURSING CONSIDERATIONS

BASELINE ASSESSMENT
Obtain baseline serum electrolyte levels.

INTERVENTION/EVALUATION
Ensure rotation of injection sites; check for inflammation. Assess vertebral bone mass (document stabilization/improvement). Assess for allergic response: rash, urticaria, swelling, dyspnea, tachycardia, hypotension. Monitor serum electrolytes, calcium, alkaline phosphatase.

PATIENT/FAMILY TEACHING
• Instruct pt/family on aseptic technique, proper injection method of subcutaneous medication, including rotation of sites, proper administration of nasal medication. • Nausea is transient and usually decreases over time. • Immediately report rash, itching, shortness of breath, significant nasal irritation. • Improvement

C

in biochemical abnormalities and bone pain usually occurs in the first few months of treatment. • Improvement of neurologic lesions may take more than a year.

calcium acetate
(Eliphos, PhosLo)

calcium carbonate
(Apo-Cal ✱, Caltrate 600 ✱, OsCal ✱, Titralac, Tums)

calcium chloride
(Cal-Citrate, Citracal, Osteocit ✱)

calcium glubionate

calcium gluconate

kal-si-um

Do not confuse Citracal with Citrucel, OsCal with Asacol, or PhosLo with ProSom.

◆**CLASSIFICATION**

PHARMACOTHERAPEUTIC: Electrolyte replenisher. **CLINICAL:** Antacid, antihypocalcemic, antihyperkalemic, antihypermagnesemic, antihyperphosphatemic.

USES

Parenteral (calcium chloride): Treatment of hypocalcemia and conditions secondary to hypocalcemia (e.g., seizures, arrhythmias), emergency treatment of severe hypermagnesemia; **(calcium gluconate):** Treatment of hypocalcemia and conditions secondary to hypocalcemia (e.g., seizures, arrhythmias), cardiac disturbances secondary to hyperkalemia; adjunctive treatment of rickets, osteomalacia, and magnesium sulfate overdose; used to decrease capillary permeability in allergic conditions, nonthrombocytopenic purpura, and exudative dermatoses. **Calcium carbonate:** Antacid, dietary supplement. **Calcium acetate:** Controls hyperphosphatemia in end-stage renal disease. **OFF-LABEL (Calcium chloride):** Calcium channel blocker overdose, severe hyperkalemia, malignant arrhythmias associated with hypermagnesemia.

PRECAUTIONS

Contraindications: Hypersensitivity to calcium formulation. **All preparations:** Calcium-based renal calculi, hypercalcemia, ventricular fibrillation. **Calcium chloride:** Digoxin toxicity. **Calcium gluconate: Neonates:** Concurrent IV use with cefTRIAXone. **Cautions:** Chronic renal impairment, hypokalemia, concurrent use with digoxin.

ACTION

Essential for function, integrity of nervous, muscular, skeletal systems. Plays an important role in normal cardiac/renal function, respiration, blood coagulation, cell membrane and capillary permeability. Assists in regulating release/storage of hormones/neurotransmitters. Neutralizes/reduces gastric acid (increases pH). **Calcium acetate:** Binds with dietary phosphate, forming insoluble calcium phosphate. **Therapeutic Effect:** Replaces calcium in deficiency states; controls hyperphosphatemia in end-stage renal disease; relieves heartburn, indigestion.

PHARMACOKINETICS

Moderately absorbed from small intestine (absorption depends on presence of vitamin D metabolites, pH). Primarily eliminated in feces.

⧗ LIFESPAN CONSIDERATIONS

Pregnancy/Lactation: Distributed in breast milk. Unknown whether calcium chloride or calcium gluconate is distributed in breast milk. **Children:** Risk of extreme irritation, possible tissue necrosis or sloughing with IV calcium preparations. Restrict IV use due to small vasculature. **Elderly:** Oral absorption may be decreased.

INTERACTIONS

DRUG: Hypercalcemia may increase **digoxin** toxicity. Oral form may decrease absorption of **biphosphonates** (e.g., **risedronate**), **calcium channel blockers** (e.g., **amlodipine, diltiazem, verapamil**), **tetracycline derivatives, thyroid products. HERBAL:** None significant. **FOOD:** Food may increase calcium absorption. **LAB VALUES:** May increase serum pH, calcium, gastrin. May decrease serum phosphate, potassium.

AVAILABILITY (Rx)

CALCIUM ACETATE (667 mg = 169 mg calcium)

Gelcap (PhosLo): 667 mg. **Tablets (Eliphos):** 667 mg.

CALCIUM CARBONATE (1 g = 400 mg calcium)

Tablets: 500 mg, 600 mg, 1,250 mg, 1,500 mg. **Tablets (Chewable):** 500 mg, 750 mg, 1,000 mg.

CALCIUM CHLORIDE

Injection Solution: 10% (100 mg/mL) equivalent to 27.2 mg elemental calcium per mL.

CALCIUM GLUCONATE (1 g = 93 mg calcium)

Injection Solution: 10%.

ADMINISTRATION/HANDLING

 IV

Dilution

Calcium Chloride • May give undiluted or may dilute with 0.9% NaCl or Sterile Water for Injection.

Calcium Gluconate • May give undiluted or may dilute with 100 mL 0.9% NaCl or D5W.

Rate of Administration

Calcium Chloride • Note: Rapid administration may produce bradycardia, metallic/chalky taste, hypotension, sensation of heart, peripheral vasodilation. • **IV push:** Infuse slowly at maximum rate of 50–100 mg/min (in cardiac arrest, may administer over 10–20

sec). • **IV infusion:** Dilute to maximum final concentration of 20 mg/mL and infuse over 1 hr or no faster than 45–90 mg/kg/hr. Give via a central line. Do **NOT** use scalp, small hand or foot veins. Stop infusion if pt complains of pain or discomfort.

Calcium Gluconate • Note: Rapid administration may produce vasodilation, hypotension, arrhythmias, syncope, cardiac arrest. • **IV push:** Infuse slowly over 3–5 min or at maximum rate of 50–100 mg/min (in cardiac arrest, may administer over 10–20 sec). • **IV infusion:** Dilute 1–2 g in 100 mL 0.9% NaCl or D5W and infuse over 1 hr.

Storage • Store at room temperature. • Once diluted, stable for 24 hrs at room temperature.

PO

Calcium Acetate • Administer with plenty of fluids during meals to optimize effectiveness.

Calcium Carbonate • Administer with or immediately following meals with plenty of water (give with meals if used for phosphate binding). Instruct pt to thoroughly chew chewable tablets before swallowing.

🔲 IV INCOMPATIBILITIES

Calcium chloride: Amphotericin B complex (Abelcet, AmBisome, Amphotec), pantoprazole (Protonix), phosphate-containing solutions, propofol (Diprivan), sodium bicarbonate. **Calcium gluconate:** Amphotericin B complex (Abelcet, AmBisome, Amphotec), fluconazole (Diflucan).

🔲 IV COMPATIBILITIES

Calcium chloride: Amikacin (Amikin), DOBUTamine (Dobutrex), lidocaine, milrinone (Primacor), morphine, norepinephrine (Levophed). **Calcium gluconate:** Ampicillin, aztreonam (Azactam), ceFAZolin (Ancef), cefepime (Maxipime), ciprofloxacin (Cipro), DOBUTamine (Dobutrex), enalapril (Vasotec), famotidine (Pepcid), furosemide (Lasix), heparin, lidocaine, lipids, magnesium sulfate, meropenem (Merrem IV), midazolam (Versed), milrinone (Primacor), norepinephrine (Levophed), piperacillin and tazobactam (Zosyn), potassium chloride, propofol (Diprivan).

INDICATIONS/ROUTES/DOSAGE

Hyperphosphatemia

PO *(Calcium Acetate):* **ADULTS, ELDERLY:** Initially, 2 tablets 3 times/day with meals. May increase gradually (q2–3wks) to decrease serum phosphate level to less than 6 mg/dL as long as hypercalcemia does not develop. Usual dose: 2001–2668 mg with each meal.

Hypocalcemia

IV *(Calcium chloride):* **ADULTS, ELDERLY:** (Acute, symptomatic): 200–1,000 mg at intervals of q1–3 days. (Severe, symptomatic): 1 g over 10 min; may repeat q60min if symptoms resolve. **CHILDREN, NEONATES:** 2.7–5 mg/kg q4–6h as needed (**Maximum:** 1,000 mg).

IV *(Calcium Gluconate):* **ADULTS, ELDERLY:** (Mild): 1–2 g over 2 hrs; (Moderate to severe, asymptomatic): 4 g over 4 hrs; (Severe, symptomatic): 1–2 g over 10 min; may repeat q60min until symptoms resolve. **CHILDREN:** 200–500 mg/kg/day as a continuous infusion or in 4 divided doses. (**Maximum:** 1,000 mg). **NEONATES:** 200 mg/kg q6–12h or 400 mg/kg/day as a continuous infusion.

Antacid

PO *(Calcium Carbonate):* **ADULTS, ELDERLY:** 1–4 tabs as needed. **Maximum:** 8,000 mg/day. **CHILDREN 6–11 YRS:** 750–800 mg. **Maximum:** 3,000 mg/day. **CHILDREN 2–5 YRS:** 375–400 mg. **Maximum:** 1,500 mg/day.

Cardiac Arrest

IV *(Calcium Chloride):* **ADULTS, ELDERLY:** 500–1,000 mg over 2–5 min. May repeat as necessary. **CHILDREN, NEONATES:** 20 mg/kg. May repeat in 10 min if necessary. If effective, consider IV infusion of 20–50 mg/kg/hr.

Supplement

PO *(Calcium carbonate):* **ADULTS, ELDERLY:** 500 mg–4 g/day in 1–3 divided doses. **CHILDREN OLDER THAN 4 YRS:** 750 mg 3 times/day. **CHILDREN 2–4 YRS:** 750 mg 2 times/day. *(Calcium Citrate):* **ADULTS, ELDERLY:** 0.5–2 g 2–4 times/day. **CHILDREN:** 45–65 mg/kg/day in 4 divided doses.

Dosage in Renal/Hepatic Impairment

No dose adjustment.

SIDE EFFECTS

Frequent: PO: Chalky taste. **Parenteral:** Pain, rash, redness, burning at injection site; flushing, nausea, vomiting, diaphoresis, hypotension. **Occasional: PO:** Mild constipation, fecal impaction, peripheral edema, metabolic alkalosis (muscle pain, restlessness, slow respirations, altered taste). **Calcium carbonate:** Milk-alkali syndrome (headache, decreased appetite, nausea, vomiting, unusual fatigue). **Rare:** Urinary urgency, painful urination.

ADVERSE EFFECTS/TOXIC REACTIONS

Hypercalcemia: Early signs: Constipation, headache, dry mouth, increased thirst, irritability, decreased appetite, metallic taste, fatigue, weakness, depression. **Later signs:** Confusion, drowsiness, hypertension, photosensitivity, arrhythmias, nausea, vomiting, painful urination.

NURSING CONSIDERATIONS

BASELINE ASSESSMENT

Assess B/P, EKG and cardiac rhythm, renal function, serum magnesium, phosphate, calcium, ionized calcium.

INTERVENTION/EVALUATION

Monitor serum BMP, calcium, ionized calcium, magnesium, phosphate; B/P, cardiac rhythm, renal function. Monitor for signs of hypercalcemia.

C

• Do not take within 1–2 hrs of other oral medications, fiber-containing foods. • Avoid excessive use of alcohol, tobacco, caffeine.

canagliflozin

kan-a-gli-**floe**-zin
(Invokana)
■ BLACK BOX ALERT ■ May increase risk of lower limb amputations, including the toe, midfoot, and leg. Some pts had multiple amputations, including both legs. Monitor for new pain, tenderness, ulcers of lower legs.

FIXED-COMBINATION(S)

Invokamet: canagliflozin/metFOR-MIN (an antidiabetic): 50 mg/500 mg, 50 mg/1,000 mg, 150 mg/500 mg, 150 mg/1,000 mg.

◆CLASSIFICATION

PHARMACOTHERAPEUTIC: Sodium-glucose co-transporter 2 (SGLT2) inhibitor. **CLINICAL:** Antidiabetic.

USES

Adjunctive treatment to diet and exercise to improve glycemic control in pts with type 2 diabetes mellitus.

PRECAUTIONS

Contraindications: History of hypersensitivity to canagliflozin, other SGLT2 inhibitors, severe renal impairment, end-stage renal disease, dialysis. **Cautions:** Not recommended in type 1 diabetes, diabetic ketoacidosis. Concurrent use of diuretics, ACE inhibitors, angiotensin receptor blockers (ARB), other hypoglycemic or nephrotoxic medications; mild to moderate renal impairment; hypovolemia (dehydration/anemia), elderly, episodic hypotension, hyperkalemia, genital mycotic infection.

ACTION

Increases excretion of urinary glucose by inhibiting reabsorption of filtered glucose in kidney. Inhibits SGLT2 in proximal renal tubule. **Therapeutic Effect:** Lowers serum glucose levels.

PHARMACOKINETICS

Readily absorbed following PO administration. Metabolized in liver. Peak plasma concentration: 1–2 hrs. Protein binding: 99%. Excreted in feces (42%), urine (33%). **Half-life:** 11–13 hrs.

⧗ LIFESPAN CONSIDERATIONS

Pregnancy/Lactation: Unknown if distributed in breast milk. Must either discontinue drug or discontinue breastfeeding. **Children:** Safety and efficacy not established in pts younger than 18 yrs. **Elderly:** May have increased risk for adverse reactions (e.g., hypotension, syncope, dehydration).

INTERACTIONS

DRUG: Phenytoin, rifAMPin may decrease concentration/effect. **Potassium-sparing diuretics (e.g., spironolactone, triamterene)** may increase serum potassium level. **Antihypertensives (e.g., amLO-DIPine, lisinopril), beta blockers (e.g., carvedilol, metoprolol), diuretics (e.g., furosemide, HCTZ)** may increase risk of hypotension. **Insulin, oral hypoglycemics** may increase risk of hypoglycemia. May increase concentration/effects of digoxin. **HERBAL:** Herbs with hypoglycemic properties **(e.g., fenugreek, garlic, ginger, ginseng, gotu)** may increase risk of hypoglycemia. **FOOD:** None known. **LAB VALUES:** May increase serum low-density lipoprotein-cholesterol (LDL-C), Hgb, creatinine, magnesium, phosphate, potassium. May decrease glomerular filtration rate.

AVAILABILITY (Rx)

Tablets: 100 mg, 300 mg.

C

ADMINISTRATION/HANDLING

PO
• Give before first meal of the day.

INDICATIONS/ROUTES/DOSAGE

Type 2 Diabetes Mellitus
PO: ADULTS/ELDERLY: 100 mg daily before first meal. May increase to 300 mg daily if glomerular filtration rate (GFR) greater than 60 mL/min.

Dosage in Renal Impairment
GFR 45–60 mL/min: 100 mg daily (maximum). **GFR less than 45 mL/min:** Permanently discontinue.

Dosage in Hepatic Impairment
No dose adjustment.

SIDE EFFECTS

Occasional (5%): Increased urination. **Rare (3%–2%):** Thirst, nausea, constipation.

ADVERSE EFFECTS/TOXIC REACTIONS

Symptomatic hypotension (postural dizziness, orthostatic hypotension, syncope) may occur. Genital mycotic (yeast) infections reported in 10% of pts. Hypoglycemic events reported in 1.5% of pts (5% in elderly). Concomitant use of hypoglycemic medications may increase hypoglycemic risk. Hypersensitivity reactions, including angioedema, urticaria, rash, pruritus, erythema, occurred in 3%–4% of pts. May cause hyperkalemia. May increase risk of ketoacidosis.

NURSING CONSIDERATIONS

BASELINE ASSESSMENT

Assess hydration status. Obtain BMP, capillary blood glucose, hemoglobin A1c, LDL-C, digoxin level (if applicable). Assess pt's understanding of diabetes management, routine blood glucose monitoring. Receive full medication history, including minerals, herbal products. Question history of co-morbidities, esp. renal or hepatic impairment.

INTERVENTION/EVALUATION

Monitor serum potassium, cholesterol; capillary blood glucose, hepatic/renal function tests. Assess for hypoglycemia, hypersensitivity reaction. Monitor for signs of hyperkalemia. Screen for glucose-altering conditions: fever, increased activity or stress, surgical procedures. Obtain dietary consult for nutritional education. Encourage PO intake. Diligently monitor for new leg ulcers, sores, pain; wound may lead to amputation.

PATIENT/FAMILY TEACHING

• Diabetes mellitus requires lifelong control. • Diet and exercise are principal parts of treatment; do not skip or delay meals. • Test blood sugar regularly. • When taking combination drug therapy or when glucose demands are altered (fever, infection, trauma, stress), have low blood sugar treatment available (glucagon, oral dextrose). • Report suspected pregnancy or plans of breastfeeding. • Monitor daily calorie intake. • Go from lying to standing slowly to prevent dizziness. • Genital itching may indicate yeast infection. • Therapy may increase risk for dehydration/low blood pressure. • Report any palpitations or muscle weakness. • Treatment may cause loss of limbs; immediately report new leg ulcers, pain, tenderness.

candesartan

kan-de-**sar**-tan
(Apo-Candesartan ✹, Atacand)
■ **BLACK BOX ALERT** ■ May cause fetal injury, mortality. Discontinue as soon as possible once pregnancy is detected.

FIXED-COMBINATION(S)

Atacand HCT: candesartan/hydro-CHLOROthiazide (a diuretic): 16 mg/12.5 mg, 32 mg/12.5 mg.

◆CLASSIFICATION

PHARMACOTHERAPEUTIC: Angiotensin II receptor antagonist. **CLINICAL:** Antihypertensive.

USES

Treatment of hypertension alone or in combination with other antihypertensives, HF: NYHA class II–IV.

PRECAUTIONS

Contraindications: Hypersensitivity to candesartan. Concomitant use with aliskiren in pts with diabetes mellitus. **Cautions:** Significant aortic/mitral stenosis, renal/hepatic impairment, unstented (unilateral/bilateral) renal artery stenosis, HF (may induce hypotension when treatment initiated).

ACTION

Blocks vasoconstriction, aldosterone-secreting effects of angiotensin II, inhibiting binding of angiotensin II to AT_1 receptors. **Therapeutic Effect:** Produces vasodilation; decreases peripheral resistance, B/P.

PHARMACOKINETICS

Route	Onset	Peak	Duration
PO	2–3 hrs	6–8 hrs	Greater than 24 hrs

Rapidly, completely absorbed. Protein binding: greater than 99%. Undergoes minor hepatic metabolism to inactive metabolite. Excreted unchanged in urine and in feces through biliary system. Not removed by hemodialysis. **Half-life:** 9 hrs.

⧗ LIFESPAN CONSIDERATIONS

Pregnancy/Lactation: Unknown if distributed in breast milk. May cause fetal/neonatal morbidity/mortality. **Children:** Safety and efficacy not established in pts younger than 1 yr. **Elderly:** No age-related precautions noted.

INTERACTIONS

DRUG: May increase risk of **lithium** toxicity. **NSAIDs (e.g., ibuprofen,** **ketorolac, naproxen)** may decrease effects. **HERBAL: Ephedra, ginseng, yohimbe** may worsen hypertension. **Garlic** may increase antihypertensive effect. **FOOD:** None known. **LAB VALUES:** May increase serum BUN, alkaline phosphatase, bilirubin, creatinine, ALT, AST. May decrease Hgb, Hct.

AVAILABILITY (Rx)

Tablets: 4 mg, 8 mg, 16 mg, 32 mg.

ADMINISTRATION/HANDLING

PO
• Give without regard to food.

INDICATIONS/ROUTES/DOSAGE

Hypertension
Note: Antihypertensive effect usually seen in 2 wks. Maximum effect within 4–6 wks.
PO: ADULTS, ELDERLY: Initially, 16 mg once daily. Titrate to response. Range: 8–32 mg/day in 1–2 divided doses. **CHILDREN 6–16 YRS, GREATER THAN 50 KG:** Initially, 8–16 mg/day in 1–2 divided doses. Range: 4–32 mg. **Maximum:** 32 g/day. **50 KG OR LESS:** Initially, 4–8 mg in 1–2 divided doses. Range: 2–16 mg/day. **Maximum:** 32 mg/day. **CHILDREN 1–5 YRS:** Initially, 0.2 mg/kg/day in 1–2 divided doses. Range: 0.05–0.4 mg/kg/day. **Maximum:** 0.4 mg/kg/day.

HF
PO: ADULTS, ELDERLY: Initially, 4 mg once daily. May double dose at approximately 2-wk intervals up to a target dose of 32 mg/day.

Dosage in Renal/Hepatic Impairment
Mild to moderate impairment: No dose adjustment. **Severe impairment:** Use caution.

SIDE EFFECTS

Occasional (6%–3%): Upper respiratory tract infection, dizziness, back/leg pain. **Rare (2%–1%):** Pharyngitis, rhinitis, headache, fatigue, diarrhea, nausea, dry cough, peripheral edema.

ADVERSE EFFECTS/TOXIC REACTIONS

Overdosage may manifest as hypotension, tachycardia. Bradycardia occurs less often. May increase risk of renal failure, hyperkalemia.

NURSING CONSIDERATIONS

BASELINE ASSESSMENT

Obtain B/P, apical pulse immediately before each dose in addition to regular monitoring (be alert to fluctuations). Question for possibility of pregnancy. Assess medication history (esp. diuretic). Question for history of hepatic/renal impairment, renal artery stenosis. Obtain serum BUN, creatinine, LFT; Hgb, Hct.

INTERVENTION/EVALUATION

Maintain hydration (offer fluids frequently). Assess for evidence of upper respiratory infection. Assist with ambulation if dizziness occurs. Monitor electrolytes, renal function, urinalysis. Assess B/P for hypertension/hypotension. If excessive reduction in B/P occurs, place pt in supine position, feet slightly elevated.

PATIENT/FAMILY TEACHING

• Hypertension requires lifelong control. • Inform female pts regarding potential for fetal injury, mortality with second- and third-trimester exposure to candesartan. • Report suspected pregnancy. • Avoid tasks that require alertness, motor skills until response to drug is established. • Report any sign of infection (sore throat, fever). • Do not stop taking medication. • Caution against exercising during hot weather (risk of dehydration, hypotension).

cangrelor

kan-grel-or
(Kengreal)
Do not confuse cangrelor with ticagrelor.

◆**CLASSIFICATION**

PHARMACOTHERAPEUTIC: $P2Y_{12}$ platelet inhibitor. **CLINICAL:** Antiplatelet.

USES

Adjunct to percutaneous coronary intervention (PCI) for reducing risk of periprocedural myocardial infarction, repeat coronary revascularization, and stent thrombosis in pts who have not been treated with a $P2Y_{12}$ platelet inhibitor and are not being given a glycoprotein IIb/IIIa inhibitor.

PRECAUTIONS

Contraindications: Major active bleeding. Hypersensitivity to cangrelor. **Cautions:** Renal impairment; history of intracranial hemorrhage, GI bleeding.

ACTION

Blocks adenosine diphosphate (ADP)-induced platelet activation and aggregation. Binds selectively and reversibly to $P2Y_{12}$ receptor to prevent further signaling and platelet activation. **Therapeutic Effect:** Reduces platelet aggregation.

PHARMACOKINETICS

Widely distributed. Metabolized rapidly in circulatory system via dephosphorylation. Protein binding: 97%–98%. Peak plasma concentration: 2 min. Platelet function returns to baseline within 1 hr after discontinuing infusion. Eliminated in urine (58%), feces (35%). **Half-Life:** 3–6 min.

⧖ **LIFESPAN CONSIDERATIONS**

Pregnancy/Lactation: Unknown if distributed in breast milk. **Children:** Safety and efficacy not established. **Elderly:** No age-related precautions noted.

INTERACTIONS

DRUG: Clopidogrel, prasugrel have no antiplatelet effect if administered during cangrelor infusion. **HERBAL:** None

C

significant. **FOOD:** None known. **LAB VALUES:** May increase serum creatinine (in pts with severe renal impairment).

AVAILABILITY (Rx)

Injection, Lyophilized Power for Reconstitution: 50 mg/10 mL vial.

ADMINISTRATION/HANDLING

 IV

Reconstitution • Obtain weight in kg. • For each 50 mg/mL vial, reconstitute with 5 mL of Sterile Water for Injection. • Swirl gently until fully dissolved. Do not shake or agitate. Allow foam to settle. • Visually inspect for particulate matter or discoloration. Solution should appear clear, colorless to pale yellow in color. • Further dilute with 250 mL 0.9% NaCl or 5% Dextrose Injection. • Gently invert bag to mix. • Final concentration of diluted solution: 200 mcg/mL.
Rate of Administration • Administer bolus rapidly (less than 1 min) from diluted bag via manual IV push or infusion pump. Ensure that bolus dose is completely administered before starting PCI. • Start infusion immediately via dedicated line after administration of bolus.
Storage • Diluted solution is stable up to 12 hrs in 5% dextrose or up to 24 hrs in 0.9% NaCl at room temperature.

INDICATIONS/ROUTES/DOSAGE

Coronary Revascularization/Cardiac Stent Thrombosis
IV Infusion: ADULTS, ELDERLY: 30 mcg/kg bolus, then 4 mcg/kg/min infusion. Maintenance infusion should be continued for at least 2 hrs or for the duration of PCI (whichever is longer).

Transition to Oral P2Y$_{12}$ Therapy
To maintain platelet inhibition after discontinuation, one oral P2Y$_{12}$ platelet inhibitor should be administered as follows: • Ticagrelor 180 mg PO at any time during infusion or immediately after discontinuation. • Prasugrel 60 mg PO immediately after discontinuation (do not administer prasugrel prior to discontinuing infusion). • Clopidogrel 600 mg PO immediately after discontinuation (do not administer clopidogrel prior to discontinuing infusion).

Dosage in Renal/Hepatic Impairment
No dose adjustment.

SIDE EFFECTS

None known (see Adverse Effects/Toxic Reactions).

ADVERSE EFFECTS/TOXIC REACTIONS

Bleeding complications, including intracranial hemorrhage, other life-threatening/severe/moderate bleeding events, occurred in less than 1% of pts. Mild bleeding reported in 15% of pts. Coronary artery dissection, coronary artery perforation, and dyspnea were the most common events leading to discontinuation. Serious hypersensitivity reactions, including angioedema, anaphylaxis, anaphylactic shock, bronchospasm, stridor, occurred in less than 1% of pts. Worsening renal function was reported in 3% of pts with severe renal impairment. Dyspnea occurred in less than 2% of pts.

NURSING CONSIDERATIONS

BASELINE ASSESSMENT

Obtain renal function test in pts with renal impairment. Cross-check dose with co-worker. Question history of renal impairment; colon polyps, gastric/duodenal ulcers, GI bleeding; CVA, head trauma, recent intracranial hemorrhage; hypersensitivity to drug class.

INTERVENTION/EVALUATION

Report hematuria, epistaxis, coffee ground emesis, black/tarry stools. Assess for headache, altered mental status, stroke-like symptoms, hypertension (may indicate intracranial hemorrhage). Assess peripheral pulses; skin for ecchymosis, petechiae; gums for erythema, gingival bleeding.

C

• It may take longer to stop bleeding during therapy. • Use soft toothbrush, electric razor to decrease risk of bleeding. • Report any sign of red or dark urine, black or tarry stools, coffee-ground vomitus, blood-tinged mucus, nosebleeds. • Do not vigorously blow nose. • Report any confusion, headache, lethargy, one-sided weakness, trouble speaking.

---

capecitabine

kap-e-**sye**-ta-bine
(Xeloda)

█ BLACK BOX ALERT █ May increase anticoagulant effect of warfarin.

Do not confuse capecitabine with decitabine or emtricitabine, or Xeloda with Xenical.

◆CLASSIFICATION

PHARMACOTHERAPEUTIC: Antimetabolite. **CLINICAL:** Antineoplastic.

USES

Treatment of metastatic breast cancer, metastatic colorectal cancer. Adjuvant (postsurgical) treatment of Dukes C colon cancer. **OFF-LABEL:** Gastric cancer, pancreatic cancer, esophageal cancer, ovarian cancer, neuroendocrine tumors, hepatobiliary cancer.

PRECAUTIONS

Contraindications: Severe renal impairment (CrCl less than 30 mL/min), dihydropyrimidine dehydrogenase (DPD) deficiency, hypersensitivity to capecitabine, 5-fluorouracil (5-FU). **Cautions:** Existing bone marrow depression, hepatic impairment, mild to moderate renal impairment, previous cytotoxic therapy/radiation therapy, elderly (60 yrs of age or older).

ACTION

Enzymatically converted to 5-fluorouracil (5-FU). Inhibits enzymes necessary for synthesis of essential cellular components. **Therapeutic Effect:** Interferes with DNA synthesis, RNA processing, protein synthesis.

PHARMACOKINETICS

Readily absorbed from GI tract. Protein binding: less than 60%. Metabolized in liver. Primarily excreted in urine. **Half-life:** 45 min.

⧖ LIFESPAN CONSIDERATIONS

Pregnancy/Lactation: May cause fetal harm. Unknown if distributed in breast milk. **Children:** Safety and efficacy not established in pts younger than 18 yrs. **Elderly:** May be more sensitive to GI side effects.

INTERACTIONS

DRUG: May increase concentration, toxicity of **warfarin, phenytoin.** Myelosuppression may be enhanced when given concurrently with **bone marrow depressants. Live virus vaccines** may potentiate virus replication, increase vaccine side effects, decrease pt's antibody response to vaccine. **HERBAL: Echinacea** may decrease level/effects. **FOOD:** None known. **LAB VALUES:** May increase serum alkaline phosphatase, bilirubin, ALT, AST. May decrease Hgb, Hct, WBC. May increase PT/INR.

AVAILABILITY (Rx)

Tablets: 150 mg, 500 mg.

ADMINISTRATION/HANDLING

• Give within 30 min after meals with water. • Administer whole; do not cut, crush.

INDICATIONS/ROUTES/DOSAGE

Metastatic Breast Cancer (as monotherapy or in combination with docetaxel), Metastatic Colorectal Cancer, Adjuvant (Postsurgery) Treatment of Dukes C Colon Cancer
PO: ADULTS, ELDERLY: Initially, 2,500 mg/m²/day in 2 equally divided doses approximately q12h apart for 2 wks. Follow with a 1-wk rest period; given in 3-wk cycles.

Dosage in Renal Impairment
CrCl 51–80 mL/min: No adjustment.
CrCl 30–50 mL/min: 75% of normal dose. **CrCl less than 30 mL/min:** Contraindicated.

Dosage in Hepatic Impairment
No dose adjustment at start of therapy; interrupt therapy for grade 3 or 4 hyperbilirubinemia until bilirubin is 3 times ULN or less.

SIDE EFFECTS

Frequent (55%–25%): Diarrhea, nausea, vomiting, stomatitis, fatigue, anorexia, dermatitis. **Occasional (24%–10%):** Constipation, dyspepsia, headache, dizziness, insomnia, edema, myalgia, pyrexia, dehydration, dyspnea, back pain. **Rare (less than 10%):** Mood changes, depression, sore throat, epistaxis, cough, visual abnormalities.

ADVERSE EFFECTS/TOXIC REACTIONS

Serious reactions include myelosuppression (neutropenia, thrombocytopenia, anemia), cardiovascular toxicity (angina, cardiomyopathy, DVT), respiratory toxicity (dyspnea, epistaxis, pneumonia), lymphedema. Palmar-plantar erythrodysesthesia syndrome (PPES), presenting as redness, swelling, numbness, skin sloughing of hands and feet, may occur.

NURSING CONSIDERATIONS

BASELINE ASSESSMENT

Assess sensitivity to capecitabine or 5-fluorouracil. Obtain baseline Hgb, Hct, serum chemistries, renal function.

INTERVENTION/EVALUATION

Monitor for severe diarrhea, nausea, vomiting; if dehydration occurs, fluid and electrolyte replacement therapy should be initiated. Assess hands/feet for PPES. Monitor CBC for evidence of bone marrow depression. Monitor renal/hepatic function. Monitor for blood dyscrasias (fever, sore throat, signs of local infection, unusual bruising/bleeding from any

site), symptoms of anemia (excessive fatigue, weakness).

PATIENT/FAMILY TEACHING
• Report nausea, vomiting, diarrhea, hand-and-foot syndrome, stomatitis. • Do not have immunizations without physician's approval (drug lowers body's resistance). • Avoid contact with those who have recently received live virus vaccine. • Promptly report fever higher than 100.5°F, sore throat, signs of local infection, unusual bruising/bleeding from any site.

---

captopril

kap-toe-pril
(Apo-Capto ✦)

■ **BLACK BOX ALERT** ■ May cause injury/death to developing fetus. Discontinue as soon as possible once pregnancy is detected.
Do not confuse captopril with calcitriol, Capitrol, carvedilol, enalapril, fosinopril, lisinopril, Monopril, or quinapril.

FIXED-COMBINATION(S)

Capozide: captopril/hydroCHLOROthiazide (a diuretic): 25 mg/15 mg, 25 mg/25 mg, 50 mg/15 mg, 50 mg/25 mg.

◆CLASSIFICATION

PHARMACOTHERAPEUTIC: Angiotensin-converting enzyme (ACE) inhibitor. **CLINICAL:** Antihypertensive, vasodilator.

USES

Treatment of hypertension, HF, diabetic nephropathy, post-MI for prevention of ventricular failure.

PRECAUTIONS

Contraindications: Hypersensitivity to captopril. History of angioedema from

---

previous treatment with ACE inhibitors, concomitant use with aliskiren in pts with diabetes mellitus. **Cautions:** Renal impairment; hypertrophic cardiomyopathy with outflow obstruction, before, during, or immediately after major surgery. Unstented unilateral/bilateral renal artery stenosis. Concomitant use of potassium-sparing diuretics, potassium supplements.

ACTION

Suppresses renin-angiotensin-aldosterone system (prevents conversion of angiotensin I to angiotensin II, a potent vasoconstrictor; may inhibit angiotensin II at local vascular and renal sites). Decreases plasma angiotensin II, increases plasma renin activity, decreases aldosterone secretion. **Therapeutic Effect:** Reduces peripheral arterial resistance, pulmonary capillary wedge pressure; improves cardiac output, exercise tolerance.

PHARMACOKINETICS

Route	Onset	Peak	Duration
PO	0.25 hr	0.5–1.5 hrs	Dose-related

Rapidly, well absorbed from GI tract (absorption decreased in presence of food). Protein binding: 25%–30%. Metabolized in liver. Primarily excreted in urine. Removed by hemodialysis. **Half-life:** Less than 3 hrs (increased in renal impairment).

⏳ LIFESPAN CONSIDERATIONS

Pregnancy/Lactation: Crosses placenta; distributed in breast milk. May cause fetal/neonatal mortality/morbidity. **Children:** Safety and efficacy not established. **Elderly:** May be more sensitive to hypotensive effects.

INTERACTIONS

DRUG: Antihypertensives (e.g., amLODIPine, metoprolol, valsartan), diuretics (e.g., furosemide, HCTZ) may increase hypotensive effects. May increase **lithium** concentration, toxicity.

NSAIDs (e.g., ibuprofen, ketorolac, naproxen) may decrease antihypertensive effect. **Potassium-sparing diuretics (e.g., spironolactone, triamterene), potassium supplements** may cause hyperkalemia. **HERBAL: Ephedra, ginseng, yohimbe** may worsen hypertension. **Garlic** may increase antihypertensive effect. **FOOD: Licorice** may cause sodium and water retention, hypokalemia. **LAB VALUES:** May increase serum BUN, alkaline phosphatase, bilirubin, creatinine, potassium, ALT, AST. May decrease serum sodium. May cause positive ANA titer.

AVAILABILITY (Rx)

Tablets: 12.5 mg, 25 mg, 50 mg, 100 mg.

ADMINISTRATION/HANDLING

PO
• Administer 1 hr before or 2 hrs after meals for maximum absorption (food may decrease drug absorption). • Tablets may be crushed.

INDICATIONS/ROUTES/DOSAGE

Hypertension
PO: ADULTS, ELDERLY: Initially, 12.5–25 mg 2–3 times/day. May increase by 12.5–25 mg/dose at 1–2-wk intervals up to 50 mg 3 times/day. Add diuretic before further increase in dose. **Maximum:** 450 mg/day in 3 divided doses. **CHILDREN, ADOLESCENTS:** 0.3–0.5 mg 3 times/day. **Maximum:** 6 mg/kg/day in 2–4 divided doses. **INFANTS:** 0.15–0.3 mg/kg/dose. May titrate up to maximum of 6 mg/kg/day in 1–4 divided doses. Usual range: 2.5–6 mg/kg/day in 2–4 divided doses. **NEONATES:** 0.01–0.1 mg/kg/dose q8–24h. **Maximum:** 0.5 mg/kg/dose q6–24h.

HF
PO: ADULTS, ELDERLY: Initially, 6.25–25 mg 3 times/day. **Target dose:** 50 mg 3 times/day.

Post-MI
PO: ADULTS, ELDERLY: Initially, 6.25 mg. If tolerated, then 12.5 mg 3 times/day. Increase to 25 mg 3 times/day over several

days, up to target dose of 50 mg 3 times/day over several wks.

Diabetic Nephropathy
PO: ADULTS, ELDERLY: 25 mg 3 times/day.

Dosage in Renal Impairment
CrCl 10–50 mL/min: 75% of normal dosage. **CrCl less than 10 mL/min:** 50% of normal dosage.

Dosage in Hepatic Impairment
No dose adjustment.

SIDE EFFECTS

Frequent (7%–4%): Rash. **Occasional (4%–2%):** Pruritus, dysgeusia. **Rare (less than 2%):** Headache, cough, insomnia, dizziness, fatigue, paresthesia, malaise, nausea, diarrhea or constipation, dry mouth, tachycardia.

ADVERSE EFFECTS/TOXIC REACTIONS

Hypotension ("first-dose syncope") may occur in pts with HF and in those who are severely sodium/volume depleted. Angioedema, hyperkalemia occur rarely. Agranulocytosis, neutropenia noted in those with collagen vascular disease (scleroderma, systemic lupus erythematosus), renal impairment. Nephrotic syndrome noted in those with history of renal disease.

NURSING CONSIDERATIONS

BASELINE ASSESSMENT

Obtain B/P immediately before each dose in addition to regular monitoring (be alert to fluctuations). If hypotension occurs, place pt in supine position with legs elevated. In pts with prior renal disease or receiving dosages greater than 150 mg/day, test urine for protein by dipstick method with first urine of day before therapy begins and periodically thereafter. In pts with renal impairment, autoimmune disease, or taking drugs that affect leukocytes or immune response, obtain CBC before beginning therapy, q2wks for 3 mos, then periodically thereafter.

INTERVENTION/EVALUATION

Assess skin for rash, pruritus. Assist with ambulation if dizziness occurs. Monitor urinalysis for proteinuria. Monitor serum potassium levels in pts on concurrent diuretic therapy. Monitor B/P, serum BUN, creatinine, CBC. Discontinue medication, contact physician if angioedema occurs.

PATIENT/FAMILY TEACHING

• Full therapeutic effect of B/P reduction may take several wks. • Skipping doses or voluntarily discontinuing drug may produce severe rebound hypertension. • Limit alcohol intake. • Immediately report if swelling of face, lips, or tongue; difficulty breathing, vomiting, diarrhea, excessive perspiration, dehydration, persistent cough, sore throat, fever occur. • Inform physician if pregnant or planning to become pregnant. • Rise slowly from sitting/lying position.

carBAMazepine

kar-ba-**maz**-e-peen
(Apo-CarBAMazepine ✦, Carbatrol, Carnexiv, Epitol, Equetro, TEGretol, TEGretol XR)

■**BLACK BOX ALERT** ■ Potentially fatal aplastic anemia, agranulocytosis reported. Potentially fatal, severe dermatologic reactions (e.g., Stevens-Johnson syndrome, toxic epidermal necrolysis) may occur. Risk increased in pts with the variant HLA-β* 1502 allele, almost exclusively in pts of Asian ancestry. **Do not confuse carBAMazepine with OXcarbazepine, eslicarbazepine, or TEGretol with Mebaral, Toprol XL, Toradol, or TRENtal.**

◆CLASSIFICATION

PHARMACOTHERAPEUTIC: Iminostilbene derivative. **CLINICAL:** Anticonvulsant, antineuralgic, antimanic, antipsychotic.

USES

Carbatrol, Epitol, TEGretol, TEGretol XR: Treatment of partial seizures with complex symptomatology, generalized tonic-clonic seizures, mixed seizure patterns, pain relief of trigeminal, glossopharyngeal neuralgia. **Carnexiv:** Replacement when oral therapy not feasible in adults with seizures. **Equetro:** Acute manic and mixed episodes associated with bipolar disorder. **OFF-LABEL:** Neuropathic pain in critically ill pts.

PRECAUTIONS

Contraindications: Concomitant use or within 14 days of use of MAOIs, myelosuppression. Concomitant use of delavirdine or other NNRT inhibitors, hypersensitivity to carBAMazepine, tricyclic antidepressants. **Cautions:** High risk of suicide, increased IOP, hepatic or renal impairment, history of cardiac impairment, EKG abnormalities, elderly.

ACTION

Decreases sodium ion influx into neuronal membranes, reducing post-tetanic potentiation at synapses. **Therapeutic Effect:** Produces anticonvulsant effect.

PHARMACOKINETICS

Slowly, completely absorbed from GI tract. Protein binding: 75%–90%. Metabolized in liver. Primarily excreted in urine. Not removed by hemodialysis. **Half-life:** 25–65 hrs (decreased with chronic use).

⧗ LIFESPAN CONSIDERATIONS

Pregnancy/Lactation: Crosses placenta; distributed in breast milk. Accumulates in fetal tissue. **Children:** Behavioral changes more likely to occur. **Elderly:** More susceptible to confusion, agitation, AV block, bradycardia, syndrome of inappropriate antidiuretic hormone (SIADH).

INTERACTIONS

DRUG: CYP3A4 inhibitors (e.g., **cimetidine, clarithromycin, azole antifungals, protease inhibitors**) may increase concentration. **CYP3A4 inducers** (e.g., **rifAMPin, phenytoin**) may decrease concentration/effects. May decrease concentration/effects of **hormonal contraceptives, warfarin, traZODone. HERBAL:** Evening primrose may decrease seizure threshold. **Gotu kola, kava kava, St. John's wort, valerian** may increase CNS depression. **FOOD:** Grapefruit products may increase absorption, concentration. **LAB VALUES:** May increase serum BUN, glucose, alkaline phosphatase, bilirubin, ALT, AST, cholesterol, HDL, triglycerides. May decrease serum calcium, thyroid hormone (T_3, T_4 index) levels. **Therapeutic serum level:** 4–12 mcg/mL; **toxic serum level:** greater than 12 mcg/mL.

AVAILABILITY (Rx)

Injection, Solution (Carnexiv): 200 mg/20 mL single-use vial. **Suspension (Tegretol):** 100 mg/5 mL. **Tablets (Epitol, Tegretol):** 200 mg. **Tablets (Chewable [Tegretol]):** 100 mg.

🍃 **Capsules (Extended-Release [Carbatrol, Equetro]):** 100 mg, 200 mg, 300 mg. **Tablets (Extended-Release [Tegretol XR]):** 100 mg, 200 mg, 400 mg.

ADMINISTRATION/HANDLING

PO

• Store oral suspension, tablets at room temperature. • Give with meals to reduce GI distress. • May give extended-release capsules without regard to food. • Extended-release tablets should be given with meals. • Shake oral suspension well. Do not administer simultaneously with other liquid medicine. • Do not crush or open extended-release capsules or tablets. • Extended-release capsules may be opened and sprinkled over food (e.g., applesauce).

 IV

Must be diluted with 100 mL 0.9% NaCl or D_5W. Solution stable for 4 hrs at room temperature, 24 hrs refrigerated.

INDICATIONS/ROUTES/DOSAGE

◀**ALERT**▶ Suspension must be given on a 3–4 times/day schedule; tablets on a 2–4 times/day schedule; extended-release capsules 2 times/day. **Carnexiv:** 70% of total oral dose given as four 30-min infusions separated by 6 hrs.

Seizure Control
PO: ADULTS, ELDERLY, CHILDREN OLDER THAN 12 YRS: Initially, 200 mg twice daily (tablet or extended-release or in 4 divided doses as suspension). May increase dosage by 200 mg/day at wkly intervals. Usual dose: 800–1,200 mg/day in 2–4 divided doses. **Maximum: ADULTS, ELDERLY:** 1,600 mg/day; **CHILDREN OLDER THAN 15 YRS:** 1,200 mg/day; **CHILDREN 13–15 YRS:** 1,000 mg/day. **CHILDREN 6–12 YRS:** Initially, 100 mg twice daily (tablets) or 4 times/day (oral suspension). May increase by 100 mg/day at wkly intervals. Usual dose: 400–800 mg/day. **Maximum:** 1,000 mg/day. **CHILDREN YOUNGER THAN 6 YRS:** Initially, 10–20 mg/kg/day 2–3 times/day (tablets) or 4 times/day (suspension). May increase at wkly intervals until optimal response and therapeutic levels are achieved. **Maximum:** 35 mg/kg/day.

Trigeminal, Glossopharyngeal Neuralgia, Diabetic Neuropathy
PO: ADULTS, ELDERLY: Initially, 100 mg twice a day (tablets or extended-release) or 4 times/day (oral suspension). May increase by 100 mg twice daily up to 400–800 mg/day. **Maximum:** 1,200 mg/day.

Bipolar Disorder
PO: ADULTS, ELDERLY (Equetro): Initially, 400 mg/day in 2 divided doses. May adjust dose in 200-mg increments. **Maximum:** 1,600 mg/day in divided doses.

Dosage in Renal Impairment
CrCl less than 10 mL/min: 75% of normal dose. **HD:** 75% of normal dose. **CRRT:** 75% of normal dose.

Dosage in Hepatic Impairment
Use caution.

SIDE EFFECTS

Frequent (greater than 10%): Vertigo, somnolence, ataxia, fatigue, leukopenia, rash, urticaria, nausea, vomiting. **Occasional (10%–1%):** Headache, diplopia, blurred vision, thrombocytopenia, dry mouth, edema, fluid retention, increased weight. **Rare (less than 1%):** Tremors, visual disturbances, lymphadenopathy, jaundice, involuntary muscle movements, nystagmus, dermatitis.

ADVERSE EFFECTS/TOXIC REACTIONS

Toxic reactions appear as blood dyscrasias (aplastic anemia, agranulocytosis, thrombocytopenia, leukopenia, leukocytosis, eosinophilia), cardiovascular disturbances (HF, hypotension/hypertension, thrombophlebitis, arrhythmias), dermatologic effects (rash, urticaria, pruritus, photosensitivity). Abrupt withdrawal may precipitate status epilepticus.

NURSING CONSIDERATIONS

BASELINE ASSESSMENT
CBC, serum iron determination, urinalysis, BUN should be performed before therapy begins and periodically during therapy. **Seizures:** Review history of seizure disorder (intensity, frequency, duration, level of consciousness [LOC]). Initiate seizure precautions. **Neuralgia:** Assess facial pain, stimuli that may cause facial pain. **Bipolar:** Assess mental status, cognitive abilities.

INTERVENTION/EVALUATION
Seizures: Observe frequently for recurrence of seizure activity. Monitor therapeutic levels. Assess for clinical improvement (decrease in intensity, frequency of seizures). Assess for clinical evidence of early toxicity (fever, sore throat, mouth ulcerations, unusual bruising/bleeding, joint pain). **Neuralgia:** Avoid triggering tic douloureux (draft, talking, washing face, jarring bed, hot/warm/cold food or liquids). **Bipolar:** Monitor for suicidal ideation, behavioral changes. Observe

for excessive sedation. **Therapeutic serum level:** 4–12 mcg/mL; **toxic serum level:** greater than 12 mcg/mL.

PATIENT/FAMILY TEACHING

• Do not abruptly discontinue medication after long-term use (may precipitate seizures). • Strict maintenance of therapy is essential for seizure control. • Avoid tasks that require alertness, motor skills until response to drug is established. • Report visual disturbances. • Blood tests should be repeated frequently during first 3 mos of therapy and at monthly intervals thereafter for 2–3 yrs. • Do not take oral suspension simultaneously with other liquid medicine. • Do not ingest grapefruit products. • Report serious skin reactions.

---

carbidopa/levodopa

kar-bi-doe-pa/**lee**-voe-doe-pa
(Apo-Levocarb ✤, Duopa, Rytary, Sinemet, Sinemet CR)
Do not confuse Sinemet with Serevent.

FIXED-COMBINATION(S)

Stalevo: carbidopa/levodopa/entacapone (antiparkinson agent): 12.5 mg/50 mg/200 mg, 18.75 mg/75 mg/200 mg, 25 mg/100 mg/200 mg, 31.25 mg/125 mg/200 mg, 37.5 mg/150 mg/200 mg, 50 mg/200 mg/200 mg.

◆CLASSIFICATION

PHARMACOTHERAPEUTIC: DOPamine precursor. **CLINICAL:** Antiparkinson agent.

USES

Treatment of Parkinson's disease, postencephalitic parkinsonism, symptomatic parkinsonism following CNS injury by carbon monoxide poisoning, manganese intoxication. **Duopa:** Treatment of motor fluctuations in advanced Parkinson's disease. **OFF-LABEL:** Restless legs syndrome.

PRECAUTIONS

Contraindications: Hypersensitivity to carbidopa/levodopa. Concurrent use with MAOIs or use within 14 days. (Tablets only): Narrow-angle glaucoma. **Cautions:** History of MI, arrhythmias, bronchial asthma, emphysema, severe cardiac, pulmonary, renal/hepatic impairment; active peptic ulcer, treated open-angle glaucoma, seizure disorder, pts at risk for hypotension, elderly.

ACTION

Converted to DOPamine in basal ganglia, increasing DOPamine concentration in brain, inhibiting hyperactive cholinergic activity. Carbidopa prevents peripheral breakdown of levodopa, making more levodopa available for transport into brain. **Therapeutic Effect:** Reduces tremor.

PHARMACOKINETICS

Rapidly and completely absorbed from GI tract. Widely distributed. Excreted primarily in urine. Levodopa is converted to DOPamine. Excreted primarily in urine. **Half-life:** 1–2 hrs (carbidopa); 1–3 hrs (levodopa).

⧖ LIFESPAN CONSIDERATIONS

Pregnancy/Lactation: Unknown if drug crosses placenta or is distributed in breast milk. May inhibit lactation. Breastfeeding not recommended. **Children:** Safety and efficacy not established in pts younger than 18 yrs. **Elderly:** More sensitive to effects of levodopa. Anxiety, confusion, nervousness more common when receiving anticholinergics.

INTERACTIONS

DRUG: Isoniazid, antipsychotics, phenytoin, pyridoxine may decrease effects. **MAOIs (e.g., selegiline, phenelzine)** may increase concentration, effects of orthostatic hypotension. **Antihypertensives (e.g., amlodipine, lisinopril, valsartan)** may increase risk of orthostatic hypotension. **HERBAL: Kava kava** may decrease effect. **FOOD: High-protein** diets may cause decreased or erratic response to levodopa. **LAB VALUES:** May increase serum BUN, LDH, alkaline phosphatase, bilirubin, ALT, AST. May decrease Hgb, Hct, WBC.

AVAILABILITY (Rx)

Enteral Suspension (Duopa): 100-mL cassette containing 4.63 mg carbidopa and 20 mg levodopa per mL. **Tablets (Immediate-Release [Sinemet]):** 10 mg carbidopa/100 mg levodopa, 25 mg carbidopa/100 mg levodopa, 25 mg carbidopa/250 mg levodopa. **Tablets (Orally Disintegrating Immediate-Release):** 10 mg carbidopa/100 mg levodopa, 25 mg carbidopa/100 mg levodopa, 25 mg carbidopa/250 mg levodopa.

🌶 **Capsules (Extended-Release [Rytary]):** carbidopa/levodopa: 23.75 mg/95 mg, 36.25 mg/145 mg, 48.75 mg/195 mg, 61.25 mg/245 mg. **Tablets (Extended-Release [Sinemet CR]):** 25 mg carbidopa/100 mg levodopa, 50 mg carbidopa/200 mg levodopa.

ADMINISTRATION/HANDLING

Note: Space doses evenly over waking hours.

Enteral Suspension
Refrigerate. Remove 20 min prior to administration.

PO
• Scored tablets may be crushed. • Give with meals to decrease GI upset. • Do not crush or chew extended-release tablets.

PO (Parcopa)
• Place orally disintegrating tablet on top of tongue. Tablet will dissolve in seconds; pt to swallow with saliva. Not necessary to administer with liquid.

INDICATIONS/ROUTES/DOSAGE

Parkinsonism
PO: ADULTS, ELDERLY (IMMEDIATE-RELEASE ORALLY DISINTEGRATING TABLET): Initially, 25/100 mg 3 times/day.

May increase daily or every other day by 1 tablet up to 200/2,000 mg daily. **(EXTENDED-RELEASE):** (Sinemet CR) 50/200 mg 2 times/day at least 6 hrs apart. Intervals between doses of Sinemet CR should be 4–8 hrs while awake, with smaller doses at end of day if doses are not equal. May adjust q3days. **Maximum:** 8 tablets/day. **(RYTARY):** Initially, 23.75/95 mg 3 times/day for 3 days, then to 36.25/145 mg 3 times/day. Frequency may be increased to maximum of 5 times/day if needed and tolerated. **Maximum daily dose:** 612.5/2450 mg/day. **(ENTERAL SUSPENSION): Maximum:** 2000 mg (1 container) over 16 hrs through NJ or PEG tube via infusion pump. Also take oral immediate-release in evening after disconnecting pump. Refer to manufacturer's guidelines for morning dose, continuous dose escalculation, titration instructions.

Dosage in Renal/Hepatic Impairment
Use caution.

SIDE EFFECTS

Frequent (80%–50%): Involuntary movements of face, tongue, arms, upper body; nausea/vomiting; anorexia. **Occasional:** Depression, anxiety, confusion, nervousness, urinary retention, palpitations, dizziness, light-headedness, decreased appetite, blurred vision, constipation, dry mouth, flushed skin, headache, insomnia, diarrhea, unusual fatigue, darkening of urine and sweat. **Rare:** Hypertension, ulcer, hemolytic anemia (marked by fatigue).

ADVERSE EFFECTS/TOXIC REACTIONS

High incidence of involuntary choreiform, dystonic, dyskinetic movements in those on long-term therapy. Numerous mild to severe CNS and psychiatric disturbances may occur (reduced attention span, anxiety, nightmares, daytime drowsiness, euphoria, fatigue, paranoia, psychotic episodes, depression, hallucinations).

NURSING CONSIDERATIONS

BASELINE ASSESSMENT

Assess symptoms of Parkinson's disease (e.g., rigidity, pill rolling, gait). Receive full medication history and screen for interactions.

INTERVENTION/EVALUATION

Be alert to neurologic effects (headache, lethargy, mental confusion, agitation). Monitor for evidence of dyskinesia (difficulty with movement). Assess for clinical reversal of symptoms (improvement of tremor of head and hands at rest, mask-like facial expression, shuffling gait, muscular rigidity). Monitor B/P (standing, sitting, supine).

PATIENT/FAMILY TEACHING

• Avoid tasks that require alertness, motor skills until response to drug is established. • Sugarless gum, sips of water may relieve dry mouth. • Take with food to minimize GI upset. • Effects may be delayed from several wks to mos. • May cause darkening of urine or sweat (not harmful). • Report any uncontrolled movement of face, eyelids, mouth, tongue, arms, hands, legs; mental changes; palpitations; severe or persistent nausea/vomiting; difficulty urinating. • Report exacerbations of asthma, underlying depression, psychosis.

CARBOplatin   HIGH ALERT

kar-boe-**plat**-in
(CARBOplatin Injection)
■ **BLACK BOX ALERT** ■ Must be administered by personnel trained in administration/handling of chemotherapeutic agents (high potential for severe reactions, including anaphylaxis [may occur within minutes of administration] and sudden death). Profound myelosuppression (anemia, thrombocytopenia) has occurred. Vomiting may occur.

Do not confuse CARBOplatin with CISplatin or oxaliplatin, or with Platinol.

◆CLASSIFICATION

PHARMACOTHERAPEUTIC: Alkylating agent. **CLINICAL:** Antineoplastic.

USES

Treatment of advanced ovarian carcinoma. Palliative treatment of recurrent ovarian cancer. **OFF-LABEL:** Brain tumors, Hodgkin's and non-Hodgkin's lymphomas, malignant melanoma, retinoblastoma; treatment of breast, bladder, cervical, endometrial, esophageal, small-cell lung, non–small-cell lung, head and neck, testicular carcinomas; germ cell tumors, osteogenic sarcoma.

PRECAUTIONS

Contraindications: Hypersensitivity to CARBOplatin. History of severe allergic reaction to CISplatin, platinum compounds, mannitol; severe bleeding, severe myelosuppression. **Cautions:** Moderate bone marrow depression, renal impairment, elderly.

ACTION

Inhibits DNA synthesis by cross-linking with DNA strands, preventing cell division. **Therapeutic Effect:** Interferes with DNA function.

PHARMACOKINETICS

Protein binding: Low. Hydrolyzed in solution to active form. Primarily excreted in urine. **Half-life:** 2.6–5.9 hrs.

⊠ LIFESPAN CONSIDERATIONS

Pregnancy/Lactation: If possible, avoid use during pregnancy, esp. first trimester. May cause fetal harm. Unknown if distributed in breast milk. Breastfeeding not recommended. **Children:** Safety and efficacy not established. **Elderly:** Peripheral neurotoxicity increased, myelotoxicity may be more severe. Age-related renal impairment may require decreased dosage, careful monitoring of blood counts.

INTERACTIONS

DRUG: Bone marrow depressants may increase myelosuppression. **Live virus vaccines** may potentiate virus replication, increase vaccine side effects, decrease pt's antibody response to vaccine. **Nephrotoxic, ototoxic medications (e.g., gentamicin, ketorolac, furosemide)** may increase risk of toxicity. **HERBAL:** Avoid **black cohosh, dong quai** in estrogen-dependent tumors. **Echinacea** may decrease level/effects. **FOOD:** None known. **LAB VALUES:** May decrease serum calcium, magnesium, potassium, sodium. May increase serum BUN, alkaline phosphatase, bilirubin, creatinine, AST.

AVAILABILITY (Rx)

Injection Solution: 10 mg/mL.

ADMINISTRATION/HANDLING

◀ **ALERT** ▶ May be carcinogenic, mutagenic, teratogenic. Handle with extreme care during preparation/administration.

 IV

Reconstitution • Dilute with D₅W or 0.9% NaCl to a final concentration as low as 0.5 mg/mL.
Rate of Administration • Infuse over 15–60 min. • Rarely, anaphylactic reaction occurs minutes after administration. Use of epinephrine, corticosteroids alleviates symptoms.
Storage • Store vials at room temperature. • After dilution, solution is stable for 8 hrs.

🔅 IV INCOMPATIBILITY

Amphotericin B complex (Abelcet, AmBisome, Amphotec).

🔅 IV COMPATIBILITIES

Etoposide (VePesid), granisetron (Kytril), ondansetron (Zofran), PACLitaxel (Taxol), palonosetron (Aloxi).

INDICATIONS/ROUTES/DOSAGE

Note: Doses commonly calculated by target AUC.

Ovarian Carcinoma
IV: ADULTS: 360 mg/m² on day 1, every 4 wks (as single agent), or 300 mg/m² q4 wks (in combination with cyclophosphamide) or target AUC 4–6 (single agent; in previously treated pts). Do not repeat dose until neutrophil and platelet counts are within acceptable levels.

Dose Modification
Platelets less than 50,000 cells/mm³ or ANC less than 500 cells/mm³: Give 75% of dose.

Dosage in Renal Impairment
Initial dosage is based on creatinine clearance; subsequent dosages are based on pt's tolerance, degree of myelosuppression.

Creatinine Clearance	Dosage Day 1
60 mL/min or greater	360 mg/m²
41–59 mL/min	250 mg/m²
16–40 mL/min	200 mg/m²

Dosage in Hepatic Impairment
No dose adjustment.

SIDE EFFECTS

Frequent (80%–65%): Nausea, vomiting. **Occasional (17%–4%):** Generalized pain, diarrhea/constipation, peripheral neuropathy. **Rare (3%–2%):** Alopecia, asthenia, hypersensitivity reaction (erythema, pruritus, rash, urticaria).

ADVERSE EFFECTS/TOXIC REACTIONS

Myelosuppression may be severe, resulting in anemia, infection (sepsis, pneumonia), major bleeding. Prolonged treatment may result in peripheral neurotoxicity.

NURSING CONSIDERATIONS

BASELINE ASSESSMENT
Obtain EKG, CBC, serum chemistries, renal function test. Offer emotional

---

support. Do not repeat treatment until WBC recovers from previous therapy. Transfusions may be needed in pts receiving prolonged therapy (myelosuppression increased in those with previous therapy, renal impairment).

INTERVENTION/EVALUATION

Monitor pulmonary function studies, hepatic/renal function tests, CBC, serum electrolytes. Monitor for fever, sore throat, signs of local infection, unusual bruising/bleeding from any site, symptoms of anemia (excessive fatigue, weakness).

PATIENT/FAMILY TEACHING

• Nausea, vomiting generally abate within 24 hrs. • Do not have immunizations without physician's approval (drug lowers body's resistance). • Avoid contact with those who have recently received live virus vaccine.

---

carfilzomib

kar-**fil**-zoh-mib
(Kyprolis)
Do not confuse carfilzomib with crizotinib, ixazomib, PAZOpanib.

◆CLASSIFICATION

PHARMACOTHERAPEUTIC: Proteasome inhibitor. **CLINICAL:** Antineoplastic.

USES

Treatment of pts with multiple myeloma who have received at least 2 prior therapies including bortezomib and an immunomodulatory agent and have demonstrated disease progression on or within 60 days of completion of last therapy. In combination with dexamethasone or lenalidomide and dexamethasone for treatment of relapsed multiple myeloma who have received 1 to 3 prior therapies.

PRECAUTIONS

Contraindications: Hypersensitivity to carfilzomib. **Cautions:** Preexisting HF, decreased left ventricular ejection fraction, myocardial abnormalities, complications of pulmonary hypertension (e.g., dyspnea), hepatic impairment, thrombocytopenia.

ACTION

Blocks action of proteasomes, intracellular proteins to induce cell death in rapidly dividing cells. **Therapeutic Effect:** Produces cell cycle arrest and apoptosis.

PHARMACOKINETICS

Protein binding: 97%. Rapidly, extensively metabolized. Excreted primarily extrahepatically. Minimal removal by hemodialysis. **Half-life:** Equal to or less than 1 hr on day 1 of cycle 1. Proteasome inhibition was maintained for 48 hrs or longer following first dose of carfilzomib for each week of dosing.

⏳ LIFESPAN CONSIDERATIONS

Pregnancy/Lactation: Avoid pregnancy. May cause fetal harm. Unknown if excreted in breast milk. **Children:** Safety and efficacy not established. **Elderly:** No age-related precautions noted.

INTERACTIONS

DRUG: None significant. **HERBAL:** None significant. **FOOD:** None known. **LAB VALUES:** May increase serum creatinine, glucose, creatinine, ALT, AST, bilirubin, calcium. May decrease RBC, Hgb, Hct, absolute neutrophil count (ANC), platelet count; serum magnesium, phosphate, potassium, sodium.

AVAILABILITY (Rx)

Injection Powder for Reconstitution (Single-Use Vial): 30 mg, 60 mg.

ADMINISTRATION/HANDLING

 IV

Reconstitution • Reconstitute 60-mg vial with 29 mL Sterile Water for Injection,

(30-mg vial with 15 mL), directing solution to inside wall of vial (minimizes foaming). • Swirl and invert vial slowly for 1 min or until completely dissolved. • Do not shake. • If foaming occurs, rest vial for 2–5 min until subsided. • Withdraw calculated dose from vial and dilute into 50–100 mL D₅W (depending on dose and infusion duration). • Final concentration of reconstituted solution: 2 mg/mL.

Rate of administration • Infuse over 10–30 min (depending on the dose regimen) via dedicated IV line. Flush line before and after with NaCl or D₅W. • Do not administer as a bolus.

Storage • Refrigerate undiluted vials. • Reconstituted solution may be refrigerated up to 24 hrs. • At room temperature, use diluted solution within 4 hrs.

▦ IV INCOMPATIBILITIES

Do not mix with other IV medications or additives. Flush IV administration line with NaCl or D₅W immediately before and after carfilzomib administration.

INDICATIONS/ROUTES/DOSAGE

◀ALERT▶ Dose is calculated using pt's actual body surface area at baseline. Pts with a body surface area greater than 2.2 m² should receive dose based on a body surface area of 2.2 m². No dose adjustment needed for weight changes of less than or equal to 20%.

◀ALERT▶ Prior to each dose in cycle 1, give 250 mL to 500 mL NaCl bolus. Give an additional 250 mL to 500 mL IV fluid following administration. Continue IV hydration in subsequent cycles (reduces risk of renal toxicity, tumor lysis syndrome).

Premedicate with dexamethasone 4 mg PO or IV prior to all doses during cycle 1 and prior to all doses during first cycle of dose escalation to 27 mg/m² (reduces incidence, severity of infusion reactions). Reinstate dexamethasone premedication (4 mg PO or IV) if symptoms develop or reappear during subsequent cycles.

Multiple Myeloma, Relapsed/Refractory (Single-Agent 20/27 mg/m² regimen)
IV infusion: ADULTS, ELDERLY: Cycle 1: 20 mg/m² over 10 min on days 1 and 2. If tolerated, increase to 27 mg/m² over 10 min on days 8, 9, 15, and 16 of a 28-day cycle. Cycles 2–12: 27 mg/m² over 10 min on days 1, 2, 8, 9, 15, and 16 of a 28-day cycle. Cycles 13 and beyond: 27 mg/m² over 10 min on days 1, 2, 15, and 16 of a 28-day cycle. Continue until disease progression or unacceptable toxicity.

Multiple Myeloma, Relapsed/Refractory (Single-Agent 20/56 mg/m² regimen)
IV infusion: ADULTS, ELDERLY: Cycle 1: 20 mg/m² over 30 min on days 1 and 2. If tolerated, increase to 56 mg/m² over 30 min on days 8, 9, 15, and 16 of a 28-day cycle. Cycles 2–12: 56 mg/m² over 30 min on days 1, 2, 8, 9, 15, and 16 of a 28-day cycle. Cycles 13 and beyond: 56 mg/m² over 30 min on days 1, 2, 15, and 16 of a 28-day cycle. Continue until disease progression or unacceptable toxicity.

Multiple Myeloma, Relapsed/Refractory (In Combination with Lenalidomide and Dexamethasone)
IV infusion: ADULTS, ELDERLY: Cycle 1: 20 mg/m² over 10 min on days 1 and 2. If tolerated, increase to 27 mg/m² over 10 min on days 8, 9, 15, and 16 of a 28-day cycle. Cycles 2–12: 27 mg/m² over 10 min on days 1, 2, 8, 9, 15, and 16 of a 28-day cycle. Cycles 13–18: 27 mg/m² over 10 min on days 1, 2, 15, and 16 of a 28-day cycle. Beginning with cycle 19, lenalidomide and dexamethasone may be continued (until disease progression or unacceptable toxicity) without carfilzomib.

Multiple Myeloma, Relapsed/Refractory (In Combination with Dexamethasone)
IV infusion: ADULTS, ELDERLY: Cycle 1: 20 mg/m² over 30 min on days 1 and 2. If tolerated, increase to 56 mg/m² over 30 min on days 8, 9, 15, and 16 of a 28-day cycle. Cycle 2 and beyond: 56 mg/m² over 30 min on days 1, 2, 8, 9, 15, and 16 of a 28-day cycle. Continue until disease progression or unacceptable toxicity.

Dose Modification
Hematologic
Grade 3 or 4 neutropenia: Withhold dose. Continue at same dose if fully recovered prior to next scheduled dose. If recovered to grade 2, reduce dose by one dose level. If dose tolerated, may escalate to previous dose. **Grade 4 thrombocytopenia:** Withhold dose. Continue at same dose if fully recovered prior to next scheduled dose. If recovered to grade 3, reduce dose by one dose level. If dose tolerated, may escalate to previous dose.

Cardiac
Grade 3 or 4, new onset or worsening of HF, decreased LVF, myocardial ischemia: Withhold dose until resolved or at baseline. After resolution, restart at reduced dose level. If dose tolerated, may escalate to previous dose.

Hepatic
Grade 3 or 4 elevation of bilirubin, transaminases: Withhold dose until resolved or at baseline. After resolution, restart at reduced dose level. If dose tolerated, may escalate to previous dose.

Peripheral Neuropathy
Grade 3 or 4: Withhold dose until resolved or at baseline. After resolution, restart at reduced dose level. If dose tolerated, may escalate to previous dose.

Pulmonary Toxicity
Pulmonary hypertension: Withhold dose until resolved or at baseline. After resolution, restart at reduced dose level. If dose tolerated, may escalate to previous dose. **Grade 3 or 4 pulmonary complications:** Withhold dose until resolved or at baseline. After resolution, restart at reduced dose level. If dose tolerated, may escalate to previous dose.

Renal
Serum creatinine 2 times or greater from baseline: Withhold dose until renal function improves to grade 1 or baseline. Withhold dose until resolved or at baseline. After resolution, restart at reduced dose level. If dose tolerated, may escalate to previous dose.

Dosage in Renal/Hepatic Impairment
No dose adjustment.

SIDE EFFECTS
Frequent (56%–20%): Fatigue, anemia, nausea, exertional dyspnea, diarrhea, fever, headache, cough, peripheral edema, vomiting, constipation, back pain. **Occasional (18%–14%):** Insomnia, chills, arthralgia, muscle spasms, hypertension, asthenia, extremity pain, dizziness, hypoesthesia (decreased sensitivity to touch), anorexia.

ADVERSE EFFECTS/TOXIC REACTIONS
Pneumonia (10% of pts), acute renal failure (4% of pts), pyrexia (3% of pts), and HF (3% of pts) were reported. Adverse reactions leading to discontinuation occurred in 15% of pts. Upper respiratory tract infection reported in 28% of pts. HF, pulmonary edema, decrease in ejection fraction were reported in 7% of pts. Infusion reaction characterized by chills, fever, wheezing, facial flushing, dyspnea, vomiting, chest tightness can occur immediately following or up to 24 hrs after administration. Tumor lysis syndrome occurs rarely.

NURSING CONSIDERATIONS
BASELINE ASSESSMENT
Obtain accurate height and weight. Obtain full history of home medications including vitamins, herbal products. Ensure hydration status and maintain throughout treatment. Obtain CBC, serum chemistries. Assess vital signs, O_2 saturation. Platelet nadirs occur around day 8 of each 28-day cycle and recover to baseline by start of the next 28-day cycle.

INTERVENTION/EVALUATION
Monitor for fluid overload. Monitor platelet count frequently; adjust dose according to grade of thrombocytopenia. Obtain serum ALT, AST, bilirubin for evidence of

hepatotoxicity. Monitor vital signs, O_2 saturation routinely. Monitor cardiac function and manage as needed. Assess for palpitations, tachycardia. Assess for anemia-related dizziness, exertional dyspnea, fatigue, weakness, syncope. Report decreases in Hgb, Hct, platelets, neutrophils. Monitor for acute infection (fever, diaphoresis, lethargy, oral mucosal changes, productive cough), bloody stools, bruising, hematuria, DVT, pulmonary embolism. Encourage nutritional intake and assess anorexia, weight loss. Reinforce birth control compliance. Monitor daily pattern of bowel activity, stool consistency. Offer antiemetics if nausea, vomiting occur. Monitor for symptoms of neutropenia.

PATIENT/FAMILY TEACHING

• Blood tests will be drawn routinely. • Immediately report any newly prescribed medications. • May alter taste of food or decrease appetite. • Report bloody stool/urine, increased bruising, difficulty breathing, weakness, dizziness, palpitations, weight loss. • Maintain strict oral hygiene. • Do not have immunizations without physician approval (drug lowers body's resistance). • Avoid those who have recently taken live virus vaccine. • Avoid crowds, those with symptoms of viral illness.

cariprazine

kar-**ip**-ra-zeen
(Vraylar)

■ BLACK BOX ALERT ■ Elderly pts treated with antipsychotic drugs are at an increased risk of death. Treatment not approved in pts with dementia-related psychosis.
Do not confuse cariprazine with Compazine or mirtazapine.

◆CLASSIFICATION

PHARMACOTHERAPEUTIC: Serotonin receptor antagonist. **CLINICAL:** Antipsychotic.

USES

Treatment of schizophrenia. Acute treatment of manic or mixed episodes associated with bipolar I disorder.

PRECAUTIONS

Contraindications: Hypersensitivity to cariprazine. **Cautions:** Baseline leukopenia, neutropenia; hx of drug-induced leukopenia, neutropenia; debilitated, diabetes mellitus, dyslipidemia, elderly, hepatic impairment, Parkinson's disease, pts at risk for hypotension (dehydration, hypovolemia, concomitant use of antihypertensives), pts at risk for aspiration, dysphagia; history of cardiovascular disease (e.g., ischemic heart disease, HF, cardiac arrhythmias); pts at risk for CVA, TIA; hx of seizures. Concomitant use of medications that lower seizure threshold. Avoid concomitant use of CYP3A inducers.

ACTION

Exact mechanism unknown. Partial agonist of central DOPamine D_2 and serotonin 5-HT_{1A} receptors and antagonist of serotonin 5-HT_{2A} receptors. **Therapeutic Effect:** Diminishes symptoms of psychotic behavior.

PHARMACOKINETICS

Widely distributed. Metabolized in liver. Protein binding: 91%–97%. Peak plasma concentration: 3–6 hrs. Mean plasma concentrations decrease approx. 50% after 1 wk from last dose. Excreted primarily in urine (21%). **Half-Life:** 2–4 days.

⌛ LIFESPAN CONSIDERATIONS

Pregnancy/Lactation: Avoid pregnancy; may cause fetal harm. May increase risk of extrapyramidal symptoms and/or withdrawal syndrome in neonates. Unknown if distributed in breast milk. Must either discontinue drug or discontinue breastfeeding. **Children:** Safety and efficacy not established. **Elderly:** May increase risk of adverse effects due to age-related cardiac/hepatic/renal impairment.

INTERACTIONS

DRUG: **Strong CYP3A inhibitors** (e.g., **clarithromycin, ketoconazole, ritonavir**) may increase concentration/effect. **Strong CYP3A inducers** (e.g., **carBAMazepine, rifampin**), **moderate CYP3A inducers** (e.g., **nafcillin**) may decrease concentration/effect; avoid use. **Alcohol, antidepressants** (e.g., **sertraline, nortriptyline**), **benzodiazepines** (e.g., **diazePAM, LORazepam**), **opioids** (e.g., **morphine**), **phenothiazines** (e.g., **thioridazine**), **sedative/hypnotics** (e.g., **zolpidem**) may increase CNS depression. **Antihypertensives** (e.g., **amLODIPine, enalapril, valsartan**) may increase hypotensive effect. **HERBAL: St. John's wort** may decrease concentration/effect. **FOOD: Grapefruit products** may increase concentration/effect. **LAB VALUES:** May increase serum ALT, AST; CPK. May decrease serum sodium.

AVAILABILITY (Rx)

Capsules: 1.5 mg, 3 mg, 4.5 mg, 6 mg.

ADMINISTRATION/HANDLING

PO
• Give without regard to food. • Administer whole; do not break, crush, cut, or open capsule.

INDICATIONS/ROUTES/DOSAGE

Schizophrenia
PO: ADULTS, ELDERLY: Initially, 1.5 mg once daily. May increase to 3 mg on day 2 if tolerated. May further increase in increments of 1.5–3 mg based on clinical response and tolerability. **Range:** 1.5–6 mg once daily.

Bipolar I Disorder
PO: ADULTS, ELDERLY: 1.5 mg once on day 1, then increase to 3 mg once daily on day 2. May further increase in increments of 1.5–3 mg based on clinical response and tolerability. **Range:** 3–6 mg once daily.

Concomitant Use of Strong CYP3A Inhibitors
Pts starting strong CYP3A inhibitor while on stable dose of cariprazine: Reduce maintenance cariprazine dose by 50%. Pts taking cariprazine 4.5 mg/day should reduce dosage to 1.5 mg/day or 3 mg/day. Pts taking 1.5 mg/day, adjust dosing to every other day. If the strong CYP3A inhibitor is discontinued, cariprazine may need to be increased. **Pts starting cariprazine while on CYP3A inhibitor:** 1.5 mg once on day 1; no dose on day 2; 1.5 mg once on day 3. After day 3, increase dose to 3 mg once daily as tolerated. If strong CYP3A inhibitor is discontinued, cariprazine may need to be increased.

Dosage in Renal Impairment
Mild to moderate impairment: No dose adjustment. **Severe impairment:** Treatment not recommended.

Dosage in Hepatic Impairment
Mild to moderate impairment: No dose adjustment. **Severe impairment:** Treatment not recommended.

SIDE EFFECTS

Frequent (26%–11%): Bradykinesia, cogwheel rigidity, drooling, dyskinesia, masked faces, muscle rigidity, dystonia, tremor, salivary hypersecretion, torticollis, trismus, insomnia, akathisia, headache. **Occasional (5%–3%):** Nausea, constipation, restlessness, vomiting, dizziness, agitation, anxiety, dyspepsia, abdominal pain, diarrhea, fatigue, asthenia, back pain, toothache, hypertension, decreased appetite. **Rare (2%–1%):** Dry mouth, weight gain, extremity pain, somnolence, sedation, cough, tachycardia, arthralgia.

ADVERSE EFFECTS/TOXIC REACTIONS

May increase risk of hypotension, orthostatic hypotension, syncope; diabetes mellitus, DKA, hyperglycemia, hyperglycemic hyperosmolar nonketotic coma; leukopenia, neutropenia, febrile neutropenia;

aspiration, dysphagia, gastritis, gastric reflux; extrapyramidal symptoms including akathisia, dystonia, parkinsonism, tardive dyskinesia; suicidal ideation. May cause neuroleptic malignant syndrome (NMS), manifested by altered mental status, cardiac arrhythmias, diaphoresis, labile blood pressure, malignant hyperthermia, muscle rigidity, rhabdomyolysis, renal failure. May increase risk of death in pts with dementia-related psychosis. Cognitive and motor impairment reported in 7% of pts. May increase seizure-like activity related to decrease in seizure threshold. Infectious processes including nasopharyngitis, urinary tract infection reported in 1% of pts. Hypersensitivity reactions including angioedema, rash, pruritus have occurred.

NURSING CONSIDERATIONS

BASELINE ASSESSMENT

Obtain baseline fasting lipid profile, fasting plasma glucose level, vital signs; Hgb A1c in pts with diabetes; ANC, CBC in pts with baseline leukopenia, neutropenia. Receive full medication history, including herbal products, and screen for interactions. Assess appearance, behavior, speech pattern, levels of interest. Verify pregnancy status. Question history of diabetes, cardiovascular disease, CVA, dysphagia, hepatic impairment, hypersensitivity reaction, TIA, seizures.

INTERVENTION/EVALUATION

Monitor ANC, CBC, fasting lipid profile, fasting plasma glucose levels periodically. Assess mental status for anxiety, depression, suicidal ideation (esp. at initiation and with change in dosage), social function. Due to long half-life, any change in dosage will not be fully reflected for several wks; monitor closely for adverse effects during the following wks. Monitor for hypersensitivity reaction, dysphagia, tardive dyskinesia, extrapyramidal symptoms, metabolic changes including hyperglycemia. Screen for infection. Monitor for neuroleptic malignant syndrome.

PATIENT/FAMILY TEACHING

• Immediately report thoughts of suicide or plans to commit suicide. • Avoid tasks that require alertness until response to drug is established. • Therapy may increase blood sugar levels. Monitor for blurry vision, confusion, frequent urination, fruity-smelling breath, thirst, weakness. • Treatment may cause fetal harm. Avoid pregnancy. Do not breastfeed. • Treatment may lower ability to fight infection. • Swallow capsules whole; do not chew, crush, cut, or open capsules. • Do not ingest grapefruit products or herbal products. Report drooling, muscle rigidity, lockjaw, tremors, or inability to control muscle movements. • Treatment may increase risk of seizures. • Report confusion, palpitations, profuse sweating, fluctuating blood pressure, unusually high core body temperature, muscle rigidity, dark-colored urine or decreased urine output; may indicate life-threatening neurologic event called neuroleptic malignant syndrome (NMS).

carmustine
HIGH ALERT

kar-**mus**-teen
(BiCNU, Gliadel Wafer)

■ **BLACK BOX ALERT** ■ Profound myelosuppression (leukopenia, thrombocytopenia) is major toxicity. High risk of pulmonary toxicity. Must be administered by personnel trained in administration/handling of chemotherapeutic agents (high potential for severe reactions, including anaphylaxis, sudden death).
Do not confuse carmustine with bendamustine or lomustine.

◆CLASSIFICATION

PHARMACOTHERAPEUTIC: Alkylating agent, nitrosourea. **CLINICAL:** Antineoplastic.

USES

BiCNU: Treatment of brain tumors, Hodgkin's lymphomas, non-Hodgkin's lymphomas, multiple myeloma. **Gliadel**

Wafer: Adjunct to surgery and radiation in treatment of newly diagnosed high-grade malignant glioma. Adjunct to surgery to prolong survival in recurrent glioblastoma multiforme. **OFF-LABEL:** Treatment of mycosis fungoides (topical).

PRECAUTIONS

Contraindications: Hypersensitivity to carmustine. **Cautions:** Thrombocytopenia, leukopenia, anemia, renal/hepatic impairment.

ACTION

Inhibits DNA, RNA synthesis by crosslinking with DNA, RNA strands, preventing cell division. Cell cycle–phase nonspecific. **Therapeutic Effect:** Interferes with DNA, RNA function.

PHARMACOKINETICS

Crosses blood-brain barrier. Metabolized in liver. Excreted in urine. **Half-life:** 15–30 min.

⌛ LIFESPAN CONSIDERATIONS

Pregnancy/Lactation: Avoid pregnancy, particularly first trimester; may cause fetal harm. Unknown if distributed in breast milk. Breastfeeding not recommended. **Children:** Safety and efficacy not established. **Elderly:** No age-related precautions noted.

INTERACTIONS

DRUG: Bone marrow depressants, cimetidine may enhance myelosuppressive effect. **Hepatotoxic, nephrotoxic medications** (e.g., **furosemide, gentamicin, ketorolac**) may increase risk of hepatotoxicity, nephrotoxicity. **Live virus vaccines** may potentiate virus replication, increase vaccine side effects, decrease pt's antibody response to vaccine. **HERBAL:** Echinacea may decrease effects. **FOOD:** None known. **LAB VALUES:** May increase serum BUN, alkaline phosphatase, bilirubin, ALT, AST.

AVAILABILITY (Rx)

Injection, Powder for Reconstitution (BiCNU): 100 mg. **Implant Device (Gliadel Wafer):** 7.7 mg.

ADMINISTRATION/HANDLING

◄**ALERT**► May be carcinogenic, mutagenic, teratogenic. Wear protective gloves during preparation of drug; may cause transient burning, brown staining of skin.

 IV

Reconstitution • Reconstitute 100-mg vial with 3 mL sterile dehydrated (absolute) alcohol, followed by 27 mL Sterile Water for Injection to provide concentration of 3.3 mg/mL. • Further dilute with 50–250 mL D₅W to final concentration of 0.2–1 mg/mL.
Rate of Administration • Infuse over 1–2 hrs (shorter duration may produce intense burning pain at injection site, intense flushing of skin, conjunctiva). • Flush IV line with 5–10 mL 0.9% NaCl or D₅W before and after administration to prevent irritation at injection site.
Storage • Refrigerate unused vials. • Reconstituted vials are stable for 8 hrs at room temperature or 24 hrs if refrigerated. • Solutions further diluted with D₅W are stable for 8 hrs at room temperature. • Solutions appear clear, colorless to yellow. • Discard if precipitate forms, color change occurs, or oily film develops on bottom of vial. • **Gliadel Wafers:** Store at or below −20°C (−4°F). Unopened pouches may be kept at room temperature for maximum of 6 hrs.

🔲 IV INCOMPATIBILITIES

Allopurinol (Aloprim), sodium bicarbonate.

🔲 IV COMPATIBILITIES

Granisetron (Kytril), ondansetron (Zofran).

INDICATIONS/ROUTES/DOSAGE

◄**ALERT**► Refer to individual oncology protocols.

Usual Dosage (Refer to Individual Protocols)
IV *(BiCNU):* **ADULTS, ELDERLY:** 150–200 mg/m² as a single dose q6wks or 75–100 mg/m² on 2 successive days q6wks.

◄ALERT► Next dosage is based on clinical and hematologic response to previous dose (platelets greater than 100,000/mm³ and leukocytes greater than 4,000/mm³).

Implantation (Gliadel Wafer):
ADULTS, ELDERLY, CHILDREN: Up to 8 wafers (62.6 mg) may be placed in resection cavity.

Dosage Modification

Leukocytes 2,000–2,999 cells/mm³ or platelets 25,000–74,999 cells/mm³: Give 70% of dose. **Leukocytes less than 2,000 cells/mm³ or platelets less than 25,000 cells/mm³:** Give 50% of dose.

Dosage in Renal Impairment

Creatinine

Clearance (mL/min)	Dosage
46–60	80% of dose
31–45	75% of dose
Less than 31	Not recommended

Dosage in Hepatic Impairment

Use caution.

SIDE EFFECTS

Frequent: Nausea, vomiting (may last up to 6 hrs). **Occasional:** Diarrhea, esophagitis, anorexia, dysphagia, hyperpigmentation. **Rare:** Thrombophlebitis, burning sensation, pain at injection site.

ADVERSE EFFECTS/TOXIC REACTIONS

Hematologic toxicity due to myelosuppression occurs frequently. Thrombocytopenia occurs approximately 4 wks after treatment begins and lasts 1–2 wks. Leukopenia is evident 5–6 wks after treatment begins and lasts 1–2 wks. Anemia occurs less frequently. Mild, reversible hepatotoxicity occurs frequently. Prolonged, high-dose therapy may produce impaired renal function, pulmonary toxicity (pulmonary infiltrate/fibrosis).

NURSING CONSIDERATIONS

BASELINE ASSESSMENT

Obtain CBC, renal/hepatic function studies before initiation and periodically thereafter. Offer emotional support.

INTERVENTION/EVALUATION

Monitor renal/hepatic function tests. Obtain CBC wkly during and for at least 6 wks after therapy ends. Monitor for hematologic toxicity (fever, sore throat, signs of local infection, unusual bruising/bleeding from any site), symptoms of anemia (excessive fatigue, weakness). Monitor for pulmonary toxicity; observe for dyspnea, adventitious breath sounds.

PATIENT/FAMILY TEACHING

• Maintain adequate hydration (may protect against renal impairment). • Do not have immunizations without physician's approval (drug lowers body's resistance). • Avoid contact with those who have recently received live virus vaccine. • Report nausea, vomiting, fever, sore throat, chills, unusual bleeding/bruising.

---

carvedilol

kar-ve-dil-ole
(Apo-Carvedilol ♣, Coreg, Coreg CR, Novo-Carvedilol ♣)
Do not confuse carvedilol with atenolol or carteolol, or Coreg with Corgard, Cortef, or Cozaar.

◆ CLASSIFICATION

PHARMACOTHERAPEUTIC: Beta-adrenergic blocker. **CLINICAL:** Antihypertensive.

USES

Treatment of mild to severe HF, left ventricular dysfunction following MI, hypertension. **OFF-LABEL:** Treatment of angina pectoris, idiopathic cardiomyopathy.

PRECAUTIONS

Contraindications: Hypersensitivity to carvedilol. Bronchial asthma or related bronchospastic conditions, cardiogenic shock, decompensated HF requiring intravenous inotropic therapy, severe hepatic impairment, second- or third-degree AV block, severe bradycardia, or sick sinus syndrome (except in pts with pacemaker). **Cautions:** Diabetes, myasthenia gravis, mild to moderate hepatic impairment. Withdraw gradually to avoid acute tachycardia, hypertension, and/or ischemia. Pts suspected of having Prinzmetal's angina, pheochromocytoma, hx of severe anaphylaxis to allergens.

ACTION

Possesses nonselective beta-blocking and alpha-adrenergic blocking activity. Causes vasodilation. **Therapeutic Effect: Hypertension:** Reduces cardiac output, exercise-induced tachycardia, reflex orthostatic tachycardia; reduces peripheral vascular resistance. **HF:** Decreases pulmonary capillary wedge pressure, heart rate, systemic vascular resistance; increases stroke volume index.

PHARMACOKINETICS

Route	Onset	Peak	Duration
PO	30 min	1–2 hrs	24 hrs

Rapidly, extensively absorbed from GI tract. Protein binding: 98%. Metabolized in liver. Excreted primarily via bile into feces. Minimally removed by hemodialysis. **Half-life:** 7–10 hrs. Food delays rate of absorption.

⏳ LIFESPAN CONSIDERATIONS

Pregnancy/Lactation: Unknown if drug crosses placenta or is distributed in breast milk. May produce bradycardia, apnea, hypoglycemia, hypothermia during delivery; may contribute to low birth-weight infants. **Children:** Safety and efficacy not established. **Elderly:** Incidence of dizziness may be increased.

INTERACTIONS

DRUG: Calcium channel blockers (e.g., diltiaZEM, verapamil), digoxin, CYP2C9 inhibitors (e.g., amiodarone, fluconazole) increase risk of cardiac conduction disturbances. **Diuretics (e.g., furosemide, HCTZ), other antihypertensives (e.g., amlodipine, lisinopril, valsartan)** may potentiate hypotensive effects. **Cimetidine** may increase concentration. May increase concentration of **cycloSPORINE, digoxin. CYP2D6 inhibitors (e.g., FLUoxetine, PARoxetine)** may increase concentration/side effects; may enhance slowing of HR or cardiac conduction. May increase effects of **insulin, oral hypoglycemics (e.g., glyburide, metformin). RifAMPin** decreases concentration. **HERBAL: Ephedra, ginseng, yohimbe** may worsen hypertension. **Garlic** may increase antihypertensive effect. **FOOD:** None known. **LAB VALUE:** May increase serum creatinine, bilirubin, ALT, AST, PT.

AVAILABILITY (Rx)

Tablets (Immediate-Release): 3.125 mg, 6.25 mg, 12.5 mg, 25 mg.

🔖 **Capsules (Extended-Release [Coreg CR]):** 10 mg, 20 mg, 40 mg, 80 mg.

ADMINISTRATION/HANDLING

PO

• Give with food (slows rate of absorption, reduces risk of orthostatic effects). • Do not crush or cut extended-release capsules. • Capsules may be opened and sprinkled on applesauce for immediate use.

INDICATIONS/ROUTES/DOSAGE

Hypertension

PO *(Immediate-Release):* **ADULTS, ELDERLY:** Initially, 6.25 mg twice daily. May double at intervals of 1–2 wks to 12.5 mg twice daily, then to 25 mg twice daily. **Maximum:** 25 mg twice daily. *(Extended-Release):* Initially, 20 mg once daily. May increase to 40 mg once daily after 1–2 wks. **Maximum:** 80 mg once daily.

HF

PO *(Immediate-Release):* **ADULTS, ELDERLY:** Initially, 3.125 mg twice daily. May double at 2-wk intervals to highest tolerated dosage. **Maximum: Greater than 85 kg:** 50 mg twice daily; **Less than 85 kg:** 25 mg twice daily. *(Extended-Release):* Initially, 10 mg once daily for 2 wks. May increase to 20 mg, 40 mg, and 80 mg over successive intervals of at least 2 wks. **Maximum:** 80 mg/day.

Left Ventricular Dysfunction Following MI
PO *(Immediate-Release):* **ADULTS, ELDERLY:** Initially, 3.125–6.25 mg twice daily. May increase at intervals of 3–10 days up to 25 mg twice daily. **Maximum:** 50 mg twice daily. *(Extended-Release):* Initially, 10–20 mg once daily. May increase incrementally in intervals of 3–10 days. Target dose: 80 mg once daily.

Dosage in Renal Impairment
No dose adjustment.

Dosage in Hepatic Impairment
Contraindicated in severe impairment.

SIDE EFFECTS

Frequent (6%–4%): Fatigue, dizziness. **Occasional (2%):** Diarrhea, bradycardia, rhinitis, back pain. **Rare (less than 2%):** Orthostatic hypotension, drowsiness, UTI, viral infection.

ADVERSE EFFECTS/TOXIC REACTIONS

Overdose may produce profound bradycardia, hypotension, bronchospasm, cardiac insufficiency, cardiogenic shock, cardiac arrest. Abrupt withdrawal may result in diaphoresis, palpitations, headache, tremors. May precipitate HF, MI in pts with cardiac disease; thyroid storm in pts with thyrotoxicosis; peripheral ischemia in pts with existing peripheral vascular disease. Hypoglycemia may occur in pts with previously controlled diabetes. May mask symptoms of hypoglycemia.

NURSING CONSIDERATIONS

BASELINE ASSESSMENT

Assess B/P, apical pulse immediately before drug is administered (if pulse is 60 beats/min or less or systolic B/P is less than 90 mm Hg, withhold medication, contact physician). Receive full medication history and screen for interactions.

INTERVENTION/EVALUATION

Monitor B/P for hypotension, respirations for dyspnea. Take standing systolic B/P 1 hr after dosing as guide for tolerance. Assess pulse for quality, regularity, rate; monitor for bradycardia. Monitor EKG for cardiac arrhythmias. Assist with ambulation if dizziness occurs. Assess for evidence of HF: dyspnea (particularly on exertion or lying down), night cough, peripheral edema, distended neck veins. Monitor I&O (increase in weight, decrease in urine output may indicate HF). Monitor renal/hepatic function tests.

PATIENT/FAMILY TEACHING

• Full therapeutic effect of B/P may take 1–2 wks. • Contact lens wearers may experience decreased lacrimation. • Take with food. • Abruptly stopping treatment or missing multiple doses may cause betablocker withdrawal symptoms (fast heart rate, high blood pressure, palpitations, sweating, tremors). • Compliance with therapy regimen is essential to control hypertension. • Report excessive fatigue, prolonged dizziness. • Do not use nasal decongestants, OTC cold preparations (stimulants) without physician's approval. • Monitor B/P, pulse before taking medication. • Restrict salt, alcohol intake.

caspofungin

kas-poe-**fun**-jin
(Cancidas)

◆CLASSIFICATION

PHARMACOTHERAPEUTIC: Echinocandin antifungal. **CLINICAL:** Antifungal.

USES

Treatment of invasive aspergillosis, candidemia, *Candida* infection (intra-abdominal abscess, peritonitis, esophageal, pleural space) in pts aged 3 months and older. Empiric therapy for presumed fungal infections in febrile neutropenia.

PRECAUTIONS

Contraindications: Hypersensitivity to caspofungin. **Cautions:** Concurrent use of cycloSPORINE, hepatic impairment.

ACTION

Inhibits synthesis of glucan, a vital component of fungal cell wall formation, damaging fungal cell membrane. **Therapeutic Effect:** Fungistatic.

PHARMACOKINETICS

Distributed in tissue. Protein binding: 97%. Metabolized in liver. Excreted in urine (50%), feces (30%). Not removed by hemodialysis. **Half-life:** 40–50 hrs.

⧗ LIFESPAN CONSIDERATIONS

Pregnancy/Lactation: May be embryotoxic. Crosses placental barrier. Distributed in breast milk. **Children:** Safety and efficacy not established. **Elderly:** Age-related moderate renal impairment may require dosage adjustment.

INTERACTIONS

DRUG: CycloSPORINE may increase concentration. **RifAMPin** may decrease concentration. May decrease concentration/effect of **tacrolimus**. **HERBAL:** None significant. **FOOD:** None known. **LAB VALUES:** May increase serum alkaline phosphatase, bilirubin, creatinine, ALT, AST, urine protein. May decrease serum albumin, bicarbonate, potassium, magnesium; Hgb, Hct.

AVAILABILITY (Rx)

Injection, Powder for Reconstitution: 50-mg, 70-mg vials.

ADMINISTRATION/HANDLING

 IV

Reconstitution • Reconstitute 50-mg or 70-mg vial with 0.9% NaCl, Sterile Water for Injection, or Bacteriostatic Water for Injection. Further dilute in 0.9% NaCl or D₅W to maximum concentration of 0.5 mg/mL.
Rate of Administration • Infuse over 60 min.
Storage • Refrigerate vials but warm to room temperature before preparing with diluent. • Reconstituted solution, diluted solution, may be stored at room temperature for 1 hr before infusion. • Final infusion solution can be stored at room temperature for 24 hrs or 48 hrs if refrigerated. • Discard if solution contains particulate or is discolored.

▨ IV COMPATIBILITIES

Aztreonam (Azactam), DAPTOmycin (Cubicin), fluconazole (Diflucan), linezolid (Zyvox), meropenem (Merrem IV), piperacillin/tazobactam (Zosyn), vancomycin.

▨ IV INCOMPATIBILITIES

Cefepime (Maxipime), ceftaroline (Teflaro), cefTAZidime (Fortaz), cefTRIAXone (Rocephin), furosemide (Lasix).

INDICATIONS/ROUTES/DOSAGE
Aspergillosis

Note: Continue for minimum of 6–12 wks.
IV: ADULTS, ELDERLY: Give single 70-mg loading dose on day 1, followed by 50 mg/day thereafter. **CHILDREN 3 MOS–17 YRS:** 70 mg/m² on day 1, then 50 mg/m² daily. **Maximum:** 70-mg loading dose, 50-mg daily dose.

Candidemia

Note: Continue for at least 14 days after last positive culture.

IV: **ADULTS, ELDERLY:** Initially, 70 mg followed by 50 mg daily. **CHILDREN 3 MOS–17 YRS:** 70 mg/m^2 on day 1, then 50 mg/m^2 daily. **Maximum:** 70-mg loading dose, 50-mg daily dose.

Esophageal Candidiasis
Note: Continue for 7–14 days after symptom resolution.
IV: **ADULTS, ELDERLY:** 50 mg/day. **CHILDREN 3 MOS–17 YRS:** 50 mg/m^2 daily. **Maximum:** 50 mg.

Empiric Therapy
Note: Continue for minimum 14 days if fungal infection confirmed (continue for 7 days after resolution of neutropenia/clinical symptoms).
IV: **ADULTS, ELDERLY:** Initially 70 mg, then 50 mg/day. May increase to 70 mg/day. **CHILDREN 3 MOS–17 YRS:** 70 mg/m^2 on day 1, then 50 mg/m^2 daily. **Maximum:** 70 mg.

Dosage in Renal Impairment
No dose adjustment.

Dosage in Hepatic Impairment
Mild: No adjustment. **Moderate: Child-Pugh score 7–9:** Decrease dose to 35 mg/day.
Severe: No clinical experience.

SIDE EFFECTS

Frequent (26%): Fever. **Occasional (11%–4%):** Headache, nausea, phlebitis. **Rare (3% or less):** Paresthesia, vomiting, diarrhea, abdominal pain, myalgia, chills, tremor, insomnia.

ADVERSE EFFECTS/TOXIC REACTIONS

Hypersensitivity reaction (rash, facial edema, pruritus, sensation of warmth), including anaphylaxis, may occur. May cause hepatic dysfunction, hepatitis (drug-induced), or hepatic failure.

NURSING CONSIDERATIONS

BASELINE ASSESSMENT
Obtain baseline CBC, BMP, LFT, serum magnesium. Determine baseline temperature. Question history of prior hypersensitivity reaction.

INTERVENTION/EVALUATION
Assess for signs/symptoms of hepatic dysfunction. Monitor LFT in pts with preexisting hepatic impairment. Monitor CBC, serum potassium. Monitor for fever, hypersensitivity reaction.

PATIENT/FAMILY TEACHING
• Report rash, facial swelling, itching, difficulty breathing, abdominal pain, yellowing of skin or eyes, dark-colored urine, nausea.

cefaclor

sef-a-klor
(Apo-Cefaclor ✦, Ceclor ✦, Novo-Cefaclor ✦)
Do not confuse cefaclor with cephalexin.

◆CLASSIFICATION

PHARMACOTHERAPEUTIC: Second-generation cephalosporin. **CLINICAL:** Antibiotic.

USES

Treatment of susceptible infections due to *S. pneumoniae, S. pyogenes, S. aureus, H. influenzae, E. coli, M. catarrhalis, Klebsiella* spp., *P. mirabilis*, including acute otitis media, bronchitis, pharyngitis/tonsillitis, respiratory tract, skin/skin structure, UTIs.

PRECAUTIONS

Contraindications: History of hypersensitivity/anaphylactic reaction to cefaclor, cephalosporins. **Cautions:** Severe renal impairment, history of penicillin allergy. Extended release not approved in children younger than 16 yrs.

ACTION

Binds to bacterial cell membranes, inhibits cell wall synthesis. **Therapeutic Effect:** Bactericidal.

PHARMACOKINETICS

Well absorbed from GI tract. Protein binding: 25%. Widely distributed. Partially metabolized in liver. Primarily excreted in urine. Moderately removed by hemodialysis. **Half-life:** 0.6–0.9 hr (increased in renal impairment).

⧗ LIFESPAN CONSIDERATIONS

Pregnancy/Lactation: Readily crosses placenta. Distributed in breast milk. **Children:** No age-related precautions noted in pts older than 1 mo. **Elderly:** Age-related renal impairment may require dosage adjustment.

INTERACTIONS

DRUG: Probenecid may increase concentration. **HERBAL:** None significant. **FOOD:** None known. **LAB VALUES:** May increase serum BUN, alkaline phosphatase, bilirubin, creatinine, LDH, ALT, AST. May cause positive direct/indirect Coombs' test.

AVAILABILITY (Rx)

🖋 **Capsules:** 250 mg, 500 mg. **Powder for Oral Suspension:** 125 mg/5 mL, 250 mg/5 mL, 375 mg/5 mL.
Tablets (Extended-Release): 500 mg.

ADMINISTRATION/HANDLING

PO
• After reconstitution, oral solution is stable for 14 days if refrigerated. • Shake oral suspension well before using. • Give without regard to food; if GI upset occurs, give with food, milk.

INDICATIONS/ROUTES/DOSAGE

Usual Dosage
PO: ADULTS, ELDERLY: 250–500 mg q8h or 500 mg q12h (extended-release). **CHILDREN:** 20–40 mg/kg/day divided q8–12h. **Maximum:** 1 g/day.

Otitis Media
PO: CHILDREN: 40 mg/kg/day divided q12h. **Maximum:** 1 g/day.

Pharyngitis
CHILDREN: 20 mg/kg/day divided q12h. **Maximum:** 1 g/day.

Dosage in Renal Impairment
Use caution.

Dosage in Hepatic Impairment
No dose adjustment.

SIDE EFFECTS

Frequent: Oral candidiasis, mild diarrhea, mild abdominal cramping, vaginal candidiasis. **Occasional:** Nausea, serum sickness–like reaction (fever, joint pain; usually occurs after second course of therapy and resolves after drug is discontinued). **Rare:** Allergic reaction (pruritus, rash, urticaria).

ADVERSE EFFECTS/TOXIC REACTIONS

Antibiotic-associated colitis, (abdominal cramps, severe watery diarrhea, fever) other superinfections may result from altered bacterial balance in GI tract. Nephrotoxicity may occur, esp. in pts with preexisting renal disease. Pts with history of penicillin allergy are at increased risk for developing a severe hypersensitivity reaction (severe pruritus, angioedema, bronchospasm, anaphylaxis).

NURSING CONSIDERATIONS

BASELINE ASSESSMENT
Obtain baseline CBC, renal function tests. Question for history of allergies, particularly cephalosporins, penicillins.

INTERVENTION/EVALUATION
Assess oral cavity for white patches on mucous membranes, tongue (thrush). Monitor daily pattern of bowel activity, stool consistency. Mild GI effects may be tolerable (increasing severity may indicate onset of antibiotic-associated colitis). Monitor I&O, renal function tests for nephrotoxicity. Be alert for superinfection: fever, vomiting, diarrhea, anal/

genital pruritus, oral mucosal changes (ulceration, pain, erythema).

PATIENT/FAMILY TEACHING

• Continue therapy for full length of treatment. • Doses should be evenly spaced. • May cause GI upset (may take with food, milk). • Chewable tablets must be chewed; do not swallow whole. • Refrigerate oral suspension. • Report persistent diarrhea.

cefadroxil

sef-a-**drox**-il
(Apo-Cefadroxil ✦)

◆CLASSIFICATION

PHARMACOTHERAPEUTIC: First-generation cephalosporin. **CLINICAL:** Antibiotic.

USES

Treatment of susceptible infections due to group A streptococci, staphylococci, *S. pneumoniae, H. influenzae, Klebsiella* spp., *E. coli, P. mirabilis*, including impetigo, pharyngitis/tonsillitis, skin/skin structure, UTIs. **OFF-LABEL:** Chronic suppression of prosthetic joint infection.

PRECAUTIONS

Contraindications: History of hypersensitivity/anaphylactic reaction to cefadroxil, cephalosporins. **Cautions:** Severe renal impairment, history of penicillin allergy. History of GI disease (colitis).

ACTION

Binds to bacterial cell membranes, inhibits cell wall synthesis. **Therapeutic Effect:** Bactericidal.

PHARMACOKINETICS

Well absorbed from GI tract. Protein binding: 15%–20%. Widely distributed. Primarily excreted in urine. Removed by hemodialysis. **Half-life:** 1.2–1.5 hrs (increased in renal impairment).

⧗ LIFESPAN CONSIDERATIONS

Pregnancy/Lactation: Readily crosses placenta. Distributed in breast milk. **Children:** No age-related precautions noted. **Elderly:** Age-related renal impairment may require dosage adjustment.

INTERACTIONS

DRUG: Probenecid may increase concentration. **HERBAL:** None significant. **FOOD:** None known. **LAB VALUES:** May increase serum BUN, alkaline phosphatase, bilirubin, creatinine, LDH, ALT, AST. May cause positive direct/indirect Coombs' test.

AVAILABILITY (Rx)

Capsules: 500 mg. **Powder for Oral Suspension:** 250 mg/5 mL, 500 mg/5 mL. **Tablets:** 1 g.

ADMINISTRATION/HANDLING

PO

• After reconstitution, oral solution is stable for 14 days if refrigerated. • Shake oral suspension well before using. • Give without regard to meals; if GI upset occurs, give with food, milk.

INDICATIONS/ROUTES/DOSAGE

Usual Dosage
PO: ADULTS, ELDERLY: 1–2 g/day as single dose or in 2 divided doses. **CHILDREN:** 30 mg/kg/day in 2 divided doses. **Maximum:** 2 g/day.

Dosage in Renal Impairment
After initial 1-g dose, dosage and frequency are modified based on creatinine clearance and severity of infection.

Creatinine Clearance	Dosage
26–50 mL/min	q12h
10–25 mL/min	q24h
Less than 10 mL/min	q36h

Dosage in Hepatic Impairment
No dose adjustment.

C

SIDE EFFECTS

Frequent: Oral candidiasis, mild diarrhea, mild abdominal cramping, vaginal candidiasis. **Occasional:** Nausea, unusual bruising/bleeding, serum sickness–like reaction (fever, joint pain; usually occurs after second course of therapy and resolves after drug is discontinued). **Rare:** Allergic reaction (rash, pruritus, urticaria), thrombophlebitis (pain, redness, swelling at injection site).

ADVERSE EFFECTS/TOXIC REACTIONS

Antibiotic-associated colitis, other superinfections (abdominal cramps, severe watery diarrhea, fever) may result from altered bacterial balance in GI tract. Nephrotoxicity may occur, esp. in pts with preexisting renal disease. Pts with history of penicillin allergy are at increased risk for developing a severe hypersensitivity reaction (severe pruritus, angioedema, bronchospasm, anaphylaxis).

NURSING CONSIDERATIONS

BASELINE ASSESSMENT

Obtain CBC, renal function tests. Question for history of allergies, particularly cephalosporins, penicillins.

INTERVENTION/EVALUATION

Assess oral cavity for white patches on mucous membranes, tongue (thrush). Monitor daily pattern of bowel activity, stool consistency. Mild GI effects may be tolerable (increasing severity may indicate onset of antibiotic-associated colitis). Monitor I&O, renal function tests for nephrotoxicity. Be alert for superinfection: fever, vomiting, diarrhea, anal/genital pruritus, oral mucosal changes (ulceration, pain, erythema).

PATIENT/FAMILY TEACHING

• Continue therapy for full length of treatment. • Doses should be evenly spaced. • May cause GI upset (may take with food, milk). • Refrigerate oral suspension. • Report persistent diarrhea.

cefAZolin

sef-a-**zoe**-lin
Do not confuse ceFAZolin with cefOXitin, cefprozil, cefTRIAXone, or cephalexin.

◆CLASSIFICATION

PHARMACOTHERAPEUTIC: First-generation cephalosporin. **CLINICAL:** Antibiotic.

USES

Treatment of susceptible infections due to *S. aureus, S. epidermidis,* group A beta-hemolytic streptococci, *S. pneumoniae, E. coli, P. mirabilis, Klebsiella* spp., *H. influenzae,* including biliary tract, bone and joint, genital, respiratory tract, skin/skin structure infections; UTIs, endocarditis, perioperative prophylaxis, septicemia. **OFF-LABEL:** Prophylaxis against infective endocarditis.

PRECAUTIONS

Contraindications: History of hypersensitivity/anaphylactic reaction to ceFAZolin, cephalosporins. **Cautions:** Severe renal impairment, history of penicillin allergy, history of seizures.

ACTION

Binds to bacterial cell membranes, inhibits cell wall synthesis. **Therapeutic Effect:** Bactericidal.

PHARMACOKINETICS

Widely distributed. Protein binding: 85%. Primarily excreted unchanged in urine. Moderately removed by hemodialysis. **Half-life:** 1.4–1.8 hrs (increased in renal impairment).

⧖ LIFESPAN CONSIDERATIONS

Pregnancy/Lactation: Readily crosses placenta; distributed in breast milk. **Children:** No age-related precautions noted. **Elderly:** Age-related renal impairment may require reduced dosage.

INTERACTIONS

DRUG: Probenecid may increase concentration. **HERBAL:** None significant. **FOOD:** None known. **LAB VALUES:** May increase serum BUN, alkaline phosphatase, bilirubin, creatinine, LDH, ALT, AST. May cause positive direct/indirect Coombs' test.

AVAILABILITY (Rx)

Injection, Powder for Reconstitution: 500 mg, 1 g. **Ready-to-Hang Infusion:** 1 g/50 mL, 2 g/100 mL.

ADMINISTRATION/HANDLING

 IV

Reconstitution • Reconstitute each 1 g with at least 10 mL Sterile Water for Injection or 0.9% NaCl. • May further dilute in 50–100 mL D_5W or 0.9% NaCl (decreases incidence of thrombophlebitis).
Rate of Administration • For IV push, administer over 3–5 min (**maximum concentration:** 100 mg/mL). • For intermittent IV infusion (piggyback), infuse over 30–60 min (**maximum concentration:** 20 mg/mL).
Storage • Solution appears light yellow to yellow in color. • Reconstituted solution stable for 24 hrs at room temperature or for 10 days if refrigerated. • IV infusion (piggyback) stable for 48 hrs at room temperature or for 14 days if refrigerated.

IM

• To minimize discomfort, inject deep IM slowly. • Less painful if injected into gluteus maximus rather than lateral aspect of thigh.

▓ IV INCOMPATIBILITIES

Amikacin (Amikin), amiodarone (Cordarone), HYDROmorphone (Dilaudid).

▓ IV COMPATIBILITIES

Calcium gluconate, dexamethasone (Decadron), diltiaZEM (Cardizem), famotidine (Pepcid), heparin, insulin (regular), lidocaine, LORazepam (Ativan), magnesium sulfate, meperidine (Demerol), metoclopramide (Reglan), midazolam (Versed), morphine, multivitamins, ondansetron (Zofran), potassium chloride, propofol (Diprivan).

INDICATIONS/ROUTES/DOSAGE

Usual Dosage Range
IV, IM: ADULTS: 1–1.5 g q6–12h (usually q8h). **Maximum:** 12 g/day. **CHILDREN OLDER THAN 1 MO:** 25–100 mg/kg/day divided q6–8h. **Maximum:** 6 g/day. **NEONATES:** 25 mg/kg/dose q8–12h.

Dosage in Renal Impairment
Dosing frequency is modified based on creatinine clearance.

Creatinine Clearance	Dosage
11–34 mL/min	50% usual dose q12h
10 mL/min or less	50% usual dose q18–24h
HD	500 mg–1 g q24h
PD	500 mg q12h
CRRT	
CVVH	Loading dose 2 g, then 1–2 g q12h
CVVHD/ CVVHDF	Loading dose 2 g, then 1 g q8h or 2 g q12h

Dosage in Hepatic Impairment
No dose adjustment.

SIDE EFFECTS

Frequent: Discomfort with IM administration, oral candidiasis (thrush), mild diarrhea, mild abdominal cramping, vaginal candidiasis. **Occasional:** Nausea, serum sickness–like reaction (fever, joint pain; usually occurs after second course of therapy and resolves after drug is discontinued). **Rare:** Allergic reaction (rash, pruritus, urticaria), thrombophlebitis (pain, redness, swelling at injection site).

ADVERSE EFFECTS/TOXIC REACTIONS

Antibiotic-associated colitis, other superinfections (abdominal cramps, severe watery diarrhea, fever) may result from altered bacterial balance in GI tract. Nephrotoxicity may occur, esp. in pts with preexisting renal disease. Pts with history of penicillin allergy are at increased risk for developing severe hypersensitivity reaction (severe pruritus, angioedema, bronchospasm, anaphylaxis).

NURSING CONSIDERATIONS

BASELINE ASSESSMENT
Obtain CBC, renal function tests. Question for history of allergies, particularly cephalosporins, penicillins.

INTERVENTION/EVALUATION
Evaluate IM site for induration and tenderness. Assess oral cavity for white patches on mucous membranes, tongue (thrush). Monitor daily pattern of bowel activity, stool consistency. Mild GI effects may be tolerable (increasing severity may indicate onset of antibiotic-associated colitis). Monitor I&O, renal function tests for nephrotoxicity. Be alert for superinfection: fever, vomiting, diarrhea, anal/genital pruritus, oral mucosal changes (ulceration, pain, erythema).

PATIENT/FAMILY TEACHING
• Discomfort may occur with IM injection.

cefdinir

sef-di-neer

◆CLASSIFICATION
PHARMACOTHERAPEUTIC: Third-generation cephalosporin. **CLINICAL:** Antibiotic.

USES
Treatment of susceptible infections due to *S. pyogenes, S. pneumoniae, H. influenzae, H. parainfluenzae, M. catarrhalis,* including community-acquired pneumonia, acute exacerbation of chronic bronchitis, acute maxillary sinusitis, pharyngitis, tonsillitis, uncomplicated skin/skin structure infections, otitis media.

PRECAUTIONS
Contraindications: Hypersensitivity to cefdinir. History of anaphylactic reaction to cephalosporins. **Cautions:** Hypersensitivity to penicillins; renal impairment.

ACTION
Binds to bacterial cell membranes, inhibits cell wall synthesis. **Therapeutic Effect:** Bactericidal.

PHARMACOKINETICS
Moderately absorbed from GI tract. Protein binding: 60%–70%. Widely distributed. Not appreciably metabolized. Primarily excreted in urine. Minimally removed by hemodialysis. **Half-life:** 1–2 hrs (increased in renal impairment).

⌛ LIFESPAN CONSIDERATIONS
Pregnancy/Lactation: Crosses placenta. Not detected in breast milk. **Children:** Newborns, infants may have lower renal clearance. **Elderly:** Age-related renal impairment may require decreased dosage or increased dosing interval.

INTERACTIONS
DRUG: Antacids, iron preparations may interfere with absorption. **Probenecid** increases concentration. **HERBAL:** None significant. **FOOD:** None known. **LAB VALUES:** May produce false-positive reaction for urine ketones. May increase serum alkaline phosphatase, bilirubin, LDH, ALT, AST.

AVAILABILITY (Rx)

🖐 **Capsules:** 300 mg. **Powder for Oral Suspension:** 125 mg/5 mL, 250 mg/5 mL.

ADMINISTRATION/HANDLING
PO
• Give without regard to food. Give at least 2 hrs before or after antacids or iron supplements. • Twice-daily doses should be given 12 hrs apart. • Shake

oral suspension well before administering. • Store mixed suspension at room temperature for 10 days.

INDICATIONS/ROUTES/DOSAGE

Usual Dosage Range
PO: ADULTS, ELDERLY: 300 mg q12h or 600 mg once daily. **CHILDREN 6 MOS–12 YRS:** 7 mg/kg q12h or 14 mg/kg once daily. **Maximum:** 600 mg/day.

Dosage in Renal Impairment
CrCl less than 30 mL/min: 300 mg/day or 7 mg/kg as single daily dose. **Maximum:** 300 mg. **Hemodialysis pts:** 300 mg or 7 mg/kg/dose every other day. **Maximum:** 300 mg.

Dosage in Hepatic Impairment
No dose adjustment.

SIDE EFFECTS

Frequent: Oral candidiasis, mild diarrhea, mild abdominal cramping, vaginal candidiasis. **Occasional:** Nausea, serum sickness–like reaction (fever, joint pain; usually occurs after second course of therapy and resolves after drug is discontinued). **Rare:** Allergic reaction (rash, pruritus, urticaria).

ADVERSE EFFECTS/TOXIC REACTIONS

Antibiotic-associated colitis, other superinfections (abdominal cramps, severe watery diarrhea, fever) may result from altered bacterial balance in GI tract. Nephrotoxicity may occur, esp. in pts with preexisting renal disease. Pts with history of penicillin allergy are at increased risk for developing a severe hypersensitivity reaction (severe pruritus, angioedema, bronchospasm, anaphylaxis).

NURSING CONSIDERATIONS

BASELINE ASSESSMENT
Obtain CBC, renal function tests. Question for hypersensitivity to cefdinir or other cephalosporins, penicillins.

INTERVENTION/EVALUATION
Observe for rash. Monitor daily pattern of bowel activity, stool consistency. Mild GI effects may be tolerable (increasing severity may indicate onset of antibiotic-associated colitis). Be alert for superinfection: fever, vomiting, diarrhea, anal/genital pruritus, oral mucosal changes (ulceration, pain, erythema). Monitor hematology reports.

PATIENT/FAMILY TEACHING
• Take antacids 2 hrs before or following medication. • Continue medication for full length of treatment; do not skip doses. • Doses should be evenly spaced. • Report persistent severe diarrhea, rash, muscle aches, fever, enlarged lymph nodes, joint pain.

cefepime

sef-e-**peem**
(Maxipime)
Do not confuse cefepime with cefixime or cefTAZidime.

◆**CLASSIFICATION**

PHARMACOTHERAPEUTIC: Fourth-generation cephalosporin. **CLINICAL:** Antibiotic.

USES

Susceptible infections due to aerobic gram-negative organisms including *P. aeruginosa,* gram-positive organisms including *S. aureus.* Treatment of empiric febrile neutropenia, intra-abdominal infections, skin/skin structure infections, UTIs, pneumonia. **OFF-LABEL:** Brain abscess, malignant otitis externa, septic lateral/cavernous sinus thrombus.

PRECAUTIONS

Contraindications: History of anaphylactic reaction to penicillins, hypersensitivity to cefepime, cephalosporins. **Cautions:** Renal impairment, history of seizure disorder, GI disease (colitis), elderly.

c

ACTION

Binds to bacterial cell wall membranes, inhibits cell wall synthesis. **Therapeutic Effect:** Bactericidal.

PHARMACOKINETICS

Well absorbed after IM administration. Protein binding: 20%. Widely distributed. Primarily excreted in urine. Removed by hemodialysis. **Half-life:** 2–2.3 hrs (increased in renal impairment, elderly pts).

⧗ LIFESPAN CONSIDERATIONS

Pregnancy/Lactation: Unknown if distributed in breast milk. **Children:** No age-related precautions noted in pts older than 2 mos. **Elderly:** Age-related renal impairment may require reduced dosage or increased dosing interval.

INTERACTIONS

DRUG: **Probenecid** may increase concentration. May increase **aminoglycoside** concentration. **HERBAL:** None significant. **FOOD:** None known. **LAB VALUES:** May increase serum BUN, alkaline phosphatase, bilirubin, LDH, ALT, AST. May cause positive direct/indirect Coombs' test.

AVAILABILITY (Rx)

Injection, Powder for Reconstitution: 1 g, 2 g. **Injection, Premix:** 1 g (50 mL), 2 g (50 mL).

ADMINISTRATION/HANDLING

 IV

Reconstitution • Add 10 mL of diluent for 1-g and 2-g vials. • Further dilute with 50–100 mL 0.9% NaCl or D_5W. **Rate of Administration** • For intermittent IV infusion (piggyback), infuse over 30 min. For direct IV, administer over 5 min. **Storage** • Solution is stable for 24 hrs at room temperature, 7 days if refrigerated.

IM

• Add 2.4 mL Sterile Water for Injection, 0.9% NaCl, or D_5W to 1-g and 2-g vials. • Inject into a large muscle mass (e.g., upper gluteus maximus).

▦ IV INCOMPATIBILITIES

Acyclovir (Zovirax), amphotericin (Fungizone), cimetidine (Tagamet), ciprofloxacin (Cipro), CISplatin (Platinol), dacarbazine (DTIC), DAUNOrubicin (Cerubidine), diazePAM (Valium), diphenhydrAMINE (Benadryl), DOBUTamine (Dobutrex), DOPamine (Intropin), DOXOrubicin (Adriamycin), droperidol (Inapsine), famotidine (Pepcid), ganciclovir (Cytovene), haloperidol (Haldol), magnesium, magnesium sulfate, mannitol, metoclopramide (Reglan), morphine, ofloxacin (Floxin), ondansetron (Zofran), vancomycin (Vancocin).

▦ IV COMPATIBILITIES

Bumetanide (Bumex), calcium gluconate, furosemide (Lasix), HYDROmorphone (Dilaudid), LORazepam (Ativan), propofol (Diprivan).

INDICATIONS/ROUTES/DOSAGE

Usual Dosage Range

IV: ADULTS, ELDERLY: 1–2 g q8–12h. **CHILDREN:** 50 mg/kg q8–12h not to exceed adult dosing. **NEONATES:** 30 mg/kg q12h up to 50 mg/kg q8–12h.

Dosage in Renal Impairment

Dosage and frequency are modified based on creatinine clearance and severity of infection.

Creatinine Clearance	Dosage
30–60 mL/min	500 mg q24h–2 g q12h
11–29 mL/min	500 mg–2 g q24h
10 mL/min or less	250 mg–1 g q24h
Hemodialysis	Initially, 1 g, then 0.5–1 g q24h or 1–2 g q48–72h
Peritoneal dialysis	Normal dose q48h
Continuous renal replacement therapy	Initially, 2 g, then 1 g q8h or 2 g q12h

Dosage in Hepatic Impairment
No dose adjustment.

SIDE EFFECTS

Frequent: Discomfort with IM administration, oral candidiasis (thrush), mild diarrhea, mild abdominal cramping, vaginal candidiasis. **Occasional:** Nausea, serum sickness–like reaction (fever, joint pain; usually occurs after second course of therapy and resolves after drug is discontinued). **Rare:** Allergic reaction (rash, pruritus, urticaria), thrombophlebitis (pain, redness, swelling at injection site).

ADVERSE EFFECTS/TOXIC REACTIONS

Antibiotic-associated colitis, other superinfections (abdominal cramps, severe watery diarrhea, fever) may result from altered bacterial balance in GI tract. Nephrotoxicity may occur, esp. in pts with preexisting renal disease. Pts with history of penicillin allergy are at increased risk for developing a severe hypersensitivity reaction (severe pruritus, angioedema, bronchospasm, anaphylaxis).

NURSING CONSIDERATIONS

BASELINE ASSESSMENT

Obtain CBC, renal function tests. Question for history of allergies, particularly cephalosporins, penicillins.

INTERVENTION/EVALUATION

Evaluate IM site for induration and tenderness. Assess oral cavity for white patches on mucous membranes, tongue (thrush). Monitor daily pattern of bowel activity, stool consistency. Mild GI effects may be tolerable (increasing severity may indicate onset of antibiotic-associated colitis). Monitor I&O, CBC, renal function tests for nephrotoxicity. Be alert for superinfection: fever, vomiting, diarrhea, anal/genital pruritus, oral mucosal changes (ulceration, pain, erythema).

PATIENT/FAMILY TEACHING

• Discomfort may occur with IM injection. • Continue therapy for full length of treatment. • Doses should be evenly spaced. • Report persistent diarrhea.

cefixime

sef-**ix**-eem
(Suprax)
Do not confuse cefixime with cefepime, or Suprax with Sporanox or Surbex.

◆CLASSIFICATION

PHARMACOTHERAPEUTIC: Third-generation cephalosporin. **CLINICAL:** Antibiotic.

USES

Treatment of susceptible infections due to *S. pneumoniae, S. pyogenes, M. catarrhalis, H. influenzae, E. coli, P. mirabilis,* including otitis media, acute bronchitis, acute exacerbations of chronic bronchitis, pharyngitis, tonsillitis, uncomplicated UTI.

PRECAUTIONS

Contraindications: History of hypersensitivity/anaphylactic reaction to cefixime, cephalosporins. **Cautions:** History of penicillin allergy, renal impairment.

ACTION

Binds to bacterial cell membranes, inhibits cell wall synthesis. **Therapeutic Effect:** Bactericidal.

PHARMACOKINETICS

Moderately absorbed from GI tract. Protein binding: 65%–70%. Widely distributed. Primarily excreted in urine. Minimally removed by hemodialysis. **Half-life:** 3–4 hrs (increased in renal impairment).

⧗ LIFESPAN CONSIDERATIONS

Pregnancy/Lactation: Not recommended during labor and delivery. Unknown if distributed in breast milk. **Children:** Safety and efficacy not established in pts younger than 6 mos. **Elderly:** Age-related renal impairment may require dosage adjustment.

INTERACTIONS

DRUG: Probenecid may increase concentration. May increase **aminoglycoside** (e.g., **gentamicin, tobramycin**) concentration. **HERBAL:** None significant. **FOOD:** None known. **LAB VALUES:** May increase serum BUN, alkaline phosphatase, bilirubin, creatinine, LDH, ALT, AST. May cause a positive direct/indirect Coombs' test.

AVAILABILITY (Rx)

Oral Suspension: 100 mg/5 mL, 200 mg/5 mL, 500 mg/5 mL. **Capsules:** 400 mg. **Tablets: (Chewable):** 100 mg, 200 mg.

ADMINISTRATION/HANDLING

PO

• Give without regard to food. • After reconstitution, oral suspension is stable for 14 days at room temperature or refrigerated. • Shake oral suspension well before administering. Chewable tablets must be chewed or crushed before swallowing.

INDICATIONS/ROUTES/DOSAGE

Usual Dosage
PO: ADULTS, ELDERLY, CHILDREN 12 YRS AND OLDER WEIGHING MORE THAN 45 KG: 400 mg/day as a single dose or in 2 divided doses. **CHILDREN 6 MOS–12 YRS WEIGHING 45 KG OR LESS:** 8 mg/kg/day as a single dose or in 2 divided doses. **Maximum:** 400 mg.

Dosage in Renal Impairment
Dosage is modified based on creatinine clearance.

Creatinine Clearance	Dosage
21–60 mL/min	260 mg/day
20 mL/min or less	200 mg/day
Hemodialysis	260 mg/day

Dosage in Hepatic Impairment
No dose adjustment.

SIDE EFFECTS

Frequent: Oral candidiasis (thrush), mild diarrhea, mild abdominal cramping, vaginal candidiasis. **Occasional:** Nausea, serum sickness–like reaction (arthralgia, fever; usually occurs after second course of therapy and resolves after drug is discontinued). **Rare:** Allergic reaction (rash, pruritus, urticaria).

ADVERSE EFFECTS/TOXIC REACTIONS

Antibiotic-associated colitis, other superinfections (abdominal cramps, severe watery diarrhea, fever) may result from altered bacterial balance in GI tract. Nephrotoxicity may occur, esp. in pts with preexisting renal disease. Pts with history of penicillin allergy are at increased risk for developing a severe hypersensitivity reaction (severe pruritus, angioedema, bronchospasm, anaphylaxis).

NURSING CONSIDERATIONS

BASELINE ASSESSMENT
Obtain CBC, renal function tests. Question for hypersensitivity to cefixime or other cephalosporins, penicillins.

INTERVENTION/EVALUATION
Assess oral cavity for white patches on mucous membranes, tongue (thrush). Monitor daily pattern of bowel activity, stool consistency. Mild GI effects may be tolerable (increasing severity may indicate onset of antibiotic-associated colitis). Monitor renal function tests for evidence of nephrotoxicity. Be alert for superinfection: fever, vomiting, diarrhea, anal/genital pruritus, oral mucosal changes (ulceration, pain, erythema).

PATIENT/FAMILY TEACHING
• Continue medication for full length of treatment; do not skip doses. • Doses should be evenly spaced. • May cause GI upset (may take with food or milk). • Report persistent diarrhea.

cefotaxime

sef-oh-**tax**-eem
(Claforan)

Do not confuse cefotaxime with cefOXitin, ceftizoxime, or cefuroxime, or Claforan with Claritin.

◆ CLASSIFICATION

PHARMACOTHERAPEUTIC: Third-generation cephalosporin. **CLINICAL:** Antibiotic.

USES

Treatment of susceptible infections (active vs. most gram-negative [not *Pseudomonas*] and gram-positive cocci [not *Enterococcus*]), including bone, joint, GU, gynecologic, intra-abdominal, lower respiratory tract, skin/skin structure infections; septicemia, meningitis, perioperative prophylaxis. **OFF-LABEL:** Surgical prophylaxis.

PRECAUTIONS

Contraindications: History of hypersensitivity/anaphylactic reaction to cefotaxime, cephalosporins. **Cautions:** History of penicillin allergy, colitis, renal impairment with CrCl less than 30 mL/min.

ACTION

Binds to bacterial cell membranes, inhibits cell wall synthesis. **Therapeutic Effect:** Bactericidal.

PHARMACOKINETICS

Widely distributed to CSF. Protein binding: 30%–50%. Partially metabolized in liver. Primarily excreted in urine. Moderately removed by hemodialysis. **Half-life:** 1 hr (increased in renal impairment).

⧗ LIFESPAN CONSIDERATIONS

Pregnancy/Lactation: Readily crosses placenta. Distributed in breast milk. **Children:** No age-related precautions noted. **Elderly:** Age-related renal impairment may require dosage adjustment.

INTERACTIONS

DRUG: Probenecid may increase concentration. May increase **aminoglycoside** (e.g., **gentamicin, tobramycin**) concentration. **HERBAL:** None significant. **FOOD:** None known. **LAB VALUES:** May cause positive direct/indirect Coombs' test. May increase serum BUN, creatinine, ALT, AST, alkaline phosphatase.

AVAILABILITY (Rx)

Injection, Powder for Reconstitution: 500 mg, 1 g, 2 g. **Intravenous Solution (Premix):** 1 g/50 mL, 2 g/50 mL.

ADMINISTRATION/HANDLING

 IV

Reconstitution • Reconstitute with 10 mL Sterile Water for Injection or 0.9% NaCl to provide a maximum concentration of 100 mg/mL. • May further dilute with 50–100 mL 0.9% NaCl or D_5W.
Rate of Administration • For IV push, administer over 3–5 min. • For intermittent IV infusion (piggyback), infuse over 15–30 min.
Storage • Solution appears light yellow to amber. • IV infusion (piggyback) is stable for 24 hrs at room temperature, 5 days if refrigerated. • Discard if precipitate forms.

IM
• Reconstitute with Sterile Water for Injection or Bacteriostatic Water for Injection to provide a concentration of 230–330 mg/mL. • To minimize discomfort, inject deep IM slowly. Less painful if injected into gluteus maximus than lateral aspect of thigh. For 2-g IM dose, give at 2 separate sites.

▥ IV INCOMPATIBILITIES

Allopurinol (Aloprim), filgrastim (Neupogen), fluconazole (Diflucan), vancomycin (Vancocin).

▥ IV COMPATIBILITIES

DiltiaZEM (Cardizem), famotidine (Pepcid), HYDROmorphone (Dilaudid), LORazepam (Ativan), magnesium sulfate, midazolam (Versed), morphine, propofol (Diprivan).

INDICATIONS/ROUTES/DOSAGE

Usual Dosage Range
IV, IM: ADULTS, ELDERLY, CHILDREN WEIGHING 50 KG OR MORE: 1–2 g q4–12h. **Maximum:** 12 g/day. **CHILDREN 1 MO–12 YRS WEIGHING LESS THAN 50 KG:** 50–180 mg/kg/day in divided doses q4–6h. **Maximum:** 12 g/day. **NEONATES:** 50 mg/kg/dose q8–12h.

Dosage in Renal Impairment

Creatinine Clearance	Dosage Interval
10–50 mL/min	6–12 hrs
Less than 10 mL/min	24 hrs
Hemodialysis	1–2g q24h
Peritoneal dialysis	1g q24h
CVVH	1–2 g q8–12h
CVVHD	1–2g q8h
CVVHDF	1–2g q6–8h

Dosage in Hepatic Impairment
No dose adjustment.

SIDE EFFECTS

Frequent: Discomfort with IM administration, oral candidiasis (thrush), mild diarrhea, mild abdominal cramping, vaginal candidiasis. **Occasional:** Nausea, serum sickness–like reaction (fever, joint pain; usually occurs after second course of therapy and resolves after drug is discontinued). **Rare:** Allergic reaction (rash, pruritus, urticaria), thrombophlebitis (pain, redness, swelling at injection site).

ADVERSE EFFECTS/TOXIC REACTIONS

Antibiotic-associated colitis, other superinfections (abdominal cramps, severe watery diarrhea, fever) may result from altered bacterial balance in GI tract. Nephrotoxicity may occur, esp. in pts with preexisting renal disease. Pts with history of penicillin allergy are at increased risk for developing a severe hypersensitivity reaction (severe pruritus, angioedema, bronchospasm, anaphylaxis).

NURSING CONSIDERATIONS

BASELINE ASSESSMENT

Question for history of allergies, particularly cephalosporins, penicillins.

INTERVENTION/EVALUATION

Check IM injection sites for induration, tenderness. Assess oral cavity for white patches on mucous membranes, tongue (thrush). Monitor daily pattern of bowel activity, stool consistency. Mild GI effects may be tolerable (increasing severity may indicate onset of antibiotic-associated colitis). Monitor I&O, renal function tests for nephrotoxicity. Be alert for superinfection: fever, vomiting, diarrhea, anal/genital pruritus, oral mucosal changes (ulceration, pain, erythema).

PATIENT/FAMILY TEACHING

• Discomfort may occur with IM injection. • Doses should be evenly spaced. • Continue antibiotic therapy for full length of treatment.

cefpodoxime

sef-poe-**dox**-eem

♦**CLASSIFICATION**

PHARMACOTHERAPEUTIC: Third-generation cephalosporin. **CLINICAL:** Antibiotic.

USES

Treatment of susceptible infections due to *S. pneumoniae, S. pyogenes, S. aureus, H. influenzae, M. catarrhalis, E. coli, Proteus, Klebsiella* spp., including acute maxillary sinusitis, chronic bronchitis, community-acquired pneumonia, gonorrhea, otitis media, pharyngitis, tonsillitis, skin/skin structure infections, UTIs.

PRECAUTIONS

Contraindications: History of hypersensitivity/anaphylactic reaction to cefpodoxime, cephalosporins. **Cautions:** Renal impairment, history of penicillin allergy.

ACTION

Binds to bacterial cell membranes, inhibits cell wall synthesis. **Therapeutic Effect:** Bactericidal.

PHARMACOKINETICS

Well absorbed from GI tract (food increases absorption). Protein binding: 18%–23%. Widely distributed. Primarily excreted unchanged in urine. Partially removed by hemodialysis. **Half-life:** 2.3 hrs (increased in renal impairment, elderly pts).

⧖ LIFESPAN CONSIDERATIONS

Pregnancy/Lactation: Readily crosses placenta. Distributed in breast milk. **Children:** Safety and efficacy not established in pts younger than 6 mos. **Elderly:** Age-related renal impairment may require dosage adjustment.

INTERACTIONS

DRUG: High doses of **antacids containing aluminum, H₂ antagonists (e.g., famotidine, ranitidine)** may decrease absorption. **Probenecid** may increase concentration. **HERBAL:** None significant. **FOOD: Food** enhances absorption. **LAB VALUES:** May increase serum BUN, alkaline phosphatase, bilirubin, creatinine, LDH, ALT, AST. May cause positive direct/indirect Coombs' test.

AVAILABILITY (Rx)

Oral Suspension: 50 mg/5 mL, 100 mg/5 mL. **Tablets:** 100 mg, 200 mg.

ADMINISTRATION/HANDLING
PO

• Administer tablet with food (enhances absorption). • Administer suspension without regard to food. • After reconstitution, oral suspension is stable for 14 days if refrigerated.

INDICATIONS/ROUTES/DOSAGE
Usual Dosage Range

PO: ADULTS, ELDERLY, CHILDREN OLDER THAN 12 YRS: 100–400 mg q12h. **CHILDREN 2 MOS–12 YRS:** 10 mg/kg/day in 2 divided doses. **Maximum:** 200 mg/dose.

Dosage in Renal Impairment

For pts with CrCl less than 30 mL/min, usual dose is given q24h. For pts on hemodialysis, usual dose is given 3 times/wk after dialysis.

Dosage in Hepatic Impairment

No dose adjustment.

SIDE EFFECTS

Frequent: Oral candidiasis (thrush), mild diarrhea, mild abdominal cramping, vaginal candidiasis. **Occasional:** Nausea, serum sickness–like reaction (fever, joint pain; usually occurs after second course of therapy and resolves after drug is discontinued). **Rare:** Allergic reaction (pruritus, rash, urticaria).

ADVERSE EFFECTS/TOXIC REACTIONS

Antibiotic-associated colitis, other superinfections (abdominal cramps, severe watery diarrhea, fever) may result from altered bacterial balance in GI tract. Nephrotoxicity may occur, esp. in pts with preexisting renal disease. Pts with history of penicillin allergy are at increased risk for developing a severe hypersensitivity reaction (severe pruritus, angioedema, bronchospasm, anaphylaxis).

NURSING CONSIDERATIONS

BASELINE ASSESSMENT

Obtain CBC, renal function tests. Question for history of allergies, particularly cephalosporins, penicillins.

INTERVENTION/EVALUATION

Assess oral cavity for white patches on mucous membranes, tongue (thrush). Monitor daily pattern of bowel activity, stool consistency. Mild GI effects may

C

be tolerable (increasing severity may indicate onset of antibiotic-associated colitis). Monitor I&O, renal function tests for nephrotoxicity. Be alert for superinfection: fever, vomiting, diarrhea, anal/genital pruritus, oral mucosal changes (ulceration, pain, erythema).

PATIENT/FAMILY TEACHING

• Doses should be evenly spaced. • Shake oral suspension well before using. • Take tablets with food (enhances absorption). • Continue antibiotic therapy for full length of treatment. • Refrigerate oral suspension. • Report persistent diarrhea.

---

cefprozil

sef-proe-zil
(Apo-Cefprozil ✦, Cefzil ✦)
Do not confuse cefprozil with ceFAZolin, or Cefzil with Cefol, Ceftin, or Kefzol.

◆CLASSIFICATION

PHARMACOTHERAPEUTIC: Second-generation cephalosporin. **CLINICAL:** Antibiotic.

USES

Treatment of susceptible infections due to *S. pneumoniae, S. pyogenes, S. aureus, H. influenzae, M. catarrhalis,* including pharyngitis, tonsillitis, otitis media, secondary bacterial infection of acute bronchitis, acute bacterial exacerbation of chronic bronchitis, uncomplicated skin/skin structure infections, acute sinusitis.

PRECAUTIONS

Contraindications: History of hypersensitivity/anaphylactic reaction to cefprozil, cephalosporins. **Cautions:** Severe renal impairment, history of penicillin allergy.

ACTION

Binds to bacterial cell membranes, inhibits cell wall synthesis. **Therapeutic Effect:** Bactericidal.

PHARMACOKINETICS

Well absorbed from GI tract. Protein binding: 36%–45%. Widely distributed. Primarily excreted in urine. Moderately removed by hemodialysis. **Half-life:** 1.3 hrs (increased in renal impairment).

⊠ LIFESPAN CONSIDERATIONS

Pregnancy/Lactation: Readily crosses placenta. Distributed in breast milk. **Children:** Safety and efficacy not established in pts younger than 6 mos. **Elderly:** Age-related renal impairment may require dosage adjustment.

INTERACTIONS

DRUG: Probenecid may increase concentration. May increase **aminoglycoside** (e.g., **gentamicin, tobramycin**) concentration. **HERBAL:** None significant. **FOOD:** None known. **LAB VALUES:** May cause positive direct/indirect Coombs' test. May increase serum BUN, creatinine, alkaline phosphatase, ALT, AST.

AVAILABILITY (Rx)

Oral Suspension: 125 mg/5 mL, 250 mg/5 mL. **Tablets:** 250 mg, 500 mg.

ADMINISTRATION/HANDLING

PO

• Give without regard to food; if GI upset occurs, give with food, milk. • After reconstitution, oral suspension is stable for 14 days if refrigerated. • Shake oral suspension well before using.

INDICATIONS/ROUTES/DOSAGE

Usual Dosage Range
PO: ADULTS, ELDERLY, CHILDREN OLDER THAN 12 YRS: 250–500 mg q12h or 500 mg q24h. **CHILDREN OLDER THAN 6 MOS–12 YRS:** 7.5–15 mg/kg/day in 2 divided doses. **Maximum:** 500 mg/dose. Do not exceed adult dose.

Dosage in Renal Impairment
CrCl less than 30 mL/min: 50% of usual dose at usual interval. **Hemodialysis:** Administer dose after completion of dialysis.

Dosage in Hepatic Impairment
No dose adjustment.

SIDE EFFECTS

Frequent: Oral candidiasis (thrush), mild diarrhea, mild abdominal cramping, vaginal candidiasis. **Occasional:** Nausea, serum sickness–like reaction (fever, joint pain; usually occurs after second course of therapy and resolves after drug is discontinued). **Rare:** Allergic reaction (pruritus, rash, urticaria).

ADVERSE EFFECTS/TOXIC REACTIONS

Antibiotic-associated colitis, other superinfections (abdominal cramps, severe watery diarrhea, fever) may result from altered bacterial balance in GI tract. Nephrotoxicity may occur, esp. in pts with preexisting renal disease. Pts with history of penicillin allergy are at increased risk for developing a severe hypersensitivity reaction (severe pruritus, angioedema, bronchospasm, anaphylaxis).

NURSING CONSIDERATIONS

BASELINE ASSESSMENT
Obtain CBC, renal function tests. Question for history of allergies, particularly cephalosporins, penicillins.

INTERVENTION/EVALUATION
Assess oral cavity for evidence of stomatitis. Monitor daily pattern of bowel activity, stool consistency. Mild GI effects may be tolerable (but increasing severity may indicate onset of antibiotic-associated colitis). Monitor I&O, renal function tests for nephrotoxicity. Be alert for superinfection: fever, vomiting, diarrhea, anal/genital pruritus, oral mucosal changes (ulceration, pain, erythema).

PATIENT/FAMILY TEACHING
• Doses should be evenly spaced. • Continue antibiotic therapy for full length of treatment. • May cause GI upset (may take with food or milk). • Report persistent diarrhea.

ceftaroline

sef-**tar**-o-leen
(Teflaro)

◆CLASSIFICATION
PHARMACOTHERAPEUTIC: Fifth-generation cephalosporin. **CLINICAL:** Antibiotic.

USES
Treatment of susceptible infections due to gram-positive and gram-negative organisms, including *S. pneumoniae, S. aureus* (methicillin-susceptible only), *H. influenzae, Klebsiella pneumoniae, E. coli,* including acute bacterial skin and skin structure infections, community-acquired bacterial pneumonia.

PRECAUTIONS
Contraindications: History of hypersensitivity/anaphylactic reaction to ceftaroline, cephalosporins. **Cautions:** History of allergy to penicillin, severe renal impairment with CrCl less than 50 mL/min, elderly.

ACTION
Binds to bacterial cell membranes, inhibits cell wall synthesis. **Therapeutic Effect:** Bactericidal.

PHARMACOKINETICS
Protein binding: 20%. Widely distributed in plasma. Not metabolized. Primarily excreted in urine. Hemodialyzable. **Half-life:** 1.6 hrs (increased in renal impairment).

⊠ LIFESPAN CONSIDERATIONS
Pregnancy/Lactation: Unknown if distributed in breast milk. **Children:** Safety

---

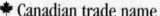 ✽ Canadian trade name   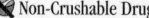 Non-Crushable Drug   **HIGH ALERT** High Alert drug

and efficacy not established in pts younger than 18 yrs. **Elderly:** Age-related renal impairment may require dose adjustment.

INTERACTIONS

DRUG: Probenecid may increase concentration. **HERBAL:** None significant. **FOOD:** None known. **LAB VALUES:** May cause positive direct/indirect Coombs' test. May increase serum BUN, creatinine. May decrease serum potassium.

AVAILABILITY (Rx)

Injection, Powder for Reconstitution: 400-mg, 600-mg single-use vial.

ADMINISTRATION/HANDLING

◀**ALERT**▶ Give by intermittent IV infusion (piggyback). Do not give IV push.
Reconstitution • Reconstitute either 400-mg or 600-mg vial with 20 mL Sterile Water for Injection. • Mix gently to dissolve powder. • Further dilute with 50–250 mL D₅W, 0.9% NaCl.
Rate of Administration • Infuse over 5–60 min.
Storage • Discard if particulate is present. • Following reconstitution, solution should appear clear, light to dark yellow. • Solution is stable for 6 hrs at room temperature or 24 hrs if refrigerated.

▩ IV INCOMPATIBILITIES

Fluconazole (Diflucan), vancomycin (Vancocin).

▩ IV COMPATIBILITIES

Famotidine (Pepcid), HYDROmorphone (Dilaudid), LORazepam (Ativan), magnesium sulfate, midazolam (Versed), morphine, propofol (Diprivan).

INDICATIONS/ROUTES/DOSAGE

Usual Dosage
IV: ADULTS, ELDERLY: 600 mg q12h. **CHILDREN 2–18 YRS (WEIGHING MORE THAN 33 KG):** 400 mg q8h or 600 mg q12h. **(WEIGHING 33 KG OR LESS):** 12 mg/kg q8h. **CHILDREN 2 MOS TO LESS THAN 2 YRS:** 8 mg/kg q8h.

Dosage in Renal Impairment

Creatinine Clearance	Dosage
30–50 mL/min	400 mg q12h
15–29 mL/min	300 mg q12h
End-stage renal disease, hemodialysis	200 mg every 12 hrs (give after dialysis)

Dosage in Hepatic Impairment
No dose adjustment.

SIDE EFFECTS

Occasional (5%–4%): Diarrhea, nausea. **Rare (3%–2%):** Allergic reaction (rash, pruritus, urticaria), phlebitis.

ADVERSE EFFECTS/TOXIC REACTIONS

Antibiotic-associated colitis, other super infections (abdominal cramps, severe watery diarrhea, fever) may result from altered bacterial balance in GI tract. Nephrotoxicity may occur, esp. with preexisting renal disease. Pts with history of penicillin allergy are at increased risk for developing a severe hypersensitivity reaction (severe pruritus, angioedema, bronchospasm, anaphylaxis).

NURSING CONSIDERATIONS

BASELINE ASSESSMENT

Obtain CBC, renal function tests. Question for hypersensitivity to other cephalosporins, penicillins. For pts on hemodialysis, administer medication after dialysis.

INTERVENTION/EVALUATION

Assess oral cavity for white patches on mucous membranes, tongue (thrush). Monitor daily pattern of bowel activity, stool consistency. Mild GI effects may be tolerable, but increasing severity may indicate onset of antibiotic-associated colitis. Monitor I&O, renal function tests for evidence of nephrotoxicity. Be alert for superinfection: fever, vomiting, severe genital/anal pruritus, moderate to severe diarrhea, oral mucosal changes (ulceration, pain, erythema).

• Continue medication for full length of treatment. • Doses should be evenly spaced.

cefTAZidime

sef-**taz**-i-deem
(Fortaz, Tazicef)
Do not confuse cefTAZidime with ceFAZolin, cefepime, or cefTRIAXone.

◆CLASSIFICATION

PHARMACOTHERAPEUTIC: Third-generation cephalosporin. **CLINICAL:** Antibiotic.

USES

Treatment of susceptible infections due to gram-negative organisms (including *Pseudomonas* and *Enterobacteriaceae*), including bone, joint, CNS (including meningitis), gynecologic, intra-abdominal, lower respiratory tract, skin/skin structure infections; UTI, septicemia. Treatment of CNS infections due to *H. influenzae, N. meningitidis,* including meningitis. **OFF-LABEL:** Bacterial endophthalmitis.

PRECAUTIONS

Contraindications: History of hypersensitivity/anaphylactic reaction to cefTAZidime, cephalosporins. **Cautions:** Severe renal impairment, history of penicillin allergy, seizure disorder.

ACTION

Binds to bacterial cell membranes, inhibits cell wall synthesis. **Therapeutic Effect:** Bactericidal.

PHARMACOKINETICS

Widely distributed, including to CSF. Protein binding: 5%–17%. Primarily excreted in urine. Removed by hemodialysis. **Half-life:** 2 hrs (increased in renal impairment).

⌛ LIFESPAN CONSIDERATIONS

Pregnancy/Lactation: Readily crosses placenta. Distributed in breast milk. **Children:** No age-related precautions noted. **Elderly:** Age-related renal impairment may require dosage adjustment.

INTERACTIONS

DRUG: Probenecid may increase concentration. May increase **aminoglycoside (e.g., gentamicin, tobramycin)** concentration. **HERBAL:** None significant. **FOOD:** None known. **LAB VALUES:** May increase serum BUN, alkaline phosphatase, creatinine, LDH, ALT, AST. May cause positive direct/indirect Coombs' test.

AVAILABILITY (Rx)

Injection, Powder for Reconstitution (Fortaz, Tazicef): 500 mg, 1 g, 2 g. **Injection, Premix:** 1 g/50 mL, 2 g/50 mL.

ADMINISTRATION/HANDLING

◀**ALERT▶** Give by IM injection, direct IV injection (IV push), or intermittent IV infusion (piggyback).

 IV

Reconstitution • Add 10 mL Sterile Water for Injection to each 1 g to provide concentration of 90 mg/mL. • May further dilute with 50–100 mL 0.9% NaCl, D_5W, or other compatible diluent.

Rate of Administration • For IV push, administer over 3–5 min (**maximum concentration:** 180 mg/mL). • For intermittent IV infusion (piggyback), infuse over 15–30 min.

Storage • Solution appears light yellow to amber, tends to darken (color change does not indicate loss of potency). • IV infusion (piggyback) stable for 12 hrs at room temperature or 3 days if refrigerated. • Discard if precipitate forms.

IM

• For reconstitution, add 1.5 mL Sterile Water for Injection or lidocaine 1% to 500-mg vial or 3 mL to 1-g vial to provide a concentration of 280 mg/mL. • To minimize discomfort, inject deep IM slowly. Less painful if injected into gluteus maximus than lateral aspect of thigh.

▨ IV INCOMPATIBILITIES

Amphotericin B complex (Abelcet, AmBisome, Amphotec), fluconazole (Diflucan), IDArubicin, midazolam (Versed), vancomycin (Vancocin).

▨ IV COMPATIBILITIES

DiltiaZEM (Cardizem), famotidine (Pepcid), heparin, HYDROmorphone (Dilaudid), lipids, morphine, propofol (Diprivan).

INDICATIONS/ROUTES/DOSAGE

Usual Dosage Range
IV, IM: ADULTS, ELDERLY: 500 mg–2 g q8–12h.
IV: CHILDREN 1 MO–12 YRS: 90–150 mg/kg/day in divided doses q8h. **Maximum:** 6 g/day. **NEONATES 0–4 WKS:** 50 mg/kg/dose q8–12h.

Dosage in Renal Impairment
Dosage and frequency are modified based on creatinine clearance and severity of infection.

Creatinine Clearance	Dosage
31–50 mL/min	1 g q12h
16–30 mL/min	1 g q24h
6–15 mL/min	500 mg q24h
Less than 6 mL/min	500 mg q48h
Hemodialysis	0.5–1 g q24h or 1–2 g q48–72h (give post hemodialysis on dialysis days)
Peritoneal dialysis	Initially, 1 g, then 0.5 g q24h
Continuous renal replacement therapy	Initially, 2 g, then 1 g q8h or 2 g q12h

Dosage in Hepatic Impairment
No dose adjustment.

SIDE EFFECTS

Frequent: Discomfort with IM administration, oral candidiasis (thrush), mild diarrhea, mild abdominal cramping, vaginal candidiasis. **Occasional:** Nausea, serum sickness–like reaction (fever, joint pain; usually occurs after second course of therapy and resolves after drug is discontinued). **Rare:** Allergic reaction (pruritus, rash, urticaria), thrombophlebitis (pain, redness, swelling at injection site).

ADVERSE EFFECTS/TOXIC REACTIONS

Antibiotic-associated colitis, other superinfections (abdominal cramps, severe watery diarrhea, fever) may result from altered bacterial balance in GI tract. Nephrotoxicity may occur, esp. in pts with preexisting renal disease. Pts with history of penicillin allergy are at increased risk for developing a severe hypersensitivity reaction (severe pruritus, angioedema, bronchospasm, anaphylaxis).

NURSING CONSIDERATIONS

BASELINE ASSESSMENT
Obtain CBC, renal function tests. Question for history of allergies, particularly cephalosporins, penicillins.

INTERVENTION/EVALUATION
Evaluate IV site for phlebitis (heat, pain, red streaking over vein). Assess IM injection sites for induration, tenderness. Check oral cavity for white patches on mucous membranes, tongue (thrush). Monitor daily pattern of bowel activity, stool consistency. Mild GI effects may be tolerable (increasing severity may indicate onset of antibiotic-associated colitis). Monitor I&O, renal function tests for nephrotoxicity. Be alert for superinfection: fever, vomiting, diarrhea, anal/genital pruritus, oral mucosal changes (ulceration, pain, erythema).

PATIENT/FAMILY TEACHING
• Discomfort may occur with IM injection. • Doses should be evenly spaced. • Continue antibiotic therapy for full length of treatment.

cefTAZidime/ avibactam

sef-**taz**-i-deem/**a**-vi-**bak**-tam (Avycaz)
Do not confuse cefTAZidime with ceFAZolin or cefepime, or avibactam with sulbactam or tazobactam.

◆CLASSIFICATION

PHARMACOTHERAPEUTIC: Cephalosporin/beta-lactamase inhibitor. **CLINICAL:** Antibacterial.

USES

Used in combination with metroNIDAZOLE for treatment of complicated intra-abdominal infections caused by the following susceptible microorganisms: *E. cloacae, E. coli, K. pneumoniae, K. oxytoca, P. mirabilis, P. stuartii,* and *P. aeruginosa* in pts 18 yrs or older. Treatment of complicated urinary tract infections, including pyelonephritis, caused by the following susceptible microorganisms: *C. freundii, C. koseri, E. aerogenes, E. cloacae, E. coli, K. pneumoniae, Proteus spp.,* and *P. aeruginosa* in pts 18 yrs or older.

PRECAUTIONS

Contraindications: Hypersensitivity to avibactam-containing products, cefTAZidime, cephalosporins. **Cautions:** History of renal impairment, seizure disorder, encephalopathy, recent *C. difficile* (C-diff) infection or antibiotic-associated colitis. Hypersensitivity to penicillins, other beta-lactams.

ACTION

Inhibits cell wall synthesis by binding to bacterial cell membrane. Bacterial action of cefTAZidime is mediated through binding to essential penicillin-binding proteins. Avibactam inactivates some beta-lactamases and protects cefTAZidime from degradation by certain beta-lactamases. **Therapeutic Effect:** Bactericidal.

PHARMACOKINETICS

Widely distributed. Excreted unchanged as parent drug; not significantly metabolized in liver. Protein binding: less than 10%. Removed extensively by hemodialysis (55% of dose). Eliminated in urine (80%–90% unchanged). **Half-life:** 2.7 hrs (dependent on dose and severity of renal impairment).

⏳ LIFESPAN CONSIDERATIONS

Pregnancy/Lactation: CefTAZidime is excreted in breast milk in low concentrations. Unknown if avibactam is excreted in breast milk. **Children:** Safety and efficacy not established. **Elderly:** May have increased risk of adverse effects (due to renal impairment).

INTERACTIONS

DRUG: None significant. **HERBAL:** None significant. **FOOD:** None known. **LAB VALUES:** May increase serum alkaline phosphatase, ALT, GGT, LDH. May decrease platelets, eosinophils, leukocytes, lymphocytes, serum potassium. May result in positive Coombs' test or false-positive elevated urine glucose.

AVAILABILITY (Rx)

◄**ALERT**► CefTAZidime/avibactam is a combination product.
Injection, Powder for Reconstitution: 2 gm cefTAZidime/0.5 gm avibactam.

ADMINISTRATION/HANDLING

 IV

Reconstitution • Reconstitute vial with 10 mL of one of the following solutions: 0.9% NaCl, Sterile Water for Injection, or 5% Dextrose Injection. • Shake gently until powder is completely dissolved. • Visually inspect for particulate matter or discoloration. Solution should appear clear to slightly yellow in color. • Final concentration of vial will equal approx. 0.167 g/mL of cefTAZidime and 0.042 g/mL of avibactam. • Further dilute with 50 mL to 250 mL 0.9% NaCl or 5% Dextrose Injection. **Rate of Administration** • Infuse over 2 hrs.

Storage • Diluted solution may be stored at room temperature up to 12 hrs or refrigerated up to 24 hrs. • Infuse within 12 hrs once removed from refrigerator. • Do not freeze.

INDICATIONS/ROUTES/DOSAGE

Complicated Intra-Abdominal Infections
IV: ADULTS, ELDERLY: 2.5 g (cefTAZidime 2 g/avibactam 0.5 g) q8h for 5–14 days (in combination with metroNIDAZOLE).

Complicated Urinary Tract Infections Including Pyelonephritis
IV: ADULTS, ELDERLY: 2.5 g (2 g ceftazidime/0.5 g avibactam) q8h for 7–14 days.

Dosage in Renal Impairment
Note: Infuse after hemodialysis on hemodialysis days.
Dosage is modified based on creatinine clearance.

Creatinine Clearance	Dosage
Greater than 50 mL/min	2.5 g (2 g/0.5 g) q8h
31–50 mL/min	1.25 g (1 g/0.25 g) q8h
16–30 mL/min	0.94 g (0.75 g/ 0.19 g) q12h
6–15 mL/min	0.94 g (0.75 g/ 0.19 g) q24h
Less than or equal to 5 mL/min	0.94 g (0.75 g/ 0.19 g) q48h

Dosage in Hepatic Impairment
No dose adjustment.

SIDE EFFECTS

Occasional (14%–5%): Vomiting, nausea, abdominal pain, anxiety, rash. **Rare (4%–2%):** Constipation, dizziness.

ADVERSE EFFECTS/TOXIC REACTIONS

May cause worsening of renal function or acute renal failure in pts with renal impairment. Clinical cure rates were lower in pts with CrCl 30–50 mL/min compared with those with CrCl greater than 50 mL/min, and in pts receiving metroNIDAZOLE combination therapy. Blood and lymphatic disorders such as agranulocytosis, hemolytic anemia, leukopenia, lymphocytosis, neutropenia, thrombocytopenia were reported. Hypersensitivity reactions, including anaphylaxis or severe skin reactions, have been reported in pts treated with beta-lactam antibacterial drugs. *C. difficile* (C-diff)–associated diarrhea, with severity ranging from mild diarrhea to fatal colitis, was reported. C-diff infection may occur more than 2 mos after treatment completion. Central nervous system reactions including asterixis, coma, encephalopathy, neuromuscular excitability, myoclonus, nonconvulsive status epilepticus, seizures have been reported in pts receiving cefTAZidime, esp. in pts with renal impairment. May increase risk of development of drug-resistant bacteria when used in the absence of a proven or strongly suspected bacterial infection. Skin and subcutaneous tissue disorders such as angioedema, erythema multiforme, pruritus, Stevens-Johnson syndrome, toxic epidermal necrolysis were reported in pts receiving cefTAZidime. Other reported adverse effects, including infusion site inflammation/hematoma/thrombosis, jaundice, candidiasis, dysgeusia, paresthesia, tubulointerstitial nephritis, vaginal inflammation, occur rarely.

NURSING CONSIDERATIONS

BASELINE ASSESSMENT

Obtain baseline CBC, BUN, serum creatinine, potassium; CrCl, GFR, LFT; bacterial culture and sensitivity; vital signs. Question history of recent *C. difficile* infection, renal impairment, seizure disorder; hypersensitivity reaction to beta-lactams, carbapenem, cephalosporins, PCN. Assess skin for wounds; assess hydration status. Question pt's usual stool characteristics (color, frequency, consistency).

INTERVENTION/EVALUATION

Monitor CBC, BMP, renal function periodically. For pts with changing renal function, monitor renal function test daily and adjust dose accordingly. Diligently monitor I&Os. Observe daily pattern of bowel activity, stool consistency (increased severity may indicate antibiotic-associated colitis). If frequent diarrhea occurs, obtain *C. difficile* toxin screen and initiate isolation precautions until test result confirmed; manage proper fluids levels/PO intake, electrolyte levels, protein intake. Antibacterial drugs that are not directed against *C. difficile* infection may need to be discontinued. Report any sign of hypersensitivity reaction.

PATIENT/FAMILY TEACHING

• It is essential to complete drug therapy despite symptom improvement. Early discontinuation may result in antibacterial resistance or increased risk of recurrent infection. • Report any episodes of diarrhea, esp. in the mos following treatment completion. Frequent diarrhea, fever, abdominal pain, blood-streaked stool may indicate infectious diarrhea and may be contagious to others. • Report abdominal pain, black/tarry stools, bruising, yellowing of skin or eyes; dark urine, decreased urine output; skin problems such as development of sores, rash, skin bubbling/necrosis. • Drink plenty of fluids. • Report any nervous system changes such as anxiety, confusion, hallucinations, muscle jerking, or seizure-like activity. • Severe allergic reactions such as hives, palpitations, shortness of breath, rash, tongue-swelling may occur.

ceftolozane/ tazobactam

cef-**tol**-oh-zane/tay-zoe-**bak**-tam
(Zerbaxa)

Do not confuse ceftolozane with cefTAZidime, or tazobactam with avibactam or sulbactam.

◆CLASSIFICATION

PHARMACOTHERAPEUTIC: Cephalosporin/beta-lactamase inhibitor. **CLINICAL:** Antibacterial.

USES

Used in combination with metroNIDAZOLE for treatment of complicated intra-abdominal infections caused by the following susceptible gram-negative and gram-positive microorganisms: *B. fragilis, E. cloacae, E. coli, K. oxytoca, K. pneumoniae, P. mirabilis, P. aeruginosa, S. anginosus, S. constellatus,* and *S. salivarius* in pts 18 yrs or older. Treatment of complicated urinary tract infections, including pyelonephritis, caused by the following susceptible gram-negative microorganisms: *E. coli, K. pneumoniae, P. mirabilis, and P. aeruginosa* in pts 18 yrs or older.

PRECAUTIONS

Contraindications: Hypersensitivity to ceftolozane/tazobactam, piperacillin/tazobactam, or other beta-lactams. **Cautions:** History of atrial fibrillation, electrolyte imbalance–associated arrhythmias, recent *C. difficile* (C-diff) infection or antibiotic-associated colitis, renal/hepatic impairment, seizure disorder; prior hypersensitivity to penicillins, other cephalosporins.

ACTION

Inhibits cell wall synthesis by binding to bacterial cell membrane. Bacterial action of ceftolozane is mediated through binding to essential penicillin-binding proteins. Tazobactam inactivates certain beta-lactamases and binds to certain chromosomal and plasmid-mediated bacterial beta-lactamases. **Therapeutic Effect:** Bactericidal.

PHARMACOKINETICS

Widely distributed. Excreted unchanged as parent drug; not significantly metabolized in liver. Protein binding: 16%–30%. Eliminated in urine (95% unchanged). Removed extensively by hemodialysis. **Half-life:** 2.7 hrs (dependent on dose and severity of renal impairment).

⧗ LIFESPAN CONSIDERATIONS

Pregnancy/Lactation: Unknown if distributed in breast milk. **Children:** Safety and efficacy not established. **Elderly:** May have increased risk of adverse effects (due to renal impairment).

INTERACTIONS

DRUG: None significant. **FOOD:** None known. **LAB VALUES:** May increase serum alkaline phosphatase, ALT, AST, GGT. May decrease Hgb, Hct, platelets; serum potassium, magnesium, phosphate. May result in positive Coombs' test.

AVAILABILITY (Rx)

◄**ALERT**► Ceftolozane/tazobactam is a combination product.

Injection, Powder for Reconstitution: 1 g ceftolozane/0.5 g tazobactam.

ADMINISTRATION/HANDLING
 IV

Reconstitution • Reconstitute vial with 10 mL of Sterile Water for Injection or 0.9% NaCl. • Shake gently until powder is completely dissolved. • Final volume of vial will equal approx. 11.4 mL. • Visually inspect for particulate matter or discoloration. Solution should appear clear, colorless to slightly yellow in color. • Withdraw required volume from reconstituted vial and inject into diluent bag containing 100 mL 0.9% NaCl or 5% dextrose injection as follows:

Ceftolozane/ Tazobactam	Volume to Withdraw from Reconstituted Vial
1.5 g (1 g/0.5 g)	11.4 mL
750 mg (500 mg/250 mg)	5.7 mL
375 mg (250 mg/125 mg)	2.9 mL
150 mg (100 mg/50 mg)	1.2 mL

Rate of Administration • Infuse over 60 min.

Storage • Refrigerate intact vials. • Reconstituted vial may be held for 1 hr prior to transfer to diluent bag. • May refrigerate diluted solution up to 7 days or store at room temperature up to 24 hrs. • Do not freeze.

INDICATIONS/ROUTES/DOSAGE

Complicated Intra-Abdominal Infections
IV: ADULTS, ELDERLY: 1.5 g (ceftolozane 1 g/tazobactam 0.5 g) q8h for 4–14 days (in combination with metroNIDAZOLE).

Complicated Urinary Tract Infections Including Pyelonephritis
IV: ADULTS, ELDERLY: 1.5 g (ceftolozane 1 g/tazobactam 0.5 g) q8h for 7 days.

Dosage in Renal Impairment
CrCl 30–50 mL/min: 750 mg (500 mg/250 mg) q8h. **CrCl 15–29 mL/min:** 375 mg (250 mg/125 mg) q8h.
End-Stage Renal Disease or on Hemodialysis: 750 mg (500 mg/250 mg) loading dose, then 150 mg (100 mg/50 mg) maintenance dose q8h for the remainder of the treatment period.
Note: Administer after hemodialysis on hemodialysis days.

Dosage in Hepatic Impairment
No dose adjustment.

SIDE EFFECTS

Occasional (6%–3%): Nausea, diarrhea, pyrexia, insomnia, headache, vomiting.
Rare (2%–1%): Constipation, anxiety, hypotension, rash, abdominal pain, dizziness, tachycardia, dyspnea, urticaria, gastritis, abdominal distention, dyspepsia, flatulence.

ADVERSE EFFECTS/TOXIC REACTIONS

Clinical cure rates were lower in pts with CrCl 30–50 mL/min compared with those with CrCl greater than 50mL/min, and in pts receiving metroNIDAZOLE combination therapy. Hypersensitivity reactions including anaphylaxis or severe skin reactions have been reported with use of beta-lactam antibacterial drugs. *Clostridium difficile* (C-diff)–associated diarrhea, with severity ranging from mild diarrhea to fatal colitis, was reported. C-diff infection may occur more than 2 mos after treatment completion. May increase risk of development of drug-resistant bacteria when used in the absence of a proven or strongly suspected bacterial infection. Atrial fibrillation reported in 1.2% of pts. Other reported adverse events such as angina pectoris, infections (candidiasis, oropharyngeal infection, fungal urinary tract infection), paralytic ileus, venous thrombosis occur rarely.

NURSING CONSIDERATIONS

BASELINE ASSESSMENT

Obtain baseline CBC, serum BUN, creatinine; CrCl, GFR, LFT; bacterial culture and sensitivity; vital signs. Question history of atrial fibrillation, recent *C. difficile* infection, hepatic/renal impairment, hypersensitivity reaction to beta-lactams, cephalosporins, penicillins, carbapenem. Assess skin for wounds; assess hydration status. Question pt's usual stool characteristics (color, frequency, consistency).

INTERVENTION/EVALUATION

Monitor CBC, BMP, renal function test periodically; serum magnesium, ionized calcium in pts at risk for arrhythmias. For pts with changing renal function, monitor renal function test daily and adjust dose accordingly. Diligently monitor I&Os. Observe daily pattern of bowel activity, stool consistency (increased severity may indicate antibiotic-associated colitis). If frequent diarrhea occurs, obtain *C. difficile* toxin screen and initiate isolation precautions until test result confirmed; manage proper fluids levels/PO intake, electrolyte levels, protein intake. Antibacterial drugs that are not directed against C-diff infection may need to be discontinued. Report any signs of hypersensitivity reaction.

PATIENT/FAMILY TEACHING

• It is essential to complete drug therapy despite symptom improvement. Early discontinuation may result in antibacterial resistance or increased risk of recurrent infection. • Report any episodes of diarrhea, esp. the following mos after treatment completion. Frequent diarrhea, fever, abdominal pain, blood-streaked stool may indicate infectious diarrhea and may be contagious to others. • Report abdominal pain, black/tarry stools, bruising, yellowing of skin or eyes; dark urine, decreased urine output. • Drink plenty of fluids. • Severe allergic reactions such as hives, palpitations, rash, shortness of breath, tongue swelling may occur.

cefTRIAXone

sef-trye-**ax**-own
Do not confuse cefTRIAXone with ceFAZolin, cefOXitin, or ceftazidime.

◆CLASSIFICATION

PHARMACOTHERAPEUTIC: Third-generation cephalosporin. **CLINICAL:** Antibiotic.

USES

Treatment of susceptible infections due to gram-negative aerobic organisms, some gram-positive organisms, including respiratory tract, GU tract, skin and skin structure, bone and joint, intra-abdominal, pelvic inflammatory disease (PID), biliary tract/urinary tract infections; bacterial septicemia, meningitis, perioperative prophylaxis, acute bacterial otitis media. **OFF-LABEL:** Complicated gonococcal infections, STDs, Lyme disease, salmonellosis, shigellosis, atypical community-acquired pneumonia.

◆ Canadian trade name   🦥 Non-Crushable Drug   HIGH ALERT High Alert drug

PRECAUTIONS

Contraindications: History of hypersensitivity/anaphylactic reaction to cefTRIAXone, cephalosporins. Hyperbilirubinemic neonates, esp. premature infants, should not be treated with cefTRIAXone (can displace bilirubin from its binding to serum albumin, causing bilirubin encephalopathy). Do not administer with calcium-containing IV solutions, including continuous calcium-containing infusion such as parenteral nutrition (in neonates) due to the risk of precipitation of cefTRIAXone-calcium salt. **Cautions:** Hepatic impairment, history of GI disease (esp. ulcerative colitis, antibiotic-associated colitis). History of penicillin allergy.

ACTION

Binds to bacterial cell membranes, inhibits cell wall synthesis. **Therapeutic Effect:** Bactericidal.

PHARMACOKINETICS

Widely distributed, including to CSF. Protein binding: 83%–96%. Primarily excreted in urine. Not removed by hemodialysis. **Half-life: IV:** 4.3–4.6 hrs; **IM:** 5.8–8.7 hrs (increased in renal impairment).

⧗ LIFESPAN CONSIDERATIONS

Pregnancy/Lactation: Readily crosses placenta. Distributed in breast milk. **Children:** May displace bilirubin from serum albumin. Contraindicated in hyperbilirubinemic neonates. **Elderly:** Age-related renal impairment may require dosage adjustment.

INTERACTIONS

DRUG: Probenecid may increase excretion. May increase **aminoglycoside (e.g., gentamicin, tobramycin)** concentration. **HERBAL:** None significant. **FOOD:** None known. **LAB VALUES:** May increase serum BUN, alkaline phosphatase, bilirubin, creatinine, LDH, ALT, AST. May cause positive direct/indirect Coombs' test.

AVAILABILITY (Rx)

Injection, Powder for Reconstitution (Rocephin): 250 mg, 500 mg, 1 g, 2 g. **Intravenous Solution (Rocephin):** 1 g/50 mL, 2 g/50 mL.

ADMINISTRATION/HANDLING

 IV

Reconstitution • Add 2.4 mL Sterile Water for Injection to each 250 mg to provide concentration of 100 mg/mL. • May further dilute with 50–100 mL 0.9% NaCl, D_5W.
Rate of Administration • For IV push, administer over 1–4 min (**maximum concentration:** 40 mg/mL). • For intermittent IV infusion (piggyback), infuse over 30 min.
Storage • Solution appears light yellow to amber. • IV infusion (piggyback) is stable for 2 days at room temperature, 10 days if refrigerated. • Discard if precipitate forms.

IM
• Add 0.9 mL Sterile Water for Injection, 0.9% NaCl, D_5W, or lidocaine to each 250 mg to provide concentration of 250 mg/mL. • To minimize discomfort, inject deep IM slowly. Less painful if injected into gluteus maximus than lateral aspect of thigh.

▦ IV INCOMPATIBILITIES

Amphotericin B complex (Abelcet, AmBisome, Amphotec), famotidine (Pepcid), fluconazole (Diflucan), labetalol (Normodyne), vancomycin (Vancocin).

▦ IV COMPATIBILITIES

DiltiaZEM (Cardizem), heparin, lidocaine, metroNIDAZOLE (Flagyl), morphine, propofol (Diprivan).

INDICATIONS/ROUTES/DOSAGE

Usual Dosage Range
IM/IV: ADULTS, ELDERLY: 1–2 g q12–24h. **CHILDREN:** 50–100 mg/kg/day in 1–2 divided doses. **Maximum:** 4 g/day

---

(meningitis), 2 g/day (other). **NEONATES:** 25–50 mg/kg/dose given once daily.

Dosage in Renal/Hepatic Impairment

Dosage modification is usually unnecessary, but hepatic/renal function test results should be monitored in pts with renal and hepatic impairment or severe renal impairment.

SIDE EFFECTS

Frequent: Discomfort with IM administration, oral candidiasis (thrush), mild diarrhea, mild abdominal cramping, vaginal candidiasis. **Occasional:** Nausea, serum sickness–like reaction (fever, joint pain; usually occurs after second course of therapy and resolves after drug is discontinued). **Rare:** Allergic reaction (rash, pruritus, urticaria), thrombophlebitis (pain, redness, swelling at injection site).

ADVERSE EFFECTS/TOXIC REACTIONS

Antibiotic-associated colitis, other superinfections (abdominal cramps, severe watery diarrhea, fever) may result from altered bacterial balance in GI tract. Nephrotoxicity may occur, esp. in pts with preexisting renal disease. Pts with history of penicillin allergy are at increased risk for developing a severe hypersensitivity reaction (severe pruritus, angioedema, bronchospasm, anaphylaxis).

NURSING CONSIDERATIONS

BASELINE ASSESSMENT

Obtain CBC, renal function tests. Question for history of allergies, particularly cephalosporins, penicillins.

INTERVENTION/EVALUATION

Assess oral cavity for white patches on mucous membranes, tongue (thrush). Monitor daily pattern of bowel activity, stool consistency. Mild GI effects may be tolerable (increasing severity may indicate onset of antibiotic-associated colitis). Monitor I&O, renal function tests for nephrotoxicity, CBC. Be alert for superinfection: fever, vomiting, diarrhea, anal/genital pruritus, oral mucosal changes (ulceration, pain, erythema).

PATIENT/FAMILY TEACHING

• Discomfort may occur with IM injection. • Doses should be evenly spaced. • Continue antibiotic therapy for full length of treatment.

---

cefuroxime

sef-ue-**rox**-eem
(Apo-Cefuroxime ✸, Ceftin, Zinacef)
Do not confuse Ceftin with Cefzil or Cipro, cefuroxime with cefotaxime, cefprozil, or deferoxamine, or Zinacef with Zithromax.

◆CLASSIFICATION

PHARMACOTHERAPEUTIC: Second-generation cephalosporin. **CLINICAL:** Antibiotic.

USES

Treatment of susceptible infections due to group B streptococci, pneumococci, staphylococci, *H. influenzae, E. coli, Enterobacter, Klebsiella,* including acute/chronic bronchitis, gonorrhea, impetigo, early Lyme disease, otitis media, pharyngitis/tonsillitis, sinusitis, skin/skin structure, UTI, perioperative prophylaxis.

PRECAUTIONS

Contraindications: History of hypersensitivity/anaphylactic reaction to cefuroxime, cephalosporins. **Cautions:** Severe renal impairment, history of penicillin allergy. Pts with hx of colitis, GI malabsorption, seizures.

ACTION

Binds to bacterial cell membranes, inhibits cell wall synthesis. **Therapeutic Effect:** Bactericidal.

C

PHARMACOKINETICS

Rapidly absorbed from GI tract. Protein binding: 33%–50%. Widely distributed, including to CSF. Primarily excreted unchanged in urine. Moderately removed by hemodialysis. **Half-life:** 1.3 hrs (increased in renal impairment).

⌛ LIFESPAN CONSIDERATIONS

Pregnancy/Lactation: Readily crosses placenta. Distributed in breast milk. **Children:** No age-related precautions noted. **Elderly:** Age-related renal impairment may require dosage adjustment.

INTERACTIONS

DRUG: Probenecid may increase concentration. **Antacids, H$_2$-receptor antagonists (e.g, cimetidine, famotidine)** may decrease absorption. **HERBAL:** None significant. **FOOD:** None known. **LAB VALUES:** May increase serum BUN, creatinine, alkaline phosphatase, bilirubin, LDH, ALT, AST. May cause positive direct/indirect Coombs' test.

AVAILABILITY (Rx)

Injection, Powder for Reconstitution: 750 mg, 1.5 g. **Injection, Solution:** 1.5 g/50 mL. **Oral Suspension (Ceftin):** 125 mg/5 mL, 250 mg/5 mL. **Tablets (Ceftin):** 250 mg, 500 mg.

ADMINISTRATION/HANDLING

 IV

Reconstitution • Reconstitute 750 mg in 8 mL (1.5 g in 14 mL) Sterile Water for Injection to provide a concentration of 100 mg/mL. • For intermittent IV infusion (piggyback), further dilute with 50–100 mL 0.9% NaCl or D$_5$W.
Rate of Administration • For IV push, administer over 3–5 min. • For intermittent IV infusion (piggyback), infuse over 15–30 min.
Storage • Solution appears light yellow to amber (may darken, but color change does not indicate loss of potency). • IV infusion (piggyback) is stable for 24 hrs at

room temperature, 7 days if refrigerated.
• Discard if precipitate forms.

IM
• To minimize discomfort, inject deep IM slowly in large muscle mass.

PO
• Give tablets without regard to food (give 400-mg dose with food). • If GI upset occurs, give with food, milk. • Avoid crushing tablets due to bitter taste. • Suspension must be given with food. • Suspension stable at room temperature or refrigerated for 10 days.

▦ IV INCOMPATIBILITIES

Fluconazole (Diflucan), midazolam (Versed), vancomycin (Vancocin).

▦ IV COMPATIBILITIES

DiltiaZEM (Cardizem), HYDROmorphone (Dilaudid), morphine, propofol (Diprivan).

INDICATIONS/ROUTES/DOSAGE
Usual Dosage
IV, IM: ADULTS, ELDERLY, CHILDREN 12 YRS AND OLDER: 750 mg–1.5 g q8h up to 1.5 g q6h for severe infections. **CHILDREN 3 MOS TO YOUNGER THAN 12 YRS:** 75–150 mg/kg/day divided q8h up to 100–200 mg/kg/day divided in 3–4 doses. **Maximum:** 6 g/day. **NEONATES:** 50 mg/kg/dose q8–12h.
PO: ADULTS, ELDERLY, CHILDREN 12 YRS AND OLDER: 250–500 mg twice a day. **CHILDREN 3 MOS TO YOUNGER THAN 12 YRS:** 20–30 mg/kg/day in 2 divided doses. **Maximum:** 1 g/day.

Dosage in Renal Impairment
Adult dosage frequency is modified based on creatinine clearance and severity of infection.

Creatinine Clearance	Dosage
IV	
Greater than 20 mL/min	q8h
10–20 mL/min	q12h
Less than 10 mL/min	q24h
Peritoneal dialysis	Dose q24h
Continuous renal replacement therapy	1 g q12h

Creatinine Clearance	Dosage
PO	
Greater than 30 mL/min	No adjustment
10–29 mL/min	q24h
Less than 10 mL/min	q48h

Dosage in Hepatic Impairment
No dose adjustment.

SIDE EFFECTS

Frequent: Discomfort with IM adminis-tration, oral candidiasis (thrush), mild diarrhea, mild abdominal cramping, vaginal candidiasis. **Occasional:** Nausea, serum sickness–like reaction (fever, joint pain; usually occurs after second course of therapy and resolves after drug is dis-continued). **Rare:** Allergic reaction (rash, pruritus, urticaria), thrombophlebitis (pain, redness, swelling at injection site).

ADVERSE EFFECTS/TOXIC REACTIONS

Antibiotic-associated colitis, other super-infections (abdominal cramps, severe watery diarrhea, fever) may result from altered bacterial balance in GI tract. Nephrotoxicity may occur, esp. in pts with preexisting renal disease. Pts with history of penicillin allergy are at increased risk for developing a severe hypersensitivity reaction (severe pruritus, angioedema, bronchospasm anaphylaxis).

NURSING CONSIDERATIONS

BASELINE ASSESSMENT

Obtain CBC, renal function tests. Ques-tion for history of allergies, particularly cephalosporins, penicillins.

INTERVENTION/EVALUATION

Assess oral cavity for white patches on mucous membranes, tongue (thrush). Monitor daily pattern of bowel activity, stool consistency. Mild GI effects may be tolerable (increasing severity may indicate onset of antibiotic-associated colitis). Monitor I&O, renal function tests for nephrotoxicity. Be alert for superin-fection: fever, vomiting, diarrhea, anal/genital pruritus, oral mucosal changes (ulceration, pain, erythema).

PATIENT/FAMILY TEACHING

• Discomfort may occur with IM injec-tion. • Doses should be evenly spaced. • Continue antibiotic therapy for full length of treatment. • May cause GI upset (may take with food, milk).

---

celecoxib

TOP 100

sel-e-**kox**-ib
(Apo-Celecoxib ✤, CeleBREX)
■ **BLACK BOX ALERT** ■ Increased risk of serious cardiovascular thrombotic events, including MI, CVA. Increased risk of severe GI reactions, including ulceration, bleeding, perforation of stomach, intestines.
Do not confuse CeleBREX with CeleXA, Cerebyx, or Clarinex.

◆CLASSIFICATION

PHARMACOTHERAPEUTIC: NSAID, COX-2 selective. **CLINICAL:** Anti-inflammatory.

USES

Relief of signs/symptoms of osteoarthri-tis, rheumatoid arthritis (RA) in adults. Treatment of acute pain, primary dys-menorrhea. Relief of signs/symptoms associated with ankylosing spondylitis. Treatment of juvenile rheumatoid arthri-tis (JRA).

PRECAUTIONS

◀**ALERT**▶ May increase cardiovascu-lar risk when high doses are given to prevent colon cancer.
Contraindications: Hypersensitivity to celecoxib, sulfonamides. Active GI bleed-ing. Pts experiencing asthma, urticaria, or allergic reactions to aspirin, other NSAIDs. Treatment of perioperative pain in coronary artery bypass graft (CABG) surgery. **Cautions:** History of GI disease

---

(bleeding/ulcers); concurrent use with aspirin, anticoagulants, smoking; alcohol, elderly, debilitated pts, hypertension, asthma, renal/hepatic impairment. Pts with edema, cerebrovascular disease, ischemic heart disease, HF, known or suspected deficiency of cytochrome P450 isoenzyme 2C9. Pediatric pts with systemic-onset juvenile idiopathic arthritis.

ACTION

Inhibits cyclooxygenase-2, the enzyme responsible for prostaglandin synthesis. **Therapeutic Effect:** Reduces inflammation, relieves pain.

PHARMACOKINETICS

Rapidly absorbed from GI tract. Widely distributed. Protein binding: 97%. Metabolized in liver. Primarily eliminated in feces. **Half-life:** 11.2 hrs.

⧗ LIFESPAN CONSIDERATIONS

Pregnancy/Lactation: Unknown if drug crosses placenta or is distributed in breast milk. Avoid use during third trimester (may adversely affect fetal cardiovascular system: premature closure of ductus arteriosus). **Children:** Safety and efficacy not established in pts younger than 18 yrs. **Elderly:** No age-related precautions noted.

INTERACTIONS

DRUG: May decrease antihypertensive effect of **ACE inhibitors (e.g., enalapril, lisinopril, ramipril), angiotensin II antagonists (e.g., losartan, valsartan). Fluconazole** may significantly increase concentration. May increase **lithium** concentration. **Warfarin** may increase risk of bleeding. **Aspirin** may increase risk of celecoxib-induced GI ulceration, other GI complications. **HERBAL:** Avoid herbs with anticoagulant or antiplatelet activity **(e.g., evening primrose, garlic, ginger, ginseng).** **FOOD:** None known. **LAB VALUES:** May increase serum ALT, AST, alkaline phosphatase, creatinine, BUN. May decrease serum phosphate.

AVAILABILITY (Rx)

🖉 **Capsules:** 50 mg, 100 mg, 200 mg, 400 mg.

ADMINISTRATION/HANDLING

PO
• May give without regard to meals.
• Capsules may be swallowed whole or opened and mixed with applesauce.

INDICATIONS/ROUTES/DOSAGE

Note: Consider reduced initial dose of 50% in poor CYP2C9 metabolizers.

Osteoarthritis
PO: ADULTS, ELDERLY: 200 mg/day as a single dose or 100 mg twice daily.

Rheumatoid Arthritis (RA)
PO: ADULTS, ELDERLY: 100–200 mg twice daily.

Juvenile Rheumatoid Arthritis (JRA)
PO: CHILDREN 2 YRS AND OLDER, WEIGHING MORE THAN 25 KG: 100 mg twice daily. **WEIGHING 10–25 KG:** 50 mg twice daily.

Acute Pain, Primary Dysmenorrhea
PO: ADULTS, ELDERLY: Initially, 400 mg with additional 200 mg on day 1, if needed. **Maintenance:** 200 mg twice daily as needed.

Ankylosing Spondylitis
PO: ADULTS, ELDERLY: 200 mg/day as a single dose or in 2 divided doses. May increase to 400 mg/day if no effect is seen after 6 wks.

Dosage in Renal Impairment
Not recommended in severe renal impairment.

Dosage in Hepatic Impairment
Decrease dose by 50% in pts with moderate hepatic impairment. Not recommended in severe hepatic impairment.

SIDE EFFECTS

Frequent (16%–5%): Diarrhea, dyspepsia, headache, upper respiratory tract infection.

C

Occasional (less than 5%): Abdominal pain, flatulence, nausea, back pain, peripheral edema, dizziness, insomnia, rash.

ADVERSE EFFECTS/TOXIC REACTIONS

Increased risk of cardiovascular events (MI, CVA), serious, potentially life-threatening GI bleeding.

NURSING CONSIDERATIONS

BASELINE ASSESSMENT

Assess onset, type, location, duration of pain/inflammation. Inspect appearance of affected joints for immobility, deformity, skin condition. Assess for allergy to sulfa, aspirin, or NSAIDs (contraindicated).

INTERVENTION/EVALUATION

Assess for therapeutic response: pain relief; decreased stiffness, swelling; increased joint mobility; reduced joint tenderness; improved grip strength. Observe for bleeding, bruising, weight gain.

PATIENT/FAMILY TEACHING

• If GI upset occurs, take with food. • Avoid aspirin, alcohol (increases risk of GI bleeding). • Immediately report chest pain, jaw pain, sweating, confusion, difficulty speaking, one-sided weakness (may indicate heart attack or stroke).

cephalexin

sef-a-**lex**-in
(Apo-Cephalex ✤, Keflex)
Do not confuse cephalexin with cefaclor, ceFAZolin, or ciprofloxacin.

◆CLASSIFICATION

PHARMACOTHERAPEUTIC: First-generation cephalosporin. **CLINICAL:** Antibiotic.

USES

Treatment of susceptible infections due to staphylococci, group A *streptococcus, K. pneumoniae, E. coli, P. mirabilis, H. influenzae, M. catarrhalis,* including respiratory tract, genitourinary tract, skin, soft tissue, bone infections; otitis media; rheumatic fever prophylaxis; follow-up to parenteral therapy. **OFF-LABEL:** Suppression of prosthetic joint infection.

PRECAUTIONS

Contraindications: History of hypersensitivity/anaphylactic reaction to cephalexin, cephalosporins. **Cautions:** Renal impairment, history of GI disease (esp. ulcerative colitis, antibiotic-associated colitis), history of penicillin allergy.

ACTION

Binds to bacterial cell membranes, inhibits cell wall synthesis. **Therapeutic Effect:** Bactericidal.

PHARMACOKINETICS

Rapidly absorbed from GI tract (delayed in young children). Protein binding: 10%–15%. Widely distributed. Primarily excreted unchanged in urine. Moderately removed by hemodialysis. **Half-life:** 0.9–1.2 hrs (increased in renal impairment).

⌛ LIFESPAN CONSIDERATIONS

Pregnancy/Lactation: Readily crosses placenta. Distributed in breast milk. **Children:** No age-related precautions noted. **Elderly:** Age-related renal impairment may require dosage adjustment.

INTERACTIONS

DRUG: Probenecid may increase concentration. **HERBAL:** None significant. **FOOD:** None known. **LAB VALUES:** May increase serum BUN, creatinine, alkaline phosphatase, bilirubin, LDH, ALT, AST. May cause positive direct/indirect Coombs' test.

✤ Canadian trade name   🐢 Non-Crushable Drug   🔲 High Alert drug

C

AVAILABILITY (Rx)

🦋 **Capsules:** 250 mg, 500 mg, 750 mg. **Powder for Oral Suspension:** 125 mg/5 mL, 250 mg/5 mL. **Tablets:** 250 mg, 500 mg.

ADMINISTRATION/HANDLING

PO

• After reconstitution, oral suspension is stable for 14 days if refrigerated. • Shake oral suspension well before using. • Give without regard to food. If GI upset occurs, give with food, milk.

INDICATIONS/ROUTES/DOSAGE

Usual Dosage Range

PO: ADULTS, ELDERLY: 250–1,000 mg q6h or 500 mg q12h. **Maximum:** 4 g/day. **CHILDREN 1 YR AND OLDER:** 25–100 mg/kg/day in 3–4 divided doses. **Maximum:** 4 g/day.

Dosage in Renal Impairment

After usual initial dose, dosing frequency is modified based on creatinine clearance and severity of infection.

Creatinine Clearance	Dosage
60 mL/min or greater	No adjustment
30–59 mL/min	Maximum: 1,000 mg/day
15–29 mL/min	250 mg q8-12h
5–14 mL/min	250 mg q24h
1–4 mL/min	250 mg q48-60h
Hemodialysis	250–500 mg q12–24h (administer after dialysis session)

Dosage in Hepatic Impairment

No dose adjustment.

SIDE EFFECTS

Frequent: Oral candidiasis, mild diarrhea, mild abdominal cramping, vaginal candidiasis. **Occasional:** Nausea, serum sickness–like reaction (fever, joint pain; usually occurs after second course of therapy and resolves after drug is discontinued). **Rare:** Allergic reaction (rash, pruritus, urticaria).

ADVERSE EFFECTS/TOXIC REACTIONS

Antibiotic-associated colitis, other super-infections (abdominal cramps, severe watery diarrhea, fever) may result from altered bacterial balance in GI tract. Nephrotoxicity may occur, esp. in pts with preexisting renal disease. Pts with history of penicillin allergy are at increased risk for developing a severe hypersensitivity reaction (severe pruritus, angioedema, bronchospasm, anaphylaxis).

NURSING CONSIDERATIONS

BASELINE ASSESSMENT

Obtain CBC, renal function tests. Question for history of allergies, particularly cephalosporins, penicillins.

INTERVENTION/EVALUATION

Assess oral cavity for white patches on mucous membranes, tongue (thrush). Monitor daily pattern of bowel activity, stool consistency. Mild GI effects may be tolerable (increasing severity may indicate onset of antibiotic-associated colitis). Monitor I&O, renal function tests for nephrotoxicity. Be alert for superinfection: fever, vomiting, diarrhea, anal/genital pruritus, oral mucosal changes (ulceration, pain, erythema). With prolonged therapy, monitor renal/hepatic function tests.

PATIENT/FAMILY TEACHING

• Doses should be evenly spaced. • Continue therapy for full length of treatment. • May cause GI upset (may take with food, milk). • Refrigerate oral suspension. • Report persistent diarrhea.

ceritinib

se-**ri**-ti-nib
(Zykadia)
Do not confuse ceritinib with crizotinib, gefitinib, imatinib, or lapatinib.

◆CLASSIFICATION

PHARMACOTHERAPEUTIC: Kinase inhibitor. **CLINICAL:** Antineoplastic.

USES

Treatment of pts with anaplastic lymphoma kinase (ALK)–positive metastatic non–small-cell lung cancer (NSCLC).

PRECAUTIONS

Contraindications: Hypersensitivity to ceritinib. **Cautions:** Bradyarrhythmias/ventricular arrhythmias, diabetes, dehydration, electrolyte imbalance (e.g., hypomagnesemia, hypokalemia), hepatic impairment, HF, ocular disease, pulmonary disease. Medications that prolong QT interval. Not recommended in pts with congenital long QT syndrome. Avoid use of medications that cause bradycardia.

ACTION

Inhibits tyrosine kinase activity and tumor cell proliferation. Inhibits autophosphorylation of ALK and ALK-dependent signaling proteins. **Therapeutic Effect:** Inhibits lung cancer growth and metastasis.

PHARMACOKINETICS

Well absorbed after PO administration. Metabolized in liver. Peak plasma concentration: 4–6 hrs. Protein binding: 97%. Eliminated in feces (92%), urine (1.3%). **Half-life:** 41 hrs.

⌛ LIFESPAN CONSIDERATIONS

Pregnancy/Lactation: Avoid pregnancy; may cause fetal harm. Do not initiate therapy until pregnancy status confirmed. Contraception recommended during treatment and for at least 2 wks after discontinuation. Unknown if distributed in breast milk. Must either discontinue drug or discontinue breastfeeding. **Children:** Safety and efficacy not established. **Elderly:** No age-related precautions noted.

INTERACTIONS

DRUG: Strong CYP3A inhibitors (e.g., ketoconazole, ritonavir) may increase concentration/effect; avoid use. **Strong CYP3A inducers (e.g., carBA-Mazepine, phenytoin, rifAMPin)** may decrease concentration/effect; avoid use. **HERBAL: St. John's wort** may decrease effectiveness. **FOOD: All food** may increase absorption/effect. **Grapefruit products** may increase concentration/effect; avoid use. **LAB VALUES:** May decrease Hgb, phosphate. May increase serum ALT, AST, bilirubin, creatinine, glucose, lipase.

AVAILABILITY (Rx)

 Capsules: 150 mg.

ADMINISTRATION/HANDLING

PO

• Give on empty stomach only. Do not administer within 2 hrs of meal. • Administer whole; do not break, cut, or open. • If a dose is missed, take dose unless next dose due within 12 hrs. If vomiting occurs, do not administer an additional dose.

INDICATIONS/ROUTES/DOSAGE

Non–Small-Cell Lung Cancer
PO: ADULTS/ELDERLY: 750 mg once daily until disease progression or unacceptable toxicity.

Dosage in Renal Impairment
Mild to moderate impairment (CrCl 30-90 mL/min): No dose adjustment. **Severe impairment:** Not specified; use caution.

Dosage in Hepatic Impairment
Mild to Moderate impairment: No dose adjustment. **Severe impairment:** Decrease dose by 1/3 (round to nearest 150 mg).

Dosage Modification
Cardiac
QTc interval greater than 500 msec on at least 2 separate EKGs: Withhold until QTc interval is less than 481 msec, or recovery to baseline (if baseline QTc interval is greater than or equal to 481 msec), then resume with a 150-mg dose reduction.

QTc prolongation in combination with torsades de pointes or polymorphic ventricular tachycardia or serious arrhythmia: Permanently discontinue.

Severe or intolerable diarrhea, nausea, vomiting despite optimal antiemetic or antidiarrheal therapy: Withhold until improved, then resume with a 150-mg dose reduction.

Symptomatic, non–life-threatening bradycardia: Withhold until recovery to asymptomatic bradycardia or heart rate of 60 beats/min or greater. Evaluate concomitant medications known to cause bradycardia and adjust dose as tolerated (reduction not specified).

Clinically significant, life-threatening bradycardia requiring intervention or life-threatening bradycardia in pts taking concomitant medications known to cause bradycardia or hypotension: Withhold until recovery to asymptomatic bradycardia or heart rate of 60 beats/min or greater. If concomitant medication can be adjusted or discontinued, then resume with a 150-mg dose reduction.

Life-threatening bradycardia in pts who are not taking concomitant medications known to cause bradycardia or hypotension: Permanently discontinue.

Concomitant use of strong CYP3A inhibitors: If concomitant use unavoidable, reduce ceritinib dose by one third, rounded to the nearest 150-mg dose strength. After discontinuation of a strong CYP3A inhibitor, resume ceritinib dose that was taken prior to initiating strong CYP3A inhibitor.

Endocrine
Persistent hyperglycemia greater than 250 mL/dL despite optimal antihyperglycemic therapy: Withhold until hyperglycemia is adequately controlled, then resume with a 150-mg dose reduction. If adequate control cannot be achieved with optimal medical management, then permanently discontinue.

Hepatic (During Treatment)
ALT, AST greater than 5 times upper limit of normal (ULN) with total

bilirubin elevation less than or equal to 2 times ULN: Withhold until recovery to baseline or less than or equal to 2 times ULN, then resume with a 150-mg dose reduction.
ALT, AST greater than 3 times ULN with total bilirubin elevation greater than or equal to 2 times ULN in the absence of cholestasis or hemolysis: Permanently discontinue.

Pulmonary
Any grade treatment related to interstitial lung disease/pneumonitis: Permanently discontinue.

Intolerability/Toxicity
If unable to tolerate 300-mg dose: Permanently discontinue.

SIDE EFFECTS

Frequent (86%–52%): Diarrhea, nausea, vomiting, abdominal pain, fatigue, asthenia.
Occasional (34%–9%): Decreased appetite, constipation, paresthesia, muscular weakness, gait disturbance, peripheral motor/sensory neuropathy, hypotonia, polyneuropathy, dyspepsia, gastric reflux disease, dysphagia, rash, maculopapular rash, acneiform dermatitis, vision impairment, blurred vision, photopsia, presbyopia, reduced visual acuity.

ADVERSE EFFECTS/TOXIC REACTIONS

Approximately 60% of pts required at least one dose reduction. Median time to first dose reduction was approximately 7 wks. Decreased Hgb levels reported in 84% of pts. Severe or persistent GI toxicity including nausea, vomiting, diarrhea occurred in 96% of pts; severe cases reported in 14% of pts. Drug-induced hepatotoxicity with elevation of serum ALT 5 times ULN occurred in 27% of pts. Bradycardia, severe interstitial lung disease (ILD), QT interval prolongation, ILD reported in 3% of pts. Grade 3–4 hyperglycemia reported in 13% of pts; diabetics have a sixfold increase in risk; pts receiving corticosteroids have twofold increase in risk. Fatal adverse reactions including pneumonia, respiratory failure, ILD/pneumonitis, pneumothorax, gastric hemorrhage, general physical health deterioration, tuberculosis, cardiac tamponade, sepsis occurred in 5% of pts.

NURSING CONSIDERATIONS

BASELINE ASSESSMENT

Obtain baseline CBC, BMP, LFT; serum ionized calcium, magnesium, phosphate; capillary blood glucose, O_2 saturation, urine pregnancy, vital signs. Obtain baseline EKG in pts with history of arrhythmias, HF, electrolyte imbalance, or concurrent use of medications known to prolong QTc interval. Question possibility of pregnancy or plans of breastfeeding. Assess hydration status. Screen for history/co-morbidities. Receive full medication history including herbal products; esp. CYP3A inhibitors or inducers, medications that prolong QT interval. Assess visual acuity. Verify ALK-positive NSCLC test prior to initiation.

INTERVENTION/EVALUATION

Monitor CBC routinely; LFT monthly (or more frequently in pts with elevated hepatic enzymes). Obtain BMP, serum ionized calcium, magnesium if arrhythmia or dehydration occurs. Monitor vital signs (esp. heart rate). Obtain EKG for bradycardia, chest pain, dyspnea; chest X-ray if ILD, pneumonitis, pneumothorax suspected. Worsening cough, fever, or shortness of breath may indicate pneumonitis. Monitor for hepatic dysfunction, hyperglycemia, sepsis, vision changes. Assess hydration status. Encourage PO intake. Offer antidiarrheal medication for loose stool, antiemetic for nausea, vomiting.

PATIENT/FAMILY TEACHING

• Blood levels, EKGs will be monitored routinely. • Most pts experience diarrhea, nausea, vomiting, which may lead to dehydration; drink plenty of fluids. • Report history of heart problems, including extremity swelling, HF, congenital long QT syndrome, palpitations, syncope. Therapy may decrease your heart rate; report dizziness, chest pain, palpitations, or fainting. • Worsening cough, fever, or shortness of breath may indicate severe lung inflammation. • Avoid pregnancy; contraception recommended during treatment and up to 2 wks after final dose. Do not breastfeed. • Blurry vision, confusion, frequent urination, increased thirst, fruity breath may indicate high blood sugar levels. • Report any yellowing of skin or eyes, upper abdominal pain, bruising, black/tarry stools, dark urine. • Immediately report any newly prescribed medications. • Take on empty stomach only; do not eat 2 hrs before or 2 hrs after any dose. • Avoid alcohol. Do not consume grapefruit products.

certolizumab pegol

ser-toe-**liz**-ue-mab
(Cimzia)

■ **BLACK BOX ALERT** ■ Serious, sometimes fatal cases of tuberculosis, invasive fungal infections, or other opportunistic infections, including viral and bacterial infection, have been reported. Lymphoma reported in children/adolescents receiving other TNF-blocking medications.

◆CLASSIFICATION

PHARMACOTHERAPEUTIC: Tumor necrosis factor (TNF) blocker. **CLINICAL:** Anti-inflammatory agent.

USES

Treatment of moderate to severe active rheumatoid arthritis, moderate to severe active Crohn's disease, active ankylosing spondylitis, active psoriatic arthritis.

PRECAUTIONS

Contraindications: Hypersensitivity to certolizumab. **Cautions:** Chronic, latent, or localized infection; preexisting or recent-onset CNS demyelinating disorders, moderate to severe HF, underlying hematologic disorders, elderly. Pts who have resided in regions where TB is endemic, pts who are hepatitis B virus carriers. Use of live vaccines.

ACTION

Binds specifically to TNF-alpha cell, a protein in the immune system that causes inflammation. **Therapeutic Effect:** Reduces signs and symptoms of Crohn's disease and joint destruction associated with rheumatoid arthritis.

PHARMACOKINETICS

Higher clearance with increasing body weight. Peak plasma concentrations: 54–171 hrs. **Half-life:** 14 days.

⧖ LIFESPAN CONSIDERATIONS

Pregnancy/Lactation: Unknown if distributed in breast milk. **Children:** Safety and efficacy not established. **Elderly:** Use cautiously due to higher rate of infection.

INTERACTIONS

DRUG: Anakinra, other TNF antagonists (e.g., adalimumab, etanercept, inFLIXimab) may increase risk of infection. **Live virus vaccines** may decrease immune response. **HERBAL: Echinacea** may decrease effect. **FOOD:** None known. **LAB VALUES:** May increase serum alkaline phosphatase, ALT, AST, bilirubin; aPTT.

AVAILABILITY (Rx)

Injection, Powder for Reconstitution: 200 mg. **Injection, Solution:** 200 mg/mL in a single-use prefilled syringe.

ADMINISTRATION/HANDLING

Subcutaneous
Reconstitution • Bring to room temperature before reconstitution. • Reconstitute with 1 mL Sterile Water for Injection. • Gently swirl without shaking, using syringe with 20-gauge needle. • Leave undisturbed to fully reconstitute (may take as long as 30 min). • Using a new 20-gauge needle, withdraw reconstituted solution into syringe

for final concentration of 1 mL (200 mg). Use separate syringes for multiple vials. • Switch each 20-gauge needle to a 23-gauge needle and inject full contents of each syringe subcutaneously into separate sites on the abdomen or thigh.

Storage • Store vial in refrigerator. • Once powder reconstituted, solution should appear clear to opalescent, colorless to pale yellow. • Discard if solution is discolored or contains precipitate. • Reconstituted solution is stable for up to 2 hrs at room temperature or 24 hrs if refrigerated.

INDICATIONS/ROUTES/DOSAGE

Note: Each 400-mg dose is given as two injections of 200 mg each.

Crohn's Disease
Subcutaneous: Initially, 400 mg (given as two subcutaneous injections of 200 mg) and at weeks 2 and 4. **Maintenance:** In pts who obtain a therapeutic response, 400 mg q4wks.

Rheumatoid Arthritis, Ankylosing Spondylitis, Psoriatic Arthritis
Subcutaneous: ADULTS, ELDERLY: Initially, 400 mg and at weeks 2 and 4. **Maintenance:** 200 mg q2wks or 400 mg q4wks.

Dosage Modification
Discontinue for hypersensitivity reaction, lupus-like syndrome, serious infection, sepsis, hepatitis B virus reactivation.

Dosage in Renal/Hepatic Impairment
No dose adjustment.

SIDE EFFECTS

Occasional (6%): Arthralgia. **Rare (less than 1%):** Abdominal pain, diarrhea.

ADVERSE EFFECTS/TOXIC REACTIONS

Upper respiratory tract infection occurs in 20% of pts. UTI occurs in 7% of pts. Serious infections such as pneumonia, pyelonephritis occur in 3% of pts.

Hypersensitivity reaction (rash, urticaria, hypotension, dyspnea) occurs rarely. May increase risk of malignancies (e.g., lymphoma).

NURSING CONSIDERATIONS

BASELINE ASSESSMENT

Obtain baseline CBC, urinalysis, C-reactive protein. Do not initiate treatment in pts with active infections, including chronic or localized infection. TB test should be obtained before initiation.

INTERVENTION/EVALUATION

Monitor pts for infection during and after treatment. If pt develops an infection, treatment should be discontinued. Monitor lab results, especially WBC count, urinalysis, C-reactive protein for evidence of infection.

PATIENT/FAMILY TEACHING

• Report cough, fever, flu-like symptoms.
• Do not receive live virus vaccine during treatment or within 3 mos after last dose.

---

cetirizine

se-**teer**-i-zeen
(Apo-Cetirizine ✦, Reactine ✦, ZyrTEC)
Do not confuse cetirizine with levocetirizine, or ZyrTEC with Xanax, Zantac, Zocor, or ZyPREXA.

FIXED-COMBINATION(S)

ZyrTEC D 12 Hour Tablets: cetirizine/pseudoephedrine: 5 mg/120 mg.

◆CLASSIFICATION

PHARMACOTHERAPEUTIC: Second-generation piperazine. **CLINICAL:** Antihistamine.

USES

Relief of symptoms (sneezing, rhinorrhea, postnasal discharge, nasal pruritus, ocular pruritus, tearing) of upper respiratory allergies; relieves itching due to urticaria.

PRECAUTIONS

Contraindications: Hypersensitivity to cetirizine, hydrOXYzine. **Cautions:** Elderly, hepatic/renal impairment.

ACTION

Competes with histamine for H₁-receptor sites on effector cells in GI tract, blood vessels, respiratory tract. **Therapeutic Effect:** Prevents allergic response, produces mild bronchodilation, blocks histamine-induced bronchitis.

PHARMACOKINETICS

Route	Onset	Peak	Duration
PO	Less than 1 hr	4–8 hrs	Less than 24 hrs

Well absorbed from GI tract. Protein binding: 93%. Undergoes low first-pass metabolism; not extensively metabolized. Primarily excreted in urine. **Half-life:** 6.5–10 hrs.

⚖ LIFESPAN CONSIDERATIONS

Pregnancy/Lactation: Not recommended during first trimester of pregnancy. Distributed in breast milk. Breastfeeding not recommended. **Children:** Less likely to cause anticholinergic effects. **Elderly:** More sensitive to anticholinergic effects (e.g., dry mouth, urinary retention). Dizziness, sedation, confusion may occur.

INTERACTIONS

DRUG: Alcohol, other CNS depressants may increase CNS depression. **Anticholinergics (e.g., glycopyrrolate, hyoscyamine, oxybutynin)** may increase anticholinergic effects. **HERBAL:** None significant. **FOOD:** None known. **LAB VALUES:** May suppress wheal and flare reactions to antigen skin testing unless drug is discontinued 4 days before testing.

AVAILABILITY (Rx)

🖊 **Capsule:** 10 mg. **Oral solution:** 5 mg/5 mL. **Syrup:** 5 mg/5 mL. **Tablets:** 5 mg, 10 mg. **Tablets (Chewable):** 5 mg, 10 mg. **Tablet (Dispersible):** 10 mg.

ADMINISTRATION/HANDLING

PO
• Give without regard to food.

INDICATIONS/ROUTES/DOSAGE

◄**ALERT**► May cause drowsiness at dosage greater than 10 mg/day.

Upper Respiratory Allergies, Urticaria
PO: ADULTS, CHILDREN OLDER THAN 5 YRS: Initially, 5–10 mg/day as single dose. **ELDERLY:** 5 mg once/day. **Maximum:** 5 mg/day. **CHILDREN 2–5 YRS:** 2.5 mg/day. May increase up to 5 mg/day as a single dose or in 2 divided doses. **CHILDREN 12–23 MOS:** Initially, 2.5 mg/day. May increase up to 5 mg/day in 2 divided doses. **CHILDREN 6–11 MOS:** 2.5 mg once daily.

Dosage in Renal Impairment
Adult: GFR 50 mL/min or less: 5 mg once daily. **Children: GFR 10–29 mL/min:** reduce dose by 50 %. **GFR <10 mL/min:** Not recommended.

Dosage in Hepatic Impairment
No dose adjustment.

SIDE EFFECTS

Occasional (10%–2%): Pharyngitis, dry mucous membranes, nausea, vomiting, abdominal pain, headache, dizziness, fatigue, thickening of mucus, drowsiness, photosensitivity, urinary retention.

ADVERSE EFFECTS/TOXIC REACTIONS

Children may experience paradoxical reaction (restlessness, insomnia, euphoria, nervousness, tremor). Dizziness, sedation, confusion more likely to occur in elderly.

NURSING CONSIDERATIONS

BASELINE ASSESSMENT
Assess lung sounds. Assess severity of rhinitis, urticaria, other symptoms.

INTERVENTION/EVALUATION
For upper respiratory allergies, increase fluids to maintain thin secretions and offset thirst. Monitor symptoms for therapeutic response.

PATIENT/FAMILY TEACHING
• Avoid tasks that require alertness, motor skills until response to drug is established. • Avoid alcohol.

---

cetuximab

se-**tux**-i-mab
(Erbitux)

■ **BLACK BOX ALERT** ■ Severe infusion reactions (bronchospasm, stridor, urticaria, hypotension, cardiac arrest) have occurred, especially with first infusion in pts with head and neck cancer. Cardiopulmonary arrest reported in pts receiving radiation in combination with cetuximab. **Do not confuse cetuximab with bevacizumab.**

◆CLASSIFICATION

PHARMACOTHERAPEUTIC: Monoclonal antibody. **CLINICAL:** Antineoplastic, epidermal growth factor receptor (EGFR) inhibitor.

USES

As a single agent or in combination with irinotecan for treatment of KRAS wild type, EGFR-expressing, metastatic colorectal carcinoma in pts who are refractory or intolerant to irinotecan-based chemotherapy. Treatment of advanced squamous cell cancer of head/neck (with radiation). Treatment of recurrent or metastasized squamous cell carcinoma of head/neck progressing after platinum-based therapy. First-line treatment of squamous cell

---

carcinoma of head and neck in combination with platinum-based therapy with 5-FU. **OFF-LABEL:** EGFR-expressing advanced non–small-cell lung cancer (NSCLC). Treatment of unresectable squamous cell skin cancer.

PRECAUTIONS

Contraindications: Hypersensitivity to cetuximab. **Cautions:** Preexisting IgE antibodies to cetuximab, coronary artery disease, HF, arrhythmias, pulmonary disease.

ACTION

Binds to the epidermal growth factor receptor (EGFR), a glycoprotein on normal and tumor cells. **Therapeutic Effect:** Inhibits tumor cell growth, inducing apoptosis (cell death).

PHARMACOKINETICS

Reaches steady-state levels by the third wkly infusion. Clearance decreases as dose increases. **Half-life:** 114 hrs (range: 75–188 hrs).

LIFESPAN CONSIDERATIONS

Pregnancy/Lactation: Crosses placental barrier; may cause fetal harm; abortifacient. Breastfeeding not recommended. **Children:** Safety and efficacy not established. **Elderly:** No age-related precautions noted.

INTERACTIONS

DRUG: None significant. **HERBAL:** None significant. **FOOD:** None known. **LAB VALUES:** May decrease WBCs; serum calcium, magnesium, potassium.

AVAILABILITY (RX)

Injection Solution: 2 mg/mL (50 mL, 100 mL).

ADMINISTRATION/HANDLING

IV

◄ALERT► Do not give by IV push or bolus.

Reconstitution • Does not require reconstitution. • Solution should appear clear, colorless; may contain a small amount of visible, white particulates. • Do not shake or dilute. • Infuse with a low protein-binding 0.22-micron inline filter.

Rate of Administration • First dose should be given as a 120-min infusion. • Maintenance infusion should be infused over 60 min. • Maximum infusion rate should not exceed 5 mL/min.

Storage • Refrigerate vials. • Infusion containers are stable for up to 12 hrs if refrigerated, up to 8 hrs at room temperature. • Discard unused portions.

IV COMPATIBILITY

Irinotecan (Camptosar).

INDICATIONS/ROUTES/DOSAGE

Head/Neck Cancer, Metastatic Colorectal Carcinoma

IV: ADULTS, ELDERLY: Initially, 400 mg/m^2 as a loading dose. **Maintenance:** 250 mg/m^2 infused over 60 min wkly.

Dosage in Renal/Hepatic Impairment
No dose adjustment.

SIDE EFFECTS

Frequent (90%–25%): Acneiform rash, malaise, fever, nausea, diarrhea, constipation, headache, abdominal pain, anorexia, vomiting. **Occasional (16%–10%):** Nail disorder, back pain, stomatitis, peripheral edema, pruritus, cough, insomnia. **Rare (9%–5%):** Weight loss, depression, dyspepsia, conjunctivitis, alopecia.

ADVERSE EFFECTS/TOXIC REACTIONS

Anemia occurs in 10% of pts. Severe infusion reaction (rapid onset of airway obstruction, hypotension, severe urticaria) occurs rarely. Dermatologic toxicity, pulmonary embolus, leukopenia, renal failure occur rarely.

C

NURSING CONSIDERATIONS

BASELINE ASSESSMENT

Monitor Hgb, Hct, serum potassium, magnesium. Assess for evidence of anemia. Question possibility of pregnancy. Question history of hypersensitivity reaction.

INTERVENTION/EVALUATION

Monitor for evidence of infusion reaction (rapid onset of bronchospasm, stridor, hoarseness, urticaria, hypotension) during infusion and for at least 1 hr postinfusion. Pts may experience first severe infusion reaction during later infusions. Assess skin for evidence of dermatologic toxicity (development of inflammatory sequelae, dry skin, exfoliative dermatitis, rash). Monitor CBC, serum electrolytes, acute onset or worsening pulmonary symptoms.

PATIENT/FAMILY TEACHING

• Do not have immunizations without physician's approval (drug lowers resistance). • Avoid contact with anyone who recently received a live virus vaccine. • Avoid crowds, those with infection. • Wear sunscreen, limit sun exposure (sunlight can exacerbate skin reactions). • Avoid pregnancy. • Report cardiac or lung symptoms, severe rash.

---

chlorambucil **HIGH ALERT**

klor-**am**-bue-sil
(Leukeran)

■ **BLACK BOX ALERT** ■ May cause myelosuppression. Affects fertility; potential for carcinogenic, mutagenic, teratogenic effects. May cause azoospermia.
Do not confuse Leukeran with Alkeran, Leukine, or Myleran.

◆CLASSIFICATION

PHARMACOTHERAPEUTIC: Alkylating agent, nitrogen mustard. **CLINICAL:** Antineoplastic.

USES

Treatment of chronic lymphocytic leukemia (CLL), Hodgkin's and non-Hodgkin's lymphomas (NHL). **OFF-LABEL:** Nephrotic syndrome in children, Waldenström's macroglobulinemia.

PRECAUTIONS

Contraindications: Hypersensitivity to chlorambucil. Previous allergic reaction to other alkylating agents, prior resistance to chlorambucil, pregnancy. **Extreme Cautions:** Treatment within 4 wks after full-course radiation therapy or myelosuppressive drug regimen. **Cautions:** History of bone marrow suppression, head trauma, hepatic impairment, nephrotic syndrome, seizure disorder; administration of live vaccines to immunocompromised pts.

ACTION

Inhibits DNA, RNA synthesis by cross-linking with DNA, RNA strands. **Therapeutic Effect:** Interferes with DNA replication and RNA transcription.

PHARMACOKINETICS

Rapidly, completely absorbed from GI tract. Protein binding: 99%. Metabolized in liver to active metabolite. Not removed by hemodialysis. **Half-life:** 1.5 hrs; metabolite, 2.5 hrs.

LIFESPAN CONSIDERATIONS

Pregnancy/Lactation: If possible, avoid use during pregnancy, esp. first trimester. Breastfeeding not recommended. **Children:** No age-related precautions noted. When taken for nephrotic syndrome, may increase risk of seizures. **Elderly:** No age-related precautions noted.

INTERACTIONS

DRUG: Bone marrow depressants may increase myelosuppression. **Other immunosuppressants (e.g., steroids)** may increase risk of infection or development of neoplasms. **Live virus vaccines** may potentiate virus replication, decrease antibody response to vaccine. **HERBAL: Echinacea** may decrease effects. **FOOD: Acidic foods, spicy foods** may delay absorption. **LAB VALUES:** May increase serum alkaline phosphatase, AST, uric acid.

AVAILABILITY (Rx)

Tablets: 2 mg.

ADMINISTRATION/HANDLING

PO

• Give 30–60 min before food.

INDICATIONS/ROUTES/DOSAGE

Chronic Lymphocytic Leukemia (CLL)
PO: ADULTS, ELDERLY: 0.1 mg/kg/day for 3–6 wks or 0.4 mg/kg pulsed doses administered intermittently, biweekly or monthly (increased by 0.1 mg/kg/dose until response/toxicity observed).

Hodgkin's Lymphoma (HL)
PO: ADULTS, ELDERLY: 0.2 mg/kg/day for 3–6 wks.

Non-Hodgkin's Lymphoma (NHL)
PO: ADULTS, ELDERLY: 0.1 mg/kg/day for 3–6 wks.

Dosage in Renal Impairment
CrCl 10–50 mL/min: 75% of dose. **CrCl less than 10 mL/min:** 50% of dose.

Dosage in Hepatic Impairment
Use caution.

SIDE EFFECTS

Expected: GI effects (nausea, vomiting, anorexia, diarrhea, abdominal distress), generally mild, last less than 24 hrs, occur only if single dose exceeds 20 mg. **Occasional:** Rash, dermatitis, pruritus, oral ulcerations. **Rare:** Alopecia, urticaria, erythema, hyperuricemia.

ADVERSE EFFECTS/TOXIC REACTIONS

Hematologic toxicity due to severe myelosuppression occurs frequently, manifested as neutropenia, anemia, thrombocytopenia. After discontinuation of therapy, thrombocytopenia, neutropenia usually last for 1–2 wks, but may persist for 3–4 wks. Neutrophil count may continue to decrease for up to 10 days after last dose. Toxicity appears to be less severe with intermittent drug administration. Overdosage may produce seizures in children. Excessive serum uric acid level, hepatotoxicity occur rarely.

NURSING CONSIDERATIONS

BASELINE ASSESSMENT

Obtain CBC before therapy and wkly during therapy, WBC count 3–4 days following each wkly, CBC during first 3–6 wks of therapy (4–6 wks if pt on intermittent dosing schedule).

INTERVENTION/EVALUATION

Monitor CBC, serum uric acid, LFT. Monitor for hematologic toxicity (fever, sore throat, signs of local infection, unusual bruising/bleeding from any site), symptoms of anemia (excessive fatigue, weakness). Assess skin for rash, pruritus, urticaria.

PATIENT/FAMILY TEACHING

• Increase fluid intake (may protect against hyperuricemia). • Avoid acidic or spicy foods; may delay absorption of medication. • Do not have immunizations without physician's approval (drug lowers resistance). • Avoid contact with those who have recently received live virus vaccine. • Promptly report fever, sore throat, signs of local infection, unusual bruising/bleeding from any site, nausea, vomiting, rash.

---

cilostazol

sil-**o**-sta-zol
(Pletal)
■ **BLACK BOX ALERT** ■ Contraindicated in pts with HF of any severity, active bleeding.
Do not confuse Pletal with Plendil.

◆ CLASSIFICATION

PHARMACOTHERAPEUTIC: Phosphodiesterase enzyme inhibitor. **CLINICAL:** Antiplatelet.

USES

Reduces symptoms of intermittent claudication (increases walking distance).

PRECAUTIONS

Contraindications: Hypersensitivity to cilostazol. HF of any severity. **Cautions:** Hemostatic disorders or active bleeding (bleeding peptic ulcer, intracranial bleeding). Severe underlying heart disease, thrombocytopenia, pts receiving other platelet aggregation inhibitors, moderate to severe hepatic impairment, severe renal impairment.

ACTION

Inhibits phosphodiesterase, increasing cAMP, leading to inhibition of platelet aggregation. **Therapeutic Effect:** Improves walking distance in pts with intermittent claudication.

PHARMACOKINETICS

Moderately absorbed from GI tract. Protein binding: 95%–98%. Metabolized in liver. Excreted in urine (74%), feces (20%). Not removed by hemodialysis. **Half-life:** 11–13 hrs.

⌧ LIFESPAN CONSIDERATIONS

Pregnancy/Lactation: Unknown if drug crosses placenta or is distributed in breast milk. **Children:** Safety and efficacy not established. **Elderly:** No age-related precautions noted.

INTERACTIONS

DRUG: **Aspirin** may potentiate inhibition of platelet aggregation. **CYP3A4 inhibitors** (e.g., **clarithromycin, diltiaZEM, fluconazole**), **CYP2C19 inhibitors** (e.g., **omeprazole**) may increase concentration/effect. **HERBAL:** **St. John's wort** may decrease effect. Avoid herbs with antiplatelet activity (e.g., **garlic,**

ginger, ginkgo). **FOOD:** **Grapefruit products** may increase concentration, toxicity. **LAB VALUES:** May increase serum BUN, glucose, uric acid. May decrease platelet count, WBC.

AVAILABILITY (Rx)

Tablets: 50 mg, 100 mg.

ADMINISTRATION/HANDLING

PO
• Give at least 30 min before or 2 hrs after meals. • Do not give with grapefruit products.

INDICATIONS/ROUTES/DOSAGE

Intermittent Claudication
PO: **ADULTS, ELDERLY:** 100 mg twice daily (in combination with aspirin or clopidogrel) at least 30 min before or 2 hrs after meals. Decrease to 50 mg twice daily during concurrent therapy with CYP3A4 or CYP2C19 inhibitors (e.g., clarithromycin, diltiaZEM, erythromycin, fluconazole, FLUoxetine, omeprazole, sertraline).

Dosage in Renal/Hepatic Impairment
No dose adjustment.

SIDE EFFECTS

Frequent (34%–10%): Headache, diarrhea, palpitations, dizziness, pharyngitis. **Occasional (7%–3%):** Nausea, rhinitis, back pain, peripheral edema, dyspepsia, abdominal pain, tachycardia, cough, flatulence, myalgia. **Rare (2%–1%):** Leg cramps, paresthesia, rash, vomiting.

ADVERSE EFFECTS/TOXIC REACTIONS

Overdose noted as severe headache, diarrhea, hypotension, cardiac arrhythmias. May increase risk of endocardial hemorrhage, fibrosis of left ventricle, intimal thickening of coronary artery.

NURSING CONSIDERATIONS

BASELINE ASSESSMENT

Assess CBC (esp. platelet count), BMP, LFT before treatment and periodically

---

C

during treatment. Assess walking distance prior to initiation.

INTERVENTION/EVALUATION

Monitor for improvement of symptoms (e.g., improved walking distance). Monitor lab tests periodically. Monitor for bleeding events, cardiovascular toxicity, or lesions.

PATIENT/FAMILY TEACHING

• Take on an empty stomach (at least 30 min before or 2 hrs after meals). • Do not take with grapefruit products. • Report severe bleeding of any kind.

---

cinacalcet

TOP 100

sin-a-**kal**-set
(Sensipar)

◆CLASSIFICATION

PHARMACOTHERAPEUTIC: Calcium receptor agonist. **CLINICAL:** Calcimimetic.

USES

Treatment of severe hypercalcemia in pts with primary parathyroid carcinoma. Treatment of secondary hyperparathyroidism in pts with chronic renal disease on dialysis. Treatment of severe hypercalcemia in pts with primary hyperparathyroidism unable to undergo parathyroidectomy.

PRECAUTIONS

Contraindications: Hypersensitivity to cinacalcet. Serum calcium lower than the lower limit of normal range. **Cautions:** Cardiovascular disease, moderate to severe hepatic impairment, seizure disorder.

ACTION

Increases sensitivity of calcium-sensing receptor on parathyroid gland to activation by extracellular calcium, thus lowering parathyroid hormone (PTH) levels.

Therapeutic Effect: Decreases serum calcium, PTH levels.

PHARMACOKINETICS

Extensively distributed after PO administration. Protein binding: 93%–97%. Metabolized in liver. Excreted in urine (80%), feces (15%). **Half-life:** 30–40 hrs.

 LIFESPAN CONSIDERATIONS

Pregnancy/Lactation: May cross placental barrier; unknown if distributed in breast milk. Safe usage during lactation not established (potential adverse reaction in infants). **Children:** Safety and efficacy not established. **Elderly:** No age-related precautions noted.

INTERACTIONS

DRUG: Strong CYP3A4 inhibitors (e.g., erythromycin, ketoconazole) increase concentration/effects. Concurrent administration of drugs metabolized by **CYP2D6 enzyme (e.g., flecainide, tricyclic antidepressants, metoprolol, carvedilol)** may require dosage adjustment. **HERBAL:** None significant. **FOOD: High-fat meals** increase plasma concentration. **LAB VALUES:** May decrease serum calcium, phosphorus.

AVAILABILITY (Rx)

Tablets: 30 mg, 60 mg, 90 mg.

ADMINISTRATION/HANDLING

PO

• Store at room temperature. • Do not break, crush, dissolve, or divide film-coated tablets. • Administer with food or shortly after a meal.

INDICATIONS/ROUTES/DOSAGE

Hypercalcemia in Parathyroid Carcinoma; Primary Hyperparathyroidism

PO: ADULTS, ELDERLY: Initially, 30 mg twice daily. Titrate dosage sequentially (60 mg twice daily, 90 mg twice daily, and 90 mg 3–4 times/day) every 2–4 wks as needed to normalize serum calcium level. **Maximum:** 360 mg/day (as 90 mg 4 times/day).

Secondary Hyperparathyroidism in Pts on Dialysis
PO: ADULTS, ELDERLY: Initially, 30 mg once daily. Titrate dosage sequentially (60, 90, 120, and 180 mg once daily) every 2–4 wks to maintain iPTH level between 150 and 300 pg/mL. **Maximum:** 180 mg/day.

Dosage in Renal Impairment
No dose adjustment.

Dosage in Hepatic Impairment
Moderate to severe impairment: Use caution.

SIDE EFFECTS

Frequent (31%–21%): Nausea, vomiting, diarrhea. **Occasional (15%–10%):** Myalgia, dizziness. **Rare (7%–5%):** Asthenia, hypertension, anorexia, noncardiac chest pain.

ADVERSE EFFECTS/TOXIC REACTIONS

Overdose may lead to hypocalcemia, seizures, worsening of HF.

NURSING CONSIDERATIONS

BASELINE ASSESSMENT

Establish baseline serum electrolyte levels (esp. serum calcium, phosphate, ionized calcium).

INTERVENTION/EVALUATION

Monitor serum calcium, phosphate, ionized calcium for hyperparathyroidism. Monitor daily pattern of bowel activity, stool consistency. Obtain order for antidiarrhea, antiemetic medication to prevent serum electrolyte imbalance. Assess for evidence of dizziness; institute fall risk precautions.

PATIENT/FAMILY TEACHING

• Take with food or shortly after a meal. • Do not chew, crush, dissolve, divide film-coated tablets. • Notify physician if vomiting, diarrhea, cramping, muscle pain, numbness occurs.

ciprofloxacin

sip-roe-**flox**-a-sin
(Apo-Ciproflox ✱, Cetraxal, Ciloxan, Cipro, Cipro XR)

■ **BLACK BOX ALERT** ■ May increase risk of tendonitis, tendon rupture. May exacerbate myasthenia gravis.
Do not confuse Ciloxan with Cytoxan, or Cipro with Ceftin, or ciprofloxacin with cephalexin.

FIXED-COMBINATION(S)

Cipro HC Otic: ciprofloxacin/hydrocortisone (a steroid): 0.2%/1%.
CiproDex Otic: ciprofloxacin/dexamethasone (a corticosteroid): 0.3%/0.1%.

◆CLASSIFICATION

PHARMACOTHERAPEUTIC: Fluoroquinolone. **CLINICAL:** Antibiotic.

USES

Treatment of susceptible infections due to *E. coli, K. pneumoniae, E. cloacae, P. mirabilis, P. vulgaris, P. aeruginosa, H. influenzae, M. catarrhalis, S. pneumoniae, S. aureus* (methicillin susceptible), *S. epidermidis, S. pyogenes, C. jejuni, Shigella* spp., *S. typhi* including intra-abdominal, bone, joint, lower respiratory tract, skin/skin structure infections; UTIs, infectious diarrhea, prostatitis, sinusitis, typhoid fever, febrile neutropenia. **Ophthalmic:** Treatment of superficial ocular infections. **Otic:** Treatment of acute otitis externa due to susceptible strains of *P. aeruginosa* or *S. aureus*. **OFF-LABEL:** Treatment of chancroid. Acute pulmonary exacerbations in cystic fibrosis, disseminated gonococcal infections, prophylaxis to *Neisseria meningitidis* following close contact with infected person. Infectious diarrhea (children); periodontitis.

PRECAUTIONS

Contraindications: Hypersensitivity to ciprofloxacin, other quinolones. Concurrent use of tiZANidine. **Cautions:** Renal impairment, CNS disorders, seizures, rheumatoid arthritis, history of QT prolongation, uncorrected hypokalemia, hypomagnesemia, myasthenia gravis. Suspension not used through feeding or gastric tubes. Use in children (due to adverse events to joints/surrounding tissue).

ACTION

Inhibits enzyme, DNA gyrase, in susceptible bacteria, interfering with bacterial cell replication. **Therapeutic Effect:** Bactericidal.

PHARMACOKINETICS

Well absorbed from GI tract. Protein binding: 20%–40%. Widely distributed including to CSF. Metabolized in liver. Primarily excreted in urine. Minimal removal by hemodialysis. **Half-life:** 3–5 hrs (increased in renal impairment, elderly).

⧗ LIFESPAN CONSIDERATIONS

Pregnancy/Lactation: Unknown if distributed in breast milk. If possible, do not use during pregnancy/lactation (risk of arthropathy to fetus/infant). **Children:** Arthropathy may occur if given to children younger than 18 yrs. **Elderly:** Age-related renal impairment may require dosage adjustment.

INTERACTIONS

DRUG: Antacids, calcium, magnesium, zinc, iron preparations, sucralfate may decrease absorption. May increase effects of **caffeine, oral anticoagulants (e.g., warfarin).** May decrease concentration of **fosphenytoin, phenytoin.** May increase concentration, toxicity of **theophylline. HERBAL: Dong quai, St. John's wort** may increase photosensitization. **FOOD:** None known. **LAB VALUES:** May increase serum alkaline phosphatase, creatine kinase (CK), LDH, ALT, AST.

AVAILABILITY (Rx)

Infusion, Solution: 200 mg/100 mL, 400 mg/200 mL. **Injection, Solution (Cipro):** 10 mg/mL. **Ophthalmic Ointment**

(Ciloxan): 0.3%. **Ophthalmic Solution (Ciloxan):** 0.3%. **Otic Solution (Cetraxal):** 0.2% (single-dose container: 0.25 mL). **Suspension, Oral:** 250 mg/5 mL, 500 mg/5 mL. **Tablets (Cipro):** 100 mg, 250 mg, 500 mg, 750 mg.

 Tablets (Extended-Release): 500 mg, 1,000 mg.

ADMINISTRATION/HANDLING

💧 IV

Reconstitution • Available prediluted in infusion container ready for use. Final concentration not to exceed 2 mg/mL. **Rate of Administration** • Infuse over 60 min (reduces risk of venous irritation). **Storage** • Store at room temperature. • Solution appears clear, colorless to slightly yellow.

PO

• May be given with food to minimize GI upset. • Give at least 2 hrs before or 6 hrs after antacids, calcium, iron, zinc-containing products. • Do not administer suspension through feeding or gastric tubes. • **NG tube:** Crush immediate-release tablet and mix with water. Flush tube before/after administration.

Ophthalmic

• Place gloved finger on lower eyelid and pull out until a pocket is formed between eye and lower lid. • Place ointment or drops into pocket. • Instruct pt to close eye gently for 1–2 min (so that medication will not be squeezed out of the sac). • Instruct pt using ointment to roll eyeball to increase contact area of drug to eye. • Instruct pt using solution to apply digital pressure to lacrimal sac at inner canthus for 1 min to minimize systemic absorption. • Do not use ophthalmic solution for injection.

🟦 IV INCOMPATIBILITIES

Ampicillin and sulbactam (Unasyn), cefepime (Maxipime), dexamethasone (Decadron), furosemide (Lasix), heparin,

C

hydrocortisone (Solu-Cortef), methyl-PREDNISolone (Solu-Medrol), phenytoin (Dilantin), sodium bicarbonate.

▦ IV COMPATIBILITIES

Calcium gluconate, diltiaZEM (Cardizem), DOBUTamine (Dobutrex), DOPamine (Intropin), lidocaine, LORazepam (Ativan), magnesium, midazolam (Versed), potassium chloride.

INDICATIONS/ROUTES/DOSAGE

Note: Not recommended as first choice in pregnancy/lactation or in children younger than 18 yrs due to adverse events related to joints/surrounding tissue.

Usual Dosage Range
PO: ADULTS, ELDERLY: 250–750 mg q12h. **CHILDREN: (Mild to moderate infections):** 10 mg/kg twice daily. **Maximum:** 500 mg/dose. **(Severe infections):** 15-20 mg/kg twice daily. **Maximum:** 750 mg/dose. **IV: ADULTS, ELDERLY:** 200–400 mg q12h. **CHILDREN:** 10 mg/kg q8–12h. **Maximum:** 400 mg/dose.

Usual Ophthalmic Dosage
ADULTS, ELDERLY, CHILDREN: (Solution): 1–2 drops q2h while awake for 2 days, then 1–2 drops q4h while awake for 5 days. **(Ointment):** Apply 3 times/day for 2 days, then 2 times/day for 5 days.

Usual Otic Dosage
ADULTS, ELDERLY, CHILDREN: Otic solution 0.2%. Instill 0.25 mL (0.5 mg) 2 times/day for 7 days.

Dosage in Renal Impairment
Dosage and frequency are modified based on creatinine clearance and the severity of the infection.

Creatinine Clearance	Dosage
Immediate-Release	
30–50 mL/min	PO: 250–500 mg q12h
5–29 mL/min	250–500 mg q18h
ESRD, HD, PD	250–500 mg q24h
Extended-Release	
< 30 mL/min	500 mg q24h
ESRD, HD, PD	500 mg q24h
IV 5–29 mL/min	200–400 mg q18–24h

Dosage in Hepatic Impairment
No dose adjustment.

SIDE EFFECTS

Frequent (5%–2%): Nausea, diarrhea, dyspepsia, vomiting, constipation, flatulence, confusion, crystalluria. **Ophthalmic:** Burning, crusting in corner of eye. **Occasional (less than 2%):** Abdominal pain/discomfort, headache, rash. **Ophthalmic:** Altered taste, sensation of foreign body in eye, eyelid redness, itching. **Rare (less than 1%):** Dizziness, confusion, tremors, hallucinations, hypersensitivity reaction, insomnia, dry mouth, paresthesia.

ADVERSE EFFECTS/TOXIC REACTIONS

Superinfection (esp. enterococcal, fungal), nephropathy, cardiopulmonary arrest, cerebral thrombosis may occur. Hypersensitivity reaction (rash, pruritus, blisters, edema, burning skin), photosensitivity have occurred. Sensitization to ophthalmic form may contraindicate later systemic use of ciprofloxacin. May exacerbate muscle weakness in pts with myasthenia gravis. Dermatologic conditions such as toxic epidermal necrolysis, Stevens-Johnson syndrome have been reported. Cases of severe hepatotoxicity have occurred. May increase risk of tendonitis, tendon rupture.

NURSING CONSIDERATIONS

BASELINE ASSESSMENT

Question for history of hypersensitivity to ciprofloxacin, quinolones; myasthenia gravis, renal/hepatic impairment.

INTERVENTION/EVALUATION

Obtain urinalysis for microscopic analysis for crystalluria prior to and during treatment. Evaluate food tolerance. Monitor daily pattern of bowel activity, stool consistency. Encourage hydration (reduces risk of crystalluria). Monitor for dizziness, headache, visual changes, tremors. Assess for chest, joint pain.

Ophthalmic: Observe therapeutic response.

PATIENT/FAMILY TEACHING

• Do not skip doses; take full course of therapy. • Maintain adequate hydration to prevent crystalluria. • Do not take antacids within 2 hrs of ciprofloxacin (reduces/destroys effectiveness). • Shake suspension well before using; do not chew microcapsules in suspension. • Sugarless gum, hard candy may relieve bad taste. • Avoid caffeine. • Report tendon pain or swelling. • Avoid exposure to sunlight/artificial light (may cause photosensitivity reaction). • Report persistent diarrhea.

CISplatin

HIGH ALERT

sis-**pla**-tin

■ **BLACK BOX ALERT** ■ Cumulative renal toxicity may be severe. Dose-related toxicities include myelosuppression, nausea, vomiting. Ototoxicity, especially pronounced in children, noted by tinnitus, loss of high-frequency hearing, deafness. Must be administered by personnel trained in administration/handling of chemotherapeutic agents. Anaphylactic reaction can occur within minutes of administration. Avoid confusion between CISplatin and CARBOplatin.

Do not confuse CISplatin with CARBOplatin or oxaliplatin.

◆CLASSIFICATION

PHARMACOTHERAPEUTIC: Alkylating agent. **CLINICAL:** Antineoplastic.

USES

Treatment of metastatic testicular cancers, metastatic ovarian cancers, advanced bladder cancer. **OFF-LABEL:** Breast, cervical, endometrial, esophageal, gastric, head and neck, lung (small-cell, non–small-cell) carcinomas; Hodgkin's and non-Hodgkin's lymphomas; malignant melanoma, neuroblastoma, osteosarcoma, soft tissue sarcoma, Wilms' tumor.

PRECAUTIONS

Contraindications: Hypersensitivity to CISplatin. Hearing impairment, myelosuppression, preexisting renal impairment. **Cautions:** Elderly, renal impairment.

ACTION

Inhibits DNA and, to a lesser extent, RNA protein synthesis by cross-linking with DNA strands. Cell cycle–phase nonspecific. **Therapeutic Effect:** Prevents cellular division.

PHARMACOKINETICS

Widely distributed. Protein binding: greater than 90%. Undergoes rapid nonenzymatic conversion to inactive metabolite. Excreted in urine. Removed by hemodialysis. **Half-life:** 58–73 hrs (increased in renal impairment).

⧗ LIFESPAN CONSIDERATIONS

Pregnancy/Lactation: If possible, avoid use during pregnancy, esp. first trimester. Breastfeeding not recommended. **Children:** Ototoxic effects may be more severe. **Elderly:** Age-related renal impairment may require dosage adjustment.

INTERACTIONS

DRUG: May decrease effects of **anticonvulsant medications. Bone marrow depressants (e.g., PACLitaxel)** may increase myelosuppression. **Live virus vaccines** may potentiate virus replication, increase vaccine side effects, decrease pt's antibody response to vaccine. **Nephrotoxic, ototoxic agents (e.g., gentamicin, furosemide, NSAIDs)** may increase risk of toxicity. **HERBAL:** Avoid **black cohosh, dong quai** with estrogen-dependent tumors. **Echinacea** may decrease effects. **FOOD:** None known. **LAB VALUES:** May increase serum BUN,

---

creatinine, uric acid, AST. May decrease CrCl, serum calcium, magnesium, phosphate, potassium, sodium. May cause positive Coombs' test.

AVAILABILITY (Rx)

Injection Solution: 1 mg/mL (50 mL, 100 mL, 200 mL).

ADMINISTRATION/HANDLING

◄ALERT► Wear protective gloves during handling. May be carcinogenic, mutagenic, teratogenic. Handle with extreme care during preparation/administration.

 IV

Dilution • Dilute desired dose in 250–1,000 mL 0.9% NaCl, D$_5$/0.45% NaCl, or D$_5$/0.9% NaCl to concentration of 0.05–2 mg/mL. Solution should have final NaCl concentration of 0.2% or greater.
Rate of Administration • Infuse over 6–8 hrs (per protocol). • Avoid rapid infusion (increases risk of nephrotoxicity, ototoxicity). • Monitor for anaphylactic reaction during first few minutes of infusion.
Storage • Protect from sunlight. • Do not refrigerate (may precipitate). Discard if precipitate forms. IV infusion: Stable for 72 hrs at 39°F–77°F.

🚫 IV INCOMPATIBILITIES

Amphotericin B complex (Abelcet, AmBisome, Amphotec), cefepime (Maxipime), piperacillin and tazobactam (Zosyn), sodium bicarbonate.

🚫 IV COMPATIBILITIES

Etoposide (VePesid), granisetron (Kytril), heparin, HYDROmorphone (Dilaudid), lipids, LORazepam (Ativan), magnesium sulfate, mannitol, morphine, ondansetron (Zofran), palonosetron (Aloxi).

INDICATIONS/ROUTES/DOSAGE

Note: Pretreatment hydration with 1–2 liters of fluid recommended. Adequate hydration, urine output greater than 100 mL/hr should be maintained for 24 hrs after administration. Verify any cisplatin dose exceeding 100 mg/m^2/course.

Bladder Cancer
IV: ADULTS, ELDERLY: (Single agent): 50–70 mg/m^2 q3–4wks.

Ovarian Cancer
IV: ADULTS, ELDERLY: 75–100 mg/m^2 q3–4wks (combination therapy) or 100 mg/m^2 q4wks (single agent).

Testicular Cancer
IV: ADULTS, ELDERLY: 20 mg/m^2 daily for 5 days repeated q3wks (in combination with bleomycin and etoposide).

Dosage in Renal Impairment
Dosage is modified based on CrCl, BUN.
◄ALERT► Repeated courses of CISplatin should not be given until serum creatinine is less than 1.5 mg/100 mL and/or BUN is less than 25 mg/100 mL.

Creatinine Clearance	Dosage
10–50 mL/min	75% of normal dose
Less than 10 mL/min	50% of normal dose
Hemodialysis	50% of dose post dialysis
Peritoneal dialysis	50% of dose
Continuous renal replacement therapy	75% of dose

Dosage in Hepatic Impairment
No dose adjustment.

SIDE EFFECTS

Frequent: Nausea, vomiting (occurs in more than 90% of pts, generally beginning 1–4 hrs after administration and lasting up to 24 hrs); myelosuppression (affecting 25%–30% of pts, with recovery generally occurring in 18–23 days). **Occasional:** Peripheral neuropathy (with prolonged therapy [4–7 mos]). Pain/redness at injection site, loss of taste, appetite.

Rare: Hemolytic anemia, blurred vision, stomatitis.

ADVERSE EFFECTS/TOXIC REACTIONS

Anaphylactic reaction (angioedema, wheezing, tachycardia, hypotension) may occur in first few minutes of administration in pt previously exposed to CISplatin. Nephrotoxicity occurs in 28%–36% of pts treated with a single dose, usually during second wk of therapy. Ototoxicity (tinnitus, hearing loss) occurs in 31% of pts treated with a single dose (more severe in children). Symptoms may become more frequent, severe with repeated doses.

NURSING CONSIDERATIONS

BASELINE ASSESSMENT

Obtain baseline CBC, BMP, LFT. Pts should be well hydrated before and 24 hrs after medication to ensure adequate urinary output (100 mL/hr), decrease risk of nephrotoxicity.

INTERVENTION/EVALUATION

Measure all emesis, urine output (general guideline requiring immediate notification of physician: 750 mL/8 hrs, urinary output less than 100 mL/hr). Monitor I&O q1–2h beginning with pretreatment hydration, continue for 48 hrs after dose. Assess vital signs q1–2h during infusion. Monitor urinalysis, serum electrolytes, LFT, renal function tests, CBC, platelet count for changes from baseline.

PATIENT/FAMILY TEACHING

• Report signs of ototoxicity (tinnitus, hearing loss). • Do not have immunizations without physician's approval (lowers body's resistance). • Avoid contact with those who have recently taken oral polio vaccine. • Report if nausea/vomiting continues at home. • Report signs of peripheral neuropathy.

citalopram

sye-**tal**-o-pram
(Apo-Citalopram ✤, CeleXA)

■ **BLACK BOX ALERT** ■ Increased risk of suicidal thinking and behavior in children, adolescents, young adults 18–24 yrs with major depressive disorder, other psychiatric disorders.
Do not confuse CeleXA with CelebREX, Cerebyx, Ranexa, or ZyPREXA.

◆CLASSIFICATION

PHARMACOTHERAPEUTIC: Serotonin reuptake inhibitor. **CLINICAL:** Antidepressant.

USES

Treatment of depression. **OFF-LABEL:** Treatment of alcohol abuse, diabetic neuropathy, obsessive-compulsive disorder, smoking cessation, GAD, panic disorder.

PRECAUTIONS

Contraindications: Hypersensitivity to citalopram, use of MAOIs intended to treat psychiatric disorders (concurrently or within 14 days of discontinuing either citalopram or MAOI), initiation in pts receiving linezolid or methylene blue. Concurrent use with pimozide. **Cautions:** Elderly, hepatic/renal impairment, seizure disorder. Not recommended in pts with congenital long QT syndrome, bradycardia, recent MI, uncompensated HF, hypokalemia, or hypomagnesemia; pts at high risk of suicide.

ACTION

Blocks uptake of the neurotransmitter serotonin at CNS presynaptic neuronal membranes, increasing its availability at postsynaptic receptor sites. **Therapeutic Effect:** Relieves symptoms of depression.

PHARMACOKINETICS

Well absorbed after PO administration. Protein binding: 80%. Extensively metabolized in liver. Excreted in urine. **Half-life:** 35 hrs.

⧗ LIFESPAN CONSIDERATIONS

Pregnancy/Lactation: Distributed in breast milk. **Children:** May cause increased anticholinergic effects, hyperexcitability. **Elderly:** More sensitive to anticholinergic effects (e.g., dry mouth), more likely to experience dizziness, sedation, confusion, hypotension, hyperexcitability.

INTERACTIONS

DRUG: CYP2C19 inhibitors (e.g., **fluconazole**), other medications prolonging QT interval (e.g., **amiodarone, azithromycin, ciprofloxacin, haloperidol**) may increase risk of QT prolongation. **Linezolid, MAOIs** (e.g., **phenelzine, selegiline**), **triptans** may cause serotonin syndrome (excitement, diaphoresis, rigidity, hyperthermia, autonomic hyperactivity, coma). **HERBAL: Gotu kola, kava kava, SAMe, St. John's wort, valerian** may increase CNS depression. **St. John's wort** may increase risk of serotonin syndrome. **FOOD:** None known. **LAB VALUES:** May decrease serum sodium.

AVAILABILITY (Rx)

Oral Solution: 10 mg/5 mL. **Tablets:** 10 mg, 20 mg, 40 mg.

ADMINISTRATION/HANDLING

PO
• Give without regard to food.

INDICATIONS/ROUTES/DOSAGE

Note: Doses greater than 40 mg not recommended.

Depression
PO: ADULTS (less than 60 yrs of age): Initially, 20 mg once daily in the morning or evening. May increase in 20-mg increments at intervals of no less than 1 wk. **Maximum:** 40 mg/day. **ELDERLY (60 yrs of age or older):** 20 mg once daily. **Maximum:** 20 mg/day.

Dose Modification
Hepatic impairment; poor metabolizers of CYP2C19; concomitant use of CYP2C19 inhibitors: 20 mg once daily. **Maximum:** 20 mg/day.

Dosage in Renal Impairment
Mild to moderate impairment: No dose adjustment. **Severe impairment:** Use caution.

SIDE EFFECTS

Frequent (21%–11%): Nausea, dry mouth, drowsiness, insomnia, diaphoresis. **Occasional (8%–4%):** Tremor, diarrhea, abnormal ejaculation, dyspepsia, fatigue, anxiety, vomiting, anorexia. **Rare (3%–2%):** Sinusitis, sexual dysfunction, menstrual disorder, abdominal pain, agitation, decreased libido.

ADVERSE EFFECTS/TOXIC REACTIONS

Overdose manifested as dizziness, drowsiness, tachycardia, confusion, seizures, torsades de pointes, ventricular tachycardia, sudden death. Serotonin syndrome or neuroleptic malignant syndrome (NMS)–like reactions have been reported.

NURSING CONSIDERATIONS

BASELINE ASSESSMENT

Hepatic/renal function tests, blood counts should be performed periodically for pts on long-term therapy. Observe, record behavior. Assess psychological status, thought content, sleep pattern, appearance, interest in environment. Screen for bipolar disorder.

INTERVENTION/EVALUATION

Supervise suicidal-risk pt closely during early therapy (as depression lessens, energy level improves, increasing suicide potential). Assess appearance, behavior, speech pattern, level of interest, mood.

PATIENT/FAMILY TEACHING

• Do not stop taking medication or increase dosage. • Avoid alcohol. • Avoid tasks that require alertness,

---

motor skills until response to drug is established. • Report worsening depression, suicidal ideation, unusual changes in behavior.

clarithromycin

kla-**rith**-roe-**mye**-sin
(Apo-Clarithromycin ✦, Biaxin, Biaxin XL, PMS-Clarithromycin ✦)
Do not confuse clarithromycin with Claritin, clindamycin, or erythromycin.

◆CLASSIFICATION

PHARMACOTHERAPEUTIC: Macrolide. **CLINICAL:** Antibiotic.

USES

Treatment of susceptible infections due to *C. pneumoniae, H. influenzae, H. parainfluenzae, H. pylori, M. catarrhalis, M. avium, M. pneumoniae, S. aureus, S. pneumoniae, S. pyogenes,* including bacterial exacerbation of bronchitis, otitis media, acute maxillary sinusitis, *Mycobacterium avium* complex (MAC), pharyngitis, tonsillitis, *H. pylori* duodenal ulcer, community-acquired pneumonia, skin and soft tissue infections. Prevention of MAC disease. **OFF-LABEL:** Prophylaxis of infective endocarditis, pertussis, Lyme disease.

PRECAUTIONS

Contraindications: Hypersensitivity to clarithromycin, other macrolide antibiotics. History of QT prolongation or ventricular arrhythmias, including torsades de pointes. History of cholestatic jaundice or hepatic impairment with prior use of clarithromycin. Concomitant use with colchicine (in pts with renal/hepatic impairment), lovastatin, simvastatin, pimozide, ergotamine, dihydroergotamine. **Cautions:** Hepatic/renal impairment, elderly with severe renal impairment, myasthenia gravis, coronary artery disease. Pts at risk of prolonged cardiac repolarization. Avoid use with uncorrected electrolytes (e.g., hypokalemia, hypomagnesemia), clinically significant bradycardia, class IA or III antiarrhythmics (see Classification).

ACTION

Binds to ribosomal receptor sites of susceptible organisms, inhibiting protein synthesis of bacterial cell wall. **Therapeutic Effect:** Bacteriostatic; may be bactericidal with high dosages or very susceptible microorganisms.

PHARMACOKINETICS

Well absorbed from GI tract. Protein binding: 65%–75%. Widely distributed (except CNS). Metabolized in liver. Primarily excreted in urine. Not removed by hemodialysis. **Half-life:** 3–7 hrs; metabolite, 5–9 hrs (increased in renal impairment).

⧗ LIFESPAN CONSIDERATIONS

Pregnancy/Lactation: Unknown if distributed in breast milk. **Children:** Safety and efficacy not established in pts younger than 6 mos. **Elderly:** Age-related renal impairment may require dosage adjustment.

INTERACTIONS

DRUG: May increase concentrations, toxicity of **carBAMazepine, colchicine, digoxin, ergotamine, theophylline, sildenafil, tadalafil, vardenafil. Atorvastatin, efavirenz, rifabutin, rifAMPin** may decrease plasma concentration. May increase effect of **warfarin**. May decrease concentration of **zidovudine. Atazanavir, ritonavir** may increase concentration of clarithromycin. **HERBAL: St. John's wort** may decrease plasma concentration. **FOOD:** None known. **LAB VALUES:** May increase serum BUN, ALT, AST, alkaline phosphatase, LDH, creatinine, PT. May decrease WBC.

AVAILABILITY (Rx)

Oral Suspension (Biaxin): 125 mg/5 mL, 250 mg/5 mL. **Tablets (Biaxin):** 250 mg, 500 mg.

✦ Canadian trade name   🔖 Non-Crushable Drug   🔳 High Alert drug

C

🔖 **Tablets (Extended-Release [Biaxin XL]):** 500 mg.

ADMINISTRATION/HANDLING
PO
• Give immediate-release tablets, oral suspension without regard to food. • Give q12h (rather than twice daily). • Shake suspension well before each use. • Extended-release tablets should be given with food. • Do not break, crush, dissolve, or divide extended-release tablets.

INDICATIONS/ROUTES/DOSAGE
Usual Dosage Range
PO: ADULTS, ELDERLY: 250–500 mg q12h or 1,000 mg once daily (extended-release tablets). **CHILDREN 6 MOS AND OLDER:** *(Immediate-Release):* 7.5 mg/kg q12h. **Maximum:** 500 mg/dose.

Dosage in Renal Impairment
CrCl less than 30 mL/min: Reduce dose by 50% and administer once or twice daily. **HD:** Administer dose after dialysis complete.

Combination with atazanavir or ritonavir

| CrCl 30–60 mL/min | Decrease dose by 50% |
| CrCl less than 30 mL/min | Decrease dose by 75% |

Dosage in Hepatic Impairment
No dose adjustment.

SIDE EFFECTS
Occasional (6%–3%): Diarrhea, nausea, altered taste, abdominal pain. **Rare (2%–1%):** Headache, dyspepsia.

ADVERSE EFFECTS/TOXIC REACTIONS
Antibiotic-associated colitis, other superinfections (abdominal cramps, severe watery diarrhea, fever) may result from altered bacterial balance in GI tract. Hepatotoxicity, thrombocytopenia occur rarely.

NURSING CONSIDERATIONS
BASELINE ASSESSMENT
Question pt for allergies to clarithromycin, erythromycins.

INTERVENTION/EVALUATION
Monitor daily pattern of bowel activity, stool consistency. Mild GI effects may be tolerable, but increasing severity may indicate onset of antibiotic-associated colitis. Be alert for superinfection: fever, vomiting, diarrhea, anal/genital pruritus, oral mucosal changes (ulceration, pain, erythema).

PATIENT/FAMILY TEACHING
• Continue therapy for full length of treatment. • Doses should be evenly spaced. • Biaxin may be taken without regard to food. Take Biaxin XL with food. • Report severe diarrhea.

clevidipine

clev-eye-di-peen
(Cleviprex)
Do not confuse clevidipine with amlodipine, cladribine, clofarabine, clozapine, or Cleviprex with Claravis.

◆CLASSIFICATION
PHARMACOTHERAPEUTIC: Dihydropyridine calcium channel blocker. **CLINICAL:** Antihypertensive.

USES
Management of hypertension when oral therapy is not feasible or not desirable.

PRECAUTIONS
Contraindications: Hypersensitivity to clevidipine. Allergy to soy or egg products; abnormal lipid metabolism (e.g., acute pancreatitis, lipoid nephrosis, pathologic hyperlipidemia if accompanied by hyperlipidemia), severe aortic stenosis. **Cautions:** HF; pt with disorders of lipid metabolism.

ACTION

Causes potent arterial vasodilation by inhibiting the influx of calcium during depolarization in arterial smooth muscle. **Therapeutic Effect:** Decreases mean arterial pressure (MAP) by reducing systemic vascular resistance.

PHARMACOKINETICS

Widely and rapidly distributed. Full recovery of therapeutic B/P occurs 5–15 min. after discontinuation. Onset of effects: 2–4 min. Metabolized via hydrolysis by esterases in blood and extravascular tissue. Protein binding: 99.5%. Excreted in urine (74%), feces (22%). **Half-life:** 15 min.

⧗ LIFESPAN CONSIDERATIONS

Pregnancy/Lactation: Unknown if distributed in breast milk. May depress uterine contractions during labor and delivery. **Children:** Safety and efficacy not established in pts younger than 18. **Elderly:** Start at low end of dosing range. May experience greater hypotensive effect.

INTERACTIONS

DRUG: Diuretics (e.g., furosemide, HCTZ, spironolactone), other **antihypertensives (e.g., hydralazine, lisinopril, metoprolol, valsartan)** may increase hypotensive effect. **NSAIDs (e.g., ibuprofen, naproxen, ketorolac)** may decrease antihypertensive effect. **HERBAL:** Herbs with hypotensive properties **(e.g., garlic, ginger, hawthorn)** may enhance effect. **Yohimbe** may decrease effect. **FOOD:** None known. **LAB VALUES:** May increase serum BUN, potassium, triglycerides, uric acid.

AVAILABILITY (Rx)

Injection, Emulsion: 50 mL (0.5 mg/mL), 100 mL (0.5 mg/mL), 250-mL vial (0.5 mg/mL).

ADMINISTRATION/HANDLING

 IV

Preparation • Do not dilute. • To ensure uniformity of emulsion, gently invert vial several times before use. • Visually inspect for particulate matter or discoloration. Emulsion should appear milky white. Discard if discoloration or particulate matter is observed.

Rate of Administration • Titrate to desired effect using infusion pump via peripheral or central line.

Storage • Refrigerate unused vial in original carton. • May store at controlled room temperature (77°F) for up to 2 mos. • Do not freeze. • Do not return to refrigerator once warmed to room temperature. Once the stopper is punctured, use within 12 hrs. • Discard unused portions.

▦ IV INCOMPATIBILITIES

May be administered with, but not diluted in, solutions including Sterile Water for Injection, 0.9% NaCl, dextrose-containing solutions, lactated Ringer's, 10% amino acid. Do not administer with other medications.

INDICATIONS/ROUTES/DOSAGE

Note: Individualize dosage depending on desired B/P and pt response. See manufacturer guidelines for dose conversion.

Hypertension

IV: ADULTS, ELDERLY: Initiate infusion at 1–2 mg/hr. **Titration:** Initially, dosage may be doubled at short (90-sec) intervals. As B/P approaches goal, an increase in dosage should be less than double, and time intervals between dose adjustments should be lengthened to q5–10 min. **Maintenance:** Desired therapeutic effect generally occurs at a rate of 4–6 mg/hr (pts with severe hypertension may require limited doses up to 32 mg/hr). **Maximum:** 16 mg/hr (no more than 21 mg/hr or 1000 mL is recommended per 24 hrs due to lipid load).

Dosage in Renal Impairment
No dose adjustment.

Dosage in Hepatic Impairment
Not specified; use caution.

C

SIDE EFFECTS

Occasional (6%-3%): Headache, insomnia, nausea, vomiting. **Rare (less than 1%):** Syncope, dyspnea.

ADVERSE EFFECTS/TOXIC REACTIONS

May cause atrial fibrillation, hypotension, reflex tachycardia. Rebound hypertension may occur in pts who are not transitioned to oral antihypertensives after discontinuation. Dihydropyridine calcium channel blockers are known to have negative inotropic effects, which may exacerbate HF. Rebound hypertension may cause emergent hypertensive crisis, which may cause CVA, myocardial infarction, renal failure, HF, seizures.

NURSING CONSIDERATIONS

BASELINE ASSESSMENT

Screen for history of defective lipid metabolism, pancreatitis, hypertriglyceridemia, severe aortic stenosis; allergy to soy products, eggs products. Assess B/P, apical pulse immediately before initiation.

INTERVENTION/EVALUATION

Monitor B/P, pulse rate. Generally, an increase of 1–2 mg/hour will produce an additional 2–4 mm Hg decrease in systolic B/P. If an oral antihypertensive is required to wean off infusion, consider the delay of onset of oral medication's effect. Pts who receive prolonged IV infusions and are not changed to other antihypertensives should be monitored for rebound hypertension for at least 8 hrs after discontinuation. Obtain serum triglyceride level in pts receiving prolonged infusions. Monitor for atrial fibrillation, hypotension, reflex tachycardia; exacerbation of HF in pts with history of HF. Beta blockers should be discontinued only after a gradual reduction in dose.

PATIENT/FAMILY TEACHING

• In some pts, an oral blood pressure medication may need to be started; compliance is essential to control high blood pressure. • Life-threatening high blood pressure crisis may occur up to 8 hrs after stopping infusion; report severe anxiety, chest pain, difficulty breathing, headache, stroke-like symptoms (confusion, difficulty speaking, paralysis, one-sided weakness, vision loss).

clindamycin

klin-da-**mye**-sin
(Apo-Clindamycin ✦, Cleocin, Cleocin T, Cleocin Vaginal, Clindagel, Clindamax, Clindesse)

■ **BLACK BOX ALERT** ■ May cause severe, potentially fatal colitis characterized by severe, persistent diarrhea, severe abdominal cramps, passage of blood and mucus.

Do not confuse Cleocin with Clinoril or Cubicin, or clindamycin with clarithromycin, Claritin, or vancomycin.

◆CLASSIFICATION

PHARMACOTHERAPEUTIC: Lincosamide. **CLINICAL:** Antibiotic.

USES

Systemic: Treatment of aerobic gram-positive staphylococci and streptococci (not enterococci), *Fusobacterium, Bacteroides* spp., and *Actinomyces* for treatment of respiratory tract infections, skin/soft tissue infections, sepsis, intra-abdominal infections, infections of female pelvis and genital tract, bacterial endocarditis prophylaxis for dental and upper respiratory procedures in penicillin-allergic pts, perioperative prophylaxis. **Topical:** Treatment of acne vulgaris. **Intravaginal:** Treatment of bacterial vaginosis. **OFF-LABEL:** Treatment of actinomycosis, babesiosis, erysipelas, malaria, otitis media, *Pneumocystis jiroveci* pneumonia (PCP), sinusitis, toxoplasmosis. **PO:** Bacterial vaginosis.

PRECAUTIONS

Contraindications: Hypersensitivity to clindamycin. **Cautions:** Severe hepatic dysfunction; history of GI disease (especially colitis).

ACTION

Inhibits protein synthesis of bacterial cell wall by binding to bacterial ribosomal receptor sites. Topically, decreases fatty acid concentration on skin. **Therapeutic Effect:** Bacteriostatic or bacteriocidal.

PHARMACOKINETICS

Rapidly absorbed from GI tract. Protein binding: 92%–94%. Widely distributed. Metabolized in liver. Primarily excreted in urine. Not removed by hemodialysis. **Half-life:** 1.6–5.3 hrs (increased in renal/hepatic impairment, premature infants).

⧗ LIFESPAN CONSIDERATIONS

Pregnancy/Lactation: Readily crosses placenta. Distributed in breast milk. **Topical/vaginal:** Unknown if distributed in breast milk. **Children:** Caution in pts younger than 1 mo. **Elderly:** No age-related precautions noted.

INTERACTIONS

DRUG: Adsorbent antidiarrheals may delay absorption. **Erythromycin** may increase effect. May increase effects of **neuromuscular blockers (e.g., rocuronium, vecuronium). HERBAL:** St. John's wort may decrease concentration/effect. **FOOD:** None known. **LAB VALUES:** May increase serum alkaline phosphatase, ALT, AST.

AVAILABILITY (Rx)

🍶 **Capsules:** 75 mg, 150 mg, 300 mg. **Cream, Vaginal:** 2%. **Gel, Topical:** 1%. **Infusion, Premix:** 300 mg/50 mL, 600 mg/50 mL, 900 mg/50 mL. **Injection Solution:** 150 mg/mL. **Lotion:** 1%. **Oral Solution:** 75 mg/5 mL. **Suppositories, Vaginal:** 100 mg. **Swabs, Topical:** 1%.

ADMINISTRATION/HANDLING

 IV

Reconstitution • Dilute 300–600 mg with 50 mL D_5W or 0.9% NaCl (900–1,200 mg with 100 mL).
Rate of Administration • Infuse over at least 10–60 min at rate not exceeding 30 mg/min. Severe hypotension, cardiac arrest can occur with rapid administration. • No more than 1.2 g should be given in a single infusion.
Storage • Reconstituted IV infusion (piggyback) is stable for 16 days at room temperature, 32 days if refrigerated.

IM
• Do not exceed 600 mg/dose. • Administer deep IM.

PO
• Store capsules at room temperature. • After reconstitution, oral solution is stable for 2 wks at room temperature. • Do not refrigerate oral solution (avoids thickening). • Give with at least 8 oz water (minimizes esophageal ulceration). • Give without regard to food.

Topical
• Wash skin; allow to dry completely before application. • Shake topical lotion well before each use. • Apply liquid, solution, or gel in thin film to affected area. • Avoid contact with eyes or abraded areas.

Vaginal, Cream or Suppository
• Use one applicatorful or suppository at bedtime. • Fill applicator that comes with cream or suppository to indicated level. • Instruct pt to lie on back with knees drawn upward and spread apart. • Insert applicator into vagina and push plunger to release medication. • Withdraw, wash applicator with soap and warm water. • Wash hands promptly to avoid spreading infection.

▦ IV INCOMPATIBILITIES

Allopurinol (Aloprim), fluconazole (Diflucan).

▓ IV COMPATIBILITIES

Amiodarone (Cordarone), diltiaZEM (Cardizem), heparin, HYDROmorphone (Dilaudid), magnesium sulfate, midazolam (Versed), morphine, multivitamins, propofol (Diprivan).

INDICATIONS/ROUTES/DOSAGE

Usual Dosage

IV, IM: ADULTS, ELDERLY: 600–2,700 mg/day in 2–4 divided doses. **Maximum:** 4,800 mg/day. **CHILDREN 1 MO–16 YRS:** 20–40 mg/kg/day in 3–4 divided doses. **Maximum:** 2,700 mg/day. **CHILDREN YOUNGER THAN 1 MO:** 5 mg/kg/dose q6–12h.

PO: ADULTS, ELDERLY: 150–450 mg q6h. **Maximum:** 1,800 mg/day. **CHILDREN 1 MO–16 YRS:** *(Capsule):* 8–40 mg/kg/day in divided doses q6–8h. **Maximum:** 1,800 mg/day. *(Oral Solution):* 8–25 mg/kg/day in 3–4 divided doses. Minimum dose: 37.5 mg 3 times/day. **CHILDREN YOUNGER THAN 1 MO:** 5 mg/kg/dose q6–12h.

Bacterial Vaginosis

Intravaginal *(Cream):* **ADULTS:** One applicatorful at bedtime for 3–7 days or 1 suppository at bedtime for 3 days. *(Clindesse):* **ADULTS:** One applicatorful once daily.

Acne Vulgaris

Topical: **ADULTS:** Apply thin layer to affected area twice daily.

Dosage in Renal/Hepatic Impairment

No dose adjustment.

SIDE EFFECTS

Frequent: Systemic: Abdominal pain, nausea, vomiting, diarrhea. **Topical:** Dry, scaly skin. **Vaginal:** Vaginitis, pruritus. **Occasional: Systemic:** Phlebitis; pain, induration at IM injection site; allergic reaction, urticaria, pruritus. **Topical:** Contact dermatitis, abdominal pain, mild diarrhea, burning, stinging. **Vaginal:** Headache, dizziness, nausea, vomiting, abdominal pain. **Rare: Vaginal:** Hypersensitivity reaction.

ADVERSE EFFECTS/TOXIC REACTIONS

Antibiotic-associated colitis, other super-infections (abdominal cramps, severe watery diarrhea, fever) may occur during and several wks after clindamycin therapy (including topical form). Blood dyscrasias (leukopenia, thrombocytopenia), nephrotoxicity (proteinuria, azotemia, oliguria) occur rarely. Thrombophlebitis with IV administration.

NURSING CONSIDERATIONS

BASELINE ASSESSMENT

Obtain baseline WBC. Question pt for history of allergies. Avoid, if possible, concurrent use of neuromuscular blocking agents.

INTERVENTION/EVALUATION

Monitor daily pattern of bowel activity, stool consistency. Report diarrhea promptly due to potential for serious colitis (even with topical or vaginal administration). Assess skin for rash (dryness, irritation) with topical application. With all routes of administration, be alert for superinfection: fever, vomiting, diarrhea, anal/genital pruritus, oral mucosal changes (ulceration, pain, erythema).

PATIENT/FAMILY TEACHING

• Continue therapy for full length of treatment. • Doses should be evenly spaced. • Take oral doses with at least 8 oz water. • Use caution when applying topical clindamycin concurrently with peeling or abrasive acne agents, soaps, alcohol-containing cosmetics to avoid cumulative effect. • Do not apply topical preparations near eyes, abraded areas. • Report severe persistent diarrhea, cramps, bloody stool. • **Vaginal:** In event of accidental contact with eyes, rinse with large amounts of cool tap water. • Do not engage in sexual intercourse during treatment. • Wear sanitary pad to protect clothes against stains. Tampons should not be used.

cloBAZam

kloe-**ba**-zam
(Apo-CloBAZam ✦, Novo-CloBAZam ✦, Onfi)

Do not confuse cloBAZam with clonazePAM or cloZAPine.

◆CLASSIFICATION

PHARMACOTHERAPEUTIC: Benzodiazepine (Schedule IV). **CLINICAL:** Anticonvulsant.

USES

Adjunctive treatment of seizures associated with Lennox-Gastaut syndrome in pts 2 yrs of age and older. **OFF-LABEL:** Catamenial epilepsy; epilepsy (monotherapy).

PRECAUTIONS

Contraindications: Hypersensitivity to cloBAZam. **Cautions:** Elderly, debilitated, mild to moderate hepatic impairment, preexisting muscle weakness or ataxia, concomitant CNS depressants, impaired gag reflex, respiratory disease, sleep apnea, concomitant poor CYP2C19 metabolizers, pts at risk for falls, myasthenia gravis, narrow-angle glaucoma.

ACTION

Potentiates neurotransmission of gamma-aminobutyric acid (GABA) by binding to GABA receptor. Depresses nerve impulse transmission in motor cortex. **Therapeutic Effect:** Decreases seizure activity.

PHARMACOKINETICS

Rapidly absorbed after PO administration. Metabolized in liver. Peak plasma concentration: 0.5–4 hrs. Protein binding: 80–90%. Primarily excreted in urine. Unknown if removed by dialysis. **Half-life:** 36–42 hrs.

⧗ LIFESPAN CONSIDERATIONS

Pregnancy/Lactation: Excreted in breast milk. Hormonal contraceptives may have decreased effectiveness. Nonhormonal contraception recommended. **Children:** Safety and efficacy not established in pts younger than 2 yrs. **Elderly:** May have decreased clearance levels (initial dose 5 mg/day).

INTERACTIONS

DRUG: CYP2C19 inhibitors (e.g., fluconazole, fluvoxaMINE, omeprazole, ticlopidine) may increase concentration/effects. **Alcohol, other CNS depressants (e.g., lorazepam, morphine, zolpidem)** may increase CNS depression. May decrease effects of **hormonal contraceptives. HERBAL: Gotu kola, kava kava, St. John's wort, valerian** may increase CNS depression. **St. John's wort** may decrease effects. **FOOD:** None known. **LAB VALUES:** None significant.

AVAILABILITY (Rx)

Suspension, Oral: 2.5 mg/mL. **Tablets:** 5 mg, 10 mg, 20 mg.

ADMINISTRATION/HANDLING

• May give without regard to food. • Tablets may be crushed and mixed with applesauce. • Shake suspension well. Use oral syringe supplied with suspension.

INDICATIONS/ROUTES/DOSAGE

Seizure Control (Lennox-Gastaut Syndrome)

PO: ADULTS, CHILDREN WEIGHING 30 KG OR LESS: Initially, 5 mg once daily for at least 7 days, then increase to 5 mg twice for at least 7 days, then increase to 10 mg twice daily. **Maximum:** 20 mg/day. **ADULTS, CHILDREN WEIGHING MORE THAN 30 KG:** Initially, 5 mg twice daily for at least 7 days, then increase to 10 mg twice daily for at least 7 days, then increase to 20 mg twice daily. **Maximum:** 40 mg/day. **ELDERLY WEIGHING MORE THAN 30 KG, HEPATIC IMPAIRMENT, CYP2C19 POOR METABOLIZERS:** Initially, 5 mg once daily for at least 7 days, then increase to 5 mg twice daily for at least 7 days, then increase to

C

10 mg twice daily. After 1 wk, may increase to 20 mg twice daily.
ELDERLY WEIGHING 30 KG OR LESS, HEPATIC IMPAIRMENT, CYP2C19 POOR METABOLIZERS: Initially, 5 mg once daily for at least 2 wks, then 5 mg twice daily for at least 1 wk, then 10 mg twice daily.

Dosage in Renal Impairment
No dose adjustment.

SIDE EFFECTS

Frequent (26%–10%): Sleepiness, URI, lethargy. **Occasional (9%–5%):** Drooling, nausea, vomiting, constipation, irritability, ataxia, insomnia, cough, fatigue. **Rare (4%–2%):** Psychomotor hyperactivity, UTI, decreased/increased appetite, dysarthria, pyrexia, dysphagia, bronchitis.

ADVERSE EFFECTS/TOXIC REACTIONS

May increase risk of suicidal behavior/ideation (less than 1%). Physical dependence can increase with higher doses or concomitant alcohol/drug abuse. Abrupt benzodiazepine withdrawal may present as profuse sweating, cramping, nausea, vomiting, muscle pain, convulsions, psychosis, hallucinations, aggression, tremor, anxiety, insomnia. Overdose may result in confusion, lethargy, diminished reflexes, respiratory depression, coma. **Antidote:** Flumazenil (see Appendix J for dosage). Decreased mobility may potentiate higher risk of pneumonia.

NURSING CONSIDERATIONS

BASELINE ASSESSMENT

Offer emotional support. Review history of seizure disorder (frequency, duration, intensity, level of consciousness [LOC]). Question history of alcohol use. Obtain baseline vital signs. Assess history of depression/suicidal ideation.

INTERVENTION/EVALUATION

Monitor for excess sedation, respiratory depression, suicidal ideation. Implement seizure precautions, observe frequently for seizure activity. Assist with ambulation if drowsiness, dizziness occurs. Evaluate for therapeutic response. Encourage turning, coughing, deep breathing for pts with decreased mobility or who are bedridden.

PATIENT/FAMILY TEACHING

• Avoid tasks that require alertness, motor skills until response to drug is established. • Do not abruptly discontinue medication. • If tapering, monitor for drug withdrawal symptoms. • Avoid alcohol. • Report depression, aggression, thoughts of suicide/self-harm, excessive drowsiness.

clofarabine

kloe-**far**-a-bine
(Clolar)
Do not confuse clofarabine with cladribine or clevidipine.

◆CLASSIFICATION

PHARMACOTHERAPEUTIC: Antimetabolite. **CLINICAL:** Antineoplastic.

USES

Treatment of pediatric pts (1–21 yrs) with relapsed or refractory acute lymphoblastic leukemia (ALL). **OFF-LABEL:** Acute myeloid leukemia (AML) in adults 60 yrs or older. Treatment of relapsed/refractory ALL.

PRECAUTIONS

Contraindications: Hypersensitivity to clofarabine. **Cautions:** Dehydration, hypotension, concomitant nephrotoxic or hepatotoxic medications, renal/hepatic impairment.

ACTION

Metabolized intracellularly to ribonucleotide reductase. Alters mitochondrial membrane necessary in DNA synthesis. **Therapeutic Effect:** Decreases cell replication, inhibits cell repair. Produces cell death.

PHARMACOKINETICS

Protein binding: 47%. Metabolized intracellularly. Primarily excreted in urine (40%–60% unchanged). **Half-life:** 5.2 hrs.

⧗ LIFESPAN CONSIDERATIONS

Pregnancy/Lactation: May cause fetal harm. Breastfeeding not recommended. **Children:** Safety and efficacy not established in pts younger than 1 yr. **Elderly:** No age-related precautions noted.

INTERACTIONS

DRUG: Hepatotoxic, nephrotoxic medications (e.g., gentamicin, furosemide, NSAIDs) may increase risk of hepatic/renal toxicity. **HERBAL: Echinacea** may decrease effect. **FOOD:** None known. **LAB VALUES:** May increase serum creatinine, uric acid, ALT, AST, bilirubin.

AVAILABILITY (Rx)

Injection, Solution: 1 mg/mL (20-mL vial).

ADMINISTRATION/HANDLING
📮 IV

Reconstitution • Filter clofarabine through sterile, 0.2-micrometer syringe filter prior to dilution with D_5W or 0.9% NaCl to final concentration of 0.15–0.4 mg/mL.
Rate of Administration • Administer over 1–2 hrs. • Continuously infuse IV fluids to decrease risk of tumor lysis syndrome, other adverse events.
Storage • Store undiluted or diluted solution at room temperature. • Use diluted solution within 24 hrs.

🔲 IV INCOMPATIBILITIES

Do not administer any other medication through same IV line.

INDICATIONS/ROUTES/DOSAGE

Acute Lymphoblastic Leukemia (ALL)
IV: CHILDREN 1–21 YRS: 52 mg/m² over 2 hrs once daily for 5 consecutive days; repeat q2–6wks following recovery or return to baseline organ function. (Subsequent cycles should begin no sooner than 14 days from day 1 of previous cycle and when ANC is 750 cells/mm³ or greater.)

Dosage in Renal Impairment
Dosage is modified based on creatinine clearance.

Creatinine Clearance	Dosage
30–60 mL/min	Decrease dose by 50%
Less than 30 mL/min	Use with caution

Dosage in Hepatic Impairment
Baseline impairment: No dose adjustment. **Hepatotoxicity during treatment; grade 3 or higher increase in bilirubin:** Discontinue. May restart at 25% dose reduction following recovery to baseline.

SIDE EFFECTS

Frequent (83%–20%): Vomiting, nausea, diarrhea, pruritus, headache, fever, dermatitis, rigors, abdominal pain, fatigue, tachycardia, epistaxis, anorexia, petechiae, limb pain, hypotension, anxiety, constipation, edema. **Occasional (19%–11%):** Cough, mucosal inflammation, erythema, flushing, hematuria, dizziness, gingival bleeding, injection site pain, respiratory distress, pharyngitis, back pain, palmar-plantar erythrodysesthesia syndrome, myalgia, oral candidiasis, hypertension, depression, irritability, arthralgia, anorexia. **Rare (10%):** Tremor, weight gain, drowsiness.

ADVERSE EFFECTS/TOXIC REACTIONS

Neutropenia occurred in 57% of pts; pericardial effusion in 35%; left ventricular systolic dysfunction in 27%; hepatomegaly, jaundice in 15%; pleural effusion, pneumonia, bacteremia in 10%; capillary leak syndrome in less than 10%.

NURSING CONSIDERATIONS

BASELINE ASSESSMENT

Question possibility of pregnancy. Obtain CBC, BMP, LFT, CrCl prior to therapy.

INTERVENTION/EVALUATION

Monitor CBC, renal function test, LFT, serum uric acid. Monitor respiratory status, cardiac function. Monitor daily pattern of bowel activity, stool consistency. Assess for GI disturbances. Assess skin for pruritus, dermatitis, petechiae, erythema on palms of hands and soles of feet. Assess for fever, sore throat; obtain blood cultures to detect evidence of infection. Ensure adequate hydration.

PATIENT/FAMILY TEACHING

• Do not have immunizations without physician's approval (drug lowers resistance). • Avoid contact with anyone who recently received a live virus vaccine. • Avoid crowds, those with infection. • Avoid pregnancy; pts of childbearing potential should use effective contraception. • Maintain strict oral hygiene and frequent handwashing. • Report fever, respiratory distress, prolonged nausea, vomiting, diarrhea, easy bruising.

clomiPRAMINE

kloe-**mip**-rah-meen
(Anafranil, Apo-ClomiPRAMINE ✦,
Novo-ClomiPRAMINE ✦)

■ **BLACK BOX ALERT** ■ Increased risk of suicidal ideation and behavior in children, adolescents, young adults 18–24 yrs with major depressive disorder, other psychiatric disorders.
Do not confuse Anafranil with enalapril, or clomiPRAMINE with chlorproMAZINE, clevidipine, clomiPHENE, or desipramine.

◆CLASSIFICATION

PHARMACOTHERAPEUTIC: Tricyclic.
CLINICAL: Antidepressant.

USES

Treatment of obsessive-compulsive disorder. **OFF-LABEL:** Depression, panic attacks.

PRECAUTIONS

Contraindications: Hypersensitivity to clomiPRAMINE, other tricyclic agents. Acute recovery period after MI, use of MAOIs intended for psychiatric disorders (concurrently or within 14 days of discontinuing either clomipramine or MAOI). Initiation in pts receiving linezolid or methylene blue. **Cautions:** Pts at high risk for suicide, prostatic hypertrophy, history of urinary retention/obstruction, narrow-angle glaucoma, seizures, cardiovascular/hepatic/renal disease, hyperthyroidism, alcoholism, xerostomia, visual problems, elderly, constipation, history of bowel obstruction. Tumors of the adrenal medulla (e.g., pheochromocytoma).

ACTION

Blocks reuptake of neurotransmitters (norepinephrine, serotonin) at CNS presynaptic membranes, increasing availability at postsynaptic receptor sites. **Therapeutic Effect:** Reduces obsessive-compulsive behavior.

PHARMACOKINETICS

Rapidly absorbed. Metabolized in liver. Eliminated in urine (51%–60%), feces (24%–32%). **Half-life:** 20–30 hrs.

⌛ LIFESPAN CONSIDERATIONS

Pregnancy/Lactation: Distributed in breast milk. **Children:** Increased risk of suicidal ideation, behavior noted in children, adolescents. Safety and effectiveness in pts younger than 10 yrs not established. **Elderly:** Not recommended in elderly due to anticholinergic effects, potential for sedation, orthostatic hypotension.

INTERACTIONS

DRUG: Alcohol, other CNS depressants (e.g., lorazepam, morphine, zolpidem) may increase CNS, respiratory depression, hypotensive effect. **Cimetidine, haloperidol** may increase concentration, risk of toxicity. May decrease effects of **cloNIDine. PHE-Nobarbital** may decrease concentration, antidepressant effect. **MAOIs (e.g., phenelzine, selegiline)** may increase risk of neuroleptic malignant syndrome, seizures, hyperpyresis, hypertensive crisis. **Phenothiazines (e.g., chlorpromazine, thioridazine)** may increase anticholinergic, sedative effects. **Sympathomimetics (e.g., dopamine, norepinephrine)** may increase the risk of cardiac effects. **HERBAL:** Gota kola, kava kava, SAMe, St. John's wort, valerian may increase CNS depression. **FOOD:** Grapefruit products may increase concentration, toxicity. **LAB VALUES:** May alter serum glucose, ECG readings.

AVAILABILITY (Rx)

Capsules: 25 mg, 50 mg, 75 mg.

ADMINISTRATION/HANDLING

PO

• May give with food to decrease risk of GI disturbance. • Recommend bedtime administration.

INDICATIONS/ROUTES/DOSAGE

NOTE: Following dose titration, may give once-daily dose at bedtime.

Obsessive-Compulsive Disorder (OCD)
PO: ADULTS, ELDERLY: Initially, 25 mg/day. May gradually increase to 100 mg/day in divided doses in the first 2 wks. **Maximum:** 250 mg/day. **CHILDREN 10 YRS AND OLDER:** Initially, 25 mg/day. May gradually increase up to maximum of 3 mg/kg/day or 100 mg in divided doses (whichever is lowest). **Maintenance:** May further increase to 3 mg/kg or 200 mg/day (whichever is less).

Dosage in Renal/Hepatic Impairment
Use caution.

SIDE EFFECTS

Frequent (30%–15%): Ejaculatory failure, dry mouth, somnolence, tremors, dizziness, headache, constipation, fatigue, nausea. **Occasional (14%–5%):** Impotence, diaphoresis, dyspepsia, sexual dysfunction, dysmenorrhea, nervousness, weight gain, pharyngitis. **Rare (less than 5%):** Diarrhea, myalgia, rhinitis, increased appetite, paresthesia, memory impairment, anxiety, rash, pruritus, anorexia, abdominal pain, vomiting, flatulence, flushing, UTI, back pain.

ADVERSE EFFECTS/TOXIC REACTIONS

Overdose may produce seizures, cardiovascular effects (severe orthostatic hypotension, dizziness, tachycardia, palpitations, arrhythmias), altered temperature regulation (hyperpyrexia, hypothermia). Abrupt discontinuation after prolonged therapy may produce headache, malaise, nausea, vomiting, vivid dreams. Anemia, agranulocytosis have been noted.

NURSING CONSIDERATIONS

BASELINE ASSESSMENT

Assess psychological status, thought content, level of interest, mood, behavior, suicidal ideation.

INTERVENTION/EVALUATION

Supervise suicidal-risk pt closely during early therapy (as depression lessens, energy level improves, increasing suicide potential). Assess appearance, behavior, speech pattern, level of interest, mood.

PATIENT/FAMILY TEACHING

• May cause dry mouth, constipation, blurred vision. Avoid tasks that require alertness, motor skills until response to drug is established. • Tolerance to postural hypotension, sedative, anticholinergic effects usually develop during early therapy. • Maximum therapeutic effect may be noted in 2–4 wks. • Do not abruptly discontinue medication. • Daily dose may be given at bedtime to minimize daytime sedation. • Avoid alcohol. • Report worsening depression, suicidal ideation, change in behavior.

C

clonazePAM

kloe-**naz**-e-pam
(Apo-ClonazePAM ✦, KlonoPIN, Rivotril ✦)

■ **BLACK BOX ALERT** ■ Concomitant use with opioids may result in profound sedation, respiratory depression, coma, and death.
Do not confuse clonazePAM or KlonoPIN with cloBAZam, cloNIDine, cloZAPine, or LORazepam.

◆CLASSIFICATION

PHARMACOTHERAPEUTIC: Benzodiazepine (Schedule IV). **CLINICAL:** Anticonvulsant, antianxiety.

USES

Adjunct in treatment of Lennox-Gastaut syndrome (petit mal variant epilepsy); akinetic, myoclonic seizures; absence seizures (petit mal) unresponsive to succinimides. Treatment of panic disorder. **OFF-LABEL:** Burning mouth syndrome, REM sleep behavior disorder, essential tremor.

PRECAUTIONS

Contraindications: Hypersensitivity to clonazePAM. Active narrow-angle glaucoma, severe hepatic disease, pregnancy. **Cautions:** Renal/hepatic impairment, impaired gag reflex, chronic respiratory disease, elderly, debilitated pts, depression, pts at risk of suicide or drug dependence, concomitant use of other CNS depressants.

ACTION

Depresses all levels of CNS; depresses nerve impulse transmission in motor cortex. Suppresses abnormal discharge in petit mal seizures. **Therapeutic Effect:** Produces anxiolytic, anticonvulsant effects.

PHARMACOKINETICS

Route	Onset	Peak	Duration
PO	20–60 min	—	12 hrs or less

Well absorbed from GI tract. Protein binding: 85%. Metabolized in liver. Excreted in urine. Not removed by hemodialysis. **Half-life:** 18–50 hrs.

⧗ LIFESPAN CONSIDERATIONS

Pregnancy/Lactation: Crosses placenta. May be distributed in breast milk. Chronic ingestion during pregnancy may produce withdrawal symptoms, CNS depression in neonates. **Children:** Long-term use may adversely affect physical/mental development. **Elderly:** Not recommended in elderly due to anticholinergic effects, potential for sedation, orthostatic hypotension.

INTERACTIONS

DRUG: Alcohol, other CNS depressants (e.g., lorazepam, morphine, zolpidem) may increase CNS depressant effect. **CYP3A4 inhibitors (e.g., azole antifungals)** may increase concentration, toxicity. **HERBAL:** Gotu kola, kava kava, SAMe, St. John's wort, valerian may increase CNS depression. **St. John's wort** may decrease concentration/effects. **FOOD:** None known. **LAB VALUES:** None significant.

AVAILABILITY (Rx)

Tablets (KlonoPIN): 0.5 mg, 1 mg, 2 mg.
Tablets (Orally Disintegrating): 0.125 mg, 0.25 mg, 0.5 mg, 1 mg, 2 mg.

ADMINISTRATION/HANDLING

PO
• Give without regard to food. • Swallow whole with water.

Orally Disintegrating Tablet
• Open pouch, peel back foil; do not push tablet through foil. • Remove tablet with dry hands, place in mouth. • Swallow with or without water. • Use immediately after removing from package.

INDICATIONS/ROUTES/DOSAGE

Seizures
PO: ADULTS, ELDERLY, CHILDREN 10 YRS AND OLDER: Initial dose not to exceed 1.5 mg/day in 3 divided doses; may be increased

in 0.5- to 1-mg increments every 3 days until seizures are controlled or adverse effects occur. **Maintenance:** 2–8 mg/day in 1–2 divided doses. **Maximum:** 20 mg/day. **INFANTS, CHILDREN YOUNGER THAN 10 YRS OR WEIGHING LESS THAN 30 KG:** 0.01–0.03 mg/kg/day (maximum initial dose: 0.05 mg/kg/day) in 2–3 divided doses; may be increased by no more than 0.25–0.5 mg every 3 days until seizures are controlled or adverse effects occur. **Maintenance:** 0.1–0.2 mg/kg/day in 3 divided doses. **Maximum:** 0.2 mg/kg/day.

Panic Disorder

PO: ADULTS, ELDERLY: Initially, 0.25 mg twice daily. Increase in increments of 0.125–0.25 mg twice daily every 3 days. **Target dose:** 1 mg/day. **Maximum:** 4 mg/day. **Note:** Discontinue gradually by 0.125 mg twice daily q3days until completely withdrawn.

Dosage in Renal Impairment
Use caution.

Dosage in Hepatic Impairment
Mild to moderate impairment: Use with caution. **Severe impairment:** Contraindicated.

SIDE EFFECTS

Frequent (37%–11%): Mild, transient drowsiness; ataxia, behavioral disturbances (aggression, irritability, agitation), esp. in children. **Occasional (10%–5%):** Dizziness, ataxia, URI, fatigue. **Rare (4% or less):** Impaired memory, dysarthria, nervousness, sinusitis, rhinitis, constipation, allergic reaction.

ADVERSE EFFECTS/TOXIC REACTIONS

Abrupt withdrawal may result in pronounced restlessness, irritability, insomnia, hand tremors, abdominal/muscle cramps, diaphoresis, vomiting, status epilepticus. Overdose results in drowsiness, confusion, diminished reflexes, coma. **Antidote:** Flumazenil (see Appendix J for dosage).

NURSING CONSIDERATIONS

BASELINE ASSESSMENT
Review history of seizure disorder (frequency, duration, intensity, level of consciousness [LOC]). For panic attack, assess motor responses (agitation, trembling, tension), autonomic responses (cold/clammy hands, diaphoresis).

INTERVENTION/EVALUATION
Observe for excess sedation, respiratory depression, suicidal ideation. Assess children, elderly for paradoxical reaction, particularly during early therapy. Initiate seizure precautions, observe frequently for recurrence of seizure activity. Assist with ambulation if drowsiness, ataxia occur. For pts on long-term therapy, CBC, BMP, LFT should be performed periodically. Evaluate for therapeutic response: decreased intensity and frequency of seizures or, if used in panic attack, calm facial expression, decreased restlessness.

PATIENT/FAMILY TEACHING
• Avoid tasks that require alertness, motor skills until response to drug is established. • Do not abruptly discontinue medication after long-term therapy. • Strict maintenance of drug therapy is essential for seizure control. • Avoid alcohol. • Report depression, thoughts of suicide/self-harm, excessive drowsiness, GI symptoms, worsening or loss of seizure control.

cloNIDine

klon-i-deen
(Apo-CloNIDine ✦, Catapres, Catapres-TTS, Dixarit ✦, Duraclon, Kapvay, Novo-CloNIDine ✦)
■ **BLACK BOX ALERT** ■ Epidural: Not to be used for perioperative, obstetric, or postpartum pain. Must dilute concentrated epidural injectable (500 mcg/mL) prior to use.

C

Do not confuse Catapres with
Cataflam, or cloNIDine with
clomiPHENE, clonazepam,
KlonoPIN, or quiNIDine.

◆CLASSIFICATION

PHARMACOTHERAPEUTIC: Alpha₂-adrenergic agonist. **CLINICAL:** Antihypertensive.

USES

Immediate-Release, Transdermal Patch: Treatment of hypertension alone or in combination with other antihypertensive agents. **Kapvay:** Treatment of attention-deficit hyperactivity disorder (ADHD). **Epidural:** Combined with opiates for relief of severe cancer pain. **OFF-LABEL:** Opioid or nicotine withdrawal, prevention of migraine headaches, treatment of diarrhea in diabetes mellitus, treatment of dysmenorrhea, menopausal flushing, alcohol dependence, glaucoma, cloZAPine-induced sialorrhea, Tourette's syndrome, insomnia in children.

PRECAUTIONS

Contraindications: Hypersensitivity to cloNIDine. **Epidural:** Contraindicated in pts with bleeding diathesis or infection at the injection site; pts receiving anticoagulation therapy. **Cautions:** Depression, elderly. Severe coronary insufficiency, recent MI, cerebrovascular disease, chronic renal impairment, preexisting bradycardia, sinus node dysfunction, conduction disturbances; concurrent use with digoxin, diltiaZEM, metoprolol, verapamil.

ACTION

Stimulates alpha₂-adrenergic receptors, reducing sympathetic CNS response. **Epidural:** Prevents pain signal transmission to brain and produces analgesia at pre- and post-alpha-adrenergic receptors in spinal cord. **ADHD:** Mechanism of action unknown. **Therapeutic Effect:** Reduces peripheral resistance; decreases B/P, heart rate. Produces analgesia.

PHARMACOKINETICS

Route	Onset	Peak	Duration
PO	0.5–1 hr	2–4 hrs	6–10 hrs

Well absorbed from GI tract. Transdermal best absorbed from chest and upper arm; least absorbed from thigh. Protein binding: 20%–40%. Metabolized in liver. Primarily excreted in urine. Minimally removed by hemodialysis. **Half-life:** 6–20 hrs (increased in renal impairment).

⧗ LIFESPAN CONSIDERATIONS

Pregnancy/Lactation: Crosses placenta. Distributed in breast milk. **Children:** More sensitive to effects; use caution. **Elderly:** Not recommended in elderly due to high risk of CNS adverse effects, orthostatic hypotension. Avoid as first-line antihypertensive.

INTERACTIONS

DRUG: Discontinuation of concurrent **beta-blocker (e.g., carvedilol, metoprolol)** therapy may increase risk of cloNIDine-withdrawal hypertensive crisis. **Tricyclic antidepressants (e.g., amitriptyline, doxepin, nortriptyline)** may decrease effect (may require increased dose of cloNIDine). **Digoxin, diltiaZEM, metoprolol, verapamil** may increase risk of serious bradycardia. **HERBAL: Gotu kola, kava kava, SAMe, St. John's wort, valerian** may increase CNS depression. **Ephedra, ginseng, yohimbe** may decrease antihypertensive effect. **FOOD:** None known. **LAB VALUES:** None significant.

AVAILABILITY (Rx)

Injection Solution (Duraclon): 100 mcg/mL, 500 mcg/mL. **Tablets (Catapres):** 0.1 mg, 0.2 mg, 0.3 mg. **(Kapvay):** 0.1 mg, 0.2 mg. **Transdermal Patch (Catapres-TTS):** 2.5 mg (release at 0.1 mg/24 hrs), 5 mg (release at 0.2 mg/24 hrs), 7.5 mg (release at 0.3 mg/24 hrs).

 Extended-Release Tablets: (Kapvay): 0.1 mg.

ADMINISTRATION/HANDLING

PO

• Give without regard to food. • Tablets may be crushed. • Give last oral dose just before bedtime. • Swallow extended-release tablets whole; do not break, crush, dissolve, or divide.

Transdermal

• Apply transdermal system to dry, hairless area of intact skin on upper arm or chest. • Rotate sites (prevents skin irritation). • Do not trim patch to adjust dose.

Epidural

• Must be administered only by medical personnel trained in epidural management.

▧ IV INCOMPATIBILITIES

None known.

▧ IV COMPATIBILITIES

Bupivacaine (Marcaine, Sensorcaine), fentaNYL (Sublimaze), heparin, ketamine (Ketalar), lidocaine, LORazepam (Ativan).

INDICATIONS/ROUTES/DOSAGE

Hypertension

PO: ADULTS: (Immediate Release): Initially, 0.1 mg twice a day. Increase by 0.1–0.2 mg q2–4days. **Maintenance:** 0.2–1.2 mg/day in 2–4 divided doses up to maximum of 2.4 mg/day. **ELDERLY:** Initially, 0.1 mg at bedtime. May increase gradually. **CHILDREN 12 YRS AND OLDER:** Initially, 0.2 mg/day in 2 divided doses. May increase gradually at 5- to 7-day intervals in 0.1 mg/day increments. **Maximum:** 2.4 mg/day. **Transdermal: ADULTS, ELDERLY:** Initially, system delivering 0.1 mg/24 hrs applied once q7days. May increase by 0.1 mg at 1- to 2-wk intervals. Usual dosage range: 0.1–0.3 mg once wkly.

Acute Hypertension

PO: ADULTS: Initially, 0.1–0.2 mg followed by 0.1 mg every hr if necessary, up to maximum total dose of 0.7 mg.

Attention-Deficit Hyperactivity Disorder (ADHD)

PO: CHILDREN 45 KG OR LESS: (Immediate Release): Initially 0.05 mg/day at bedtime. May increase in increments of 0.05 mg/day q3–7days up to 0.2 mg/day (27–40.5 kg), 0.3 mg/day (40.5–45 kg). **GREATER THAN 45 KG: (Immediate Release):** 0.1 mg at bedtime. May increase 0.1 mg/day q3–7 days. **Maximum:** 0.4 mg/day. **Extended-Release Tablet** *(Kapvay):* **CHILDREN 6 YRS AND OLDER:** Initially, 0.1 mg daily at bedtime. May increase in increments of 0.1 mg/day at wkly intervals (**Maximum:** 0.4 mg/day). Doses should be taken twice daily with higher split dose given at bedtime.

Severe Pain

Epidural: ADULTS, ELDERLY: 30–40 mcg/hr. **CHILDREN:** Range: 0.5–2 mcg/kg/hr, not to exceed adult dose.

Dosage in Renal/Hepatic Impairment

No dose adjustment.

SIDE EFFECTS

Frequent (40%–10%): Dry mouth, drowsiness, dizziness, sedation, constipation. **Occasional (5%–1%): Tablets, Injection:** Depression, pedal edema, loss of appetite, decreased sexual function, itching eyes, dizziness, nausea, vomiting, nervousness. **Transdermal:** Pruritus, redness or darkening of skin. **Rare (less than 1%):** Nightmares, vivid dreams, feeling of coldness in distal extremities (esp. the digits).

ADVERSE EFFECTS/TOXIC REACTIONS

Overdose produces profound hypotension, irritability, bradycardia, respiratory depression, hypothermia, miosis (pupillary constriction), arrhythmias, apnea. Abrupt withdrawal may result in rebound hypertension associated with nervousness, agitation, anxiety, insomnia, paresthesia, tremor, flushing, diaphoresis. May produce sedation in pts with acute CVA.

NURSING CONSIDERATIONS

BASELINE ASSESSMENT

Obtain B/P immediately before each dose is administered, in addition to regular monitoring (be alert to B/P fluctuations).

INTERVENTION/EVALUATION

Monitor B/P, pulse, mental status. Monitor daily pattern of bowel activity, stool consistency. If cloNIDine is to be withdrawn, discontinue concurrent beta-blocker therapy several days before discontinuing cloNIDine (prevents cloNIDine withdrawal hypertensive crisis). Slowly reduce cloNIDine dosage over 2–4 days.

PATIENT/FAMILY TEACHING

• Sugarless gum, sips of water may relieve dry mouth. • Avoid tasks that require alertness, motor skills until response to drug is established. • To reduce hypotensive effect, rise slowly from lying to standing. • Skipping doses or voluntarily discontinuing drug may produce severe rebound hypertension. • Avoid alcohol. • If patch loosens during 7-day application period, secure with adhesive cover.

---

clopidogrel TOP 100　HIGH ALERT

kloe-**pid**-oh-grel
(Apo-Clopidogrel ✦, <u>Plavix</u>)

■ **BLACK BOX ALERT** ■ Diminished effectiveness in CYP2C19 metabolizers increases risk for cardiovascular events. Pts with CYP2C19*2 and/or CYP2C19*3 alleles may have reduced platelet inhibition. **Do not confuse Plavix with Elavil or Paxil.**

◆CLASSIFICATION

PHARMACOTHERAPEUTIC: Thienopyridine derivative. **CLINICAL:** Antiplatelet.

USES

To decrease rate of MI and stroke in pts with non–ST-segment elevation acute coronary syndrome (ACS), acute ST-elevation MI (STEMI); pts with history of recent MI or stroke, established peripheral arterial disease (PAD). **OFF-LABEL:** Graft patency (saphenous vein), stable coronary artery disease (in combination with aspirin). Initial treatment of ACS in pts allergic to aspirin.

PRECAUTIONS

Contraindications: Hypersensitivity to clopidogrel. Active bleeding (e.g., peptic ulcer, intracranial hemorrhage). **Cautions:** Severe hepatic/renal impairment, pts at risk of increased bleeding (e.g., trauma), concurrent use of anticoagulants. Avoid concurrent use of CYP2C19 inhibitors (e.g., omeprazole).

ACTION

Inhibits binding of enzyme adenosine phosphate (ADP) to its platelet receptor and subsequent ADP-mediated activation of a glycoprotein complex. **Therapeutic Effect:** Inhibits platelet aggregation.

PHARMACOKINETICS

Route	Onset	Peak	Duration
PO	2 hrs	5–7 days (with repeated doses of 75 mg/day)	5 days after last dose

Rapidly absorbed. Protein binding: 98%. Metabolized in liver. Eliminated equally in the urine and feces. **Half-life:** 8 hrs.

⌛ LIFESPAN CONSIDERATIONS

Pregnancy/Lactation: Unknown if drug crosses placenta or is distributed in breast milk. **Children:** Safety and efficacy not established. **Elderly:** No age-related precautions noted.

INTERACTIONS

DRUG: Aspirin, NSAIDs (e.g., ibuprofen, ketorolac, naproxen), warfarin may increase risk of bleeding. **Proton pump inhibitors (e.g., omeprazole, pantoprazole) may decrease efficacy, increase risk of cardiovascular events.** **HERBAL: Cat's claw, dong quai, evening**

primrose, **feverfew, garlic, ginger, ginkgo, ginseng, green tea, red clover** may have additive antiplatelet effects. **FOOD: Grapefruit products** may decrease effects. **LAB VALUES:** May increase serum bilirubin, ALT, AST, cholesterol, uric acid. May decrease neutrophil count, platelet count.

AVAILABILITY (Rx)

Tablets: 75 mg, 300 mg.

ADMINISTRATION/HANDLING

PO
• Give without regard to food. • Avoid grapefruit products.

INDICATIONS/ROUTES/DOSAGE

Recent MI, Stroke, PAD
PO: ADULTS, ELDERLY: 75 mg once daily.

Acute Coronary Syndrome (ACS), Unstable Angina/NSTEMI
PO: ADULTS, ELDERLY: Initially, loading dose of 300–600 mg, then 75 mg once daily (in combination with aspirin for up to 12 months, then aspirin indefinitely).

ACS (STEMI)
Note: Continue for at least 14 days up to 12 months.
PO: ADULTS, ELDERLY 75 YRS OR YOUNGER: Initially 300-mg loading dose, then 75 mg once daily. **ELDERLY OLDER THAN 75 YRS:** 75 mg once daily.

ACS (PCI)
PO: ADULTS, ELDERLY: Initially, 600 mg, then 75 mg once daily (in combination with aspirin) for at least 12 months.

Dosage in Renal Impairment
No dose adjustment.

Dosage in Hepatic Impairment
Use caution.

SIDE EFFECTS

Frequent (15%): Skin disorders. **Occasional (8%–6%):** Upper respiratory tract infection, chest pain, flu-like symptoms, headache, dizziness, arthralgia. **Rare (5%–3%):** Fatigue, edema, hypertension, abdominal pain, dyspepsia, diarrhea, nausea, epistaxis, dyspnea, rhinitis.

ADVERSE EFFECTS/TOXIC REACTIONS

Agranulocytosis, aplastic anemia/pancytopenia, thrombotic thrombocytopenic purpura (TTP) occur rarely. Hepatitis, hypersensitivity reaction, anaphylactoid reaction have been reported.

NURSING CONSIDERATIONS

BASELINE ASSESSMENT

Obtain baseline chemistries, platelet count, PFA. Perform platelet counts before drug therapy, q2days during first wk of treatment, and wkly thereafter until therapeutic maintenance dose is reached. Abrupt discontinuation of drug therapy produces elevated platelet count within 5 days.

INTERVENTION/EVALUATION

Monitor platelet count for evidence of thrombocytopenia. Assess Hgb, Hct, for evidence of bleeding; serum ALT, AST, bilirubin, BUN, creatinine; signs/symptoms of hepatic insufficiency during therapy.

PATIENT/FAMILY TEACHING

• It may take longer to stop bleeding during drug therapy. • Report any unusual bleeding. • Inform physicians, dentists if clopidogrel is being taken, esp. before surgery is scheduled or before taking any new drug.

cloZAPine

kloe-za-peen
(Apo-CloZAPine ✤, Clozaril, FazaClo, Versacloz)

■ **BLACK BOX ALERT** ■ Significant risk of life-threatening agranulocytosis, increased risk of potentially fatal cardiovascular events, particularly myocarditis, in elderly pts with dementia-related psychosis. May cause severe orthostatic hypotension,

C

bradycardia, syncope, cardiac arrest, dose-dependent seizures.

Do not confuse cloZAPine with clonazePAM, cloNIDine, or KlonoPIN, or Clozaril with Clinoril or Colazal.

◆CLASSIFICATION

PHARMACOTHERAPEUTIC: Second-generation (atypical) antipsychotic. **CLINICAL:** Antipsychotic.

USES

Management of severely ill schizophrenic pts who have failed to respond to other antipsychotic therapy. Treatment of recurrent suicidal behavior in schizophrenia or schizoaffective disorder. **OFF-LABEL:** Schizoaffective disorder, bipolar disorder, childhood psychosis, obsessive-compulsive disorder, agitation related to Alzheimer's dementia.

PRECAUTIONS

Contraindications: Hypersensitivity to cloZAPine. History of cloZAPine-induced agranulocytosis or severe granulocytopenia. **Cautions:** History of seizures, cardiovascular disease, myocarditis, respiratory/hepatic/renal impairment, alcohol withdrawal, high risk of suicide, paralytic ileus, myasthenia gravis, pts at risk for aspiration pneumonia, urinary retention, narrow-angle glaucoma, prostatic hypertrophy, xerostomia, visual disturbances, constipation, history of bowel obstruction, diabetes mellitus. History of long QT prolongation/ventricular arrhythmias; concomitant use of medications that prolong QT interval; hypokalemia, hypomagnesemia.

ACTION

Interferes with binding of DOPamine and serotonin receptor sites. **Therapeutic Effect:** Diminishes schizophrenic behavior.

PHARMACOKINETICS

Readily absorbed from GI tract. Protein binding: 97%. Metabolized in liver. Excreted in urine. **Half-life:** 12 hrs.

LIFESPAN CONSIDERATIONS

Pregnancy/Lactation: Crosses placenta. Avoid use during pregnancy. Distributed in breast milk. Breastfeeding not recommended. **Children:** Not recommended for use. **Elderly:** Avoid use in pts with dementia.

INTERACTIONS

DRUG: Antihypertensive medications (e.g., amLODIPine, lisinopril, valsartan) may increase risk of hypotension. **Alcohol, other CNS depressants (e.g., lorazepam, morphine, zolpidem)** may increase CNS depressant effects. **Bone marrow depressants** may increase myelosuppression. **Cimetidine, citalopram, ciprofloxacin, erythromycin** may increase concentration, risk of adverse effects. **SSRIs (e.g., PARoxetine)** may increase concentration. **Lithium** may increase risk of confusion, dyskinesia, seizures. **Medications prolonging QT interval (e.g., amiodarone, azithromycin, ciprofloxacin, haloperidol)** may increase risk of QT prolongation. **CYP3A4 inducers (e.g., phenytoin, carBAMazepine, rifAMPin)** may decrease concentration/effects. **HERBAL: St. John's wort** may decrease concentration/therapeutic effects. **Kava kava, gotu kola, valerian, St. John's wort** may increase risk of CNS depression. **FOOD:** None known. **LAB VALUES:** May increase serum glucose, cholesterol (rare), triglycerides (rare).

AVAILABILITY (Rx)

Suspension, Oral (Versacloz): 50 mg/mL (100 mL). **Tablets (Clozaril):** 25 mg, 50 mg, 100 mg, 200 mg. **Tablets (Orally Disintegrating [FazaClo]):** 12.5 mg, 25 mg, 100 mg, 150 mg, 200 mg.

ADMINISTRATION/HANDLING

PO
• Give without regard to food. • **Suspension:** Use oral syringes (provided). Shake well, administer dose immediately after preparing. Suspension stable for 100 days after initial bottle opening.

Orally Disintegrating Tablets
• Remove from foil blister; do not push tablet through foil. • Remove tablet with dry hands, place in mouth. • Allow to dissolve in mouth; swallow with saliva. • If dose requires splitting tablet, discard unused portion.

INDICATIONS/ROUTES/DOSAGE

Schizophrenic Disorders
◄ALERT► For initiation of therapy, must have WBC equal to or greater than 3,500 cells/mm³ and ANC equal to or greater than 1,500 cells/mm³. 1,000 cells/mm³ or greater in pts with documented benign ethnic neutropenia (BEN).

PO: ADULTS: Initially, 12.5 mg once or twice daily. May increase by 25–50 mg/day over 2 wks until target dose of 300–450 mg/day is achieved. May further increase by 50–100 mg/day no more than once or twice wkly. Range: 200–600 mg/day. **Maximum:** 900 mg/day. **ELDERLY:** Initially, 12.5 mg/day for 3 days, then 25 mg/day for 3 days. May further increase in increments of 12.5–25 mg daily q3days. **Mean dose:** 300 mg/day. **Maximum:** 700 mg/day.

Suicidal Behavior in Schizophrenia or Schizoaffective Disorder
PO: ADULTS: Initially, 12.5 mg 1–2 times/day. May increase in increments of 25–50 mg/day to a target dose of 300–450 mg/day after 2 wks. **Mean dose:** 300 mg/day. **Maximum:** 900 mg/day.

Dose Modification
Leukopenia/granulocytopenia: Mild: (WBC 3,000–3,500 cells/mm³ and/or ANC 1,500–2,000 cells/mm³): Continue treatment, monitor WBC and ANC twice wkly until WBC greater than 3,500 cells/mm³ and ANC greater than 2,000 cells/mm³. **Moderate: (WBC 2,000–3,000 cells/mm³ and/or ANC greater than 1,000 cells/mm³–1,500 cells/mm³):** Interrupt therapy, monitor WBC and ANC daily until WBC greater than 3,000 cells/mm³ and ANC

greater than 1,500 cells/mm³, then twice wkly until WBC greater than 3,500 cells/mm³ and ANC greater than 2,000 cells/mm³. **Severe: (WBC less than 2,000 cells/mm³ and/or ANC less than 1,500 cells/mm³):** Discontinue treatment. **Discontinue:** QT$_C$ interval greater than 500 msec, cardiomyopathy/myocarditis, hepatotoxicity, or neuroleptic malignant syndrome.

Dosage in Renal/Hepatic Impairment
No dose adjustment.

SIDE EFFECTS

Frequent (39%–14%): Drowsiness, salivation, tachycardia, dizziness, constipation. **Occasional (9%–4%):** Hypotension, headache, tremor, syncope, diaphoresis, dry mouth, nausea, visual disturbances, nightmares, restlessness, akinesia, agitation, hypertension, abdominal discomfort, heartburn, weight gain. **Rare:** Rigidity, confusion, fatigue, insomnia, diarrhea, rash.

ADVERSE EFFECTS/TOXIC REACTIONS

Seizures occur occasionally (3% of pts). Overdose produces CNS depression (sedation, delirium, coma), respiratory depression, hypersalivation. Blood dyscrasias, particularly agranulocytosis, mild leukopenia, may occur.

NURSING CONSIDERATIONS

BASELINE ASSESSMENT
Obtain baseline weight, glucose, Hgb A1c, WBC, absolute neutrophil count (ANC) before initiating treatment. Assess behavior, appearance, emotional status, response to environment, speech pattern, thought content.

INTERVENTION/EVALUATION
Monitor B/P for hypertension/hypotension. Assess pulse for tachycardia (common side effect). Monitor CBC for blood dyscrasias. Monitor ANC, WBC count every wk for first 6 mos, then biweekly for 6 mos. If CBC and ANC are normal after 12 mos, then monthly monitoring of CBC and ANC is recommended. Supervise

C

suicidal-risk pt closely during early therapy (as depression lessens, energy level improves, increasing suicide potential). Assess for therapeutic response (interest in surroundings, improvement in self-care, increased ability to concentrate, relaxed facial expression).

PATIENT/FAMILY TEACHING

• Do not abruptly discontinue long-term drug therapy. • Avoid tasks that require alertness, motor skills until response to drug is established. • Drowsiness generally subsides during continued therapy. • Avoid alcohol, caffeine. • Report fever, sore throat, flu-like symptoms.

cobicistat

koe-bi-**sye**-stat
(Tybost)

FIXED-COMBINATION(S)

Evotaz: cobicistat (antiretroviral booster)/atazanavir (antiretroviral): 150 mg/300 mg. **Genvoya:** cobicistat (antiretroviral booster)/emtricitabine/elvitegravir/tenofovir (TAF) (antiretroviral agents): 150 mg/200 mg/150 mg/25 mg. **Prezcobix:** cobicistat (antiretroviral booster)/darunavir (antiretroviral): 150 mg/800 mg. **Stribild:** cobicistat (antiretroviral booster)/emtricitabine/elvitegravir/tenofovir (TDF) (antiretroviral agents): 150 mg/200 mg/150 mg/300 mg.

◆CLASSIFICATION

PHARMACOTHERAPEUTIC: CYP3A inhibitor. **CLINICAL:** Antiretroviral booster.

USES

Indicated to increase systemic exposure of atazanavir or darunavir (once-daily dosing regimen), in combination with other antiretroviral agents for treatment of HIV-1 infection.

PRECAUTIONS

Contraindications: Concomitant use with atazanavir or darunavir with alfuzosin, carbamazepine, colchicine (in pts with renal or hepatic impairment), dihydroergotamine, dronedarone, ergotamine, indinavir, irinotecan, lovastatin, methylergonovine, midazolam (oral), phenobarbital, phenytoin, pimozide, ranolazine, rifAMPin, sildenafil (use in PAH), simvastatin, St. John's wort. Concomitant use with atazanavir with indinavir, irinotecan, or nevirapine. **Cautions:** Renal impairment, hypercholesterolemia. Avoid use with nephrotoxic medications. Do not initiate in pts with CrCl less than 70 mL/min. Use with HIV-1 protease inhibitors other than atazanavir or darunavir (once daily) or more than 1 antiretroviral requiring kinetic enhancement is NOT recommended. Co-administration of cobicistat and ritonavir. Cobicistat is not interchangeable with ritonavir.

ACTION

Inhibits cytochrome P450 3A (CYP3A). **Therapeutic Effect:** Boosts exposure of atazanavir or darunavir. Does not exhibit antiviral activity.

PHARMACOKINETICS

Readily absorbed after PO administration. Metabolized in liver. Protein binding: 97%–98%. Peak plasma concentration: 3.5 hrs. Eliminated in feces (86%), urine (8%). **Half-life:** 3–4 hrs.

⊠ LIFESPAN CONSIDERATIONS

Pregnancy/Lactation: Breastfeeding not recommended due to risk of postnatal HIV transmission. **Children:** Safety and efficacy not established in pts younger than 18 yrs. **Elderly:** Safety and efficacy not established in pts older than 65 yrs. May have increased risk of side effects/adverse reactions, renal failure.

INTERACTIONS

DRUG: Note: See contraindications. **Nephrotoxic medications (e.g.,**

gentamicin, NSAIDs) may increase risk of acute renal failure. **Efavirenz, etravirine, nevirapine** may decrease cobicistat effectiveness. May increase concentration/effect of **antiarrhythmics (e.g., amiodarone, digoxin), antifungals (e.g., ketoconazole), atorvastatin, benzodiazepines, beta blockers (e.g., carvedilol, metoprolol), calcium channel blockers (e.g., amLODIPine, diltiaZEM), clarithromycin, colchicine, cycloSPORINE, fluticasone, maraviroc, neuroleptics (e.g., risperiDONE, thioridazine), opioids (e.g., morphine), PDE-5 inhibitors (e.g., sildenafil), SSRIs, tricyclic antidepressants. Antacids, anticonvulsants (e.g., carBAMazepine, phenytoin), famotidine, omeprazole** may decrease absorption/effect. **HERBAL: St. John's wort** contraindicated; may decrease effectiveness. **FOOD:** None known. **LAB VALUES:** May increase serum amylase, ALT, AST, bilirubin, BUN, cholesterol (LDL/HDL), creatine kinase (CK), creatinine, GGT, triglycerides, urine glucose; urine protein, urine RBC. May decrease CrCl.

AVAILABILITY (Rx)

Film-Coated Tablets: 150 mg.

ADMINISTRATION/HANDLING

PO
• Give with food. • Must be administered simultaneously with atazanavir or darunavir. • If pt receiving antacid with cobicistat/atazanavir regimen, do not give aluminum- or magnesium-containing antacids within 2 hrs, H₂-receptor antagonists (e.g., famotidine) within 10 hrs, or proton pump inhibitors (e.g., omeprazole) within 12 hrs of antiretroviral dose.

INDICATIONS/ROUTES/DOSAGE

HIV Infection
Note: Must be given with atazanavir or darunavir and other antiretroviral medications.

PO: ADULTS/ELDERLY: 150 mg once daily (see Uses).

Dosage in Renal Impairment
No dose adjustment. Not recommended in pts with CrCl less than 70 mL/min when used with tenofovir (TDF).

Dosage in Hepatic Impairment
Mild to moderate impairment: No dose adjustment; use caution. **Severe impairment:** Not recommended.

SIDE EFFECTS

Occasional (5%): Jaundice, dermatitis, pruritus, pustular folliculitis, rash, urticaria. **Rare (3%–2%):** Ocular icterus, nausea, diarrhea, headache, depression, abnormal dreams, insomnia.

ADVERSE EFFECTS/TOXIC REACTIONS

May cause acute renal failure or Fanconi syndrome when administered with tenofovir. Nephrolithiasis reported in 2% of pts. Pts co-infected with hepatitis B or C virus have increased risk for viral reactivation, worsening of hepatic function, or may experience hepatic decompensation and/or failure if therapy is discontinued.

NURSING CONSIDERATIONS

BASELINE ASSESSMENT
Obtain CBC, BMP, CrCl, GFR, lipid panel, LFT, serum phosphate (baseline renal impairment), urine glucose, urine protein, vital signs; CD4+ count, viral load. Screen for hepatitis B or C virus coinfection, hypercholesterolemia. Receive full medication history, including herbal products, and screen for contraindications. Question possibility of pregnancy.

INTERVENTION/EVALUATION
Diligently monitor hepatic/renal function tests. An increase in serum creatinine greater than 0.4 mg/dL from baseline may indicate renal impairment. Monitor CD4+ count, viral load for treatment effectiveness. Assess skin for urticaria, pruritus, rash. Cough, dyspnea, fever, excess of band cells on CBC may indicate acute infection (WBC test may be unreliable in pts with uncontrolled HIV infection).

• Offer emotional support. • Take cobicistat with atazanavir or darunavir at the same time each day with food (optimizes absorption). • Antacids may decrease drug effectiveness. • Drug resistance can form if therapy is interrupted; do not run out of supply. • Cobicistat does not cure HIV infection nor reduce risk of transmission. • As immune system strengthens, it may respond to dormant infections hidden within the body. Report body aches, chills, cough, fever, night sweats, shortness of breath. • Treatment may cause kidney failure if used with tenofovir regimen. Report abdominal pain, darkened urine, decreased urine output. • Clay-colored stools, significant weight loss, or yellowing of skin or eyes may indicate liver problem. • Do not take any new medications, including over-the-counter drugs or herbal products, unless approved by your doctor.

---

cobimetinib

koe-bi-**me**-ti-nib
(Cotellic)
Do not confuse cobimetinib with cabozantinib, imatinib, or trametinib.

◆CLASSIFICATION

PHARMACOTHERAPEUTIC: Kinase inhibitor. **CLINICAL:** Antineoplastic.

USES

Treatment of pts with unresectable or metastatic melanoma with a BRAF V600E or V600K mutation, in combination with vemurafenib.

PRECAUTIONS

Contraindications: Hypersensitivity to cobimetinib. **Cautions:** Baseline anemia, lymphopenia, thrombocytopenia; cardiomyopathy, hepatic/renal impairment, HF, hypertension, ocular disorders; pts at risk for bleeding (history of gastrointestinal, genitourinary, intracranial, reproductive system bleeding), electrolyte imbalance. Not recommended in pts taking moderate or strong CYP3A inhibitors.

ACTION

Inhibits mitogen-activated protein kinase/extracellular signal regulated kinase 1 (MEK1) and MEK2. Cobimetinib also prevents vemurafenib-mediated growth enhancement of a wild-type BRAF tumor cell line. **Therapeutic Effect:** Inhibits tumor cell growth and metastasis.

PHARMACOKINETICS

Widely distributed. Metabolized in liver. Protein binding: 95%. Peak plasma concentration: 2.4 hrs. Steady state reached in 9 days. Eliminated in feces (76%), urine (18%). **Half-life:** 44 hrs.

⊠ LIFESPAN CONSIDERATIONS

Pregnancy/Lactation: Avoid pregnancy; may cause fetal harm/malformations. Female pts of reproductive potential should use effective contraception during treatment and up to 2 wks after discontinuation. Unknown if distributed in breast milk. Breastfeeding not recommended. May reduce fertility in females and males. **Children:** Safety and efficacy not established. **Elderly:** Safety and efficacy not established.

INTERACTIONS

DRUG: Strong CYP3A inhibitors (e.g., clarithromycin, ketoconazole, ritonavir), moderate CYP3A inhibitors (e.g., atazanavir, ciprofloxacin) may increase concentration/effect. **Strong CYP3A inducers (e.g., carBAMazepine, rifampicin), moderate CYP3A inducers (e.g., bosentan, nafcillin)** may decrease concentration/effect. **HERBAL: St. John's wort** may decrease concentration/effect. **FOOD:** None known. **LAB VALUES:** Many increase serum alkaline phosphatase, ALT, AST, creatine phosphokinase, creatinine, GGT.

May decrease Hct, Hgb, lymphocytes, platelets, RBCs; serum albumin, calcium, sodium. May increase or decrease serum potassium.

AVAILABILITY (Rx)

Tablets: 20 mg.

ADMINISTRATION/HANDLING

PO
• Give without regard to food. • If dose is missed or vomiting occurs during administration, give next dose at regularly scheduled time.

INDICATIONS/ROUTES/DOSAGE

Metastatic Melanoma
PO: ADULTS, ELDERLY: 60 mg (three 20-mg tablets) once daily for first 21 days of 28-day cycle. Continue until disease progression or unacceptable toxicity.

Concomitant Use of CYP3A Inhibitors
Reduce dose to 20 mg once daily if short-term (14 days or less) use of moderate CYP3A inhibitors is unavoidable. May resume 60-mg once-daily dose once the short-term CYP3A inhibitor is discontinued. Use an alternative strong or moderate CYP3A inhibitor in pts already taking reduced dose of 20 mg or 40 mg daily.

Dose Modification
Based on Common Terminology Criteria for Adverse Events (CTCAE) grading 1–4. See prescribing information for vemurafenib for recommended dose modification.

Dose Reduction Schedule
First dose reduction: 40 mg once daily. **Second dose reduction:** 20 mg once daily. Permanently discontinue if unable to tolerate 20 mg once daily.

Cardiomyopathy
Asymptomatic decrease in left ventricular ejection fraction (LVEF) greater than 10% from baseline and less than institutional lower limit of normal (LLN): Withhold treatment for 2 wks, then reassess LVEF. Resume at next lower dose level if LVEF is at or above LLN and the decrease from baseline is 10% or less. Permanently discontinue if LVEF is less than LLN or the decrease from baseline LVEF is more than 10%. **Symptomatic decrease of LVEF from baseline:** Withhold treatment for up to 4 wks, then reassess LVEF. Resume at next lower dose level if symptoms resolve, LVEF is at or above LLN, and the decrease from baseline LVEF is 10% or less. Permanently discontinue if symptoms persist, LVEF is less than LLN, or the decrease from baseline LVEF is more than 10%.

Dermatologic Reactions
Grade 2 (intolerable); grade 3 or 4: Withhold or reduce dose.

Hepatotoxicity or Hepatic Laboratory Abnormalities
First occurrence, grade 4: Withhold treatment for up to 4 wks. If improved to grade 0 or 1, resume at next lower dose level. If not improved to grade 0 or 1 within 4 wks, permanently discontinue. **Recurrent grade 4:** Permanently discontinue.

Hemorrhage
Grade 3: Withhold treatment for up to 4 wks. If not improved to grade 0 or 1, resume at next lower dose level. If not improved within 4 wks, permanently discontinue. **Grade 4:** Permanently discontinue.

New Primary Malignancies (Cutaneous or Noncutaneous)
No dose adjustment.

Nonspecific Adverse Effects
Any intolerable grade 2; any grade 3: Withhold for up to 4 wks. If improved to grade 0 or 1, resume at next lower dose level. If not improved within 4 wks, permanently discontinue. **First occurrence of any grade 4:** Permanently discontinue.

Ocular Toxicities
Serious retinopathy: Withhold treatment for up to 4 wks. If signs and symptoms improve, resume at next lower dose level. If not improved or symptoms recur at the lower dose within 4 wks, permanently discontinue. **Retinal vein occlusion:** Permanently discontinue.

Photosensitivity
Grade 2 (intolerable); grade 3 or 4: Withhold treatment for up to 4 wks. If improved to grade 0 or 1, resume at next lower dose level. If not improved within 4 wks, permanently discontinue.

Rhabdomyolysis, CPK Level Elevations
Grade 4 CPK elevation or any CPK elevation with myalgia: Withhold treatment for up to 4 wks. If improved to grade 3 or lower, resume at next lower dose level. If not improved within 4 wks, permanently discontinue.

Severe Hypersensitivity Reaction
Permanently discontinue.

Renal Impairment
Mild to moderate impairment: No dose adjustment. **Severe impairment:** Not specified; use caution.

Hepatic Impairment
Mild impairment: No dose adjustment. **Moderate to severe impairment:** Not specified; use caution.

SIDE EFFECTS

Frequent (60%–24%): Diarrhea, photosensitivity, sunburn, solar dermatitis, nausea, pyrexia, vomiting. **Occasional (16%–10%):** Acneiform dermatitis, stomatitis, aphthous stomatitis, mouth ulceration, mucosal inflammation, alopecia, hypertension, vision impairment, blurred vision, reduced visual acuity, hyperkeratosis, erythema, chills.

ADVERSE EFFECTS/TOXIC REACTIONS

Anemia, lymphopenia, thrombocytopenia is an expected response to therapy. New primary malignancies, including squamous cell carcinoma, keratoacanthoma, secondary-primary melanomas, were reported. Serious, sometimes fatal hemorrhagic events, including GI bleeding (4% of pts), intracranial bleeding (1% of pts), hematuria (2% of pts), reproductive system hemorrhage (2% of pts), have occurred. Other hemorrhagic events may include cerebral/conjunctival/intracranial/gingival/hemorrhoidal/ovarian/pulmonary/rectal/uterine/vaginal bleeding; ecchymosis, epistaxis. Grade 3 or 4 cardiomyopathy reported in 26% of pts. Grade 3 or 4 skin reactions including severe rash occurred in 16% of pts. Ocular toxicities, including retinopathy, chorioretinopathy, retinal detachment, reported in 26% of pts. Grade 3 or 4 CPK level elevations occurred in 14% of pts and may lead to rhabdomyolysis. Hepatotoxicity reported in 7%–11% of pts. Severe photosensitivity reported in 47% of pts.

NURSING CONSIDERATIONS

BASELINE ASSESSMENT

Confirm presence of BRAF V600E or V600K mutation in tumor specimen prior to initiation. Obtain baseline CBC, BMP, LFT, CPK; serum albumin, magnesium, phosphate, ionized calcium; urine pregnancy; vital signs. Obtain ophthalmologic exam with visual acuity; EKG, echocardiogram for LVEF. Assess skin for moles, lesions, papillomas. Verify use of effective contraception in female pts of reproductive potential. Receive full medication history, including herbal products. Question history as listed in Precautions. Assess hydration status.

INTERVENTION/EVALUATION

Monitor CBC, BMP, LFT, CPK; serum albumin, magnesium, phosphate, ionized calcium; vital signs. Assess skin for new lesions, dermal toxicities at least q2mos during treatment and for least 6 mos after discontinuation. Assess LVEF by

C

echocardiogram 1 mo after initiation, then q3mos thereafter until discontinuation. If treatment interrupted due to change in LVEF, monitor LVEF at 2 wks, 4 wks, 10 wks, and 16 wks, and then as indicated. Conduct ophthalmologic examinations regularly, esp. with any new or worsening visual disturbances. Assess for eye pain, visual changes. Immediately report GI bleeding, hematuria, unusual reproductive system hemorrhage; symptoms of intracranial bleeding (aphasia, blindness, confusion, facial droop, hemiplegia, seizures). Monitor for hepatotoxicity; monitor for signs of rhabdomyolysis, such as dark-colored urine, flank pain, decreased urine output, muscle aches. Due to high risk of diarrhea, strictly monitor I&O.

PATIENT/FAMILY TEACHING

• Blood levels monitoring, cardiac function tests, eye exams, skin exams will be conducted frequently. • Treatment may lead to severe anemia, HF, kidney failure, new cancers, severe light sensitivity, liver dysfunction, skin toxicities (such as severe rash, peeling), vision changes. • Report bloody stools, bloody urine, unusual reproductive system bleeding, nose bleeds, coughing up blood; abdominal or flank pain, dark-colored urine, decreased urinary output; strokelike symptoms; new skin moles or lesions, rash; eye pain, vision changes; heart problems such as shortness of breath, dizziness, fainting, palpitations. • Report any newly prescribed medications. • Avoid sunlight, tanning beds. Wear protective clothing, high-SPF sunscreen, and lip balm when outdoors. • Treatment may cause fetal harm. Women of childbearing potential should use effective contraception during treatment and up to 2 wks after last dose. Immediately report suspected pregnancy. Do not breastfeed. Treatment may reduce fertility.

codeine

koe-deen
(Codeine Contin ✤)

■ **BLACK BOX ALERT** ■ Respiratory depression, death have occurred in children following tonsillectomy and/or adenoidectomy.
Do not confuse codeine with Cardene or Lodine.

FIXED-COMBINATION(S)

Capital with Codeine, Tylenol with Codeine: acetaminophen/codeine: 120 mg/12 mg per 5 mL. **Tylenol with Codeine:** acetaminophen/codeine: 300 mg/15 mg, 300 mg/30 mg, 300 mg/60 mg.

◆CLASSIFICATION

PHARMACOTHERAPEUTIC: Opioid agonist. **Schedule II** (single entity). **Schedule III** (Fixed combination). **CLINICAL:** Analgesic.

USES

Relief of mild to moderate pain. **OFF-LABEL:** Short-term relief of cough.

PRECAUTIONS

Contraindications: Hypersensitivity to codeine. Respiratory depression in absence of resuscitative equipment, acute or severe bronchial asthma or hypercarbia, paralytic ileus. Postoperative pain management in children following tonsillectomy/adenoidectomy. **Cautions:** Adrenal insufficiency, biliary tract impairment, CNS depression/coma, morbid obesity, prostatic hyperplasia, urinary stricture, thyroid dysfunction, severe renal/hepatic impairment, COPD, respiratory disease, cardiovascular disease, hypovolemia, GI obstruction, head injury, elevated intracranial pressure, history of drug abuse, patients with 2 or more copies of variant CYP2D6*2 allele (may have extensive conversion to morphine), elderly, debilitated pts, seizure disorder, acute alcoholism.

ACTION

Binds to opioid receptors in CNS. Inhibits ascending pain pathways. **Therapeutic Effect:** Alters perception, emotional response to pain; suppresses cough reflex.

PHARMACOKINETICS

Route	Onset	Peak	Duration
PO	30–60 min	1–1.5 hrs	4–6 hrs
IM	10–30 min	0.5–1 hr	4–6 hrs

Well absorbed following PO administration. Protein binding: 7%–25%. Metabolized in liver. Excreted in urine. **Half-life:** 2.5–3.5 hrs.

LIFESPAN CONSIDERATIONS

Pregnancy/Lactation: Birth defects associated with maternal use of codeine during first trimester. Excreted in breast milk. Breastfeeding not recommended. Nonopioid analgesics recommended for postpartum pain. **Children:** Efficacy not established in pts younger than 2 yrs. **Elderly:** May cause confusion, oversedation; use lower dosing range.

INTERACTIONS

DRUG: **Alcohol, other CNS depressants (e.g., lorazepam, morphine, zolpidem)** may increase CNS, respiratory depression, hypotension. **Anticholinergics** may increase risk of urinary retention, severe constipation. **MAOIs (e.g., phenelzine, selegiline)** may produce a severe, sometimes fatal reaction (reduce dosage to ¼ usual dose). **HERBAL: St. John's wort** may decrease concentration. **Gotu kola, kava kava, SAMe, St. John's wort, valerian** may increase CNS depression. **FOOD:** None known. **LAB VALUES:** May increase serum amylase, lipase.

AVAILABILITY (Rx)

Tablets: 15 mg, 30 mg, 60 mg.

ADMINISTRATION/HANDLING

PO
• May give without regard to food.
• Take with food or milk to decrease adverse GI effects.

INDICATIONS/ROUTES/DOSAGE

◄**ALERT**► Reduce initial dosage in pts with hypothyroidism, Addison's disease, renal insufficiency, pts using other CNS depressants concurrently. Respiratory depression and death have occurred in children receiving codeine following tonsillectomy and/or adenoidectomy and found to have evidence of being ultrarapid metabolizers of codeine due to a CYP2D6 polymorphism.

Analgesia
PO: ADULTS, ELDERLY: 15–60 mg q4h as needed. **Maximum total daily dose:** 360 mg. **CHILDREN:** 0.5–1 mg/kg q4–6h. **Maximum:** 60 mg/dose.

Dosage in Renal Impairment
Dosage is modified based on creatinine clearance.

Creatinine Clearance	Dosage
10–50 mL/min	75% of usual dose
Less than 10 mL/min	50% of usual dose
CRRT	75% of usual dose

Dosage in Hepatic Impairment
Use caution.

SIDE EFFECTS

◄**ALERT**► Ambulatory pts, pts not in severe pain may experience dizziness, nausea, vomiting, hypotension more frequently than those in supine position or with severe pain. **Frequent:** Constipation, drowsiness, nausea, vomiting. **Occasional:** Paradoxical excitement, confusion, palpitations, facial flushing, decreased urination, blurred vision, dizziness, dry mouth, headache, hypotension (including orthostatic hypotension), decreased appetite, injection site redness, burning, or pain. **Rare:** Hallucinations, depression, abdominal pain, insomnia.

ADVERSE EFFECTS/TOXIC REACTIONS

Chronic use may result in paralytic ileus. Overdose may produce cold/clammy skin, confusion, seizures, decreased B/P, restlessness, pinpoint pupils, bradycardia, respiratory depression, decreased

LOC, severe weakness. Tolerance to drug's analgesic effect, physical dependence may occur with chronic use.

NURSING CONSIDERATIONS

BASELINE ASSESSMENT

Analgesic: Assess onset, type, location, duration of pain. Effect of medication is reduced if full pain response recurs before next dose. **Antitussive:** Assess type, severity, frequency of cough, sputum production.

INTERVENTION/EVALUATION

Monitor daily pattern of bowel activity, stool consistency. Increase fluid intake, environmental humidity to improve viscosity of lung secretions. Initiate deep breathing, coughing exercises. Assess for clinical improvement; record onset of relief of pain, cough.

PATIENT/FAMILY TEACHING

• Change positions slowly to avoid orthostatic hypotension. • Avoid tasks that require alertness, motor skills until response to drug is established. • Tolerance, dependence may occur with prolonged use of high dosages. • Avoid alcohol.

---

colchicine ![HIGH ALERT]

kol-chi-seen
(Colcrys, Mitigare)
Do not confuse colchicine with Cortrosyn.

◆**CLASSIFICATION**

PHARMACOTHERAPEUTIC: Alkaloid.
CLINICAL: Antigout.

USES

Prevention, treatment of acute gouty arthritis. Used to reduce frequency of recurrence of familial Mediterranean fever (FMF). **OFF-LABEL:** Treatment of biliary cirrhosis, recurrent pericarditis.

PRECAUTIONS

Contraindications: Hypersensitivity to colchicine. Concomitant use of a P-glycoprotein (e.g., cycloSPORINE) or strong CYP3A4 inhibitor (e.g., clarithromycin) in presence of renal or hepatic impairment. **Mitigare:** Pts with both renal/hepatic impairment. **Cautions:** Hepatic impairment, elderly, debilitated pts, renal impairment. Concomitant use of cycloSPORINE, diltiaZEM, verapamil, fibrates, statins may increase risk of myopathy.

ACTION

Decreases leukocyte motility, phagocytosis, lactic acid production. **Therapeutic Effect:** Reduces inflammatory process.

PHARMACOKINETICS

Rapidly absorbed from GI tract. Oral bioavailability: 45%. Highest concentration is in liver, spleen, kidney. Protein binding: 30%–50%. Re-enters intestinal tract by biliary secretion and is reabsorbed from intestines. Partially metabolized in liver via CYP3A4. Eliminated primarily in feces. **Half-life:** 27–31 hrs.

▧ LIFESPAN CONSIDERATIONS

Pregnancy/Lactation: Drug crosses placenta and is distributed in breast milk. **Children:** Safety and efficacy not established. **Elderly:** May be more susceptible to cumulative toxicity. Age-related renal impairment may increase risk of myopathy.

INTERACTIONS

DRUG: May increase concentration of **statins** and increase risk of rhabdomyolysis. **Atazanavir, clarithromycin, cycloSPORINE, diltiaZEM, erythromycin, fluconazole, fosamprenavir, indinavir, ketoconazole, ranolazine, ritonavir, saquinavir, verapamil** may increase colchicine concentration, toxicity. **HERBAL:** None significant. **FOOD: Grapefruit products** may increase concentration/toxicity. **LAB VALUES:** May increase serum alkaline phosphatase, AST. May decrease platelet count.

AVAILABILITY (Rx)

Tablets (Colcrys): 0.6 mg. **Capsule (Mitigare):** 0.6 mg.

ADMINISTRATION/HANDLING
PO
• Give without regard to food. • For FMF, give in 1 or 2 divided doses. • Give with adequate water and maintain fluid intake.

INDICATIONS/ROUTES/DOSAGE
Acute Gouty Arthritis (Colcrys)
PO: ADULTS, ELDERLY: Initially, 1.2 mg at first sign of gout flare, then 0.6 mg 1 hr later. **Maximum:** 1.8 mg within 1 hr. **Coadministration with strong CYP3A4 inhibitors:** Initially, 0.6 mg, then 0.3 mg dose 1 hr later. Do not repeat for at least 3 days. **Coadministration with moderate CYP3A4 inhibitors:** 1.2 mg once. Do not repeat for at least 3 days. **Coadministration with P-glycoprotein inhibitors:** 0.6 mg once. Do not repeat for at least 3 days.

Gout Prophylaxis (Colcrys, Mitigare)
Note: Duration of prophylaxis is 6 mos or 3 mos (pts without tophi) to 6 mos (pts with 1 or more tophi)
PO: ADULTS, ELDERLY: 0.6 mg 1–2 times/day. **Maximum:** 1.2 mg/day. **Coadministration with strong CYP3A4 inhibitors:** If dose is 0.6 mg 2 times/day, adjust dose to 0.3 mg once daily; if dose is 0.6 mg once daily, adjust dose to 0.3 mg every other day. **Coadministration with moderate CYP3A4 inhibitors:** If dose is 0.6 mg 2 times/day, adjust dose to 0.3 mg twice daily or 0.6 mg once daily; if dose is 0.6 mg once daily, adjust dose to 0.3 mg once daily. **Coadministration with P-glycoprotein inhibitors:** If dose is 0.6 mg 2 times/day, adjust dose to 0.3 mg once daily; if dose is 0.6 mg once daily, adjust dose to 0.3 mg every other day.

FMF (Colcrys)
PO: ADULTS, ELDERLY, CHILDREN OLDER THAN 12 YRS: 1.2–2.4 mg/day in 1–2 divided doses. Titrate dose in 0.3-mg increments. **Coadministration with strong CYP3A4 inhibitors: Maximum:** 0.6 mg once daily (or 0.3 mg twice daily). **Coadministration with moderate CYP3A4 inhibitors:** 1.2 mg/day (0.6 mg twice daily). **Coadministration with P-glycoprotein inhibitors:** 0.6 mg once daily (or 0.3 mg twice daily). **CHILDREN 6–12 YRS:** 0.9–1.8 mg/day in 1–2 divided doses. **CHILDREN 4–5 YRS:** 0.3–1.8 mg/day in 1–2 divided doses. **Note:** Increase or decrease dose by 0.3 mg/day, not to exceed maximum dose.

Pericarditis
PO: ADULTS, ELDERLY: 0.6 mg 2 times/day.

Dosage in Renal Impairment

Creatinine Clearance	Dosage
Less than 30 mL/min	
FMF	0.3 mg initially
Gout prophylaxis	0.3 mg/day
Gout flare	No reduction
HD	
FMF	0.3 mg as single dose
Gout prophylaxis	0.3 mg 2–4 times/wk

Dosage in Hepatic Impairment
Use caution.

SIDE EFFECTS
Frequent: Nausea, vomiting, abdominal discomfort. **Occasional:** Anorexia. **Rare:** Hypersensitivity reaction, including angioedema.

ADVERSE EFFECTS/TOXIC REACTIONS

Bone marrow depression (aplastic anemia, agranulocytosis, thrombocytopenia) may occur with long-term therapy. Overdose initially causes burning feeling in skin/throat; severe diarrhea, abdominal pain. Second stage manifests as fever, seizures, delirium, renal impairment (hematuria, oliguria). Third stage causes hair loss, leukocytosis, stomatitis.

C

NURSING CONSIDERATIONS

BASELINE ASSESSMENT

Obtain baseline laboratory studies. **Gout:** Assess involved joints for pain, mobility, edema. **Mediterranean fever:** Assess abdominal pain, fever, chills, erythema, swollen skin lesions.

INTERVENTION/EVALUATION

Discontinue medication immediately if GI symptoms occur. Encourage high fluid intake (3,000 mL/day). Monitor I&O (output should be at least 2,000 mL/day), CBC, hepatic/renal function tests. Monitor serum uric acid. Assess for therapeutic response: relief of pain, stiffness, swelling; increased joint mobility; reduced joint tenderness; improved grip strength.

PATIENT/FAMILY TEACHING

• Drink 8–10 (8-oz) glasses of fluid daily while taking medication. • Report skin rash, sore throat, fever, unusual bruising/bleeding, weakness, fatigue, numbness. • Stop medication as soon as gout pain is relieved or at first sign of nausea, vomiting, diarrhea. • Avoid grapefruit products.

conjugated estrogens

kon-joo-gate-ed **ess**-troe-jenz (Premarin)

■ **BLACK BOX ALERT** ■ Risk of dementia may be increased in post-menopausal women. Do not use to prevent cardiovascular disease. May increase risk of endometrial carcinoma or invasive breast cancer in postmenopausal women.

Do not confuse Premarin with Primaxin, Provera, or Remeron.

FIXED-COMBINATION(S)

Duavee: conjugated estrogen/bazedoxifene (estrogen agonist/antagonist): 0.45 mg/20 mg.

◆CLASSIFICATION

PHARMACOTHERAPEUTIC: Estrogen. **CLINICAL:** Hormone.

USES

Management of moderate to severe vasomotor symptoms associated with menopause. Treatment of hypoestrogenism due to hypogonadism, castration, or primary ovarian failure. Prevention of osteoporosis in postmenopausal women. Palliative treatment of inoperable, progressive cancer of the prostate and breast in men, and of the breast in postmenopausal women. Abnormal uterine bleeding (injection only). Treatment of moderate to severe vulvar and vaginal atrophy due to menopause. **OFF-LABEL:** Prevention of estrogen deficiency–induced premenopausal osteoporosis. **Cream:** Prevention of nosebleeds.

PRECAUTIONS

Contraindications: Hypersensitivity to estrogens. Breast cancer (except in pts being treated for metastatic disease), hepatic disease, history of or current thrombophlebitis, undiagnosed abnormal vaginal bleeding, pregnancy, DVT or PE (current or history of), angioedema or anaphylactic reaction to estrogens, estrogen-dependent tumors. Known protein C, protein S, antithrombin deficiency or other thrombophilic disorder. **Cautions:** Asthma, epilepsy, migraine headaches, diabetes, cardiac/renal dysfunction, history of severe hypocalcemia, lupus erythematosus, porphyria, endometriosis, gallbladder disease, familial defects of lipoprotein metabolism. Hypoparathyroidism, history of cholestatic jaundice.

ACTION

Responsible for development and maintenance of female reproductive system and secondary sexual characteristics; modulates release of gonadotropin-releasing hormone, reduces follicle-stimulating hormone (FSH), luteinizing hormone (LH). **Therapeutic Effect:** Reduces elevated levels of gonadotropins, LH, and FSH.

PHARMACOKINETICS

Well absorbed from GI tract. Widely distributed. Protein binding: 50%–80%. Metabolized in liver. Primarily excreted in urine. **Half-life (total estrone):** 27 hrs.

⌛ LIFESPAN CONSIDERATIONS

Pregnancy/Lactation: Distributed in breast milk. May cause fetal harm. Breastfeeding not recommended. **Children:** Safety and efficacy not established. **Elderly:** No age-related precautions noted.

INTERACTIONS

DRUG: None significant. **HERBAL: Black cohosh, dong quai** may increase estrogenic activity. **Ginseng, red clover, saw palmetto** may increase hormonal effects. **St. John's wort** may decrease concentration. **FOOD: Grapefruit products** may increase concentration/toxicity. **LAB VALUES:** May increase serum glucose, HDL, calcium, triglycerides. May decrease serum cholesterol, LDH. May affect serum metaprone testing, thyroid function tests.

AVAILABILITY (Rx)

Cream, Vaginal (Premarin): 0.625 mg/g.
Injection, Powder for Reconstitution: 25 mg. **Tablet:** 0.3 mg, 0.45 mg, 0.625 mg, 0.9 mg, 1.25 mg.

ADMINISTRATION/HANDLING

 IV

Reconstitution • Reconstitute with Sterile Water for Injection. • Slowly add diluent, shaking gently. • Avoid vigorous shaking.
Rate of Administration • Give slowly to prevent flushing reaction.
Storage • Refrigerate vials for IV use. • Use immediately following reconstitution.

PO

• Administer at same time each day. • Give with milk, food if nausea occurs.

🖩 IV INCOMPATIBILITIES

No information available on Y-site administration.

INDICATIONS/ROUTES/DOSAGE

Note: Cyclic administration is either 3 wks on, 1 wk off or 25 days on, 5 days off.

Vasomotor Symptoms Associated with Menopause
PO: ADULTS, ELDERLY: 0.3 mg/day cyclically or daily. May titrate up to 1.25 mg/day.

Vulvar and Vaginal Atrophy
PO: ADULTS, ELDERLY: 0.3 mg/day cyclically or daily.
Intravaginal: ADULTS, ELDERLY: 0.5–2 g/day cyclically.

Female Hypogonadism
PO: ADULTS: 0.3–0.625 mg/day given cyclically. Dose may be titrated in 6- to 12-mo intervals. Progestin treatment should be added to maintain bone mineral density once skeletal maturity is achieved.

Female Castration, Primary Ovarian Failure
PO: ADULTS: Initially, 1.25 mg/day cyclically. Adjust dosage, upward or downward, according to severity of symptoms and pt response. For maintenance, adjust dosage to lowest level that will provide effective control.

Postmenopausal Osteoporosis Prevention
PO: ADULTS, ELDERLY: 0.3 daily or cyclically.

Breast Cancer
PO: ADULTS, ELDERLY: 10 mg 3 times/day for at least 3 mos.

Prostate Cancer
PO: ADULTS, ELDERLY: 1.25–2.5 mg 3 times/day.

Abnormal Uterine Bleeding
IV, IM: ADULTS: 25 mg; may repeat once in 6–12 hrs.

Dyspareunia
Intravaginal: ADULTS, ELDERLY: 0.5 g cyclically (21 days on, 7 days off) or 0.5 g twice weekly.

Dosage in Renal Impairment
No dose adjustment.

Dosage in Hepatic Impairment
Contraindicated.

SIDE EFFECTS

Frequent: Vaginal bleeding (spotting, breakthrough bleeding), breast pain/tenderness, gynecomastia. **Occasional:** Headache, hypertension, intolerance to contact lenses. **High doses:** Anorexia, nausea. **Rare:** Loss of scalp hair, depression.

ADVERSE EFFECTS/TOXIC REACTIONS

Prolonged administration may increase risk of breast, cervical, endometrial, hepatic, vaginal carcinoma; cerebrovascular disease, coronary heart disease, gallbladder disease, hypercalcemia.

NURSING CONSIDERATIONS

BASELINE ASSESSMENT

Question for hypersensitivity to estrogen, hepatic impairment, thromboembolic disorders associated with pregnancy, estrogen therapy. Assess frequency/severity of vasomotor symptoms. Review results of baseline mammogram in pts with breast cancer.

INTERVENTION/EVALUATION

Assess B/P periodically. Assess for edema; weigh daily. Monitor for loss of vision, diplopia, migraine, thromboembolic disorder, sudden onset of proptosis.

PATIENT/FAMILY TEACHING

• Avoid smoking due to increased risk of heart attack, blood clots. • Avoid grapefruit products. • Diet, exercise important part of therapy when used to retard osteoporosis. • Promptly report signs/symptoms of thromboembolic, thrombotic disorders: sudden severe headache, shortness of breath, vision/speech disturbance, weakness/numbness of an extremity, loss of coordination; pain in chest, groin, leg. • Report abnormal vaginal bleeding, depression.

• Teach female pts to perform breast self-exam. • Report weight gain of more than 5 lbs a wk. • Stop taking medication, contact physician if pregnancy is suspected.

crizotinib

kriz-**o**-ti-nib
(Xalkori)

◆CLASSIFICATION

PHARMACOTHERAPEUTIC: Tyrosine kinase inhibitor. **CLINICAL:** Antineoplastic.

USES

Treatment of locally advanced or metastatic non–small-cell lung cancer (NSCLC) that is anaplastic lymphoma kinase (ALK) positive. Metastatic NSCLC in pts whose tumors are ROS1 positive.

PRECAUTIONS

Contraindications: Hypersensitivity to crizotinib. **Cautions:** Baseline hepatic impairment, congenital long QT interval syndrome. Pregnancy (avoid use). Concomitant use of CYP3A4 inducers/inhibitors, medications known to cause bradycardia, renal impairment.

ACTION

Inhibits receptor tyrosine kinases including anaplastic lymphoma kinase (ALK), hepatocyte growth factor receptors (HGFR, c-Met), receptor d'origine nantais (RON). **Therapeutic Effect:** Inhibits tumor cell proliferation and survival.

PHARMACOKINETICS

Well absorbed after PO administration. Peak plasma concentration: 4–6 hrs. Protein binding: 91%. Metabolized in liver. Excreted in feces (63%) and urine (22%). **Half-life:** 42 hrs.

⏳ LIFESPAN CONSIDERATIONS

Pregnancy/Lactation: Avoid pregnancy. May cause fetal harm. Contraception should be considered during therapy and for at least 12 wks after discontinuation. Do not initiate therapy until pregnancy status confirmed. Unknown if crosses placenta or distributed in breast milk. Nursing mothers must discontinue either nursing or drug therapy. **Children:** Safety and efficacy not established. **Elderly:** No age-related precautions noted.

INTERACTIONS

DRUG: Strong CYP3A inhibitors, including **atazanavir, clarithromycin, itraconazole, ketoconazole, ritonavir, saquinavir, voriconazole,** may increase concentration. **Strong CYP3A inducers,** including **carBAMazepine, phenytoin, rifabutin, rifAMPin,** may decrease concentration. May alter plasma levels of **alfentanil, cycloSPORINE, dihydroergotamine, ergotamine, fentaNYL, pimozide, sirolimus. Proton pump inhibitors, H₂ blockers, antacids** may decrease solubility. May increase plasma levels of **colchicine, dexamethasone, DOXOrubicin, etoposide, non-nucleoside reverse transcriptase inhibitors, protease inhibitors, quiNIDine, tacrolimus, vinBLAStine. HERBAL:** St. John's wort may decrease effectiveness. **FOOD:** Grapefruit products may increase concentration/toxicity (potential for torsades, myelotoxicity). **LAB VALUES:** May increase serum ALT, AST, alkaline phosphatase, bilirubin. May decrease neutrophils, platelets, lymphocytes.

AVAILABILITY (Rx)

✂ **Capsules:** 200 mg, 250 mg.

ADMINISTRATION/HANDLING

• May give without regard to meals.
• Avoid grapefruit products. • Do not break, crush, dissolve, or divide capsules.

INDICATIONS/ROUTES/DOSAGE

Non–Small-Cell Lung Cancer (ALK Positive), Metastatic NSCLC, ROS-1 Positive

PO: ADULTS: 250 mg twice daily. Continue until disease progression or unacceptable toxicity. **Dosage Modification:** Interrupt and/or reduce to 200 mg twice daily based on graded protocol, including hematologic toxicity (grade 4), elevated LFT with bilirubin elevation (grade 1), QT prolongation (grade 3). May reduce to 250 mg once daily if indicated. Discontinue treatment for QT prolongation (grade 4), elevated LFT with bilirubin elevation (grades 2, 3, 4), pneumonitis of any grade.

Dosage in Renal Impairment
CrCl less than 30 mL/min: 250 mg once daily.

Dosage in Hepatic Impairment
No dose adjustment (see dose for hepatotoxicity during treatment).

Dose Modification
Hematologic
Grade 3 toxicity (WBC 1,000–2,000 cells/mm³, ANC 500–1,000 cells/mm³, platelets 25,000–50,000 cells/mm³), grade 3 anemia: Withhold treatment until recovery to grade 2 or less, then resume at same dosage. **Grade 4 toxicity (WBC less than 1,000 cells/mm³, ANC less than 500 cells/mm³, platelets less than 25,000 cells/mm³), grade 4 anemia:** Withhold treatment until recovery to grade 2 or less, then resume at 200 mg twice daily. **Grade 4 toxicity on 200 mg twice daily:** Withhold treatment until recovery to grade 2 or less, then resume at 250 mg once daily. **Recurrent grade 4 toxicity on 250 mg once daily:** Permanently discontinue.

Cardiac
Grade 3 QTc prolongation on at least 2 separate EKGs: Withhold treatment until recovery to baseline or grade 1 or less. Resume at 200 mg twice daily. **Recurrent grade 3 QTc prolongation on**

200 mg twice daily: Withhold treatment until recovery to baseline or grade 1 or less. Resume at 250 mg once daily. **Recurrent Grade 3 QTc prolongation on 250 mg once daily:** Permanently discontinue.

Bradycardia
Grades 2 or 3: Withhold until recovery to asymptomatic bradycardia or heart rate 60 or more beats/min, evaluate concomitant medications, then resume at 200 mg twice daily. **Grade 4 due to crizotinib:** Permanently discontinue. **Grade 4 associated with concurrent medications known to cause bradycardia/hypotension:** Withhold until recovery to asymptomatic bradycardia or heart rate 60 or more beats/min, and if concurrent medications can be stopped, resume at 250 mg once daily.

Pulmonary
Pulmonary toxicity: Permanently discontinue.

SIDE EFFECTS

Frequent (62%–27%): Diplopia, photopsia, photophobia, blurry vision, visual field defect, vitreous floaters, reduced visual acuity, nausea, diarrhea, vomiting, peripheral/localized edema, constipation. **Occasional (20%–4%):** Fatigue, decreased appetite, dizziness, neuropathy, paresthesia, dysgeusia, dyspepsia, dysphagia, esophageal obstruction/pain/spasm/ulcer, odynophagia, reflux esophagitis, rash, abdominal pain/tenderness, stomatitis, glossodynia, glossitis, cheilitis, mucosal inflammation, oropharyngeal pain/discomfort, bradycardia, headache, cough. **Rare (3%–1%):** Musculoskeletal chest pain, insomnia, dyspnea, arthralgia, nasopharyngitis, rhinitis, pharyngitis, URI, back pain, complex renal cysts, chest pain/tightness.

ADVERSE EFFECTS/TOXIC REACTIONS

Severe, sometimes fatal treatment-related pneumonitis, pneumonia, dyspnea, pulmonary embolism in less than 2% of pts was noted. Grade 3–4 elevation of hepatic enzymes, increased QT prolongation may require discontinuation. May cause thrombocytopenia, neutropenia, lymphopenia. Severe/worsening vitreous floaters, photopsia may indicate retinal hole, retinal detachment.

NURSING CONSIDERATIONS

BASELINE ASSESSMENT

Assess vital signs, O_2 saturation. Obtain baseline CBC with differential, serum chemistries, LFT, PT/INR, EKG. Question possibility of pregnancy or plans for breastfeeding. Obtain full medication history including vitamins, herbal products. Detection of ALK-positive NSCLC test needed prior to treatment. Assess history of tuberculosis, HIV, HF, bradyarrhythmias, electrolyte imbalance, medications that prolong QT interval. Assess visual acuity, history of vitreous floaters. Offer emotional support.

INTERVENTION/EVALUATION

Assess vital signs, O_2 saturation routinely. Monitor CBC with differential monthly, LFT, monthly; increase testing for grades 2, 3, 4 adverse effects. Obtain EKG for bradycardia, electrolyte imbalance, chest pain, difficulty breathing. Monitor for bruising, hematuria, jaundice, right upper abdominal pain, weight loss, or acute infection (fever, diaphoresis, lethargy, oral mucosal changes, productive cough). Report decrease in RBC, Hgb, Hct, platelets, neutrophils, lymphocytes. Worsening cough, fever, or shortness of breath may indicate pneumonitis. Consider ophthalmological evaluation for vision changes. Reinforce birth control compliance.

PATIENT/FAMILY TEACHING

• Blood levels will be drawn routinely. • Report urine changes, bloody or clay-colored stools, upper abdominal pain, nausea, vomiting, bruising, fever, cough, difficulty breathing. • Report history of liver abnormalities or heart problems, including long QT syndrome, syncope, palpitations, extremity swelling. • Immediately report any newly prescribed medications, suspected pregnancy, or vision changes, including light flashes, blurred vision, photophobia, or new or increased floaters. • Contraception recommended during treatment and for at least 3 mos after treatment. • Avoid alcohol, grapefruit products.

cyanocobalamin (vitamin B$_{12}$)

sye-an-oh-koe-**bal**-a-min
(Nascobal)

◆CLASSIFICATION
PHARMACOTHERAPEUTIC: Coenzyme. **CLINICAL:** Vitamin, antianemic.

USES
Treatment of pernicious anemia, vitamin B$_{12}$ deficiency due to malabsorption diseases, increased B$_{12}$ requirement due to pregnancy, thyrotoxicosis, hemorrhage, malignancy, hepatic/renal disease.

PRECAUTIONS
Contraindications: Hypersensitivity to cyanocobalamin. Hereditary optic nerve atrophy. **Cautions:** Folic acid deficiency, anemia, premature neonates.

ACTION
Coenzyme for metabolic functions (fat, carbohydrate metabolism, protein synthesis). **Therapeutic Effect:** Necessary for cell growth and replication, hematopoiesis, myelin synthesis.

PHARMACOKINETICS
In presence of calcium, absorbed systemically in lower half of ileum. Initially, bound to intrinsic factor; this complex passes down intestine, binding to receptor sites on ileal mucosa. Protein binding: High. Metabolized in liver. Primarily eliminated unchanged in urine. **Half-life:** 6 days.

⧖ LIFESPAN CONSIDERATIONS
Pregnancy/Lactation: Crosses placenta. Distributed in breast milk. **Children/Elderly:** No age-related precautions noted.

INTERACTIONS
DRUG: None significant. **HERBAL:** None significant. **FOOD:** None known. **LAB VALUES:** None significant.

AVAILABILITY (Rx)
Injection Solution: 1,000 mcg/mL. **Nasal Spray (Nascobal):** 500 mcg/spray. **Tablets:** 50 mcg, 100 mcg, 250 mcg, 500 mcg, 1,000 mcg. **Tablets (Extended-Release):** 1,000 mcg. **Tablets (Sublingual):** 2,500 mcg.

ADMINISTRATION/HANDLING
IM, Subcutaneous
• Avoid IV route.

PO
• May give without regard to food.

Intranasal
• Clear both nostrils. • Pull clear cover off top of pump. • Press down firmly and quickly on pump's finger grips until a droplet of gel appears at top. Then press down on finger grips two more times. • Place the tip halfway into nostril, pointing tip toward back of nose. • Press down firmly and quickly on finger grips to release medication into one nostril while pressing other nostril closed. • Massage medicated nostril for a few seconds. • Administer nasal preparation at least 1 hr before or 1 hr after hot foods or liquids are consumed (hot foods can cause nasal secretion, resulting in loss of medication).

INDICATIONS/ROUTES/DOSAGE
Pernicious Anemia
IM, Subcutaneous: ADULTS, ELDERLY: 100 mcg/day for 7 days, then every other day for 7 doses, then every 3–4 days for 2–3 wks. **Maintenance:** 100 mcg/mo

(PO 1,000–2,000 mcg/day). **CHILDREN:** 30–50 mcg/day for 2 or more wks (to a total dose of 1,000–5,000 mcg). **Maintenance:** 100 mcg/mo. **NEONATES:** 0.2 mcg/kg for 2 days, then 1,000 mcg/day for 2–7 days. **Maintenance:** 100 mcg/mo.

Vitamin Deficiency

IM, Subcutaneous: ADULTS, ELDERLY: 100 mcg daily for 6–7 days; if improvement, 100 mcg q other day for 7 doses, then q3–4 days for 2–3 wks. **Maintenance:** 100 mcg monthly.
PO: ADULTS, ELDERLY: 1,000–2,000 mcg daily for 1–2 wks. **Maintenance:** 1,000 mcg daily.
Intranasal: ADULTS, ELDERLY: (NASCOBAL): 500 mcg in one nostril once wkly.

Dosage in Renal/Hepatic Impairment
No dose adjustment.

SIDE EFFECTS

Occasional: Diarrhea, pruritus.

ADVERSE EFFECTS/TOXIC REACTIONS

Impurities in preparation may cause rare allergic reaction. Peripheral vascular thrombosis, pulmonary edema, hypokalemia, HF occur rarely.

NURSING CONSIDERATIONS

BASELINE ASSESSMENT

Assess for signs, symptoms of vitamin B$_{12}$ deficiency (anorexia, ataxia, fatigue, hyporeflexia, insomnia, irritability, loss of positional sense, pallor, palpitations on exertion).

INTERVENTION/EVALUATION

Assess for HF, pulmonary edema, hypokalemia in cardiac pts receiving subcutaneous/IM therapy. Monitor serum potassium, serum B$_{12}$, rise in reticulocyte count (peaks in 5–8 days). Assess for reversal of deficiency symptoms (hyporeflexia, loss of positional sense, ataxia, fatigue, irritability, insomnia, anorexia, pallor, palpitations on exertion). Therapeutic response usually dramatic within 48 hrs.

PATIENT/FAMILY TEACHING

• Lifetime treatment may be necessary with pernicious anemia. • Report symptoms of infection. • Foods rich in vitamin B$_{12}$ include clams, oysters, herring, red snapper, muscle meats, fermented cheese, dairy products, egg yolks. • Use nasal preparation at least 1 hr before or 1 hr after consuming hot foods, liquids.

cyclobenzaprine

sye-kloe-**ben**-za-preen
(Amrix, Apo-Cyclobenzaprine ❧, Fexmid, Novo-Cycloprine ❧)
Do not confuse cyclobenzaprine with cycloSERINE or cyproheptadine, or Flexeril with Floxin.

◆CLASSIFICATION

PHARMACOTHERAPEUTIC: Centrally acting muscle relaxant. **CLINICAL:** Skeletal muscle relaxant.

USES

Treatment of muscle spasm associated with acute, painful musculoskeletal conditions. **OFF-LABEL:** Treatment of muscle spasms associated with temporomandibular joint pain (TMJ).

PRECAUTIONS

Contraindications: Hypersensitivity to cyclobenzaprine. Acute recovery phase of MI, arrhythmias, HF, heart block, conduction disturbances, hyperthyroidism, use within 14 days of MAOIs. **Cautions:** Hepatic impairment, history of urinary hesitancy or retention, angle-closure glaucoma, increased intraocular pressure (IOP), elderly.

ACTION

Centrally acting skeletal muscle relaxant that reduces tonic somatic muscle activity at level of brainstem. Influences both alpha and gamma motor neurons.

❧ Canadian trade name　　🔰 Non-Crushable Drug　　🔲 High Alert drug

Therapeutic Effect: Relieves local skeletal muscle spasm.

PHARMACOKINETICS

Route	Onset	Peak	Duration
PO	1 hr	3–4 hrs	12–24 hrs

Well but slowly absorbed from GI tract. Protein binding: 93%. Metabolized in GI tract and liver. Primarily excreted in urine. **Half-life:** 8–37 hrs.

LIFESPAN CONSIDERATIONS

Pregnancy/Lactation: Unknown if drug crosses placenta or is distributed in breast milk. **Children:** Safety and efficacy not established. **Elderly:** Increased sensitivity to anticholinergic effects (e.g., confusion, urinary retention). Increased risk of falls, fractures. Not recommended.

INTERACTIONS

DRUG: Alcohol, other CNS depressant medications (e.g., lorazepam, morphine, zolpidem) may increase CNS depression. **MAOIs (e.g., phenelzine, selegiline)** may increase risk of hypertensive crisis, seizures. **TraMADol** may increase risk of seizures. **HERBAL: Gotu kola, kava kava, SAMe, St. John's wort, valerian** may increase CNS depression. **FOOD:** None known. **LAB VALUES:** None significant.

AVAILABILITY (Rx)

Tablets: 5 mg, 7.5 mg, 10 mg.

Capsules (Extended-Release [Amrix]): 15 mg, 30 mg.

ADMINISTRATION/HANDLING

PO
• Give without regard to food. • Do not break, crush, dissolve, or divide extended-release capsule. • Give extended-release capsule at same time each day.

INDICATIONS/ROUTES/DOSAGE

◄ALERT► Do not use longer than 2–3 wks.

Acute, Painful Musculoskeletal Conditions
PO: ADULTS, ELDERLY, CHILDREN 15 YRS AND OLDER: Initially, 5 mg 3 times/day. May increase to 7.5–10 mg 3 times/day. **PO** *(Extended-Release)*: **ADULTS:** 15–30 mg once daily. Not recommended in elderly.

Dosage in Renal Impairment
No dose adjustment.

Dosage in Hepatic Impairment
Note: Extended-release capsule not recommended in hepatic impairment. **Mild impairment:** 5 mg 3 times/day. **Moderate to severe impairment:** Not recommended.

SIDE EFFECTS

Frequent (39%–11%): Drowsiness, dry mouth, dizziness. **Rare (3%–1%):** Fatigue, asthenia, blurred vision, headache, anxiety, confusion, nausea, constipation, dyspepsia, unpleasant taste.

ADVERSE EFFECTS/TOXIC REACTIONS

Overdose may result in visual hallucinations, hyperactive reflexes, muscle rigidity, vomiting, hyperpyrexia.

NURSING CONSIDERATIONS

BASELINE ASSESSMENT
Record onset, type, location, duration of muscular spasm. Check for immobility, stiffness, swelling.

INTERVENTION/EVALUATION
Assist with ambulation. Assess for therapeutic response: relief of pain; decreased stiffness, swelling; increased joint mobility; reduced joint tenderness; improved grip strength.

PATIENT/FAMILY TEACHING
• Avoid tasks that require alertness, motor skills until response to drug is established. • Drowsiness usually diminishes with continued therapy. • Avoid alcohol, other depressants while taking

medication. • Avoid sudden changes in posture. • Sugarless gum, sips of water may relieve dry mouth.

HIGH ALERT

cyclophosphamide

sye-kloe-**foss**-fa-mide
(Procytox)
Do not confuse cyclophospha-mide with cycloSPORINE or ifosfamide.

◆CLASSIFICATION

PHARMACOTHERAPEUTIC: Alkylating agent. **CLINICAL:** Antineoplastic.

USES

Treatment of acute lymphocytic, acute nonlymphocytic, chronic myelocytic, chronic lymphocytic leukemias; ovarian, breast carcinomas; neuroblastoma; retinoblastoma; Hodgkin's, non-Hodgkin's lymphomas; multiple myeloma; mycosis fungoides; nephrotic syndrome in children. **OFF-LABEL:** Treatment of adrenocortical, bladder, cervical, endometrial, prostatic, testicular carcinomas; Ewing's sarcoma; multiple sclerosis; non–small-cell, small-cell lung cancer; organ transplant rejection; osteosarcoma; ovarian germ cell, primary brain, trophoblastic tumors; rheumatoid arthritis; soft-tissue sarcomas; systemic dermatomyositis; systemic lupus erythematosus; Wilms' tumor.

PRECAUTIONS

Contraindications: Hypersensitivity to cyclophosphamide. Urinary outflow obstruction. **Cautions:** Severe leukopenia, thrombocytopenia, tumor infiltration of bone marrow, previous therapy with other antineoplastic agents, radiation, renal/hepatic/cardiac impairment, active UTI.

ACTION

Inhibits DNA, RNA protein synthesis by cross-linking with DNA, RNA strands. Cell cycle–phase nonspecific. **Therapeutic Effect:** Prevents cell growth. Potent immunosuppressant.

PHARMACOKINETICS

Well absorbed from GI tract. Protein binding: 10%–60%. Crosses blood-brain barrier. Metabolized in liver. Primarily excreted in urine. Removed by hemodialysis. **Half-life:** 3–12 hrs.

☒ LIFESPAN CONSIDERATIONS

Pregnancy/Lactation: If possible, avoid use during pregnancy. Use of effective contraception during therapy and up to 1 yr after completion of therapy is recommended. May cause fetal malformations (limb abnormalities, cardiac anomalies, hernias). Distributed in breast milk. Breastfeeding not recommended. **Children:** No age-related precautions noted. **Elderly:** Age-related renal impairment may require dosage adjustment.

INTERACTIONS

DRUG: CYP2D6 inducers (e.g., car-BAMazepine, PHENobarbital) may decrease concentration; **CYP2D6 inhibitors** (e.g., PARoxetine, amiodarone) may increase concentration. **Anthracycline agents** (e.g., DOXOrubicin, epiRUBicin) may increase risk of cardiomyopathy. **CYP3A4 inhibitors** (e.g., ketoconazole) may increase concentration, risk of adverse effects. **Live virus vaccines** may potentiate virus replication, increase vaccine side effects, decrease pt's antibody response to vaccine. **HERBAL:** Pts with an estrogen-dependent tumor should avoid **black cohosh, dong quai. FOOD:** None known. **LAB VALUES:** May increase serum uric acid.

AVAILABILITY (Rx)

Capsules: 25 mg, 50 mg. **Injection, Powder for Reconstitution:** 500 mg, 1 g, 2 g.

ADMINISTRATION/HANDLING

◄**ALERT**► May be carcinogenic, mutagenic, teratogenic. Handle with extreme care during preparation/administration.

📋 IV

Reconstitution • Reconstitute each 100 mg with 5 mL Sterile Water for Injection, 0.9% NaCl, or D₅W to provide concentration of 20 mg/mL. • Shake to dissolve. • Allow to stand until clear.
Rate of Administration • Infusion rates vary based on protocol. May give by direct IV injection, IV piggyback, or continuous IV infusion.
Storage • Reconstituted solution in 0.9% NaCl is stable for 24 hrs at room temperature or up to 6 days if refrigerated.

PO
• Give on an empty stomach. If GI upset occurs, give with food. • Do not cut or crush. • To minimize risk of bladder irritation, do not give at bedtime.

🔲 IV INCOMPATIBILITY

Amphotericin B complex (Abelcet, AmBisome, Amphotec).

🔲 IV COMPATIBILITIES

Granisetron (Kytril), heparin, HYDROmorphone (Dilaudid), LORazepam (Ativan), morphine, ondansetron (Zofran), propofol (Diprivan).

INDICATIONS/ROUTES/DOSAGE

Note: Hematologic toxicity may require dose reduction.

Usual Dosage (Refer to Individual Protocols)
IV: ADULTS, ELDERLY, CHILDREN: (Single agent): 40–50 mg/kg in divided doses over 2–5 days or 10–15 mg/kg q7–10 days or 3–5 mg/kg twice wkly.
PO: ADULTS, ELDERLY, CHILDREN: 1–5 mg/kg/day.

Nephrotic Syndrome
PO: ADULTS, CHILDREN: 2 mg/kg/day for 60–90 days. **Maximum cumulative dose:** 168 mg/kg.

Dosage in Renal/Hepatic Impairment
No dose adjustment. Use caution.

SIDE EFFECTS

Expected: Marked leukopenia 8–15 days after initiation. **Frequent:** Nausea, vomiting (beginning about 6 hrs after administration and lasting about 4 hrs); alopecia (33%). **Occasional:** Diarrhea, darkening of skin/fingernails, stomatitis, headache, diaphoresis. **Rare:** Pain/redness at injection site.

ADVERSE EFFECTS/TOXIC REACTIONS

Myelosuppression resulting in blood dyscrasias (leukopenia, anemia, thrombocytopenia, hypoprothrombinemia) has been noted. Expect leukopenia to resolve in 17–28 days. Anemia generally occurs after large doses or prolonged therapy. Thrombocytopenia may occur 10–15 days after drug initiation. Hemorrhagic cystitis occurs commonly in long-term therapy (esp. in children). Pulmonary fibrosis, cardiotoxicity noted with high doses. Amenorrhea, azoospermia, hyperkalemia may occur.

NURSING CONSIDERATIONS

BASELINE ASSESSMENT
Obtain CBC wkly during therapy or until maintenance dose is established, then at 2- to 3-wk intervals. Question history of urinary outlet flow obstruction, hepatic/renal impairment, active infections. Obtain urine/serum pregnancy test.

INTERVENTION/EVALUATION
Monitor CBC, serum BUN, creatinine, electrolytes; urine output. Monitor WBC counts closely during initial therapy. Monitor for hematologic toxicity (fever, sore throat, signs of local infection, unusual bruising/bleeding from any site),

symptoms of anemia (excessive fatigue, weakness). Recovery from marked leukopenia due to myelosuppression can be expected in 17–28 days.

PATIENT/FAMILY TEACHING

• Encourage copious fluid intake, frequent voiding (assists in preventing cystitis) at least 24 hrs before, during, after therapy. • Do not have immunizations without physician's approval (drug lowers resistance). • Avoid contact with those who have recently received live virus vaccine. • Promptly report fever, sore throat, signs of local infection, difficulty or pain with urination, unusual bruising/bleeding from any site. • Hair loss is reversible, but new hair growth may have different color, texture. • Avoid pregnancy for up to 1 yr after completion of treatment.

cycloSPORINE

sye-kloe-**spor**-in
(Apo-CycloSPORINE ✦, Gengraf, Neoral, Restasis, SandIMMUNE)

■ **BLACK BOX ALERT** ■ Only physicians experienced in management of immunosuppressive therapy and organ transplant pts should prescribe. Renal impairment may occur with high dosage. Increased risk of neoplasia, susceptibility to infections. May cause hypertension, nephrotoxicity. Psoriasis pts: Increased risk of developing skin malignancies. The modified/non-modified formulations are not bioequivalent and cannot be used interchangeably without close monitoring.
Do not confuse cycloSPORINE with cycloSERINE or cyclophosphamide, Gengraf with ProGraf, Neoral with Neurontin or Nizoral, or SandIMMUNE with SandoSTATIN.

◆CLASSIFICATION

PHARMACOTHERAPEUTIC: Calcineurin inhibitor. **CLINICAL:** Immunosuppressant.

USES

Modified, Non-Modified: Prevents organ rejection of kidney, liver, heart in combination with steroid therapy and/or azaTHIOprine. **Non-Modified:** Treatment of chronic allograft rejection in those previously treated with other immunosuppressives. **Modified:** Treatment of severe, active rheumatoid arthritis, severe recalcitrant plaque psoriasis in nonimmunocompromised adults. **Ophthalmic:** Chronic dry eyes. **OFF-LABEL:** Allogenic stem cell transplants for prevention/treatment of graft-vs-host disease; focal segmental glomerulosclerosis, lupus nephritis, severe ulcerative colitis.

PRECAUTIONS

Contraindications: History of hypersensitivity to cycloSPORINE, polyoxyethylated castor oil; uncontrolled hypertension, renal impairment, or malignancies in treatment of psoriasis or rheumatoid arthritis. **Cautions:** Hepatic/renal impairment. History of seizures. Avoid live vaccines.

ACTION

Inhibits cellular, humoral immune responses by inhibiting interleukin-2, a proliferative factor needed for T-cell activity. **Therapeutic Effect:** Prevents organ rejection, relieves symptoms of psoriasis, arthritis.

PHARMACOKINETICS

Variably absorbed from GI tract. Protein binding: 90%. Metabolized in liver. Eliminated primarily by biliary or fecal excretion. Not removed by hemodialysis. **Half-life:** Adults, 10–27 hrs; children, 7–19 hrs.

⧖ LIFESPAN CONSIDERATIONS

Pregnancy/Lactation: Readily crosses placenta. Distributed in breast milk. Breastfeeding not recommended. **Children:** No age-related precautions noted in transplant pts. **Elderly:** Increased risk of hypertension, increased serum creatinine.

INTERACTIONS

DRUG: Allopurinol, bromocriptine, cimetidine, clarithromycin, danazol, diltiaZEM, oral contraceptives, erythromycin, fluconazole, ketoconazole may increase concentration, risk of hepatic/renal toxicity. RifAMPin, carBAMazepine, phenytoin may decrease cycloSPORINE concentration. ACE inhibitors (e.g., enalapril, lisinopril), potassium-sparing diuretics (e.g., spironolactone, triamterene), potassium supplements may cause hyperkalemia. Immunosuppressants may increase risk of infection, lymphoproliferative disorders. Lovastatin, simvastatin, atorvastatin, pravastatin may increase risk of rhabdomyolysis. Live virus vaccines may potentiate virus replication, increase vaccine side effects, decrease pt's response to vaccine. May increase concentration/toxicity of digoxin, colchicine. **HERBAL:** Avoid cat's claw, echinacea (possess immunostimulant properties). St. John's wort may decrease plasma concentration. **FOOD:** Grapefruit products may increase absorption/immunosuppression, risk of toxicity. **LAB VALUES:** May increase serum BUN, alkaline phosphatase, amylase, bilirubin, creatinine, potassium, uric acid, ALT, AST. May decrease serum magnesium. Therapeutic peak serum level: 50–400 ng/mL; toxic serum level: greater than 400 ng/mL.

AVAILABILITY (Rx)

Capsules (Gengraf, Neoral [Modified], SandIMMUNE [Nonmodified]): 25 mg, 50 mg, 100 mg. Injection, Solution (SandIMMUNE): 50 mg/mL. Ophthalmic Emulsion (Restasis): 0.05%. Oral Solution (Gengraf, Neoral [Modified], SandIMMUNE [Nonmodified]): 100 mg/mL.

ADMINISTRATION/HANDLING

◀**ALERT**▶ Oral solution available in bottle form with calibrated liquid measuring device. Oral form should replace IV administration as soon as possible.

 IV

Reconstitution • Dilute each mL (50 mg) concentrate with 20–100 mL 0.9% NaCl or D5W (**maximum concentration:** 2.5 mg/mL).

Rate of Administration • Infuse over 2–6 hrs. • Monitor pt continuously for hypersensitivity reaction (facial flushing, dyspnea).

Storage • Store parenteral form at room temperature. • Protect IV solution from light. • After diluted, stable for 6 hrs in PVC; 24 hrs in Excel or glass.

PO

• Administer consistently with relation to time of day and meals. • Oral solution may be mixed in glass container with milk, chocolate milk, orange juice, or apple juice (preferably at room temperature). Stir well. • Drink immediately. • Add more diluent to glass container. Mix with remaining solution to ensure total amount is given. • Dry outside of calibrated liquid measuring device before replacing cover. • Do not rinse with water. • Avoid refrigeration of oral solution (solution may separate). • Discard oral solution after 2 mos once bottle is opened.

Ophthalmic

• Invert vial several times to obtain uniform suspension. • Instruct pt to remove contact lenses before administration (may reinsert 15 min after administration). • May use with artificial tears.

▓ IV INCOMPATIBILITIES

Acyclovir (Zovirax), amphotericin B complex (Abelcet, AmBisome, Amphotec), magnesium.

▓ IV COMPATIBILITY

Propofol (Diprivan).

INDICATIONS/ROUTES/DOSAGE

Note: The modified/non-modified formulations are not bioequivalent and cannot be used interchangeably without close monitoring.

Transplantation, Prevention of Organ Rejection

Note: Initial dose given 4–12 hrs prior to transplant or postoperatively.

PO: ADULTS, ELDERLY, CHILDREN: NOT MODIFIED: Initially, 10–12 mg/kg daily for 1–2 wks, then taper by 5% each wk to maintenance dose of 5–10 mg/kg daily. **MODIFIED:** (dose dependent upon type of transplant). **Renal:** 6–12 mg/kg/day in 2 divided doses. **Hepatic:** 4–12 mg/kg/day in 2 divided doses. **Heart:** 4–10 mg/kg/day in 2 divided doses.

IV: ADULTS, ELDERLY, CHILDREN: NOT MODIFIED: Initially, 5–6 mg/kg/dose daily. Switch to oral as soon as possible.

Rheumatoid Arthritis

PO: ADULTS, ELDERLY: MODIFIED: Initially, 2.5 mg/kg a day in 2 divided doses. May increase by 0.5–0.75 mg/kg/day after 8 wks with additional increases made at 12 wks. **Maximum:** 4 mg/kg/day.

Psoriasis

PO: ADULTS, ELDERLY: MODIFIED: Initially, 2.5 mg/kg/day in 2 divided doses. May increase by 0.5 mg/kg/day after 4 wks; additional increases may be made q2wks. **Maximum:** 4 mg/kg/day.

Dry Eye

Ophthalmic: ADULTS, ELDERLY: Instill 1 drop in each affected eye q12h.

Dosage in Renal Impairment

Modify dose if serum creatinine levels 25% or above pretreatment levels.

Dosage in Hepatic Impairment

Mild to moderate impairment: No dose adjustment. **Severe impairment:** Use caution.

SIDE EFFECTS

Frequent (26%–12%): Mild to moderate hypertension, hirsutism, tremor. **Occasional (4%–2%):** Acne, leg cramps, gingival hyperplasia (red, bleeding, tender gums), paresthesia, diarrhea, nausea, vomiting, headache. **Rare (less than 1%):** Hypersensitivity reaction, abdominal discomfort, gynecomastia, sinusitis.

ADVERSE EFFECTS/TOXIC REACTIONS

Mild nephrotoxicity occurs in 25% of renal transplants, 38% of cardiac transplants, 37% of liver transplants, generally 2–3 mos after transplantation (more severe toxicity may occur soon after transplantation). Hepatotoxicity occurs in 4% of renal, 7% of cardiac, and 4% of liver transplants, generally within first mo after transplantation. Both toxicities usually respond to dosage reduction. Severe hyperkalemia, hyperuricemia occur occasionally.

NURSING CONSIDERATIONS

BASELINE ASSESSMENT

Obtain baseline serum chemistries, esp. renal function, LFT. If nephrotoxicity occurs, mild toxicity is generally noted 2–3 mos after transplantation; more severe toxicity noted early after transplantation; hepatotoxicity may be noted during first mo after transplantation.

INTERVENTION/EVALUATION

Diligently monitor serum BUN, creatinine, bilirubin, ALT, AST, LDH levels for evidence of hepatotoxicity/nephrotoxicity (mild toxicity noted by slow rise in serum levels; more overt toxicity noted by rapid rise in levels; hematuria also noted in nephrotoxicity). Monitor serum potassium for evidence of hyperkalemia. Encourage diligent oral hygiene (gingival hyperplasia). Monitor B/P for evidence of hypertension. **Note:** Reference ranges dependent on organ transplanted, organ function, cycloSPORINE toxicity. Trough levels should be obtained immediately prior to next dose. **Therapeutic serum level:** 50–400 ng/mL; **toxic serum level:** greater than 400 ng/mL.

PATIENT/FAMILY TEACHING

• Blood levels will be drawn routinely. • Report severe headache, persistent nausea/vomiting, unusual swelling of extremities, chest pain. • Avoid grapefruit products (increases concentration/effects), St. John's wort (decreases concentration). • Do not take any newly prescribed or OTC medications unless approved by the prescriber who originally started treatment.

---

cytarabine HIGH ALERT

sye-**tar**-a-bine
(Ara-C, Cytosar-U ✚, Depo-Cyt)

■ **BLACK BOX ALERT** ■ Must be administered by personnel trained in administration/handling of chemotherapeutic agents. **Conventional:** Potent myelosuppressant. High risk of multiple toxicities (GI, CNS, pulmonary, cardiac). **Liposomal:** Chemical arachnoiditis, manifested by profound nausea, vomiting, fever, may be fatal if untreated.

Do not confuse cytarabine with Cytoxan or vidarabine, or Cytosar with Cytoxan or Neosar.

◆CLASSIFICATION

PHARMACOTHERAPEUTIC: Antimetabolite. **CLINICAL:** Antineoplastic.

USES

Conventional: Remission induction in acute myeloid leukemia (AML), treatment of acute lymphocytic leukemia (ALL) and chronic myelocytic leukemia (CML), prophylaxis and treatment of meningeal leukemia. **Liposomal:** Treatment of lymphomatous meningitis. **OFF-LABEL:** Ara-C: Carcinomatous meningitis, Hodgkin's and non-Hodgkin's lymphomas, myelodysplastic syndrome.

PRECAUTIONS

Contraindications: Hypersensitivity to cytarabine. (Liposomal): Active meningeal infection. **Cautions:** Renal/hepatic impairment, prior drug-induced bone marrow suppression.

ACTION

Inhibits DNA polymerase. Cell cycle–specific for S phase of cell division. **Therapeutic Effect:** Appears to inhibit DNA synthesis. Potent immunosuppressive activity.

PHARMACOKINETICS

Widely distributed; moderate amount crosses blood-brain barrier. Protein binding: 15%. Primarily excreted in urine. **Half-life:** 1–3 hrs.

⧗ LIFESPAN CONSIDERATIONS

Pregnancy/Lactation: If possible, avoid use during pregnancy. May cause fetal malformations. Unknown if distributed in breast milk. Breastfeeding not recommended. **Children:** No age-related precautions noted. **Elderly:** Age-related renal impairment may require dosage adjustment.

INTERACTIONS

DRUG: May decrease concentration of **digoxin, flucytosine. Live virus vaccines** may potentiate virus replication, increase vaccine side effects, decrease pt's response to vaccine. **HERBAL:** Echinacea may decrease therapeutic effect. **FOOD:** None known. **LAB VALUES:** May increase serum alkaline phosphatase, bilirubin, uric acid, AST.

AVAILABILITY (Rx)

Injection, Powder for Reconstitution (Conventional): 100 mg, 500 mg, 1 g. **Injection, Solution (Conventional):** 20 mg/mL, 100 mg/mL. **Injection, Suspension (Liposomal):** 10 mg/mL.

ADMINISTRATION/HANDLING

◀**ALERT**▶ May give by subcutaneous, IV push, IV infusion, intrathecal routes at concentration not to exceed 100 mg/mL. May be carcinogenic, mutagenic, teratogenic (embryonic deformity). Handle with extreme care during preparation/administration. Liposomal for intrathecal use only.

IV, Intrathecal
 IV

Reconstitution • Conventional: Reconstitute with Bacteriostatic Water for Injection. • Dose may be further diluted with 250–1,000 mL D_5W or 0.9% NaCl for IV infusion. • For intrathecal use, reconstitute vial with preservative-free 0.9% NaCl or pt's spinal fluid. Dose usually administered in 5–15 mL of solution, after equivalent volume of CSF removed. • Liposomal: No reconstitution required.
Rate of Administration • Conventional: For IV infusion, give over 1–3 hrs or as continuous infusion.
Storage • Conventional: Store at room temperature. • Reconstituted solution is stable for 48 hrs at room temperature. • Use diluted solution within 24 hrs. • Discard if slight haze develops. • Liposomal: Refrigerate; use within 4 hrs following withdrawal from vial.

🕸 IV INCOMPATIBILITIES

Amphotericin B complex (Abelcet, AmBisome, Amphotec), ganciclovir (Cytovene), heparin, insulin (regular).

🕸 IV COMPATIBILITIES

Dexamethasone (Decadron), diphenhydrAMINE (Benadryl), filgrastim (Neupogen), granisetron (Kytril), HYDROmorphone (Dilaudid), LORazepam (Ativan), morphine, ondansetron (Zofran), potassium chloride, propofol (Diprivan).

INDICATIONS/ROUTES/DOSAGE

Usual Dosage for Induction (Conventional) (Refer to Individual Protocols)
IV: **ADULTS, ELDERLY, CHILDREN:** (Induction): 100 mg/m²/day continuous infusion for 7 days or 200 mg/m²/day continuous infusion (as 100 mg/m² over 12 hrs q12h) for 7 days.

Intrathecal: ADULTS, ELDERLY, CHILDREN: Usual dose: 30 mg/m² q4days. Range: 5–75 mg/m² daily for 4 days or once q4days until CNS findings normalize, followed by one additional treatment.

Usual Maintenance Dosage (Conventional)
IV: **ADULTS, ELDERLY, CHILDREN:** 70–200 mg/m²/day for 2–5 days q mo.

Usual Dosage for Depo-Cyt (Liposomal)
Intrathecal: **ADULTS, ELDERLY:** (**Induction):** 50 mg q14 days for 2 doses (wks 1, 3). (**Consolidation):** 50 mg q14 days for 3 doses (wks 5, 7, 9) followed by additional dose at wk 13. (**Maintenance):** 50 mg q28days for 4 doses (wks 17, 21, 25, 29).

Dosage in Renal/Hepatic Impairment
No dose adjustment.

SIDE EFFECTS

Frequent: IV, (33%–16%): Asthenia, fever, pain, altered taste/smell, nausea, vomiting (risk greater with IV push than with continuous IV infusion). **Intrathecal (28%–11%):** Headache, asthenia, altered taste/smell, confusion, drowsiness, nausea, vomiting. **Occasional: IV, (11%–7%):** Abnormal gait, drowsiness, constipation, back pain, urinary incontinence, peripheral edema, headache, confusion. **Intrathecal (7%–3%):** Peripheral edema, back pain, constipation, abnormal gait, urinary incontinence.

ADVERSE EFFECTS/TOXIC REACTIONS

Myelosuppression resulting in blood dyscrasias (leukopenia, anemia, thrombocytopenia, megaloblastosis, reticulocytopenia), occurring minimally after single IV dose. Leukopenia, anemia, thrombocytopenia should be expected with daily or continuous IV therapy. Cytarabine syndrome (fever, myalgia, rash, conjunctivitis, malaise, chest pain), hyperuricemia may

C

occur. High-dose therapy may produce severe CNS, GI, pulmonary toxicity.

NURSING CONSIDERATIONS

BASELINE ASSESSMENT

Obtain baseline CBC, renal function, LFT. Leukocyte count decreases within 24 hrs after initial dose, continues to decrease for 7–9 days followed by brief rise at 12 days, decreases again at 15–24 days, then rises rapidly for next 10 days. Platelet count decreases 5 days after drug initiation to its lowest count at 12–15 days, then rises rapidly for next 10 days.

INTERVENTION/EVALUATION

Monitor BMP, LFT; serum uric acid. Monitor CBC for evidence of myelosuppression. Monitor for blood dyscrasias (fever, sore throat, signs of local infection, unusual bruising/bleeding from any site), symptoms of anemia (excessive fatigue, weakness). Monitor for signs of neuropathy (gait disturbances, handwriting difficulties, paresthesia).

PATIENT/FAMILY TEACHING

• Increase fluid intake (may protect against hyperuricemia). • Do not have immunizations without physician's approval (drug lowers resistance). • Avoid contact with those who have recently received live virus vaccine. • Promptly report fever, sore throat, signs of local infection, unusual bruising/bleeding from any site.

dabigatran

dab-i-**gah**-tran
(Pradaxa)

■ BLACK BOX ALERT ■ Risk of thrombotic events (e.g., stroke) increased if discontinued for a reason other than pathological bleeding. Spinal or epidural hematoma may occur with neuraxial anesthesia.

◆CLASSIFICATION

PHARMACOTHERAPEUTIC: Thrombin inhibitor. **CLINICAL:** Anticoagulant.

USES

Indicated to reduce risk of stroke, systemic embolism in pts with nonvalvular atrial fibrillation. Treatment and reduction of risk of deep vein thrombosis (DVT) and pulmonary embolism (PE). Prophylaxis of DVT and PE in pts who have undergone hip replacement surgery.

PRECAUTIONS

Contraindications: Severe hypersensitivity to dabigatran. Active major bleeding, pts with mechanical prosthetic heart valves. **Cautions:** Renal impairment (CrCl 15–30 mL/min), moderate hepatic impairment, invasive procedures, spinal anesthesia, major surgery, pts with congenital or acquired bleeding disorders, elderly, concurrent use of medications that increase risk of bleeding, valvular heart disease.

ACTION

Direct thrombin inhibitor that inhibits coagulation by preventing thrombin effects (e.g., inhibition of thrombin-induced platelet aggregation). **Therapeutic Effect:** Produces anticoagulation, preventing development of thrombus.

PHARMACOKINETICS

Metabolized in liver. Protein binding: 35%. Eliminated primarily in urine. **Half-life:** 12–17 hrs.

☒ LIFESPAN CONSIDERATIONS

Pregnancy/Lactation: Unknown if distributed in breast milk. **Children:** Safety and efficacy not established in pts younger than 18 yrs. **Elderly:** Severe renal impairment may require dosage adjustment.

INTERACTIONS

DRUG: RifAMPin may decrease concentration. **Antacids, proton pump inhibitors (e.g., omeprazole, pantoprazole)** may decrease level, effect. **Antiplatelet agents (e.g., aspirin, clopidogrel), NSAIDs (e.g., ibuprofen, ketorolac, naproxen), thrombolytics (e.g., tPA)** may increase risk of bleeding. **HERBAL: Feverfew, ginkgo biloba, green tea, red clover** may increase risk of bleeding. **St. John's wort** may decrease concentration/effect. **FOOD: High-fat meal** delays absorption approx. 2 hrs. **LAB VALUES:** May increase aPTT, PT, INR.

AVAILABILITY (Rx)

Capsules: 75 mg, 110 mg, 150 mg.

ADMINISTRATION/HANDLING

PO
• May be given without regard to food. Administer with water. • Do not break, cut, open capsules.

INDICATIONS/ROUTES/DOSAGE

◀ALERT▶ Medication should be discontinued prior to invasive or surgical procedures.

Treatment/Prevention of DVT/PE
PO: ADULTS, ELDERLY: 150 mg twice daily (after 5–10 days of treatment with parenteral anticoagulants).

Nonvalvular Atrial Fibrillation
PO: ADULTS, ELDERLY: 150 mg twice daily (to reduce risk of stroke/systemic embolism).

Prophylaxis following Hip Surgery
PO: ADULTS, ELDERLY: 110 mg on day one (1–4 hr postoperative and established

hemostasis), then 220 mg daily for up to 35 days.

Dosage in Renal Impairment (Nonvalvular Atrial Fibrillation)

CrCl 15–30 mL/min: 75 mg twice daily. **CrCl less than 15, or HD:** Not recommended (HD removes ~60% over 2–3 hrs).

Dosage in Hepatic Impairment

No dosage adjustment.

SIDE EFFECTS

Frequent (less than 16%): Dyspepsia (heartburn, nausea, indigestion), diarrhea, upper abdominal pain.

ADVERSE EFFECTS/TOXIC REACTIONS

Severe, sometimes fatal, hemorrhagic events, including intracranial hemorrhage, hemorrhagic stroke, GI bleeding, may occur. Hypersensitivity reactions, including anaphylaxis, reported in less than 1% of pts.

NURSING CONSIDERATIONS

BASELINE ASSESSMENT

Obtain CBC (esp. platelet count), renal function test, PT, aPTT. Question history of mechanical heart valve, recent surgery; hepatic, renal impairment; recent spinal, epidural procedures. Receive full medication history and screen for interactions.

INTERVENTION/EVALUATION

Assess for any sign of bleeding (hematuria, melena, bleeding from gums, petechiae, bruising), decrease in B/P, increase in pulse rate, complaint of abdominal pain, diarrhea. Obtain aPTT, PT, platelet count. Question for increase in discharge during menses. Monitor for hematoma. Use care in removing any dressing, tape. Monitor for symptoms of intracranial hemorrhage (e.g., altered mental status, aphagia, lethargy, one-sided weakness, seizures, vision changes).

PATIENT/FAMILY TEACHING

• Do not chew, crush, open, or divide capsules. • Use electric razor, soft toothbrush to prevent bleeding. • Report any sign of red or dark urine, black or red stool, coffee-ground vomitus, red-speckled mucus from cough. • Keep in original container. • Once bottle is opened, must be used within 60 days. • Open blister pack at time of use. • Treatment may increase risk of bleeding into the brain; report difficulty speaking, headache, numbness, paralysis, vision changes, seizures.

dabrafenib

da-**braf**-e-nib
(Tafinlar)
Do not confuse dabrafenib with dasatinib.

◆CLASSIFICATION

PHARMACOTHERAPEUTIC: Kinase inhibitor. **CLINICAL:** Antineoplastic.

USES

Treatment of unresectable or metastatic melanoma with BRAF V600E mutation as detected by FDA-approved test. ◀**ALERT**▶ Not indicated for treatment of wild-type BRAF melanomas.

PRECAUTIONS

Contraindications: Hypersensitivity to dabrafenib. **Cautions:** Diabetes, hepatic/renal impairment, dehydration, glucose-6-phosphate dehydrogenase (G6PD) deficiency, pts at increased risk for arrhythmias.

ACTION

Inhibits BRAF kinase gene mutation, a main cause of tumor cell growth, in the absence of growth factors that are normally required for proliferation. **Therapeutic Effect:** Inhibits tumor cell growth and metastasis.

PHARMACOKINETICS

Readily absorbed after PO administration. Protein binding: 99.7%. Peak plasma concentration: 2 hrs. Metabolized in liver. Excreted in feces (71%), urine (23%). **Half-life:** 8 hrs.

☒ LIFESPAN CONSIDERATIONS

Pregnancy/Lactation: Avoid pregnancy. May cause fetal harm. Must use effective nonhormonal contraception during treatment and for at least 2 wks after treatment (intrauterine device, barrier methods). Unknown if distributed in breast milk. Must either discontinue breastfeeding or discontinue therapy. **Children:** Safety and efficacy not established. **Elderly:** May have increased risk of adverse effects, skin lesions.

INTERACTIONS

DRUG: Antacids, H_2-receptors blockers (e.g., famotidine, raNITIdine), proton pump inhibitors (e.g., omeprazole, pantoprazole) may decrease concentration/effect. **CYP3A4 inducers** (e.g., carBAMazepine, phenytoin, rifAMPin) may decrease concentration/effect. **CYP3A4 inhibitors** (e.g., clarithromycin, gemfibrozil, ketoconazole) may increase concentration. May decrease effectiveness of **hormonal contraceptives, warfarin.** **HERBAL:** St. John's wort may decrease concentration/effect. **FOOD:** High-fat meals may decrease absorption/effect. **LAB VALUES:** May increase serum glucose, alkaline phosphatase. May decrease serum phosphate, sodium.

AVAILABILITY (Rx)

🖌 **Capsules:** 50 mg, 75 mg.

ADMINISTRATION/HANDLING

PO

• Give at least 1 hr before or at least 2 hrs after meal. • Do not break, crush, open, or divide capsule. • Missed dose may be given up to 6 hrs prior to next dose.

INDICATIONS/ROUTES/DOSAGE

Metastatic Melanoma

PO: ADULTS/ELDERLY: 150 mg twice daily (about 12 hrs apart) until disease progression or unacceptable toxicity.

Dose Modification

Based on Common Terminology Criteria for Adverse Events (CTCAE) grading 1–4.

Reduction Levels	Dose
1st dose reduction	100 mg twice daily
2nd dose reduction	75 mg twice daily
3rd dose reduction	50 mg twice daily

Fever Greater Than 101.3°F or Any Grade 2 or Grade 3 Adverse Event

Withhold until fever or adverse event resolves to grade 1 or less, then reduce dose by one level. May further decrease each dose level based on tolerability.

Recurrent Grade 4 Adverse Event or 50-mg Dose Intolerability or Hemodynamic Instability

Permanently discontinue.

Dosage in Renal Impairment

No dosage adjustment.

Dosage in Hepatic Impairment

Mild to moderate impairment: No dosage adjustment. **Severe impairment:** Use with caution.

SIDE EFFECTS

Frequent (37%–17%): Hyperkeratosis, headache, pyrexia, arthralgia, alopecia, rash. **Occasional (12%–10%):** Back pain, cough, myalgia, constipation, nasopharyngitis, fatigue.

ADVERSE EFFECTS/TOXIC REACTIONS

Cutaneous squamous cell carcinoma (cuSCC) and keratocanthomas reported in 11% of pts (esp. elderly, prior skin cancer, chronic sun exposure). Skin reactions including palmar-plantar erythrodysesthesia syndrome (PPES), papilloma have occurred. May increase cell proliferation of wild-type BRAF melanoma or new

---

D

malignant melanomas. Eye conditions including uveitis, iritis reported. Hyperglycemia reported in 6% of pts. Serious febrile drug reactions including hypotension, rigors, dehydration reported in 4% of pts. Pts with G6PD deficiency have increased risk of hemolytic anemia. Pancreatitis, interstitial nephritis, bullous rash reported in less than 10% of pts.

NURSING CONSIDERATIONS

BASELINE ASSESSMENT

Obtain BMP, LFT, serum magnesium, phosphate, blood glucose level. Confirm presence of BRAF V600E mutation, negative urine pregnancy before initiating treatment. Assess skin for moles, lesions, papillomas. Baseline ophthalmologic exam, visual acuity. Question current breastfeeding status. Receive full medication history including herbal products. Offer emotional support.

INTERVENTION/EVALUATION

Monitor serum electrolytes, blood glucose routinely. Obtain CBC if hemolytic anemia suspected. Monitor for signs of hyperglycemia. Assess for skin lesions every 2 mos during treatment and at least 6 mos after discontinuation. Immediately report any vision changes, eye pain/swelling, febrile events, renal impairment. Monitor urinary output.

PATIENT/FAMILY TEACHING

• Treatment may cause hair loss. • Do not breastfeed. • Avoid pregnancy; non-hormonal contraception should be used during treatment and up to 4 wks after last dose. • Take capsule at least 1 hr before or at least 2 hrs after meal. Swallow whole; do not chew, crush, open, or divide. • Report any increased urination, thirst, confusion, vision changes, eye pain, fever, skin changes including moles or lesions, rash, hematuria, weight gain from water retention. • Minimize exposure to sunlight. • Males may experience a decreased sperm count. • Report any newly prescribed medications.

daclatasvir

dak-**lat**-as-vir
(Daklinza)
Do not confuse daclatasvir with ombitasvir, or Daklinza with Zolinza.

◆CLASSIFICATION

PHARMACOTHERAPEUTIC: NS5A inhibitor. **CLINICAL:** Antiviral.

USES

Treatment of chronic hepatitis C virus (HCV) genotypes 1 or 3 infection, in combination with other antiviral therapy.

PRECAUTIONS

Contraindications: Hypersensitivity to daclatasvir. Concomitant use of strong CYP3A inducers (e.g., phenytoin, carBAMazepine, rifAMPin, St. John's wort). **Cautions:** Concomitant use of strong or moderate CYP3A inhibitors, moderate CYP3A inducers. Concomitant use of amiodarone is not recommended. History of bradycardia, bradyarrhythmias, cardiovascular disease, severe hepatic disease.

ACTION

Inhibits NS5A, a nonstructural protein encoded by HCV. Binds to N-terminus of NS5A and inhibits both viral RNA replication and virion assembly. **Therapeutic Effect:** Inhibits viral replication of hepatitis C virus.

PHARMACOKINETICS

Widely distributed. Metabolized in liver. Protein binding: 99%. Peak plasma concentration: 2 hrs. Eliminated in feces (88%), urine (7%). **Half-life:** 12–15 hrs.

⧗ LIFESPAN CONSIDERATIONS

Pregnancy/Lactation: Unknown if distributed in breast milk. **Children:** Safety and efficacy not established in pts younger than 18 yrs. **Elderly:** No age-related precautions noted.

INTERACTIONS

DRUG: **Amiodarone, beta blockers (e.g., carvedilol, metoprolol)** may increase risk of symptomatic bradycardia. **Strong CYP3A inhibitors (e.g., clarithromycin, itraconazole, saquinavir), moderate CYP3A inhibitors (e.g., ciprofloxacin, diltiaZEM, fosamprenavir)** may increase concentration/effect. **Moderate CYP3A inducers (e.g., dexamethasone, efavirenz, nafcillin)** may decrease concentration/effect. May increase concentration/effect, anticoagulant effect of **dabigatran.** May increase concentration/effect of **digoxin.** May increase risk of myopathy, concentration/effects of **HMG-CoA reductase inhibitors (e.g., atorvastatin, simvastatin). HERBAL: St. John's wort** may decrease concentration/effect; use contraindicated. **FOOD: High-fat, high-caloric meal** may decrease absorption by 28%. **LAB VALUES:** May increase serum lipase.

AVAILABILITY (Rx)

Tablets: 30 mg, 60 mg, 90 mg.

ADMINISTRATION/HANDLING

PO
• Give without regard to meals.

INDICATIONS/ROUTES/DOSAGE

Note: Cirrhotic pts with genotype 1a should undergo testing for presence of virus with NSA5A-resistance–associated polymorphisms.

Genotype 1
PO: ADULTS, ELDERLY: (Without cirrhosis or with compensated Child-Pugh A cirrhosis): 60 mg once daily with sofosbuvir for 12 wks. (With decompensated Child-Pugh B or C cirrhosis or post–liver transplant): 60 mg once daily with sofosbuvir and ribavirin for 12 wks.

Genotype 3
PO: ADULTS, ELDERLY: (Without cirrhosis): 60 mg once daily with sofosbuvir for 12 wks. (With compensated Child-Pugh

A or decompensated Child-Pugh B or C cirrhosis or post–liver transplant: 60 mg once daily with sofosbuvir and ribavirin for 12 wks.

Dose Modification
Concomitant use of strong CYP3A inhibitors
30 mg once daily, in combination with sofosbuvir, with or without riboflavin for 12 wks.
Concomitant use of moderate CYP3A inducers
90 mg once daily, in combination with sofosbuvir, with or without riboflavin for 12 wks.
Discontinuation
If sofosbuvir is permanently discontinued, then daclatasvir should also be discontinued.
Concomitant use of digoxin
Consider decreasing digoxin dose by 30%–50%, or use lowest dose possible to maintain adequate response.

Dosage in Renal Impairment
No dose adjustment.

Dosage in Hepatic Impairment
No dose adjustment. Safety and efficacy not established in pts with decompensated hepatic cirrhosis or in liver transplant pts.

SIDE EFFECTS

Occasional (14%–8%): Headache, fatigue, nausea. **Rare (5%):** Diarrhea.

ADVERSE EFFECTS/TOXIC REACTIONS

Symptomatic bradycardia and some cases requiring pacemaker intervention have been reported when amiodarone is coadministered with sofosbuvir, in combination with another HCV direct-acting antiviral, including daclatasvir. Bradycardia generally occurred within hrs to days, but may extend up to 2 wks after initiation. Pts taking beta blockers (e.g., metoprolol), those with underlying cardiac disease, or pts with advanced hepatic disease are at increased

D

risk of bradycardia when treated with amiodarone. Transient, asymptomatic elevations of serum lipase levels greater than 3 times upper limit of normal reported in 2% of pts.

NURSING CONSIDERATIONS

BASELINE ASSESSMENT

Obtain HCV-RNA level, LFT. Receive full medication history, including herbal products, and screen for contraindications/interactions, esp. concomitant use of amiodarone or digoxin. Confirm HCV genotype. Question history of bradycardia, arrhythmias. Assess hydration status.

INTERVENTION/EVALUATION

Monitor HCV-RNA level, LFT. Pts requiring treatment with amiodarone should be monitored with a cardiac monitor in an inpatient setting for the first 48 hrs of initiation. Further outpatient monitoring or self-monitoring of the heart rate should occur on a daily basis for at least the first 2 wks of treatment. Due to amiodarone's long half-life, pts discontinuing amiodarone just prior to starting sofosbuvir, in combination with daclatasvir, should have similar cardiac monitoring as listed earlier. Immediately report symptoms of bradycardia.

PATIENT/FAMILY TEACHING

• There is an increased risk of drug interactions with other medications. • Do not take any new medications unless approved by physician. • Treatment with amiodarone, an antiarrhythmic drug, may increase the risk of a slow heartbeat and is not recommended during drug therapy. If taking amiodarone, seek immediate medical attention if chest pain, confusion, dizziness, fainting, lethargy, or shortness of breath occurs after starting therapy. • Do not take herbal products, esp. St. John's wort. • Daclatasvir must be used in combination with sofosbuvir (an antiviral drug) and should not be used alone.

daclizumab

dac-**klye**-zue-mab
(Zinbryta)

■ **BLACK BOX ALERT** ■ May cause severe, sometimes life-threatening, hepatic injury, including hepatic failure and autoimmune hepatitis. Hepatic injury, including autoimmune hepatitis, may occur at any time during treatment and up to 4 mos after discontinuation. Contraindicated in pts with preexisting hepatic disease or impairment. Immune-mediated disorders, including toxic skin reactions, lymphadenopathy, noninfectious colitis, were reported.
Do not confuse daclizumab with certolizumab, eculizumab, efalizumab, natalizumab, tocilizumab, vedolizumab.

◆CLASSIFICATION

PHARMACOTHERAPEUTIC: Interleukin-2 receptor blocking antibody. **CLINICAL:** Multiple sclerosis agent.

USES

Treatment of adult pts with relapsing forms of multiple sclerosis (MS). Therapy should generally be reserved for pts who have had an inadequate response to 2 or more medications indicated for the treatment of MS.

PRECAUTIONS

Contraindications: Hypersensitivity to daclizumab; preexisting hepatic disease or impairment, including serum ALT or AST at least 2 times upper limit of normal (ULN), history of autoimmune hepatitis or other autoimmune disorders involving the liver. **Cautions:** History of chronic opportunistic infections (esp. fungal infections, viral infections, tuberculosis); history of autoimmune disorders (demyelinating polyneuropathy, Crohn's disease, Guillain-Barré syndrome, Hashimoto's thyroiditis, hyperthyroidism, myasthenia gravis, psoriasis, rheumatoid arthritis, systemic lupus erythematosus, type 1 diabetes, vasculitis); concomitant use of other immunosuppressants;

conditions predisposing to infection (e.g., diabetes, kidney failure, open wounds), elderly, HIV infection, hematologic cytopenias; history of depression, suicidal ideation. Concomitant use of live vaccines not recommended during treatment and up to 4 mos after treatment. Avoid use during severe active infection.

ACTION

Exact mechanism of action unknown. May involve modulation of interleukin-2 mediated activation of lymphocytes, reducing the number of lymphocytes available to CNS. **Therapeutic Effect:** May reduce lymphocyte migration into CNS, which reduces central inflammation.

PHARMACOKINETICS

Widely distributed. Bioavailability: 90%. Degraded into small peptides and amino acids via catabolic pathway. Peak plasma concentration: 5–7 days. Elimination not specified. **Half-life:** 21 days.

⧗ LIFESPAN CONSIDERATIONS

Pregnancy/Lactation: Unknown if distributed in breast milk. Monoclonal antibodies are known to cross the placenta. **Children:** Safety and efficacy not established in pts younger than 17 yrs. **Elderly:** Not specified; use caution.

INTERACTIONS

DRUG: None known. **Note:** Use caution with other **hepatotoxic medications (e.g., acetaminophen, ketoconazole, methotrexate, simvastatin).** **HERBAL: Echinacea** may decrease effect. **FOOD:** None known. **LAB VALUES:** May increase serum alkaline phosphatase, ALT, AST, bilirubin. May decrease ANC, Hgb, Hct, lymphocytes, RBC.

AVAILABILITY (Rx)

Injection Solution: 150 mg/mL in prefilled syringe.

ADMINISTRATION/HANDLING

Subcutaneous

• 30 min prior to injection, remove syringe from the refrigerator to allow to warm to room temperature. • Do not use external heat sources (e.g., hot water, heating plate). • Visually inspect for particulate matter or discoloration. • Solution should appear colorless to slightly yellow, clear to slightly opalescent in color. Discard if solution is cloudy or discolored or if visible particles are observed.

Administration

• Insert needle subcutaneously into upper arms, outer thigh, or abdomen and inject solution. • Do not inject into areas of active skin disease or injury such as sunburns, rashes, inflammation, skin infections, or active psoriasis. • Rotate injection sites.

Storage

• Refrigerate until time of use. • If unable to refrigerate, may store protected from light at room temperature (no more than 30°C [86°F]) up to 30 days. • Do not place syringe back in refrigerator after allowing it to warm to room temperature. • Do not freeze.

INDICATIONS/ROUTES/DOSAGE

Multiple Sclerosis, Relapsing

SQ: ADULTS: 150 mg once monthly. If a dose is missed, inject missed dose as soon as possible if no more than 2 wks have passed. If more than 2 wks have passed, skip missed dose and administer the next dose on schedule.

Dose Modification

Hepatic Impairment

Serum ALT or AST greater than 5 times ULN; total serum bilirubin greater than 2 times ULN; serum ALT or AST 3 to less than 5 times ULN with total serum bilirubin 1.5 to less than 2 times ULN: Withhold treatment and investigate for other etiologies of abnormal LFT values. If none are identified, discontinue treatment. If other etiologies are identified, use clinical judgment and consider if it is appropriate to resume treatment when both serum ALT or AST are less than 2 times ULN and total serum bilirubin is less than or equal to ULN.

Suspected autoimmune hepatitis: Permanently discontinue.

Immune-Mediated Disorders
Dermatologic toxicity, serious diffuse or inflammatory rashes; lymphadenopathy, lymphadenitis; noninfectious colitis; other single-organ or multiorgan inflammatory events: Consider interrupting treatment or permanent discontinuation.

Other Toxicities
Allergic reaction, anaphylaxis: Permanently discontinue. **Severe depression, suicidal ideation:** Consider permanent discontinuation. **Infection:** Withhold treatment until infection fully resolved.

Dosage in Renal Impairment
Not specified; use caution.

SIDE EFFECTS

Occasional (11%–5%): Rash, oropharyngeal pain, eczema. **Rare (3%–2%):** Acne, pyrexia, diarrhea, dry skin, erythema.

ADVERSE EFFECTS/TOXIC REACTIONS

Serious, sometimes life-threatening, hepatic injury, including autoimmune hepatitis, may occur (less than 1% of pts). Serum ALT or AST elevation reported in 6% of pts. Infections occurred in up to 60% of pts. Respiratory tract infections, including nasopharyngitis, upper respiratory tract infection, influenza, bronchitis, pharyngitis, tonsillitis, rhinitis, laryngitis, pneumonia, reported in 29%–4% of pts. Dermatitis, folliculitis, skin exfoliation, toxic skin eruption may occur. Lymphadenopathy, lymphadenitis reported in 5%–2% of pts. Other immune-mediated disorders may include immune hemolytic anemia, glomerulonephritis, noninfectious colitis, pancreatitis, rheumatoid arthritis, sarcoidosis, sialadenitis thyroiditis. Depression occurred in 7% of pts. Severe hypersensitivity reactions, including anaphylaxis, angioedema, may occur any time during treatment. Immunogenicity (auto-daclizumab antibodies) reported in 8%–19% of pts.

NURSING CONSIDERATIONS

BASELINE ASSESSMENT
Obtain baseline LFT, vital signs. Screen for hepatitis B and C virus infection, active infection. Pts should be evaluated for active tuberculosis and tested for latent infection prior to initiating treatment and periodically during therapy. Induration of 5 mm or greater with tuberculin skin testing should be considered a positive test result when assessing for latent tuberculosis infection. Antifungal therapy should be considered for pts who reside in or travel to regions where mycoses are endemic. Question history of autoimmune diseases (as listed in Precautions), depression or suicidal ideation, demyelinating disorders, HIV infection, prior hypersensitivity reactions. Conduct neurologic and dermatologic exam. Assess motor function and speech characteristics. Assess pt's willingness to self-administer medication.

INTERVENTION/EVALUATION
Monitor LFT monthly during treatment and for at least 6 mos after discontinuation. If autoimmune hepatitis is suspected or severe immune-mediated disorder occurs, consider referral to specialist; may require treatment with corticosteroids and other immunosuppressant agents. Monitor for symptoms of tuberculosis, including those who tested negative for latent tuberculosis infection at baseline. Interrupt or discontinue treatment if serious infection, opportunistic infection, or sepsis occurs, and initiate appropriate antimicrobial therapy. Diligently monitor for depression or suicidal ideation, hepatotoxicity, hypersensitivity reaction (esp. anaphylaxis, angioedema), lymphadenopathy, noninfectious colitis, other immune-mediated disorders, reactivation of latent infection, toxic skin reactions. Assess neurologic status for symptom improvement. Assess skin for rash, lesions.

PATIENT/FAMILY TEACHING
• A health care provider will show you how to properly prepare and inject your

---

medication. You must demonstrate correct preparation and injection techniques before using medication at home. • Treatment may depress immune system and reduce ability to fight infection. Report symptoms of infection such as body aches, chills, cough, fatigue, fever. Avoid those with active infection. • Report travel plans to possible endemic areas. • Do not receive live vaccines during treatment and up to 4 mos following last dose. • Expect frequent tuberculosis screening. • Treatment may cause signs of a common cold or flu-like symptoms. • Allergic reactions such as difficulty breathing, hives, rash, swelling of the face or tongue, wheezing can happen at any time. If allergic reaction occurs, seek immediate medical attention. • Treatment may cause worsening of chronic autoimmune disorders; inflammatory disorders such as toxic skin reactions, inflammation of the lymph nodes or colon, or life-threatening inflammation of the liver. • Report abdominal pain, diarrhea, easy bruising, clay-colored stools, dark-amber urine, fatigue, loss of appetite, yellowing of skin or eyes; swelling or pain of lymph nodes. • Immediately report thoughts of suicide or worsening of depression.

dalbavancin

dal-ba-**van**-sin
(Dalvance)
Do not confuse dalbavancin with oritavancin or telavancin.

◆CLASSIFICATION

PHARMACOTHERAPEUTIC: Glycopeptide. **CLINICAL:** Antibiotic.

USES

Treatment of adult pts with acute bacterial skin and skin structure infections (ABSSSI) caused by susceptible strains of gram-positive microorganisms, including *S. aureus* (methicillin-susceptible and methicillin-resistant strains), *S. pyogenes, S. agalactiae,* and *S. anginosus* group (including *S. anginosus, S. intermedius, S. constellatus*).

PRECAUTIONS

Contraindications: Known hypersensitivity reaction to dalbavancin. **Cautions:** Hepatic/renal impairment, chronic hepatitis, hx alcohol abuse, hx hypersensitivity reaction to glycopeptides (e.g., vancomycin), recent *C. difficile* infection or antibiotic-associated colitis.

ACTION

Inhibits cell wall synthesis by binding to bacterial cell membrane. **Therapeutic Effect:** Bactericidal.

PHARMACOKINETICS

Widely distributed. Metabolism not defined. Protein binding: 93%. Primarily eliminated in urine. **Half-life:** 14.4 days.

⧗ LIFESPAN CONSIDERATIONS

Pregnancy/Lactation: Unknown if distributed in breast milk; use caution. **Children:** Safety and efficacy not established. **Elderly:** No age-related precautions noted.

INTERACTIONS

DRUG: None known. **HERBAL:** None known. **FOOD:** None significant. **LAB VALUES:** May increase serum ALT, AST, bilirubin.

AVAILABILITY (Rx)

Injection, Powder for Reconstitution: 500 mg.

ADMINISTRATION/HANDLING

 IV

◀**ALERT**▶ Must be reconstituted with Sterile Water for Injection and subsequently diluted with 5% Dextrose Injection only.

D

Reconstitution • Reconstitute each 500-mg vial with 25 mL of Sterile Water for Injection for final concentration of 20 mg/mL. • To avoid foaming, alternate between gentle swirling and inversion of vial until completely dissolved. Do not shake. • Visually inspect for particulate matter. Solution should appear clear, colorless to yellow. Do not use if particulate matter observed. • Aseptically transfer required dose into 5% dextrose to a final concentration of 1–5 mg/mL.

Rate of Administration • Infuse over 30 min.

Storage • Store unused vials at room temperature. • Reconstituted vials/diluted bag may be refrigerated or stored at room temperature for up to 48 hrs. • Do not freeze.

▦ IV INCOMPATIBILITIES

Do not infuse with other medications or electrolytes. Saline-based solutions may cause precipitate formation. If using single IV access, flush IV with 5% dextrose before and after each use.

INDICATIONS/ROUTES/DOSAGE

Acute Bacterial Skin and Skin Structure Infection
IV: ADULTS/ELDERLY: *(Two-Dose Regimen):* 1,000 mg once, followed by 500 mg once 7 days later. *(Single-Dose Regimen):* 1,500 mg.

Dosage in Renal Impairment
CrCl less than 30 mL/min in pts who are not receiving regularly scheduled hemodialysis: *(Two-Dose Regimen):* 750 mg once, followed by 375 mg once 7 days later. *(Single-Dose Regimen):* 1,125 mg. **Pts receiving regularly scheduled hemodialysis:** No dose adjustment necessary.

Dosage in Hepatic Impairment
Mild impairment: No dose adjustment. **Moderate to severe impairment:** Not defined; use caution.

SIDE EFFECTS

Occasional (6%–4%): Nausea, vomiting, diarrhea, headache. **Rare (3%–2%):** Rash, pruritus.

ADVERSE EFFECTS/TOXIC REACTIONS

Serious hypersensitivity reactions including anaphylaxis or severe skin reactions have been reported with glycopeptide antibacterial agents. Too-rapid infusion may cause "red-man syndrome" reaction, characterized by flushing of upper body, urticaria, pruritus, rash. *C. difficile*–associated diarrhea with severity ranging from mild diarrhea to fatal colitis has occurred. Drug-induced hepatotoxicity with hepatic enzymes greater than 3 times upper limit of normal has been reported. Treatment in the absence of proven or strongly suspected bacterial infection may increase risk of drug-resistant bacteria.

NURSING CONSIDERATIONS

BASELINE ASSESSMENT

Obtain baseline CBC, BMP, LFT, wound culture and sensitivity, vital signs. Question history of recent *C. difficile* infection, hepatic/renal impairment, hypersensitivity reaction. Assess skin wound characteristics, hydration status. Question pt's usual stool characteristics (color, frequency, consistency).

INTERVENTION/EVALUATION

Assess skin infection/wound for improvement. Monitor daily pattern of bowel activity, stool consistency; increasing severity may indicate antibiotic-associated colitis. If frequent diarrhea occurs, obtain *C. difficile* toxin screen and initiate isolation precautions until result confirmed. Encourage PO intake. Monitor I&O. Monitor for "red-man syndrome" during infusion; stopping or slowing infusion may decrease reaction.

PATIENT/FAMILY TEACHING

• It is essential to complete drug therapy despite symptom improvement. Early discontinuation may result in antibacterial resistance or increased risk of recurrent infection. • Report any episodes of diarrhea, esp. following weeks after treatment completion. Frequent diarrhea, fever, abdominal pain, blood-streaked stool may indicate infectious diarrhea, which may be contagious to others. • Report abdominal pain, black/tarry stools, bruising, yellowing of skin or eyes, dark urine, decreased urine output. • Do not breastfeed. • Drink plenty of fluids.

dalfampridine

dal-**fam**-pri-deen
(Ampyra, Fampyra ✦)
Do not confuse Ampyra with anakinra, or dalfampridine with desipramine.

◆ CLASSIFICATION

PHARMACOTHERAPEUTIC: Potassium channel blocker. **CLINICAL:** Multiple sclerosis agent.

USES

Indicated to improve ambulation in pts with MS.

PRECAUTIONS

Contraindications: Hypersensitivity to dalfampridine. History of seizures, moderate to severe renal impairment (CrCl equal to or less than 50 mL/min). **Cautions:** Mild renal impairment (CrCl equal to 51–80 mL/min).

ACTION

Increases conduction of action potentials in demyelinated axons, inhibiting potassium channels. **Therapeutic Effect:** Improves ambulation in pts with multiple sclerosis (MS).

PHARMACOKINETICS

Rapidly absorbed from GI tract. Minimally metabolized in liver. Primarily excreted in urine. **Half-life:** 5.2–6.5 hrs.

⧗ LIFESPAN CONSIDERATIONS

Pregnancy/Lactation: Unknown if drug crosses placenta or is distributed in breast milk. **Children:** Safety and efficacy not established in pts younger than 18. **Elderly:** Age-related renal impairment may require dosage adjustment.

INTERACTIONS

DRUG: None significant. **HERBAL:** None significant. **FOOD:** None known. **LAB VALUES:** May increase creatinine clearance.

AVAILABILITY (Rx)

Tablet, Film-Coated, Extended-Release: 10 mg.

ADMINISTRATION/HANDLING

PO
• May give without regard to food.
• Do not break, crush, dissolve, or divide tablets.

INDICATIONS/ROUTES/DOSAGE

Multiple Sclerosis
PO: ADULTS 18 YRS AND OLDER, ELDERLY: 10 mg twice daily.

Dosage in Renal Impairment
CrCl 50 mL/min or less: Contraindicated.

Dosage in Hepatic Impairment
No dose adjustment.

SIDE EFFECTS

Frequent (9%–5%): Insomnia, dizziness, headache, nausea, asthenia, back pain. **Rare (4%–2%):** Paresthesia, nasopharyngitis, constipation, dyspepsia, pharyngolaryngeal pain.

ADVERSE EFFECTS/TOXIC REACTIONS

Urinary tract infection occurs in 12% of pts.

D

NURSING CONSIDERATIONS

BASELINE ASSESSMENT

Obtain CBC, BUN, creatinine clearance, serum chemistries prior to treatment and routinely thereafter. Conduct baseline neurologic exam. Assess motor function, speech characteristics, gait, ability to ambulate.

INTERVENTION/EVALUATION

Monitor CBC, serum chemistries, renal function tests, particularly creatinine clearance. Monitor for urinary, respiratory infection. Assess for therapeutic response (improvement in walking as demonstrated by increase in walking speed).

PATIENT/FAMILY TEACHING

• Avoid tasks that require alertness, motor skills until response to drug is established. • Report difficulty in sleeping, dizziness, headache, nausea, back pain, loss of strength or energy. • Do not chew, crush, dissolve, or divide tablets. • Inform physician if ambulation does not improve or worsens.

---

dalteparin **HIGH ALERT**

dal-te-par-in
(Fragmin)

■ **BLACK BOX ALERT** ■ Epidural or spinal anesthesia greatly increases potential for spinal or epidural hematoma, subsequent long-term or permanent paralysis. **Do not confuse dalteparin with heparin.**

◆CLASSIFICATION

PHARMACOTHERAPEUTIC: Low molecular weight heparin. **CLINICAL:** Anticoagulant.

USES

Prevention of ischemic complications in pts with unstable angina or non–Q-wave MI. Prevention of deep vein thrombosis

(DVT) in pts undergoing hip replacement surgery or in pts undergoing abdominal surgery who are at risk for thromboembolic complications (e.g., pts older than 40 yrs, obese, pts with malignancy, history of DVT or PE, surgery requiring general anesthesia and lasting more than 30 min). Extended treatment of symptomatic venous thromboembolism (VTE) to reduce recurrence of VTE in cancer pts. Prevention of DVT or pulmonary embolism in acutely ill pts with severely restricted mobility.

PRECAUTIONS

Contraindications: Active major bleeding; concurrent heparin therapy; hypersensitivity to dalteparin, heparin, pork products; unstable angina; history of heparin-induced thrombocytopenia (HIT), or HIT with thrombosis; non–Q-wave MI; prolonged venous thromboembolism undergoing epidural/neuraxial anesthesia. **Cautions:** Conditions with increased risk for hemorrhage, bacterial endocarditis, renal/hepatic impairment, uncontrolled hypertension, history of recent GI ulceration/hemorrhage, peptic ulcer disease, pericarditis, preexisting thrombocytopenia, recent childbirth, concurrent use of aspirin.

ACTION

Antithrombin in presence of low molecular weight heparin inhibits factor Xa, thrombin. Only slightly influences platelet aggregation, PT, aPTT. **Therapeutic Effect:** Produces anticoagulation.

PHARMACOKINETICS

Route	Onset	Peak	Duration
Subcutaneous	N/A	4 hrs	N/A

Protein binding: less than 10%. **Half-life:** 3–5 hrs.

⧗ LIFESPAN CONSIDERATIONS

Pregnancy/Lactation: Use with caution, particularly during last trimester, immediate postpartum period (increased risk of maternal hemorrhage). Unknown if distributed in breast milk. **Children:** Safety and efficacy not established. **Elderly:** No age-related precautions noted.

INTERACTIONS

DRUG: Anticoagulants (e.g., warfarin), NSAIDs (e.g., ibuprofen, ketorolac, naproxen), platelet inhibitors (e.g., clopidogrel), thrombolytic agents (e.g., tPA) may increase risk of bleeding. **HERBAL:** Cat's claw, dong quai, evening primrose, garlic, ginseng, other herbs with anticoagulant/antiplatelet activity may increase antiplatelet activity. **FOOD:** None known. **LAB VALUES:** May increase serum ALT, AST. May decrease serum triglycerides.

AVAILABILITY (Rx)

Injection, Solution: 2,500 units/0.2 mL, 5,000 units/0.2 mL, 7,500 units/0.3 mL, 10,000 units/mL, 12,500 units/0.5 mL, 15,000 units/0.6 mL, 18,000 units/0.72 mL.

ADMINISTRATION/HANDLING

Subcutaneous
• Visually inspect for particulate matter or discoloration. • Subcutaneously insert needle into abdomen, outer thigh, or upper arm region and inject solution. • Do not inject into areas of active skin disease or injury such as sunburns, rashes, inflammation, or infection. Rotate injection sites.

INDICATIONS/ROUTES/DOSAGE

Abdominal Surgery
SQ: ADULTS, ELDERLY: *(Low DVT Risk):* 2,500 units 1–2 hrs before surgery, then daily for 5–10 days. *(High DVT Risk):* 5,000 units evening before surgery or 2,500 units 1–2 hrs before surgery, 2,500 units 12 hrs later, then 5,000 units daily for 5–10 days.

Total Hip Surgery
SQ: ADULTS, ELDERLY: 2,500 units 1–2 hrs before surgery, then 2,500 units 4–8 hrs after surgery, then 5,000 units/day (starting at least 6 hrs after postsurgical dose) for 10–14 days.

Unstable Angina, Non–Q-Wave MI
SQ: ADULTS, ELDERLY: 120 units/kg q12h for up to 5–8 days (**maximum: 10,000 units/dose**) given with aspirin. Discontinue dalteparin once clinically stable.

Venous Thromboembolism (Cancer Pts)
SQ: ADULTS, ELDERLY: Initially (1 mo), 200 units/kg (**maximum: 18,000 units**) daily for 30 days. **Maintenance (2–6 mos):** 150 units/kg once daily (**maximum: 18,000 units**). If platelet count 50,000–100,000 cells/mm^3, reduce dose by 2,500 units until platelet count recovers to 100,000 cells/mm^3 or more. If platelet count less than 50,000 cells/mm^3, discontinue until platelet count recovers to more than 50,000 cells/mm^3.

Prevention of DVT, Acutely Ill Pt, Immobile Pt
SQ: ADULTS, ELDERLY: 5,000 units once daily.

Dosage in Renal Impairment
For CrCl less than 30 mL/min, monitor anti-Xa levels to determine appropriate dose.

Dosage in Hepatic Impairment
No dose adjustment.

SIDE EFFECTS

Occasional (7%–3%): Hematoma at injection site. **Rare (less than 1%):** Hypersensitivity reaction (chills, fever, pruritus, urticaria, asthma, rhinitis, lacrimation, headache); mild, local skin irritation.

ADVERSE EFFECTS/TOXIC REACTIONS

Overdose may lead to bleeding complications ranging from local ecchymoses to major hemorrhage. Thrombocytopenia occurs rarely.

NURSING CONSIDERATIONS

BASELINE ASSESSMENT
Obtain baseline coagulation studies, CBC, esp. platelet count. Determine baseline B/P. Screen for risk factors as listed in Precautions.

D

INTERVENTION/EVALUATION

Periodically monitor CBC, stool for occult blood (no need for daily monitoring in pts with normal presurgical coagulation parameters). Assess for any sign of bleeding (bleeding at surgical site, hematuria, blood in stool, bleeding from gums, petechiae, bruising/bleeding at injection sites). Monitor for DVT (extremity pain, swelling, redness), pulmonary embolism (chest pain, dyspnea, hypoxia, tachycardia).

PATIENT/FAMILY TEACHING

• Usual length of therapy is 5–10 days. • Do not take any OTC medication (esp. aspirin) without consulting physician. • Report bleeding, bruising, dizziness, light-headedness, rash, itching, fever, swelling, breathing difficulty. • Rotate injection sites daily. • Teach proper injection technique. • Excessive bruising at injection site may be lessened by ice massage before injection. • Monitor for symptoms of blood clots in the leg (extremity pain, swelling, redness) or blood clots in the lungs (chest pain, difficulty breathing, shortness of breath, fast heart rate).

dantrolene

dan-troe-leen
(Dantrium, Revonto, Ryanodex)
■ **BLACK BOX ALERT** ■ Potential for hepatotoxicity.
Do not confuse Dantrium with danazol or Daraprim, or Revonto with Revatio.

◆CLASSIFICATION

PHARMACOTHERAPEUTIC: Calcium release blocker. **CLINICAL:** Skeletal muscle relaxant.

USES

PO: Relief of symptoms of spasticity due to spinal cord injuries, stroke, cerebral palsy, multiple sclerosis, esp. flexor spasms, concomitant pain, clonus, muscular rigidity. Management of malignant hyperthermia (MH), prevention of MH in susceptible individuals. **Parenteral:** Management of malignant hyperthermia. Prevention of malignant hyperthermia (preoperative/postoperative administration). **OFF-LABEL:** Neuroleptic malignant syndrome.

PRECAUTIONS

Contraindications: Hypersensitivity to dantrolene. **IV:** None known. **PO:** When spasticity used to maintain posture/balance during locomotion or to obtain increased motor function. Active hepatic disease. **Cautions:** Cardiac/pulmonary impairment, history of previous hepatic disease.

ACTION

Interferes with release of calcium from sarcoplasmic reticulum of skeletal muscle. **Therapeutic Effect:** Dissociates excitation-contraction coupling. Interferes with catabolic process associated with malignant hyperthermia.

PHARMACOKINETICS

Poorly absorbed from GI tract. Protein binding: High. Metabolized in liver. Primarily excreted in urine. **Half-life: IV:** 4–8 hrs; **PO:** 8.7 hrs.

⌛ LIFESPAN CONSIDERATIONS

Pregnancy/Lactation: Readily crosses placenta. Breastfeeding not recommended. **Children:** No age-related precautions noted in pts 5 yrs and older. **Elderly:** No precautions specified.

INTERACTIONS

DRUG: CNS depressants (e.g., lorazepam, morphine, zolpidem) may increase CNS depression with short-term use. **Hepatotoxic medications (e.g., acetaminophen, ketoconazole, methotrexate, simvastatin)** may increase risk of hepatic toxicity with chronic use. **CYP3A4 inhibitors (e.g., clarithromycin)** may increase concentration.

HERBAL: Gotu kola, kava kava, St. John's wort, valerian may increase CNS depression. **FOOD:** None known. **LAB VALUES:** May alter serum ALT, AST.

AVAILABILITY (Rx)

Capsules: 25 mg, 50 mg, 100 mg. **Injection, Powder for Reconstitution:** 20-mg vial. **Injection Suspension:** 250 mg powder.

ADMINISTRATION/HANDLING

 IV

Reconstitution • Reconstitute 20-mg vial with 60 mL Sterile Water for Injection (**not** Bacteriostatic Water for Injection). *(Ryanodex):* 250-mg vial with 5 mL Sterile Water for Injection.
Rate of Administration • For therapeutic or emergency dose, give IV over 2–3 min. • For IV infusion, administer over 1 hr. • Diligently monitor for extravasation (high pH of IV preparation). May produce severe complications. *(Ryanodex):* Do not dilute; infuse into IV catheter or indwelling catheter. Infuse over 1 min.
Storage • Store at room temperature. • Use within 6 hrs after reconstitution. • Solution is clear, colorless. Discard if cloudy, precipitate forms.

PO
• Give without regard to food.

🔲 IV INCOMPATIBILITIES

D₅W, 0.9% NaCl.

INDICATIONS/ROUTES/DOSAGE

Spasticity
PO: ADULTS, ELDERLY: Initially, 25 mg once daily for 7 days; then 25 mg 3 times/day for 7 days; then 50 mg 3 times/day for 7 days; then 100 mg 3 times/day. **Maximum:** 400 mg/day. **CHILDREN:** Initially, 0.5 mg/kg/dose once daily for 7 days; then 0.5 mg/kg/dose 3 times/day for 7 days; then 1 mg/kg/dose 3 times/day for 7 days; then 2 mg/kg/dose 3 times/day. Some pts may require dosing 4 times/day. **Maximum:** 400 mg/day.

Perioperative Prophylaxis for Malignant Hyperthermic Crisis
PO: ADULTS, ELDERLY, CHILDREN: 4–8 mg/kg/day in 3–4 divided doses beginning 1–2 days before surgery; give last dose 3–4 hrs before surgery.
IV: ADULTS, ELDERLY, CHILDREN: 2.5 mg/kg about 1.25 hrs before surgery with additional doses as needed.

Management of Malignant Hyperthermic Crisis
IV: ADULTS, ELDERLY, CHILDREN: Initially, a minimum of 2.5 mg/kg rapid IV; may repeat up to total cumulative dose of 10 mg/kg. May follow with 4–8 mg/kg/day PO in 4 divided doses up to 3 days after crisis.

Dosage in Renal/Hepatic Impairment
No dose adjustment. Contraindicated with active hepatic disease.

SIDE EFFECTS

Frequent: Drowsiness, dizziness, weakness, general malaise, diarrhea (mild). **Occasional:** Confusion, diarrhea (severe), headache, insomnia, constipation, urinary frequency. **Rare:** Paradoxical CNS excitement or restlessness, paresthesia, tinnitus, slurred speech, tremor, blurred vision, dry mouth, nocturia, impotence, rash, pruritus.

ADVERSE EFFECTS/TOXIC REACTIONS

Risk of hepatotoxicity, most notably in females, pts 35 yrs and older, pts taking other hepatotoxic medications concurrently. Overt hepatitis noted most frequently between 3rd and 12th mo of therapy. Overdose results in vomiting, muscular hypotonia, muscle twitching, respiratory depression, seizures.

NURSING CONSIDERATIONS

BASELINE ASSESSMENT
Obtain baseline LFT. Record onset, type, location, duration of muscular spasm. Check for immobility, stiffness, swelling.

INTERVENTION/EVALUATION

Assist with ambulation. For pts on long-term therapy, hepatic/renal function tests, CBC should be performed periodically. Assess for therapeutic response: relief of pain, stiffness, spasm.

PATIENT/FAMILY TEACHING

• Drowsiness usually diminishes with continued therapy. • Avoid tasks that require alertness, motor skills until response to drug is established. • Avoid alcohol/other depressants. • Report continued weakness, fatigue, nausea, diarrhea, skin rash, itching, bloody/tarry stools.

DAPTOmycin

dap-toe-mye-sin
(Cubicin)
Do not confuse Cubicin with Cleocin, or DAPTOmycin with DACTINomycin.

◆CLASSIFICATION

PHARMACOTHERAPEUTIC: Lipopeptide antibacterial agent. **CLINICAL:** Antibiotic.

USES

Treatment of complicated skin/skin structure infections caused by susceptible strains of gram-positive pathogens, including *S. aureus* (methicillin susceptible and methicillin resistant [MRSA]), *S. pyogenes, S. agalactiae.* Treatment of *S. aureus* systemic infections caused by methicillin-susceptible and methicillin-resistant *S. aureus.* **OFF-LABEL:** Severe infections caused by MRSA or vancomycin-resistant *Enterococcus* (VRE); treatment of prosthetic joint infection caused by staphylococci or *Enterococcus.*

PRECAUTIONS

Contraindications: Hypersensitivity to daptomycin. **Cautions:** Severe renal impairment (CrCl less than 30 mL/min), concurrent use of other medications associated with myopathy (e.g., statins).

ACTION

Binds to bacterial membranes and causes rapid depolarization of membrane potential. Inhibits protein, DNA, RNA synthesis. **Therapeutic Effect:** Bactericidal.

PHARMACOKINETICS

Widely distributed. Protein binding: 90%. Primarily excreted unchanged in urine. Moderately removed by hemodialysis. **Half-life:** 7–8 hrs (increased in renal impairment).

⌛ LIFESPAN CONSIDERATIONS

Pregnancy/Lactation: Unknown if drug is distributed in breast milk. **Children:** Safety and efficacy not established in pts younger than 18 yrs. **Elderly:** No age-related precautions noted.

INTERACTIONS

DRUG: Concurrent use with **HMG-CoA reductase inhibitors (e.g., simvastatin)** may cause myopathy. **HERBAL:** None significant. **FOOD:** None known. **LAB VALUES:** May increase CPK, serum potassium. May alter LFT results.

AVAILABILITY (Rx)

Injection, Powder for Reconstitution: 500 mg/vial.

ADMINISTRATION/HANDLING

 IV

Reconstitution • Reconstitute 500-mg vial with 10 mL 0.9% NaCl to provide a concentration of 50 mg/mL. May further dilute in 0.9% NaCl. • Do not shake or agitate vial.
Rate of Administration • For IV injection, give over 2 min (concentration: 50 mg/mL). • For intermittent IV infusion (piggyback), infuse over 30 min.
Storage • Refrigerate. • Appears as pale yellow to light brown lyophilized

cake. • Reconstituted solution is stable for 12 hrs at room temperature or up to 48 hrs if refrigerated. • Discard if particulate forms.

▦ IV INCOMPATIBILITIES

Diluents containing dextrose. If same IV line is used to administer different drugs, flush line with 0.9% NaCl.

▦ IV COMPATIBILITIES

0.9% NaCl, lactated Ringer's, aztreonam (Azactam), DOPamine, fluconazole (Diflucan), gentamicin, heparin, levoFLOXacin (Levaquin).

INDICATIONS/ROUTES/DOSAGE

Complicated Skin/Skin Structure Infections
IV: ADULTS, ELDERLY: 4 mg/kg every 24 hrs for 7–14 days.

Systemic Infections
IV: ADULTS, ELDERLY: 6–8 mg/kg once daily for 2–6 wks.

Dosage in Renal Impairment
CrCl less than 30 mL/min, hemodialysis (HD), peritoneal dialysis (PD): Dosage is 4 mg/kg q48h for skin and soft tissue infections; 6 mg/kg q48h for staphylococcal bacteremia. **Hemodialysis (HD):** Give dose after dialysis. **Continuous renal replacement therapy: Continuous Venovenous Hemodialysis (CVVHD):** 8 mg/kg q48h, **Continuous Venovenous Hemofiltration (CVVH)** or **Continuous Venovenous Hemodiafiltration (CVVHDF):** 8 mg/kg q48h or 4–6 mg/kg q24h.

Dosage in Hepatic Impairment
No dose adjustment.

SIDE EFFECTS

Frequent (6%–5%): Constipation, nausea, peripheral injection site reactions, headache, diarrhea. **Occasional (4%–3%):** Insomnia, rash, vomiting. **Rare (less than 3%):** Pruritus, dizziness, hypotension.

ADVERSE EFFECTS/TOXIC REACTIONS

Skeletal muscle myopathy (muscle pain/weakness, particularly of distal extremities) occurs rarely. Antibiotic-associated colitis (abdominal cramps, severe diarrhea, fever), other superinfections may result from altered bacterial balance in GI/GU tract.

NURSING CONSIDERATIONS

BASELINE ASSESSMENT

Obtain CPK, blood cultures before first dose (therapy may begin before results are known). Question history of renal impairment. Screen for concomitant use of statins.

INTERVENTION/EVALUATION

Assess oral cavity for white patches on mucous membranes, tongue (thrush). Monitor for myopathy (muscle pain, weakness), CPK levels, renal function tests. Monitor daily pattern of bowel activity, stool consistency. Mild GI effects may be tolerable, but increasing severity may indicate onset of antibiotic-associated colitis. Be alert for superinfection: fever, vomiting, diarrhea, anal/genital pruritus, oral mucosal changes (ulceration, pain, erythema). Monitor for dizziness; institute appropriate measures.

PATIENT/FAMILY TEACHING

• Report rash, headache, nausea, dizziness, constipation, diarrhea, muscle pain, or any other new symptom.

daratumumab

dar-a-toom-ue-mab
(Darzalex)
Do not confuse daratumumab with adalimumab, ofatumumab, panitumumab, or necitumumab.

◆CLASSIFICATION

PHARMACOTHERAPEUTIC: Monoclonal antibody. **CLINICAL:** Antineoplastic.

USES

Monotherapy for the treatment of pts with multiple myeloma who have received at least three prior lines of therapy including a proteasome inhibitor and an immunomodulatory agent or who are double-refractory to a proteasome inhibitor and an immunomodulatory agent. In combination with dexamethasone and either lenalidomide or bortezomib for treatment of multiple myeloma in pts who have received at least one prior therapy. In combination with pomalidomide and dexamethasone for treatment of multiple myeloma in pts who have received at least two prior therapies including lenalidomide and a proteasome inhibitor.

PRECAUTIONS

Contraindications: Hypersensitivity to daratumumab. **Cautions:** Obstructive pulmonary disorders (e.g., COPD, emphysema), baseline cytopenias, herpes zoster infection, elderly.

ACTION

Binds to cell surface glycoprotein CD38 on CD38-expressing tumor cells. Inhibits tumor cell proliferation and induces apoptosis. **Therapeutic Effect:** Inhibits tumor cell growth and metastasis. Promotes tumor cell death.

PHARMACOKINETICS

Widely distributed. Metabolism not specified. Steady state reached approx. 5 mos into the q4wk dosing period (by 21st infusion). Elimination not specified. **Half-life:** 18 ± 9 days.

LIFESPAN CONSIDERATIONS

Pregnancy/Lactation: Avoid pregnancy; may cause fetal harm/malformations. Monoclonal antibodies are known to cross the placenta. Females of reproductive potential should use effective contraception during treatment and up to 3 mos after discontinuation. Unknown if distributed in breast milk. However, human immunoglobulin G is present in breast milk. **Children:** Safety and efficacy not established. **Elderly:** No age-related precautions noted.

INTERACTIONS

DRUG: May decrease effect of **BCG vaccine.** **HERBAL:** None significant. **FOOD:** None known. **LAB VALUES:** Drug may be detected on both serum protein electrophoresis and immunofixation assays used to monitor multiple myeloma endogenous M protein. May affect the determination of complete response and disease progression of some pts with immunoglobulin G kappa myeloma protein. May cause positive Coombs' test. Expected to decrease Hgb, Hct, lymphocytes, neutrophils, platelets, RBCs.

AVAILABILITY (Rx)

Injection Solution: 100 mg/5 mL, 400 mg/20 mL.

ADMINISTRATION/HANDLING

🖥 IV

Preparation for Administration • Calculate the dose and number of vials required based on weight in kg. • Solution should appear colorless to pale yellow. Do not use if opaque particles, discoloration, or foreign particles are observed. • Remove a volume from the 0.9% NaCl infusion bag that is equal to the required volume of the dose solution. • Dilute in 1000 mL (first infusion) or 500 mL (subsequent infusions) 0.9% NaCl bag. • Mix by gentle inversion. Do not shake or agitate. • Infusion bags must be made of polyvinylchloride, polypropylene, polyethylene, or polyolefin blend. • Diluted solution may develop very small translucent to white proteinaceous particles; do not use if diluted solution is discolored or if visibly opaque or foreign particles are observed. • Discard used portions of vials.

Infusion Guidelines • Prior to administration, premedicate with an IV corticosteroid, acetaminophen, and an IV or

oral antihistamine approx. 60 min before each infusion (see manufacturer guidelines). • Infuse using an in-line, sterile, nonpyrogenic, low protein-binding polyethersulfone filter (0.22 or 0.2 μm). • Infuse via dedicated line using infusion pump. • Do not administer as IV push or bolus. • Infusion should be completed within 15 hrs. • If infusion cannot be completed for any reason, do not save unused portions for reuse. • Postinfusion, administer an oral corticosteroid on the first and second day after each infusion to reduce risk of delayed infusion reactions (see manufacturer guidelines). • In pts with a history of obstructive pulmonary disease, consider short-acting and long-acting bronchodilators and an inhaled corticosteroid postinfusion (may discontinue if no infusion reaction occurs after the first four infusions).
Rate of Administration • First infusion (1000 mL volume): Infuse at 50 mL/hr for the first 60 min. Increase in increments of 50 mL/hr q1hr if no infusion reactions occur. **Maximum:** 200 mL/hr. • **Second infusion (500 mL volume):** Infuse at 50 mL/hr for the first 60 min. Increase in increments of 50 mL/hr q1hr if there were no grade 1 or greater infusion reactions during the first 3 hrs of first infusion. **Maximum:** 200 mL/hr. • **Subsequent infusions (500 mL volume):** Infuse at 100 mL/hr if there were no grade 1 or greater infusion reactions during a final infusion rate of greater than or equal to 100 mL/hr in the first two infusions. Increase in increments of 50 mL/hr q1hr if tolerated. **Maximum:** 200 mL/hr.
Storage • Refrigerate unused vials. • Do not shake. • May refrigerate diluted solution up to 24 hrs. • If diluted solution is refrigerated, allow solution to warm to room temperature before use. • Protect from light.

▒ IV INCOMPATIBILITIES
Do not mix with other medications.

INDICATIONS/ROUTES/DOSAGE
Multiple Myeloma
IV: ADULTS, ELDERLY: (Monotherapy or combination with lenalidomide or pomalidomide/dexamethasone) Wks 1–8: 16 mg/kg once wkly. **Wks 9–24:** 16 mg/kg once q2wks. **Wk 25 and beyond:** 16 mg/kg once q4wks until disease progression. **(Combination with bortezomib/dexamethasone) Wks 1–9):** 16 mg/kg once wkly. **Wks 10–24):** 16 mg/kg q3wks. **Wk 25 and beyond:** 16 mg/kg q4wks until disease progression.

Dose Modification
Infusion Reactions
Promptly interrupt infusion if any reaction occurs.
Grade 1 or 2 reaction: Once symptoms resolve, resume infusion at a decreased rate that is 50% (or less) of previous rate. If no further reactions are observed, may increase infusion rate as appropriate.
Grade 3 reaction: If symptoms resolve to grade 2 or less, consider resuming infusion at a decreased rate that is 50% (or less) of previous rate. If no further reactions are observed, may increase rate as appropriate. If a grade 3 reaction recurs, decrease rate as outlined earlier. If grade 3 reaction occurs for a third time, permanently discontinue.
Grade 4 reaction: Permanently discontinue.

Dosage in Renal Impairment
No dose adjustment.

Dosage in Hepatic Impairment
Mild impairment: No dose adjustment.
Moderate to severe impairment: Not specified; use caution.

SIDE EFFECTS
Frequent (37%–14%): Fatigue, back pain, nausea, pyrexia, cough, nasal congestion, arthralgia, diarrhea, dyspnea, decreased appetite, extremity pain, constipation, vomiting. **Occasional (12%–10%):** Headache, musculoskeletal chest pain, chills, hypertension.

D

ADVERSE EFFECTS/TOXIC REACTIONS

Anemia, leukopenia, neutropenia, thrombocytopenia are expected responses to therapy. Infusion reactions occurred in approx. 50% of pts (mostly during first infusion). Infusion reactions can also occur with subsequent infusions (mainly during the infusion or within 4 hrs of completion). Severe infusion reactions may include cough, dyspnea, bronchospasm, hypertension, hypoxia, laryngeal edema, pulmonary edema, wheezing. Less common reactions may include chills, headache, hypotension, rash, nausea, pruritus, urticaria, vomiting. Infections including pneumonia, upper respiratory tract infection, nasopharyngitis reported in 20%–11% of pts. Herpes zoster reported in 3% of pts. Thrombocytopenia may increase risk of bleeding.

NURSING CONSIDERATIONS

BASELINE ASSESSMENT

Obtain CBC, blood type and screen; vital signs. Obtain pregnancy test in female pts of reproductive potential. Question history of COPD, emphysema, herpes infection; prior hypersensitivity reaction to any drug in treatment regimen; prior infusion reaction. Assess nutritional status. Screen for active infection. Offer emotional support.

INTERVENTION/EVALUATION

Monitor CBC, vital signs periodically. Administer in an environment equipped to monitor for and manage infusion reactions. If infusion reaction of any grade/severity occurs, immediately interrupt infusion and manage symptoms. Accurately record characteristics of infusion reactions (severity, type, time of onset). Reactions may affect future infusion rates. To prevent herpes zoster reactivation in pts with prior history, consider antiviral prophylaxis within 1 wk of starting treatment and continue for 3 mos following discontinuation. Monitor for infection. Monitor daily pattern of bowel activity, stool consistency.

PATIENT/FAMILY TEACHING

• Blood levels will be monitored periodically. • Treatment may depress your immune system and reduce your ability to fight infection. Report symptoms of infection such as body aches, chills, cough, fatigue, fever. Avoid those with active infection. • Avoid pregnancy. Do not breastfeed. • Effective contraception is recommended during treatment and for at least 3 mos after final dose. • Severe infusion reactions can occur at any time. Immediately report symptoms of infusion reactions such as chills, cough, difficulty breathing, headache, hives, itching, nausea, rash, stuffy or runny nose, throat tightness, vomiting, wheezing.

darbepoetin alfa ^{TOP 100}

dar-be-poe-e-tin al-fa
(Aranesp)
■ **BLACK BOX ALERT** ■ Increased risk of serious cardiovascular events, thromboembolic events, mortality, time-to-tumor progression when administered to a target hemoglobin greater than 11 g/dL. Shortened overall survival and/or increased risk of tumor progression has been reported with breast, cervical, head/neck, NSCL cancers. **Do not confuse Aranesp with Aricept, or darbepoetin with dalteparin or epoetin.**

◆CLASSIFICATION

PHARMACOTHERAPEUTIC: Erythropoiesis stimulating agent (ESA). **CLINICAL:** Hematopoietic agent.

USES

Treatment of anemia associated with chronic renal failure (including pts on dialysis and pts not on dialysis), treatment of anemia caused by concurrent myelosuppressive chemotherapy in pts planned to receive chemotherapy for minimum of 2 additional months. **OFF-LABEL:** Treatment of symptomatic anemia in myelodysplastic syndrome (MDS).

PRECAUTIONS

Contraindications: Hypersensitivity to darbepoetin. Pure red cell aplasia that begins after treatment with darbepoetin alfa or other erythropoietin protein medication. **Cautions:** History of seizures, hypertension. Not recommended in pts with mild to moderate anemia and HF or CAD.

ACTION

Stimulates formation of RBCs in bone marrow. **Therapeutic Effect:** Induces erythropoiesis, release of reticulocytes from bone marrow into bloodstream.

PHARMACOKINETICS

Well absorbed after subcutaneous administration. **Half-life:** 48.5 hrs.

⏳ LIFESPAN CONSIDERATIONS

Pregnancy/Lactation: Unknown if drug crosses placenta or is distributed in breast milk. **Children:** Safety and efficacy not established. **Elderly:** Age-related renal impairment may require dosage adjustment.

INTERACTIONS

DRUG: Contraceptives (e.g., estradiol, levonorgestrel), estrogens may increase risk of thrombosis. **HERBAL:** None significant. **FOOD:** None known. **LAB VALUES:** May decrease serum ferritin, serum transferrin saturation.

AVAILABILITY (Rx)

Injection Solution: 10 mcg/0.4 mL, 25 mcg/mL, 40 mcg/mL, 60 mcg/mL, 100 mcg/mL, 150 mcg/0.75 mL, 200 mcg/mL, 300 mcg/mL. **Prefilled Syringe:** 25 mcg/0.42 mL, 40 mcg/0.4 mL, 60 mcg/0.3 mL, 100 mcg/0.5 mL, 150 mcg/0.3 mL, 200 mcg/0.4 mL, 300 mcg/0.6 mL, 500 mcg/mL.

ADMINISTRATION/HANDLING

 IV

Preparation • Avoid excessive agitation of vial; do not shake (will cause foaming). Do not dilute.

Rate of Administration • May be given as IV bolus.

Storage • Refrigerate. • Do not shake. Vigorous shaking may denature medication, rendering it inactive.

Subcutaneous
• Use 1 dose per vial; do not reenter vial. Discard unused portion.

▒ IV INCOMPATIBILITIES

Do not mix with other medications.

INDICATIONS/ROUTES/DOSAGE

Anemia in Chronic Renal Failure
◄ **ALERT** ► Individualize dosing and use lowest dose to reduce need for RBC transfusions. **ON DIALYSIS:** Initiate when Hgb less than 10 g/dL; reduce or stop dose when Hgb approaches or exceeds 11 g/dL. **NOT ON DIALYSIS:** Initiate when Hgb less than 10 g/dL and Hgb decline would likely result in RBC transfusion; reduce dose or stop if Hgb exceeds 10 g/dL.

IV, SQ: ADULTS, ELDERLY: ON DIALYSIS: Initially, 0.45 mcg/kg once wkly or 0.75 mcg/kg once q2wks. **NOT ON DIALYSIS:** 0.45 mcg/kg q4wks.

Decrease dose by 25%: If Hgb approaches 12 g/dL or increases greater than 1 g/dL in any 2-wk period.

Increase dose by 25%: If Hgb does not increase by 1 g/dL after 4 wks of therapy and Hgb is below target range (with adequate iron stores). Do not increase dose more frequently than every 4 wks.

Note: If pt does not attain Hgb range of 10–12 g/dL after appropriate dosing over 12 wks, do not increase dose and use minimum effective dose to maintain Hgb level that will avoid red blood cell transfusions. Discontinue

D

D

treatment if responsiveness does not improve.

Anemia Associated with Chemotherapy
◀**ALERT**▶ Initiate only if Hgb less than 10 g/dL and anticipated duration of myelosuppression is 2 months or longer. Titrate dose to maintain Hgb level and avoid RBC transfusions. Discontinue upon completion of chemotherapy.

SQ: ADULTS, ELDERLY: 2.25 mcg/kg once wkly or 500 mcg every 3 wks.

Increase dose: If Hgb does not increase by 1 g/dL after 6 wks and remains below 10 g/dL, increase dose to 4.5 mcg/kg once wkly. No dose adjustment if using q3wk dosing.

Decrease dose: Decrease dose by 40% if Hgb increases greater than 1 g/dL in any 2-wk period or Hgb reaches level that will avoid red blood cell transfusions. **Note:** Withhold dose when Hgb exceeds a level needed to avoid RBC transfusions; resume at dose 40% lower when Hgb approaches a level where transfusions may be required.

Dosage in Renal/Hepatic Impairment
No dose adjustment.

SIDE EFFECTS

Frequent: Myalgia, hypertension/hypotension, headache, diarrhea. **Occasional:** Fatigue, edema, vomiting, reaction at injection site, asthenia, dizziness.

ADVERSE EFFECTS/TOXIC REACTIONS

Cardiovascular events, including CVA, MI, venous thromboembolism, vascular access device thrombosis, mortality, may occur when given to target hemoglobin greater than 11 g/dL or during rapid rise in hemoglobin. Hypersensitivity reactions, including anaphylaxis, may occur. Cases of anemia and pure red cell aplasia may occur in pts with chronic renal disease when given subcutaneously.

NURSING CONSIDERATIONS

BASELINE ASSESSMENT

Establish baseline CBC (esp. note Hgb, Hct). Assess B/P before drug administration. B/P often rises during early therapy in pts with history of hypertension. Assess serum iron (transferrin saturation should be greater than 20%), serum ferritin (greater than 100 ng/mL) before and during therapy. Consider supplemental iron therapy.

INTERVENTION/EVALUATION

Monitor CBC, Hgb, reticulocyte count, serum BUN, creatinine, ferritin, potassium, phosphate. Monitor B/P aggressively for increase (25% of pts taking medication require antihypertension therapy, dietary restrictions).

PATIENT/FAMILY TEACHING

• Frequent blood tests needed to determine correct dose. • Report swollen extremities, breathing difficulty, extreme fatigue, or severe headache. • Avoid tasks requiring alertness, motor skills until response to drug is established.

darifenacin

dare-i-**fen**-a-sin
(Enablex)

◆**CLASSIFICATION**

PHARMACOTHERAPEUTIC: Muscarinic receptor antagonist. **CLINICAL:** Urinary antispasmodic.

USES

Management of symptoms of bladder overactivity (urge incontinence, urinary urgency/frequency).

PRECAUTIONS

Contraindications: Hypersensitivity to darifenacin. Uncontrolled narrow-angle glaucoma, paralytic ileus, GI/GU obstruction, urine retention. **Cautions:** Bladder outflow obstruction, hepatic impairment, nonobstructive prostatic hyperplasia, decreased GI motility, constipation, hiatal hernia, reflux esophagitis, ulcerative colitis, controlled narrow-angle glaucoma, myasthenia gravis, concurrent use of strong CYP3A4 inhibitors. Hot weather and/or exercise.

ACTION

Acts as a direct antagonist at muscarinic receptor sites in cholinergically innervated organs; limits bladder contractions. **Therapeutic Effect:** Reduces symptoms of bladder irritability/overactivity (urge incontinence, urinary urgency/frequency), improves bladder capacity.

PHARMACOKINETICS

Well absorbed following PO administration. Protein binding: 98%. Metabolized in liver. Excreted in urine (60%), feces (40%). **Half-life:** 13–19 hrs.

⧖ LIFESPAN CONSIDERATIONS

Pregnancy/Lactation: Unknown if drug crosses placenta or is distributed in breast milk. **Children:** Safety and efficacy not established. **Elderly:** No age-related precautions noted.

INTERACTIONS

DRUG: CYP3A4 inhibitors (clarithromycin, erythromycin, protease inhibitors) may increase concentration/effects. **Anticholinergics** may increase side effects (e.g., dry mouth, constipation). **HERBAL: St. John's wort** may decrease concentration/effects. **FOOD:** None known. **LAB VALUES:** None known.

AVAILABILITY (Rx)

⧖ **Tablets (Extended-Release):** 7.5 mg, 15 mg.

ADMINISTRATION/HANDLING

PO
• Give without regard to food. • Administer extended-release tablets whole; do not break, crush, dissolve, or divide tablet.

INDICATIONS/ROUTES/DOSAGE

Overactive Bladder
PO: ADULTS, ELDERLY: Initially, 7.5 mg once daily. If response is not adequate after at least 2 wks, may increase to 15 mg once daily. Do not exceed 7.5 mg once daily in moderate hepatic impairment or concurrent use with CYP3A4 inhibitors (e.g., clarithromycin, fluconazole, protease inhibitors).

Dosage in Renal Impairment
No dose adjustment.

Dosage Hepatic Impairment
Moderate impairment: Maximum dose: 7.5 mg. **Severe impairment:** Not recommended.

SIDE EFFECTS

Frequent (35%–21%): Dry mouth, constipation. **Occasional (8%–4%):** Dyspepsia, headache, nausea, abdominal pain. **Rare (3%–2%):** Asthenia, diarrhea, dizziness, ocular dryness.

ADVERSE EFFECTS/TOXIC REACTIONS

UTI occurs occasionally.

NURSING CONSIDERATIONS

BASELINE ASSESSMENT
Monitor voiding pattern, assess signs/symptoms of overactive bladder prior to therapy as baseline.

INTERVENTION/EVALUATION
Monitor I&O. Palpate bladder and use bladder scanner to assess for urine retention. Monitor daily pattern of bowel activity, stool consistency for evidence

D

of constipation. Dry mouth may be relieved with sips of water. Assess for relief of symptoms of overactive bladder (urge incontinence, urinary frequency/urgency).

PATIENT/FAMILY TEACHING
• Swallow tablet whole; do not chew, crush, dissolve, or divide. • Increase fluid intake to reduce risk of constipation. • Avoid tasks that require alertness, motor skills until response to drug is established.

---

darunavir

dar-**ue**-na-veer
(Prezista)

FIXED-COMBINATION(S)

Prezcobix: Darunavir/cobicistat (antiretroviral booster): 800 mg/150 mg.

◆CLASSIFICATION

PHARMACOTHERAPEUTIC: Protease inhibitor. **CLINICAL:** Antiretroviral.

USES

Treatment of HIV infection in combination with ritonavir and other antiretroviral agents in adults and children 3 yrs and older.

PRECAUTIONS

Contraindications: Hypersensitivity to darunavir. Concurrent therapy with alfuzosin, colchicine (in pts with renal and/or hepatic impairment), dihydroergotamine, dronedarone, ergonovine, ergotamine, lovastatin, lurasidone, methylergonovine, oral midazolam, pimozide, ranolazine, rifAMPin, sildenafil (for treatment of PAH), simvastatin, St. John's wort, triazolam. **Cautions:** Diabetes mellitus, hemophilia, known sulfonamide allergy, hepatic impairment.

ACTION

Binds to site of HIV-I protease activity, inhibiting cleavage of viral precursors into functional proteins required for infectious HIV. **Therapeutic Effect:** Prevents formation of mature viral cells.

PHARMACOKINETICS

Readily absorbed following PO administration. Protein binding: 95%. Metabolized in liver. Eliminated in feces (79.5%), urine (13.9%). Not significantly removed by hemodialysis. **Half-life:** 15 hrs.

⧖ LIFESPAN CONSIDERATIONS

Pregnancy/Lactation: Unknown if drug crosses placenta or is distributed in breast milk. Breastfeeding not recommended. **Children:** Safety and efficacy not established. **Elderly:** No age-related precautions noted.

INTERACTIONS

DRUG: May increase concentration/effects of **amiodarone, bepridil, lidocaine, desipramine, colchicine, beta blockers, midazolam, PARoxetine, sertraline, atorvastatin, clarithromycin, cycloSPORINE, felodipine, inhaled fluticasone, lovastatin, niCARdipine, NIFEdipine, pravastatin, simvastatin, sirolimus, tacrolimus, traZODone, sildenafil, tadalafil, vardenafil. CYP3A4 inhibitors (e.g., itraconazole, ketoconazole, voriconazole)** may increase concentration. May decrease effects of **methadone, oral contraceptives. HERBAL: St. John's wort** may lead to loss of virologic response, potential resistance to darunavir. **FOOD: Food** increases plasma concentration. **LAB VALUES:** May increase aPTT, PT, serum alkaline phosphatase, bilirubin, amylase, lipase, cholesterol, triglycerides, uric acid. May decrease lymphocytes/neutrophil count, platelets, WBC count; serum bicarbonate, albumin, calcium. May alter serum glucose, sodium.

AVAILABILITY (Rx)

Suspension, oral (Prezista): 100 mg/mL

Tablets (Prezista): 75 mg, 150 mg, 400 mg, 600 mg, 800 mg.

ADMINISTRATION/HANDLING

PO
• Give with food (increases plasma concentration). • Coadministration with ritonavir required. • Do not break, crush, dissolve, or divide film-coated tablets. • Shake suspension prior to each dose. Use provided oral dosing syringe.

INDICATIONS/ROUTES/DOSAGE

Note: Genotypic testing recommended in therapy-experienced pts.

HIV Infection, Treatment Experienced
PO: ADULTS, ELDERLY: *(With 1 or more darunavir resistance–associated substitution):* 600 mg administered twice daily with 100 mg ritonavir twice daily. *(With no darunavir resistance–associated substitutions):* 800 mg with 100 mg ritonavir or 150 mg cobicistat once daily.

HIV Infection, Treatment Naive
PO: ADULTS, ELDERLY: 800 mg administered with 100 mg ritonavir or 150 mg cobicistat once daily.

Usual Dosage During Pregnancy
PO: ADULTS: 600 mg administered twice daily with 100 mg ritonavir twice daily.

Usual Pediatric Dose
Treatment naive or treatment experienced with no darunavir resistance–associated substitutions: *(Once-daily dosing) (Suspension only):* **14 kg:** 490 mg with 96 mg ritonavir. **13 kg:** 455 mg with 80 mg ritonavir. **12 kg:** 420 mg with 80 mg ritonavir. **11 kg:** 385 mg with 64 mg ritonavir. **10 kg:** 350 mg with 64 mg ritonavir.
(Suspension or Tablets): **40 kg or greater:** 800 mg with 100 mg ritonavir. **30–39 kg:** 675 mg with 100 mg ritonavir. **15–29 kg:** 600 mg with 100 mg ritonavir.

Treatment Experienced with 1 or More Darunavir Resistance–Associated Substitution
Use Tablet or Suspension
PO: CHILDREN WEIGHING 40 KG OR MORE: 600 mg twice daily with 100 mg ritonavir. **WEIGHING 30–39 KG:** 450 mg twice daily with 60 mg ritonavir. **WEIGHING 15–29 KG:** 375 mg twice daily with 48 mg ritonavir.

Use Oral Suspension Only
14 KG TO LESS THAN 15 KG: 280 mg (48 mg ritonavir) twice daily. **13 KG TO LESS THAN 14 KG:** 260 mg (40 mg ritonavir) twice daily. **12 KG TO LESS THAN 13 KG:** 240 mg (40 mg ritonavir) twice daily. **11 KG TO LESS THAN 12 KG:** 220 mg (32 mg ritonavir) twice daily. **10 KG TO LESS THAN 11 KG:** 200 mg (32 mg ritonavir) twice daily.

Dosage in Renal Impairment
No dose adjustment.

Dosage in Hepatic Impairment
Not recommended in severe impairment.

SIDE EFFECTS

Frequent (19%–13%): Diarrhea, nausea, headache, nasopharyngitis. **Occasional (3%–2%):** Constipation, abdominal pain, vomiting. **Rare (less than 2%):** Allergic dermatitis, dyspepsia, flatulence, abdominal distention, anorexia, arthralgia, myalgia, paresthesia, memory impairment.

ADVERSE EFFECTS/TOXIC REACTIONS

Hypertension, MI, transient ischemic attack occur in less than 2% of pts. Acute renal failure, diabetes mellitus, dyspnea, worsening of hepatic impairment, skin reactions (including Stevens-Johnson syndrome, toxic epidermal necrolysis) occur rarely.

NURSING CONSIDERATIONS

BASELINE ASSESSMENT

Obtain baseline LFT before beginning therapy and at periodic intervals during therapy. Perform blood testing for HIV genotype and viral load. Offer emotional support. Obtain full medication history.

INTERVENTION/EVALUATION

Closely monitor for GI discomfort. Monitor daily pattern of bowel activity, stool consistency. Assess skin for rash, other skin reactions, chemistries, laboratory abnormalities, particularly hepatic profile, glucose, cholesterol, triglycerides. Assess for opportunistic infections (onset of fever, oral mucosa changes, cough, other respiratory symptoms).

PATIENT/FAMILY TEACHING

• Take medication with food. • Continue therapy for full length of treatment. • Doses should be evenly spaced. • Darunavir is not a cure for HIV infection, nor does it reduce risk of transmission to others. • Pt may continue to experience illnesses, including opportunistic infections. • Diarrhea can be controlled with OTC medication. • Report any skin reactions.

---

dasatinib

da-**sa**-ti-nib
(Sprycel)
Do not confuse dasatinib with erlotinib, imatinib, or lapatinib.

◆CLASSIFICATION

PHARMACOTHERAPEUTIC: Protein-tyrosine kinase inhibitor. **CLINICAL:** Antineoplastic.

USES

Chronic myeloid leukemia (CML): Treatment of adults with chronic, accelerated, myeloid or lymphoid blast phase of CML with resistance, intolerance to prior therapy, including imatinib. Treatment of Philadelphia chromosome–positive (Ph+) CML in chronic phase of newly diagnosed pt. **Acute lymphoblastic leukemia:** Treatment of adults with Ph+ acute lymphoblastic leukemia (ALL) with resistance or intolerance to prior therapy, including imatinib. **OFF-LABEL:** Post–stem cell transplant follow-up treatment of CML. Treatment of GI stromal tumor.

PRECAUTIONS

Contraindications: Hypersensitivity to dasatinib. **Cautions:** Hepatic impairment, myelosuppression (particularly thrombocytopenia), pts prone to fluid retention, those with prolonged QT interval, cardiovascular/pulmonary disease. Concomitant use of anticoagulants, CYP3A4 inducers/inhibitors may increase risk of pulmonary arterial hypertension.

ACTION

Reduces activity of proteins responsible for uncontrolled growth of leukemia cells by binding to most imatinib-resistant BCR-ABL mutations of pts with CML or ALL. **Therapeutic Effect:** Inhibits proliferation, tumor growth of CML and ALL cancer cell lines.

PHARMACOKINETICS

Extensively distributed in extravascular space. Protein binding: 96%. Metabolized in liver. Eliminated primarily in feces. **Half-life:** 3–5 hrs.

⌛ LIFESPAN CONSIDERATIONS

Pregnancy/Lactation: Has potential for severe teratogenic effects, fertility impairment. Breastfeeding not recommended. **Children:** Safety and efficacy not established in pts younger than 18 yrs. **Elderly:** No age-related precautions noted.

INTERACTIONS

DRUG: CYP3A4 inhibitors (e.g., clarithromycin, ketoconazole, saquinavir) may increase concentration. CYP3A4 inducers (e.g., carBAMazepine, phenytoin, rifAMPin) may decrease concentration. **Antacids** alter pH-dependent solubility of dasatinib. **Famotidine, omeprazole** may reduce dasatinib absorption. **HERBAL:** St. John's wort, echinacea may decrease concentration. **FOOD:** Grapefruit products may increase concentration/toxicity (increased risk of torsades, myelotoxicity). **LAB VALUES:** May decrease WBC, platelets, Hgb, Hct, RBC; serum calcium, phosphates. May increase serum ALT, AST, bilirubin, creatinine.

AVAILABILITY (Rx)

Tablets (Film-Coated): 20 mg, 50 mg, 70 mg, 80 mg, 100 mg, 140 mg.

ADMINISTRATION/HANDLING

PO
• Give without regard to food. • Take with food or large glass of water if GI upset occurs. • Avoid grapefruit products. • Do not break, crush, dissolve, or divide film-coated tablets. • Do not give antacids either 2 hrs prior to or within 2 hrs after dasatinib administration.

INDICATIONS/ROUTES/DOSAGE

Note: CYP3A4 Inhibitors: Consider decreasing dose from 100 mg to 20 mg or 140 mg to 40 mg.
CYP3A4 Inducers: Consider increasing dose with monitoring.

CML (Resistant or Intolerant)
PO: ADULTS, ELDERLY: (Chronic phase): 100 mg once daily. May increase to 140 mg once daily in pts not achieving cytogenetic response. **(Accelerated or blast phase):** 140 mg once daily. May increase to 180 mg once daily in pts not achieving cytogenetic response.

CML (Newly Diagnosed in Chronic Phase)
PO: ADULTS, ELDERLY: 100 mg once daily. May increase to 140 mg/day in pts not achieving cytogenetic response.

CHILDREN (1 YR AND OLDER): 45 kg or greater: 100 mg once daily. May increase to 120 mg once daily. **30–44 kg:** 70 mg once daily. May increase to 90 mg once daily. **20–29 kg:** 60 mg once daily. May increase to 70 mg once daily. **10–19 kg:** 40 mg once daily. May increase to 50 mg once daily.

Ph+ ALL
PO: ADULTS, ELDERLY: 140 mg once daily. May increase to 180 mg once daily in pts not achieving cytogenetic response.

Dosage in Renal/Hepatic Impairment
No dose adjustment.

SIDE EFFECTS

Frequent (50%–32%): Fluid retention, diarrhea, headache, fatigue, musculoskeletal pain, fever, rash, nausea, dyspnea. **Occasional (28%–12%):** Cough, abdominal pain, vomiting, anorexia, asthenia, arthralgia, stomatitis, dizziness, constipation, peripheral neuropathy, myalgia. **Rare (less than 12%):** Abdominal distention, chills, weight increase, pruritus.

ADVERSE EFFECTS/TOXIC REACTIONS

Pleural effusion occurred in 8% of pts, febrile neutropenia in 7%, GI bleeding, pneumonia in 6%, thrombocytopenia in 5%, dyspnea in 4%; anemia, cardiac failure in 3%.

NURSING CONSIDERATIONS

BASELINE ASSESSMENT

Obtain CBC weekly for first mo, biweekly for second mo, and periodically thereafter. Monitor LFT before treatment begins and monthly thereafter. Obtain baseline weight. Offer emotional support.

INTERVENTION/EVALUATION

Assess lower extremities for pedal edema, early evidence of fluid retention. Weigh daily, monitor for unexpected rapid weight gain. Offer antiemetics to control nausea, vomiting. Monitor daily pattern of bowel activity, stool consistency. Assess oral mucous membranes for evidence of stomatitis. Monitor CBC for neutropenia, thrombocytopenia; monitor hepatic function tests for hepatotoxicity.

PATIENT/FAMILY TEACHING

• Avoid crowds, those with known infection. • Avoid contact with anyone who recently received live virus vaccine; do not receive vaccinations. • Antacids may be taken up to 2 hrs before or 2 hrs after taking dasatinib. • Avoid grapefruit products. • Do not chew, crush, dissolve, or divide tablets.

DAUNOrubicin HIGH ALERT

daw-noe-**roo**-bi-sin
(Cerubidine, DaunoXome)

■ **BLACK BOX ALERT** ■ Irreversible cardiotoxicity may occur. Myelosuppressant. Lipid component may cause infusion-related effects (back pain, flushing, chest tightness) within first 5 min of infusion. Must be administered by personnel trained in administration/handling of chemotherapeutic agents. Caution in renal impairment or hepatic dysfunction. Potent vesicant.

Do not confuse DAUNOrubicin with DACTINomycin, DOXOrubicin, epiRUBicin, IDArubicin, or valrubicin.

◆CLASSIFICATION

PHARMACOTHERAPEUTIC: Anthracycline antibiotic. **CLINICAL:** Antineoplastic.

USES

Cerubidine: Treatment of leukemias (acute lymphocytic [ALL], acute myeloid [AML]) in combination with other agents. **DaunoXome:** Advanced HIV-related Kaposi's sarcoma.

PRECAUTIONS

Contraindications: Hypersensitivity to DAUNOrubicin. **Cautions:** Preexisting heart disease or bone marrow suppression, hypertension, concurrent chemotherapeutic agents, elderly, infants, radiation therapy.

ACTION

Inhibits DNA and RNA synthesis by intercalation between DNA base pairs and by steric obstruction. Cell cycle–phase nonspecific. **Therapeutic Effect:** Prevents cell division.

PHARMACOKINETICS

Widely distributed. Protein binding: High. Does not cross blood-brain barrier. Metabolized in liver. Excreted in urine (40%); biliary excretion (40%). **Half-life:** 18.5 hrs; metabolite: 26.7 hrs.

⧗ LIFESPAN CONSIDERATIONS

Pregnancy/Lactation: If possible, avoid use during pregnancy, esp. first trimester. May cause fetal harm. Breastfeeding not recommended. **Children:** Safety and efficacy not established. **Elderly:** Cardiotoxicity may be more frequent; reduced bone marrow reserves require caution. Age-related renal impairment may require dosage adjustment.

INTERACTIONS

DRUG: Previous use of **DOXOrubicin,** concurrent use of **cyclophosphamide** increases risk of cardiotoxicity. **Hepatotoxic medications (e.g., acetaminophen, ketoconazole, methotrexate, simvastatin)** increase risk of hepatotoxicity. **Bone marrow depressants** may enhance myelosuppression. **Live virus vaccines** may potentiate virus replication, increase vaccine side effects, decrease pt's antibody response to vaccine. **HERBAL:** Echinacea may decrease level/effects. **FOOD:** None known. **LAB VALUES:** May increase serum alkaline phosphatase, bilirubin, uric acid, AST.

AVAILABILITY (Rx)

Injection Solution (Cerubidine): 5 mg/mL.
Injection Solution (DaunoXome): 2 mg/mL.

ADMINISTRATION/HANDLING

 IV

◀ALERT▶ **Cerubidine:** Give by IV push or IV infusion. **DaunoXome:** Give by IV infusion. May be carcinogenic, mutagenic, teratogenic. Handle with extreme care during preparation/administration.

Reconstitution

Cerubidine • May further dilute with 100 mL D_5W or 0.9% NaCl.

DaunoXome • Must dilute with equal part D_5W to provide concentration of 1 mg/mL. • Do not use any other diluent.

Rate of Administration

Cerubidine • For IV push, withdraw desired dose into syringe containing 10–15 mL 0.9% NaCl. Inject over 1–5 min into tubing of rapidly infusing IV solution of D_5W or 0.9% NaCl. • For IV infusion, further dilute with 100 mL D_5W or 0.9% NaCl. Infuse over 15–30 min. • Extravasation produces immediate pain, severe local tissue damage. Aspirate as much infiltrated drug as possible, then infiltrate area with hydrocortisone sodium succinate injection (50–100 mg hydrocortisone) and/ or isotonic sodium thiosulfate injection or ascorbic acid injection (1 mL of 5% injection). Apply cold compresses.

DaunoXome • Infuse over 60 min. • Do not use in-line filter.

Storage

Cerubidine • Refrigerate intact vials. • Protect from light. • Solutions prepared for infusion stable for 24 hrs at room temperature.

DaunoXome • Refrigerate unopened vials. • Reconstituted solution is stable for 6 hrs if refrigerated. • Do not use if opaque.

🕸 IV INCOMPATIBILITIES

Allopurinol (Aloprim), aztreonam (Azactam), cefepime (Maxipime), dexamethasone (Decadron), heparin, piperacillin and tazobactam (Zosyn). **DaunoXome:** Do not mix with any other solution, esp. NaCl or bacteriostatic agents (e.g., benzyl alcohol).

🕸 IV COMPATIBILITIES

Granisetron (Kytril), ondansetron (Zofran).

INDICATIONS/ROUTES/DOSAGE

◀ALERT▶ Refer to individual protocols. **Cerubidine:** Cumulative dose should not exceed 550 mg/m² in adults (increased risk of cardiotoxicity) or 400 mg/m² in those receiving chest irradiation.

Acute Lymphoblastic Leukemia

IV: *(Cerubidine):* **ADULTS, ELDERLY:** 45 mg/m² on days 1, 2, and 3 (in combination with vinCRIStine, predniSONE, asparaginase). **CHILDREN 2 YRS AND OLDER AND BODY SURFACE AREA 0.5 m² OR GREATER:** 25 mg/m² on day 1 of every wk for up to 4–6 cycles (in combination with vinCRIStine, predniSONE). **CHILDREN YOUNGER THAN 2 YRS, OR BODY SURFACE AREA LESS THAN 0.5 m²:** 1 mg/kg/dose on day 1 of every wk for up to 4 to 6 cycles (in combination with vinCRIStine, predniSONE).

Acute Myeloid Leukemia

IV: *(Cerubidine):* **ADULTS YOUNGER THAN 60 YRS:** 45 mg/m² on days 1, 2, and 3 of induction course, then on days 1 and 2 of subsequent courses (in combination with cytarabine). **ADULTS 60 YRS AND OLDER:** 30 mg/m² on days 1, 2, and 3 of induction course, then on days 1 and 2 of subsequent courses (in combination with cytarabine).

Kaposi's Sarcoma

IV: *(DaunoXome):* **ADULTS:** 40 mg/m² over 1 hr repeated q2wks until disease progression.

Dosage in Renal Impairment

Cerubidine: Serum creatinine greater than 3 mg/dL: 50% of normal dose.

DaunoXome: Serum creatinine greater than 3 mg/dL: 50% of normal dose.

Dosage in Hepatic Impairment
Cerubidine: Bilirubin 1.2–3 mg/dL: 75% of normal dose. **Bilirubin 3.1–5 mg/dL:** 50% of normal dose. **Bilirubin greater than 5 mg/dL:** DAUNOrubicin is not recommended for use in this pt population.
DaunoXome: Bilirubin 1.2–3 mg/dL: 75% of normal dose. **Bilirubin greater than 3 mg/dL:** 50% of normal dose.

SIDE EFFECTS

Frequent: Complete alopecia (scalp, axillary, pubic), nausea, vomiting (beginning a few hrs after administration and lasting 24–48 hrs). **DaunoXome:** Mild to moderate nausea, fatigue, fever. **Occasional:** Diarrhea, abdominal pain, esophagitis, stomatitis, transverse pigmentation of fingernails, toenails. **Rare:** Transient fever, chills.

ADVERSE EFFECTS/TOXIC REACTIONS

Myelosuppression manifested as hematologic toxicity (severe leukopenia, anemia, thrombocytopenia). Decrease in platelet count, WBC count occurs in 10–14 days, returns to normal level by third week. Cardiotoxicity noted as either acute, transient, abnormal. EKG findings and/or cardiomyopathy manifested as HF (risk increases when cumulative dose exceeds 550 mg/m^2 in adults, 300 mg/m^2 in children 2 yrs and older, or total dosage greater than 10 mg/kg in children younger than 2 yrs).

NURSING CONSIDERATIONS

BASELINE ASSESSMENT

Obtain WBC, platelet, erythrocyte counts before and at frequent intervals during therapy. EKG should be obtained before therapy. Antiemetics may be effective in preventing, treating nausea. Obtain accurate height and weight for dose calculation. Offer emotional support.

INTERVENTION/EVALUATION

Monitor for stomatitis. May lead to ulceration within 2–3 days. Assess skin, nailbeds for hyperpigmentation. Monitor hematologic status, renal/hepatic function, serum uric acid. Monitor daily pattern of bowel activity, stool consistency. Monitor for hematologic toxicity (fever, sore throat, signs of local infection, unusual bruising/bleeding from any site), symptoms of anemia (excessive fatigue, weakness).

PATIENT/FAMILY TEACHING

• Urine may turn reddish color for 1–2 days after beginning therapy. • Hair loss is reversible, but new hair growth may have different color, texture. • New hair growth resumes about 5 wks after last therapy dose. • Maintain strict oral hygiene. • Do not have immunizations without physician's approval (drug lowers resistance). • Avoid contact with those who have recently received live virus vaccine. • Promptly report fever, sore throat, signs of local infection, unusual bruising/bleeding from any site, yellowing of whites of eyes/skin, difficulty breathing. • Increase fluid intake (may protect against hyperuricemia). • Report for persistent nausea, vomiting.

deferasirox

dee-**fur**-a-sir-ox
(Exjade, Jadenu)
■ **BLACK BOX ALERT** ■ May cause renal/hepatic failure, hepatotoxicity, gastrointestinal hemorrhage.
Do not confuse deferasirox with deferoxamine.

◆CLASSIFICATION

PHARMACOTHERAPEUTIC: Iron-chelating agent. **CLINICAL:** Iron reduction agent.

USES

Treatment of chronic iron overload due to blood transfusions (transfusional hemosiderosis) or due to non–transfusion-dependent thalassemia syndrome.

PRECAUTIONS

Contraindications: Hypersensitivity to deferasirox. Platelet counts less than 50,000 cells/mm³; poor performance status, high-risk myelodysplastic syndromes or advanced malignancies; CrCl less than 40 mL/min or serum creatinine greater than 2 times the upper limit of normal. **Cautions:** Renal/hepatic impairment, elderly, concurrent medications that may increase GI effects (e.g., NSAIDs).

ACTION

Selective for iron. Binds iron with high affinity in a 2:1 ratio. **Therapeutic Effect:** Induces iron excretion.

PHARMACOKINETICS

Well absorbed following PO administration. Protein binding: 99%. Metabolized in liver. Excreted in feces (84%), urine (8%). **Half-life:** 8–16 hrs.

⌛ LIFESPAN CONSIDERATIONS

Pregnancy/Lactation: Unknown if drug crosses placenta or is distributed in breast milk. **Children:** Not recommended for pts younger than 2 yrs. **Elderly:** No age-related precautions noted.

INTERACTIONS

DRUG: Antacids containing aluminium, cholestyramine, PHENobarbital, phenytoin, rifAMPin, ritonavir decrease concentration/effects. May decrease effects of **cycloSPORINE, simvastatin, oral contraceptives.** May increase concentration of **cyclobenzaprine, OLANZapine, tiZANidine. HERBAL:** None significant. **FOOD:** Bioavailability is variably increased when given with **food.**

LAB VALUES: Decreases serum ferritin. May increase serum ALT, AST, creatinine; urine protein.

AVAILABILITY (Rx)

Tablets (Jadenu): 90 mg, 180 mg, 360 mg. **Tablets, Soluble (Exjade):** 125 mg, 250 mg, 500 mg.

ADMINISTRATION/HANDLING

PO
• Give on empty stomach 30 min before food. • Do not give simultaneously with aluminum-containing antacids, cholestyramine. • Tablets for suspension should not be chewed or swallowed whole. • Disperse tablet by stirring in water, apple juice, orange juice until fine suspension is achieved. • Dosage less than 1 g should be dispersed in 3.5 oz of liquid, dosage more than 1 g should be dispersed in 7 oz of liquid. If any residue remains in glass, resuspend with a small amount of liquid. • Give regular tablets whole with water.

INDICATIONS/ROUTES/DOSAGE

Iron Overload Due to Transfusions
PO: ADULTS, ELDERLY, CHILDREN 2 YRS AND OLDER: *(Exjade):* Initially, 20 mg/kg once daily. **Maintenance:** (Titrate to individual response and goals.) Adjust dosage by 5 or 10 mg/kg/day every 3–6 mos based on serum ferritin levels. Consider holding for serum ferritin less than 500 mcg/L. **Maximum:** 40 mg/kg once daily. *(Jadenu):* Initially, 14 mg/kg once daily. **Maintenance:** (Titrate to individual response and goals.) Adjust dosage by 3.5 or 7 mg/kg/day based on serum ferritin levels. Consider holding for serum ferritin less than 500 mcg/L. **Maximum:** 28 mcg/kg once daily.

Thalassemia Syndromes
PO: ADULTS, ELDERLY, CHILDREN 10 YRS AND OLDER: *(Exjade):* Initially, 10 mg/kg once daily. May increase to 20 mg/kg

once daily after 4 wks if baseline iron is greater than 15 mg Fe/g dry wgt. *(Jadenu):* Initially, 7 mg/kg once daily. May increase to 14 mg/kg/day after 4 wks if baseline iron greater than 15 mg Fe/g dry wgt. **Maintenance: *(Exjade/Jadenu):*** Dose adjustments based on serum ferritin and hepatic iron concentrations.

Dosage in Renal Impairment
Note: See Contraindications.
ADULTS: For increase in serum creatinine greater than 33% on 2 consecutive measures, reduce daily dose by 10 mg/kg. **CHILDREN:** For increase in serum creatinine above age-appropriate upper limit of normal on 2 consecutive measures, reduce daily dose by 10 mg/kg. **CrCl 40–60 mL/min:** Reduce starting dose by 50%.

Dosage in Hepatic Impairment
For severe or persistent elevations in hepatic function tests, consider dose reduction or discontinuation. **Moderate impairment:** Reduce initial dose by 50%.

SIDE EFFECTS

Frequent (19%–10%): Fever, headache, abdominal pain, cough, nasopharyngitis, diarrhea, nausea, vomiting. **Occasional (9%–4%):** Rash, arthralgia, fatigue, back pain, urticaria. **Rare (1%):** Edema, sleep disorder, dizziness, anxiety.

ADVERSE EFFECTS/TOXIC REACTIONS

Bronchitis, pharyngitis, acute tonsillitis, ear infection occur occasionally. Hepatitis, auditory disturbances, ocular abnormalities occur rarely. Acute renal failure, cytopenias (e.g., agranulocytosis, neutropenia, thrombocytopenia) may occur.

NURSING CONSIDERATIONS

BASELINE ASSESSMENT
Obtain baseline serum CBC, ferritin, iron, creatinine, ALT, AST, urine protein, then monthly thereafter. Auditory, ophthalmic testing should be obtained before therapy and annually thereafter.

INTERVENTION/EVALUATION
Treatment should be interrupted if serum ferritin levels are consistently less than 500 mcg/L. Suspend treatment if severe rash occurs.

PATIENT/FAMILY TEACHING
• Take on empty stomach 30 min before food. • Do not chew or swallow soluble tablets; disperse tablet completely in water, apple juice, orange juice; drink resulting suspension immediately. • Do not take aluminum-containing antacids concurrently. • Report severe skin rash, changes in vision/hearing, or yellowing of skin/eyes.

delafloxacin

del-a-**floks**-a-sin
(Baxdela)
Do not confuse delafloxacin with ciprofloxacin, gatifloxacin, moxifloxacin, norfloxacin, levofloxacin, or Baxdela with Pradaxa.

■ **BLACK BOX ALERT** ■ May increase risk of tendonitis, tendon rupture, peripheral neuropathy, central nervous system effects. May exacerbate muscle weakness in pts with myasthenia gravis (avoid use).

◆**CLASSIFICATION**

PHARMACOTHERAPEUTIC: Fluoroquinolone. **CLINICAL:** Antibiotic.

USES

Treatment of adult pts with acute bacterial skin and skin structure infections

D

(ABSSSI) caused by susceptible strains of gram-positive microorganisms including *S. aureus* (including methicillin-susceptible [MSSA] and methicillin-resistant [MRSA] strains), *S. haemolyticus, S. lugdunensis, S. agalactiae, S. anginosus group (including S. anginosus, S. intermedius, S. constellatus), S. pyogenes,* and *E. faecalis; gram-negative microorganisms E. coli, E. cloacae, K. pneumoniae, P. aeruginosa.*

PRECAUTIONS

Contraindications: Known hypersensitivity to delafloxacin, other fluoroquinolones. **Cautions:** Pts with known or suspected CNS disorders, risk factors predisposing to seizures or lowering seizure threshold, diabetes, elderly, renal impairment; pts at risk for tendon rupture, tendonitis (e.g., renal failure, concomitant use of corticosteroids; solid organ transplant recipient, elderly pts). Avoid use in pts who previously experienced peripheral neuropathy; pts with history of myasthenia gravis.

ACTION

Inhibits the DNA enzyme gyrase in susceptible microorganisms, interfering with bacterial cell replication and repair. **Therapeutic Effect:** Bactericidal.

PHARMACOKINETICS

Widely distributed following PO, IV administration. Protein binding: 84%. Peak plasma concentration: 1 hr. Excreted in urine (IV: 65%, PO: 50%), feces (IV: 28%, PO: 48%). Partially removed by hemodialysis. **Half-life:** IV: 3.7 hrs, PO: 4.2–8.5 hrs.

⌛ LIFESPAN CONSIDERATIONS

Pregnancy/Lactation: Unknown if distributed in breast milk; however, other fluoroquinolones are known to be distributed in breast milk. **Children:** Safety and efficacy not established. **Elderly:** May have increased risk of tendon rupture, tendonitis. Age-related renal impairment may require dosage adjustment.

INTERACTIONS

DRUG: Aluminum-, calcium-, or **magnesium-containing antacids, iron preparations, sucralfate, or sevelamer** may decrease absorption. May decrease concentration/effect of **BCG vaccine, didanosine; quinapril** may decrease concentration/effect. **HERBAL:** None significant. **FOOD:** None known. **LAB VALUES:** May increase serum alkaline phosphatase, ALT, AST, CPK, creatinine. May increase or decrease serum glucose.

AVAILABILITY (Rx)

Injection, Powder for Reconstitution: 300 mg. **Tablets:** 450 mg.

ADMINISTRATION/HANDLING
PO

• Do not give antacids (aluminum, magnesium), sucralfate, iron, multivitamin preparations with zinc, didanosine (buffered tablets for oral suspension, pediatric powder for oral solution) at least 2 hrs before or 6 hrs after administration (significantly reduces absorption). • Give tablet with or without food. • Administer tablets whole; do not cut, crush, or divide. • If a dose is missed, administer as soon as possible up to 8 hrs before next scheduled dose. If less than 8 hrs remain until next scheduled dose or if vomiting occurs after administration, give dose at next regularly scheduled time.

IV

Reconstitution • Reconstitute vial with 10.5 mL D_5W or 0.9% NaCl for a concentration of 300 mg/12 mL (25 mg/mL). • Shake until completely dissolved. • Visually inspect for particulate matter or discoloration. Solution should appear clear yellow to amber in color. • Withdraw proper dose volume from vial (12 mL for 300-mg dose or 8 mL for 200-mg dose), and dilute in 250 mL D_5W or 0.9% NaCl.

Rate of Administration
• Infuse over 60 min.

Storage
• Store unused vials at room temperature. • Reconstituted vials/diluted solution may be refrigerated or stored at room temperature for up to 24 hrs.
• Do not freeze.

▦ IV INCOMPATIBILITIES

Do not infuse with other solutions containing calcium, magnesium, other multivalent cations. Do not infuse with other medications.

INDICATIONS/ROUTES/DOSAGE

Acute Bacterial Skin and Skin Structure Infections

IV: ADULTS, ELDERLY: 300 mg q12hrs for 5–14 days (or transition to PO for total of 5–14 days).
PO: ADULTS, ELDERLY: 450 mg q12hrs for total duration of 5–14 days (which includes switching from IV to PO).

Dosage in Renal Impairment
Dosage and frequency are modified based on creatinine clearance and severity of the infection.

GFR	Dosage
30–89 mL/min	PO/IV: No dose adjustment
15–29 mL/min	PO: No dose adjustment
	IV: 200 mg q12hrs or switch to 450 mg PO at physician discretion
Less than 15 mL/min, ESRD, HD, PD	PO/IV: Not recommended

Dosage in Hepatic Impairment
No dose adjustment.

SIDE EFFECTS

Occasional (8%): Nausea, diarrhea. **Rare (3%-2%):** Headache, vomiting.

ADVERSE EFFECTS/TOXIC REACTIONS

C. difficile–associated diarrhea or colitis, with severity ranging from mild diarrhea to fatal colitis, was reported; may occur greater than 2 mos after discontinuation. May increase risk of development of drug-resistant bacteria when used in the absence of a proven or strongly suspected bacterial infection. Superinfection (genital/anal pruritus, ulceration/changes to oral mucosa, moderate to severe diarrhea) may occur from altered bacterial balance in GI tract. May increase risk of tendonitis, tendon rupture, irreversible peripheral neuropathy; CNS effects including agitation, anxiety, confusion, depression, dizziness, hallucinations, nightmares, paranoia, tremors, vertigo. May exacerbate muscle weakness in pts with myasthenia gravis. Hypersensitivity reactions, including anaphylaxis, have occurred in pts receiving fluoroquinolones.

NURSING CONSIDERATIONS

BASELINE ASSESSMENT

Obtain BUN, serum creatinine; CrCl, GFR in pts with renal impairment; LFT in pts with hepatic impairment. Obtain bacterial culture and sensitivity prior to administration. Question pt's usual stool characteristics (color, frequency, consistency). Question medical history as listed in Precautions, esp. cardiac conduction disorders, CNS disorders; prior hypersensitivity reaction.

INTERVENTION/EVALUATION

Monitor for CNS reactions (agitation, anxiety, convulsions, depression, hallucinations, increased ICP, insomnia, nightmares, suicidal ideation and behavior), peripheral neuropathy; hypersensitivity reactions (angioedema, dyspnea, itching, hypotension, urticaria); muscle weakness, voice dystonia in pts with myasthenia gravis; pain, swelling, bruising, popping of tendons. Be alert for superinfections. Obtain EKG if palpitations occur or cardiac arrhythmia suspected. Observe daily pattern of bowel activity, stool consistency (increased severity may indicate antibiotic-associated colitis). If frequent diarrhea occurs, obtain *C. difficile* toxin screen, and initiate isolation precautions until test result confirmed. Antibacterial drugs that are not directed against *C. difficile* infection may need to be discontinued. Monitor I&O.

PATIENT/FAMILY TEACHING

• It is essential to complete drug therapy despite symptom improvement. Early discontinuation may result in antibacterial resistance or increase risk of recurrent infection. • Report any episodes of diarrhea, esp. in the first few mos after final dose. Frequent abdominal pain, blood-streaked stool, foul-smelling diarrhea, fever may indicate infectious diarrhea, which may be contagious to others. • Severe allergic reactions such as hives, palpitations, rash, shortness of breath, tongue swelling may occur. • Tendon inflammation/swelling, tendon rupture may occur; report bruising, pain, swelling, snapping, or popping of tendons. • Immediately report nervous system problems such as anxiety, confusion, dizziness, nervousness, nightmares, thoughts of suicide, seizures, tremors, trouble sleeping. • Treatment may cause heart problems such as low heart rate, palpitations; permanent nerve damage such as burning, numbness, tingling, weakness. • Do not take aluminum- or magnesium-containing antacids, multivitamins, zinc or iron products at least 2 hrs before or 6 hrs after dose. • Drink plenty of fluids.

---

denosumab

den-**oh**-sue-mab
(Prolia, Xgeva)
Do not confuse denosumab with daclizumab, or Prolia with Avandia or Zebeta.

◆CLASSIFICATION

PHARMACOTHERAPEUTIC: Monoclonal antibody (with affinity for RANKL). **CLINICAL:** Bone-modifying agent.

USES

Prolia: Treatment of osteoporosis in postmenopausal women at high risk for fracture. Treatment to increase bone mass in men at high risk for fractures; treatment of bone loss in men receiving androgen deprivation therapy for nonmetastatic prostate cancer and in women at high risk for fractures receiving adjuvant aromatase inhibitor therapy for breast cancer. **Xgeva:** Prevention of skeletal-related events (e.g., fracture, spinal cord compression) in pts with bone metastases from solid tumor. Treatment of giant cell tumor of bone in adults and skeletally mature adolescents. Treatment of hypercalcemia of malignancy refractory to biphosphonate therapy. **OFF-LABEL:** Treatment of bone destruction caused by rheumatoid arthritis.

PRECAUTIONS

Contraindications: Hypersensitivity to denosumab. **Prolia:** Preexisting hypocalcemia, pregnancy. **Cautions:** History of hypoparathyroidism, thyroid/parathyroid surgery, malabsorption syndromes, excision of small intestine, immunocompromised pts. Pts with severe renal impairment or receiving dialysis (greater risk for developing hypocalcemia). Pts with impaired immune system or immunosuppressive therapy.

ACTION

Binds to RANK ligand (transmembrane protein), preventing osteoclast formation. **Therapeutic Effect:** Decreases bone resorption; increases bone mass in osteoporosis; decreases skeletal-related events and tumor-induced bone destruction in solid tumors. Inhibits tumor growth.

PHARMACOKINETICS

Serum level detected 1 hr after administration. **Half-life:** 32 days.

⧖ LIFESPAN CONSIDERATIONS

Pregnancy/Lactation: Approved for use only in postmenopausal women. **Children:** Approved for use only in postmenopausal women. **Elderly:** No age-related precautions noted.

INTERACTIONS

DRUG: None significant. **HERBAL:** None significant. **FOOD:** None known. **LAB VALUES:** May decrease serum calcium. May increase serum cholesterol.

AVAILABILITY (Rx)

Injection, Solution (Prolia): 60 mg/mL. **(Xgeva):** 120 mg/1.7 mL.

ADMINISTRATION/HANDLING

Subcutaneous
• Administer in upper arm, upper thigh, or abdomen.
Storage • Refrigerate. Use within 14 days once at room temperature. • Solution appears as clear, colorless to pale yellow.

INDICATIONS/ROUTES/DOSAGE

Note: Administer calcium and vitamin D to prevent/treat hypocalcemia.

Prolia
Androgen Deprivation, Bone Loss, Osteoporosis
SQ: ADULTS, ELDERLY: 60 mg every 6 mos.

Xgeva
Prevention of Skeletal-Related Events from Solid Tumors
SQ: ADULTS, ELDERLY: 120 mg q4wks.

Xgeva
Giant Cell Tumor of Bone, Hypercalcemia of Malignancy
SQ: ADULTS, ELDERLY, MATURE ADOLESCENTS: 120 mg q4wks with additional doses on days 8 and 15 of first mo of therapy.

Dosage in Renal/Hepatic Impairment
No dose adjustment.

SIDE EFFECTS

Frequent (35%–12%): Back pain, extremity pain. **Occasional (8%–5%):** Musculoskeletal pain, vertigo, peripheral edema, sciatica. **Rare (4%–2%):** Bone pain, upper abdominal pain, rash, insomnia, flatulence, pruritus, myalgia, asthenia, GI reflux.

ADVERSE EFFECTS/TOXIC REACTIONS

Increases risk of infection, specifically cystitis, upper respiratory tract infection, pneumonia, pharyngitis, herpes zoster (shingles) occur in 2%–6% of pts. Osteonecrosis of the jaw (OJN) was reported. Suppression of bone turnover, pancreatitis have been reported.

NURSING CONSIDERATIONS

BASELINE ASSESSMENT

Hypocalcemia must be corrected prior to treatment. Calcium 1,000 mg/day and vitamin D at least 400 international units/day should be given. Dental exam should be provided prior to treatment. Recommend baseline bone density scan.

INTERVENTION/EVALUATION

Monitor serum magnesium, calcium, ionized calcium, phosphate. In pts predisposed with hypocalcemia and disturbances of mineral metabolism, clinical monitoring of calcium, mineral levels is highly recommended. Adequately supplement all pts with calcium and vitamin D. Monitor for delayed fracture healing.

PATIENT/FAMILY TEACHING

• Report rash, new-onset eczema. • Seek prompt medical attention if signs, symptoms of severe infection (rash, itching, reddened skin, cellulitis) occur. • Report muscle stiffness, numbness, cramps, spasms (signs of hypocalcemia); swelling or drainage from jaw, mouth, or teeth.

desmopressin

des-moe-**press**-in
(Apo-Desmopressin ✦, DDAVP,
DDAVP Rhinal Tube, Stimate)

◆CLASSIFICATION

PHARMACOTHERAPEUTIC: Synthetic
pituitary hormone. **CLINICAL:** Antidiuretic.

USES

DDAVP Nasal: (DDAVP Rhinal Tube):
Antidiuretic replacement therapy in
managing central cranial diabetes insipidus. Management of temporary polyuria
and polydipsia following head trauma or
surgery in the pituitary region. **Parenteral:** Antidiuretic replacement therapy
in managing central cranial diabetes
insipidus. Manage polyuria and polydipsia following head trauma or surgery in
pituitary region. Maintain hemostasis and
control bleeding in hemophilia A, von
Willebrand's disease (type I). **Stimate
intranasal:** Maintain hemostasis and
control bleeding due to spontaneous or
trauma-induced injuries in hemophilia
A, von Willebrand's disease (type I).
PO: Antidiuretic replacement therapy
in managing central cranial diabetes
insipidus, primary management of nocturnal enuresis, management of temporary polyuria, polydipsia following
pituitary surgery or head trauma. **OFF-LABEL:** Uremic bleeding occurring with
acute/chronic renal failure; prevent surgical bleeding in pts with uremia.

PRECAUTIONS

Contraindications: Hypersensitivity to
desmopressin. Hyponatremia, history of
hyponatremia, moderate to severe renal
impairment. **Cautions:** Predisposition
to thrombus formation; conditions with
fluid, electrolyte imbalance; coronary artery disease; hypertensive cardiovascular
disease, elderly pts, cystic fibrosis, HF,
renal impairment, polydipsia. Avoid use

in hemophilia A with factor VIII levels less
than 5%; hemophilia B; severe type I, type
IIB, platelet-type von Willebrand's disease.

ACTION

Increases cAMP in renal tubular cells,
which increases water permeability, decreasing urine volume. Increases levels
of von Willebrand factor, factor VIII, tissue plasminogen activator (tPA). **Therapeutic Effect:** Shortens activated partial
thromboplastin time (aPTT), bleeding
time. Decreases urinary output.

PHARMACOKINETICS

Route	Onset	Peak	Duration
PO	1 hr	2–7 hrs	8–12 hrs
IV	15–30 min	1.5–3 hrs	8–12 hrs
Intranasal	15 min–1 hr	1–5 hrs	8–12 hrs

Poorly absorbed after PO, nasal administration. Metabolism: Unknown.
Half-life: PO: 1.5–2.5 hrs. **Intranasal:** 3.3–3.5 hrs. **IV:** 0.4–4 hrs.

⌛ LIFESPAN CONSIDERATIONS

Pregnancy/Lactation: Unknown if distributed in breast milk. **Children:** Caution in neonates, pts younger than 3 mos
(increased risk of fluid balance problems). Careful fluid restrictions recommended in infants. **Elderly:** Increased
risk of hyponatremia, water intoxication.

INTERACTIONS

DRUG: CarBAMazepine, lamoTRIgine, NSAIDs (e.g., ibuprofen, ketorolac, naproxen), SSRIs (e.g.,
citalopram, sertraline), tricyclic
antidepressants (e.g., amitriptyline,
doxepin, nortriptyline) may increase
effect. **Demeclocycline, lithium** may
decrease effect. **HERBAL:** None significant. **FOOD:** None known. **LAB VALUES:** May decrease serum sodium.

AVAILABILITY (Rx)

Injection Solution (DDAVP): 4 mcg/mL.
**Nasal Solution (DDAVP Rhinal Tube
0.01%):** 100 mcg/mL (10 mcg/spray).

Nasal Spray (Stimate): 1.5 mg/mL (150 mcg/spray). **Tablets (DDAVP):** 0.1 mg, 0.2 mg.

ADMINISTRATION/HANDLING

 IV

Reconstitution • For IV infusion, dilute in 10–50 mL 0.9% NaCl (10 mL for children 10 kg or less; 50 mL for adults, children greater than 10 kg).
Rate of Administration• Infuse over 15–30 min.
Storage • Refrigerate.

Subcutaneous
• Withdraw dose from vial. Further dilution not required.

Intranasal
• Refrigerate DDAVP Rhinal Tube solution, Stimate nasal spray. • Rhinal Tube solution, Stimate nasal spray are stable for 3 wks at room temperature. • DDAVP nasal spray is stable at room temperature. • Calibrated catheter (rhinyle) is used to draw up measured quantity of desmopressin; with one end inserted in nose, pt blows on other end to deposit solution deep in nasal cavity. • For infants, young children, obtunded pts, air-filled syringe may be attached to catheter to deposit solution.

INDICATIONS/ROUTES/DOSAGE

Primary Nocturnal Enuresis
PO: CHILDREN 6 YRS AND OLDER: 0.2–0.6 mg once before bedtime. Limit fluid intake 1 hr prior and at least 8 hrs after dose.

Central Cranial Diabetes Insipidus
◀**ALERT**▶ Fluid restriction should be observed.
PO: ADULTS, ELDERLY, CHILDREN 4 YRS AND OLDER: Initially, 0.05 mg twice daily. Titrate to desired response. Range: 0.1–1.2 mg/day in 2–3 divided doses.
IV, SQ: ADULTS, ELDERLY, CHILDREN 12 YRS AND OLDER: 2–4 mcg/day in 2 divided doses or 1/10 of maintenance intranasal dose.

Intranasal: *(Use 100 mcg/mL Concentration):* **ADULTS, ELDERLY, CHILDREN OLDER THAN 12 YRS:** 10–40 mcg (0.1–0.4 mL) in 1–3 doses/day. Usual dose: 10 mcg 2 times/day. **CHILDREN 3 MOS–12 YRS:** Initially, 5 mcg (0.05 mL)/day. Range: 5–30 mcg (0.05–0.3 mL)/day as a single or 2 divided doses.

Hemophilia A, Von Willebrand's Disease (Type I)
IV Infusion: ADULTS, ELDERLY, CHILDREN: 0.3 mcg/kg as slow infusion.
Intranasal: *(Use 1.5 mg/mL Concentration Providing 150 mcg/Spray):* **ADULTS, ELDERLY, CHILDREN MORE THAN 50 KG:** 300 mcg; use 1 spray in each nostril. **ADULTS, ELDERLY, CHILDREN WEIGHING 50 KG OR LESS:** 150 mcg as a single spray. Repeat use based on clinical conditions/laboratory work.

Dosage in Renal Impairment
CrCl less than 50 mL/min: Not recommended.

Dosage in Hepatic Impairment
No dose adjustment.

SIDE EFFECTS

Occasional: IV: Pain, redness, swelling at injection site; headache, abdominal cramps, vulvular pain, flushed skin, mild B/P elevation, nausea with high dosages. **Nasal:** Rhinorrhea, nasal congestion, slight B/P elevation.

ADVERSE EFFECTS/ TOXIC REACTIONS

Water intoxication, hyponatremia (headache, drowsiness, confusion, decreased urination, rapid weight gain, seizures, coma) may occur in overhydration. Children, elderly pts, infants are esp. at risk.

NURSING CONSIDERATIONS

BASELINE ASSESSMENT

Establish baselines for B/P, pulse, weight, serum electrolytes, urine specific gravity. Check lab values for factor VIII coagulant concentration for hemophilia A, von Willebrand's disease; bleeding times.

INTERVENTION/EVALUATION

Check B/P, pulse with IV infusion. Monitor pt weight, fluid intake; urine volume, urine specific gravity, osmolality, serum electrolytes for diabetes insipidus. Assess factor VIII antigen levels, aPTT, factor VIII activity level for hemophilia.

PATIENT/FAMILY TEACHING

• Avoid overhydration. • Follow guidelines for proper intranasal administration. • Report headache, shortness of breath, heartburn, nausea, abdominal cramps.

---

dexamethasone

dex-a-**meth**-a-sone
(Apo-Dexamethasone ♣, Dexamethasone Intensol, DexPak, Maxidex)
Do not confuse Decadron with Percodan, or dexamethasone with dextroamphetamine, or Maxidex with Maxzide.

FIXED-COMBINATION(S)

Ciprodex Otic: dexamethasone/ciprofloxacin (antibiotic): 0.1%/0.3%.
Dexacidin, Maxitrol: dexamethasone/neomycin/polymyxin (anti-infectives): 0.1%/3.5 mg/10,000 units per g or mL.

◆CLASSIFICATION

PHARMACOTHERAPEUTIC: Long-acting glucocorticoid. **CLINICAL:** Corticosteroid.

USES

Used primarily as an anti-inflammatory or immunosuppressant agent in a variety of diseases (e.g., allergic, inflammatory, autoimmune). **OFF-LABEL:** Antiemetic, treatment of croup, dexamethasone suppression test (indicator consistent with suicide and/or depression), accelerate fetal lung maturation. Treatment of acute mountain sickness, high-altitude cerebral edema.

PRECAUTIONS

Contraindications: Hypersensitivity to dexamethasone. Systemic fungal infections, cerebral malaria. **Cautions:** Thyroid disease, renal/hepatic impairment, cardiovascular disease, diabetes, glaucoma, cataracts, myasthenia gravis, pts at risk for seizures, osteoporosis, post-MI, elderly.

ACTION

Suppresses neutrophil migration, decreases production of inflammatory mediators, reverses increased capillary permeability. **Therapeutic Effect:** Decreases inflammation. Suppresses normal immune response.

PHARMACOKINETICS

Rapidly absorbed from GI tract after PO administration. Widely distributed. Protein binding: High. Metabolized in liver. Primarily excreted in urine. Minimally removed by hemodialysis. **Half-life:** 3–4.5 hrs.

▨ LIFESPAN CONSIDERATIONS

Pregnancy/Lactation: Crosses placenta. Distributed in breast milk. **Children:** Prolonged treatment with high-dose therapy may decrease short-term growth rate, cortisol secretion. **Elderly:** Higher risk for developing hypertension, osteoporosis.

INTERACTIONS

DRUG: Amphotericin may increase hypokalemia. May increase **digoxin** toxicity caused by hypokalemia. **CYP3A4 inducers (e.g., carBAMazepine, phenytoin,**

---

rifAMPin) may decrease concentration. **CYP3A4 inhibitors (e.g., ketoconazole), macrolide antibiotics** may increase concentration. May decrease effects of **oral antidiabetic agents (e.g., glyburide, metformin). Live virus vaccines** may decrease pt's antibody response to vaccine, increase vaccine side effects, potentiate virus replication. **HERBAL: Cat's claw, echinacea** may increase immunosuppressant effect. **FOOD:** Interferes with **calcium** absorption. **LAB VALUES:** May increase serum glucose, lipids, sodium levels. May decrease serum calcium, potassium, thyroxine, WBC.

AVAILABILITY (Rx)

Elixir: 0.5 mg/5 mL. **Injection, Solution:** 4 mg/mL, 10 mg/mL. **Ophthalmic Solution:** 0.1%. **Ophthalmic Suspension (Maxidex):** 0.1%. **Solution, Oral:** 0.5 mg/5 mL. **Solution, Oral Concentrate (Dexamethasone Intensol):** 1 mg/mL. **Tablets:** 0.5 mg, 0.75 mg, 1 mg, 1.5 mg, 2 mg, 4 mg, 6 mg. **Tablets (TaperPak [DexPak]):** 1.5 mg (35 or 51 tablets on taper dose card).

ADMINISTRATION/HANDLING

 IV

◄**ALERT**► Dexamethasone sodium phosphate may be given by IV push or IV infusion. Rapid injection may cause genital burning sensation in females.
• For IV push, give over 1–4 min if dose is less than 10 mg. • For IV infusion, mix with 50–100 mL 0.9% NaCl or D₅W and infuse over 15–30 min. • For neonates, solution must be preservative free. • IV solution must be used within 24 hrs.

IM
• Give deep IM, preferably in gluteus maximus.

PO
• Give with milk, food (to decrease GI effect).

Ophthalmic Solution, Suspension
• Place gloved finger on lower eyelid and pull out until a pocket is formed between eye and lower lid. • Place prescribed number of drops or ¼–½ inch ointment into pocket. • Instruct pt to close eye gently for 1–2 min (so that medication will not be squeezed out of the sac). • Instruct pt to apply digital pressure to lacrimal sac at inner canthus for 1–2 min to minimize systemic absorption.

▨ IV INCOMPATIBILITIES

Ciprofloxacin (Cipro), DAUNOrubicin (Cerubidine), IDArubicin (Idamycin), midazolam (Versed).

▨ IV COMPATIBILITIES

Cimetidine (Tagamet), CISplatin (Platinol), cyclophosphamide (Cytoxan), cytarabine (Cytosar), DOCEtaxel (Taxotere), DOXOrubicin (Adriamycin), etoposide (VePesid), furosemide (Lasix), granisetron (Kytril), heparin, HYDROmorphone (Dilaudid), LORazepam (Ativan), morphine, ondansetron (Zofran), PACLitaxel (Taxol), palonosetron (Aloxi), potassium chloride, propofol (Diprivan).

INDICATIONS/ROUTES/DOSAGE

Anti-Inflammatory
PO, IV, IM: ADULTS, ELDERLY: 0.5–9 mg/day in divided doses q6–12h. **CHILDREN:** 0.08–0.3 mg/kg/day in divided doses q6–12h. **INTRA-ARTICULAR: ADULTS, ELDERLY:** 0.4–6 mg/day.

Cerebral Edema
IV: ADULTS, ELDERLY: Initially, 10 mg, then 4 mg (IV or IM) q6h.
PO, IV, IM: CHILDREN: Loading dose of 1–2 mg/kg, then 1–1.5 mg/kg/day in divided doses q4–6h.

Nausea/Vomiting in Chemotherapy Pts
Note: Refer to individual protocols and emetogenic potential.

IV: **ADULTS, ELDERLY:** 8–20 mg 15–30 min before treatment. **CHILDREN:** 6 mg/m²/dose on days of chemotherapy.

Physiologic Replacement
PO, IV, IM: **ADULTS, ELDERLY, CHILDREN:** 0.03–0.15 mg/kg/day in divided doses q6–12h.

Usual Ophthalmic Dosage, Ocular Inflammatory Conditions
ADULTS, ELDERLY, CHILDREN: (Solution): Initially, 2 drops q1h while awake and q2h at night for 1 day, then reduce to 3–4 times/day. (**Suspension**): 1–2 drops up to 4–6 times/day.

Dosage in Renal/Hepatic Impairment
No dose adjustment.

SIDE EFFECTS

Frequent: Inhalation: Cough, dry mouth, hoarseness, throat irritation. **Intranasal:** Burning, mucosal dryness. **Ophthalmic:** Blurred vision. **Systemic:** Insomnia, facial edema (cushingoid appearance ["moon face"]), moderate abdominal distention, indigestion, increased appetite, nervousness, facial flushing, diaphoresis. **Occasional: Inhalation:** Localized fungal infection (thrush). **Intranasal:** Crusting inside nose, epistaxis, sore throat, ulceration of nasal mucosa. **Ophthalmic:** Decreased vision; lacrimation; eye pain; burning, stinging, redness of eyes; nausea; vomiting. **Systemic:** Dizziness, decreased/blurred vision. **Rare: Inhalation:** Increased bronchospasm, esophageal candidiasis. **Intranasal:** Nasal/pharyngeal candidiasis, eye pain. **Systemic:** Generalized allergic reaction (rash, urticaria); pain, redness, swelling at injection site; psychological changes; false sense of well-being; hallucinations; depression.

ADVERSE EFFECTS/ TOXIC REACTIONS

Long-term therapy: Muscle wasting (esp. arms, legs), osteoporosis, spontaneous fractures, amenorrhea, cataracts, glaucoma, peptic ulcer disease, HF. **Ophthalmic:** Glaucoma, ocular hypertension, cataracts. **Abrupt withdrawal following long-term therapy:** Severe joint pain, severe headache, anorexia, nausea, fever, rebound inflammation, fatigue, weakness, lethargy, dizziness, orthostatic hypotension.

NURSING CONSIDERATIONS

BASELINE ASSESSMENT

Question for hypersensitivity to any corticosteroids. Obtain baselines for height, weight, B/P, serum glucose, electrolytes. Question medical history as listed in Precautions.

INTERVENTION/EVALUATION

Monitor I&O, daily weight, serum glucose. Assess for edema. Evaluate food tolerance. Monitor daily pattern of bowel activity, stool consistency. Report hyperacidity promptly. Check vital signs at least twice daily. Be alert to infection (sore throat, fever, vague symptoms). Monitor serum electrolytes, esp. for hypercalcemia, hypokalemia, paresthesia (esp. lower extremities, nausea/vomiting, irritability), Hgb, occult blood loss. Assess emotional status, ability to sleep. Abrupt withdrawal may cause adrenal insufficiency; taper dose gradually.

PATIENT/FAMILY TEACHING

• Do not change dose/schedule or stop taking drug. • **Must** taper off gradually under medical supervision. • Report fever, sore throat, muscle aches, sudden weight gain, edema, exposure to measles/chickenpox. • Severe stress (serious infection, surgery, trauma) may require increased dosage. • Inform dentist, other physicians of dexamethasone therapy within past 12 mos. • Avoid alcohol, limit caffeine.

dexmedetomidine

dex-med-e-**toe**-mye-deen
(Precedex)
Do not confuse Precedex with Percocet or Peridex.

◆CLASSIFICATION

PHARMACOTHERAPEUTIC: Alpha$_2$ agonist. **CLINICAL:** Nonbarbiturate sedative, hypnotic.

USES

Sedation of initially intubated, mechanically ventilated adults in intensive care setting. Use in nonintubated pts requiring sedation before and/or during surgical and other procedures. **OFF-LABEL:** Treatment of shivering, use in children. Awake craniotomy.

PRECAUTIONS

Contraindications: Hypersensitivity to dexmedetomidine. **Cautions:** Heart block, bradycardia, hepatic impairment, hypovolemia, diabetes, hypotension, chronic hypertension, severe ventricular dysfunction, elderly, use of vasodilators or drugs decreasing heart rate.

ACTION

Selective alpha$_2$-adrenergic agonist. Inhibits norepinephrine release. **Therapeutic Effect:** Produces analgesic, hypnotic, sedative effects.

PHARMACOKINETICS

Protein binding: 94%. Metabolized in liver. Excreted in urine. **Half-life:** 2 hrs.

INTERACTIONS

DRUG: Sedatives (e.g., **midazolam, LORazepam**), opioids (e.g., **fentaNYL, morphine, HYDROmorphone**), hypnotics (e.g., **zolpidem, temazepam**) may enhance effects. **Antihypertensives** (e.g., **amlodipine, clonidine, lisinopril, valsartan**) may increase risk of hypotension. **Beta blockers** (e.g., **carvedilol, metoprolol**), **calcium channel blockers** (e.g., **diltiazem, verapamil**) may increase risk of bradycardia, hypotension. **HERBAL:** None significant. **FOOD:** None known. **LAB VALUES:** May increase serum alkaline phosphatase, potassium, ALT, AST.

AVAILABILITY (Rx)

Injection Solution: 80 mcg/20 mL, 200 mcg/2 mL vials, 4 mcg/mL solutions (50 mL, 100 mL).

ADMINISTRATION/HANDLING
 IV

Reconstitution • Dilute 2 mL of dexmedetomidine with 48 mL 0.9% NaCl.
Rate of Administration • Individualized, titrated to desired effect. Use controlled infusion pump.
Storage • Store at room temperature.

▨ IV INCOMPATIBILITIES

Do not mix with any other medications.

▨ IV COMPATIBILITIES

Amiodarone (Cordarone), bumetanide (Bumex), calcium gluconate, cisatracurium (Nimbex), dexamethasone, DOBUTamine, DOPamine, magnesium sulfate, norepinephrine (Levophed), propofol (Diprivan).

INDICATIONS/ROUTES/DOSAGE

Sedation
IV: ADULTS: Loading dose of 1 mcg/kg over 10 min followed by maintenance infusion of 0.2–0.7 mcg/kg/hr. **ELDERLY:** May require decreased dosage.

Dosage in Renal Impairment
No dose adjustment.

Dosage in Hepatic Impairment
Use caution.

SIDE EFFECTS

Frequent (30%–11%): Hypotension, nausea. **Occasional (3%–2%):** Pain, fever, oliguria, thirst.

ADVERSE EFFECTS/ TOXIC REACTIONS

Bradycardia, atrial fibrillation, hypoxia, anemia, pain, pleural effusion may occur with too-rapid IV infusion.

NURSING CONSIDERATIONS

BASELINE ASSESSMENT

Obtain baseline B/P, heart rate and assess mental status prior to initiation. Obtain full medication history; screen for medications known to cause hypotension, bradycardia, sedation.

INTERVENTION/EVALUATION

Assess cardiac monitor for arrhythmia, pulse for bradycardia, B/P for hypotension, level of sedation. Assess respiratory rate, rhythm. Monitor ventilator settings. Discontinue once pt is extubated.

TOP 100

dextroamphetamine and amphetamine

dex-troe-am-**fet**-ah-meen/am-**fet**-ah-meen
(Adderall, <u>Adderall-XR</u>)
■ **BLACK BOX ALERT** ■ High potential for abuse. Prolonged administration may lead to drug dependence. Severe cardiovascular events including CVA/MI reported. **Do not confuse Adderall with Inderal.**

◆CLASSIFICATION

PHARMACOTHERAPEUTIC: Amphetamine (Schedule II). **CLINICAL:** CNS stimulant.

USES

Treatment of narcolepsy; treatment of ADHD.

PRECAUTIONS

Contraindications: Hypersensitivity to dextroamphetamine, amphetamine, or sympathomimetics. Advanced arteriosclerosis, agitated mental states, glaucoma, history of alcohol or drug abuse, hypersensitivity to sympathomimetic amines, hyperthyroidism, moderate to severe hypertension, symptomatic cardiovascular disease, use of MAOIs within 14 days. **Cautions:** Elderly, debilitated pts, history of seizures, mild hypertension. Preexisting psychotic or bipolar disorder.

ACTION

Enhances action of DOPamine, norepinephrine by blocking reuptake from synapses. Inhibits monoamine oxidase, facilitates release of catecholamines. **Therapeutic Effect:** Increases motor activity, mental alertness; decreases drowsiness, fatigue; suppresses appetite.

PHARMACOKINETICS

Well absorbed following PO administration. Widely distributed including CNS. Metabolized in liver. Excreted in urine. Removed by hemodialysis. **Half-life:** 10–13 hrs.

⏳ LIFESPAN CONSIDERATIONS

Pregnancy/Lactation: Distributed in breast milk. **Children:** Safety and efficacy not established in pts younger than 3 yrs. **Elderly:** Age-related cardiovascular, cerebrovascular disease, hepatic/renal impairment may increase risk of side effects.

INTERACTIONS

DRUG: May enhance effects of **tricyclic antidepressants (e.g., amitriptyline, doxepin, nortriptyline), sympathomimetics. MAOIs (e.g., phenelzine, selegiline)** may prolong, intensify effects. May antagonize effects of **hypotensive agents. HERBAL:** None significant. **FOOD:** None known. **LAB VALUES:** May increase plasma corticosteroid.

AVAILABILITY (Rx)

Tablets (Adderall): 5 mg, 7.5 mg, 10 mg, 12.5 mg, 15 mg, 20 mg, 30 mg.

📎 **Capsules (Extended-Release [Adderall-XR]):** 5 mg, 10 mg, 15 mg, 20 mg, 25 mg, 30 mg.

ADMINISTRATION/HANDLING

PO

• Give tablets at least 6 hrs before bedtime. • Extended-release capsules should be swallowed whole; do not break, crush, or cut. • Avoid afternoon doses to prevent insomnia. • May open capsules and sprinkle on applesauce. Instruct pt not to chew sprinkled beads; take immediately.

INDICATIONS/ROUTES/DOSAGE

Narcolepsy

PO: ADULTS, CHILDREN OLDER THAN 12 YRS: Initially, 10 mg/day. Increase by 10 mg/day at wkly intervals until therapeutic response is achieved. **Maximum:** 60 mg/day given in 1–3 divided doses with interval of 4–6 hrs between doses. **CHILDREN 6–12 YRS:** Initially, 5 mg/day. Increase by 5 mg/day at wkly intervals until therapeutic response is achieved. **Maximum:** 60 mg/day given in 1–3 divided doses with interval of 4–6 hrs between doses.

ADHD

ADULTS, ELDERLY: (ADDERALL): Initially, 5 mg 1–2 times/day. May increase by 5-mg increments at wkly intervals. **Maximum:** 40 mg/day in 1–3 divided doses (usual intervals of 4–6 hrs). **(ADDERALL-XR):** Initially, 20 mg once daily in the morning. May increase up to 60 mg/day. **CHILDREN 13–17 YRS: (ADDERALL):** Initially, 5 mg 1–2 times/day. May increase by 5 mg at wkly intervals. **Maximum:** 40 mg/day in 1–3 divided doses (usual intervals of 4–6 hrs). **(ADDERALL-XR):** Initially, 10 mg once daily in the morning. May increase to 20 mg/day after 1 wk if symptoms are not controlled. May increase up to 60 mg/day. **CHILDREN 6–12 YRS: (ADDERALL):** Initially, 5 mg 1–2 times/day. May increase in 5-mg increments at wkly intervals until optimal response is obtained. **Maximum:** 40 mg/day given in 1–3 divided doses (use intervals of 4–6 hrs between additional doses). **(ADDERALL-XR):** Initially, 5–10 mg once daily in the morning. May increase daily dose in 5- to 10-mg increments at wkly intervals. **Maximum:** 30 mg/day. **CHILDREN 3–5 YRS: (ADDERALL):** Initially, 2.5 mg/day given every morning. May increase daily dose in 2.5-mg increments at wkly intervals until optimal response is obtained. **Maximum:** 40 mg/day given in 1–3 divided doses (use intervals of 4–6 hrs between additional doses). Not recommended in children younger than 3 yrs.

Dosage in Renal/Hepatic Impairment
No dose adjustment.

SIDE EFFECTS

Frequent: Increased motor activity, talkativeness, nervousness, mild euphoria, insomnia. **Occasional:** Headache, chills, dry mouth, GI distress, worsening depression in pts who are clinically depressed, tachycardia, palpitations, chest pain, dizziness, decreased appetite.

ADVERSE EFFECTS/ TOXIC REACTIONS

Overdose may produce skin pallor/flushing, arrhythmias, psychosis. Abrupt withdrawal after prolonged use of high doses may produce lethargy (may last for wks). Prolonged administration to children with ADHD may temporarily suppress normal weight/height pattern.

NURSING CONSIDERATIONS

BASELINE ASSESSMENT

Assess attention span, impulse control, interaction with others. Screen for drug-seeking behavior, past drug abuse. Obtain baseline B/P. Assess sleep pattern.

INTERVENTION/EVALUATION

Monitor for CNS overstimulation, increase in B/P, growth rate, change in pulse rate, respirations, weight loss. **Narcolepsy:** Observe/document frequency of narcoleptic episodes. **ADHD:** Observe for improved attention span.

PATIENT/FAMILY TEACHING

• Normal dosage levels may produce tolerance to drug's anorexic mood-elevating effects within a few wks. • Dry mouth may be relieved with sugarless gum, sips of water. • Take early in day. • Do not break, chew, or crush extended-release capsules. • May mask extreme fatigue. • Report pronounced anxiety, dizziness, decreased appetite, dry mouth, new or worsening behavior, chest pain, palpitations. • Avoid alcohol, caffeine.

---

diazePAM

dye-**az**-e-pam
(Apo-DiazePAM ♣, Diastat,
DiazePAM Intensol, Novo-Dipam ♣,
Valium)
Do not confuse diazePAM with diazoxide, diltiaZEM, Ditropan, or LORazepam, or Valium with Valcyte.

◆CLASSIFICATION

PHARMACOTHERAPEUTIC: Benzodiazepine (Schedule IV). **CLINICAL:** Antianxiety, skeletal muscle relaxant, anticonvulsant.

USES

Short-term relief of anxiety symptoms, relief of acute alcohol withdrawal. Adjunct for relief of acute musculoskeletal conditions, treatment of seizures (IV route used for termination of status epilepticus). **Gel:** Control of increased seizure activity in refractory epilepsy in pts on stable regimens.

OFF-LABEL: Treatment of panic disorder. Short-term treatment of spasticity in children with cerebral palsy. Sedation for mechanically vented pts in ICU.

PRECAUTIONS

Contraindications: Hypersensitivity to diazePAM. Acute narrow-angle glaucoma, untreated open-angle glaucoma, severe respiratory depression, severe hepatic insufficiency, sleep apnea syndrome, myasthenia gravis. Children younger than 6 mos (oral). **Cautions:** Pts receiving other CNS depressants or psychoactive agents, depression, history of drug and alcohol abuse, renal/hepatic impairment, respiratory disease, impaired gag reflex, concurrent use of strong CYP3A4 inhibitors or inducers.

ACTION

Depresses all levels of CNS by enhancing action of gamma-aminobutyric acid (GABA), a major inhibitory neurotransmitter in the brain. **Therapeutic Effect:** Produces anxiolytic effect, elevates seizure threshold, produces skeletal muscle relaxation.

PHARMACOKINETICS

Well absorbed from GI tract. Widely distributed. Protein binding: 98%. Excreted in urine. Minimally removed by hemodialysis. **Half-life:** 20–70 hrs (increased in hepatic dysfunction, elderly).

⧖ LIFESPAN CONSIDERATIONS

Pregnancy/Lactation: Crosses placenta. Distributed in breast milk. May increase risk of fetal abnormalities if administered during first trimester of pregnancy. Chronic ingestion during pregnancy may produce withdrawal symptoms, CNS depression in neonates. **Children/Elderly:** Use small initial doses with gradual increases to avoid ataxia, excessive sedation. Elderly at increased risk of impaired cognition, delirium, falls, fractures.

INTERACTIONS

DRUG: Alcohol, CNS depressants (e.g., gabapentin, morphine, zolpidem) may increase CNS depression. CYP3A4 inducers (e.g., carBAMazepine, rifAMPin) may decrease concentration. CYP3A4 inhibitors (e.g., itraconazole, ketoconazole) may increase concentration. **HERBAL:** Gotu kola, kava kava, St. John's wort, valerian may increase CNS depression. St. John's wort may decrease concentration/effects. **FOOD:** Grapefruit products may increase concentration/effects. **LAB VALUES:** None significant. **Therapeutic serum level:** 0.5–2 mcg/mL; **toxic serum level:** greater than 3 mcg/mL.

AVAILABILITY (Rx)

Injection, Solution: 5 mg/mL. **Oral Concentrate (DiazePAM Intensol):** 5 mg/mL. **Oral Solution:** 5 mg/5 mL. **Rectal Gel (Diastat):** 2.5 mg, 10 mg, 20 mg. **Tablet (Valium):** 2 mg, 5 mg, 10 mg.

ADMINISTRATION/HANDLING

 IV

Rate of Administration • Give by IV push into tubing of flowing IV solution as close as possible to vein insertion point. • Administer directly into large vein (reduces risk of thrombosis/phlebitis). Do not use small veins (e.g., wrist/dorsum of hand). • Administer IV at rate not exceeding 5 mg/min for adults. For children, give 1–2 mg/min (too-rapid IV may result in hypotension, respiratory depression). • Monitor respirations q5–15 min for 2 hrs.
Storage • Store at room temperature.

IM

• Injection may be painful. Inject deeply into large muscle mass.

PO

• Give without regard to meals. • Dilute oral concentrate with water, juice, carbonated beverages; may be mixed in semisolid food (applesauce, pudding). • Tablets may be crushed.

GEL

• Insert rectal tip and gently push plunger over 3 sec. Remove tip after 3 additional sec. • Buttocks should be held together for 3 sec after removal.

▨ IV INCOMPATIBILITIES

Amphotericin B complex (Abelcet, AmBisome, Amphotec), cefepime (Maxipime), diltiaZEM (Cardizem), fluconazole (Diflucan), foscarnet (Foscavir), furosemide (Lasix), heparin, hydrocortisone (SOLU-Cortef), HYDROmorphone (Dilaudid), meropenem (Merrem IV), potassium chloride, propofol (Diprivan), vitamins.

▨ IV COMPATIBILITIES

DOBUTamine (Dobutrex), fentaNYL, morphine.

INDICATIONS/ROUTES/DOSAGE

Anxiety
PO: ADULTS: 2–10 mg 2–4 times/day. **ELDERLY:** Initially, 1–2 mg 1–2 times/day. **CHILDREN:** 0.12–0.8 mg/kg/day in divided doses q6–8h.
IV, IM: ADULTS: 2–10 mg; may repeat in 3–4 hrs if needed. **CHILDREN:** 0.04–0.3 mg/kg/dose q2–4h. **Maximum:** 0.6 mg/kg within 8-hr period.

Skeletal Muscle Relaxation
PO: ADULTS: 2–10 mg 2–4 times/day. **ELDERLY:** Initially, 1–2 mg 1–2 times/day. **CHILDREN:** 0.12–0.8 mg/kg/day in divided doses q6–8h.

Alcohol Withdrawal
IM, IV: ADULTS, ELDERLY: Initially, 10 mg, then 5–10 mg 3–4 hrs later. **PO: ADULTS, ELDERLY:** 10 mg 3–4 times during first 24 hrs, then reduce to 5 mg 3–4 times/day as needed.

Status Epilepticus
IV: ADULTS, ELDERLY: 5–10 mg q10–15 min. **Maximum Total Dose:** 30 mg.

May repeat in 2–4 hrs. **INFANTS, CHILDREN:** 0.1–0.3 mg/kg over 2 min; may repeat after 5–10 min. **Maximum:** 10 mg/dose.

Control of Increased Seizure Activity (Breakthrough Seizures) in Pts with Refractory Epilepsy Who Are on Stable Regimens of Anticonvulsants
PO: ADULTS, ELDERLY: 2–10 mg 2–4 times/day. **Note:** Do not use gel for more than 5 episodes/mo or more than 1 episode q5days. **Rectal Gel: ADULTS, CHILDREN 12 YRS AND OLDER:** 0.2 mg/kg; may be repeated in 4–12 hrs. **CHILDREN 6–11 YRS:** 0.3 mg/kg; may be repeated in 4–12 hrs. **CHILDREN 2–5 YRS:** 0.5 mg/kg; may be repeated in 4–12 hrs.

Dosage in Renal Impairment
Use caution.

Dosage in Hepatic Impairment
Use caution. Oral tablets contraindicated in severe hepatic impairment.

SIDE EFFECTS

Frequent: Pain with IM injection, drowsiness, fatigue, ataxia. **Occasional:** Slurred speech, orthostatic hypotension, headache, hypoactivity, constipation, nausea, blurred vision. **Rare:** Paradoxical CNS reactions (hyperactivity/nervousness in children, excitement/restlessness in elderly/debilitated pts) generally noted during first 2 wks of therapy, particularly in presence of uncontrolled pain.

ADVERSE EFFECTS/ TOXIC REACTIONS

IV route may produce pain, swelling, thrombophlebitis, carpal tunnel syndrome. Abrupt or too-rapid withdrawal may result in pronounced restlessness, irritability, insomnia, hand tremor, abdominal/muscle cramps, diaphoresis, vomiting, seizures. Abrupt withdrawal in pts with epilepsy may produce increase in frequency/severity of seizures. Overdose results in drowsiness, confusion, diminished reflexes, CNS depression, coma. **Antidote:** Flumazenil (see Appendix J for dosage).

NURSING CONSIDERATIONS

BASELINE ASSESSMENT

Assess B/P, pulse, respirations immediately before administration. **Anxiety:** Assess autonomic response (cold, clammy hands; diaphoresis), motor response (agitation, trembling, tension). **Musculoskeletal spasm:** Record onset, type, location, duration of pain. Check for immobility, stiffness, swelling. **Seizures:** Review history of seizure disorder (length, intensity, frequency, duration, LOC). Observe frequently for recurrence of seizure activity.

INTERVENTION/EVALUATION

Monitor heart rate, respiratory rate, B/P, mental status. Assess children, elderly for paradoxical reaction, particularly during early therapy. Evaluate for therapeutic response (decrease in intensity/frequency of seizures; calm facial expression, decreased restlessness; decreased intensity of skeletal muscle pain). **Therapeutic serum level:** 0.5–2 mcg/mL; **toxic serum level:** greater than 3 mcg/mL.

PATIENT/FAMILY TEACHING

• Avoid alcohol. • Limit caffeine. • May cause drowsiness; avoid tasks that require alertness, motor skills until response to drug is established. • May be habit forming. • Avoid abrupt discontinuation after prolonged use.

diclofenac

dye-**kloe**-fen-ak
(Apo-Diclo ♣, Cambia, Cataflam, Dyloject, Flector, Pennsaid, Solaraze, Voltaren Gel, Zipsor, Zorvolex)

■ **BLACK BOX ALERT** ■ Increased risk of serious cardiovascular thrombotic events, including myocardial infarction, CVA. Increased risk of severe GI reactions, including ulceration, bleeding, perforation of stomach, intestines. Contraindicated for treatment of perioperative pain in setting of CABG surgery.

Do not confuse Cataflam with Catapres, diclofenac with Diflucan or Duphalac, or Voltaren with traMADol, Ultram, or Verelan.

FIXED-COMBINATION(S)

Arthrotec: diclofenac/miSOPROStol (an antisecretory gastric protectant): 50 mg/200 mcg, 75 mg/200 mcg.

◆CLASSIFICATION

PHARMACOTHERAPEUTIC: NSAID (nonselective). **CLINICAL:** Analgesic, anti-inflammatory.

USES

PO: (Immediate-release): Treatment of rheumatoid arthritis, osteoarthritis, mild to moderate pain, primary dysmenorrhea. **(Zipsor):** Mild to moderate pain. **(Zorvolex):** Mild to moderate pain, osteoarthritic pain. **(Delayed-release):** Treatment of rheumatoid arthritis, osteoarthritis, ankylosing spondylitis. **(Extended-release):** Treatment of rheumatoid arthritis, osteoarthritis. **Oral Solution (Cambia):** Treatment of migraine. **Injection:** Treatment of mild to moderate acute pain and moderate to severe acute pain in adults. **Topical Patch:** Treatment of acute pain due to minor strains, sprains, contusions. **OFF-LABEL:** Treatment of juvenile idiopathic arthritis.

PRECAUTIONS

Contraindications: Hypersensitivity to diclofenac. Pts experiencing asthma, urticaria after taking aspirin, other NSAIDs. Pts with moderate to severe renal impairment in perioperative period who are at risk for volume depletion (injection only); perioperative pain in setting of CABG surgery. **Cautions:** HF, hypertension, renal/hepatic impairment, hepatic porphyria, history of GI disease (e.g., bleeding, ulcers), concomitant use of aspirin or anticoagulants, elderly, debilitated pts.

ACTION

Reversibly inhibits cyclo-oxygenase-1 and -2 (COX-1 and COX-2) enzymes, resulting in decreased formation of prostaglandin precursors. **Therapeutic Effect:** Produces analgesic, antipyretic, anti-inflammatory effects.

PHARMACOKINETICS

Route	Onset	Peak	Duration
PO	30 min	2–3 hrs	Up to 8 hrs

Completely absorbed from GI tract. Protein binding: greater than 99%. Widely distributed. Metabolized in liver. Primarily excreted in urine. Minimally removed by hemodialysis. **Half-life:** 1.2–2 hrs.

⌛ LIFESPAN CONSIDERATIONS

Pregnancy/Lactation: Crosses placenta. Unknown if distributed in breast milk. Avoid use during third trimester (may adversely affect fetal cardiovascular system: premature closure of ductus arteriosus). **Children:** Safety and efficacy not established. **Elderly:** GI bleeding, ulceration more likely to cause serious adverse effects. Age-related renal impairment may increase risk of hepatic/renal toxicity; reduced dosage recommended.

INTERACTIONS

DRUG: May decrease effects of **acetylcholine**, **antihypertensives** (e.g., **amlodipine**, **hydralazine**, **valsartan**), **carbachol**, **diuretics** (e.g., **furosemide**, **HCTZ**). **Aspirin**, **other salicylates**, **warfarin** may increase risk of GI side effects/bleeding. **CYP2C9 inhibitors** (e.g., **voriconazole**) may increase concentration/risk of toxicity. **CYP2C9 inducers** (e.g., **rifAMPin**) may decrease effect. May increase **cycloSPORINE** concentration/toxicity. **Ophthalmic:** May decrease antiglaucoma effects of **antiglaucoma agents**, **EPINEPHrine**. **HERBAL:** Cat's claw, dong quai, evening primrose, garlic, ginseng may increase antiplatelet activity. **FOOD:** None known. **LAB VALUES:** May increase urine protein, serum BUN, alkaline phosphatase, creatinine, LDH, potassium, ALT, AST. May decrease serum uric acid.

AVAILABILITY (Rx)

Adhesive Patch (Flector): 10×14-cm patch containing 180 mg diclofenac. **Capsules (Zipsor):** 25 mg. **(Zorvolex):** 18 mg, 35 mg. **Intravenous Solution (Dyloject):** 37.5 mg/mL. **Oral Solution (Cambia):** 50-mg packets. **Tablets:** 50 mg. **Tablets (Delayed-Release):** 25 mg, 50 mg, 75 mg. **Tablets (Extended-Release):** 100 mg.

ADMINISTRATION/HANDLING

PO
• Do not break, crush, dissolve, or divide enteric-coated tablets. • May give with food, milk, antacids if GI distress occurs. • **Cambia:** Mix one packet in 1–2 oz water, stir well, and instruct pt to drink immediately.

IV
Administer as IV bolus over 15 sec.

Transdermal Patch
• Apply to intact skin; avoid contact with eyes. • Do not wear when bathing/showering. • Wash hands after handling.

INDICATIONS/ROUTES/DOSAGE

Osteoarthritis
PO: *(Immediate-Release):* **ADULTS, ELDERLY:** 50 mg 2–3 times/day.
PO: *(Extended-Release):* **ADULTS, ELDERLY:** 100 mg/day as a single dose. May increase to 200 mg/day in 2 divided doses. *(Zorvolex):* 35 mg 3 times/day.
PO: *(Delayed-Release):* **ADULTS, ELDERLY:** 50 mg 2–3 times/day or 75 mg twice daily.

Rheumatoid Arthritis (RA)
PO: *(Immediate-Release):* **ADULTS, ELDERLY:** 50 mg 3–4 times/day.
PO: *(Extended-Release):* **ADULTS, ELDERLY:** 100 mg once daily. May increase to 200 mg/day in 2 divided doses.
PO: *(Delayed-Release):* **ADULTS, ELDERLY:** 50 mg 3–4 times/day or 75 mg twice daily.

Ankylosing Spondylitis
PO: *(Delayed-Release):* **ADULTS, ELDERLY:** 100–125 mg/day in 4–5 divided doses.

Primary Dysmenorrhea
PO: *(Immediate-Release):* **ADULTS, ELDERLY:** 50 mg 3 times/day.

Pain
PO: ADULTS, ELDERLY: *(Immediate-Release):* 100 mg once, then 50 mg 3 times/day. *(Zipsor):* 25 mg 4 times/day. *(Zorvolex):* 18–35 mg 3 times/day.
IV: 37.5 mg q6h prn. **Maximum:** 150 mg/day.
Topical Patch: *(Flector):* Apply 2 times/day.

Migraine (Oral Solution)
PO: ADULTS, ELDERLY: 50 mg (one packet) once.

Dosage in Renal Impairment
Not recommended in severe impairment.

Dosage in Hepatic Impairment
May require dose adjustment. Use caution.

D

SIDE EFFECTS

Frequent (9%–4%): PO: Headache, abdominal cramps, constipation, diarrhea, nausea, dyspepsia. **Ophthalmic:** Burning, stinging on instillation, ocular discomfort. **Occasional (3%–1%): PO:** Flatulence, dizziness, epigastric pain. **Ophthalmic:** Ocular itching, tearing. **Rare (less than 1%): PO:** Rash, peripheral edema, fluid retention, visual disturbances, vomiting, drowsiness.

ADVERSE EFFECTS/ TOXIC REACTIONS

Overdose may result in acute renal failure. In pts treated chronically, peptic ulcer, GI bleeding, gastritis, severe hepatic reaction (jaundice), nephrotoxicity (hematuria, dysuria, proteinuria), severe hypersensitivity reaction (bronchospasm, angioedema) occur rarely.

NURSING CONSIDERATIONS

BASELINE ASSESSMENT

Obtain baseline B/P. **Anti-inflammatory:** Assess onset, type, location, duration of pain, inflammation. Inspect appearance of affected joints for immobility, deformities, skin condition.

INTERVENTION/EVALUATION

Monitor CBC, renal function, LFT, urine output, occult blood test, B/P. Monitor for headache, dyspepsia. Monitor daily pattern of bowel activity, stool consistency. Assess for therapeutic response: relief of pain, stiffness, swelling; increased joint mobility; reduced joint tenderness; improved grip strength.

PATIENT/FAMILY TEACHING

• Swallow tablets whole; do not chew, crush, dissolve, or divide. • Avoid aspirin, alcohol during therapy (increases risk of GI bleeding). • If GI upset occurs, take with food, milk. • Report skin rash, itching, weight gain, changes in vision, black stools, bleeding, jaundice, upper quadrant pain, persistent headache. • **Ophthalmic:** Do not use hydrogel soft contact lenses. • **Topical:** Avoid exposure to sunlight, sunlamps. • Report rash.

digoxin

di-**jox**-in
(Apo-Digoxin ✦, Digitek, Digox, Lanoxin)
Do not confuse digoxin with Desoxyn or doxepin, or Lanoxin with Lasix, Levoxyl, Levsinex, Lonox, or Mefoxin.

◆CLASSIFICATION

PHARMACOTHERAPEUTIC: Cardiac glycoside. **CLINICAL:** Antiarrhythmic, cardiotonic.

USES

Treatment of mild to moderate HF. Control ventricular response rate in pts with chronic atrial fibrillation. **OFF-LABEL:** Fetal tachycardia with or without hydrops; decrease ventricular rate in supraventricular tachyarrhythmias.

PRECAUTIONS

Contraindications: Hypersensitivity to digoxin. Ventricular fibrillation. **Cautions:** Renal impairment, sinus nodal disease, acute MI (within 6 mos), second- or third-degree heart block (unless functioning pacemaker), concurrent use of strong inducers or inhibitors of P-glycoprotein (e.g., cycloSPORINE), hyperthyroidism, hypothyroidism, hypokalemia, hypocalcemia.

ACTION

HF: Inhibits sodium/potassium ATPase pump in myocardial cells. Promotes calcium influx. **Supraventricular Arrhythmias:** Suppresses AV node conduction. **Therapeutic Effect: HF:** Increases contractility. **Supraventricular Arrhythmias:** Increases effective refractory period/decreases conduction velocity, decreases heart rate.

PHARMACOKINETICS

Route	Onset	Peak	Duration
PO	0.5–2 hrs	2–8 hrs	3–4 days
IV	5–30 min	1–4 hrs	3–4 days

Readily absorbed from GI tract. Widely distributed. Protein binding: 30%. Partially metabolized in liver. Primarily excreted in urine. Minimally removed by hemodialysis. **Half-life:** 36–48 hrs (increased in renal impairment, elderly).

⧗ LIFESPAN CONSIDERATIONS

Pregnancy/Lactation: Crosses placenta. Distributed in breast milk. **Children:** Premature infants more susceptible to toxicity. **Elderly:** Age-related hepatic/renal impairment may require dosage adjustment. Increased risk of loss of appetite. Avoid use as first-line therapy for atrial fibrillation or HF.

INTERACTIONS

DRUG: Amiodarone may increase concentration/toxicity. **Beta blockers (e.g., metoprolol), calcium channel blockers (e.g., diltiaZEM)** may have additive effect on slowing AV nodal conduction. **Potassium-depleting diuretics (e.g., furosemide)** may increase toxicity due to hypokalemia. **Sympathomimetics (e.g., norepinephrine)** may increase risk of arrhythmias. **HERBAL: Ephedra** may increase risk of arrhythmias. **Licorice** may cause sodium and water retention, loss of potassium. **FOOD: Meals with increased fiber (bran) or high in pectin** may decrease absorption. **LAB VALUES:** None known.

AVAILABILITY (Rx)

Oral Solution (Lanoxin): 50 mcg/mL. **Injection Solution (Lanoxin):** 100 mcg/mL, 250 mcg/mL. **Tablets (Lanoxin):** 62.5 mcg, 125 mcg, 187.5 mcg, 250 mcg.

ADMINISTRATION/HANDLING

◄ALERT► IM rarely used (produces severe local irritation, erratic absorption). If no other route possible, give deep into muscle followed by massage. Give no more than 2 mL at any one site.

 IV

• May give undiluted or dilute with at least a 4-fold volume of Sterile Water for Injection or D$_5$W (less may cause precipitate). • Use immediately. • Give IV slowly over at least 5 min.

PO

• May give without regard to meals.
• Tablets may be crushed.

▦ IV INCOMPATIBILITIES

Amphotericin B complex (Abelcet, AmBisome, Amphotec), fluconazole (Diflucan), foscarnet (Foscavir), propofol (Diprivan).

▦ IV COMPATIBILITIES

DiltiaZEM (Cardizem), furosemide (Lasix), heparin, insulin regular, lidocaine, midazolam (Versed), milrinone (Primacor), morphine, potassium chloride.

INDICATIONS/ROUTES/DOSAGE

Note: Loading dose not recommended in HF.

Loading Dose
PO: ADULTS,ELDERLY: 0.75–1.5 mg. **CHILDREN 10 YRS AND OLDER:** 10–15 mcg/kg. **CHILDREN 5–9 YRS:** 20–35 mcg/kg. **CHILDREN 2–4 YRS:** 30–40 mcg/kg. **CHILDREN 1–23 MOS:** 35–60 mcg/kg. **NEONATE, FULL-TERM:** 25–35 mcg/kg. **NEONATE, PREMATURE:** 20–30 mcg/kg.
IV: ADULTS, ELDERLY: 0.5–1 mg. **CHILDREN 10 YRS AND OLDER:** 8–12 mcg/kg. **CHILDREN 5–9 YRS:** 15–30 mcg/kg. **CHILDREN 2–4 YRS:** 25–35 mcg/kg. **CHILDREN 1–23 MOS:** 30–50 mcg/kg. **NEONATES,**

✦ Canadian trade name   🐮 Non-Crushable Drug   🔲 High Alert drug

FULL-TERM: 20–30 mcg/kg. **NEONATES, PREMATURE:** 15–25 mcg/kg.

Maintenance Dosage

	PO	IV/IM
Preterm infant	5–7.5 mcg/kg	4–6 mcg/kg
Full-term infant	6–10 mcg/kg	5–8 mcg/kg
1 mo–2 yrs	10–15 mcg/kg	7.5–12 mcg/kg
2–5 yrs	7.5–10 mcg/kg	6–9 mcg/kg
5–10 yrs	5–10 mcg/kg	4–8 mcg/kg

Note: Avoid doses greater than 0.125 mg/day in elderly due to decreased renal clearance.

HF
PO: ADULTS, ELDERLY: 0.125–0.25 mg once daily.

Supraventricular Arrhythmias
PO: ADULTS, ELDERLY: Digitalizing dose: 0.125–1.5 mg. **Maintenance dose:** 0.125–0.5 mg once daily. **IV: Digitalizing dose:** 0.5–1 mg. **Maintenance dose:** 0.1–0.4 mg once daily.

Dosage in Renal Impairment
Dosage adjustment is based on creatinine clearance. **Loading dose:** Decrease by 50% in end-stage renal disease.

Maintenance Dose

eGFR	Dosage
10–50 mL/min	25%–75% of usual dose or q36h (0.0625 mg q24–36hrs)
Less than 10 mL/min (HD, PD, CRRT)	10%–25% of usual dose or q48h (0.0625 mg q48h)

Dosage in Hepatic Impairment
No dose adjustment.

SIDE EFFECTS

Dizziness, headache, diarrhea, rash, visual disturbances.

ADVERSE EFFECTS/ TOXIC REACTIONS

The most common early manifestations of digoxin toxicity are GI disturbances (anorexia, nausea, vomiting), neurologic abnormalities (fatigue, headache, depression, weakness, drowsiness, confusion, nightmares). Facial pain, personality change, ocular disturbances (photophobia, light flashes, halos around bright objects, yellow or green color perception) may occur. Sinus bradycardia, AV block, ventricular arrhythmias noted. **Antidote:** Digoxin immune FAB (see Appendix J for dosage).

NURSING CONSIDERATIONS

BASELINE ASSESSMENT

Assess apical pulse. If pulse is 60 or less/min (70 or less/min for children), withhold drug, contact physician. Blood samples are best taken 6–8 hrs after dose or just before next dose.

INTERVENTION/EVALUATION

Monitor pulse for bradycardia, EKG for arrhythmias for 1–2 hrs after administration (excessive slowing of pulse may be first clinical sign of toxicity). Assess for GI disturbances, neurologic abnormalities (signs of toxicity) q2–4h during loading dose (daily during maintenance). Monitor serum potassium, magnesium, calcium, renal function. **Therapeutic serum level:** 0.8–2 ng/mL; **toxic serum level:** greater than 2 ng/mL.

PATIENT/FAMILY TEACHING

• Follow-up visits, blood tests are an important part of therapy. • Follow guidelines to take apical pulse and report pulse of 60 or less/min (or as indicated by physician). • Wear/carry identification of digoxin therapy and inform dentist, other physician of taking digoxin. • Do not increase or skip doses. • Do not take OTC medications without consulting physician. • Report decreased appetite, nausea/vomiting, diarrhea, visual changes.

---

dihydroergotamine

dye-**hye**-droe-er-**got**-a-meen
(D.H.E. 45, Migranal)

■ **BLACK BOX ALERT** ■ Concurrent use with CYP3A4 inhibitors (macrolide antibiotics, azole antifungals, protease inhibitors) increases risk of vasospasm, producing ischemia of brain and peripheral extremities.
Do not confuse Cafergot with Carafate.

FIXED-COMBINATION(S)

Cafergot, Wigraine: ergotamine/caffeine (stimulant): 1 mg/100 mg, 2 mg/100 mg.

◆CLASSIFICATION

PHARMACOTHERAPEUTIC: Ergotamine derivative. **CLINICAL:** Antimigraine.

USES

Treatment of migraine headache with or without aura. Injection also used to treat cluster headache.

PRECAUTIONS

Contraindications: Hypersensitivity to dihydroergotamine. Uncontrolled hypertension, ischemic heart disease, coronary artery vasospasm (including Prinzmetal's angina), angina pectoris, history of MI following vascular surgery, concurrent use of peripheral and central vasoconstrictors, hemiplegic or basilar migraine, peripheral vascular disease, sepsis, severe renal/hepatic impairment, use of MAOIs within 14 days, use of sumatriptan, zolmitriptan, other serotonin agonists, or ergot-like agents within 24 hrs, potent CYP3A4 inhibitors (e.g., azole antifungals, macrolide antibiotics, protease inhibitors), pregnancy, breastfeeding. **Cautions:** Elderly.

ACTION

Directly stimulates vascular smooth muscle, resulting in peripheral and cerebral vasoconstriction. May have antagonist effects on serotonin. **Therapeutic Effect:** Suppresses vascular headaches, migraine headaches.

PHARMACOKINETICS

Slowly, incompletely absorbed from GI tract; rapidly and extensively absorbed after rectal administration. Protein binding: greater than 90%. Eliminated in feces by the biliary system. **Half-life:** 21 hrs.

⧖ LIFESPAN CONSIDERATIONS

Pregnancy/Lactation: Contraindicated in pregnancy (produces uterine stimulant action, resulting in possible fetal death or retarded fetal growth); increases vasoconstriction of placental vascular bed. Drug distributed in breast milk. May produce diarrhea, vomiting in neonate. May prohibit lactation. **Children:** No precautions in pts 6 yrs and older, but use only when unresponsive to other medication. **Elderly:** Age-related occlusive peripheral vascular disease increases risk of peripheral vasoconstriction. Age-related renal impairment may require dosage adjustment.

INTERACTIONS

DRUG: Beta blockers (e.g., carvedilol, metoprolol), erythromycin may increase risk of peripheral vasoconstriction. Ergot alkaloids, 5-HT$_B$ agonists (e.g., SUMAtriptan), systemic vasoconstrictors may increase vasopressor effect. **HERBAL:** None significant. **FOOD:** Coffee, cola, tea may increase absorption. Grapefruit products may increase concentration, toxicity. **LAB VALUES:** None significant.

AVAILABILITY (Rx)

Dihydroergotamine Injection, Solution: 1 mg/mL. **Intranasal Spray, Solution (Migranal):** 4 mg/mL (0.5 mg/spray).

INDICATIONS/ROUTES/DOSAGE

Migraine Headache

IM/SQ: ADULTS, ELDERLY: 1 mg at onset of headache; repeat hourly. **Maximum:** 3 mg/day; 6 mg/wk.

IV: ADULTS, ELDERLY: (Give slowly over 2–3 min) 1 mg at onset of headache; repeat hourly. **Maximum:** 2 mg/day; 6 mg/wk.

Intranasal: ADULTS, ELDERLY: 1 spray (0.5 mg) into each nostril; repeat in 15 min up to a total of 4 sprays (2 mg). Do not exceed 6 sprays (3 mg) in 24-hr period or 8 sprays (4 mg) in a wk.

Dosage in Renal/Hepatic Impairment

Contraindicated in severe impairment.

SIDE EFFECTS

Occasional (5%–2%): Cough, dizziness. **Rare (less than 2%):** Myalgia, fatigue, diarrhea, upper respiratory tract infection, dyspepsia.

ADVERSE EFFECTS/ TOXIC REACTIONS

Prolonged administration, excessive dosage may produce ergotamine poisoning, manifested as nausea, vomiting, paresthesia of extremities, muscle pain/ weakness, precordial pain, significant changes in pulse rate and blood pressure. Vasoconstriction of peripheral arteries/arterioles may result in localized edema, pruritus; feet, hands will become cold, pale. Muscle pain will occur when walking and later, even at rest. Other rare effects include confusion, depression, drowsiness, seizures, gangrene.

NURSING CONSIDERATIONS

BASELINE ASSESSMENT

Question for history of peripheral vascular disease, renal/hepatic impairment, possibility of pregnancy. Question onset, location, duration of migraine, possible precipitating symptoms. Obtain full medication history and screen for interactions. Obtain B/P.

INTERVENTION/EVALUATION

Monitor closely for evidence of ergotamine overdosage as result of prolonged administration or excessive dosage. Monitor B/P.

PATIENT/FAMILY TEACHING

• Initiate therapy at first sign of migraine headache. • Report if there is need to progressively increase dose to relieve vascular headaches or if palpitations, nausea, vomiting, paresthesia, pain or weakness of extremities, chest pain. Avoid grapefruit products. • Female pts should avoid pregnancy; if suspected, immediately report. • Do not use triptans for 24 hrs after last dose of dihydroergotamine.

---

dilTIAZEM　　TOP 100

dil-**tye**-a-zem
(Apo-Diltiaz , <u>Cardizem</u>, Cardizem CD, Cardizem LA, Cartia XT, Dilt-XR, Matzim LA, Taztia XT, Tiazac)
Do not confuse Cardizem with Cardene or Cardene SR, Cartia XT with Procardia XL, diltiaZEM with Calan, diazePAM, or Dilantin, or Tiazac with Ziac.

FIXED-COMBINATION(S)

Teczem: diltiaZEM/enalapril (ACE inhibitor): 180 mg/5 mg.

◆CLASSIFICATION

PHARMACOTHERAPEUTIC: Calcium channel blocker. **CLINICAL:** Antianginal, antihypertensive, class IV antiarrhythmic.

USES

PO: Treatment of angina due to coronary artery spasm (Prinzmetal's variant angina), chronic stable angina (effort-associated angina). Treatment of hypertension. **Parenteral:** Temporary control of rapid ventricular rate in atrial fibrillation/flutter. Rapid conversion of paroxysmal supraventricular tachycardia (PSVT) to normal sinus rhythm.

PRECAUTIONS

Contraindications: PO: Acute MI, pulmonary congestion, hypersensitivity to diltiaZEM, second- or third-degree AV block (except in presence of pacemaker), severe hypotension (less than 90 mm Hg, systolic), sick sinus syndrome (except in presence of pacemaker). **IV:** Hypersensitivity to diltiaZEM. Sick sinus syndrome or second- or third-degree block (except with functioning pacemaker), cardiogenic shock, administration of IV beta blocker within several hours, atrial fibrillation/flutter associated with accessory bypass tract, severe hypotension, ventricular tachycardia. **Cautions:** Renal/hepatic impairment, HF, concurrent use with beta blocker, hypertrophic obstructive cardiomyopathy.

ACTION

Inhibits calcium movement across cardiac, vascular smooth-muscle cell membranes (causes dilation of coronary arteries, peripheral arteries, arterioles). **Therapeutic Effect:** Relaxes coronary vascular smooth muscle, increases myocardial oxygen delivery in pts with vasospastic angina, decreases heart rate.

PHARMACOKINETICS

Route	Onset	Peak	Duration
PO	0.5–1 hr	N/A	N/A
PO (extended-release)	2–3 hrs	N/A	N/A
IV	3 min	N/A	N/A

Well absorbed from GI tract. Protein binding: 70%–80%. Primarily excreted in urine. Not removed by hemodialysis. **Half-life:** 3–8 hrs.

⊠ LIFESPAN CONSIDERATIONS

Pregnancy/Lactation: Distributed in breast milk. **Children:** No age-related precautions noted. **Elderly:** Age-related renal impairment may require dosage adjustment.

INTERACTIONS

DRUG: **Beta blockers (e.g., carvedilol, metoprolol), digoxin** may have additive effect on prolonging AV conduction. May increase concentration, risk of toxicity with **carBAMazepine, benzodiazepines.** May increase serum **digoxin** concentration. **RifAMPin** may decrease concentration/effects. May increase concentration of **statins** and risk of myopathy/rhabdomyolysis. **HERBAL:** **Ephedra** may worsen arrhythmias, hypertension. **Garlic** may increase antihypertensive effect. **Ginseng, yohimbe** may worsen hypertension. **St. John's wort** may decrease concentration. **FOOD:** None known. **LAB VALUES:** EKG: May increase PR interval.

AVAILABILITY (Rx)

Injection, Solution: 25 mg/5 mL, 50 mg/10 mL, 125 mg/25 mL. **Tablets, Immediate-Release:** 30 mg, 60 mg, 90 mg, 120 mg.
 Capsules, Extended-Release, 24 Hour: 120 mg, 180 mg, 240 mg, 300 mg, 360 mg, 420 mg. **Capsules, Extended-Release, 12 Hour:** 60 mg, 90 mg, 120 mg. **Tablets, Extended-Release, 24 Hour:** 120 mg, 180 mg, 240 mg, 300 mg, 360 mg, 420 mg.

ADMINISTRATION/HANDLING

⊞ IV

Reconstitution • Add 125 mg to 100 mL D₅W, 0.9% NaCl to provide concentration of 1 mg/mL.
Rate of Administration • Infuse per dilution/rate chart provided by manufacturer.
Storage • Refrigerate vials. • After dilution, stable for 24 hrs.

PO

• Give immediate-release tablets before meals and at bedtime. • Tablets may be crushed. • Do not break, crush, dissolve, or divide sustained-release capsules or extended-release capsules or tablets. • Taztia XT capsules may be

D

opened and mixed with applesauce; follow with glass of water. • Cardizem CD, Cardizem LA, Cartia XT, Matzim LA may be given without regard to meals. • Dilacor XR, Dilt-XR to be given on empty stomach.

🞖 IV INCOMPATIBILITIES

AcetaZOLAMIDE (Diamox), acyclovir (Zovirax), ampicillin, ampicillin/sulbactam (Unasyn), diazePAM (Valium), furosemide (Lasix), heparin, insulin, nafcillin, phenytoin (Dilantin), rifAMPin (Rifadin), sodium bicarbonate.

🞖 IV COMPATIBILITIES

Albumin, aztreonam (Azactam), bumetanide (Bumex), ceFAZolin (Ancef), cefotaxime (Claforan), cefTAZidime (Fortaz), cefTRIAXone (Rocephin), cefuroxime (Zinacef), ciprofloxacin (Cipro), clindamycin (Cleocin), dexmedetomidine (Precedex), digoxin (Lanoxin), DOBUTamine (Dobutrex), DOPamine (Intropin), gentamicin, HYDROmorphone (Dilaudid), lidocaine, LORazepam (Ativan), metoclopramide (Reglan), metroNIDAZOLE (Flagyl), midazolam (Versed), morphine, multivitamins, nitroglycerin, norepinephrine (Levophed), potassium chloride, potassium phosphate, tobramycin (Nebcin), vancomycin (Vancocin).

INDICATIONS/ROUTES/DOSAGE

Angina
PO: *(Immediate-Release)* **ADULTS, ELDERLY:** Initially, 30 mg 4 times/day. Range: 120–320 mg/day.
PO: *(Extended-Release)* *(Cardizem CD, Cartia XT, DILT-XR):* **ADULTS, ELDERLY:** Initially, 120–180 mg once daily. May increase at 7- to 14-day intervals. Range: 120–320 mg. **Maximum:** 480 mg/day.
(Extended-Release) *(Tiazac, Taztia XT):* **ADULTS, ELDERLY:** Initially, 120–180 mg once daily. May increase at 7- to 14-day intervals. Range: 120–320 mg/day. **Maximum:** 540 mg/day.
(Extended-Release) *(Cardizem LA, Matzim LA):* Initially, 180 mg/day. May increase at 7- to 14-day intervals. Range: 120–320 mg. **Maximum:** 360 mg daily.

Hypertension
PO Capsule Extended-Release (once-daily dosing): *(Cardizem CD, Cartia XT):* Initially, 180–240 mg/day. May increase after 14 days. Usual dose: 240–360 mg/day. **Maximum:** 480 mg/day. *(Dilt-XR):* Initially, 180–240 mg/day. May increase after 14 days. Usual dose: 240–360 mg/day. **Maximum:** 540 mg/day. *(Tiazac, Taztia XT):* Initially, 120–240 mg/day. Usual dose: 240–360 mg/day. **Maximum:** 540 mg/day.
PO Capsule Extended-Release (twice-daily dosing): **ADULTS, ELDERLY:** Initially, 60–120 mg twice daily. May increase at 14-day intervals. **Maintenance:** 240–360 mg/day.
PO Tablet Extended-Release (once-daily dosing): *(Cardizem LA, Matzim LA):* **ADULTS, ELDERLY:** Initially, 180–240 mg/day. May increase at 14-day intervals. Range: 120–540 mg/day. 240–360 mg/day. **Maximum:** 540 mg/day.

Temporary Control of Rapid Ventricular Rate in Atrial Fibrillation/Flutter; Rapid Conversion of Paroxysmal Supraventricular Tachycardia to Normal Sinus Rhythm
IV Push: ADULTS, ELDERLY: Initially, 0.25 mg/kg (average dose: 20 mg) actual body weight over 2 min. May repeat in 15 min at dose of 0.35 mg/kg (average dose: 25 mg) actual body weight. Subsequent doses individualized.
IV Infusion: ADULTS, ELDERLY: After initial bolus injection, may begin infusion at 5–10 mg/hr; may increase by 5 mg/hr up to a maximum of 15 mg/hr. Continuous infusion longer than 24 hrs or infusion rate greater than 15 mg/hr are not recommended. Attempt conversion to PO therapy as soon as possible.

Dosage in Renal/Hepatic Impairment
Use with caution.

SIDE EFFECTS

Frequent (10%–5%): Peripheral edema, dizziness, light-headedness, headache, bradycardia, asthenia. **Occasional (5%–2%):** Nausea, constipation, flushing, EKG changes. **Rare (less than 2%):** Rash, micturition disorder (polyuria, nocturia, dysuria, frequency of urination), abdominal discomfort, drowsiness.

ADVERSE EFFECTS/ TOXIC REACTIONS

Abrupt withdrawal may increase frequency, duration of angina, HF; second- or third-degree AV block occurs rarely. Overdose produces nausea, drowsiness, confusion, slurred speech, profound bradycardia. **Antidote:** Glucagon, insulin drip with continuous calcium infusion (see Appendix J for dosage).

NURSING CONSIDERATIONS

BASELINE ASSESSMENT

Record onset, type (sharp, dull, squeezing), radiation, location, intensity, duration of anginal pain, precipitating factors (exertion, emotional stress). Assess baseline renal/hepatic function tests. Assess B/P, apical pulse immediately before drug is administered. Obtain baseline EKG in pts with history of arrhythmia.

INTERVENTION/EVALUATION

Assist with ambulation if dizziness occurs. Assess for peripheral edema. Monitor pulse rate for bradycardia. Assess B/P, renal function, LFT, EKG with IV therapy. Question for asthenia, headache.

PATIENT/FAMILY TEACHING

• Do not abruptly discontinue medication. • Compliance with therapy regimen is essential to control anginal pain. • To avoid postural dizziness, go from lying to standing slowly. • Avoid tasks that require alertness, motor skills until response to drug is established. • Report palpitations, shortness of breath, pronounced dizziness, nausea, constipation. • Avoid alcohol (may increase risk of hypotension or vasodilation).

---

dimethyl fumarate ㅤ TOP 100

dye-**meth**-il-**fue**-ma-rate
(Tecfidera)

◆CLASSIFICATION

PHARMACOTHERAPEUTIC: Fumaric acid ester. **CLINICAL:** Multiple sclerosis agent.

USES

Treatment of relapsing-remitting multiple sclerosis.

PRECAUTIONS

Contraindications: Hypersensitivity to dimethyl fumarate. **Cautions:** Hepatic impairment (may increase hepatic transaminases, lymphopenia (may decrease lymphocyte count).

ACTION

Exact mechanism of action unknown. May include anti-inflammatory action and cytoprotective properties. **Therapeutic Effect:** Modifies disease progression.

PHARMACOKINETICS

Undergoes rapid hydrolysis into active metabolite, monomethyl fumarate. Peak concentration: 2–2½ hrs. Protein binding: 27%–45%. Extensively metabolized by esterases. Primarily eliminated as exhaled carbon dioxide (60%). **Half-life:** 1 hr.

⏳ LIFESPAN CONSIDERATIONS

Pregnancy/Lactation: Unknown if distributed in breast milk. **Children:** Safety and efficacy not established in pts younger than 18 yrs. **Elderly:** No age-related precautions noted.

✦ Canadian trade name ㅤ 🍴 Non-Crushable Drug ㅤ 🔲 High Alert drug

INTERACTIONS

DRUG: None known. **HERBAL:** None known. **FOOD:** None significant. **LAB VALUES:** May decrease lymphocytes. May increase serum ALT, AST; eosinophils; urine albumin.

AVAILABILITY (Rx)

Capsules, Delayed-Release: 120 mg, 240 mg.

ADMINISTRATION/HANDLING

PO
• Give capsule whole; do not break, crush, dissolve, or divide. • May give without regard to meal. May give with food to decrease flushing reaction and GI effects. • Protect from light.

INDICATIONS/ROUTES/DOSAGE

Relapsing-Remitting Multiple Sclerosis
PO: ADULTS/ELDERLY: Initially, 120 mg twice daily for 7 days. Then, increase to 240 mg twice daily.

Dosage in Renal/Hepatic Impairment
No dose adjustment.

SIDE EFFECTS

Frequent (40%): Flushing. **Occasional (18%–5%):** Abdominal pain, diarrhea, nausea, vomiting, dyspepsia, pruritus, rash, erythema.

ADVERSE EFFECTS/ TOXIC REACTIONS

Lymphopenia may increase risk for infection. Severe flushing may lead to noncompliance of therapy.

NURSING CONSIDERATIONS

BASELINE ASSESSMENT

Obtain baseline CBC, CMP, urine pregnancy if applicable. Question any plans of breastfeeding. Assess hydration status (urine output, skin turgor). Question history of hepatic impairment, lymphopenia.

INTERVENTION/EVALUATION

Monitor CBC, LFT. Encourage PO intake. Offer antiemetics for nausea, vomiting. Question any episodes of noncompliance due to flushing, GI symptoms. Monitor for infectious process (fever, malaise, chills, body aches, cough).

PATIENT/FAMILY TEACHING

• Pts will most likely experience abdominal pain, diarrhea, nausea, and flushing. Side effects may decrease over time. • Take with meals to decrease flushing reaction. • Swallow capsule whole; do not chew, crush, dissolve, or divide. • Two dosage strengths will be provided for starting dose and maintenance dose. • Report any yellowing of skin or eyes, upper abdominal pain, bruising, dark-colored urine, fever, body aches, cough, dehydration.

dinutuximab

din-ue-**tux**-i-mab
(Unituxin)
■ **BLACK BOX ALERT** ■
Life-threatening infusion-related reactions have occurred. Administer required prehydration and premedication, including antihistamines, prior to each infusion. Treatment causes severe neuropathic pain. Administer IV opioids prior to each infusion and for 2 hrs following completion of infusion. Severe peripheral sensory neuropathy occurred in pts with neuroblastoma. Severe motor neuropathy was observed. Discontinue therapy if severe unresponsive pain, severe sensory neuropathy, or moderate to severe peripheral motor neuropathy occurs.
Do not confuse dinutuximab with brentuximab, cetuximab, riTUXimab, or siltuximab.

◆**CLASSIFICATION**

PHARMACOTHERAPEUTIC: GD2-binding monoclonal antibody. **CLINICAL:** Antineoplastic.

USES

Used in combination with granulocyte-macrophage colony-stimulating factor (GM-CSF), interleukin-2 (IL-2), and 13-cis-retinoic acid, for the treatment of pediatric pts with high-risk neuroblastoma who achieve at least a partial response to prior fine-line multiagent, multimodality therapy.

PRECAUTIONS

Contraindications: History of anaphylaxis to dinutuximab. **Cautions:** Active infection; baseline cytopenias; diabetes, dehydration, electrolyte imbalance, hepatic/renal impairment, peripheral or generalized edema; intolerance of opioids, antipyretics, antihistamines; history of arrhythmias, hypotension, neuropathy, optic disorders.

ACTION

Binds to glycolipid GD2 expressed on neuroblastoma cells and on normal cells of neuroectodermal origin, including CNS and peripheral nerves. Induces cell lysis of GD2-expressing cells through antibody-dependent cell-mediated cytotoxicity and complement-dependent cytotoxicity. **Therapeutic Effect:** Inhibits tumor cell growth and metastasis.

PHARMACOKINETICS

Widely distributed. Metabolism not specified. Protein binding: not specified. Elimination not specified. **Half-life:** 10 days.

⧖ LIFESPAN CONSIDERATIONS

Pregnancy/Lactation: Avoid pregnancy; may cause fetal harm, esp. in third trimester. Unknown if distributed in breast milk. However, human immunoglobulin G is present in human breast milk. Must either discontinue drug or discontinue breastfeeding. Females of reproductive potential must use effective contraception during treatment and for at least 2 mos following discontinuation. **Children:** No age-related precautions noted. **Elderly:** Safety and efficacy not established.

INTERACTIONS

DRUG: None known (not studied). **HERBAL:** None significant. **FOOD:** None known. **LAB VALUES:** May decrease Hgb, Hct, lymphocytes, neutrophils, platelets, RBCs; serum albumin, calcium, magnesium, phosphate, potassium, sodium. May increase serum ALT, AST, bilirubin, creatinine, glucose; urine protein.

AVAILABILITY (Rx)

Injection Solution: 17.5 mg/5 mL (3.5 mg/mL).

ADMINISTRATION/HANDLING

 IV

Pretreatment Guidelines

IV Hydration • Administer bolus of 0.9% NaCl 10 mL/kg IV over 1 hr prior to initiation. **Analgesics** • Administer morphine sulfate 50 mcg/kg IV immediately prior to initiation and then continue as morphine sulfate drip at rate of 20–50 mcg/kg/hr during and for 2 hrs following completion of infusion. • Administer additional doses of morphine sulfate 25–50 mcg/kg IV once every 2 hrs as needed for pain, followed by an increase in morphine infusion rate, if clinically stable. • Consider use of fentaNYL or HYDROmorphone if morphine sulfate not tolerated. • If pain is inadequately controlled with opioids, consider use of gabapentin or lidocaine in addition with IV morphine.

Antihistamines and Antipyretics • Administer an antihistamine such as diphenhydrAMINE 0.5–1 mg/kg (maximum dose 50 mg) IV over 10–15 min, starting 20 min prior to initiation and as tolerated every 4–6 hrs during infusion. • Administer acetaminophen 10–15 mg/kg (maximum dose 650 mg) 20 minutes prior to each infusion and every 4–6 hrs as needed for fever/pain. • May administer ibuprofen 5–10 mg/kg every 6 hrs as needed for persistent fever/pain.

Preparation of Infusion • Visually inspect for particulate matter or discoloration. Do not use if solution is cloudy or contains particulate matter. • Withdraw required volume from vial and inject into 100 mL 0.9% NaCl. • Mix by gentle inversion. Do not shake or agitate. • Discard unused portions of vial.

Rate of Administration • Initiate infusion rate at 0.875 mg/m^2/hr for 30 min via dedicated IV line. May gradually increase rate to maximum rate of 1.75/m^2/hr as tolerated. • Do not infuse as IV push or bolus.

Storage • Refrigerate vials. • Protect from light by storing in outer carton. • May refrigerate diluted solution up to 4 hrs. • Discard diluted solution 24 hrs after preparation.

▦ IV INCOMPATIBILITIES
Do not mix with other medications.

INDICATIONS/ROUTES/DOSAGE
Neuroblastoma
IV: PEDIATRIC: 17.5 mg/m^2/day over 10–20 hrs for 4 consecutive days for maximum of 5 cycles (Tables 1 and 2).

TABLE 1 SCHEDULE OF DINUTUXIMAB ADMINISTRATION FOR CYCLES 1, 3, AND 5

Cycle Day	1 through 3	4	5	6	7	8 through 24*
dinutuximab		X	X	X	X	

*Cycles 2 and 4 are 32 days in duration.

TABLE 2 SCHEDULE OF DINUTUXIMAB ADMINISTRATION FOR CYCLES 2 AND 4

Cycle Day	1 through 7	8	9	10	11	12 through 32*
dinutuximab		X	X	X	X	

*Cycles 2 and 4 are 32 days in duration.

Dose Modification
Infusion-Related Reactions
Mild to moderate adverse reactions such as transient rash, fever, rigors, or localized urticaria that respond promptly to symptomatic treatment: *Onset of Reaction:* Decrease infusion rate to 50% of the previous rate. *After Resolution:* Gradually increase infusion rate up to maximum rate 1.75 mg/m^2/hr. **Prolonged or severe adverse reactions such as mild bronchospasm without other symptoms, angioedema that does not affect the airway:** *Onset of Reaction:* Immediately interrupt infusion. *After Resolution:* If symptoms resolve rapidly, restart infusion at 50% of the previous rate. *First Recurrence:* Discontinue treatment until the following day. If symptoms resolve and continued treatment is warranted, premedicate with hydrocortisone 1 mg/kg (maximum dose 50 mg) IV and administer

dinutuximab infusion at a rate of 0.875 mg/m^2/hr in an intensive care unit. *Second Recurrence:* Permanently discontinue.
Capillary Leak Syndrome
Moderate to severe, non–life-threatening capillary leak syndrome: *Onset of Reaction:* Interrupt infusion. *After Resolution:* Resume infusion rate at 50% of previous rate. **Life-threatening capillary leak syndrome:** *Onset of Reaction:* Discontinue for the current cycle. *After Resolution:* In subsequent cycles, administer at 50% of the previous rate. *First Recurrence:* Permanently discontinue.
Hypotension Requiring Medical Intervention
Onset of Reaction: Interrupt infusion. *After Resolution:* Resume infusion at 50% of the previous rate. If blood pressure remains stable for at least 2 hrs, increase infusion rate as tolerated up to maximum rate of 1.75 mg/m^2/hr.

Severe Systemic Infection or Sepsis
Onset of Reaction: Discontinue treatment until resolution of infection, then proceed with subsequent cycles of therapy.
Neurologic Disorders of the Eye
Onset of Reaction: Discontinue infusion until resolution of disorder. *After Resolution:* Reduce dose by 50%. *First Recurrence or if Accompanied by Visual Impairment:* Permanently discontinue.
Adverse Reactions Requiring Permanent Discontinuation (using CTCAE Grading 1–5)
Grade 3 or 4 anaphylaxis, serum sickness; grade 3 pain unresponsive to maximum supportive measures; grade 4 sensory neuropathy or grade 3 sensory neuropathy that interferes with daily activities for more than 2 wks; grade 2 peripheral motor neuropathy, subtotal or total vision loss; grade 4 hyponatremia despite appropriate fluid management.

Dosage in Renal/Hepatic Impairment
Not specified; use caution.

SIDE EFFECTS

Frequent (85%–24%): Pain (abdominal, back, bladder, bone, chest, neck, facial, gingival, musculoskeletal, oropharyngeal, extremity), arthralgia, myalgia, neuralgia, proctalgia, pyrexia, hypotension, vomiting, diarrhea, urticaria, hypoxia. **Occasional (19%–10%):** Tachycardia, edema, hypertension, peripheral neuropathy, weight gain, nausea.

ADVERSE EFFECTS/ TOXIC REACTIONS

Anemia, neutropenia, lymphopenia, thrombocytopenia are expected results of therapy. Severe bone marrow suppression occurred in up to 39% of pts. Serious infusion-related reactions, such as bronchospasm, dyspnea, facial and upper airway edema, hypotension, or stridor, may require urgent interventions, including bronchodilator therapy, blood pressure support, corticosteroids, infusion interruption, infusion rate reduction, or permanent treatment discontinuation. Severe infusion-related reactions were reported in 26% of pts. Infusion-related

reactions usually occurred during or within 24 hrs of infusion completion. Other serious adverse effects may include: severe urticaria (13% of pts); anaphylaxis, cardiac arrest (1% or less of pts); pain despite pretreatment with analgesics including morphine sulfate infusion (85% of pts); grade 3 pain (51% of pts); grade 3 peripheral sensory/motor neuropathy (1% of pts); grade 3–5 capillary leak syndrome (23% of pts); grade 3 hypotension (16% of pts); grade 3 or 4 bacteremia requiring IV antibiotics or other urgent interventions (13% of pts); sepsis (18% of pts); neurologic disorders of the eye, including blurred vision, photophobia, mydriasis, fixed or unequal pupils, optic nerve disorder, eyelid ptosis, papilledema (2%–13% of pts); grade 3 or 4 electrolyte abnormalities, including hyponatremia, hypokalemia, hypocalcemia (37%–23% of pts); atypical hemolytic uremic syndrome resulting in anemia, electrolyte imbalance, hypertension, renal insufficiency. Bleeding events, including GI/rectal/renal/respiratory/urinary tract/catheter site hemorrhage, disseminated intravascular coagulation, epistaxis, hematemesis, hematochezia, hematuria, were reported. Immunogenicity (anti-dinutuximab antibodies) reported in 18% of pts.

NURSING CONSIDERATIONS

BASELINE ASSESSMENT

Obtain baseline CBC, BMP, LFT; serum magnesium, ionized calcium, prealbumin, phosphate triglyceride level; capillary blood glucose, urinalysis, urine protein, urine pregnancy test, vital signs. Verify that pts have adequate hematologic/hepatic/ophthalmic/respiratory/renal function and proper hydration status prior to start of each infusion. Ensure proper resuscitative equipment/medications are readily available. Obtain baseline visual acuity, pupillary response, neurologic status. Question history of anaphylaxis; intolerance of opioids, antipyretics, antihistamines. Screen for active infection. Offer emotional support.

INTERVENTION/EVALUATION

Frequently monitor CBC, BMP, LFT, other serum electrolytes, vital signs. Monitor I&O. Administer required prehydration and premedication with antihistamine, antipyretics, opioids prior to each infusion and during infusion as indicated. Diligently monitor for infusion-related reactions as listed in Adverse Effects/Toxic Reactions and institute medical support as needed. Monitor for bleeding events of any kind. Consider administration of naloxone if narcotic overdose is suspected. Routinely assess visual acuity, hydration status. Offer emotional support. Initiate fall precautions.

PATIENT/FAMILY TEACHING

• Serious infusion reactions, including anaphylaxis, difficulty breathing, facial swelling, itching, rash, and wheezing, may occur during or within 24 hrs of each infusion. • Immediately report any allergic reactions; bleeding of any kind; decreased urine output or dark urine; disorders of the eye including blurry vision, double vision, unequal pupil size, sensitivity to light, eyelid drooping; fever; palpitations; seizures (related to electrolyte imbalance); severe nerve pain or loss of motor function; signs of low blood pressure such as confusion, fainting, pallor; swelling of face, arms, or legs. • Moderate to severe generalized pain is an expected side effect. Medications for pain, fever, and mild allergic reactions will need to be provided before or during each infusion; report any intolerance to such medications. • Therapy is expected to lower blood counts/immune system and may increase risk of bleeding or infection. • Drink plenty of fluids. • Treatment may be harmful to fetuses. Contraception is recommended during therapy and for at least 2 mos after discontinuation in females of childbearing potential.

diphenhydrAMINE

dye-fen-**hye**-dra-meen
(Allerdryl ✤, Banophen, Benadryl, Benadryl Children's Allergy, Diphen, Diphenhist, Genahist, Nytol)
Do not confuse Benadryl with benazepril, Bentyl, or Benylin, or diphenhydrAMINE with desipramine, dicyclomine, or dimenhyDRINATE.

FIXED-COMBINATION(S)

Advil PM: diphenhydrAMINE/ibuprofen (NSAID): 38 mg/200 mg. With calamine, an astringent, and camphor, a counterirritant **(Caladryl).**

◆CLASSIFICATION

PHARMACOTHERAPEUTIC: Histamine-1 antagonist, first generation. **CLINICAL:** Antihistamine, anticholinergic, antipruritic, antitussive, antiemetic, antidyskinetic.

USES

Treatment of allergic reactions, including nasal allergies and allergic dermatoses; parkinsonism, including drug-induced extrapyramidal symptoms; prevention/treatment of nausea, vomiting, or vertigo due to motion sickness; antitussive; short-term management of insomnia; adjunct to EPINEPHrine in treatment of anaphylaxis. Topical form used for relief of pruritus from insect bites, skin irritations.

PRECAUTIONS

Contraindications: Hypersensitivity to diphenhydrAMINE. Neonates or premature infants, breastfeeding. **Cautions:** Narrow-angle glaucoma, stenotic peptic ulcer, prostatic hypertrophy, pyloroduodenal/bladder neck obstruction, asthma, COPD, increased IOP, cardiovascular disease, hyperthyroidism, elderly.

ACTION

Competes with histamine for H-1 receptor site on effector cells in GI tract, blood vessels, respiratory tract. **Therapeutic Effect:** Produces anticholinergic, antipruritic, antitussive, antiemetic, antidyskinetic, sedative effects.

PHARMACOKINETICS

Route	Onset	Peak	Duration
PO	15–30 min	1–4 hrs	4–6 hrs
IV, IM	Less than 15 min	1–4 hrs	4–6 hrs

Well absorbed after PO, parenteral administration. Protein binding: 98%–99%. Widely distributed. Metabolized in liver. Primarily excreted in urine. **Half-life:** 1–4 hrs. Adults: 7–12 hrs, elderly: 9–18 hrs, children: 4–7 hrs.

⏳ LIFESPAN CONSIDERATIONS

Pregnancy/Lactation: Crosses placenta. Detected in breast milk (may produce irritability in breastfed infants). Increased risk of seizures in neonates, premature infants if used during third trimester of pregnancy. May prohibit lactation. **Children:** Not recommended in newborns, premature infants (increased risk of paradoxical reaction, seizures). **Elderly:** Potentially inappropriate due to potent anticholinergic effects. Increased risk for dizziness, sedation, confusion, hypotension, hyperexcitability.

INTERACTIONS

DRUG: Alcohol, other CNS depressants (e.g., lorazepam, morphine, zolpidem) may increase CNS depressant effects. **Anticholinergics** may increase anticholinergic effects. **HERBAL: Gotu kola, kava kava, St. John's wort, valerian** may increase CNS depression. **FOOD:** None known. **LAB VALUES:** May suppress wheal/flare reactions to antigen skin testing unless drug is discontinued 4 days before testing.

AVAILABILITY (OTC)

Capsules: 25 mg, 50 mg. **Cream:** 1%, 2%. **Injection Solution:** 50 mg/mL. **Syrup:** 12.5 mg/5 mL. **Tablets:** 25 mg, 50 mg. **Tablets, Chewable:** 12.5 mg.

ADMINISTRATION/HANDLING

IV

• May be given undiluted. • Give IV injection over at least 1 min. **Maximum rate:** 25 mg/min.

IM

• Give deep IM into large muscle mass.

PO

• Give with food to decrease GI distress. • Scored tablets may be crushed.

🚫 IV INCOMPATIBILITIES

Allopurinol (Aloprim), cefepime (Maxipime), dexamethasone (Decadron), foscarnet (Foscavir).

🚫 IV COMPATIBILITIES

Atropine, CISplatin (Platinol), cyclophosphamide (Cytoxan), cytarabine (Ara-C), fentaNYL, glycopyrrolate (Robinul), heparin, hydrocortisone (SOLU-Cortef), HYDROmorphone (Dilaudid), hydrOXYzine (Vistaril), lidocaine, metoclopramide (Reglan), ondansetron (Zofran), potassium chloride, promethazine (Phenergan), propofol (Diprivan).

INDICATIONS/ROUTES/DOSAGE

Allergic Reaction
PO: ADULTS, ELDERLY: 25–50 mg q4–8h. **Maximum:** 300 mg/day. **IM, IV:** 10–50 mg/dose. **Maximum:** 400 mg/day. **PO, IV, IM: CHILDREN:** 5 mg/kg/day in divided doses q6–8h. **Maximum:** 300 mg/day.

Motion Sickness
Note: When used for prophylaxis, give 30 min before motion.
PO: *(Prophylaxis/treatment):* ADULTS, ELDERLY: 25–50 mg q6–8h. **CHILDREN:** 5 mg/kg/day in 3–4 divided doses. **Maximum:** 300 mg/day. **IV/IM: *(Treatment):* ADULTS, ELDERLY:** 10–50 mg/dose. **Maximum:** 400 mg/day. **CHILDREN:** 5 mg/kg/day in 4 divided doses. **Maximum:** 300 mg/day.

D

Antitussive
PO: ADULTS, ELDERLY, CHILDREN 12 YRS AND OLDER: 25 mg q4h. **Maximum:** 150 mg/day.

Nighttime Sleep Aid
PO: ADULTS, ELDERLY, CHILDREN 12 YRS AND OLDER: 25–50 mg at bedtime. **CHILDREN 2–11 YRS:** 1 mg/kg/dose. **Maximum Single Dose:** 50 mg.

Pruritus
Topical: ADULTS, ELDERLY, CHILDREN 12 YRS AND OLDER: Apply 1% or 2% cream or spray 3–4 times/day. **CHILDREN 2–11 YRS:** Apply 1% cream or spray 3–4 times/day.

Dosage in Renal/Hepatic Impairment
No dose adjustment.

SIDE EFFECTS

Frequent: Drowsiness, dizziness, muscle weakness, hypotension, urinary retention, thickening of bronchial secretions, dry mouth, nose, throat, lips; in elderly: sedation, dizziness, hypotension. **Occasional:** Epigastric distress, flushing, visual/hearing disturbances, paresthesia, diaphoresis, chills.

ADVERSE EFFECTS/TOXIC REACTIONS

Hypersensitivity reactions (eczema, pruritus, rash, cardiac disturbances, photosensitivity) may occur. Overdose symptoms may vary from CNS depression (sedation, apnea, hypotension, cardiovascular collapse, death) to severe paradoxical reactions (hallucinations, tremors, seizures). Children, infants, neonates may experience paradoxical reactions (restlessness, insomnia, euphoria, nervousness, tremors). Overdosage in children may result in hallucinations, seizures, death.

NURSING CONSIDERATIONS

BASELINE ASSESSMENT

If pt is having acute allergic reaction, obtain history of recently ingested foods, drugs, environmental exposure, emotional stress. Monitor B/P rate; depth, rhythm, type of respiration; quality, rate of pulse. Assess lung sounds for rhonchi, wheezing, rales.

INTERVENTION/EVALUATION

Monitor B/P, esp. in elderly (increased risk of hypotension). Monitor children closely for paradoxical reaction. Monitor for sedation.

PATIENT/FAMILY TEACHING

• Tolerance to antihistaminic effect generally does not occur; tolerance to sedative effect may occur. • Avoid tasks that require alertness, motor skills until response to drug is established. • Dry mouth, drowsiness, dizziness may be an expected response to drug. • Avoid alcohol.

diphenoxylate with atropine

dye-fen-**ox**-i-late **at**-roe-peen
(Lomotil)
Do not confuse Lomotil with LaMICtal, LamISIL, Lamotrigine, Lanoxin, or Lasix

FIXED-COMBINATION(S)

Lomotil: diphenoxylate/atropine (anticholinergic, antispasmodic): 2.5 mg/0.025 mg.

◆CLASSIFICATION

PHARMACOTHERAPEUTIC: Opioid/anticholinergic **(Schedule V). CLINICAL:** Antidiarrheal.

USES

Adjunctive treatment of acute, chronic diarrhea.

PRECAUTIONS

Contraindications: Hypersensitivity to diphenoxylate, atropine. Obstructive jaundice, diarrhea associated with pseudomembranous colitis or enterotoxin-producing bacteria. **Cautions:** Children (not recommended in children less than 2 yrs of age), acute ulcerative colitis, renal/hepatic impairment.

ACTION

Acts locally and centrally on gastric mucosa. **Therapeutic Effect:** Reduces excessive GI motility and GI propulsion.

PHARMACOKINETICS

	Onset	Peak	Duration
Antidiar-rheal	45–60 min	—	3–4 hrs

Well absorbed from GI tract. Metabolized in liver. Primarily eliminated in feces. **Half-life:** 2.5 hrs; metabolite: 12–24 hrs.

⧗ LIFESPAN CONSIDERATIONS

Pregnancy/Lactation: Unknown if drug crosses placenta or is distributed in breast milk. **Children:** Not recommended (increased susceptibility to toxicity, including respiratory depression). **Elderly:** More susceptible to anticholinergic effects, confusion, respiratory depression.

INTERACTIONS

DRUG: Alcohol, other CNS depressants (e.g., lorazepam, morphine, zolpidem) may increase CNS depressant effects. **Anticholinergics** may increase effects of atropine. **MAOIs** (e.g., phenelzine, selegiline) may precipitate hypertensive crisis. **HERBAL:** None significant. **FOOD:** None known. **LAB VALUES:** May increase serum amylase.

AVAILABILITY (Rx)

Liquid (Lomotil): 2.5 mg diphenoxylate/ 0.025 mg atropine/5 mL. **Tablets (Lomotil):** 2.5 mg diphenoxylate/0.025 mg atropine.

ADMINISTRATION/HANDLING

PO
• Give without regard to meals. If GI irritation occurs, give with food. • Use liquid for children 2–12 yrs (use graduated dropper for administration of liquid medication).

INDICATIONS/ROUTES/DOSAGE

Diarrhea
PO: **ADULTS, ELDERLY:** Initially, 5 mg (2 tabs or 10 mL) 3–4 times/day. **Maximum:** 20 mg/day. Then reduce dose as needed. **CHILDREN:** 0.3–0.4 mg/kg/day in 4 divided doses (**Maximum:** 10 mg/ day); then reduce dose as needed.

Dosage in Renal/Hepatic Impairment
No dose adjustment. Use caution with severe renal/hepatic disease.

SIDE EFFECTS

Frequent: Drowsiness, light-headedness, dizziness, nausea. **Occasional:** Headache, dry mouth. **Rare:** Flushing, tachycardia, urinary retention, constipation, paradoxical reaction (marked by restlessness, agitation), blurred vision.

ADVERSE EFFECTS/TOXIC REACTIONS

Dehydration may predispose pt to diphenoxylate toxicity. Paralytic ileus, toxic megacolon (constipation, decreased appetite, abdominal pain with nausea/ vomiting) occur rarely. Severe anticholinergic reaction (severe lethargy, hypotonic reflexes, hyperthermia) may result in severe respiratory depression, coma.

NURSING CONSIDERATIONS

BASELINE ASSESSMENT

Check baseline hydration status: skin turgor, mucous membranes for dryness, urinary status. Assess usual stool frequency, consistency.

INTERVENTION/EVALUATION

Encourage adequate fluid intake. Assess bowel sounds for peristalsis. Monitor daily pattern of bowel activity, stool consistency. Record time of evacuation. Assess for abdominal disturbances. Discontinue medication if abdominal distention occurs.

✦ Canadian trade name   🐢 Non-Crushable Drug   ▦ High Alert drug

PATIENT/FAMILY TEACHING

• Avoid tasks that require alertness, motor skills until response to drug is established. • Avoid alcohol. • Report persistent fever, palpitations, diarrhea. • Report abdominal distention.

DOBUTamine

doe-**bue**-ta-meen
(Dobutrex ❦)
Do not confuse DOBUTamine with DOPamine.

✦CLASSIFICATION

PHARMACOTHERAPEUTIC: Adrenergic agonist. **CLINICAL:** Cardiac stimulant.

USES

Short-term management of cardiac decompensation.

PRECAUTIONS

Contraindications: Hypersensitivity to DOBUTamine. Hypertrophic cardiomyopathy with outflow obstruction. **Cautions:** Atrial fibrillation, hypovolemia, post-MI, concurrent use of MAOIs, elderly.

ACTION

Direct-action inotropic agent acting primarily on beta$_1$-adrenergic receptors. **Therapeutic Effect:** Enhances myocardial contractility, increases heart rate.

PHARMACOKINETICS

Route	Onset	Peak	Duration
IV	1–2 min	10 min	Length of infusion

Metabolized in liver. Primarily excreted in urine. Not removed by hemodialysis. **Half-life:** 2 min.

⧗ LIFESPAN CONSIDERATIONS

Pregnancy/Lactation: Unknown if drug crosses placenta or is distributed in breast milk. **Children/Elderly:** No age-related precautions noted.

INTERACTIONS

DRUG: Sympathomimetics (e.g., norepinephrine, phenylephrine) may increase effects. **HERBAL:** None significant. **FOOD:** None known. **LAB VALUES:** May decrease serum potassium.

AVAILABILITY (Rx)

Infusion (Ready-to-Use): 1 mg/mL (250 mL), 2 mg/mL (250 mL), 4 mg/mL (250 mL). **Injection Solution:** 12.5-mg/mL vial.

ADMINISTRATION/HANDLING

◀**ALERT**▶ Correct hypovolemia with volume expanders before DOBUTamine infusion. Pts with atrial fibrillation should be digitalized before infusion. Administer by IV infusion only.

🖐 IV

Reconstitution • Dilute vial in 0.9% NaCl or D$_5$W to maximum concentration of 5,000 mcg/mL (5 mg/mL).
Rate of Administration • Use infusion pump to control flow rate. • Titrate dosage to individual response. • Infiltration causes local inflammatory changes. • Extravasation may cause dermal necrosis.
Storage • Store at room temperature. • Pink discoloration of solution (due to oxidation) does not indicate significant loss of potency if used within recommended time period. • Further diluted solution for infusion is stable for 48 hrs at room temperature, 7 days if refrigerated.

▦ IV INCOMPATIBILITIES

Acyclovir (Zovirax), alteplase (Activase), amphotericin B complex (Abelcet, AmBisome, Amphotec), bumetanide (Bumex), cefepime (Maxipime), foscarnet (Foscavir), furosemide (Lasix), heparin, piperacillin/tazobactam (Zosyn), sodium bicarbonate.

🔲 IV COMPATIBILITIES

Amiodarone (Cordarone), calcium chloride, calcium gluconate, diltiaZEM (Cardizem), DOPamine (Intropin), enalapril (Vasotec), EPINEPHrine, famotidine (Pepcid), HYDROmorphone (Dilaudid), insulin (regular), lidocaine, LORazepam (Ativan), magnesium sulfate, midazolam (Versed), milrinone (Primacor), morphine, nitroglycerin, nitroprusside (Nipride), norepinephrine (Levophed), potassium chloride, propofol (Diprivan).

INDICATIONS/ROUTES/DOSAGE

◀**ALERT**▶ Dosage determined by severity of decompensation.

Cardiac Decompensation
IV Infusion: ADULTS, ELDERLY, CHILDREN: Initially, 0.5–2.5 mcg/kg/min. **Maintenance:** 2–20 mcg/kg/min titrated to desired response. May be infused at a rate of up to 40 mcg/kg/min to increase cardiac output. **NEONATES:** 2–20 mcg/kg/min titrated to desired response. (Also maintenance dose).

Dosage in Renal/Hepatic Impairment
No dose adjustment.

SIDE EFFECTS

Frequent (greater than 5%): Increased heart rate, B/P. **Occasional (5%–3%):** Pain at injection site. **Rare (3%–1%):** Nausea, headache, anginal pain, shortness of breath, fever.

ADVERSE EFFECTS/TOXIC REACTIONS

Overdose may produce severe tachycardia, severe hypertension.

NURSING CONSIDERATIONS

BASELINE ASSESSMENT
Pt must be on continuous cardiac monitoring. Determine weight (for dosage calculation). Obtain initial B/P, heart rate, respirations. Correct hypovolemia before drug therapy.

INTERVENTION/EVALUATION
Continuously monitor for cardiac rate, arrhythmias. Maintain accurate I&O; measure urinary output frequently. Assess serum potassium, plasma DOBUTamine (therapeutic range: 40–190 ng/mL). Monitor B/P continuously (hypertension risk greater in pts with preexisting hypertension). Check cardiac output, pulmonary wedge pressure/central venous pressure (CVP) frequently. Immediately notify physician of decreased urinary output, cardiac arrhythmias, significant increase in B/P, heart rate, or less commonly, hypotension.

DOCEtaxel

doe-se-**tax**-el
(Docefrez, <u>Taxotere</u>)
■ **BLACK BOX ALERT** ■ Avoid use with serum bilirubin more than upper limit of normal (ULN) or serum ALT, AST more than 1.5 times ULN in conjunction with serum alkaline phosphatase more than 2.5 times ULN. Severe hypersensitivity reaction (rash, hypotension, bronchospasm, anaphylaxis) may occur. Fluid retention syndrome (pleural effusions, ascites, edema, dyspnea at rest) has been reported. Pts with abnormal hepatic function, receiving higher doses, and pts with non–small-cell lung carcinoma (NSCLC) and history of prior platinum treatment receiving DOCEtaxel dose of 100 mg/m^2 at higher risk for mortality. Avoid use with ANC less than 1,500 cells/mm^3.
Do not confuse DOCEtaxel with PACLitaxel or Taxotere with Taxol.

◆CLASSIFICATION

PHARMACOTHERAPEUTIC: Antimitotic agent, taxoid. **CLINICAL:** Antineoplastic.

USES

Treatment of locally advanced or metastatic breast carcinoma after failure of prior chemotherapy. Treatment of metastatic non–small-cell lung cancer. Treatment of metastatic prostate cancer, head and neck cancer (with predniSONE). Treatment of advanced gastric adenocarcinoma. **OFF-LABEL:** Bladder, esophageal, ovarian, small-cell lung carcinoma; soft tissue carcinoma, cervical cancer, Ewing's sarcoma, osteosarcoma.

PRECAUTIONS

Contraindications: Hypersensitivity to DOCEtaxel. History of severe hypersensitivity to drugs formulated with polysorbate 80, neutrophil count less than 1,500 cells/mm³. **Cautions:** Hepatic impairment, myelosuppression, concomitant CYP3A4 inhibitors/inducers, fluid retention, pulmonary disease, HF, active infection.

ACTION

Disrupts microtubular cell network, essential for cellular function. **Therapeutic Effect:** Inhibits cellular mitosis.

PHARMACOKINETICS

Widely distributed. Protein binding: 94%. Extensively metabolized in liver. Excreted in feces (75%), urine (6%). **Half-life:** 11.1 hrs.

⏳ LIFESPAN CONSIDERATIONS

Pregnancy/Lactation: May cause fetal harm. Unknown if distributed in breast milk. Breastfeeding not recommended. **Children:** Safety and efficacy not established in pts younger than 16 yrs. **Elderly:** No age-related precautions noted.

INTERACTIONS

DRUG: CYP3A4 inhibitors (e.g., erythromycin, ketoconazole) may increase concentration/toxicity. **CYP3A4 inducers (e.g., rifAMPin)** may decrease concentration/effects. **Live virus vaccines** may potentiate replication, increase vaccine side effects, decrease pt's antibody response to vaccine. **HERBAL: Echinacea** may decrease concentration. **FOOD:** None known. **LAB VALUES:** May increase serum alkaline phosphatase, bilirubin, ALT, AST. Reduces neutrophil, platelet count, Hgb, Hct.

AVAILABILITY (Rx)

Injection, Powder for Reconstitution: 20 mg, 80 mg. **Injection Solution:** 10 mg/mL, 20 mg/mL.

ADMINISTRATION/HANDLING

 IV

Reconstitution (Solution) • Withdraw dose and add to 250–500 mL 0.9% NaCl or D₅W in glass or polyolefin container to provide a final concentration of 0.3–0.74 mg/mL. **(Powder)** Add 1 mL diluent provided to 20-mg vial to provide a concentration of 20 mg/0.8 mL (4 mL to 80-mg vial to provide a concentration of 24 mg/mL). Shake well. Further dilute in 250 mL NaCl or D₅W to a final concentration of 0.3–0.74 mg/mL.

Rate of Administration • Administer as a 1-hr infusion. • Monitor closely for hypersensitivity reaction (flushing, localized skin reaction, bronchospasm [may occur within a few min after beginning infusion]).

Storage • Store vials between 36°F–77°F. • Protect from bright light. • If refrigerated, stand vial at room temperature for 5 min before administering (do not store in PVC bags). • Diluted solution should be used within 4 hrs (including infusion time).

🔲 IV INCOMPATIBILITIES

Amphotericin B (Fungizone), methyl-PREDNISolone (SOLU), nalbuphine (Nubain).

🔲 IV COMPATIBILITIES

Bumetanide (Bumex), calcium gluconate, dexamethasone (Decadron), diphenhydrAMINE (Benadryl), DOBUTamine (Dobutrex), DOPamine (Intropin), furosemide

---

(Lasix), granisetron (Kytril), heparin, HY-DROmorphone (Dilaudid), LORazepam (Ativan), magnesium sulfate, mannitol, morphine, ondansetron (Zofran), palonosetron (Aloxi), potassium chloride.

INDICATIONS/ROUTES/DOSAGE

◄ALERT► Pt should be premedicated with oral corticosteroids (e.g., dexamethasone 16 mg/day for 5 days beginning day 1 before DOCEtaxel therapy); reduces severity of fluid retention, hypersensitivity reaction.

Breast Carcinoma
IV: ADULTS: Locally advanced or metastatic: 60–100 mg/m^2 given over 1 hr q3wks as a single agent. Operable, node positive: 75 mg/m^2 q3wks for 6 courses (in combination with DOXOrubicin and cyclophosphamide).

Non–Small-Cell Lung Carcinoma
IV: ADULTS: 75 mg/m^2 q3wks (as monotherapy or in combination with CISplatin).

Prostate Cancer
IV: ADULTS, ELDERLY: 75 mg/m^2 q3wks with concurrent administration of predniSONE.

Head/Neck Cancer
IV: ADULTS, ELDERLY: 75 mg/m^2 q3wks (in combination with CISplatin and fluorouracil) for 3–4 cycles, followed by radiation therapy.

Gastric Adenocarcinoma
IV: ADULTS, ELDERLY: 75 mg/m^2 q3wks (in combination with CISplatin and fluorouracil).

Dose Modification for Gastric or Head/Neck Cancer

ALT, AST 2.5 to 5 times ULN and alkaline phosphatase less than or equal to 2.5 times ULN	80% of dose
ALT, AST 1.5 to 5 times ULN and alkaline phosphatase 2.5 to 5 times ULN	80% of dose
ALT, AST greater than 5 times ULN and/or alkaline phosphatase greater than 5 times ULN	Discontinue DOCEtaxel

Note: Toxicity includes febrile neutropenia, neutrophils less than 500 cells/mm^3 for longer than 1 wk, severe cutaneous reactions. Also, for NSCLC, platelet nadir less than 25,000 cells/mm^3, any CTCAE grade 3 or 4 nonhematologic toxicity.

Breast Cancer
Reduce dose to 75 mg/m^2; if toxicity persists, reduce to 55 mg/m^2.

Breast Cancer Adjuvant
Administer when neutrophils are less than 1,500 cells/mm^3. If toxicity persists, or grade 3 or 4 stomatitis, reduce dose to 60 mg/m^2.

Non–Small-Cell Lung Cancer
Monotherapy
Hold dose until toxicity resolves, then reduce dose to 55 mg/m^2. Discontinue if grade 3 or 4 neuropathy occurs.
Combination Therapy
Reduce dose to 65 mg/m^2; may further reduce to 50 mg/m^2 if needed.

Prostate Cancer
Reduce dose to 60 mg/m^2; discontinue if toxicity persists.

Gastric or Head and Neck Cancer
Reduce dose to 60 mg/m^2; if neutropenic toxicity persists, further reduce to 45 mg/m^2. For grade 3 or 4 thrombocytopenia, reduce dose from 75 mg/m^2 to 60 mg/m^2; discontinue if toxicity persists.

Dosage in Renal Impairment
No dose adjustment.

Dosage in Hepatic Impairment
Total bilirubin more than ULN, or ALT, AST more than 1.5 times ULN with alkaline phosphatase more than 2.5 times ULN: Use not recommended.

✦ Canadian trade name   🦊 Non-Crushable Drug   🔺 High Alert drug

D

SIDE EFFECTS

Frequent (80%–19%:) Alopecia, asthenia, hypersensitivity reaction (e.g., dermatitis), which is decreased in pts pretreated with oral corticosteroids; fluid retention, stomatitis, nausea, diarrhea, fever, nail changes, vomiting, myalgia. **Occasional:** Hypotension, edema, anorexia, headache, weight gain, infection (urinary tract, injection site, indwelling catheter tip), dizziness. **Rare:** Dry skin, sensory disorders (vision, speech, taste), arthralgia, weight loss, conjunctivitis, hematuria, proteinuria.

ADVERSE EFFECTS/TOXIC REACTIONS

In pts with normal hepatic function, neutropenia (ANC count less than 1,500 cells/mm^3), leukopenia (WBC count less than 4,000 cells/mm^3) occur in 96% of pts; anemia (hemoglobin level less than 11 g/dL) occurs in 90% of pts; thrombocytopenia (platelet count less than 100,000 cells/mm^3) occurs in 8% of pts; infection occurs in 28% of pts. Neurosensory, neuromotor disturbances (distal paresthesia, weakness) occur in 54% and 13% of pts, respectively.

NURSING CONSIDERATIONS

BASELINE ASSESSMENT

Obtain baseline ANC, CBC, serum chemistries. Offer emotional support to pt, family. Antiemetics may be effective in preventing, treating nausea/vomiting. Pt should be pretreated with corticosteroids to reduce fluid retention, hypersensitivity reaction.

INTERVENTION/EVALUATION

Frequently monitor blood counts, particularly ANC count (less than 1,500 cells/mm^3 requires discontinuation of therapy). Monitor LFT, serum uric acid levels. Observe for cutaneous reactions (rash with eruptions, mainly on hands, feet). Assess for extravascular fluid accumulation: rales in lungs, dependent edema, dyspnea at rest, pronounced abdominal distention (due to ascites).

PATIENT/FAMILY TEACHING

• Hair loss is reversible, but new hair growth may have different color or texture. • New hair growth resumes 2–3 mos after last therapy dose. • Maintain strict oral hygiene. • Do not have immunizations without physician's approval (drug lowers resistance). • Avoid those who have recently taken any live virus vaccine. • Report persistent nausea, diarrhea, respiratory difficulty, chest pain, fever, chills, unusual bleeding, bruising.

dofetilide

doe-**fet**-i-lide
(Tikosyn)
■ BLACK BOX ALERT ■ Pt must be placed in a setting with continuous cardiac monitoring for minimum of 3 days and monitored by staff familiar with treatment of life-threatening arrhythmias.

◆CLASSIFICATION

PHARMACOTHERAPEUTIC: Potassium channel blocker. **CLINICAL:** Antiarrhythmic: Class III.

USES

Maintenance of normal sinus rhythm (NSR) in pts with chronic atrial fibrillation/atrial flutter of longer than 1-wk duration who have been converted to NSR. Conversion of atrial fibrillation/flutter to NSR.

PRECAUTIONS

Contraindications: Hypersensitivity to dofetilide. Congenital or acquired prolonged QT syndrome (do not use if baseline QT interval or QTc is greater than 440 msec), severe renal impairment, concurrent use of drugs that may prolong QT interval, hypokalemia, hypomagnesemia, concurrent use with verapamil, dolutegravir, itraconazole, ketoconazole, prochlorperazine, megestrol, cimetidine, hydroCHLOROthiazide, trimethoprim. Severe renal impairment (CrCl less than 20 mL/min). **Cautions:** Severe hepatic impairment, renal impairment, pts previously taking amiodarone, elderly. Concurrent use of other agents that prolong QT interval. Pts with sick sinus syndrome or second- or third-degree heart block unless functional pacemaker in place.

ACTION

Prolongs repolarization without affecting conduction velocity by blocking one or more time-dependent potassium currents. No effect on sodium channels, alpha-adrenergic, beta-adrenergic receptors. **Therapeutic Effect:** Terminates reentrant tachyarrhythmias, preventing reinduction.

PHARMACOKINETICS

Well absorbed following PO administration. 80% eliminated in urine as unchanged drug, 20% excreted as minimally active metabolites. Protein binding: 60%–70%. **Half-life:** 2–3 hrs.

⧗ LIFESPAN CONSIDERATIONS

Pregnancy/Lactation: Unknown if drug is distributed in breast milk. **Children:** No age-related precautions noted. **Elderly:** Age-related renal impairment may require dosage adjustment.

INTERACTIONS

DRUG: **Cimetidine, verapamil, itraconazole, ketoconazole, trimethoprim, hydroCHLOROthiazide** may increase concentration, toxicity. **HERBAL:** **St. John's wort** may decrease concentration. **Ephedra** may worsen arrhythmias. **FOOD:** None known. **LAB VALUES:** None significant.

AVAILABILITY (Rx)

Capsules: 125 mcg, 250 mcg, 500 mcg.

ADMINISTRATION/HANDLING

PO

• Give without regard to meals. • Do not break, crush, or open capsules.

INDICATIONS/ROUTES/DOSAGE

◀**ALERT**▶ EKG interval measurements (esp. Qtc intervals), creatinine clearance, must be determined prior to first dose. Correct hypokalemia, hypomagnesemia prior to starting.

Antiarrhythmias
PO: ADULTS, ELDERLY: Initially, 500 mcg twice daily. Modify dose in response to QTc interval.

Dosage in Renal Impairment

Creatinine Clearance	Dosage
Greater than 60 mL/min	500 mcg twice daily
40–60 mL/min	250 mcg twice daily
20–39 mL/min	125 mcg twice daily
Less than 20 mL/min	Contraindicated

Dosage in Hepatic Impairment
No dose adjustment.

SIDE EFFECTS

Rare (less than 2%): Headache, chest pain, dizziness, dyspnea, nausea, insomnia, back/abdominal pain, diarrhea, rash.

ADVERSE EFFECTS/TOXIC REACTIONS

Angioedema, bradycardia, cerebral ischemia, facial paralysis, serious arrhythmias (ventricular, various forms of block) have been noted.

NURSING CONSIDERATIONS

BASELINE ASSESSMENT

Assess baseline serum electrolytes (esp. potassium, magnesium). Prior to initiating treatment, QTc intervals must be determined. Do not use if heart rate less than 50 beats/min. Provide continuous EKG monitoring, calculation of creatinine clearance, equipment for resuscitation available for minimum of 3 days. Anticipate proarrhythmic events.

D

INTERVENTION/EVALUATION

Assess for conversion of cardiac dysrhythmias and absence of new arrhythmias. Constantly monitor EKG. Provide emotional support. Monitor renal function for electrolyte imbalance (prolonged or excessive diarrhea, sweating, vomiting, thirst).

PATIENT/FAMILY TEACHING

• Instruct pt on need for compliance and requirement for periodic monitoring of EKG and renal function. • Do not break, crush, or open capsule.

---

donepezil

doe-**nep**-e-zil
(Apo-Donepezil ✱, Aricept)
Do not confuse Aricept with Aciphex, Ascriptin, or Azilect.

FIXED-COMBINATION(S)

Namzaric: donepezil/memantine (NMDA receptor antagonist): 10 mg/14 mg, 10 mg/28 mg.

◆CLASSIFICATION

PHARMACOTHERAPEUTIC: Acetylcholinesterase inhibitor. **CLINICAL:** Cholinergic.

USES

Treatment of mild, moderate, or severe dementia of Alzheimer's disease. **OFF-LABEL:** Treatment of behavioral syndromes in dementia, dementia associated with Parkinson's disease, Lewy body dementia.

PRECAUTIONS

Contraindications: History of hypersensitivity to donepezil, other piperidine derivatives. **Cautions:** Asthma, COPD, bradycardia, bladder outflow obstruction, history of ulcer disease, those taking concurrent NSAIDs, supraventricular cardiac conduction disturbances (e.g.,

"sick sinus syndrome," Wolff-Parkinson-White syndrome), seizure disorder.

ACTION

Inhibits enzyme acetylcholinesterase, increasing concentration of acetylcholine at cholinergic synapses, enhancing cholinergic function in CNS. **Therapeutic Effect:** Slows progression of Alzheimer's disease.

PHARMACOKINETICS

Well absorbed after PO administration. Protein binding: 96%. Extensively metabolized. Eliminated in urine, feces. **Half-life:** 70 hrs.

⧖ LIFESPAN CONSIDERATIONS

Pregnancy/Lactation: Unknown if drug is distributed in breast milk. **Children:** Safety and efficacy not established. **Elderly:** No age-related precautions noted.

INTERACTIONS

DRUG: May decrease effect of **anticholinergics** (e.g., **glycopyrrolate, scopolamine**). May increase synergistic effects of **cholinergic agonists, neuromuscular blockers** (e.g., **rocuronium, succinylcholine**). **Ketoconazole** may inhibit metabolism. **CYP3A4 inducers** (e.g., **carBAMazepine, rifAMPin**) may decrease concentration/effects. **HERBAL: St. John's wort** may decrease concentration. **Ginkgo** may increase adverse effects. **FOOD:** None known. **LAB VALUES:** None significant.

AVAILABILITY (Rx)

Tablets: 5 mg, 10 mg, 23 mg. **Tablets (Orally Disintegrating):** 5 mg, 10 mg.

ADMINISTRATION/HANDLING

PO

• May be given at bedtime without regard to meals. • Swallow tablets whole; do not break, crush, dissolve, or divide. • Follow dose with water.

INDICATIONS/ROUTES/DOSAGE

Alzheimer's Disease

PO: ADULTS, ELDERLY: For mild to moderate, initially 5 mg/day at bedtime. May increase at 4- to 6-wk intervals to 10 mg/day at bedtime. Range: 5–10 mg/day. For moderate to severe Alzheimer's, a dose of 23 mg once daily can be administered once pt has been taking 10 mg once daily for at least 3 mos. Range: 10–23 mg/day.

Dosage in Renal/Hepatic Impairment

No dose adjustment.

SIDE EFFECTS

Frequent (11%–8%): Nausea, diarrhea, headache, insomnia, nonspecific pain, dizziness. **Occasional (6%–3%):** Mild muscle cramps, fatigue, vomiting, anorexia, ecchymosis. **Rare (3%–2%):** Depression, abnormal dreams, weight loss, arthritis, drowsiness, syncope, frequent urination.

ADVERSE EFFECTS/TOXIC REACTIONS

Overdose may result in cholinergic crisis (severe nausea, increased salivation, diaphoresis, bradycardia, hypotension, flushed skin, abdominal pain, respiratory depression, seizures, cardiorespiratory collapse). Increasing muscle weakness may occur, resulting in death if muscles of respiration become involved. **Antidote:** Atropine sulfate 1–2 mg IV with subsequent doses based on therapeutic response.

NURSING CONSIDERATIONS

BASELINE ASSESSMENT

Assess cognitive function (e.g., memory, attention, reasoning). Obtain baseline vital signs. Assess history for peptic ulcer, urinary obstruction, asthma, COPD, seizure disorder, cardiac conduction disturbances.

INTERVENTION/EVALUATION

Monitor behavior, mood/cognitive function, activities of daily living. Monitor for cholinergic reaction (GI discomfort/cramping, feeling of facial warmth, excessive salivation/diaphoresis), lacrimation, pallor, urinary urgency, dizziness. Monitor for nausea, diarrhea, headache, insomnia.

PATIENT/FAMILY TEACHING

• Report nausea, vomiting, diarrhea, diaphoresis, increased salivary secretions, severe abdominal pain, dizziness. • May take without regard to food (best taken at bedtime). • Not a cure for Alzheimer's disease but may slow progression of symptoms.

DOPamine **HIGH ALERT**

dope-a-meen

■ **BLACK BOX ALERT** ■ If extravasation occurs, infiltrate area with phentolamine (5–10 mL 0.9% NaCl) as soon as possible, no later than 12 hrs after extravasation.
Do not confuse DOPamine with DOBUTamine or Dopram.

◆CLASSIFICATION

PHARMACOTHERAPEUTIC: Sympathomimetic (adrenergic agonist). **CLINICAL:** Cardiac stimulant, vasopressor.

USES

Adjunct in treatment of shock (e.g., MI, trauma, renal failure, cardiac decompensation, open heart surgery, persisting after adequate fluid volume replacement). **OFF-LABEL:** Symptomatic bradycardia or heart block unresponsive to atropine or cardiac pacing.

PRECAUTIONS

Contraindications: Hypersensitivity to DOPamine, sulfites. Pheochromocytoma, ventricular fibrillation. Uncorrected tachyarrhythmias. **Cautions:** Ischemic heart disease, occlusive vascular disease, hypovolemia, recent use of MAOIs (within 2–3 weeks), ventricular arrhythmias, post-MI.

ACTION

Stimulates adrenergic and dopaminergic receptors. Effects are dose dependent. Lower dosage stimulates dopaminergic receptors, causing renal vasodilation. Higher doses stimulate both dopaminergic and beta$_1$-adrenergic receptors, causing cardiac stimulation and renal vasodilation. Higher doses stimulate alpha-adrenergic receptors, causing vasoconstriction, increased B/P. **Therapeutic Effect: Low dosage (1–3 mcg/kg/min):** Increases renal blood flow, urinary flow, sodium excretion. **Low to moderate dosage (4–10 mcg/kg/min):** Increases myocardial contractility, stroke volume, cardiac output. **High dosage (greater than 10 mcg/kg/min):** Increases peripheral resistance, vasoconstriction, B/P.

PHARMACOKINETICS

Route	Onset	Peak	Duration
IV	1–2 min	N/A	Less than 10 min

Widely distributed. Does not cross blood-brain barrier. Metabolized in liver, kidneys, plasma. Primarily excreted in urine. Not removed by hemodialysis. **Half-life:** 2 min.

🕱 LIFESPAN CONSIDERATIONS

Pregnancy/Lactation: Unknown if drug crosses placenta or is distributed in breast milk. **Children:** Recommended close hemodynamic monitoring (gangrene due to extravasation reported). **Elderly:** No age-related precautions noted.

INTERACTIONS

DRUG: May have increased effects with **vasopressors (e.g., midodrine, norepinephrine, phenylephrine).** **COMT inhibitors (e.g., entacapone, tolcapone)** may increase level/effects. **HERBAL:** None significant. **FOOD:** None known. **LAB VALUES:** None significant.

AVAILABILITY (Rx)

Injection Solution: 40 mg/mL, 80 mg/mL, 160 mg/mL. **Injection (Premix with Dextrose):** 0.8 mg/mL (250 mL, 500 mL), 1.6 mg/mL (250 mL, 500 mL), 3.2 mg/mL (250 mL).

ADMINISTRATION/HANDLING

◀**ALERT**▶ Fluid volume depletion must be corrected before administering DOPamine (may be used concurrently with fluid replacement).

IV

Reconstitution • Available prediluted in 250 or 500 mL D$_5$W or dilute in 250–500 mL 0.9% NaCl or D$_5$W, to maximum concentration of 3,200 mcg/mL (3.2 mg/mL). **Rate of Administration** • Administer into large vein (antecubital fossa, central line preferred) to prevent extravasation. • Use infusion pump to control flow rate. • Titrate drug to desired hemodynamic, renal response (optimum urinary flow determines dosage). **Storage** • Do not use solutions darker than slightly yellow or discolored to yellow, brown, pink to purple (indicates decomposition of drug). • Stable for 24 hrs after dilution.

🕮 IV INCOMPATIBILITIES

Acyclovir (Zovirax), amphotericin B complex (Abelcet, AmBisome, Amphotec), cefepime (Maxipime), furosemide (Lasix), insulin, sodium bicarbonate.

🕮 IV COMPATIBILITIES

Amiodarone (Cordarone), calcium chloride, dexmedetomidine (Precedex), diltiaZEM (Cardizem), DOBUTamine (Dobutrex), enalapril (Vasotec), EPINEPHrine, heparin, HYDROmorphone (Dilaudid), labetalol (Trandate), levoFLOXacin (Levaquin), lidocaine, LORazepam (Ativan), methylPREDNISolone (Solu-Medrol), midazolam (Versed), milrinone (Primacor), morphine, niCARdipine (Cardene), nitroglycerin, norepinephrine (Levophed), piperacillin/

tazobactam (Zosyn), potassium chloride, propofol (Diprivan).

INDICATIONS/ROUTES/DOSAGE

◄ALERT► Effects of DOPamine are dose dependent. Titrate to desired response. Doses greater than 20 mcg/kg/min may not have beneficial effect on BP and may increase risk of tachyarrhythmias.

Hemodynamic Support

IV Infusion: ADULTS, ELDERLY, CHILDREN: Range: 2–20 mcg/kg/min. Titrate to desired response. May gradually increase by 5–10 mcg/kg/min increments. **Maximum:** 50 mcg/kg/min. **NEONATES:** 1–20 mcg/kg/min. Titrate to desired response.

SIDE EFFECTS

Frequent: Headache, arrhythmias, tachycardia, anginal pain, palpitations, vasoconstriction, hypotension, nausea, vomiting, dyspnea. **Occasional:** Piloerection (goose bumps), bradycardia, widening of QRS complex.

ADVERSE EFFECTS/TOXIC REACTIONS

High doses may produce ventricular arrhythmias, tachycardia. Pts with occlusive vascular disease are at high risk for further compromise of circulation to extremities, which may result in gangrene. Tissue necrosis with sloughing may occur with extravasation of IV solution.

NURSING CONSIDERATIONS

BASELINE ASSESSMENT

Pt must be on continuous cardiac monitoring. Determine weight (for dosage calculation). Obtain initial B/P, heart rate, respirations. Assess patency of IV access.

INTERVENTION/EVALUATION

Continuously monitor for cardiac arrhythmias. Measure urinary output frequently. If extravasation occurs, immediately infiltrate affected tissue with 10–15 mL 0.9% NaCl solution containing 5–10

mg phentolamine mesylate. Monitor B/P, heart rate, respirations q15min during administration (more often if indicated). Assess cardiac output, pulmonary wedge pressure, or central venous pressure (CVP) frequently. Assess peripheral circulation (palpate pulses, note color/temperature of extremities). Immediately notify physician of decreased urinary output, cardiac arrhythmias, significant changes in B/P, heart rate, or failure to respond to increase or decrease in infusion rate, decreased peripheral circulation (cold, pale, mottled extremities). Taper dosage before discontinuing (abrupt cessation of therapy may result in marked hypotension). Be alert to excessive vasoconstriction (decreased urine output, increased heart rate, arrhythmias, disproportionate increase in diastolic B/P, decrease in pulse pressure); slow or temporarily stop infusion, notify physician.

doripenem

dor-i-**pen**-em
(Doribax)
Do not confuse Doribax with Zovirax, or doripenem with ertapenem, imipenem, or meropenem.

◆CLASSIFICATION

PHARMACOTHERAPEUTIC: Carbapenem. **CLINICAL:** Antibiotic.

USES

Treatment of complicated intra-abdominal infections, complicated UTIs (including pyelonephritis) due to susceptible gram-positive, gram-negative (including *P. aeruginosa*), and anaerobic bacteria. **OFF-LABEL:** Treatment of intravascular catheter-related bloodstream infection due to ESBL-producing *E. coli* and *Klebsiella* spp. pneumonia, including ventilator-associated.

PRECAUTIONS

Contraindications: History of serious hypersensitivity to doripenem or other carbapenems (meropenem, imipenem-cilastatin, ertapenem). Anaphylactic reactions to beta-lactam antibiotics. **Cautions:** Hypersensitivity to penicillins, cephalosporins. Pts with renal impairment, CNS disorders (e.g., stroke, history of seizures).

ACTION

Inactivates penicillin-binding proteins, resulting in inhibition of cell wall synthesis. **Therapeutic Effect:** Produces bacterial cell death.

PHARMACOKINETICS

Penetrates into body fluids, tissues. Widely distributed. Protein binding: 8%. Primarily excreted in urine. Removed by dialysis. **Half-life:** 1 hr.

⧖ LIFESPAN CONSIDERATIONS

Pregnancy/Lactation: Distributed in breast milk. **Children:** Safety and efficacy not established in pts younger than 18 yrs. **Elderly:** Advanced renal insufficiency, end-stage renal insufficiency may require dosage adjustment.

INTERACTIONS

DRUG: Probenecid reduces renal excretion of doripenem. May decrease **valproic acid** concentration (do not use concurrently). **HERBAL:** None significant. **FOOD:** None known. **LAB VALUES:** May increase serum alkaline phosphatase, ALT, AST. May decrease Hgb, Hct, platelet count; serum potassium.

AVAILABILITY (Rx)

Injection, Powder for Reconstitution: 250 mg, 500 mg.

ADMINISTRATION/HANDLING

 IV

Reconstitution • Reconstitute 250-mg or 500-mg vial with 10 mL Sterile Water for Injection or 0.9% NaCl. • Shake well to dissolve. • Further dilute with 100 mL 0.9% NaCl or D₅W.

Rate of Administration • Give by intermittent IV infusion (piggyback). • Do not give IV push. • Infuse over 60 min.

Storage • Stable for 12 hrs at room temperature, 72 hrs if refrigerated when diluted in 0.9% NaCl; 4 hrs at room temperature, 24 hrs if refrigerated when diluted in D₅W.

🖩 IV INCOMPATIBILITIES

DiazePAM (Valium), potassium phosphate, propofol (Diprivan).

🖩 IV COMPATIBILITIES

Amiodarone, bumetanide (Bumex), calcium gluconate, dexamethasone, diltiaZEM (Cardizem), diphenhydrAMINE (Benadryl), furosemide (Lasix), heparin, hydrocortisone (SOLU-Cortef), HYDROmorphone (Dilaudid), insulin, labetalol (Trandate), LORazepam (Ativan), magnesium sulfate, methylPREDNISolone (SOLU-Medrol), metoclopramide (Reglan), milrinone, morphine, ondansetron (Zofran), pantoprazole (Protonix), potassium chloride.

INDICATIONS/ROUTES/DOSAGE

Intra-Abdominal Infections
IV: ADULTS, ELDERLY: 500 mg q8h for 5–14 days.

Urinary Tract Infections
IV: ADULTS, ELDERLY: 500 mg q8h for 10–14 days.

Dosage in Renal Impairment

Creatinine Clearance	Dosage
Greater than 50 mL/min	No adjustment
30–50 mL/min	250 mg q8h
11–29 mL/min	250 mg q12h
Hemodialysis	250 mg q24h; if treating infection caused by *Pseudomonas aeruginosa:* 500 mg q12h on day 1, then 500 g q24h

Creatinine Clearance	Dosage
Continuous renal replacement therapy	250 mg q12h

Dosage in Hepatic Impairment
No dose adjustment.

SIDE EFFECTS

Frequent (10%–6%): Diarrhea, nausea, headache. **Occasional (5%–2%):** Altered mental status, insomnia, rash, abdominal pain, constipation, vomiting, edema, fever. **Rare (less than 2%):** Dizziness, cough, oral candidiasis, anxiety, tachycardia, phlebitis at IV site.

ADVERSE EFFECTS/TOXIC REACTIONS

Antibiotic-associated colitis, other superinfections (abdominal cramps, severe watery diarrhea, fever) may occur. Anaphylactic reactions in pts receiving beta-lactams have occurred. Seizures may occur in those with CNS disorders (brain lesions, history of seizures) or with bacterial meningitis or severe impaired renal function.

NURSING CONSIDERATIONS

BASELINE ASSESSMENT
Question pt for history of allergies, particularly to beta-lactams, penicillins, cephalosporins. Inquire about history of seizures.

INTERVENTION/EVALUATION
Monitor for signs of hypersensitivity reaction during first dose. Monitor daily pattern of bowel activity, stool consistency. Monitor for nausea, vomiting. Evaluate hydration status. Evaluate for inflammation at IV injection site. Assess skin for rash. Check mental status; be alert to tremors, possible seizures. Assess sleep pattern for evidence of insomnia.

PATIENT/FAMILY TEACHING
• Report tremors, seizures, rash, diarrhea, or other new symptoms.

doxazosin

dox-a-**zoe**-sin
(Apo-Doxazosin ✤, Cardura, Cardura XL)
Do not confuse Cardura with Cardene, Cordarone, Coumadin, K-Dur, or Ridaura, or doxazosin with doxapram, doxepin, or DOXOrubicin.

◆CLASSIFICATION

PHARMACOTHERAPEUTIC: Alpha-adrenergic blocker. **CLINICAL:** Antihypertensive.

USES

Cardura: Treatment of mild to moderate hypertension. Used alone or in combination with other antihypertensives. Treatment of urinary outflow obstruction and/or obstruction and irritation associated with benign prostatic hyperplasia *(BPH)*. **Cardura XL:** Treatment of urinary outflow obstruction and/or obstruction and irritation associated with benign prostatic hyperplasia. **OFF-LABEL:** Pediatric hypertension. Facilitate distal ureteral stone expulsion. Erectile dysfunction in pts with BPH.

PRECAUTIONS

Contraindications: Hypersensitivity to doxazosin or other quinazolines (prazosin, terazosin). **Cautions:** Constipation, ileus, GI obstruction, hepatic impairment.

ACTION

Hypertension: Selectively blocks alpha$_1$-adrenergic receptors, decreasing peripheral vascular resistance. **BPH:** Inhibits postsynaptic alpha-adrenergic receptors in prostatic stromal and bladder neck tissues. **Therapeutic Effect: Hypertension:** Causes peripheral vasodilation, lowering B/P. **BPH:** Relaxes smooth muscle of bladder, prostate, reducing BPH symptoms.

✤ Canadian trade name   🍁 Non-Crushable Drug   📕 High Alert drug

D

PHARMACOKINETICS

Route	Onset	Peak	Duration
PO (antihypertensive)	1–2 hrs	2–6 hrs	24 hrs

Well absorbed from GI tract. Protein binding: 98%–99%. Metabolized in liver. Primarily eliminated in feces. Not removed by hemodialysis. **Half-life:** 19–22 hrs.

⧗ LIFESPAN CONSIDERATIONS

Pregnancy/Lactation: Unknown if drug crosses placenta or is distributed in breast milk. **Children:** Safety and efficacy not established. **Elderly:** May be more sensitive to hypotensive effects.

INTERACTIONS

DRUG: NSAIDs (e.g., ibuprofen, ketorolac, naproxen) may decrease effect. **Hypotension-producing medications (e.g., antihypertensives, diuretics)** may increase effect. **CYP3A4 inhibitors (e.g., atazanavir, ketoconazole)** may increase hypotensive effect. **Phosphodiesterase inhibitors (e.g., sildenafil)** may produce additive hypotension. **HERBAL: Ephedra, ginseng, yohimbe** may worsen hypertension. **Garlic** may increase antihypertensive effect. Avoid **saw palmetto** (limited experience with this combination). **FOOD:** None known. **LAB VALUES:** None significant.

AVAILABILITY (Rx)

Tablets: 1 mg, 2 mg, 4 mg, 8 mg.

🔖 **Tablets, Extended-Release:** 4 mg, 8 mg.

ADMINISTRATION/HANDLING

PO
• Give without regard to food. • Do not break, crush, dissolve, or divide extended-release tablet. • Immediate-release tablets given morning or evening; extended-release tablets given with morning meal.

INDICATIONS/ROUTES/DOSAGE

Hypertension
PO: *(Immediate-Release):* **ADULTS, ELDERLY:** Initially, 1 mg once daily. May be increased to 2 mg once daily. Thereafter, may increase upward over several weeks to a maximum of 16 mg/day.

Benign Prostatic Hyperplasia
PO: *(Immediate-Release):* **ADULTS, ELDERLY:** Initially, 1 mg/day. May be increased to 2 mg once daily. Thereafter, may increase q1–2wks. **Maximum:** 8 mg/day. *(Extended-Release):* Initially, 4 mg/day. May increase to 8 mg in 3–4 wks. **Note:** When switching to extended-release, omit evening dose prior to starting morning dose.

Dosage in Renal Impairment
No dose adjustment.

Dosage in Hepatic Impairment
Mild to moderate impairment: Use caution. **Severe Impairment:** Avoid use.

SIDE EFFECTS

Frequent (20%–10%): Dizziness, asthenia, headache, edema. **Occasional (9%–3%):** Nausea, pharyngitis, rhinitis, pain in extremities, drowsiness. **Rare (2%–1%):** Palpitations, diarrhea, constipation, dyspnea, myalgia, altered vision, anxiety.

ADVERSE EFFECTS/TOXIC REACTIONS

First-dose syncope (hypotension with sudden loss of consciousness) may occur 30–90 min following initial dose of 2 mg or greater, too-rapid increase in dosage, addition of another antihypertensive agent to therapy. First-dose syncope may be preceded by tachycardia (pulse rate 120–160 beats/min).

NURSING CONSIDERATIONS

BASELINE ASSESSMENT

Give first dose at bedtime. If initial dose is given during daytime, pt must remain recumbent for 3–4 hrs. Assess B/P, pulse immediately before each dose and q15–30 min until B/P is stabilized (be alert to fluctuations).

INTERVENTION/EVALUATION

Monitor B/P, I&O. Monitor pulse diligently (first-dose syncope may be preceded by tachycardia). Assess for edema, headache. Assist with ambulation if dizziness, light-headedness occurs.

PATIENT/FAMILY TEACHING

• Full therapeutic effect may not occur for 3–4 wks. • May cause syncope (fainting); go from lying to standing slowly. • Avoid tasks that require alertness, motor skills until response to drug is established.

---

doxepin

dox-e-pin
(Apo-Doxepin ✦, Novo-Doxepin ✦, Prudoxin, Silenor, **SINE**quan ✦, Zonalon)

■ **BLACK BOX ALERT** ■ Increased risk of suicidal ideation and behavior in children, adolescents, young adults 18–24 yrs with major depressive disorder, other psychiatric disorders.
Do not confuse doxepin with digoxin, doxapram, doxazosin, Doxidan, or doxycycline, or SINEquan with SEROquel, or Singulair.

◆CLASSIFICATION

PHARMACOTHERAPEUTIC: Tricyclic. **CLINICAL:** Antidepressant, antianxiety, antineuralgic, antipruritic.

USES

Treatment of depression and/or anxiety. **Silenor (only):** Treatment of insomnia in pts with difficulty staying asleep. **Topical:** Treatment of pruritus associated with atopic dermatitis. **OFF-LABEL:** Treatment of neurogenic pain, treatment of anxiety.

PRECAUTIONS

Contraindications: Hypersensitivity to doxepin. Glaucoma, hypersensitivity to other tricyclic antidepressants, urinary retention, use of MAOIs within 14 days. **Cautions:** Cardiac/hepatic/renal disease, pts at risk for suicidal ideation, respiratory compromise, sleep apnea, history of bowel obstruction, increased IOP, glaucoma, history of seizures, history of urinary retention/obstruction, hyperthyroidism, prostatic hypertrophy, hiatal hernia, elderly.

ACTION

Increases synaptic concentrations of norepinephrine, serotonin. **Therapeutic Effect:** Produces antidepressant, anxiolytic effects.

PHARMACOKINETICS

PO: Rapidly absorbed from GI tract. Protein binding: 80%–85%. Metabolized in liver. Primarily excreted in urine. Not removed by hemodialysis. **Half-life:** 6–8 hrs. **Topical:** Absorbed through skin. Distributed to body tissues. Metabolized to active metabolite. Excreted in urine.

⧗ LIFESPAN CONSIDERATIONS

Pregnancy/Lactation: Crosses placenta. Distributed in breast milk. **Children:** Safety and efficacy not established in pts younger than 12 yrs. **Elderly:** Increased risk of toxicity (lower dosages recommended). Avoid doses greater than 6 mg/day due to anticholinergic effects, sedation, and orthostatic hypotension.

INTERACTIONS

DRUG: Alcohol, other CNS depressants (e.g., lorazepam, morphine, zolpidem) may increase CNS, respiratory depression, hypotensive effects. **Cimetidine** may increase concentration, risk of toxicity. **MAOIs (e.g., phenelzine, selegiline)** may increase risk of seizures, hyperpyrexia, hypertensive crisis (discontinue at least 2 wks prior to starting doxepin). **Phenothiazines** may increase anticholinergic, sedative effects. **HERBAL:** Kava kava, SAMe, St. John's wort, valerian may increase sedation, risk of serotonin syndrome. **St. John's wort** may decrease concentration/effects. **FOOD:** None known. **LAB VALUES:** May alter serum glucose,

---

EKG readings. **Therapeutic serum level:** 110–250 ng/mL; **toxic serum level:** greater than 300 ng/mL.

AVAILABILITY (Rx)

Capsules: 10 mg, 25 mg, 50 mg, 75 mg, 100 mg, 150 mg. **Cream (Prudoxin, Zonalon):** 5%. **Oral Concentrate:** 10 mg/mL. **Tablets (Silenor):** 3 mg, 6 mg.

ADMINISTRATION/HANDLING

PO
• Give with food, milk if GI distress occurs. • Dilute concentrate in 4-oz glass of water, milk, or orange, tomato, prune, pineapple juice. Incompatible with carbonated drinks. • Give larger portion of daily dose at bedtime.

Topical
• Apply thin film of cream on affected areas of skin. • Do not use for more than 8 days. • Do not use occlusive dressing.

INDICATIONS/ROUTES/DOSAGE

Depression, Anxiety
PO: ADULTS: Initially, 25–50 mg/day at bedtime or in 2–3 divided doses. May increase gradually to usual dose of 150 mg–300 mg/day (single dose should not exceed 150 mg). **ELDERLY:** Initially, 10–25 mg at bedtime. May increase by 10–25 mg/day every 3–7 days.

Insomnia (Silenor only)
PO: ADULTS: 3–6 mg. **ELDERLY:** 3 mg (give within 30 min of bedtime). May increase to 6 mg once daily.

Pruritus Associated with Atopic Dermatitis
Topical: ADULTS, ELDERLY: Apply thin film 4 times/day at 3- to 4-hr intervals. Not recommended for more than 8 days.

Dosage in Renal Impairment
No dose adjustment.

Dosage in Hepatic Impairment
Use lower initial dose; adjust gradually. **Silenor:** Initially, 3 mg once daily.

SIDE EFFECTS

Frequent: PO: Orthostatic hypotension, drowsiness, dry mouth, headache, increased appetite, weight gain, nausea, unusual fatigue, unpleasant taste. **Topical:** Edema, increased pruritus, eczema, burning, tingling, stinging at application site, altered taste, dizziness, drowsiness, dry skin, dry mouth, fatigue, headache, thirst. **Occasional: PO:** Blurred vision, confusion, constipation, hallucinations, difficult urination, eye pain, irregular heartbeat, fine muscle tremors, nervousness, impaired sexual function, diarrhea, diaphoresis, heartburn, insomnia. **Silenor:** Nausea, upper respiratory infection. **Topical:** Anxiety, skin irritation/cracking, nausea. **Rare: PO:** Allergic reaction, alopecia, tinnitus, breast enlargement. **Topical:** Fever, photosensitivity.

ADVERSE EFFECTS/TOXIC REACTIONS

Abrupt or too-rapid withdrawal may result in headache, malaise, nausea, vomiting, vivid dreams. Overdose may produce confusion, severe drowsiness, agitation, tachycardia, arrhythmias, shortness of breath, vomiting.

NURSING CONSIDERATIONS

BASELINE ASSESSMENT
Assess B/P, pulse, EKG (those with history of cardiovascular disease). Perform CBC, serum electrolyte tests before long-term therapy. Assess pt's appearance, behavior, level of interest, mood, suicidal ideation, sleep pattern.

INTERVENTION/EVALUATION
Monitor B/P, pulse, weight. Perform CBC, serum electrolyte tests periodically to assess renal/hepatic function. Monitor mental status, suicidal ideation. Supervise suicidal-risk pt closely during early therapy (as depression lessens, energy level improves, increasing suicide potential). Assess appearance, behavior, speech pattern, level of interest, mood. **Therapeutic serum level:** 110–250 ng/mL; **toxic serum level:** greater than 300 ng/mL.

PATIENT/FAMILY TEACHING

• Do not discontinue abruptly.
• Change positions slowly to avoid dizziness. • Avoid tasks that require alertness, motor skills until response to drug is established. • Do not cover affected area with occlusive dressing after applying cream. • May cause dry mouth. • Avoid alcohol, limit caffeine. • May increase appetite. • Avoid exposure to sunlight/artificial light source. • Therapeutic effect may be noted within 2–5 days, maximum effect within 2–3 wks. • Report worsening depression, suicidal ideation, unusual changes in behavior (esp. at initiation of therapy or with changes in dosage).

DOXOrubicin ▪HIGH ALERT▪

dox-o-**rue**-bi-sin
(Adriamycin, Caelyx ✿, Doxil, Lipodox)

■ **BLACK BOX ALERT** ■ May cause concurrent or cumulative myocardial toxicity. Acute allergic or anaphylaxis-like infusion reaction may be life threatening. Severe myelosuppression may occur. Must be administered by personnel trained in administration/handling of chemotherapeutic agents. Secondary acute myelogenous leukemia and myelodysplastic syndrome have been reported. Potent vesicant.

Do not confuse DOXOrubicin with dactinomycin, DAUNOrubicin, doxazosin, epiRUBicin, IDArubicin, or valrubicin, or Adriamycin with Aredia or idamycin.

◆CLASSIFICATION

PHARMACOTHERAPEUTIC: Anthracycline antibiotic. **CLINICAL:** Antineoplastic.

USES

Adriamycin: Treatment of acute lymphocytic leukemia (ALL), acute myeloid leukemia (AML), Hodgkin's lymphoma, malignant lymphoma; breast, gastric, small-cell lung, ovarian, epithelial, thyroid, bladder carcinomas; neuroblastoma, Wilms tumor, osteosarcoma, soft tissue sarcoma. **Doxil, Lipodox:** Treatment of AIDS-related Kaposi's sarcoma, advanced ovarian cancer. Used with bortezomib to treat multiple myeloma in pts who have not previously received bortezomib and have received at least one previous treatment. **OFF-LABEL: Adriamycin:** Multiple myeloma, endometrial carcinoma, uterine sarcoma; head and neck cancer, liver, kidney cancer. **Doxil:** Metastatic breast cancer, Hodgkin's lymphoma, cutaneous T-cell lymphomas, advanced soft tissue sarcomas, recurrent or metastatic cervical cancer, advanced or metastatic uterine sarcoma.

PRECAUTIONS

Contraindications: Hypersensitivity to DOXOrubicin. **Adriamycin:** Severe hepatic impairment, severe myocardial insufficiency, recent MI (within 4–6 wks), severe arrhythmias. Previous or concomitant treatment with high accumulative doses of DOXOrubicin, DAUNOrubicin, IDArubicin, or other anthracyclines or anthracenediones; severe, persistent drug-induced myelosuppression or baseline ANC count less than 1,500 cells/mm^3. **Doxil:** Breastfeeding (Canada). **Cautions:** Hepatic impairment. Cardiomyopathy, preexisting myelosuppression, severe HF. Pts who received radiation therapy.

ACTION

Inhibits DNA, DNA-dependent RNA synthesis by binding with DNA strands. Liposomal encapsulation increases uptake by tumors, prolongs drug action, may decrease toxicity. **Therapeutic Effect:** Prevents cell division.

D

PHARMACOKINETICS

Widely distributed. Protein binding: 74%–76%. Does not cross blood-brain barrier. Metabolized in liver. Primarily eliminated by biliary system. Not removed by hemodialysis. **Half-life:** 20–48 hrs.

LIFESPAN CONSIDERATIONS

Pregnancy/Lactation: If possible, avoid use during pregnancy, esp. first trimester. Breastfeeding not recommended. **Children/Elderly:** Cardiotoxicity may be more frequent in pts younger than 2 yrs or older than 70 yrs.

INTERACTIONS

DRUG: CycloSPORINE may increase risk of hematologic toxicity. **Bone marrow depressants** may increase myelosuppression. **DAUNOrubicin** may increase risk of cardiotoxicity. **Live virus vaccines** may potentiate virus replication, increase vaccine side effects, decrease pt's antibody response to vaccine. **HERBAL: St. John's wort** may decrease concentration. Avoid **black cohosh, dong quai** in estrogen-dependent tumors. **FOOD:** None known. **LAB VALUES:** May cause EKG changes, increase serum uric acid. May reduce neutrophil, RBC counts.

AVAILABILITY (Rx)

Injection, Powder for Reconstitution: 10 mg, 20 mg, 50 mg. **Injection Solution (Adriamycin):** 2 mg/mL (5-mL, 10-mL, 25-mL, 100-mL vial). **Lipid Complex (Doxil, Lipodox):** 2 mg/mL (10 mL, 25 mL).

ADMINISTRATION/HANDLING

◀**ALERT**▶ Wear gloves. If powder or solution comes into contact with skin, wash thoroughly. Avoid small veins; swollen/edematous extremities; areas overlying joints, tendons. **Doxil:** Do not use with in-line filter or mix with any diluent except D_5W. May be carcinogenic, mutagenic, teratogenic. Handle with extreme care during preparation/administration.

 IV

Reconstitution • Reconstitute vials of powder with 0.9% NaCl to provide concentration of 2 mg/mL. • Shake vial; allow contents to dissolve. • Withdraw appropriate volume of air from vial during reconstitution (avoids excessive pressure buildup). • May be further diluted with 50–1,000 mL D_5W or 0.9% NaCl and given as continuous infusion. • **Doxil:** Dilute each dose in 250 mL D_5W (doses greater than 90 mg in 500 mL D_5W).

Rate of Administration (Adriamycin) • For IV push, administer into tubing of freely running IV infusion of D_5W or 0.9% NaCl, preferably via butterfly needle over 3–5 min (avoids local erythematous streaking along vein and facial flushing). • Must test for flashback q30sec to be certain needle remains in vein during injection. IV piggyback over 15–60 min or continuous infusion. • Extravasation produces immediate pain, severe local tissue damage. Terminate administration immediately; withdraw as much medication as possible, obtain extravasation kit, follow protocol. **Doxil:** Give as infusion over 60 min. Do not use in-line filter.

Storage • **Adriamycin powder:** Store at room temperature. • Reconstituted vials stable for 7 days at room temperature, 15 days if refrigerated. Infusions stable for 48 hrs at room temperature. • Protect from prolonged exposure to sunlight; discard unused solution. • **Adriamycin solution:** Refrigerate vials. Solutions diluted in D_5W or 0.9% NaCl stable for 48 hrs at room temperature. • **Doxil:** Refrigerate unopened vials. After solution is diluted, use within 24 hrs.

IV INCOMPATIBILITIES

DOXOrubicin: Allopurinol (Aloprim), amphotericin B complex (Abelcet, Am-Bisome, Amphotec), cefepime (Maxipime), furosemide (Lasix), ganciclovir (Cytovene), heparin, piperacillin/tazobactam (Zosyn), propofol (Diprivan).

D

Doxil: Do not mix with any other medications.

🔲 IV COMPATIBILITIES

Dexamethasone (Decadron), diphenhydrAMINE (Benadryl), granisetron (Kytril), HYDROmorphone (Dilaudid), LORazepam (Ativan), morphine, ondansetron (Zofran).

INDICATIONS/ROUTES/DOSAGE
◀**ALERT**▶ Refer to individual protocols.

Usual Dosage
IV: *(Adriamycin):* **ADULTS: (Single-agent Therapy):** 60–75 mg/m² as a single dose every 21 days, 20 mg/m² once wkly. **(Combination Therapy):** 40–75 mg/m² q21–28 days. Because of risk of cardiotoxicity, do not exceed cumulative dose of 550 mg/m² (400–450 mg/m² for those previously treated with related compounds or irradiation of cardiac region). **CHILDREN: (Single-agent Therapy):** 60–75 mg/m² q3wks. **(Combination Therapy):** 40–75 mg/m² q21–28 days.

Kaposi's Sarcoma
IV: *(Doxil, Lipodox):* **ADULTS:** 20 mg/m² q3wks infused over 30 min. Continue until disease progression or unacceptable toxicity.

Ovarian Cancer
IV: *(Doxil, Lipodox):* **ADULTS:** 50 mg/m² q4wks. Continue until disease progression or unacceptable toxicity.

Multiple Myeloma
IV: *(Doxil, Lipodox):* **ADULTS:** 30 mg/m²/dose on day 4 q3wks (in combination with bortezomib). Continue until disease progression or unacceptable toxicity.

Dosage in Renal Impairment
No dose adjustment.

Dose Modifications
Adriamycin
Neutropenic Fever/Infection: Reduce dose to 75%. **ANC less than 1,000 cells/mm³:** Delay treatment until ANC 1,000 cells/mm³ or more. **Platelets less than 100,000/mm³:** Delay treatment until platelets 100,000 cells/mm³ or more.
Doxil
Adjustments for Hand-Foot Syndrome, Stomatitis, Hematologic Toxicities: Refer to manufacturer's guidelines.

Dosage in Hepatic Impairment
ADRIAMYCIN

Hepatic Function	Dosage
ALT, AST 2–3 times ULN	75% of normal dose
ALT, AST greater than 3 times ULN or bilirubin 1.2–3 mg/dL	50% of normal dose
Bilirubin 3.1–5 mg/dL	25% of normal dose
Bilirubin greater than 5 mg/dL	Not recommended

ULN = upper limit of normal.

DOXIL

Hepatic Function	Dosage
Bilirubin 1.2–3 mg/dL	50% of normal dose
Bilirubin greater than 3 mg/dL	25% of normal dose

SIDE EFFECTS

Frequent: Complete alopecia (scalp, axillary, pubic hair), nausea, vomiting, stomatitis, esophagitis (esp. if drug is given on several successive days), reddish urine. **Doxil:** Nausea. **Occasional:** Anorexia, diarrhea; hyperpigmentation of nailbeds, phalangeal, dermal creases. **Rare:** Fever, chills, conjunctivitis, lacrimation.

ADVERSE EFFECTS/ TOXIC REACTIONS

Myelosuppression manifested as hematologic toxicity (principally leukopenia and, to lesser extent, anemia, thrombocytopenia) generally occurs within 10–15 days, returns to normal levels by third wk. Cardiotoxicity (either acute, manifested as transient EKG abnormalities, or chronic, manifested as HF) may occur.

NURSING CONSIDERATIONS

BASELINE ASSESSMENT

Obtain ANC, CBC, erythrocyte counts before and at frequent intervals during therapy. Obtain EKG before therapy, LFT before each dose. Antiemetics may be effective in preventing, treating nausea. Offer emotional support.

INTERVENTION/EVALUATION

Monitor for stomatitis (burning or erythema of oral mucosa at inner margin of lips, difficulty swallowing). Observe IV injection site for infiltration, vein irritation. May lead to ulceration of mucous membranes within 2–3 days. Assess dermal creases, nailbeds for hyperpigmentation. Monitor hematologic status, renal/hepatic function studies, serum uric acid levels. Monitor daily pattern of bowel activity, stool consistency. Monitor for hematologic toxicity (fever, sore throat, signs of local infection, unusual bruising/bleeding from any site), symptoms of anemia (excessive fatigue, weakness).

PATIENT/FAMILY TEACHING

• Hair loss is reversible, but new hair growth may have different color, texture. New hair growth resumes 2–3 mos after last therapy dose. • Maintain strict oral hygiene. • Do not have immunizations without physician's approval (drug lowers resistance). • Avoid contact with those who have recently received live virus vaccine. • Promptly report fever, sore throat, signs of local infection, unusual bruising/bleeding from any site. • Report persistent nausea/vomiting. • Avoid alcohol (may cause GI irritation, a common side effect with liposomal DOXOrubicin).

---

doxycycline   TOP 100

dox-i-**sye**-kleen
(Acticlate, Adoxa, Apo-Doxy ✚,
Avidoxy, Doryx, Doxy-100, Monodox,
Oracea, Vibramycin)

Do not confuse doxycycline with dicyclomine or doxepin, Monodox with Maalox, Oracea with Orencia, Vibramycin with Vancomycin or Vibativ, or Vibra-Tabs with Vibativ.

◆CLASSIFICATION

PHARMACOTHERAPEUTIC: Tetracycline. **CLINICAL:** Antibiotic.

USES

Treatment of susceptible infections due to *H. ducreyi, Pasteurella pestis, P. tularensis, Bacteroides* spp., *V. cholerae, Brucella* spp., *Rickettsiae, Y. pestis, Francisella tularensis, M. pneumoniae,* including brucellosis, chlamydia, cholera, granuloma inguinale, lymphogranuloma venereum, malaria prophylaxis, nongonococcal urethritis, pelvic inflammatory disease (PID), plague, psittacosis, relapsing fever, rickettsia infections, primary and secondary syphilis, tularemia. **(Oracea):** Treatment of inflammatory lesions in adults with rosacea. **OFF-LABEL:** Sclerosing agent for pleural effusion; vancomycin-resistant enterococci (VRE); alternative for MRSA, treatment of refractory periodontitis, juvenile periodontitis.

PRECAUTIONS

Contraindications: Hypersensitivity to doxycycline, other tetracyclines. **Cautions:** History or predisposition to oral candidiasis (Oracea). Avoid use during pregnancy, during tooth development in children. Avoid prolonged exposure to sunlight.

ACTION

Inhibits bacterial protein synthesis by binding to ribosomes. **Therapeutic Effect:** Bacteriostatic.

PHARMACOKINETICS

Rapidly absorbed after PO administration. Protein binding: 90%. Partially excreted in urine; partially eliminated in bile. **Half-life:** 15–24 hrs.

⧖ LIFESPAN CONSIDERATIONS

Pregnancy/Lactation: Crosses placenta; distributed in breast milk. **Children:** May cause permanent discoloration of teeth, enamel hypoplasia. **Elderly:** No age-related precautions noted.

INTERACTIONS

DRUG: Antacids containing aluminum, calcium, magnesium; laxatives containing magnesium, oral iron preparations decrease absorption. **Barbiturates, carBAMazepine, phenytoin** may decrease concentration. **Cholestyramine, colestipol** may decrease absorption. May decrease effects of **oral contraceptives. HERBAL: Dong quai, St. John's wort** may increase photosensitization. **St. John's wort** may decrease concentration/effects. **FOOD:** None known. **LAB VALUES:** May increase serum alkaline phosphatase, amylase, bilirubin, ALT, AST. May alter CBC.

AVAILABILITY (Rx)

Capsules: 40 mg, 50 mg, 75 mg, 100 mg, 150 mg. **Injection, Powder for Reconstitution:** 100 mg. **Oral Suspension:** 25 mg/5 mL. **Syrup:** 50 mg/5 mL. **Tablets:** 20 mg, 50 mg, 75 mg, 100 mg, 150 mg.

🦮 **Tablets, delayed release:** 50 mg, 75 mg, 100 mg, 150 mg, 200 mg.

ADMINISTRATION/HANDLING

◀**ALERT**▶ Do not administer IM or subcutaneous. Space doses evenly around clock.

 IV

Reconstitution • Reconstitute each 100-mg vial with 10 mL Sterile Water for Injection for concentration of 10 mg/mL. • Further dilute each 100 mg with at least 100 mL D₅W, 0.9% NaCl, lactated Ringer's.
Rate of Administration • Give by intermittent IV infusion (piggyback). • Infuse over 1–4 hrs.
Storage • After reconstitution, IV infusion (piggyback) is stable for 12 hrs at room temperature or 72 hrs if refrigerated. • Protect from direct sunlight. Discard if precipitate forms.

PO
• Oral suspension is stable for 2 wks at room temperature. • Give with full glass of fluid. • Instruct pt to sit up for 30 min after taking to reduce risk of esophageal irritation and ulceration. • Give without regard to food. Oracea should be given 1 hr before or 2 hrs after meals. • Avoid concurrent use of antacids, milk; separate by 2 hrs.

▦ IV INCOMPATIBILITIES

Allopurinol (Aloprim), heparin, piperacillin/tazobactam (Zosyn).

▦ IV COMPATIBILITIES

Acyclovir (Zovirax), amiodarone (Cordarone), dexmedetomidine (Precedex), diltiaZEM (Cardizem), granisetron (Kytril), HYDROmorphone (Dilaudid), magnesium sulfate, meperidine (Demerol), morphine, ondansetron (Zofran), propofol (Diprivan).

INDICATIONS/ROUTES/DOSAGE

Usual Dosage
IV/PO: ADULTS, ELDERLY, CHILDREN OLDER THAN 8 YRS; WEIGHING MORE THAN 45 KG: 100–200 mg/day in 1–2 divided doses. **CHILDREN OLDER THAN 8 YRS; WEIGHING 45 KG OR LESS:** 2–4 mg/kg/day (**Maximum:** 200 mg/day) in 1–2 divided doses.

Dosage in Renal/Hepatic Impairment
No dose adjustment.

SIDE EFFECTS

Frequent: Anorexia, nausea, vomiting, diarrhea, dysphagia, photosensitivity (may be severe). **Occasional:** Rash, urticaria.

ADVERSE EFFECTS/TOXIC REACTIONS

Superinfection (esp. fungal), benign intracranial hypertension (headache, visual changes) may occur. Hepatotoxicity, fatty degeneration of liver, pancreatitis occur rarely.

D

NURSING CONSIDERATIONS

BASELINE ASSESSMENT

Question for history of allergies, esp. to tetracyclines, sulfites.

INTERVENTION/EVALUATION

Monitor daily pattern of bowel activity, stool consistency. Assess skin for rash. Monitor LOC due to potential for increased intracranial pressure (ICP). Be alert for superinfection: fever, vomiting, diarrhea, anal/genital pruritus, oral mucosal changes (ulceration, pain, erythema).

PATIENT/FAMILY TEACHING

• Avoid unnecessary exposure to sunlight. • Do not take with antacids, iron products. • Complete full course of therapy. • After application of dental gel, avoid brushing teeth, flossing the treated areas for 7 days. • Report severe diarrhea. • May cause nausea, vomiting. If GI upset occurs, may take with small amount food; however, Oracea should be taken on an empty stomach.

---

dronabinol

droe-**nab**-i-nol
(Marinol, Syndros)
Do not confuse dronabinol with droperidol.

◆CLASSIFICATION

PHARMACOTHERAPEUTIC: Cannabinoid **(Schedule III). CLINICAL:** Antinausea, antiemetic, appetite stimulant.

USES

Prevention, treatment of nausea/vomiting due to cancer chemotherapy; appetite stimulant in AIDS. **OFF-LABEL:** Cancer-related anorexia.

PRECAUTIONS

Contraindications: Hypersensitivity to dronabinol, sesame oil (capsule), alcohol (oral solution), tetrahydrocannabinol products, marijuana; receiving or recently received disulfiram- or metronidazole-containing products within 14 days (oral solution). **Cautions:** History of psychiatric illness, schizophrenia, history of substance abuse, mania, depression, seizure disorder, hepatic impairment, elderly.

ACTION

Exact mechanism unknown. May inhibit endorphins in brain's emetic center, suppress prostaglandins synthesis or effect on cannabinoid receptor in CNS. **Therapeutic Effect:** Inhibits nausea/vomiting, stimulates appetite.

PHARMACOKINETICS

Well absorbed after PO administration, only 10%–20% reaches systemic circulation. Protein binding: 97%. Undergoes first-pass metabolism. Highly lipid soluble. Primarily excreted in feces. **Half-life:** 25–36 hrs.

⧖ LIFESPAN CONSIDERATIONS

Pregnancy/Lactation: Unknown if drug crosses placenta. Distributed in breast milk. **Children:** Not recommended. **Elderly:** Monitor carefully during therapy.

INTERACTIONS

DRUG: Alcohol, other CNS suppressants (e.g., lorazepam, morphine, zolpidem) may increase CNS depression. **Sympathomimetics, tricyclic antidepressants (e.g., amitriptyline, doxepin, nortriptyline)** may increase risk of hypertension, tachycardia. **Anticholinergics (e.g., glycopyrrolate, scopolamine)** may increase drowsiness, tachycardia. **HERBAL: St. John's wort** may decrease concentration. **FOOD:** None known. **LAB VALUES:** None significant.

AVAILABILITY (Rx)

Capsules (Gelatin [Marinol]): 2.5 mg, 5 mg, 10 mg. **Oral Solution (Syndros):** 5 mg/mL.

ADMINISTRATION/HANDLING

PO
• Store in cool environment. May refrigerate capsules. • May administer without regard to meals. Give before meals if used for appetite stimulant. • **Oral solution:** Always use enclosed calibrated syringe. Take each dose with a full glass of water.

INDICATIONS/ROUTES/DOSAGE

Prevention of Chemotherapy-Induced Nausea and Vomiting
PO: ADULTS, ELDERLY, CHILDREN: *(Marinol):* Initially, 5 mg/m^2 1–3 hrs before chemotherapy, then q2–4h after chemotherapy for total of 4–6 doses/day. May increase by 2.5 mg/m^2 up to 15 mg/m^2 per dose. *(Syndros):* Initially, 2.1–4.2 mg/m^2 1–2 hrs prior to chemotherapy, then q2–4 hrs after chemotherapy for total of 4–6 doses/day. May increase in increments of 2.1 mg/m^2. **Maximum:** 12.6 mg/m^2/dose and 4 to 6 doses per day.

Appetite Stimulant
PO: ADULTS, ELDERLY: *(Marinol):* Initially, 2.5 mg twice daily (before lunch and dinner). Range: 2.5–20 mg/day. *(Syndros):* Initially, 2.1 mg twice daily. May gradually increase dose in 2.1-mg increments. **Maximum:** 8.4 mg twice daily.

Dosage in Renal/Hepatic Impairment
No dose adjustment.

SIDE EFFECTS

Frequent (24%–3%): Euphoria, dizziness, paranoid reaction, drowsiness. **Occasional (less than 3%–1%):** Asthenia, ataxia, confusion, abnormal thinking, depersonalization. **Rare (less than 1%):** Diarrhea, depression, nightmares, speech difficulties, headache, anxiety, tinnitus, flushed skin.

ADVERSE EFFECTS/TOXIC REACTIONS

Mild intoxication may produce increased sensory awareness (taste, smell, sound), altered time perception, reddened conjunctiva, dry mouth, tachycardia. Moderate intoxication may produce memory impairment, urinary retention. Severe intoxication may produce lethargy, decreased motor coordination, slurred speech, orthostatic hypotension.

NURSING CONSIDERATIONS

BASELINE ASSESSMENT
Assess dehydration status if excessive vomiting occurs (skin turgor, mucous membranes, urinary output).

INTERVENTION/EVALUATION
Supervise closely for serious mood, behavioral responses, esp. in pts with history of psychiatric illness. Monitor B/P, heart rate.

PATIENT/FAMILY TEACHING
• Change positions slowly to avoid dizziness. • Relief from nausea/vomiting generally occurs within 15 min of drug administration. • Do not take any other medications, including OTC, without physician approval. • Avoid alcohol, barbiturates. • Avoid tasks that require alertness, motor skills until response to drug is established. • For appetite stimulation, take before lunch and dinner.

dulaglutide

doo-la-**gloo**-tide
(Trulicity)

■ **BLACK BOX ALERT** ■ Contraindicated in pts with a personal/family history of medullary thyroid carcinoma (MTC) or in pts with multiple endocrine neoplasia syndrome type 2 (MEN2). Unknown if dulaglutide causes thyroid cell tumors in humans.

Do not confuse dulaglutide with albiglutide or liraglutide.

◆CLASSIFICATION

PHARMACOTHERAPEUTIC: GLP-1 receptor agonist. **CLINICAL:** Antidiabetic.

D

USES

Adjunct to diet and exercise to improve glycemic control in pts with type 2 diabetes mellitus.

PRECAUTIONS

Contraindications: Hypersensitivity to dulaglutide, other GLP-1 receptor agonists. Personal/family history of medullary thyroid carcinoma or multiple endocrine neoplasia syndrome type 2. **Cautions:** Pts with increased serum calcitonin, thyroid nodules, hx pancreatitis, renal/hepatic impairment. Not recommended in pts with severe GI disease, diabetic ketoacidosis, or type 1 diabetes.

ACTION

Activates GLP-1 receptors in pancreatic beta cells increasing intracellular cyclic AMP. **Therapeutic Effect:** Augments glucose-dependent insulin release, slows gastric emptying. Improves glycemic control.

PHARMACOKINETICS

Readily absorbed following subcutaneous administration. Degraded into amino acids by general protein catabolism. Peak plasma concentration: 24–72 hrs. Steady state reached in 2–4 wks. Elimination not specified. **Half-life:** 5 days.

⌛ LIFESPAN CONSIDERATIONS

Pregnancy/Lactation: Unknown if distributed in breast milk. Must either discontinue drug or discontinue breastfeeding. **Children:** Safety and efficacy not established in pts younger than 18 yrs. **Elderly:** No age-related precautions noted.

INTERACTIONS

DRUG: Insulin, insulin secretagogues (e.g., glyBURIDE) may increase risk of hypoglycemia. May reduce rate of absorption of oral medications. **HERBAL: Garlic,** other herbs with hypoglycemic activity may increase the risk of hypoglycemia. **FOOD:** None known. **LAB VALUES:** Expected to decrease serum glucose, Hgb A1c. May increase amylase, lipase.

AVAILABILITY (Rx)

Prefilled Injector Pen or Syringe: 0.75 mg/0.5 mL, 1.5 mg/0.5 mL.

ADMINISTRATION/HANDLING

Subcutaneous
• Administer any time of day, without regard to meals, on same day each week. • May change administration day if last dose was given more than 3 days prior. If dose missed, administer within 3 days of missed dose. If more than 3 days have passed after missed dose, wait until next regularly scheduled dose to administer.
Administrations • Subcutaneously insert needle into abdomen, thigh, or upper arm region and inject solution. • Do not reuse needle. • Rotate injection sites each week.
Storage • Refrigerate unused pens/syringes; do not freeze. • May store at room temperature for up to 14 days. • Protect from light.

INDICATIONS/ROUTES/DOSAGE

Type 2 Diabetes Mellitus
SQ: ADULTS/ELDERLY: 0.75 mg once wkly. May increase to 1.5 mg once wkly if glycemic response inadequate. **Maximum:** 1.5 mg wkly.

Dose Modification
Concomitant Use with Insulin Secretagogue (e.g., Sulfonylurea) or Insulin: Consider reduced dose of insulin secretagogue or insulin based on glycemic goal.

Dosage in Renal Impairment
No dose adjustment.

Dosage in Hepatic Impairment
Use caution.

SIDE EFFECTS

Occasional (12%–6%): Nausea, diarrhea, vomiting, abdominal pain. **Rare (4% or less):** Decreased appetite, dyspepsia, fatigue, asthenia.

ADVERSE EFFECTS/ TOXIC REACTIONS

May increase risk of acute renal failure or worsening of chronic renal impairment (esp. with dehydration), severe gastroparesis, pancreatitis, thyroid C-cell tumors. May increase risk of hypoglycemia when used with other hypoglycemic agents or insulin. Dyspnea, pruritus, rash may indicate hypersensitivity reaction. May prolong PR interval by 2–3 msec or may rarely cause first-degree AV block, tachycardia. Immunogenicity (antidulaglutide antibody formation) reported. Some pts with antibody formation also tested positive for antibodies to GLP-1 and human albumin.

NURSING CONSIDERATIONS

BASELINE ASSESSMENT

Obtain baseline fasting glucose level, Hgb A1c, BMP. Question history of medullary thyroid carcinoma, multiple endocrine neoplasia syndrome type 2, pancreatitis, renal impairment; first-degree AV block, PR interval prolongation. Receive full medication history and screen for use of other hypoglycemic agents or insulin. Assess pt's understanding of diabetes management, routine home glucose monitoring, medication self-administration. Assess hydration status.

INTERVENTION/EVALUATION

Monitor capillary blood glucose levels, Hgb A1c; renal function test in pts with renal impairment reporting severe GI reactions, including diarrhea, gastroparesis, vomiting. Screen for thyroid tumors (dysphagia, dyspnea, persistent hoarseness, neck mass). If tumor suspected, consider endocrinologist consultation. Clinical significance of serum calcitonin level or thyroid ultrasound with

GLP-1–associated thyroid tumors is debated/unknown. Assess for hypoglycemia, hyperglycemia, hypersensitivity/ allergic reaction. Screen for glucose-altering conditions: fever, stress, surgical procedures, trauma. Obtain dietary consult for nutritional education. Encourage PO intake.

PATIENT/FAMILY TEACHING

• Diabetes requires lifelong control. Diet and exercise are principal parts of treatment; do not skip or delay meals. Test blood sugar regularly. Monitor daily calorie intake. • When taking additional medications to lower blood sugar or when glucose demands are altered (fever, infection, stress, trauma), have low blood sugar treatment available (glucagon, oral dextrose). • Report suspected pregnancy or plans for breastfeeding. • Therapy may increase risk of thyroid cancer; report lumps or swelling of the neck; hoarseness, shortness of breath, trouble swallowing. • Persistent, severe abdominal pain that radiates to the back (with or without vomiting) may indicate acute pancreatitis. • Rash, itching, hives may indicate allergic reaction.

DULoxetine ^{TOP 100}

du-**lox**-e-teen
(Apo-Duloxetine ♣, <u>Cymbalta</u>, Irenka)
■ **BLACK BOX ALERT** ■ Increased risk of suicidal thinking and behavior in children, adolescents, young adults 18–24 yrs with major depressive disorder, other psychiatric disorders.
Do not confuse DULoxetine with FLUoxetine or PARoxetine.

◆CLASSIFICATION

PHARMACOTHERAPEUTIC: Serotonin norepinephrine reuptake inhibitor (SNRI). **CLINICAL:** Antidepressant.

D

USES

Treatment of major depression. Management of pain associated with diabetic neuropathy or chronic musculoskeletal pain. Treatment of generalized anxiety disorder. **Cymbalta only:** Treatment of fibromyalgia. **OFF-LABEL:** Treatment of stress urinary incontinence in women.

PRECAUTIONS

Contraindications: Hypersensitivity to DULoxetine. Uncontrolled narrow-angle glaucoma. Use of MAOI intended to treat psychiatric disorder (concurrent or within 14 days of discontinuing MAOI). Initiation of MAOI intended to treat psychiatric disorder within 5 days of discontinuing DULoxetine. Initiation of DULoxetine in pt receiving linezolid or IV methylene blue. **Cautions:** Renal impairment, history of alcoholism, chronic hepatic disease, history of mania, pts with suicidal ideation or behavior. Concurrent use with inhibitors of CYP1A2 or thioridazine, CNS depressants. Hypertension, controlled narrow-angle glaucoma, pts with impaired GI motility. Concomitant use of NSAIDs (may increase risk of bleeding), history of seizures. Use of medications that lower seizure threshold; elderly; pts at high risk for suicide.

ACTION

Appears to inhibit serotonin and norepinephrine reuptake at CNS neuronal presynaptic membranes; is a less potent inhibitor of DOPamine reuptake. **Therapeutic Effect:** Produces antidepressant effect.

PHARMACOKINETICS

Well absorbed from GI tract. Protein binding: greater than 90%. Metabolized in liver. Excreted in urine (70%), feces (20%). **Half-life:** 8–17 hrs.

⌛ LIFESPAN CONSIDERATIONS

Pregnancy/Lactation: May produce neonatal adverse reactions (constant crying, feeding difficulty, hyperreflexia, irritability). Unknown if distributed in breast milk. Breastfeeding not recommended. **Children:** Safety and efficacy not established. **Elderly:** Caution required when increasing dosage.

INTERACTIONS

DRUG: Alcohol increases risk of hepatic injury. **CYP1A2** and **CYP2D6 inhibitors (e.g., FLUoxetine, fluvoxaMINE, PARoxetine, quiNIDine, quinolone antimicrobials)** may increase plasma concentration. **MAOIs** may cause serotonin syndrome (autonomic hyperactivity, coma, diaphoresis, excitement, hyperthermia, rigidity). **Aspirin, NSAIDs (e.g., ibuprofen, ketorolac, naproxen)** may increase risk of bleeding. May increase concentration, potential toxicity of **tricyclic antidepressants. Serotonergic drugs (e.g., triptans, lithium, traMADol)** may increase risk of serotonin syndrome. **HERBAL: Gotu kola, kava kava, St. John's wort, valerian** may increase CNS depression. **St. John's wort** may increase risk of serotonin syndrome. **FOOD:** None known. **LAB VALUES:** May increase serum bilirubin, ALT, AST, alkaline phosphatase.

AVAILABILITY (Rx)

🖋 **Capsules (Delayed-Release, Enteric-Coated Pellets):** 20 mg, 30 mg, 40 mg, 60 mg.

ADMINISTRATION/HANDLING

◀**ALERT**▶ Allow at least 14 days to elapse between use of MAOIs and DULoxetine.

PO
• Give without regard to meals. Give with food, milk if GI distress occurs. • Do not break, crush, cut delayed-release capsules. • Contents of capsule may be sprinkled on applesauce or mixed in apple juice and swallowed (without chewing) immediately.

INDICATIONS/ROUTES/DOSAGE

Fibromyalgia
PO: ADULTS, ELDERLY: Initially, 30 mg/day for 1 wk. Increase to 60 mg/day.

Major Depressive Disorder
PO: ADULTS, ELDERLY: Initially, 40–60 mg/day in 1 or 2 divided doses. For doses greater than 60 mg/day, titrate in increments of 30 mg/day over 1 wk. **Maximum:** 120 mg/day.

Diabetic Neuropathy Pain
PO: ADULTS, ELDERLY: 60 mg once daily. **Maximum:** 60 mg/day. Consider lower dose with renal impairment or if tolerability is a concern.

Generalized Anxiety Disorder
PO: ADULTS, ELDERLY: Initially, 30–60 mg once daily. May increase up to 120 mg/day in 30-mg increments wkly. **CHILDREN 7–17 YRS:** Initially, 30 mg once daily. After 2 wks, may increase to 60 mg once daily. May further increase in increments of 30 mg/day at wkly intervals. **Maximum:** 120 mg/day.

Chronic Musculoskeletal Pain
PO: ADULTS, ELDERLY: 30 mg once daily for 1 wk, then increase to 60 mg once daily. **Maximum:** 60 mg/day.

Dosage in Renal/Hepatic Impairment
Renal: Not recommended with CrCl less than 30 mL/min or ESRD. **Hepatic:** Not recommended.

SIDE EFFECTS

Frequent (20%–11%): Nausea, dry mouth, constipation, insomnia. **Occasional (9%–5%):** Dizziness, fatigue, diarrhea, drowsiness, anorexia, diaphoresis, vomiting. **Rare (4%–2%):** Blurred vision, erectile dysfunction, delayed or failed ejaculation, anorgasmia, anxiety, decreased libido, hot flashes.

ADVERSE EFFECTS/TOXIC REACTIONS

May slightly increase heart rate. Colitis, dysphagia, gastritis, irritable bowel syndrome occur rarely.

NURSING CONSIDERATIONS

BASELINE ASSESSMENT

Assess appearance, behavior, speech pattern, level of interest, mood, sleep pattern, suicidal tendencies. Question pain level, intensity, location of pain.

INTERVENTION/EVALUATION

For pts on long-term therapy, serum chemistry profile to assess hepatic/renal function should be performed periodically. Supervise suicidal-risk pt closely during early therapy (as depression lessens, energy level improves, increasing suicide potential). Monitor B/P, mental status, anxiety, social functioning, serum glucose levels.

PATIENT/FAMILY TEACHING

• Therapeutic effect may be noted within 1–4 wks. • Do not abruptly discontinue medication. • Avoid tasks that require alertness, motor skills until response to drug is established. • Inform physician of intention of pregnancy or if pregnancy occurs. • Report anxiety, agitation, panic attacks, worsening of depression. • Avoid heavy alcohol intake (associated with severe hepatic injury).

durvalumab

dur-**val**-ue-mab
(Imfinzi)
Do not confuse durvalumab with daclizumab, dupilumab, or nivolumab.

◆CLASSIFICATION

PHARMACOTHERAPEUTIC: Anti-programmed death ligand-1 (PD-L1). Monoclonal antibody. **CLINICAL:** Antineoplastic.

USES

Treatment of pts with locally advanced or metastatic urothelial carcinoma who have disease progression during or following platinum-containing chemotherapy or have disease progression within 12 mos of neoadjuvant or adjuvant treatment with platinum-containing chemotherapy.

PRECAUTIONS

Contraindications: Hypersensitivity to durvalumab. **Cautions:** Active infection, conditions predisposing to infection (e.g., diabetes, immunocompromised pts, renal failure, open wounds); corticosteroid intolerance, baseline hematologic cytopenias, elderly pts, hepatic impairment, interstitial lung disease, renal insufficiency; history of autoimmune disorders (Crohn's disease, demyelinating polyneuropathy, Guillain-Barré syndrome, Hashimoto's thyroiditis, hyperthyroidism, myasthenia gravis, rheumatoid arthritis, Type I diabetes, vasculitis); diabetes, pancreatitis.

ACTION

Blocks programmed cell death ligand 1 (PD-L1) binding to PD-1 and CD80 (B7.1). PD-L1 blockade increases T-cell activation allowing T-cells to kill tumor cells. Restores antitumor T-cell function. **Therapeutic Effect:** Inhibits tumor cell growth and metastasis.

PHARMACOKINETICS

Widely distributed. Metabolism not specified. Steady state reached in 16 wks. Excretion not specified. **Half-life:** 17 days.

⧗ LIFESPAN CONSIDERATIONS

Pregnancy/Lactation: Avoid pregnancy; may cause fetal harm. Females of reproductive potential should use effective contraception during treatment and for at least 3 mos after discontinuation. Unknown if distributed in breast milk; however, human immunoglobulin G (IgG) is present in breast milk and is known to cross the placenta. Breastfeeding not recommended during treatment and for at least 3 mos after discontinuation. **Children:** Safety and efficacy not established. **Elderly:** May have increased risk of toxic reactions; use caution.

INTERACTIONS

DRUG: May enhance adverse effects/ toxicity of **belimumab**. **HERBAL:** None significant. **FOOD:** None known. **LAB VALUES:** May increase serum albumin, alkaline phosphatase, ALT, AST, bilirubin, calcium, creatinine, glucose, magnesium. May decrease serum sodium; Hgb, Hct, lymphocytes, neutrophils, RBCs. May increase or decrease serum potassium.

AVAILABILITY (Rx)

Injection: 120 mg/2.4 mL (50 mg/mL), 500 mg/10 mL (50 mg/mL).

ADMINISTRATION/HANDLING
💉 IV

Preparation • Visually inspect vial for particulate matter or discoloration. Solution should appear clear to opalescent, colorless to slightly yellow in color. • Do not use if solution is cloudy, discolored, or if visible particles are observed. • Do not shake. • Withdraw proper volume from vial and dilute in 0.9% NaCl or D_5W to a final concentration of 1–15 mg/ mL. • Gently invert to mix; do not shake. • Diluted solution should appear clear, colorless, and free of particles.
Rate of Administration • Infuse over 60 mins via dedicated IV line using a sterile, low protein-binding 0.2- or 0.22-micron in-line filter.
Storage • Refrigerate unused vials in original carton. • Protect from light. May refrigerate diluted solution for no more than 24 hrs or store at room temperature for no more than 4 hrs. If refrigerated, allow diluted solution to warm to room temperature before use. • Do not freeze or shake.

▓ IV INCOMPATIBILITIES

Do not infuse with other medications.

INDICATIONS/ROUTES/DOSAGE
Urothelial Carcinoma
IV: ADULTS, ELDERLY: 10 mg/kg q2wks. Continue until disease progression or unacceptable toxicity.

Dose Modification

Note: Withhold and/or discontinue durvalumab to manage adverse reactions. Based on severity of adverse reactions, withhold durvalumab and administer systemic corticosteroids. Initiate corticosteroid taper when adverse reactions improve to below grade 1, and continue taper over at least 1 mo. If treatment is not permanently discontinued due to adverse reactions, resume therapy when adverse reactions return to grade 1 or lower and the corticosteroid dose has been reduced to less than 10 mg prednisone (or equivalent) per day. No dose reductions of durvalumab are recommended.

Colitis (GI Toxicity)

Grade 2 diarrhea or colitis: Withhold dose. Start prednisone 1–2 mg/kg/day (or equivalent) followed by taper. **Grade 3 or 4 diarrhea or colitis:** Permanently discontinue. Start prednisone 1–2 mg/kg/day (or equivalent), followed by taper.

Dermatitis

Grade 2 rash or dermatitis (for greater than 1 wk); grade 3 rash or dermatitis: Withhold dose. Consider starting prednisone 1–2 mg/kg/day (or equivalent), followed by taper. **Grade 4 rash or dermatitis:** Permanently discontinue. Consider starting prednisone 1–2 mg/kg/day (or equivalent), followed by taper.

Endocrinopathies

Grade 2–4 adrenal insufficiency (hypophysitis, hypopituitarism): Withhold dose until clinically stable. Start prednisone 1–2 mg/kg/day (or equivalent), followed by taper. Consider hormone replacement therapy as clinically indicated. **Grade 2–4 hyperthyroidism:** Withhold dose until clinically stable and manage symptoms. **Grade 2–4 hypothyroidism:** Consider hormone replacement therapy. **Grade 2–4 type 1 diabetes:** Withhold dose until clinically stable. Start insulin therapy as clinically indicated.

Hepatitis (Hepatotoxicity During Treatment)

Grade 2 hepatitis (serum ALT or AST greater than 3 and up to 5 times upper limit of normal [ULN] or serum bilirubin greater than 1.5 and up to 3 times ULN); grade 3 hepatitis (serum ALT or AST less than or equal to 8 times ULN or serum bilirubin less than or equal to 5 times ULN): Withhold dose. Start prednisone 1–2 mg/kg/day (or equivalent), followed by taper. **Grade 3 hepatitis (serum ALT or AST greater than 8 times ULN or serum bilirubin greater than 5 times ULN; transaminase elevation (concurrent serum ALT or AST greater than 3 times ULN and serum bilirubin greater than 2 times ULN) with no known cause:** Permanently discontinue. Start prednisone 1–2 mg/kg/day (or equivalent), followed by taper.

Infection

Grade 3 or 4 infection: Withhold dose and manage symptoms. Start anti-infectives for suspected or confirmed infections.

Infusion-Related Reactions

Grade 1 or 2 infusion reactions: Interrupt or decrease rate of infusion. Consider premedication for subsequent infusions. **Grade 3 or 4 infusion reactions:** Permanently discontinue.

Nephritis (Renal Toxicity During Treatment)

Grade 2 nephritis (serum creatinine greater than 1.5 and up to 3 times ULN): Withhold dose. Start prednisone 1–2 mg/kg/day (or equivalent), followed by taper. **Grade 3 nephritis (serum creatinine greater than 3 and up to 6 times ULN); grade 4 nephritis (serum creatinine greater than 6 times ULN):** Permanently discontinue. Start prednisone 1–2 mg/kg/day (or equivalent), followed by taper.

Other Toxic Reactions

Any other grade 3 reactions: Withhold dose and manage symptoms. **Any other grade 4 reactions:** Permanently discontinue. Start prednisone 1–4 mg/kg/day (or equivalent), followed by taper.

Pneumonitis
Grade 2 pneumonitis: Withhold dose. Start prednisone 1–2 mg/kg/day (or equivalent), followed by taper. **Grade 3 or grade 4 pneumonitis:** Permanently discontinue. Start prednisone 1–4 mg/kg/day (or equivalent) followed by taper.

Dosage in Renal/Hepatic Impairment (Prior to Treatment Initiation)
Not specified; use caution.

SIDE EFFECTS

Frequent (39%–19%): Fatigue, asthenia, malaise, back/musculoskeletal/neck pain, myalgia, constipation, decreased appetite. **Occasional (16%–11%):** Nausea, peripheral edema, scrotal edema, lymphedema, abdominal/flank pain, diarrhea, pyrexia, dyspnea, cough, dermatitis, dermatitis acneiform, dermatitis psoriasiform, psoriasis, maculopapular rash, pustular rash, eczema, erythema, erythema multiforme, erythematous rash, acne, lichen planus.

ADVERSE EFFECTS/TOXIC REACTIONS

Anemia, neutropenia, lymphopenia are expected responses to therapy. May cause severe, sometimes fatal immune-mediated reactions such as adrenal insufficiency (1% of pts), colitis (2% of pts), hepatitis (1% of pts), hypothyroidism (9% of pts), hyperthyroidism (6% of pts), hypophysitis, nephritis (less than 1% of pts), pneumonitis (2% of pts), type 1 diabetes (less than 1% of pts), rash (15% of pts); aseptic meningitis, hemolytic anemia, keratitis, myocarditis, myositis, thrombocytopenic purpura, uveitis. Urinary tract infections including candiduria, cystitis, urosepsis occurred in 15% of pts. Immunogenicity (auto-durvalumab antibodies) reported in 3% of pts.

NURSING CONSIDERATIONS

BASELINE ASSESSMENT

Obtain CBC, BMP, LFT, serum ionized calcium, magnesium; thyroid function test; urine pregnancy; vital signs. Question medical history as listed in Precautions; prior infusion reactions. Question intolerance to corticosteroids. Verify use of effective contraception in females of reproductive potential. Screen for active infection. Assess nutritional/hydration status. Conduct neurologic/dermatologic exam. Offer emotional support.

INTERVENTION/EVALUATION

Monitor CBC, BMP, LFT, serum ionized calcium, magnesium; thyroid function test periodically. Monitor for infusion reactions including angioedema, back or neck pain, dyspnea, flushing, pruritus, pyrexia, rash, syncope. Consider increasing corticosteroid dose if toxic effects worsen or do not improve. Assess skin for rash, lesions. Diligently monitor for immune-mediated adverse effects as listed in Adverse Effects/Toxic Reactions. Notify physician if any CTCAE toxicities occur and initiate proper treatment. If immune-mediated reactions occur, consider referral to specialist. Obtain CXR if interstitial lung disease, pneumonitis suspected. Interrupt or discontinue treatment if serious infection, opportunistic infection, sepsis occurs, and initiate appropriate antimicrobial therapy. If corticosteroid therapy is started, monitor capillary blood glucose and screen for corticosteroid side effects or intolerance. Report neurologic changes including nuchal rigidity with fever, positive Kernig's sign, positive Brudzinski's sign, altered mental status, seizures (related to aseptic meningitis). Strictly monitor I&O. Encourage fluid intake.

PATIENT/FAMILY TEACHING

• Treatment may depress your immune system and reduce your ability to fight infection. Report symptoms of infection such as body aches, chills, cough, fatigue, fever. Avoid those with active infection. • Avoid pregnancy; treatment may cause birth defects. Do not breastfeed. Females of childbearing potential should use effective contraception during treatment and for at least 3 mos after final dose. • Treatment may cause serious or life-threatening inflammatory reactions. Report signs and symptoms of treatment-related inflammatory events in the following body systems: brain (confusion, headache, fever, rigid neck, seizures), colon (severe abdominal pain or diarrhea), eye (blurry vision, double vision, unequal pupil size, sensitivity to light, drooping eyelid), lung (chest pain, cough, shortness of breath), liver (bruising easily, amber-colored urine, clay-colored/tarry stools, yellowing of skin or eyes), nerves (severe nerve pain or loss of motor function), pituitary (persistent or unusual headache, dizziness, extreme weakness, fainting, vision changes), thyroid (trouble sleeping, high blood pressure, fast heart rate [overactive thyroid] or fatigue, goiter, weight gain [underactive thyroid]). Immediately report infusion reactions such as neck or back pain, dizziness, fever, flushing, itching, shortness of breath, swelling of the face. • Treatment may cause severe diarrhea. Drink plenty of fluids.

edoxaban

e-**dox**-a-ban
(Savaysa)

■ **BLACK BOX ALERT** ■ Avoid use in nonvalvular atrial fibrillation pts with creatinine clearance (CrCl) greater than 95 mL/min (increased risk of ischemic stroke). Premature discontinuation of oral anticoagulant in the absence of alternative anticoagulation may increase risk of ischemic events. If treatment is discontinued for any reason other than pathologic bleeding or completion of course of therapy, consider coverage with another anticoagulant as described in transition guideline. Epidural or spinal hematomas may occur in pts who are receiving neuraxial anesthesia or undergoing spinal puncture, which may result in long-term or permanent paralysis. **Do not confuse edoxaban with apixaban or rivaroxaban.**

◆CLASSIFICATION

PHARMACOTHERAPEUTIC: Factor Xa inhibitor. **CLINICAL:** Anticoagulant.

USES

To reduce risk of stroke and systemic embolism (SE) in pts with nonvalvular atrial fibrillation (NVAF). Treatment of deep vein thrombosis (DVT) and pulmonary embolism (PE) following 5–10 days of initial therapy with a parenteral anticoagulant.

PRECAUTIONS

Contraindications: Hypersensitivity to edoxaban. Major active bleeding. **Cautions:** Elderly, pts at increased risk of bleeding (e.g., prior CVA, thrombocytopenia, severe uncontrolled hypertension; history of bleeding ulcers, upper or lower GI bleeding), recent surgery, renal/hepatic impairment. Avoid concomitant use with aspirin, heparin, low molecular weight heparin (LMWH), NSAIDs, P-gp inducers (e.g., rifAMPin). Not recommended in pts with CrCl greater than 95 mL/min (increased risk of ischemic stroke); mechanical heart valves; moderate to severe mitral stenosis.

ACTION

Selectively blocks active site of factor Xa, a key factor in the intrinsic and extrinsic pathway of blood coagulation cascade. Inhibits platelet activation and fibrin clot formation. **Therapeutic Effect:** Inhibits blood coagulation.

PHARMACOKINETICS

Readily absorbed after PO administration. Peak plasma concentration: 1–2 hrs. Steady state reached within 3 days. Protein binding: 55%. Primarily excreted in urine (50%), biliary/intestinal excretion (remaining %). Not removed by hemodialysis. **Half-life:** 10–14 hrs.

⧖ LIFESPAN CONSIDERATIONS

Pregnancy/Lactation: Unknown if excreted in breast milk. **Children:** Safety and efficacy not established. **Elderly:** May have increased risk of bleeding due to age-related renal impairment.

INTERACTIONS

DRUG: Anticoagulants (e.g., warfarin), antiplatelets (e.g., clopidogrel), NSAIDs **(e.g., ibuprofen, ketorolac, naproxen), fibrinolytic therapy (e.g., TPA)** may increase concentration/effect; may increase risk of bleeding. **HERBAL:** None significant. **FOOD:** None known. **LAB VALUES:** May increase serum AST, ALT. May prolong aPTT, PT/INR.

AVAILABILITY (Rx)

🏷 **Tablets:** 15 mg, 30 mg, 60 mg.

ADMINISTRATION/HANDLING

PO
• Give without regard to meals. • Do not administer within 2 hrs of removal of epidural or intrathecal catheters.

INDICATIONS/ROUTES/DOSAGE

Nonvalvular Atrial Fibrillation
PO: ADULTS, ELDERLY: 60 mg once daily.

DVT/PE
PO: ADULTS, ELDERLY: 60 mg once daily following 5–10 days of initial therapy with a parenteral anticoagulant.

Dose Modification
Body weight less than or equal to 60 kg or concomitant use of certain P-gp inhibitors: 30 mg once daily.

Dosage in Renal Impairment
DVT/PE
CrCl 15–50 mL/min: 30 mg once daily. **CrCl less than 15 mL/min:** Not recommended.

NVAF
CrCl greater than 95 mL/min: Not recommended. **CrCl 51–95 mL/min:** No dose adjustment. **CrCl 15–50 mL/min:** 30 mg once daily. **CrCl less than 15 mL/min:** Not recommended.

Dosage in Hepatic Impairment
Mild impairment: No dose adjustment. **Moderate to severe impairment:** Not recommended.

Discontinuation for Surgery or Other Interventions
Discontinue at least 24 hrs before invasive surgical procedures. May restart as soon as adequate hemostasis is achieved, noting that the time of onset of pharmacodynamic effect is 1–2 hrs.

Transition Guideline to Edoxaban
From warfarin or other vitamin K antagonists: Discontinue warfarin and start edoxaban when INR is less than or equal to 2.5. **From oral anticoagulants other than warfarin or other vitamin K antagonists:** Discontinue current oral anticoagulant and start edoxaban at the time of the next scheduled dose of the other oral anticoagulant. **From LMWH:** Discontinue LMWH and start edoxaban at the time of the next scheduled dose of LMWH. **From low unfractionated heparin:** Discontinue infusion and start edoxaban 4 hrs later.

Transition Guideline from Edoxaban to Other Anticoagulant
To Warfarin: Oral option: For pts taking edoxaban 60 mg, reduce to 30 mg and begin warfarin concomitantly. For pts taking edoxaban 30 mg, reduce dose to 15 mg and begin warfarin concomitantly. Once stable INR greater than or equal to 2, discontinue edoxaban and continue warfarin. **Parenteral option:** Discontinue edoxaban and administer parenteral anticoagulant and warfarin at the time of next scheduled edoxaban dose. Once stable INR greater than or equal to 2, discontinue parenteral anticoagulant and continue warfarin. **To non–vitamin K-dependent oral anticoagulant or parenteral anticoagulant:** Discontinue edoxaban and start other oral anticoagulant at the time of the next scheduled dose.

SIDE EFFECTS

Rare (4%): Rash.

ADVERSE EFFECTS/TOXIC REACTIONS

Hemorrhagic events including intracranial hemorrhage, hemorrhagic stroke, cutaneous/GI/GU/oral/pharyngeal/urethral/vaginal bleeding, epistaxis, epidural/spinal hematoma (esp. with epidural catheters, spinal trauma) were reported. Discontinuation in the absence of other adequate anticoagulants may increase the risk of ischemic events, stroke. May increase risk of epidural or spinal hematomas, which can lead to long-term or permanent paralysis. Protamine sulfate, vitamin K, tranexamic acid are not expected to reverse anticoagulant effect. Interstitial lung disease was reported in less than 1% of pts.

NURSING CONSIDERATIONS

BASELINE ASSESSMENT

Obtain baseline renal function test, esp. creatinine clearance; PT/INR in pts transitioning on or off warfarin therapy. Do not initiate if CrCl greater than 95 mL/min. Question history of bleeding disorders, recent surgery, spinal procedures,

E

intracranial hemorrhage, bleeding ulcers, open wounds, anemia, renal/hepatic impairment, trauma. Receive full medication history including herbal products.

INTERVENTION/EVALUATION

Monitor renal function test; occult urine/stool, urine output. Monitor for symptoms of hemorrhage: abdominal/back pain, headache, altered mental status, weakness, paresthesia, aphasia, vision changes, GI bleeding. Question for increase in menstrual bleeding/discharge. Assess peripheral pulses; skin for ecchymosis, petechiae. Assess urine output for hematuria.

PATIENT/FAMILY TEACHING

• Do not discontinue current blood thinning regimen or take any newly prescribed medication unless approved by physician who started anticoagulant therapy. • Suddenly stopping therapy may increase risk of stroke or blood clots. Refill prescriptions so that next scheduled dose is not missed. • Immediately report bleeding of any kind. • Avoid alcohol, aspirin, NSAIDs. • Consult physician before surgery/dental work. • Use electric razor, soft toothbrush to prevent bleeding. • Report any numbness, muscular weakness, signs of stroke (confusion, headache, one-sided weakness, trouble speaking), bloody stool or urine, nosebleeds. • Monitor changes in urine output.

efavirenz

e-fav-ir-enz
(Sustiva)

FIXED-COMBINATION(S)

Atripla: efavirenz/emtricitabine (an antiretroviral)/tenofovir (an antiretroviral): 600 mg/200 mg/300 mg.

◆CLASSIFICATION

PHARMACOTHERAPEUTIC: Nonnucleoside reverse transcriptase inhibitor. **CLINICAL:** Antiretroviral.

USES

Treatment of HIV infection, in combination with at least two other appropriate antiretroviral agents, in adults and children 3 mos and older weighing at least 3.5 kg.

PRECAUTIONS

Contraindications: Hypersensitivity to efavirenz. **Cautions:** History of mental illness, seizures, suspected hepatitis B or C virus infection, history of substance abuse, hepatic impairment (class A). Avoid pregnancy.

ACTION

Binds to reverse transcriptase, blocking RNA and DNA-dependent DNA polymerase activity, including HIV-1 replication. **Therapeutic Effect:** Interrupts HIV replication, slowing progression of HIV infection.

PHARMACOKINETICS

Rapidly absorbed after PO administration. Protein binding: 99%. Metabolized in liver. Excreted in feces (16%–61%), urine (14%–34%). **Half-life:** 40–55 hrs.

⌛ LIFESPAN CONSIDERATIONS

Pregnancy/Lactation: Avoid pregnancy during treatment and up to 12 wks after discontinuation. Breastfeeding not recommended. **Children:** Safety and efficacy not established in pts younger than 3 yrs; may have increased incidence of rash. **Elderly:** No age-related precautions noted.

INTERACTIONS

DRUG: Ergot derivatives, midazolam, triazolam may cause serious or life-threatening reactions (cardiac arrhythmias, prolonged sedation, respiratory depression). Decreases plasma concentrations of **amprenavir, atazanavir, boceprevir, telaprevir, indinavir, saquinavir.** Increases plasma concentrations of **ritonavir.** CYP3A4 inducers (e.g., **PHENobarbital, rifabutin, rifAMPin**) decrease concentration/effects. May alter **warfarin** plasma concentration.

HERBAL: St. John's wort may decrease concentration/effects. **FOOD: High-fat meals** may increase drug absorption. **LAB VALUES:** May produce false-positive urine test results for cannabinoid. May increase serum ALT, AST, GGT, amylase, glucose, triglycerides, cholesterol. May decrease neutrophils.

AVAILABILITY (Rx)

Capsules: 50 mg, 200 mg.

 **Tablets:** 600 mg.

ADMINISTRATION/HANDLING

PO

• Give with water at bedtime (decreases CNS adverse effects). • Avoid high-fat meals (may increase absorption). • Capsules may be opened and added to small amount of food/liquid. Administer within 30 min. • Do not break, crush, dissolve, or divide tablets.

INDICATIONS/ROUTES/DOSAGE

HIV Infection
PO: ADULTS, ELDERLY, CHILDREN WEIGHING 40 KG OR MORE: 600 mg once daily at bedtime. **CHILDREN WEIGHING 32.5 KG–LESS THAN 40 KG:** 400 mg once daily. **CHILDREN WEIGHING 25 KG–LESS THAN 32.5 KG:** 350 mg once daily. **CHILDREN WEIGHING 20 KG–LESS THAN 25 KG:** 300 mg once daily. **CHILDREN WEIGHING 15 KG–LESS THAN 20 KG:** 250 mg once daily. **CHILDREN WEIGHING 7.5 KG–LESS THAN 15 KG:** 200 mg once daily. **CHILDREN WEIGHING 5 KG–LESS THAN 7.5 KG:** 150 mg once daily. **CHILDREN WEIGHING 3.5 KG–LESS THAN 5 KG:** 100 mg once daily.

Dosage: Concurrent RifAMPin
PO: ONLY IF PT WEIGHS 50 KG OR GREATER: 800 mg once daily.

Dosage: Concurrent Voriconazole
PO: Reduce efavirenz to 300 mg once daily; increase voriconazole to 400 mg q12h.

Dosage in Renal Impairment
No dose adjustment.

Dosage in Hepatic Impairment
Mild impairment: Use caution. **Moderate to severe impairment:** Not recommended.

SIDE EFFECTS

Frequent (52%): Mild to severe: Dizziness, vivid dreams, insomnia, confusion, impaired concentration, amnesia, agitation, depersonalization, hallucinations, euphoria. **Occasional: Mild to moderate:** Maculopapular rash (27%); nausea, fatigue, headache, diarrhea, fever, cough (less than 26%).

ADVERSE EFFECTS/ TOXIC REACTIONS

Serious adverse psychiatric experiences (aggressive reactions, agitation, delusions, emotional lability, mania, neurosis, paranoia, psychosis, suicide) have been reported. Grade 4 rash, Stevens-Johnson syndrome, erythema multiforme occurs rarely. Hepatotoxicity with serum ALT, AST elevation greater than 5 times upper limit of normal reported in 5% of pts. May induce immune reconstitution syndrome (inflammatory response to dormant opportunistic infections or acceleration of autoimmune disorders).

NURSING CONSIDERATIONS

BASELINE ASSESSMENT

Offer emotional support. Obtain baseline serum cholesterol, triglycerides; pregnancy test in females of reproductive potential before initiating therapy. Obtain LFT in pts with history of hepatitis B or C virus infection. Receive full medication history including herbal products (high risk of drug interaction).

INTERVENTION/EVALUATION

Monitor for CNS, psychological symptoms: severe acute depression (including suicidal ideation or attempts), dizziness, impaired concentration, drowsiness, abnormal dreams, insomnia (begins during first or second day of therapy, generally resolves in 2–4 wks). Assess for evidence of rash (common side effect). Monitor LFT for abnormalities. Assess for headache, nausea, diarrhea. Obtain pregnancy test in females of reproductive potential at regular intervals during therapy.

PATIENT/FAMILY TEACHING

• Avoid high-fat meals during therapy. • Report appearance of skin rash immediately. • CNS, psychological symptoms occur in more than half of pts (dizziness, impaired concentration, delusions, depression). • Take medication every day as prescribed. • Do not alter dose or discontinue medication without informing physician. • Do not chew, crush, dissolve, or divide tablets. • Avoid tasks that require alertness, motor skills until response to drug is established. • Avoid alcohol. • Efavirenz is not a cure for HIV infection, nor does it reduce risk of transmission to others. • Recommend effective contraception during treatment and up to 12 wks after last dose. Do not breastfeed.

---

elbasvir/grazoprevir

el-bas-vir/graz-**oh**-pre-vir
(Zepatier)
Do not confuse elbasvir with daclatasvir, ombitasvir or grazoprevir with boceprevir or simeprevir.

♦CLASSIFICATION

PHARMACOTHERAPEUTIC: NS5A inhibitor/protease inhibitor. **CLINICAL:** Antihepaciviral.

USES

Treatment of chronic hepatitis C virus genotypes 1 or 4 infection in adults, with or without ribavirin.

PRECAUTIONS

Contraindications: Hypersensitivity to elbasvir or grazoprevir, decompensated hepatic cirrhosis, moderate or severe hepatic impairment; concomitant use of organic anion transporting polypeptides 1B1/3 (OATP1B1/3) inhibitors, strong CYP3A inducers. Concomitant use of atazanavir, carBAMazepine, cycloSPORINE, darunavir, efavirenz, lopinavir, phenytoin, rifAMPin, saquinavir, St. John's wort, tipranavir. Any contraindications or hypersensitivity to ribavirin (if used with treatment regimen). **Cautions:** HIV infection, mild hepatic impairment. Safety and efficacy not established in pts with hepatitis B virus coinfection, liver transplant recipients.

ACTION

Elbasvir inhibits hepatitis C virus (HCV) NS5A protein, which is essential for viral RNA replication and virion assembly. Grazoprevir inhibits HCV NS3/4A protease needed for processing HCV-encoded polyproteins, which is essential for viral replication. **Therapeutic Effect:** Inhibits viral replication of hepatitis C virus.

PHARMACOKINETICS

Widely distributed. Metabolized in liver. Protein binding: elbasvir (99.9%), grazoprevir (98.8%). Peak plasma concentration: 3 hrs. Steady state reached in approx. 6 days. Excreted in feces (greater than 90%), urine (less than 1%). **Half-life:** elbasvir: 24 hrs; grazoprevir: 31 hrs.

⧗ LIFESPAN CONSIDERATIONS

Pregnancy/Lactation: Use caution in pregnancy. Unknown if distributed in breast milk. When used with ribavirin, breastfeeding and pregnancy are contraindicated during treatment and up to 6 mos after discontinuation. **Children:** Safety and efficacy not established in pts younger than 18 yrs. **Elderly:** May have increased risk of hepatotoxicity.

INTERACTIONS

DRUG: Anticonvulsants (e.g., **carBAMazepine, phenytoin**), antimycobacterials (e.g., **rifabutin, rifAMPin**), **efavirenz** may significantly decrease concentration/effect; use

---

contraindicated. **Atazanavir, darunavir, lopinavir, tipranavir, cycloSPORINE** may significantly increase risk of hepatotoxicity; use contraindicated. **Moderate CYP3A inducers (e.g., etravirine, modafinil, nafcillin)** may decrease concentration/effect. **Elvitegravir/cobicistat/emtricitabine/tenofovir (disoproxil or alafenamide), ketoconazole** may increase concentration/effect. May increase concentration/effect of **atorvastatin, fluvastatin, HYDROcodone, lovastatin, niMODipine, rosuvastatin, simvastatin, tacrolimus. Acetaminophen** may increase risk of hepatotoxicity. **HERBAL:** St. John's wort may decrease concentration/effect; use contraindicated. **FOOD:** Grapefruit products may increase grazoprevir concentration/effect. **LAB VALUES:** May decrease Hgb. May increase serum ALT, bilirubin.

AVAILABILITY (Rx)

Fixed-Dose Combination Tablets: elbasvir 50 mg/grazoprevir 100 mg.

ADMINISTRATION/HANDLING

PO
• Give without regard to meals.

INDICATIONS/ROUTES/DOSAGE

Note: NS5A resistance testing recommended in HCV genotype 1a infected pts prior to initiating treatment with Zepatier.

Chronic Hepatitis C Virus Infection
PO: ADULTS, ELDERLY: 1 tablet once daily (with or without ribavirin).

Treatment Regimen and Duration
PO: ADULTS, ELDERLY: Genotype 1a: Treatment-naïve or peginterferon alfa (PegIFN)/ribavirin (RBV)–experienced without baseline NS5A polymorphisms: 1 tablet once daily for 12 wks. **Genotype 1a: Treatment-naïve or PegIFN/RBV–experienced with baseline NS5A polymorphisms:** 1 tablet once daily with ribavirin for 16 wks. **Genotype**

1b: Treatment-naïve or PegIFV/RBV–experienced: 1 tablet once daily for 12 wks. **Genotype 1a or 1b: PegIFV/RBV/ protease inhibitor–experienced:** 1 tablet once daily with ribavirin for 12 wks. **Genotype 4: Treatment-naïve:** 1 tablet once daily for 12 wks. **Genotype 4: PegIFN/RBV–experienced:** 1 tablet once daily with ribavirin for 16 wks.

Treatment-Induced Hepatotoxicity
Consider discontinuation in pts with persistent serum ALT elevation greater than 10 times upper limit of normal (ULN). Permanently discontinue if serum ALT elevation is accompanied with elevated alkaline phosphatase, conjugated bilirubin, prolonged INR, or signs of acute hepatic inflammation.

Dosage in Renal Impairment
No dose adjustment.

Dosage in Hepatic Impairment
Mild impairment: No dose adjustment. **Moderate to severe impairment:** Contraindicated.

SIDE EFFECTS

Occasional (11%–3%): Fatigue, headache, diarrhea, nausea, insomnia, dyspnea, rash, pruritus, irritability. **Rare (2%):** Abdominal pain, arthralgia.

ADVERSE EFFECTS/TOXIC REACTIONS

Serum ALT elevation up to 5 times ULN reported in 1% of pts. Serum bilirubin elevation greater than 2.5 times ULN occurred in 6% of pts. Serum ALT elevation occurred more frequently in the elderly, female pts, and pts of Asian ancestry.

NURSING CONSIDERATIONS

BASELINE ASSESSMENT
Obtain CBC, LFT, HCV-RNA level; pregnancy test in female pts of reproductive potential. Confirm hepatitis C genotype. In pts with HCV genotype 1a, recommend testing for the presence of NS5A resistance-associated polymorphisms prior to initiation. Receive full medication history

including herbal products; screen for contraindications. Question history of chronic anemia, hepatitis B virus infection, HIV infection, liver transplantation.

INTERVENTION/EVALUATION

Obtain LFT at wk 8, then as clinically indicated. For pts receiving 16 wks of therapy, obtain additional LFT at wk 12. Monitor CBC periodically; HCV-RNA levels at wks 4, 8, 12, 16 and as clinically indicated. Monitor for hepatotoxicity. Assess for anemia-related dizziness, exertional dyspnea, fatigue, weakness, syncope. Encourage nutritional intake. Assess for decreased appetite, weight loss. Obtain monthly pregnancy tests in females of reproductive potential if treated with ribavirin.

PATIENT/FAMILY TEACHING

• Blood levels will be drawn routinely. • Treatment may be used in combination with ribavirin (inform pt of side effects/toxic reactions). If therapy includes ribavirin, female pts of reproductive potential should avoid pregnancy during treatment and up to 6 mos after last dose. • Do not take newly prescribed medication unless approved by the doctor who originally started treatment. • Do not take herbal products, esp. St. John's wort. • Avoid alcohol, grapefruit products. • Report signs of treatment-induced liver injury such as abdominal pain, clay-colored stool, dark amber urine, decreased appetite, fatigue, weakness, yellowing of the skin or eyes. • Maintain proper nutritional intake.

eletriptan

el-e-**trip**-tan
(Relpax)

◆CLASSIFICATION

PHARMACOTHERAPEUTIC: Serotonin receptor agonist. **CLINICAL:** Antimigraine.

USES

Treatment of acute migraine headache with or without aura.

PRECAUTIONS

Contraindications: Hypersensitivity to eletriptan. Arrhythmias associated with conduction disorders, cerebrovascular syndrome including strokes and transient ischemic attacks (TIAs), coronary artery disease, hemiplegic or basilar migraine, ischemic heart disease, peripheral vascular disease including ischemic bowel disease, severe hepatic impairment, uncontrolled hypertension; use within 24 hrs of treatment with another 5-HT_1 agonist, an ergotamine-containing or ergot-type medication such as dihydroergotamine (DHE) or methysergide. Recent use (within 72 hrs) of strong CYP3A4 inhibitors (e.g., clarithromycin, ketoconazole, itraconazole, ritonavir). **Cautions:** Mild to moderate renal/hepatic impairment, controlled hypertension, history of CVA.

ACTION

Selective agonist for serotonin in cranial arteries; causes vasoconstriction and reduces inflammation. **Therapeutic Effect:** Relieves migraine headache.

PHARMACOKINETICS

Well absorbed after PO administration. Metabolized by liver. Excreted in urine. **Half-life:** 4.4 hrs (increased in hepatic impairment, elderly [older than 65 yrs]).

⧗ LIFESPAN CONSIDERATIONS

Pregnancy/Lactation: May decrease possibility of ovulation. Distributed in breast milk. **Children:** Safety and efficacy not established in pts younger than 18 yrs. **Elderly:** Increased risk of hypertension in those older than 65 yrs.

INTERACTIONS

DRUG: CYP3A4 inhibitors (e.g., **clarithromycin, ketoconazole, ritonavir**) may decrease metabolism. **Ergotamine-containing medications** may produce vasospastic reaction. **SSRIs (e.g., escitalopram, paroxetine, sertraline), SNRIs (e.g., duloxetine, venlafaxine), tricyclic antidepressants (e.g., amitriptyline, nortriptyline), MAOIs (e.g., phenelzine, selegiline)** may cause serotonin syndrome. **HERBAL:** None significant. **FOOD:** None known. **LAB VALUES:** None significant.

AVAILABILITY (Rx)

 Tablets: 20 mg, 40 mg.

ADMINISTRATION/HANDLING
PO
• May take without regard to food. • Do not break, crush, dissolve, or divide film-coated tablets.

INDICATIONS/ROUTES/DOSAGE
Acute Migraine Headache
PO: **ADULTS, ELDERLY:** 20–40 mg. **Maximum:** 40 mg. If headache improves but then returns, dose may be repeated after 2 hrs. **Maximum:** 80 mg/day.

Dosage in Renal/Hepatic Impairment
No dose adjustment. Not recommended in severe hepatic impairment.

SIDE EFFECTS
Occasional (6%–5%): Dizziness, drowsiness, asthenia, nausea. **Rare (3%–2%):** Paresthesia, headache, dry mouth, warm or hot sensation, dyspepsia, dysphagia.

ADVERSE EFFECTS/TOXIC REACTIONS
Cardiac reactions (ischemia, coronary artery vasospasm, MI), noncardiac vasospasm-related reactions (hemorrhage, CVA) occur rarely, particularly in pts with hypertension, obesity, diabetes, strong family history of coronary artery disease; smokers; males older than 40 yrs; postmenopausal women. May cause GI ischemia, bowel infarction, non–cardiac-related vasospasms including peripheral vascular ischemia, Raynaud's syndrome. Overuse may increase frequency, occurrence of headaches.

NURSING CONSIDERATIONS
BASELINE ASSESSMENT
Question pt regarding onset, location, duration of migraine, possible precipitating symptoms. Obtain baseline B/P or evidence of uncontrolled hypertension (contraindication).

INTERVENTION/EVALUATION
Assess for relief of migraine headache, potential for photophobia, phonophobia (sound sensitivity), nausea, vomiting. Monitor for cardiac arrhythmia, coronary events, hypertension, hypersensitivity reaction.

PATIENT/FAMILY TEACHING
• Take a single dose as soon as symptoms of an actual migraine attack appear. • Medication is intended to relieve migraine headaches, not to prevent or reduce number of attacks. • Avoid tasks that require alertness, motor skills until response to drug is established. • Immediately report palpitations, pain/tightness in chest/throat, sudden or severe abdominal pain, pain/weakness of extremities.

elotuzumab
el-oh-**tooz**-ue-mab
(Empliciti)
Do not confuse elotuzumab with alemtuzumab, eculizumab, evolocumab, pertuzumab, gemtuzumab, trastuzumab.

◆CLASSIFICATION
PHARMACOTHERAPEUTIC: Monoclonal antibody. **CLINICAL:** Antineoplastic.

USES
Treatment of multiple myeloma (in combination with lenalidomide and dexamethasone) in pts who have received one to three prior therapies.

E

PRECAUTIONS

Contraindications: Hypersensitivity to elotuzumab. **Cautions:** Diabetes, baseline cytopenias, hypertension; history of chronic opportunistic infections (esp. viral infections, fungal infections), conditions predisposing to infection (e.g., diabetes, kidney failure, open wounds). Concomitant use of medications known to cause bradycardia (e.g., antiarrhythmics, beta blockers, calcium channel blockers). Concomitant use of live vaccines not recommended during treatment and up to 3 mos after discontinuation. Avoid use during severe active infection.

ACTION

Binds to and specifically targets signaling lymphocytic activation molecule family member 7 (SLAMF7), a protein that is expressed on most myeloma and natural killer cells. Directly activates natural killer cells and facilitates cellular death. **Therapeutic Effect:** Inhibits tumor cell growth and metastasis.

PHARMACOKINETICS

Widely distributed. Metabolism not specified. Elimination not specified. **Half-life:** Not specified; 97% of steady-state concentration is expected to be eliminated within 82 days.

⏳ LIFESPAN CONSIDERATIONS

Pregnancy/Lactation: Avoid pregnancy; may cause fetal harm/malformations/fetal demise when used with lenalidomide. Unknown if distributed in breast milk. However, immunoglobulin G (IgG) is present in breast milk. Breastfeeding contraindicated when used with concomitant lenalidomide treatment. **Men:** Lenalidomide is present in semen. Recommend use of barrier methods during sexual activity. **Children:** Safety and efficacy not established. **Elderly:** No age-related precautions noted.

INTERACTIONS

DRUG: May increase immunosuppressant/toxic effects of **immunosuppressants** (e.g., **fingolimod, leflunomide, nivolumab**). **Roflumilast** may increase immunosuppressant effect. May enhance adverse/toxic effect of **live vaccines;** may decrease therapeutic effect of **vaccines. HERBAL:** Echinacea may decrease effect. **FOOD:** None known. **LAB VALUES:** May be detected on both serum protein electrophoresis and immunofixation assays used to monitor multiple myeloma endogenous M-protein. May affect the determination of complete response and disease progression of some pts with IgG kappa myeloma protein. Expected to decrease lymphocytes, leukocytes, platelets. May decrease serum albumin, bicarbonate, calcium. May increase serum alkaline phosphatase, ALT, AST, glucose, potassium.

AVAILABILITY (Rx)

Injection, Powder for Reconstitution: 300 mg, 400 mg.

ADMINISTRATION/HANDLING
 IV

Reconstitution • Calculate the dose and number of vials required based on weight in kg. • Reconstitute the 300-mg vial with 13 mL of Sterile Water for Injection or the 400-mg vial with 17 mL of Sterile Water for Injection using an 18-g or lower (e.g., 17, 16, or 15) needle. • Gently roll vial upright to mix. To dissolve any powder left on top of vial or stopper, gently invert vial several times. • Do not shake or agitate. • The powder should dissolve in less than 10 mins. • After dissolution, allow vials to stand for 5–10 mins. • Visually inspect solution for particulate matter or discoloration. Solution should appear clear, colorless to slightly yellow. Discard if solution is cloudy or discolored or if foreign particles are observed. Each vial contains an overfill volume to allow for a specific withdrawal of 12 mL (300-mg vial) or 16 mL (400-mg vial). • Final concentration of withdrawn volume (without overfill) will equal 25 mg/mL. • Dilute in 230 mL of 0.9% NaCl or 5% Dextrose injection in polyvinyl chloride or polyolefin infusion bag. • Mix by gentle inversion; do not shake or agitate. • The volume may be adjusted in order to not exceed 5 mL/kg of pt weight at any given dose.

Infusion Guidelines • Prior to administration, premedicate with dexamethasone, acetaminophen, antihistamine (H_1 antagonist, plus H_2 antagonist) approx. 45–90 mins before each infusion (see manufacturer guidelines). • Use an in-line, sterile, nonpyrogenic, low protein-binding filter (0.2–1.2 mm). • Infuse via dedicated line using an infusion pump.

Rate of Administration • First Infusion (Cycle 1, Dose 1): Infuse at 0.5 mL/min for the first 30 mins. If no infusion reactions occur, may increase to 1 mL/min for next 30 mins. If tolerated, may increase to 2 mL/min. **Maximum rate: 2 mL/min. • Second Infusion (Cycle 1, Dose 2):** Initiate at 1 mL/min for first 30 mins if no infusion reactions occurred during first infusion. If tolerated, may increase to 2 mL/min until infusion completed. **Maximum rate: 2 mL/min. • Subsequent Infusions (Cycle 1, Doses 3 and 4, All Subsequent Infusions):** Initiate at 2 mL/min until completion if no infusion reactions occurred during prior infusion. **Maximum rate: 2 mL/min.** In pts who have received four cycles of treatment, infusion rate may be increased to maximum rate of 5 mL/min.

Storage • Refrigerate intact vials until time of use. • Do not freeze or shake. • Refrigerate diluted solution up to 24 hrs. • May store at room temperature up to 8 hrs (of the total 24 hrs). • Diluted solution must be administered within 24 hrs of reconstitution. • Protect from light.

▦ IV INCOMPATIBILITIES

Do not mix with other medications.

INDICATIONS/ROUTES/DOSAGE

Multiple Myeloma
IV: ADULTS, ELDERLY: Cycles 1 and 2: 10 mg/kg once wkly on days 1, 8, 15, 22

of 28-day cycle (in combination with lenalidomide and dexamethasone).

Cycles 3 and beyond: 10 mg/kg once q2wks on days 1 and 15 of 28-day cycle (in combination with lenalidomide and dexamethasone). Continue until disease progression or unacceptable toxicity.

Dose Modification
Infusion Reactions
Grade 2 or higher reaction: Interrupt infusion until symptoms improve. Once resolved to Grade 1 or 0, resume infusion at 0.5 mL/min. If tolerated, increase in increments of 0.5 mL/min q30mins back to previous rate. May further increase rate as indicated if no reaction recurs. If infusion reaction recurs, stop infusion and do not restart for that day.

Dosage in Renal/Hepatic Impairment
Not specified; use caution.

SIDE EFFECTS

Frequent (61%–20%): Fatigue, diarrhea, pyrexia, constipation, cough, peripheral neuropathy, decreased appetite. **Occasional (16%–10%):** Extremity pain, headache, vomiting, decreased weight, oropharyngeal pain, hypoesthesia, mood change, night sweats.

ADVERSE EFFECTS/TOXIC REACTIONS

All cases were reported in combination with lenalidomide and dexamethasone. Infusion reactions reported in 10% of pts. Most infusion reactions were Grade 3 and lower. Lymphopenia, leukopenia, thrombocytopenia are expected responses to therapy. Infections were reported in 81% of pts. Grade 3 or 4 infections occurred in 28% of pts. Nasopharyngitis (25% of pts), upper respiratory tract infection (23% of pts), opportunistic infection (22% of pts), herpes zoster (14% of pts), fungal infection (10% of pts), influenza; second primary malignancies, skin malignancies, solid tumors, malignant neoplasms; tachycardia, bradycardia, systolic or diastolic hypertension, hypotension;

pulmonary embolism may occur. Hepatotoxicity with elevation of serum alkaline phosphatase greater than 2 times upper limit of normal (ULN), serum ALT/AST greater than 3 times ULN, total bilirubin greater than 2 times ULN reported in 3% of pts. Other adverse effects may include cataracts (12% of pts), hyperglycemia (89% of pts), hypersensitivity reaction (greater than 5% of pts). Immunogenicity (auto-elotuzumab antibodies) occurred in 19% of pts. Thrombocytopenia may increase risk of bleeding.

NURSING CONSIDERATIONS

BASELINE ASSESSMENT

Obtain CBC, BMP, LFT; serum ionized calcium; capillary blood glucose, vital signs; pregnancy test in female pts of reproductive potential. Obtain baseline EKG in pts concurrently using medications known to cause bradycardia. Question history of chronic opportunistic infections, diabetes, hepatic impairment, pulmonary embolism; prior infusion or hypersensitivity reactions. Screen for medications known to cause bradycardia, hyperglycemia. Screen for active infection. Offer emotional support.

INTERVENTION/EVALUATION

Obtain CBC, BMP, LFT, ionized calcium periodically. Administer in an environment equipped to monitor for and manage infusion reactions. If infusion reaction of any grade/severity occurs, immediately interrupt infusion and manage symptoms. Accurately record characteristics of infusion reactions (severity, type, time of onset). Infusion reactions may affect future infusion rates. Monitor HR, BP q30mins during infusion and for at least 2 hrs after completion in pts with prior hemodynamic reactions. Cough, dyspnea, hypoxia, tachycardia may indicate pulmonary embolism. Monitor for bradycardia, cataracts, hyperglycemia, hyperkalemia, hypersensitivity reaction, hepatotoxicity, neuropathy, tachycardia. Assess for new primary malignancies (solid tumors, skin cancers); skin for new lesions, moles. Monitor daily pattern

bowel activity, stool consistency. Obtain urine, serum pregnancy test periodically throughout therapy.

PATIENT/FAMILY TEACHING

• Blood levels, EKGs will be monitored routinely. • Treatment may depress your immune system and reduce your ability to fight infection. Report symptoms of infection such as body aches, chills, cough, fatigue, fever. Avoid those with active infection. • Therapy may decrease your heart rate, esp. in those taking medications that lower heart rate; report dizziness, chest pain, palpitations, or fainting. • Avoid pregnancy. Do not breastfeed. • Male pts should use condoms during sexual activity. • Treatment includes a steroid that may raise blood sugar levels; report dehydration, blurry vision, confusion, frequent urination, increased thirst, fruity breath. • Report allergic reactions of any kind. • Abdominal pain, easy bruising, clay-colored stools, dark-amber urine, fatigue, loss of appetite, yellowing of skin or eyes may indicate liver problem.

eltrombopag

el-**trom**-boe-pag
(Promacta, Revolade ✦)

■ **BLACK BOX ALERT** ■ May cause hepatotoxicity. Measure serum ALT, AST, bilirubin prior to initiation of eltrombopag, every 2 wks during dose adjustment phase, and monthly following establishment of a stable dose. If bilirubin is elevated, perform fractionation. Discontinue if serum ALT levels increase to 3 times or greater upper limit of normal and are progressive, persistent for 4 or more wks, accompanied by increased direct bilirubin, clinical symptoms of hepatic injury, or evidence of hepatic decompensation.

◆ CLASSIFICATION

PHARMACOTHERAPEUTIC: Thrombopoietin receptor agonist. **CLINICAL:** Prevents thrombocytopenia.

USES

Treatment of thrombocytopenia in pts with chronic immune (idiopathic) thrombocytopenic purpura (ITP) with insufficient response with corticosteroids, immunoglobulins, or splenectomy. Use only in pts who are at increased risk for bleeding; should not be used to normalize platelet counts. Treatment of thrombocytopenia in pts with chronic hepatitis C virus infection to allow the initiation and maintenance of interferon-based therapy. Treatment of severe aplastic anemia in pts having an insufficient response to immunosuppressive therapy.

PRECAUTIONS

Contraindications: Hypersensitivity to eltrombopag. **Cautions:** Preexisting hepatic impairment, renal impairment (any degree), myelodysplastic syndrome (may increase risk for hematologic malignancies). Pts with known risk for thromboembolism, risk for cataracts.

ACTION

Interacts with the human thrombopoietin receptor and initiates signaling cascades. **Therapeutic Effect:** Induces proliferation and differentiation of megakaryocytes from bone marrow progenitor cells.

PHARMACOKINETICS

Readily absorbed from gastrointestinal tract. Primarily distributed in blood cells. Protein binding: 99%. Extensively metabolized including oxidation, conjugation with glucuronic acid or cysteine. Excreted primarily in feces. **Half-life:** 26–35 hrs.

⌛ LIFESPAN CONSIDERATIONS

Pregnancy/Lactation: Unknown if distributed in breast milk. **Children:** Safety and efficacy not established. **Elderly:** Use caution due to increased frequency of hepatic, renal, cardiac dysfunction.

INTERACTIONS

DRUG: May increase concentration/toxicity of **atorvastatin, fluvastatin, methotrexate, nateglinide, pravastatin, repaglinide, rifAMPin, rosuvastatin. Aluminum, antacids, calcium, iron, magnesium** may decrease concentration/effects. **HERBAL:** None significant. **FOOD: Dairy products** may decrease concentration/effects. **LAB VALUES:** May increase serum ALT, AST.

AVAILABILITY (Rx)

Tablets: 12.5 mg, 25 mg, 50 mg, 75 mg, 100 mg. **Oral Suspension:** 25 mg.

ADMINISTRATION/HANDLING

PO

• Give on an empty stomach, either 1 hr before or 2 hrs after meal. • Give at least 4 hrs before or 4 hrs after ingestion of antacids, food high in calcium or minerals, or calcium-fortified juices.

INDICATIONS/ROUTES/DOSAGE

Aplastic Anemia
PO: ADULTS, ELDERLY: 50 mg once daily (25 mg for pts of East Asian ancestry or hepatic impairment). Titrate dose based on platelet response. Adjust dose to maintain platelets more than 50,000/mm³. **Maximum:** 150 mg/day.

ITP
PO: ADULTS, ELDERLY, CHILDREN 6 YRS AND OLDER: Initially, 50 mg once daily (25 mg for pts of East Asian ancestry or moderate to severe hepatic insufficiency or children 1 to 5 yrs of age). Then, adjust dose (25 mg to 75 mg once daily) to achieve and maintain platelet count of 50,000 cells/mm³ or greater as necessary to reduce risk of bleeding. **Maximum:** 75 mg once daily.

Chronic Hepatitis C–associated Thrombocytopenia
PO: ADULTS, ELDERLY: Initially, 25 mg once daily. Titrate dose based on platelet response. **Maximum:** 100 mg once daily.

E

Dosage Adjustment Based on Platelet Response

Less than 50,000/mm³ (after at least 2 wks)	Increase by 25 mg q2wks up to 100 mg/day
200,000/mm³ or more and 400,000/mm³ or less	Decrease by 25 mg
More than 400,000/mm³	Withhold; when less than 150,000/mm³, resume with dose reduced by 25 mg
More than 400,000/mm³ after 2 wks at lowest dose	Discontinue

Dosage in Renal Impairment
No dose adjustment.

Dosage in Hepatic Impairment
ITP

Mild to severe	Initial: 25 mg/day
East Asian ancestry	Initial: 12.5 mg/day

Chronic Hepatitis C
No dose adjustment.

Aplastic Anemia
Initial dose 25 mg once daily.

SIDE EFFECTS

Frequent (6%–4%): Nausea, vomiting, menorrhagia. **Occasional (3%–2%):** Myalgia, paresthesia, dyspepsia, ecchymosis, cataract, conjunctival hemorrhage.

ADVERSE EFFECTS/TOXIC REACTIONS

May cause hepatotoxicity. Increases risk of reticulin fiber deposits within bone marrow (may lead to bone marrow fibrosis). May produce hematologic malignancies. May cause excessive increase in platelets, leading to thrombotic complications.

NURSING CONSIDERATIONS

BASELINE ASSESSMENT
Assess CBC and peripheral blood smears, LFT. Examine peripheral blood smear to establish extent of RBC and WBC abnormalities. Conduct ocular examination. Screen for hepatic/renal impairment, myelodysplastic syndrome, history of thromboembolism. Question use of antacids or herbal products.

INTERVENTION/EVALUATION
Monitor CBC, platelet counts, peripheral blood smears, LFT throughout and following discontinuation. Monitor for cataracts, hepatotoxicity during therapy.

PATIENT/FAMILY TEACHING
• Lab values will be closely monitored throughout therapy and for at least 4 wks after last dose. • Report any yellowing of the skin or eyes, unusual darkening of the urine, unusual tiredness, pain in right upper stomach area. • Do not take antacids, magnesium, or calcium products 4 hrs before or after dose. • Report changes in vision.

eluxadoline

el-ux-**ad**-oh-leen
(Viberzi)

◆CLASSIFICATION
PHARMACOTHERAPEUTIC: Mu-opioid receptor agonist. Schedule IV. **CLINICAL:** Antidiarrheal.

USES
Treatment of irritable bowel syndrome with diarrhea in adults.

PRECAUTIONS
Contraindications: Hypersensitivity to eluxadoline. Known or suspected biliary duct obstruction, sphincter of Oddi disease or dysfunction; pts without a gallbladder; severe hepatic impairment;

severe constipation or sequelae from constipation, or known or suspected mechanical GI obstruction. History of alcoholism, alcohol abuse, alcohol addiction, or consumption of more than 3 alcoholic beverages/day. History of pancreatitis; structural disease of the pancreas, including known or suspected pancreatic duct obstruction. **Cautions:** Mild to moderate hepatic impairment, respiratory disease.

ACTION

Affects mu-opioid receptors involved with gut motility, pain sensations, and secretion of liquids within the digestive tract. **Therapeutic Effect:** Reduces abdominal pain and diarrhea (without causing constipation).

PHARMACOKINETICS

Metabolism not specified. Protein binding: 81%. Peak plasma concentration: 1.5 hrs. Primarily excreted in feces (82%), urine (less than 1%). **Half-life:** 3.7–6 hrs.

⏳ LIFESPAN CONSIDERATIONS

Pregnancy/Lactation: Unknown if distributed in breast milk. **Children:** Safety and efficacy not established. **Elderly:** No age-related precautions noted.

INTERACTIONS

DRUG: **OATP1B1 inhibitors** (e.g., cycloSPORINE, ritonavir, rifAMPin), **strong CYP inhibitors** (e.g., ciprofloxacin, gemfibrozil, fluconazole, clarithromycin) may increase concentration/effect. **Drugs that cause constipation** (e.g., alosetron, anticholinergics [e.g., diphenhydrAMINE], loperamide, opioids [e.g., morphine] may increase risk of serious constipation-associated adverse effects. May increase concentration of **rosuvastatin**, increasing risk of myopathy/rhabdomyolysis. May increase effects of **CYP3A substrates with narrow therapeutic index** (e.g., cycloSPORINE, sirolimus, tacrolimus). **HERBAL:** None significant. **FOOD:** **High-fat meals** may

decrease absorption. **LAB VALUES:** May increase serum ALT, AST, lipase.

AVAILABILITY (Rx)

📋 **Tablets:** 75 mg, 100 mg.

ADMINISTRATION/HANDLING

PO
• Administer with food. • If scheduled dose is missed, give next dose at the regular time; do not give 2 doses at once.

INDICATIONS/ROUTES/DOSAGE

Irritable Bowel Syndrome–Associated Diarrhea
PO: ADULTS, ELDERLY: 100 mg twice daily. May decrease to 75 mg twice daily if unable to tolerate 100-mg dose.

Dose Modification
Pts who are unable to tolerate 100-mg dose, or are receiving concomitant OATP1B1 inhibitors: 75 mg twice daily.
Pts who develop severe constipation for more than 4 days: Permanently discontinue.

Dosage in Renal Impairment
Not specified; use caution.

Dosage in Hepatic Impairment
Mild to moderate impairment: 75 mg twice daily. **Severe impairment:** Contraindicated.

SIDE EFFECTS

Occasional (8%–4%): Constipation, nausea, abdominal pain (upper or lower), upper respiratory tract infection, vomiting. **Rare (3%–1%):** Abdominal distention, dizziness, flatulence, rash, urticaria, fatigue, sedation, somnolence, euphoric mood.

ADVERSE EFFECTS/TOXIC REACTIONS

May increase risk of sphincter of Oddi spasm (esp. in pts without a gallbladder), resulting in pancreatitis or hepatic enzyme elevation that may be associated

E

with or without acute abdominal pain, or nausea/vomiting; 80% of pts reported sphincter of Oddi spasm within the first week of treatment. May also increase risk of pancreatitis that is not associated with sphincter of Oddi spasm. Infectious processes including upper respiratory tract infection, bronchitis, nasopharyngitis, viral gastroenteritis were reported. May cause hypersensitivity reaction including asthma, bronchospasm, respiratory failure, wheezing. Recreational abuse may produce feelings of euphoria, which may lead to physical dependence.

NURSING CONSIDERATIONS

BASELINE ASSESSMENT

Obtain baseline LFT in pts with baseline hepatic impairment. Receive full medication history and screen for interactions requiring lower dosage. Question pt's usual stool characteristics (color, frequency, consistency). Question history of alcoholism, biliary duct obstruction, cholecystectomy, mechanical GI obstruction, hepatic impairment, hypersensitivity reaction, pancreatic disease, respiratory disease, sphincter of Oddi disease or spasm. Assess hydration status.

INTERVENTION/EVALUATION

Monitor for abdominal pain that radiates to the back or shoulder, with or without nausea or vomiting (esp. during first few weeks of treatment). Obtain LFT, serum lipase level if acute pancreatitis, sphincter of Oddi spasm, biliary tract obstruction suspected. Monitor for hypersensitivity reaction including dyspnea, rash, wheezing. Observe and record daily pattern of bowel activity, stool consistency. Encourage PO intake. If an acute overdose occurs, a narcotic mu-opioid antagonist such as naloxone may be considered if reversal of overdose-related adverse effects is needed.

PATIENT/FAMILY TEACHING

• Therapy may cause inflammation of the pancreas (pancreatitis) or elevated liver-associated abdominal pain, esp. during the first few weeks of treatment. Report any new or worsening abdominal pain that radiates to the back or shoulder, with or without nausea/vomiting. • Avoid chronic or acute excessive use of alcohol; may increase risk of liver or pancreas injury. • If a dose is missed, take the next dose at the regular time; do not take 2 doses at once. • Report constipation lasting longer than 4 days. • Avoid medications that cause constipation (e.g., antidiarrheals, narcotics). • Report signs of allergic reaction; respiratory problems such as worsening of asthma, bronchitis, wheezing. • Drink plenty of fluids.

elvitegravir

el-vi-**teg**-ra-vir
(Vitekta)
Do not confuse elvitegravir with dolutegravir or raltegravir.

FIXED-COMBINATION(S)

Genvoya, Stribild: elvitegravir (an integrase inhibitor)/cobicistat (an antiretroviral booster)/emtricitabine/ tenofovir (antiretroviral agents): 150 mg/150 mg/200 mg/300 mg.

◆CLASSIFICATION

PHARMACOTHERAPEUTIC: Integrase strand transfer inhibitor. **CLINICAL:** Antiretroviral agent.

USES

Used in combination with an HIV protease inhibitor, coadministered with ritonavir and other antiretroviral medications for the treatment of HIV-1 infection in antiretroviral treatment–experienced adults.

PRECAUTIONS

Contraindications: Hypersensitivity to elvitegravir. **Cautions:** Diabetes, hepatic impairment, hypercholesterolemia. Not recommended with a HIV protease inhibitor and cobicistat combination; coadministration of HIV-1 protease inhibitors other than atazanavir, darunavir, fosamprenavir, lopinavir, and tipranavir.

ACTION

Inhibits HIV integrase by preventing integration of HIV-1 DNA into host DNA, blocking formation of HIV-1 provirus. **Therapeutic Effect:** Interferes with HIV replication, slowing progression of HIV infection.

PHARMACOKINETICS

Readily absorbed after PO administration. Metabolized in liver. Protein binding: 98%–99%. Peak plasma concentration: 4 hrs. Excreted in feces (95%), urine (7%). **Half-life:** 8.7 hrs.

⧗ LIFESPAN CONSIDERATIONS

Pregnancy/Lactation: Breastfeeding not recommend due to risk of postnatal HIV transmission. Unknown if distributed in human breast milk. **Children:** Safety and efficacy not established in pts younger than 18 yrs. **Elderly:** Safety and efficacy not established in pts older than 65 yrs. May have increased risk of adverse reactions, hepatic impairment.

INTERACTIONS

DRUG: Antacids, aluminum/calcium/magnesium/iron supplements, antiretrovirals (e.g., efavirenz, nevirapine), corticosteroids (e.g., dexamethasone), anticonvulsants (e.g., carBAMazepine, phenytoin), rifAMPin may decrease concentration/effect. May increase concentrations/effects of **ketoconazole, rifAMPin. Antifungals (e.g., ketoconazole), atazanavir, lopinavir** may increase concentration/effect. May decrease concentration/effect of **hormonal contraceptives. HERBAL:** St John's wort may decrease effectiveness. **FOOD:** None known. **LAB VALUES:** May increase serum ALT, AST, amylase bilirubin, cholesterol, creatine kinase (CK), GGT, glucose, lipase, triglycerides, urine glucose, urine RBC. May decrease neutrophils.

AVAILABILITY (Rx)

🍳 **Tablets:** 85 mg, 150 mg.

ADMINISTRATION/HANDLING

PO
• Must be taken with food. • Must be administered with a protease inhibitor, in combination with ritonavir and another antiretroviral drug. • If pt receiving antacid, do not give aluminum- or magnesium-containing antacids within 2 hrs of dose.

INDICATIONS/ROUTES/DOSAGE

HIV Infection
PO: ADULTS, ELDERLY: *(Coadministered with darunavir/ritonavir, fosamprenavir/ritonavir or tipranavir/ritonavir):* 150 mg once daily. *(Coadministered with atazanavir/ritonavir or lopinavir/ritonavir):* **PO: ADULTS, ELDERLY:** 85 mg once daily.

Dosage in Renal Impairment
No dose adjustment.

Dosage in Hepatic Impairment
Mild to moderate impairment: No dose adjustment. **Severe impairment:** Not recommended.

SIDE EFFECTS

Occasional (7%–4%): Diarrhea, nausea. **Rare (3%):** Headache.

ADVERSE EFFECTS/TOXIC REACTIONS

May induce immune recovery syndrome (inflammatory response to dormant opportunistic infections such as *Mycobacterium avium,* cytomegalovirus, *Pneumocystis carinii* pneumonia [PCP], tuberculosis, or acceleration of autoimmune disorders such as Graves' disease, polymyositis, Guillain-Barré). Pts coinfected with hepatitis B or C virus have increased risk for viral reactivation and worsening of hepatic function and may

---

✦ Canadian trade name   🍳 Non-Crushable Drug   🔲 High Alert drug experience hepatic decompensation and/or failure if therapy is discontinued. Elevation of hepatic enzymes greater than 5 times upper limit of normal reported in 2% of pts.

NURSING CONSIDERATIONS

BASELINE ASSESSMENT

Obtain BMP, CBC, lipid panel, LFT, urine glucose, vital signs; CD4+ count, viral load level. Screen for hepatitis B or C coinfection, hypercholesterolemia. Receive full medication history including herbal products. Question possibility of pregnancy; history of diabetes, hypercholesterolemia.

INTERVENTION/EVALUATION

Monitor CBC, LFT, lipid levels. Monitor CD4+ count, viral load for treatment effectiveness. Cough, dyspnea, fever, excess of band cells on CBC may indicate acute infection (WBC count may be unreliable in pts with uncontrolled HIV infection). Screen for immune reconstitution syndrome.

PATIENT/FAMILY TEACHING

• Offer emotional support. • Take elvitegravir with an HIV protease inhibitor, combined with ritonavir at the same time each day with food (optimizes absorption). • Antacids may decrease drug effectiveness; do not take within 2 hrs of dose • Treatment regimen does not cure HIV infection, nor reduce risk of transmission. • Drug resistance can form if therapy is interrupted; do not run out of supply. • As immune system strengthens, it may respond to dormant infections hidden within the body. Report body aches, chills, cough, fever, night sweats, shortness of breath. • Treatment may cause liver dysfunction; report abdominal pain, darkened urine, clay-colored stools, significant weight loss, or yellowing of skin or eyes. • Do not take any new medications, including over-the-counter drugs or herbal products, unless approved by your doctor. • Do not breastfeed.

empagliflozin

em-pa-gli-**floe**-zin
(Jardiance)
Do not confuse empagliflozin with canagliflozin or dapagliflozin.

FIXED-COMBINATION(S)

Glyxambi: empagliflozin/linagliptin (an antidiabetic): 10 mg/5 mg, 25 mg/5 mg. **Synjardy:** Empagliflozin/metFORMIN (an antidiabetic): 5 mg/500 mg, 5 mg/1000 mg, 12.5 mg/500 mg, 12.5 mg/1000 mg.

◆CLASSIFICATION

PHARMACOTHERAPEUTIC: Sodium-glucose co-transporter 2 (SGLT2) inhibitor. **CLINICAL:** Antidiabetic.

USES

Adjunctive treatment to diet and exercise to improve glycemic controls in pts with type 2 diabetes mellitus. Reduce risk of cardiovascular death in pts with type 2 diabetes and cardiovascular disease.

PRECAUTIONS

Contraindications: History of hypersensitivity to empagliflozin, other SGLT2 inhibitors, severe renal impairment, end-stage renal disease, dialysis. **Cautions:** Not recommended in type 1 diabetes, diabetic ketoacidosis. Concurrent use of diuretics, other hypoglycemic medications, mild to moderate renal impairment, hypovolemia (dehydration/anemia), elderly, those with low systolic B/P, hyperlipidemia, history of genital mycotic infection. May cause ketoacidosis.

ACTION

Increases excretion of urinary glucose by inhibiting reabsorption of filtered glucose in kidney. Inhibits SGLT2 in proximal renal tubule. **Therapeutic Effect:** Lowers serum glucose levels.

PHARMACOKINETICS

Readily absorbed following PO administration. Metabolized in liver by glucuronidation. Peak plasma concentration: 1.5 hrs. Protein binding: 86%. Excreted in urine (54%) and feces (41%). **Half-life:** 12.4 hrs.

⏳ LIFESPAN CONSIDERATIONS

Pregnancy/Lactation: Avoid use during second or third trimester. Unknown if distributed in breast milk. Must either discontinue drug or discontinue breast-feeding. **Children:** Safety and efficacy not established in pts younger than 18 yrs. **Elderly:** May have increased risk for adverse reactions (e.g., hypotension, syncope, dehydration).

INTERACTIONS

DRUG: Diuretics (e.g., furosemide, HCTZ) may increase risk of hypotension/volume depletion. Insulin, insulin secretagogues (e.g., glyBURIDE) may increase risk of hypoglycemia. May increase concentration/effect of digoxin. **HERBAL:** Fenugreek, garlic, ginger, ginseng, gotu may increase risk of hypoglycemia. **FOOD:** None known. **LAB VALUES:** May increase low-density lipoprotein cholesterol (LDL-C), serum creatinine. May decrease glomerular filtration rate.

AVAILABILITY (Rx)

🍷 **Tablets:** 10 mg, 25 mg.

ADMINISTRATION/HANDLING

PO

May give without regard to food in the morning.

INDICATIONS/ROUTES/DOSAGE

Type 2 Diabetes Mellitus, Reduce Risk of Cardiovascular Death

PO: ADULTS/ELDERLY: Initially, 10 mg once daily in the morning. May increase to 25 mg once daily.

Dosage in Renal Impairment

GFR 45 mL/min or greater: No dose adjustment. **GFR less than 45 mL/min:** Discontinue. Do not initiate.

Dosage in Hepatic Impairment

No dose adjustment.

SIDE EFFECTS

Rare (4%–1.1%): Increased urination, dyslipidemia, arthralgia, nausea.

ADVERSE EFFECTS/TOXIC REACTIONS

Symptomatic hypotension (postural dizziness, orthostatic hypotension, syncope) may occur. Hypoglycemic events reported (concomitant use of hypoglycemic medications may increase hypoglycemic risk). Infections including urosepsis, pyelonephritis, UTI, genital mycotic infections (male and female), upper respiratory tract infection may occur. May increase risk of acute kidney injury, renal impairment. Fatal cases of ketoacidosis have been reported.

NURSING CONSIDERATIONS

BASELINE ASSESSMENT

Assess hydration status. Obtain serum chemistries, capillary blood glucose, hemoglobin A1c, LDL-C. Assess pt's understanding of diabetes management, routine home glucose monitoring. Receive full medication history including minerals, herbal products. Question history of co-morbidities, esp. renal or hepatic impairment.

INTERVENTION/EVALUATION

Monitor serum cholesterol, blood glucose, renal function, LFT. Assess for hypoglycemia, infection (esp. sepsis, mycotic infections, UTI), decreased urinary output, amber-colored urine, edema, fever, flank pain, hypersensitivity reaction. Screen for glucose-altering conditions: fever, increased activity or stress, surgical procedures. Obtain dietary consult for nutritional education. Encourage fluid intake.

E

PATIENT/FAMILY TEACHING

• Diabetes mellitus requires lifelong control. • Diet and exercise are principal parts of treatment; do not skip or delay meals. • Test blood sugar regularly. When taking combination drug therapy or when glucose demands are altered (fever, infection, trauma, stress), have low blood sugar treatment available (glucagon, oral dextrose). • Report suspected pregnancy or plans of breastfeeding. • Monitor daily calorie intake. • Slowly go from lying to standing to prevent dizziness. • Therapy may increase risk for dehydration/low blood pressure, which may cause kidney failure. • Genital itching may indicate yeast infection. Report any signs of UTI (e.g., burning while urinating, cloudy urine, pelvic pain, back pain).

emtricitabine

em-tri-**sye**-ta-bine
(Emtriva)

■ **BLACK BOX ALERT** ■ Serious, sometimes fatal, hypersensitivity reaction, lactic acidosis, severe hepatomegaly with steatosis (fatty liver) have occurred. May exacerbate hepatitis B virus infection after completing treatment.

FIXED-COMBINATION(S)

Descovy: emtricitabine/tenofovir alafenamide (TAF) (a nucleotide reverse transcriptase inhibitor): 200 mg/25 mg. **Atripla:** emtricitabine/efavirenz (an antiretroviral)/tenofovir disoproxil fumarate (TDF) (an antiretroviral): 200 mg/600 mg/300 mg. **Complera:** emtricitabine/rilpivirine (an antiretroviral)/tenofovir disoproxil fumarate (TDF) (an antiretroviral): 200 mg/25 mg/300 mg. **Genvoya:** emtricitabine/elvitegravir (an integrase inhibitor)/cobicistat (a pharmacokinetic enhancer)/tenofovir alafenamide (TAF) (a nucleotide reverse transcriptase inhibitor):

200 mg/150 mg/150 mg/10 mg. **Truvada:** emtricitabine/tenofovir disoproxil fumarate (TDF) (an antiretroviral): 200 mg/300 mg. **Stribild:** emtricitabine/elvitegravir (an integrase inhibitor)/cobicistat (a pharmacokinetic enhancer)/tenofovir disoproxil fumarate (TDF) (a nucleotide reverse transcriptase inhibitor): 200 mg/150 mg/150 mg/300 mg.
Odefsey: emtricitabine/rilpivirine (non-nucleoside reverse transcriptase inhibitor [NNRTI])/tenofovir alafenamide (TAF) (a nucleotide reverse transcriptase inhibitor): 200 mg/25 mg/25 mg.

◆CLASSIFICATION

PHARMACOTHERAPEUTIC: Nucleoside reverse transcriptase inhibitor. **CLINICAL:** Antiretroviral agent.

USES

Used in combination with at least two other antiretroviral agents for treatment of HIV-1 infection.

PRECAUTIONS

Contraindications: Hypersensitivity to emtricitabine. **Cautions:** Renal impairment, history of hepatitis, diabetes.

ACTION

Inhibits HIV-1 reverse transcriptase by incorporating itself into viral DNA, resulting in chain termination. **Therapeutic Effect:** Impairs HIV replication, slowing progression of HIV infection.

PHARMACOKINETICS

Rapidly, extensively absorbed from GI tract. Protein binding: less than 4%. Excreted primarily in urine. **Half-life:** 10 hrs.

⧖ LIFESPAN CONSIDERATIONS

Pregnancy/Lactation: Breastfeeding not recommended. **Children:** Safety and efficacy not established. **Elderly:** Age-related renal impairment may require dosage adjustment.

INTERACTIONS

DRUG: None significant. **HERBAL:** None significant. **FOOD:** None known. **LAB VALUES:** May increase serum amylase, lipase, ALT, AST, triglycerides. May alter serum glucose.

AVAILABILITY (Rx)

Capsules: 200 mg. **Oral Solution:** 10 mg/mL.

ADMINISTRATION/HANDLING

PO
• Give without regard to food.

INDICATIONS/ROUTES/DOSAGE

HIV
Capsules
PO: ADULTS, ELDERLY, CHILDREN 3 MOS–17 YRS, WEIGHING MORE THAN 33 KG: 200 mg once daily.
Oral Solution
PO: ADULTS, ELDERLY: 240 mg once daily. **CHILDREN 3 MOS–17 YRS WEIGHING MORE THAN 33 KG:** 6 mg/kg once daily. **Maximum:** 240 mg once daily. **CHILDREN 0–3 MOS:** 3 mg/kg/day.

Dosage in Renal Impairment

Creatinine Clearance	Capsule	Oral Solution
30–49 mL/min	200 mg q48h	120 mg q24h
15–29 mL/min	200 mg q72h	80 mg q24h
Less than 15 mL/min; hemodialysis pts	200 mg q96h	60 mg q24h (administer after dialysis)

Administer after dialysis on dialysis days.

Dosage in Hepatic Impairment
No dose adjustment.

SIDE EFFECTS

Frequent (23%–13%): Headache, rhinitis, rash, diarrhea, nausea. **Occasional (14%–4%):** Cough, vomiting, abdominal pain, insomnia, depression, paresthesia, dizziness, peripheral neuropathy, dyspepsia, myalgia. **Rare (3%–2%):** Arthralgia, abnormal dreams.

ADVERSE EFFECTS/TOXIC REACTIONS

Lactic acidosis, hepatomegaly with steatosis (excess fat in liver) occur rarely; may be severe. May cause immune reconstitution syndrome, reactivation of hepatitis B virus infection.

NURSING CONSIDERATIONS

BASELINE ASSESSMENT

Obtain LFT, serum triglycerides before beginning and at periodic intervals during therapy. Offer emotional support.

INTERVENTION/EVALUATION

Monitor daily pattern of bowel activity, stool consistency. Question for evidence of nausea, pruritus. Assess skin for rash, urticaria. Monitor serum chemistry tests, LFT for marked abnormalities; signs/symptoms of lactic acidosis. Monitor for immune reconstitution syndrome, Hepatitis B virus reactivation.

PATIENT/FAMILY TEACHING

• May cause redistribution of body fat. • Continue therapy for full length of treatment. • Emtricitabine is not a cure for HIV infection, nor does it reduce risk of transmission to others. • Pts may continue to acquire illnesses associated with advanced HIV infection. • Avoid tasks that require alertness, motor skills until response to drug is established. • Report persistent or severe abdominal pain, nausea, vomiting, numbness.

enalapril

en-**al**-a-pril
(Apo-Enalapril ✦, Epaned, Novo-Enalapril ✦, Vasotec)
■ **BLACK BOX ALERT** ■ May cause fetal injury. Discontinue as soon as possible once pregnancy is detected.
Do not confuse enalapril with Anafranil, Elavil, Eldepryl, lisinopril, or ramipril.

E

FIXED-COMBINATION(S)

Lexxel: enalapril/felodipine (calcium channel blocker): 5 mg/2.5 mg, 5 mg/5 mg. **Teczem:** enalapril/diltiaZEM (calcium channel blocker): 5 mg/180 mg. **Vaseretic:** enalapril/hydroCHLOROthiazide (diuretic): 5 mg/12.5 mg, 10 mg/25 mg.

◆CLASSIFICATION

PHARMACOTHERAPEUTIC: Angiotensin-converting enzyme (ACE) inhibitor. **CLINICAL:** Antihypertensive, vasodilator.

USES

Treatment of hypertension alone or in combination with other antihypertensives. Adjunctive therapy for symptomatic HF. Treatment of asymptomatic left ventricular dysfunction. **(Epaned):** Treatment of hypertension in adults and children older than 1 mo. **OFF-LABEL:** Proteinuria in steroid-resistant nephrotic syndrome.

PRECAUTIONS

Contraindications: Hypersensitivity to enalapril. History of angioedema from previous treatment with ACE inhibitors. Idiopathic/hereditary angioedema. Concomitant use of aliskiren in pts with diabetes. **Cautions:** Renal impairment, hypertrophic cardiomyopathy with outflow tract obstruction; severe aortic stenosis; before, during, or immediately after major surgery. Concomitant use of potassium supplement; unstented unilateral or bilateral renal artery stenosis.

ACTION

Suppresses renin-angiotensin-aldosterone system (prevents conversion of angiotensin I to angiotensin II, a potent vasoconstrictor; may inhibit angiotensin II at local vascular, renal sites). Decreases plasma angiotensin II, increases plasma renin activity, decreases aldosterone secretion. **Therapeutic Effect:** In hypertension, reduces peripheral arterial resistance. In HF, increases cardiac output; decreases peripheral vascular resistance, B/P, pulmonary capillary wedge pressure, heart size.

PHARMACOKINETICS

Route	Onset	Peak	Duration
PO	1 hr	4–6 hrs	24 hrs
IV	15 min	1–4 hrs	6 hrs

Readily absorbed from GI tract. Prodrug undergoes hepatic biotransformation to enalaprilat. Protein binding: 50%–60%. Primarily excreted in urine. Removed by hemodialysis. **Half-life:** 11 hrs (increased in renal impairment).

⏳ LIFESPAN CONSIDERATIONS

Pregnancy/Lactation: Crosses placenta. Distributed in breast milk. May cause fetal/neonatal mortality, morbidity. **Children:** Safety and efficacy not established. **Elderly:** May be more susceptible to hypotensive effects.

INTERACTIONS

DRUG: Alcohol, antihypertensives (e.g., amLODIPine, cloNIDine, valsartan), diuretics (e.g., furosemide, torsemide) may increase effects. **NSAIDs (e.g., ibuprofen, ketorolac, naproxen)** may decrease antihypertensive effect, increase risk of possible acute renal failure. **Potassium-sparing diuretics (e.g., spironolactone, triamterene), potassium supplements** may cause hyperkalemia. May increase **lithium** concentration, toxicity. **HERBAL: Ephedra, ginseng, yohimbe** may worsen hypertension. **Garlic** may increase antihypertensive effect. **Licorice** may cause sodium/water retention, loss of potassium. **FOOD:** None known. **LAB VALUES:** May increase serum BUN, alkaline phosphatase, bilirubin, creatinine, potassium, ALT, AST. May decrease serum sodium. May cause positive ANA titer.

AVAILABILITY (Rx)

Injection Solution: 1.25 mg/mL. **Powder for Oral Solution (Epaned):** 1 mg/mL (after reconstitution). **Tablets:** 2.5 mg, 5 mg, 10 mg, 20 mg.

ADMINISTRATION/HANDLING

 IV

Reconstitution • May give undiluted or dilute with D₅W or 0.9% NaCl.
Rate of Administration • For IV push, give undiluted over 5 min. • For IV piggyback, infuse over 10–15 min.
Storage • Store parenteral form at room temperature. • Use only clear, colorless solution. • Diluted IV solution is stable for 24 hrs at room temperature.

PO

• Give without regard to food. • Tablets may be crushed.

Epaned

• Reconstitute with 150 mL Ora-Sweet SF (provided) to produce a 1 mg/mL concentration. Stable for 60 days after reconstitution.

🔲 IV INCOMPATIBILITIES

Amphotericin B (Fungizone), amphotericin B complex (Abelcet, AmBisome, Amphotec), cefepime (Maxipime), phenytoin (Dilantin).

🔲 IV COMPATIBILITIES

Calcium gluconate, dexmedetomidine (Precedex), DOBUTamine (Dobutrex), DOPamine (Intropin), fentaNYL (Sublimaze), heparin, lidocaine, magnesium sulfate, morphine, nitroglycerin, potassium chloride, potassium phosphate, propofol (Diprivan).

INDICATIONS/ROUTES/DOSAGE

Hypertension

PO: ADULTS, ELDERLY: Initially, 2.5–5 mg/day (2.5 mg if pt taking a diuretic). May increase at 1–2 wk intervals. Range: 10–40 mg/day in 1–2 divided doses. **CHILDREN 1 MO–16 YRS:** Initially, 0.08 mg/kg once daily. Adjust dose based on pt response. **Maximum:** 5 mg/day. **NEONATES:** 0.04–0.1 mg/kg/day given q24h. **Epaned: ADULTS, ELDERLY:** Initially, 5 mg once daily.

CHILDREN: Initially, 0.08 mg/kg once daily. Adjust dose on pt response. **Maximum:** 5 mg.
IV: ADULTS, ELDERLY: 0.625–1.25 mg q6h up to 5 mg q6h.

Adjunctive Therapy for HF

PO: ADULTS, ELDERLY: Initially, 2.5 mg twice daily. Titrate slowly at 1–2 wk intervals. Range: 5–40 mg/day in 2 divided doses. Target: 10–20 mg twice daily.

Asymptomatic Left Ventricular Dysfunction

PO: ADULTS, ELDERLY: 2.5 mg twice daily. Titrate up to 20 mg/day.

Dosage in Renal Impairment

CrCl greater than 30 mL/min: No dosage adjustment. **CrCl 30 mL/min or less: (HTN):** Initially, 2.5 mg/day. Titrate until B/P controlled. **(HF):** Initially, 2.5 mg twice daily. May increase by 2.5 mg/dose at greater than 4-day intervals. **Maximum:** 40 mg/day.
Hemodialysis: Initially, 2.5 mg on dialysis days; adjust dose on non-dialysis days depending on B/P.

Dosage in Hepatic Impairment

No dose adjustment.

SIDE EFFECTS

Frequent (7%–5%): Headache, dizziness. **Occasional (3%–2%):** Orthostatic hypotension, fatigue, diarrhea, cough, syncope. **Rare (less than 2%):** Angina, abdominal pain, vomiting, nausea, rash, asthenia.

ADVERSE EFFECTS/TOXIC REACTIONS

Excessive hypotension ("first-dose syncope") may occur in pts with HF, severe salt or volume depletion. Angioedema (facial, lip swelling), hyperkalemia occur rarely. Agranulocytosis, neutropenia may be noted in pts with renal impairment, collagen vascular diseases (scleroderma, systemic lupus erythematosus). Nephrotic syndrome may be noted in those with history of renal disease.

NURSING CONSIDERATIONS

BASELINE ASSESSMENT

Obtain BUN, serum creatinine, CrCL. Receive full medication history, esp. potassium-sparing diuretics. Obtain B/P immediately before each dose (be alert to fluctuations). In pts with renal impairment, autoimmune disease, or taking drugs that affect leukocytes/immune response, CBC should be performed before beginning therapy, q2wks for 3 mos, then periodically thereafter.

INTERVENTION/EVALUATION

Assist with ambulation if dizziness occurs. Monitor CBC, serum BUN, potassium, creatinine, B/P. Monitor daily pattern of bowel activity, stool consistency.

PATIENT/FAMILY TEACHING

• To reduce hypotensive effect, go from lying to standing slowly. • Several wks may be needed for full therapeutic effect of B/P reduction. • Skipping doses or voluntarily discontinuing drug may produce severe rebound hypertension. • Limit alcohol intake. • Report vomiting, diarrhea, diaphoresis, persistent cough, difficulty in breathing; swelling of face, lips, tongue.

---

enoxaparin

en-**ox**-a-par-in
(Lovenox)
■ **BLACK BOX ALERT** ■ Epidural or spinal anesthesia greatly increases potential for spinal or epidural hematoma, subsequent long-term or permanent paralysis.

Do not confuse Lovenox with Lasix, Levaquin, Lotronex, or Protonix, or enoxaparin with dalteparin or heparin.

◆CLASSIFICATION

PHARMACOTHERAPEUTIC: Low molecular weight heparin. **CLINICAL:** Anticoagulant.

USES

DVT prophylaxis following hip or knee replacement surgery, abdominal surgery, or pts with severely restricted mobility during acute illness. Treatment of acute coronary syndrome (ACS): unstable angina, non–Q-wave MI, acute ST-segment elevation MI (STEMI). Treatment of DVT with or without pulmonary embolism (PE) (inpatient); without PE (outpatient). **OFF-LABEL:** DVT prophylaxis following moderate-risk general surgery, gynecologic surgery; management of venous thromboembolism (VTE) during pregnancy. Bariatric surgery, mechanical heart valve to bridge anticoagulation, percutaneous coronary intervention (PCI) adjunctive therapy.

PRECAUTIONS

Contraindications: Hypersensitivity to enoxaparin. Active major bleeding, concurrent heparin therapy, hypersensitivity to heparin, pork products, thrombocytopenia associated with positive in vitro test for antiplatelet antibodies. Not for IM use. **Cautions:** Conditions with increased risk of hemorrhage, platelet defects, renal impairment (renal failure), elderly, uncontrolled arterial hypertension, history of recent GI ulceration or hemorrhage. When neuraxial anesthesia (epidural or spinal anesthesia) or spinal puncture is used, pts anticoagulated or scheduled to be anticoagulated with enoxaparin for prevention of thromboembolic complications are at risk for developing an epidural or spinal hematoma that can result in long-term or permanent paralysis. Bacterial endocarditis, hemorrhagic stroke, history of heparin-induced thrombocytopenia (HIT), severe hepatic disease.

ACTION

Potentiates action of antithrombin III, inactivates coagulation factor Xa. **Therapeutic Effect:** Produces anticoagulation. Does not significantly influence PT, aPTT.

PHARMACOKINETICS

Route	Onset	Peak	Duration
Subcutaneous	N/A	3–5 hrs	12 hrs

Well absorbed after subcutaneous administration. Excreted primarily in urine. Not removed by hemodialysis. **Half-life:** 4.5–7 hrs.

⧗ LIFESPAN CONSIDERATIONS

Pregnancy/Lactation: Use with caution, particularly during third trimester, immediate postpartum period (increased risk of maternal hemorrhage). Unknown if distributed in breast milk. Pregnant women with mechanical heart valves (and their fetuses) may have increased risk of bleeding. **Children:** Safety and efficacy not established. **Elderly:** May be more susceptible to bleeding.

INTERACTIONS

DRUG: Antiplatelet agents (e.g., **clopidogrel**), **aspirin**, NSAIDs (e.g., **ibuprofen, ketorolac, naproxen**), **thrombolytics** (e.g., **tPA**) may increase risk of bleeding. **HERBAL:** Cat's claw, dong quai, evening primrose, feverfew, garlic, ginger, ginkgo, ginseng may increase antiplatelet action. **FOOD:** None known. **LAB VALUES:** Increases serum alkaline phosphatase, ALT, AST. May decrease Hgb, Hct, platelets, RBCs.

AVAILABILITY (Rx)

Injection Solution: 30 mg/0.3 mL, 40 mg/0.4 mL, 60 mg/0.6 mL, 80 mg/0.8 mL, 100 mg/mL, 120 mg/0.8 mL, 150 mg/mL in prefilled syringes.

ADMINISTRATION/HANDLING

◀**ALERT**▶ Do not mix with other injections, infusions. Do not give IM.
Subcutaneous
Preparation • Visually inspect for particulate matter or discoloration. Solution should appear clear, colorless to pale yellow in color. Do not use if solution is cloudy, discolored, or if visible particles are observed.

Administration • Flick syringe so that the air bubble rises toward the plunger. • Insert needle subcutaneously into abdomen or outer thigh and inject solution (including air bubble). • Do not inject into areas of active skin disease or injury such as sunburns, skin rashes, inflammation, skin infections, or active psoriasis. • Rotate injection sites.
Storage • Store at room temperature.

INDICATIONS/ROUTES/DOSAGE

Prevention of Deep Vein Thrombosis (DVT) After Hip and Knee Surgery
SQ: ADULTS, ELDERLY: 30 mg twice daily, generally for 7–10 days, with initial dose given within 12–24 hrs following surgery. **Hip surgery:** An initial dose of 40 mg, given 9–15 hrs before surgery, may be considered for some pts. Following hip surgery, recommend continuing 40 mg once daily for 3 wks (if 40 mg dose was initially given).

Prevention of DVT After Abdominal Surgery
SQ: ADULTS, ELDERLY: 40 mg/day for 7–10 days, with initial dose given 2 hrs prior to surgery.

Prevention of DVT After Bariatric Surgery
BMI 50 or less (kg/m²): 40 mg q12h. **BMI greater than 50 kg/m²:** 60 mg q12h.

Prevention of Long-Term DVT in Nonsurgical Acute Illness
SQ: ADULTS, ELDERLY: 40 mg once daily; continue until risk of DVT has diminished (usually 6–11 days).

Prevention of Ischemic Complications of Unstable Angina, Non–Q-Wave MI (with Oral Aspirin Therapy)
SQ: ADULTS, ELDERLY: 1 mg/kg q12h (with oral aspirin).

STEMI
SQ: ADULTS YOUNGER THAN 75 YRS: 30 mg IV once plus 1 mg/kg q12h (**maximum:** 100 mg first 2 doses only). **ADULTS 75 YRS OR OLDER:** 0.75 mg/kg (**maximum:** 75 mg first 2 doses only) q12h.

E

Acute DVT

SQ: ADULTS, ELDERLY: (Inpatient): 1 mg/kg q12h or 1.5 mg/kg once daily. **(Outpatient):** 1 mg/kg q12h.

Usual Pediatric Dosage

SQ: CHILDREN 2 MOS AND OLDER: 0.5 mg/kg q12h (prophylaxis); 1 mg/kg q12h (treatment). **NEONATES, INFANTS YOUNGER THAN 2 MOS:** 0.75/mg/kg/dose q12h (prophylaxis); 1.5 mg/kg/dose q12h (treatment).

Dosage in Renal Impairment

Elimination is decreased when CrCl is less than 30 mL/min. Monitor and adjust dosage as necessary.

Use	Dosage
Abdominal surgery, pts with acute illness	30 mg once/day
Hip, knee surgery	30 mg once/day
DVT, angina, MI	1 mg/kg once/day
STEMI (<75 yrs)	30 mg IV once plus 1 mg/kg q24h
STEMI (75 yrs or greater)	1 mg/kg q24h
NSTEMI	1 mg/kg q24h

Dosage in Hepatic Impairment

Use caution.

SIDE EFFECTS

Occasional (4%–1%): Injection site hematoma, nausea, peripheral edema.

ADVERSE EFFECTS/TOXIC REACTIONS

May lead to bleeding complications ranging from local ecchymoses to major hemorrhage. May cause heparin-induced thrombocytopenia (HIT). **Antidote:** IV injection of protamine sulfate (1% solution) equal to dose of enoxaparin injected. 1 mg protamine sulfate neutralizes 1 mg enoxaparin. One additional dose of 0.5 mg protamine sulfate per 1 mg enoxaparin may be given if aPTT tested 2–4 hrs after first injection remains prolonged.

NURSING CONSIDERATIONS

BASELINE ASSESSMENT

Obtain baseline CBC. Note platelet count. Question medical history as listed in Precautions. Ensure that pt has not received spinal anesthesia, spinal procedures. Assess for active bleeding. Assess pt's willingness to self-inject medication. Assess potential risk of bleeding.

INTERVENTION/EVALUATION

Periodically monitor CBC, platelet count, stool for occult blood (no need for daily monitoring in pts with normal presurgical coagulation parameters). A decrease in the platelet count of more than 50% from baseline may indicate heparin-induced thrombocytopenia. Ensure active hemostasis of puncture site following PCI. Assess for any sign of bleeding (bleeding at surgical site, hematuria, blood in stool, bleeding from gums, petechiae, bruising, bleeding from injection sites).

PATIENT/FAMILY TEACHING

• Usual length of therapy is 7–10 days. • A health care provider will show you how to properly prepare and inject your medication. You must demonstrate correct preparation and injection techniques before using medication at home. • Do not discontinue current blood thinning regimen or take any newly prescribed medications unless approved by the prescriber who originally started treatment. • Suddenly stopping therapy may increase the risk of blood clots or stroke. • Report bleeding of any kind (bloody urine, stool; nosebleeds; increased menstrual bleeding). If bleeding occurs, it may take longer to stop bleeding. • Immediately report signs of stroke (confusion, headache, numbness, one-sided weakness, trouble speaking, loss of vision). • Minor blunt force trauma to the head, chest, or abdomen can be life-threatening. • Do not take aspirin, herbal supplements, OTC nonsteroidal anti-inflammatories (may increase risk of bleeding). • Consult physician before any surgery/dental work. • Use electric razor, soft toothbrush to prevent bleeding.

entecavir

en-**tek**-a-veer
(Baraclude, Apo-Entecavir ✦)

■ **BLACK BOX ALERT** ■ Serious, sometimes fatal hypersensitivity reaction, lactic acidosis, severe hepatomegaly with steatosis (fatty liver) have occurred. May cause HIV resistance in chronic hepatitis B pts. Severe acute exacerbations of hepatitis B virus infection may occur upon discontinuation of entecavir.

◆CLASSIFICATION

PHARMACOTHERAPEUTIC: Reverse transcriptase inhibitor, nucleoside. **CLINICAL:** Antihepadnaviral agent.

USES

Treatment of chronic hepatitis B virus (HBV) infection with evidence of active viral replication and evidence of either persistent transaminase elevations or histologically active disease or evidence of decompensated hepatic disease. **OFF-LABEL:** HBV reinfection prophylaxis, post–liver transplant, HIV/HBV coinfection.

PRECAUTIONS

Contraindications: Hypersensitivity to entecavir. **Cautions:** Renal impairment, pts receiving concurrent therapy that may reduce renal function. Pts at risk for hepatic disease. Cross resistance may develop with lamivudine.

ACTION

Inhibits hepatitis B viral polymerase, an enzyme blocking reverse transcriptase activity. **Therapeutic Effect:** Interferes with viral DNA synthesis.

PHARMACOKINETICS

Poorly absorbed from GI tract. Protein binding: 13%. Extensively distributed into tissues. Partially metabolized in liver. Excreted primarily in urine. **Half-life:** 5–6 days (increased in renal impairment).

⌛ LIFESPAN CONSIDERATIONS

Pregnancy/Lactation: Unknown if drug crosses placenta or is distributed in breast milk. **Children:** Safety and efficacy not established in pts younger than 16 yrs. **Elderly:** Age-related renal impairment may require dosage adjustment.

INTERACTIONS

DRUG: Ganciclovir, ribavirin, valGANciclovir may increase concentration. **HERBAL:** None significant. **FOOD: Food** delays absorption, decreases concentration. **LAB VALUES:** May increase serum amylase, lipase, bilirubin, ALT, AST, creatinine, glucose. May decrease serum albumin; platelets.

AVAILABILITY (Rx)

Oral Solution: 0.05 mg/mL. **Tablets:** 0.5 mg, 1 mg.

ADMINISTRATION/HANDLING

PO

• Administer tablets on an empty stomach (at least 2 hrs after a meal and 2 hrs before the next meal). • Do not dilute, mix oral solution with water or any other liquid. • Each bottle of oral solution is accompanied by a dosing spoon. Before administering, hold spoon in vertical position, fill it gradually to mark corresponding to prescribed dose.

Storage • Store tablets, oral solution at room temperature.

INDICATIONS/ROUTES/DOSAGE

Chronic Hepatitis B Virus Infection (No Previous Nucleoside Treatment)
PO: ADULTS, ELDERLY, CHILDREN 16 YRS AND OLDER: 0.5 mg once daily. **CHILDREN 2 YRS AND OLDER: (Weighing more than 30 kg):** 0.5 mg once daily (tablet or solution). **(27–30 kg):** 0.45 mg once daily (solution). **(24–26 kg):** 0.4 mg once daily (solution). **(21–23 kg):** 0.35 mg once

E

daily (solution). **(18–20 kg):** 0.3 mg once daily (solution). **(15–17 kg):** 0.25 mg once daily (solution). **(12–14 kg):** 0.2 mg once daily (solution). **(10–11 kg):** 0.15 mg once daily (solution).

Chronic Hepatitis B Virus Infection (Receiving LamiVUDine, Known LamiVUDine Resistance, Decompensated Liver Disease)
PO: **ADULTS, ELDERLY, CHILDREN 16 YRS AND OLDER:** 1 mg once daily. **CHILDREN 2 YRS AND OLDER: (Weighing more than 30 kg):** 1 mg once daily (tablet or solution). **(27–30 kg):** 0.9 mg once daily (solution). **(24–26 kg):** 0.8 mg once daily (solution). **(21–23 kg):** 0.7 mg once daily (solution). **(18–20 kg):** 0.6 mg once daily (solution). **(15–17 kg):** 0.5 mg once daily (solution). **(12–14 kg):** 0.4 mg once daily (solution). **(10–11 kg):** 0.3 mg once daily (solution).

Dosage in Renal Impairment

Creatinine Clearance	Dosage
50 mL/min and greater	0.5 mg once daily
30–49 mL/min	0.25 mg once daily
10–29 mL/min	0.15 mg once daily
9 mL/min and less	0.05 mg once daily

Dosage in Hepatic Impairment
No dose adjustment.

SIDE EFFECTS

Occasional (4%–3%): Headache, fatigue. **Rare (less than 1%):** Diarrhea, dyspepsia, nausea, vomiting, dizziness, insomnia.

ADVERSE EFFECTS/TOXIC REACTIONS

Lactic acidosis, severe hepatomegaly with steatosis have been reported. Severe, acute exacerbations of hepatitis B virus infection have been reported in pts who have discontinued therapy; reinitiation of antihepatitis B therapy may be required. Hematuria occurs occasionally. May cause development of HIV resistance if HIV untreated.

NURSING CONSIDERATIONS

BASELINE ASSESSMENT

Obtain LFT before beginning therapy and at periodic intervals during therapy. Offer emotional support. Obtain full medication history.

INTERVENTION/EVALUATION

Hepatic function should be monitored closely with both clinical and laboratory follow-up for at least several mos in pts who discontinue antihepatitis B therapy. For pts on therapy, closely monitor serum amylase, lipase, bilirubin, ALT, AST, creatinine, glucose, albumin; platelet count. Assess for evidence of GI discomfort.

PATIENT/FAMILY TEACHING

• Take medication at least 2 hrs after a meal and 2 hrs before the next meal. • Avoid transmission of hepatitis B infection to others through sexual contact, blood contamination. • Immediately report unusual muscle pain, abdominal pain with nausea/vomiting, cold feeling in extremities, dizziness (signs and symptoms signaling onset of lactic acidosis).

enzalutamide

en-za-**loo**-ta-mide
(XTANDI)
Do not confuse enzalutamide with bicalutamide, flutamide, or nilutamide.

◆CLASSIFICATION

PHARMACOTHERAPEUTIC: Antiandrogen renal inhibitor. **CLINICAL:** Antineoplastic.

USES

Treatment of metastatic castration-resistant prostate cancer.

PRECAUTIONS

Contraindications: Hypersensitivity to enzalutamide. Women who are pregnant or may become pregnant (not indicated in female population). **Cautions:** History of seizure disorder, underlying brain injury with loss of consciousness, transient ischemic attack within past 12 mos, CVA, brain metastases, brain arteriovenous abnormality, use of concurrent medications that may lower seizure threshold.

ACTION

Inhibits androgen binding to androgen receptors in target tissue, and inhibits interaction with DNA. **Therapeutic Effect:** Decreases proliferation, induces cell death of prostate cancer cells.

PHARMACOKINETICS

Readily absorbed in GI tract. Maximum plasma concentration achieved in 0.5–3 hrs. Metabolized in liver. Protein binding: (97%–98%). Primarily excreted in urine. **Half-life:** 5.8 days (Range: 2.8–10.2 days).

LIFESPAN CONSIDERATIONS

Pregnancy/Lactation: Not used in female population. **Children:** Safety and efficacy not established. **Elderly:** No age-related precautions noted.

INTERACTIONS

DRUG: Strong CYP2C8, CYP3A4 inhibitors (e.g., gemfibrozil, itraconazole) may increase concentration. **CYP3A4 inducers (e.g., carBAMazepine, phenytoin, rifAMPin)** may decrease concentration/effect. **HERBAL:** None significant. **FOOD:** None known. **LAB VALUES:** May increase serum ALT, AST, bilirubin. May decrease Hgb, Hct, platelets, WBC count.

AVAILABILITY (Rx)

Capsules: 40 mg.

ADMINISTRATION/HANDLING

PO • May give with or without food. Take at same time each day. Swallow whole. • Do not break, crush, dissolve, or open capsules.

INDICATIONS/ROUTES/DOSAGE

Metastatic Castration-Resistant Prostate Cancer
PO: ADULTS, ELDERLY: 160 mg (4 × 40 mg capsules) given once daily.

Dose Modification
If CTCAE Grade 3 or greater toxicity or an intolerable side effect occurs, withhold dosing for 1 week or until symptoms improve to Grade 2 or less, then resume at same dose or a reduced dose (120 mg or 80 mg). **Concurrent use of strong CYP2C8 inhibitors:** Avoid use (if possible). If concurrent use is necessary, reduce the enzalutamide dose to 80 mg once daily. **Concurrent use of strong CYP3A4 inducers:** Increase dose to 240 mg once daily.

Dosage in Renal/Hepatic Impairment
No dose adjustment.

SIDE EFFECTS

Common (51%): Asthenia. **Frequent (26%–15%):** Back pain, diarrhea, arthralgia, hot flashes, peripheral edema, musculoskeletal pain. **Occasional (12%–6%):** Headache, dizziness, insomnia, hematuria, paresthesia, anxiety, hypertension. **Rare (4%–2%):** Mental impairment disorders (includes amnesia, memory impairment, cognitive disorder, attention deficit), hematuria (includes pollakiuria, pruritus, dry skin).

ADVERSE EFFECTS/TOXIC REACTIONS

Upper respiratory tract infection occurs in 11% of pts; lower respiratory tract and lung infection (includes pneumonia, bronchitis) occur in slightly less (9% of pts). Spinal cord compression and cauda equina syndrome occur in 7% of pts.

NURSING CONSIDERATIONS

BASELINE ASSESSMENT

Offer emotional support. Obtain LFT at baseline and periodically throughout therapy. Assess bowel activity, stool consistency. If coadministered with warfarin

---

(CYP2C9 substrate), perform additional INR monitoring.

INTERVENTION/EVALUATION

Assess for peripheral edema. Question level of fatigue, weakness. Question presence of back pain, arthralgia, or headache. Assess level of anxiety. Monitor B/P for hypertension. Assess for hematuria. Question pt regarding sleeping pattern.

PATIENT/FAMILY TEACHING

• Sexually active men must wear condom during treatment and for 1 wk after treatment due to potential risks to fetus. • Women who are pregnant or are planning pregnancy may not touch medication without gloves. • Dizziness, headache, muscle weakness, leg swelling/discomfort should be reported. • Immediately report fever or cough. • Routine lab testing will occur during treatment.

EPINEPHrine   [HIGH ALERT]

ep-i-**nef**-rin
(Adrenalin, EpiPen, EpiPen Jr., Twinject)
Do not confuse EPINEPHrine with ePHEDrine.

FIXED-COMBINATION(S)

LidoSite: EPINEPHrine/lidocaine (anesthetic): 0.1%/10%.

◆CLASSIFICATION

PHARMACOTHERAPEUTIC: Sympathomimetic (alpha-, beta-adrenergic agonist). **CLINICAL:** Antiglaucoma, bronchodilator, cardiac stimulant, antiallergic, antihemorrhagic, priapism reversal agent.

USES

Treatment of allergic reactions (including anaphylactic reactions). Treatment of hypotension associated with septic shock. Added to local anesthetics to decrease systemic absorption and increase duration of activity of local anesthetic. Decreases superficial hemorrhage. **OFF-LABEL:** Ventricular fibrillation or pulseless ventricular tachycardia unresponsive to initial defibrillatory shocks; pulseless electrical activity, asystole, hypotension unresponsive to volume resuscitation; bradycardia/hypotension unresponsive to atropine or pacing; inotropic support.

PRECAUTIONS

Contraindications: Hypersensitivity to EPINEPHrine. **Note:** There are no absolute contraindications with injectable EPINEPHrine in a life-threatening situation. **IV:** Narrow-angle glaucoma, thyrotoxicosis, diabetes, hypertension, other cardiovascular disorders. **Inhalation:** Concurrent use or within 2 wks of MAOIs. **Cautions:** Elderly, diabetes mellitus, hypertension, Parkinson's disease, thyroid disease, cerebrovascular or cardiovascular disease, concurrent use of tricyclic antidepressants. History of prostate enlargement, urinary retention.

ACTION

Stimulates alpha-adrenergic receptors (vasoconstriction, pressor effects), beta$_1$-adrenergic receptors (cardiac stimulation), beta$_2$-adrenergic receptors (bronchial dilation, vasodilation). **Therapeutic Effect:** Relaxes smooth muscle of bronchial tree, produces cardiac stimulation, dilates skeletal muscle vasculature.

PHARMACOKINETICS

Route	Onset	Peak	Duration
IM	5–10 min	20 min	1–4 hrs
Subcutaneous	5–10 min	20 min	1–4 hrs
Inhalation	3–5 min	20 min	1–3 hrs

Well absorbed after parenteral administration; minimally absorbed after inhalation. Metabolized in liver, other tissues, sympathetic nerve endings. Excreted in urine. Ophthalmic form may be systemically absorbed as a result of drainage into nasal pharyngeal passages. Mydriasis occurs within several min and persists several hrs; vasoconstriction occurs within 5 min and lasts less than 1 hr.

⧖ LIFESPAN CONSIDERATIONS

Pregnancy/Lactation: Crosses placenta. Distributed in breast milk. **Children/Elderly:** No age-related precautions noted.

INTERACTIONS

DRUG: May decrease effects of **beta blockers** (e.g., **carvedilol, metoprolol**). **Digoxin, sympathomimetics** (e.g., **dopamine, norepinephrine**) may increase risk of arrhythmias. **Ergonovine, methergine, oxytocin** may increase vasoconstriction. **MAOIs** (e.g., **phenelzine, selegiline**), **tricyclic antidepressants** (e.g., **amitriptyline, doxepin, nortriptyline**) may increase cardiovascular effects. **HERBAL:** Ephedra, yohimbe may increase CNS stimulation. **FOOD:** None known. **LAB VALUES:** May decrease serum potassium.

AVAILABILITY (Rx)

Injection, Solution (Prefilled Syringes): *(EpiPen):* 0.3 mg/0.3 mL, *(EpiPen Jr.):* 0.15 mg/0.3 mL, *(Twinject):* 0.15 mg/0.15 mL. **Injection, Solution:** 0.1 mg/mL (1:10,000), 1 mg/mL (1:1,000).

Solution for Oral Inhalation *(Adrenalin):* 2.25% (0.5 mL).

ADMINISTRATION/HANDLING

 IV

Reconstitution • For injection, dilute each 1 mg of 1:1,000 solution with 10 mL 0.9% NaCl to provide 1:10,000 solution and inject each 1 mg or fraction thereof over 1 min or more (except in cardiac arrest). • For infusion, further dilute with 250–500 mL D₅W. Maximum concentration 64 mcg/mL.
Rate of Administration • For IV infusion, give at 1–10 mcg/min (titrate to desired response).

Storage • Store parenteral forms at room temperature. • Do not use if solution appears discolored or contains a precipitate.

Subcutaneous
• Shake ampule thoroughly. • Use tuberculin syringe for injection into lateral deltoid region. • Massage injection site (minimizes vasoconstriction effect). Use only 1:1,000 solution.

Nebulizer
• No more than 10 drops Adrenalin Chloride solution 1:100 should be placed in reservoir of nebulizer. • Place nozzle just inside pt's partially opened mouth. • As bulb is squeezed once or twice, instruct pt to inhale deeply, drawing vaporized solution into lungs. • Rinse mouth with water immediately after inhalation (prevents mouth/throat dryness). • When nebulizer is not in use, replace stopper, keep in upright position.

▣ IV INCOMPATIBILITIES

Ampicillin, pantoprazole (Protonix), sodium bicarbonate.

▣ IV COMPATIBILITIES

Calcium chloride, calcium gluconate, dexmedetomidine (Precedex), diltiaZEM (Cardizem), DOBUTamine (Dobutrex), DOPamine (Intropin), fentaNYL (Sublimaze), heparin, HYDROmorphone (Dilaudid), LORazepam (Ativan), midazolam (Versed), milrinone (Primacor), morphine, nitroglycerin, norepinephrine (Levophed), potassium chloride, propofol (Diprivan).

INDICATIONS/ROUTES/DOSAGE

Anaphylaxis
IM, SQ: ADULTS, ELDERLY: 0.2–0.5 mg (0.2–0.5 mL of 1:1,000 solution). May repeat q5–15 min if anaphylaxis persists. **CHILDREN:** 0.01 mg/kg (0.01 mL/kg of a 1:1,000 solution) q5–15 min. **Maximum single dose:** 0.3 mg.

E

Hypotension (Shock)
IV INFUSION: **ADULTS, ELDERLY:** 0.05–2 mcg/kg/min. Titrate to desired mean arterial pressure (MAP). May adjust dose by 0.05–0.2 mcg/kg/min.

Cardiac Arrest
IV: **ADULTS, ELDERLY:** Initially, 1 mg. May repeat q3–5min as needed. **CHILDREN:** Initially, 0.01 mg/kg (0.1 mL/kg of a 1:10,000 solution). May repeat q3–5min as needed.
Endotracheal: **ADULTS, ELDERLY:** 2–2.5 mg q3–5 min as needed. **CHILDREN:** 0.1 mg/kg (0.1 mL/kg of a 1:1,000 solution). May repeat q3–5min as needed.

Dosage in Renal/Hepatic Impairment
No dose adjustment.

SIDE EFFECTS

Frequent: **Systemic:** Tachycardia, palpitations, anxiety. **Ophthalmic:** Headache, eye irritation, watering of eyes. **Occasional:** **Systemic:** Dizziness, lightheadedness, facial flushing, headache, diaphoresis, increased B/P, nausea, trembling, insomnia, vomiting, fatigue. **Ophthalmic:** Blurred/decreased vision, eye pain. **Rare:** **Systemic:** Chest discomfort/pain, arrhythmias, bronchospasm, dry mouth/throat.

ADVERSE EFFECTS/TOXIC REACTIONS

Excessive doses may cause acute hypertension, arrhythmias. Prolonged/excessive use may result in metabolic acidosis due to increased serum lactic acid. Metabolic acidosis may cause disorientation, fatigue, hyperventilation, headache, nausea, vomiting, diarrhea.

NURSING CONSIDERATIONS

INTERVENTION/EVALUATION
Monitor changes of B/P, HR. Assess lung sounds for rhonchi, wheezing, rales. Monitor ABGs. In cardiac arrest, adhere to ACLS protocols.

PATIENT/FAMILY TEACHING
• Avoid excessive use of caffeine.
• Report any new symptoms (tachycardia, shortness of breath, dizziness) immediately: may be systemic effects.

eplerenone

ep-**ler**-e-none
(Inspra)
Do not confuse Inspra with Spiriva.

◆CLASSIFICATION

PHARMACOTHERAPEUTIC: Aldosterone receptor antagonist. **CLINICAL:** Antihypertensive.

USES

Treatment of hypertension alone or in combination with other antihypertensive agents. Treatment of HF following acute myocardial infarction (AMI).

PRECAUTIONS

Contraindications: Hypersensitivity to eplerenone. Concurrent use with strong CYP3A4 inhibitors (e.g., ketoconazole, itraconazole), CrCl less than 30 mL/min, serum potassium level greater than 5.5 mEq/L at initiation. **Hypertension (Additional):** Type 2 diabetes with microalbuminuria; CrCl less than 50 mL/min; serum creatinine greater than 2 mg/dL in men, greater than 1.8 mg/dL in women; concomitant use of potassium supplements or potassium-sparing diuretics. **Cautions:** Hyperkalemia, HF, post-MI, diabetes, mild renal impairment.

ACTION

Binds to mineralocorticoid receptors in kidney, heart, blood vessels, brain, blocking binding of aldosterone. **Therapeutic Effect:** Reduces B/P.

PHARMACOKINETICS

Absorption unaffected by food. Protein binding: 50%. Metabolized in liver.

Excreted in urine (67%), feces (32%). Not removed by hemodialysis. **Half-life:** 4–6 hrs.

⊠ LIFESPAN CONSIDERATIONS

Pregnancy/Lactation: Unknown if drug crosses placenta or is distributed in breast milk. **Children:** Safety and efficacy not established. **Elderly:** No age-related precautions noted.

INTERACTIONS

DRUG: ACE inhibitors (e.g., enalapril, lisinopril), angiotensin II antagonists (e.g., losartan, valsartan), potassium-sparing diuretics (e.g., spironolactone), potassium supplements increase risk of hyperkalemia. CYP3A4 inhibitors (e.g., itraconazole, ketoconazole) increase concentration five-fold (use is contraindicated). NSAIDs may decrease antihypertensive effect. **HERBAL:** St. John's wort decreases effectiveness. **FOOD:** Grapefruit products may increase potential for hyperkalemia, arrhythmias. **LAB VALUES:** May increase serum potassium, ALT, AST, cholesterol, triglycerides, serum creatinine, uric acid. May decrease serum sodium.

AVAILABILITY (Rx)

 Tablets: 25 mg, 50 mg.

ADMINISTRATION/HANDLING

• Do not break, crush, dissolve, or divide film-coated tablets. • May give without regard to food.

INDICATIONS/ROUTES/DOSAGE

Hypertension
PO: ADULTS, ELDERLY: Initially, 50 mg once daily. If 50 mg once daily produces an inadequate B/P response, may increase dosage to 50 mg twice daily. If pt is concurrently receiving CYP3A4 inhibitors (e.g., erythromycin, saquinavir, verapamil, or fluconazole), reduce initial dose to 25 mg once daily.

HF Following MI
PO: ADULTS, ELDERLY: Initially, 25 mg once daily. If tolerated, titrate up to 50 mg once daily within 4 wks.

Dosage Adjustment for Serum Potassium Concentrations in HF
Less than 5 mEq/L: Increase dose from 25 mg daily to 50 mg daily or increase dose from 25 mg every other day to 25 mg daily.
5–5.4 mEq/L: No adjustment needed.
5.5–5.9 mEq/L: Decrease dose from 50 mg daily to 25 mg daily or from 25 mg daily to 25 mg every other day. Decrease dose from 25 mg every other day to withhold medication.
6 mEq/L or Greater: Withhold medication until potassium is less than 5.5 mEq/L, then restart at 25 mg every other day.

Dosage in Renal Impairment
Contraindicated in pts with hypertension with CrCl less than 50 mL/min or serum creatinine greater than 2 mg/dL in males or greater than 1.8 mg/dL in females. All other indications, CrCl less than 30 mL/min, use is contraindicated.

Dosage in Hepatic Impairment
No dose adjustment.

SIDE EFFECTS

Rare (3%–1%): Dizziness, diarrhea, cough, fatigue, flu-like symptoms, abdominal pain.

ADVERSE EFFECTS/TOXIC REACTIONS

Hyperkalemia may occur, particularly in pts with type 2 diabetes mellitus and microalbuminuria.

NURSING CONSIDERATIONS

BASELINE ASSESSMENT

Obtain serum potassium level. Obtain B/P, apical pulse immediately before each dose, in addition to regular monitoring (be alert to fluctuations). If excessive reduction in B/P occurs, place pt in supine position, feet slightly elevated.

E

INTERVENTION/EVALUATION

Assist with ambulation if dizziness occurs. Monitor serum potassium levels. Assess B/P for hypertension/hypotension. Monitor daily pattern of bowel activity, stool consistency. Assess for evidence of flu-like symptoms.

PATIENT/FAMILY TEACHING

• Avoid tasks that require alertness, motor skills until response to drug is established (possible dizziness effect).
• Hypertension requires lifelong control.
• Avoid exercising during hot weather (risk of dehydration, hypotension).
• Do not use salt substitutes containing potassium.

---

epoetin alfa   TOP 100

e-poe-e-tin **al**-fa
(Epogen, Eprex ♥, Procrit)

■ **BLACK BOX ALERT** ■ Increased risk of serious cardiovascular events, thromboembolic events, mortality, time-to-tumor progression in pts with head and neck cancer, metastatic breast cancer, non–small-cell lung cancer when administered to a target hemoglobin of more than 11 g/dL. Increases rate of deep vein thrombosis in perioperative pts not receiving anticoagulant therapy.
Do not confuse epoetin with darbepoetin, or Epogen with Neupogen.

◆CLASSIFICATION

PHARMACOTHERAPEUTIC: Erythropoiesis-stimulating agent (ESA). **CLINICAL:** Erythropoietin.

USES

Treatment of anemia in pts receiving or who have received myelosuppressive chemotherapy for a planned minimum of 2 mos of chemotherapy; pts with chronic renal failure to decrease need for RBC transfusion; HIV-infected pts on zidovudine (AZT) therapy when endogenous erythropoietin levels are 500 mUnits/mL or less; pts scheduled for elective noncardiac, nonvascular surgery, reducing need for allogenic blood transfusions when perioperative Hgb is greater than 10 or less than or equal to 13 g/dL and high risk for blood loss. **OFF-LABEL:** Anemia in myelodysplastic syndromes.

PRECAUTIONS

Contraindications: Hypersensitivity to epoetin. Pure red cell aplasia, uncontrolled hypertension. **Cautions:** History of seizures or controlled hypertension. **Cancer pts:** Tumor growth, shortened survival may occur when Hgb levels of 11 g/dL or greater are achieved with epoetin alfa. **Chronic renal failure pts:** Increased risk for serious cardiovascular reactions (e.g., stroke, MI) when Hgb levels greater than 11 g/dL are achieved with epoetin alfa.

ACTION

Stimulates division, differentiation of erythroid progenitor cells in bone marrow. **Therapeutic Effect:** Induces erythropoiesis, releases reticulocytes from bone marrow.

PHARMACOKINETICS

Well absorbed after subcutaneous administration. Following administration, an increase in reticulocyte count occurs within 10 days, and increases in Hgb, Hct, and RBC count are seen within 2–6 wks. **Half-life:** 4–13 hrs.

⧗ LIFESPAN CONSIDERATIONS

Pregnancy/Lactation: Unknown if drug crosses placenta or is distributed in breast milk. **Children:** Safety and efficacy not established in pts 12 yrs and younger. **Elderly:** No age-related precautions noted.

INTERACTIONS

DRUG: None significant. **HERBAL:** None significant. **FOOD:** None known. **LAB VALUES:** May increase serum BUN, phosphorus, potassium, creatinine, uric acid, sodium. May decrease bleeding time, iron concentration, serum ferritin.

AVAILABILITY (Rx)

Injection Solution (Epogen, Procrit): 2,000 units/mL, 3,000 units/mL, 4,000 units/mL, 10,000 units/mL, 20,000 units/mL, 40,000 units/mL.

ADMINISTRATION/HANDLING

◄**ALERT**► Avoid excessive agitation of vial; do not shake (foaming).

 IV

Reconstitution • No reconstitution necessary.
Rate of Administration • May be given as an IV bolus.
Storage • Refrigerate. • Vigorous shaking may denature medication, rendering it inactive.

Subcutaneous
• Mix in syringe with bacteriostatic 0.9% NaCl with benzyl alcohol 0.9% (bacteriostatic saline) at a 1:1 ratio (benzyl alcohol acts as local anesthetic; may reduce injection site discomfort). • Use 1 dose per vial; do not reenter vial. Discard unused portion.

IV INCOMPATIBILITIES

Do not mix injection form with other medications.

INDICATIONS/ROUTES/DOSAGE

Anemia Associated with Chemotherapy
◄**ALERT**► Begin therapy only if Hgb less than 10 g/dL and anticipated duration of myelosuppressive chemotherapy is greater than 2 mos. Use minimum effective dose to maintain Hgb level that will avoid red blood cell transfusions. Discontinue upon completion of chemotherapy.
SQ: ADULTS, ELDERLY: Initially, 150 units/kg 3 times/wk (commonly used dose of 10,000 units 3 times/wk) or 40,000 units once wkly. **IV: CHILDREN 5 YRS AND OLDER:** 600 units/kg once wkly. **Maximum:** 40,000 units.

Increase dose: **ADULTS, ELDERLY:** If Hgb does not increase by greater than 1 g/dL and remains below 10 g/dL after initial 4 wks, may increase to 300 units/kg 3 times/wk or 60,000 units once wkly. **CHILDREN:** If Hgb does not increase by greater than 1 g/dL and remains less than 10 g/dL after initial 4 wks of once-wkly dosing, may increase dose to 900 units/kg/wk. **Maximum:** 60,000 units once wkly.
Decrease dose: Decrease dose by 25% if Hgb increases greater than 1 g/dL in any 2-wk period or Hgb level reaches level that will avoid red blood cell transfusions.

Reduction of Allogenic Blood Transfusions in Elective Surgery
SQ: ADULTS, ELDERLY: 300 units/kg/day for 10 days before and 4 days after surgery or 600 units/kg once weekly for 4 doses given 21, 14, 7 days before surgery and on the day of surgery.

Anemia in Chronic Renal Failure
◄**ALERT**► Individualize dose, using lowest dose to reduce need for RBC transfusions. **ON DIALYSIS:** Initiate when Hgb less than 10 g/dL; reduce dose or discontinue if Hgb approaches or exceeds 11 g/dL. **NOT ON DIALYSIS:** Initiate when Hgb less than 10 g/dL; reduce dose or stop if Hgb exceeds 10 g/dL.
IV, SQ: ADULTS, ELDERLY: 50–100 units/kg 3 times/wk. **CHILDREN:** 50 units/kg 3 times/wk.
Maintenance: *Decrease dose by 25%:* If Hgb increases greater than 1 g/dL in any 2-wk period. *Increase dose by 25%:* If Hgb does not increase by greater than 1 g/dL after 4 wks of therapy. Do not increase dose more frequently than every 4 wks.
Note: If pt does not attain adequate response after appropriate dosing over 12 wks, do not continue to increase dose, and use minimum effective dose to maintain Hgb level that will avoid red blood cell transfusions.

E

HIV Infection in Pts Treated with Zidovudine (AZT)

IV, SQ: ADULTS: Initially, 100 units/kg 3 times/wk for 8 wks; may increase by 50–100 units/kg 3 times/wk. Evaluate response q4–8wks thereafter. Adjust dosage by 50–100 units/kg 3 times/wk. If dosages larger than 300 units/kg 3 times/wk are not eliciting response, it is unlikely pt will respond. **Maintenance:** Titrate to maintain desired Hgb level. Hgb levels should not exceed 12 g/dL. If Hgb greater than 12 g/dL, resume treatment with 25% dose reduction when Hgb drops below 11 g/dL. Discontinue if Hgb increase not attained with 300 units/kg for 8 wks.

Dosage in Renal/Hepatic Impairment

No dose adjustment.

SIDE EFFECTS

Pts Receiving Chemotherapy

Frequent (20%–17%): Fever, diarrhea, nausea, vomiting, edema. **Occasional (13%–11%):** Asthenia, shortness of breath, paresthesia. **Rare (5%–3%):** Dizziness, trunk pain.

Pts with Chronic Renal Failure

Frequent (24%–11%): Hypertension, headache, nausea, arthralgia. **Occasional (9%–7%):** Fatigue, edema, diarrhea, vomiting, chest pain, skin reactions at administration site, asthenia, dizziness.

Pts with HIV Infection Treated with AZT

Frequent (38%–15%): Fever, fatigue, headache, cough, diarrhea, rash, nausea. **Occasional (14%–9%):** Shortness of breath, asthenia, skin reaction at injection site, dizziness.

ADVERSE EFFECTS/TOXIC REACTIONS

Hypertensive encephalopathy, thrombosis, cerebrovascular accident, MI, seizures occur rarely. Hyperkalemia occurs occasionally in pts with chronic renal failure, usually in those who do not comply with medication regimen, dietary guidelines, frequency of dialysis regimen.

NURSING CONSIDERATIONS

BASELINE ASSESSMENT

Assess B/P before initiation (80% of pts with chronic renal failure have history of hypertension). B/P often rises during early therapy in pts with history of hypertension. Consider that all pts eventually need supplemental iron therapy. Assess serum iron (should be greater than 20%), serum ferritin (should be greater than 100 ng/mL) before and during therapy. Establish baseline CBC (esp. note Hct).

INTERVENTION/EVALUATION

Assess CBC routinely (esp. Hgb, Hct). Monitor aggressively for increased B/P (25% of pts require antihypertensive therapy, dietary restrictions). Monitor temperature, esp. in cancer pts on chemotherapy and zidovudine-treated HIV pts. Monitor serum BUN, uric acid, creatinine, phosphorus, potassium, esp. in chronic renal failure pts.

PATIENT/FAMILY TEACHING

• Frequent laboratory assessments needed to determine correct dosage. • Immediately report any severe headache. • Avoid potentially hazardous activity during first 90 days of therapy (increased risk of seizures in pts with chronic renal failure during first 90 days). • Specific dietary regimen must be maintained.

eprosartan

ep-roe-**sar**-tan
(Teveten)

■ **BLACK BOX ALERT** ■ May cause fetal injury, mortality. Discontinue as soon as possible once pregnancy is detected.

FIXED-COMBINATION(S)

Teveten HCT: eprosartan/hydro-CHLOROthiazide (a diuretic): 400 mg/12.5 mg.

◆CLASSIFICATION

PHARMACOTHERAPEUTIC: Angiotensin II receptor antagonist. **CLINICAL:** Antihypertensive.

USES

Treatment of hypertension (alone or in combination with other medications).

PRECAUTIONS

Contraindications: Hypersensitivity to eprosartan. Concomitant use with aliskiren in pts with diabetes. **Cautions:** Unstented unilateral/bilateral renal artery stenosis, preexisting renal insufficiency. Concomitant use of potassium-sparing medications (e.g., spironolactone), potassium supplements, pts who are volume depleted.

ACTION

Potent vasodilator. Blocks vasoconstrictor, aldosterone-secreting effects of angiotensin II, inhibiting binding of angiotensin II to AT_1 receptors. **Therapeutic Effect:** Causes vasodilation, decreases peripheral resistance, decreases B/P.

PHARMACOKINETICS

Rapidly absorbed after PO administration. Protein binding: 98%. Minimally metabolized in liver. Primarily excreted via urine, biliary system. Minimally removed by hemodialysis. **Half-life:** 5–9 hrs.

☒ LIFESPAN CONSIDERATIONS

Pregnancy/Lactation: Has caused fetal and neonatal morbidity and mortality. Potential for adverse effects on breastfeeding infant. Breastfeeding not recommended. **Children:** Safety and efficacy not established. **Elderly:** No age-related precautions noted.

INTERACTIONS

DRUG: Potassium-sparing diuretics (e.g., spironolactone, triamterene), potassium supplements may increase risk of hyperkalemia. May produce additive effect with **antihypertensive agents** (e.g., **amlodipine, clonidine, lisinopril**). **HERBAL:** Ephedra, ginseng, yohimbe may worsen hypertension. **Garlic** may increase antihypertensive effect. **FOOD:** None known. **LAB VALUES:** May increase serum BUN, alkaline phosphatase, bilirubin, creatinine, ALT, AST. May decrease Hgb, Hct.

AVAILABILITY (Rx)

📎 **Tablets:** 400 mg, 600 mg.

ADMINISTRATION/HANDLING

PO
• Give without regard to food. • Do not break, crush, dissolve, or divide tablets.

INDICATIONS/ROUTES/DOSAGE

Hypertension
PO: ADULTS, ELDERLY: Initially, 600 mg/day. Range: 400–800 mg/day as single dose or 2 divided doses.

Dosage in Renal Impairment
Mild impairment: No dose adjustment. **Moderate to severe impairment: Maximum:** 600 mg/day.

Dosage in Hepatic Impairment
No dose adjustment. **Severe impairment: Maximum:** 600 mg/day.

SIDE EFFECTS

Occasional (5%–2%): Headache, cough, dizziness. **Rare (less than 2%):** Muscle pain, fatigue, diarrhea, upper respiratory tract infection, dyspepsia.

ADVERSE EFFECTS/TOXIC REACTIONS

Overdosage may manifest as hypotension, tachycardia. Bradycardia occurs less often.

NURSING CONSIDERATIONS

BASELINE ASSESSMENT

Obtain B/P, apical pulse immediately before each dose, in addition to regular monitoring (be alert to fluctuations). Question for possibility of pregnancy, history of hepatic/renal impairment, renal artery stenosis. Obtain urine pregnancy test. Assess medication history (esp. diuretics).

INTERVENTION/EVALUATION

Monitor B/P, pulse, serum BUN, creatinine, electrolytes, urinalysis.

PATIENT/FAMILY TEACHING

• Inform female pt regarding consequences of second- and third-trimester exposure to medication. • Avoid tasks that require alertness, motor skills until response to drug is established. • Restrict sodium, alcohol intake. • Follow diet, control weight. • Do not stop taking medication; hypertension requires lifelong control. • Check B/P regularly. • Do not chew, crush, dissolve, or divide tablets; take whole.

---

eptifibatide
HIGH ALERT

ep-ti-**fye**-ba-tide
(<u>Integrilin</u>)

◆CLASSIFICATION

PHARMACOTHERAPEUTIC: Glycoprotein IIb/IIIa inhibitor. **CLINICAL:** Antiplatelet, antithrombotic.

USES

Treatment of pts with acute coronary syndrome (ACS), including those managed medically and those undergoing percutaneous coronary intervention (PCI). **OFF-LABEL:** Support PCI during ST-elevation myocardial infarction (STEMI).

PRECAUTIONS

Contraindications: Hypersensitivity to eptifibatide. Active abnormal bleeding within previous 30 days; history of bleeding diathesis; history of stroke within 30 days or history of hemorrhagic stroke; severe hypertension (systolic B/P greater than 200 mm Hg or diastolic B/P greater than 110 mm Hg); major surgery within previous 6 wks; dependency on hemodialysis. **Cautions:** Renal impairment, hemorrhagic retinopathy, platelet count less than 100,000 cells/mm³, elderly, history of bleeding disorder. Medications that increase risk of bleeding (e.g., oral anticoagulants, NSAIDs).

ACTION

Blocks platelet glycoprotein IIb/IIIa receptor (binding site for fibrinogen, von Willebrand factor). **Therapeutic Effect:** Prevents thrombus formation within coronary arteries. Prevents platelet aggregation.

LIFESPAN CONSIDERATIONS

Pregnancy/Lactation: Unknown if excreted in breast milk. **Children/Elderly:** No age-related precautions noted.

PHARMACOKINETICS

Protein binding: 25%. Excreted in urine. **Half-life:** 2.5 hrs.

INTERACTIONS

DRUG: Anticoagulants (e.g., **warfarin**), **heparin**, NSAIDs (e.g., **ibuprofen**, **ketorolac**, **naproxen**), antiplatelets (e.g., **clopidogrel**), thrombolytic agents (e.g., **alteplase**) may increase risk of bleeding. **HERBAL: Cat's claw, dong quai, evening primrose, feverfew, garlic, ginger, ginkgo, ginseng** may increase antiplatelet effects. **FOOD:** None known. **LAB VALUES:** Increases PT, aPTT. Decreases platelet count. Prolongs clotting time.

AVAILABILITY (Rx)

Injection Solution: 0.75 mg/mL, 2 mg/mL.

ADMINISTRATION/HANDLING

📋 **IV**

Reconstitution • Withdraw bolus dose from 10-mL vial (2 mg/mL); for IV infusion, withdraw from 100-mL vial (0.75 mg/mL). • IV push and infusion administration may be given undiluted.

Rate of Administration • Give bolus dose IV push over 1–2 min.

Storage • Store vials in refrigerator.
• Solution appears clear, colorless. • Do
not shake. • Discard any unused portion
left in vial; discard if preparation contains any opaque particles.

▦ IV INCOMPATIBILITIES

Administer via dedicated line; do not add
other medications to infusion solution.

▦ IV COMPATIBILITIES

Amiodarone (Cordarone), argatroban,
bivalirudin, metoprolol (Lopressor).

INDICATIONS/ROUTES/DOSAGE

**Adjunct to Percutaneous Coronary
Intervention (PCI)**
IV Bolus, IV Infusion: ADULTS, ELDERLY:
180 mcg/kg (**maximum: 22.6 mg**)
before PCI initiation; then continuous
drip of 2 mcg/kg/min and a second 180
mcg/kg (**maximum: 22.6 mg**) bolus
10 min after the first. **Maximum: 15
mg/hr.** Continue until hospital
discharge or for up to 18–24 hrs. Minimum 12 hrs is recommended. Concurrent aspirin and heparin therapy is
recommended.

Acute Coronary Syndrome (ACS)
IV Bolus, IV Infusion: ADULTS, ELDERLY:
180 mcg/kg over 1–2 min (**maximum:
22.6 mg**) bolus then 2 mcg/kg/min until discharge or coronary artery bypass
graft, up to 72 hrs. **Maximum: 15 mg/
hr.** Concurrent aspirin and heparin therapy is recommended.

Dosage in Renal Impairment
CrCl Less than 50 mL/min: Use 180
mcg/kg bolus (**maximum: 22.6 mg**)
and 1 mcg/kg/min infusion (**maximum:
7.5 mg/hr**). **End-Stage Renal Disease
(Dialysis):** Contraindicated.

Dosage in Hepatic Impairment
No dose adjustment.

SIDE EFFECTS

Occasional (7%): Hypotension.

ADVERSE EFFECTS/TOXIC REACTIONS

Minor to major bleeding complications
may occur, most commonly at arterial access site for cardiac catheterization.

NURSING CONSIDERATIONS

BASELINE ASSESSMENT

Assess platelet count, Hgb, Hct before
treatment and during therapy. If platelet
count less than 90,000 cells/mm^3, additional platelet counts should be obtained
routinely to avoid thrombocytopenia.

INTERVENTION/EVALUATION

Diligently monitor for potential bleeding,
particularly at other arterial, venous puncture sites. If possible, urinary catheters,
nasogastric tubes should be avoided.

E

---

eriBULin

er-i-**bue**-lin
(Halaven)
**Do not confuse eriBULin with
epiRUBicin or erlotinib.**

◆CLASSIFICATION

PHARMACOTHERAPEUTIC: Microtubule inhibitor. **CLINICAL:** Antineoplastic.

USES

Treatment of metastatic breast cancer in
pts who previously received at least 2 chemotherapeutic regimens for treatment.
Treatment of metastatic liposarcoma in
pts who received a prior anthracycline-
containing regimen.

PRECAUTIONS

Contraindications: Hypersensitivity to eriBULin. **Cautions:** Prolonged QTc (congenital, other medications that prolong
QT interval), hypokalemia, hypomagnesemia, hepatic/renal impairment, moderate to severe neuropathy, HF.

E

ACTION

Binds directly on microtubules during active stage of G_2 and M phases of cell cycle, preventing formation of microtubules, an essential part of process of separation of chromosomes. **Therapeutic Effect:** Blocks cells in mitotic phase of cell division, leading to cell death.

PHARMACOKINETICS

Extensively metabolized in liver. Protein binding: 49%–65%. Excreted in feces (82%), urine (9%). **Half-life:** 40 hrs.

⧗ LIFESPAN CONSIDERATIONS

Pregnancy/Lactation: May cause embryo-fetal toxicity. Unknown if distributed in breast milk. **Children:** Safety and efficacy not established in pts younger than 18 yrs. **Elderly:** No age-related precautions noted.

INTERACTIONS

DRUG: None significant. **FOOD:** None known. **HERBAL:** None significant. **LAB VALUES:** May decrease WBC, Hgb, Hct, platelet count, potassium. May increase ALT.

AVAILABILITY (Rx)

Injection, Solution: 1 mg/2 mL (0.5-mg/mL).

ADMINISTRATION/HANDLING
 IV

Reconstitution • May administer undiluted or dilute in 100 mL 0.9% NaCl.
Rate of Administration • Administer over 2–5 min.
Storage • Store at room temperature. • Once diluted, syringe or diluted solution may be stored for up to 4 hrs at room temperature or up to 24 hrs if refrigerated.

▦ IV INCOMPATIBILITIES

Do not dilute with D_5W or administer through IV line containing solutions with dextrose or in same IV line with other medications.

INDICATIONS/ROUTES/DOSAGE

Metastatic Breast Cancer, Liposarcoma
IV: ADULTS, ELDERLY: 1.4 mg/m² over 2–5 min on days 1 and 8 of 21-day cycle.

Dosage in Renal Impairment
Mild: No dose adjustment. **Moderate to severe impairment (CrCl 15–49 mL/min):** 1.1 mg/m²/dose.

Dosage in Hepatic Impairment
Mild: 1.1 mg/m²/dose. **Moderate impairment:** 0.7 mg/m²/dose. **Severe impairment:** Use not recommended.

Recommended Dose Delays
Do not administer day 1 or day 8 of treatment for any of the following: ANC less than 1,000 cells/mm³, platelets less than 75,000 cells/mm³, Grade 3 or 4 nonhematologic toxicities. Day 8 dose may be delayed for maximum of 1 wk. If toxicities do not resolve or improve to Grade 2 severity by day 15, omit dose. If toxicities resolve or improve to Grade 2 severity by day 15, continue treatment at reduced dose and initiate next cycle no sooner than 2 wks later. Do not re-escalate dose after it has been reduced.

SIDE EFFECTS

Common (54%–35%): Fatigue, asthenia, alopecia, peripheral sensory neuropathy, nausea. **Frequent (25%–18%):** Constipation, arthralgia/myalgia, decreased weight, anorexia, pyrexia, headache, diarrhea, vomiting. **Occasional (16%–9%):** Back pain, dyspnea, cough, bone pain, extremity pain, urinary tract infection, oral mucosal inflammation.

ADVERSE EFFECTS/TOXIC REACTIONS

Neutropenia occurs in 82% of pts, with 57% developing grade 3 neutropenia. Severe neutropenia (ANC less than 500 cells/mm³) lasting more than 1 wk occurred in 12%. Anemia occurs in 58% of pts. Peripheral neuropathy occurs in 8% of pts but is the most common adverse reaction requiring discontinuation of therapy. Prolonged QTc may be noted on or after day 8 of treatment.

NURSING CONSIDERATIONS

BASELINE ASSESSMENT

Question for possibility of pregnancy. Obtain baseline CBC, serum chemistries before treatment begins. Obtain CBC prior to each dose. Offer emotional support.

INTERVENTION/EVALUATION

Diligently monitor for neutropenia, peripheral neuropathy (most frequent cause of drug discontinuation). Monitor for symptoms of neuropathy (burning sensation, hyperesthesia, hypoesthesia, paresthesia, discomfort, neuropathic pain). Assess hands, feet for erythema. Monitor CBC for evidence of neutropenia, thrombocytopenia. Assess mouth for stomatitis (erythema, ulceration, mucosal burning).

PATIENT/FAMILY TEACHING

• Avoid crowds, those with known infection. • Avoid contact with anyone who recently received live virus vaccine. • Do not have immunizations without physician's approval (drug lowers body resistance). • Promptly report fever over 100.5°F, chills, cough, burning or pain urinating, numbness, tingling, burning sensation, erythema of hands/feet. • Women of reproductive potential should use effective contraception during and for 2 wks following last dose of eribulin; males with female partners of reproductive potential should use effective contraception during and for 3.5 mos following last dose of eribulin.

erlotinib HIGH ALERT

er-**loe**-ti-nib
(Tarceva)
Do not confuse erlotinib with dasatinib, eriBULin, gefitinib, imatinib, or lapatinib.

◆CLASSIFICATION

PHARMACOTHERAPEUTIC: Epidermal growth factor receptor (EGFR) inhibitor; kinase inhibitor. **CLINICAL:** Antineoplastic.

E

USES

Treatment of locally advanced or metastatic non–small-cell lung cancer (NSCLC) after failure of at least one prior chemotherapy regimen (as monotherapy). First-line treatment of locally advanced, unresectable, or metastatic pancreatic cancer (in combination with gemcitabine).

PRECAUTIONS

Contraindications: Hypersensitivity to erlotinib. **Cautions:** Severe hepatic/renal impairment, cardiovascular disease. Concurrent use of strong CYP3A4 inhibitors and inducers or CYP1A2 inhibitors, pts at risk for GI perforation (e.g., peptic ulcer disease, diverticular disease). Total serum bilirubin greater than 3 times upper limit of normal.

ACTION

Reversibly inhibits overall epidermal growth factor receptor (EGFR)–tyrosine kinase activity. **Therapeutic Effect:** Produces tumor cell death.

PHARMACOKINETICS

About 60% is absorbed after PO administration; bioavailability is increased by food to almost 100%. Protein binding: 93%. Extensively metabolized in liver. Primarily excreted in feces (83%), urine (8%). **Half-life:** 24–36 hrs.

⌛ LIFESPAN CONSIDERATIONS

Pregnancy/Lactation: Unknown if drug crosses placenta or is distributed in breast milk. **Children:** Safety and efficacy not established. **Elderly:** No age-related precautions noted.

E

INTERACTIONS

DRUG: CYP3A4 inhibitors (e.g., atazanavir, clarithromycin, ketoconazole, ritonavir) may increase concentration/effects. **CYP3A4 inducers (e.g., carBAMazepine, phenytoin, rifAMPin)** may decrease concentration/effects. **Proton pump inhibitors (e.g., omeprazole), H₂ antagonists (e.g., raNITIdine)** may decrease absorption/effects. (Avoid use of **proton pump inhibitors.** Give erlotinib 10 hrs after or 2 hrs prior to **H₂ antagonists.**) **HERBAL: St. John's wort** may decrease concentration/effects. **FOOD: Grapefruit products** may increase potential for myelotoxicity. **LAB VALUES:** May increase serum bilirubin, ALT, AST.

AVAILABILITY (Rx)

Tablets: 25 mg, 100 mg, 150 mg.

ADMINISTRATION/HANDLING

PO

• Give at least 1 hr before or 2 hrs after ingestion of food. • Avoid grapefruit products. • May dissolve in 3–4 oz water and give orally or via feeding tube.

INDICATIONS/ROUTES/DOSAGE

◄**ALERT**► Dosage adjustment for toxicity: Reduce dose in 50-mg increments.

NSCLC

PO: ADULTS, ELDERLY: 150 mg/day until disease progression or unacceptable toxicity occurs.

Pancreatic Cancer

PO: ADULTS, ELDERLY: 100 mg/day, in combination with gemcitabine, until disease progression or unacceptable toxicity occurs.

Dosage in Renal Impairment

Interrupt dosing for Grade 3 or 4 renal toxicity during treatment.

Dosage in Hepatic Impairment

Use extreme caution. Reduce starting dose to 75 mg and individualize dose escalation if tolerated.

SIDE EFFECTS

Frequent (greater than 10%): Fatigue, anxiety, headache, depression, insomnia, rash, pruritus, dry skin, erythema, diarrhea, anorexia, nausea, vomiting, mucositis, constipation, dyspepsia, weight loss, dysphagia, abdominal pain, arthralgia, dyspnea, cough. **Occasional (10%–1%):** Keratitis. **Rare (less than 1%):** Corneal ulceration.

ADVERSE EFFECTS/TOXIC REACTIONS

UTI occurs occasionally. Pneumonitis, GI bleeding occur rarely.

NURSING CONSIDERATIONS

BASELINE ASSESSMENT

Obtain CBC, serum electrolytes, hepatic enzyme levels before beginning therapy. Obtain pregnancy test. Offer emotional support.

INTERVENTION/EVALUATION

Assess LFT and CBC, renal function, serum electrolytes, hydration status periodically.

PATIENT/FAMILY TEACHING

• Take drug on empty stomach. • Report rash, blood in stool, diarrhea, irritated eyes, fever. • Avoid grapefruit products. • Do not breastfeed. • Use effective contraception during therapy and for at least 1 mo after final dose.

---

ertapenem

er-ta-**pen**-em
(INVanz)
Do not confuse ertapenem with doripenem, imipenem, or meropenem, or INVanz with AVINza.

◆CLASSIFICATION

PHARMACOTHERAPEUTIC: Carbapenem. **CLINICAL:** Antibiotic.

USES

Treatment of susceptible infections due to *S. aureus* (methicillin-susceptible only), *S. agalactiae, S. pneumoniae* (penicillin-susceptible only), *S. pyogenes, E. coli, H. influenzae* (beta-lactamase negative strains only), *K. pneumoniae, M. catarrhalis, Bacteroides* spp., *C. clostridioforme, Peptostreptococcus* spp., including moderate to severe intra-abdominal, skin/skin structure infections; community-acquired pneumonia; complicated UTI; acute pelvic infection; adult diabetic foot infections without osteomyelitis. Prevention of surgical site infection. **OFF-LABEL:** Treatment of IV catheter–related bloodstream infection; prosthetic joint infection.

PRECAUTIONS

Contraindications: Hypersensitivity to ertapenem. History of anaphylactic hypersensitivity to beta-lactams (e.g., imipenem and cilastatin, meropenem), hypersensitivity to amide-type local anesthetics (IM). **Cautions:** Hypersensitivity to penicillins, cephalosporins, renal impairment, CNS disorders (brain lesions or history of seizure disorder), elderly.

ACTION

Penetrates bacterial cell wall of microorganisms, binds to penicillin-binding proteins, inhibiting cell wall synthesis. **Therapeutic Effect:** Produces bacterial cell death.

PHARMACOKINETICS

Almost completely absorbed after IM administration. Protein binding: 85%–95%. Widely distributed. Primarily excreted in urine (80%), feces (10%). Removed by hemodialysis. **Half-life:** 4 hrs.

⧗ LIFESPAN CONSIDERATIONS

Pregnancy/Lactation: Distributed in breast milk. **Children:** Safety and efficacy not established in pts younger than 18 yrs. **Elderly:** Advanced or end-stage renal insufficiency may require dosage adjustment.

INTERACTIONS

DRUG: Probenecid may increase concentration/effect. May decrease concentration/effect of **valproic acid. HERBAL:** None significant. **FOOD:** None known. **LAB VALUES:** May increase serum alkaline phosphatase, ALT, AST, bilirubin, BUN, creatinine, glucose, PT, aPTT, sodium. May decrease platelet count, Hgb, Hct, WBC.

AVAILABILITY (Rx)

Injection, Powder for Reconstitution: 1 g.

ADMINISTRATION/HANDLING

 IV

Reconstitution • Dilute 1-g vial with 10 mL 0.9% NaCl or Bacteriostatic Water for Injection. • Shake well to dissolve. • Further dilute with 50 mL 0.9% NaCl **(maximum concentration: 20 mg/mL).**
Rate of Administration • Give by intermittent IV infusion (piggyback). Do not give IV push. • Infuse over 30 min.
Storage • Solution appears colorless to yellow (variation in color does not affect potency). • Discard if solution contains precipitate. • Reconstituted solution is stable for 6 hrs at room temperature or 24 hrs if refrigerated.

IM
• Reconstitute with 3.2 mL 1% lidocaine HCl injection (without EPINEPHrine). • Shake vial thoroughly. • Inject deep in large muscle mass (gluteal or lateral part of thigh). • Administer suspension within 1 hr after preparation.

▨ IV INCOMPATIBILITIES

Do not mix or infuse with any other medications. Do not use diluents or IV solutions containing dextrose.

▨ IV COMPATIBILITIES

Heparin, potassium chloride, tigecycline (Tygacil), Sterile Water for Injection, 0.9% NaCl.

INDICATIONS/ROUTES/DOSAGE

Usual Dosage Range
IM, IV: ADULTS, ELDERLY, CHILDREN 13 YRS AND OLDER: 1 g/day. **CHILDREN 3 MOS–12 YRS:** 15 mg/kg 2 times/day. **Maximum:** 1 g/day.

Dosage in Renal Impairment

CrCl 30 mL/min or less	500 mg once daily
Hemodialysis	If daily dose given within 6h prior to HD, give 150 mg dose after HD.
Peritoneal dialysis	500 mg once daily

Dosage in Hepatic Impairment
No dose adjustment.

SIDE EFFECTS

Frequent (10%–6%): Diarrhea, nausea, headache. **Occasional (5%–2%):** Altered mental status, insomnia, rash, abdominal pain, constipation, chest pain, vomiting, edema, fever. **Rare (less than 2%):** Dizziness, cough, oral candidiasis, anxiety, tachycardia, phlebitis at IV site.

ADVERSE EFFECTS/TOXIC REACTIONS

Antibiotic-associated colitis, other superinfections (abdominal cramps, severe watery diarrhea, fever) may result from altered bacterial balance in GI tract. Anaphylactic reactions have been reported. Seizures may occur in pts with CNS disorders (brain lesions, history of seizures), bacterial meningitis, severe renal impairment.

NURSING CONSIDERATIONS

BASELINE ASSESSMENT

Question for history of allergies, particularly to beta-lactams, penicillins, cephalosporins. Inquire about history of seizures.

INTERVENTION/EVALUATION

Monitor WBC count. Monitor renal/hepatic function. Monitor daily pattern of bowel activity, stool consistency. Monitor for nausea, vomiting. Evaluate hydration status. Evaluate for inflammation at IV injection site. Assess skin for rash. Observe mental status; be alert to tremors, possible seizures. Assess sleep pattern for evidence of insomnia.

PATIENT/FAMILY TEACHING

• Report tremors, seizures, rash, prolonged diarrhea, chest pain, other new symptoms.

erythromycin

er-**ith**-roe-**mye**-sin
(Akne-Mycin, Apo-Erythro Base ✦, EES, Erybid ✦, Eryc, EryDerm, EryPed, Ery-Tab, Erythrocin, PCE Dispertab)
Do not confuse Eryc with Emcyt, or erythromycin with azithromycin or clarithromycin.

FIXED-COMBINATION(S)

Eryzole, Pediazole: erythromycin/sulfiSOXAZOLE (sulfonamide): 200 mg/600 mg per 5 mL.

◆CLASSIFICATION

PHARMACOTHERAPEUTIC: Macrolide. **CLINICAL:** Antibiotic, antiacne.

USES

Treatment of susceptible infections due to *S. pyogenes, S. pneumoniae, S. aureus, M. pneumoniae, Legionella, Chlamydia, N. gonorrheae, E. histolytica,* including syphilis, nongonococcal urethritis, diphtheria, pertussis, chancroid, *Campylobacter* gastroenteritis. **Topical:** Treatment of acne vulgaris. **Ophthalmic:** Prevention of gonococcal ophthalmia neonatorum, superficial ocular infections. **OFF-LABEL: Systemic:** Treatment of acne vulgaris, chancroid, *Campylobacter* enteritis, gastroparesis, Lyme disease, preoperative gut sterilization. **Topical:** Treatment of minor bacterial skin infections. **Ophthalmic:** Treatment of blepharitis, conjunctivitis, keratitis, chlamydial trachoma.

PRECAUTIONS

Contraindications: Hypersensitivity to erythromycin. Concomitant administration with ergot derivatives, lovastatin, pimozide, simvastatin. **Cautions:** Elderly, myasthenia gravis, strong CYP3A4 inhibitor, hepatic impairment, pts with prolonged QT intervals, uncorrected hypokalemia or hypomagnesemia, concurrent use of class IA or III antiarrhythmics.

ACTION

Penetrates bacterial cell membranes, reversibly binds to bacterial ribosomes, inhibiting protein synthesis. **Therapeutic Effect:** Bacteriostatic.

PHARMACOKINETICS

Variably absorbed from GI tract (depending on dosage form used). Protein binding: 70%–90%. Widely distributed. Metabolized in liver. Primarily eliminated in feces by bile. Not removed by hemodialysis. **Half-life:** 1.4–2 hrs (increased in renal impairment).

⌛ LIFESPAN CONSIDERATIONS

Pregnancy/Lactation: Crosses placenta. Distributed in breast milk. Erythromycin estolate may increase hepatic enzymes in pregnant women. **Children/Elderly:** No age-related precautions noted. High dosage in pts with decreased hepatic/renal function increases risk of hearing loss.

INTERACTIONS

DRUG: May increase concentration of busPIRone, cycloSPORINE, calcium channel blockers (e.g., diltiaZEM, verapamil), statins (e.g., atorvastatin, simvastatin). May inhibit metabolism of carBAMazepine. Hepatotoxic medications (e.g., acetaminophen, ketoconazole, methotrexate, simvastatin) may increase risk of hepatotoxicity. May increase risk of theophylline toxicity. May increase effects of warfarin. **HERBAL:** St. John's wort may decrease concentration. **FOOD:** Grapefruit may increase potential for torsades. **LAB VALUES:** May increase serum alkaline phosphatase, bilirubin, ALT, AST.

AVAILABILITY (Rx)

Gel, Topical: 2%. **Injection, Powder for Reconstitution:** 500 mg, 1 g. **Ointment, Ophthalmic:** 0.5%. **Ointment, Topical (Akne-Mycin):** 2%. **Oral Suspension (EES, EryPed):** 100 mg/2.5 mL, 200 mg/5 mL, 400 mg/5 mL. **Tablet as Base:** 250 mg, 333 mg, 500 mg. **Tablet as Ethylsuccinate (EES):** 400 mg.

 Capsules, Delayed-Release (Eryc): Capsules, Delayed-Release (Eryc): 250 mg. **Tablets, Delayed-Release (Ery-Tab):** 250 mg, 333 mg, 500 mg.

ADMINISTRATION/HANDLING

💉 IV

Reconstitution • Reconstitute each 500 mg with 10 mL Sterile Water for Injection without preservative to provide a concentration of 50 mg/mL. • Further dilute with 100–250 mL D₅W or 0.9% NaCl to maximum concentration of 5 mg/mL.
Rate of Administration • For intermittent IV infusion (piggyback), infuse over 20–60 min.
Storage • Store parenteral form at room temperature. • Initial reconstituted solution in vial is stable for 2 wks refrigerated or 24 hrs at room temperature. • Diluted IV solution stable for 8 hrs at room temperature or 24 hrs if refrigerated. • Discard if precipitate forms.

PO

• May give with food to decrease GI upset. Do not give with milk or acidic beverages. • Oral suspension is stable for 35 days at room temperature. • Do not crush delayed-release capsules, tablets.

E

Ophthalmic

• Place gloved finger on lower eyelid and pull out until a pocket is formed between eye and lower lid. • Place ¼–½ inch of ointment into pocket. • Instruct pt to close eye gently for 1–2 min (so that medication will not be squeezed out of the sac) and to roll eyeball to increase contact area of drug to eye.

▨ IV INCOMPATIBILITIES

Fluconazole (Diflucan), furosemide (Lasix), heparin, metoclopramide (Reglan).

▨ IV COMPATIBILITIES

Amiodarone (Cordarone), diltiaZEM (Cardizem), HYDROmorphone (Dilaudid), lidocaine, LORazepam (Ativan), magnesium sulfate, midazolam (Versed), morphine, multivitamins, potassium chloride.

INDICATIONS/ROUTES/DOSAGE

Usual Dosage Range
PO: ADULTS, ELDERLY: BASE: 250–500 mg q6–12h. **CHILDREN:** 30–50 mg/kg/day in 2–4 divided doses. **Maximum:** 2 g/day. **ETHYLSUCCINATE: ADULTS, ELDERLY:** 400–800 mg q6–12h. **Maximum:** 4 g/day. **CHILDREN:** 30–50 mg/kg/day in divided doses. **Maximum:** 3.2 g/day. **NEONATES:** 10 mg/kg/dose q8–12h.
IV: ADULTS, ELDERLY: 15–20 mg/kg/day divided q6h. **Maximum:** 4 g/day. **CHILDREN, INFANTS:** 15–20 mg/kg/day divided q6h. **Maximum:** 4 g/day. **NEONATES:** 10 mg/kg/dose q8–12h.

Dosage in Renal/Hepatic Impairment
No dose adjustment.

SIDE EFFECTS

Frequent: IV: Abdominal cramping/discomfort, phlebitis/thrombophlebitis. **Topical:** Dry skin (50%). **Occasional:** Nausea, vomiting, diarrhea, rash, urticaria. **Rare: Ophthalmic:** Sensitivity reaction with increased irritation, burning, itching, inflammation. **Topical:** Urticaria.

ADVERSE EFFECTS/TOXIC REACTIONS

Antibiotic-associated colitis, other superinfections (abdominal cramps, severe watery diarrhea, fever), reversible cholestatic hepatitis may occur. High dosage in pts with renal impairment may lead to reversible hearing loss. Anaphylaxis occurs rarely. Ventricular arrhythmias, prolonged QT interval occur rarely with IV form.

NURSING CONSIDERATIONS

BASELINE ASSESSMENT

Question for history of allergies (particularly erythromycins), hepatitis. Receive full medication history and screen for interactions.

INTERVENTION/EVALUATION

Monitor daily pattern of bowel activity, stool consistency. Assess skin for rash. Assess for hepatotoxicity (malaise, fever, abdominal pain, GI disturbances). Be alert for superinfection: fever, vomiting, diarrhea, anal/genital pruritus, oral mucosal changes (ulceration, pain, erythema). Check for phlebitis (heat, pain, red streaking over vein). Monitor for high-dose hearing loss.

PATIENT/FAMILY TEACHING

• Continue therapy for full length of treatment. • Doses should be evenly spaced. • Take medication with 8 oz water 1 hr before or 2 hrs following food or beverage. • **Ophthalmic:** Report burning, itching, inflammation. • **Topical:** Report excessive skin dryness, itching, burning. • Improvement of acne may not occur for 1–2 mos; maximum benefit may take 3 mos; therapy may last mos or yrs. • Use caution if using other topical acne preparations containing peeling or abrasive agents, medicated or abrasive soaps, cosmetics containing alcohol (e.g., astringents, aftershave lotion).

escitalopram

es-sye-**tal**-o-pram
(Apo-Escitalopram, Cipralex ✦,
Lexapro)

■ **BLACK BOX ALERT** ■ Increased risk of suicidal ideation and behavior in children, adolescents, young adults 18–24 yrs with major depressive disorder, other psychiatric disorders.

◆CLASSIFICATION

PHARMACOTHERAPEUTIC: Selective serotonin reuptake inhibitor. **CLINICAL:** Antidepressant.

USES

Treatment of major depressive disorder. Treatment of generalized anxiety disorder (GAD). **OFF-LABEL:** Seasonal affective disorder (SAD) in children and adolescents, pervasive developmental disorders (e.g., autism), vasomotor symptoms associated with menopause.

PRECAUTIONS

Contraindications: Hypersensitivity to escitalopram. Use of MAOI intended to treat psychiatric disorders (concurrent or within 14 days of discontinuing either escitalopram or MAOI). Initiation in pts receiving linezolid or IV methylene blue. Concurrent use with pimozide. **Cautions:** Hepatic/renal impairment, history of seizure disorder, concurrent use of CNS depressants, pts at high risk of suicide, concomitant aspirin, NSAIDs, warfarin (may potentiate bleeding risk), elderly, metabolic disease; recent history of MI, cardiovascular disease.

ACTION

Blocks uptake of neurotransmitter serotonin at neuronal presynaptic membranes, increasing its availability at postsynaptic receptor sites. **Therapeutic Effect:** Antidepressant effect.

PHARMACOKINETICS

Well absorbed after PO administration. Protein binding: 56%. Primarily metabolized in liver. Primarily excreted in feces, with a lesser amount eliminated in urine. **Half-life:** 35 hrs.

⧖ LIFESPAN CONSIDERATIONS

Pregnancy/Lactation: Distributed in breast milk. **Children:** May cause increased anticholinergic effects or hyperexcitability. **Elderly:** More sensitive to anticholinergic effects (e.g., dry mouth), more likely to experience dizziness, sedation, confusion, hypotension, hyperexcitability.

INTERACTIONS

DRUG: Alcohol, other CNS depressants (e.g., LORazepam, morphine, zolpidem) may increase CNS depression. Linezolid, aspirin, NSAIDs (e.g., ibuprofen, ketorolac, naproxen), warfarin may increase risk of bleeding. MAOIs may cause serotonin syndrome (autonomic hyperactivity, diaphoresis, excitement, hyperthermia, rigidity, neuroleptic malignant syndrome, coma). SUMAtriptan may cause weakness, hyperreflexia, poor coordination. **HERBAL:** Gotu kola, kava kava, SAMe, St. John's wort, valerian may increase CNS depression. Ginkgo biloba, St. John's wort may increase risk of serotonin syndrome. **FOOD:** None known. **LAB VALUES:** May decrease serum sodium.

AVAILABILITY (Rx)

Oral Solution: 5 mg/5 mL.

Tablets: 5 mg, 10 mg, 20 mg.

ADMINISTRATION/HANDLING

PO
• Give without regard to food. • Do not break, crush, dissolve, or divide tablets.

INDICATIONS/ROUTES/DOSAGE

Depression
PO: ADULTS: Initially, 10 mg once daily in the morning or evening. May increase

E

to 20 mg after a minimum of 1 wk. **ELDERLY:** 10 mg/day. **CHILDREN 12–17 YRS:** Initially, 10 mg once daily. May increase to 20 mg/day after at least 3 wks. **Maximum:** 20 mg once daily. Recommended: 10 mg once daily.

Generalized Anxiety Disorder
PO: ADULTS: Initially, 10 mg once daily in morning or evening. May increase to 20 mg after minimum of 1 wk. **ELDERLY:** 10 mg/day.

Dosage in Renal Impairment
Mild to moderate impairment: No dose adjustment. **Severe impairment:** Use caution in pts with CrCl less than 20 mL/min.

Dosage in Hepatic Impairment
10 mg/day.

SIDE EFFECTS

Frequent (21%–11%): Nausea, dry mouth, drowsiness, insomnia, diaphoresis. **Occasional (8%–4%):** Tremor, diarrhea, abnormal ejaculation, dyspepsia, fatigue, anxiety, vomiting, anorexia. **Rare (3%–2%):** Sinusitis, sexual dysfunction, menstrual disorder, abdominal pain, agitation, decreased libido.

ADVERSE EFFECTS/TOXIC REACTIONS

Overdose manifested as dizziness, drowsiness, tachycardia, confusion, seizures.

NURSING CONSIDERATIONS

BASELINE ASSESSMENT

For pts on long-term therapy, LFT, renal function tests, blood counts should be performed periodically. Observe, record behavior. Assess psychological status, thought content, sleep pattern, appearance, interest in environment.

INTERVENTION/EVALUATION

Supervise suicidal-risk pt closely during early therapy (as depression lessens, energy level improves, suicide potential increases). Assess appearance, behavior,

speech pattern, level of interest, mood. Monitor for suicidal ideation (esp. at beginning of therapy or when doses are increased or decreased), social interaction, mania, panic attacks.

PATIENT/FAMILY TEACHING

• Do not stop taking medication or increase dosage. • Avoid alcohol. • Avoid tasks that require alertness, motor skills until response to drug is established. • Report worsening depression, suicidal ideation, unusual changes in behavior.

---

esmolol

es-moe-lol
(Brevibloc)
Do not confuse Brevibloc with Bumex or Buprenex, or esmolol with Osmitrol.

◆CLASSIFICATION

PHARMACOTHERAPEUTIC: Beta$_1$-adrenergic blocker. **CLINICAL:** Antiarrhythmic.

USES

Rapid, short-term control of ventricular rate in supraventricular tachycardia (SVT), atrial fibrillation or flutter; treatment of tachycardia and/or hypertension (esp. intraop or postop). Treatment of noncompensatory sinus tachycardia. **OFF-LABEL:** Postoperative hypertension or SVT in children. Arrhythmia and/or rate control in ACS, intubation, thyroid storm, pheochromocytoma, electroconvulsive therapy.

PRECAUTIONS

Contraindications: Hypersensitivity to esmolol. Cardiogenic shock, uncompensated cardiac failure, second- or third-degree heart block (except in pts with pacemaker), severe sinus bradycardia, sick sinus syndrome, IV administration of calcium blockers in close proximity to esmolol, pulmonary hypertension.

Cautions: Compensated HF; concurrent use of digoxin, verapamil, diltiaZEM. Diabetes, myasthenia gravis, renal impairment, history of anaphylaxis to allergens. Hypovolemia, hypertension, bronchospastic disease, peripheral vascular disease, Raynaud's disease.

ACTION

Selectively blocks beta$_1$-adrenergic receptors. **Therapeutic Effect:** Slows sinus heart rate, decreases cardiac output, reducing B/P.

PHARMACOKINETICS

Rapidly metabolized primarily by esterase in cytosol of red blood cells. Protein binding: 55%. Less than 1%–2% excreted in urine. **Half-life:** 9 min.

⏳ LIFESPAN CONSIDERATIONS

Pregnancy/Lactation: Crosses placenta; distributed in breast milk. **Children:** Safety and efficacy not established. **Elderly:** No age-related precautions noted.

INTERACTIONS

DRUG: Opioids (e.g., fentaNYL, morphine), calcium channel blockers (e.g., diltiaZEM, verapamil), MAOIs (e.g., phenelzine, selegiline) may increase level/effects. **HERBAL:** Yohimbe may decrease effects. **FOOD:** None known. **LAB VALUES:** None significant.

AVAILABILITY (Rx)

Injection Solution: 10 mg/mL (10 mL, 250 mL), 20 mg/mL (100 mL).

ADMINISTRATION/HANDLING

◀**ALERT**▶ Give by IV infusion. Avoid butterfly needles, very small veins (can cause thrombophlebitis).

💧 IV

Rate of Administration • Administer by controlled infusion device; titrate to tolerance and response. • Infuse IV loading dose over 1–2 min. • Hypotension

(systolic B/P less than 90 mm Hg) is greatest during first 30 min of IV infusion.

Storage • Use only clear and colorless to light yellow solution. • Discard solution if discolored or precipitate forms.

▨ IV INCOMPATIBILITIES

Amphotericin B complex (Abelcet, AmBisome, Amphotec), furosemide (Lasix).

▨ IV COMPATIBILITIES

Amiodarone (Cordarone), dexmedetomidine (Precedex), diltiaZEM (Cardizem), DOPamine (Intropin), heparin, magnesium, midazolam (Versed), potassium chloride, propofol (Diprivan).

INDICATIONS/ROUTES/DOSAGE

Rate Control in Supraventricular Arrhythmias
IV: ADULTS, ELDERLY: Initially, loading dose of 500 mcg/kg/min for 1 min, followed by 50 mcg/kg/min for 4 min. If optimum response is not attained in 5 min, give second loading dose of 500 mcg/kg/min for 1 min, followed by infusion of 100 mcg/kg/min for 4 min. A third (and final) loading dose can be given and infusion increased by 50 mcg/kg/min, up to 200 mcg/kg/min, for 4 min. Once desired response is attained, increase infusion by no more than 25 mcg/kg/min. Infusion usually administered over 24–48 hrs in most pts. Range: 50–200 mcg/kg/min (average dose 100 mcg/kg/min).

Intraop/Postop Tachycardia Hypertension (Immediate Control)
IV: ADULTS, ELDERLY: Initially, 1,000 mcg/kg over 30 sec, then 150 mcg/kg/min infusion up to 300 mcg/kg/min.

Dosage in Renal/Hepatic Impairment
No dose adjustment.

SIDE EFFECTS

Generally well tolerated, with transient, mild side effects. **Frequent:** Hypotension (systolic B/P less than 90 mm Hg)

E

manifested as dizziness, nausea, diaphoresis, headache, cold extremities, fatigue. **Occasional:** Anxiety, drowsiness, flushed skin, vomiting, confusion, inflammation at injection site, fever.

ADVERSE EFFECTS/TOXIC REACTIONS

Overdose may produce profound hypotension, bradycardia, dizziness, syncope, drowsiness, breathing difficulty, bluish fingernails or palms of hands, seizures. May potentiate insulin-induced hypoglycemia in diabetic pts.

NURSING CONSIDERATIONS

BASELINE ASSESSMENT

Assess B/P, apical pulse immediately before drug is administered (if pulse is 60 or less/min or systolic B/P is 90 mm Hg or less, withhold medication, contact physician).

INTERVENTION/EVALUATION

Monitor B/P for hypotension, EKG, heart rate, respiratory rate, development of diaphoresis, dizziness (usually first sign of impending hypotension). Assess pulse for quality, irregular rate, bradycardia, extremities for coldness. Assist with ambulation if dizziness occurs. Assess for nausea, diaphoresis, headache, fatigue.

esomeprazole

es-o-**mep**-ra-zole
(Apo-Esomeprazole ✦, NexIUM, NexIUM 24 HR, Nexium IV)
Do not confuse esomeprazole with ARIPiprazole or omeprazole, or NexIUM with NexAVAR.

FIXED-COMBINATION(S)

Vimovo: esomeprazole/naproxen (NSAID): 20 mg/375 mg, 20 mg/500 mg.

♦**CLASSIFICATION**

PHARMACOTHERAPEUTIC: Proton pump inhibitor. **CLINICAL:** Gastric acid inhibitor.

USES

PO: Short-term treatment (4–8 wks) of erosive esophagitis; maintenance treatment of healing of erosive esophagitis; symptomatic gastroesophageal reflux disease (GERD). Treatment of pathologic hypersecretory conditions, including Zollinger-Ellison syndrome. Used in triple therapy with amoxicillin and clarithromycin for treatment of *H. pylori* infection in pts with duodenal ulcer. Reduces risk of NSAID-induced gastric ulcer. **OTC:** Treatment of frequent heartburn (2 or more days/wk). **IV:** Treatment of GERD with erosive esophagitis. Reduce risk of ulcer re-bleeding postprocedures.

PRECAUTIONS

Contraindications: Hypersensitivity to esomeprazole, other proton pump inhibitors. **Cautions:** May increase risk of hip, wrist, spine fractures; hepatic impairment; elderly; Asian populations. Concurrent use of CYP3A4 inducers (e.g., rifAMPin).

ACTION

Converted to active metabolites that irreversibly bind to, inhibit enzymes on surface of gastric parietal cells. Inhibits hydrogen ion transport into gastric lumen. **Therapeutic Effect:** Increases gastric pH; reduces gastric acid secretion.

PHARMACOKINETICS

Well absorbed after PO administration. Protein binding: 97%. Extensively metabolized in liver. Primarily excreted in urine. **Half-life:** 1–1.5 hrs.

⧖ LIFESPAN CONSIDERATIONS

Pregnancy/Lactation: Unknown if drug crosses placenta or is distributed in breast milk. **Children:** Safety and efficacy not established. **Elderly:** No age-related precautions noted.

INTERACTIONS

DRUG: May decrease concentration/ effects of **atazanavir, digoxin, iron, ketoconazole.** May increase effect of **warfarin.** May decrease effect of **clopidogrel.** CYP3A4 inducers (e.g., **carbamazepine, phenytoin, rifAMPin**) may decrease concentration/effects. **HERBAL:** St. John's wort may decrease concentration/effects. **FOOD:** None known. **LAB VALUES:** None significant.

AVAILABILITY (Rx)

Injection, Powder for Reconstitution: 20 mg, 40 mg. **Oral Suspension, Delayed-Release Packets:** 2.5 mg, 5 mg, 10 mg, 20 mg, 40 mg.

 Capsules (Delayed-Release [NexIUM]): 20 mg, 40 mg. [NexIUM 24 HR]: 20 mg.

ADMINISTRATION/HANDLING

 IV

Reconstitution • For IV push, add 5 mL of 0.9% NaCl to esomeprazole vial.
Infusion • For IV infusion, dissolve contents of one vial in 50 mL 0.9% NaCl, or D₅W.
Rate of Administration • For IV push, administer over not less than 3 min. For intermittent infusion (piggyback) infuse over 10–30 min. • Flush line with 0.9% NaCl, or D₅W, both before and after administration.
Storage • Use only clear and colorless to very slightly yellow solution. • Discard solution if particulate forms. • IV infusion stable for 12 hrs in 0.9% NaCl or lactated Ringer's; 6 hrs in D₅W.

PO (Capsules)

• Give 1 hr or more before eating (best before breakfast). • Do not crush, cut capsule; administer whole. • For pts with difficulty swallowing capsules, open capsule and mix pellets with 1 tbsp applesauce. Swallow immediately without chewing.

PO (Oral Suspension)

• Empty contents into 5 mL water for 2.5 mg, 5 mg; 15 mL for 10 mg, 20 mg, 40 mg and stir. • Let stand 2–3 min to thicken. • Stir and drink within 30 min.

⊞ IV INCOMPATIBILITIES

Do not mix esomeprazole with any other medications through the same IV line or tubing.

⊞ IV COMPATIBILITIES

Ceftaroline (Teflaro), doripenem (Doribax).

INDICATIONS/ROUTES/DOSAGE

Erosive Esophagitis
PO: ADULTS, ELDERLY, CHILDREN 12 YRS AND OLDER: 20–40 mg once daily for 4–8 wks. May continue for additional 4–8 wks. **CHILDREN 1–11 YRS, WEIGHING 20 KG OR MORE:** 10–20 mg/day for up to 8 wks. **WEIGHING LESS THAN 20 KG:** 10 mg/day for up to 8 wks. **CHILDREN 1-11 MONTHS: (GREATER THAN 7.5 kg–12 kg):** 10 mg/day for up to 6 wks. **(6–7.5 kg):** 5 mg/ day for up to 6 wks. **(3–5 kg):** 2.5 mg/day for up to 6 wks.

Maintenance Therapy for Erosive Esophagitis
PO: ADULTS, ELDERLY: 20 mg/day.

Treatment of NSAID-Induced Gastric Ulcers
PO: ADULTS, ELDERLY: 20 mg/day for 4–8 wks.

Prevention of NSAID-Induced Gastric Ulcer
PO: ADULTS, ELDERLY: 20–40 mg once daily for up to 6 mos.

Gastroesophageal Reflux Disease (GERD)
IV: ADULTS, ELDERLY: 20 or 40 mg once daily for up to 10 days. **CHILDREN 1–17 YRS, WEIGHING 55 KG OR MORE:** 20 mg once daily; **1–17 YRS, WEIGHING LESS THAN 55 KG:** 10 mg once daily; **1 MO TO LESS THAN 1 YR:** 0.5 mg/kg once daily.

E

PO: ADULTS, ELDERLY, CHILDREN, 12–17 YRS: 20 mg once daily for up to 8 wks. **CHILDREN 1–11 YRS:** 10 mg/day for up to 8 wks.

Zollinger-Ellison Syndrome
PO: ADULTS, ELDERLY: 40 mg 2 times/day. Doses up to 240 mg/day have been used.

Duodenal Ulcer Caused by *Helicobacter Pylori*
PO: ADULTS, ELDERLY: 40 mg (esomeprazole) once daily, with amoxicillin 1,000 mg and clarithromycin 500 mg twice daily for 10 days.

Heartburn (OTC)
PO: ADULTS, ELDERLY: 20 mg/day for 14 days. May repeat after 4 mos if needed.

Dosage in Renal Impairment
No dose adjustment.

Dosage in Hepatic Impairment
Mild to moderate impairment: No dose adjustment. **Severe impairment:** Doses should not exceed 20 mg/day.

SIDE EFFECTS

Frequent (7%): Headache. **Occasional (3%–2%):** Diarrhea, abdominal pain, nausea. **Rare (less than 2%):** Dizziness, asthenia, vomiting, constipation, rash, cough.

ADVERSE EFFECTS/TOXIC REACTIONS

Pancreatitis, hepatotoxicity, interstitial nephritis occur rarely.

NURSING CONSIDERATIONS

BASELINE ASSESSMENT

Assess epigastric/abdominal pain. Question history of hepatic impairment, pathologic bone fractures.

INTERVENTION/EVALUATION

Evaluate for therapeutic response (relief of GI symptoms). Question if GI discomfort, nausea, diarrhea occur. Monitor for occult blood, observe for hemorrhage in pts with peptic ulcer.

PATIENT/FAMILY TEACHING

• Report headache. • Take at least 1 hr before eating. • If swallowing capsules is difficult, open capsule and mix pellets with 1 tbsp applesauce. Swallow immediately without chewing.

estradiol

es-tra-**dye**-ole
(Alora, Climara, Delestrogen, Depo-Estradiol, Divigel, Elestrin, Estrogel, Evamist, Femring, Menostar, Minivelle, Vivelle-Dot)

■ **BLACK BOX ALERT** ■ Increased risk of dementia when given to women 65 yrs and older. Use of estrogen without progestin increases risk of endometrial cancer in postmenopausal women with intact uterus. Increased risk of invasive breast cancer in postmenopausal women using conjugated estrogens with medroxyPROGESTERone. Do not use to prevent cardiovascular disease or dementia.
Do not confuse Alora with Aldara, or Estraderm with Testoderm.

FIXED-COMBINATION(S)

Activella: estradiol/norethindrone (hormone): 1 mg/0.5 mg. **Climara PRO:** estradiol/levonorgestrel (progestin): 0.045 mg/24 hr, 0.015 mg/24 hr. **Combi-patch:** estradiol/norethindrone (hormone): 0.05 mg/0.14 mg, 0.05 mg/0.25 mg. **Femhrt:** estradiol/norethindrone (hormone): 5 mcg/1 mg. **Lunelle:** estradiol/medroxyprogesterone (progestin): 5 mg/25 mg per 0.5 mL.

◆CLASSIFICATION

PHARMACOTHERAPEUTIC: Estrogen.
CLINICAL: Estrogen, antineoplastic.

USES

Treatment of moderate to severe vasomotor symptoms associated with menopause, vulvar and vaginal atrophy associated with menopause, hypoestrogenism (due to castration, hypogonadism, primary ovarian failure), metastatic breast cancer (palliation) in men and postmenopausal women, advanced prostate cancer (palliation), prevention of osteoporosis in postmenopausal women.

PRECAUTIONS

Contraindications: Hypersensitivity to estradiol, angioedema, hepatic dysfunction or disease, undiagnosed abnormal vaginal bleeding, active or history of arterial thrombosis, estrogen-dependent cancer (known, suspected, or history of), known or suspected breast cancer (except for pts being treated for metastatic disease), pregnancy, thrombophlebitis or thromboembolic disorders (current or history of), known protein C, protein S, antithrombin deficiency or other known thrombophilic disorder. **Cautions:** Renal insufficiency, diabetes mellitus, endometriosis, severe hypocalcemia, hyperlipidemias, asthma, epilepsy, migraines, SLE, hypertension, hypocalcemia, hypothyroidism, history of jaundice due to past estrogen use or pregnancy, cardiovascular disease, obesity, porphyria, severe hypocalcemia.

ACTION

Modulates pituitary secretion of gonadotropins; follicle-stimulating hormone (FSH), luteinizing hormone (LH). **Therapeutic Effect:** Promotes normal growth/development of female sex organs.

PHARMACOKINETICS

Well absorbed from GI tract. Widely distributed. Protein binding: 50%–80%. Metabolized in liver. Primarily excreted in urine. **Half-life:** Unknown.

⌛ LIFESPAN CONSIDERATIONS

Pregnancy/Lactation: Contraindicated during pregnancy. Breastfeeding not recommended. **Children:** Caution in pts for whom bone growth is not complete (may accelerate epiphyseal closure). **Elderly:** May increase risk of new-onset dementia.

INTERACTIONS

DRUG: CYP3A4 inducers (e.g., car-BAMazepine, rifAMPin) may decrease concentration/effects. **CYP3A4 inhibitors (e.g., ketoconazole, ritonavir)** may increase concentration/effect. **HERBAL:** Avoid **black cohosh, dong quai, saw palmetto;** may enhance toxic/adverse effects. **St. John's wort** may decrease concentration/effects of estrogens. **FOOD:** None known. **LAB VALUES:** May increase serum glucose, calcium, HDL, triglycerides. May decrease serum cholesterol, LDL. May affect metapyrone testing, thyroid function tests.

AVAILABILITY (Rx)

Cream, Topical: 0.4%, 0.6%. **Emulsion, Topical (Estrasorb):** 4.35 mg estradiol/1.74 g pouch (contents of 2 pouches deliver estradiol 0.05 mg/day). **Gel, Topical: (Divigel):** 0.1% (0.25-g packet delivers estradiol 0.25 mg, 0.5 g-packet delivers estradiol 0.5 mg, 1-g packet delivers 1 mg). **(Elestrin):** 0.06% delivers 0.52 mg estradiol/actuation. **(Estrogel):** 0.06% delivers 0.75 mg/actuation. **Injection (Cypionate):** Depo-Estradiol: 5 mg/mL. **(Valerate):** Delestrogen: 10 mg/mL, 20 mg/mL, 40 mg/mL. **Tablets:** 0.5 mg, 1 mg, 2 mg. **Topical Spray (Evamist):** 1.53 mg/spray. **Transdermal System (Alora):** twice wkly: 0.025 mg/24 hrs, 0.05 mg/24 hrs, 0.075 mg/24 hrs, 0.1 mg/24 hrs. **Transdermal System (Climara):** once wkly: 0.025 mg/24 hrs, 0.0375 mg/24 hrs, 0.05 mg/24 hrs, 0.06 mg/24 hrs, 0.075 mg/24 hrs, 0.1 mg/24 hrs. **Transdermal System (Menostar):** once wkly: 0.014 mg/24 hrs. **Transdermal System (Minivelle, Vivelle-Dot):** twice wkly: 0.025 mg/24 hrs, 0.0375 mg/24 hrs, 0.05 mg/24 hrs, 0.075 mg/24 hrs, 0.1 mg/24 hrs. **Vaginal Cream (Estrace):** 0.1 mg/g. **Vaginal Ring (Estring):** 2 mg (releases 7.5 mcg/day over 90 days). **Vaginal Ring (Femring):** 0.05

mg/day (total estradiol 12.4 mg-release 0.05 mg/day over 3 mos); 0.1 mg/day (total estradiol 24.8 mg-release 0.1 mg/day over 3 mos). **Vaginal Tablet (Vagifem):** 10 mcg.

ADMINISTRATION/HANDLING

E

IM
• Rotate vial to disperse drug in solution. • Inject deep IM in large muscle mass.

PO
• Administer at same time each day. • Administer with food.

Transdermal
• Remove old patch; select new site (buttocks are alternative application site). • Peel off protective strip to expose adhesive surface. • Apply to clean, dry, intact skin on trunk of body (area with as little hair as possible). • Press in place for at least 10 sec (do not apply to breasts or waistline).

Vaginal
• Apply at bedtime for best absorption. • Insert end of filled applicator into vagina, directed slightly toward sacrum; push plunger down completely. • Avoid skin contact with cream (prevents skin absorption).

INDICATIONS/ROUTES/DOSAGE

Prostate Cancer
IM *(Delestrogen)*: ADULTS, ELDERLY: 30 mg or more q1–2wks.
PO: ADULTS, ELDERLY: 1–2 mg tid for at least 3 mos.

Breast Cancer
PO: ADULTS, ELDERLY: 10 mg 3 times/day for at least 3 mos.

Osteoporosis Prophylaxis in Postmenopausal Females
PO: ADULTS, ELDERLY: 0.5 mg/day cyclically (3 wks on, 1 wk off).
Transdermal *(Climara)*: ADULTS, ELDERLY: Initially, 0.025 mg/24 hrs wkly; adjust dose as needed.

Transdermal *(Alora, Minivelle, Vivelle-Dot)*: ADULTS, ELDERLY: Initially, 0.025 mg/24 hrs patch twice wkly; adjust dose as needed.
Transdermal *(Menostar)*: ADULTS, ELDERLY: 0.014 mg/24 hrs patch wkly.

Female Hypoestrogenism
PO: ADULTS, ELDERLY: 1–2 mg/day; adjust dose as needed.
IM *(Depo-Estradiol)*: ADULTS, ELDERLY: 1.5–2 mg monthly.
IM *(Delestrogen)*: ADULTS, ELDERLY: 10–20 mg q4wks.
Transdermal *(Alora, Climara, Vivelle-Dot)*: See dose in Availability section.

Vasomotor Symptoms Associated with Menopause
PO: ADULTS, ELDERLY: 1–2 mg/day cyclically (3 wks on, 1 wk off); adjust dose as needed.
IM *(Depo-Estradiol)*: ADULTS, ELDERLY: 1–5 mg q3–4wks.
IM *(Delestrogen)*: ADULTS, ELDERLY: 10–20 mg q4wks.
Topical Emulsion *(Estrasorb)*: ADULTS, ELDERLY: 3.48 g (contents of 2 pouches) once daily in the morning.
Topical Gel *(Estrogel)*: ADULTS, ELDERLY: 1.25 g/day.
Transdermal Spray *(Evamist)*: Initially, 1 spray daily. May increase to 2–3 sprays daily.
Transdermal *(Climara)*: ADULTS, ELDERLY: 0.025 mg/24 hrs wkly. Adjust dose as needed.
Transdermal: ADULTS, ELDERLY: *(Alora)*: 0.05 mg/24 hrs twice wkly. ***(Vivelle-Dot)*:** 0.0375 mg/24 hrs twice wkly.
Vaginal Ring *(Femring)*: ADULTS, ELDERLY: 0.05 mg. May increase to 0.1 mg if needed.

Vulvar and Vaginal Atrophy Associated with Menopause
IM *(Delestrogen)*: ADULTS, ELDERLY: 10–20 mg q4wks.
Vaginal Ring *(Femring)*: Initially 0.05 mg. Usual dose: 0.05–0.1 mg q3mos.

PO *(Estrace):* 1–2 mg/day 3 wks on and 1 wk off.

Topical Gel *(Estrogel):* 1.25 g/day at same time each day.

Transdermal *(Alora, Climara, Vivelle-Dot):* See dose in availability section).

Vaginal Ring *(Estring):* ADULTS, ELDERLY: 2 mg.

Vaginal Cream *(Estrace):* Insert 2–4 g/day intravaginally for 2 wks, then reduce dose to half of initial dose for 2 wks, then maintenance dose of 1 g 1–3 times/wk.

Vaginal Tablet *(Vagifem):* ADULTS, ELDERLY: Initially, 1 tablet/day for 2 wks. **Maintenance:** 1 tablet twice wkly.

Dosage in Renal Impairment
No dose adjustment.

Dosage in Hepatic Impairment
Contraindicated.

SIDE EFFECTS

Frequent: Anorexia, nausea, swelling of breasts, peripheral edema marked by swollen ankles and feet. **Transdermal:** Skin irritation, redness. **Occasional:** Vomiting (esp. with high doses), headache (may be severe), intolerance to contact lenses, hypertension, glucose intolerance, brown spots on exposed skin. **Vaginal:** Local irritation, vaginal discharge, changes in vaginal bleeding (spotting, breakthrough, prolonged bleeding). **Rare:** Chorea (involuntary movements), hirsutism (abnormal hairiness), loss of scalp hair, depression.

ADVERSE EFFECTS/TOXIC REACTIONS

Prolonged administration increases risk of gallbladder disease, thromboembolic disease, breast/cervical/vaginal/endometrial/hepatic carcinoma. Cholestatic jaundice occurs rarely.

NURSING CONSIDERATIONS

BASELINE ASSESSMENT

Assess frequency/severity of vasomotor symptoms. Question medical history as listed in Precautions. Question for possibility of pregnancy (contraindicated).

INTERVENTION/EVALUATION

Monitor B/P, weight, serum calcium, glucose, LFT. Monitor for loss of vision, sudden onset of proptosis, diplopia, migraine, thromboembolic disorders.

PATIENT/FAMILY TEACHING

• Limit alcohol, caffeine. • Avoid grapefruit products. • Immediately report sudden headache, vomiting, disturbance of vision/speech, numbness/weakness of extremities, chest pain, calf pain, shortness of breath, severe abdominal pain, mental depression, unusual bleeding. • Avoid smoking. • Report abnormal vaginal bleeding. • Never place patch on breast or waistline.

eszopiclone

e-**zop**-i-klone
(Lunesta)
Do not confuse Lunesta with Neulasta.

◆ CLASSIFICATION

PHARMACOTHERAPEUTIC: Nonbenzodiazepine **(Schedule IV). CLINICAL:** Hypnotic.

USES

Treatment of insomnia.

PRECAUTIONS

Contraindications: Hypersensitivity to eszopiclone. **Cautions:** Hepatic impairment, compromised respiratory function, COPD, sleep apnea, clinical depression, suicidal ideation, history of drug dependence; concomitant CNS depressants, strong CYP3A4 inhibitors (e.g., ketoconazole); elderly.

E

ACTION

May interact with GABA-receptor complexes at binding domains located close to or allosterically coupled to benzodiazepine receptors. **Therapeutic Effect:** Prevents insomnia, difficulty maintaining normal sleep.

PHARMACOKINETICS

Rapidly absorbed following PO administration. Protein binding: 52%–59%. Metabolized in liver. Excreted in urine. **Half-life:** 5–6 hrs.

⧗ LIFESPAN CONSIDERATIONS

Pregnancy/Lactation: Unknown if drug crosses placenta or is distributed in breast milk. **Children:** Safety and efficacy not established. **Elderly:** Pts with impaired motor or cognitive performance may require dosage adjustment.

INTERACTIONS

DRUG: Alcohol, anticonvulsants (e.g., **carBAMazepine, phenytoin**), antihistamines (e.g., **diphenhydrAMINE**), other CNS depressants may increase CNS depression. **CYP3A4 inhibitors (e.g., clarithromycin, ketoconazole, ritonavir)** may increase concentration/toxicity. **HERBAL: Gotu kola, kava kava, St. John's wort, valerian** may increase CNS depression. **FOOD:** Onset of action may be reduced if taken with or immediately after a **high-fat meal. LAB VALUES:** None known.

AVAILABILITY (Rx)

▒ **Tablets, Film-Coated:** 1 mg, 2 mg, 3 mg.

ADMINISTRATION/HANDLING

PO
• Should be administered immediately before bedtime. • Do not give with or immediately following a high-fat or heavy meal. • Do not break, crush, dissolve, or divide tablet.

INDICATIONS/ROUTES/DOSAGE

Insomnia
PO: ADULTS: 1 mg before bedtime. **Maximum:** 3 mg. **Concurrent use with CYP3A4 inhibitors (e.g., clarithromycin, erythromycin, azole antifungals):** 1 mg before bedtime; if needed, dose may be increased to 2 mg. **ELDERLY, DEBILITATED PTS:** Initially, 1 mg before bedtime. **Maximum:** 2 mg.

Sleep Maintenance Difficulty
PO: ADULTS: 2 mg before bedtime.

Dosage in Renal Impairment
No dose adjustment.

Dosage in Hepatic Impairment
Use caution. Initially, 1 mg immediately before bedtime. **Maximum:** 2 mg.

SIDE EFFECTS

Frequent (34%–21%): Unpleasant taste, headache. **Occasional (10%–4%):** Drowsiness, dry mouth, dyspepsia, dizziness, nervousness, nausea, rash, pruritus, depression, diarrhea. **Rare (3%–2%):** Hallucinations, anxiety, confusion, abnormal dreams, decreased libido, neuralgia.

ADVERSE EFFECTS/TOXIC REACTIONS

Chest pain, peripheral edema occur occasionally.

NURSING CONSIDERATIONS

BASELINE ASSESSMENT

Assess B/P, pulse, respirations. Raise bed rails, provide call light. Provide environment conducive to sleep (quiet environment, low or no lighting). Question usual sleep patterns. Initiate fall precautions. Screen for other conditions affecting sleep (e.g., stress, depression, hyperactivity, drug abuse).

INTERVENTION/EVALUATION

Assess sleep pattern of pt. Evaluate for therapeutic response (decrease in number of nocturnal awakenings, increase in length of sleep).

PATIENT/FAMILY TEACHING

• Take only when experiencing insomnia. Do not take when insomnia is not present. • Do not break, chew, crush, dissolve, or divide tablet. Take whole. • Avoid alcohol. • At least 8 hrs must be devoted for sleep time before daily activity begins. • Take immediately before bedtime. • Report insomnia that worsens or persists longer than 7–10 days, abnormal thoughts or behavior, memory loss, anxiety.

---

etanercept   TOP 100

e-**tan**-er-sept
(Enbrel, Enbrel SureClick)

■ **BLACK BOX ALERT** ■ Serious, potentially fatal infections, including bacterial sepsis, tuberculosis, have occurred. Lymphomas, other malignancies may occur (reported in children/adolescents).

Do not confuse Enbrel with Levbid.

◆CLASSIFICATION

PHARMACOTHERAPEUTIC: Protein, TNF inhibitor. **CLINICAL:** Antiarthritic.

USES

Treatment of moderate to severely active rheumatoid arthritis (RA). Treatment of moderately to severely active polyarticular juvenile idiopathic arthritis (JIA), ankylosing spondylitis, psoriatic arthritis. Treatment of chronic, moderate to severe plaque psoriasis. **OFF-LABEL:** Treatment of acute graft-versus-host disease.

PRECAUTIONS

Contraindications: Hypersensitivity to etanercept. Serious active infection or sepsis. **Cautions:** History of recurrent infections, illnesses that predispose to infection (e.g., diabetes, travel from areas of endemic mycosis). History of HF, decreased left ventricular function, significant hematologic abnormalities; moderate to severe alcoholic hepatitis, elderly, preexisting or recent-onset CNS demyelinating disorder.

ACTION

Binds to tumor necrosis factor (TNF), blocking its interaction with cell surface receptors. Elevated levels of TNF, involved in inflammatory and immune responses, are found in synovial fluid of rheumatoid arthritis pts. **Therapeutic Effect:** Relieves symptoms of arthritis, psoriasis, spondylitis.

PHARMACOKINETICS

Well absorbed after subcutaneous administration. **Half-life:** 72–132 hrs.

⧗ LIFESPAN CONSIDERATIONS

Pregnancy/Lactation: Unknown if distributed in breast milk. **Children:** No age-related precautions noted in pts 4 yrs and older. **Elderly:** No age-related precautions noted.

INTERACTIONS

DRUG: Anakinra may increase risk of infection. Use of **live virus vaccines** may potentiate virus replication, increase vaccine side effect, decrease pt's antibody response to vaccine. **HERBAL: Echinacea** may decrease effects. **FOOD:** None known. **LAB VALUES:** May increase serum alkaline phosphatase, ALT, AST, bilirubin.

AVAILABILITY (Rx)

Injection, Solution (Prefilled Syringe): 25 mg/0.5 mL, 50 mg/mL. **Injection, Solution (Autoinjector):** 50 mg/mL. **Solution, Reconstituted:** 25 mg.

ADMINISTRATION/HANDLING

◄**ALERT**► Do not add other medications to solution. Do not use filter during reconstitution or administration.

Subcutaneous

• Refrigerate prefilled syringes. • Inject into thigh, abdomen, upper arm.

Rotate injection sites. • Give new injection at least 1 inch from an old site and never into area where skin is tender, bruised, red, hard. • Once reconstituted, may be stored in vial for up to 14 days refrigerated.

INDICATIONS/ROUTES/DOSAGE

Rheumatoid Arthritis (RA), Psoriatic Arthritis, Ankylosing Spondylitis
SQ: ADULTS, ELDERLY: 25 mg twice wkly given 72–96 hrs apart or 50 mg once wkly. **Maximum:** 50 mg/wk.

Juvenile Rheumatoid Arthritis (JIA)
SQ: CHILDREN 2–17 YRS: (63 kg or greater): 50 mg once weekly. (Less than 63 kg): 0.8 mg/kg once weekly. **Maximum:** 50 mg/dose.

Plaque Psoriasis
SQ: ADULTS, ELDERLY: 50 mg twice wkly (give 3–4 days apart) for 3 mos. (25 mg or 50 mg once wkly have also been used.) **Maintenance:** 50 mg once wkly. **CHILDREN 4 YRS AND OLDER (63 kg or greater):** 50 mg once weekly. **(Less than 63 kg):** 0.8 mg/kg once wkly. **Maximum dose:** 50 mg/wk.

Dosage in Renal/Hepatic Impairment
No dose adjustment.

SIDE EFFECTS

Frequent (37%): Injection site erythema, pruritus, pain, swelling; abdominal pain, vomiting (more common in children than adults). **Occasional (16%–4%):** Headache, rhinitis, dizziness, pharyngitis, cough, asthenia, abdominal pain, dyspepsia. **Rare (less than 3%):** Sinusitis, allergic reaction.

ADVERSE EFFECTS/TOXIC REACTIONS

Infection (pyelonephritis, cellulitis, osteomyelitis, wound infection, leg ulcer, septic arthritis, diarrhea, bronchitis, pneumonia) occurs in 29%–38% of pts. Rare adverse effects include heart failure, hypertension, hypotension, pancreatitis, GI hemorrhage.

NURSING CONSIDERATIONS

BASELINE ASSESSMENT
Assess onset, type, location, duration of pain, inflammation. If significant exposure to varicella virus has occurred during treatment, therapy should be temporarily discontinued and treatment with varicella-zoster immune globulin should be considered. Screen for active infection. Question history as listed in Precautions. Question travel history.

INTERVENTION/EVALUATION
Assess for improvement of joint swelling, pain, tenderness. Monitor erythrocyte sedimentation rate (ESR), C-reactive protein level, CBC with differential, platelet count. Observe for signs of infection.

PATIENT/FAMILY TEACHING
• Instruct pt in subcutaneous injection technique, including areas of body acceptable as injection sites. • Injection site reaction generally occurs in first mo of treatment and decreases in frequency during continued therapy. • Do not receive live vaccines during treatment. • Report persistent fever, bruising, bleeding, pallor.

ethambutol

eth-**am**-bue-tol
(Etibi ✚, Myambutol)

◆CLASSIFICATION
PHARMACOTHERAPEUTIC: Isonicotinic acid derivative. **CLINICAL:** Antitubercular.

USES

In conjunction with other antitubercular agents for treatment of pulmonary tuberculosis. **OFF-LABEL:** Treatment of atypical mycobacterial infections (e.g., *Mycobacterium avium* complex [MAC]).

PRECAUTIONS

Contraindications: Hypersensitivity to ethambutol. Optic neuritis (risk-versus-benefit decision). Use in young children, unconscious pts, or anyone unable to report visual changes. **Cautions:** Renal/hepatic dysfunction, ocular defects (diabetic retinopathy, cataracts), recurrent ocular inflammatory conditions. Not recommended for children 13 yrs and younger (unless benefit outweighs risk).

ACTION

Inhibits arabinosyl transferase, causing impaired mycobacterial cell wall synthesis. **Therapeutic Effect:** Suppresses multiplication of mycobacteria.

PHARMACOKINETICS

Rapidly, well absorbed from GI tract. Protein binding: 20%–30%. Widely distributed. Metabolized in liver. Primarily excreted in urine. Removed by hemodialysis. **Half-life:** 3–4 hrs (increased in renal impairment).

⏳ LIFESPAN CONSIDERATIONS

Pregnancy/Lactation: Crosses placenta. Distributed in breast milk. **Children:** Safety and efficacy not established in pts younger than 13 yrs. **Elderly:** Age-related renal impairment may require dosage adjustment.

INTERACTIONS

DRUG: Aluminum hydroxide may decrease concentration/effect. **HERBAL:** None significant. **FOOD:** None known. **LAB VALUES:** May increase serum uric acid.

AVAILABILITY (Rx)

Tablets: 100 mg, 400 mg.

ADMINISTRATION/HANDLING

PO
• May be crushed and mixed with apple juice or applesauce. • Administer at least 4 hrs before giving aluminum hydroxide. • Give with food (decreases GI upset).

INDICATIONS/ROUTES/DOSAGE

Tuberculosis
PO: ADULTS, ELDERLY: Initially, 15 mg/kg once daily. (**maximum:** 1.5 g/day). Retreatment: 25 mg/kg once daily (**maximum:** 2.5 g/day) for 60 days or until bacteriologic smears/cultures become negative, then 15 mg/kg once daily. **CHILDREN: (HIV negative):** 15–20 mg/kg/day (**maximum:** 1 g/day) or 50 mg/kg twice wkly (**maximum:** 2.5 g/dose). **(HIV exposed/infected):** 15–25 mg/kg/day. **Maximum:** 2.5 g/day.

Dosage in Renal Impairment
Dosage interval is modified based on creatinine clearance.

Creatinine Clearance	Dosage
10–50 mL/min	q24–36h
Less than 10 mL/min	q48h
Hemodialysis	Administer post HD
Peritoneal dialysis	Administer q48h
Continuous renal replacement therapy	Administer q24–36h

Dosage in Hepatic Impairment
Use caution.

SIDE EFFECTS

Occasional: Acute gouty arthritis (chills, pain, swelling of joints with hot skin), confusion, abdominal pain, nausea, vomiting, anorexia, headache. **Rare:** Rash, fever, blurred vision, red-green color blindness.

ADVERSE EFFECTS/TOXIC REACTIONS

Optic neuritis (more common with high-dosage, long-term therapy), peripheral neuritis, thrombocytopenia, anaphylactoid reaction occur rarely.

NURSING CONSIDERATIONS

BASELINE ASSESSMENT
Evaluate baseline CBC, renal function, LFT, and monitor periodically. Obtain baseline visual acuity.

🍁 Canadian trade name   🦫 Non-Crushable Drug   🔲 High Alert drug

INTERVENTION/EVALUATION

Assess for vision changes (altered color perception, decreased visual acuity may be first signs). Give with food if GI distress occurs. Monitor serum uric acid. Assess for hot, painful, swollen joints, esp. great toe, ankle, knee (gout). Report numbness, tingling, burning of extremities (peripheral neuritis).

PATIENT/FAMILY TEACHING

• Do not skip doses; take for full length of therapy (may take mos or yrs). • Immediately report any visual changes (visual effects generally reversible with discontinuation of ethambutol but in rare cases may take up to 1 yr to disappear or may be permanent). • Promptly report swelling or pain of joints, numbness or tingling/burning of extremities, fever, chills.

---

etoposide, VP-16 **HIGH ALERT**

e-toe-poe-side
(Etopophos, Toposar, VePesid ✦)
■ **BLACK BOX ALERT** ■ Severe myelosuppression with resulting infection, bleeding may occur. Must be administered by personnel trained in administration/handling of chemotherapeutic agents.
Do not confuse etoposide with etidronate, or VePesid with Pepcid or Versed.

◆CLASSIFICATION

PHARMACOTHERAPEUTIC: Topoisomerase II inhibitor. **CLINICAL:** Antineoplastic.

USES

Treatment of refractory testicular tumors, small-cell lung carcinoma. **OFF-LABEL:** Acute lymphocytic, acute nonlymphocytic leukemias; Ewing's and Kaposi's sarcoma; Hodgkin's and non-Hodgkin's lymphomas; endometrial, gastric, non–small-cell lung carcinomas; multiple myeloma; myelodysplastic syndromes; neuroblastoma; osteosarcoma; ovarian germ cell tumors; primary brain, gestational trophoblastic tumors; soft tissue sarcomas; Wilms tumor.

PRECAUTIONS

Contraindications: Hypersensitivity to etoposide. **Cautions:** Hepatic/renal impairment, myelosuppression, elderly, pts with low serum albumin.

ACTION

Induces single- and double-stranded breaks in DNA. Cell cycle–dependent and phase-specific; most effective in S and G_2 phases of cell division. **Therapeutic Effect:** Inhibits, alters DNA synthesis.

PHARMACOKINETICS

Variably absorbed from GI tract. Rapidly distributed, low concentrations in CSF. Protein binding: 97%. Metabolized in liver. Primarily excreted in urine. Not removed by hemodialysis. **Half-life:** 3–12 hrs.

▧ LIFESPAN CONSIDERATIONS

Pregnancy/Lactation: If possible, avoid use during pregnancy, esp. first trimester. May cause fetal harm. Breastfeeding not recommended. **Children:** Safety and efficacy not established. **Elderly:** Age-related renal impairment may require dosage adjustment.

INTERACTIONS

DRUG: Bone marrow depressants may increase myelosuppression. **Live-virus vaccines** may potentiate virus replication, increase vaccine side effects, decrease pt's antibody response to vaccine. **HERBAL: Echinacea, St. John's wort** may decrease concentration. **FOOD:** None known. **LAB VALUES:** Expected decrease of leukocytes, platelets, RBC, Hgb, Hct.

AVAILABILITY (Rx)

Capsules: 50 mg. **Injection, Powder for Reconstitution (Etopophos):** 100 mg. **Injection Solution (Toposar):** 20 mg/mL (5 mL, 25 mL, 50 mL).

ADMINISTRATION/HANDLING

◀ALERT▶ Administer by slow IV infusion. Wear gloves when preparing solution. If powder or solution comes in contact with skin, wash immediately and thoroughly with soap, water. May be carcinogenic, mutagenic, teratogenic. Handle with extreme care during preparation, administration.

 IV

Reconstitution

Toposar • Dilute to a concentration of 0.2–0.4 mg/mL in D_5W or 0.9% NaCl.

Etopophos • Reconstitute each 100 mg with 5–10 mL Sterile Water for Injection, D_5W, or 0.9% NaCl to provide concentration of 20 mg/mL or 10 mg/mL, respectively. • May give without further dilution or further dilute to concentration as low as 0.1 mg/mL with 0.9% NaCl or D_5W.

Rate of administration

Toposar • Infuse slowly, at least 30–60 min (rapid IV may produce marked hypotension) at a rate not to exceed 100 mg/m²/hr. • Monitor for anaphylactic reaction during infusion (chills, fever, dyspnea, diaphoresis, lacrimation, sneezing, throat, back, chest pain).

Etopophos • May give over as little as 5 min up to 210 min.

Storage

Toposar • Store injection at room temperature before dilution. • Concentrate for injection is clear, yellow. • Diluted solution is stable at room temperature for 96 hrs at 0.2 mg/mL, 24 hrs at 0.4 mg/mL. • Discard if crystallization occurs.

Etopophos • Refrigerate vials. • Stable at room temperature for 24 hrs or for 7 days if refrigerated after reconstitution.

PO

Storage • Refrigerate gelatin capsules.

▧ IV INCOMPATIBILITIES

VePesid: Cefepime (Maxipime), filgrastim (Neupogen). **Etopophos:** Amphotericin B (Fungizone), cefepime (Maxipime), chlorproMAZINE (Thorazine), methylPREDNISolone (Solu-Medrol), prochlorperazine (Compazine).

▧ IV COMPATIBILITIES

VePesid: CARBOplatin (Paraplatin), CISplatin (Platinol), cytarabine (Cytosar), DAUNOrubicin (Cerubidine), DOXOrubicin (Adriamycin), granisetron (Kytril), mitoXANTRONE (Novantrone), ondansetron (Zofran). **Etopophos:** CARBOplatin (Paraplatin), CISplatin (Platinol), cytarabine (Cytosar), dacarbazine (DTIC-Dome), DAUNOrubicin (Cerubidine), dexamethasone (Decadron), diphenhydrAMINE (Benadryl), DOXOrubicin (Adriamycin), granisetron (Kytril), magnesium sulfate, mannitol, mitoXANTRONE (Novantrone), ondansetron (Zofran), potassium chloride.

INDICATIONS/ROUTES/DOSAGE

◀ALERT▶ Dosage individualized based on clinical response, tolerance to adverse effects. Treatment repeated at 3- to 4-wk intervals. Refer to individual protocols.

Refractory Testicular Tumors

IV: ADULTS: 50–100 mg/m²/day on days 1–5, or 100 mg/m²/day on days 1, 3, 5 (as combination therapy). Give q3–4wks for 3–4 courses.

Small-Cell Lung Carcinoma

PO: ADULTS: Twice the IV dose rounded to nearest 50 mg. Give once daily for doses 200 mg or less, in divided doses for dosages greater than 200 mg.

IV: ADULTS: 35 mg/m²/day for 4 consecutive days up to 50 mg/m²/day for 5 consecutive days q3–4wks (as combination therapy).

Dosage in Renal Impairment

Creatinine Clearance	Dosage
15–50 mL/min	75% of normal dose
Less than 15 mL/min	Consider further dose reduction.

E

E

Dosage in Hepatic Impairment
No dose adjustment.

SIDE EFFECTS

Frequent (66%–43%): Mild to moderate nausea/vomiting, alopecia. **Occasional (13%–6%):** Diarrhea, anorexia, stomatitis. **Rare (2% or less):** Hypotension, peripheral neuropathy.

ADVERSE EFFECTS/TOXIC REACTIONS

Myelosuppression manifested as hematologic toxicity, principally anemia, leukopenia (occurring 7–14 days after drug administration), thrombocytopenia (occurring 9–16 days after administration), and, to lesser extent, pancytopenia. Bone marrow recovery occurs by day 20. Hepatotoxicity occurs occasionally.

NURSING CONSIDERATIONS

BASELINE ASSESSMENT

Obtain CBC before and at frequent intervals during therapy. Antiemetics readily control nausea, vomiting. Offer emotional support.

INTERVENTION/EVALUATION

Monitor CBC, B/P, hepatic/renal function tests. Monitor daily pattern of bowel activity, stool consistency. Monitor for hematologic toxicity (fever, sore throat, signs of local infection, unusual bruising/bleeding from any site), symptoms of anemia (excessive fatigue, weakness). Assess for paresthesia (peripheral neuropathy). Monitor for stomatitis.

PATIENT/FAMILY TEACHING

• Hair loss is reversible, but new hair growth may have different color, texture. • Do not have immunizations without physician's approval (drug lowers resistance). • Avoid contact with those who have recently received live virus vaccine. • Promptly report fever, sore throat, signs of local infection, unusual bruising or bleeding from any site, burning or pain with urination, numbness in extremities, yellowing of skin or eyes.

everolimus

e-**veer**-oh-li-mus
(Afinitor, Afinitor Disperz, Zortress)
■ **BLACK BOX ALERT** ■ Immunosuppressant (may result in infection, malignancy including lymphoma or skin cancer); increased risk of nephrotoxicity in renal transplants (avoid standard doses of cycloSPORINE); increased risk of renal arterial or venous thrombosis in renal transplants.
Do not confuse Afinitor with Lipitor, or everolimus with sirolimus, tacrolimus, or temsirolimus.

◆CLASSIFICATION

PHARMACOTHERAPEUTIC: Enzyme inhibitor. **CLINICAL:** Antineoplastic, immunosuppressant.

USES

Afinitor: Treatment of advanced renal cell carcinoma after failure of treatment with SUNItinib or SORAfenib. Treatment of subependymal giant cell astrocytoma (SEGA) associated with tuberous sclerosis. Treatment of progressive neuroendocrine tumors of pancreatic origin and progressive, well-differentiated, non-functional neuroendocrine tumors of GI or lung origin. Treatment of advanced hormone receptor–positive, HER2-negative breast cancer in postmenopausal women. Treatment of tuberous sclerosis complex (TSC) not requiring immediate surgery. **Afinitor Disperz:** Treatment of SEGA associated with TSC requiring intervention but that cannot be curatively resected. **Zortress:** Prophylaxis of organ rejection after kidney/liver transplant at low to moderate immunologic risk. **OFF-LABEL:** Relapsed or refractory Waldenström's macroglobulinemia. Treatment of progressive advanced carcinoid tumors.

PRECAUTIONS

Contraindications: Hypersensitivity to everolimus, sirolimus, other rapamycin derivatives. **Cautions:** Noninfectious pneumonitis; viral, fungal, or bacterial infection; oral ulceration; mucositis; current immunosuppression; hereditary galactose intolerance; renal/hepatic impairment; hyperlipidemia; concurrent use of CYP3A4 inducers and inhibitors. Medications known to cause angioedema.

ACTION

Binds to the FK binding protein, reducing protein synthesis and cell proliferation. Also reduces lipoma volume. **Therapeutic Effect:** Reduces cell proliferation, produces cell death.

PHARMACOKINETICS

Peak concentration occurs in 1–2 hrs following administration, with steady-state levels achieved in 2 wks. Undergoes extensive hepatic metabolism. Protein binding: 74%. Eliminated in feces (80%), urine (5%). **Half-life:** 30 hrs.

⧗ LIFESPAN CONSIDERATIONS

Pregnancy/Lactation: Avoid pregnancy during treatment and for up to 8 wks after discontinuation. Breastfeeding not recommended during treatment and for up to 2 wks after discontinuation. May cause fetal harm. Unknown if distributed in breast milk. **Children:** Safety and efficacy not established. **Elderly:** No age-related precautions noted.

INTERACTIONS

DRUG: CYP3A4 inhibitors (e.g., **clarithromycin, ketoconazole, ritonavir**) may increase concentration. **CYP3A4 inducers** (e.g., **carBAMazepine, dexamethasone, phenytoin, rifAMPin**) may decrease concentration. **P-gp inhibitors** (e.g., **cycloSPORINE**) may increase everolimus concentration, toxicity. **Statins** (e.g., **simvastatin**) may increase risk of rhabdomyolysis. **FOOD: High-fat meals** may reduce plasma concentration. **Grapefruit products** may increase concentration (potential for myelotoxicity, nephrotoxicity). **HERBAL: St. John's wort** may decrease plasma concentration. **LAB VALUES:** May increase serum BUN,

creatinine, glucose, triglycerides, lipids. May decrease neutrophils, Hgb, platelets.

AVAILABILITY (Rx)

🔖 **Tablets (Zortress):** 🔖 0.25 mg, 0.5 mg, 0.75 mg. **Tablets (Afinitor):** 2.5 mg, 5 mg, 7.5 mg, 10 mg. **Tablets for Oral Suspension (Afinitor Disperz):** 2 mg, 3 mg, 5 mg.

ADMINISTRATION/HANDLING

• Give without regard to food. • Swallow tablets whole; do not crush/cut Afinitor or Zortress. • If pt unable to swallow Afinitor tablets, may disperse in water with gentle stirring; give immediately. • Administer Afinitor Disperz as suspension only. Disperse in water until dissolved. • Avoid direct contact of dispersed tablet or oral solution with skin or mucous membranes.

INDICATIONS/ROUTES/DOSAGE

◀ **ALERT** ▶ If pt requires coadministration of a strong CYP3A4 inducer (e.g., carBAMazepine, dexamethasone, PHENobarbital, phenytoin, rifabutin, rifAMPin), consider doubling the dose. If strong inducer is discontinued, reduce everolimus to dose used prior to initiation. If moderate CYP3A4 inhibitors are required, reduce dose by 50%.

Renal Carcinoma, Neuroendocrine Tumors, Breast Cancer, TSC
PO: ADULTS, ELDERLY: (Afinitor): 10 mg once daily. **Coadministration with CYP3A4 inhibitors or P-gp inhibitors:** 2.5 mg once daily. May increase to 5 mg/day. **Coadministration with CYP3A4 inducers:** Increase by 5-mg increments up to 20 mg/day.

Renal Transplant Rejection Prophylaxis
PO: ADULTS, ELDERLY: (Zortress): Initially, 0.75 mg 2 times/day. Give in combination with basiliximab and concurrently with reduced doses of cycloSPORINE and corticosteroids.

Liver Transplant Rejection Prophylaxis (begin at least 30 days post-transplant)
PO: ADULTS, ELDERLY: (Zortress): Initially, 1 mg 2 times/day. Adjust dose at

4–5-day intervals based on serum concentration, tolerability, and response.

SEGA

PO: ADULTS, ELDERLY: Initially, 4.5 mg/m² once daily, titrated to attain trough concentration of 5–15 ng/mL. **If trough greater than 15 ng/mL:** reduce dose by 2.5 mg/day (tablets) or 2 mg/day (tablets for oral suspension). **If trough less than 15 ng/mL:** increase dose by 2.5 mg/day (tablets) or 2 mg/day (tablets for oral suspension).

Dosage in Renal Impairment

No dose adjustment.

Dosage in Hepatic Impairment

	Mild	Moderate	Severe
Breast Cancer PNET, RCC, renal angiomyolipoma	7.5 mg/day or 5 mg/day	5 mg/day or 2.5 mg/day	2.5 mg/day
Liver/ Renal transplant	Reduce dose by 33%	Reduce dose by 50%	Reduce dose by 50%
SEGA	No change	No change	Initial dose 2.5 mg/m²/day

SIDE EFFECTS

Common (44%–26%): Stomatitis, asthenia. Diarrhea, cough, rash, nausea. **Frequent (25%–20%):** Peripheral edema, anorexia, dyspnea, vomiting, pyrexia. **Occasional (19%–10%):** Mucosal inflammation, headache, epistaxis, pruritus, dry skin, epigastric distress, extremity pain. **Rare (less than 10%):** Abdominal pain, insomnia, dry mouth, dizziness, paresthesia, eyelid edema, hypertension, nail disorder, chills.

ADVERSE EFFECTS/TOXIC REACTIONS

Noninfectious pneumonitis characterized as hypoxia, pleural effusion, cough, or dyspnea was reported in 14% of pts; Grade 3 noninfectious pneumonitis reported in 4%. Localized and systemic infections, including pneumonia, other bacterial infections, and invasive fungal infections, have occurred due to everolimus immunosuppressive properties. Renal failure occurs in 3% of pts.

NURSING CONSIDERATIONS

BASELINE ASSESSMENT

Assess medical history, esp. renal function, use of other immunosuppressants. Obtain CBC, BMP, LFT before treatment begins and routinely thereafter. Offer emotional support.

INTERVENTION/EVALUATION

Offer antiemetics to control nausea, vomiting. Monitor daily pattern of bowel activity, stool consistency. Assess skin for evidence of rash, edema. Monitor CBC, particularly Hgb, platelet, neutrophil count; BUN, creatinine, LFT. Monitor for shortness of breath, fatigue, hypertension. Assess mouth for stomatitis, mucositis.

PATIENT/FAMILY TEACHING

• Take dose at same time each day. • Avoid crowds, those with known infection. • Avoid contact with anyone who recently received live virus vaccine. • Do not have immunizations without physician's approval (drug lowers body resistance). • Promptly report fever, unusual bruising/bleeding from any site. • Avoid direct contact of crushed tablets with skin or mucous membrane (wash thoroughly if contact occurs). • Avoid grapefruit products.

exemestane

ex-e-**mes**-tane
(Aromasin)
Do not confuse Aromasin with Arimidex, or exemestane with estramustine.

◆CLASSIFICATION

PHARMACOTHERAPEUTIC: Aromatase inhibitor. **CLINICAL:** Antineoplastic.

USES

Treatment of advanced breast cancer in postmenopausal women whose disease has progressed following tamoxifen therapy. Adjuvant treatment of postmenopausal women with estrogen-receptor positive early breast cancer after 2–3 yrs of tamoxifen therapy for completion of 5 consecutive yrs of adjuvant hormonal therapy. **OFF-LABEL:** Reduces risk of invasive breast cancer in postmenopausal women; treatment of endometrial cancer, uterine sarcoma.

PRECAUTIONS

Contraindications: Hypersensitivity to exemestane. **Cautions:** Not indicated for use in premenopausal women. Concomitant use of estrogen-containing agents, strong CYP3A4 inducers.

ACTION

Inactivates aromatase, the principal enzyme that converts androgens to estrogens in both premenopausal and postmenopausal women, lowering circulating estrogen level. **Therapeutic Effect:** Inhibits growth of breast cancers stimulated by estrogens.

PHARMACOKINETICS

Rapidly absorbed after PO administration. Protein binding: 90%. Distributed extensively into tissues. Metabolized in liver. Excreted in urine and feces. **Half-life:** 24 hrs.

⧗ LIFESPAN CONSIDERATIONS

Pregnancy/Lactation: Indicated for postmenopausal women. **Children:** Not indicated for use in this pt population. **Elderly:** No age-related precautions noted.

INTERACTIONS

DRUG: CYP3A4 inducers (e.g., PHENobarbital, rifAMPin) may decrease concentration/effect. **HERBAL: St. John's wort** may decrease concentration. Avoid **black cohosh, dong quai** in estrogen-dependent tumors. **FOOD:** None known. **LAB VALUES:** May increase serum alkaline phosphatase, ALT, AST.

AVAILABILITY (Rx)

Tablets: 25 mg.

ADMINISTRATION/HANDLING

PO
• Give after meals.

INDICATIONS/ROUTES/DOSAGE

Breast Cancer (Early)
PO: POSTMENOPAUSAL WOMEN: 25 mg once daily after a meal (following 2–3 yrs tamoxifen therapy) for total duration of 5 yrs (in absence of recurrence or contralateral breast cancer).

Breast Cancer (Advanced)
PO: POSTMENOPAUSAL WOMEN: 25 mg once daily after a meal. 50 mg/day when used concurrently with potent CYP3A4 inducers (e.g., rifAMPin, phenytoin). Continue until tumor progression.

Dosage in Renal/Hepatic Impairment
No dose adjustment.

SIDE EFFECTS

Frequent (22%–10%): Fatigue, nausea, depression, hot flashes, pain, insomnia, anxiety, dyspnea. **Occasional (8%–5%):** Headache, dizziness, vomiting, peripheral edema, abdominal pain, anorexia, flu-like symptoms, diaphoresis, constipation, hypertension. **Rare (4%):** Diarrhea.

ADVERSE EFFECTS/TOXIC REACTIONS

MI has been reported.

NURSING CONSIDERATIONS

BASELINE ASSESSMENT

Question history of cardiac disease. Receive full medication history and screen for interactions. Offer emotional support.

INTERVENTION/EVALUATION

Monitor for onset of depression. Assess sleep pattern. Monitor for and assist with ambulation if dizziness occurs. Assess for headache. Offer antiemetic for nausea/vomiting.

PATIENT/FAMILY TEACHING
• Report if nausea, hot flashes become unmanageable. • Avoid tasks that require alertness, motor skills until response to drug is established. • Best taken after meals and at same time each day.

---

exenatide
HIGH ALERT

ex-**en**-a-tide
(Bydureon, Bydureon BCise, Byetta, 5 mcg Pen, 10 mcg Pen)
■ **BLACK BOX ALERT** ■ (Bydureon): Risk of thyroid C-cell tumors.

◆CLASSIFICATION
PHARMACOTHERAPEUTIC: Glucagon-like peptide-1 (GLP-1) receptor agonist. **CLINICAL:** Antidiabetic.

USES
Adjunct to diet, exercise to improve glycemic control in pts with type 2 diabetes mellitus.

PRECAUTIONS
Contraindications: Hypersensitivity to exenatide. Bydureon only: History of medullary thyroid carcinoma. Pts with multiple endocrine neoplasia syndrome type 2 (MEN2). **Cautions:** Diabetic ketoacidosis, type 1 diabetes mellitus. Pts with renal transplantation or moderate renal impairment. Not recommended in severe renal impairment, severe GI disease, pancreatitis.

ACTION
Stimulates release of insulin from beta cells of pancreas, mimics enhancement of glucose-dependent insulin secretion, suppresses elevated glucagon secretion, slows gastric emptying (central action increases satiety). **Therapeutic Effect:** Improves glycemic control by increasing postmeal insulin secretion, decreasing postmeal glucagon levels, delaying gastric emptying, and increasing satiety.

PHARMACOKINETICS
Minimal systemic metabolism. Eliminated by glomerular filtration with subsequent proteolytic degradation. **Half-life:** 2.4 hrs.

⌛ LIFESPAN CONSIDERATIONS
Pregnancy/Lactation: Unknown if distributed in breast milk. **Children:** Safety and efficacy not established. **Elderly:** No age-related precautions noted.

INTERACTIONS
DRUG: May decrease effects of **digoxin, lovastatin.** May increase bleeding time, risk of bleeding when used with **warfarin.** **HERBAL:** None significant. **FOOD:** None known. **LAB VALUES:** None known.

AVAILABILITY (Rx)
Injection, Solution (Prefilled Pen): (Byetta) 10 mcg/0.04 mL (2.4 mL); 5 mcg/0.02 mL (1.2 mL). **Injection, Suspension (Bydureon):** 2 mg. **Injection Prefilled single dose Auto-injector (Bydureon BCise):** 2 mg in 0.85 ml vehicle.

ADMINISTRATION/HANDLING
Subcutaneous
• May be given in thigh, abdomen, upper arm. • Rotation of injection sites is essential; maintain careful injection site record. • Give within 60 min before morning and evening meals. Give suspension immediately after powder is suspended.
Storage • Refrigerate prefilled pens. • Discard if freezing occurs. • May be stored at room temperature after first use. • Discard pen 30 days after initial use.

INDICATIONS/ROUTE/DOSAGE
Diabetes Mellitus
SQ: ADULTS, ELDERLY: (Byetta) 5 mcg per dose given twice daily at any time within the 60-min period before the morning and evening meals. Dose may be increased to 10 mcg twice daily after 1 mo of therapy. (Bydureon): 2 mg once q7days.

Dosage in Renal Impairment
Mild impairment: No dose adjustment. **Moderate impairment:** Use caution. **Severe impairment (CrCl less than 30 mL/min or ESRD):** Not recommended.

Dosage in Hepatic Impairment
No dose adjustment.

SIDE EFFECTS

(Byetta) Frequent (44%): Nausea. **Occasional (13%–6%):** Diarrhea, vomiting, dizziness, anxiety, dyspepsia. **Rare (less than 6%):** Weakness. **(Bydureon) 5% or greater:** Nausea, diarrhea, headache, constipation, vomiting, dyspepsia, injection site pruritus or nodule.

ADVERSE EFFECTS/TOXIC REACTIONS

With concurrent sulfonylurea, hypoglycemia occurs in 36% when given a 10-mcg dose of exenatide, 16% when given a 5-mcg dose. May cause acute pancreatitis.

NURSING CONSIDERATIONS

BASELINE ASSESSMENT

Check serum glucose before administration. Discuss lifestyle to determine extent of learning, emotional needs. Ensure follow-up instruction if pt or family does not thoroughly understand diabetes management, glucose-testing technique. At least 1 mo should elapse to assess response to drug before new dose adjustment is made.

INTERVENTION/EVALUATION

Monitor serum glucose, food intake, renal function. Assess for hypoglycemia (cool wet skin, tremors, dizziness, anxiety, headache, tachycardia, numbness in mouth, hunger, diplopia), hyperglycemia (polyuria, polyphagia, polydipsia, nausea, vomiting, dim vision, fatigue, deep rapid breathing). Be alert to conditions that alter glucose requirements (fever, increased activity or stress, surgical procedure).

PATIENT/FAMILY TEACHING

• Diabetes mellitus requires lifelong control. • Prescribed diet and exercise are principal parts of treatment. Do not skip, delay meals. • Continue to adhere to dietary instructions, regular exercise program, regular testing of serum glucose. • When taking combination therapy with a sulfonylurea, have source of glucose available to treat symptoms of hypoglycemia. • Report any unexplained severe abdominal pain with or without nausea or vomiting.

---

ezetimibe

e-**zet**-i-mib
(Apo-Ezetimibe ♣, Ezetrol ♣, Zetia)
Do not confuse Zetia with Zebeta or Zestril.

FIXED-COMBINATION(S)

Liptruzet: ezetimibe/atorvastatin (statin): 10 mg/10 mg, 10 mg/20 mg, 10 mg/40 mg, 10 mg/80 mg. **Vytorin:** ezetimibe/simvastatin (statin): 10 mg/10 mg, 10 mg/20 mg, 10 mg/40 mg, 10 mg/80 mg.

◆CLASSIFICATION

PHARMACOTHERAPEUTIC: Antihyperlipidemic. **CLINICAL:** Anticholesterol agent.

USES

Adjunct to diet for treatment of primary hypercholesterolemia (monotherapy or in combination with HMG-CoA reductase inhibitors [statins]), homozygous sitosterolemia, homozygous familial hypercholesterolemia (combined with atorvastatin or simvastatin). Mixed hyperlipidemia (in combination with fenofibrate).

PRECAUTIONS

Contraindications: Hypersensitivity to ezetimibe. Concurrent use of an HMG-CoA reductase inhibitor (atorvastatin, fluvastatin, lovastatin, pravastatin, simvastatin) in pts with active hepatic disease

---

E

or unexplained persistent elevations in serum transaminase; pregnancy and breastfeeding (when used with a statin). **Cautions:** Severe renal or mild hepatic impairment. Not recommended in those with moderate or severe hepatic impairment.

ACTION

Inhibits cholesterol absorption in brush border of small intestine, leading to decrease in delivery of intestinal cholesterol to liver. **Therapeutic Effect:** Reduces total serum cholesterol, LDL, triglycerides; increases HDL.

PHARMACOKINETICS

Well absorbed following PO administration. Protein binding: greater than 90%. Metabolized in small intestine and liver. Excreted in feces (78%), urine (11%). **Half-life:** 22 hrs.

⧗ LIFESPAN CONSIDERATIONS

Pregnancy/Lactation: Unknown if drug crosses placenta or is distributed in breast milk. **Children:** Safety and efficacy not established in pts 10 yrs or younger. **Elderly:** Age-related mild hepatic impairment may require dosage adjustment.

INTERACTIONS

DRUG: Antacids containing aluminum or magnesium, cycloSPORINE**, fenofibrate, gemfibrozil** increase concentration. **Cholestyramine resin** decreases effectiveness. **HERBAL:** None significant. **FOOD:** None known. **LAB VALUES:** May increase serum alkaline phosphatase, bilirubin, ALT, AST.

AVAILABILITY (Rx)

Tablets: 10 mg.

ADMINISTRATION/HANDLING

• Give without regard to food. • May give at same time as statins. Give at least 2 hrs before or 4 hrs after bile acid sequestrants.

INDICATIONS/ROUTES/DOSAGE

Hypercholesterolemia
PO: ADULTS, ELDERLY, CHILDREN 10 YRS AND OLDER: Initially, 10 mg once daily, given with or without food. If pt is also receiving a bile acid sequestrant, give ezetimibe at least 2 hrs before or at least 4 hrs after bile acid sequestrant.

Dosage in Renal Impairment
No dose adjustment.

Dosage in Hepatic Impairment
Mild impairment: No dose adjustment. **Moderate to severe impairment:** Not recommended.

SIDE EFFECTS

Occasional (4%–3%): Back pain, diarrhea, arthralgia, sinusitis, abdominal pain. **Rare (2%):** Cough, pharyngitis, fatigue, depression.

ADVERSE EFFECTS/TOXIC REACTIONS

Hepatitis, hypersensitivity reaction, myopathy, rhabdomyolysis occur rarely.

NURSING CONSIDERATIONS

BASELINE ASSESSMENT

Obtain diet history, esp. fat consumption. Obtain serum cholesterol, triglycerides, hepatic function tests, blood counts during initial therapy and periodically during treatment. Treatment should be discontinued if hepatic enzyme levels persist more than 3 times normal limit. Receive full medication history and screen for interactions. Question history of hepatic/renal impairment.

INTERVENTION/EVALUATION

Monitor daily pattern of bowel activity, stool consistency. Question pt for signs/symptoms of back pain, abdominal disturbances. Monitor serum cholesterol, triglycerides for therapeutic response.

PATIENT/FAMILY TEACHING

• Periodic laboratory tests are essential part of therapy. • Do not stop medication without consulting physician. • Report muscular or bone pain. • May take at same time as statins. Take at least 2 hrs before or 4 hrs after cholestyramine, colestipol, colesevelam.

ezogabine

e-**zog**-a-bine
(Potiga)
■ **BLACK BOX ALERT** ■ Retinal abnormalities may progress to vision loss.

◆CLASSIFICATION

PHARMACOTHERAPEUTIC: Potassium channel opener **(Schedule V). CLINICAL:** Anticonvulsant.

USES

Adjunctive therapy for treatment of partial-onset seizures in pts 18 yrs of age and older.

PRECAUTIONS

Contraindications: Hypersensitivity to ezogabine. **Cautions:** Hepatic/renal impairment, BPH, urinary retention, chronic cognitive impairment, prolonged QT interval, psychiatric history, pts at risk for suicide. Hypokalemia, hypomagnesemia, familial long-QT syndrome, medications that prolong QT interval, hypothyroidism, HF, ventricular arrhythmias, elderly.

ACTION

Binds to voltage-gated potassium channels, stabilizing the channels in open formation and enhancing the M current. **Therapeutic Effect:** Regulates neuronal excitability, suppressing seizure activity.

PHARMACOKINETICS

Rapidly absorbed after PO administration. Peak concentration: 0.5–2 hrs. Protein binding: 80%. Metabolized by glucuronidation and acetylation. Primarily excreted in urine (85%), feces (14%). **Half-life:** 7–11 hrs.

⌛ LIFESPAN CONSIDERATIONS

Pregnancy/Lactation: Unknown if drug crosses placenta or is distributed in breast milk. Must either discontinue breastfeeding or discontinue drug regimen. **Children:** Safety and efficacy not established in pts under 18 yrs of age. **Elderly:** Dosage adjustment recommended for pts older than 65 yrs.

INTERACTIONS

DRUG: Phenytoin, car**BAMaz**epine may decrease plasma concentration/effects. **Alcohol** may increase concentration/adverse effects. May inhibit clearance of **digoxin. HERBAL:** None known. **FOOD:** None significant. **LAB VALUES:** May create falsely elevated urine bilirubin level.

AVAILABILITY (Rx)

Tablets: 50 mg, 200 mg, 300 mg, 400 mg.

ADMINISTRATION/HANDLING

• May give without regard to food. Swallow tablets whole.

INDICATIONS/ROUTES/DOSAGE

Partial Seizures
◄ **ALERT** ► Increase at wkly intervals by no more than 50 mg 3 times daily (150 mg/day).
PO: ADULTS: Initially, 100 mg 3 times daily. May increase to maintenance dose of 200–400 mg 3 times daily (600–1,200 mg daily). **Maximum:** 1,200 mg/day. **ELDERLY:** Initially, 50 mg 3 times/day. May increase wkly to therapeutic level. **Maximum:** 250 mg 3 times/day (750 mg/day). Discontinuation: Reduce gradually over period of at least 3 wks.

Dosage in Renal Impairment
CrCl less than 50 mL/min or ESRD: 50 mg 3 times/day for 7 days, then increase dose to therapeutic level. **Maximum:** 200 mg 3 times/day (600 mg/day).

Dosage in Hepatic Impairment

Mild Impairment (Child-Pugh score less than 9): 50 mg 3 times/day for 7 days, then increase dose to therapeutic level. **Maximum:** 250 mg 3 times/day (750 mg/day). **Severe Hepatic Impairment (Child-Pugh score greater than 9):** 50 mg 3 times/day for 7 days, then increase dose to therapeutic level. **Maximum:** 200 mg 3 times/day (600 mg/day).

SIDE EFFECTS

Frequent (23%–15%): Dizziness, somnolence, fatigue. **Occasional (8%–4%):** Tremor, vertigo, abnormal coordination, nausea, diplopia, attention disturbance, memory impairment, asthenia, blurred vision, gait disturbance, aphasia, dysarthria, balance disorder. **Rare (3%–1%):** Constipation, anxiety, weight gain, dyspepsia, amnesia, dysphasia, disorientation, dysuria, urinary hesitation, hematuria, urine discoloration, psychotic behavior.

ADVERSE EFFECTS/TOXIC REACTIONS

Urinary retention requiring catheterization, prolonged QT interval, myoclonus, peripheral edema, hypokinesia, dysphasia, hyperhidrosis, malaise reported in less than 2% of pts. Hydronephrosis associated with baseline renal impairment, increased risk of psychosis, hallucinations, suicidal ideation, depression, aggression, mania noted.

NURSING CONSIDERATIONS

BASELINE ASSESSMENT

Review history of seizure disorder (intensity, frequency, duration, LOC). Question history of BPH, urinary retention, cognitive impairment, psychiatric disorder, hepatic/renal impairment, alcoholism, prolonged QT syndrome. Obtain full medication history including digoxin, antiarrhythmics, adjunct anticonvulsant therapy. Obtain baseline EKG, digoxin level if applicable. Question possibility of pregnancy or current breastfeeding.

INTERVENTION/EVALUATION

Initiate seizure precautions and observe for seizure activity. Assist with ambulation if dizziness occurs. Monitor for depression, suicidal ideation, unusual behavior, mania, anxiety. Routinely monitor digoxin levels. Monitor QT interval for pts with HF, ventricular hypertrophy, hypokalemia, hypomagnesemia.

PATIENT/FAMILY TEACHING

• Monitor closely for seizure activity. • Immediately report any new medications, trouble urinating, palpitations, pregnancy, or plans to breastfeed. • Avoid alcohol. • Report any thoughts of suicide, aggressive behavior, depression, anxiety, trouble sleeping, impulsiveness, unusual behavior. • Noncompliance may lead to increased risk of seizures.

famciclovir

fam-**sye**-klo-veer
(Apo-Famciclovir ✦, Famvir)
**Do not confuse famciclovir
with acyclovir, ganciclovir, or
valGANciclovir; or Famvir with
Femara.**

◆CLASSIFICATION
PHARMACOTHERAPEUTIC: Synthetic
nucleoside. **CLINICAL:** Antiviral.

USES
Treatment of acute herpes zoster (shingles) in immunocompetent pts, treatment and suppression of recurrent genital herpes in immunocompetent pts, treatment of recurrent mucocutaneous herpes simplex in HIV-infected pts. Treatment of recurrent herpes labialis (cold sores) in immunocompetent pts.

PRECAUTIONS
Contraindications: Hypersensitivity to famciclovir, penciclovir. **Cautions:** Renal impairment. Avoid use in galactose intolerance, severe lactose deficiency, or glucose-galactose malabsorption syndromes.

ACTION
Inhibits HSV-2 polymerase, inhibiting herpes viral DNA synthesis and replication. **Therapeutic Effect:** Suppresses replication of herpes simplex virus, varicella-zoster virus. Shortens healing time of herpes zoster lesions. Reduces symptom severity of genital herpes.

PHARMACOKINETICS
Rapidly absorbed. Protein binding: 20%–25%. Rapidly metabolized to penciclovir by enzymes in GI tract, liver, plasma. Excreted unchanged in urine. Removed by hemodialysis.

Half-life: 2–3 hrs (increased in severe renal failure).

⧗ LIFESPAN CONSIDERATIONS
Pregnancy/Lactation: Unknown if excreted in breast milk. **Children:** Safety and efficacy not established. **Elderly:** Age-related renal impairment may require dosage adjustment.

INTERACTIONS
DRUG: Probenecid, methotrexate may increase adverse effects. **HERBAL:** None significant. **FOOD:** None known. **LAB VALUES:** May increase serum ALT, AST, amylase, bilirubin, lipase. May decrease neutrophils, platelets.

AVAILABILITY (Rx)
Tablets: 125 mg, 250 mg, 500 mg.

ADMINISTRATION/HANDLING
PO
• Give without regard to meals. • Give with food to decrease GI distress.

INDICATIONS/ROUTES/DOSAGE
Herpes Zoster (Shingles)
PO: ADULTS: 500 mg q8h for 7 days. Begin as soon as possible after diagnosis and within 72 hrs of rash onset. **(HIV pts):** 500 mg 3 times/day for 7–10 days.

Genital Herpes Simplex (Initial)
PO: ADULTS: 250 mg 3 times/day for 7–10 days.

Genital Herpes Simplex (Recurrence)
PO: ADULTS: 1,000 mg twice daily for 1 day; or 125 mg 2 times/day for 5 days; or 500 mg once, then 250 mg 2 times/ day for 2 days.

Genital Herpes Simplex (Suppression)
PO: ADULTS: 250 mg twice daily for up to 1 yr.

Genital Herpes Simplex in HIV Pts
PO: ADULTS: 500 mg twice daily for 7 days or 5–10 days.

F

Herpes Labialis (Cold Sores)
PO: ADULTS, ELDERLY: (Immunocompetent): 1,500 mg as a single dose. Initiate at first sign or symptoms. **(HIV pts):** 500 mg 2 times/day for 5–10 days.

Dosage in Renal Impairment
Dosage and frequency are modified based on creatinine clearance and disease process.

Creatinine Clearance	Herpes Zoster	Recurrent Genital Herpes (single-day regimen)	Recurrent Genital Herpes (suppression)	Recurrent Herpes Labialis Treatment (single-day regimen)	Recurrent Orolabial or Genital Herpes in HIV Pts
40–59 mL/min	500 mg q12h	500 mg q12h	—	750 mg	—
20–39 mL/min	500 mg q24h	500 mg	125 mg q12h	500 mg	500 mg q24h
Less than 20 mL/min	250 mg q24h	250 mg	125 mg q24h	250 mg	250 mg q24h
Hemodialysis	250 mg after each hemodialysis session	250 mg after each hemodialysis session	125 mg after each hemodialysis session	250 mg after each hemodialysis session	250 mg after each hemodialysis session

Dosage in Hemodialysis Pts
Herpes zoster: 250 mg after each dialysis treatment. **Genital herpes:** 125 mg after each dialysis treatment.

Dosage in Hepatic Impairment
No dose adjustment.

SIDE EFFECTS

Frequent (23%–12%): Headache, nausea. **Occasional (10%–2%):** Dizziness, drowsiness, paresthesia (esp. feet), diarrhea, vomiting, constipation, decreased appetite, fatigue, fever, pharyngitis, sinusitis, pruritus. **Rare (less than 2%):** Insomnia, abdominal pain, dyspepsia, flatulence, back pain, arthralgia.

ADVERSE EFFECTS/TOXIC REACTIONS

Urticaria, severe skin rash, hallucinations, confusion (delirium, disorientation occur predominantly in elderly) has been reported.

NURSING CONSIDERATIONS

BASELINE ASSESSMENT

Obtain baseline chemistry tests, esp. renal function. Question history of galactose intolerance, severe lactose deficiency, glucose-galactose malabsorption, renal impairment. Assess herpetic lesions.

INTERVENTION/EVALUATION

Evaluate cutaneous lesions. Be alert to neurologic effects: headache, dizziness. Provide analgesics, comfort measures. Monitor renal function, hepatic enzymes, CBC.

PATIENT/FAMILY TEACHING

• Drink adequate fluids. • Fingernails should be kept short, hands clean. • Do not touch lesions with fingers to avoid spreading infection to new site. • **Genital herpes:** Continue therapy for full length of treatment. • Avoid contact with lesions during duration of outbreak to prevent cross-contamination. • Use condoms during sexual activity. • Report if lesions recur or do not improve. • Slowly go from lying to standing to avoid dizziness. • Avoid tasks that require alertness, motor skills until response to drug is established.

famotidine

fa-**moe**-ta-deen
(Acid Reducer Maximum Strength, Apo-Famotidine 🍁, Pepcid, Ulcidine 🍁)

Do not confuse famotidine with cimetidine, ranitidine, fluoxetine, or furosemide.

FIXED-COMBINATION(S)

Duexis: famotidine/ibuprofen (an NSAID): 26.6 mg/800 mg. **Pepcid Complete:** famotidine/calcium chloride/magnesium hydroxide (antacids): 10 mg/800 mg/165 mg.

◆CLASSIFICATION

PHARMACOTHERAPEUTIC: H_2 receptor antagonist. **CLINICAL:** Antiulcer, gastric acid secretion inhibitor.

USES

Short-term treatment of active duodenal ulcer. Prevention, maintenance of duodenal ulcer recurrence. Treatment of active benign gastric ulcer, pathologic GI hypersecretory conditions. Short-term treatment of gastroesophageal reflux disease (GERD). OTC formulation for relief of heartburn, acid indigestion, sour stomach. **OFF-LABEL:** *H. pylori* eradication, risk reduction of duodenal ulcer recurrence (part of multidrug regimen), stress ulcer prophylaxis in critically ill pts, relief of gastritis.

PRECAUTIONS

Contraindications: Hypersensitivity to famotidine, other H_2 antagonists. **Cautions:** Renal/hepatic impairment, elderly, thrombocytopenia.

ACTION

Inhibits histamine action of H_2 receptors of parietal cells. **Therapeutic Effect:** Inhibits gastric acid secretion (fasting, nocturnal, or stimulated by food, caffeine, insulin).

PHARMACOKINETICS

Route	Onset	Peak	Duration
PO	1 hr	1–4 hrs	10–12 hrs
IV	0.5 hr	0.5–3 hrs	10–12 hrs

Rapidly, incompletely absorbed from GI tract. Protein binding: 15%–20%. Partially metabolized in liver. Primarily excreted in urine. Not removed by hemodialysis. **Half-life:** 2.5–3.5 hrs (increased in renal impairment).

⧖ LIFESPAN CONSIDERATIONS

Pregnancy/Lactation: Unknown if drug crosses placenta or is distributed in breast milk. **Children:** No age-related precautions noted. **Elderly:** Confusion more likely to occur, esp. in pts with renal/hepatic impairment.

INTERACTIONS

DRUG: May decrease absorption of **atazanavir, itraconazole, ketoconazole.** **HERBAL:** None significant. **FOOD:** None known. **LAB VALUES:** Interferes with skin tests using allergen extracts. May increase serum alkaline phosphatase, ALT, AST. May decrease platelet count.

AVAILABILITY (Rx)

Infusion, Premix: 20 mg in 50 mL 0.9% NaCl. **Injection, Solution:** 10 mg/mL (2-mL vial). **Powder for Oral Suspension:** 40 mg/5 mL. **Tablets:** 10 mg. 20 mg, 40 mg.

ADMINISTRATION/HANDLING

 IV

Reconstitution • For IV push, dilute 20 mg with 5–10 mL 0.9% NaCl. • For intermittent IV infusion (piggyback), dilute with 50–100 mL D_5W, or 0.9% NaCl. **Rate of Administration** • Give IV push over at least 2 min. • Infuse piggyback over 15–30 min.

Storage • Refrigerate unused vials. • IV solution appears clear, colorless. • After dilution, IV solution is stable for 48 hrs if refrigerated.

PO

• Store tablets, suspension at room temperature. • Following reconstitution, oral suspension is stable for 30 days at room temperature. • Give without

---

✦ Canadian trade name   🗑 Non-Crushable Drug   🔲 High Alert drug regard to meals. • Shake suspension well before use.

🔲 IV INCOMPATIBILITIES

Amphotericin B complex (Abelcet, AmBisome, Amphotec), piperacillin/tazobactam (Zosyn).

🔲 IV COMPATIBILITIES

Calcium gluconate, dexamethasone (Decadron), dexmedetomidine (Precedex), DOBUTamine (Dobutrex), DOPamine (Intropin), DOXOrubicin (Adriamycin), furosemide (Lasix), heparin, HYDROmorphone (Dilaudid), insulin (regular), lidocaine, LORazepam (Ativan), magnesium sulfate, midazolam (Versed), morphine, nitroglycerin, norepinephrine (Levophed), ondansetron (Zofran), potassium chloride, potassium phosphate, propofol (Diprivan).

INDICATIONS/ROUTES/DOSAGE

Duodenal Ulcer
PO: ADULTS, ELDERLY: Acute therapy: 40 mg/day at bedtime or 20 mg twice daily for 4–8 wks. **Maintenance:** 20 mg/day at bedtime.

Peptic Ulcer
PO: CHILDREN 1–16 YRS: 0.5 mg/kg/day at bedtime or 2 divided doses. **Maximum:** 40 mg/day.

Gastric Ulcer
PO: ADULTS, ELDERLY: (Acute therapy): 40 mg/day at bedtime.

Gastroesophageal Reflux Disease (GERD)
PO: ADULTS, ELDERLY: 20 mg twice daily for 6 wks. **CHILDREN 1–16 YRS:** 1 mg/kg/day in 2 divided doses. **Maximum:** 40 mg 2 times/day. **CHILDREN 3 MOS–11 MOS:** 0.5 mg/kg/dose twice daily. **CHILDREN YOUNGER THAN 3 MOS, NEONATES:** 0.5 mg/kg/dose once daily.

Esophagitis
PO: ADULTS, ELDERLY, CHILDREN 12 YRS AND OLDER: 20–40 mg twice daily for up to 12 wks.

Hypersecretory Conditions
PO: ADULTS, ELDERLY, CHILDREN 12 YRS AND OLDER: Initially, 20 mg q6h. May increase up to 160 mg q6h.

Acid Indigestion, Heartburn (OTC Use)
PO: ADULTS, ELDERLY, CHILDREN 12 YRS AND OLDER: 10–20 mg q12h. May take 15–60 min before eating. **Maximum:** 2 doses/day.

Usual Parenteral Dosage
IV: ADULTS, ELDERLY, CHILDREN OLDER THAN 12 YRS: 20 mg q12h. **CHILDREN 1–12 YRS:** 0.25–0.5 mg/kg q12h. **Maximum:** 40 mg/day.

Dosage in Renal Impairment

Creatinine Clearance	Dosage
Less than 50 mL/min	50% normal dose or increase dosing interval to 48 hrs

Dosage in Hepatic Impairment
No dose adjustment.

SIDE EFFECTS

Occasional (5%): Headache. **Rare (2% or less):** Confusion, constipation, diarrhea, dizziness.

ADVERSE EFFECTS/TOXIC REACTIONS

Agranulocytosis, pancytopenia, thrombocytopenia occur rarely.

NURSING CONSIDERATIONS

BASELINE ASSESSMENT
Assess epigastric/abdominal pain. Verify platelet count in critically ill pts.

INTERVENTION/EVALUATION
Monitor daily pattern of bowel activity, stool consistency. Monitor for headache. Assess for confusion in elderly. Consider interrupting treatment in pts who develop thrombocytopenia.

PATIENT/FAMILY TEACHING

• May take without regard to meals, antacids. • Report headache. • Avoid excessive amounts of coffee, aspirin. • Report persistent symptoms of heartburn, acid indigestion, sour stomach.

febuxostat

fe-**bux**-oh-stat
(Uloric)
Do not confuse febuxostat with panobinostat or Femstat.

♦CLASSIFICATION

PHARMACOTHERAPEUTIC: Xanthine oxidase inhibitor. **CLINICAL:** Antigout agent.

USES

Management of hyperuricemia in pts with gout. Not recommended for treatment of asymptomatic hyperuricemia.

PRECAUTIONS

Contraindications: Hypersensitivity to febuxostat. Concomitant use with azaTHIOprine, mercaptopurine. **Cautions:** Severe renal/hepatic impairment, history of heart disease or stroke. Hypersensitivity to allopurinol. Pts at risk for urate formation.

ACTION

Decreases uric acid production by inhibiting the enzyme xanthine oxidase. **Therapeutic Effect:** Reduces uric acid concentrations in serum and urine.

PHARMACOKINETICS

Well absorbed from GI tract. Widely distributed. Protein binding: 99%. Metabolized in liver. Excreted in urine (49%), feces (45%). Removed by hemodialysis. **Half-life:** 5–8 hrs.

⊠ LIFESPAN CONSIDERATIONS

Pregnancy/Lactation: Unknown if drug crosses placenta or is distributed in breast milk. **Children:** Safety and efficacy not established. **Elderly:** No age-related precautions noted.

INTERACTIONS

DRUG: May increase concentration, toxicity of **azaTHIOprine, mercaptopurine, theophylline. HERBAL:** None significant. **FOOD:** None known. **LAB VALUES:** May increase serum alkaline phosphatase, ALT, AST, LDH, amylase, sodium, potassium, cholesterol, triglycerides, BUN, creatinine. May decrease platelets, Hgb, Hct, neutrophils. May prolong prothrombin time.

AVAILABILITY (Rx)

Tablets: 40 mg, 80 mg.

ADMINISTRATION/HANDLING

PO
• Give without regard to meals or antacids.

INDICATIONS/ROUTES/DOSAGE

◀**ALERT**▶ Recommended concomitant NSAID or colchicine with initiation of therapy and continue for up to 6 mos to prevent exacerbations of gout.

Hyperuricemia
PO: ADULTS, ELDERLY: Initially, 40 mg once daily. If pt does not achieve serum uric acid level less than 6 mg/dL after 2 wks with 40 mg, may give 80 mg once daily. **Maximum:** 120 mg/day.

Dosage in Renal/Hepatic Impairment
Mild to moderate impairment: No dose adjustment. **Severe impairment:** Use caution.

SIDE EFFECTS

Rare (1%): Nausea, arthralgia, rash, dizziness.

ADVERSE EFFECTS/TOXIC REACTIONS

Hepatic function abnormalities occur in 6% of pts. May increase risk of thromboembolic events including CVA, MI.

NURSING CONSIDERATIONS

BASELINE ASSESSMENT

Assess baseline renal function, LFT; concomitant use with azaTHIOprine, mercaptopurine, theophylline (contraindicated).

INTERVENTION/EVALUATION

Discontinue medication immediately if rash appears. Encourage high fluid intake (3,000 mL/day). Monitor I&O (output should be at least 2,000 mL/day). Monitor CBC, serum uric acid, renal function, LFT. Assess urine for cloudiness, unusual color, odor. Assess for therapeutic response (reduced joint tenderness, swelling, redness, limitation of motion). Monitor for symptoms of CVA, MI.

PATIENT/FAMILY TEACHING

• Encourage drinking 8–10 (8-oz) glasses of fluid daily while taking medication. • Report rash, chest pain, shortness of breath, symptoms suggestive of stroke. • Gout attacks may occur for several months after starting treatment (medication is not a pain reliever). • Continue taking even if gout attack occurs.

---

felodipine

fe-**loe**-di-peen
(Plendil ✦)
Do not confuse Plendil with Isordil, Pletal, PriLOSEC, or Prinivil, or Renedil with Prinivil.

FIXED-COMBINATION(S)

Lexxel: felodipine/enalapril (ACE inhibitor): 2.5 mg/5 mg, 5 mg/5 mg.

◆CLASSIFICATION

PHARMACOTHERAPEUTIC: Calcium channel blocker. **CLINICAL:** Antihypertensive.

USES

Management of hypertension. May be used alone or with other antihypertensives. **OFF-LABEL:** Management of pediatric hypertension.

PRECAUTIONS

Contraindications: Hypersensitivity to felodipine or other calcium channel blocker. **Cautions:** Severe left ventricular dysfunction, HF, hepatic impairment, hypertrophic cardiomyopathy with outflow tract obstruction, peripheral edema, severe aortic stenosis, elderly. Concomitant CYP3A4 inhibitors.

ACTION

Inhibits calcium movement across cardiac, vascular smooth muscle cell membranes. **Therapeutic Effect:** Relaxes coronary vascular smooth muscle and causes vasodilation. Increases myocardial oxygen delivery.

PHARMACOKINETICS

Route	Onset	Peak	Duration
PO	2–5 hrs	N/A	24 hrs

Rapidly, completely absorbed from GI tract. Protein binding: greater than 99%. Metabolized in liver. Primarily excreted in urine. Not removed by hemodialysis. **Half-life:** 11–16 hrs.

☒ LIFESPAN CONSIDERATIONS

Pregnancy/Lactation: Unknown if drug crosses placenta or is distributed in breast milk. **Children:** Safety and efficacy not established. **Elderly:** May experience greater hypotensive response. Constipation may be more problematic.

INTERACTIONS

DRUG: CYP3A4 inhibitors (e.g., keto-conazole, erythromycin, cimetidine) may increase concentration. **HERBAL:** St. John's wort may decrease concentration. **Ephedra, ginseng, yohimbe** may worsen hypertension. **Garlic** may increase antihypertensive effect. **FOOD: Grapefruit products** may increase absorption, concentration. **LAB VALUES:** None significant.

AVAILABILITY (Rx)

Tablets (Extended-Release): 2.5 mg, 5 mg, 10 mg.

ADMINISTRATION/HANDLING

PO

• Give with or without food. • Do not break, crush, dissolve, or divide extended-release tablets. Swallow whole.

INDICATIONS/ROUTES/DOSAGE

Hypertension

PO: ADULTS: Initially, 5 mg once daily. Increase by 5 mg at 2-wk intervals. Usual dose: 5–10 mg once daily. **ELDERLY:** Initially, 2.5 mg/day. Adjust dosage at no less than 2-wk intervals. Usual dose: 2.5–10 mg once daily. **CHILDREN 6 YRS AND OLDER:** Initially, 2.5 mg once daily. May increase at 2-wk intervals. **Maximum:** 10 mg/day.

Dosage in Renal Impairment

No dose adjustment.

Dosage in Hepatic Impairment

Initially, 2.5 mg once daily. Titrate carefully.

SIDE EFFECTS

Frequent (22%–18%): Headache, peripheral edema. **Occasional (6%–4%):** Flushing, respiratory infection, dizziness, light-headedness, asthenia. **Rare (less than 3%):** Angina, gingival hyperplasia, paresthesia, abdominal discomfort, anxiety, muscle cramping, cough, diarrhea, constipation.

ADVERSE EFFECTS/TOXIC REACTIONS

Overdose produces nausea, drowsiness, confusion, slurred speech, hypotension, bradycardia.

NURSING CONSIDERATIONS

BASELINE ASSESSMENT

Assess B/P, apical pulse immediately before drug administration (if pulse is 60 or less/min or systolic B/P is less than 90 mm Hg, withhold medication, contact physician). Question history of HF, hepatic impairment, valvular disease.

INTERVENTION/EVALUATION

Assist with ambulation if dizziness occurs. Assess for peripheral edema. Monitor pulse rate for bradycardia. Assess skin for flushing. Monitor hepatic function. Question for headache, asthenia.

PATIENT/FAMILY TEACHING

• Do not abruptly discontinue medication. • Compliance with therapy regimen is essential to control hypertension. • To avoid hypotensive effect, go from lying to standing slowly. • Avoid tasks that require alertness, motor skills until response to drug is established. • Report palpitations, shortness of breath, pronounced dizziness, nausea. • Swallow tablet whole; do not chew, crush, dissolve, or divide. • Avoid grapefruit products, alcohol. • Report exacerbation of angina.

---

fenofibrate

fen-o-**fye**-brate
(Antara, Apo-Fenofibrate ✤, Fenoglide, Fibricor, Lipofen, Lofibra, Novo-Fenofibrate ✤, Tricor, Triglide, Trilipix)
Do not confuse Tricor with Fibricor or Tracleer.

◆CLASSIFICATION

PHARMACOTHERAPEUTIC: Fibric acid derivative. **CLINICAL:** Antihyperlipidemic.

USES

Adjunct to diet for reduction of low-density lipoprotein cholesterol (LDL-C), total cholesterol, triglycerides (types IV and V hyperlipidemia), apo-lipoprotein B, and to increase high-density lipoprotein cholesterol (HDL-C) in pts with primary hypercholesterolemia, mixed dyslipidemia.

PRECAUTIONS

Contraindications: Hypersensitivity to fenofibrate. Active hepatic disease, preexisting gallbladder disease, severe renal/hepatic dysfunction (including primary biliary cirrhosis, unexplained persistent hepatic function abnormality), breastfeeding. **Cautions:** Anticoagulant therapy (e.g., warfarin), history of hepatic disease, venous thromboembolism, mild to moderate renal impairment, substantial alcohol consumption, statin or colchicine therapy (increased risk of myopathy, rhabdomyolysis), elderly.

ACTION

Downregulates apoprotein C-III and upregulates apoprotein A-I, increasing VLDL catabolism. **Therapeutic Effect:** Decreases triglycerides, increases HDL.

PHARMACOKINETICS

Well absorbed from GI tract. Absorption increased when given with food. Protein binding: 99%. Metabolized in liver. Excreted in urine (60%), feces (25%). Not removed by hemodialysis. **Half-life:** 10–35 hrs.

⏳ LIFESPAN CONSIDERATIONS

Pregnancy/Lactation: Safety in pregnancy not established. Breastfeeding not recommended. **Children:** Safety and efficacy not established. **Elderly:** No age-related precautions noted.

INTERACTIONS

DRUG: Potentiates effects of **anticoagulants (e.g., warfarin). Bile acid sequestrants** may impede absorption. **CycloSPORINE** may increase concentration, risk of nephrotoxicity. **Colchicine, HMG-CoA reductase inhibitors (statins)** may increase risk of severe myopathy, rhabdomyolysis, acute renal failure. **HERBAL:** None significant. **FOOD: All foods** increase absorption. **LAB VALUES:** May increase serum creatine kinase (CK), ALT, AST. May decrease Hgb, Hct, WBC; serum uric acid.

AVAILABILITY (Rx)

Capsules: *(Antara):* 30 mg, 90 mg. *(Lipofen):* 50 mg, 150 mg. *(Lofibra):* 67 mg, 134 mg, 200 mg. *(Trilipix):* 45 mg, 135 mg. **Tablets:** *(Fenoglide):* 40 mg, 120 mg. *(Fibricor):* 35 mg, 105 mg. *(Lofibra):* 54 mg, 160 mg. *(Tricor):* 48 mg, 145 mg. *(Triglide):* 160 mg.

ADMINISTRATION/HANDLING

PO

• Give Fenoglide, Lipofen, Lofibra with meals. • Antara, Fibricor, Tricor, Triglide, and Trilipix may be given without regard to food. Antara, Fenoglide, Lipofen: Swallow whole; do not open (capsules), crush, dissolve, or cut.

INDICATIONS/ROUTES/DOSAGE

Hypertriglyceridemia
PO *(Antara):* ADULTS, ELDERLY: 30–90 mg/day.
PO *(Fenoglide):* ADULTS, ELDERLY: 40–120 mg/day with meals.
PO *(Fibricor):* ADULTS, ELDERLY: 35–105 mg/day.
PO *(Lipofen):* ADULTS, ELDERLY: 50–150 mg/day with meals.
PO *(Lofibra):* ADULTS, ELDERLY: 67–200 mg/day with meals.
PO *(Tricor):* ADULTS, ELDERLY: 48–145 mg/day.
PO *(Triglide):* ADULTS, ELDERLY: 160 mg/day.
PO *(Trilipix):* ADULTS, ELDERLY: 45–135 mg/day.

Hypercholesterolemia, Mixed Hyperlipidemia
PO *(Antara):* ADULTS, ELDERLY: 90 mg/day.
PO *(Fenoglide):* ADULTS, ELDERLY: 120 mg/day with meals.
PO *(Fibricor):* ADULTS, ELDERLY: 105 mg/day.
PO *(Lipofen):* ADULTS, ELDERLY: 150 mg/day with meals.
PO *(Lofibra):* ADULTS, ELDERLY: 200 mg/day with meals.
PO *(Tricor):* ADULTS, ELDERLY: 145 mg/day.

PO *(Triglide):* **ADULTS, ELDERLY:** 160 mg/day.

PO *(Trilipix):* **ADULTS, ELDERLY:** 135 mg/day.

Dosage in Renal Impairment

Monitor renal function before adjusting dose. Decrease dose or increase dosing interval for pts with renal failure.

Initial doses:	Antara: 30 mg/day	Lofibra: 67 mg/day
	Fenoglide: 40 mg/day	Tricor: 48 mg/day
	Lipofen: 50 mg/day	Triglide: 50 mg/day

Dosage in Hepatic Impairment

Contraindicated.

SIDE EFFECTS

Frequent (8%–4%): Pain, rash, headache, asthenia, fatigue, flu-like symptoms, dyspepsia, nausea/vomiting, rhinitis. **Occasional (3%–2%):** Diarrhea, abdominal pain, constipation, flatulence, arthralgia, decreased libido, dizziness, pruritus. **Rare (less than 2%):** Increased appetite, insomnia, polyuria, cough, blurred vision, eye floaters, earache.

ADVERSE EFFECTS/TOXIC REACTIONS

May increase cholesterol excretion into bile, leading to cholelithiasis. Pancreatitis, hepatitis, thrombocytopenia, agranulocytosis occur rarely.

NURSING CONSIDERATIONS

BASELINE ASSESSMENT

Obtain diet history, esp. fat consumption. Obtain serum cholesterol, triglycerides, LFT, CBC during initial therapy and periodically during treatment. Treatment should be discontinued if hepatic enzyme levels persist greater than 3 times normal limit. Question medical history as listed in Precautions.

INTERVENTION/EVALUATION

For pts on concurrent therapy with HMG-CoA reductase inhibitors, monitor for complaints of myopathy (muscle pain, weakness). Monitor serum creatine kinase (CK). Monitor serum cholesterol, triglyceride for therapeutic response.

PATIENT/FAMILY TEACHING

• Report severe diarrhea, constipation, nausea. • Report skin rash/irritation, insomnia, muscle pain, tremors, dizziness.

fentaNYL

fen-ta-nil

(Abstral, Actiq, Apo-FentaNYL ♦ Duragesic, Fentora, Ionsys, Lazanda, Sublimaze, Subsys)

■ **BLACK BOX ALERT** ■ Physical and psychological dependence may occur with prolonged use. Must be alert to abuse, misuse, or diversion. May cause life-threatening hypoventilation, respiratory depression, or death. Use with strong or moderate CYP3A4 inhibitors may result in potentially fatal respiratory depression. **Buccal:** Tablet and lozenge contain enough medication to potentially be fatal to children. **Transdermal patch:** Serious or life-threatening hypoventilation has occurred. Limit use to children 2 yrs of age and older. Exposure to direct heat source increases drug release, resulting in overdose/death.

Do not confuse fentaNYL with alfentanil or SUFentanil.

♦CLASSIFICATION

PHARMACOTHERAPEUTIC: Opioid, narcotic agonist **(Schedule II). CLINICAL:** Analgesic.

USES

Injection: (FentaNYL): Pain relief, preop medication; adjunct to general or regional anesthesia. **Abstral:** Treatment of breakthrough pain in cancer pts 18 yrs of age and older. **Actiq:** Treatment of breakthrough pain in chronic cancer or AIDS-related pain. **Duragesic:** Management of chronic pain *(transdermal)*. **Fentora:** Breakthrough pain in pts on chronic opioids. **Ionsys:** Short-term management of acute postoperative pain in adults. **Lazanda:** Management of breakthrough pain in cancer. **Onsolis:** Breakthrough pain in pts with cancer currently receiving opioids and tolerant to opioid therapy. **Subsys:** Treatment of breakthrough cancer pain.

PRECAUTIONS

Contraindications: Hypersensitivity to fentaNYL. **Transdermal: Device (additional):** Significant respiratory depression, acute/severe bronchial asthma, paralytic ileus, GI obstruction. **Transdermal patch (additional):** Significant respiratory depression, acute/severe bronchial asthma, paralytic ileus, short-term therapy for acute or postoperative pain, pts who are not opioid tolerant. **Transmucosal buccal, buccal films, lozenges, sublingual tablets/spray, nasal spray (additional):** Management of acute or postoperative pain, pts who are not opioid tolerant. **Cautions:** Bradycardia; renal, hepatic, respiratory disease; head injuries; altered LOC; biliary tract disease; acute pancreatitis; cor pulmonale; significant COPD; increased ICP; use of MAOIs within 14 days; elderly; morbid obesity.

ACTION

Binds to opioid receptors in CNS, reducing stimuli from sensory nerve endings; inhibits ascending pain pathways. **Therapeutic Effect:** Alters pain reception, increases pain threshold.

PHARMACOKINETICS

Route	Onset	Peak	Duration
IV	1–2 min	3–5 min	0.5–1 hr
IM	7–15 min	20–30 min	1–2 hrs
Transdermal	6–8 hrs	24 hrs	72 hrs
Transmucosal	5–15 min	20–30 min	1–2 hrs

Well absorbed after IM or topical administration. Transmucosal form absorbed through buccal mucosa and GI tract. Protein binding: 80%–85%. Metabolized in liver. Primarily excreted by biliary system.

Half-life: 2–4 hrs IV; 17 hrs transdermal; 6.6 hrs transmucosal.

⌛ LIFESPAN CONSIDERATIONS

Pregnancy/Lactation: Readily crosses placenta. Unknown if distributed in breast milk. May prolong labor if administered in latent phase of first stage of labor or before cervical dilation of 4–5 cm has occurred. Respiratory depression may occur in neonate if mother received opiates during labor. **Children:** Neonates more susceptible to respiratory depressant effects. Patch: Safety and efficacy not established in pts younger than 12 yrs. **Elderly:** May be more susceptible to respiratory depressant effects. Age-related renal impairment may require dosage adjustment.

INTERACTIONS

DRUG: CYP3A4 inducers (e.g., ri- **fAMPin,** modafinil) may decrease concentration, effects. **Alcohol, CNS depressant** (e.g., **LORazepam, gabapentin, zolpidem**) may increase CNS depression. **CYP3A4 inhibitors (e.g., erythromycin, ketoconazole, protease inhibitors [e.g., ritonavir])** may increase effects and potential for respiratory depression. **HERBAL: Gotu kola, kava kava, St. John's wort,** valerian may increase CNS depression. **St. John's wort** may decrease concentration, effects. **FOOD: Grapefruit products** may increase potential for respiratory depression with oral, transmucosal forms. **LAB VALUES:** May increase serum amylase, lipase.

AVAILABILITY (Rx)

Buccal Tablet (Fentora): 100 mcg, 200 mcg, 400 mcg, 600 mcg, 800 mcg. **Buccal Soluble Film (Onsolis):** 200 mcg, 400 mcg, 600 mcg, 800 mcg, 1,200 mcg. **Injection Solution:** 50 mcg/mL. **Nasal Spray (Lazanda):** 100 mcg/spray, 400 mcg/spray. **Sublingual Tablets (Abstral):** 100 mcg, 200 mcg, 300 mcg, 400 mcg, 600 mcg, 800 mcg. **Sublingual Spray (Subsys):** 100 mcg, 200 mcg, 400 mcg, 600 mcg, 800 mcg. **Transdermal Patch (Duragesic):** 12 mcg/hr, 25 mcg/hr, 50 mcg/hr,

75 mcg/hr, 100 mcg/hr. **Transmucosal Lozenges (Actiq):** 200 mcg, 400 mcg, 600 mcg, 800 mcg, 1,200 mcg, 1,600 mcg.

ADMINISTRATION/HANDLING

 IV

Rate of Administration • Give by slow IV injection (over 1–2 min). • Too-rapid injection increases risk of severe adverse reactions (skeletal/thoracic muscle rigidity resulting in apnea, laryngospasm, bronchospasm, peripheral circulatory collapse, anaphylactoid effects, cardiac arrest).
Storage • Store parenteral form at room temperature. • Opiate antagonist (naloxone) should be readily available.

Transdermal
• Apply to hairless area of intact skin of upper torso. • Use flat, nonirritated site. • Firmly press evenly and hold for 30 sec, ensuring that adhesion is in full contact with skin and that edges are completely sealed. • Use only water to cleanse site before application (soaps, oils may irritate skin). • Rotate sites of application. • Carefully fold used patches so that system adheres to itself; discard in toilet. • If patch becomes loose, cover with a transparent adhesive dressing; if patch comes off, apply new patch, rotating sites (this starts a new dosing interval). Normal exposure to water may loosen the adhesive.

Buccal Film
• Wet inside of cheek. • Place film inside mouth with pink side of unit against cheek. • Press film against cheek and hold for 5 sec. • Leave in place until dissolved (15–30 min). • Do not chew, swallow, cut film. • Liquids may be given after 5 min of application; food after film dissolves.

Buccal Tablets
• Place tablet above a rear molar between upper cheek and gum. • Dissolve over 30 min. • Swallow remaining pieces with water. • Do not split tablet.

Sublingual Spray
• Open blister pack with scissors immediately prior to use. • Spray contents underneath tongue.

Sublingual Tablets
• Place under tongue. • Dissolves rapidly. • Do not suck, chew, or swallow tablet.

Nasal
• Prime device before use by spraying into pouch. • Insert nozzle about ½ inch into nose, pointing toward bridge of nose, tilting bottle slightly. • Press down firmly until hearing a "click" and number on counting window advances by one. Do not blow nose for at least 30 min following administration.

Transmucosal
• Suck lozenge vigorously. • Allow to dissolve over 15 min. • Do not chew.

IV INCOMPATIBILITIES

Azithromycin (Zithromax), pantoprazole (Protonix), phenytoin (Dilantin).

IV COMPATIBILITIES

Atropine, bupivacaine (Marcaine, Sensorcaine), cloNIDine (Duraclon), dexmedetomidine (Precedex), diltiaZEM (Cardizem), diphenhydrAMINE (Benadryl), DOBUTamine (Dobutrex), DOPamine (Intropin), droperidol (Inapsine), heparin, HYDROmorphone (Dilaudid), ketorolac (Toradol), LORazepam (Ativan), metoclopramide (Reglan), midazolam (Versed), milrinone (Primacor), morphine, nitroglycerin, norepinephrine (Levophed), ondansetron (Zofran), potassium chloride, propofol (Diprivan).

INDICATIONS/ROUTES/DOSAGE

Note: Doses titrated to desired effect dependent upon degree of analgesia, pt status.

Acute Pain Management (FentaNYL)
IM/IV: ADULTS, ELDERLY: 25–100 mcg/dose q0.5–2h as needed. **CHILDREN:** 0.5–2

mcg/kg/dose q1–2h as needed. **INFANTS (IV push):** 1–4 mcg/kg/dose q2–4h.

Continuous IV Infusion (FentaNYL)
ADULTS, ELDERLY: 1–2 mcg/kg/hr. **CHILDREN:** 0.5–3 mcg/kg/hr.

Usual Buccal Dose (Fentora)
ADULTS, ELDERLY: Initially, 100 mcg. Titrate dose, providing adequate analgesia with tolerable side effects.

Usual Buccal Soluble Film Dose (Onsolis)
Note: All pts must initiate with 200 mcg. **ADULTS, ELDERLY:** Initially, 200 mcg up to 1,200 mcg. **Maximum:** No more than 4 doses/day; separate by at least 2 hrs.

Usual Nasal Dose (Lazanda)
Nasal: ADULTS, ELDERLY: Initially, 100 mcg. Titrate from 100 mcg to 200 mcg to 400 mcg to 800 mcg **(maximum).** Wait at least 2 hrs between doses; no more than 4 doses in 24 hrs.

Usual Sublingual Tablet Dose (Abstral)
ADULTS, ELDERLY: Initially, 100 mcg, then titrate to desired dose/effect. Wait at least 2 hrs between doses; no more than 4 doses in 24 hrs.

Usual Sublingual Spray Dose (Subsys)
ADULTS, ELDERLY: Initially, 100 mcg. May repeat in 30 min if pain not relieved. Must wait at least 4 hours before treating another episode of pain.

Usual Transdermal Dose (Duragesic)
ADULTS, ELDERLY, CHILDREN 12 YRS AND OLDER: Initially, 12–25 mcg/hr. May increase after 3 days.

Usual Transmucosal Dose (Actiq)
ADULTS, CHILDREN: 200–1200 mcg for breakthrough pain. Limit to 4 applications/day.

Dosage in Renal/Hepatic Impairment
Injection: No dose adjustment.
Transdermal patch: Mild to moderate impairment: Reduce dose by 50%.

Severe impairment: Not recommended.

SIDE EFFECTS

Frequent: IV: Postop drowsiness, nausea, vomiting. **Transdermal (10%–3%):** Headache, pruritus, nausea, vomiting, diaphoresis, dyspnea, confusion, dizziness, drowsiness, diarrhea, constipation, decreased appetite. **Occasional: IV:** Postop confusion, blurred vision, chills, orthostatic hypotension, constipation, difficulty urinating. **Transdermal (3%–1%):** Chest pain, arrhythmias, erythema, pruritus, syncope, agitation, skin irritations.

ADVERSE EFFECTS/TOXIC REACTIONS

Overdose or too-rapid IV administration may produce severe respiratory depression, skeletal/thoracic muscle rigidity (may lead to apnea, laryngospasm, bronchospasm, cold/clammy skin, cyanosis, coma). Tolerance to analgesic effect may occur with repeated use. **Antidote:** Naloxone (see Appendix J for dosage). Abrupt stoppage of prolonged high-dose, continuous infusions may induce opiate withdrawal.

NURSING CONSIDERATIONS

BASELINE ASSESSMENT

Resuscitative equipment, opiate antagonist (naloxone 0.5 mcg/kg) should be available for initial use. Establish baseline B/P, respirations. Assess type, location, intensity, duration of pain. Determine daily morphine equivalency in cancer pts who are being transitioned to chronic therapy.

INTERVENTION/EVALUATION

Assist with ambulation. Encourage postop pt to turn, cough, deep breathe q2h. Monitor respiratory rate, B/P, heart rate, oxygen saturation. Assess for relief of pain. In pts with prolonged high-dose, continuous infusions (critical care, ventilated pts), consider weaning drip gradually or transition to a fentanyl patch to decrease symptoms of opiate withdrawal.

F

PATIENT/FAMILY TEACHING

• Avoid alcohol; do not take other medications without consulting physician. • Avoid tasks that require alertness, motor skills until response to drug is established. • Teach pt proper transdermal, buccal, lozenge administration. • **Transdermal:** Avoid saunas (increases drug release time). • Use as directed to avoid overdosage; potential for physical dependence with prolonged use. • Report constipation, absence of pain relief. • Taper slowly after long-term use.

ferric gluconate

fer-ick **gloo**-koe-nate
(Ferrlecit)

ferrous fumarate

fer-us **fue**-ma-rate
(Ferrocite, Palafer ✦)

ferrous gluconate

fer-us **gloo**-koe-nate
(Apo-Ferrous Gluconate ✦, Ferate)

ferrous sulfate

fer-us **sul**-fate
(Apo-Ferrous Sulfate ✦, Fer-In-Sol, Fer-Iron, Slow-Fe)

◆CLASSIFICATION

PHARMACOTHERAPEUTIC: Enzymatic mineral. **CLINICAL:** Iron preparation.

USES

Ferrous fumarate, gluconate, sulfate: Prevention, treatment of iron deficiency anemia. **Ferric gluconate:** Treatment of microcytic, hypochromic anemia in combination with erythropoietin in HD pts when iron administration is not feasible or is ineffective.

PRECAUTIONS

Contraindications: Hypersensitivity to iron salts. Hemochromatosis, hemolytic anemias. **Cautions:** Peptic ulcer, regional enteritis, ulcerative colitis, pts receiving frequent blood transfusions.

ACTION

Essential component in formation of Hgb, myoglobin, enzymes. Promotes effective erythropoiesis and transport, utilization of oxygen. **Therapeutic Effect:** Prevents iron deficiency.

PHARMACOKINETICS

Absorbed in duodenum and upper jejunum. Ten percent absorbed in pts with normal iron stores; increased to 20%–30% in pts with inadequate iron stores. Primarily bound to serum transferrin. Excreted in urine, sweat, sloughing of intestinal mucosa, menses. **Half-life:** 6 hrs.

⧗ LIFESPAN CONSIDERATIONS

Pregnancy/Lactation: Crosses placenta; distributed in breast milk. **Children/Elderly:** No age-related precautions noted.

INTERACTIONS

DRUG: Antacids, calcium supplements, pancreatin, pancrelipase may decrease absorption of ferrous compounds. May decrease absorption of **etidronate, quinolones, tetracyclines. HERBAL:** None significant. **FOOD: Cereal, coffee, dietary fiber, eggs, milk, tea** decrease absorption. **LAB VALUES:** May increase serum bilirubin, iron. May decrease serum calcium.

AVAILABILITY (OTC)

Ferric Gluconate
Injection, solution: 12.5 mg/mL.

Ferrous Fumarate
Tablets: 90 mg (29.5 mg elemental iron), 324 mg (106 mg elemental iron).

Ferrous Gluconate
Tablets: 240 mg (27 mg elemental iron) (Fergon), 325 mg (36 mg elemental iron).

✦ Canadian trade name   🐾 Non-Crushable Drug   ▨ High Alert drug

Ferrous Sulfate
Oral Solution: 75 mg/mL (15 mg/mL elemental iron). **Tablets:** 325 mg (65 mg elemental iron). **Syrup:** 300 mg/5 mL (60 mg elemental iron per 5 mL).

⬥ **Tablets (Timed-Release):** 160 mg (50 mg elemental iron).

ADMINISTRATION/HANDLING

PO
• Store all forms (tablets, capsules, suspension, drops) at room temperature. • Ideally, give between meals with water or juice but may give with meals if GI discomfort occurs. • Transient staining of mucous membranes, teeth occurs with liquid iron preparation. To avoid staining, place liquid on back of tongue via dropper or straw. • Do not give with milk or milk products. • Do not break, crush, dissolve, or divide timed-release tablets.

INDICATIONS/ROUTES/DOSAGE

Iron Deficiency Anemia
Dosage is expressed in terms of milligrams of elemental iron. Assess degree of anemia, pt weight, presence of any bleeding. Expect to use periodic hematologic determinations as guide to therapy.
IV *(Ferric Gluconate):* ADULTS, ELDERLY: 125 mg/dose. Usual dose: 1,000 mg given over 8 sessions.
PO *(Ferrous Fumarate):* ADULTS, ELDERLY: 100–200 mg/day in 2–3 divided doses. **CHILDREN:** 3–6 mg/kg/day in 2–3 divided doses.
PO *(Ferrous Gluconate):* ADULTS, ELDERLY: 100–200 mg/day in 2–3 divided doses. **CHILDREN:** 3–6 mg/kg/day in 2–3 divided doses.
PO *(Ferrous Sulfate):* ADULTS, ELDERLY: 100–200 mg/day in 2–3 divided doses. **CHILDREN:** 3–6 mg/kg/day in 2–3 divided doses.

Prevention of Iron Deficiency
PO *(Ferrous Fumarate):* ADULTS, ELDERLY: 60 mg/day. **CHILDREN:** 30 mg/day with folic acid.

PO *(Ferrous Gluconate):* ADULTS, ELDERLY: 60 mg/day. **CHILDREN:** 30 mg/day with folic acid.
PO *(Ferrous Sulfate):* ADULTS, ELDERLY: 60 mg/day. **CHILDREN:** 30 mg/day with folic acid.

SIDE EFFECTS

⬥ **Occasional:** Mild, transient nausea. **Rare:** Heartburn, anorexia, constipation, diarrhea.

ADVERSE EFFECTS/TOXIC REACTIONS

Large doses may aggravate existing GI tract disease (peptic ulcer, regional enteritis, ulcerative colitis). Severe iron poisoning occurs most often in children, manifested as vomiting, severe abdominal pain, diarrhea, dehydration, followed by hyperventilation, pallor, cyanosis, cardiovascular collapse.

NURSING CONSIDERATIONS

BASELINE ASSESSMENT
Assess nutritional status, dietary history. Question history of hemochromatosis, hemolytic anemia, ulcerative colitis. Question use of antacids, calcium supplements.

INTERVENTION/EVALUATION
Monitor serum iron, total iron-binding capacity, reticulocyte count, Hgb, ferritin. Monitor daily pattern of bowel activity, stool consistency. Assess for clinical improvement, record relief of iron deficiency symptoms (fatigue, irritability, pallor, paresthesia of extremities, headache).

PATIENT/FAMILY TEACHING
• Expect stool color to darken. • Oral liquid may stain teeth. • To prevent mucous membrane and teeth staining with liquid preparation, use dropper or straw and allow solution to drop on back of tongue. • If GI discomfort occurs, take after meals or with food. • Do not take within 2 hrs of other medication or eggs, milk, tea, coffee, cereal. • Do not take antacids or OTC calcium supplements.

fesoterodine

fes-oh-**ter**-oh-deen
(Toviaz)
Do not confuse fesoterodine with fexofenadine or tolterodine.

◆CLASSIFICATION

PHARMACOTHERAPEUTIC: Muscarinic receptor antagonist. **CLINICAL:** Antispasmodic.

USES

Treatment of overactive bladder with symptoms including urinary incontinence, urgency, frequency.

PRECAUTIONS

Contraindications: Hypersensitivity to fesoterodine. Gastric retention, uncontrolled narrow-angle glaucoma, urinary retention. **Cautions:** Severe renal impairment, severe hepatic impairment, clinically significant bladder outflow obstruction (risk of urinary retention), GI obstructive disorders (e.g., pyloric stenosis [risk of gastric retention], treated narrow-angle glaucoma, myasthenia gravis, concurrent therapy with strong CYP3A4 inhibitors, elderly, use in hot weather.

ACTION

Exhibits antimuscarinic activity by interceding via cholinergic muscarinic receptors, thereby mediating urinary bladder contraction. **Therapeutic Effect:** Decreases urinary frequency, urgency.

PHARMACOKINETICS

Well absorbed following PO administration. Protein binding: 50%. Rapidly and extensively hydrolyzed to its active metabolite. Primarily excreted in urine. **Half-life:** 7 hours.

⧗ LIFESPAN CONSIDERATIONS

Pregnancy/Lactation: Unknown if distributed in breast milk. **Children:** Safety and efficacy not established.

Elderly: Increased incidence of antimuscarinic adverse events, including dry mouth, constipation, dyspepsia; increase in residual urine, dizziness, urinary tract infections higher in pts 75 yrs of age and older.

INTERACTIONS

DRUG: CYP3A4 inhibitors (e.g., clarithromycin, erythromycin, ketoconazole) may increase concentration. **HERBAL:** None significant. **FOOD: Grapefruit products** may increase potential for urinary retention, constipation. **LAB VALUES:** May increase serum ALT, GGT.

AVAILABILITY (Rx)

🖋 **Tablets, Extended-Release:** 4 mg, 8 mg.

ADMINISTRATION/HANDLING

PO
• May be administered with or without food. • Swallow whole; do not break, crush, dissolve, or divide tablet.

INDICATIONS/ROUTES/DOSAGE

Overactive Bladder
PO: ADULTS, ELDERLY: Initially, 4 mg once daily. May increase to 8 mg once daily. Maximum dose for pts with concurrent use of strong CYP3A4 inhibitors (e.g., erythromycin, ketoconazole) is 4 mg once daily.

Dosage in Renal Impairment
PO: ADULTS, ELDERLY: Maximum dose: 4 mg with CrCl less than 30 mL/min.

Dosage in Hepatic Impairment
Mild to moderate impairment: No dose adjustment. **Severe impairment:** Not recommended.

SIDE EFFECTS

Frequent (34%–18%): Dry mouth. **Occasional (6%–3%):** Constipation, urinary tract infection, dry eyes. **Rare (2% or less):** Nausea, dysuria, back pain, rash, insomnia, peripheral edema.

F

◆ Canadian trade name   🖋 Non-Crushable Drug   🄷🄸 High Alert drug

ADVERSE EFFECTS/TOXIC REACTIONS

Severe anticholinergic effects including abdominal cramps, facial warmth, excessive salivation/lacrimation, diaphoresis, pallor, urinary urgency, blurred vision.

NURSING CONSIDERATIONS

BASELINE ASSESSMENT

Assess urinary pattern (e.g., urinary frequency, urgency). Obtain baseline chemistries. Question history as listed in Precautions. Receive full medication history.

INTERVENTION/EVALUATION

Assist with ambulation if dizziness occurs. Question for visual changes. Monitor incontinence, postvoid residuals. Monitor daily pattern of bowel activity, stool consistency.

PATIENT/FAMILY TEACHING

• May produce constipation and urinary retention. • Blurred vision may occur; use caution until drug effects have been determined. • Heat prostration (due to decreased sweating) can occur if used in a hot environment. • Do not ingest grapefruit products.

---

fexofenadine

fex-oh-**fen**-a-deen
(Allegra, Allegra Allergy, Allegra Children's)
Do not confuse Allegra with Viagra, or fexofenadine with fesoterodine.

FIXED-COMBINATION(S)

Allegra-D 12 Hour: fexofenadine/pseudoephedrine (sympathomimetic): 60 mg/120 mg. **Allegra-D 24 Hour:** fexofenadine/pseudoephedrine (sympathomimetic): 180 mg/240 mg.

◆CLASSIFICATION

PHARMACOTHERAPEUTIC: Histamine H_1 antagonist. **CLINICAL:** Antihistamine.

USES

Relief of symptoms associated with hayfever or other upper respiratory allergies.

PRECAUTIONS

Contraindications: Hypersensitivity to fexofenadine. **Cautions:** Renal impairment, hypertension (if drug combined with pseudoephedrine). Orally disintegrating tablet not recommended in children younger than 6 yrs.

ACTION

Competes with histamine-1 receptor site on effector cells in GI tract, blood vessels, and respiratory tract. **Therapeutic Effect:** Relieves hayfever/upper respiratory symptoms.

PHARMACOKINETICS

	Onset	Peak	Duration
PO	60 min	—	12 hrs or greater

Rapidly absorbed after PO administration. Protein binding: 60%–70%. Does not cross blood-brain barrier. Minimally metabolized. Excreted in feces (80%), urine (11%). Not removed by hemodialysis. **Half-life:** 14.4 hrs (increased in renal impairment).

⧖ LIFESPAN CONSIDERATIONS

Pregnancy/Lactation: Unknown if drug crosses placenta or is distributed in breast milk. **Children:** Safety and efficacy not established in pts younger than 12 yrs. **Elderly:** No age-related precautions noted.

INTERACTIONS

DRUG: Aluminum- and **magnesium-containing antacids** may decrease absorption if given within 15 min of fexofenadine. May increase concentrations of **erythromycin, ketoconazole. HERBAL: St. John's wort** may decrease concentration. **FOOD: Fruit juices** may decrease bioavailability. **LAB VALUES:** May suppress wheal, flare reactions to antigen skin testing unless drug is discontinued at least 4 days before testing.

AVAILABILITY (Rx)

Oral Suspension: 30 mg/5 mL. **Tablets:** 60 mg, 180 mg. **Tablets (Orally Disintegrating):** 30 mg.

ADMINISTRATION/HANDLING

PO

• Give without regard to food. • Avoid giving with fruit juices (apple, grapefruit, orange). Administer with water only. • Shake suspension well before use.

PO (Orally Disintegrating Tablet)

• Take on empty stomach. • Remove from blister pack; immediately place on tongue. • May take with or without liquid. • Do not split or cut.

INDICATIONS/ROUTES/DOSAGE

Hayfever, Upper Respiratory Symptoms
PO: ADULTS, ELDERLY, CHILDREN 12 YRS AND OLDER: 60 mg twice daily or 180 mg once daily. **CHILDREN 2–11 YRS:** 30 mg twice daily.

Dosage in Renal Impairment
PO: ADULTS, ELDERLY, CHILDREN 12 YRS AND OLDER: 60 mg once daily. **CHILDREN 2–11 YRS:** 30 mg once daily. **CHILDREN 6 MOS–LESS THAN 2 YRS:** 15 mg once daily.

CrCl	Adults	Children
>50 mL/min	No adjustment	No adjustment
10–50 mL/min	60 mg q24h	60 mg q24h
<10 mL/min	30 mg q24h	30 mg q24h

Dosage in Hepatic Impairment
No dose adjustment.

SIDE EFFECTS

Rare (less than 2%): Drowsiness, headache, fatigue, nausea, vomiting, abdominal distress, dysmenorrhea.

ADVERSE EFFECTS/TOXIC REACTIONS

Hypersensitivity reaction occurs rarely.

NURSING CONSIDERATIONS

BASELINE ASSESSMENT

Assess severity of congestion, rhinitis, urticaria, watery eyes. If pt is having an allergic reaction, obtain history of recently ingested foods, drugs, environmental exposure, emotional stress. Monitor rate, depth, rhythm, type of respiration; quality, rate of pulse. Assess lung sounds for rhonchi, wheezing, rales.

INTERVENTION/EVALUATION

Assess for therapeutic response; relief from allergy: itching, red, watery eyes, rhinorrhea, sneezing.

PATIENT/FAMILY TEACHING

• Avoid tasks that require alertness, motor skills until response to drug is established. • Avoid alcohol during antihistamine therapy. • Coffee, tea may help reduce drowsiness. • Do not take with any fruit juices.

fidaxomicin

fye-**dax**-oh-**mye**-sin
(Dificid)

◆CLASSIFICATION

PHARMACOTHERAPEUTIC: Macrolide. **CLINICAL:** Antibiotic.

USES

Treatment of *C. difficile*–associated diarrhea.

PRECAUTIONS

Contraindications: Hypersensitivity to fidaxomicin. **Cautions:** History of anemia, neutropenia, macrolide allergy.

ACTION

Binds to ribosomal sites of susceptible organisms, inhibiting RNA-dependent protein synthesis by RNA polymerase. **Therapeutic Effect:** Bactericidal against *C. difficile*.

PHARMACOKINETICS

Minimal systemic absorption following PO administration. Mainly confined to GI tract. Excreted primarily in feces (92%). **Half-life:** 9 hrs.

⧗ LIFESPAN CONSIDERATIONS

Pregnancy/Lactation: Unknown if distributed in breast milk. **Children:** Safety and efficacy not established. **Elderly:** No age-related precautions noted.

INTERACTIONS

DRUG: CycloSPORINE may increase serum concentration, effects. **HERBAL:** None known. **FOOD:** None significant. **LAB VALUES:** May increase serum ALT, AST, bilirubin, alkaline phosphatase.

AVAILABILITY (Rx)

Tablets: 200 mg.

ADMINISTRATION/HANDLING

• Give without regard to food.

INDICATIONS/ROUTES/DOSAGE

Clostridium Difficile–Associated Diarrhea
PO: ADULTS: 200 mg twice daily for 10 days.

Dosage in Renal/Hepatic Impairment
No dose adjustment.

SIDE EFFECTS

Frequent (62%–33%): Nausea, vomiting, abdominal pain. **Rare (less than 2%):** Pruritus, rash.

ADVERSE EFFECTS/TOXIC REACTIONS

Less than 2% reported events most likely related to diarrhea-associated illness including volume loss, dehydration, GI bleeding, bloating, megacolon, abdominal distention/tenderness, flatulence, dyspepsia, dysphagia, intestinal obstruction, bicarbonate loss, hyperglycemia, metabolic acidosis, and increased hepatic function tests. GI tract infection may cause bleeding, decreased platelets, decreased RBC count.

NURSING CONSIDERATIONS

BASELINE ASSESSMENT

Verify positive *C. difficile* toxin test before initiating treatment. Implement infection control measures. Obtain baseline CBC, electrolytes, renal function, fecal occult blood test. Assess abdominal pain, bowel sounds, and stool characteristics (color, frequency, consistency). Assess hydration status.

INTERVENTION/EVALUATION

Monitor for volume loss, dehydration, hypotension, abdominal pain, pyrexia. Encourage nutrition/fluid intake. Monitor daily pattern of bowel activity, stool consistency. Routinely assess bowel sounds. Screen for intestinal obstruction (increased nausea, abdominal pain, hyperactive bowel sounds) and consider abdominal X-ray if suspected.

PATIENT/FAMILY TEACHING

• Complete drug therapy, despite symptom improvement. Early discontinuation may result in antibacterial resistance and increased risk of recurrent infection. • Report weakness, fatigue, pale skin, dizziness, or red/dark, tarry stools relating to GI bleeding. • *C. difficile* infection is extremely contagious to others. Wash hands frequently with soap and water, esp. after bowel movements. *C. difficile* spores can live on objects for months. Use bleach products to cleanse bathroom, doorknobs, other high-touch surfaces. If possible, use a separate bathroom away from others. • Drink plenty of fluids.

filgrastim ^{TOP 100}

fil-**gras**-tim
(Granix, <u>Neupogen</u>, Zarxio)
**Do not confuse Neupogen with
Epogen, Neulasta, Neumega, or
Nutramigen.**

◆CLASSIFICATION

PHARMACOTHERAPEUTIC: Biologic
modifier. **CLINICAL:** Granulocyte
colony-stimulating factor (G-CSF).

USES

Granix: Decreases duration of severe
neutropenia in pts with malignancies
receiving chemotherapy associated with
severe neutropenia, fever. **Neupogen,
Zarxio:** Reduces neutropenia duration,
sequelae in pts with nonmyeloid malignancies having myeloablative therapy followed by bone marrow transplant (BMT).
Mobilization of hematopoietic progenitor
cells into peripheral blood for collection by apheresis. Treatment of chronic,
severe neutropenia. Decreases incidence
of infection in pts with malignancies receiving chemotherapy associated with
increased incidence of severe neutropenia with fever. Reduces time to neutrophil
recovery/duration of fever after induction/consolidation chemotherapy in AML
pts. **Neupogen:** Increases survival in
pts acutely exposed to myelosuppressive
doses of radiation. **OFF-LABEL:** Treatment of AIDS-related neutropenia in
pts receiving zidovudine; drug-induced
neutropenia; anemia in myelodysplastic syndrome; hepatitis C virus infection
treatment-associated neutropenia.

PRECAUTIONS

Contraindications: Hypersensitivity to
filgrastim. **Neupogen, Zarxio (additional):**
History of serious allergic reaction to
human granulocyte colony-stimulating
factors. **Cautions:** Malignancy with myeloid characteristics (due to G-CSF's
potential to act as growth factor), gout,

psoriasis, neutrophil count greater than
50,000 cells/mm³, sickle cell disease,
concomitant use of other drugs that may
result in thrombocytopenia. Do not use
24 hrs before or after cytotoxic chemotherapy.

ACTION

Stimulates production, maturation, activation of neutrophils. **Therapeutic Effect:** Increases migration and cytotoxicity of neutrophils.

PHARMACOKINETICS

Readily absorbed. Onset of action: 24
hrs (plateaus in 3–5 days). WBC return
to normal in 4–7 days. Not removed by
hemodialysis. **Half-life:** 3.5 hrs.

⌛ LIFESPAN CONSIDERATIONS

Pregnancy/Lactation: Unknown if
drug crosses placenta or is distributed in
breast milk. **Children/Elderly:** No age-related precautions noted.

INTERACTIONS

DRUG: None significant. **HERBAL:** None
significant. **FOOD:** None known. **LAB
VALUES:** May increase LDH, leukocyte
alkaline phosphatase (LAP) scores, serum alkaline phosphatase, uric acid.

AVAILABILITY (Rx)

Injection Solution: (Neupogen): 300 mcg/
mL, 480 mcg/1.6 mL **Injection, Prefilled
Syringe: (Granix, Neupogen, Zarxio):** 300
mcg/0.5 mL, 480 mcg/0.8 mL.

ADMINISTRATION/HANDLING

◀**ALERT**▶ May be given by subcutaneous injection, short IV infusion (15–30
min), or continuous IV infusion. Do not
dilute with normal saline.

 **IV**

Reconstitution • Allow vial to warm
to room temperature (approx. 30
mins). • Visually inspect for particulate
matter or discoloration. • Dilute in
D₅W from concentration of 300 mcg/mL
to 5 mcg/mL (do not dilute to a final

F

concentration less than 5 mcg/mL). Diluted solutions of 5–15 mcg/mL should have addition of albumin to a final concentration of 2 mg/mL. • Do not dilute with saline.

Rate of Administration • For intermittent infusion (piggyback), infuse over 15–30 min. • For continuous infusion, give single dose over 4–24 hrs. • In all situations, flush IV line with D5W before and after administration.

Storage • Refrigerate vials and syringes. • Stable for up to 24 hrs at room temperature (provided vial contents are clear and contain no particulate matter).

Subcutaneous

• Aspirate syringe before injection (avoid intra-arterial administration).

Storage • Store in refrigerator, but remove before use and allow to warm to room temperature.

▦ IV INCOMPATIBILITIES

Amphotericin (Fungizone), cefepime (Maxipime), cefotaxime (Claforan), cefOXitin (Mefoxin), ceftizoxime (Cefizox), cefTRIAXone (Rocephin), clindamycin (Cleocin), DACTINomycin (Cosmegen), etoposide (VePesid), fluorouracil, furosemide (Lasix), heparin, mannitol, methylPREDNISolone (Solu-Medrol), mitoMYcin (Mutamycin), prochlorperazine (Compazine).

▦ IV COMPATIBILITIES

Bumetanide (Bumex), calcium gluconate, HYDROmorphone (Dilaudid), LORazepam (Ativan), morphine, potassium chloride.

INDICATIONS/ROUTES/DOSAGE

◀ALERT▶ Begin therapy at least 24 hrs after last dose of chemotherapy and at least 24 hrs after bone marrow infusion. Dosing based on actual body weight.

Chemotherapy-Induced Neutropenia
Neupogen, Zarxio
IV or SQ Infusion, SQ Injection:
ADULTS, ELDERLY, CHILDREN: Initially,

5 mcg/kg/day. May increase by 5 mcg/kg for each chemotherapy cycle based on duration/severity of neutropenia; continue for up to 14 days or until absolute neutrophil count (ANC) reaches 10,000 cells/mm^3.

Granix
SQ: ADULTS, ELDERLY: 5 mcg/kg/day. Continue until nadir has passed and neutrophil count recovered to normal range.

Bone Marrow Transplant
IV or SQ Infusion: *(Neupogen, Zarxio)*
ADULTS, ELDERLY, CHILDREN: 10 mcg/kg/day. Administer >24 hrs after chemotherapy or bone marrow transfusion. Adjust dosage daily during period of neutrophil recovery based on neutrophil response.

Mobilization of Progenitor Cells
IV or SQ Infusion: *(Neupogen, Zarxio)*
ADULTS: 10 mcg/kg/day in donors beginning at least 4 days before first leukapheresis and continuing until last leukapheresis (usually for 6–7 days). Discontinue for WBC greater than 100,000 cells/mm^3.

Chronic Neutropenia,
Congenital Neutropenia
SQ: *(Neupogen, Zarxio)* **ADULTS, CHILDREN:** Initially, 6 mcg/kg/dose twice daily. Adjust dose based on ANC/clinical response.

Idiopathic or Cyclic Neutropenia
SQ: *(Neupogen, Zarxio)* **ADULTS, CHILDREN:** Initially, 5 mcg/kg/dose once daily. Adjust dose based on ANC/clinical response.

Radiation Injury Syndrome
SQ: ADULTS, ELDERLY: 10 mcg/kg once daily. Continue until ANC remains greater than 1,000 cells/mm^3 for 3 consecutive CBCs or ANC exceeds 10,000 cells/mm^3 after radiation-induced nadir.

Dosage in Renal/Hepatic Impairment
No dose adjustment.

SIDE EFFECTS

Frequent (57%–11%): Nausea/vomiting, mild to severe bone pain (more frequent with high-dose IV form, less frequent with low-dose subcutaneous form), alopecia, diarrhea, fever, fatigue. **Occasional (9%–5%):** Anorexia, dyspnea, headache, cough, rash. **Rare (less than 5%):** Psoriasis, hematuria, proteinuria, osteoporosis.

ADVERSE EFFECTS/TOXIC REACTIONS

Long-term administration occasionally produces chronic neutropenia, splenomegaly. Acute respiratory distress syndrome, alveolar hemorrhage and hemoptysis (pts undergoing peripheral blood progenitor cell collection mobilization), capillary leak syndrome, cutaneous vasculitis, glomerulonephritis, leukocytosis, MI, thrombocytopenia, sickle cell crisis, splenic rupture may occur.

NURSING CONSIDERATIONS

BASELINE ASSESSMENT

CBC, platelet count should be obtained before therapy initiation and twice wkly thereafter.

INTERVENTION/EVALUATION

In septic pts, be alert for adult respiratory distress syndrome. Closely monitor those with preexisting cardiac conditions. Monitor B/P (transient decrease in B/P may occur), temperature, CBC with differential, platelet count, serum uric acid, hepatic function tests.

PATIENT/FAMILY TEACHING

• Report fever, chills, severe bone pain, chest pain, palpitations, difficulty breathing; left upper abdominal pain/tightness; flank pain.

finasteride

fin-**as**-ter-ide
(Apo-Finasteride ✦, Propecia, Proscar)
Do not confuse finasteride with furosemide, or Proscar with ProSom, Provera, or PROzac.

◆CLASSIFICATION

PHARMACOTHERAPEUTIC: Androgen hormone inhibitor. **CLINICAL:** Benign prostatic hyperplasia agent.

USES

Proscar: Reduces risk of acute urinary retention, need for surgery in symptomatic benign prostatic hyperplasia (BPH) alone or in combination with doxazosin (Cardura). **Propecia:** Treatment of male pattern hair loss. **OFF-LABEL:** Treatment of female hirsutism.

PRECAUTIONS

Contraindications: Hypersensitivity to finasteride, pregnancy or women of childbearing potential. **Cautions:** Hepatic impairment, urinary outflow obstruction, urinary retention. Women who are attempting to conceive should avoid exposure to crushed or broken tablets.

ACTION

Inhibits 5-alpha reductase, an intracellular enzyme that converts testosterone into dihydrotestosterone (DHT) in prostate gland, resulting in decreased serum DHT. **Therapeutic Effect:** Reduces size of prostate gland.

PHARMACOKINETICS

Route	Onset	Peak	Duration
PO (reduction of DHT)	8 hrs	—	24 hrs

Rapidly absorbed from GI tract. Protein binding: 90%. Widely distributed. Metabolized in liver. **Half-life:** 6–8 hrs. Onset of clinical effect: 3–6 mos of continued therapy.

⧗ LIFESPAN CONSIDERATIONS

Pregnancy/Lactation: Physical handling of tablet by those who are or may become pregnant may produce abnormalities of external genitalia of male fetus. **Children:** Not indicated for use in children. **Elderly:** No age-related precautions noted.

INTERACTIONS

DRUG: None significant. **HERBAL: St. John's wort** may decrease concentration. Avoid concurrent use with **saw palmetto** (not adequately studied). **FOOD:** None known. **LAB VALUES:** Decreases serum prostate-specific antigen (PSA) level, even in presence of prostate cancer. Decreases dihydrotestosterone (DHT). Increases follicle-stimulating hormone (FSH), luteinizing hormone (LH), testosterone.

AVAILABILITY (Rx)

🖋 **Tablets:** 1 mg (Propecia), 5 mg (Proscar).

ADMINISTRATION/HANDLING

PO

• Do not break, crush, dissolve, or divide film-coated tablets. • Give without regard to meals.

INDICATIONS/ROUTES/DOSAGE

Benign Prostatic Hyperplasia (BPH)
PO: ADULTS, ELDERLY: *(Proscar):* 5 mg once daily (as single agent or in combination with doxazosin). 6 months of treatment usually needed to assess benefit.

Hair Loss
PO: ADULTS: *(Propecia):* 1 mg/day.

Dosage in Renal Impairment
No dose adjustment.

Dosage in Hepatic Impairment
Use caution.

SIDE EFFECTS

Rare (4%–2%): Gynecomastia, sexual dysfunction (impotence, decreased libido, decreased volume of ejaculate).

ADVERSE EFFECTS/TOXIC REACTIONS

Hypersensitivity reaction, circumoral swelling, testicular pain occur rarely.

NURSING CONSIDERATIONS

BASELINE ASSESSMENT

Digital rectal exam, serum prostate-specific antigen (PSA) determination should be performed in pts with benign prostatic hyperplasia (BPH) before initiating therapy and periodically thereafter. Assess usual urinary characteristics (frequency, ability to empty bladder, urinary flow). Assess degree of urinary retention with baseline bladder scan.

INTERVENTION/EVALUATION

Diligently monitor I&O, esp. in pts with large residual urinary volume, severely diminished urinary flow, or obstructive uropathy. Obtain periodic bladder scan to assess treatment effectiveness (or to assess for acute urinary retention).

PATIENT/FAMILY TEACHING

• Treatment may cause impotence, decreased volume of ejaculate. • May not notice improved urinary flow even if prostate gland shrinks. • Must take medication longer than 6 mos, and it is unknown if medication decreases need for surgery. • Because of potential risk to male fetus, women who are or may become pregnant should not handle tablets or be exposed to pt's semen. • Immediately report inability to urinate or severe bladder pain.

fingolimod   TOP 100

fin-**goe**-li-mod
(Gilenya)

◆CLASSIFICATION

PHARMACOTHERAPEUTIC: Immunomodulator. **CLINICAL:** Multiple sclerosis agent.

USES

Treatment of pts with relapsing forms of multiple sclerosis (MS) to reduce frequency of clinical exacerbations, delay accumulation of physical disability.

PRECAUTIONS

Contraindications: Hypersensitivity to fingolimod. Sick sinus syndrome, second-degree or higher conduction block (unless pt has functioning pacemaker). Baseline QT interval 500 msec or greater. Concurrent use of class Ia or III antiarrhythmic. Recent (within 6 mos) MI, unstable angina, stroke, TIA, decompensated requiring hospitalization or NYHA class III/IV HF. **Cautions:** Concomitant use of antiarrhythmics, beta blockers, calcium channel blockers, immunosuppressants, immune modulators, antineoplastics, QT interval–prolonging medications (e.g., amiodarone, ciprofloxacin); bradycardia, severe hepatic impairment, ischemic heart disease, diabetes, hypokalemia, hypomagnesemia; history of syncope, uveitis; pts at risk for developing bradycardia or heart block.

ACTION

Blocks capacity of lymphocytes to move out from lymph nodes, reducing number of lymphocytes available to the CNS. **Therapeutic Effect:** May involve reduction of lymphocyte migration into central nervous system, which reduces central inflammation.

PHARMACOKINETICS

Metabolized by the enzyme sphingosine kinase to active metabolite. Highly distributed in red blood cells (85%). Minimally metabolized in liver. Protein binding: 99.7%. Primarily excreted in urine. **Half-life:** 6–9 days.

⌛ LIFESPAN CONSIDERATIONS

Pregnancy/Lactation: May cause fetal harm. Unknown if distributed in breast milk. **Children:** Safety and efficacy not established in pts younger than 18 yrs.

Elderly: Age-related severe hepatic impairment may increase risk of adverse reactions.

INTERACTIONS

DRUG: Beta blockers (e.g., carvedilol, metoprolol), bretylium, calcium channel blockers (e.g., diltiazem, verapamil), ceritinib, esmolol, lacosamide may increase risk of bradycardia. May increase effects of **antiarrhythmics** (e.g., amiodarone, sotalol). **CarBAMazepine** may decrease concentration/ effect. **Ketoconazole** may increase concentration/effect. May increase effects of **QT interval–prolonging medications** (e.g., amiodarone, azithromycin, ciprofloxacin, haloperidol). May increase toxic effects of **denosumab, leflunomide, natalizumab, tacrolimus.** May decrease effect of **nivolumab, sipuleucel-T, tertomotide.** May increase immunosuppressive effect of **tofacitinib, other immunosuppressants.** May increase neutropenic effect of **trastuzumab.** May decrease therapeutic effect of **vaccines,** increase toxic effects of **live vaccines. HERBALS:** Echinacea may decrease concentration. **FOOD:** None known. **LAB VALUES:** Expect decrease in neutrophil count. May increase serum alkaline phosphatase, ALT, AST, bilirubin, triglycerides. May reduce diagnostic effect of *Coccidioides immitis* skin test.

AVAILABILITY (Rx)

Capsules: 0.5 mg.

ADMINISTRATION/HANDLING

PO
• May give without regard to food.

INDICATIONS/ROUTES/DOSAGE

Multiple Sclerosis
PO: ADULTS 18 YRS AND OLDER, ELDERLY: 0.5 mg once daily.

Dosage in Renal/Hepatic Impairment
Mild to moderate impairment: No dose adjustment. **Severe impairment:** Use caution.

SIDE EFFECTS

Frequent (25%–10%): Headache, diarrhea, back pain, cough. **Occasional (8%–5%):** Dyspnea, clinical depression, dizziness, hypertension, migraine, paresthesia, decreased weight. **Rare (4%–2%):** Blurred vision, alopecia, eye pain, asthenia, eczema, pruritus.

ADVERSE EFFECTS/TOXIC REACTIONS

May increase risk of infections (influenza, herpes viral infection, bronchitis, sinusitis, gastroenteritis, ear infection) in 13%–4% of pts. Pts with diabetes or history of uveitis are at increased risk for developing macular edema. Cases of skin cancer, lymphoma, basal cell carcinoma have been reported. Progressive multifocal leukoencephalopathy (PML) (weakness, paralysis, vision loss, aphasia, cognition impairment) may occur. Neurotoxicity, posterior reversible encephalopathy may evolve into cerebral hemorrhage, CVA. May increase risk of hypertension.

NURSING CONSIDERATIONS

BASELINE ASSESSMENT

Obtain baseline CBC, serum chemistries prior to initial treatment. At initial treatment (within first 4–6 hrs after dose), medication reduces heart rate, AV conduction, followed by progressive increase after first day of treatment. Obtain baseline vitals, with particular attention to pulse rate. Perform ophthalmologic evaluation prior to treatment and 3–4 mos after initiation of treatment. Question medical history as listed in Precautions. Obtain full medication history and screen for interactions.

INTERVENTION/EVALUATION

Monitor for bradycardia for 6 hrs after first dose, then as appropriate. Periodically monitor CBC, serum chemistries, particularly lymphocyte count (expected to decrease approximately 80% from baseline with continued treatment).

Monitor for signs of systemic or local infection. Diligently monitor for hypersensitivity reaction, neurological changes, symptoms of posterior reversible encephalopathy (altered mental status, seizures, visual disturbances), PML, QT interval prolongation. Assess for new skin lesions, malignancies. Conduct ophthalmologic exams q3–4 mos after initiation, during treatment, and with any changes in vision.

PATIENT/FAMILY TEACHING

• Obtain regular eye examinations during and for 2 mos following treatment. • Use effective methods of contraception during and for 3 mos following treatment. • Immediately report neurological changes such as confusion, severe headache, seizure activity, vision changes, trouble speaking, one-sided weakness, paralysis. • Treatment may increase risk of certain cancers; report new skin lesions, fever, chills, night sweats, generalized weakness, weight loss, or pain or swelling of the lymph nodes. • Report allergic reactions such as itching, rash, swelling of the face or tongue. • Report symptoms of infection, visual changes, yellowing of skin, eyes, dark urine. • Due to high risk for drug interactions, do not take newly prescribed medication unless approved by prescriber who originally started treatment.

fluconazole

flu-**kon**-a-zole
(Apo-Fluconazole ✤, Diflucan, Novo-Fluconazole ✤)
Do not confuse Diflucan with diclofenac, Diprivan, or disulfiram, or fluconazole with itraconazole, ketoconazole, omeprazole, or pantoprazole.

◆**CLASSIFICATION**

PHARMACOTHERAPEUTIC: Synthetic azole. **CLINICAL:** Systemic antifungal.

USES

Antifungal prophylaxis in pts undergoing bone marrow transplant; candidiasis (esophageal, oropharyngeal, urinary tract, vaginal); systemic Candida infections (e.g., candidemia); treatment of cryptococcal meningitis. **OFF-LABEL:** Cryptococcal pneumonia, candidal intertrigo.

PRECAUTIONS

Contraindications: Hypersensitivity to fluconazole. Concomitant administration of QT-prolonging medications (e.g., erythromycin, pimozide). **Cautions:** Hepatic/renal impairment, hypokalemia, hypersensitivity to other triazoles (e.g., itraconazole, terconazole), imidazoles (e.g., butoconazole, ketoconazole). Medications or conditions known to cause arrhythmias.

ACTION

Interferes with cytochrome P-450 activity, an enzyme necessary for ergosterol formation. **Therapeutic Effect:** Directly damages fungal membrane, altering its function. Fungistatic.

PHARMACOKINETICS

Well absorbed from GI tract. Widely distributed, including to CSF. Protein binding: 11%. Partially metabolized in liver. Excreted unchanged primarily in urine. Partially removed by hemodialysis. **Half-life:** 20–30 hrs (increased in renal impairment).

⏳ LIFESPAN CONSIDERATIONS

Pregnancy/Lactation: Secreted in human breast milk. Use caution in breastfeeding females. **Children:** No age-related precautions noted. **Elderly:** Age-related renal impairment may require dosage adjustment.

INTERACTIONS

DRUG: Increases concentration/effect of **calcium channel blockers (e.g., amlodipine, nifedipine, verapamil),** celecoxib, cyclosporine, midazolam, methadone, NSAIDS (e.g., ibuprofen, ketorolac, naproxen), rifabutin, sirolimus, tacrolimus, theophylline, tofacitinib, zidovudine. May increase concentration/effect, risk of myopathy of **HMG-CoA reductase inhibitors (e.g. atorvastatin, simvastatin). HCTZ** may increase concentration/effect. **Cimetidine, rifampin** may decrease concentration/effect. May increase concentration/effect of **oral hypoglycemics (e.g., glipizide, glyburide), phenytoin.** May further prolong prothrombin time of **warfarin. Quinidine** may increase QT prolongation; risk of torsades de pointes. **HERBAL:** None significant. **FOOD:** None known. **LAB VALUES:** May increase serum alkaline phosphatase, bilirubin, ALT, AST.

AVAILABILITY (Rx)

Injection, Solution, Pre-Mix: 100 mg (50 mL), 200 mg (100 mL), 400 mg (200 mL). **Powder for Oral Suspension:** 10 mg/mL, 40 mg/mL. **Tablets:** 50 mg, 100 mg, 150 mg, 200 mg.

ADMINISTRATION/HANDLING

 IV

Rate of Administration • Do not exceed maximum flow rate of 200 mg/hr.
Storage • Store at room temperature. • Do not remove from outer wrap until ready to use. • Squeeze inner bag to check for leaks. • Do not use parenteral form if solution is cloudy, precipitate forms, seal is not intact, or it is discolored. • Do not add supplementary medication.

PO
• Give without regard to meals.

🖵 IV INCOMPATIBILITIES

Amphotericin B (Fungizone), amphotericin B complex (Abelcet, AmBisome, Amphotec), ampicillin (Polycillin), calcium gluconate, cefotaxime (Claforan), cefTRIAXone

(Rocephin), cefuroxime (Zinacef), chloramphenicol (Chloromycetin), clindamycin (Cleocin), co-trimoxazole (Bactrim), diazePAM (Valium), digoxin (Lanoxin), erythromycin (Erythrocin), furosemide (Lasix), haloperidol (Haldol), hydrOXYzine (Vistaril), imipenem and cilastatin (Primaxin).

⊞ IV COMPATIBILITIES

Dexmedetomidine (Precedex), diltiaZEM (Cardizem), DOBUTamine (Dobutrex), DOPamine (Intropin), heparin, lipids, LORazepam (Ativan), midazolam (Versed), propofol (Diprivan).

INDICATIONS/ROUTES/DOSAGE

◀ **ALERT** ▶ PO and IV therapy equally effective; IV therapy recommended for pt intolerant of drug or unable to take orally. Oral suspension stable for 14 days at room temperature or refrigerated.

Usual Dosage
Note: Duration and dose dependent on location/severity of infection.
PO/IV: ADULTS, ELDERLY: 150 mg once or **loading dose:** 200–800 mg. **Maintenance dose:** 200–800 mg once daily. **CHILDREN AND NEONATES: Loading dose:** 6–12 mg/kg. **Maintenance dose:** 3–12 mg/kg once daily. **Maximum:** 600 mg/day.

Dosage in Renal Impairment
After a loading dose of 400 mg, daily dosage is based on creatinine clearance.

Creatinine Clearance	Dosage
Greater than 50 mL/min	100%
50 mL/min or less	50%
Dialysis	50%
CCRT	400–800 mg as loading dose
CVVH	then 200–800 mg/day
CVVHDF	400–800 mg as loading dose, then 400–800 mg/day

Dosage in Hepatic Impairment
Use caution.

SIDE EFFECTS

Occasional (4%–1%): Hypersensitivity reaction (chills, fever, pruritus, rash), dizziness, drowsiness, headache, constipation, diarrhea, nausea, vomiting, abdominal pain.

ADVERSE EFFECTS/TOXIC REACTIONS

Exfoliative skin disorders, serious hepatic injury, blood dyscrasias (eosinophilia, thrombocytopenia, anemia, leukopenia) have been reported rarely. May increase risk of QT prolongation, torsades de pointes. Skin disorders including Stevens-Johnson syndrome, toxic epidermal necrolysis may occur.

NURSING CONSIDERATIONS

BASELINE ASSESSMENT

Obtain CBC, LFT; serum potassium in critically ill pts. Receive full medication history and screen for interactions. Assess areas of infection. Assess infected area.

INTERVENTION/EVALUATION

Assess for hypersensitivity reaction (chills, fever). Monitor CBC, BMP, LFT. Report rash, itching promptly. Monitor temperature at least daily. Monitor daily pattern of bowel activity, stool consistency. Assess for dizziness; provide assistance as needed.

PATIENT/FAMILY TEACHING

• Report dark urine, pale stool, jaundiced skin or sclera of eyes, rash, pruritus. • Pts with oropharyngeal infections should maintain fastidious oral hygiene. • Consult physician before taking any other medication.

---

fluorouracil, 5-FU HIGH ALERT

flure-oh-**ue**-ra-sil
(Adrucil, Carac, Efudex, Fluoroplex, Tolak)

■ **BLACK BOX ALERT** ■ Must be administered by personnel trained in administration/handling of chemotherapeutic agents.

F

Do not confuse Efudex with Efidac.

◆**CLASSIFICATION**

PHARMACOTHERAPEUTIC: Antimetabolite. **CLINICAL:** Antineoplastic.

USES

Parenteral: Treatment of carcinoma of colon, rectum, breast, stomach, pancreas. **Topical:** Treatment of multiple actinic or solar keratoses, superficial basal cell carcinomas. **OFF-LABEL: Parenteral:** Treatment of carcinoma of: bladder, cervical, endometrial, head/neck, anal, esophageal, renal cell, unknown primary cancer.

PRECAUTIONS

Contraindications: Hypersensitivity to fluorouracil. Myelosuppression, poor nutritional status, potentially serious infections. **Cautions:** History of high-dose pelvic irradiation, hepatic/renal impairment, palmar-plantar erythrodysesthesia syndrome (hand and foot syndrome), previous use of alkylating agents. Pts with widespread metastatic marrow involvement.

ACTION

Blocks formation of thymidylic acid. Cell cycle–specific for S phase of cell division. **Therapeutic Effect:** Inhibits DNA, RNA synthesis. **Topical:** Destroys rapidly proliferating cells.

PHARMACOKINETICS

Widely distributed. Crosses blood-brain barrier. Metabolized in liver. Primarily excreted by lungs as carbon dioxide. Removed by hemodialysis. **Half-life:** 16 min.

⌛ LIFESPAN CONSIDERATIONS

Pregnancy/Lactation: If possible, avoid use during pregnancy, esp. first trimester. May cause fetal harm. Unknown if distributed in breast milk. Breastfeeding not recommended. **Children:** No age-related precautions noted. **Elderly:** Age-related

renal impairment may require dosage adjustment.

INTERACTIONS

DRUG: Bone marrow depressants may increase risk of myelosuppression. **Live virus vaccines** may potentiate virus replication, increase vaccine side effects, decrease pt's antibody response to vaccine. **HERBAL: Echinacea** may decrease effects. Avoid use of **black cohosh, dong quai** in pts with estrogen-dependent tumors. **FOOD:** None known. **LAB VALUES:** May decrease serum albumin. **Topical:** May cause eosinophilia, leukocytosis, thrombocytopenia, toxic granulation.

AVAILABILITY (Rx)

Cream, Topical (Carac): 0.5%. **(Tolak):** 4%, **(Efudex):** 5%. **(Fluoroplex):** 1%. **Injection Solution (Adrucil):** 50 mg/mL. **Solution, Topical (Efudex):** 2%, 5%.

ADMINISTRATION/HANDLING

◀**ALERT**▶ Give by IV injection or IV infusion. Do not add to other IV infusions. Avoid small veins, swollen/edematous extremities, areas overlying joints, tendons. May be carcinogenic, mutagenic, teratogenic. Handle with extreme care during preparation/administration.

 IV

Reconstitution • IV push does not need to be diluted or reconstituted. • Inject through Y-tube or 3-way stopcock of free-flowing solution. • For IV infusion, further dilute with 50–1,000 mL D₅W or 0.9% NaCl.
Rate of Administration • Give IV push slowly over 1–2 min. • IV infusion is administered over 30 min–24 hrs (refer to individual protocols). • Extravasation produces immediate pain, severe local tissue damage.
Storage • Store at room temperature. • Solution appears colorless to faint yellow. Slight discoloration does not adversely affect potency or safety. • If precipitate forms, redissolve by heating,

F

shaking vigorously; allow to cool to body temperature. • Diluted solutions stable for 72 hrs at room temperature.

🔳 IV INCOMPATIBILITIES

Amphotericin B complex (Abelcet, AmBisome, Amphotec), filgrastim (Neupogen), ondansetron (Zofran), vinorelbine (Navelbine).

🔳 IV COMPATIBILITIES

Granisetron (Kytril), heparin, HYDROmorphone (Dilaudid), leucovorin, morphine, potassium chloride, propofol (Diprivan).

INDICATIONS/ROUTES/DOSAGE

Note: Refer to individual protocols.

Usual Range
IV Bolus: ADULTS, ELDERLY: 200–1000 mg/m^2/day for 1–21 days or 500–600 mg/m^2/dose q3–4wks.
IV Infusion: ADULTS, ELDERLY: 15 mg/kg/day or 500 mg/m^2/day over 4 hrs for 5 days or 800–1200 mg/m^2 over 24–120 hrs.

Multiple Actinic or Solar Keratoses
Topical *(Carac):* ADULTS, ELDERLY: Apply once daily for up to 4 wks.
Topical *(Efudex):* ADULTS, ELDERLY: Apply twice daily for 2–4 wks.
Topical *(Fluoroplex):* Apply twice daily for 2–6 wks.
Topical *(Tolak):* Apply once daily for 4 wks.

Basal Cell Carcinoma
Topical *(Efudex 5%):* ADULTS, ELDERLY: Apply twice daily for 3–6 wks up to 10–12 wks.

Dosage in Renal Impairment
No dose adjustment.

Dosage in Hepatic Impairment
Use extreme caution.

SIDE EFFECTS

Parenteral: Frequent (greater than 10%): Alopecia, dermatitis, anorexia, diarrhea, esophagitis, dyspepsia, stomatitis. **Occasional (10%–1%):** Cardiotoxicity (angina,

EKG changes), skin dryness, epithelial fissuring, nausea, vomiting, excessive lacrimation, blurred vision. **Rare (less than 1%):** Headache, photosensitivity, somnolence, allergic reaction, dyspnea, hypotension, MI, pulmonary edema. **Topical: Occasional:** Erythema, skin ulceration, pruritus, hyperpigmentation, dermatitis, insomnia, stomatitis, irritability, photosensitivity, excessive lacrimation, blurred vision.

ADVERSE EFFECTS/TOXIC REACTIONS

Earliest sign of toxicity (4–8 days after beginning therapy) is stomatitis (dry mouth, burning sensation, mucosal erythema, ulceration at inner margin of lips). Most common dermatologic toxicity is pruritic rash (generally on extremities, less frequently on trunk). Leukopenia (WBC less than 3500 cells/mm^3) generally occurs within 9–14 days after drug administration but may occur as late as 25th day. Thrombocytopenia (platelets less than 100,000 cells/mm^3) occasionally occurs within 7–17 days after administration. Pancytopenia, agranulocytosis occur rarely.

NURSING CONSIDERATIONS

BASELINE ASSESSMENT

Obtain baseline CBC with differential, serum renal function, LFT and monitor during therapy. Question history of hypersensitivity reaction, hepatic/renal impairment.

INTERVENTION/EVALUATION

Monitor for rapidly falling WBC, platelet count; intractable diarrhea, GI bleeding (bright red or tarry stool). Assess oral mucosa for stomatitis. Drug should be discontinued if intractable diarrhea, stomatitis, GI bleeding occurs. Assess skin for rash.

PATIENT/FAMILY TEACHING

• Maintain strict oral hygiene. • Report signs/symptoms of infection, unusual bruising/bleeding, visual changes, nausea, vomiting, diarrhea, chest pain, palpitations. • Avoid sunlight, artificial light sources; wear protective clothing, sunglasses, sunscreen. • **Topical:** Apply only to affected area. • Do not use occlusive coverings. • Be careful near eyes, nose, mouth. • Wash hands thoroughly after application. • Treated areas may be unsightly for several weeks after therapy.

FLUoxetine

floo-**ox**-e-teen
(Apo-FLUoxetine ♣, Novo-FLUoxetine ♣, PROzac, PROzac Weekly, Sarafem)

■ BLACK BOX ALERT ■ Increased risk of suicidal thinking and behavior in children, adolescents, young adults 18–24 yrs of age with major depressive disorder, other psychiatric disorders.

Do not confuse FLUoxetine with DULoxetine, famotidine, fluvastatin, fluvoxaMINE, furosemide, or PARoxetine, or PROzac with Paxil, PriLOSEC, Prograf, Proscar, or ProSom, or Sarafem with Serophene.

FIXED-COMBINATION(S)

Symbyax: FLUoxetine/OLANZapine (an antipsychotic): 25 mg/6 mg, 25 mg/12 mg, 50 mg/6 mg, 50 mg/12 mg.

◆CLASSIFICATION

PHARMACOTHERAPEUTIC: Selective serotonin reuptake inhibitor (SSRI). **CLINICAL:** Antidepressant, antiobsessional agent, antibulimic.

USES

Treatment of major depressive disorder (MDD), obsessive-compulsive disorder (OCD), binge-eating and vomiting in moderate to severe bulimia nervosa, premenstrual dysphoric disorder (PMDD), panic disorder with or without agoraphobia. Treatment of resistant or bipolar 1 depression (with OLANZapine). **OFF-LABEL:** Treatment of fibromyalgia, post-traumatic stress disorder (PTSD), Raynaud's phenomena, social anxiety disorder, selective mutism.

PRECAUTIONS

Contraindications: Hypersensitivity to **FLU**oxetine. Use of MAOIs within 5 wks of discontinuing FLUoxetine or within 14 days of discontinuing MAOIs. Initiation in pts receiving linezolid or methylene blue. Use with pimozide or thioridazine. **Note:** Do not initiate thioridazine until 5 wks after discontinuing fluoxetine. **Cautions:** Seizure disorder, cardiac dysfunction (e.g., history of MI), diabetes, pts with risk factors for QT prolongation, concurrent use of medication that increases QT interval, renal/hepatic impairment, pts at high risk for suicide, in pts where weight loss is undesirable, elderly. Pts at risk of acute narrow-angle glaucoma or with increased intraocular pressure.

ACTION

Selectively inhibits serotonin uptake in CNS, enhancing serotonergic function. **Therapeutic Effect:** Relieves depression; reduces obsessive-compulsive, bulimic behavior.

PHARMACOKINETICS

Well absorbed from GI tract. Crosses blood-brain barrier. Protein binding: 94%. Metabolized in liver. Primarily excreted in urine. Not removed by hemodialysis. **Half-life:** 2–3 days; metabolite, 7–9 days.

⧖ LIFESPAN CONSIDERATIONS

Pregnancy/Lactation: Unknown whether drug crosses placenta or is distributed in breast milk. **Children:** May be more sensitive to behavioral side effects (e.g., insomnia, restlessness). **Elderly:** No age-related precautions noted.

INTERACTIONS

DRUG: NSAIDs (e.g., ibuprofen, ketorolac, naproxen), antiplatelets (e.g., clopidogrel), anticoagulants (e.g., warfarin) may increase risk of bleeding. Alcohol, other CNS depressants (e.g., lorazepam, morphine, zolpidem) may increase CNS depression. MAOIs (e.g., phenelzine, selegiline)

F

---

may produce serotonin syndrome and neuroleptic malignant syndrome. May increase concentration/toxicity of **phenytoin, tricyclic antidepressants (e.g., amitriptyline, doxepin, nortriptyline). HERBAL: Gotu kola, kava kava, St. John's wort, valerian** may increase CNS depression. **St. John's wort** may increase effects, risk of serotonin syndrome. **FOOD:** None known. **LAB VALUES:** May decrease serum sodium. May increase serum ALT, AST.

AVAILABILITY (Rx)

Capsules: 10 mg, 20 mg, 40 mg. **Oral Solution:** 20 mg/5 mL. **Tablets:** 10 mg, 20 mg, 60 mg.

🦚 **Capsules (Delayed-Release):** 90 mg.

ADMINISTRATION/HANDLING

PO
• Give without regard to food, but give with food, milk if GI distress occurs. • **Bipolar disorder:** Give once daily in evening. • **Depression, OCD:** Give once daily in morning or twice daily (morning and noon). • **Bulimia:** Give once daily in morning.

INDICATIONS/ROUTES/DOSAGE

◀ **ALERT** ▶ Use lower or less frequent doses in pts with renal/hepatic impairment, pts with concurrent disease or multiple medications, the elderly.

Depression
PO: **ADULTS, ELDERLY:** Initially, 5–20 mg each morning. May increase after several wks by 20 mg/day. **Maximum:** 80 mg/day as single or 2 divided doses. **Prozac Weekly:** 90 mg/wk, begin 7 days after last dose of 20 mg in pts maintained on 20 mg/day. **CHILDREN 8–18 YRS:** Initially, 10–20 mg/day. Lower-weight children may be started at 10 mg/day and increased to 20 mg/day after 1 wk if needed.

Panic Disorder
PO: **ADULTS, ELDERLY:** Initially, 10 mg/day. May increase to 20 mg/day after

1 wk. May further increase dose after several wks. **Maximum:** 60 mg/day.

Bulimia Nervosa
PO: **ADULTS:** 60 mg each morning. May titrate to 60 mg over several days.

Obsessive-Compulsive Disorder (OCD)
PO: **ADULTS, ELDERLY:** Initially, 20 mg/day. May increase after several wks. Usual dose: 20–60 mg/day. **Maximum:** 80 mg/day. **CHILDREN 7–18 YRS:** Initially, 10 mg/day. May increase to 20 mg/day after 2 wks. Range: 20–60 mg/day.

Depression Associated with Bipolar Disorder
PO: **ADULTS, ELDERLY, CHILDREN 10–17 YRS:** *(with olanzapine):* Initially, 20 mg/day. May increase after several wks. Range: 20–50 mg/day.

Premenstrual Dysphoric Disorder (PMDD) (Sarafem)
PO: **ADULTS:** 20 mg/day continuously **or** 20 mg/day beginning 14 days prior to menstruation and continuing through first full day of menses (repeated with each cycle).

Dosage in Renal/Hepatic Impairment
Use caution.

SIDE EFFECTS

Frequent (greater than 10%): Headache, asthenia, insomnia, anxiety, drowsiness, nausea, diarrhea, decreased appetite. **Occasional (9%–2%):** Dizziness, tremor, fatigue, vomiting, constipation, dry mouth, abdominal pain, nasal congestion, diaphoresis, rash. **Rare (less than 2%):** Flushed skin, light-headedness, impaired concentration.

ADVERSE EFFECTS/TOXIC REACTIONS

May increase risk of suicide. Agitation, coma, diarrhea, delirium, hallucinations, hyperreflexia, hyperthermia, tachycardia, seizures may indicate life-threatening serotonin syndrome.

NURSING CONSIDERATIONS

BASELINE ASSESSMENT

Assess appearance, behavior, mood, suicidal tendencies. For pts on long-term therapy, baseline renal function, LFT, blood counts should be performed at baseline and periodically thereafter.

INTERVENTION/EVALUATION

Supervise suicidal-risk pt closely during early therapy (as depression lessens, energy level improves, increasing suicide potential). Monitor mental status, anxiety, social functioning, appetite, nutritional intake. Monitor daily pattern of bowel activity, stool consistency. Assess skin for rash. Monitor serum LFT, glucose, sodium; weight.

PATIENT/FAMILY TEACHING

• Maximum therapeutic response may require 4 or more wks of therapy. • Do not abruptly discontinue medication. • Avoid tasks that require alertness, motor skills until response to drug is established. • Avoid alcohol. • To avoid insomnia, take last dose of drug before 4 PM.

---

fluticasone

floo-**tik**-a-sone
(Apo-Fluticasone ✦, Arnuity Ellipta, Cutivate, <u>Flonase</u>, Flonase Allergy Relief, Flovent Diskus, Flovent HFA, Veramyst, Xhance)
Do not confuse Cutivate with Ultravate, or Flonase with Flovent, Beconase.

FIXED-COMBINATION(S)

Advair, Advair Diskus, Advair HFA: fluticasone/salmeterol (bronchodilator): 100 mcg/50 mcg, 250 mcg/50 mcg, 500 mcg/50 mcg. **Breo Ellipta:** fluticasone/vilanterol (bronchodilator): 100 mcg/25 mcg. **Dymista:** fluticasone/azelastine (an antihistamine): 50 mcg/137 mcg per spray.

Trelegy Ellipta: fluticasone/umeclidium (anticholinergic)/vilanterol (bronchodilator): 100 mcg/62.5 mcg/ 25 mcg.

◆CLASSIFICATION

PHARMACOTHERAPEUTIC: Corticosteroid. **CLINICAL:** Anti-inflammatory, antipruritic.

USES

Nasal: (Flonase): Management of nasal symptoms of perennial nonallergic rhinitis in adults and children 4 yrs and older. **(Veramyst):** Management of seasonal and perennial allergic rhinitis in adults, children 2 yrs and older. **Topical:** Relief of inflammation/pruritus associated with steroid-responsive disorders (e.g., contact dermatitis, eczema), atopic dermatitis. **Inhalation:** Maintenance treatment of bronchial asthma. Assists in reducing, discontinuing oral corticosteroid therapy.

PRECAUTIONS

Contraindications: Hypersensitivity to fluticasone. (Arnuity Ellipta, Flovent Diskus): Severe hypersensitivity to milk proteins or lactose. **Inhalation:** Primary treatment of status asthmaticus, acute exacerbation of asthma, other acute asthmatic conditions. **Cautions:** Untreated systemic ocular herpes simplex; untreated fungal, bacterial infection; active or quiescent tuberculosis. Thyroid disease, cardiovascular disease, diabetes, glaucoma, hepatic/renal impairment, cataracts, myasthenia gravis, seizures, GI disease, risk for osteoporosis, untreated localized infection of nasal mucosa. Following acute MI; concurrent use with strong CYP3A4 inhibitors.

ACTION

Controls rate of protein synthesis, depresses migration of polymorphonuclear leukocytes, reverses capillary permeability, stabilizes lysosomal membranes. **Therapeutic Effect:** Prevents, controls inflammation.

PHARMACOKINETICS

Inhalation/intranasal: Protein binding: 91%. Metabolized in liver. Excreted in urine. **Half-life:** 3–7.8 hrs. **Topical:** Amount absorbed depends on affected area and skin condition (absorption increased with fever, hydration, inflamed or denuded skin).

⌛ LIFESPAN CONSIDERATIONS

Pregnancy/Lactation: Unknown if drug crosses placenta or is distributed in breast milk. **Children:** Safety and efficacy not established in pts younger than 4 yrs. Children 4 yrs and older may experience growth suppression with prolonged or high doses. **Elderly:** No age-related precautions noted.

INTERACTIONS

DRUG: CYP3A4 inhibitors (carBAMazepine, ketoconazole, phenytoin, rifAMPin) may increase concentration. **Ritonavir** may reduce serum cortisol concentration. **HERBAL:** Echinacea, St. John's wort may decrease concentration/effects. **FOOD:** None known. **LAB VALUES:** None significant.

AVAILABILITY (Rx)

Aerosol for Oral Inhalation (Flovent HFA): 44 mcg/inhalation, 110 mcg/inhalation, 220 mcg/inhalation. **Cream (Cutivate):** 0.05%. **Ointment (Cutivate):** 0.005%. **Powder for Oral Inhalation (Flovent Diskus):** 50 mcg/blister, 100 mcg/blister, 250 mcg/blister. **(Arnuity Ellipta):** 100 mcg/actuation, 200 mcg/actuation. **Suspension Intranasal Spray: (Flonase, Flonase Allergy Relief):** 50 mcg/inhalation. **(Veramyst):** 27.5 mcg/spray. **(Xhance):** 93 mcg/actuation.

ADMINISTRATION/HANDLING

Inhalation
Flovent HFA
• Shake container well. Prime before first use. Instruct pt to exhale completely. Place mouthpiece fully into mouth, inhale, and hold breath as long as possible before exhaling. • Allow 30–60 seconds between inhalations. • Rinsing mouth after each use decreases dry mouth, hoarseness.

Flovent Diskus
• Do not shake or prime before use. Place mouthpiece fully into mouth, inhale quickly and deeply, remove device, and hold breath up to 10 seconds.

Arnuity Ellipta
• Do not shake or prime before use; put mouthpiece between lips, breathe deeply and slowly through the mouth, remove inhaler, and hold breath for 3–4 seconds.

Intranasal
• Instruct pt to clear nasal passages as much as possible before use (topical nasal decongestants may be needed 5–15 min before use). Tilt head slightly forward. • Insert spray tip into 1 nostril, pointing toward inflamed nasal turbinates, away from nasal septum. • Pump medication into 1 nostril while pt holds other nostril closed, concurrently inspires through nose.

INDICATIONS/ROUTES/DOSAGE

Allergic Rhinitis
Intranasal *(Flonase):* **ADULTS, ELDERLY:** Initially, 200 mcg (2 sprays in each nostril once daily or 1 spray in each nostril q12h). **Maintenance:** 1 spray in each nostril once daily. May increase to 100 mcg (2 sprays) in each nostril. **Maximum:** 200 mcg/day. **CHILDREN 4 YRS AND OLDER:** Initially, 100 mcg (1 spray in each nostril once daily). **Maximum:** 200 mcg/day (2 sprays each nostril).

(Veramyst): **ADULTS, ELDERLY, CHILDREN 12 YRS AND OLDER:** 110 mcg (2 sprays in each nostril) once daily. **Maintenance:** 55 mcg (1 spray in each nostril) once daily. **CHILDREN 2–11 YRS:** 55 mcg (1 spray in each nostril) once daily. May increase to 110 mcg (2 sprays each nostril) once daily.

(Xhance): **ADULTS, ELDERLY:** 93 mcg (1 spray) per nostril twice daily. May increase to 2 sprays twice daily.

Usual Topical Dosage
Note: Ointment for adults only.
Topical: ADULTS, ELDERLY, CHILDREN 3 MOS AND OLDER: Apply sparingly to affected area once or twice daily.

Maintenance Treatment of Asthma
Inhalation Powder *(Arnuity Ellipta):*
ADULTS, ELDERLY, CHILDREN 12 YRS AND
OLDER: 100–200 mcg once daily. **Maximum:** 200 mcg/day.

**Maintenance Treatment for Asthma
(Previously Treated with Bronchodilators)**
Inhalation Powder *(Flovent Diskus):*
ADULTS, ELDERLY, CHILDREN 12 YRS AND
OLDER: Initially, 100 mcg twice daily.
Maximum: 500 mcg twice daily.
Inhalation *(Flovent HFA):* ADULTS,
ELDERLY, CHILDREN 12 YRS AND OLDER: 88
mcg twice daily. **Maximum:** 440 mcg
twice daily.

**Maintenance Treatment for Asthma
(Previously Treated with Inhaled Steroids)**
Inhalation Powder *(Flovent Diskus):*
ADULTS, ELDERLY, CHILDREN 12 YRS AND
OLDER: Initially, 100–250 mcg twice
daily. **Maximum:** 500 mcg twice daily.
Inhalation *(Flovent HFA):* ADULTS, EL-
DERLY, CHILDREN 12 YRS AND OLDER: 88–
220 mcg twice daily. **Maximum:** 440
mcg twice daily.

**Maintenance Treatment for Asthma
(Previously Treated with Oral Steroids)**
Inhalation Powder *(Flovent Dis-
kus):* ADULTS, ELDERLY, CHILDREN 12 YRS
AND OLDER: 500–1,000 mcg twice daily.
Inhalation *(Flovent HFA):* ADULTS,
ELDERLY, CHILDREN 12 YRS AND OLDER:
440–880 mcg twice daily.

Usual Pediatric Dose (4–11 Yrs)
Flovent Diskus: Initially, 50 mcg twice
daily. May increase to 100 mcg twice
daily. **Flovent HFA:** 88 mcg twice daily.

Dosage in Renal/Hepatic Impairment
No dose adjustment. *(Arnuity Ellipta):*
Use caution in hepatic impairment.

SIDE EFFECTS

Frequent: Inhalation: Throat irritation, hoarseness, dry mouth, cough, temporary wheezing, oropharyngeal candidiasis (particularly if mouth is not rinsed
with water after each administration).

Intranasal: Mild nasopharyngeal irritation, nasal burning, stinging, dryness,
rebound congestion, rhinorrhea, altered
sense of taste. **Occasional: Inhalation:** Oral candidiasis. **Intranasal:**
Nasal/pharyngeal candidiasis, headache.
Topical: Stinging, burning of skin.

ADVERSE EFFECTS/TOXIC REACTIONS

None known.

NURSING CONSIDERATIONS

BASELINE ASSESSMENT

Establish baseline history of skin disorder,
asthma, rhinitis. Question hypersensitivity,
esp. milk products or lactose. Question
medical history as listed in Precautions.

INTERVENTION/EVALUATION

Monitor rate, depth, rhythm, type of
respiration; quality/rate of pulse. Assess
lung sounds for rhonchi, wheezing, rales.
Assess oral mucous membranes for evidence of candidiasis. Monitor growth in
pediatric pts. **Topical:** Assess involved
area for therapeutic response to irritation.

PATIENT/FAMILY TEACHING

• Pts receiving bronchodilators by inhalation concomitantly with steroid inhalation
therapy should use bronchodilator several
min before corticosteroid aerosol (enhances penetration of steroid into bronchial
tree). • Do not change dose/schedule or
stop taking drug; must taper off gradually
under medical supervision. • Maintain
strict oral hygiene. • Rinse mouth with
water immediately after inhalation (prevents mouth/throat dryness, oral fungal
infection). • Increase fluid intake (decreases lung secretion viscosity). • **Intranasal:** Clear nasal passages before
use. • Report if no improvement in symptoms or if sneezing/nasal irritation occurs. • Improvement noted in several
days. • **Topical:** Rub film gently into
affected area. • Use only for prescribed
area and no longer than ordered. • Avoid
contact with eyes.

F

fluvoxaMINE

floo-**vox**-a-meen
(Apo-Fluvoxamine ✦, Luvox CR,
Novo-FluvoxaMINE ✦)

■ BLACK BOX ALERT ■ Increased
risk of suicidal ideation and behavior in children, adolescents, young
adults 18–24 yrs with major depressive disorder, other psychiatric
disorders.
**Do not confuse fluvoxaMINE with
flavoxATE or FLUoxetine, or Luvox
with Lasix, Levoxyl, or Lovenox.**

◆ CLASSIFICATION

PHARMACOTHERAPEUTIC: Selective
serotonin reuptake inhibitor. **CLINI-
CAL:** Antidepressant, antiobsessive.

USES

Immediate-Release: Treatment of
obsessive-compulsive disorder (OCD)
in adults and children 8–17 yrs of age.
Extended-Release: Treatment of OCD
in adults. **OFF-LABEL:** Treatment of social
anxiety disorder (SAD), post-traumatic
stress disorder (PTSD).

PRECAUTIONS

Contraindications: Hypersensitivity to fluvoxaMINE. Use of MAOIs concurrently or
within 14 days of discontinuing MAOIs or
fluvoxaMINE. Concomitant use with alosetron, pimozide, ramelteon, thioridazine,
or tiZANidine. Initiation of fluvoxaMINE
in pts receiving linezolid or methylene
blue. **Cautions:** Renal/hepatic impairment; elderly; impaired platelet aggregation; concurrent use of NSAIDs, aspirin;
seizure disorder; pts that are volume
depleted; third trimester of pregnancy;
pts with high suicide risk; risk of bleeding or receiving concurrent anticoagulant
therapy. May precipitate a shift to mania or
hypomania in pts with bipolar disorder.

ACTION

Selectively inhibits neuronal reuptake of
serotonin. **Therapeutic Effect:** Relieves
depression, symptoms of obsessive-compulsive disorder (OCD).

PHARMACOKINETICS

Well absorbed following PO administration. Protein binding: 77%. Metabolized
in liver. Excreted in urine. **Half-life:**
15–20 hrs.

⧗ LIFESPAN CONSIDERATIONS

Pregnancy/Lactation: Unknown if
drug crosses the placenta; distributed
in breast milk. **Children:** Safety and efficacy not established in pts younger than
8 yrs. **Elderly:** Potential for reduced serum clearance; maintain caution.

INTERACTIONS

DRUG: May increase concentration, risk
of toxicity of **benzodiazepines (e.g.,
ALPRAZolam, LORazepam), carBA-
Mazepine, cloZAPine, theophylline.
Lithium, tryptophan** may enhance fluvoxaMINE's serotonergic effects. **MAOIs (e.g.,
phenelzine, selegiline)** may increase
risk of serotonin syndrome (hyperthermia,
rigidity, myoclonus). **Tricyclic antidepressants (e.g., amitriptyline)** may
increase concentration. May increase effects of **warfarin. HERBAL: Valerian, St.
John's wort, SAMe, kava kava** may increase risk of serotonin syndrome or CNS
depression. Avoid **herbs with antiplatelet
activity (e.g., cat's claw, feverfew, ginger). FOOD:** None known. **LAB VALUES:**
May decrease serum sodium.

AVAILABILITY (Rx)

Tablets: 25 mg, 50 mg, 100 mg.

🖎 **Capsules (Extended-Release):** 100
mg, 150 mg.

ADMINISTRATION/HANDLING

• Do not break, crush, dissolve, or divide extended-release capsules. • May
give with or without food.

INDICATIONS/ROUTES/DOSAGE

Obsessive-Compulsive Disorder (OCD)
PO (Immediate-Release): ADULTS: Initially, 50 mg at bedtime; may increase by

50 mg every 4–7 days. Dosages greater than 100 mg/day should be given in 2 divided doses with larger dose given at bedtime. Usual dose: 100–300 mg/day. **Maximum:** 300 mg/day. *(Extended-Release)* Initially, 100 mg once daily at bedtime. May increase by 50 mg at no less than 1-wk intervals. Range: 100–300 mg/day. **Maximum:** 300 mg/day. **CHILDREN 8–17 YRS** *(Immediate-Release):* Initially, 25 mg at bedtime; may increase by 25 mg every 4–7 days. Dosages greater than 50 mg/day should be given in 2 divided doses with larger dose given at bedtime. **Maximum: (CHILDREN 8–11 YRS):** 200 mg/day. **(CHILDREN 12–17 YRS):** 300 mg/day.

Dosage in Renal/Hepatic Impairment
No dose adjustment.

SIDE EFFECTS

Frequent (40%–21%): Nausea, headache, drowsiness, insomnia. **Occasional (14%–8%):** Dizziness, diarrhea, dry mouth, asthenia, dyspepsia, constipation, abnormal ejaculation. **Rare (6%–3%):** Anorexia, anxiety, tremor, vomiting, flatulence, urinary frequency, sexual dysfunction, altered taste.

ADVERSE EFFECTS/TOXIC REACTIONS

Agitation, coma, diarrhea, delirium, hallucinations, hyperreflexia, hyperthermia, tachycardia, seizures may indicate life-threatening serotonin syndrome.

NURSING CONSIDERATIONS

BASELINE ASSESSMENT

Obtain LFT, BUN, serum creatinine; CrCl; urine/serum pregnancy test. Receive full medication history in screen for interactions, esp. contraindicated use of concomitant medications. Question history of seizure disorder. Assess hydration status.

INTERVENTION/EVALUATION

Supervise suicidal-risk pt closely during early therapy (as depression lessens, energy level improves, increasing suicide potential). Assess appearance, behavior, speech pattern, level of interest, mood. Assist with ambulation if dizziness, drowsiness occurs. Monitor daily pattern of bowel activity, stool consistency.

PATIENT/FAMILY TEACHING

• Maximum therapeutic response may require 4 wks or more of therapy. • Dry mouth may be relieved by sugarless gum, sips of water. • Do not abruptly discontinue medication. • Avoid tasks that require alertness, motor skills until response to drug is established.

folic acid

foe-lik as-id
(Apo-Folic ✦)
Do not confuse folic acid with folinic acid.

✦CLASSIFICATION

PHARMACOTHERAPEUTIC: Vitamin, water soluble. **CLINICAL:** Nutritional supplement.

USES

Treatment of megaloblastic and macrocytic anemias due to folate deficiency. Treatment of anemias due to folate deficiency in pregnant women. Folate supplementation during periconceptual period decreases risk of neural tube defects.

PRECAUTIONS

Contraindications: Hypersensitivity to folic acid. **Cautions:** Anemias (aplastic, normocytic, pernicious, refractory) when anemia present with vitamin B_{12} deficiency.

ACTION

Stimulates production of platelets, RBCs, WBCs in folate deficiency anemia. **Therapeutic Effect:** Essential for nucleoprotein synthesis, maintenance of normal erythropoiesis.

PHARMACOKINETICS

PO form almost completely absorbed from GI tract (upper duodenum). Protein binding: High. Metabolized in liver. Excreted in urine. Removed by hemodialysis.

 LIFESPAN CONSIDERATIONS

Pregnancy/Lactation: Distributed in breast milk. **Children/Elderly:** No age-related precautions noted.

INTERACTIONS

DRUG: May decrease effects of **PHE-Nobarbital, phenytoin, primidone, raltitrexed. HERBAL: Green tea** may increase concentration. **FOOD:** None known. **LAB VALUES:** May decrease vitamin B_{12} concentration.

AVAILABILITY (Rx)

Capsules: 0.8 mg, 5 mg, 20 mg. **Injection Solution:** 5 mg/mL. **Tablets:** 0.4 mg (OTC), 0.8 mg (OTC), 1 mg.

ADMINISTRATION/HANDLING

PO
• May give without regard to food.

IV

May give 5 mg or less undiluted over at least 1 min, or dilute with 50 mL 0.9% NaCl or D_5W and infuse over 30 min.

INDICATIONS/ROUTES/DOSAGE

Anemia
IM/IV/SQ/PO: ADULTS, ELDERLY, CHILDREN 4 YRS AND OLDER: 0.4 mg/day. **CHILDREN YOUNGER THAN 4 YRS:** Up to 0.3 mg/day. **INFANTS:** 0.1 mg/day. **PREGNANT/LACTATING WOMEN:** 0.8 mg/day.

Prevention of Neural Tube Defects
PO: WOMEN OF CHILDBEARING AGE: 400–800 mcg/day. **WOMEN AT HIGH RISK OR FAMILY HISTORY OF NEURAL TUBE DEFECTS:** 4 mg/day.

SIDE EFFECTS

None known.

ADVERSE EFFECTS/TOXIC REACTIONS

Allergic hypersensitivity occurs rarely with parenteral form. Oral folic acid is nontoxic.

NURSING CONSIDERATIONS

BASELINE ASSESSMENT

Pernicious anemia should be ruled out with Schilling test and vitamin B_{12} blood level before initiating therapy (may produce irreversible neurologic damage). Resistance to treatment may occur if decreased hematopoiesis, alcoholism, antimetabolic drugs, deficiency of vitamin B_6, B_{12}, C, E is evident.

INTERVENTION/EVALUATION

Assess for therapeutic improvement: improved sense of well-being, relief from iron deficiency symptoms (fatigue, shortness of breath, sore tongue, headache, pallor).

PATIENT/FAMILY TEACHING

• Eat foods rich in folic acid, including fruits, vegetables, organ meats.

---

fondaparinux

fon-**dap**-a-rin-ux
(Arixtra)
■ **BLACK BOX ALERT** ■ Epidural or spinal anesthesia greatly increases potential for spinal or epidural hematoma, subsequent long-term or permanent paralysis.

◆CLASSIFICATION

PHARMACOTHERAPEUTIC: Factor Xa inhibitor. **CLINICAL:** Antithrombotic.

USES

Prevention of venous thromboembolism in pts undergoing total hip replacement, hip fracture surgery, knee replacement surgery, abdominal surgery. Treatment of acute deep vein thrombosis (DVT), acute pulmonary embolism. **OFF-LABEL:** Prophylaxis of DVT in pts with history of heparin-induced thrombocytopenia (HIT), acute symptomatic superficial vein thrombosis of the legs.

PRECAUTIONS

Contraindications: Hypersensitivity to fondaparinux, active major bleeding, bacterial endocarditis, prophylaxis treatment in pts with body weight less than 50 kg, severe renal impairment (CrCl less than 30 mL/min), thrombocytopenia associated with antiplatelet antibody formation in presence of fondaparinux. **Cautions:** Conditions with increased risk of bleeding, bacterial endocarditis, active ulcerative GI disease, hemorrhagic stroke; shortly after brain, spinal, or ophthalmologic surgery; concurrent platelet inhibitors, severe uncontrolled hypertension, history of CVA, history of heparin-induced thrombocytopenia, renal/hepatic impairment, elderly, indwelling epidural catheter use.

ACTION

Factor Xa inhibitor that selectively binds to antithrombin and increases its affinity for factor Xa, inhibiting factor Xa, stopping blood coagulation cascade. **Therapeutic Effect:** Indirectly prevents formation of thrombin and subsequently fibrin clot.

PHARMACOKINETICS

Well absorbed after subcutaneous administration. Undergoes minimal, if any, metabolism. Highly bound to antithrombin III. Distributed mainly in blood and to a minor extent in extravascular fluid. Excreted unchanged in urine. Removed by hemodialysis. **Half-life:** 17–21 hrs (increased in renal impairment).

⧗ LIFESPAN CONSIDERATIONS

Pregnancy/Lactation: Use with caution, particularly during third trimester, immediate postpartum period (increased risk of maternal hemorrhage). Unknown if excreted in breast milk. **Children:** Safety

and efficacy not established. **Elderly:** Age-related renal impairment may increase risk of bleeding.

INTERACTIONS

DRUG: Anticoagulants (e.g., heparin, warfarin), antiplatelet medications (e.g., clopidogrel), aspirin, drotrecogin alfa, NSAIDs (e.g., ibuprofen, ketorolac, naproxen), thrombolytics may increase risk of bleeding. **HERBAL: Cat's claw, dong quai, evening primrose, feverfew, garlic, ginger, ginkgo, ginseng, horse chestnut, red clover, Omega-3** may increase antiplatelet activity. **FOOD:** None known. **LAB VALUES:** May cause reversible increases in serum creatinine, ALT, AST. May decrease Hgb, Hct, platelet count.

AVAILABILITY (Rx)

Injection, Solution: 2.5 mg/0.5 mL, 5 mg/0.4 mL, 7.5 mg/0.6 mL, 10 mg/0.8 mL.

ADMINISTRATION/HANDLING

Subcutaneous
• Parenteral form appears clear, colorless. Discard if discoloration or particulate matter is noted. • Store at room temperature. • Do not expel air bubble from prefilled syringe before injection. • Insert needle subcutaneously into upper arms, outer thigh, or abdomen and inject solution. • Do not inject into areas of active skin disease or injury such as sunburns, rashes, inflammation, skin infections, or active psoriasis. • Rotate injection sites.

INDICATIONS/ROUTES/DOSAGE

◀**ALERT**▶ For subcutaneous administration only.

Prevention of Venous Thromboembolism
SQ: ADULTS WEIGHING 50 KG OR MORE: 2.5 mg once daily for 5–9 days after surgery (up to 10 days following abdominal surgery; 11 days following hip or knee replacement). Initial dose should be given no earlier than 6–8h

F

after surgery. Initiate dose once hemostasis established. **WEIGHING LESS THAN 50 KG:** Contraindicated.

Treatment of Venous Thromboembolism, Pulmonary Embolism

Note: Start warfarin on first treatment day and continue fondaparinux until INR reaches 2 to 3 for at least 24 hr. Usual duration of fondaparinux: 5–9 days.

SQ: ADULTS, ELDERLY WEIGHING MORE THAN 100 KG: 10 mg once daily. **ADULTS, ELDERLY WEIGHING 50–100 KG:** 7.5 mg once daily. **ADULTS, ELDERLY WEIGHING LESS THAN 50 KG:** 5 mg once daily.

Dosage in Renal Impairment

CrCl greater than 50 mL/min: No dose adjustment. **CrCl 30–50 mL/min:** Use caution (50% dose reduction or use of low-dose heparin). **CrCl less than 30 mL/min:** Contraindicated.

Dosage in Hepatic Impairment

Mild to moderate impairment: No dose adjustment. **Severe impairment:** Use caution.

SIDE EFFECTS

Frequent (19%–11%): Anemia, fever, nausea. **Occasional (10%–4%):** Edema, constipation, rash, vomiting, insomnia, increased wound drainage, hypokalemia. **Rare (less than 4%):** Dizziness, hypotension, confusion, urinary retention, injection site hematoma, diarrhea, dyspepsia, headache.

ADVERSE EFFECTS/TOXIC REACTIONS

Accidental overdose may lead to bleeding complications ranging from local ecchymoses to major hemorrhage. Thrombocytopenia occurs rarely.

NURSING CONSIDERATIONS

BASELINE ASSESSMENT

Assess CBC, renal function test. Evaluate potential risk for bleeding. Question history of recent surgery, trauma, intracranial hemorrhage, GI bleeding. Question medical history as listed in Precautions. Ensure

that pt has not received spinal anesthesia, spinal procedures.

INTERVENTION/EVALUATION

Periodically monitor CBC, esp. platelet count, stool for occult blood (no need for daily monitoring in pts with normal presurgical coagulation parameters). Assess for any signs of bleeding: bleeding at surgical site, hematuria, blood in stool, bleeding from gums, petechiae, ecchymosis, bleeding from injection sites. Monitor B/P, pulse; hypotension, tachycardia may indicate bleeding, hypovolemia.

PATIENT/FAMILY TEACHING

• Usual length of therapy is 5–9 days. • Do not take any OTC medication (esp. aspirin, NSAIDs). • Report swelling of hands/feet, unusual back pain, unusual bleeding/bruising. Treatment may increase risk of bleeding into the brain; report confusion, one-sided weakness, trouble speaking, seizures. Treatment may increase risk of GI bleeding; report bloody stool, vomiting up blood; dark, tarry stools.

fosinopril

foe-**sin**-oh-pril ✤
(Apo-Fosinopril ✤, Monopril)
■ **BLACK BOX ALERT** ■ May cause fetal injury, mortality. Discontinue as soon as possible once pregnancy is detected. **Do not confuse fosinopril with Fosamax or lisinopril, or Monopril with Accupril, minoxidil, moexipril, or ramipril.**

◆CLASSIFICATION

PHARMACOTHERAPEUTIC: ACE inhibitor. **CLINICAL:** Antihypertensive.

USES

Treatment of hypertension, used alone or in combination with other antihypertensives. Treatment of HF.

PRECAUTIONS

Contraindications: Hypersensitivity to fosinopril. History of angioedema from previous treatment with ACE inhibitors. Concomitant use with aliskiren in pts with diabetes. **Cautions:** Renal/hepatic impairment, pts with sodium depletion or on diuretic therapy, dialysis, hypovolemia, hypertrophic cardiomyopathy with outflow tract obstruction, hyperkalemia, concomitant use of potassium supplements, unstented unilateral/bilateral renal stenosis, diabetes, severe aortic stenosis. Before, during, or immediately after major surgery.

ACTION

Suppresses renin-angiotensin-aldosterone system (prevents conversion of angiotensin I to angiotensin II, a potent vasoconstrictor; may inhibit angiotensin II at local vascular, renal sites). Decreases plasma angiotensin II, increases plasma renin activity, decreases aldosterone secretion. **Therapeutic Effect:** Reduces B/P.

PHARMACOKINETICS

Route	Onset	Peak	Duration
PO	1 hr	2–6 hrs	24 hrs

Slowly absorbed from GI tract. Protein binding: 97%–98%. Metabolized in liver and GI mucosa. Primarily excreted in urine. Minimal removal by hemodialysis. **Half-life:** 11.5 hrs.

⌛ LIFESPAN CONSIDERATIONS

Pregnancy/Lactation: Crosses placenta. Distributed in breast milk. May cause fetal or neonatal mortality or morbidity. **Children:** Safety and efficacy not established. Neonates, infants may be at increased risk for oliguria, neurologic abnormalities. **Elderly:** May be more sensitive to hypotensive effects.

INTERACTIONS

DRUG: Alcohol, antihypertensive agents (e.g., amLODIPine, valsartan), diuretics (e.g., furosemide, HCTZ), NSAIDs may increase effects. **Potassium-sparing diuretics (e.g., spironolactone), potassium supplements** may cause hyperkalemia. May increase **lithium** concentration/toxicity. **Antacids** may decrease absorption. **HERBAL: Ephedra, ginseng, yohimbe** may worsen hypertension. **Garlic** may increase antihypertensive effect. **Licorice** may cause sodium/water retention, loss of potassium. **FOOD:** None known. **LAB VALUES:** May increase serum BUN, alkaline phosphatase, bilirubin, creatinine, potassium, ALT, AST. May decrease serum sodium. May cause positive antinuclear antibody titer (ANA).

AVAILABILITY (Rx)

Tablets: 10 mg, 20 mg, 40 mg.

ADMINISTRATION/HANDLING

PO
• Give without regard to food. • Tablets may be crushed.

INDICATIONS/ROUTES/DOSAGE

Hypertension
PO: ADULTS, ELDERLY: Initially, 10 mg once daily. **Maintenance:** 20–40 mg once daily. **Maximum:** 80 mg once daily. **CHILDREN 6–16 YRS WEIGHING MORE THAN 50 KG:** Initially, 5–10 mg once daily. **Maximum:** 40 mg once daily.

HF
PO: ADULTS, ELDERLY: Initially, 5–10 mg once daily. May increase dose over several wks. **Maintenance:** 20–40 mg once daily. **Maximum:** 40 mg once daily.

Dosage in Renal Impairment
Reduce initial dose to 5 mg in pts with HF.

Dosage in Hepatic Impairment
No dose adjustment.

SIDE EFFECTS

Frequent (12%–9%): Dizziness, cough. **Occasional (4%–2%):** Hypotension, nausea, vomiting, upper respiratory tract infection.

ADVERSE EFFECTS/TOXIC REACTIONS

Excessive hypotension ("first-dose syncope") may occur in pts with HF, severely salt/volume depleted. Angioedema (swelling of face/lips), hyperkalemia occur rarely. Agranulocytosis, neutropenia may be noted in pts with renal impairment, collagen vascular disease (scleroderma, systemic lupus erythematosus). Nephrotic syndrome may be noted in those with history of renal disease.

NURSING CONSIDERATIONS

BASELINE ASSESSMENT

Obtain B/P immediately before each dose, in addition to regular monitoring (be alert to fluctuations). Renal function tests should be performed before beginning therapy. In pts with renal impairment, autoimmune disease, or taking drugs that affect leukocytes or immune response, CBC, differential count should be performed before therapy begins and q2wks for 3 mos, then periodically thereafter. Question medical history as listed in Precautions. Question history of hypersensitivity reaction, angioedema.

INTERVENTION/EVALUATION

If excessive reduction in B/P occurs, place pt in supine position with legs elevated. Assist with ambulation if dizziness occurs. Assess for urinary frequency. Auscultate lung sounds for rales, wheezing in pts with HF. Monitor renal function tests, CBC, urinalysis for proteinuria. Observe for angioedema (swelling of face, lips, tongue). Monitor serum potassium in those on concurrent diuretic therapy.

PATIENT/FAMILY TEACHING

• Report any sign of infection (sore throat, fever). • Several wks may be needed for full therapeutic effect of B/P reduction. • Skipping doses or voluntarily discontinuing drug may produce severe rebound hypertension. • To reduce hypotensive effect, go from lying to standing slowly. • Immediately report swelling of face, lips, tongue, difficulty breathing, vomiting, excessive perspiration, persistent cough. • Avoid potassium salt substitutes.

fosphenytoin

fos-**fen**-i-toyn
(Cerebyx)
Do not confuse Cerebyx with CeleBREX or CeleXA, or fosphenytoin with fospropofol.

◆CLASSIFICATION

PHARMACOTHERAPEUTIC: Hydantoin. **CLINICAL:** Anticonvulsant.

USES

Acute treatment, control of generalized convulsive status epilepticus; prevention, treatment of seizures occurring during neurosurgery; short-term substitution for oral phenytoin.

PRECAUTIONS

Contraindications: Hypersensitivity to fosphenytoin, phenytoin, other hydantoins. Adams-Stokes syndrome; second- or third-degree AV block; sinus bradycardia; SA block; concurrent use of delavirdine. **Cautions:** Porphyria, diabetes, hypothyroidism, hypotension, severe myocardial insufficiency, renal/hepatic disease, hypoalbuminemia.

ACTION

Stabilizes neuronal membranes, limits spread of seizure activity. Decreases sodium, calcium ion influx into neurons. Decreases post-tetanic potentiation, repetitive discharge. **Therapeutic Effect:** Decreases seizure activity.

PHARMACOKINETICS

Completely absorbed after IM administration. Protein binding: 95%–99%. Rapidly and completely hydrolyzed to phenytoin after IM or IV administration. Time of complete conversion to phenytoin: 4 hrs after IM injection; 2 hrs after IV infusion. **Half-life:** 8–15 min (for conversion to phenytoin). (Phenytoin: 12–29 hrs.)

☒ LIFESPAN CONSIDERATIONS

Pregnancy/Lactation: May increase frequency of seizures during pregnancy. Increased risk of congenital malformations. Unknown if excreted in breast milk. **Children:** Safety and efficacy not established. **Elderly:** Lower dosage recommended.

INTERACTIONS

DRUG: Alcohol, other **CNS depressants (e.g., LORazepam, morphine, zolpidem)** may increase CNS depression. **Amiodarone, anticoagulants (e.g., warfarin), cimetidine, disulfiram, FLUoxetine, isoniazid, sulfonamides** may increase concentration/effects, risk of toxicity. **CYP3A4 inhibitors (e.g., fluconazole, ketoconazole, miconazole)** may increase concentration. **HERBAL:** None significant. **FOOD:** None known. **LAB VALUES:** May increase serum glucose, GGT, alkaline phosphatase.

AVAILABILITY (Rx)

Injection Solution: 75 mg/mL (equivalent to 50 mg phenytoin equivalents (PE)/mL phenytoin).

ADMINISTRATION/HANDLING

 IV

Reconstitution • Dilute in D_5W or 0.9% NaCl to a concentration ranging from 1.5–25 mg PE/mL.
Rate of Administration • Administer at rate less than 150 mg PE/min (decreases risk of hypotension, arrhythmias). Children: 1–3 mg PE/kg/min. **Maximum:** 150 mg PE/min.
Storage • Refrigerate. • Do not store at room temperature for longer than 48 hrs. • After dilution, solution is stable for 8 hrs at room temperature or 24 hrs if refrigerated.

▨ IV INCOMPATIBILITY

Midazolam (Versed).

▨ IV COMPATIBILITIES

LORazepam (Ativan), PHENobarbital, potassium chloride.

INDICATIONS/ROUTES/DOSAGE

◀ **ALERT** ▶ 150 mg fosphenytoin yields 100 mg phenytoin. Dosage, concentration solution, infusion rate of fosphenytoin are expressed in terms of phenytoin equivalents (PE).

Status Epilepticus
IV: ADULTS: Loading dose: 15–20 mg PE/kg infused at rate of 100–150 mg PE/min. Follow with maintenance dose of either fosphenytoin or phenytoin.

Nonemergent Seizures
IV, IM: ADULTS: Loading dose: 10–20 mg PE/kg. **Maintenance:** 4–6 mg PE/kg/day in divided doses.

Short-Term Substitution
for Oral Phenytoin
IV, IM: ADULTS: May substitute for oral phenytoin at same total daily dose.

Dosage in Renal/Hepatic Impairment
No dose adjustment.

SIDE EFFECTS

Frequent: Dizziness, paresthesia, tinnitus, pruritus, headache, drowsiness. **Occasional:** Morbilliform rash.

ADVERSE EFFECTS/TOXIC REACTIONS

Toxic fosphenytoin serum concentration may produce ataxia (muscular incoordination), nystagmus (rhythmic oscillation of eyes), diplopia, lethargy, slurred speech, nausea, vomiting, hypotension. As drug level increases, extreme lethargy may progress to coma.

NURSING CONSIDERATIONS

BASELINE ASSESSMENT

Review history of seizure disorder (intensity, frequency, duration, LOC). Initiate seizure precautions. Obtain vital signs, medication history (esp. use of phenytoin, other anticonvulsants). Observe clinically.

INTERVENTION/EVALUATION

Monitor EKG, measure cardiac function, respiratory function, B/P during and immediately following infusion (10–20 min). Discontinue if skin rash appears. Interrupt or decrease rate if hypotension, arrhythmias are detected. Assess pt postinfusion (may feel dizzy, ataxic, drowsy). Monitor free and total dilantin levels (2 hrs after IV infusion or 4 hrs after IM injection).

PATIENT/FAMILY TEACHING

• If noncompliance is cause of acute seizures, discuss and address reasons for noncompliance. • Avoid tasks that require alertness, motor skills until response to drug is established.

---

frovatriptan

froe-va-**trip**-tan
(Frova)

◆CLASSIFICATION

PHARMACOTHERAPEUTIC: Serotonin 5-HT$_1$ receptor agonist. **CLINICAL:** Antimigraine.

USES

Acute treatment of migraine headache with or without aura in adults.

PRECAUTIONS

Contraindications: Hypersensitivity to frovatriptan. Management of basilar or hemiplegic migraine, cerebrovascular or peripheral vascular disease, coronary artery disease, ischemic heart disease (angina pectoris, history of MI, silent ischemia, Prinzmetal's angina), severe hepatic impairment (Child-Pugh grade C), uncontrolled hypertension, use within 24 hrs of ergotamine-containing preparations or another serotonin receptor agonist. **Cautions:** Mild to moderate hepatic impairment, pt profile

suggesting cardiovascular risks. History of seizures or structural brain lesions.

ACTION

Selective agonist for serotonin in cranial arteries causing vasoconstriction and reduction of inflammation. **Therapeutic Effect:** Relieves migraine headache.

PHARMACOKINETICS

Well absorbed after PO administration. Protein binding: 15%. Metabolized in liver. Primarily eliminated in feces (62%), urine (32%). **Half-life:** 26 hrs (increased in hepatic impairment).

⧖ LIFESPAN CONSIDERATIONS

Pregnancy/Lactation: Unknown if drug is excreted in breast milk. **Children:** Safety and efficacy not established. **Elderly:** Not recommended for use in this pt population.

INTERACTIONS

DRUG: Ergotamine-containing medications may produce vasospastic reaction. **SSRI, SNRI (e.g., DULoxetine, FLUoxetine, fluvoxaMINE, PARoxetine, sertraline, venlafaxine)** may produce weakness, hyperreflexia, uncoordination. **HERBAL:** None significant. **FOOD:** None known. **LAB VALUES:** None significant.

AVAILABILITY (Rx)

Tablets: 2.5 mg.

ADMINISTRATION/HANDLING

PO

• Give with fluids as soon as symptoms appear. • Do not break, crush, dissolve, or divide film-coated tablets.

INDICATIONS/ROUTES/DOSAGE

Acute Migraine Headache
PO: ADULTS, ELDERLY: Initially, 2.5 mg. If headache improves but then returns, dose may be repeated after at least 2 hrs. **Maximum:** 7.5 mg/day.

Dosage in Renal Impairment
No dose adjustment.

Dosage in Hepatic Impairment

Mild to moderate impairment: No dose adjustment. **Severe impairment:** Use caution.

SIDE EFFECTS

Occasional (8%–4%): Dizziness, paresthesia, fatigue, flushing. **Rare (3%–2%):** Hot/cold sensation, dry mouth, dyspepsia.

ADVERSE EFFECTS/TOXIC REACTIONS

Cardiac reactions (ischemia, coronary artery vasospasm, MI), noncardiac vasospasm-related reactions (cerebral hemorrhage, CVA) occur rarely, particularly in pts with hypertension, obesity, smokers, diabetes, strong family history of coronary artery disease; males older than 40 yrs; postmenopausal women.

NURSING CONSIDERATIONS

BASELINE ASSESSMENT

Question for history of peripheral vascular disease, renal/hepatic impairment, possibility of pregnancy. Question regarding onset, location, duration of migraine, possible precipitating factors.

INTERVENTION/EVALUATION

Assess for relief of migraine headache, potential for photophobia, phonophobia (sound sensitivity), nausea, vomiting.

PATIENT/FAMILY TEACHING

• Take a single dose as soon as symptoms of an actual migraine attack appear. • Medication is intended to relieve migraine headaches, not to prevent or reduce number of attacks. • Avoid tasks that require alertness, motor skills until response to drug is established. • Immediately report palpitations, pain, tightness in chest or throat, sudden or severe abdominal pain, pain or weakness of extremities.

furosemide

fur-**oh**-se-myde
(Apo-Furosemide ✚, Lasix, Novo-Semide ✚)

■ **BLACK BOX ALERT** ■ Large amounts can lead to profound diuresis with water and electrolyte depletion.

Do not confuse furosemide with famotidine, finasteride, fluconazole, FLUoxetine, loperamide, or torsemide, or Lasix with Lidex, Lovenox, Luvox, or Luxiq.

◆CLASSIFICATION

PHARMACOTHERAPEUTIC: Loop diuretic. **CLINICAL:** Diuretic.

USES

Treatment of edema associated with HF and renal/hepatic disease; acute pulmonary edema. Treatment of hypertension (not recommended as initial treatment).

PRECAUTIONS

Contraindications: Hypersensitivity to furosemide. Anuria. **Cautions:** Hepatic cirrhosis, hepatic coma, severe electrolyte depletion, prediabetes, diabetes, systemic lupus erythematosus. Pts with prostatic hyperplasia/urinary stricture.

ACTION

Enhances excretion of sodium, chloride, potassium by direct action at ascending limb of loop of Henle. **Therapeutic Effect:** Produces diuresis, lowers B/P.

PHARMACOKINETICS

Route	Onset	Peak	Duration
PO	30–60 min	1–2 hrs	6–8 hrs
IV	5 min	20–60 min	2 hrs
IM	30 min	N/A	N/A

Moderately absorbed from GI tract. Protein binding: greater than 98%. Partially metabolized in liver. Primarily excreted in urine (nonrenal clearance increases in severe renal impairment). Not removed

---

✚ Canadian trade name   🗲 Non-Crushable Drug   📋 High Alert drug by hemodialysis. **Half-life:** 30–90 min (increased in renal/hepatic impairment, neonates).

⏳ LIFESPAN CONSIDERATIONS

Pregnancy/Lactation: Crosses placenta. Distributed in breast milk. **Children:** Half-life increased in neonates; may require increased dosage interval. **Elderly:** May be more sensitive to hypotensive, electrolyte effects, developing circulatory collapse, thromboembolic effect. Age-related renal impairment may require dosage adjustment.

INTERACTIONS

DRUG: Amphotericin B, nephrotoxic ototoxic medications (e.g., lisinopril, IV contrast dye, vancomycin) may increase risk of nephrotoxicity, ototoxicity. May increase risk of **lithium** toxicity. **Other medications causing hypokalemia (e.g., HCTZ, laxatives)** may increase risk of hypokalemia. **HERBAL: Ephedra, ginseng, yohimbe** may worsen hypertension. **Garlic** may increase antihypertensive effect. **FOOD:** None known. **LAB VALUES:** May increase serum glucose, BUN, uric acid. May decrease serum calcium, chloride, magnesium, potassium, sodium.

AVAILABILITY (Rx)

Injection Solution: 10 mg/mL. **Oral Solution:** 10 mg/mL, 40 mg/5 mL. **Tablets:** 20 mg, 40 mg, 80 mg.

ADMINISTRATION/HANDLING

 IV

Rate of Administration• May give undiluted but is compatible with D₅W or 0.9% NaCl. • May be diluted for infusion to 1–2 mg/mL (**maximum:** 10 mg/mL). • Administer each 40 mg or fraction by IV push over 1–2 min. Do not exceed administration rate of 4 mg/min for short-term intermittent infusion.

Storage • Solution appears clear, colorless. • Discard yellow solutions. • Stable for 24 hrs at room temperature when mixed with 0.9% NaCl or D₅W.

IM

• Temporary pain at injection site may be noted.

PO

• Administer on empty stomach. • Give with food to avoid GI upset, preferably with breakfast (may prevent nocturia). • Food may decrease diuretic effect.

⚕ IV INCOMPATIBILITIES

Ciprofloxacin (Cipro), diltiaZEM (Cardizem), DOBUTamine (Dobutrex), DOPamine (Intropin), DOXOrubicin (Adriamycin), droperidol (Inapsine), esmolol (Brevibloc), famotidine (Pepcid), filgrastim (Neupogen), fluconazole (Diflucan), gemcitabine (Gemzar), gentamicin (Garamycin), IDArubicin (Idamycin), labetalol (Trandate), metoclopramide (Reglan), midazolam (Versed), milrinone (Primacor), niCARdipine (Cardene), ondansetron (Zofran), quiNIDine, thiopental (Pentothal), vinBLAStine (Velban), vinCRIStine (Oncovin), vinorelbine (Navelbine).

⚕ IV COMPATIBILITIES

Amiodarone (Cordarone), bumetanide (Bumex), calcium gluconate, cimetidine (Tagamet), dexmedetomidine (Precedex), heparin, HYDROmorphone (Dilaudid), lidocaine, lipids, morphine, nitroglycerin, norepinephrine (Levophed), potassium chloride, propofol (Diprivan).

INDICATIONS/ROUTES/DOSAGE

Edema, HF
PO: ADULTS, ELDERLY: Initially, 20–80 mg/dose; may increase by 20–40 mg/dose q6–8h. May titrate up to 600 mg/day in severe edematous states. **CHILDREN:** Initially, 2 mg/kg/dose. May increase by 1–2 mg/kg/dose at 6–8 hr intervals. **Maximum:** 6 mg/kg/dose. **NEONATES:** 1 mg/kg/dose 1–2 times/day.
IV, IM: ADULTS, ELDERLY: 20–40 mg/dose; may increase by 20 mg/dose q1–2h. **Maximum single dose:** 160–200 mg. **CHILDREN:** Initially, 1 mg/kg/dose.

May increase by 1 mg/kg/dose no sooner than 2 hrs after previous dose. **Maximum:** 6 mg/kg/dose. **NEONATES:** 1–2 mg/kg/dose q12–24h.

IV Infusion: ADULTS, ELDERLY: Loading dose bolus of 40–100 mg over 1–2 min, followed by infusion of 10–40 mg/hr; repeat loading dose before increasing infusion rate. **Maximum:** 80–160 mg/hr. **CHILDREN:** 0.05 mg/kg/hr; titrate to desired effect. **NEONATES:** Initially, 0.2 mg/kg/hr. May increase by 0.1 mg/kg/hr q12–24h. **Maximum:** 0.4 mg/kg/hr.

Hypertension
PO: **ADULTS, ELDERLY:** 40 mg twice daily

Dosage in Renal Impairment
Avoid use in oliguric states.

Dosage in Hepatic Impairment
No dose adjustment. Decreased effect, increased sensitivity to hypokalemia/volume depletion in cirrhosis.

SIDE EFFECTS

Expected: Increased urinary frequency/volume. **Frequent:** Nausea, dyspepsia, abdominal cramps, diarrhea or constipation, electrolyte disturbances. **Occasional:** Dizziness, light-headedness, headache, blurred vision, paresthesia, photosensitivity, rash, fatigue, bladder spasm, restlessness, diaphoresis. **Rare:** Flank pain.

ADVERSE EFFECTS/TOXIC REACTIONS

Vigorous diuresis may lead to profound water loss/electrolyte depletion, resulting in hypokalemia, hyponatremia, dehydration. Sudden volume depletion may result in increased risk of thrombosis, circulatory collapse, sudden death. Acute hypotensive episodes may occur, sometimes several days after beginning therapy. Ototoxicity (deafness, vertigo, tinnitus) may occur, esp. in pts with severe renal impairment. Can exacerbate diabetes mellitus, systemic lupus erythematosus, gout, pancreatitis. Blood dyscrasias have been reported.

NURSING CONSIDERATIONS

BASELINE ASSESSMENT

Check vital signs, esp. B/P, pulse, for hypotension before administration. Assess baseline renal function, serum electrolytes, esp. serum sodium, potassium. Assess skin turgor, mucous membranes for hydration status; observe for edema. Assess muscle strength, mental status. Note skin temperature, moisture. Obtain baseline weight. Initiate I&O monitoring. Auscultate lung sounds. In pts with hepatic cirrhosis and ascites, consider giving initial doses in a hospital setting.

INTERVENTION/EVALUATION

Monitor B/P, vital signs, serum electrolytes, I&O, weight. Note extent of diuresis. Watch for symptoms of electrolyte imbalance: Hypokalemia may result in changes in muscle strength, tremor, muscle cramps, altered mental status, cardiac arrhythmias; hyponatremia may result in confusion, thirst, cold/clammy skin. Consider potassium supplementation if hypokalemia occurs.

PATIENT/FAMILY TEACHING

• Expect increased frequency, volume of urination. • Report palpitations, signs of electrolyte imbalances (noted previously), hearing abnormalities (sense of fullness in ears, tinnitus). • Eat foods high in potassium such as whole grains (cereals), legumes, meat, bananas, apricots, orange juice, potatoes (white, sweet), raisins. • Avoid sunlight, sunlamps.

F

gabapentin

ga-ba-**pen**-tin
(Apo-Gabapentin ✦, Fanatrex
FusePaq, Gralise, Horizant, Neurontin)
**Do not confuse Neurontin with
Motrin, Neoral, nitrofurantoin,
Noroxin, or Zarontin.**

◆CLASSIFICATION

PHARMACOTHERAPEUTIC: Gamma-
aminobutyric acid analogue. **CLINICAL:**
Anticonvulsant, antineuralgic.

USES

Neurontin: Adjunct in treatment of partial seizures (with or without secondary
generalized seizures) in children 13 yrs
and older and adults. Adjunct to treatment of partial seizures in children 3–12
yrs; management of postherpetic neuralgia (PHN). **Horizant:** Treatment of moderate to severe primary restless legs
syndrome (RLS), PHN. **Gralise:** Management of PHN. **OFF-LABEL:** Treatment of
neuropathic pain, diabetic peripheral
neuropathy, vasomotor symptoms, fibromyalgia, postoperative pain adjunct.

PRECAUTIONS

Contraindications: Hypersensitivity to gabapentin. **Cautions:** Severe renal impairment, elderly, history of suicidal behavior;
substance abuse.

ACTION

Binds to gabapentin binding sites in brain
and may modulate release of excitatory
neurotransmitters, which participates in
epileptogenesis and nociception. **Therapeutic Effect:** Reduces seizure activity,
neuropathic pain.

PHARMACOKINETICS

Well absorbed from GI tract (not affected by
food). Protein binding: less than 5%. Widely
distributed. Crosses blood-brain barrier.
Primarily excreted unchanged in urine. Removed by hemodialysis. **Half-life:** 5–7 hrs
(increased in renal impairment, elderly).

⧗ LIFESPAN CONSIDERATIONS

Pregnancy/Lactation: Crosses placenta,
excreted in breast milk. **Children:** Safety
and efficacy not established in pts 3 yrs and
younger. **Elderly:** Age-related renal impairment may require dosage adjustment.

INTERACTIONS

DRUG: Antacids decrease absorption.
**Benzodiazepines (e.g., ALPRAZolam,
LORazepam), opiates (e.g., morphine,
fentaNYL), other CNS depressants
(e.g., carisoprodol, zolpidem)** may
increase CNS depression. **HERBAL: Evening primrose** may decrease seizure
threshold. **Gotu kola, kava kava, St.
John's wort, valerian** may increase
CNS depression. **FOOD:** None known.
LAB VALUES: May alter serum glucose;
WBC count. May increase serum alkaline
phosphatase, ALT, AST, bilirubin.

AVAILABILITY (Rx)

Capsules: 100 mg, 300 mg, 400 mg.
Oral Solution: 250 mg/5 mL. **Oral Sus-
pension (Fanatrex FusePaq):** 25 mg/mL.
Tablets: 600 mg, 800 mg. **Tablets
(Gralise):** 300 mg, 600 mg.

▨ **Tablets, Extended-Release:** (Horizant)
300 mg, 600 mg.

ADMINISTRATION/HANDLING

PO
Immediate-Release/Solution • Give
without regard to meals; may give with
food to avoid, reduce GI upset. • Swallow extended-release tablets whole; do not
break, crush, dissolve, or divide. Take with
evening meal.

INDICATIONS/ROUTES/DOSAGE

Note: When given 3 times/day, maximum time between doses should not exceed 12 hrs. If treatment is discontinued
or anticonvulsant therapy is added, do so
gradually over at least 1 wk (reduces risk
of loss of seizure control).

Adjunctive Therapy for Seizure Control
**PO: ADULTS, ELDERLY, CHILDREN 13 YRS
AND OLDER:** Initially, 300 mg 3 times/day.

G

May titrate dosage. Range: 900–1,800 mg/day in 3 divided doses. **Maximum:** 3,600 mg/day. **CHILDREN 3–12 YRS:** Initially, 10–15 mg/kg/day in 3 divided doses. May titrate up to 25–35 mg/kg/day (for children 5–12 yrs) and 40 mg/kg/day (for children 3–4 yrs). **Maximum:** 50 mg/kg/day.

Adjunctive Therapy for Neuropathic Pain
PO: ADULTS, ELDERLY: Initially, 100 mg 3 times/day; may increase by 300 mg/day at wkly intervals. **Maximum:** 3,600 mg/day in 3 divided doses. **CHILDREN:** Initially, 5 mg/kg/dose at bedtime, followed by 5 mg/kg/dose for 2 doses on day 2, then 5 mg/kg/dose for 3 doses on day 3. **Maximum:** 300 mg. Range: 8–35 mg/kg/day in 3 divided doses.

Postherpetic Neuralgia
PO: ADULTS, ELDERLY: *(Neurontin):* 300 mg once on day 1, 300 mg twice daily on day 2, and 300 mg 3 times/day on day 3 as needed. Range: 1,800–3,600 mg/day. *(Gralise):* 300 mg once on day 1; 600 mg once on day 2; 900 mg once daily on days 3–6; 1,200 mg once daily on days 7–10; 1,500 mg once daily on days 11–14; then 1,800 mg once daily. *(Horizant):* 600 mg once daily in AM for 3 days, then increase to 600 mg twice daily.

RLS
PO: ADULTS, ELDERLY (HORIZANT): 600 mg once daily at about 5 PM.

Dosage in Renal Impairment
Dosage and frequency are modified based on creatinine clearance:

Dosage in Hepatic Impairment
No dose adjustment.

SIDE EFFECTS

Frequent (19%–10%): Fatigue, drowsiness, dizziness, ataxia. **Occasional (8%–3%):** Nystagmus, tremor, diplopia, rhinitis, weight gain, peripheral edema. **Rare (less than 2%):** Anxiety, dysarthria, memory loss, dyspepsia, pharyngitis, myalgia.

ADVERSE EFFECTS/TOXIC REACTIONS

Abrupt withdrawal may increase seizure frequency, increase risk of suicidal behavior/thoughts. Overdosage may result in slurred speech, drowsiness, lethargy, diarrhea. Drug reaction with eosinophilia and systemic symptoms (multiorgan hypersensitivity) was reported. Hypersensitivity reaction, including anaphylaxis and angioedema, can occur at any time.

NURSING CONSIDERATIONS

BASELINE ASSESSMENT

Review history of seizure disorder (type, onset, intensity, frequency, duration, LOC). Assess location, intensity of neuralgia/neuropathic pain. Question history of renal impairment.

INTERVENTION/EVALUATION

Provide safety measures as needed. Monitor seizure frequency/duration, renal function, weight, behavior in children. Monitor for signs/symptoms of depression, suicidal tendencies, other unusual behavior; hypersensitivity reaction.

Creatinine Clearance	Neurontin Dosage (Immediate-release)	Gralise Dosage (Extended-release)	Horizant Dosage	
			RLS	**PHN**
30–59 mL/min	200–700 mg q12h	600–1,800 mg once/day	300–600 mg/day	Same
16–29 mL/min	200–700 mg once daily	Not recommended	300 mg/day	Same
Less than 16 mL/min	100–300 mg once daily	Not recommended	300 mg q48 h	Same
Hemodialysis	125–350 mg following HD	Not recommended	Not recommended	300–600 mg following HD

♣ Canadian trade name   🐢 Non-Crushable Drug   High Alert drug

G

PATIENT/FAMILY TEACHING

• Use only as prescribed; do not abruptly stop taking drug (may increase seizure frequency). • Avoid tasks that require alertness, motor skills until response to drug is established. • Avoid alcohol. • Carry identification card/bracelet to note seizure disorder/anticonvulsant therapy. • Report suicidal ideation, depression, unusual behavioral changes (esp. with changes in dosage), worsening of seizure activity or loss of seizure control. Seek medical attention for allergic reactions including difficulty breathing, coughing, wheezing, throat tightness, swelling of face or tongue.

galantamine

gal-**an**-ta-meen
(Razadyne, Razadyne ER, Reminyl ER ✹)
Do not confuse Razadyne with Rozerem, or Reminyl with Amaryl.

◆CLASSIFICATION

PHARMACOTHERAPEUTIC: Cholinesterase inhibitor. **CLINICAL:** Antidementia.

USES

Treatment of mild to moderate dementia of Alzheimer's type. **OFF-LABEL:** Diabetic neuropathy, neuropathic pain, postoperative pain (adjunct), hot flashes.

PRECAUTIONS

Contraindications: Hypersensitivity to galantamine. **Cautions:** Moderate renal/hepatic impairment (not recommended in severe impairment), history of ulcer disease, asthma, COPD, bladder outflow obstruction, supraventricular cardiac conduction conditions (except with pacemaker), seizure disorder, concurrent medications that slow cardiac conduction through SA or AV node. Elderly with low body weight and/or serious co-morbidities.

ACTION

Elevates acetylcholine concentrations by slowing degeneration of acetylcholine released by still intact cholinergic neurons. May increase serotonin levels. **Therapeutic Effect:** Slows progression of Alzheimer's disease.

PHARMACOKINETICS

Rapidly, completely absorbed from GI tract. Protein binding: 18%. Distributed to blood cells; binds to plasma proteins, mainly albumin. Metabolized in liver. Excreted in urine. **Half-life:** 7 hrs.

⏳ LIFESPAN CONSIDERATIONS

Pregnancy/Lactation: Unknown if drug crosses placenta or is distributed in breast milk. **Children:** Not prescribed for this pt population. **Elderly:** No age-related precautions noted, but use is not recommended in those with severe hepatic/renal impairment (CrCl less than 9 mL/min).

INTERACTIONS

DRUG: Anticholinergic agents may decrease levels/effects. **HERBAL: St. John's wort** may decrease concentration. **FOOD:** None known. **LAB VALUES:** None significant.

AVAILABILITY (Rx)

Oral Solution (Razadyne): 4 mg/mL. **Tablets (Razadyne):** 4 mg, 8 mg, 12 mg.

💊 **Capsules (Extended-Release [Razadyne ER]):** 8 mg, 16 mg, 24 mg.

ADMINISTRATION/HANDLING

PO

• Give tablet or solution with morning and evening meals. • Mix oral solution with nonalcoholic beverage, take immediately. • Extended-release capsule should be given with breakfast. Swallow whole. Do not break, crush, cut, or divide.

INDICATIONS/ROUTES/DOSAGE

Note: If therapy interrupted for 3 or more days, restart at lowest dose; then increase gradually.

Alzheimer's Disease

PO *(Immediate-Release Tablets, Oral Solution):* **ADULTS, ELDERLY:** Initially, 4 mg twice daily (8 mg/day). After a minimum of 4 wks (if well tolerated), may increase to 8 mg twice daily (16 mg/day). After another 4 wks, may increase to 12 mg twice daily (24 mg/day). Range: 16–24 mg/day in 2 divided doses.

PO *(Extended-Release):* **ADULTS, ELDERLY:** Initially, 8 mg once daily for 4 wks; then increase to 16 mg once daily for 4 wks or longer. If tolerated, may increase to 24 mg once daily. Range: 16–24 mg once daily.

Dosage in Renal/Hepatic Impairment

Moderate impairment: Maximum dosage is 16 mg/day. **Severe impairment:** Not recommended.

SIDE EFFECTS

Frequent (17%–7%): Nausea, vomiting, diarrhea, anorexia, weight loss. **Occasional (5%–4%):** Abdominal pain, insomnia, depression, headache, dizziness, fatigue, rhinitis. **Rare (less than 3%):** Tremors, constipation, confusion, cough, anxiety, urinary incontinence.

ADVERSE EFFECTS/TOXIC REACTIONS

Overdose may cause cholinergic crisis (increased salivation, lacrimation, urination, defecation, bradycardia, hypotension, muscle weakness). Treatment aimed at generally supportive measures, use of anticholinergics (e.g., atropine).

NURSING CONSIDERATIONS

BASELINE ASSESSMENT

Assess cognitive, behavioral, functional deficits of pt. Obtain baseline serum renal function, LFT. Question history as listed in Precautions, esp. cardiac conduction disorders.

INTERVENTION/EVALUATION

Monitor cognitive, behavioral, functional status of pt. Evaluate EKG, periodic rhythm strips in pts with underlying arrhythmias. Assess for evidence of GI disturbances (nausea, vomiting, diarrhea, anorexia, weight loss).

PATIENT/FAMILY TEACHING

• Take with meals (reduces risk of nausea). • Avoid tasks that require alertness, motor skills until response to drug is established. • Report persistent GI disturbances, excessive salivation, diaphoresis, excessive tearing, excessive fatigue, insomnia, depression, dizziness, increased muscle weakness, palpitations.

G

ganciclovir

gan-**sye**-kloe-veer
(Cytovene)

■ **BLACK BOX ALERT** ■ Toxicity presents as neutropenia, thrombocytopenia, anemia. Studies suggest carcinogenic and teratogenic effects, inhibition of spermatogenesis. **Do not confuse Cytovene with Cytosar, or ganciclovir with famciclovir or acyclovir.**

◆CLASSIFICATION

PHARMACOTHERAPEUTIC: Synthetic nucleoside. **CLINICAL:** Antiviral.

USES

Treatment of cytomegalovirus (CMV) retinitis in immunocompromised pts (e.g., HIV), prophylaxis of CMV infection in transplant pts. **OFF-LABEL:** CMV retinitis.

PRECAUTIONS

Contraindications: Hypersensitivity to acyclovir, ganciclovir. **Cautions:** Neutropenia, thrombocytopenia, renal impairment, children (long-term safety not determined due to potential for long-term carcinogenic, adverse reproductive effects), pregnancy. Absolute neutrophil count less than 500 cells/mm^3, platelet count less than 25,000 cells/mm^3.

ACTION

Competes with viral DNA polymerase and incorporation into growing viral DNA chains. **Therapeutic Effect:** Interferes with DNA synthesis, viral replication.

PHARMACOKINETICS

Widely distributed (including CSF and ocular tissue). Protein binding: 1%–2%. Excreted primarily in urine. Removed by hemodialysis. **Half-life:** 1.7–5.8 hrs (increased in renal impairment).

⧖ LIFESPAN CONSIDERATIONS

Pregnancy/Lactation: Avoid pregnancy. Female pts of reproductive potential should use effective contraception during treatment and for 30 days after discontinuation; male pts should use a barrier contraceptive during and for at least 90 days after discontinuation. Do not breastfeed. May resume breastfeeding no sooner than 72 hrs after the last dose. **Children:** Safety and efficacy not established in pts younger than 12 yrs. **Elderly:** Age-related renal impairment may require dosage adjustment.

INTERACTIONS

DRUG: Bone marrow depressants may increase myelosuppression. **Imipenem** may increase risk for seizures. **HERBAL:** None significant. **FOOD:** None known. **LAB VALUES:** May increase serum alkaline phosphatase, ALT, AST, bilirubin, BUN, creatinine.

AVAILABILITY (Rx)

Injection, Powder for Reconstitution (Cytovene): 500 mg.

ADMINISTRATION/HANDLING

 IV

Reconstitution • Reconstitute 500-mg vial with 10 mL Sterile Water for Injection to provide concentration of 50 mg/mL; do **not** use Bacteriostatic Water (contains parabens, which is incompatible with ganciclovir). • Further dilute with 100 mL D_5W, 0.9% NaCl to provide a concentration of 10 mg/mL or less for infusion.
Rate of Administration • Administer only by IV infusion over at least 1 hr. • Do not give by IV push or rapid IV infusion (increases risk of toxicity). Flush line with 0.9% NaCl before and after administration.

Storage • Store vials at room temperature. Do not refrigerate. • Reconstituted solution in vial is stable for 12 hrs at room temperature. • After dilution, use within 24 hrs. • Discard if precipitate forms, discoloration occurs. • Avoid exposure to skin, eyes, mucous membranes. • Use latex gloves, safety glasses during preparation/handling of solution. • Avoid inhalation. • If solution contacts skin or mucous membranes, wash thoroughly with soap and water; rinse eyes thoroughly with plain water.

▦ IV INCOMPATIBILITIES

Aldesleukin (Proleukin), amifostine (Ethyol), aztreonam (Azactam), cefepime (Maxipime), cytarabine (ARA-C), DOXOrubicin (Adriamycin), fludarabine (Fludara), foscarnet (Foscavir), gemcitabine (Gemzar), ondansetron (Zofran), piperacillin and tazobactam (Zosyn), sargramostim (Leukine), vinorelbine (Navelbine).

▦ IV COMPATIBILITIES

Amphotericin B, enalapril (Vasotec), filgrastim (Neupogen), fluconazole (Diflucan), granisetron (Kytril), propofol (Diprivan).

INDICATIONS/ROUTES/DOSAGE

Cytomegalovirus (CMV) Retinitis
IV: ADULTS, CHILDREN 3 MOS AND OLDER: 5 mg/kg/dose q12h for 14–21 days, then 5 mg/kg/day as a single daily dose or 6 mg/kg 5 days/wk.

Prevention of CMV in Transplant Pts
IV: ADULTS, CHILDREN: 5 mg/kg/dose q12h for 7–14 days, then 5 mg/kg/day as a single daily dose or 6 mg/kg 5 days/wk. Duration dependent on clinical condition and degree of immunosuppression.

Congenital CMV
IV: NEONATES: 6 mg/kg/dose q12h for 6 wks (if HIV positive, longer duration may be considered).

Dosage in Renal Impairment
Dosage and frequency are modified based on creatinine clearance (see table).

| Creatinine Clearance | Dosage | |
	IV Induction	IV Maintenance
50–69 mL/min	2.5 mg/kg q12h	2.5 mg/kg q24h
25–49 mL/min	2.5 mg/kg q24h	1.25 mg/kg q24h
10–24 mL/min	1.25 mg/kg q24h	0.625 mg/kg q24h
Less than 10 mL/min	1.25 mg/kg 3 times/wk	0.625 mg/kg 3 times/wk
Hemodialysis (give after HD on HD days)	1.25 mg/kg q48–72h	0.625 mg/kg q48–72h
Peritoneal dialysis	1.25 mg/kg 3 times/wk	0.625 mg/kg 3 times/wk
Continuous renal replacement therapy		
Continuous venovenous hemofiltration	2.5 mg/kg q24h	1.25 mg/kg q24h
Continuous venovenous hemodialysis/ continuous venovenous hemodiafiltration	2.5 mg/kg q12h	2.5 mg/kg q24h

Dosage in Hepatic Impairment
No dose adjustment.

SIDE EFFECTS

Frequent (41%–13%): Diarrhea, fever, nausea, abdominal pain, vomiting. **Occasional (11%–6%):** Diaphoresis, infection, paresthesia, flatulence, pruritus. **Rare (4%–2%):** Headache, stomatitis, dyspepsia, phlebitis.

ADVERSE EFFECTS/TOXIC REACTIONS

Hematologic toxicity occurs commonly: leukopenia (41%–29% of pts), anemia (25%–19% of pts). Intraocular implant occasionally results in visual acuity loss, vitreous hemorrhage, retinal detachment. GI hemorrhage occurs rarely.

NURSING CONSIDERATIONS

BASELINE ASSESSMENT

Obtain baseline CBC, BMP, LFT. Perform baseline ophthalmic exam. Obtain specimens for support of differential diagnosis (urine, feces, blood, throat) since retinal infection is usually due to hematogenous dissemination.

INTERVENTION/EVALUATION

Monitor I&O, ensure adequate hydration (minimum 1,500 mL/24 hrs). Diligently evaluate hematology reports for neutropenia, thrombocytopenia, leukopenia. Obtain periodic ophthalmic examinations. Question pt regarding visual acuity, therapeutic improvement, complications. Assess for rash, pruritus.

PATIENT/FAMILY TEACHING

• Ganciclovir provides suppression, not cure, of cytomegalovirus (CMV) retinitis. • Frequent blood tests, eye exams are necessary during therapy due to toxic nature of drug. • Report any new symptom promptly. • May temporarily or permanently inhibit sperm production in men, suppress fertility in women. • Barrier contraception should be used during and for 90 days after therapy due to mutagenic potential.

gefitinib

ge-fi-ti-nib
(Iressa)
Do not confuse gefitinib with erlotinib, dasatinib, imatinib, or lapatinib.

◆CLASSIFICATION

PHARMACOTHERAPEUTIC: Tyrosine kinase inhibitor. **CLINICAL:** Antineoplastic.

G

USES

First-line treatment of metastatic non–small-cell lung cancer (NSCLC) whose tumors have epidermal growth factor receptor (EGFR) exon 19 deletions or exon 21 substitution mutations.

PRECAUTIONS

Contraindications: Hypersensitivity to gefitinib. **Cautions:** Hepatic impairment, lung disease, ocular disease, concurrent administration of CYP3A4 inducers and inhibitors.

ACTION

Inhibits epidermal growth factor receptor–tyrosine kinase (EGFR-TK), a key driver in tumor cell growth. Interrupts angiogenesis and metastasis. **Therapeutic Effect:** Inhibits tumor cell proliferation and survival.

PHARMACOKINETICS

Slowly absorbed following PO administration. Peak plasma levels in 3–7 hrs. Protein binding: 90%. Metabolized in liver. Excreted primarily in feces (86%). **Half-life:** 48 hrs.

⧗ LIFESPAN CONSIDERATIONS

Pregnancy/Lactation: Avoid pregnancy. Use effective contraception during treatment and for at least 2 wks after discontinuation. Unknown if crosses placenta or distributed in breast milk. Must either discontinue breastfeeding or discontinue therapy. **Children:** Safety and efficacy not established in those younger than 18 yrs. **Elderly:** No age-related precautions noted.

INTERACTIONS

DRUG: **CYP3A4 inhibitors** (e.g., **clarithromycin, ketoconazole**) may increase concentration. **CYP3A4 inducers** (e.g., **phenytoin, rifAMPin**) may decrease concentration. **H_2 antagonists** (e.g., **famotidine**), **proton pump inhibitors** (e.g., **pantoprazole**) may decrease concentration. May increase bleeding risk with **warfarin**. **HERBAL:** St. John's wort may decrease effectiveness. **FOOD:** Avoid grapefruit products.

LAB VALUES: May increase serum AST, ALT, bilirubin, urine protein.

AVAILABILITY (Rx)

Tablets: 250 mg.

ADMINISTRATION/HANDLING

• May give without regard to meals. • Avoid grapefruit products. • Do not crush or cut. Swallow whole or administer as dispersion in water. Gently swirl glass for up to 20 min and immediately ingest once dispersed.

INDICATIONS/ROUTES/DOSAGE

NSCLC
PO: ADULTS, ELDERLY: 250 mg once daily, with or without food. (Concurrent CYP3A4 inducers: consider increasing dose to 500 mg once daily.) Continue until disease progression or unacceptable toxicity.

Dosage in Renal Impairment
No dose adjustment.

Dosage in Hepatic Impairment
Mild impairment: No dose adjustment. **Moderate to severe impairment:** Use with caution.

SIDE EFFECTS

Frequent (47%–15%): Skin reactions (e.g., acne, pruritus, rash, xeroderma), diarrhea, decreased appetite, vomiting. **Occasional** (7%–5%): Stomatitis, conjunctivitis, blepharitis, dry eye, nail disorders (e.g., infection).

ADVERSE EFFECTS/TOXIC REACTIONS

Hepatotoxicity, interstitial lung disease, gastrointestinal perforation, severe or persistent diarrhea, ocular disorders including keratitis, bullous and exfoliative skin disorders.

NURSING CONSIDERATIONS

BASELINE ASSESSMENT
Obtain baseline CBC with differential, serum chemistries, LFT, thyroid function test, PT/INT (if taking warfarin), EGFR

mutation serostatus. Question possibility of pregnancy or plans of breastfeeding. Receive full medication history including vitamins, minerals, herbal products. Assess visual acuity.

INTERVENTION/EVALUATION

Assess vital signs, oxygen saturation routinely. Routinely monitor CBC with differential, LFT. Worsening cough, fever, or shortness of breath may indicate interstitial lung disease. Consider ophthalmologic evaluation for vision changes. Monitor for bruising, hematuria, jaundice, right upper abdominal pain, weight loss, or acute infection (fever, diaphoresis, lethargy, productive cough). Monitor for skin lesions.

PATIENT/FAMILY TEACHING

• Blood levels will be drawn routinely. Report urine changes, bloody or clay-colored stools, upper abdominal pain, nausea, vomiting, bruising, fever, cough, difficulty breathing. • Immediately report any newly prescribed medications, suspected pregnancy, vision changes (eye pain, bleeding, sensitivity to light), or persistent diarrhea, dehydration. • Avoid alcohol. • Avoid grapefruit products.

gemcitabine [HIGH ALERT]

jem-**sye**-ta-been
(Gemzar)
Do not confuse gemcitabine with gemtuzumab, Gemzar with Zinecard.

◆CLASSIFICATION

PHARMACOTHERAPEUTIC: Antimetabolite. **CLINICAL:** Antineoplastic.

USES

Metastatic breast cancer in combination with PACLitaxel. Treatment of locally advanced (stage II, III) or metastatic (stage IV) adenocarcinoma of pancreas. In combination with CISplatin for treatment of locally advanced or metastatic non–small-cell lung cancer (NSCLC). Treatment of advanced ovarian cancer (in combination with CARBOplatin) that has relapsed. **OFF-LABEL:** Treatment of biliary tract carcinoma, bladder carcinoma, germ cell tumors (e.g., testicular), Hodgkin's lymphoma, non-Hodgkin's lymphoma, cervical cancer.

PRECAUTIONS

Contraindications: Hypersensitivity to gemcitabine. **Cautions:** Renal/hepatic impairment, pregnancy, elderly, concurrent radiation therapy, impaired pulmonary function.

ACTION

Inhibits ribonucleotide reductase, the enzyme necessary for catalyzing DNA synthesis. Cell-cycle specific for the S-phase. **Therapeutic Effect:** Produces death of cells undergoing DNA synthesis.

PHARMACOKINETICS

Not extensively distributed after IV infusion (increased with length of infusion). Protein binding: less than 10%. Metabolized intracellularly by nucleoside kinases. Excreted primarily in urine. **Half-life:** Influenced by duration of infusion. Infusion 1 hr or less: 42–94 min; infusion 3–4 hrs: 4–10.5 hrs.

⧖ LIFESPAN CONSIDERATIONS

Pregnancy/Lactation: If possible, avoid use during pregnancy, esp. first trimester. May cause fetal harm. Unknown if distributed in breast milk. Breastfeeding not recommended. **Children:** Safety and efficacy not established. **Elderly:** Increased risk of hematologic toxicity.

INTERACTIONS

DRUG: Bone marrow depressants may increase risk of myelosuppression. **Live virus vaccines** may potentiate virus replication, increase vaccine side effects, decrease pt's antibody response to vaccine. **HERBAL: Echinacea** may decrease effects. **FOOD:** None known. **LAB VALUES:** May increase serum BUN, alkaline phosphatase, bilirubin, creatinine, ALT, AST. May decrease Hgb, Hct, leukocyte count, platelet count.

AVAILABILITY (Rx)

Injection, Powder for Reconstitution: 200-mg, 1-g, 2-g vials. **Injection, Solution:** 38 mg/mL.

ADMINISTRATION/HANDLING

 IV

Reconstitution • Use gloves when handling/preparing. • Reconstitute with 0.9% NaCl injection without preservative to provide concentration of 38 mg/mL. • Shake to dissolve. Further diluted with 50–500 mL 0.9% NaCl to a concentration as low as 0.1 mg/mL.
Rate of Administration • Infuse over 30 min. • Infusion time greater than 60 min increases toxicity.
Storage • Store at room temperature (refrigeration may cause crystallization). • Reconstituted vials or diluted solutions are stable for 24 hrs at room temperature. Do not refrigerate.

▓ IV INCOMPATIBILITIES

Acyclovir (Zovirax), amphotericin B (Fungizone), cefotaxime (Claforan), furosemide (Lasix), ganciclovir (Cytovene), imipenem/cilastatin (Primaxin), irinotecan (Camptosar), methotrexate, methylPREDNISolone (SOLU-Medrol), mitoMYcin (Mutamycin), piperacillin/tazobactam (Zosyn), prochlorperazine (Compazine).

▓ IV COMPATIBILITIES

Bumetanide (Bumex), calcium gluconate, dexamethasone (Decadron), diphenhydrAMINE (Benadryl), DOBUTamine (Dobutrex), DOPamine (Intropin), granisetron (Kytril), heparin, hydrocortisone (Solu-Cortef), LORazepam (Ativan), ondansetron (Zofran), potassium chloride.

INDICATIONS/ROUTES/DOSAGE

◀**ALERT**▶ Dosage is individualized based on clinical response, tolerance to adverse effects. When used in combination therapy, consult specific protocols for optimum dosage, sequence of drug administration.

Breast Cancer
IV: ADULTS, ELDERLY: (in combination with PACLitaxel): 1,250 mg/m² over 30 min on days 1 and 8 of each 21-day cycle.

Non–Small-Cell Lung Cancer (NSCLC)
IV: ADULTS, ELDERLY, CHILDREN: (in combination with CISplatin): 1,000 mg/m² on days 1, 8, and 15, repeated every 28 days; or 1,250 mg/m² on days 1 and 8. Repeat every 21 days.

Ovarian Cancer
IV: ADULTS, ELDERLY: (in combination with CARBOplatin): 1,000 mg/m² on days 1 and 8 of each 21-day cycle.

Pancreatic Cancer
IV: ADULTS: 1,000 mg/m² once wkly for up to 7 wks or until toxicity necessitates decreasing dosage or withholding the dose, followed by 1 wk of rest. Subsequent cycles should consist of once-wkly dose for 3 consecutive wks out of every 4 wks.

Dosage in Renal/Hepatic Impairment
No dose adjustment.

Dosage Reduction Guidelines
Pancreatic Cancer, Non–Small-Cell Lung Cancer (NSCLC)
Dosage adjustments should be based on granulocyte count and platelet count, as follows:

Absolute Granulocyte Counts (cells/mm³)	Platelet Count (cells/mm³)	% of Full Dose
1,000	100,000	100
500–999	50,000–99,000	75
Less than 500 or	Less than 50,000	Hold

Breast Cancer Absolute Granulocyte Counts (cells/mm³)	Platelet Count (cells/mm³)	% of Full Dose
Equal to or greater than 1,200 and	Greater than 75,000	100
1,000–1,199 or	50,000–75,000	75
700–999 and	Equal to or greater than 50,000	50
Less than 700 or	Less than 50,000	Hold

Ovarian Cancer Absolute Granulocyte Counts (cells/mm³)	Platelet Count (cells/mm³)	% of Full Dose
1,500 or greater and	100,000 or greater	100
1,000–1,499 and/or	75,000–99,999	50
Less than 1,000 and/or	Less than 75,000	Hold

SIDE EFFECTS

Frequent (69%–20%): Nausea, vomiting, generalized pain, fever, mild to moderate pruritic rash, mild to moderate dyspnea, constipation, peripheral edema. **Occasional (19%–10%):** Diarrhea, petechiae, alopecia, stomatitis, infection, drowsiness, paresthesia. **Rare:** Diaphoresis, rhinitis, insomnia, malaise.

ADVERSE EFFECTS/TOXIC REACTIONS

Severe myelosuppression (anemia, thrombocytopenia, leukopenia) occurs commonly.

NURSING CONSIDERATIONS

BASELINE ASSESSMENT

Obtain baseline CBC, renal function, LFT, and periodically thereafter (CBC, platelets before each dose). Drug should be suspended or dosage modified if myelosuppression is detected. Question history of pulmonary disease, hepatic/renal impairment. Offer emotional support.

INTERVENTION/EVALUATION

Assess all lab results prior to each dose. Monitor for dyspnea, fever, pruritic rash, dehydration. Assess oral mucosa for erythema, ulceration at inner margin of lips, sore throat, difficulty swallowing (stomatitis). Assess skin for rash. Monitor daily pattern of bowel activity, stool consistency. Provide antiemetics as needed.

PATIENT/FAMILY TEACHING

• Avoid crowds, exposure to infection. • Maintain strict oral hygiene. • Promptly report fever, sore throat, signs of local infection, easy bruising, rash, yellowing of skin or eyes. • Report nausea or vomiting that continues at home.

gemfibrozil

jem-**fye**-broe-zil
(Apo-Gemfibrozil ✦, Lopid, Novo-Gemfibrozil ✦)
Do not confuse Lopid with Levbid, Lipitor, Lodine, or Slo-Bid.

◆CLASSIFICATION

PHARMACOTHERAPEUTIC: Fibric acid derivative. **CLINICAL:** Antihyperlipidemic.

USES

Treatment of hypertriglyceridemia in types IV and V hyperlipidemia in pts who are at greater risk for pancreatitis and those who have not responded to dietary intervention. Reduce risk of coronary heart disease (CHD) development in pts without symptoms who have decreased HDL, increased LDL, increased triglycerides.

PRECAUTIONS

Contraindications: Hypersensitivity to gemfibrozil. Hepatic impairment (including primary biliary cirrhosis), preexisting gallbladder disease, severe renal impairment, concurrent use with dasabuvir, repaglinide or simvastatin. **Cautions:** Concurrent use

---

✦ Canadian trade name   🦬 Non-Crushable Drug   🔲 High Alert drug

with statins, mild to moderate renal impairment. anticoagulant therapy (e.g., warfarin).

ACTION

Exact mechanism of action unknown. Can inhibit lipolysis of fat in adipose tissue, decrease hepatic uptake of free fatty acids (reduces hepatic triglyceride production), or inhibit hepatic secretion of very low-density lipoprotein (VLDL). **Therapeutic Effect:** Lowers serum cholesterol, triglycerides (decreases VLDL, LDL; increases HDL).

PHARMACOKINETICS

Well absorbed from GI tract. Protein binding: 99%. Metabolized in liver. Primarily excreted in urine. Not removed by hemodialysis. **Half-life:** 1.5 hrs.

⌛ LIFESPAN CONSIDERATIONS

Pregnancy/Lactation: Unknown if drug crosses placenta or is distributed in breast milk. Decision to discontinue breastfeeding or drug should be based on potential for serious adverse effects. **Children:** Not recommended in pts younger than 2 yrs (cholesterol necessary for normal development). **Elderly:** Age-related renal impairment may require dosage adjustment.

INTERACTIONS

DRUG: Statins (e.g., atorvastatin, simvastatin) may increase risk for myopathy/rhabdomyolysis. May increase effects of **repaglinide, warfarin. Bile acid–binding resins (e.g., colestipol)** may decrease concentration. **HERBAL:** None significant. **FOOD:** None known. **LAB VALUES:** May increase serum alkaline phosphatase, bilirubin, creatine kinase, LDH, ALT, AST. May decrease Hgb, Hct, leukocyte counts, serum potassium.

AVAILABILITY (Rx)

Tablets: 600 mg.

ADMINISTRATION/HANDLING

PO
• Give 30 min before morning and evening meals.

INDICATIONS/ROUTES/DOSAGE

Hyperlipidemia/Hypertriglyceridemia
PO: ADULTS, ELDERLY: 600 mg twice daily 30 min before breakfast and dinner.

Dosage in Renal Impairment
Use caution. Contraindicated in severe impairment.

Dosage in Hepatic Impairment
Contraindicated.

SIDE EFFECTS

Frequent (20%): Dyspepsia. **Occasional (10%–2%):** Abdominal pain, diarrhea, nausea, vomiting, fatigue. **Rare (less than 2%):** Constipation, acute appendicitis, vertigo, headache, rash, pruritus, altered taste.

ADVERSE EFFECTS/TOXIC REACTIONS

Cholelithiasis, cholecystitis, acute appendicitis, pancreatitis, malignancy occur rarely.

NURSING CONSIDERATIONS

BASELINE ASSESSMENT

Obtain diet history, esp. fat/alcohol consumption. Obtain serum glucose, triglyceride, cholesterol, LFT. Question history of hepatic/renal impairment, cholecystectomy. Receive full medication history and screen for contraindications.

INTERVENTION/EVALUATION

Monitor LDL, VLDL, serum triglycerides, cholesterol lab results for therapeutic response. Monitor daily pattern of bowel activity, stool consistency. Assess for rash, pruritus. Question for headache, dizziness. Monitor LFT, hematology tests. Assess for abdominal pain, esp. right upper quadrant or epigastric pain suggestive of adverse gallbladder effects. Monitor serum glucose in pts receiving insulin, oral antihyperglycemics.

PATIENT/FAMILY TEACHING

• Follow special diet (important part of treatment). • Take before meals. • Periodic lab tests are essential part of therapy. • Report pronounced dizziness, blurred vision, abdominal pain, diarrhea, nausea, vomiting.

gentamicin

jen-ta-**mye**-sin
(Gentak)

■ **BLACK BOX ALERT** ■ Aminoglycoside antibiotics may cause neurotoxicity, nephrotoxicity. Risk of ototoxicity directly proportional to dosage, duration of treatment; ototoxicity usually is irreversible, precipitated by tinnitus, vertigo. May cause fetal harm if given during pregnancy.
Do not confuse gentamicin with vancomycin.

◆CLASSIFICATION

PHARMACOTHERAPEUTIC: Aminoglycoside. **CLINICAL:** Antibiotic.

USES

Parenteral: Treatment of infections susceptible to *Pseudomonas, Proteus, Serratia,* and other gram-negative organisms and gram-positive *Staphylococcus* including skin/skin structure, bone, joint, respiratory tract, intra-abdominal, complicated urinary tract, acute pelvic infections; burns; septicemia; meningitis. **Ophthalmic:** Ophthalmic infections caused by susceptible bacteria. **OFF-LABEL:** Surgical (preoperative) prophylaxis.

PRECAUTIONS

Contraindications: Hypersensitivity to gentamicin, other aminoglycosides (cross-sensitivity) or their components. **Cautions:** Elderly, neonates due to renal insufficiency or immaturity, neuromuscular disorders (potential for respiratory depression), vestibular or cochlear impairment, renal impairment, hypocalcemia, myasthenia gravis. Pediatric pts on extracorporeal membrane oxygenation.

ACTION

Irreversibly binds to protein of bacterial ribosomes. **Therapeutic Effect:** Interferes with protein synthesis of susceptible microorganisms. Bactericidal.

PHARMACOKINETICS

Rapid, complete absorption after IM administration. Protein binding: less than 30%. Widely distributed (does not cross blood-brain barrier, low concentrations in CSF). Excreted unchanged in urine. Removed by hemodialysis. **Half-life:** 2–4 hrs (increased in renal impairment, neonates; decreased in cystic fibrosis, burn, or febrile pts).

⧗ LIFESPAN CONSIDERATIONS

Pregnancy/Lactation: Readily crosses placenta; unknown if distributed in breast milk. **Children:** Caution in neonates: Immature renal function increases half-life and toxicity. **Elderly:** Age-related renal impairment may require dosage adjustment.

INTERACTIONS

DRUG: Nephrotoxic (e.g., lisinopril, IV contrast dye), ototoxic medications (e.g., CISplatin, furosemide) may increase risk of nephrotoxicity, ototoxicity. May increase neuromuscular blockade with concurrent use of **neuromuscular blockers (e.g., succinylcholine). HERBAL:** None significant. **FOOD:** None known. **LAB VALUES:** May increase serum BUN, creatinine, bilirubin, LDH, ALT, AST. May decrease serum calcium, magnesium, potassium, sodium. **Therapeutic serum level:** peak: 4–10 mcg/mL; trough: 0.5–2 mcg/mL. **Toxic serum level:** peak: greater than 10 mcg/mL; trough: greater than 2 mcg/mL.

AVAILABILITY (Rx)

Injection, Infusion: 60 mg/50 mL, 80 mg/50 mL, 80 mg/100 mL, 100 mg/50 mL, 100 mg/100 mL, 120 mg/100 mL. **Injection, Solution:** 10 mg/mL, 40 mg/mL. **Ointment, Ophthalmic:** 0.3%. **Solution, Ophthalmic (Gentak):** 0.3%.

G

ADMINISTRATION/HANDLING

 IV

Reconstitution • Dilute with 50–100 mL D$_5$W or 0.9% NaCl. Amount of diluent for infants, children depends on individual needs.

Rate of Administration • Infuse over 30–60 min for adults, older children; over 60–120 min for infants, young children.

Storage • Store vials at room temperature. • Solution appears clear or slightly yellow. • Intermittent IV infusion (piggyback) is stable for 48 hrs at room temperature or refrigerated. • Discard if precipitate forms.

IM

• To minimize discomfort, give deep IM slowly. • Less painful if injected into gluteus maximus than lateral aspect of thigh.

Ophthalmic

• Place gloved finger on lower eyelid and pull out until a pocket is formed between eye and lower lid. • Place prescribed number of drops or ¼–½ inch ointment into pocket. Instruct pt to close eye gently for 1–2 min (so that medication will not be squeezed out of the sac). • **Solution:** Instruct pt to apply digital pressure to lacrimal sac at inner canthus for 1 min to minimize systemic absorption. • **Ointment:** Instruct pt to roll eyeball to increase contact area of drug to eye. • Remove excess solution or ointment around eye with tissue.

▨ IV INCOMPATIBILITIES

Allopurinol (Aloprim), amphotericin B complex (Abelcet, AmBisome, Amphotec), furosemide (Lasix), heparin, heta-starch (Hespan), IDArubicin (Idamycin), indomethacin (Indocin), propofol (Diprivan).

▨ IV COMPATIBILITIES

Amiodarone (Cordarone), dexmedetomidine (Precedex), diltiaZEM (Cardizem), enalapril (Vasotec), filgrastim (Neupogen), HYDROmorphone (Dilaudid), insulin, LORazepam (Ativan), magnesium sulfate, midazolam (Versed), morphine, multivitamins.

INDICATIONS/ROUTES/DOSAGE

◄ALERT► Space parenteral doses evenly around the clock. Dosage based on ideal body weight. Peak, trough levels are determined periodically to maintain desired serum concentrations and minimize risk of toxicity.

Usual Parenteral Dosage

IM, IV: ADULTS, ELDERLY: (Conventional): 3–5 mg/kg/day in divided doses q8h. **(Once Daily):** 5–7 mg/kg/dose q24h. **CHILDREN 5 YRS AND OLDER:** 2–2.5 mg/kg/dose q8h. **INFANTS, CHILDREN YOUNGER THAN 5 YRS:** 2.5 mg/kg/dose q8h. **NEONATES (GREATER THAN 2 KG) PNA 8–28 days:** 4–5 mg/kg/dose q24h; **PNA 7 days or less:** 4 mg/kg/dose q24h. **(1–2 KG) PNA 8–28 days:** 5 mg/kg/dose q36h; **PNA 7 days or less:** 5 mg/kg/dose q48h. **(LESS THAN 1 KG) PNA 15–28 days:** 5 mg/kg/dose q36h; **PNA 14 days or less:** 5 mg/kg/dose q48h.

Hemodialysis (HD)

Note: Administer after HD on dialysis days.

Loading dose: 2–3 mg/kg, then 1 mg/kg q48–72h for mild UTI or synergy (consider redose for pre- or post-HD concentrations less than 1 mg/L); 1–1.5 mg/kg q48–72h for moderate to severe UTI (consider redose for pre-HD concentration less than 1.5–2 mg/L or post-HD concentrations less than 1 mg/L); 1.5–2 mg/kg q48–72h for systemic gram-negative rod infection (consider redose for pre-HD concentration less than 3–5 mg/L or post-HD concentrations less than 2 mg/L).

Continuous Renal Replacement Therapy (CRRT)

Loading dose: 2–3 mg/kg, then 1 mg/kg q24–36h for mild UTI or synergy (redose when concentration less than 1 mg/L); 1–1.5 mg/kg q24–36h for moderate to severe UTI (redose when concentration less than 1.5–2 mg/L); 1.5–2 mg/kg q24–48h for systemic gram-negative infection (redose when concentration less than 3–5 mg/L).

Usual Ophthalmic Dosage

Ophthalmic Ointment: ADULTS, ELDERLY: Apply ½-inch strip to conjunctival sac 2–3 times/day.

Ophthalmic Solution: ADULTS, ELDERLY, CHILDREN: 1–2 drops q2–4h up to 2 drops/hr.

Dosage in Renal Impairment
Adults

Creatinine Clearance	Conventional Dosage	Once-Daily Dosage
Greater than 60 mL/mil	q8h	q24h
41–60 mL/min	q12h	q36h
20–40 mL/min	q24h	q48h
Less than 20 mL/min	Loading dose, then monitor levels to determine dosage interval	Monitor levels

Children

Creatinine Clearance	Conventional Dosage
Greater than 50 mL/min	q8h
30–50 mL/min	q12–18h
10–29 mL/min	q18–24h
Less than 10 mL/min	q48–72h

Dosage in Hepatic Impairment
Monitor plasma concentrations.

SIDE EFFECTS

Occasional: IM: Pain, induration at injection site. **IV:** Phlebitis, thrombophlebitis, hypersensitivity reactions (fever, pruritus, rash, urticaria). **Ophthalmic:** Burning, tearing, itching, blurred vision. **Rare:** Alopecia, hypertension, fatigue.

ADVERSE EFFECTS/TOXIC REACTIONS

Nephrotoxicity (increased serum BUN, creatinine; decreased creatinine clearance)

may be reversible if drug is stopped at first sign of symptoms. Irreversible ototoxicity (tinnitus, dizziness, diminished hearing), neurotoxicity (headache, dizziness, lethargy, tremor, visual disturbances) occur occasionally. Risk increases with higher dosages, prolonged therapy, or if solution is applied directly to mucosa. Superinfections, particularly with fungi, may result from bacterial imbalance via any route of administration. Ophthalmic application may cause paresthesia of conjunctiva, mydriasis.

G

NURSING CONSIDERATIONS

BASELINE ASSESSMENT

Dehydration must be treated before beginning parenteral therapy. Establish baseline hearing acuity. Question for history of allergies, esp. aminoglycosides, sulfites (parabens for topical/ophthalmic routes). Screen for risk of acute kidney injury, esp. pts at risk for renal failure (baseline renal insufficiency, elderly, HF, hypertension, septic shock).

INTERVENTION/EVALUATION

Monitor I&O (maintain hydration), urinalysis, BUN, creatinine. Be alert to ototoxic, neurotoxic symptoms (see Adverse Effects/Toxic Reactions). Check IM injection site for induration. Evaluate IV site for phlebitis (heat, pain, red streaking over vein). Assess for rash **(Ophthalmic:** redness, burning, itching, tearing). Be alert for superinfection (genital/anal pruritus, changes in oral mucosa, diarrhea). When treating pts with neuromuscular disorders, assess respiratory response carefully. **Therapeutic serum level:** peak: 4–10 mcg/mL; peak levels are 2–3 times greater with once-daily dosing; trough: 0.5–2 mcg/mL. **Toxic serum level:** peak: greater than 10 mcg/mL; trough: greater than 2 mcg/mL.

G

PATIENT/FAMILY TEACHING
• Discomfort may occur with IM injection. • Blurred vision, tearing may occur briefly after each ophthalmic dose. • Report any hearing, visual, balance, urinary problems, even after therapy is completed. • **Ophthalmic:** Report if tearing, redness, irritation continues.

---

glatiramer

gla-**tir**-a-mer
(Copaxone, Glatopa)
Do not confuse Copaxone with Compazine.

◆CLASSIFICATION
PHARMACOTHERAPEUTIC: Immunosuppressive. **CLINICAL:** Neurologic agent for multiple sclerosis.

USES
Treatment of relapsing, remitting multiple sclerosis.

PRECAUTIONS
Contraindications: Hypersensitivity to glatiramer, mannitol. **Cautions:** Pts exhibiting immediate postinjection reaction (flushing, chest pain, palpitations, anxiety, dyspnea, urticaria).

ACTION
Induces/activates T-lymphocyte suppressor cells specific to myelin antigens. May also interfere with the antigen-presenting function of immune cells. **Therapeutic Effect:** Slows progression of multiple sclerosis.

PHARMACOKINETICS
Substantial fraction of glatiramer is hydrolyzed locally. Some fraction of injected material enters lymphatic circulation, reaching regional lymph nodes; some may enter systemic circulation intact.

⧗ LIFESPAN CONSIDERATIONS
Pregnancy/Lactation: Unknown if distributed in breast milk. **Children:** Safety and efficacy not established. **Elderly:** Safety and efficacy not established.

INTERACTIONS
DRUG: None significant. **HERBAL: Echinacea** may decrease effects. **FOOD:** None known. **LAB VALUES:** None significant.

AVAILABILITY (Rx)
Injection Solution: (Copaxone, Glatopa) 20 mg/mL in prefilled syringes, (Copaxone) 40 mg/mL in prefilled syringes.

ADMINISTRATION/HANDLING
Subcutaneous
• Refrigerate syringes (bring to room temperature before use). • May be stored at room temperature for up to 1 mo. • Avoid heat, intense light. • Inject into deltoid region, abdomen, gluteus maximus, or lateral aspect of thigh. • Prefilled syringe suitable for single use only; discard unused portions.

INDICATIONS/ROUTES/DOSAGE
Multiple Sclerosis
SQ: ADULTS, ELDERLY: 20 mg once daily or 40 mg 3 times/wk.

Dosage in Renal/Hepatic Impairment
No dose adjustment.

SIDE EFFECTS
Expected (73%–40%): Pain, erythema, inflammation, pruritus at injection site, asthenia. **Frequent (27%–18%):** Arthralgia, vasodilation, anxiety, hypertonia, nausea, transient chest pain, dyspnea, flu-like symptoms, rash, pruritus. **Occasional (17%–10%):** Palpitations, back pain, diaphoresis, rhinitis, diarrhea, urinary urgency. **Rare (less than 9%):** Anorexia, fever, neck pain, peripheral edema, ear pain, facial edema, vertigo, vomiting.

ADVERSE EFFECTS/TOXIC REACTIONS
Infection occurs commonly. Lymphadenopathy occurs occasionally.

NURSING CONSIDERATIONS

BASELINE ASSESSMENT

Assess baseline muscle strength, gait, voice quality, pain level; ability to conduct activities of daily living. Question other baseline symptoms including bowel/bladder dysfunction, depression, dizziness, fatigue, paresthesia, spasticity, sexual dysfunction, tremors.

INTERVENTION/EVALUATION

Observe injection site for reaction. Monitor for fever, chills (evidence of infection). Observe for improvement of symptoms, neurologic function.

PATIENT/FAMILY TEACHING

• Report difficulty in breathing/swallowing, rash, itching, swelling of lower extremities, fatigue. • Avoid pregnancy.

---

glimepiride `HIGH ALERT`

glye-**mep**-ir-ide
(Amaryl, Apo-Glimepiride ✦,
Novo-Glimepiride ✦)
Do not confuse Amaryl with Altace, Amerge, or Reminyl, or Avandaryl with Benadryl, or glimepiride with glipiZIDE or glyBURIDE.

FIXED-COMBINATION(S)

Avandaryl: glimepiride/rosiglitazone (an antidiabetic): 1 mg/4 mg, 2 mg/ 4 mg, 4 mg/4 mg.
Duetact: glimepiride/pioglitazone (an antidiabetic): 2 mg/30 mg, 4 mg/30 mg.

◆CLASSIFICATION

PHARMACOTHERAPEUTIC: Sulfonylurea. **CLINICAL:** Antidiabetic agent.

USES

Adjunct to diet, exercise in the management of type 2 diabetes mellitus.

PRECAUTIONS

Contraindications: Hypersensitivity to glimepiride, sulfonamides. Diabetic ketoacidosis (with or without coma). **Cautions:** Renal/hepatic impairment, glucose-altering conditions (fever, trauma, infection), G6PD deficiency, elderly, malnourished. Allergy to sulfa.

ACTION

Promotes release of insulin from beta cells of pancreas, decreases glucose output from liver, increases insulin sensitivity at peripheral sites. **Therapeutic Effect:** Lowers serum glucose.

PHARMACOKINETICS

Route	Onset	Peak	Duration
PO	N/A	2–3 hrs	24 hrs

Completely absorbed from GI tract. Protein binding: greater than 99%. Metabolized in liver. Excreted in urine (60%), feces (40%). **Half-life:** 5–9.2 hrs.

⧖ LIFESPAN CONSIDERATIONS

Pregnancy/Lactation: Avoid pregnancy. Unknown if distributed in breast milk. **Children:** Safety and efficacy not established. **Elderly:** Hypoglycemia may be difficult to recognize. Age-related renal impairment may increase sensitivity to glucose-lowering effect.

INTERACTIONS

DRUG: Beta blockers (e.g., **carvedilol, metoprolol**) may increase hypoglycemic effect, mask signs of hypoglycemia. **Cimetidine, ciprofloxacin, fluconazole, raNITIdine,** large doses of **salicylates** may increase effect. **Corticosteroids** (e.g., **dexamethasone, predniSONE**), **thiazide diuretics** (e.g., **HCTZ**) may decrease effect. **HERBAL: Garlic** may worsen hypoglycemia. **FOOD: Alcohol** may cause rare disulfiram reaction. **LAB VALUES:** May increase LDH concentrations, serum alkaline phosphatase, ALT, AST, bilirubin, C-peptide.

G

AVAILABILITY (Rx)

Tablets: 1 mg, 2 mg, 4 mg.

ADMINISTRATION/HANDLING

PO

• Give with breakfast or first main meal.

INDICATIONS/ROUTES/DOSAGE

Diabetes Mellitus

PO: ADULTS: Initially, 1–2 mg once daily with breakfast or first main meal. May increase by 1–2 mg q1–2wks, based on serum glucose response. **Maximum:** 8 mg/day. **ELDERLY:** Initially, 1 mg/day. Titrate dose to avoid hypoglycemia.

Dosage in Renal Impairment

Initially, 1 mg/day, then titrate dose based on fasting serum glucose levels.

Dosage in Hepatic Impairment

No dose adjustment (not studied).

SIDE EFFECTS

Rare (less than 3%): Altered taste, dizziness, drowsiness, weight gain, constipation, diarrhea, heartburn, nausea, vomiting, stomach fullness, headache, photosensitivity, peeling of skin, pruritus, rash.

ADVERSE EFFECTS/TOXIC REACTIONS

Overdose or insufficient food intake may produce hypoglycemia (esp. with increased glucose demands). GI hemorrhage, cholestatic hepatic jaundice, leukopenia, thrombocytopenia, pancytopenia, agranulocytosis, aplastic or hemolytic anemia occur rarely.

NURSING CONSIDERATIONS

BASELINE ASSESSMENT

Check serum glucose level. Discuss lifestyle to determine extent of learning, emotional needs. Ensure follow-up instruction if pt or family does not thoroughly understand diabetes management or serum glucose testing technique.

INTERVENTION/EVALUATION

Monitor serum glucose level, food intake. Assess for hypoglycemia (cool/wet skin, tremors, dizziness, anxiety, headache, tachycardia, perioral numbness, hunger, diplopia), hyperglycemia (polyuria, polyphagia, polydipsia, nausea, vomiting, dim vision, fatigue, deep or rapid breathing). Be alert to conditions that alter glucose requirements (fever, increased activity or stress, trauma, surgical procedure).

PATIENT/ FAMILY TEACHING

• Diet and exercise are principal parts of treatment; do not skip or delay meals. • Avoid alcohol. • Carry candy, sugar packets, other quick-acting sugar supplements for immediate response to hypoglycemia. • Wear medical alert identification. • Check with physician when glucose demands are altered (fever, infection, trauma, stress, heavy physical activity). • Avoid direct exposure to sunlight.

---

glipiZIDE

glip-i-zide
(Glucotrol, Glucotrol XL)
Do not confuse glipiZIDE with glimepiride or glyBURIDE, or Glucotrol with Glucophage or Glucotrol XL.

FIXED-COMBINATION(S)

GlipiZIDE/metFORMIN (an antidiabetic): 2.5 mg/250 mg, 2.5 mg/500 mg, 5 mg/500 mg.

◆Classification

PHARMACOTHERAPEUTIC: Sulfonylurea. **CLINICAL:** Antidiabetic agent.

USES

Adjunct to diet, exercise in management of type 2 diabetes mellitus.

PRECAUTIONS

Contraindications: Hypersensitivity to glipiZIDE, sulfonamides. Diabetic ketoacidosis with or without coma, type 1 diabetes mellitus. **Cautions:** Elderly, malnourished, concomitant use of beta blockers, pts with G6PD deficiency, hepatic/renal impairment. Avoid use of extended-release tablets in pts with stricture/narrowing of GI tract.

ACTION

Promotes release of insulin from beta cells of pancreas, decreases glucose output from liver, increases insulin sensitivity at peripheral sites. **Therapeutic Effect:** Lowers serum glucose.

PHARMACOKINETICS

Route	Onset	Peak	Duration
PO	15–30 min	2–3 hrs	12–24 hrs
Extended-release	2–3 hrs	6–12 hrs	24 hrs

Well absorbed from GI tract. Protein binding: 92%–99%. Metabolized in liver. Excreted in urine. **Half-life:** 2–4 hrs.

⧗ LIFESPAN CONSIDERATIONS

Pregnancy/Lactation: Agents other than glipizide are recommended to treat diabetes in pregnant women. GlipiZIDE given within 1 mo of delivery may produce neonatal hypoglycemia. Drug crosses placenta. Distributed in breast milk. **Children:** Safety and efficacy not established. **Elderly:** Hypoglycemia may be difficult to recognize. Age-related renal impairment may increase sensitivity to glucose-lowering effect.

INTERACTIONS

DRUG: Beta blockers (e.g., **carvedilol, metoprolol**) may increase hypoglycemic effect, mask signs of hypoglycemia. **Corticosteroids** (e.g., **dexamethasone, predniSONE**), **thiazide diuretics** (e.g., **HCTZ**) may decrease effect. **HERBAL: Garlic** may worsen hypoglycemia. **FOOD:** None known. **LAB VALUES:** May increase serum alkaline phosphatase, LDH, ALT, AST, bilirubin, C-peptide.

AVAILABILITY (Rx)

Tablets: 5 mg, 10 mg.

🦄 **Tablets (Extended-Release):** 2.5 mg, 5 mg, 10 mg.

ADMINISTRATION/HANDLING

PO
• Give immediate-release tablets 30 min before meals. Give extended-release tablets with breakfast. • Do not crush, cut, dissolve, or divide extended-release tablets.

INDICATIONS/ROUTES/DOSAGE

Diabetes Mellitus
PO: ADULTS: (Immediate-Release): Initially, 5 mg/day. Adjust dosage in 2.5- to 5-mg increments at intervals of several days. Immediate-release: **Maximum once-daily dose:** 15 mg. **Maximum dose/day:** 40 mg. **(Extended-Release):** Initially, 5 mg/day. May increase dose no more frequently than q7days. **Maximum dose:** 20 mg/day. **ELDERLY: (Immediate-Release):** Initially, 2.5–5 mg/day. May increase by 2.5–5 mg/day q1–2wks. **(Extended-Release):** Initially, 2.5 mg/day. Dosing should be on lower end of adult dosing.

Dosage in Renal Impairment
For CrCl of 50 mL/min or less, reduce dose by 50%.

Dosage in Hepatic Impairment
(Immediate-Release): Initial dose: 2.5 mg/day.

SIDE EFFECTS

Rare (less than 3%): Altered taste, dizziness, drowsiness, weight gain, constipation, diarrhea, heartburn, nausea, vomiting, headache, photosensitivity, peeling of skin, pruritus, rash.

ADVERSE EFFECTS/TOXIC REACTIONS

Overdose or insufficient food intake may produce hypoglycemia (esp. with increased glucose demands). GI hemorrhage, cholestatic hepatic jaundice, leukopenia, thrombocytopenia, pancytopenia, agranulocytosis, aplastic or hemolytic anemia occur rarely.

NURSING CONSIDERATIONS

BASELINE ASSESSMENT

Check serum glucose level. Discuss lifestyle to determine extent of learning, emotional needs. Ensure follow-up instruction if pt or family does not thoroughly understand diabetes management or serum glucose testing technique.

INTERVENTION/EVALUATION

Monitor serum glucose level, food intake. Assess for hypoglycemia (cool/wet skin, tremors, dizziness, anxiety, headache, tachycardia, perioral numbness, hunger, diplopia), hyperglycemia (polyuria, polyphagia, polydipsia, nausea, vomiting, dim vision, fatigue, deep or rapid breathing). Be alert to conditions that alter glucose requirements (fever, increased activity or stress, trauma, surgical procedure).

PATIENT/ FAMILY TEACHING

• Diet and exercise are principal parts of treatment; do not skip or delay meals. • Avoid alcohol. • Carry candy, sugar packets, other quick-acting sugar supplements for immediate response to hypoglycemia. • Wear medical alert identification. • Check with physician when glucose demands are altered (fever, infection, trauma, stress, heavy physical activity). • Avoid direct exposure to sunlight.

glucagon

gloo-ka-gon
(GlucaGen, GlucaGen Diagnostic Kit, Glucagon Emergency Kit)

◆CLASSIFICATION

PHARMACOTHERAPEUTIC: Glucose elevating agent. **CLINICAL:** Antidote for hypoglycemia, diagnostic agent.

USES

Treatment of severe hypoglycemia in diabetic pts. Diagnostic aid in radiographic examination to temporarily inhibit GI tract movement. **OFF-LABEL:** Hypoglycemia secondary to insulin or oral hypoglycemic therapy. Toxicity associated with beta blockers, calcium channel blockers.

PRECAUTIONS

Contraindications: Hypersensitivity to glucagon. Known insulinoma, pheochromocytoma, glucagonoma (except GlucaGen). **Cautions:** History of insulinoma, pheochromocytoma, prolonged fasting, starvation, adrenal insufficiency, chronic hypoglycemia. Avoid use in pts with hereditary galactose intolerance.

ACTION

Promotes hepatic glycogenolysis, gluconeogenesis. Stimulates cAMP, an enzyme, resulting in increased serum glucose concentration. **Therapeutic Effect:** Increases serum glucose level.

PHARMACOKINETICS

Route	Onset	Peak	Duration
IV	5–20 min	—	60–90 min
IM	30 min	—	60–90 min
SQ	30–45 min	—	60–90 min

Metabolized in liver. **Half-life:** 3–10 min.

⌛ LIFESPAN CONSIDERATIONS

Pregnancy/Lactation: Unknown if drug crosses placenta or is distributed in breast milk. **Children/Elderly:** No age-related precautions noted.

INTERACTIONS

DRUG: May increase effects of **anticoagulants.** **HERBAL:** None significant. **FOOD:** None known. **LAB VALUES:** May decrease serum potassium.

AVAILABILITY (Rx)

Injection Powder (GlucaGen, GlucaGen Diagnostic Kit, Glucagon Emergency Kit): 1 mg.

ADMINISTRATION/HANDLING

◄**ALERT**► Place pt in side-lying position to prevent aspiration (glucagon, hypoglycemia may produce nausea/vomiting).

IV, IM, SQ

Reconstitution • Reconstitute with 1 mL sterile diluent to provide concentration of 1 mg/mL.

Rate of Administration • Pt usually awakens in 5–20 min. Although 1–2 additional doses may be administered, concern for effects of continuing cerebral hypoglycemia requires consideration of parenteral glucose. • When pt awakens, give supplemental carbohydrate to restore hepatic glycogen and prevent secondary hypoglycemia. If pt fails to respond to glucagon, IV dextrose is necessary.

Storage • Store vial at room temperature. • After reconstitution, is stable for 48 hrs if refrigerated. If reconstituted with Sterile Water for Injection, use immediately. Do not use glucagon solution unless clear.

🔲 IV INCOMPATIBILITIES

Do not mix glucagon with any other medications.

INDICATIONS/ROUTES/DOSAGE

Hypoglycemia

◄**ALERT**► Administer IV dextrose if pt fails to respond to glucagon.

IV, IM, SQ: ADULTS, ELDERLY, CHILDREN WEIGHING MORE THAN 20 KG: 1 mg. May repeat in 15 min. **CHILDREN WEIGHING 20 KG OR LESS:** 0.5 mg. May repeat in 15 min. **NEONATES:** 0.02–0.2 mg/kg/dose. **Maximum:** 1 mg. May repeat in 20 min if needed.

Diagnostic Aid

IV: ADULTS, ELDERLY: 0.25–2 mg 10 min prior to procedure. **IM:** 1–2 mg 10 minutes prior to procedure.

Dosage in Renal/Hepatic Impairment

No dose adjustment.

SIDE EFFECTS

Occasional: Nausea, vomiting. **Rare:** Allergic reaction (urticaria, respiratory distress, hypotension).

ADVERSE EFFECTS/TOXIC REACTIONS

Overdose may produce persistent nausea/vomiting, hypokalemia (severe fatigue, decreased appetite, palpitations, muscle cramps).

NURSING CONSIDERATIONS

BASELINE ASSESSMENT

Obtain immediate assessment, including history, clinical signs/symptoms. If presence of hypoglycemic coma is established, give glucagon promptly. Immediately evaluate for other life-threatening conditions that mimic hypoglycemia (CVA, delirium, postictal state, toxicity).

INTERVENTION/EVALUATION

Monitor serum glucose, B/P, pulse, mental status. Monitor response time carefully. Have IV dextrose readily available in event pt does not respond. Assess for possible allergic reaction (urticaria, respiratory difficulty, hypotension). When pt is conscious, give oral carbohydrate.

PATIENT/FAMILY TEACHING

• Identify symptoms of low blood sugar (pale, cool skin; anxiety, confusion, difficulty concentrating, headache, nausea, passing out, seizures, sweating). • Report any episodes of low blood sugar to health care provider; medications, diet, lifestyle may need to be changed. • If symptoms of hypoglycemia develop, give sugar form first (orange juice, honey, hard candy, sugar cubes, table sugar dissolved in water or juice) followed by cheese and crackers, half a sandwich, glass of milk.

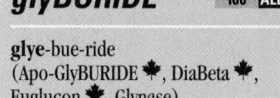

glyBURIDE TOP 100 HIGH ALERT

glye-bue-ride
(Apo-GlyBURIDE ✸, DiaBeta ✸, Euglucon ✸, Glynase)

Do not confuse DiaBeta with Zebeta, glyBURIDE with glimepiride, glipiZIDE, or Glucotrol.

FIXED-COMBINATION(S)

Glucovance: glyBURIDE/metFORMIN (an antidiabetic): 1.25 mg/250 mg, 2.5 mg/500 mg, 5 mg/500 mg.

◆CLASSIFICATION

PHARMACOTHERAPEUTIC: Sulfonylurea. **CLINICAL:** Antidiabetic agent.

USES

Adjunct to diet, exercise in management of stable, mild to moderately severe type 2 diabetes mellitus.

PRECAUTIONS

Contraindications: Hypersensitivity to glyBURIDE. Diabetic ketoacidosis with or without coma, type 1 diabetes mellitus, concurrent use with bosentan. **Cautions:** Stress, elderly, debilitated pts, malnourished, severe hepatic/renal impairment, G6PD deficiency, adrenal and/or pituitary insufficiency.

ACTION

Promotes release of insulin from beta cells of pancreas, decreases glucose output from liver, increases insulin sensitivity at peripheral sites. **Therapeutic Effect:** Lowers serum glucose level.

PHARMACOKINETICS

Route	Onset	Peak	Duration
PO	0.25–1 hr	1–2 hrs	12–24 hrs

Well absorbed from GI tract. Protein binding: 99%. Metabolized in liver. Primarily excreted in urine. Not removed by hemodialysis. **Half-life:** 5–16 hrs.

⏳ LIFESPAN CONSIDERATIONS

Pregnancy/Lactation: Crosses placenta. Distributed in breast milk. May produce neonatal hypoglycemia if given within 2 wks of delivery. **Children:** Safety and efficacy not established. **Elderly:** Hypoglycemia may be difficult to recognize. Age-related renal impairment may increase sensitivity to glucose-lowering effect.

INTERACTIONS

DRUG: Beta blockers (e.g., carvedilol, metoprolol) may increase hypoglycemic effect, mask signs of hypoglycemia. **Corticosteroids (e.g., dexamethasone, predniSONE), thiazide diuretics (e.g., HCTZ)** may decrease effect. **HERBAL: Garlic,** other herbs with hypoglycemic properties may enhance effect. **FOOD:** None known. **LAB VALUES:** May increase serum alkaline phosphatase, LDH, ALT, AST, bilirubin, C-peptide.

AVAILABILITY (Rx)

Tablets: 1.25 mg, 2.5 mg, 5 mg. **Tablets, Micronized:** 1.5 mg, 3 mg, 6 mg.

ADMINISTRATION/HANDLING

PO
• May give with food at same time each day.

INDICATIONS/ROUTES/DOSAGE

Diabetes Mellitus
PO *(Tablets):* **ADULTS:** Initially, 1.25–5 mg. May increase by 2.5 mg/day at wkly intervals. **Maintenance:** 1.25–20 mg/day as single or divided doses. **Maximum:** 20 mg/day. **ELDERLY:** Initially, 1.25 mg daily. Conservative initial and maintenance doses are recommended to avoid hypoglycemic reactions.
PO *(Tablets, Micronized):* **ADULTS:** Initially 0.75–3 mg/day. May increase by 1.5 mg/day at wkly intervals. **Maintenance:** 0.75–12 mg/day as a single dose or in divided doses. **Maximum:** 12 mg/day. **ELDERLY:** Initially, 0.75 mg daily. Conservative initial and maintenance doses are recommended to avoid hypoglycemic reactions.

Dosage in Renal Impairment
Not recommended for pts with CrCl less than 60 mL/min.

G

Dosage in Hepatic Impairment
No dose adjustment.

SIDE EFFECTS

Rare (less than 3%): Altered taste, dizziness, drowsiness, weight gain, constipation, diarrhea, heartburn, nausea, vomiting, headache, photosensitivity, peeling of skin, pruritus, rash.

ADVERSE EFFECTS/TOXIC REACTIONS

Overdose or insufficient food intake may produce hypoglycemia (esp. in pts with increased glucose demands). Cholestatic jaundice, leukopenia, thrombocytopenia, pancytopenia, agranulocytosis, aplastic or hemolytic anemia occur rarely.

NURSING CONSIDERATIONS

BASELINE ASSESSMENT

Check serum glucose level. Discuss lifestyle to determine extent of learning, emotional needs. Ensure follow-up instruction if pt or family does not thoroughly understand diabetes management or glucose testing technique.

INTERVENTION/EVALUATION

Monitor serum glucose level, food intake. Assess for hypoglycemia (cool/wet skin, tremors, dizziness, anxiety, headache, tachycardia, perioral numbness, hunger, diplopia); hyperglycemia (polyuria, polyphagia, polydipsia, nausea, vomiting, dim vision, fatigue, deep or rapid breathing). Be alert to conditions that alter glucose requirements (fever, increased activity or stress, trauma, surgical procedure).

PATIENT/ FAMILY TEACHING

• Diet and exercise are principal parts of treatment; do not skip or delay meals. • Avoid alcohol. • Carry candy, sugar packets, other quick-acting sugar supplements for immediate response to hypoglycemia. • Wear medical alert identification. • Check with physician when glucose demands are altered (fever, infection, trauma, stress, heavy physical activity). • Avoid direct exposure to sunlight.

golimumab

goe-**lim**-ue-mab
(Simponi, Simponi Aria)

■ **BLACK BOX ALERT** ■ Tuberculosis (TB), invasive fungal infections, other opportunistic infections reported. Discontinue treatment if active infection or sepsis occurs. Test for TB prior to and during treatment, regardless of initial result; if positive, start treatment for TB prior to initiating therapy. Lymphoma, other malignancies reported in pts treated with tumor necrosis factor blockers.
Do not confuse Simponi (subcutaneous) with Simponi Aria (intravenous).

◆CLASSIFICATION

PHARMACOTHERAPEUTIC: Monoclonal antibody. **CLINICAL:** Immune modulator, antirheumatic, tumor necrosis factor (TNF) blocking agent.

USES

Simponi, Simponi Aria: Used alone or in combination with methotrexate for the treatment of adult pts with active psoriatic arthritis. Used in combination with methotrexate for the treatment of adult pts with moderately to severely active rheumatoid arthritis. Used alone or in combination with methotrexate for the treatment of adult pts with active ankylosing spondylitis. **Simponi:** Treatment of moderate to severe active ulcerative colitis in pts with corticosteroid dependence or who are refractory/intolerant to aminosalicylates, oral steroids, azathioprine, or 6-mercaptopurine.

PRECAUTIONS

Contraindications: Hypersensitivity to golimumab. **Cautions:** Elderly, concomitant immunosuppressants, co-morbid conditions predisposing to infections (e.g., diabetes). Residence or travel from areas of endemic mycosis; tuberculosis, underlying hematologic disorders, preexisting or recent-onset demyelinating disorders (e.g., multiple sclerosis, polyneuropathy), pts with HF or decreased left ventricular function. Avoid concomitant use with live vaccines, abatacept, or anakinra (increased incidence of serious infections). Do not start during an active infection.

ACTION

Binds specifically to tumor necrosis factor (TNF) alpha, blocking its interaction with cell surface TNF receptors. **Therapeutic Effect:** Alters biologic activity of TNF alpha, reduces inflammation, may alter pathophysiology of rheumatoid arthritis.

PHARMACOKINETICS

Serum concentration reaches steady state by wk 12. Elimination pathway not specified. **Half-life:** 12–14 days.

⏳ LIFESPAN CONSIDERATIONS

Pregnancy/Lactation: Unknown if distributed in breast milk. Must either discontinue drug or discontinue breastfeeding. **Children:** Safety and efficacy not established in pts younger than 18 yrs. **Elderly:** May have increased risk of serious infections, malignancy.

INTERACTIONS

DRUG: Anakinra, abatacept, riTUXimab, natalizumab, immunosuppressive therapy may increase risk of infections. May decrease efficacy of immune response of **vaccines.** **HERBAL:** Echinacea may decrease effects. **FOOD:** None known. **LAB VALUES:** May increase ALT, AST. May decrease Hgb, leukocytes, neutrophils, platelets.

AVAILABILITY (Rx)

Injection Solution (Simponi): 50 mg/0.5 mL, 100 mg/mL in single-dose prefilled autoinjector or prefilled syringe. **Injection Solution (Simponi Aria):** 50 mg/4 mL per single-use vial (12.5 mg/mL).

ADMINISTRATION/HANDLING

Simponi Subcutaneous

• Remove prefilled syringe or autoinjector from refrigerator. Allow to sit at room temperature for 30 min; do not warm in any other way. • Avoid areas where skin is scarred, tender, bruised, red, scaly, hard. Recommended injection site is front of middle thighs, although lower abdomen 2 inches below navel or outer, upper arms are acceptable. • Inject within 5 min after cap has been removed. **Autoinjector** • Push open end of autoinjector firmly against skin at 90-degree angle. • Do not pull autoinjector away from skin until a first "click" sound is heard and then a second "click" sound (injection is finished and needle is pulled back). This usually takes 3 to 6 sec but may take up to 15 sec for the second "click" to be heard. If autoinjector is pulled away from skin before injection is completed, full dose may not be administered. **Prefilled Syringe** • Gently pinch skin and hold firmly. Use a quick, dart-like motion to insert needle into pinched skin at a 45-degree angle. **Storage** • Refrigerate; do not freeze. Do not shake. • Solution appears slightly opalescent, colorless to light yellow. Discard if cloudy or contains particulate.

Simponi Aria

◀ **ALERT** ▶ Use in-line 0.22-micron filter.

 IV

Reconstitution • Calculate dosage and number of vials needed based on pt weight. • Visually inspect for particulate matter. • Dilute in 100 mL 0.9% NaCl. • Prior to mixing, withdraw and discard volume of 0.9% NaCl equal to the volume of patient-dosed solution. • Slowly inject solution into bag and gently mix. • Do not shake. **Rate of Administration** • Infuse over 30 min using an in-line low protein-binding 0.22-micron filter.

Storage • Refrigerate vials, prefilled syringes • Vial solution should be colorless to light yellow and opalescent. • It is normal for solution to develop fine translucent particles since drug is a protein. • Do not use if opaque particles, discoloration, or other foreign particles are present. • May store diluted solution at room temperature up to 4 hrs.

▓ IV INCOMPATIBILITIES

Do not infuse concomitantly with other drugs.

INDICATIONS/ROUTES/DOSAGE

Active Psoriatic Arthritis
SQ: *(Simponi):* **ADULTS, ELDERLY:** 50 mg once monthly. Use alone or in combination with methotrexate or other non-biologic DMARD.
IV Infusion: *(Simponi Aria):* **ADULTS, ELDERLY:** 2 mg/kg at wk 0, 4 then q8wks thereafter.

Moderate to Severe Active Rheumatoid Arthritis (with Methotrexate)
SQ: *(Simponi):* **ADULTS, ELDERLY:** 50 mg once monthly.
IV Infusion: *(Simponi Aria):* **ADULTS, ELDERLY:** 2 mg/kg at wk 0 and wk 4. Then, decrease frequency to q8wks.

Active Ankylosing Spondylitis
SQ: *(Simponi):* **ADULTS, ELDERLY:** 50 mg once monthly. Use alone or in combination with methotrexate or other non-biologic DMARD.
IV Infusion: *(Simponi Aria):* **ADULTS, ELDERLY:** 2 mg/kg at wk 0, 4 then q8wks thereafter.

Ulcerative Colitis
SQ: *(Simponi):* **ADULTS, ELDERLY:** Initially, 200 mg, then 100 mg 2 wks later, and then 100 mg q4wks thereafter.

Dosage in Renal/Hepatic Impairment
No dose adjustment.

SIDE EFFECTS

Frequent (13%): Laryngitis, nasopharyngitis, pharyngitis, rhinitis, upper respiratory tract infection. **Occasional (3%–2%):** Bronchitis, hypertension, rash, pyrexia. **Rare (less than 1%):** Dizziness, paresthesia, constipation.

ADVERSE EFFECTS/TOXIC REACTIONS

Neutropenia, lymphopenia may increase risk of infection. New-onset psoriasis, exacerbation of preexisting psoriasis have been reported. Serious infections including sepsis, pneumonia, cellulitis, TB, invasive fungal infections reported. May increase risk of lymphoma, melanoma, new malignancies. New onset or exacerbation of CNS demyelinating disorders, including multiple sclerosis, or worsening of HF have occurred. Viral reactivation of herpes zoster, HIV, hepatitis B virus infection may occur. Pts who receive TNF blockers have risk of autoantibody formation (immunogenicity). Hypersensitivity reactions including anaphylaxis reported. May induce lupus-like symptoms (butterfly rash, new joint pain, peripheral edema, UV sensitivity).

NURSING CONSIDERATIONS

BASELINE ASSESSMENT

Obtain baseline LFT, CBC, vital signs, urine pregnancy. Obtain B-type natriuretic peptide (BNP) level and review echocardiogram in pts with history of HF. Do not initiate therapy if active infection suspected. Evaluate for active TB and test for latent infection prior to and during treatment. Induration of 5 mm or greater with tuberculin skin test should be considered a positive result when assessing for latent TB. Antifungal therapy should be considered for those who reside or travel to regions where mycoses are endemic. Question history of anemia, HF, CNS disorders, hepatic impairment, HIV, malignancies. Assess skin for moles, lesions. Receive full medication history including herbal products.

INTERVENTION/EVALUATION

Monitor CBC, LFT every 4–8 wks, then periodically. Screen pts for TB (night sweats,

G

hemoptysis, weight loss, fever) regardless of baseline tuberculin skin test result. Monitor hepatitis B virus carriers during treatment and several mos after treatment. If any viral reactivation occurs, interrupt treatment and consider antiviral therapy. Discontinue treatment if acute infection, opportunistic infection, or sepsis occurs, and initiate appropriate antimicrobial therapy. Routinely assess skin for new lesions. Peripheral edema, difficulty breathing, coarse crackles on lung auscultation, elevated BNP may indicate worsening HF. Monitor for hypersensitivity reactions.

PATIENT/FAMILY TEACHING

• Treatment may depress your immune system and reduce your ability to fight infection. Report symptoms of infection such as body aches, chills, cough, fatigue, fever. Avoid those with active infection. • Do not receive live vaccines. • Report history of HIV, fungal infections, HF, hepatitis B, multiple sclerosis, TB, or close relatives who have active TB. Report travel plans to possible endemic areas. Blood levels, TB screening will be routinely monitored. • Hives, swelling of face, difficulty breathing may indicate allergic reaction. • Do not breastfeed. • Abdominal pain, yellowing of skin or eyes, dark-amber urine, clay-colored stools, fatigue, loss of appetite may indicate liver problems. • Decreased platelet count may increase risk of bleeding. • Swelling of hands or feet, difficulty breathing may indicate HF.

---

goserelin   HIGH ALERT

goe-se-**rel**-in
(Zoladex, Zoladex LA ✦)

◆CLASSIFICATION

PHARMACOTHERAPEUTIC: Gonadotropin-releasing hormone analogue.
CLINICAL: Antineoplastic.

USES

Treatment of locally confined prostate cancer. Palliative treatment of advanced carcinoma of prostate as alternative when orchiectomy, estrogen therapy is either not indicated or unacceptable. In combination with an antiestrogen before and during radiation therapy for early stages of prostate cancer. Management of endometriosis. Treatment of advanced breast cancer in premenopausal and perimenopausal women. Endometrial thinning before ablation for dysfunctional uterine bleeding.

PRECAUTIONS

Contraindications: Hypersensitivity to goserelin. Pregnancy (except when used for palliative treatment of advanced breast cancer). **Cautions:** Women of childbearing potential until pregnancy has been excluded. Pts at risk for decreased bone density; diabetes.

ACTION

Stimulates release of luteinizing hormone (LH) and follicle-stimulating hormone (FSH) from anterior pituitary. **Therapeutic Effect:** In females, reduces ovarian, uterine, mammary gland size; regresses hormone-responsive tumors. In males, decreases testosterone level, reduces growth of abnormal prostate tissue.

PHARMACOKINETICS

Protein binding: 27%. Metabolized in liver. Excreted in urine. **Half-life:** 4.2 hrs (male); 2.3 hrs (female).

⧖ LIFESPAN CONSIDERATIONS

Pregnancy/Lactation: Crosses placenta; unknown if distributed in breast milk. **Children:** Safety and efficacy not established. **Elderly:** No age-related precautions noted.

INTERACTIONS

DRUG: Anticoagulants (e.g., rivaroxaban, warfarin) may increase risk of severe injection site injury. **Medications prolonging the QT interval**

(e.g., **amiodarone, azithromycin, ceritinib, haloperidol, moxifloxacin**) may increase risk of QT interval prolongation, cardiac arrhythmias. **HERBAL:** None significant. **FOOD:** None known. **LAB VALUES:** May increase serum prostatic acid phosphatase, testosterone, calcium; Hgb A1c.

AVAILABILITY (Rx)

Injection, Implant (Zoladex): 3.6 mg, 10.8 mg.

ADMINISTRATION/HANDLING

Subcutaneous Implant

• Administer implant by inserting needle at 30- to 45-degree angle into anterior abdominal wall below the navel line. Do not attempt to eliminate air bubbles or aspirate prior to injection. Do not penetrate into muscle or peritoneum.

INDICATIONS/ROUTES/DOSAGE

Prostatic Carcinoma, Advanced
SQ: ADULTS OLDER THAN 18 YRS, EL-DERLY: 3.6 mg every 28 days or 10.8 mg q12wks subcutaneously into upper abdominal wall.

Prostate Carcinoma, Locally Confined
SQ: ADULTS, ELDERLY: (in combination with an antiestrogen and radiotherapy, begin 8 wks prior to radiotherapy): 3.6 mg once. 28 days after initial dose, give 10.8 mg or 3.6 mg q28days for 4 doses.

Breast Carcinoma, Endometriosis
SQ: ADULTS: 3.6 mg every 28 days subcutaneously into upper abdominal wall.

Endometrial Thinning
SQ: ADULTS: 3.6 mg subcutaneously into upper abdominal wall as a single dose or in 2 doses 4 wks apart.

Endometriosis
SQ: ADULTS: 3.6 mg every 28 days for 6 mos.

Dosage in Renal/Hepatic Impairment
No dose adjustment.

SIDE EFFECTS

Frequent (60%–13%): Headache, hot flashes, depression, diaphoresis, sexual dysfunction, impotence, lower urinary tract symptoms. **Occasional (10%–5%):** Pain, lethargy, dizziness, insomnia, anorexia, nausea, rash, upper respiratory tract infection, hirsutism, abdominal pain. **Rare:** Pruritus.

ADVERSE EFFECTS/TOXIC REACTIONS

Arrhythmias, HF, hypertension occur rarely. Ureteral obstruction, spinal cord compression have been observed (immediate orchiectomy may be necessary). Hypersensitivity reactions, including anaphylaxis, may occur. Hyperglycemia, new-onset diabetes occurred in men taking GnRH antagonists. Increased risk of MI, sudden cardiac death was reported. Injection site injuries including hematoma, hemorrhage, hemorrhagic shock may require blood transfusion or surgical intervention.

NURSING CONSIDERATIONS

BASELINE ASSESSMENT

Question history of diabetes, cardiovascular disease, recent MI, prior hypersensitivity reaction. Receive full medication history; screen for QT interval–prolonging medications, anticoagulant medications. Screen for conditions predisposing to QT interval prolongation. In males, question history of urethral obstruction, urinary retention, spinal cord compression, spinal stenosis. Obtain urine pregnancy. If applicable, obtain bone density test.

INTERVENTION/EVALUATION

Monitor pt closely for worsening signs/symptoms of prostatic cancer, esp. during first mo of therapy.

PATIENT/FAMILY TEACHING

• Use nonhormonal methods of contraception during therapy. • Report suspected pregnancy or if regular menstruation

G

does not cease. • Breakthrough menstrual bleeding may occur if dose is missed. • Immediately report sudden weakness, paralysis, numbness, tingling; difficulty urinating, bladder distention. • Do not take newly prescribed medications unless approved by prescriber who originally started treatment. • Severe bleeding may occur at the injection site, esp. in pts who take blood-thinning medication. • Pts with heart disease are at an increased risk of heart attack or sudden death.

granisetron

gra-**nis**-e-tron
(Sancuso, Sustol)
Do not confuse granisetron with dolasetron, ondansetron, or palonosetron.

◆CLASSIFICATION

PHARMACOTHERAPEUTIC: Serotonin receptor antagonist (5-HT$_3$). **CLINICAL:** Antiemetic.

USES

Prevention of nausea/vomiting associated with emetogenic cancer therapy and cancer radiation therapy. **OFF-LABEL:** Prevention, treatment of postop nausea, vomiting. Breakthrough treatment of chemotherapy-associated nausea/vomiting.

PRECAUTIONS

Contraindications: Hypersensitivity to granisetron. Hypersensitivity to other 5-HT$_3$ receptor antagonists. **Cautions:** Congenital QT prolongation, concomitant administration of medications that prolong QT interval, electrolyte abnormalities, cumulative high-dose anthracycline therapy. Following abdominal surgery or in chemotherapy-induced nausea, vomiting (may mask progressive ileus or gastric distention), hepatic disease.

ACTION

Selectively blocks serotonin stimulation at receptor sites at chemoreceptor trigger zone, vagal nerve terminals. **Therapeutic Effect:** Prevents nausea/vomiting.

PHARMACOKINETICS

Route	Onset	Peak	Duration
IV	1–3 min	N/A	24 hrs

Rapidly, widely distributed to tissues. Protein binding: 65%. Metabolized in liver. Excreted in urine (48%), feces (38%). **Half-life:** 10–12 hrs (increased in elderly).

⌛ LIFESPAN CONSIDERATIONS

Pregnancy/Lactation: Unknown if distributed in breast milk. **Children:** Safety and efficacy not established in pts younger than 2 yrs. **Elderly:** No age-related precautions noted.

INTERACTIONS

DRUG: QT interval–prolonging medications (e.g., **amiodarone, azithromycin, ceritinib, haloperidol, moxifloxacin**) may increase risk of QT interval prolongation, cardiac arrhythmias. **SSRIs (e.g., escitalopram, paroxetine, sertraline), SNRIs (e.g., duloxetine, venlafaxine)** may increase risk of serotonin syndrome. **HERBAL:** None significant. **FOOD:** None known. **LAB VALUES:** May increase serum ALT, AST.

AVAILABILITY (Rx)

Injection, Extended Release (Sustol): 10 mg/0.4 mL single-dose syringe. **Injection Solution:** 0.1 mg/mL, 1 mg/mL. **Tablets:** 1 mg. **Transdermal Patch (Sancuso):** 52-cm^2 patch containing 34.3 mg granisetron delivering 3.1 mg/24 hrs.

ADMINISTRATION/HANDLING

 IV

Reconstitution • May be given undiluted or dilute with 20–50 mL 0.9% NaCl or D$_5$W. Do not mix with other medications.

Rate of Administration • May give undiluted as IV push over 30 sec. • For IV piggyback, infuse over 5–10 min depending on volume of diluent used.

Storage • Appears as a clear, colorless solution. • Store at room temperature. • After dilution, stable for 3 days at room temperature or 7 days if refrigerated. • Inspect for particulates, discoloration.

PO

• Give 30 min to 1 hr prior to initiating chemotherapy.

Subcutaneous

Administer in skin of back of upper arm, abdomen (at least 1 inch away from umbilicus). Avoid areas of compromised skin. Administer over 20–30 sec.

Transdermal

• Apply to clean, dry intact skin on upper outer arm. • Remove immediately from pouch before application. • Do not cut patch.

▧ IV INCOMPATIBILITY

Amphotericin B (Fungizone).

▧ IV COMPATIBILITIES

Allopurinol (Aloprim), bumetanide (Bumex), calcium gluconate, CARBOplatin (Paraplatin), CISplatin (Platinol), cyclophosphamide (Cytoxan), cytarabine (Ara-C), dacarbazine (DTIC-Dome), dexamethasone (Decadron), dexmedetomidine (Precedex), diphenhydrAMINE (Benadryl), DOCEtaxel (Taxotere), DOXOrubicin (Adriamycin), etoposide (VePesid), gemcitabine (Gemzar), magnesium, mitoXANTRONE (Novantrone), PACLitaxel (Taxol), potassium.

INDICATIONS/ROUTES/DOSAGE

Prevention of Chemotherapy-Induced Nausea/Vomiting

PO: ADULTS, ELDERLY: 2 mg up to 1 hr before chemotherapy or 1 mg up to 1 hr before chemotherapy, with a second dose 12 hrs later.

IV: ADULTS, ELDERLY, CHILDREN 2 YRS AND OLDER: 10 mcg/kg/dose (**Maximum:** 1 mg/dose) within 30 min of chemotherapy. **Maximum:** 1 mg.

Subcutaneous: ADULTS, ELDERLY: (In combination with dexamethasone): 10 mg at least 30 min before chemotherapy. Do not repeat more frequently than 7 days.

Transdermal: ADULTS, ELDERLY: Apply 24–48 hrs prior to chemotherapy. Remove minimum 24 hrs after completion of chemotherapy. May be worn up to 7 days, depending on chemotherapy duration.

Prevention of Radiation-Induced Nausea/Vomiting

PO: ADULTS, ELDERLY: 2 mg once daily, given 1 hr before radiation therapy.

Postop Nausea/Vomiting

IV: ADULTS, ELDERLY: 0.35–3 mg (5–20 mcg/kg) given at end of surgery.

Dosage in Renal/Hepatic Impairment

No dose adjustment. **(Sustol) Moderate:** No more frequently than 14 days. **Severe:** Not recommended.

SIDE EFFECTS

Frequent (21%–14%): Headache, constipation, asthenia. **Occasional (8%–6%):** Diarrhea, abdominal pain. **Rare (less than 2%):** Altered taste, fever.

ADVERSE EFFECTS/TOXIC REACTIONS

Hypersensitivity reaction, hypertension, hypotension, arrhythmias (sinus bradycardia, atrial fibrillation, AV block, ventricular ectopy), EKG abnormalities occur rarely. Increased risk of serotonin syndrome reported in pts taking concomitant serotonergic drugs (e.g., SSRIs, SNRIs). May prolong QTc interval.

NURSING CONSIDERATIONS

BASELINE ASSESSMENT

Assess hydration status. Ensure that granisetron is given within 30 min of starting chemotherapy. Receive full medication history and screen for interactions. Screen for QT interval–prolonging conditions.

INTERVENTION/EVALUATION

Monitor for therapeutic effect. Assess for headache. Monitor for dehydration due to recurrent vomiting. Monitor daily pattern of bowel activity, stool consistency.

PATIENT/FAMILY TEACHING

• Granisetron is effective shortly following administration; prevents nausea/vomiting. • Transitory taste disorder may occur.

---

guselkumab

gue-sel-**koo**-mab
(Tremfya)
Do not confuse guselkumab with golimumab, infliximab, secukinumab.

◆CLASSIFICATION

PHARMACOTHERAPEUTIC: Interleukin-23 inhibitor. Monoclonal antibody. **CLINICAL:** Antipsoriasis agent.

USES

Treatment of moderate to severe plaque psoriasis in adult pts who are candidates for systemic therapy or phototherapy.

PRECAUTIONS

Contraindications: Hypersensitivity to guselkumab. **Cautions:** Hepatic impairment, active infection until resolved, history of chronic or recurrent infections, conditions predisposing to infection (e.g., diabetes, immunocompromised pts, open wounds), prior tuberculosis exposure (do not give to pts with active TB infection). Concomitant use of live vaccines not recommended.

ACTION

Selectively binds to interleukin-23 receptor reducing levels of IL-17A, IL-17F, IL-22. IL-23 is a cytokine that is involved in inflammatory and immune responses. **Therapeutic Effect:** Inhibits release of pro-inflammatory cytokines and chemokines.

PHARMACOKINETICS

Widely distributed. Degraded into small peptides and amino acids via catabolic pathways. Peak plasma concentration: 5.5 days. Elimination not specified. **Half-life:** 15–18 days.

⌛ LIFESPAN CONSIDERATIONS

Pregnancy/Lactation: Unknown if distributed in breast milk; however, human immunoglobulin G (IgG) is present in breast milk and is known to cross placenta. **Children:** Safety and efficacy not established in pts younger than 18 yrs. **Elderly:** No age-related precautions noted.

INTERACTIONS

DRUG: May enhance adverse/toxic effects, diminish therapeutic effects of **vaccines (line and attenuated)**. May decrease therapeutic effect of **BCG**. May increase adverse effects/toxicity of **natalizumab, pimecrolimus, tacrolimus**. **HERBAL:** Echinacea may decrease effect. **FOOD:** None known. **LAB VALUES:** May increase serum ALT, AST.

AVAILABILITY (Rx)

Injection, Solution: 100 mg/mL in prefilled syringe.

ADMINISTRATION/HANDLING

Subcutaneous

Preparation • Remove prefilled syringe from refrigerator and allow to warm to room temperature (approx. 30 mins) with needle cap intact. • Visually inspect for particulate matter or discoloration. Solution should appear clear, colorless to slightly yellow in color; may contain small translucent particles. Do

---

not use if solution is cloudy, discolored, or if large particles are observed. • Discard unused portions.

Administration • Insert needle subcutaneously into back of upper arms, front of thighs, or into lower abdomen (except for 2 inches around navel), and inject solution. • Do not inject into areas of the skin where it is tender, bruised, red, hard, thick, scaly, or affected by psoriasis. • Rotate injection sites.

Storage • Refrigerate prefilled syringes in original carton until time of use. • Do not freeze. • Do not shake. • Protect from light.

INDICATIONS/ROUTES/DOSAGE

Plaque Psoriasis
SQ: ADULTS, ELDERLY: 100 mg at wk 0, wk 4, and then q8wks thereafter.

Dosage in Renal/Hepatic Impairment
Not specified; use caution.

SIDE EFFECTS

Occasional (5%–2%): Headache, tension headache, arthralgia, diarrhea.

ADVERSE EFFECTS/TOXIC REACTIONS

May increase risk of tuberculosis infection. Other infections including upper respiratory tract infection, nasopharyngitis, pharyngitis, viral upper respiratory tract infection (14% of pts), gastroenteritis, viral gastroenteritis (1% of pts), tinea infections (1% of pts), herpes simplex virus (1% of pts) may occur. Mild to moderate elevated serum ALT, AST reported in 3% of pts. Immunogenicity (auto-guselkumab antibodies) occurred in 6% of pts.

NURSING CONSIDERATIONS

BASELINE ASSESSMENT

Obtain LFT in pts with hepatic impairment. Question history of hepatic impairment, herpes zoster infection, parasitic infection. Screen for active infection. Pts should be evaluated for active tuberculosis and tested for latent infection prior to initiating treatment and periodically during therapy. Induration of 5 mm or greater with tuberculin skin testing should be considered a positive test result when assessing if treatment for latent tuberculosis is necessary. Conduct dermatologic exam; record characteristics of psoriatic lesions. Assess pt's willingness to self-inject medication.

INTERVENTION/EVALUATION

Monitor LFT periodically. Monitor for symptoms of tuberculosis, including those who tested negative for latent tuberculosis infection prior to initiating therapy. Interrupt or discontinue treatment if serious infection, opportunistic infection, or sepsis occurs, and initiate appropriate antimicrobial therapy. Assess skin for improvement of lesions.

PATIENT/FAMILY TEACHING

• A health care provider will show you how to properly prepare and inject your medication. You must demonstrate correct preparation and injection techniques before using medication at home. • Treatment may depress your immune system response and reduce your ability to fight infection. Report symptoms of infection such as body aches, chills, cough, fatigue, fever. Avoid those with active infection. • Do not receive live vaccines. • Expect frequent tuberculosis screening. Report travel plans to possible endemic areas. • Report liver problems such as abdominal pain, bruising, clay-colored stool, yellowing of the skin or eyes.

haloperidol

hal-o-per-i-dol
(Apo-Haloperidol ✤, Haldol, Haldol Decanoate, Novo-Peridol ✤)

■ BLACK BOX ALERT ■ Increased risk of mortality in elderly pts with dementia-related psychosis with use of injections.

Do not confuse Haldol with Halcion or Stadol.

◆CLASSIFICATION

PHARMACOTHERAPEUTIC: First-generation (typical) antipsychotic. **CLINICAL:** Antipsychotic, antiemetic, antidyskinetic.

USES

Treatment of schizophrenia, Tourette's disorder (controls tics and vocal utterances), severe behavioral problems in children with combative explosive hyperexcitability without immediate provocation. Management of psychotic disorder, short-term treatment of hyperactive children. **OFF-LABEL:** Treatment of nonschizophrenic psychosis, alcohol dependence, psychosis/agitation related to Alzheimer's dementia, emergency sedation of severely agitated/psychotic pts.

PRECAUTIONS

Contraindications: Hypersensitivity to haloperidol, CNS depression, coma, Parkinson's disease, severe cardiac/hepatic disease. **Cautions:** Renal/hepatic impairment, cardiovascular disease, history of seizures, prolonged QT syndrome, medications that prolong QT interval, hypothyroidism, thyrotoxicosis, electrolyte imbalance (e.g., hypokalemia, hypomagnesemia), EEG abnormalities, narrow–angle glaucoma, elderly, pts at risk for pneumonia, decreased GI motility, urinary retention, BPH, visual disturbances, myelosuppression. Pts at risk for orthostatic hypotension (e.g., cerebrovascular disease).

ACTION

Competitively blocks postsynaptic DOPamine receptors in brain. **Therapeutic Effect:** Produces tranquilizing effect. Strong extrapyramidal, antiemetic effects; weak anticholinergic, sedative effects.

PHARMACOKINETICS

Readily absorbed from GI tract. Protein binding: 92%. Metabolized in liver. Excreted in urine. Not removed by hemodialysis. **Half-life:** 20 hrs.

⧖ LIFESPAN CONSIDERATIONS

Pregnancy/Lactation: Crosses placenta. Distributed in breast milk. **Children:** More susceptible to dystonias; not recommended in pts younger than 3 yrs. **Elderly:** More susceptible to orthostatic hypotension, anticholinergic effects, sedation; increased risk for extrapyramidal effects. Decreased dosage recommended.

INTERACTIONS

DRUG: Alcohol, other CNS depressants (e.g., diphenhydrAMINE, gabapentin, LORazepam, morphine) may increase CNS depression. **CYP3A4 inducers** (e.g., carBAMazepine) may decrease concentration. **Medications prolonging QT interval** (e.g., amiodarone, ciprofloxacin, ondansetron) may increase risk of QT prolongation. **Medications producing extrapyramidal symptoms (EPS)** (e.g., diphenhydrAMINE, benztropine) may increase EPS. **HERBAL:** Gotu kola, kava kava, St. John's wort, valerian may increase CNS depression. **FOOD:** None known. **LAB VALUES:** None significant. **Therapeutic serum level:** 0.2–1 mcg/mL; **toxic serum level:** Greater than 1 mcg/mL.

AVAILABILITY (Rx)

Injection, Oil (Decanoate): 50 mg/mL, 100 mg/mL. **Injection, Solution (Lactate):** 5 mg/mL. **Oral Concentrate:** 2 mg/mL. **Tablets:** 0.5 mg, 1 mg, 2 mg, 5 mg, 10 mg, 20 mg.

ADMINISTRATION/HANDLING

 IV

◀ALERT▶ Only haloperidol lactate is given IV.

Note: For IV administration, ECG monitoring for QT prolongation/arrhythmias is recommended.

Reconstitution • May give undiluted. • May add to 50–100 mL of D₅W.
Rate of Administration • Give IV push at rate of 5 mg/min. • Infuse IV piggyback over 30 min. • For IV infusion, up to 25 mg/hr has been used (titrated to pt response).

Storage • Discard if precipitate forms, discoloration occurs. • Store at room temperature; do not freeze. • Protect from light.

IM

Parenteral Administration • Pt should remain recumbent for 30–60 min to minimize hypotensive effect. • Prepare Decanoate IM injection using 21-gauge needle. • Do not exceed maximum volume of 3 mL per IM injection site. • Inject slow, deep IM into upper outer quadrant of gluteus maximus.

PO

• Give without regard to meals. • Scored tablets may be crushed. • Dilute oral concentrate with water or juice. • Avoid skin contact with oral concentrate; may cause contact dermatitis.

▦ IV INCOMPATIBILITIES

Allopurinol (Aloprim), amphotericin B complex (Abelcet, AmBisome, Amphotec), cefepime (Maxipime), fluconazole (Diflucan), foscarnet (Foscavir), heparin, nitroprusside (Nipride), piperacillin/tazobactam (Zosyn).

▦ IV COMPATIBILITIES

DOBUTamine (Dobutrex), DOPamine (Intropin), fentaNYL (Sublimaze), HYDROmorphone (Dilaudid), lidocaine, LORazepam (Ativan), midazolam (Versed), morphine, nitroglycerin, norepinephrine (Levophed), propofol (Diprivan).

INDICATIONS/ROUTES/DOSAGE
Usual Dosage

IM *(Lactate):* **ADULTS, ELDERLY:** 2–5 mg q1–8 as needed. **CHILDREN 6–12 YRS:** 1–3 mg/dose q4–8h as needed. **Maximum:** 0.15 mg/kg/day. Change to PO as soon as possible. *(Decanoate):* **ADULTS, ELDERLY:** Initially, 10–20 times stabilized oral dose. **Maximum:** 100 mg. **Maintenance:** 10–15 times daily oral dose or 50–200 mg q4wks.

PO: ADULTS: 0.5–5 mg 2–3 times/day. **Usual dose:** 5–20 mg/day. **Maximum:** 100 mg/day. **ELDERLY:** 0.2–2 mg/day. **Usual dose:** 5–20 mg/day. **Maximum:** 100 mg/day. **CHILDREN WEIGHING MORE THAN 40 KG, ADOLESCENTS:** 0.5–15 mg/day in 2–3 divided doses. May increase at no less than 5–7 days. **Maximum:** 15 mg/day. **CHILDREN 3–12 YRS (15–40 KG):** 0.5 mg/day. May increase by 0.5 mg q5–7days. Range: 0.05–0.15 mg/kg/day in 2–3 divided doses. **Maximum:** 15 mg/day.

Tourette's Disorder

PO: CHILDREN 3–12 YRS: 15–40 KG: Initially, 0.25–0.5 mg/day in 2–3 divided doses. May increase by 0.5 mg/day every 5–7 days to usual dose of 1–4 mg/day. **CHILDREN GREATER THAN 40 KG, ADOLESCENTS:** Initially, 0.25–0.5 mg/day in 2–3 divided doses. May increase as needed every 5–7 days to usual dose of 1–4 mg/day.

Dosage in Renal/Hepatic Impairment
No dose adjustment.

SIDE EFFECTS

Frequent: Blurred vision, constipation, orthostatic hypotension, dry mouth, swelling or soreness of female breasts, peripheral edema. **Occasional:** Allergic reaction, difficulty urinating, decreased thirst, dizziness, diminished sexual function, drowsiness, nausea, vomiting, photosensitivity, lethargy.

H

ADVERSE EFFECTS/TOXIC REACTIONS

Extrapyramidal symptoms (EPS) appear to be dose related and typically occur in first few days of therapy. Marked drowsiness/lethargy, excessive salivation, fixed stare may be mild to severe in intensity. Less frequently noted are severe akathisia (motor restlessness), acute dystonias: torticollis (neck muscle spasm), opisthotonos (rigidity of back muscles), oculogyric crisis (rolling back of eyes). Tardive dyskinesia (tongue protrusion, puffing of cheeks, chewing/puckering of the mouth) may occur during long-term therapy or after drug discontinuance and may be irreversible. Elderly female pts have greater risk of developing this reaction. May increase risk of QT interval prolongation, cardiac arrhythmias.

NURSING CONSIDERATIONS

BASELINE ASSESSMENT

Assess behavior, appearance, emotional status, response to environment, speech pattern, thought content. Assess LOC. Screen for co-morbidities as listed in Precautions (esp. seizure disorder, long QT syndrome).

INTERVENTION/EVALUATION

Monitor B/P, heart rate/rhythm, QT interval. Supervise suicidal-risk pt closely during early therapy (as depression lessens, energy level improves, increasing suicide potential). Monitor for rigidity, tremor, mask-like facial expression, fine tongue movement. Assess for therapeutic response (interest in surroundings, improvement in self-care, increased ability to concentrate, relaxed facial expression). Monitor EKG and QT interval. **Therapeutic serum level:** 0.2–1 mcg/mL; **toxic serum level:** greater than 1 mcg/mL.

PATIENT/FAMILY TEACHING

• Full therapeutic effect may take up to 6 wks. • Do not abruptly withdraw from long-term drug therapy. • Sugarless gum, sips of water may relieve dry mouth. • Drowsiness generally subsides during continued therapy. • Avoid tasks that require alertness, motor skills until response to drug is established. • Avoid alcohol. • Report muscle stiffness. • Avoid exposure to sunlight, overheating, dehydration (increased risk of heatstroke).

---

heparin

hep-a-rin
(Hepalean Leo ✦)
Do not confuse heparin with Hespan.

◆CLASSIFICATION

PHARMACOTHERAPEUTIC: Blood modifier. **CLINICAL:** Anticoagulant.

USES

Prophylaxis and treatment of thromboembolic disorders and thromboembolic complications associated with atrial fibrillation; anticoagulant for extracorporeal and dialysis procedures; maintain patency of IV devices. **OFF-LABEL:** STEMI, non-STEMI, unstable angina, anticoagulant used during percutaneous coronary intervention.

PRECAUTIONS

Contraindications: Hypersensitivity to heparin. Severe thrombocytopenia, uncontrolled active bleeding (unless secondary to disseminated intravascular coagulation [DIC]), history of heparin-induced thrombocytopenia (HIT), heparin-induced thrombocytopenia with thrombosis (HITT), or pts who test positive for HIT antibody. **Cautions:** Allergy to pork. Pts at risk for bleeding (e.g., congenital/acquired bleeding disorders, active GI ulcerative disease, hemophilia, concomitant platelet inhibitors, severe hypertension, menses, recent lumbar puncture or spinal anesthesia; recent major surgery, trauma). Use of preservative-free heparin recommended in neonates, infants, pregnant or nursing mothers.

ACTION

Interferes with blood coagulation by blocking conversion of prothrombin to thrombin and fibrinogen to fibrin. **Therapeutic Effect:** Prevents further extension of existing thrombi or new clot formation. No effect on existing clots.

PHARMACOKINETICS

Well absorbed following subcutaneous administration. Protein binding: Very high. Metabolized in liver. Removed from circulation via uptake by reticuloendothelial system. Primarily excreted in urine. Not removed by hemodialysis. Half-life: 1–6 hrs.

⧗ LIFESPAN CONSIDERATIONS

Pregnancy/Lactation: Use with caution, particularly during last trimester, immediate postpartum period (increased risk of maternal hemorrhage). Does not cross placenta. Not distributed in breast milk. **Children:** No age-related precautions noted. Benzyl alcohol preservative may cause gasping syndrome in infants. **Elderly:** More susceptible to hemorrhage. Age-related renal impairment may increase risk of bleeding.

INTERACTIONS

DRUG: Other anticoagulants (e.g., **dabigatran, warfarin**), platelet aggregation inhibitors (e.g., **aspirin, clopidogrel**), thrombolytics (e.g., **tissue plasminogen activator [TPA]**) may increase risk of bleeding. **HERBAL: Cat's claw, dong quai, evening primrose, feverfew, garlic, ginkgo, ginseng, horse chestnut, red clover** have additional antiplatelet activity. **FOOD:** None known. **LAB VALUES:** May increase free fatty acids, serum ALT, AST, aPTT. May decrease serum cholesterol.

AVAILABILITY (Rx)

Injection Solution: 10 units/mL, 100 units/mL, 1,000 units/mL, 5,000 units/mL, 10,000 units/mL, 20,000 units/mL. **Premix Solution for Infusion:** 25,000 units/250 mL infusion, 25,000 units/500 mL infusion.

ADMINISTRATION/HANDLING

◄**ALERT**► Do not give by IM injection (pain, hematoma, ulceration, erythema).

 IV

◄**ALERT**► Used in full-dose therapy. Intermittent IV dosage produces higher incidence of bleeding abnormalities. Continuous IV route preferred.
Reconstitution • Premix solution requires no reconstitution.
Rate of Administration • Infuse and titrate per protocol using infusion pump.
Storage • Store at room temperature.

Subcutaneous

◄**ALERT**► Used in low-dose therapy. • After withdrawal of heparin from vial, change needle before injection (prevents leakage along needle track). • Inject above iliac crest or in abdominal fat layer. Do not inject within 2 inches of umbilicus or any scar tissue. • Withdraw needle rapidly, apply prolonged pressure at injection site. Do not massage or apply heat/cold to injection site. • Rotate injection sites.

▦ IV INCOMPATIBILITIES

Amiodarone (Cordarone), amphotericin B complex (Abelcet, AmBisome, Amphotec), ciprofloxacin (Cipro), dacarbazine (DTIC), diazePAM (Valium), DOBUTamine (Dobutrex), DOXOrubicin (Adriamycin), filgrastim (Neupogen), gentamicin (Garamycin), haloperidol (Haldol), IDArubicin (Idamycin), labetalol (Trandate), niCARdipine (Cardene), phenytoin (Dilantin), quiNIDine (Quinidine), tobramycin (Nebcin), vancomycin (Vancocin).

▦ IV COMPATIBILITIES

Ampicillin/sulbactam (Unasyn), aztreonam (Azactam), calcium gluconate, ceFAZolin (Ancef), cefTAZidime (Fortaz), cefTRIAXone (Rocephin), dexmedetomidine (Precedex), digoxin (Lanoxin), diltiaZEM (Cardizem), DOPamine (Intropin), enalapril (Vasotec), famotidine (Pepcid), fentaNYL (Sublimaze), furosemide (Lasix), HYDROmorphone (Dilaudid), insulin, lidocaine, LORazepam (Ativan), magnesium sulfate, methylPREDNISolone (Solu-Medrol), midazolam (Versed), milrinone (Primacor), morphine, nitroglycerin, norepinephrine (Levophed), oxytocin (Pitocin), piperacillin/tazobactam (Zosyn), procainamide (Pronestyl), propofol (Diprivan).

INDICATIONS/ROUTES/DOSAGE

Line Flushing
IV: ADULTS, ELDERLY, CHILDREN: 100 units as needed. **INFANTS WEIGHING LESS THAN 10 KG:** 10 units as needed.

Acute Coronary Syndrome
IV Infusion: ADULTS, ELDERLY: 60 units/kg bolus (**Maximum:** 4,000 units), then 12 units/kg/hr (**Maximum:** 1,000 units/hr).

Treatment of DVT/PE
IV Infusion: ADULTS, ELDERLY: 80 units/kg bolus (**Maximum:** 5,000 units), then 18 units/kg/hr adjusted according to aPTT.

Usual Pediatric/Neonatal Dose
IV Infusion: 75 units/kg bolus over 10 min, then initial maintenance dose of 28 units/kg/hr. Adjust to maintain aPTT of 60–85 sec.

Thromboembolic Prophylaxis
SQ: ADULTS, ELDERLY: 5,000 units q8–12h.

Dosage in Renal/Hepatic Impairment
No dose adjustment.

SIDE EFFECTS

Occasional: Pruritus, burning (particularly on soles of feet) caused by vasospastic reaction. **Rare:** Pain, cyanosis of extremity 6–10 days after initial therapy lasting 4–6 hrs, hypersensitivity reaction (chills, fever, pruritus, urticaria, asthma, rhinitis, lacrimation, headache).

ADVERSE EFFECTS/TOXIC REACTIONS

Bleeding complications ranging from local ecchymoses to major hemorrhage (cutaneous/GI/genitourinary/intracranial/nasal/oral/pharyngeal/urethral/vaginal bleeding) occur more frequently in high-dose therapy, intermittent IV infusion, women 60 yrs and older. HIT can cause life-threatening thromboembolism such as CVA, MI, DVT, pulmonary embolism, renal artery thrombosis, mesenteric thrombosis. **Antidote:** Protamine sulfate 1–1.5 mg IV for every 100 units heparin subcutaneous within 30 min of overdose, 0.5–0.75 mg for every 100 units heparin subcutaneous if within 30–60 min of overdose, 0.25–0.375 mg for every 100 units heparin subcutaneous if 2 hrs have elapsed since overdose, 25–50 mg if heparin was given by IV infusion.

NURSING CONSIDERATIONS

BASELINE ASSESSMENT
Obtain CBC, PT/INR, aPTT. Cross-check dose with co-worker. Assess for bleeding risk. Question history of recent trauma, head injuries, GI/GU bleeding. Ensure that pt has not received spinal anesthesia, spinal procedures.

INTERVENTION/EVALUATION
Monitor CBC, PT/INR daily. Obtain aPTT 6 hrs after initiation or any change in dosage (or per clinical standards) until maintenance dose is established, then check aPTT q24hrs (or clinical standards). In long-term therapy, monitor 1–2 times/mo. Diligently assess for bleeding. If platelet count decreases more than 50% from baseline, obtain stat HIT antibody test. If HIT antibody positive, discontinue heparin and consider treatment with direct thrombin inhibitor (e.g., argatroban); avoid all heparin products and place heparin allergy on chart. Monitor urine and stool for occult blood. Assess for decrease in B/P, increase in pulse rate, complaint of abdominal/back pain, severe headache

(may be evidence of hemorrhage). Question for increase in amount of discharge during menses. Assess peripheral pulses; skin for ecchymosis, petechiae. Check for excessive bleeding from minor cuts, scratches. Assess gums for erythema, gingival bleeding. Assess urine output for hematuria. Avoid IM injections due to potential for hematomas. When converting to warfarin (Coumadin) therapy, monitor PT/INR results (will be 10%–20% higher while heparin is given concurrently).

PATIENT/FAMILY TEACHING

• Use electric razor, soft toothbrush to prevent bleeding. • Report red or dark urine, black or red stool, coffee-ground vomitus, blood-tinged mucus from cough, signs of stroke, nosebleeds, or increase in menstruation. • Do not use any OTC medication without physician approval (may interfere with platelet aggregation). • Wear or carry identification that notes anticoagulant therapy. • Inform dentist, other physicians of heparin therapy. • Limit alcohol.

---

hydrALAZINE

hye-**dral**-a-zeen
(Apresoline ✦)
Do not confuse hydrALAZINE with hydrOXYzine.

FIXED-COMBINATION(S)

Apresazide: hydralazine/hydrochlorothiazide (a diuretic): 25 mg/25 mg, 50 mg/50 mg, 100 mg/50 mg. **BiDil:** hydralazine/isosorbide (a nitrate): 37.5 mg/20 mg.

◆CLASSIFICATION

PHARMACOTHERAPEUTIC: Vasodilator. **CLINICAL:** Antihypertensive.

USES

Management of moderate to severe hypertension. **OFF-LABEL:** Hypertension secondary to eclampsia, preeclampsia. Treatment of HF with reduced ejection fraction, postoperative hypertension.

PRECAUTIONS

Contraindications: Hypersensitivity to hydrALAZINE. Coronary artery disease, mitral valvular rheumatic heart disease. **Cautions:** Advanced renal impairment, cerebrovascular accident, suspected coronary artery disease. Pts with mitral valvular disease, positive ANA titer, pulmonary hypertension.

ACTION

Direct vasodilating effects on arterioles. **Therapeutic Effect:** Decreases B/P, systemic vascular resistance.

PHARMACOKINETICS

Route	Onset	Peak	Duration
PO	20–30 min	N/A	Up to 8 hrs
IV	5–20 min	N/A	1–4 hrs

Well absorbed from GI tract. Widely distributed. Protein binding: 85%–90%. Metabolized in liver. Primarily excreted in urine. Not removed by hemodialysis. **Half-life:** 3–7 hrs (increased in renal impairment).

⌛ LIFESPAN CONSIDERATIONS

Pregnancy/Lactation: Drug crosses placenta. Unknown if distributed in breast milk. Thrombocytopenia, leukopenia, petechial bleeding, hematomas have occurred in newborns (resolved within 1–3 wks). **Children:** No age-related precautions noted. **Elderly:** More sensitive to hypotensive effects. Age-related renal impairment may require dosage adjustment.

INTERACTIONS

DRUG: Diuretics (e.g., furosemide, HCTZ), other antihypertensives (e.g., amLODIPine, cloNIDine, lisinopril, valsartan) may increase hypotensive effect. **HERBAL:** Ephedra, ginseng, yohimbe may worsen hypertension. **Garlic** may increase antihypertensive

H

effect. **FOOD:** Any **foods** may increase absorption. **LAB VALUES:** May produce positive direct Coombs' test.

AVAILABILITY (Rx)

Injection Solution: 20 mg/mL. **Tablets:** 10 mg, 25 mg, 50 mg, 100 mg.

ADMINISTRATION/HANDLING

 IV

Rate of Administration • May give undiluted. • Administer slowly: maximum rate 5 mg/min (0.2 mg/kg/min for children).
Storage • Store at room temperature.

PO
• Best given with food at regularly spaced meals. • Tablets may be crushed.

⊞ IV INCOMPATIBILITIES

Ampicillin (Polycillin), furosemide (Lasix).

⊞ IV COMPATIBILITIES

DOBUTamine (Dobutrex), heparin, hydrocortisone (Solu-Cortef), nitroglycerin, potassium chloride.

INDICATIONS/ROUTES/DOSAGE

Hypertension
PO: ADULTS, ELDERLY: Initially, 10 mg 4 times/day for first 2–4 days. May increase to 25 mg 4 times/day balance of first wk. May increase by 10–25 mg/dose gradually q2–5 days to 50 mg 4 times/day. Usual range: 25–100 mg in 2–3 divided doses. **Maximum:** 300 mg/day in divided doses. **CHILDREN:** Initially, 0.75 mg/kg/day in 2–4 divided doses. May increase over 3–4 wks. **Maximum:** 7.5 mg/kg/day (7.5 mg/kg/day in infants). **Maximum daily dose:** 200 mg/day in divided doses.
IV, IM: ADULTS, ELDERLY: Initially, 10–20 mg/dose q4–6h. May increase to 40 mg/dose. **CHILDREN:** Initially, 0.1–0.2 mg/kg/dose (**Maximum:** 20 mg) q4–6h, as needed, up to 1.7–3.5 mg/kg/day in 4–6 divided doses.

Dosage in Renal Impairment
Dosage interval is based on creatinine clearance.

Creatinine Clearance	Dosage
10–50 mL/min	q8h
Less than 10 mL/min	q12–24h

Dosage in Hepatic Impairment
No dose adjustment.

SIDE EFFECTS

Occasional: Headache, anorexia, nausea, vomiting, diarrhea, palpitations, tachycardia, angina pectoris. **Rare:** Constipation, ileus, edema, peripheral neuritis (paresthesia), dizziness, muscle cramps, anxiety, hypersensitivity reactions (rash, urticaria, pruritus, fever, chills, arthralgia), nasal congestion, flushing, conjunctivitis.

ADVERSE EFFECTS/TOXIC REACTIONS

High dosage may produce lupus erythematosus–like reaction (fever, facial rash, muscle/joint aches, glomerulonephritis, splenomegaly). Severe orthostatic hypotension, skin flushing, severe headache, myocardial ischemia, cardiac arrhythmias may develop. Profound shock may occur with severe overdosage.

NURSING CONSIDERATIONS

BASELINE ASSESSMENT
Obtain B/P, pulse immediately before each dose, in addition to regular monitoring (be alert to fluctuations).

INTERVENTION/EVALUATION
Monitor B/P, pulse. Monitor for headache, palpitations, tachycardia. Assess for peripheral edema of hands, feet.

PATIENT/FAMILY TEACHING
• To reduce hypotensive effect, go from lying to standing slowly. • Report muscle/joint aches, fever (lupus-like reaction), flu-like symptoms. • Limit alcohol use.

H

hydroCHLOROthiazide

hye-dro-**klor**-oh-**thy**-ah-zide
(Apo-Hydro ✤, Microzide)
Do not confuse Microzide with Maxzide.

FIXED-COMBINATION(S)

Accuretic: hydrochlorothiazide/quinapril (an angiotensin-converting enzyme [ACE] inhibitor): 12.5 mg/10 mg, 12.5 mg/20 mg, 25 mg/20 mg. **Aldactazide:** hydrochlorothiazide/spironolactone (a potassium-sparing diuretic): 25 mg/25 mg, 50 mg/50 mg. **Aldoril:** hydrochlorothiazide/methyldopa (an antihypertensive): 15 mg/250 mg, 25 mg/250 mg, 30 mg/500 mg, 50 mg/500 mg. **Amturnide:** hydrochlorothiazide/aliskiren (renin inhibitor)/amLODIPine (calcium channel blocker): 12.5 mg/150 mg/5 mg, 12.5 mg/300 mg/5 mg, 25 mg/300 mg/5 mg, 12.5 mg/300 mg/10 mg, 25 mg/300 mg/10 mg. **Apresazide:** hydroCHLOROthiazide/hydrALAZINE (a vasodilator): 25 mg/25 mg, 50 mg/50 mg, 50 mg/100 mg. **Atacand HCT:** hydroCHLOROthiazide/candesartan (an angiotensin II receptor antagonist): 12.5 mg/16 mg, 12.5 mg/32 mg. **Avalide:** hydroCHLOROthiazide/irbesartan (an angiotensin II receptor antagonist): 12.5 mg/150 mg, 12.5 mg/300 mg, 25 mg/300 mg. **Benicar HCT:** hydroCHLOROthiazide/olmesartan (an angiotensin II receptor antagonist): 12.5 mg/20 mg, 12.5 mg/40 mg, 25 mg/40 mg. **Capozide:** hydroCHLOROthiazide/captopril (an ACE inhibitor): 15 mg/25 mg, 15 mg/50 mg, 25 mg/25 mg, 25 mg/50 mg. **Diovan HCT:** hydroCHLOROthiazide/valsartan (an angiotensin II receptor antagonist): 12.5 mg/80 mg, 12.5 mg/160 mg. **Dutoprol:** hydroCHLOROthiazide/metoprolol (a beta blocker): 12.5 mg/25 mg, 12.5 mg/50 mg, 12.5 mg/100 mg. **Dyazide/Maxide:** hydroCHLOROthiazide/triamterene (a potassium-sparing diuretic): 25 mg/37.5 mg, 25 mg/50 mg, 50 mg/75 mg. **Exforge HCT:** hydroCHLOROthiazide/amLODIPine (a calcium channel blocker)/valsartan (an angiotensin II receptor blocker): 12.5 mg/5 mg/160 mg, 25 mg/5 mg/160 mg, 12.5 mg/10 mg/160 mg, 25 mg/10 mg/160 mg, 25 mg/10 mg/320 mg. **Hyzaar:** hydroCHLOROthiazide/losartan (an angiotensin II receptor antagonist): 12.5 mg/50 mg, 12.5 mg/100 mg, 25 mg/100 mg. **Inderide:** hydroCHLOROthiazide/propranolol (a beta blocker): 25 mg/40 mg, 25 mg/80 mg, 50 mg/80 mg, 50 mg/120 mg, 50 mg/160 mg. **Lopressor HCT:** hydroCHLOROthiazide/metoprolol (a beta blocker): 25 mg/50 mg, 25 mg/100 mg, 50 mg/100 mg. **Lotensin HCT:** hydroCHLOROthiazide/benazepril (an ACE inhibitor): 6.25 mg/5 mg, 12.5 mg/10 mg, 12.5 mg/20 mg, 25 mg/20 mg. **Micardis HCT:** hydroCHLOROthiazide/telmisartan (an angiotensin II receptor antagonist): 12.5 mg/40 mg, 12.5 mg/80 mg. **Moduretic:** hydroCHLOROthiazide/aMILoride (a potassium-sparing diuretic): 50 mg/5 mg. **Normozide:** hydroCHLOROthiazide/labetalol (a beta blocker): 25 mg/100 mg, 25 mg/300 mg. **Prinzide/Zestoretic:** hydroCHLOROthiazide/lisinopril (an ACE inhibitor): 12.5 mg/10 mg, 12.5 mg/20 mg, 25 mg/20 mg. **Tekturna HCT:** hydroCHLOROthiazide/aliskiren (a renin inhibitor): 12.5 mg/150 mg, 25 mg/300 mg. **Teveten HCT:** hydroCHLOROthiazide/eprosartan (an angiotensin II receptor antagonist): 12.5 mg/600 mg, 25 mg/600 mg. **Timolide:** hydroCHLOROthiazide/timolol (a beta blocker): 25 mg/10 mg. **Tribenzor:** hydroCHLOROthiazide/olmesartan/amLODIPine: 12.5 mg/20 mg/5 mg, 12.5 mg/40 mg/5 mg, 25 mg/40 mg/5 mg,

12.5 mg/40 mg/10 mg, 25 mg/40 mg/10 mg. **Uniretic:** hydroCHLORO-thiazide/moexipril (an ACE inhibitor): 12.5 mg/7.5 mg, 25 mg/15 mg. **Vaseretic:** hydroCHLOROthiazide/enalapril (an ACE inhibitor): 12.5 mg/5 mg, 25 mg/10 mg. **Ziac:** hydroCHLORO-thiazide/bisoprolol (a beta blocker): 6.25 mg/5 mg, 6.25 mg/10 mg.

◆CLASSIFICATION

PHARMACOTHERAPEUTIC: Sulfonamide derivative. **CLINICAL:** Thiazide diuretic, antihypertensive.

USES

Treatment of mild to moderate hypertension, edema in HF, hepatic cirrhosis, renal dysfunction (e.g., nephrotic syndrome). **OFF-LABEL:** Treatment of calcium nephrolithiasis.

PRECAUTIONS

Contraindications: Hypersensitivity to hydroCHLOROthiazide. Anuria, history of hypersensitivity to sulfonamides or thiazide diuretics. **Cautions:** Severe renal/hepatic impairment, prediabetes or diabetes, elderly or debilitated, history of gout, moderate to high serum cholesterol, hypercalcemia, hypokalemia.

ACTION

Inhibits sodium reabsorption in distal renal tubules, causing excretion of sodium, potassium, hydrogen ions, water. **Therapeutic Effect:** Promotes diuresis; reduces B/P.

PHARMACOKINETICS

Route	Onset	Peak	Duration
PO (diuretic)	2 hrs	4–6 hrs	6–12 hrs

Variably absorbed from GI tract. Primarily excreted unchanged in urine. Not removed by hemodialysis. **Half-life:** 5.6–14.8 hrs.

⧗ LIFESPAN CONSIDERATIONS

Pregnancy/Lactation: Crosses placenta. Small amount distributed in breast milk. Breastfeeding not recommended.

Children: No age-related precautions noted, except jaundiced infants may be at risk for hyperbilirubinemia. **Elderly:** May be more sensitive to hypotensive, electrolyte effects. Age-related renal impairment may require dosage adjustment.

INTERACTIONS

DRUG: Cholestyramine, colestipol may decrease absorption, effects. **Antihypertensives (e.g., amLODIPine, cloNIDine, lisinopril, valsartan)** may increase hypotensive effect. May increase risk of **digoxin** toxicity associated with hydroCHLOROthiazide-induced hypokalemia. May increase risk of **lithium** toxicity. **HERBAL: Ephedra, ginseng, yohimbe** may diminish effect. **Black cohosh, periwinkle** may increase antihypertensive effect. **FOOD:** None known. **LAB VALUES:** May increase serum glucose, cholesterol, LDL, bilirubin, calcium, creatinine, uric acid, triglycerides. May decrease urinary calcium, serum magnesium, potassium, sodium.

AVAILABILITY (Rx)

Capsules (Microzide): 12.5 mg. **Tablets:** 12.5 mg, 25 mg, 50 mg.

ADMINISTRATION/HANDLING

PO
• May take with or without food. If GI upset occurs, give with food or milk, preferably with breakfast (may prevent nocturia). • Give last dose no later than 6 PM unless instructed otherwise.

INDICATIONS/ROUTES/DOSAGE

Edema
PO: ADULTS: 25–100 mg/day in 1–2 divided doses. May give on alternate days or on 3–5 days/wk.

Hypertension
PO: ADULTS: Initially, 12.5–25 mg once daily. May increase up to 50 mg/day in 1–2 divided doses.

Usual Elderly Dosage
PO: 12.5–25 mg once daily. Titrate in 12.5-mg increments.

Usual Pediatric Dosage (Edema/HTN)

PO: CHILDREN 2–12 YRS: 1–2 mg/kg/day. **Maximum:** 100 mg/day. **CHILDREN 6 MOS–2 YRS:** 1–2 mg/kg/day in 1–2 divided doses. **Maximum:** 37.5 mg/day. **CHILDREN YOUNGER THAN 6 MOS:** 1–3 mg/kg/day in 2 divided doses. **Maximum:** 37.5 mg/day.

Dosage in Renal Impairment

CrCl less than 30 mL/min: Generally not effective. Avoid use with CrCl less than 10 mL/min.

Dosage in Hepatic Impairment

Use caution.

SIDE EFFECTS

Expected: Increased urinary frequency (diminishes with continued use), urine volume. **Frequent:** Potassium depletion. **Occasional:** Orthostatic hypotension, headache, GI disturbances, photosensitivity.

ADVERSE EFFECTS/TOXIC REACTIONS

Vigorous diuresis may lead to profound water loss/electrolyte depletion, resulting in hypokalemia, hyponatremia, dehydration. Acute hypotensive episodes may occur. Hyperglycemia may occur during prolonged therapy. Pancreatitis, blood dyscrasias, pulmonary edema, allergic pneumonitis, dermatologic reactions occur rarely. Overdose can lead to lethargy, coma without changes in electrolytes or hydration.

NURSING CONSIDERATIONS

BASELINE ASSESSMENT

Check vital signs, esp. B/P for hypotension, before administration. Assess baseline electrolytes, esp. for hypokalemia. Evaluate skin turgor, mucous membranes for hydration status. Evaluate for peripheral edema. Assess muscle strength, mental status. Note skin temperature, moisture. Obtain baseline weight. Monitor I&O.

INTERVENTION/EVALUATION

Continue to monitor B/P, vital signs, electrolytes, I&O, daily weight. Note extent of diuresis. Watch for changes from initial assessment (hypokalemia may result in weakness, tremor, muscle cramps, nausea, vomiting, altered mental status, tachycardia; hyponatremia may result in confusion, thirst, cold/clammy skin). Be esp. alert for potassium depletion in pts taking digoxin (cardiac arrhythmias). Potassium supplements are frequently ordered. Check for constipation (may occur with exercise diuresis).

PATIENT/FAMILY TEACHING

• Expect increased frequency (diminishes with continued use), volume of urination. • To reduce hypotensive effect, go from lying to standing slowly. • Eat foods high in potassium, such as whole grains (cereals), legumes, meat, bananas, apricots, orange juice, potatoes (white, sweet), raisins. • Protect skin from sun, ultraviolet light (photosensitivity may occur).

H

HYDROcodone

hye-droe-**koe**-done
(Hycodan ✤, Hysingla ER, Robidone ✤, Zohydro ER)
Do not confuse Hycodan with Vicodin.

FIXED-COMBINATION(S)

Hycet: HYDROcodone/acetaminophen: 7.5 mg/325 mg per 15 mL. **Hycodan:** HYDROcodone/homatropine (an anticholinergic): 5 mg/1.5 mg. **Hycotuss, Vitussin:** HYDROcodone/guaiFENesin (an expectorant): 5 mg/100 mg. **Norco:** HYDROcodone/acetaminophen: 5 mg/325 mg, 7.5 mg/325 mg, 10 mg/325 mg. **Reprexain CIII:** HYDROcodone/ibuprofen (an NSAID): 5 mg/200 mg. **Rezira:** HYDROcodone/pseudoephedrine (a nasal

 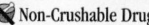

decongestant): 5 mg/60 mg per 5 mL. **Tussend:** HYDROcodone/pseudoephedrine (a sympathomimetic)/guaiFENesin (an expectorant): 2.5 mg/30 mg/100 mg per 5 mL. **Vicodin:** HYDROcodone/acetaminophen: 5 mg/300 mg. **Vicodin ES:** HYDROcodone/acetaminophen: 7.5 mg/300 mg. **Vicodin HP:** HYDROcodone/acetaminophen: 10 mg/300 mg. **Vicoprofen:** HYDROcodone/ibuprofen (an NSAID): 7.5 mg/200 mg. **Xodol:** HYDROcodone/acetaminophen: 5 mg/300 mg, 7.5 mg/300 mg, 10 mg/300 mg. **Zutripro:** HYDROcodone/chlorpheniramine (an antihistamine)/pseudoephedrine (a nasal decongestant): 5 mg/4 mg/60 mg.

◆CLASSIFICATION

PHARMACOTHERAPEUTIC: Opioid agonist **(Schedule III). CLINICAL:** Narcotic analgesic, antitussive.

USES

Relief of moderate to moderately severe pain, nonproductive cough. **Hysingla ER, Zohydro ER:** Around-the-clock management of moderate to severe chronic pain.

PRECAUTIONS

Contraindications: Hypersensitivity to HYDROcodone. Significant respiratory depression, acute or severe bronchial asthma or hypercarbia, paralytic ileus. **Cautions:** Adrenal insufficiency, biliary tract disease, pancreatitis, CNS depression/coma, acute alcoholism, hypothyroidism; severe renal, hepatic, or pulmonary impairment; urinary stricture, prostatic hypertrophy, seizures, elderly, debilitated, other CNS depressants, history of substance abuse.

ACTION

Binds with opioid receptors in CNS. **Therapeutic Effect:** Reduces intensity of incoming pain stimuli from sensory nerve endings, altering pain perception, emotional response to pain; suppresses cough reflex.

PHARMACOKINETICS

Route	Onset	Peak	Duration
PO (analgesic)	10–20 min	30–60 min	4–6 hrs
PO (antitussive)	N/A	N/A	4–6 hrs

Well absorbed from GI tract. Metabolized in liver. Primarily excreted in urine. **Half-life:** 3.8 hrs (increased in elderly).

⌛ LIFESPAN CONSIDERATIONS

Pregnancy/Lactation: Readily crosses placenta. Distributed in breast milk. May prolong labor if administered in latent phase of first stage of labor or before cervical dilation of 4–5 cm has occurred. Respiratory depression may occur in neonate if mother received opiates during labor. Regular use of opiates during pregnancy may produce withdrawal symptoms (irritability, excessive crying, tremors, hyperactive reflexes, fever, vomiting, diarrhea, yawning, sneezing, seizures) in the neonate. **Children:** Pts younger than 2 yrs may be more susceptible to respiratory depression. **Elderly:** May be more susceptible to respiratory depression, may cause paradoxical excitement. Age-related renal impairment, prostatic hypertrophy or obstruction may increase risk of urinary retention; dosage adjustment recommended.

INTERACTIONS

DRUG: Alcohol, other CNS depressants (e.g., diphenhydrAMINE, gabapentin, haloperidol LORazepam, morphine) may increase CNS or respiratory depression, hypotension. **MAOIs (e.g., phenelzine, selegiline), tricyclic antidepressants (e.g., amitriptyline, doxepin)** may alter effect of HYDROcodone. **CYP3A4 inhibitors (e.g., clarithromycin, ketoconazole)** may increase or prolong opioid effects. **HERBAL: Gotu kola, kava kava, St. John's wort, valerian** may increase CNS depression. **FOOD:** None known.

---

underlined – top prescribed drug

LAB VALUES: May increase serum amylase, lipase.

AVAILABILITY (Rx)

Capsules, Extended-Release (Zohydro ER): 10 mg, 15 mg, 20 mg, 30 mg, 40 mg, 50 mg. **Tablets, Extended-Release (Hysingla ER):** 20 mg, 30 mg, 40 mg, 60 mg, 80 mg, 100 mg, 120 mg.

ADMINISTRATION/HANDLING
PO
• Give without regard to meals. • Extended-release capsules/tablets must be swallowed whole. Do not cut, crush, or dissolve.

INDICATIONS/ROUTES/DOSAGE

Analgesia (Combination Products)
PO: ADULTS, CHILDREN WEIGHING 50 KG OR MORE: Initially, 5–10 mg q3–4h as needed. **ADULTS, CHILDREN WEIGHING LESS THAN 50 KG:** Initially, 0.1–0.2 mg/kg q3–4h as needed. **ELDERLY:** 2.5–5 mg q4–6h.

Analgesia (Extended-Release)
PO: ADULTS, ELDERLY: *(Zohydro ER):* Initially, 10 mg q12h. May increase by 10 mg q12h q3–7 days to achieve adequate analgesia. *(Hysingla ER):* Initially, 20 mg q24h. May titrate q3–5 days.

Cough (Combination Products)
PO: ADULTS, ELDERLY: 5–10 mg q4–6h as needed. **Maximum:** 15 mg/dose. **CHILDREN:** 0.6 mg/kg/day in 3–4 divided doses at intervals of at least 4 hrs. **Maximum single dose:** 10 mg (children older than 12 yrs), 5 mg (children 2–12 yrs), 1.25 mg (children younger than 2 yrs).

Dosage in Renal Impairment
No dose adjustment.

Dosage in Hepatic Impairment
Use caution.

SIDE EFFECTS
Frequent: Lethargy, hypotension, diaphoresis, facial flushing, dizziness, drowsiness.

Occasional: Urine retention, blurred vision, constipation, dry mouth, headache, nausea, vomiting, difficult/painful urination, euphoria, dysphoria.

ADVERSE EFFECTS/TOXIC REACTIONS

Overdose results in respiratory depression, skeletal muscle flaccidity, cold/clammy skin, cyanosis, extreme drowsiness progressing to seizures, stupor, coma. Tolerance to analgesic effect, physical dependence may occur with repeated use. Prolonged duration of action, cumulative effect may occur in those with hepatic/renal impairment. **Antidote:** Naloxone (see Appendix J).

NURSING CONSIDERATIONS

BASELINE ASSESSMENT
Obtain vital signs. If respirations are 12/min or less (20/min or less in children), withhold medication, contact physician. **Analgesic:** Assess onset, type, location, duration of pain. Effect of medication is reduced if full pain recurs before next dose. **Antitussive:** Assess type, severity, frequency of cough.

INTERVENTION/EVALUATION
Palpate bladder for urinary retention. Monitor daily pattern of bowel activity, stool consistency. Initiate deep breathing and coughing exercises, particularly in pts with pulmonary impairment. Assess for clinical improvement; record onset of relief of pain, cough. Monitor LOC.

PATIENT/FAMILY TEACHING
• Go from lying to standing slowly to avoid orthostatic hypotension. • Avoid tasks that require alertness, motor skills until response to drug is established. • Avoid alcohol. • Tolerance or dependence may occur with prolonged use at high dosages. • Report nausea, vomiting, constipation, shortness of breath, difficulty breathing.

---

hydrocortisone

hye-droe-**kor**-ti-sone
(Anusol HC, Caldecort, Colocort, Cortaid, SOLU-Cortef, Cortenema, Cortizone-10, Preparation H Hydrocortisone, Proctocort, Westcort.)
Do not confuse hydrocortisone with hydroCHLOROthiazide, HYDROcodone, or hydroxychloroquine, Cortef with Coreg, or SOLU-Cortef with SOLU-Medrol.

FIXED-COMBINATION(S)

Cortisporin: hydrocortisone/neomycin/polymyxin (an anti-infective): 5 mg/10,000 units/5 mg, 10 mg/10,000 units/5 mg. **Lipsovir:** hydrocortisone/acyclovir (an antiviral): 1%/5%.

◆CLASSIFICATION

PHARMACOTHERAPEUTIC: Adrenal corticosteroid. **CLINICAL:** Glucocorticoid.

USES

Systemic: Management of adrenocortical insufficiency, anti-inflammatory, immunosuppressive. **Topical:** Inflammatory dermatoses, adjunctive treatment of ulcerative colitis, atopic dermatitis, inflamed hemorrhoids. **OFF-LABEL:** Management of septic shock. Treatment of thyroid storm.

PRECAUTIONS

Contraindications: Hypersensitivity to hydrocortisone. Fungal, tuberculosis, viral skin lesions; serious infections, IM administration in idiopathic thrombocytopenia purpura. **Cautions:** Thyroid dysfunction, cirrhosis, hypertension, osteoporosis, thromboembolic tendencies or thrombophlebitis, HF, seizure disorders, diabetes, respiratory tuberculosis, untreated systemic infections, renal/hepatic impairment, acute MI, myasthenia gravis, glaucoma, cataracts, increased intraocular pressure, elderly, immunocompromised pts.

ACTION

Inhibits accumulation of inflammatory cells at inflammation sites, phagocytosis, lysosomal enzyme release, synthesis and/or release of mediators of inflammation. Reverses increased capillary permeability. **Therapeutic Effect:** Prevents/suppresses cell-mediated immune reactions. Decreases/prevents tissue response to inflammatory process.

PHARMACOKINETICS

Route	Onset	Peak	Duration
IV	N/A	4–6 hrs	8–12 hrs

Well absorbed after IM administration. Widely distributed. Metabolized in liver. **Half-life:** Plasma, 1.5–2 hrs; biologic, 8–12 hrs.

☒ LIFESPAN CONSIDERATIONS

Pregnancy/Lactation: Crosses placenta; distributed in breast milk. May produce cleft palate if used chronically during first trimester. Breastfeeding not recommended. **Children:** Prolonged treatment or high dosages may decrease short-term growth rate, cortisol secretion. **Elderly:** May be more susceptible to developing hypertension or osteoporosis.

INTERACTIONS

DRUG: May decrease effects of **diuretics (e.g., furosemide), insulin, oral hypoglycemics (e.g., glimepiride, metFORMIN, SITagliptin), potassium supplements. CYP3A4 inducers (e.g., carBAMazepine, phenytoin, rifAMPin)** may decrease effects. **Live virus vaccines** may decrease pt's antibody response to vaccine, increase vaccine side effects, potentiate virus replication. **HERBAL: St. John's wort** may decrease concentration. **Cat's claw, echinacea** may increase immunostimulant properties. **FOOD:** None known. **LAB VALUES:** May increase serum glucose, lipids, sodium. May decrease serum calcium, potassium, thyroxine; WBC count.

AVAILABILITY (Rx)

Cream, Rectal (Cortizone-10, Preparation H Hydrocortisone): 1%, 2.5%. **Cream, Topical:** 0.5%, 1%, 2.5%. **Injection, Powder for Reconstitution (Solu-Cortef):** 100 mg, 250 mg, 500 mg, 1 g. **Ointment, Topical:** 0.5%, 1%, 2.5%. **Suppository (Anusol HC):** 25 mg. **Suspension, Rectal (Colocort, Cortenema):** 100 mg/60 mL. **Tablets (Cortef):** 5 mg, 10 mg, 20 mg.

ADMINISTRATION/HANDLING

 IV

Hydrocortisone Sodium Succinate
Reconstitution • Initially, reconstitute vial per manufacturer's instructions. • May further dilute with D₅W or 0.9% NaCl. For IV push, dilute to 50 mg/mL; for intermittent infusion, dilute to 1 mg/mL. **Note:** 100–3,000 mg may be added to 50 mL D₅W or 0.9% NaCl.
Rate of Administration • Administer IV push over 3–5 min (over 10 min for doses 500 mg or greater). Give intermittent infusion over 20–30 min.
Storage • Store at room temperature. • Once reconstituted, stable for 3 days at room temperature. Once further diluted with 0.9% NaCl or D₅W, stability is concentration dependent: 1 mg/mL (24 hrs), 2–60 mg/mL (4 hrs).

PO

• Give with food or milk if GI distress occurs.

Rectal

• Shake homogeneous suspension well. • Instruct pt to lie on left side with left leg extended, right leg flexed. • Gently insert applicator tip into rectum, pointed slightly toward navel (umbilicus). Slowly instill medication.

Topical

• Gently cleanse area before application. • Use occlusive dressings only as ordered. • Apply sparingly; rub into area thoroughly.

▓ IV INCOMPATIBILITIES

Ciprofloxacin (Cipro), diazePAM (Valium), midazolam (Versed), phenytoin (Dilantin).

▓ IV COMPATIBILITIES

Amphotericin, calcium gluconate, cefepime (Maxipime), digoxin (Lanoxin), diltiaZEM (Cardizem), diphenhydrAMINE (Benadryl), DOPamine (Intropin), insulin, lidocaine, LORazepam (Ativan), magnesium sulfate, morphine, norepinephrine (Levophed), procainamide (Pronestyl), potassium chloride, propofol (Diprivan).

INDICATIONS/ROUTES/DOSAGE

Acute Adrenal Insufficiency
IV: ADULTS, ELDERLY: 100 mg IV bolus, then 50–75 mg q6h for 24 hrs, then taper slowly. **CHILDREN:** 1–2 mg/kg IV bolus, then 150–250 mg/day in divided doses q6–8h. **INFANTS:** 1–2 mg/kg/dose IV bolus, then 25–150 mg/day in divided doses q6–8h.

Anti-Inflammation, Immunosuppression
IV, IM: ADULTS, ELDERLY: 100–500 mg/dose at intervals of 2 hrs, 4 hrs, or 6 hrs. **CHILDREN:** 1–5 mg/kg/day in divided doses q12h.
PO: ADULTS, ELDERLY: 15–240 mg q12h. **CHILDREN:** 2.5–10 mg/kg/day in divided doses q6–8h.

Physiologic Replacement
PO: CHILDREN: 8–10 mg/m²/day in 3 divided doses.

Adjunctive Treatment of Ulcerative Colitis
Rectal *(Enema):* ADULTS, ELDERLY: 100 mg at bedtime for 21 nights or until clinical and proctologic remission occurs (may require 2–3 mos of therapy).
Rectal Foam: ADULTS, ELDERLY: 1 applicator 1–2 times/day for 2–3 wks, then every second day until therapy ends.
Usual Topical Dosage: ADULTS, ELDERLY: Apply sparingly 2–4 times/day.

Dosage in Renal/Hepatic Impairment
No dose adjustment.

H

SIDE EFFECTS

Frequent: Insomnia, heartburn, anxiety, abdominal distention, diaphoresis, acne, mood swings, increased appetite, facial flushing, delayed wound healing, increased susceptibility to infection, diarrhea or constipation. **Occasional:** Headache, edema, change in skin color, frequent urination. **Topical:** Pruritus, redness, irritation. **Rare:** Tachycardia, allergic reaction (rash, hives), psychological changes, hallucinations, depression. **Topical:** Allergic contact dermatitis, purpura. **Systemic:** Absorption more likely with use of occlusive dressings or extensive application in young children.

ADVERSE EFFECTS/TOXIC REACTIONS

Long-term therapy: Hypocalcemia, hypokalemia, muscle wasting (esp. arms, legs), osteoporosis, spontaneous fractures, amenorrhea, cataracts, glaucoma, peptic ulcer, HF. **Abrupt withdrawal after long-term therapy:** Nausea, fever, headache, sudden severe joint pain, rebound inflammation, fatigue, weakness, lethargy, dizziness, orthostatic hypotension.

NURSING CONSIDERATIONS

BASELINE ASSESSMENT

Obtain baseline weight, B/P, serum glucose, cholesterol, electrolytes. Screen for infections including fungal infections, TB, viral skin lesions. Question medical history as listed in Precautions.

INTERVENTION/EVALUATION

Assess for edema. Be alert to infection (reduced immune response): sore throat, fever, vague symptoms. Monitor daily pattern of bowel activity, stool consistency. Monitor electrolytes, B/P, weight, serum glucose. Monitor for hypocalcemia (muscle twitching, cramps), hypokalemia (weakness, paresthesia [esp. lower extremities], nausea/vomiting, irritability, EKG changes). Assess emotional status, ability to sleep.

PATIENT/FAMILY TEACHING

• Report fever, sore throat, muscle aches, sudden weight gain, swelling, visual disturbances, behavioral changes. • Do not take aspirin or any other medication without consulting physician. • Limit caffeine; avoid alcohol. • Inform dentist, other physicians of cortisone therapy now or within past 12 mos. • Caution against overusing joints injected for symptomatic relief. • **Topical:** Apply after shower or bath for best absorption. • Do not cover or use occlusive dressings unless ordered by physician; do not use tight diapers, plastic pants, coverings. • Avoid contact with eyes.

HYDROmorphone ■HIGH ALERT

hye-droe-**mor**-fone
(Apo-HYDROmorphone ✤, Dilaudid, Exalgo, Hydromorph Contin ✤)

■ **BLACK BOX ALERT** ■ High abuse potential, respiratory depression risk. Other opioids, alcohol, CNS depressants increase risk of potentially fatal respiratory depression. Highly concentrated (Dilaudid HP, 10 mg/mL) form not to be interchanged with less concentrated (Dilaudid) form; overdose, death may result. Exalgo: For use in opioid-tolerant pts. Do not crush, break, chew, or dissolve. Swallow whole.

Do not confuse Dilaudid with Demerol or Dilantin, or HYDROmorphone with HYDROcodone or morphine.

◆CLASSIFICATION

PHARMACOTHERAPEUTIC: Opioid agonist **(Schedule II)**. **CLINICAL:** Narcotic analgesic, antitussive.

USES

Relief of moderate to severe pain. Extended-release tablet (Exalgo): Around the clock, continuous analgesia for extended period.

PRECAUTIONS

Contraindications: Hypersensitivity to HYDROmorphone. Acute or severe asthma, severe respiratory depression. **Additional Product-Specific Contraindications: Dilaudid liquids and tablets:** Obstetric analgesia. **Dilaudid injection:** Opioid-intolerant pts, pts at risk of developing GI obstruction. **Exalgo:** Opioid-intolerant pts, preexisting GI surgery/diseases causing GI narrowing, GI obstruction, paralytic ileus. **Cautions:** Severe hepatic, renal, respiratory disease; hypothyroidism, adrenal cortical insufficiency, seizures, acute alcoholism, head injury, intracranial lesions, increased intracranial pressure, prostatic hypertrophy, Addison's disease, urethral stricture, pancreatitis, biliary tract disease, cardiovascular disease, morbid obesity, delirium tremens, toxic psychosis, pts with CNS depression or coma, pts with depleted blood volume, obstructive bowel disorder.

ACTION

Binds to opioid receptors in CNS, reducing intensity of pain stimuli from sensory nerve endings. **Therapeutic Effect:** Alters perception, emotional response to pain; suppresses cough reflex.

PHARMACOKINETICS

Route	Onset	Peak	Duration
PO	30 min	90–120 min	4 hrs
IV	10–15 min	15–30 min	2–3 hrs
IM	15 min	30–60 min	4–5 hrs
SQ	15 min	30–90 min	4 hrs
Rectal	15–30 min	N/A	N/A

Well absorbed from GI tract after IM administration. Widely distributed. Metabolized in liver. Excreted in urine. **Half-life:** 2.6–4 hrs.

⧗ LIFESPAN CONSIDERATIONS

Pregnancy/Lactation: Readily crosses placenta. Unknown if distributed in breast milk. May prolong labor if administered in latent phase of first stage of labor or before cervical dilation of 4–5 cm has occurred. Respiratory depression may occur in neonate if mother receives opiates during labor. Regular use of opiates during pregnancy may produce withdrawal symptoms in the neonate (irritability, excessive crying, tremors, hyperactive reflexes, fever, vomiting, diarrhea, yawning, sneezing, seizures). **Children:** Pts younger than 2 yrs may be more susceptible to respiratory depression. **Elderly:** May be more susceptible to respiratory depression, may cause paradoxical excitement. Age-related renal impairment, prostatic hypertrophy or obstruction may increase risk of urinary retention; dosage adjustment recommended.

INTERACTIONS

DRUG: Alcohol, other CNS depressants (e.g., diphenhydrAMINE, gabapentin, LORazepam, morphine) may increase CNS, respiratory depression, hypotension. **HERBAL:** Gotu kola, kava kava, St. John's wort, valerian may increase CNS depression. **FOOD:** None known. **LAB VALUES:** May increase serum amylase, lipase.

AVAILABILITY (Rx)

Injection, Solution: 1 mg/mL, 2 mg/mL, 4 mg/mL, 10 mg/mL. **Liquid, Oral:** 1 mg/mL. **Suppository:** 3 mg. **Tablets:** 2 mg, 4 mg, 8 mg.

⧗ **Tablets, Extended-Release (Exalgo):** 8 mg, 12 mg, 16 mg, 32 mg.

ADMINISTRATION/HANDLING

⧗ **IV**

◄**ALERT**► High-concentration injection (10 mg/mL) should be used only in pts tolerant to opiate agonists, currently receiving high doses of another opiate agonist for severe, chronic pain due to cancer. **Reconstitution** • May give undiluted. • May further dilute with 5 mL Sterile Water for Injection or 0.9% NaCl. **Rate of Administration** • Administer IV push very slowly (over 2–3 min). • Rapid IV increases risk of severe adverse reactions (chest wall rigidity, apnea, peripheral circulatory collapse, anaphylactoid effects, cardiac arrest).

Storage • Store at room temperature; protect from light. • Slight yellow discoloration of parenteral form does not indicate loss of potency.

IM, SQ

• Subcutaneously or intramuscularly insert needle and inject solution. Pulling back the plunger before IM injection may ensure that drug is not delivered directly into bloodstream (however, this topic is currently debated). • Administer slowly; rotate injection sites. • Pts with circulatory impairment experience higher risk of overdosage due to delayed absorption of repeated administration.

PO

• Give without regard to meals. • Tablets may be crushed. • Extended-release tablets must be swallowed whole; do not break, crush, dissolve, or divide.

Rectal

• Refrigerate suppositories. • Moisten suppository with cold water before inserting well up into rectum.

🔲 IV INCOMPATIBILITIES

Amphotericin B complex (Abelcet, AmBisome, Amphotec), ceFAZolin (Ancef, Kefzol), diazePAM (Valium), PHENobarbital, phenytoin (Dilantin).

🔲 IV COMPATIBILITIES

Dexmedetomidine (Precedex), diltiaZEM (Cardizem), diphenhydrAMINE (Benadryl), DOBUTamine (Dobutrex), DOPamine (Intropin), fentaNYL (Sublimaze), furosemide (Lasix), heparin, LORazepam (Ativan), magnesium sulfate, metoclopramide (Reglan), midazolam (Versed), milrinone (Primacor), morphine, propofol (Diprivan).

INDICATIONS/ROUTES/DOSAGE

Analgesia (Acute, Moderate to Severe)
PO: ADULTS: *(Immediate-Release)*: Initially 2–4 mg q4–6h prn (tablets) or 2.5–10 mg q3–6h prn (liquid).

ELDERLY: Use with caution; initiating at the low end of the dosage range is recommended. **CHILDREN, ADOLESCENTS WEIGHING MORE THAN 50 KG:** 1–2 mg q3–4h. **CHILDREN OLDER THAN 6 MOS AND WEIGHING LESS THAN 50 KG:** 0.03–0.08 mg/kg/dose q3–4h.
IV: ADULTS, ELDERLY: (For use in opiate-naive pts) 0.2–1 mg q2–3h (pts with prior opioid exposure may require higher doses). **CHILDREN, ADOLESCENTS WEIGHING MORE THAN 50 KG:** 0.2–0.6 mg/dose q2–4h as needed. **CHILDREN WEIGHING 50 KG OR LESS:** 0.015 mg/kg/dose q3–6h as needed.
Rectal: ADULTS, ELDERLY: 3 mg q6–8h.

Patient-Controlled Analgesia (PCA)
IV: ADULTS, ELDERLY: (Usual concentration: 0.2 mg/mL). Demand dose: Initially, 0.1–0.2 mg. Range: 0.05–0.4 mg. Lockout interval: 6 min. Range: 5–10 min.
Epidural: ADULTS, ELDERLY: Bolus dose of 0.4–1 mg; infusion rate: 0.03–0.3 mg/hr; demand dose: 0.02–0.05 mg. Lockout interval: 10–15 min.

Dosage in Renal/Hepatic Impairment
Decrease initial dose; use with caution.

SIDE EFFECTS

Frequent: Drowsiness, dizziness, hypotension (including orthostatic hypotension), decreased appetite. **Occasional:** Confusion, diaphoresis, facial flushing, urinary retention, constipation, dry mouth, nausea, vomiting, headache, pain at injection site. **Rare:** Allergic reaction, depression.

ADVERSE EFFECTS/TOXIC REACTIONS

Overdose results in respiratory depression, skeletal muscle flaccidity, cold/clammy skin, cyanosis, extreme drowsiness progressing to seizures, stupor, coma. Tolerance to analgesic effect, physical dependence may occur with repeated use. Prolonged duration of action, cumulative effect may occur in those with hepatic/renal impairment. **Antidote:** Naloxone (see Appendix J).

NURSING CONSIDERATIONS

BASELINE ASSESSMENT

Obtain vital signs. If respirations are 12/min or less (20/min or less in children), withhold medication, contact physician. **Analgesic:** Assess onset, type, location, duration of pain. Effect of medication is reduced if full pain recurs before next dose. **Antitussive:** Assess type, severity, frequency of cough.

INTERVENTION/EVALUATION

Monitor vital signs; assess for pain relief, cough. To prevent pain cycles, instruct pt to request pain medication as soon as discomfort begins. Monitor daily pattern of bowel activity, stool consistency (esp. in long-term use). Initiate deep breathing and coughing exercises, particularly in pts with pulmonary impairment. Assess for clinical improvement; record onset of relief of pain, cough.

PATIENT/FAMILY TEACHING

• Avoid alcohol. • Avoid tasks that require alertness/motor skills until response to drug is established. • Tolerance or dependence may occur with prolonged use at high dosages. • Change positions slowly to avoid orthostatic hypotension. • Do not chew, crush, dissolve, or divide extended-release tablets.

---

hydroxyurea   HIGH ALERT

hye-**drox**-ee-yoo-**ree**-ah
(Apo-Hydroxyurea ✦, Droxia, Hydrea)

■ **BLACK BOX ALERT** ■ Must be administered by personnel trained in administration/handling of chemotherapeutic agents or in treatment of sickle cell anemia. Carcinogenic risk; secondary leukemias reported with long-term treatment.
Do not confuse hydroxyurea with hydrOXYzine.

◆CLASSIFICATION

PHARMACOTHERAPEUTIC: Synthetic urea analogue. **CLINICAL:** Antineoplastic.

USES

Treatment of melanoma, resistant chronic myelocytic leukemia, recurrent, metastatic, inoperable ovarian carcinoma. Used in combination with radiation therapy for local control of primary squamous cell carcinoma of head/neck, excluding lip. Treatment of sickle cell anemia with at least 3 painful crises in previous 12 mos. **OFF-LABEL:** Treatment of hematologic conditions (e.g., polycythemia vera), cervical cancer, essential thrombocythemia, hyperleukocytosis due to AML, treatment of meningiomas.

PRECAUTIONS

Contraindications: Hypersensitivity to hydroxyurea. **Cautions:** WBC count less than 2,500 cells/mm³ or platelet count less than 100,000 cells/mm³, severe anemia. Previous irradiation therapy, concurrent use with other cytotoxic drugs, renal/hepatic impairment, elderly; pts with sickle cell anemia if neutrophils less than 2,000 cells/mm³, platelets less than 80,000 cells/mm³, Hgb less than 4.5 g/dL, or reticulocytes less than 80,000 cells/mm³ when Hgb less than 9 g/dL.

ACTION

Inhibits DNA synthesis without interfering with RNA synthesis or protein. In sickle cell anemia, increases RBC, Hgb levels, thereby decreasing concentration of sickled cells; alters adhesion of RBCs to endothelium. **Therapeutic Effect:** Interferes with normal repair process of cancer cells damaged by irradiation.

PHARMACOKINETICS

Well absorbed from GI tract. Protein binding: 75%–80%. Metabolized in liver. Excreted in urine as urea and unchanged drug. **Half-life:** 3–4 hrs.

✦ Canadian trade name   Non-Crushable Drug   HIGH ALERT High Alert drug

H

⌛ LIFESPAN CONSIDERATIONS

Pregnancy/Lactation: Crosses placenta; distributed in breast milk. May cause fetal harm. **Children:** Safety and efficacy not established. **Elderly:** More sensitive to hydroxyurea effects; may require lower dosage.

INTERACTIONS

DRUG: Bone marrow depressants (e.g., alemtuzumab, methotrexate) may increase myelosuppression. **Live virus vaccines** may potentiate virus replication, increase vaccine side effects, decrease the pt's antibody response to vaccine. **HERBAL: Echinacea** may decrease effect. **FOOD:** None known. **LAB VALUES:** May increase serum BUN, creatinine, uric acid.

AVAILABILITY (Rx)

Capsules: 200 mg (Droxia), 300 mg (Droxia), 400 mg (Droxia), 500 mg (Hydrea).

ADMINISTRATION/HANDLING

Do not open capsules.

INDICATIONS/ROUTES/DOSAGE

◀ALERT▶ Antineoplastic therapy interrupted when platelet count less than 100,000 cells/mm³ or WBC count less than 2,500 cells/mm³. Resume when counts return to normal.

Sickle cell anemia therapy interrupted when neutrophils less than 2,000 cells/mm³, platelets less than 80,000 cells/mm³, Hgb less than 4.5 g/dL, or reticulocytes less than 80,000 cells/mm³ with Hgb less than 9 g/dL. Reduce dose by 2.5 mg/kg/day following recovery.

CML, Head and Neck Cancer

PO: ADULTS, ELDERLY: 15 mg/kg/day. Adjust dose based on tumor type, disease state, response, pt risk factors. May give alone or in combination with other agents.

Sickle Cell Anemia

PO: ADULTS, ELDERLY: Initially, 15 mg/kg once daily. May increase by 5 mg/kg/day every 12 wks. **Maximum:** 35 mg/kg/day. **CHILDREN 6 MOS AND OLDER:** 20 mg/kg/dose once daily; increase by 5 mg/kg/day q8wk until mild myelosuppression is achieved. **Maximum:** 35 mg/kg/day.

Dosage in Renal Impairment

Reduce dose to 7.5 mg/kg/day for CrCl 60 mL/min or less.

Dosage in Hepatic Impairment

No dose adjustment.

SIDE EFFECTS

Frequent: Nausea, vomiting, anorexia, constipation or diarrhea. **Occasional:** Mild, reversible rash; facial flushing, pruritus, fever, chills, malaise. **Rare:** Alopecia, headache, drowsiness, dizziness, disorientation.

ADVERSE EFFECTS/TOXIC REACTIONS

Myelosuppression manifested as hematologic toxicity (leukopenia and, to a lesser extent, thrombocytopenia, anemia).

NURSING CONSIDERATIONS

BASELINE ASSESSMENT

Obtain bone marrow studies, renal function, LFT before therapy begins, periodically thereafter. Obtain Hgb, WBC, platelet count, serum uric acid at baseline and wkly during therapy. Pts with marked renal impairment may develop visual or auditory hallucinations, marked hematologic toxicity.

INTERVENTION/EVALUATION

Monitor CBC with differential, renal/hepatic function, uric acid. Monitor daily pattern of bowel activity, stool consistency. Monitor for hematologic toxicity (fever, sore throat, signs of local infection, unusual bleeding/bruising at any site), symptoms of anemia (excessive fatigue, weakness). Assess skin for rash, erythema.

PATIENT/FAMILY TEACHING

• Promptly report fever, sore throat, signs of local infection, unusual bleeding/bruising at any site.

hydrOXYzine

hye-**drox**-ee-zeen
(Apo-HydrOXYzine ♣, Atarax ♣,
Novo-Hydroxyzin ♣, Vistaril)
**Do not confuse hydrOXYzine with
hydrALAZINE or hydroxyurea, or
Vistaril with Restoril, Versed, or
Zestril.**

◆CLASSIFICATION

PHARMACOTHERAPEUTIC: Histamine
H_1 antagonist. **CLINICAL:** Antihistamine, antianxiety, antispasmodic,
antiemetic, antipruritic.

USES

Antiemetic, treatment of anxiety/agita-
tion, antipruritic.

PRECAUTIONS

Contraindications: Hypersensitivity to hydrOXYzine. Early pregnancy; subcutaneous, intravenous administration; pts with
prolonged QT interval. **Cautions:** Narrow-
angle glaucoma, prostatic hypertrophy,
bladder neck obstruction, asthma, COPD,
elderly.

ACTION

Competes with histamine for receptor
sites in GI tract, blood vessels, respiratory tract. **Therapeutic Effect:** Produces   anxiolytic,   anticholinergic,
antihistaminic, analgesic effects; relaxes skeletal muscle; controls nausea,
vomiting.

PHARMACOKINETICS

Route	Onset	Peak	Duration
PO	15–30 min	N/A	4–6 hrs

Well absorbed from GI tract and after
parenteral administration. Metabolized
in liver. Primarily excreted in urine.
Not removed by hemodialysis. **Half-
life:** 3–7 hrs (increased in elderly,
hepatic impairment).

⌛ LIFESPAN CONSIDERATIONS

Pregnancy/Lactation: Unknown   if
drug crosses placenta or is distributed
in breast milk. **Children:** Not recommended in newborns or premature infants (increased risk of anticholinergic
effects). Paradoxical excitement may
occur. **Elderly:** Increased risk of dizziness, sedation, confusion. Hypotension,
hyperexcitability may occur.

INTERACTIONS

DRUG: Alcohol, other CNS depressants (e.g., diphenhydrAMINE, gabapentin, LORazepam, morphine)
may increase CNS depressant effects. **QT
interval–prolonging medications (e.g.,
amiodarone, azithromycin, certinib,
haloperidol, moxifloxacin)** may increase
risk of QT interval prolongation, torsades de
pointes. **HERBAL:** Gotu kola, kava kava,
St. John's wort, valerian may increase
CNS depression. **FOOD:** None known. **LAB
VALUES:** May cause false-positive urine
17-hydroxycorticosteroid determinations.

AVAILABILITY (Rx)

Oral Solution: 10 mg/5 mL. **Syrup:** 10
mg/5 mL. **Tablets:** 10 mg, 25 mg, 50 mg.

🐲 **Capsules:** 25 mg, 50 mg, 100 mg.

ADMINISTRATION/HANDLING

PO
• May give without regard to food.
• Shake oral suspension well. • Scored
tablets may be crushed; do not break,
crush, or open capsule.

INDICATIONS/ROUTES/DOSAGE

Anxiety
Note: Initiate elderly dose at the lower
end of recommended dosage.
PO: ADULTS, ELDERLY: 50–100 mg 4 times/
day or 37.5–75 mg/day in divided doses.

Pruritus
PO: ADULTS, ELDERLY: 25 mg 3–4 times/
day. **CHILDREN 6 YRS AND OLDER:** 50–100
mg/day in divided doses. **CHILDREN**

H

♣ Canadian trade name   🐲 Non-Crushable Drug   ⚠ High Alert drug

YOUNGER THAN 6 YRS: 50 mg/day in divided doses.

Dosage in Renal/Hepatic Impairment

No dose adjustment. Change dosing interval to q24h in pts with primary biliary cirrhosis.

SIDE EFFECTS

Side effects are generally mild, transient. **Frequent:** Drowsiness, dry mouth, marked discomfort with IM injection. **Occasional:** Dizziness, ataxia, asthenia, slurred speech, headache, agitation, increased anxiety. **Rare:** Paradoxical reactions (hyperactivity, anxiety in children; excitement, restlessness in elderly or debilitated pts) generally noted during first 2 wks of therapy, particularly in presence of uncontrolled pain.

ADVERSE EFFECTS/TOXIC REACTIONS

Hypersensitivity reaction (wheezing, dyspnea, chest tightness) may occur. QT interval prolongation, torsades de pointes have been reported. Acute generalized exanthematous pustulosis (AGEP) may occur.

NURSING CONSIDERATIONS

BASELINE ASSESSMENT

Anxiety: Offer emotional support. Assess motor responses (agitation, trembling, tension), autonomic responses (cold/clammy hands, diaphoresis). **Antiemetic:** Assess for dehydration (poor skin turgor, dry mucous membranes, longitudinal furrows in tongue).

INTERVENTION/EVALUATION

For pts on long-term therapy, CBC, BMP, LFT should be performed periodically. Monitor lung sounds for signs of hypersensitivity reaction. Monitor serum electrolytes in pts with severe vomiting. Assess for paradoxical reaction, particularly during early therapy. Assist with ambulation if drowsiness, light-headedness occur. Obtain EKG if palpitations occur or cardiac arrhythmia is suspected. Assess skin for rash, pustules.

PATIENT/FAMILY TEACHING

• Marked discomfort may occur with IM injection. • Sugarless gum, sips of water may relieve dry mouth. • Drowsiness usually diminishes with continued therapy. • Avoid tasks that require alertness, motor skills until response to drug is established. • Treatment may cause life-threatening heart arrhythmias; report chest pain, difficulty breathing, palpitations, passing out. Do not take newly prescribed medications unless approved by prescriber who originally started treatment.

ibandronate

eye-**ban**-droe-nate
(Boniva)

◆CLASSIFICATION

PHARMACOTHERAPEUTIC: Bisphosphonate. **CLINICAL:** Calcium regulator.

USES

Treatment/prevention of osteoporosis in postmenopausal women. **OFF-LABEL:** Hypercalcemia of malignancy; reduces bone pain and skeletal complications from metastatic bone disease due to breast cancer.

PRECAUTIONS

Contraindications: Hypersensitivity to ibandronate, other bisphosphonates; oral tablets in pts unable to stand or sit upright for at least 60 min; pts with abnormalities of the esophagus that would delay emptying (e.g., stricture, achalasia), hypocalcemia. **Cautions:** GI diseases (duodenitis, dysphagia, esophagitis, gastritis, ulcers [drug may exacerbate these conditions]), renal impairment with CrCl less than 30 mL/min.

ACTION

Inhibits bone resorption via activity on osteoclasts. **Therapeutic Effect:** Reduces rate of bone resorption, resulting in increased bone mineral density.

PHARMACOKINETICS

Absorbed in upper GI tract. Extent of absorption impaired by food, beverages (other than plain water). Protein binding: 85%–99%. Rapidly binds to bone. Unabsorbed portion excreted in urine. **Half-life: PO:** 37–157 hrs; **IV:** 5–25 hrs.

⧗ LIFESPAN CONSIDERATIONS

Pregnancy/Lactation: May cause fetal harm/malformations. Unknown if distributed in breast milk. Breastfeeding not recommended. **Children:** Safety and efficacy not established. **Elderly:** No age-related precautions noted.

INTERACTIONS

DRUG: **Vitamin D, antacids containing aluminum, calcium, magnesium** decrease absorption. **Aspirin, NSAIDs (e.g., ibuprofen, ketorolac, naproxen)** may increase GI irritation. **HERBAL:** None significant. **FOOD:** **Beverages (other than plain water), dietary supplements, dairy products, food** interfere with absorption. **LAB VALUES:** May decrease serum alkaline phosphatase. May increase serum cholesterol.

AVAILABILITY (Rx)

Injection Solution: 3 mg/3 mL syringe.
Tablets: 150 mg.

ADMINISTRATION/HANDLING

PO

• Give 60 min before first food or beverage of the day, on an empty stomach with 6–8 oz plain water (not mineral water) while pt is standing or sitting in upright position. • Pt cannot lie down for 60 min following administration. • Instruct pt to swallow whole; do not break, crush, dissolve, or divide tablet (potential for oropharyngeal ulceration).

IV

• Give over 15–30 sec. • Give over 1 hr for metastatic bone disease; over 1–2 hrs for hypercalcemia of malignancy.

INDICATIONS/ROUTES/DOSAGE

Note: May consider discontinuing after 3–5 yrs in pts at low risk for fracture.

Osteoporosis
PO *(Prevention/Treatment):* **ADULTS, ELDERLY:** 150 mg once monthly.
IV *(Treatment):* **ADULTS, ELDERLY:** 3 mg q3mos.

Dosage in Renal Impairment
Not recommended for pts with CrCl less than 30 mL/min.

Dosage in Hepatic Impairment
No dose adjustment.

SIDE EFFECTS

Frequent (13%–6%): Back pain, dyspepsia, peripheral discomfort, diarrhea, headache, myalgia. **IV:** Abdominal pain, dyspepsia, constipation, nausea, diarrhea. **Occasional (4%–3%):** Dizziness, arthralgia, asthenia. **Rare (2% or less):** Vomiting, hypersensitivity reaction.

ADVERSE EFFECTS/TOXIC REACTIONS

Upper respiratory infection occurs occasionally. Overdose results in hypocalcemia, hypophosphatemia, significant GI disturbances.

NURSING CONSIDERATIONS

BASELINE ASSESSMENT

Hypocalcemia, vitamin D deficiency must be corrected before beginning therapy. Obtain laboratory baselines, esp. serum chemistries, renal function. Obtain results of bone density study.

INTERVENTION/EVALUATION

Monitor electrolytes, esp. serum calcium, phosphate. Monitor renal function tests.

PATIENT/FAMILY TEACHING

• Expected benefits occur only when medication is taken with full glass (6–8 oz) of plain water, first thing in the morning and at least 60 min before first food, beverage, medication of the day. Any other beverage (mineral water, orange juice, coffee) significantly reduces absorption of medication. • Do not chew, crush, dissolve, or divide tablets; swallow whole. • Do not lie down for at least 60 min after taking medication (potentiates delivery to stomach, reduces risk of esophageal irritation). • Report swallowing difficulties, pain when swallowing, chest pain, new/worsening heartburn. • Consider weight-bearing exercises; modify behavioral factors (e.g., cigarette smoking, alcohol consumption). • Calcium and vitamin D supplements should be taken if dietary intake inadequate.

ibrutinib

eye-**broo**-ti-nib
(Imbruvica)
Do not confuse ibrutinib with axitinib, dasatinib, erlotinib, gefitinib, imatinib, nilotinib, PONATinib, SORAfenib, SUNItinib, or vandetanib.

◆CLASSIFICATION

PHARMACOTHERAPEUTIC: Kinase inhibitor. **CLINICAL:** Antineoplastic.

USES

Treatment of pts with mantle cell lymphoma (MCL) who have received at least one prior therapy, chronic lymphocytic leukemia (CLL) with at least one prior therapy or with 17p deletion, first-line treatment of CLL. Waldenstrom's macroglobulinemia (WM). Marginal zone lymphoma (MZL) requiring systemic therapy and having received at least one prior anti-CD-20 based therapy. Chronic graft versus host disease (CGVHD) after failure of at least one line of systemic therapy.

PRECAUTIONS

Contraindications: Hypersensitivity to ibrutinib. **Cautions:** Hepatic/renal impairment, elderly, pregnancy, history of GI disease (e.g., bleeding, ulcers).

ACTION

Inhibits enzymatic activity of Bruton's tyrosine kinase (BTK), a signaling molecule that promotes malignant B-cell proliferation and survival. **Therapeutic Effect:** Inhibits tumor cell growth and metastasis.

PHARMACOKINETICS

Readily absorbed following PO. Metabolized in liver. Peak plasma concentration: 1–2 hrs. Protein binding: 97%. Excreted in feces (80%), urine (10%). **Half-life:** 4–6 hrs.

⊠ LIFESPAN CONSIDERATIONS

Pregnancy/Lactation: May cause fetal harm. Avoid pregnancy. Unknown if distributed in breast milk. Must either discontinue drug or discontinue breastfeeding. **Children:** Safety and efficacy not established. **Elderly:** Increased risk of cardiac events (atrial fibrillation, hypertension), infections (pneumonia, cellulitis), GI events (diarrhea, dehydration, bleeding).

INTERACTIONS

DRUG: Strong CYP3A4 inhibitors (e.g., ketoconazole, clarithromycin) may increase plasma concentration/effect; avoid use. **Strong CYP3A4 inducers (e.g., rifAMPin, phenytoin)** may decrease plasma concentration/effect; avoid use. **Anticoagulants (e.g., warfarin), antiplatelets (e.g., aspirin, clopidogrel), NSAIDs** may increase risk of bleeding. **HERBAL: St. John's wort** may decrease concentration/effect. **FOOD: Grapefruit products, Seville oranges** may increase concentration/effect. **All foods** may increase absorption/concentration. **LAB VALUES:** May decrease Hgb, Hct, neutrophils, platelets.

AVAILABILITY (Rx)

🦚 **Capsules:** 140 mg.

ADMINISTRATION/HANDLING

PO
• Give with water. • Do not break, crush, or open capsule.

INDICATIONS/ROUTES/DOSAGE

MCL, MZL
PO: ADULTS/ELDERLY: 560 mg (4 × 140-mg capsules) once daily. Continue until disease progression or unacceptable toxicity.

CLL, WM, CGVHD
PO: ADULTS, ELDERLY: 420 mg (3 × 140 mg) once daily. Continue until disease progression or unacceptable toxicity.

Dose Modification
Based on Common Terminology Criteria for Adverse Events (CTCAE).

Any Grade 3 or Greater Nonhematologic Event, Grade 3 or Greater Neutropenia with Infection or Fever, or Any Grade 4 Hematologic Toxicities
Interrupt treatment until resolution to grade 1 or baseline, then restart at initial dose. If toxicity reoccurs, interrupt treatment until resolution to grade 1 or baseline, then reduce dose to 420 mg daily (one capsule less). If toxicity reoccurs, interrupt treatment until resolution to grade 1 or baseline, then reduce dose to 280 mg once daily (one capsule less). If toxicity still occurs at 280 mg dose, discontinue treatment.

Concomitant Use of Moderate CYP3A4 Inhibitors (e.g., Fluconazole, DiltiaZEM, Verapamil)
Start at reduced dose of 140 mg daily. If toxicity occurs, either discontinue treatment or find alternate agent with less CYP3A inhibition.

Concomitant Short-Term Use of Strong CYP3A4 Inhibitors (7 days or less) (e.g., Antifungals, Antibiotics)
Interrupt treatment until strong CYP3A medications no longer needed.

Concomitant Chronic Use of Strong CYP3A4 Inhibitors or Inducers
Treatment not recommended.

Dosage in Renal Impairment
No dose adjustment.

Dosage in Hepatic Impairment
Mild impairment: Decrease dose to 140 mg. **Moderate to severe impairment:** Avoid use.

SIDE EFFECTS

Frequent (51%–23%): Diarrhea, fatigue, musculoskeletal pain, peripheral edema, nausea, bruising, dyspnea, constipation, rash, abdominal pain, vomiting. **Occasional (21%–11%):** Decreased appetite, cough, pyrexia, stomatitis, asthenia, dizziness, muscle spasms, dehydration, headache, dyspepsia, petechiae, arthralgia.

ADVERSE EFFECTS/ TOXIC REACTIONS

Anemia, lymphopenia, neutropenia, thrombocytopenia is expected response to therapy. Treatment-emergent myelosuppression (grade 3–4 CTCAE) reported in 41% of pts: neutropenia (29%), thrombocytopenia (17%), anemia (9%). Infections including upper respiratory tract infection, UTI, pneumonia, skin infection, sinusitis were reported. Hemorrhagic events including epistaxis, GI bleeding, hematuria, intracranial hemorrhage, subdural hematoma reported in 5% of pts. Serious and fatal cases of renal toxicity reported: increased serum creatinine 1.5 times upper limit of normal (ULN) (67% of pts), increased serum creatinine 1.53 times ULN (9% of pts). Second primary malignancies including skin cancer (4%), other carcinomas (1%) occurred.

NURSING CONSIDERATIONS

BASELINE ASSESSMENT

Obtain baseline vital signs, CBC, serum chemistries, LFT, PT/INR if on anticoagulants. Question history of arrhythmias, HF, GI bleed, hepatic/renal impairment, peripheral edema, pulmonary disease. Obtain negative urine pregnancy before initiating treatment. Assess hydration status. Receive full medication history including herbal products. Assess skin for open/unhealed wounds, lesions, moles. Conduct baseline neurologic exam. Offer emotional support.

INTERVENTION/EVALUATION

Monitor CBC monthly; LFT, serum chemistries, renal function routinely. Monitor stool frequency, consistency, characteristics. Immediately report hemorrhagic events: epistaxis, hematuria, hemoptysis, melena. Encourage PO intake. Obtain EKG for arrhythmias, dyspnea, palpitations. Screen for possible intracranial hemorrhage: altered mental status, aphasia, hemiparesis, unequal pupils, homonymous hemianopsia (blindness of one half of vision on same side of both eyes). Monitor for renal toxicity (anuria, hypertension, generalized edema, flank pain). Assess skin for new lesions.

PATIENT/FAMILY TEACHING

• Blood levels will be monitored routinely. • Difficulty breathing, fever, cough, burning with urination, body aches, chills may indicate acute infection. • Avoid pregnancy. • Report any black/tarry stools, bruising, nausea, RUQ abdominal pain, yellowing of skin or eyes, palpitations, nose bleeds, blood in urine or stool, decreased urine output. • Avoid alcohol. • Do not take herbal products. • Do not ingest grapefruit products. • Severe diarrhea may lead to dehydration. • Contact physician before any planned surgical/dental procedures. • Immediately report neurological changes: confusion, one-sided paralysis, difficulty speaking, partial blindness. • Do not receive live vaccines. • Do not break, crush, or open capsule.

ibuprofen

eye-bue-**pro**-fen
(Advil, Apo-Ibuprofen ✦, Caldolor, Motrin, NeoProfen, Novo-Profen ✦)

■ **BLACK BOX ALERT** ■ Increased risk of serious cardiovascular thrombotic events, including myocardial infarction, CVA. Increased risk of severe GI reactions, including ulceration, bleeding, perforation.
Do not confuse Motrin with Neurontin, or Advil with Aleve.

FIXED-COMBINATION(S)

Children's Advil Cold: ibuprofen/pseudoephedrine (a nasal decongestant): 100 mg/15 mg per 5 mL. **Combunox:** ibuprofen/oxyCODONE (a narcotic analgesic): 400 mg/5 mg. **Duexis:** ibuprofen/famotidine (an H_2 antagonist): 800 mg/26.6 mg. **Reprexain CIII:** ibuprofen/HYDROcodone (a narcotic analgesic): 200 mg/5 mg. **Vicoprofen:** ibuprofen/HYDROcodone (a narcotic analgesic): 200 mg/7.5 mg.

◆ CLASSIFICATION

PHARMACOTHERAPEUTIC: NSAID.
CLINICAL: Antirheumatic, analgesic, antipyretic, antidysmenorrheal, vascular headache suppressant.

USES

Oral: Treatment of fever, rheumatoid disorders, osteoarthritis, mild to moderate pain, primary dysmenorrhea. **Caldolor:** Mild to moderate pain; severe pain in combination with an opioid analgesic; fever. **NeoProfen:** Induces closure in clinically significant patent ductus arteriosus (PDA) in premature infants weighing between 500 and 1,500 g who are no more than 32 wks gestational age when usual medical management is ineffective. **OFF-LABEL:** Treatment of cystic fibrosis, pericarditis. Juvenile idiopathic arthritis.

PRECAUTIONS

Contraindications: History of hypersensitivity to ibuprofen, aspirin, other NSAIDs. Treatment of perioperative pain in coronary artery bypass graft (CABG) surgery. Aspirin triad (bronchial asthma, aspirin intolerance, rhinitis). **NeoProfen:** Infants with proven or suspected untreated infection, elevated total bilirubin, congenital heart disease in whom patency of the patent ductus arteriosus is necessary for satisfactory pulmonary or systemic blood flow (e.g., pulmonary atresia), bleeding, thrombocytopenia, coagulation defects, suspected necrotizing enterocolitis, significant renal impairment. **Cautions:** Pts with fluid retention, HF, dehydration, coagulation disorders, concurrent use with aspirin, anticoagulants, steroids; history of GI disease (e.g., bleeding, ulcers), smoking, use of alcohol, elderly, debilitated pts, hepatic/renal impairment, asthma.

ACTION

Reversibly inhibits COX-1 and COX-2 enzymes, resulting in decreased formation of prostaglandin precursors. **Therapeutic Effect:** Produces analgesic, antiinflammatory effects; decreases fever.

PHARMACOKINETICS

Route	Onset	Peak	Duration
PO (analgesic)	0.5 hr	N/A	4–6 hrs
PO (antirheumatic)	2 days	1–2 wks	N/A

Rapidly absorbed from GI tract. Protein binding: 90%–99%. Metabolized in liver. Primarily excreted in urine. Not removed by hemodialysis. **Half-life:** 2–4 hrs.

⏳ LIFESPAN CONSIDERATIONS

Pregnancy/Lactation: Unknown if drug crosses placenta or is distributed in breast milk. Avoid use during third trimester (may adversely affect fetal cardiovascular system: premature closure of ductus arteriosus). **Children:** Safety and efficacy not established in pts younger than 6 mos. **Elderly:** GI bleeding, ulceration more likely to cause serious adverse effects. Age-related renal impairment may increase risk of hepatic/renal toxicity; reduced dosage recommended.

INTERACTIONS

DRUG: May decrease effects of **anti-hypertensives (e.g., amLODIPine, lisinopril, valsartan), diuretics (e.g., furosemide). Aspirin, other salicylates** may increase risk of GI side effects, bleeding. May increase effects of **oral anticoagulants (e.g., warfarin).** May increase concentration, risk of toxicity of **lithium, methotrexate. HERBAL: Cat's claw, dong quai, evening primrose, feverfew, garlic, ginkgo, ginseng, horse chestnut, red clover** may increase antiplatelet activity. **FOOD:** None known. **LAB VALUES:** May prolong bleeding time. May alter serum glucose level. May increase serum BUN, creatinine, potassium, ALT, AST. May decrease serum calcium, glucose; Hgb, Hct, platelets.

AVAILABILITY (Rx)

Capsules: 200 mg. **Injection, Solution (NeoProfen):** 10 mg/mL. **(Caldolor):** 100 mg/mL. **Suspension, Oral:** 100 mg/5 mL. **Suspension, Oral Drops:** 40 mg/mL.

Tablets: 200 mg, 400 mg, 600 mg, 800 mg.
Tablets, Chewable: 100 mg.

ADMINISTRATION/HANDLING

 IV (Caldolor)

Reconstitution • Dilute with D₅W or 0.9% NaCl to final concentration of 4 mg/mL or less.
Rate of Administration • Infuse over at least 30 min.
Storage • Store at room temperature. • Stable for 24 hrs after dilution.

IV (Neoprofen)

Reconstitution • Dilute to appropriate volume with D₅W or 0.9% NaCl. • Discard any remaining medication after first withdrawal from vial.
Rate of Administration • Administer via IV port nearest the insertion site. • Infuse continuously over 15 min.
Storage • Store at room temperature. • Stable for 30 min after dilution.

PO

• Give with food, milk, antacids if GI distress occurs.

INDICATIONS/ROUTES/DOSAGE

Fever
PO: ADULTS, ELDERLY: 200–400 mg q4–6h prn. **CHILDREN 6 MOS AND OLDER:** 5–10 mg/kg q6–8h. **Maximum:** 400 mg/dose; 1,200 mg/day.
IV: ADULTS, ELDERLY: 400 mg q4–6h or 100–200 mg q4h prn. **Maximum:** 3.2 g/day.
CHILDREN 12–17 YRS: 400 mg q4–6h prn. **Maximum:** 2,400 mg/day. **CHILDREN 6 MOS–11 YRS:** 10 mg/kg q4–6h prn. **Maximum/dose:** 400 mg. **Maximum:** 40 mg/kg up to 2,400 mg/day.

Osteoarthritis, Rheumatoid Disorders
PO: ADULTS, ELDERLY: 400–800 mg 3–4 times/day. **Maximum:** 3.2 g/day.

Pain
PO: ADULTS, ELDERLY, CHILDREN 12 YRS AND OLDER: 200–400 mg q4–6h prn. **CHILDREN**

6 MOS–11 YRS: 4–10 mg/kg q6–8h prn.
Maximum: 40 mg/kg/day (400 mg/dose).
IV: ADULTS, ELDERLY: 400–800 mg q6h prn. **Maximum:** 3.2 g/day.

Primary Dysmenorrhea
PO: ADULTS: 200–800 mg q4–6h prn.
Maximum: 1,200 mg/day.

Patent Ductus Arteriosus (PDA)
IV: INFANTS: Initially, 10 mg/kg then 2 doses of 5 mg/kg, after 24 hrs and 48 hrs. All doses based on birth weight.

Dosage in Renal Impairment
Hold if anuria or oliguria evident. Avoid use in severe impairment.

Dosage in Hepatic Impairment
Avoid use in severe impairment.

SIDE EFFECTS

Occasional (9%–3%): Nausea, vomiting, dyspepsia, dizziness, rash. **Rare (less than 3%):** Diarrhea or constipation, flatulence, abdominal cramps or pain, pruritus, increased B/P.

ADVERSE EFFECTS/TOXIC REACTIONS

Overdose may result in metabolic acidosis. Rare reactions with long-term use include peptic ulcer, GI bleeding, gastritis, severe hepatic reaction (cholestasis, jaundice), nephrotoxicity (dysuria, hematuria, proteinuria, nephrotic syndrome), severe hypersensitivity reaction (particularly in pts with systemic lupus erythematosus or other collagen diseases). **NeoProfen:** Hypoglycemia, hypocalcemia, respiratory failure, UTI, edema, atelectasis may occur. **Caldolor:** Abdominal pain, anemia, cough, dizziness, dyspnea, edema, hypertension, nausea, vomiting have been reported.

NURSING CONSIDERATIONS

BASELINE ASSESSMENT

Assess onset, type, location, duration of pain, inflammation. Inspect appearance of affected joints for immobility, deformities, skin condition. Assess temperature. Question medical history as listed in Precautions.

INTERVENTION/EVALUATION

Monitor for evidence of nausea, dyspepsia. Assess skin for rash. Observe for bleeding, bruising, occult blood loss. Evaluate for therapeutic response: relief of pain, stiffness, swelling; increased joint mobility; reduced joint tenderness; improved grip strength. Monitor for fever.

PATIENT/FAMILY TEACHING

• Avoid aspirin, alcohol during therapy (increases risk of GI bleeding). • If GI upset occurs, take with food, milk, antacids. • May cause dizziness. • Report ringing in ears, persistent stomach pain, respiratory difficulty, unusual bruising/bleeding, swelling of extremities, chest pain/palpitations.

---

idelalisib

eye-**del**-a-**lis**-ib
(Zydelig)

■ **BLACK BOX ALERT** ■ Fatal and/or serious hepatotoxicity may occur. Monitor LFT prior to and during treatment. Fatal and/or serious and severe diarrhea or colitis may occur. Monitor for GI symptoms. Fatal and serious pneumonitis may occur. Monitor for pulmonary symptoms and bilateral interstitial infiltrates. Interrupt, then reduce or discontinue treatment if hepatotoxicity, severe diarrhea, or pneumonitis occurs. Fatal and serious intestinal perforation may occur. Discontinue if perforation suspected.

◆CLASSIFICATION

PHARMACOTHERAPEUTIC: Kinase inhibitor. **CLINICAL:** Antineoplastic.

USES

Treatment of relapsed chronic lymphocytic leukemia (CLL), in combination with riTUXimab, in pts for whom riTUXimab alone would not be considered appropriate therapy due to other co-morbidities. Treatment of relapsed follicular B-cell non-Hodgkin's lymphoma (FL) or relapsed small lymphocytic lymphoma (SLL) in pts who have received at least two prior systemic therapies.

PRECAUTIONS

Contraindications: History of serious allergic reactions to idelalisib (e.g., anaphylaxis, toxic epidermal necrolysis). **Cautions:** Baseline anemia, leukopenia, neutropenia, thrombocytopenia; GI bleeding, hepatic impairment. Pts with active infection, high tumor burden. Avoid concomitant use of hepatotoxic or promotility medications.

ACTION

Inhibits several cell signaling pathways including B-cell receptor signaling and CXCR4 and CXCR5 signaling, which are involved in trafficking B cells to lymph nodes and bone marrow. **Therapeutic Effect:** Inhibits tumor cell growth and metastasis.

PHARMACOKINETICS

Well absorbed following PO administration. Metabolized in liver. Protein binding: 84%. Peak plasma concentration: 1.5 hrs. Excreted in feces (78%), urine (14%). **Half-life:** 8.3 hrs.

☒ LIFESPAN CONSIDERATIONS

Pregnancy/Lactation: May cause fetal harm; avoid pregnancy. Use effective contraception during treatment and for at least 1 mo after discontinuation. Unknown if distributed in breast milk. Must either discontinue drug or discontinue breastfeeding. **Children:** Safety and efficacy not established in pts younger than 18 yrs. **Elderly:** May have increased risk of side effects/adverse reactions.

INTERACTIONS

DRUG: Strong CYP3A4 inducers (e.g., rifAMPin, phenytoin) may decrease concentration/effect. **Strong CYP3A4 inhibitors (ketoconazole, ritonavir)** may increase concentration/effect. **HERBAL: St. John's wort** may decrease concentration/effect. **FOOD:** None known. **LAB VALUES:** May increase serum ALT, AST, bilirubin, GGT;

triglycerides. May decrease Hgb, neutrophils, platelets, serum sodium. May increase or decrease lymphocytes, serum glucose.

AVAILABILITY (Rx)

Tablets: 100 mg, 150 mg.

ADMINISTRATION/HANDLING

PO
• Give without regard to meals. • Swallow tablets whole.

INDICATIONS/ROUTES/DOSAGE

Chronic Lymphocytic Leukemia (in Combination with RiTUXimab), Follicular B-cell Non-Hodgkin's Lymphoma, Small Lymphocytic Lymphoma
PO: ADULTS/ELDERLY: 150 mg twice daily. Continue until disease progression or unacceptable toxicity.

Dose Modification
Hepatotoxicity
Elevated Serum ALT, AST
3–5 Times Upper Limit of Normal (ULN): Maintain dose. **5–20 Times ULN:** Monitor serum ALT, AST wkly. Withhold until ALT, AST less than 1 times ULN, then resume at 100 mg twice daily. **Greater Than 20 Times ULN:** Permanently discontinue.

Elevated Serum Bilirubin
1.5–3 Times ULN: Monitor serum bilirubin wkly. Maintain dose.
3–10 Times ULN: Monitor serum bilirubin wkly. Withhold until bilirubin less than 1 times ULN, then resume at 100-mg dose. **Greater Than 10 Times ULN:** Permanently discontinue.

Diarrhea
Moderate Diarrhea: Maintain dose. **Severe Diarrhea or Hospitalization:** Withhold until resolved, then resume at 100-mg dose. **Life-Threatening Diarrhea:** Permanently discontinue.

Neutropenia
ANC 1,000–1,500 cells/mm³: Maintain dose. **ANC 500–1,000 cells/mm³:** Monitor ANC wkly and maintain dose. **ANC Less Than 500 cells/mm³:** Permanently discontinue.

Thrombocytopenia
Platelets 50,000–75,000 cells/mm³: Maintain dose. **Platelets 25,000–50,000 cells/mm³:** Monitor platelet count wkly and maintain dose. **Platelets Less Than 25,000 cells/mm³:** Monitor platelet count wkly. Withhold until platelets greater than 25,000 cells/mm³, then resume at 100-mg dose.

Pneumonitis
Any Symptoms: Permanently discontinue.

Dosage in Renal Impairment
No dose adjustment.

Dosage in Hepatic Impairment
Use caution. See dose modification.

SIDE EFFECTS

CLL
Frequent (35%–21%): Pyrexia, nausea, diarrhea, chills. **Occasional (10%–5%):** Headache, vomiting, generalized pain, arthralgia, stomatitis, gastric reflux, nasal congestion.

Non-Hodgkin's Lymphoma
Frequent (47%–21%): Diarrhea, fatigue, nausea, cough, pyrexia, abdominal pain, rash. **Occasional (17%–10%):** Dyspnea, decreased appetite, vomiting, asthenia, night sweats, insomnia, headache, peripheral edema.

ADVERSE EFFECTS/TOXIC REACTIONS

Thrombocytopenia, neutropenia, leukopenia, lymphopenia are expected responses to therapy, but more severe reactions, including bone marrow failure, febrile neutropenia, may occur. Fatal and/or serious events including hepatotoxicity (14% of pts), severe diarrhea or colitis (14% of pts), hypersensitivity reactions (including anaphylaxis), pneumonitis, intestinal perforation were reported. Neutropenia occurred in 31% of pts, which may greatly increase risk of infection. Severe skin reactions including toxic epidermal necrolysis, generalized rash, exfoliative rash were reported. Other infections may include bronchitis, *C.difficile* colitis, pneumonia, sepsis, UTI. Fatal and/or serious intestinal perforation may occur.

NURSING CONSIDERATIONS

BASELINE ASSESSMENT

Obtain ANC, CBC, BMP, LFT, PT/INR, vital signs, urine pregnancy. Receive full medication history including herbal products. Question possibility of pregnancy, current breastfeeding status, use of contraceptive measures in female pts of reproductive potential. Question history of hypersensitivity reaction or acute skin reactions to drug class. Perform full dermatologic exam with routine assessment. Offer emotional support.

INTERVENTION/EVALUATION

Diligently monitor blood counts (esp. ANC, CBC, platelet count) frequently. Any interruption of therapy or dosage change may require wkly lab monitoring until symptoms resolve. Obtain *C. difficile* toxin PCR if severe diarrhea occurs. Screen for acute cutaneous reactions, allergic reactions, other acute infections (sepsis, UTI), hepatic impairment, pulmonary events (dyspnea, pneumonitis, pneumonia), or tumor lysis syndrome (electrolyte imbalance, uric acid nephropathy, acute renal failure). Monitor strict I&O, hydration status, stool frequency and consistency.

PATIENT/FAMILY TEACHING

• Blood levels will be routinely monitored. Any change in dose or interruption of therapy may require blood draws every week. • Avoid pregnancy; do not breastfeed. • Report abdominal pain, amber or bloody urine, bruising, black/tarry stools, persistent diarrhea, yellowing of skin or eyes. • Fever, cough, burning with urination, body aches, chills may indicate acute infection. • Avoid alcohol. • Immediately report difficult breathing, severe coughing, chest tightness. • Therapy may cause severe allergic reactions, intestinal tearing, or skin rashes or severe diarrhea related to an infected colon. • Do not take any over-the-counter medications including herbal products unless approved by your doctor.

ifosfamide

eye-**fos**-fa-mide
(Ifex)

■ BLACK BOX ALERT ■ Hemorrhagic cystitis may occur. Severe myelosuppressant. May cause CNS toxicity, including confusion, coma. Must be administered by personnel trained in administration/handling of chemotherapeutic agents. May cause severe nephrotoxicity, resulting in renal failure.

Do not confuse ifosfamide with cyclophosphamide.

◆CLASSIFICATION

PHARMACOTHERAPEUTIC: Alkylating agent. **CLINICAL:** Antineoplastic.

USES

Treatment of germ cell testicular carcinoma (used in combination with other chemotherapy agents and with concurrent mesna for prophylaxis of hemorrhagic cystitis). **OFF-LABEL:** Small-cell lung, non–small-cell lung, ovarian, cervical, bladder cancer; soft tissue sarcomas, Hodgkin's, non-Hodgkin's lymphomas; osteosarcoma; head and neck, Ewing's sarcoma.

PRECAUTIONS

Contraindications: Hypersensitivity to ifosfamide. Urinary outflow obstruction. **Cautions:** Renal/hepatic impairment, compromised bone marrow reserve, active urinary tract infection, preexisting cardiac disease, prior radiation therapy. Avoid use in pts with WBCs less than 2,000 cells/mm³ and platelets less than 50,000 cells/mm³.

ACTION

Inhibits DNA, RNA protein synthesis by cross-linking with DNA, RNA strands, preventing cell growth. Cell cycle–phase nonspecific. **Therapeutic Effect:** Interferes with DNA, RNA function.

PHARMACOKINETICS

Metabolized in liver. Protein binding: Negligible. Crosses blood-brain barrier (to a limited extent). Primarily excreted in urine. Removed by hemodialysis. **Half-life:** 11–15 hrs (high dose); 4–7 hrs (low dose).

⚖ LIFESPAN CONSIDERATIONS

Pregnancy/Lactation: If possible, avoid use during pregnancy, esp. first trimester. Males must use effective contraception and not conceive a child during treatment and for at least 6 months after discontinuation. May cause fetal harm. Distributed in breast milk. Breastfeeding not recommended. **Children:** Not intended for this pt population. **Elderly:** Age-related renal impairment may require dosage adjustment.

INTERACTIONS

DRUG: Bone marrow depressants (e.g., alemtuzumab, methotrexate) may increase myelosuppression. **Live virus vaccines** may potentiate virus replication, increase vaccine side effects, decrease pt's antibody response to vaccine. **HERBAL: St. John's wort** may decrease concentration. **FOOD:** None known. **LAB VALUES:** May increase serum BUN, bilirubin, creatinine, uric acid, ALT, AST.

AVAILABILITY (Rx)

Injection, Powder for Reconstitution (Ifex): 1 g, 3 g. **Injection, Solution:** 50 mg/mL.

ADMINISTRATION/HANDLING

◀ALERT▶ Hemorrhagic cystitis occurs if mesna is not given concurrently. Mesna should always be given with ifosfamide.

💧 IV

Reconstitution • Reconstitute vial with Sterile Water for Injection or Bacteriostatic Water for Injection to provide concentration of 50 mg/mL. Shake to dissolve. • Further dilute with 50–1,000 mL D_5W or 0.9% NaCl to provide concentration of 0.6–20 mg/mL.
Rate of Administration • Infuse over minimum of 30 min. • Give with at least 2,000 mL PO or IV fluid (prevents bladder toxicity). • Give with protectant against hemorrhagic cystitis (i.e., mesna).

Storage • Store vials of powder at room temperature. • Refrigerate vials of solution. • After reconstitution with Bacteriostatic Water for Injection, vials and diluted solutions stable for 24 hrs if refrigerated.

▦ IV INCOMPATIBILITIES

Cefepime (Maxipime), methotrexate.

▦ IV COMPATIBILITIES

Granisetron (Kytril), ondansetron (Zofran).

INDICATIONS/ROUTES/DOSAGE

◀ALERT▶ Dosage individualized based on clinical response, tolerance to adverse effects. When used in combination therapy, consult specific protocols for optimum dosage, sequence of drug administration.

Germ Cell Testicular Carcinoma

IV: ADULTS: 1,200 mg/m²/day for 5 consecutive days. Repeat q3wks or after recovery from hematologic toxicity. Administer with mesna (to prevent bladder toxicity).

Dosage in Renal/Hepatic Impairment
Use caution.

SIDE EFFECTS

Frequent (83%–58%): Alopecia, nausea, vomiting. **Occasional (15%–5%):** Confusion, drowsiness, hallucinations, infection. **Rare (less than 5%):** Dizziness, seizures, disorientation, fever, malaise, stomatitis (mucosal irritation, glossitis, gingivitis).

ADVERSE EFFECTS/ TOXIC REACTIONS

Hemorrhagic cystitis with hematuria, dysuria occurs frequently if protective agent (mesna) is not used. Myelosuppression (leukopenia, thrombocytopenia) occurs frequently. Pulmonary toxicity, hepatotoxicity, nephrotoxicity, cardiotoxicity, CNS toxicity (confusion, hallucinations, drowsiness, coma) may require discontinuation of therapy.

NURSING CONSIDERATIONS

BASELINE ASSESSMENT

Obtain urinalysis before each dose. If hematuria occurs (greater than 10 RBCs per field), therapy should be withheld until resolution occurs. Obtain WBC, platelet count, Hgb before each dose. Offer emotional support.

INTERVENTION/EVALUATION

Monitor hematologic studies, urinalysis, renal function, LFT. Assess for fever, sore throat, signs of local infection, unusual bruising/bleeding from any site, symptoms of anemia (excessive fatigue, weakness). Monitor for toxicities.

PATIENT/FAMILY TEACHING

• Alopecia is reversible, but new hair growth may have a different color or texture. • Drink plenty of fluids (protects against cystitis). • Do not have immunizations without physician's approval (drug lowers resistance). • Avoid contact with those who have recently received live virus vaccine. • Avoid crowds, those with infections. • Report unusual bleeding/bruising, fever, chills, sore throat, joint pain, sores in mouth or on lips, yellowing skin or eyes.

---

iloperidone

eye-loe-**per**-i-doan
(Fanapt, Fanapt Titration Pack)

■ **BLACK BOX ALERT** ■ Elderly pts with dementia-related psychosis are at increased risk for mortality due to cerebrovascular events.

Do not confuse iloperidone with amiodarone or dronedarone.

◆CLASSIFICATION

PHARMACOTHERAPEUTIC: Second-generation (atypical) antipsychotic. **CLINICAL:** Antipsychotic.

USES

Acute treatment of schizophrenia in adults.

PRECAUTIONS

Contraindications: Hypersensitivity to iloperidone. **Cautions:** Cardiovascular disease (HF, history of MI, ischemia, cardiac conduction abnormalities), cerebrovascular disease (increases risk of CVA in pts with dementia, seizure disorders). Pts at risk for orthostatic hypotension. Pts with bradycardia, hypokalemia, hypomagnesemia may be at greater risk for torsades de pointes. History of seizures, conditions lowering seizure threshold, high risk of suicide, risk of aspiration pneumonia, congenital QT syndrome, concurrent use of medications that prolong QT interval, decreased GI motility, urinary retention, BPH, xerostomia, visual problems, hepatic impairment, narrow-angle glaucoma, diabetes, elderly.

ACTION

Exact mechanism mediated through combination of DOPamine type 2 (D_2) and serotonin type 2 (5-HT_2) antagonisms. **Therapeutic Effect:** Diminishes symptoms of schizophrenia and reduces incidence of extrapyramidal side effects.

PHARMACOKINETICS

Steady-state concentration occurs in 3–4 days. Well absorbed from GI tract (unaffected by food). Protein binding: 95%. Metabolized in liver. Primarily excreted in urine, with a lesser amount excreted in feces. **Half-life:** 18–33 hrs.

⧗ LIFESPAN CONSIDERATIONS

Pregnancy/Lactation: Unknown if drug crosses placenta or is excreted in breast milk. Breastfeeding not recommended. **Children:** Safety and efficacy not established. **Elderly:** More susceptible to postural hypotension. Increased risk of cerebrovascular events, mortality, including stroke in elderly pts with psychosis.

INTERACTIONS

DRUG: Alcohol, **CNS depressants** (e.g., diphenhydrAMINE, LORazepam,

---

morphine) may increase CNS depression. **Strong CYP3A4 inhibitors (e.g., clarithromycin, ketoconazole)** or **strong CYP2D6 inhibitors (e.g., FLUoxetine, PARoxetine)** may increase concentration. **Medications causing prolongation of QT interval (e.g., amiodarone, dofetilide, sotalol)** may increase effects on cardiac conduction, leading to malignant arrhythmias (torsades de pointes). **HERBAL: Gotu kola, kava kava, St. John's wort, valerian** may increase CNS depression. **St. John's wort** may decrease concentration. **FOOD:** None known. **LAB VALUES:** May increase serum prolactin levels.

AVAILABILITY (Rx)

Tablets: 1 mg, 2 mg, 4 mg, 6 mg, 8 mg, 10 mg, 12 mg.

ADMINISTRATION/HANDLING

PO
• Give without regard to food. • Tablets may be crushed.

INDICATIONS/ROUTES/DOSAGE

Note: Titrate to the proper dose range with dosage adjustments not to exceed 2 mg twice daily (4 mg/day).

Schizophrenia
PO: ADULTS: To avoid orthostatic hypotension, begin with 1 mg twice daily, then adjust dosage to 2 mg twice daily, 4 mg twice daily, 6 mg twice daily, 8 mg twice daily, 10 mg twice daily, and 12 mg twice daily on days 2, 3, 4, 5, 6, and 7, respectively, to reach target daily dose of 12–24 mg/day in 2 divided doses. **Note:** Reduce dose by 50% when receiving strong CYP2D6 or CYP3A4 inhibitors or poor metabolizers of CYP2D6 (see Interactions).

Dosage in Renal Impairment
No dose adjustment.

Dosage in Hepatic Impairment
Mild impairment: No adjustment. **Moderate impairment:** Use caution. **Severe impairment:** Not recommended.

SIDE EFFECTS

Frequent (20%–12%): Dizziness, drowsiness, tachycardia. **Occasional (10%–4%):** Nausea, dry mouth, nasal congestion, weight increase, diarrhea, fatigue, orthostatic hypotension. **Rare (3%–1%):** Arthralgia, musculoskeletal stiffness, abdominal discomfort, nasopharyngitis, tremor, hypotension, rash, ejaculatory failure, dyspnea, blurred vision, lethargy.

ADVERSE EFFECTS/ TOXIC REACTIONS

Extrapyramidal disorders, including tardive dyskinesia (protrusion of tongue, puffing of cheeks, chewing/puckering of the mouth), occur in 4% of pts. Upper respiratory infection occurs in 3% of pts. QT interval prolongation may produce torsades de pointes, a form of ventricular tachycardia. Neuroleptic malignant syndrome (e.g., hyperpyrexia, muscle rigidity, altered mental status, irregular pulse or B/P) has been noted.

NURSING CONSIDERATIONS

BASELINE ASSESSMENT
Assess pt's behavior, appearance, emotional status, response to environment, speech pattern, thought content. EKG should be obtained to assess for QT prolongation before instituting medication. Question medical history as listed in Precautions.

INTERVENTION/EVALUATION
Monitor for orthostatic hypotension; assist with ambulation. Monitor for fine tongue movement (may be first sign of tardive dyskinesia, possibly irreversible). Monitor serum potassium, magnesium in pts at risk for electrolyte disturbances. Assess for therapeutic response (greater interest in surroundings, improved self-care, increased ability to concentrate, relaxed facial expression).

PATIENT/FAMILY TEACHING
• Avoid tasks that require alertness, motor skills until response to drug is established. • Be alert to symptoms of orthostatic hypotension; slowly go from lying to

standing. • Report if feeling faint, if experiencing heart palpitations, or if fever or muscle rigidity occurs. • Report extrapyramidal symptoms (e.g., involuntary muscle movements, tics) immediately.

imatinib

im-**at**-in-ib
(Gleevec)
Do not confuse imatinib with dasatinib, erlotinib, lapatinib, nilotinib, SORAfenib, or SUNItinib.

◆CLASSIFICATION

PHARMACOTHERAPEUTIC: Protein tyrosine kinase inhibitor. **CLINICAL:** Antineoplastic.

USES

Newly diagnosed chronic-phase Philadelphia chromosome positive chronic myeloid leukemia (Ph+ CML) in children and adults. Pts in blast crisis, accelerated phase, or chronic phase Ph+ CML who have already failed interferon therapy. Adults with relapsed or refractory Ph+ acute lymphoblastic leukemia (ALL). Treatment in children with Ph+ ALL. Adults with myelodysplastic/myeloproliferative disease (MDS/MPD) associated with platelet-derived growth factor receptor (PDGFR) gene rearrangements. Adults with aggressive systemic mastocytosis (ASM) without mutation of the D816V c-Kit or unknown mutation status of the c-Kit. Adults with hypereosinophilic syndrome (HES) and/or chronic eosinophilic leukemia (CEL) with positive, negative, or unknown FIP1L1-PDGFR fusion kinase. Adults with dermatofibrosarcoma protuberans (DFSP) that is unresectable, recurrent, and/or metastatic. Pts with malignant gastrointestinal stromal tumors (GIST) that are unresectable and/or metastatic. Prevention of cancer recurrence in pts following surgical removal of GIST. **OFF-LABEL:** Treatment of desmoid

tumors (soft tissue sarcoma). Post–stem cell transplant (allogeneic), follow-up treatment in recurrent CML. Treatment of advanced or metastatic melanoma.

PRECAUTIONS

Contraindications: Hypersensitivity to imatinib. **Cautions:** Hepatic/renal impairment, thyroidectomy pts, hypothyroidism, gastric surgery pts. Pts in whom fluid accumulation is poorly tolerated (e.g., HF, hypertension, pulmonary disease).

ACTION

Inhibits Bcr-Abl tyrosine kinase, an enzyme created by Philadelphia chromosome abnormality found in pts with chronic myeloid leukemia. **Therapeutic Effect:** Suppresses tumor growth during the three stages of CML: blast crisis, accelerated phase, chronic phase. Induces apoptosis.

PHARMACOKINETICS

Well absorbed after PO administration. Protein binding: 95%. Metabolized in liver. Eliminated in feces (68%), urine (13%). **Half-life:** 18 hrs; metabolite, 40 hrs.

⌛ LIFESPAN CONSIDERATIONS

Pregnancy/Lactation: May cause fetal harm. Breastfeeding not recommended. **Children:** Safety and efficacy not established. **Elderly:** Increased frequency of fluid retention.

INTERACTIONS

DRUG: CYP3A4 inducers (e.g., carBAMazepine, phenytoin, rifAMPin) may decrease concentration. **CYP3A4 inhibitors** (e.g., clarithromycin, erythromycin, ketoconazole) may increase concentration. **Bone marrow depressants** (e.g., alemtuzumab, methotrexate) may increase myelosuppression. **Live virus vaccines** may potentiate virus replication, increase vaccine side effects, decrease pt's antibody response to vaccine. May reduce effect of **warfarin. HERBAL:** St. John's wort decreases concentration. **FOOD:** Grapefruit products may increase concentration. **LAB VALUES:** May increase serum bilirubin, ALT, AST, creatinine. May decrease platelet count, RBC, WBC count; serum potassium, albumin, calcium.

AVAILABILITY (Rx)

Tablets: 100 mg, 400 mg.

ADMINISTRATION/HANDLING

PO

• Give with a meal and large glass of water. • Tablets may be dispersed in water or apple juice (stir until dissolved; give immediately). Do not crush or chew tablets.

INDICATIONS/ROUTES/DOSAGE

Ph+ Chronic Myeloid Leukemia (CML) (Chronic Phase)

PO: ADULTS, ELDERLY: 400 mg once daily; may increase to 600 mg/day. Maximum: 800 mg. CHILDREN: 340 mg/m²/day. Maximum: 600 mg.

Ph+ CML (Accelerated Phase)

PO: ADULTS, ELDERLY: 600 mg once daily. May increase to 800 mg/day in 2 divided doses (400 mg twice daily). CHILDREN: 340 mg/m²/day. Maximum: 600 mg.

Ph+ Acute Lymphoblastic Leukemia (ALL)

PO: ADULTS, ELDERLY: 600 mg once daily.

Gastrointestinal Stromal Tumors (GIST) (Following Complete Resection)

PO: ADULTS, ELDERLY: 400 mg once daily for 3 yrs.

GIST (Unresectable)

PO: ADULTS, ELDERLY: 400 mg once daily. May increase up to 400 mg twice daily.

Aggressive Systemic Mastocytosis (ASM) with Eosinophilia

PO: ADULTS, ELDERLY: Initially, 100 mg/day. May increase up to 400 mg/day.

ASM without Mutation of the D816V C-Kit or Unknown Mutation Status of C-Kit

PO: ADULTS, ELDERLY: 400 mg once daily.

Dermatofibrosarcoma Protuberans (DFSP)

PO: ADULTS, ELDERLY: 400 mg twice daily.

Hypereosinophilic Syndrome (HES)/ Chronic Eosinophilic Leukemia (CEL)

PO: ADULTS, ELDERLY: 400 mg once daily.

HES/CEL with Positive or Unknown FIP1L1-PDGFR Fusion Kinase

PO: ADULTS, ELDERLY: Initially, 100 mg/day. May increase up to 400 mg/day.

Myelodysplastic/Myeloproliferative Disease (MDS/MPD)

PO: ADULTS, ELDERLY: 400 mg once daily.

Usual Dosage for Children (2 Yrs and Older)

Ph+ CML (Chronic Phase, Recurrent or Resistant)

PO: 340 mg/m²/day. Maximum: 600 mg/day.

Ph+ CML (Chronic Phase, Newly Diagnosed, Ph+ ALL)

PO: 340 mg/m²/day. Maximum: 600 mg/day.

Dosage with Strong CYP3A4 Inducers

Increase dose by 50% with careful monitoring.

Dosage in Renal Impairment

Creatinine Clearance	Maximum Dose
40–59 mL/min	600 mg
20–39 mL/min	400 mg
Less than 20 mL/min	100 mg

Dosage in Hepatic Impairment

Mild to moderate impairment: No adjustment. **Severe impairment:** Reduce dosage by 25%.

SIDE EFFECTS

Frequent (68%–24%): Nausea, diarrhea, vomiting, headache, fluid retention, rash, musculoskeletal pain, muscle cramps, arthralgia. Occasional (23%–10%): Abdominal pain, cough, myalgia, fatigue, fever, anorexia, dyspepsia, constipation, night sweats, pruritus, dizziness, blurred vision, somnolence. Rare (less than

10%): Nasopharyngitis, petechiae, asthenia, epistaxis.

ADVERSE EFFECTS/ TOXIC REACTIONS

Severe fluid retention (pleural effusion, pericardial effusion, pulmonary edema, ascites), hepatotoxicity occur rarely. Neutropenia, thrombocytopenia are expected responses to the therapy. Respiratory toxicity is manifested as dyspnea, pneumonia. Heart damage (left ventricular dysfunction, HF) may occur.

NURSING CONSIDERATIONS

BASELINE ASSESSMENT

Obtain baseline CBC, serum chemistries, renal function test. Monitor LFT before beginning treatment, monthly thereafter. Offer emotional support.

INTERVENTION/EVALUATION

Assess periorbital area, lower extremities for early evidence of fluid retention. Monitor for unexpected, rapid weight gain. Offer antiemetics to control nausea, vomiting. Monitor daily pattern of bowel activity, stool consistency. Monitor CBC wkly for first mo, biweekly for second mo, periodically thereafter for evidence of neutropenia, thrombocytopenia; assess hepatic function tests for hepatotoxicity. Monitor renal function, serum electrolytes. Duration of neutropenia or thrombocytopenia ranges from 2–4 wks.

PATIENT/FAMILY TEACHING

• Avoid crowds, those with known infection. • Avoid contact with anyone who recently received live virus vaccine; do not receive vaccinations. • Take with food and a full glass of water. • Avoid grapefruit products. • Report chest pain, swelling of extremities, weight gain greater than 5 lb, easy bruising/bleeding. • Avoid tasks that require alertness, motor skills until response to drug is established.

imipenem/cilastatin

im-i-**pen**-em/sye-la-**stat**-in
(Primaxin)
Do not confuse imipenem with doripenem, ertapenem, or meropenem, or Primaxin with Premarin or Primacor.

◆CLASSIFICATION

PHARMACOTHERAPEUTIC: Fixed-combination carbapenem. **CLINICAL:** Antibiotic.

USES

Treatment of susceptible infections due to gram-negative (ESBL *E. coli* and *Klebsiella*, *Enterobacter* spp. PsAs), gram-positive (MSSA, *Streptococcus* spp.), anaerobic organisms including respiratory tract, skin/skin structure, gynecologic, bone, joint, intra-abdominal, complicated or uncomplicated UTIs; endocarditis (caused by *S. aureus*); polymicrobic infections; septicemia; serious nosocomial infections. **OFF-LABEL:** Hepatic abscess, neutropenic fever, melioidosis.

PRECAUTIONS

Contraindications: Hypersensitivity to imipenem/cilastatin. **Cautions:** CNS disorders (e.g., brain lesions and history of seizures), sensitivity to beta-lactams (e.g., penicillins, cephalosporins), renal impairment, elderly.

ACTION

Imipenem: Penetrates bacterial cell membrane, inhibiting cell wall synthesis. **Cilastatin:** Competitively inhibits the enzyme dehydropeptidase, preventing renal metabolism of imipenem. **Therapeutic Effect:** Produces bacterial cell death.

PHARMACOKINETICS

Readily absorbed after IM administration. Protein binding: **Imipenem:** 20%; **Cilastatin:** 40%. Widely distributed. Metabolized in kidneys. Primarily excreted in urine. Removed by hemodialysis. **Half-life:** 1 hr (increased in renal impairment).

⏳ LIFESPAN CONSIDERATIONS

Pregnancy/Lactation: Crosses placenta. Distributed in cord blood, amniotic fluid, breast milk. **Children:** No precautions noted. **Elderly:** Age-related renal impairment may require dosage adjustment.

INTERACTIONS

DRUG: May decrease concentration of valproic acid. **Ganciclovir, probenecid** may increase concentration. **HERBAL:** None significant. **FOOD:** None known. **LAB VALUES:** May increase serum alkaline phosphatase, BUN, bilirubin, creatinine, LDH, ALT, AST. May decrease Hgb, Hct.

AVAILABILITY (Rx)

Injection, Powder for Reconstitution (Primaxin): 250 mg, 500 mg.

ADMINISTRATION/HANDLING

 IV

Reconstitution • Dilute each 250- or 500-mg vial with 100–250 mL D$_5$W or 0.9% NaCl. Final concentration not to exceed 5 mg/mL.
Rate of Administration • Give by intermittent IV infusion (piggyback). • Do not give IV push. • Infuse over 20–30 min (doses greater than 500 mg over 40–60 min). • Observe pt during initial 30 min of first-time infusion for possible hypersensitivity reaction.
Storage • Solution appears colorless to yellow; discard if solution turns brown. • IV infusion (piggyback) is stable for 4 hrs at room temperature, 24 hrs if refrigerated. • Discard if precipitate forms.

▦ IV INCOMPATIBILITIES

Allopurinol (Aloprim), amphotericin B complex (Abelcet, AmBisome, Amphotec), fluconazole (Diflucan).

▦ IV COMPATIBILITIES

DiltiaZEM (Cardizem), insulin, propofol (Diprivan).

INDICATIONS/ROUTES/DOSAGE

Usual Dosage Ranges
IV: ADULTS, ELDERLY, WEIGHING 70 KG OR MORE: 250–500 mg q6–8h. **Maximum:** 4 g/day. **60–69 KG:** 250 mg q8h up to 1 g q8h. **50–59 KG:** 125 mg q6h up to 750 mg q8h. **40–49 KG:** 125 mg q6h up to 500 mg q6h. **30–39 KG:** 125 mg q8h up to 500 mg q8h. **CHILDREN OLDER THAN 3 MOS–12 YRS:** 15–25 mg/kg q6h. **Maximum:** 4 g/day. **CHILDREN 1–3 MOS:** 15–25 mg/kg q6h. **CHILDREN 1–4 WKS:** 20–25 mg/kg q8h. **CHILDREN YOUNGER THAN 1 WK:** 20–25 mg/kg q12h.

Dosage in Renal Impairment
Dosage and frequency are modified based on creatinine clearance and severity of infection. (See table.)

Dosage in Hepatic Impairment
Consider reducing dose frequency.

Creatinine Clearance (mL/min)	70 kg or greater	60–69 kg	50–59 kg	40–49 kg	30–39 kg
41–70	250 mg q8h– 750 mg q8h	125 mg q6h– 750 mg q8h	125 mg q6h– 500 mg q6h	125 mg q6h– 500 mg q8h	125 mg q8h– 250 mg q6h
21–40	250 mg q12h– 500 mg q6h	250 mg q12h– 500 mg q8h	125 mg q8h– 500 mg q8h	125 mg q12h– 250 mg q8h	125 mg q12h– 250 mg q8h
6–20	250 mg q12h– 500 mg q12h	125 mg q12h– 500 mg q12h	125 mg q12h– 500 mg q12h	125 mg q12h– 250 mg q12h	125 mg q12h– 250 mg q12h

SIDE EFFECTS

Occasional (3%): Diarrhea, nausea, vomiting. **Rare (1%):** Rash.

ADVERSE EFFECTS/ TOXIC REACTIONS

Antibiotic-associated colitis, other superinfections (abdominal cramps, severe watery diarrhea, fever) may result from altered bacterial balance in GI tract. Anaphylactic reactions have been reported.

NURSING CONSIDERATIONS

BASELINE ASSESSMENT

Question for history of allergies, particularly to beta-lactams, penicillins, cephalosporins. Inquire about history of seizures.

INTERVENTION/EVALUATION

Monitor renal, hepatic, hematologic function tests. Evaluate for phlebitis (heat, pain, red streaking over vein), pain at IV injection site. Assess for GI discomfort, nausea, vomiting. Monitor daily pattern of bowel activity, stool consistency. Assess skin for rash. Be alert to tremors, possible seizures.

immune globulin IV (IGIV)

im-**mune glob**-u-lin
(Bivigam, Carimune NF, Flebogamma DIF, Gammagard Liquid, Gammagard S/D, Gammaplex, Gamunex-C, Hizentra, Octagam 5%, Privigen)

■ **BLACK BOX ALERT** ■ Acute renal impairment characterized by increased serum creatinine, oliguria, acute renal failure, osmotic nephrosis, particularly pts with any degree of renal insufficiency, diabetes mellitus, volume depletion, sepsis, and those older than age 65 yrs. Thrombosis may occur.

◆CLASSIFICATION

PHARMACOTHERAPEUTIC: Immune globulin, blood product. **CLINICAL:** Immunizing agent.

USES

Treatment of pts with primary humoral immunodeficiency syndromes, acute/chronic immune idiopathic thrombocytopenic purpura (ITP), prevention of coronary artery aneurysms associated with Kawasaki disease, prevention of recurrent bacterial infections in pts with hypogammaglobulinemia associated with B-cell chronic lymphocytic leukemia (CLL). Treatment of chronic inflammatory demyelinating polyneuropathies. Provide passive immunity in pts with hepatitis A, measles, rubella, varicella. **OFF-LABEL:** Guillain-Barré syndrome; myasthenia gravis; prevention of acute infections in immunosuppressed pts; prevention, treatment of infection in high-risk, preterm, low birth-weight neonates; treatment of multiple sclerosis, HIV-associated thrombocytopenia.

PRECAUTIONS

Contraindications: Hypersensitivity to immune globulin. Selective IgA deficiency, hyperprolinemia (Hizentra, Privigen), severe thrombocytopenia, coagulation disorders where IM injections contraindicated. Hypersensitivity to corn (Octagam); infants/neonates for whom sucrose or fructose tolerance has not been established (Gammaplex). **Cautions:** Cardiovascular disease, history of thrombosis, renal impairment.

ACTION

Replacement therapy for primary/secondary immunodeficiencies and IgG antibodies against bacteria, viral antigens; interferes with receptors on cells of reticuloendothelial system for autoimmune cytopenias/idiopathic thrombocytopenia purpura (ITP); increases antibody titer and antigen-antibody reaction potential. **Therapeutic Effect:** Provides passive immunity replacement for immunodeficiencies, increases antibody titer.

PHARMACOKINETICS

Evenly distributed between intravascular and extravascular space. **Half-life:** 21–23 days.

⏳ LIFESPAN CONSIDERATIONS

Pregnancy/Lactation: Unknown if drug crosses placenta or is distributed in breast milk. **Children/Elderly:** No age-related precautions noted.

INTERACTIONS

DRUG: Live virus vaccines may increase vaccine side effects, potentiate virus replication, decrease pt's antibody response to vaccine. **HERBAL:** None significant. **FOOD:** None known. **LAB VALUES:** None significant.

AVAILABILITY (Rx)

Injection, Powder for Reconstitution (Carimune NF): 3 g, 6 g, 12 g. (Gammagard S/D): 5 g, 10 g. Injection, Solution (Bivigam 10%, Flebogamma DIF 5%, 10%, Gammagard Liquid 10%, Gammaplex 5%, Gamunex-C 10%, Octagam 5%, Privigen 10%).

ADMINISTRATION/HANDLING

 IV

◀ALERT▶ Monitor vital signs, B/P diligently during and immediately after IV administration (precipitous fall in B/P may indicate anaphylactic reaction). Stop infusion immediately. EPINEPHrine should be readily available.
Reconstitution • Reconstitute only with diluent provided by manufacturer. • Discard partially used or turbid preparations.
Rate of Administration • Give by infusion only. • After reconstitution, administer via separate tubing. • Rate of infusion varies with product used.
Storage • Refer to individual IV preparations for storage requirements, stability after reconstitution.

▦ IV INCOMPATIBILITIES

Do not mix with any other medications.

INDICATIONS/ROUTES/DOSAGE

Primary Immunodeficiency Syndrome
IV: ADULTS, ELDERLY, CHILDREN: *(Privigen):* 200–800 mg/kg q3–4wks. *(Carimune NF):* 400–800 mg/kg q3–4 wks. *(Flebogamma DIF, Gammagard, Gamunex-C, Octagam):* 300–600 mg/kg/q3–4wks. *(Bivigam, Gammaplex):* 300–800 mg/kg q3–4wks.

Idiopathic Thrombocytopenic Purpura (ITP)
IV: ADULTS, ELDERLY, CHILDREN: *(Carimune NF):* 400 mg/kg/day for 2–5 days. **Maintenance:** 400–1,000 mg/kg/dose to maintain platelet count or control bleeding. *(Gammagard):* 1,000 mg/kg: up to 3 additional doses may be given on alternate days.

Kawasaki Disease
Note: Must be used with aspirin.
IV: ADULTS, ELDERLY, CHILDREN: *(Gammagard):* 1,000 mg/kg as single dose or 400 mg/kg/day for 4 consecutive days. Begin within 7 days of onset of fever. **American Heart Association Guidelines:** 2,000 mg/kg as a single dose given over 10–12 hrs within 10 days of disease onset.

Chronic Lymphocytic Leukemia (CLL)
IV: ADULTS, ELDERLY, CHILDREN: *(Gammagard):* 400 mg/kg/dose q3–4wks.

Chronic Inflammatory Demyelinating Polyneuropathy
IV: ADULTS, ELDERLY, CHILDREN: *(Gamunex-C):* **Loading Dose:** 2 g/kg divided over 2–4 days (consecutive). **Maintenance:** 1g/kg/day q3wks or 500 mg/kg for 2 consecutive days q3wks. **Privigen:** Loading Dose: 2 g/kg in divided doses over 2-5 consecutive days. **Maintenance:** 1 g/kg q3wks or 500 mg/kg for 2 consecutive days q3wks.

Dosage in Renal Impairment
Caution when giving IV.

Dosage in Hepatic Impairment
No dose adjustment.

SIDE EFFECTS

Frequent: Tachycardia, backache, headache, arthralgia, myalgia. **Occasional:** Fatigue, wheezing, injection site rash/pain, leg cramps, urticaria, bluish color of lips/nailbeds, light-headedness.

ADVERSE EFFECTS/ TOXIC REACTIONS

Anaphylactic reactions occur rarely, but incidence increases with repeated injections. EPINEPHrine should be readily available. Overdose may produce chest tightness, chills, diaphoresis, dizziness, facial flushing, nausea, vomiting, fever, hypotension. Hypersensitivity reaction (anxiety, arthralgia, dizziness, flushing, myalgia, palpitations, pruritus) occurs rarely.

NURSING CONSIDERATIONS

BASELINE ASSESSMENT

Inquire about exposure history to disease for pt/family as appropriate. Have EPINEPHrine readily available. Pt should be well hydrated prior to administration.

INTERVENTION/EVALUATION

Control rate of IV infusion carefully; too-rapid infusion increases risk of precipitous fall in B/P, signs of anaphylaxis (facial flushing, chest tightness, chills, fever, nausea, vomiting, diaphoresis). Assess pt closely during infusion, esp. first hr; monitor vital signs continuously. Stop infusion if aforementioned signs noted. For treatment of idiopathic thrombocytopenic purpura (ITP), monitor platelet count.

PATIENT/FAMILY TEACHING

• Explain rationale for therapy. • Report sudden weight gain, fluid retention, edema, decreased urine output, shortness of breath.

indacaterol

in-da-ka-ter-ol
(Arcapta Neohaler, Onbrez Breezhaler ✦)
■ **BLACK BOX ALERT** ■ Long-acting beta₂-adrenergic agonists (LABAs) have an increased risk of asthma-related deaths. Not indicated for treatment of asthma.

FIXED COMBINATION(S)

Utibron Neohaler: indacaterol/glycopyrrolate (an anticholinergic): 27.5 mcg/15.6 mcg.

◆ **CLASSIFICATION**

PHARMACOTHERAPEUTIC: Long-acting beta₂-adrenergic agonist. **CLINICAL:** Bronchodilator.

USES

Long-term maintenance treatment of airflow obstruction in pts with chronic obstructive pulmonary disease (COPD), including chronic bronchitis and emphysema.

PRECAUTIONS

◄**ALERT**► Not indicated for the treatment of asthma, acute exacerbations of COPD.
Contraindications: Hypersensitivity to indacaterol. Monotherapy in treatment of asthma. **Cautions:** Cardiovascular disease (coronary insufficiency, arrhythmias, hypertension, history of hypersensitivity to sympathomimetics), seizure disorders, hyperthyroidism, hypokalemia, diabetes. May cause paradoxical bronchospasm, severe asthma.

ACTION

Stimulates beta₂-adrenergic receptors in lungs, resulting in relaxation of bronchial smooth muscle. **Therapeutic Effect:** Relieves bronchospasm, reduces airway resistance, improves bronchodilation.

PHARMACOKINETICS

Extensive activation of systemic beta-adrenergic receptors; acts primarily in lungs. Protein binding: 94%–95%. Metabolized in liver. Steady-state level: 12–15 days. Primarily excreted in feces. **Half-life:** 45–126 hrs.

⧗ LIFESPAN CONSIDERATIONS

Pregnancy/Lactation: Unknown if drug crosses placenta or is distributed in breast milk. **Children:** Safety and efficacy not established. **Elderly:** May be more sensitive to tremor, tachycardia due to age-related increased sympathetic sensitivity.

INTERACTIONS

DRUG: May decrease effectiveness of **beta blockers** (e.g., **carvedilol, metoprolol**). **Diuretics** (e.g, **furosemide, HCTZ**), **corticosteroids** (e.g., **dexamethasone, predniSONE**), **xanthine derivatives** may increase risk of hypokalemia. **Drugs that can prolong QT interval** (e.g., **erythromycin, quiNIDine, thioridazine**), **antiarrhythmics** (e.g., **amiodarone**), **MAOIs, tricyclic antidepressants** (e.g., **amitriptyline, doxepin**) may potentiate cardiovascular effects (increased risk of ventricular arrhythmias). **Erythromycin, ketoconazole, ritonavir, verapamil** may increase serum concentration. **HERBAL:** None significant. **FOOD:** None known. **LAB VALUES:** May decrease serum potassium. May increase serum glucose.

AVAILABILITY (Rx)

Powder for Inhalation: 75 mcg (in blister packs).

ADMINISTRATION/ HANDLING

Inhalation
• Do not shake or prime. • Open cap of Neohaler by pulling upward, then open mouthpiece. • Remove capsule from blister package and place in center of chamber. Firmly close until click is heard. • Hold inhaler upright and pierce capsule by pressing side buttons once only. • Instruct pt to exhale completely. Place mouthpiece into mouth, close lips, and inhale quickly and deeply through mouth (this causes capsule to spin, dispensing the drug). A slight whirring noise should occur. If not, this may indicate capsule is stuck. Gently tap inhaler to loosen and reattempt. • Pt should hold breath as long as possible before exhaling. • Check capsule to ensure that all the powder is gone. Instruct pt to reinhale if powder remains.
Storage • Store at room temperature. • Maintain capsules within individual blister pack until time of use. • Do not store capsules in Neohaler device.

INDICATIONS/ROUTES/DOSAGE

Maintenance Therapy and Prevention of COPD
Inhalation: ADULTS, ELDERLY: 75 mcg (1 capsule) once daily via Neohaler inhalation device.

Dosage in Renal/Hepatic Impairment
No dose adjustment.

SIDE EFFECTS

Occasional (7%–5%): Cough, nasopharyngitis, headache. **Rare (2%):** Oropharyngeal pain, nausea.

ADVERSE EFFECTS/ TOXIC REACTIONS

Peripheral edema, diabetes mellitus, hyperglycemia, sinusitis, URI reported in greater than 2% of pts. Excessive sympathomimetic stimulation, hypokalemia may produce palpitations, arrhythmias, angina pectoris, tachycardia, muscle cramps, weakness. Hyperglycemia symptoms present with increased thirst, polyuria, dry mouth, drowsiness/confusion, blurred vision. Severe shortness of breath may indicate paradoxical bronchospasm, deteriorating COPD. Serious asthma-related events, including death, reported.

NURSING CONSIDERATIONS

BASELINE ASSESSMENT

Assess rate, depth, rhythm, type of respirations. Monitor EKG, serum potassium, ABG determinations, O_2 saturation, pulmonary function test. Assess lung sounds for wheezing (bronchoconstriction), rales. Obtain baseline electrolytes, blood glucose. Receive full medication history and screen for possible drug interactions. Question for history of asthma, angina pectoris, diabetes, peripheral edema.

INTERVENTION/EVALUATION

Routinely monitor serum electrolytes, blood glucose, O_2 saturation. Recommend discontinuation of short-acting beta$_2$-agonists (use only for symptomatic relief of acute respiratory symptoms). Monitor for palpitations, tachycardia, serum hypokalemia. Inspect oropharyngeal cavity for irritation.

PATIENT/FAMILY TEACHING

• Follow manufacturer guidelines for proper use of inhaler. • Increase fluid intake (decreases lung secretion viscosity). • Rinse mouth with water after inhalation to decrease mouth/throat irritation. • Avoid excessive use of caffeine derivatives (chocolate, coffee, tea, cola). • An immediate cough lasting 15 sec may occur after inhaler use. • Report any fever, productive cough, body aches, difficulty breathing.

indapamide

in-**dap**-a-mide
(Apo-Indapamide ♣, Lozide ♣)
Do not confuse indapamide with iopidine.

◆CLASSIFICATION

PHARMACOTHERAPEUTIC: Thiazide. **CLINICAL:** Diuretic, antihypertensive.

USES

Management of mild to moderate hypertension. Treatment of edema associated with HF. **OFF-LABEL:** Calcium nephrolithiasis.

PRECAUTIONS

Contraindications: Hypersensitivity to indapamide. Anuria, sulfonamide-derived drugs. **Cautions:** History of hypersensitivity to sulfonamides or thiazide diuretics. Severe renal disease, hepatic impairment, history of gout, prediabetes, diabetes, elderly, severe hyponatremia, elevated serum cholesterol.

ACTION

Diuretic: Blocks reabsorption of water, sodium, potassium at cortical diluting segment of distal renal tubule. **Antihypertensive:** Reduces plasma, extracellular fluid volume, and peripheral vascular resistance by direct effect on blood vessels. **Therapeutic Effect:** Promotes diuresis, reduces B/P.

PHARMACOKINETICS

Almost completely absorbed following PO administration. Protein binding: 71%–79%. Metabolized in liver. Excreted in urine. Half-life: 14–18 hrs.

⧖ LIFESPAN CONSIDERATIONS

Pregnancy/Lactation: Unknown if drug crosses placenta or is distributed in breast milk. **Children:** Safety and efficacy not established. **Elderly:** May be more sensitive to hypotensive, electrolyte effects.

INTERACTIONS

DRUG: May increase risk of **lithium** toxicity. **HERBAL: Ephedra, ginseng, licorice, yohimbe** may worsen hypertension. **Black cohosh** may increase antihypertensive effect. **FOOD:** None known. **LAB VALUES:** May increase uric acid, plasma renin activity. May decrease protein-bound iodine; serum calcium, potassium, sodium.

AVAILABILITY (Rx)

Tablets: 1.25 mg, 2.5 mg.

ADMINISTRATION/HANDLING

PO

• Give with food, milk if GI upset occurs, preferably with breakfast (may prevent nocturia).

INDICATIONS/ROUTES/DOSAGE

Edema
PO: ADULTS: Initially, 2.5 mg/day, may increase to 5 mg/day after 1 wk.

Hypertension
PO: ADULTS, ELDERLY: Initially, 1.25 mg. May increase to 2.5 mg/day after 4 wks or 5 mg/day after additional 4 wks. Usual dose: 1.25–2.5 mg/day.

Dosage in Renal/Hepatic Impairment
Use caution.

♣ Canadian trade name   🗟 Non-Crushable Drug   ⚠ High Alert drug

SIDE EFFECTS

Frequent (5% and greater): Fatigue, paresthesia of extremities, tension, irritability, agitation, headache, dizziness, light-headedness, insomnia, muscle cramps. **Occasional (less than 5%):** Urinary frequency, urticaria, rhinorrhea, flushing, weight loss, orthostatic hypotension, depression, blurred vision, nausea, vomiting, diarrhea, constipation, dry mouth, impotence, rash, pruritus.

ADVERSE EFFECTS/TOXIC REACTIONS

Vigorous diuresis may lead to profound water and electrolyte depletion, resulting in hypokalemia, hyponatremia, dehydration. Acute hypotensive episodes may occur. Hyperglycemia may be noted during prolonged therapy. Pancreatitis, blood dyscrasias, pulmonary edema, allergic pneumonitis, dermatologic reactions occur rarely. Overdose can lead to lethargy, coma without changes in electrolytes or hydration.

NURSING CONSIDERATIONS

BASELINE ASSESSMENT

Obtain vital signs, esp. B/P for hypotension, before administration. Assess baseline electrolytes, particularly hypokalemia. Observe for edema; assess skin turgor, mucous membranes for hydration status. Assess muscle strength, mental status. Note skin temperature, moisture. Obtain baseline weight.

INTERVENTION/EVALUATION

Continue to monitor B/P, vital signs, electrolytes, I&O, weight. Note extent of diuresis. Watch for electrolyte disturbances (hypokalemia may result in weakness, tremor, muscle cramps, nausea, vomiting, altered mental status, tachycardia; hyponatremia may result in confusion, thirst, cold/clammy skin).

PATIENT/FAMILY TEACHING

• Expect increased frequency, volume of urination (diminishes with long-term use). • To reduce hypotensive effect, go slowly from lying to standing. • Eat foods high in potassium such as whole grains (cereals), legumes, meat, bananas, apricots, orange juice, potatoes (white, sweet), raisins. • Take early in the day to avoid nocturia.

indomethacin

in-doe-**meth**-a-sin
(Indocin, Novo-Methacin ✦, Tivorbex)

■ **BLACK BOX ALERT** ■ Increased risk of serious cardiovascular thrombotic events, including myocardial infarction, CVA. Increased risk of severe GI reactions, including ulceration, bleeding, perforation.
Do not confuse Indocin with Imodium, Minocin, or Vicodin.

◆CLASSIFICATION

PHARMACOTHERAPEUTIC: NSAID. **CLINICAL:** Anti-inflammatory, analgesic.

USES

(Indocin): Treatment of active stages of rheumatoid arthritis, osteoarthritis, ankylosing spondylitis, acute gouty arthritis. Relieves acute bursitis, tendonitis. **(Tivorbex):** Treatment of mild to moderate acute pain in adults. **(IV Form):** For closure of hemodynamically significant patent ductus arteriosus of premature infants. **OFF-LABEL:** Management of preterm labor.

PRECAUTIONS

Contraindications: Hypersensitivity to aspirin, indomethacin, other NSAIDs. Perioperative pain in setting of CABG surgery. History of asthma, urticaria, allergic reactions after taking aspirin, other NSAIDs. **Suppositories:** History of proctitis, recent rectal bleeding. **Injection:** In preterm infants with untreated/systemic infection or congenital heart disease where patency of PDA necessary for pulmonary or systemic blood flow; bleeding, thrombocytopenia, coagulation defects, necrotizing enterocolitis, significant renal dysfunction. **Cautions:** Cardiac dysfunction, fluid retention, HF, hypertension, renal/hepatic impairment, epilepsy; concurrent aspirin, steroids, anticoagulant therapy. Treatment of juvenile rheumatoid arthritis in children. History of GI disease (bleeding or ulcers), elderly, debilitated, asthma, depression, Parkinson's disease.

ACTION

Produces antipyretic, analgesic, anti-inflammatory effects by inhibiting prostaglandin synthesis. **Therapeutic Effect:** Reduces inflammatory response, fever, intensity of pain. Closure of patent ductus arteriosus.

PHARMACOKINETICS

Route	Onset	Peak	Duration
PO	30 min	—	4–6 hrs

Well absorbed from GI tract. Protein binding: 99%. Metabolized in liver. Excreted in urine. **Half-life:** 4.5 hrs.

⧖ LIFESPAN CONSIDERATIONS

Pregnancy/Lactation: Crosses placenta; distributed in breast milk. Avoid use during third trimester. **Children:** Safety and efficacy not established in those younger than 14 yrs. **Elderly:** Increased risk of serious adverse effects; GI bleeding, ulceration.

INTERACTIONS

DRUG: May decrease effects of **antihypertensives** (e.g., **amLODIPine, lisinopril, valsartan**), **diuretics** (e.g., **furosemide**). **Aspirin, other salicylates** may increase risk of GI side effects, bleeding. **Bone marrow depressants** (e.g., **alemtuzumab, methotrexate**) may increase risk of hematologic reactions. May increase risk of bleeding with **heparin, anticoagulants** (e.g., **rivaroxaban, warfarin**), **thrombolytics** (e.g.,

alteplase). May increase concentration, risk of toxicity of **lithium.** May increase risk of **cycloSPORINE, methotrexate** toxicity. **HERBAL:** Cat's claw, dong quai, evening primrose, feverfew, garlic, ginkgo, ginseng, horse chestnut, red clover may increase antiplatelet activity. **FOOD:** None known. **LAB VALUES:** May prolong bleeding time. May alter serum glucose. May increase serum BUN, creatinine, potassium, ALT, AST. May decrease serum sodium, platelet count, leukocytes.

AVAILABILITY (Rx)

Capsules: 25 mg, 50 mg. **(Tivorbex):** 20 mg, 40 mg. **Injection, Powder for Reconstitution (Indocin IV):** 1 mg. **Oral Suspension (Indocin):** 25 mg/5 mL. **Suppository:** 50 mg.

🦫 **Capsules, Extended-Release:** 75 mg.

ADMINISTRATION/HANDLING

💉 IV

Reconstitution • To 1-mg vial, add 1–2 mL preservative-free Sterile Water for Injection or 0.9% NaCl to provide concentration of 1 mg/mL or 0.5 mg/mL, respectively. • Do not further dilute.

Rate of Administration • Administer over 20–30 min.

Storage • Use IV solution immediately following reconstitution. • IV solution appears clear; discard if cloudy or precipitate forms. • Discard unused portion.

PO

• Give after meals or with food, antacids. • Do not break, crush, or open extended-release capsule. Swallow whole.

▦ IV INCOMPATIBILITIES

Amino acid injection, calcium gluconate, DOBUTamine (Dobutrex), DOPamine (Intropin), gentamicin (Garamycin), tobramycin (Nebcin).

✦ Canadian trade name   🦫 Non-Crushable Drug   🔲 High Alert drug

🕸 IV COMPATIBILITIES

Insulin, potassium.

INDICATIONS/ROUTES/DOSAGE

Moderate to Severe Rheumatoid Arthritis (RA), Osteoarthritis, Ankylosing Spondylitis
PO: ADULTS, ELDERLY *(Immediate-Release):* Initially, 25–50 mg 2–3 times/day; increased by 25–50 mg/wk up to 200 mg/day. *(Extended-Release):* Initially, 75 mg once daily. May increase to 75 mg twice daily. **Maximum:** 150 mg/day.
CHILDREN 2 YRS AND OLDER *(Immediate-Release):* 1–2 mg/kg/day in 2–4 divided doses. **Maximum:** 4 mg/kg/day not to exceed 150–200 mg/day.
RECTAL: ADULTS, ELDERLY, CHILDREN: Initially, 50 mg once daily. Maintenance: 50-200 mg/day in divided doses. **Maximum:** 200mg/day (daily dose), 100 mg (single dose).

Acute Gouty Arthritis
PO: RECTAL: ADULTS, ELDERLY *(Immediate-Release):* 50 mg 3 times/day for 3–5 days until pain is tolerable, then rapidly reduce dose to complete cessation of medication.

Acute Bursitis, Tendonitis
PO: ADULTS, ELDERLY: *(Immediate-Release):* 75–150 mg/day in 3–4 divided doses for 7–14 days. *(Extended-Release):* 75–150 mg/day in 1–2 doses/day for 7–14 days.
RECTAL: ADULTS, ELDERLY, CHILDREN: 50 mg up to 3 times/day.

Acute Pain
PO: ADULTS, ELDERLY: *(Tivorbex):* 20 mg 3 times/day or 40 mg 2–3 times/day.

Patent Ductus Arteriosus
IV: NEONATES: Initially, 0.2 mg/kg. Subsequent doses are based on age, as follows: NEONATES OLDER THAN 7 DAYS: 0.25 mg/kg for 2nd and 3rd doses. NEONATES 2–7 DAYS: 0.2 mg/kg for 2nd and 3rd doses. NEONATES LESS THAN 48 HRS: 0.1 mg/kg for 2nd and 3rd doses. In general, dosing interval is 12 hrs if urine output is greater than 1 mL/kg/hr after prior dose, 24 hrs if urine output is less than 1 mL/kg/hr but greater than 0.6 mL/kg/hr. Dose is held if urine output is less than 0.6 mL/kg/hr or if neonate is anuric.

Dosage in Renal Impairment
Mild to moderate impairment: No dose adjustment. **Severe impairment:** Not recommended.

Dosage in Hepatic Impairment
Use caution.

SIDE EFFECTS

Frequent (11%–3%): Headache, nausea, vomiting, dyspepsia, dizziness. **Occasional (less than 3%):** Depression, tinnitus, diaphoresis, drowsiness, constipation, diarrhea. **Patent ductus arteriosus:** Bleeding abnormalities. **Rare:** Hypertension, confusion, urticaria, pruritus, rash, blurred vision.

ADVERSE EFFECTS/ TOXIC REACTIONS

Paralytic ileus, ulceration of esophagus, stomach, duodenum, small intestine may occur. Pts with renal impairment may develop hyperkalemia with worsening of renal impairment. May aggravate depression or other psychiatric disturbances, epilepsy, parkinsonism. Nephrotoxicity (dysuria, hematuria, proteinuria, nephrotic syndrome) occurs rarely. Metabolic acidosis/alkalosis, bradycardia occur rarely in neonates with patent ductus arteriosus.

NURSING CONSIDERATIONS

BASELINE ASSESSMENT

Assess onset, type, location, duration of pain, fever, inflammation. Inspect appearance of affected joints for immobility, deformities, skin condition. Question medical history as listed in Precautions.

INTERVENTION/EVALUATION

Monitor serum BUN, creatinine, potassium, LFT. Monitor for evidence of nausea, dyspepsia. Assist with ambulation if dizziness occurs. Evaluate for therapeutic response: relief of pain, stiffness, swelling;

increased joint mobility; reduced joint tenderness; improved grip strength. Observe for weight gain, edema, bleeding, bruising. In neonates, also monitor heart rate, heart sounds for murmur, B/P, urine output, EKG, serum sodium, glucose, platelets.

PATIENT/FAMILY TEACHING

• Avoid aspirin, alcohol during therapy (increases risk of GI bleeding). • If GI upset occurs, take with food, milk. • Avoid tasks that require alertness, motor skills until response to drug is established. • Report ringing in ears, persistent stomach pain, unusual bruising/bleeding.

---

inFLIXimab

in-**flix**-i-mab
(Remicade)

■ **BLACK BOX ALERT** ■ Risk of severe/fatal opportunistic infections (tuberculosis, sepsis, fungal), reactivation of latent infections. Rare cases of very aggressive, usually fatal hepatosplenic T-cell lymphoma reported in adolescents, young adults with Crohn's disease. **Do not confuse inFLIXimab with riTUXimab, or Remicade with Reminyl.**

◆CLASSIFICATION

PHARMACOTHERAPEUTIC: Tumor necrosis factor (TNF) blocking agent. Monoclonal antibody. **CLINICAL:** Antirheumatic, disease-modifying, GI, immunosuppressant agent.

USES

In combination with methotrexate, reduces signs/symptoms, inhibits progression of structural damage, improves physical function in moderate to severe active rheumatoid arthritis (RA), psoriatic arthritis. Reduces signs/symptoms, induces and maintains remission in moderate to severe active Crohn's disease. Reduces number of draining enterocutaneous/rectovaginal fistulas, maintains fistula closure in fistulizing Crohn's disease. Reduces sign/symptoms of active ankylosing spondylitis. Treatment of chronic severe plaque psoriasis in pts who are candidates for systemic therapy. Reduces sign/symptoms, induces and maintains clinical remission and mucosal healing, eliminates corticosteroid use in moderate to severe active ulcerative colitis.

PRECAUTIONS

Contraindications: Hypersensitivity to inFLIXimab. Moderate to severe HF (doses greater than 5 mg/kg should be avoided). Sensitivity to murine proteins, sepsis, serious active infection. **Cautions:** Hematologic abnormalities, history of COPD, preexisting or recent-onset CNS demyelinating disorders, seizures, mild HF, history of recurrent infections, conditions predisposing pt to infections (e.g., diabetes), pts exposed to tuberculosis, elderly pts, chronic hepatitis B virus infection.

ACTION

Binds to tumor necrosis factor (TNF), inhibiting functional activity of TNF (induction of proinflammatory cytokines, enhanced leukocytic migration, activation of neutrophils/eosinophils). **Therapeutic Effect:** Prevents disease and allows diseased joints to heal.

PHARMACOKINETICS

Absorbed into GI tissue; primarily distributed in vascular compartment. **Half-life:** 8–9.5 days.

⌛ LIFESPAN CONSIDERATIONS

Pregnancy/Lactation: Unknown if distributed in breast milk. **Children:** Safety and efficacy not established. **Elderly:** Use cautiously due to higher rate of infection.

INTERACTIONS

DRUG: Anakinra, abatacept may increase risk of infection. **Immunosuppressants** may reduce frequency of infusion reactions, antibodies to inFLIXimab. **Live virus vaccines** may decrease immune response (do not give concurrently). **HERBAL: Echinacea** may decrease effects. **FOOD:** None known. **LAB VALUES:** May increase serum alkaline phosphatase, ALT, AST, bilirubin.

AVAILABILITY (Rx)

Injection, Powder for Reconstitution: 100 mg.

ADMINISTRATION/HANDLING
 IV

Reconstitution • Reconstitute each vial with 10 mL Sterile Water for Injection, using 21-gauge or smaller needle. Direct stream of Sterile Water for Injection to glass wall of vial. • Swirl vial gently to dissolve contents (do not shake). • Allow solution to stand for 5 min and inject into 250-mL bag 0.9% NaCl; gently mix. Concentration should range between 0.4 and 4 mg/mL. • Begin infusion within 3 hrs after reconstitution.
Rate of Administration • Administer IV infusion over at least 2 hrs using a low protein-binding filter.
Storage • Refrigerate vials. • Solution should appear colorless to light yellow and opalescent; do not use if discolored or if particulate forms.

⬚ IV INCOMPATIBILITIES

Do not infuse in same IV line with other agents.

INDICATIONS/ROUTES/DOSAGE

◀**ALERT**▶ Premedicate with antihistamines, acetaminophen, steroids to prevent/manage infusion reactions.

Rheumatoid Arthritis (RA)
IV Infusion: ADULTS, ELDERLY: (in combination with methotrexate): 3 mg/kg followed by additional doses at 2 and 6 wks after first infusion, then q8wks thereafter. Range: 3–10 mg/kg at 4- to 8-wk intervals.

Crohn's Disease
IV Infusion: ADULTS, ELDERLY, CHILDREN 6 YRS AND OLDER: 5 mg/kg followed by additional doses at 2 and 6 wks after first infusion, then q8wks thereafter. For adults who

respond then lose response, consideration may be given to treatment with 10 mg/kg.

Ankylosing Spondylitis
IV Infusion: ADULTS, ELDERLY: 5 mg/kg followed by additional doses at 2 and 6 wks after first infusion, then q6wks thereafter.

Psoriatic Arthritis
IV Infusion: ADULTS, ELDERLY: 5 mg/kg followed by additional doses at 2 and 6 wks after first infusion, then q8wks thereafter. May be used with or without methotrexate.

Plaque Psoriasis
IV Infusion: ADULTS, ELDERLY: 5 mg/kg followed by additional doses at 2 and 6 wks after first infusion, then q8wks thereafter.

Ulcerative Colitis
IV Infusion: ADULTS, ELDERLY, CHILDREN 6 YRS AND OLDER: 5 mg/kg followed by additional doses at 2 and 6 wks after first infusion, then q8wks thereafter.

Dosage in Renal/Hepatic Impairment
No dose adjustment.

SIDE EFFECTS

Frequent (22%–10%): Headache, nausea, fatigue, fever. **Occasional (9%–5%):** Fever/chills during infusion, pharyngitis, vomiting, pain, dizziness, bronchitis, rash, rhinitis, cough, pruritus, sinusitis, myalgia, back pain. **Rare (4%–1%):** Hypotension or hypertension, paresthesia, anxiety, depression, insomnia, diarrhea, UTI.

ADVERSE EFFECTS/TOXIC REACTIONS

Serious infections, including sepsis, occur rarely. Potential for hypersensitivity reaction, lupus-like syndrome, severe hepatic reaction, HF.

NURSING CONSIDERATIONS

BASELINE ASSESSMENT

Evaluate baseline hydration status (skin turgor urinary status). Question history of CNS disorders, COPD, HF. Screen for active infection. Pts should be evaluated for active tuberculosis and tested for latent infection prior to initiating treatment and periodically during therapy. Induration of 5 mm or greater with tuberculin skin test should be considered a positive test result when assessing if treatment for latent tuberculosis is necessary. Verify that pt has not received live vaccines prior to initiation.

INTERVENTION/EVALUATION

Monitor urinalysis, erythrocyte sedimentation rate (ESR), B/P. Monitor for signs of infection. Monitor daily pattern of bowel activity, stool consistency. **Crohn's disease:** Monitor C-reactive protein, frequency of stools. Assess for abdominal pain. **Rheumatoid arthritis (RA):** Monitor C-reactive protein. Assess for decreased pain, swollen joints, stiffness.

PATIENT/FAMILY TEACHING

• Report persistent fever, cough, abdominal pain, swelling of ankles/feet. • Treatment may depress your immune system and reduce your ability to fight infection. • Report symptoms of infection such as body aches, chills, cough, fatigue, fever. Avoid those with active infection. • Do not receive live vaccines. • Expect frequent tuberculosis screening. • Report travel plans to possible endemic areas.

---

insulin

in-su-lin
Rapid-acting: (Afrezza):
INHALATION POWDER, INSULIN ASPART: (Fiasp, Novolog), **INSULIN GLULISINE:** (Apidra), **INSULIN LISPRO:** (Humalog)
Short-acting: REGULAR INSULIN: (Humulin R , Novolin R)
Intermediate-acting: NPH: (Humulin N , Novolin N)
Long-acting: INSULIN DEGLUDEC: (Tresiba), **INSULIN DETEMIR:** (Levemir), **INSULIN GLARGINE:** (Basaglar, Lantus , Toujeo)

■ **BLACK BOX ALERT** ■ (Afrezza): Acute bronchospasms reported in pts with asthma and COPD.
Do not confuse NovoLOG with HumaLOG or NovoLIN.

FIXED-COMBINATION(S)

HumaLOG Mix 75/25: lispro suspension 75% and lispro solution 25%. **HumuLIN Mix 50/50:** NPH 50% and regular 50%. **HumuLIN 70/30, NovoLIN 70/30:** NPH 70% and rapid-acting regular 30%. **NovoLOG Mix 70/30:** aspart suspension 70% and aspart solution 30%. **Ryzodeg 70/30:** degludec suspension 70% and aspart solution 30%. **Soliqua 100/33:** glargine 100 units/mL and lixisenatide (a GLP-1 receptor agonist) 33 mcg/mL. **Xultophy 100/3.6:** degludec 100 units/ mL and liraglutide (a GLP-1 receptor agonist) 3.6 mg/mL.

◆CLASSIFICATION

PHARMACOTHERAPEUTIC: Exogenous insulin. **CLINICAL:** Antidiabetic.

USES

Treatment of type 1 diabetes (insulin dependent) and type 2 diabetes (non–insulin dependent) to improve glycemic control. **OFF-LABEL: Insulin aspart, insulin lispro, insulin regular:** Gestational diabetes, mild to moderate diabetic ketoacidosis, mild to moderate hyperosmolar hyperglycemic state. **Insulin NPH:** Gestational diabetes.

PRECAUTIONS

Contraindications: Hypersensitivity to insulin, use during episodes of hypoglycemia. **Afrezza:** Chronic lung disease. **Cautions:** Pts at risk for hypokalemia; renal/hepatic impairment, elderly. **Afrezza:** Must be used with a long-acting insulin in type 1 diabetes. Not recommended for use in diabetic ketoacidosis or in smokers. Pts with active lung cancer, history of lung cancer or at risk for lung cancer.

ACTION

Acts via specific receptor to regulate metabolism of carbohydrates, protein, and fats. Acts on liver, skeletal muscle, and adipose tissue. **Liver:** Stimulates hepatic glycogen synthesis, synthesis of fatty acids. **Muscle:** Increases protein, glycogen synthesis. **Adipose tissue:** Stimulates lipoproteins to provide free fatty acids, triglyceride synthesis. **Therapeutic Effect:** Controls serum glucose levels.

PHARMACOKINETICS

Rapid-Acting

	Onset (min)	Peak (hrs)	Duration (hrs)
Fiasp	12–18	1.5–2.2	5–7
Aspart (NovoLOG)	10–20	1–3	3–5
Glulisine (Apidra)	5–15	0.75–1.25	2–4
Insulin Human (Afrezza)	15–30	1	2
Lispro (HumaLOG)	15–30	0.5–2.5	3–6.5

Short-Acting

	Onset (min)	Peak (hrs)	Duration (hrs)
Regular (HumuLIN R)	30–60	1–5	6–10
Regular (NovoLIN R)	30–60	1–5	6–10

Intermediate-Acting

	Onset (hrs)	Peak (hrs)	Duration (hrs)
NPH (HumuLIN N)	1–2	6–14	16–24+
NPH (NovoLIN N)	1–2	6–14	16–24+

Long-Acting

	Onset (hrs)	Peak (hrs)	Duration (hrs)
Degludec (Tresiba)	0.5–1.5	12	42
Detemir (Levemir)	3–4	3–9	6–23
Glargine (Lantus)	3–4	No peak	24
Glargine (Toujeo)	Over 6	No peak	Over 24

⧖ LIFESPAN CONSIDERATIONS

Pregnancy/Lactation: Insulin is the drug of choice for diabetes in pregnancy; close medical supervision is needed. Following delivery, insulin needs may drop for 24–72 hrs, then rise to pre-pregnancy levels. Not distributed in breast milk; lactation may decrease insulin requirements. **Children:** No age-related precautions noted. **Elderly:** Decreased vision, fine motor tremors may lead to inaccurate self-dosing.

INTERACTIONS

DRUG: Alcohol may increase risk of hypoglycemia. **Beta blockers (e.g., carvedilol, metoprolol)** may alter effects; may mask signs, prolong periods of hypoglycemia. **Glucocorticoids, thiazide diuretics** may increase serum glucose. **HERBAL: Garlic, ginger, ginseng** may increase risk of hypoglycemia. **FOOD:** None known. **LAB VALUES:** May decrease serum magnesium, phosphate, potassium.

AVAILABILITY (Rx)

Rapid-Acting
(Afrezza) Inhalation Powder: 4 units, 8 units, 12 units as single-use inhalation cartridges. **Aspart (Novolog):** 100 units/mL vial, 3-mL cartridge, 3-mL Flex-Pen. **Glulisine (Apidra):** 100 units/mL vial, 3-mL cartridge. **Lispro (Humalog):** 100 units/mL vial, 3-mL pen.

Short-Acting
Regular (Humulin R): 100 units/mL vial, U-500 Kwik Pen. **Regular (Novolin R):** 100 units/mL vial, 3-mL cartridge, 3-mL Innolet prefilled syringe.

Intermediate-Acting
NPH (HumuLIN N): 100 units/mL vial, 3-mL pen. **NPH (NovoLIN N):** 100 units/mL vial, 3-mL cartridge, 3-mL Innolet prefilled syringe.

Long-Acting

Detemir (Levemir): 100 units/mL vial, 3-mL Flex-Pen. Glargine (Lantus): 100 units/mL vial, 3-mL cartridge.

Intermediate- and Short-Acting Mixtures

HumuLIN 50/50, HumuLIN 70/30, HumaLOG Mix 75/25, HumaLOG Mix 50/50, NovoLIN 70/30, NovoLOG Mix 70/30.

ADMINISTRATION/HANDLING

IV Regular and Insulin Glulisine (Apidra)

• Use only if solution is clear. • May give undiluted.

Rapid-Acting

Afrezza • Administer using a single inhalation/cartridge. Give at beginning of a meal.

Aspart (NovoLOG) • May give subcutaneous, IV infusion. • Can mix with NPH (draw aspart into syringe first; inject immediately after mixing). • After first use, stable at room temperature for 28 days. • Administer 5–10 min before meals.

Glulisine (Apidra) • May mix with NPH (draw glulisine into syringe first; inject immediately after mixing). • After first use, stable at room temperature for 28 days. • Administer 15 min before or within 20 min after starting a meal.

Lispro (HumaLOG) • For subcutaneous use only. • May mix with NPH. Stable for 28 days at room temperature; syringe is stable for 14 days if refrigerated. • After first use, stable at room temperature for 28 days. • Administer 15 min before or immediately after meals.

Short-Acting

Regular (HumuLIN R, NovoLIN R) • May give subcutaneous, IM, IV. • May mix with NPH for immediate use or for storage for future use. Stable for 1 mo at room temperature, 3 mos if refrigerated. • Can mix with Sterile Water for Injection or 0.9% NaCl. • After first use, stable at room temperature for 28 days. • Administer 30 min before meals.

Intermediate-Acting

NPH (HumuLIN N, NovoLIN N) • For subcutaneous use only. • May mix with aspart (NovoLOG) or lispro (HumaLOG). Draw aspart or lispro first and use immediately. • May mix with regular (HumuLIN R, NovoLIN R) insulin. Draw regular insulin first, use immediately or may store for future use (up to 28 days). • After first use, stable at room temperature for 28 days. • Administer 15 min before meals when mixed with aspart or lispro; 30 min before meals when mixed with regular insulin.

Long-Acting

Degludec (Tresiba) • For subcutaneous use only. • Do not mix with other insulins. • After first use, stable at room temperature for 56 days. • May take once daily any time of day.

Detemir (Levemir) • For subcutaneous use only. • Do not mix with other insulins. • After first use, stable at room temperature for 42 days. • Evening dose given at dinner or at bedtime. Twice-daily regimens can be given 12 hrs after morning dose.

Glargine (Lantus, Toujeo) • For subcutaneous use only. • Do not mix with other insulins. • After first use, stable at room temperature for 28 days. • Administer once daily at same time. Meal timing is not applicable.

Subcutaneous

• Check serum glucose concentration before administration; dosage highly individualized. • Subcutaneous injections may be given in thigh, abdomen, upper arm, buttocks, upper back if there is adequate adipose tissue. • Rotation of injection sites is essential; maintain careful record. • Prefilled syringes should be stored in vertical or oblique position to avoid plugging; plunger should be pulled back slightly and syringe rocked to remix solution before injection.

IV INCOMPATIBILITIES

DiltiaZEM (Cardizem), DOPamine (Intropin), nafcillin (Nafcil).

I

▓ IV COMPATIBILITIES

Amiodarone (Cordarone), ampicillin/sulbactam (Unasyn), ceFAZolin (Ancef), digoxin (Lanoxin), DOBUTamine (Dobutrex), famotidine (Pepcid), gentamicin, heparin, magnesium sulfate, metoclopramide (Reglan), midazolam (Versed), milrinone (Primacor), morphine, nitroglycerin, potassium chloride, propofol (Diprivan), vancomycin (Vancocin).

INDICATIONS/ROUTES/DOSAGE

Note: Insulin requirements vary dramatically among pts, requiring dosage adjustment.

Type 1 Diabetes: Multiple daily injections, guided by glucose monitoring or continuous subcutaneous insulin infusions, is standard of care.
Usual initial dose: 0.2-0.6 unit/kg/day in divided doses. **Usual maintenance:** 0.5–1.2 units/kg/day in divided doses.

Type 2 Diabetes: General goal is to achieve Hgb A_{1c} less than 7% using safe medication titration. Dual therapy (metformin and a second antihyperglycemic agent) is recommended in pts who fail to achieve glycemic goals after 3 mos with lifestyle interventions and metformin monotherapy.

Afrezza: Dosage based on metabolic needs, blood glucose results, glycemic goal control.

Dosage in Renal Impairment

Creatinine Clearance	Dose
10–50 mL/min	75% normal dose
Less than 10 mL/min	25–50% normal dose

Dosage in Hepatic Impairment

Insulin requirement may be reduced.

SIDE EFFECTS

Occasional: Localized redness, swelling, itching (due to improper insulin injection technique), allergy to insulin cleansing solution. **Infrequent:** Somogyi effect (rebound hyperglycemia) with chronically excessive insulin dosages. Systemic allergic reaction (rash, angioedema, anaphylaxis), lipodystrophy (depression at injection site due to breakdown of adipose tissue), lipohypertrophy (accumulation of subcutaneous tissue at injection site due to inadequate site rotation). **Rare:** Insulin resistance.

ADVERSE EFFECTS/ TOXIC REACTIONS

Severe hypoglycemia (due to hyperinsulinism) may occur with insulin overdose, decrease/delay of food intake, excessive exercise, pts with brittle diabetes. Diabetic ketoacidosis may result from stress, illness, omission of insulin dose, long-term poor insulin control.

NURSING CONSIDERATIONS

BASELINE ASSESSMENT

Obtain serum glucose level, Hgb A1c. Discuss lifestyle to determine extent of learning, emotional needs. If given IV, obtain serum chemistries (esp. serum potassium).

INTERVENTION/EVALUATION

Assess for hypoglycemia (refer to pharmacokinetics table for peak times and duration): cool, wet skin, tremors, dizziness, headache, anxiety, tachycardia, numbness in mouth, hunger, diplopia. Assess sleeping pt for restlessness, diaphoresis. Check for hyperglycemia: polyuria (excessive urine output), polyphagia (excessive food intake), polydipsia (excessive thirst), nausea/vomiting, dim vision, fatigue, deep and rapid breathing (Kussmaul respirations). Be alert to conditions altering glucose requirements: fever, trauma, increased activity/stress, surgical procedure.

PATIENT/FAMILY TEACHING

• Instruct on proper technique for drug administration, testing of glucose, signs/symptoms of hypoglycemia and hyperglycemia. • Diet and exercise are essential parts of treatment; do not skip/delay meals. • Carry candy, sugar packets, other sugar supplements for immediate response to hypoglycemia. • Wear or carry medical alert identification. • Check with physician when insulin demands are altered (e.g., fever, infection, trauma, stress, heavy physical activity). • Do not take other medication without consulting physician. • Weight control, exercise, hygiene (including foot care), not smoking are integral parts of therapy. • Protect skin, limit sun exposure. • Inform dentist, physician, surgeon of medication before any treatment is given.

interferon alfa-2b HIGH ALERT

in-ter-**feer**-on
(Intron-A)

■ **BLACK BOX ALERT** ■ May cause or aggravate fatal or life-threatening autoimmune disorders, ischemia, neuropsychiatric symptoms (profound depression, suicidal thoughts/behaviors), infectious disorders.

Do not confuse interferon alfa-2b with interferon alfa-2a, interferon alfa-n3, or peginterferon alfa-2b, or Intron with Peg-Intron.

FIXED-COMBINATION(S)

Rebetron: interferon alfa-2b/ribavirin (an antiviral): 3 million units/200 mg.

◆CLASSIFICATION

PHARMACOTHERAPEUTIC: Biologic response modifier, immunomodulator. **CLINICAL:** Antineoplastic.

USES

Treatment of hairy cell leukemia, condylomata acuminata (genital, venereal warts), malignant melanoma, AIDS-related Kaposi's sarcoma, chronic hepatitis C virus infection (including children 3 yrs of age and older), chronic hepatitis B virus infection (including children 1 yr and older), follicular non-Hodgkin's lymphoma. **OFF-LABEL:** Treatment of bladder, cervical, renal carcinoma; chronic myelocytic leukemia; laryngeal papillomatosis; multiple myeloma; cutaneous T-cell lymphoma; mycosis fungoides; West Nile virus.

PRECAUTIONS

Contraindications: Hypersensitivity to interferon alfa-2b. Decompensated hepatic disease, autoimmune hepatitis. **In combination with ribavirin:** Women who are pregnant, males with pregnant partners, pts with hemoglobinemias (e.g., sickle cell anemia), CrCl less than 50 mL/min). **Cautions:** Renal/hepatic impairment, seizure disorder, compromised CNS function, cardiac diseases, myelosuppression, concurrent use of medications causing myelosuppression, pulmonary impairment, multiple sclerosis, diabetes, thyroid disease, coagulopathy, hypertension, preexisting eye disorders, history of psychiatric disorders. History of autoimmune disorders, MI, arrhythmias, cardiac abnormalities.

ACTION

Inhibits viral replication in virus-infected cells, suppresses cell proliferation, augments specific cytotoxicity of lymphocytes. **Therapeutic Effect:** Prevents rapid growth of malignant cells; inhibits hepatitis virus.

PHARMACOKINETICS

Well absorbed after IM, subcutaneous administration. Undergoes proteolytic degradation during reabsorption in kidneys. **Half-life:** 2–3 hrs.

⌛ LIFESPAN CONSIDERATIONS

Pregnancy/Lactation: If possible, avoid use during pregnancy. Breastfeeding not recommended. **Children:** Safety and efficacy not established. **Elderly:** Neurotoxicity, cardiotoxicity may occur more frequently. Age-related renal impairment may require dosage adjustment.

INTERACTIONS

DRUG: Bone marrow depressants (e.g., alemtuzumab, methotrexate) may increase myelosuppression. **HERBAL:** None significant. **FOOD:** None known. **LAB VALUES:** May increase PT, aPTT, LDH, serum alkaline phosphatase, ALT, AST. May decrease Hgb, Hct, leukocyte, platelet counts.

✦ Canadian trade name   🍂 Non-Crushable Drug   🔳 High Alert drug

AVAILABILITY (Rx)

Injection, Powder for Reconstitution: 10 million units, 18 million units, 50 million units.
Injection, Solution: 6 million units/mL, 10 million units/mL.

ADMINISTRATION/HANDLING

 IV

Reconstitution • Prepare immediately before use. • Reconstitute with diluent provided by manufacturer. • Withdraw desired dose and further dilute with 100 mL 0.9% NaCl to provide final concentration of at least 10 million international units/100 mL.
Rate of Administration • Administer over 20 min.
Storage • Refrigerate unopened vials. • Following reconstitution, stable for 24 hrs if refrigerated.

IM, Subcutaneous
IM • Rotate sites. Preferred sites are anterior thigh, deltoid, and superolateral buttock. Administer in evening (if possible).
SQ • Reconstitute with recommended amount of Sterile Water for Injection. Agitate gently; do not shake. Rotate sites. Preferred sites are anterior thigh, abdomen (except around navel), outer upper arm.

IV INCOMPATIBILITIES

D_5W. Do not mix with other medications via Y-site administration.

IV COMPATIBILITIES

0.9% NaCl, lactated Ringer's.

INDICATIONS/ROUTES/DOSAGE

Hairy Cell Leukemia
IM, SQ: ADULTS: 2 million units/m² 3 times/wk for up to 2–6 mos. May continue treatment for sustained response. If severe adverse reactions occur, modify dose or temporarily discontinue drug. Discontinue for disease progression or failure to respond after 6 months.

Condylomata Acuminata
Intralesional: ADULTS: 1 million units/lesion 3 times/wk for 3 wks. May administer a second course at 12–16 wks. Use only 10 million–unit vial, and reconstitute with no more than 1 mL diluent. **Maximum:** 5 lesions per treatment.

AIDS-Related Kaposi's Sarcoma
IM, SQ: ADULTS: 30 million units/m² 3 times/wk. Use only 50 million–unit vials. Continue until disease progression or maximal response achieved after 16 wks. If severe adverse reactions occur, modify dose or temporarily discontinue drug.

Chronic Hepatitis C Virus Infection
IM, SQ: ADULTS: 3 million units 3 times/wk for up to 6 mos. For pts who tolerate therapy and whose ALT level normalizes within 16 wks, therapy may be extended for up to 18–24 mos. May be used in combination with ribavirin. **CHILDREN, 3–17 YRS (WITH HIV CO-INFECTION):** 3–5 million units/m² 3 times/wk with ribavirin for 48 wks.

Chronic Hepatitis B Virus Infection
IM, SQ: ADULTS: 30–35 million units wkly, either as 5 million units/day or 10 million units 3 times/wk for 16 wks.
SQ: CHILDREN 1–17 YRS: 3 million units/m² 3 times/wk for 1 wk, then 6 million units/m² 3 times/wk for 16–24 wks. **Maximum:** 10 million units 3 times/wk.

Malignant Melanoma
IV: ADULTS: Initially, 20 million units/m² 5 times/wk for 4 wks. **Maintenance:** 10 million units subcutaneously 3 times/wk for 48 wks.

Follicular Non-Hodgkin's Lymphoma
SQ: ADULTS: 5 million units 3 times/wk for up to 18 mos.

Dosage in Renal Impairment
Do not use when combined with ribavirin.

Dosage in Hepatic Impairment
No dose adjustment (see Contraindications).

SIDE EFFECTS

Frequent: Flu-like symptoms (fever, fatigue, headache, myalgia, anorexia, chills), rash (hairy cell leukemia, Kaposi's sarcoma only). **Pts with Kaposi's sarcoma:** All previously mentioned side effects plus depression, dyspepsia, dry mouth or thirst, alopecia, rigors. **Occasional:** Dizziness, pruritus, dry skin, dermatitis, altered taste. **Rare:** Confusion, leg cramps, back pain, gingivitis, flushing, tremor, anxiety, eye pain.

ADVERSE EFFECTS/ TOXIC REACTIONS

Hypersensitivity reactions occur rarely. Severe flu-like symptoms appear dose-related.

NURSING CONSIDERATIONS

BASELINE ASSESSMENT

CBC, blood chemistries, urinalysis, renal function, LFT should be performed before initial therapy and routinely thereafter.

INTERVENTION/EVALUATION

Offer emotional support. Monitor all levels of clinical function (numerous side effects). Encourage PO intake, particularly during early therapy. Monitor for worsening depression, suicidal ideation, associated behaviors.

PATIENT/FAMILY TEACHING

• Clinical response occurs in 1–3 mos. • Flu-like symptoms tend to diminish with continued therapy. • Some symptoms may be alleviated or minimized by bedtime doses. • Do not have immunizations without physician's approval (drug lowers resistance). • Avoid contact with those who have recently received live virus vaccine. • Avoid tasks that require alertness, motor skills until response to drug is established. • Sips of tepid water may relieve dry mouth. • Report depression, thoughts of suicide, unusual behavior.

TOP
100

interferon beta-1a

in-ter-**feer**-on
(Avonex, Rebif)
Do not confuse Avonex with Avelox, or interferon beta-1a with interferon beta-1b.

◆ CLASSIFICATION

PHARMACOTHERAPEUTIC: Biologic response modifier. **CLINICAL:** Multiple sclerosis agent.

USES

Treatment of relapsing multiple sclerosis to slow progression of physical disability, decrease frequency of clinical exacerbations.

PRECAUTIONS

Contraindications: Hypersensitivity to natural or recombinant interferon, human albumin (only for albumin-containing products). **Cautions:** Depression, severe psychiatric disorders, hepatic impairment, increased serum ALT at baseline, alcohol abuse, cardiovascular disease, seizure disorders, myelosuppression.

ACTION

Alters expression and response to surface antigens and may enhance immune cell activity. **Therapeutic Effect:** Slows progression of multiple sclerosis.

PHARMACOKINETICS

Peak serum levels attained 3–15 hrs after IM administration. Biologic markers increase within 12 hrs and remain elevated for 4 days. **Half-life:** 10 hrs (Avonex); 69 hrs (Rebif).

⌛ LIFESPAN CONSIDERATIONS

Pregnancy/Lactation: Has abortifacient potential. Unknown if distributed in breast milk. **Children:** Safety and efficacy not established. **Elderly:** No information available.

◆ Canadian trade name   🦺 Non-Crushable Drug   🟥 High Alert drug

INTERACTIONS

DRUG: **Alcohol, hepatotoxic drugs (e.g., acetaminophen, simvastatin)** may increase risk of hepatic injury. **HERBAL:** None significant. **FOOD:** None known. **LAB VALUES:** May increase serum glucose, BUN, alkaline phosphatase, bilirubin, calcium, ALT, AST. May decrease Hgb, neutrophil, platelet, WBC.

AVAILABILITY (Rx)

Injection, Powder for Reconstitution (Avonex): 30 mcg. **Injection Solution (Pre-filled Syringe):** 22 mcg/0.5 mL (Rebif), 30 mcg/0.5 mL (Avonex Prefilled Syringe), 44 mcg/0.5 mL (Rebif). **Titration Pack (Prefilled Syringe [Rebif]):** 8.8 mcg/0.2 mL, 22 mcg/0.5 mL.

ADMINISTRATION/HANDLING

IM (Avonex) Syringe
• Refrigerate syringe. • Allow to warm to room temperature before use. • May store up to 7 days at room temperature.

IM (Avonex) Vial
• Refrigerate vials (may store at room temperature up to 30 days). • Following reconstitution, may refrigerate again but use within 6 hrs if refrigerated. • Reconstitute 30-mcg *MicroPin* (6.6 million international units) vial with 1.1 mL diluent (supplied by manufacturer). • Gently swirl to dissolve medication; do not shake. • Discard if discolored or particulate forms. • Discard unused portion (contains no preservative).

Subcutaneous (Rebif)
• Refrigerate. May store at room temperature up to 30 days. Avoid heat, light. • Administer at same time of day 3 days each wk. Separate doses by at least 48 hrs.

INDICATIONS/ROUTES/DOSAGE

Relapsing Multiple Sclerosis
IM *(Avonex):* ADULTS: 30 mcg once wkly.

SQ *(Rebif):* ADULTS: **(Target dose 44 mcg 3 times/wk):** Initially, 8.8 mcg 3 times/wk for 2 wks, then 22 mcg 3 times/wk for 2 wks, then 44 mcg 3 times/wk thereafter. **(Target dose 22 mcg 3 times/wk):** Initially, 4.4 mcg 3 times/wk for 2 wks, then 11 mcg 3 times/wk for 2 wks, then 22 mcg 3 times/wk thereafter.

Dosage in Renal Impairment
No dose adjustment.

Dosage in Hepatic Impairment (Rebif)
Use with caution in pts with history of active hepatic disease or ALT more than 2.5 times upper limit of normal (ULN).

SIDE EFFECTS

Frequent (67%–11%): Headache, flu-like symptoms, myalgia, upper respiratory tract infection, depression with suicidal ideation, generalized pain, asthenia, chills, sinusitis, infection. **Occasional (9%–4%):** Abdominal pain, arthralgia, chest pain, dyspnea, malaise, syncope. **Rare (3%):** Injection site reaction, hypersensitivity reaction.

ADVERSE EFFECTS/ TOXIC REACTIONS

Anemia occurs in 8% of pts. Hepatic failure has been reported.

NURSING CONSIDERATIONS

BASELINE ASSESSMENT
Obtain CBC, BMP, LFT. Assess home situation for support of therapy.

INTERVENTION/EVALUATION
Assess for headache, flu-like symptoms, myalgia. Periodically monitor lab results, re-evaluate injection technique. Assess for depression, suicidal ideation.

PATIENT/FAMILY TEACHING
• Do not change schedule, dosage without consulting physician. • Follow guidelines for reconstitution of product and administration, including aseptic technique. • Use puncture-resistant container for used needles, syringes; dispose of used needles,

---

syringes properly. • Injection site reactions may occur. These do not require discontinuation of therapy, but type and extent should be carefully noted. Report flu-like symptoms (fever, chills, fatigue, muscle aches).

TOP
100

interferon beta-1b

in-ter-**feer**-on
(Betaseron, Extavia)
Do not confuse interferon beta-1b with interferon beta-1a.

◆CLASSIFICATION

PHARMACOTHERAPEUTIC: Biologic response modifier. **CLINICAL:** Multiple sclerosis agent.

USES

Reduces frequency of clinical exacerbations in pts with relapsing-remitting multiple sclerosis (recurrent attacks of neurologic dysfunction).

PRECAUTIONS

Contraindications: Hypersensitivity to albumin, interferon. **Cautions:** Depression, severe psychiatric disorders, hepatic/renal impairment, alcohol abuse, cardiovascular disease, seizure disorders, myelosuppression, pulmonary disease.

ACTION

Exact mechanism unknown. Participates in immunoregulation by enhancing oxidative metabolism of macrophages, antibody-dependent cellular cytotoxicity and activating natural killer cells. **Therapeutic Effect:** Improves MRI lesions, decreases relapse rate and disease severity in multiple sclerosis.

PHARMACOKINETICS

Slowly absorbed following subcutaneous administration. **Half-life:** 8 min–4.3 hrs.

⌛ LIFESPAN CONSIDERATIONS

Pregnancy/Lactation: Spontaneous abortions reported. Discontinuation of the drug before conception is recommended. Unknown if distributed in breast milk. **Children:** Safety and efficacy not established. **Elderly:** No information available.

INTERACTIONS

DRUG: None significant. **HERBAL:** None significant. **FOOD:** None known. **LAB VALUES:** May increase bilirubin, ALT, AST. May decrease neutrophil, lymphocyte, WBC.

AVAILABILITY (Rx)

Injection, Powder for Reconstitution: 0.3 mg.

ADMINISTRATION/HANDLING

Subcutaneous
• Store vials at room temperature. • After reconstitution, stable for 3 hrs if refrigerated. • Use within 3 hrs of reconstitution. • Discard if discolored or precipitate forms. • Reconstitute 0.3-mg (9.6 million international units) vial with 1.2 mL diluent (supplied by manufacturer) to provide concentration of 0.25 mg/mL (8 million units/mL). • Gently swirl to dissolve medication; do not shake. • Withdraw 1 mL solution and inject subcutaneously into arms, abdomen, hips, thighs using 27-gauge needle. • Discard unused portion (contains no preservative).

INDICATIONS/ROUTES/DOSAGE

Relapsing-Remitting Multiple Sclerosis
SQ: ADULTS: Initially, 0.0625 mg every other day; gradually increase by 0.0625 mg every 2 wks. Target dose: 0.25 mg every other day.

Dosage in Renal/Hepatic Impairment
No dose adjustment.

SIDE EFFECTS

Frequent (85%–21%): Injection site reaction, headache, flu-like symptoms, fever, asthenia, myalgia, sinusitis, diarrhea,

---

dizziness, altered mental status, constipation, diaphoresis, vomiting. **Occasional (15%–4%):** Malaise, drowsiness, alopecia.

ADVERSE EFFECTS/ TOXIC REACTIONS

Seizures occur rarely.

NURSING CONSIDERATIONS

BASELINE ASSESSMENT

Obtain CBC, BMP, LFT. Assess home situation for support of therapy.

INTERVENTION/EVALUATION

Periodically monitor lab results, re-evaluate injection technique. Assess for nausea (high incidence). Monitor sleep pattern. Monitor daily pattern of bowel activity, stool consistency. Assist with ambulation if dizziness occurs. Monitor food intake.

PATIENT/FAMILY TEACHING

• Report flu-like symptoms (fever, chills, fatigue, muscle aches); occur commonly but decrease over time.
• Wear sunscreen, protective clothing if exposed to sunlight, ultraviolet light until tolerance known.

interferon gamma-1b

in-ter-**feer**-on
(Actimmune)

◆CLASSIFICATION

PHARMACOTHERAPEUTIC: Biologic response modifier. **CLINICAL:** Immunologic agent.

USES

Reduces frequency, severity of serious infections due to chronic granulomatous disease. Delays time to disease progression in pts with severe, malignant osteopetrosis.

PRECAUTIONS

Contraindications: Hypersensitivity to interferon gamma-1b, *Escherichia coli*–derived products. **Cautions:** Seizure disorders, compromised CNS function, preexisting cardiac disease (e.g., ischemia, HF, arrhythmias), hepatic disease, myelosuppression.

ACTION

Exact mechanism unknown. Enhances oxidative metabolism of macrophages, antibody-dependent cellular cytotoxicity; activates natural killer cells. **Therapeutic Effect:** Decreases signs/symptoms of serious infections in chronic granulomatous disease.

PHARMACOKINETICS

Slowly absorbed after subcutaneous administration. **Half-life:** 3–6 hrs.

⧖ LIFESPAN CONSIDERATIONS

Pregnancy/Lactation: Unknown if drug crosses placenta or is distributed in breast milk. **Children:** Safety and efficacy not established in pts younger than 1 yr. Flu-like symptoms may occur more frequently. **Elderly:** No information available.

INTERACTIONS

DRUG: Bone marrow depressants (e.g., alemtuzumab, methotrexate) may increase myelosuppression. **HERBAL:** None significant. **FOOD:** None known. **LAB VALUES:** May increase serum ALT, AST, alkaline phosphatase, LDH, triglycerides, cortisol concentrations. May decrease leukocytes, neutrophils, platelets.

AVAILABILITY (Rx)

Injection Solution: 100 mcg/0.5 mL (2 million units).

ADMINISTRATION/HANDLING

◀**ALERT**▶ Avoid excessive agitation of vial; do not shake.
Subcutaneous
• Refrigerate vials. Do not freeze. • Do not keep at room temperature for more than 12 hrs; discard after 12 hrs. • Vials are single dose; discard unused portion. • Solution is clear, colorless. Do

not use if discolored or precipitate forms. • When given 3 times/wk, rotate injection sites. • Administer into right and left deltoid or anterior thigh.

INDICATIONS/ROUTES/DOSAGE

Chronic Granulomatous Disease; Severe, Malignant Osteopetrosis

SQ: ADULTS, ELDERLY, CHILDREN OLDER THAN 1 YR: 50 mcg/m^2 (1 million units/m^2) 3 times/wk in pts with body surface area (BSA) greater than 0.5 m^2; 1.5 mcg/kg/dose 3 times/wk in pts with BSA 0.5 m^2 or less.

Dosage in Renal/Hepatic Impairment

No dose adjustment.

SIDE EFFECTS

Frequent (52%–14%): Fever, headache, rash, chills, fatigue, diarrhea. **Occasional (13%–10%):** Vomiting, nausea. **Rare (6%–3%):** Weight loss, myalgia, anorexia.

ADVERSE EFFECTS/ TOXIC REACTIONS

May exacerbate preexisting CNS dysfunction (manifested as decreased mental status, gait disturbance, dizziness), cardiac abnormalities.

NURSING CONSIDERATIONS

BASELINE ASSESSMENT

CBC, serum electrolytes, urinalysis, renal function, LFT should be performed before initial therapy and at 3-mo intervals during course of treatment.

INTERVENTION/EVALUATION

Monitor for flu-like symptoms. Assess skin for evidence of rash.

PATIENT/FAMILY TEACHING

• Flu-like symptoms (fever, chills, fatigue, muscle aches) are generally mild and tend to disappear as treatment continues. Symptoms may be minimized with bedtime administration. • Avoid tasks that require alertness, motor skills until response to drug is established. • If home use is prescribed, follow guidelines for proper technique of administration and for care in the proper disposal of needles, syringes. • Vials should remain refrigerated.

interleukin-2 (aldesleukin)   **HIGH ALERT**

in-ter-**loo**-kin
(Proleukin)

■ **BLACK BOX ALERT** ■ High-dose therapy is associated with capillary leak syndrome resulting in significant hypotension and reduced organ perfusion. Use restricted to pts with normal cardiac/pulmonary function. Increased risk of disseminated infection (sepsis, bacterial endocarditis). Withhold treatment for pts developing moderate-to-severe lethargy or drowsiness (continued treatment may result in coma). Must be administered by personnel trained in administration/handling of chemotherapeutic agents.
Do not confuse aldesleukin with oprelvekin.

◆CLASSIFICATION

PHARMACOTHERAPEUTIC: Biologic response modifier. **CLINICAL:** Antineoplastic.

USES

Treatment of metastatic renal cell carcinoma, metastatic melanoma. **OFF-LABEL:** Treatment of acute myeloid leukemia (AML).

PRECAUTIONS

Contraindications: Hypersensitivity to aldesleukin. Abnormal pulmonary function or thallium stress test results, bowel ischemia or perforation, coma or toxic psychosis lasting longer than 48 hrs, GI bleeding requiring surgery, intubation lasting more than 72 hrs, organ allografts, pericardial tamponade, renal dysfunction requiring dialysis for longer than 72 hrs, repetitive or difficult-to-control seizures; retreatment in pts who experience any of the following

---

toxicities: angina, MI, recurrent chest pain with EKG changes, sustained ventricular tachycardia, uncontrolled or unresponsive cardiac rhythm disturbances. **Extreme Caution:** Pts with normal thallium stress tests and pulmonary function tests who have history of cardiac or pulmonary disease. **Cautions:** Pts with fixed requirements for large volumes of fluid (e.g., those with hypercalcemia), history of seizures, renal/hepatic impairment, autoimmune disease, inflammatory disorders.

ACTION

Promotes proliferation, differentiation, recruitment of T and B cells, lymphokine-activated and natural killer cells, thymocytes. **Therapeutic Effect:** Enhances cytolytic activity in lymphocytes.

PHARMACOKINETICS

Primarily distributed into plasma, lymphocytes, lungs, liver, kidney, spleen. Metabolized to amino acids in cells lining the kidneys. **Half-life:** 80–120 min.

⧗ LIFESPAN CONSIDERATIONS

Pregnancy/Lactation: Avoid use in those of either sex not practicing effective contraception. **Children:** Safety and efficacy not established. **Elderly:** Age-related renal impairment may require dosage adjustment; will not tolerate toxicity.

INTERACTIONS

DRUG: Antihypertensives (e.g., amlodipine, lisinopril, valsartan) may increase hypotensive effect. **Cardiotoxic, hepatotoxic, myelotoxic, nephrotoxic medications** may increase risk of toxicity. **Glucocorticoids** may decrease effects. **HERBAL:** None significant. **FOOD:** None known. **LAB VALUES:** May increase serum BUN, alkaline phosphatase, bilirubin, creatinine, ALT, AST. May decrease serum calcium, magnesium, phosphorus, potassium, sodium.

AVAILABILITY (Rx)

Injection, Powder for Reconstitution (Proleukin): 22 million units (1.3 mg) (18

million units/mL = 1.1 mg/mL when reconstituted).

ADMINISTRATION/HANDLING

◀ **ALERT** ▶ Hold administration in pts who develop moderate to severe lethargy or drowsiness (continued administration may result in coma).

 IV

Reconstitution • Reconstitute 22 million units vial with 1.2 mL Sterile Water for Injection to provide concentration of 18 million units/mL (1.1 mg/mL). • Bacteriostatic Water for Injection or NaCl should not be used to reconstitute because of increased aggregation. • During reconstitution, direct Sterile Water for Injection at the side of vial. Swirl contents gently to avoid foaming. Do not shake.

Rate of Administration • Further dilute dose in 50 mL D_5W to a final concentration between 0.49 and 1.1 million international units/mL (30–70 mcg/mL) and infuse over 15 min. Do not use an in-line filter. • Solution should be warmed to room temperature before infusion. • Monitor diligently for drop in mean arterial B/P (sign of capillary leak syndrome [CLS]). Continued treatment may result in significant hypotension (less than 90 mm Hg or a 20 mm Hg drop from baseline systolic pressure), edema, pleural effusion, altered mental status.

Storage • Refrigerate vials; do not freeze. • Reconstituted solution is stable for 48 hrs refrigerated or at room temperature (refrigeration preferred).

▦ IV INCOMPATIBILITIES

Ganciclovir (Cytovene), pentamidine (Pentam), prochlorperazine (Compazine), promethazine (Phenergan).

▦ IV COMPATIBILITIES

Calcium gluconate, DOPamine (Intropin), heparin, LORazepam (Ativan), magnesium, potassium.

INDICATIONS/ROUTES/DOSAGE

Metastatic Melanoma, Metastatic Renal Cell Carcinoma

IV: ADULTS 18 YRS AND OLDER: 600,000 units/kg q8h for 14 doses; followed by 9 days of rest, then another 14 doses for a total of 28 doses per course. Course may be repeated if tumor shrinkage observed after rest period of at least 7 wks from date of hospital discharge.

Dosage in Renal/Hepatic Impairment

No dose adjustment. Do not initiate if serum creatinine greater than 1.5 mg/dL.

Dosage Modification for Toxicity

Withhold or interrupt therapy; do not reduce dose. Retreatment contraindicated with the following toxicities: Sustained ventricular tachycardia, uncontrolled arrhythmias; chest pain/EKG changes consistent with angina or MI; cardiac tamponade, repetitive/refractory seizures; GI bleeding; bowel ischemia/perforation; renal failure requiring dialysis; coma lasting more than 48 hrs.

SIDE EFFECTS

Side effects are generally self-limited and resolve within 2–3 days after discontinuing therapy. **Frequent (89%–48%):** Fever, chills, nausea, vomiting, hypotension, diarrhea, oliguria/anuria, altered mental status, irritability, confusion, depression, sinus tachycardia, pain (abdominal, chest, back), fatigue, dyspnea, pruritus. **Occasional (47%–17%):** Edema, erythema, rash, stomatitis, anorexia, weight gain, infection (UTI, injection site, catheter tip), dizziness. **Rare (15%–4%):** Dry skin, sensory disorders (vision, speech, taste), dermatitis, headache, arthralgia, myalgia, weight loss, hematuria, conjunctivitis, proteinuria.

ADVERSE EFFECTS/TOXIC REACTIONS

Anemia, thrombocytopenia, leukopenia occur commonly. GI bleeding, pulmonary edema occur occasionally. Capillary leak syndrome (CLS) results in hypotension (systolic pressure less than 90 mm Hg or a 20 mm Hg drop from baseline systolic pressure), extravasation of plasma proteins and fluid into extravascular space, loss of vascular tone. May result in cardiac arrhythmias, angina, MI, respiratory insufficiency. Fatal malignant hyperthermia, cardiac arrest, CVA, pulmonary emboli, bowel perforation/gangrene, severe depression leading to suicide occur in less than 1% of pts.

NURSING CONSIDERATIONS

BASELINE ASSESSMENT

Pts with bacterial infection and with indwelling central lines should be treated with antibiotic therapy before treatment begins. All pts should be neurologically stable with a negative CT scan before treatment begins. CBC, BMP, LFT, chest X-ray should be performed before therapy begins and daily thereafter.

INTERVENTION/EVALUATION

Monitor CBC with differential, amylase, electrolytes, renal function, LFT, weight, pulse oximetry. Discontinue medication at first sign of hypotension and hold for moderate to severe lethargy (physician must decide whether therapy should continue). Assess for altered mental status (irritability, confusion, depression), weight gain/loss. Maintain strict I&O. Assess for extravascular fluid accumulation (rales in lungs, edema in dependent areas).

PATIENT/FAMILY TEACHING

• Nausea may decrease during therapy. • At home, increase fluid intake (protects against renal impairment). • Do not have immunizations without physician's approval (drug lowers resistance). • Avoid exposure to persons with infection. • Report fever, chills, lower back pain, difficulty with urination, unusual bleeding/bruising, black tarry stools, blood in urine, petechial rash (pinpoint red spots on skin). • Report symptoms of depression or suicidal ideation immediately.

✤ Canadian trade name   🜲 Non-Crushable Drug   🔴 High Alert drug

ipilimumab

ip-i-**lim**-ue-mab
(Yervoy)

■ **BLACK BOX ALERT** ■ Severe and fatal immune-mediated adverse reactions due to T-cell activation and proliferation are capable of involving any organ system. Specific reactions include enterocolitis, hepatitis, dermatitis, neuropathy, endocrinopathy. Majority of immune-mediated reactions may initially manifest during treatment or weeks to months after treatment. Permanently discontinue treatment and initiate high-dose corticosteroid therapy for severe immune-mediated adverse reactions. Assess all pts for signs/symptoms of enterocolitis, hepatitis, dermatitis (including toxic epidermal necrolysis), neuropathy, endocrinopathy, and evaluate clinical chemistries, including hepatic function tests and thyroid tests at baseline and before each treatment.

◆ CLASSIFICATION

PHARMACOTHERAPEUTIC: Human cytotoxic T-lymphocyte antigen 4 (CTLA-4)-blocking antibody. **CLINICAL:** Antineoplastic.

USES

Treatment of unresectable or metastatic melanoma in adults and children 12 yrs of age and older. Adjuvant treatment of pts with cutaneous melanoma with pathologic involvement of regional lymph nodes and who have undergone complete resection, including total lymphadenectomy.

PRECAUTIONS

Contraindications: Hypersensitivity to ipilimumab. **Cautions:** Hepatic impairment, chronic peripheral neuropathy, thyroid/adrenal/pituitary dysfunction, autoimmune disorders (ulcerative colitis, Crohn's disease, lupus, sarcoidosis).

ACTION

Augments T-cell activation and proliferation. Binds to cytotoxic T-lymphocyte-associated antigen 4 (CTLA-4) and blocks interaction of CTLA-4 with its ligands. **Therapeutic Effect:** Inhibits tumor cell growth and metastasis.

PHARMACOKINETICS

Metabolized in liver. Steady state reached by third dose. **Half-life:** 14.7 days.

⧖ LIFESPAN CONSIDERATIONS

Pregnancy/Lactation: May cause fetal harm. Use effective contraception during treatment and for at least 3 mos after discontinuation. Unknown if distributed in breast milk. Discontinue drug or discontinue breastfeeding. **Children:** Safety and efficacy not established. **Elderly:** No age-related precautions noted.

INTERACTIONS

DRUG: None significant. **HERBAL:** None significant. **FOOD:** None known. **LAB VALUES:** May increase serum ALT, AST, bilirubin; eosinophils.

AVAILABILITY (Rx)

Injection, Solution: 5 mg/mL (10 mL, 40 mL vials).

ADMINISTRATION/HANDLING
 IV

◀ **ALERT** ▶ Use sterile, nonpyrogenic, low protein-binding in-line filter. Use dedicated line only.

Reconstitution • Calculate number of vials needed for injection. • Inspect for particulate matter or discoloration. • Allow vials to stand at room temperature for approximately 5 min. • Withdraw proper volume and transfer to infusion bag. Dilute in NaCl or D₅W with final concentration ranging from 1–2 mg/mL. • Mix diluted solution by gentle inversion. Do not shake or agitate.

Rate of Administration • Infuse over 90 min. Flush with 0.9% NaCl or D₅W at end of infusion.

Storage • Solution should be translucent to white or pale yellow with amorphous particles. • Discard vial if cloudy or discolored. • Refrigerate vials until time of use. • May store diluted solution either under refrigeration or at room temperature for no more than 24 hrs.

INDICATIONS/ROUTES/DOSAGE

Metastatic Melanoma

IV: **ADULTS, CHILDREN 12 YRS of AGE and OLDER:** 3 mg/kg q3wks for maximum of 4 doses. Doses may be delayed due to toxicity, but all doses must be given within 16 wks of initial dose.

◄**ALERT**► Pts who are presenting with severe immune-mediated adverse reactions must immediately discontinue drug therapy and start predniSONE 1 mg/kg/day.

Cutaneous Melanoma

IV: **ADULTS:** 10 mg/kg q3wks for 4 doses, then 10 mg/kg q12wks for up to 3 yrs. If toxicity occurs, doses are omitted (not delayed).

Dosage Modification

Hold scheduled dose for moderate immune-mediated adverse reactions. Pts with complete or partial resolution of adverse reactions and who are receiving less than 7.5 mg/day of predniSONE may resume scheduled doses. Permanently discontinue for persistent moderate adverse reactions or inability to reduce corticosteroid dose to 7.5 mg/day, failure to complete full treatment course in 16 wks, any severe or life-threatening adverse reactions.

Dosage in Renal/Hepatic Impairment

No dose adjustment.

Hepatotoxicity During Treatment

ALT/AST greater than 2.5 times upper limit of normal (ULN) or bilirubin greater than 1.5–3 times ULN: Withhold treatment. **ALT/AST greater than 5 times ULN or bilirubin greater than 3 times ULN:** Permanently discontinue.

SIDE EFFECTS

Frequent (42%): Fatigue. **Occasional (32%–29%):** Diarrhea, pruritus, rash, colitis.

ADVERSE EFFECTS/ TOXIC REACTIONS

Severe and fatal immune-mediated adverse reactions have occurred. Enterocolitis (7% of pts) may present with fever, ileus, abdominal pain, GI bleeding, intestinal perforation, severe dehydrating diarrhea. Endocrinopathies (4% of pts), including hypopituitarism, adrenal insufficiency, hypogonadism, hypothyroidism, may present with fatigue, headache, mental status change, unusual bowel habits, hypotension and may require emergent hormone replacement therapy. Dermatitis including toxic epidermal necrolysis (2% of pts) may present with full-thickness ulceration or necrotic, bullous, hemorrhagic manifestations. Hepatotoxicity (1% of pts), defined as LFT greater than 2.5–5 times ULN, may present with right upper abdominal pain, jaundice, black/tarry stools, bruising, dark-colored urine, nausea, vomiting. Neuropathy (1% of pts), including Guillain-Barré syndrome or myasthenia gravis, may present with weakness, sensory alterations, paresthesia, paralysis. Other serious adverse reactions such as pneumonitis, meningitis, nephritis, eosinophilia, pericarditis, myocarditis, angiopathy, temporal arteritis, vasculitis, polymyalgia rheumatica, conjunctivitis, blepharitis, episcleritis, scleritis, leukocytoclastic vasculitis, erythema multiforme, psoriasis, pancreatitis, arthritis, autoimmune thyroiditis reported. Anti-ipilimumab antibodies reported in 1.1% of pts. All severe immune-mediated adverse reactions require immediate high-dose corticosteroid therapy.

NURSING CONSIDERATIONS

BASELINE ASSESSMENT

Obtain baseline CBC, complete metabolic profile, LFT, TSH, free T_4, urine pregnancy. Screen for history of hepatic impairment, chronic neuropathy, thyroid/adrenal/pituitary dysfunction, autoimmune disorders. Focused assessment relating to possible adverse reactions includes abdominal area (inspection, auscultation, percussion, palpation, bowel pattern, symmetry), skin (color, lesions, mucosal inspection, edema), neurologic (mental status, gait, numbness, tingling, pain, strength, visual acuity), hormonal glands (lymph node inspection/palpation, pyrexia, goiter, palpitations). Question possibility of pregnancy or plans of breastfeeding. Receive full medication history including herbal products.

INTERVENTION/EVALUATION

Monitor vital signs, LFT, thyroid panel before each dose. Continue focused assessment and screen for life-threatening immune-mediated adverse reactions. If adverse reactions occur, immediately notify physician and initiate proper treatment. Report suspected pregnancy. Obtain CBC, blood cultures for fever, suspected infection. EKG for palpitations, chest pain, difficulty breathing, dizziness. If predniSONE therapy initiated, monitor capillary blood glucose and screen for side effects.

PATIENT/FAMILY TEACHING

• Inform pt that serious and fatal adverse reactions indicate inflammation to certain systems: intestines (diarrhea, dark/tarry stools, abdominal pain), liver (yellowing of the skin, dark-colored urine, right upper quadrant pain, bruising), skin (rash, mouth sores, blisters, ulcers), nerves (weakness, numbness, tingling, difficulty breathing, paralysis), hormonal glands (headaches, weight gain, palpitations, changes in mood or behavior, dizziness), eyes (blurry vision, double vision, eye pain/redness). • PredniSONE therapy may be started if adverse reactions occur. • May cause fetal harm, stillbirth, premature delivery. • Blood levels will be drawn before each dose. • Report any chest pain, palpitations, fever, swollen glands, stomach pain, vomiting, or any sign of adverse reactions.

ipratropium

ip-ra-**troe**-pee-um
(<u>Atrovent HFA</u>, PMS-Ipratropium ✿)
Do not confuse Atrovent with Alupent or Serevent, or ipratropium with tiotropium.

FIXED-COMBINATION(S)

Combivent, DuoNeb: ipratropium/albuterol (a bronchodilator): *Aerosol:* 18 mcg/90 mcg per actuation. *Solution:* 0.5 mg/2.5 mg per 3 mL.

◆CLASSIFICATION

PHARMACOTHERAPEUTIC: Anticholinergic. **CLINICAL:** Bronchodilator.

USES

Inhalation, Nebulization: Maintenance treatment of bronchospasm due to COPD, bronchitis, emphysema, asthma. Not indicated for immediate bronchospasm relief. **Nasal Spray:** Symptomatic relief of rhinorrhea associated with the common cold and allergic/nonallergic rhinitis.

PRECAUTIONS

Contraindications: History of hypersensitivity to ipratropium, atropine. **Cautions:** Narrow-angle glaucoma, prostatic hypertrophy, bladder neck obstruction, myasthenia gravis.

ACTION

Blocks action of acetylcholine at parasympathetic sites in bronchial smooth muscle. Application to nasal mucosa inhibits serous/seromucous gland secretions. **Therapeutic Effect:** Causes bronchodilation, inhibits nasal secretions.

PHARMACOKINETICS

Route	Onset	Peak	Duration
Inhalation	1–3 min	1.5–2 hrs	Up to 4 hrs
Nasal	5 min	1–4 hrs	4–8 hrs

Minimal systemic absorption after inhalation. Metabolized in liver (systemic absorption). Primarily excreted in feces. **Half-life:** 1.5–4 hrs (nasal).

☒ LIFESPAN CONSIDERATIONS

Pregnancy/Lactation: Unknown if distributed in breast milk. **Children/Elderly:** No age-related precautions noted.

INTERACTIONS

DRUG: Anticholinergics (e.g., glycopyrrolate, scopolamine), medications with anticholinergic properties may increase toxicity. **HERBAL:** None significant. **FOOD:** None known. **LAB VALUES:** None significant.

AVAILABILITY (Rx)

Aerosol for Oral Inhalation (Atrovent HFA): 17 mcg/actuation. **Solution, Intranasal Spray:** 0.03%; 0.06%. **Solution for Nebulization:** 0.02% (500 mcg).

ADMINISTRATION/HANDLING

Inhalation
• Do not shake. Prime before first use or if not used for more than 3 days.
• Instruct pt to exhale completely, place mouthpiece between lips, inhale deeply through mouth while fully depressing top of canister. Hold breath as long as possible before exhaling slowly. • Allow at least 1 minute between inhalations. • Rinse mouth with water immediately after inhalation (prevents mouth/throat dryness).

Nebulization
• May be administered with or without dilution in 0.9% NaCl. • Stable for 1 hr when mixed with albuterol. • Give over 5–15 min.

Nasal
• Store at room temperature. • Initial pump priming requires 7 actuations of pump. • If used regularly as recommended, no further priming is required. If not used for more than 4 hrs, pump will require 2 actuations, or if not used for more than 7 days, the pump will require 7 actuations to re-prime.

INDICATIONS/ROUTES/DOSAGE

Bronchodilator for COPD
Inhalation: ADULTS, ELDERLY, CHILDREN OLDER THAN 12 YRS: 2 inhalations 4 times/day. **Maximum:** 12 inhalations per 24 hrs.

Nebulization: ADULTS, ELDERLY, CHILDREN OLDER THAN 12 YRS: 500 mcg (1 unit dose vial) 3–4 times/day (doses 6–8 hrs apart).

Asthma Exacerbation
Note: Should be given in combination with a short-acting beta-adrenergic agonist.
Inhalation: ADULTS, ELDERLY, CHILDREN OLDER THAN 12 YRS: 8 inhalations q20min as needed for up to 3 hrs. CHILDREN 6–12 YRS: 4–8 inhalations q20min as needed for up to 3 hrs. CHILDREN 5 YRS OR YOUNGER: 2 inhalations q20 min for 1 hr.

Nebulization: ADULTS, ELDERLY, CHILDREN OLDER THAN 12 YRS: 500 mcg q20min for 3 doses, then as needed. CHILDREN 6–12 YRS: 250–500 mcg q20min for 3 doses, then as needed. CHILDREN 5 YRS OR YOUNGER: 250 mcg q20 min for 1 hr.

Rhinorrhea (Perennial Allergic/Nonallergic Rhinitis)
Intranasal *(0.03%):* ADULTS, ELDERLY, CHILDREN 6 YRS AND OLDER: 2 sprays per nostril 2–3 times/day.

Rhinorrhea (Common Cold)
Intranasal *(0.06%):* ADULTS, ELDERLY, CHILDREN 12 YRS AND OLDER: 2 sprays per nostril 3–4 times/day for up to 4 days. CHILDREN 5–11 YRS: 2 sprays per nostril 3 times/day for up to 4 days.

Rhinorrhea (Seasonal Allergy)
Intranasal *(0.06%):* ADULTS, ELDERLY, CHILDREN 5 YRS AND OLDER: 2 sprays per nostril 4 times/day for up to 3 wks.

Dosage in Renal/Hepatic Impairment
No dose adjustment.

SIDE EFFECTS

Frequent: Inhalation (6%–3%): Cough, dry mouth, headache, nausea. **Nasal:** Dry nose/mouth, headache, nasal irritation. **Occasional: Inhalation (2%):** Dizziness, transient increased bronchospasm. **Rare (less than 1%): Inhalation:** Hypotension, insomnia, metallic/unpleasant taste, palpitations, urinary retention. **Nasal:** Diarrhea, constipation, dry throat, abdominal pain, nasal congestion.

ADVERSE EFFECTS/ TOXIC REACTIONS

Worsening of angle-closure glaucoma, acute eye pain, hypotension occur rarely.

NURSING CONSIDERATIONS

BASELINE ASSESSMENT

Auscultate lung sounds. Question history of glaucoma, urinary retention, myasthenia gravis.

INTERVENTION/EVALUATION

Monitor rate, depth, rhythm, type of respiration; quality, rate of pulse. Assess lung sounds for rhonchi, wheezing, rales. Monitor ABGs. Observe for retractions (clavicular, sternal, intercostal), hand tremor. Evaluate for clinical improvement (quieter, slower respirations, relaxed facial expression, cessation of retractions). Monitor for improvement of rhinorrhea.

PATIENT/ FAMILY TEACHING

• Increase fluid intake (decreases lung secretion viscosity). • Do not take more than 2 inhalations at any one time (excessive use may produce paradoxical bronchoconstriction, decreased bronchodilating effect). • Rinsing mouth with water immediately after inhalation may prevent mouth and throat dryness. • Avoid excessive use of caffeine derivatives (chocolate, coffee, tea, cola, cocoa).

irbesartan

ir-be-**sar**-tan
(Apo-Irbesartan ✤, Avapro)
■ **BLACK BOX ALERT** ■ May cause fetal injury, mortality if used during second or third trimester of pregnancy. Discontinue as soon as possible once pregnancy is detected. **Do not confuse Avapro with Anaprox.**

FIXED-COMBINATION(S)

Avalide: irbesartan/hydroCHLOROthiazide (a diuretic): 150 mg/12.5 mg, 300 mg/12.5 mg, 300 mg/25 mg.

◆CLASSIFICATION

PHARMACOTHERAPEUTIC: Angiotensin II receptor antagonist. **CLINICAL:** Antihypertensive.

USES

Treatment of hypertension alone or in combination with other antihypertensives. Treatment of diabetic nephropathy in pts with type 2 diabetes. **OFF-LABEL:** Reduce proteinuria in children with chronic kidney disease.

PRECAUTIONS

Contraindications: Hypersensitivity to irbesartan. Concomitant use with aliskiren in pts with diabetes. **Cautions:** Renal impairment, unstented unilateral or bilateral renal artery stenosis, dehydration, HF, idiopathic or hereditary angioedema or angioedema associated with ACE inhibitor therapy.

ACTION

Blocks vasoconstriction, aldosterone-secreting effects of angiotensin II, inhibiting binding of angiotensin II to AT_1 receptors. **Therapeutic Effect:** Produces vasodilation, decreases peripheral resistance, decreases B/P.

PHARMACOKINETICS

Route	Onset	Peak	Duration
PO	—	1–2 hrs	Greater than 24 hrs

Rapidly, completely absorbed after PO administration. Protein binding: 90%. Metabolized in liver. Excreted in feces (80%), urine (20%). Not removed by hemodialysis. **Half-life:** 11–15 hrs.

☒ LIFESPAN CONSIDERATIONS

Pregnancy/Lactation: Unknown if distributed in breast milk. May cause fetal or neonatal morbidity or mortality. **Children:** Safety and efficacy not established. **Elderly:** No age-related precautions noted.

INTERACTIONS

DRUG: Diuretics (e.g., **furosemide, HCTZ**) produce additive hypotensive effects. **Potassium-sparing diuretics (e.g., spironolactone, triamterene), potassium supplements** may increase risk of hyperkalemia. **NSAIDs (e.g., ibuprofen, ketorolac, naproxen)** may decrease antihypertensive effect. **HERBAL: Ephedra, ginseng, yohimbe** may worsen hypertension. **Garlic** may increase antihypertensive effect. **FOOD:** None known. **LAB VALUES:** May slightly increase serum BUN, creatinine. May decrease Hgb.

AVAILABILITY (Rx)

Tablets: 75 mg, 150 mg, 300 mg.

ADMINISTRATION/HANDLING

PO

• Give without regard to meals.

INDICATIONS/ROUTES/DOSAGE

Hypertension
PO: ADULTS, ELDERLY, CHILDREN 13 YRS AND OLDER: Initially, 75–150 mg/day. May increase to 300 mg/day. **CHILDREN 6–12 YRS:** Initially, 75 mg/day. May increase to 150 mg/day.

Diabetic Nephropathy
PO: ADULTS, ELDERLY: Target dose of 300 mg once daily.

Dosage in Renal/Hepatic Impairment
No dose adjustment.

SIDE EFFECTS

Occasional (9%–3%): Upper respiratory tract infection, fatigue, diarrhea, cough. **Rare (2%–1%):** Heartburn, dizziness, headache, nausea, rash.

ADVERSE EFFECTS/ TOXIC REACTIONS

Overdose may manifest as hypotension, syncope, tachycardia. Bradycardia occurs less often.

NURSING CONSIDERATIONS

BASELINE ASSESSMENT

Obtain B/P, apical pulse immediately before each dose in addition to regular monitoring (be alert to fluctuations). Question possibility of pregnancy. Assess medication history (esp. diuretic therapy).

INTERVENTION/EVALUATION

Maintain hydration (offer fluids frequently). Assess for evidence of upper respiratory infection. Assist with ambulation if dizziness occurs. Monitor electrolytes, renal function, urinalysis, B/P, pulse. Assess for hypotension.

PATIENT/ FAMILY TEACHING

• May cause fetal or neonatal morbidity or mortality. • Avoid tasks that require alertness, motor skills until response to drug is established (possible dizziness effect); ensure that appropriate birth control measures are in place. • Report any sign of infection (sore throat, fever). • Avoid exercising during hot weather (risk of dehydration, hypotension).

irinotecan

eye-ri-noe-**tee**-kan
(Camptosar, Onivyde)

■ **BLACK BOX ALERT** ■
(Camptosar, Onivyde): Can induce both early and late forms of severe diarrhea. Early diarrhea (during

 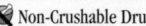

or shortly after administration) accompanied by salivation, rhinitis, lacrimation, diaphoresis, flushing. Late diarrhea (occurring more than 24 hrs after administration) can be prolonged and life-threatening. **(Camptosar):** May produce severe, profound myelosuppression. Administer under supervision of experienced cancer chemotherapy physician. **(Onivyde):** Severe, life-threatening, or fatal neutropenic fever/sepsis occurred. Withhold for ANC below 1,500/mm³ or neutropenic fever. Monitor blood cell counts.

◆CLASSIFICATION

PHARMACOTHERAPEUTIC: DNA topoisomerase inhibitor. **CLINICAL:** Antineoplastic.

USES

Camptosar: Treatment of metastatic carcinoma of colon or rectum. **Onivyde:** Treatment of metastatic adenocarcinoma of the pancreas (in combination with 5-fluorouracil and leucovorin) after disease progression following gemcitabine-based therapy. **OFF-LABEL:** Non–small-cell lung cancer; small-cell lung cancer; CNS tumor; cervical, gastric, pancreatic, ovarian, esophageal cancer; Ewing's sarcoma; brain tumor.

PRECAUTIONS

Contraindications: Hypersensitivity to irinotecan. **Cautions:** Pt previously receiving pelvic, abdominal irradiation (increased risk of myelosuppression), pts older than 65 yrs, hepatic dysfunction, hyperbilirubinemia, renal impairment, preexisting pulmonary disease.

ACTION

Interacts with topoisomerase I, an enzyme that relieves torsional strain in DNA by inducing reversible single-strand breaks. Prevents religation of these single-stranded breaks, resulting in damage to double-strand DNA, cell death. **Therapeutic Effect:** Produces cytotoxic effect on cancer cells.

PHARMACOKINETICS

Metabolized in liver. Protein binding: 95% (metabolite). Excreted in urine and eliminated by biliary route. **Half-life:** 6–12 hrs; metabolite, 10–20 hrs.

⧗ LIFESPAN CONSIDERATIONS

Pregnancy/Lactation: May cause fetal harm. Unknown if distributed in breast milk. Breastfeeding not recommended. **Children:** Safety and efficacy not established. **Elderly:** Risk of diarrhea significantly increased.

INTERACTIONS

DRUG: CYP3A4 inducers (e.g., phenytoin, PHENobarbital, carBAMazepine) may decrease concentration/effects. **CYP3A4 inhibitors (e.g., ketoconazole)** increase concentration. Avoid **live vaccines** during treatment. **HERBAL: St. John's wort** may decrease irinotecan effectiveness. **FOOD:** None known. **LAB VALUES:** May increase serum alkaline phosphatase, AST. May decrease Hgb, leukocytes, platelets.

AVAILABILITY (Rx)

Injection Solution (Conventional): 20 mg/mL (2 mL, 5 mL, 15 mL, 25 mL). **(Liposomal):** 43 mg/10 mL.

ADMINISTRATION/HANDLING

 IV

Camptosar
Reconstitution • Dilute in D₅W (preferred) or 0.9% NaCl to concentration of 0.12–2.8 mg/mL.
Rate of Administration • Administer all doses as IV infusion over 30–90 min. • Assess for extravasation (flush site with Sterile Water for Injection, apply ice if extravasation occurs).
Storage • Store vials at room temperature, protect from light. • Solution diluted with D₅W is stable for 24 hrs at room temperature or 48 hrs if refrigerated. • Solution diluted with 0.9% NaCl is stable for 24 hrs at room tem-

perature. • Do not refrigerate solution if diluted with 0.9% NaCl.

Onivyde

Reconstitution • Withdraw dose from vial and dilute with 500 mL D$_5$W or 0.9% NaCl. Mix gently.
Rate of Administration • Infuse over 90 min.
Storage • Refrigerate vials; do not freeze. • Protect from light. • Stable for 4 hrs at room temperature or 24 hrs refrigerated.

▦ IV INCOMPATIBILITY

Gemcitabine (Gemzar).

INDICATIONS/ROUTES/DOSAGE

Note: Genotyping of UGT1AI available. Pts who are homozygous for the UGT1AI*28 allele are at increased risk for neutropenia. Decreased dose is recommended.

Carcinoma of the Colon, Rectum (Camptosar)

IV (Single-Agent Therapy): ADULTS, ELDERLY: (WEEKLY REGIMEN): Initially, 125 mg/m^2 once wkly for 4 wks, followed by a rest period of 2 wks. Additional courses may be repeated q6wks. Dosage may be adjusted in 25–50 mg/m^2 increments/decrements to as high as 150 mg/m^2 or as low as 50 mg/m^2. **(THREE-WEEK REGIMEN):** 350 mg/m^2 q3wks. Dosage may be adjusted to as low as 200 mg/m^2 in decrements of 25–50 mg/m^2.
(In Combination with Leucovorin and 5-Fluorouracil): **REGIMEN ONE:** 125 mg/m^2 on days 1, 8, 15, 22. Dose may be adjusted to 100 mg/m^2, then 75 mg/m^2, then decrements of approximately 20%. **REGIMEN TWO:** 180 mg/m^2 on days 1, 15, 29. Dose may be adjusted to 150 mg/m^2, then 120 mg/m^2, then decrements of approximately 20%.

Pancreatic Cancer (Onivyde)

IV Infusion: ADULTS, ELDERLY: 70 mg/m^2 once q2wks (in combination with leucovorin and 5-fluorouracil).

Dosage in Renal Impairment

No dose adjustment.

Dosage in Hepatic Impairment

Bilirubin	Dose
More than upper limit of normal to 2 mg/dL or less:	Reduce dose one level
More than 2 mg/dL:	Not recommended

SIDE EFFECTS

Expected (64%–32%): Nausea, alopecia, vomiting, diarrhea. **Frequent (29%–22%):** Constipation, fatigue, fever, asthenia, skeletal pain, abdominal pain, dyspnea. **Occasional (19%–16%):** Anorexia, headache, stomatitis, rash.

ADVERSE EFFECTS/TOXIC REACTIONS

Hematologic toxicity characterized by anemia, leukopenia, thrombocytopenia, and neutropenia, sepsis occur frequently. Camptosar may cause severe/fatal interstitial lung disease.

NURSING CONSIDERATIONS

BASELINE ASSESSMENT

Offer emotional support. Assess hydration status, electrolytes, CBC before each dose. Premedicate with antiemetics on day of treatment, starting at least 30 min before administration. Inform pt of possibility of alopecia.

INTERVENTION/EVALUATION

Monitor daily pattern of bowel activity, stool consistency. Monitor hydration status, I&O, electrolytes, CBC, renal function, LFT. Monitor infusion site for signs of inflammation. Assess skin for rash.

PATIENT/ FAMILY TEACHING

• Report diarrhea, vomiting, fever, lightheadedness, dizziness. • Do not have immunizations without physician's approval (drug lowers resistance). • Avoid contact with those who have recently received live virus vaccine. • Avoid crowds, those with infections.

---

iron dextran

iron **dex**-tran
(Dexiron ✤, Infed, Infufer ✤, DexFerrum)

■ **BLACK BOX ALERT** ■ Potentially fatal anaphylactic-type reaction has been associated with parenteral administration. Test dose should be given prior to first therapeutic dose. **Do not confuse DexFerrum with Desferal, or iron dextran with iron sucrose.**

◆CLASSIFICATION

PHARMACOTHERAPEUTIC: Trace element. **CLINICAL:** Hematinic iron preparation.

USES

Treatment of anemia, iron deficiency. Use only when PO administration is not feasible or when rapid replenishment of iron is warranted.

PRECAUTIONS

Contraindications: Hypersensitivity to iron formulation. All anemias not associated with iron deficiency anemia (pernicious, aplastic, normocytic, refractory). **Caution:** Serious hepatic impairment. History of allergies, bronchial asthma, rheumatoid arthritis, preexisting cardiac disease. Avoid use during acute kidney infection.

ACTION

Essential component in formation of Hgb. Necessary for effective erythropoiesis, transport and utilization of oxygen. Serves as cofactor of several essential enzymes. **Therapeutic Effect:** Replenishes Hgb, depleted iron stores.

PHARMACOKINETICS

Readily absorbed after IM administration. Most absorption occurs within 72 hrs; remainder within 3–4 wks. Bound to protein to form hemosiderin, ferritin, or transferrin. No physiologic system of elimination. Small amounts lost daily in shedding of skin, hair, nails and in feces, urine, perspiration. **Half-life:** 5–20 hrs.

⧖ LIFESPAN CONSIDERATIONS

Pregnancy/Lactation: May cross placenta in some form (unknown). Trace distributed in breast milk. **Children/Elderly:** No age-related precautions noted.

INTERACTIONS

DRUG: None significant. **HERBAL:** None significant. **FOOD:** None known. **LAB VALUES:** None significant.

AVAILABILITY (Rx)

Injection Solution (Infed): 50 mg/mL.

ADMINISTRATION/HANDLING

◀ **ALERT** ▶ Test dose is generally given before full dosage; monitor pt for several min after injection due to potential for anaphylactic reaction.

 IV

Reconstitution • May give undiluted or dilute in 250–1,000 mL 0.9% NaCl for infusion. • Avoid dilution in dextrose (increased pain/phlebitis).
Rate of Administration • Do not exceed IV bolus administration rate of 50 mg/min (1 mL/min). Too-rapid IV rate may produce flushing, chest pain, hypotension, tachycardia, shock. • Infuse diluted solution over 1–6 hrs. • Pt must remain recumbent 30–45 min after IV administration (minimizes postural hypotension).
Storage • Store at room temperature.

▦ IV INCOMPATIBILITIES

Do not mix with other medications.

INDICATIONS/ROUTES/DOSAGE

0.5-mL test dose (0.25 mL in infants). Give prior to initiating iron dextran therapy.

◀ **ALERT** ▶ Discontinue oral iron preparations before administering iron dextran. Dosage expressed in terms of milligrams of elemental iron. Dosage individualized based on degree of anemia, pt weight, presence of any bleeding. Use periodic hematologic determinations as guide to therapy.

◄ALERT► Not normally given in first 4 mos of life.

Iron Deficiency Anemia
IV: ADULTS, ELDERLY, CHILDREN WEIGHING MORE THAN 15 KG: Dose in mL (50 mg elemental iron/mL) = 0.0442 (desired Hgb less observed Hgb) × lean body weight (in kg) + (0.26 × lean body weight). Give 2 mL or less once daily until total dose reached. **CHILDREN WEIGHING 5–15 KG:** Dose in mL (50 mg elemental iron/mL) = 0.0442 (desired Hgb less observed Hgb) × body weight (in kg) + (0.26 × body weight). Give 2 mL or less once daily until total dose reached.

Maximum Daily Dosages
ADULTS WEIGHING MORE THAN 50 KG: 100 mg. **CHILDREN WEIGHING MORE THAN 10 KG:** 100 mg. **CHILDREN WEIGHING 5–10 KG:** 50 mg. **CHILDREN WEIGHING LESS THAN 5 KG:** 25 mg.

Dosage in Renal/Hepatic Impairment
No dose adjustment.

SIDE EFFECTS
Frequent: Allergic reaction (rash, pruritus), backache, myalgia, chills, dizziness, headache, fever, nausea, vomiting, flushed skin, pain/redness at injection site, brown discoloration of skin, metallic taste.

ADVERSE EFFECTS/TOXIC REACTIONS
Anaphylaxis occurs rarely in first few min following injection. Leukocytosis, lymphadenopathy occur rarely.

NURSING CONSIDERATIONS
BASELINE ASSESSMENT
Do not give concurrently with oral iron form (excessive iron may produce excessive iron storage [hemosiderosis]). Be alert to pts with rheumatoid arthritis (RA),

iron deficiency anemia (acute exacerbation of joint pain, swelling may occur).

INTERVENTION/EVALUATION
Check IV site for phlebitis. Monitor serum ferritin. Monitor daily pattern of bowel activity, stool consistency.

PATIENT/FAMILY TEACHING
• Pain, brown staining may occur at injection site. • Oral iron should not be taken when receiving iron injections. • Stools often become black with iron therapy, but this is harmless unless accompanied by red streaking, sticky consistency of stool, abdominal pain/cramping, which should be reported to physician. • Oral hygiene, hard candy, gum may reduce metallic taste. • Immediately report fever, back pain, headache.

---

iron sucrose

iron **soo**-krose
(Venofer)
Do not confuse iron sucrose with iron dextran.

◆CLASSIFICATION
PHARMACOTHERAPEUTIC: Trace element. **CLINICAL:** Hematinic iron preparation.

USES
Treatment of iron deficiency anemia in chronic kidney disease. **OFF-LABEL:** Chemotherapy-associated anemia.

PRECAUTIONS
Contraindications: Hypersensitivity to iron sucrose. **Cautions:** History of allergies, bronchial asthma; hepatic impairment, rheumatoid arthritis, preexisting cardiac disease. Pts at risk for significant hypotension.

ACTION
Essential component in formation of Hgb. Necessary for effective erythropoi-

esis, transport and utilization of oxygen. Serves as cofactor of several essential enzymes. **Therapeutic Effect:** Replenishes body iron stores in pts on chronic hemodialysis who have iron deficiency anemia and are receiving erythropoietin.

PHARMACOKINETICS

Distributed mainly in blood and to some extent in extravascular fluid. Iron sucrose is dissociated into iron and sucrose by reticuloendothelial system. Sucrose component is eliminated mainly by urinary excretion. **Half-life:** 6 hrs.

⌛ LIFESPAN CONSIDERATIONS

Pregnancy/Lactation: Unknown if drug crosses placenta or is distributed in breast milk. **Children:** Safety and efficacy not established. **Elderly:** Age-related renal impairment may require dosage adjustment.

INTERACTIONS

DRUG: None significant. **HERBAL:** None significant. **FOOD:** None known. **LAB VALUES:** Increases Hgb, Hct; serum ferritin, transferrin.

AVAILABILITY (Rx)

Injection Solution: 20 mg of elemental iron/mL in 2.5-mL, 5-mL, 10-mL vials.

ADMINISTRATION/HANDLING

◀**ALERT**▶ Administer directly into dialysis line during hemodialysis.

 IV

Reconstitution • May give undiluted as slow IV injection or IV infusion. For IV infusion, dilute 100-mg (5-mL) vial in maximum of 100 mL 0.9% NaCl immediately before infusion. (Do not dilute to concentration less than 1 mg/mL in children.) • Dilute large doses in maximum of 250 mL 0.9% NaCl.
Rate of Administration • For IV injection, administer 100–200 mg (5–10 mL) over 2–5 min. • For IV infusion, administer 100 mg over at least 15 min;

300 mg over 1.5 hrs; 400 mg over 2.5 hrs; 500 mg over 3.5–4 hrs.
Storage • Store at room temperature. • Following dilution, stable for 7 days at room temperature or if refrigerated.

▨ IV INCOMPATIBILITIES

Do not mix with other medications or add to parenteral nutrition solution for IV infusion.

INDICATIONS/ROUTES/DOSAGE

Iron Deficiency Anemia
Dosage is expressed in terms of milligrams of elemental iron.
IV: ADULTS, ELDERLY (HEMODIALYSIS-DEPENDENT PTS): 5 mL iron sucrose (100 mg elemental iron) delivered during dialysis; administer 1–3 times/wk to total dose of 1,000 mg in 10 doses. Give no more than 3 times/wk. **CHILDREN 2 YRS AND OLDER:** 0.5 mg/kg/dose (**Maximum:** 100 mg) q2wks for 6 doses. **(PERITONEAL DIALYSIS–DEPENDENT PTS):** Two infusions of 300 mg over 90 min 14 days apart followed by a single 400-mg dose over 2½ hrs 14 days later. **CHILDREN 2 YRS AND OLDER:** 0.5 mg/kg/dose (**Maximum:** 100 mg) q4wks for 3 doses. **(NON–DIALYSIS-DEPENDENT PTS):** 200 mg over 2–5 min on 5 different occasions within 14 days. **CHILDREN 2 YRS AND OLDER:** 0.5 mg/kg/dose (**Maximum:** 100 mg) q4wks for 3 doses.

Dosage in Renal/Hepatic Impairment
No dose adjustment.

SIDE EFFECTS

Frequent (36%–23%): Hypotension, leg cramps, diarrhea.

ADVERSE EFFECTS/TOXIC REACTIONS

Too-rapid IV administration may produce severe hypotension, headache, vomiting, nausea, dizziness, paresthesia, abdominal/muscle pain, edema, cardiovascular collapse. Hypersensitivity reaction occurs rarely.

NURSING CONSIDERATIONS

INTERVENTION/EVALUATION

Initially, monitor Hgb, Hct, serum ferritin, transferrin monthly, then q2–3mos thereafter. Reliable serum iron values can be obtained 48 hrs following administration.

---

isavuconazonium

eye-sa-vue-**kon**-a-**zoe**-nee-um
(Cresemba)

◆CLASSIFICATION

PHARMACOTHERAPEUTIC: Azole antifungal derivative. **CLINICAL:** Antifungal.

USES

Treatment of invasive aspergillosis and invasive mucormycosis in pts 18 yrs and older.

PRECAUTIONS

Contraindications: Hypersensitivity to isavuconazonium or isavuconazole, concomitant use of strong CYP3A inhibitors (e.g., ketoconazole, ritonavir), strong CYP3A inducers (e.g., carBAMazepine, rifAMPin, St. John's wort), history of short QT syndrome. **Cautions:** Renal/hepatic impairment, hypersensitivity to other azoles. Pts at risk for acute pancreatitis; concomitant use of nephrotoxic medications; pts at risk for hypokalemia, hypomagnesemia. Concomitant use of medications that prolong QT interval.

ACTION

Isavuconazonium is the prodrug of isavuconazole. Interferes with fungal cytochrome activity, decreasing ergosterol synthesis, inhibiting fungal cell membrane formation. **Therapeutic Effect:** Damages fungal cell wall membrane.

PHARMACOKINETICS

Widely distributed. Metabolized in liver. Protein binding: greater than 99%. Peak plasma concentration: 2–3 hrs. Excreted in feces (46%), urine (46%). **Half-life:** 130 hrs.

⧗ LIFESPAN CONSIDERATIONS

Pregnancy/Lactation: May cause fetal harm. Avoid pregnancy. Avoid breastfeeding while taking Cresemba. **Children:** Safety and efficacy not established in pts younger than 18 yrs. **Elderly:** No age-related precautions noted.

INTERACTIONS

DRUG: Strong CYP3A4 inhibitors (e.g., ketoconazole, ritonavir) may increase concentration/effect. **Strong CYP3A4 inducers (e.g., carBAMazepine, rifAMPin)** may decrease concentration/effect. **Medications that prolong QT interval (e.g., amiodarone, azithromycin, ceritinib, haloperidol, moxifloxacin)** may increase the risk of QT interval prolongation, cardiac arrhythmias. May increase concentration/effects of **atorvastatin, buPROPion, cycloSPORINE, digoxin, midazolam, mycophenolate mofetil/sirolimus, tacrolimus. HERBAL: St. John's wort** may decrease concentration/effect. **FOOD:** None known. **LAB VALUES:** May increase serum alkaline phosphatase, ALT, AST, bilirubin. May decrease serum potassium, magnesium.

AVAILABILITY (Rx)

Injection Powder: 372 mg/vial (equivalent to 200 mg isavuconazole). **Capsules:** 186 mg (equivalent to 100 mg isavuconazole).

ADMINISTRATION/HANDLING

 IV

**Reconstitution • Reconstitute vial with 5 mL Sterile Water for Injection. • Gently shake until completely dissolved. • Visually inspect for particulate matter or discoloration. Solution may contain visible translucent to white particles. • Inject reconstituted solution into 250 mL 0.9% NaCl or 5% Dextrose injection. • Gently invert bag to mix. Do not shake or agitate. Do not use pneumatic transport system. • Diluted solution may also contain visible translucent to white particles (which will be removed by in-line filter).

Administration • Do not give as IV push or bolus. Flush IV line with 0.9% NaCl or 5% Dextrose injection prior to and after infusion.

Rate of Administration • Infuse over 60 min (minimum) using 0.2- to 1.2-micron in-line filter.

Storage • Diluted solution may be stored at room temperature up to 6 hrs or refrigerated up to 24 hrs. • Do not freeze.

PO

• Give without regard to meals. • Do not cut, crush, divide, or open capsules.

INDICATIONS/ROUTES/DOSAGE

Note: 372 mg is equivalent to 200 mg isavuconazole.

Invasive Aspergillosis, Invasive Mucormycosis

IV: ADULTS, ELDERLY: Loading dose: 372 mg q8h for 6 doses (48 hrs). **Maintenance:** 372 mg once daily. Start maintenance dose 12–24 hrs after last loading dose. **PO: ADULTS, ELDERLY: Loading dose:** 372 mg (2 capsules) q8h for 6 doses (48 hrs). **Maintenance:** 372 mg (2 capsules) once daily. Start maintenance dose 12–24 hrs after last loading dose.

Dosage in Renal Impairment
No dose adjustment.

Dosage in Hepatic Impairment
Mild to moderate impairment: No dose adjustment. **Severe impairment:** Not specified; use caution.

SIDE EFFECTS

Frequent (28%–17%): Nausea, vomiting, diarrhea, abdominal pain, headache, dyspnea. **Occasional (15%–6%):** Peripheral edema, constipation, fatigue, insomnia, back pain, delirium, agitation, confusion, disorientation, chest pain, rash, pruritus, hypotension, anxiety, dyspepsia, injection site reaction, decreased appetite.

ADVERSE EFFECTS/TOXIC REACTIONS

Severe hepatic injury including cholestasis, hepatitis, hepatic failure reported in pts with underlying medical conditions (e.g., hematologic malignancies). Infusion-related reactions including chills, dizziness, dyspnea, hypoesthesia, hypotension, paresthesia may occur. Acute respiratory failure, renal failure, Stevens-Johnson syndrome, serious hypersensitivity reaction (including anaphylaxis) were reported.

NURSING CONSIDERATIONS

BASELINE ASSESSMENT

Obtain baseline LFT. Confirm negative pregnancy test before initiating treatment. Specimens for fungal culture, histopathology should be obtained prior to initiating therapy. Receive full medication history and screen for interactions/contraindications. Question history of hypersensitivity reaction, hepatic impairment.

INTERVENTION/EVALUATION

Monitor BMP, LFT periodically. Monitor for infusion-related reactions, hypersensitivity reactions, anaphylaxis. Monitor I&O. Report worsening of hepatic/renal function.

PATIENT/FAMILY TEACHING

• Swallow capsule whole; do not chew, crush, cut, or open capsules. • Treatment may cause fetal harm. Females of reproductive potential should use effective contraception. Immediately report suspected pregnancy. • Do not take herbal products such as St. John's wort. • Report liver problems such as upper abdominal pain, bleeding, dark or amber-colored urine, nausea, vomiting, or yellowing of the skin or eyes. • Report decreased urinary output, extremity swelling, dark-colored urine; skin changes such as rash, skin bubbling, or sloughing.

isoniazid

eye-soe-**nye**-a-zid
(Isotamine ✦)

■ **BLACK BOX ALERT** ■ Severe, potentially fatal hepatitis may occur.

FIXED-COMBINATION(S)

Rifamate: isoniazid/rifAMPin (antitubercular): 150 mg/300 mg.
Rifater: isoniazid/pyrazinamide/rifAMPin (antitubercular): 50 mg/300 mg/120 mg.

◆CLASSIFICATION

PHARMACOTHERAPEUTIC: Isonicotinic acid derivative. **CLINICAL:** Antitubercular.

USES

Treatment of susceptible active tuberculosis due to *Mycobacterium tuberculosis*. Treatment of latent tuberculosis caused by *Mycobacterium tuberculosis*.

PRECAUTIONS

Contraindications: Hypersensitivity to isoniazid (including drug-induced hepatitis), acute hepatic disease, hepatic injury or severe adverse reactions with previous isoniazid therapy. **Cautions:** Chronic hepatic disease, alcoholism, severe renal impairment. Pregnancy, pts at risk for peripheral neuropathy, HIV infection, history of hypersensitivity reactions to latent TB infection medications.

ACTION

Inhibits mycolic acid synthesis. Causes disruption of bacterial cell wall, loss of acid-fast properties in susceptible mycobacteria. **Therapeutic Effect:** Bactericidal against actively growing intracellular, extracellular susceptible mycobacteria.

PHARMACOKINETICS

Note: Isoniazid is metabolized by acetylation. The rate of acetylation is genetically determined (e.g., 50% of black and caucasian pts are slow inactivators; Eskimo and Asian pts are rapid inactivators. Slower inactivation may lead to higher blood levels and increased adverse effects.
Readily absorbed from GI tract. Protein binding: 10%–15%. Widely distributed (including to CSF). Metabolized in liver. Primarily excreted in urine. Removed by hemodialysis. **Half-life:** (Fast acetylators): 30–100 min; (slow acetylators): 2–5 hrs.

⌛ LIFESPAN CONSIDERATIONS

Pregnancy/Lactation: Prophylaxis usually postponed until after delivery. Crosses placenta. Distributed in breast milk. **Children:** No age-related precautions noted. **Elderly:** More susceptible to developing hepatitis.

INTERACTIONS

DRUG: Alcohol may increase isoniazid metabolism, risk of hepatotoxicity. May increase toxicity of **carBAMazepine, phenytoin. Hepatotoxic medications (e.g., acetaminophen, simvastatin)** may increase risk of hepatotoxicity. May decrease **ketoconazole** concentration. **HERBAL:** None significant. **FOOD: Foods containing tyramine** may cause hypertensive crisis. **LAB VALUES:** May increase serum bilirubin, ALT, AST.

AVAILABILITY (Rx)

Oral Solution: 50 mg/5 mL. **Solution, Injection:** 100 mg/mL. **Tablets:** 100 mg, 300 mg.

ADMINISTRATION/HANDLING

PO

• Give 1 hr before or 2 hrs following meals (may give with food to decrease GI upset, but will delay absorption).

✦ Canadian trade name   🗲 Non-Crushable Drug   [HIGH ALERT] High Alert drug

• Administer at least 1 hr before antacids, esp. those containing aluminum.

INDICATIONS/ROUTES/DOSAGE

Active Tuberculosis (in Combination with One or More Antituberculars)
IM/PO: ADULTS, ELDERLY: 5 mg/kg once daily. **Usual dose:** 300 mg. **CHILDREN WEIGHING LESS THAN 40 KG:** 10–15 mg/kg once daily. **Maximum:** 300 mg.
Note: Give isoniazid with rifAMPin, pyrazinamide, and with or without ethambutol for 8 wks, then give with rifAMPin for 18 wks.

Latent Tuberculosis
Note: Give for 9 mos.
IM/PO: ADULTS, ELDERLY: 5 mg/kg once daily (**Maximum:** 300 mg) or 15 mg/kg twice wkly (**Maximum:** 900 mg). **CHILDREN:** 10–20 mg/kg/day as a single daily dose. **Maximum:** 300 mg/day or 20–40 mg/kg 2 times/wk. **Maximum:** 900 mg/dose.

Dosage in Renal Impairment
No dose adjustment.

Dosage in Hepatic Impairment
Use caution. Contraindicated with acute hepatic disease.

SIDE EFFECTS

Frequent: Nausea, vomiting, diarrhea, abdominal pain. **Rare:** Pain at injection site, hypersensitivity reaction.

ADVERSE EFFECTS/TOXIC REACTIONS

Neurotoxicity (ataxia, paresthesia), optic neuritis, hepatotoxicity occur rarely.

NURSING CONSIDERATIONS

BASELINE ASSESSMENT

Question for history of hypersensitivity reactions, hepatic injury or disease, sensitivity to nicotinic acid or chemically related medications. Ensure collection of specimens for culture, sensitivity. Evaluate initial LFT.

INTERVENTION/EVALUATION

Monitor LFT, assess for hepatitis: anorexia, nausea, vomiting, weakness, fatigue, dark urine, jaundice (withhold concurrent INH therapy and inform physician promptly). Assess for paresthesia of extremities (pts esp. at risk for neuropathy may be given pyridoxine prophylactically: malnourished, elderly, diabetics, pts with chronic hepatic disease [including alcoholics]). Be alert for fever, skin eruptions (hypersensitivity reaction).

PATIENT/FAMILY TEACHING

• Do not skip doses; continue to take isoniazid for full length of therapy (6–24 mos). • Take preferably 1 hr before or 2 hrs following meals (with food if GI upset). • Avoid alcohol during treatment. • Do not take any other medications, including antacids, without consulting physician. • Must take isoniazid at least 1 hr before antacid. • Avoid tuna, sauerkraut, aged cheeses, smoked fish (consult list of tyramine-containing foods), which may cause hypertensive reaction (red/itching skin, palpitations, light-headedness, hot or clammy feeling, headache). • Report any new symptom, immediately for vision difficulties, nausea/vomiting, dark urine, yellowing of skin/eyes (jaundice), fatigue, paresthesia of extremities.

isosorbide dinitrate

eye-soe-**sor**-bide
(ISDN ✽, IsoDitrate ER, Dilatrate-SR, Isordil)

isosorbide mononitrate

(Apo-ISMN ✽)
Do not confuse Imdur with Imuran, Inderal, or K-Dur, Isordil with Inderal, Isuprel, or Plendil.

FIXED-COMBINATION(S)

BiDil: isosorbide dinitrate/hydrALA-ZINE (a vasodilator): 20 mg/37.5 mg.

◆CLASSIFICATION

PHARMACOTHERAPEUTIC: Nitrate. **CLINICAL:** Antianginal.

USES

Dinitrate: Prevention and treatment of angina pectoris due to coronary artery disease. **Mononitrate:** Treatment (immediate release only) and prevention of angina pectoris due to coronary artery disease.

PRECAUTIONS

Contraindications: Hypersensitivity to nitrates, concurrent use of sildenafil, tadalafil, vardenafil. **Cautions:** Inferior wall MI, head trauma, increased intracranial pressure (ICP), orthostatic hypotension, blood volume depletion from diuretic therapy, systolic B/P less than 90 mm Hg, hypertrophic cardiomyopathy, alcohol consumption.

ACTION

Stimulates intracellular cyclic guanosine monophosphate. **Therapeutic Effect:** Relaxes vascular smooth muscle of arterial, venous vasculature. Decreases preload, afterload, cardiac oxygen demand.

PHARMACOKINETICS

Route	Onset	Peak	Duration
Dinitrate			
Sublingual	3 min	N/A	1–2 hrs
PO	45–60 min	N/A	up to 8 hrs
Mononitrate			
PO (extended-release)	30–60 min	N/A	12–24 hrs

Dinitrate poorly absorbed and metabolized in liver to its active metabolite isosorbide mononitrate. Mononitrate well absorbed after PO administration. Primarily excreted in urine. **Half-life:** Dinitrate, 1–4 hrs; mononitrate, 4 hrs.

⧗ LIFESPAN CONSIDERATIONS

Pregnancy/Lactation: Unknown if drug crosses placenta or is distributed in breast milk. **Children:** Safety and efficacy not established. **Elderly:** May be more sensitive to hypotensive effects. Age-related renal impairment may require dosage adjustment.

INTERACTIONS

DRUG: Alcohol, antihypertensives (e.g., amLODIPine, lisinopril, valsartan) may increase risk of orthostatic hypotension. **Sildenafil, tadalafil, vardenafil** may potentiate hypotensive effects (concurrent use of these agents is contraindicated). **HERBAL:** None significant. **FOOD:** None known. **LAB VALUES:** May increase urine catecholamine, urine vanillylmandelic acid levels.

AVAILABILITY (Rx)

Dinitrate

Tablets: 5 mg, 10 mg, 20 mg, 30 mg, 40 mg.

🐢 **Capsules, Extended-Release:** 40 mg.

🐢 **Tablets, Extended-Release:** 40 mg.

Mononitrate

Tablets: 10 mg, 20 mg.

🐢 **Tablets, Extended-Release:** 30 mg, 60 mg, 120 mg.

ADMINISTRATION/HANDLING

PO

• Best if taken on an empty stomach. • Do not administer around the clock. • Oral tablets may be crushed. • Do not crush/break sustained-, extended-release form.

INDICATIONS/ROUTES/DOSAGE

Angina

PO *(Isosorbide Dinitrate) (Immediate-Release):* **ADULTS, ELDERLY:** Initially, 5–20 mg 2–3 times/day. **Maintenance:** 10–40 mg (or between 5–80 mg) 2–3 times/day. *(Sustained-Release):* **ADULTS, ELDERLY:** 40 mg 1–2 times/day. A nitrate-free interval of greater than 18 hrs is recommended. **Maximum:** 160 mg/day.

PO *(Isosorbide Mononitrate) (Immediate-Release):* **ADULTS, ELDERLY:** 20 mg twice daily given 7 hrs apart to decrease tolerance development. In pts with small stature, may start at 5 mg twice daily and titrate to at least 10 mg twice daily in first 2–3 days of therapy.

(Sustained-Release): Initially, 30–60 mg/day in morning as a single dose. May increase dose at 3-day intervals to 120 mg once daily. **Maximum daily single dose:** 240 mg.

Dosage in Renal/Hepatic Impairment
No dose adjustment.

SIDE EFFECTS

Frequent: Headache (may be severe) occurs mostly in early therapy, diminishes rapidly in intensity, usually disappears during continued treatment. **Occasional:** Transient flushing of face/neck, dizziness, weakness, orthostatic hypotension, nausea, vomiting, restlessness. GI upset, blurred vision, dry mouth. **Sublingual: Frequent:** Burning, tingling at oral point of dissolution.

ADVERSE EFFECTS/TOXIC REACTIONS

Discontinue if blurred vision occurs. Severe orthostatic hypotension manifested by syncope, pulselessness, cold/clammy skin, diaphoresis has been reported. Tolerance may occur with repeated, prolonged therapy, but may not occur with extended-release form. Minor tolerance with intermittent use of sublingual tablets. High dosage tends to produce severe headache.

NURSING CONSIDERATIONS

BASELINE ASSESSMENT

Record onset, type (sharp, dull, squeezing), radiation, location, intensity, duration of anginal pain; precipitating factors (exertion, emotional stress). If headache occurs during management therapy, administer medication with meals.

INTERVENTION/EVALUATION

Assist with ambulation if light-headedness, dizziness occurs. Assess for facial/neck flushing. Monitor number of anginal episodes, orthostatic B/P.

PATIENT/FAMILY TEACHING

• Do not chew, crush, dissolve, or divide sublingual, extended-release, sustained-release forms. • Take sublingual tablets while sitting down. • Go from lying to standing slowly (prevents dizziness effect). • Take oral form on empty stomach (however, if headache occurs during management therapy, take medication with meals). • Dissolve sublingual tablet under tongue; do not swallow. • Avoid alcohol (intensifies hypotensive effect). • If alcohol is ingested soon after taking nitrates, possible acute hypotensive episode (marked drop in B/P, vertigo, pallor) may occur. • Report signs/symptoms of hypotension, angina.

itraconazole

it-ra-**kon**-a-zole
(Onmel, Sporanox)

■ **BLACK BOX ALERT** ■ Serious cardiovascular events, including HF, ventricular tachycardia, torsades de pointes, death, have occurred due to concurrent use with colchicine (pts with renal/hepatic impairment), dofetilide, dronedarone, eplerenone, ergot alkaloids, felodipine, fesoterodine, irinotecan, ivabradine, levomethadyl, lovastatin, lurasidone, methadone, midazolam (oral), pimozide, quiNIDine, ranolazine, simvastatin, solifenacin, ticagrelor, or triazolam. Negative inotropic effects observed following IV administration. Contraindicated for treatment of onychomycosis in pts with HF, ventricular dysfunction.
Do not confuse itraconazole with fluconazole, or Sporanox with Suprax or Topamax.

◆CLASSIFICATION

PHARMACOTHERAPEUTIC: Imidazole/triazole type antifungal. **CLINICAL:** Antifungal.

USES

Oral capsules: Treatment of aspergillosis, blastomycosis, esophageal and oropharyngeal candidiasis, empiric treatment in febrile neutropenia, histoplasmosis, onychomycosis. **Oral solution:** Treatment of oral and esophageal candidiasis. **Oral tablet:** Treatment of onychomycosis of toenail.

PRECAUTIONS

Contraindications: Hypersensitivity to itraconazole, other azoles. Treatment of onychomycosis in pts with evidence of ventricular dysfunction (e.g., HF or history of HF); concurrent use of dofetilide, dronedarone, eplerenone, ergot derivatives, felodipine, irinotecan, lovastatin, lurasidone, methadone, midazolam (oral), pimozide, ranolazine, simvastatin, ticagrelor, triazolam, quiNIDine; concurrent use with colchicine, fesoterodine, solifenacin in pts with renal/hepatic impairment; treatment of onychomycosis in women who are pregnant or are intending to become pregnant. **Cautions:** Preexisting hepatic impairment (not recommended in pts with active hepatic disease, elevated LFTs), renal impairment, pts with risk factors for HF (e.g., COPD, myocardial ischemia).

ACTION

Inhibits synthesis of ergosterol (vital component of fungal cell formation). **Therapeutic Effect:** Damages fungal cell membrane, altering its function. Fungistatic.

PHARMACOKINETICS

Moderately absorbed from GI tract. Absorption is increased when taken with food. Protein binding: 99%. Widely distributed, primarily in fatty tissue, liver, kidneys. Metabolized in liver. Primarily excreted in urine. Not removed by hemodialysis. **Half-life:** 16–26 hrs.

⌛ LIFESPAN CONSIDERATIONS

Pregnancy/Lactation: Distributed in breast milk. **Children:** Safety and efficacy not established. **Elderly:** Age-related renal impairment may require dosage adjustment.

INTERACTIONS

DRUG: May increase concentration/toxicity of **calcium channel–blocking agents** (e.g., **felodipine, NIFEdipine**), **carBAMazepine, cycloSPORINE, digoxin, ergot alkaloids, HMG-CoA reductase inhibitors** (e.g., **lovastatin, simvastatin**), **midazolam, oral antidiabetic agents** (e.g., **glyBURIDE, glipiZIDE**), **protease inhibitors** (e.g., **indinavir, ritonavir, saquinavir**), **sirolimus, tacrolimus, triazolam, warfarin. CYP3A4 inducers** (e.g., **carBAMazepine, isoniazid, PHENobarbital, phenytoin, rifAMPin**) may decrease concentration/effects. May inhibit metabolism of **busulfan, DOCEtaxel, vinca alkaloids. Erythromycin** may increase risk of cardiac toxicity. **Antacids, H₂ antagonists, proton pump inhibitors** may decrease absorption. **HERBAL: St. John's wort** may decrease concentration. **FOOD: Grapefruit products** may alter absorption. **LAB VALUES:** May increase serum alkaline phosphatase, bilirubin, ALT, AST, LDH. May decrease serum potassium.

AVAILABILITY (Rx)

Capsules: 100 mg. **Oral Solution:** 10 mg/mL. **Tablet:** 200 mg.

ADMINISTRATION/HANDLING

PO
• Give capsules and tablets with food (increases absorption). • Give solution on empty stomach. Swish vigorously in mouth, then swallow.

INDICATIONS/ROUTES/DOSAGE

Note: Capsules/tablets are not bioequivalent with oral solution.

Blastomycosis, Histoplasmosis

PO: ADULTS, ELDERLY: Initially, 200 mg once daily. May increase in increments of 100 mg/day up to 400 mg/day. **Life-threatening infections:** 200 mg 3 times/day for first 3 days of therapy. Continue for at least 3 mos.

Aspergillosis

PO: ADULTS, ELDERLY: 200–400 mg daily for 3 mos. **Life-threatening infections:** 200 mg 3 times/day for first 3 days of therapy. Continue 200–400 mg/day for at least 3 mos.

Esophageal Candidiasis

PO: ADULTS,ELDERLY: Swish 100–200mg (10–20 mL) in mouth for several seconds, then swallow once daily for a minimum of 3 wks. Continue for 2 wks after resolution of symptoms. **Maximum:** 200 mg/day.

Oropharyngeal Candidiasis

PO: ADULTS, ELDERLY: 200 mg (10 mL) oral solution, swish and swallow once daily for 7–14 days.

Onychomycosis (Fingernail)

PO: ADULTS, ELDERLY: 200 mg twice daily for 7 days, off for 21 days, repeat 200 mg twice daily for 7 days.

Onychomycosis (Toenail)

PO: ADULTS, ELDERLY: 200 mg once daily for 12 wks.

Dosage in Renal/Hepatic Impairment

Use caution.

SIDE EFFECTS

Frequent (11%–9%): Nausea, rash. **Occasional (5%–3%):** Vomiting, headache, diarrhea, hypertension, peripheral edema, fatigue, fever. **Rare (2% or less):** Abdominal pain, dizziness, anorexia, pruritus.

ADVERSE EFFECTS/TOXIC REACTIONS

Hepatitis (anorexia, abdominal pain, unusual fatigue/weakness, jaundiced skin/sclera, dark urine) occurs rarely.

NURSING CONSIDERATIONS

BASELINE ASSESSMENT

Determine baseline temperature, LFT. Assess allergies. Receive full medication history (numerous contraindications/cautions).

INTERVENTION/EVALUATION

Assess for signs, symptoms of hepatic dysfunction. Monitor LFT in pts with pre-existing hepatic impairment.

PATIENT/ FAMILY TEACHING

• Take capsules with food, liquids if GI distress occurs. • Therapy will continue for at least 3 mos, until lab tests, clinical presentation indicate infection is controlled. • Immediately report unusual fatigue, yellow skin, dark urine, pale stool, anorexia, nausea, vomiting. • Avoid grapefruit products.

ivabradine

eye-**vab**-ra-deen
(Corlanor)

◆CLASSIFICATION

PHARMACOTHERAPEUTIC: Hyperpolarization-activated cyclic nucleotide-gated (HCN) channel blocker. **CLINICAL:** Reduces risk of worsening HF.

USES

To reduce the risk of hospitalization for worsening HF in pts with stable, symptomatic chronic HF with left ventricular ejection fraction less than or equal to 35%, who are in sinus rhythm with a resting heart rate greater than or equal to 70 bpm, and either are on maximally tolerated dose of beta blockers or have a contraindication to beta blocker use.

PRECAUTIONS

Contraindications: Hypersensitivity to ivabradine. Acute decompensated HF, B/P less than 90/50 mm Hg, sick sinus syndrome; sinoatrial block or third-degree AV block (unless a functional pacemaker is present), resting heart rate less than 60 bpm prior to initiation, severe hepatic impairment, pacemaker dependence (heart rate maintained exclusively by a pacemaker), concomitant use of CYP3A4 inhibitors. **Cautions:** History of atrial fibrillation, hypertension. Avoid concomitant use of diltiaZEM or verapamil. Avoid use in pts with second-degree heart block (unless a functioning pacemaker is present). Pts at risk for bradycardia. Not recommended with pacemakers set to rate of 60 bpm or greater.

ACTION

Reduces spontaneous pacemaker activity of the cardiac sinus node by blocking HCN channels that are responsible for cardiac current, which regulates heart rate. Does not affect ventricular repolarization or myocardial contractility. Also inhibits retinal current involved in reducing bright light in retina. **Therapeutic Effect:** Reduces heart rate.

PHARMACOKINETICS

Widely distributed. Metabolized in liver and intestines. Protein binding: 70%. Peak plasma concentration: 1 hr. Eliminated in feces, urine (% not specified). **Half-life:** 6 hrs.

⌛ LIFESPAN CONSIDERATIONS

Pregnancy/Lactation: May cause fetal harm. Females of reproductive potential should use effective contraception. Unknown if distributed in breast milk. Must either discontinue drug or discontinue breastfeeding. If treatment is decided to be absolutely necessary, pregnant pts should be closely monitored for destabilizing HF, esp. during the first trimester. Pregnant women with chronic HF in the third trimester should be closely monitored for preterm birth. **Children:** Safety and efficacy not established. **Elderly:** No age-related precautions noted.

INTERACTIONS

DRUG: Beta blockers (e.g., labetalol, metoprolol), negative chronotropes (e.g., amiodarone, digoxin, diltiaZEM, verapamil) may increase risk of bradycardia. **DiltiaZEM, verapamil** may increase concentration/effect; may further increase risk of bradycardia. **Strong CYP3A4 inhibitors (e.g., clarithromycin, itraconazole)** may increase concentration/effect. **CYP3A4 inducers (e.g., phenytoin, rifAMPin)** may decrease concentration/effect. **HERBAL:** St. John's wort may decrease concentration/effect. **FOOD:** Grapefruit products may increase concentration/effect. **LAB VALUES:** None significant.

AVAILABILITY (Rx)

Tablets: 5 mg, 7.5 mg.

ADMINISTRATION/HANDLING

PO
• Give with meals. May divide 5-mg tablet, providing 2.5-mg dose.

INDICATIONS/ROUTES/DOSAGE

HF
PO: **ADULTS, ELDERLY:** Initially, 5 mg twice daily for 14 days, then adjust dose to resting heart rate of 50–60 bpm. Further adjustments based on resting heart rate and tolerability. **Maximum dose:** 7.5 mg twice daily. (See Dose Modification below.) **Pts with history of conduction defects, pts in whom bradycardia could lead to hemodynamic compromise:** Initiate therapy at 2.5 mg twice daily.

Dose Modification
Adjust dose to maintain a resting heart between 50–60 bpm as follows:

I

Heart rate	Dose Adjustment
Greater than 60 bpm	Increase by 2.5 mg (given twice daily) up to maximum dose of 7.5 mg daily.
50–60 bpm	Maintain dose.
Less than 50 bpm or symptomatic bradycardia	Decrease by 2.5 mg (given twice daily); if current dose is 2.5 mg twice daily, permanently discontinue.

Dosage in Renal Impairment
Mild to moderate impairment: No dose adjustment. **Severe impairment:** Use caution.

Dosage in Hepatic Impairment
Mild impairment: No dose adjustment. **Moderate impairment: ADULTS, ADOLESCENTS, CHILDREN 6 YRS AND OLDER:** 150 mg once daily. **CHILDREN 2–5 YRS: (14 KG OR GREATER):** 75 mg granule packet once daily. **(LESS THAN 14 KG):** 50 mg granule packet once daily. **Severe impairment: ADULTS, ADOLESCENTS, CHILDREN 6 YRS AND OLDER:** 150 mg once daily or less frequently. **CHILDREN 2–5 YRS: (14 KG OR GREATER):** 75 mg granule packet once daily or less frequently. **(LESS THAN 14 KG):** 50 mg granule packet once daily or less frequently.

SIDE EFFECTS

Occasional (10%–3%): Bradycardia, hypertension, phosphenes (visual disturbances, luminous phenomena), visual brightness.

ADVERSE EFFECTS/TOXIC REACTIONS

May increase risk of atrial fibrillation (8.3% of pts). Bradycardia, sinus arrest, or heart block may occur. Bradycardia occurred in 10% of pts. Risk factors for bradycardia may include sinus node dysfunction, conduction defects (e.g., first- or second-degree AV block, bundle branch block), ventricular dyssynchrony, or use of negative chronotropic drugs. Phosphenes, a transient enhanced brightness in the visual field (which may include halos, stroboscopic or kaleidoscopic effect, colored bright lights, or multiple images) may occur. Phosphenes are usually triggered by sudden variations in light intensity and generally occur within the first 2 mos of treatment. Other adverse reactions such as angioedema, diplopia, erythema, hypotension, pruritus, rash, syncope, urticaria, vertigo, visual impairment occur rarely. Overdose may lead to severe and prolonged bradycardia requiring temporary cardiac pacing or infusion of IV beta-stimulating agents.

NURSING CONSIDERATIONS

BASELINE ASSESSMENT
Obtain baseline HR, B/P. Confirm negative pregnancy test before initiating therapy. Receive full medication history and screen for interactions. Screen for contraindications as listed in Precautions. Question history of atrial fibrillation, bradycardia, hypertension.

INTERVENTION/EVALUATION
Frequently monitor HR, B/P. Diligently monitor for atrial fibrillation, bradycardia, syncope. If symptomatic bradycardia occurs, temporary cardiac pacing or infusion of beta-stimulating agents may be warranted. Immediately report suspected pregnancy. Monitor for hypersensitivity reaction. Monitor for visual changes. Initiate fall precautions.

PATIENT/FAMILY TEACHING
• Take medication with meals. • Avoid grapefruit products, herbal supplements such as St. John's wort. • Treatment may cause fetal harm. Female pts of reproductive potential should use effective contraception during treatment. • Report symptoms of low heart rate such as confusion, dizziness, fatigue, fainting, low blood pressure, pallor. • Report symptoms of atrial fibrillation such as chest pressure, palpitations, shortness of breath. • Treatment may cause luminous phenomena (phosphenes), a transient visual brightness that may include halos, light sensitivity, or colored bright lights. • Avoid tasks

that require alertness, motor skills until response to drug is established. • Report allergic reactions such as hives, itching, rash, tongue swelling.

ivacaftor

eye-va-kaf-tor
(Kalydeco)

FIXED-COMBINATION(S)

Orkambi: ivacaftor/lumacaftor (cystic fibrosis transmembrane conductance regulator): 125 mg/200 mg.

◆CLASSIFICATION

PHARMACOTHERAPEUTIC: Cystic fibrosis transmembrane conductance regulator potentiator. **CLINICAL:** Cystic fibrosis agent.

USES

A cystic fibrosis transmembrane regulator (CFTR) potentiator used for the treatment of cystic fibrosis (CF) in pts 2 yrs of age and older having one mutation in the CFTR gene that is responsive to ivacaftor.

PRECAUTIONS

Contraindications: Hypersensitivity to ivacaftor. **Cautions:** Moderate to severe hepatic/renal impairment.

ACTION

Potentiates a specific protein to facilitate, regulate chloride ions, water transport. In cystic fibrosis pts with a specific gene mutation (G551D), a defect in chloride and water transport results in formation of thick mucus in lungs. **Therapeutic Effect:** Improves lung function, fewer respiratory exacerbations.

PHARMACOKINETICS

Readily absorbed. Peak concentration occurs in 4 hrs. Metabolized in liver. Protein binding: 99%. Primarily excreted in feces. **Half-life:** 12 hrs.

⌛ LIFESPAN CONSIDERATIONS

Pregnancy/Lactation: Distributed in breast milk. **Children:** Safety and efficacy not established in children younger than 2 yrs. **Elderly:** No age-related precautions noted.

INTERACTIONS

DRUG: Strong CYP3A4 inducers (e.g., carBAMazepine, rifAMPin) substantially decrease concentration/effects. Concurrent use not recommended. **Strong CYP3A4 inhibitors (e.g., clarithromycin, ketoconazole)** significantly increase concentration. **Moderate CYP3A4 inhibitors (e.g., erythromycin, fluconazole)** may increase concentration and should not be given concurrently. **HERBAL: St. John's wort** decreases concentration/effects. **FOOD: Grapefruit products, Seville oranges** should be avoided (increases concentration). **High-fat meals** increase absorption. **LAB VALUES:** May increase serum ALT, AST.

AVAILABILITY (Rx)

Oral Granules: 50 mg, 75 mg. **Tablets, Film-Coated:** 150 mg.

ADMINISTRATION/HANDLING

PO
• Give with a high-fat meal (e.g., eggs, butter, peanut butter, cheese pizza).

INDICATIONS/ROUTES/DOSAGE

Cystic Fibrosis
PO: ADULTS, CHILDREN 6 YRS AND OLDER: One 150-mg tablet q12h with fat-containing food. **Total daily dose:** 300 mg. **CHILDREN 2–6 YRS, WEIGHING 14 KG OR MORE:** 75-mg packet q12hr. **CHILDREN 2–6 YRS, WEIGHING LESS THAN 14 KG:** 50-mg packet q12hr.

Concurrent Use with Moderate CYP3A4 Inhibitors (e.g., fluconazole)
PO: ADULTS, CHILDREN 6 YRS AND OLDER: 150 mg once daily.

Concurrent Use with Strong CYP3A4 Inhibitors (e.g., clarithromycin, ketoconazole)
PO: ADULTS, CHILDREN 6 YRS AND OLDER: 150 mg twice wkly.

Dosage in Renal Impairment
Mild to moderate impairment: No dose adjustment. **Severe impairment, ESRD:** Use caution.

Dosage in Hepatic Impairment
Mild impairment: No dose adjustment. **Moderate impairment: ADULTS, ELDERLY:** 150 mg once daily. **CHILDREN WEIGHING 14 KG OR MORE:** 75 mg once daily. **CHILDREN WEIGHING LESS THAN 14 KG:** 50 mg once daily. **Severe impairment:** 150 mg once daily or q48h. Use caution.

SIDE EFFECTS

Frequent (24%–10%): Headache, nasal congestion, abdominal discomfort, diarrhea, nausea, rash. **Occasional (6%–5%):** Rhinitis, dizziness, arthralgia, bacteria in sputum. **Rare (4% and Less):** Myalgia, wheezing, acne.

ADVERSE EFFECTS/TOXIC REACTIONS

Upper respiratory infection occurs in 22% of pts, nasopharyngitis in 15%. Increase in ALT, AST occurs in 6% of pts.

NURSING CONSIDERATIONS

BASELINE ASSESSMENT
If the pt's genotype is unknown, an FDA-cleared CF mutation test should be used to detect presence of a CFTR mutation. Assess LFT prior to and periodically during therapy.

INTERVENTION/EVALUATION
Patients who develop increased serum ALT, AST levels should be closely monitored until the abnormalities resolve. Dosing should be interrupted if transaminases (serum ALT or AST) are greater than 5 times upper limit of normal. Transaminases should be obtained every 3 mos during the first year of treatment and annually thereafter.

PATIENT/FAMILY TEACHING
• Always take medication with fatty food. • Avoid grapefruit products and Seville oranges. • Adhere to routine laboratory testing as a part of treatment regimen. • Report headache, diarrhea, rash, signs and symptoms of respiratory infection.

ixabepilone

ix-ab-**ep**-i-lone
(Ixempra)
■ **BLACK BOX ALERT** ■ Combination therapy with capecitabine is contraindicated in pts with serum ALT or AST greater than 2.5 times upper limit of normal (ULN) or bilirubin greater than 1 times ULN. Increased risk of toxicity, neutropenia-related mortality.

◆CLASSIFICATION

PHARMACOTHERAPEUTIC: Epothilone microtubule inhibitor, antimitotic agent. **CLINICAL:** Antineoplastic.

USES

Combination therapy with capecitabine for treatment of metastatic or locally advanced breast cancer in pts after failure of anthracycline, taxane therapy. As monotherapy, treatment of metastatic or locally advanced breast cancer in pts after failure of anthracycline, taxane, and capecitabine therapy. **OFF-LABEL:** Treatment of endometrial cancer.

PRECAUTIONS

Contraindications: Hypersensitivity to ixabepilone. Severe hypersensitivity reaction (grade 3 or 4) to Cremophor, baseline neutrophil count less than 1,500 cells/mm³ or platelet count less than 100,000 cells/mm³. **Combination Capecitabine Therapy:** Serum ALT or AST greater than 2.5 times the upper limit of normal, bilirubin greater than 1 times the upper limit of normal. **Cautions:** Diabetes, existing moderate to severe neuropathy, history of cardiovascular disease. **Monotherapy:** Serum ALT or AST greater than 5 times upper limit of normal bilirubin greater than 3 times upper limit of normal.

ACTION

Binds directly on microtubules during active stage of G2 and M phases of cell cycle, preventing formation of microtubules, an essential part of the process of separation of chromosomes. **Therapeutic Effect:** Blocks cells in mitotic phase of cell division, leading to cell death.

PHARMACOKINETICS

Metabolized in liver. Protein binding: 77%. Excreted in feces (65%), urine (21%). **Half-life:** 52 hrs.

⧗ LIFESPAN CONSIDERATIONS

Pregnancy/Lactation: May cause fetal harm. Unknown if distributed in breast milk. **Children:** Safety and efficacy not established. **Elderly:** Higher incidence of severe adverse reactions in those older than 65 yrs.

INTERACTIONS

DRUG: CYP3A4 inhibitors (e.g., atazanavir, clarithromycin, indinavir, itraconazole, ketoconazole, nefazodone, ritonavir, voriconazole) may increase concentration. **CYP3A4 inducers (e.g., carBAMazepine, dexamethasone, phenytoin, rifAMPin)** may decrease concentration. **HERBAL: St. John's wort** may decrease plasma concentration. **FOOD: Grapefruit products** may increase plasma concentration. **LAB VALUES:** May increase serum ALT, AST, bilirubin. May decrease WBCs, Hgb, platelets.

AVAILABILITY (Rx)

Injection, Solution: Kit: 15-mg kit supplied with diluent for Ixempra, 8 mL; 45 mg supplied with diluent for Ixempra, 23.5 mL.

ADMINISTRATION/HANDLING

 IV

Reconstitution • Withdraw diluent and slowly inject into vial. • Gently swirl and invert until powder is completely dissolved. • Further dilute with 250 mL lactated Ringer's. • Solution may be stored in vial for a maximum of 1 hr at room temperature. • Final concentration for infusion must be between 0.2 mg/mL and 0.6 mg/mL. • Mix infusion bag by manual rotation.
Rate of Administration • Administer through an in-line filter of 0.2 to 1.2 microns. • Infuse over 3 hrs. Administration must be completed within 6 hrs of reconstitution.
Storage • Refrigerate kit. • Prior to reconstitution, kit should be removed from refrigerator and allowed to stand at room temperature for approximately 30 min. • When vials are initially removed from refrigerator, a white precipitate may be observed in the diluent vial. • This precipitate will dissolve to form a clear solution once diluent warms to room temperature. • Once diluted with lactated Ringer's, solution is stable at room temperature and room light for a maximum of 6 hrs.

INDICATIONS/ROUTES/DOSAGE

◀**ALERT**▶ An H_1 antagonist (diphenhydrAMINE 50 mg PO or equivalent) and an H_2 antagonist (raNITIdine 150–300 mg PO or equivalent) must be given prior to beginning treatment with ixabepilone. Pts who experienced a previous hypersensitivity reaction to ixabepilone require pretreatment with corticosteroids (e.g., dexamethasone 20 mg IV 30 min before infusion, or PO 1 hr before infusion) in addition to pretreatment with H_1 and H_2 antagonists.

Breast Cancer

IV: ADULTS, ELDERLY: 40 mg/m² infused over 3 hrs q3 wks. **Maximum:** 88 mg.

Monotherapy Dosage Adjustments for Hepatic Impairment

Mild Hepatic Impairment (ALT and AST Less Than 2.5 Times Upper Limit of Normal [ULN] and Bilirubin Less Than 1 Time ULN)
IV: ADULTS, ELDERLY: 40 mg/m^2 infused over 3 hrs q3 wks.

Mild Hepatic Impairment (ALT and AST Greater Than 2.5 Times ULN and Less Than 10 Times ULN and Bilirubin Greater Than 1 Time ULN and Less Than 1.5 Times ULN)
IV: ADULTS, ELDERLY: 32 mg/m^2 infused over 3 hrs q3 wks.

Moderate Hepatic Impairment (ALT and AST Less Than 10 Times ULN and Bilirubin Greater Than 1.5 Times ULN and Less Than 3 Times ULN)
IV Infusion: ADULTS, ELDERLY: 20–30 mg/m^2 infused over 3 hrs q3 wks (initiate at 20 mg/m2; may increase up to a maximum of 30 mg/m2 in subsequent cycles if tolerated).

Dosage with Strong CYP3A4 Inhibitors/ Inducers
Inhibitors: Consider dose reduction to 20 mg/m^2.
Inducers: Consider dose increase to 60 mg/m^2.

Dosage in Renal Impairment
No dose adjustment.

Dose Modification
Dosage adjustment based on grade of neuropathy, hematologic conditions.

Hematologic
Neutrophils less than 500 cells/mm^3 for 7 days or longer: Reduce dose by 20%. **Neutropenic fever:** Reduce dose by 20%. **Platelets less than 25,000 cells/ mm^3 (less than 50,000 cells/mm^3 with bleeding):** Reduce dose by 20%.

Neuropathy
Grade 2 for 7 days or longer or grade 3 for less than 7 days: Reduce dose by 20%. **Grade 3 for 7 days or longer:** Discontinue treatment. **Grade 3**

(other than neuropathy): Reduce dose by 20%. **Grade 4:** Discontinue treatment.

SIDE EFFECTS

Common (62%): Peripheral sensory neuropathy. **Frequent (56%–46%):** Fatigue, asthenia, myalgia, arthralgia, alopecia, nausea. **Occasional (29%–11%):** Vomiting, stomatitis, mucositis, diarrhea, musculoskeletal pain, anorexia, constipation, abdominal pain, headache. **Rare (9%–5%):** Skin rash, nail disorder, edema, hand-foot syndrome (blistering/ rash/peeling of skin on palms of hands, soles of feet), pyrexia, dizziness, pruritus, gastroesophageal reflux disease (GERD), hot flashes, taste disorder, insomnia.

ADVERSE EFFECTS/TOXIC REACTIONS

Neuropathy occurs early during treatment; 75% of new onset or worsening neuropathy occurred during first 3 cycles. Diabetics may be at increased risk for severe neuropathy manifested as grade 4 neutropenia. Neutropenia, leukopenia occur commonly; anemia, thrombocytopenia occur rarely.

NURSING CONSIDERATIONS

BASELINE ASSESSMENT

Question possibility of pregnancy. Obtain baseline CBC, serum chemistries, LFT before treatment begins as baseline and monitor for hepatotoxicity, peripheral neuropathy (most frequent cause of drug discontinuation). Offer emotional support.

INTERVENTION/EVALUATION

Monitor for symptoms of neuropathy (burning sensation, hyperesthesia, hypoesthesia, paresthesia, discomfort, neuropathic pain). Assess hands and feet for erythema. Monitor CBC for evidence of neutropenia, thrombocytopenia; LFT for hepatotoxicity. Assess mouth for stomatitis, mucositis.

PATIENT/FAMILY TEACHING

• Avoid crowds, those with known infection. • Avoid contact with those who have recently received live virus vaccine. • Do not have immunizations without physician's approval (drug lowers resistance). • Promptly report fever over 100.5°F, chills, numbness, tingling, burning sensation, erythema of hands/feet.

ixazomib

ix-**az**-oh-mib
(Ninlaro)
Do not confuse ixazomib with bortezomib, carfilzomib, idelalisib, or ixekizumab.

◆CLASSIFICATION

PHARMACOTHERAPEUTIC: Proteasome inhibitor. **CLINICAL:** Antineoplastic.

USES

Treatment of multiple myeloma (in combination with lenalidomide and dexamethasone) in pts who have received at least 1 prior therapy.

PRECAUTIONS

Contraindications: Severe hypersensitivity to ixazomib. **Cautions:** Baseline neutropenia, thrombocytopenia; hepatic/renal impairment, chronic peripheral edema, predisposing factors to infection (e.g., diabetes, renal failure, open wounds). Concomitant use of strong CYP3A inducers not recommended.

ACTION

Inhibits activity of beta 5 subunit of the 20S proteasome, leading to cell cycle arrest and tumor cell death (apoptosis). **Therapeutic Effect:** Inhibits tumor cells growth and metastasis.

PHARMACOKINETICS

Well absorbed following oral administration. Widely distributed. Metabolized in liver. Protein binding: 99%. Peak plasma concentration: 1 hr. Excreted in urine (62%), feces (22%). Not removed by hemodialysis. **Half-life:** 9.5 days.

⌛ LIFESPAN CONSIDERATIONS

Pregnancy/Lactation: Avoid pregnancy; may cause fetal harm/malformations. Female and male pts of reproductive potential should use effective contraception during treatment and up to 3 mos after discontinuation. Unknown if distributed in breast milk. Breastfeeding not recommended. **Children:** Safety and efficacy not established. **Elderly:** No age-related precautions noted.

INTERACTIONS

DRUG: Strong CYP3A inducers (e.g., carBAMazepine, phenytoin, rifAMPin) may decrease concentration/effect; avoid use. **HERBAL: St. John's wort** may decrease concentration/effect. **FOOD: High-fat meals** may decrease absorption/concentration. **LAB VALUES:** Expected to decrease neutrophils, platelets.

AVAILABILITY (Rx)

Capsules: 2.3 mg, 3 mg, 4 mg.

ADMINISTRATION/HANDLING

PO
• Capsule contents are hazardous; use cytotoxic precautions during handling and disposal. • Administer capsule whole; do not break, cut, crush, or open. • Give at least 1 hr before or 2 hrs after food. • Give on the same day each wk and at the same time that day. If a dose is missed, do not administer within 72 hrs of next scheduled dose. • If vomiting occurs after dosing, do not readminister; give dose at next scheduled time.

INDICATIONS/ROUTES/DOSAGE

Multiple Myeloma
Note: ANC should be 1,000 cells/mm^3 or greater, platelets 75,000 cells/mm^3 or greater, nonhematologic toxicities at

---

baseline or grade 1 or less prior to initiating a new cycle of therapy.

PO: ADULTS, ELDERLY: 4 mg once wkly on days 1, 8, and 15 of 28-day cycle, in combination with lenalidomide 25 mg daily (on days 1–21 of 28-day cycle) and dexamethasone 40 mg (on days 1, 8, 15, and 22 of 28-day cycle). Continue until disease progression or unacceptable toxicity.

Dose Reduction Schedule
Initial dose: 4 mg. **First dose reduction:** 3 mg. **Second dose reduction:** 2.3 mg. **Unable to tolerate 2.3-mg dose:** Permanently discontinue.

Dose Modification
Based on Common Terminology Criteria for Adverse Events (CTCAE).

Thrombocytopenia
Platelet count less than 30,000 cells/mm³: Withhold ixazomib and lenalidomide until platelet count is 30,000 cells/mm³ or greater, then resume ixazomib at the same dose and resume lenalidomide at reduced dose level (see manufacturer guidelines).
Recurrence of platelet count less than 30,000 cells/mm³: Withhold ixazomib and lenalidomide until platelet count is 30,000 cells/mm³ or greater, then resume ixazomib at reduced dose level and resume lenalidomide at the same dose.
Additional occurrences: Alternate dose modification of ixazomib and lenalidomide.

Neutropenia
Absolute neutrophil count (ANC) less than 500 cells/mm³: Withhold ixazomib and lenalidomide until ANC is 500 cells/mm³ or greater, then resume ixazomib at the same dose and resume lenalidomide at reduced dose level (see manufacturer guidelines).
Recurrence of ANC less than 500 cells/mm³: Withhold ixazomib and lenalidomide until ANC is 500 cells/mm³ or greater, then resume ixazomib at reduced dose level and resume lenalidomide at the same dose.

Additional occurrences: Alternate dose modification of ixazomib and lenalidomide.

Rash
Grade 2 or 3 rash: Withhold lenalidomide until resolved to grade 1 or 0, then resume lenalidomide at next lower dose level (see manufacturer guidelines) and resume ixazomib at the same dose.
Recurrence of grade 2 or 3 rash: Withhold ixazomib and lenalidomide until recovery to grade 1 or 0, then resume ixazomib at reduced dose level and resume lenalidomide at the same dose.
Grade 4 rash: Permanently discontinue.
Additional occurrences: Alternate dose modification of ixazomib and lenalidomide.

Peripheral Neuropathy
Grade 1 (with pain) or grade 2: Withhold ixazomib until resolved to baseline or improved to grade 1 or 0 without pain (at prescriber's discretion), then resume ixazomib at the same dose.
Grade 2 (with pain) or grade 3: Withhold ixazomib until resolved to baseline or improved to grade 1 or 0 without pain (at prescriber's discretion), then resume ixazomib at reduced dose level.
Grade 4: Permanently discontinue.

Any Other Nonhematologic Toxicity
Grade 3 or 4: Withhold ixazomib until resolved to baseline or improved to grade 1 or 0 (at physician's discretion), then resume ixazomib at reduced dose level.

Dosage in Renal Impairment
Mild to moderate impairment: Not specified; use caution. **Severe impairment (CrCl less than 30 mL/min), end-stage renal disease:** Reduce starting dose to 3 mg.

Dosage in Hepatic Impairment
Mild impairment: No dose adjustment. **Moderate to severe impairment:** Reduce starting dose to 3 mg.

SIDE EFFECTS

Frequent (42%–26%): Diarrhea, constipation, nausea. **Occasional (22%–5%):** Vomiting, back pain, blurry vision, dry eye.

ADVERSE EFFECTS/TOXIC REACTIONS

Neutropenia, thrombocytopenia are expected responses to therapy. Thrombocytopenia reported in 78% of pts; neutropenia in 67% of pts. Severe diarrhea may lead to discontinuation of treatment. Peripheral neuropathy reported in 28% of pts (sensory neuropathies were the most common type). Peripheral edema occurred in 28% of pts. Dermatologic toxicities including maculopapular and macular rash may occur. Infectious processes including upper respiratory tract infection (19% of pts), conjunctivitis (6% of pts) may occur. Other toxic reactions including neutrophilic dermatosis, posterior reversible encephalopathy, Stevens-Johnson syndrome, thrombotic thrombocytopenic purpura, transverse myelitis, treatment-induced hepatotoxicity, tumor lysis syndrome, occur rarely.

NURSING CONSIDERATIONS

BASELINE ASSESSMENT

Obtain ANC, CBC (esp. platelet count), renal function test (in pts with renal impairment), LFT; pregnancy test in female pts of reproductive potential. Screen for active infection. Question history of peripheral neuropathy, peripheral edema, hepatic/renal impairment, current hemodialysis status. Receive full medication history including herbal supplements. Offer emotional support. Assess hydration status. Obtain baseline visual acuity. Obtain dietary consult for nutritional support. Offer emotional support.

INTERVENTION/EVALUATION

Monitor ANC, platelet count at least monthly, more frequently during first 3 cycles; LFT in pts with hepatic impairment. Consider concomitant granulocyte colony-stimulating factor (e.g., filgrastim, pegfilgrastim) in pts with neutropenia. Monitor for dehydration, electrolyte imbalance if diarrhea occurs. Offer antiemetics for nausea, antidiarrheals for diarrhea. Monitor for infection (esp. in pts with neutropenia); dermal toxicity, skin rashes, petechiae; peripheral neuropathy (with or without pain); peripheral edema. Monitor daily pattern bowel activity, stool consistency. Monitor for side effects of dexamethasone (e.g., hyperglycemia, weight loss, decreased appetite), lenalidomide (see prescribing information). Reversible posterior leukoencephalopathy syndrome should be considered in pts with altered mental status, confusion, headache, seizures, visual disturbances. Obtain visual acuity if vision becomes blurry.

PATIENT/FAMILY TEACHING

• Treatment may depress your immune system and reduce your ability to fight infection. Report symptoms of infection such as body aches, chills, cough, fatigue, fever. Avoid those with active infection. • Female and male pts of reproductive potential should use effective contraception during treatment and up to 3 mos after last dose. Do not breastfeed. Immediately report suspected pregnancy. • Do not take ixazomib and dexamethasone at the same time. Take dexamethasone with food to minimize GI upset. • Swallow capsules whole; do not chew, crush, or open. Take dose at least 1 hr before or 2 hrs after any food. • Do not expose the capsule contents to the skin or eyes. If eyes are exposed to the capsule powder, thoroughly flush eyes with water. If skin is exposed to the capsule powder, thoroughly wash skin with soap and water. • Treatment may cause nerve pain; extreme sensitivity to touch; muscle weakness; or prickling, tingling, numbness in your hands and feet. • Report swelling of the legs, ankles, feet. • Report neurologic changes such as blurry vision, confusion, headache, seizures; may indicate life-threatening brain swelling. • Treatment may increase risk of bleeding. • Do not take herbal supplements, esp. St. John's wort.

ixekizumab

ix-ee-**kiz**-ue-mab
(Taltz)
Do not confuse ixekizumab with daclizumab, eculizumab, gevokizumab, secukinumab, or ustekinumab.

◆CLASSIFICATION

PHARMACOTHERAPEUTIC: Human interleukin-17A antagonist. Monoclonal antibody. **CLINICAL:** Antipsoriasis agent.

USES

Treatment of moderate to severe plaque psoriasis in adults who are candidates for systemic therapy or phototherapy.

PRECAUTIONS

Contraindications: Hypersensitivity to ixekizumab. **Cautions:** Baseline neutropenia, thrombocytopenia; inflammatory bowel disease (Crohn's disease, ulcerative colitis), HIV infection, concomitant immunosuppressant therapy, conditions predisposing to infection (e.g., diabetes, renal failure, open wounds), pts who have been exposed to tuberculosis. Concomitant use of live vaccines not recommended.

ACTION

Binds to and inhibits interaction of interleukin-17A receptor, a cytokine that is involved in inflammatory and immune response. May reduce epidermal neutrophils in psoriatic plaques. **Therapeutic Effect:** Alters biologic immune response; reduces inflammation.

PHARMACOKINETICS

Widely distributed. Degraded into small peptides and amino acids via catabolic pathway. Peak plasma concentration: 4 days. Steady state reached in 8–10 wks. Elimination not specified. **Half-life:** 13 days.

⧗ LIFESPAN CONSIDERATIONS

Pregnancy/Lactation: Unknown if distributed in breast milk. However, human immunoglobulin G is present in breast milk and is known to cross placenta. **Children:** Safety and efficacy not established in pts younger than 18 yrs. **Elderly:** No age-related precautions noted.

INTERACTIONS

DRUG: Avoid use of **live vaccines.** May decrease therapeutic response. **HERBAL: Echinacea** may decrease effect. **FOOD:** None known. **LAB VALUES:** May decrease neutrophils, platelets. May decrease diagnostic effect of *Coccidioides immitis* skin test.

AVAILABILITY (Rx)

Auto-injector Pen: 80 mg/mL. **Prefilled Syringe:** 80 mg/mL.

ADMINISTRATION/HANDLING

Subcutaneous

• Follow instructions for preparation according to manufacturer guidelines. • Remove auto-injector or prefilled syringe from refrigerator and allow to warm to room temperature (approx. 30 mins) with needle cap intact. • Visually inspect for particulate matter or discoloration. Solution should appear clear, colorless to slightly yellow in color. Do not use if solution is cloudy, discolored, or if visible particles are observed.
Administration • Insert needle subcutaneously into upper arms, outer thigh, or abdomen, and inject solution. • Do not inject into areas of active skin disease or injury such as

sunburns, skin rashes, inflammation, skin infections, or active psoriasis. • Rotate injection sites. **Storage** • Refrigerate until time of use. • Do not freeze. • Do not shake. • Protect from light.

INDICATIONS/ROUTES/DOSAGE

Plaque Psoriasis

SQ: ADULTS, ELDERLY: Initially, 160 mg (two injections of 80 mg) once, then 80 mg at wks 2, 4, 6, 8, 10, 12, then 80 mg once q4wks.

Dosage in Renal Impairment
Not specified; use caution.

Dosage in Hepatic Impairment
Not specified; use caution.

SIDE EFFECTS

Occasional (17%): Injection site reactions (pain, erythema). **Rare (2%):** Nausea.

ADVERSE EFFECTS/TOXIC REACTIONS

May increase risk of infection including tuberculosis. Infections including upper respiratory tract infection (14% of pts), nasopharyngitis (14% of pts), tinea infections (2% of pts) have occurred. Cytopenias including neutropenia (11% of pts), thrombocytopenia (3% of pts) were reported. May cause exacerbation of Crohn's disease and ulcerative colitis. Hypersensitivity reactions, including angioedema, occur rarely. Immunogenicity (auto-ixekizumab antibodies) occurred in less than 9% of pts.

NURSING CONSIDERATIONS

BASELINE ASSESSMENT

Obtain CBC in pts with known history of neutropenia, thrombocytopenia. Screen for active infection. Pts should be evaluated for active tuberculosis and tested for latent infection prior to initiating treatment and periodically during therapy. Induration of 5 mm or greater with tuberculin skin testing should be considered a positive test result when assessing if treatment for latent tuberculosis is necessary. Consider administration of age-appropriate immunizations (if applicable) before initiation. Question history of Crohn's disease, ulcerative colitis, hypersensitivity reaction. Conduct dermatologic exam; record characteristics of psoriatic lesions.

INTERVENTION/EVALUATION

Monitor for symptoms of tuberculosis, including pts who tested negative for latent tuberculosis infection prior to initiating therapy. Interrupt or discontinue treatment if serious infection, opportunistic infection, or sepsis occurs, and initiate appropriate antimicrobial therapy. Assess skin for improvement of lesions. Monitor for hypersensitivity reaction, symptoms of inflammatory bowel disease.

PATIENT/FAMILY TEACHING

• A healthcare provider will show you how to properly prepare and inject your medication. You must demonstrate correct preparation and injection techniques before using medication at home. • Treatment may depress your immune system response and reduce your ability to fight infection. Report symptoms of infection such as body aches, chills, cough, fatigue, fever. Avoid people with active infection. • Do not receive live vaccines. • Expect frequent tuberculosis screening. • Report travel plans to possible endemic areas. • Immediately report difficulty breathing, itching, hives, rash, swelling of the face or tongue; may indicate allergic reaction. • Treatment may cause worsening of Crohn's disease or cause inflammatory bowel disease. Report abdominal pain, diarrhea, weight loss.

ketoconazole

kee-toe-kon-a-zole
(Apo-Ketoconazole ✦, Extina, Nizoral, Nizoral AD, Xolegel)

■ **BLACK BOX ALERT** ■
Potentially fatal hepatotoxicity has occurred; serious cardiovascular events (QT prolongation, torsades de pointes, ventricular tachycardia, ventricular fibrillation, fatalities) have occurred.

Do not confuse Nizoral with Nasarel, Neoral, or Nitrol.

◆CLASSIFICATION

PHARMACOTHERAPEUTIC: Imidazole derivative. **CLINICAL:** Antifungal.

USES

PO: Treatment of susceptible fungal infections, including histoplasmosis, blastomycosis, coccidioidomycosis, paracoccidioidomycosis, chromomycosis. **Shampoo:** Treatment of dandruff. Treatment of tinea versicolor. **Topical:** Treatment of tineas, pityriasis versicolor, cutaneous candidiasis, seborrhea dermatitis, dandruff. **Xolegel:** Treatment of seborrheic dermatitis. **OFF-LABEL: PO:** Treatment of advanced prostate cancer.

PRECAUTIONS

Contraindications: Hypersensitivity to ketoconazole. Acute or chronic liver disease; concurrent use with ALPRAZolam, colchicine, dofetilide, dronedarone, eplerenone, ergot derivatives, irinotecan, lurasidone, methadone, midazolam (oral), pimozide, quiNIDine, ranolazine, statins, tolvaptan, triazolam. **Cautions:** Hepatic impairment, concomitant use of drugs decreasing gastric acidity (e.g., antacids, H$_2$ antagonists, proton pump inhibitors), adrenal insufficiency.

ACTION

Alters cell wall permeability, inhibits phospholipids/enzymes of fungi. **Therapeutic Effect:** Damages fungal cell membrane, altering its function. Fungistatic.

PHARMACOKINETICS

Well absorbed from GI tract following PO administration (absorption decreases as pH of gastric contents increases). Protein binding: 93%–96%. Metabolized in liver. Primarily excreted in bile. Negligible systemic absorption following topical absorption. Ketoconazole is not detected in plasma after shampooing, topical administration. **Half-life:** 8 hrs.

▧ LIFESPAN CONSIDERATIONS

Pregnancy/Lactation: Oral form distributed in breast milk. Unknown if topical form crosses placenta or is distributed in breast milk. **Children: Cream, shampoo:** Safety and efficacy not established. **Oral form:** Safety and efficacy not established in pts younger than 2 yrs. **Elderly:** No age-related precautions noted.

INTERACTIONS

DRUG: May increase concentration/toxicity of **cycloSPORINE, digoxin, ergot alkaloids, midazolam, protease inhibitors (e.g., indinavir, ritonavir, saquinavir), sirolimus, tacrolimus, triazolam, warfarin.** Isoniazid, rifAMPin may decrease concentration/effects. **Antacids, H$_2$ antagonists (e.g., cimetidine, famotidine), proton pump inhibitors (e.g., omeprazole)** may decrease absorption. **HERBAL: St. John's wort** may decrease concentration. **FOOD:** None known. **LAB VALUES:** May increase serum alkaline phosphatase, bilirubin, ALT, AST. May decrease serum corticosteroid, testosterone.

AVAILABILITY (Rx)

Foam (Extina): 2%. **Gel (Xolegel):** 2%. **Shampoo (Nizoral AD [OTC]):** 1%. **Tablets (Nizoral):** 200 mg.

ADMINISTRATION/HANDLING

PO
• Give with food to minimize GI irritation.
• Tablets may be crushed. • Ketoconazole requires acidity; give antacids, anticholinergics, H$_2$ blockers at least 2 hrs following dosing.

Shampoo

• Apply to wet hair, massage for 1 min, rinse thoroughly, reapply for 3 min, rinse.

Topical

• Apply, rub gently into affected/surrounding area.

INDICATIONS/ROUTES/DOSAGE

Usual Dosage

PO: ADULTS, ELDERLY: 200–400 mg once daily. **CHILDREN 2 YRS AND OLDER:** 3.3–6.6 mg/kg once daily.

Topical: ADULTS, ELDERLY: Apply to affected area 1–2 times/day for 2–4 wks.

Shampoo: ADULTS, ELDERLY: Use twice wkly for up to 8 wks, allowing at least 3 days between shampooing. Use intermittently to maintain control.

Dosage in Renal Impairment

No dose adjustment.

Dosage in Hepatic Impairment

Use caution.

SIDE EFFECTS

Occasional (10%–3%): Nausea, vomiting. **Rare (less than 2%):** Abdominal pain, diarrhea, headache, dizziness, photophobia. **Topical:** Burning, irritation, pruritus.

ADVERSE EFFECTS/TOXIC REACTIONS

Hematologic toxicity (thrombocytopenia, hemolytic anemia, leukopenia) occurs occasionally. Hepatotoxicity may occur within first wk to several mos after starting therapy. Anaphylaxis occurs rarely.

NURSING CONSIDERATIONS

BASELINE ASSESSMENT

Confirm culture or histologic test for accurate diagnosis; therapy may begin before results known. Receive full medication history and screen for contraindications. Question history of hepatic impairment.

INTERVENTION/EVALUATION

Monitor LFT; be alert for hepatotoxicity: dark urine, pale stools, jaundice, fatigue, anorexia, nausea, or vomiting (unrelieved by giving medication with food). Monitor CBC for hematologic toxicity. Monitor daily pattern of bowel activity, stool consistency. Assess for dizziness, provide assistance as needed. Evaluate skin for rash, urticaria, pruritus. Monitor adrenal function. **Topical:** Check for localized burning, pruritus, irritation.

PATIENT/FAMILY TEACHING

• Prolonged therapy (wks or mos) is usually necessary. • Avoid alcohol. • May cause dizziness; avoid tasks that require alertness, motor skills until response to drug is established. • Take antacids, antiulcer medications at least 2 hrs after ketoconazole. • Report dark urine, pale stool, yellow skin or eyes, vomiting, increased irritation in topical use, onset of other new symptoms. • Rub well into affected areas. • Avoid contact with eyes. • Keep skin clean, dry; wear light clothing for ventilation. • Separate personal items in direct contact with affected area.

ketorolac

kee-**toe**-role-ak
(Acular, Acular LS, Acuvail, Apo-Ketorolac ♣, Novo-Ketorolac ♣, Sprix, Toradol ♣)

■ **BLACK BOX ALERT** ■ Increased risk of serious cardiovascular thrombotic events, including myocardial infarction, CVA. Increased risk of severe GI reactions, including ulceration, bleeding, perforation.
Do not confuse Acular with Acthar or Ocular, ketorolac with Ketalar, or Toradol with Foradil, Inderal, TEGretol, or traMADol.

K

◆ CLASSIFICATION

PHARMACOTHERAPEUTIC: NSAID. **CLINICAL:** Analgesic, intraocular anti-inflammatory.

USES

PO, injection, nasal: Short-term (5 days or less) relief of mild to moderate pain. **Ophthalmic:** Relief of ocular itching due to seasonal allergic conjunctivitis. Treatment postop for inflammation following cataract extraction, pain following incisional refractive surgery. **OFF-LABEL:** Prevention, treatment of ocular inflammation (ophthalmic form).

PRECAUTIONS

Contraindications: Hypersensitivity to ketorolac, aspirin or other NSAIDs. Intracranial bleeding, hemorrhagic diathesis, incomplete hemostasis, high risk of bleeding; concomitant use of aspirin, NSAIDs, probenecid or pentoxifylline; labor and delivery, advanced renal impairment or risk of renal failure, active or history of peptic ulcer disease, chronic inflammation of GI tract, recent or history of GI bleeding/ulceration. Perioperative pain in setting of CABG surgery. Prophylaxis before major surgery. **Cautions:** Hepatic impairment, history of GI tract disease, asthma, coagulation disorders, receiving anticoagulants, fluid retention, HF, renal impairment, inflammatory bowel disease, smoking, use of alcohol, elderly, debilitated.

ACTION

Inhibits prostaglandin synthesis, reduces prostaglandin levels in aqueous humor. **Therapeutic Effect:** Reduces intensity of pain stimulus, reduces intraocular inflammation.

PHARMACOKINETICS

Readily absorbed from GI tract after IM administration. Protein binding: 99%. Metabolized in liver. Primarily excreted in urine. Not removed by hemodialysis. **Half-life:** 5–9 hrs (increased in renal impairment, in elderly).

⧗ LIFESPAN CONSIDERATIONS

Pregnancy/Lactation: Unknown if distributed in breast milk. Avoid use during third trimester (may adversely affect fetal cardiovascular system: premature closure of ductus arteriosus). **Children:** Safety and efficacy not established, but doses of 0.5 mg/kg have been used. **Elderly:** GI bleeding, ulceration more likely to cause serious adverse effects. Age-related renal impairment may increase risk of hepatic/renal toxicity; decreased dosage recommended.

INTERACTIONS

DRUG: May decrease effects of **antihypertensives (e.g., amLODIPine, lisinopril), diuretics (e.g., furosemide, HCTZ). Aspirin, NSAIDs, other salicylates** may increase risk of GI side effects, bleeding. May increase risk of bleeding with **heparin, oral anticoagulants (e.g., warfarin), thrombolytics.** May increase concentration, risk of toxicity of **lithium.** May increase risk of **methotrexate** toxicity. **Probenecid** may increase concentration. **HERBAL:** **Cat's claw, dong quai, evening primrose, feverfew, garlic, ginkgo, ginseng, horse chestnut, red clover** may decrease antiplatelet activity, risk of bleeding. **FOOD:** None known. **LAB VALUES:** May prolong bleeding time. May increase serum ALT, AST, BUN, potassium, creatinine.

AVAILABILITY (Rx)

Injection Solution: 15 mg/mL, 30 mg/mL. **Nasal Spray (Sprix):** 1.7-g bottle provides 8 sprays (15.75 mg/spray). **Ophthalmic Solution:** 0.4% (Acular LS), 0.45% (Acuvail), 0.5% (Acular). **Tablets:** 10 mg.

ADMINISTRATION/HANDLING

 IV

• Give undiluted as IV push. • Give over at least 15 sec.

IM

• Give deep IM slowly into large muscle mass.

PO

• Give with food, milk, antacids if GI distress occurs.

Ophthalmic

• Place gloved finger on lower eyelid and pull out until pocket is formed between eye and lower lid. Place prescribed number of drops into pocket. • Instruct pt to close eye gently for 1–2 min (so that medication will not be squeezed out of the sac) and to apply digital pressure to lacrimal sac at inner canthus for 1 min to minimize system absorption.

IV INCOMPATIBILITY

Promethazine (Phenergan).

IV COMPATIBILITIES

FentaNYL (Sublimaze), HYDROmorphone (Dilaudid), morphine, nalbuphine (Nubain).

INDICATIONS/ROUTES/DOSAGE

Note: Total duration is 5 days (parenteral and oral). Do not increase dose/frequency; supplement with low-dose opioids if needed.

Pain Management

PO: ADULTS, ELDERLY: Initially, 20 mg (10 mg for elderly), then 10 mg q4–6h. **Maximum:** 40 mg/24 hrs.

IM: ADULTS YOUNGER THAN 65 YRS: 60 mg once or 30 mg q6h. **Maximum:** 120 mg/24 hrs. **ADULTS 65 YRS AND OLDER, PTS WITH RENAL IMPAIRMENT, PTS WEIGHING LESS THAN 50 KG:** 30 mg once or 15 mg q6h. **Maximum:** 60 mg/24 hrs.

IV: ADULTS YOUNGER THAN 65 YRS: 30 mg once or 30 mg q6h. **Maximum:** 120 mg/24 hrs. **ADULTS 65 YRS AND OLDER, PTS WITH RENAL IMPAIRMENT, PTS WEIGHING LESS THAN 50 KG:** 15 mg once or 15 mg q6h. **Maximum:** 60 mg/24 hrs.

Nasal Spray: ADULTS YOUNGER THAN 65 YRS, PTS WEIGHING 50 KG OR GREATER: 31.5 mg (1 spray each nostril) q6–8h. **Maximum daily dose:** 126 mg. **ADULTS 65 YRS AND OLDER, PTS WEIGHING LESS THAN 50 KG:** 15.75 (1 spray in one nostril) mg q6–8h. **Maximum daily dose:** 63 mg.

Allergic Conjunctivitis

Ophthalmic: ADULTS, ELDERLY, CHILDREN 2 YRS AND OLDER: 1 drop (0.5%) 4 times/day.

Cataract Extraction

Ophthalmic: ADULTS, ELDERLY: 1 drop (0.5%) 4 times/day. Begin 24 hrs after surgery and continue for 2 wks.

Corneal Refractive Surgery

Ophthalmic: ADULTS, ELDERLY: 1 drop (0.4%) 4 times/day for 3 days.

Dosage in Renal Impairment

See dosage section.

Dosage in Hepatic Impairment

Use caution.

SIDE EFFECTS

Frequent (17%–12%): Headache, nausea, abdominal cramps/pain, dyspepsia. **Occasional (9%–3%):** Diarrhea. **Nasal:** Nasal discomfort, rhinalgia, increased lacrimation, throat irritation, rhinitis. **Ophthalmic:** Transient stinging, burning. **Rare (3%–1%):** Constipation, vomiting, flatulence, stomatitis. **Ophthalmic:** Ocular irritation, allergic reactions (manifested by pruritus, stinging), superficial ocular infection, keratitis.

ADVERSE EFFECTS/TOXIC REACTIONS

Peptic ulcer, GI bleeding, gastritis, severe hepatic reaction (cholestasis, jaundice) occur rarely. Nephrotoxicity (glomerular nephritis, interstitial nephritis, nephrotic

K

syndrome) may occur in pts with preexisting renal impairment. Acute hypersensitivity reaction (fever, chills, joint pain) occurs rarely.

NURSING CONSIDERATIONS

BASELINE ASSESSMENT

Assess onset, type, location, duration of pain. Obtain baseline renal/hepatic function tests.

INTERVENTION/EVALUATION

Monitor renal function, LFT, urinary output. Monitor daily pattern of bowel activity, stool consistency. Observe for occult blood loss. Assess for therapeutic response: relief of pain, stiffness, swelling; increased joint mobility; reduced joint tenderness; improved grip strength. Monitor for bleeding (may also occur with ophthalmic route due to systemic absorption).

PATIENT/ FAMILY TEACHING

• Avoid aspirin, alcohol. • Report abdominal pain, bloody stools, or vomiting blood. • If GI upset occurs, take with food, milk. • **Ophthalmic:** Transient stinging, burning may occur upon instillation. • Do not administer while wearing soft contact lenses.

K

labetalol

la-**bayt**-a-lol
(Apo-Labetalol ✤, Trandate ✤)
Do not confuse labetalol with atenolol, betaxolol, metoprolol or propranolol, or Trandate with traMADol or TRENtal.

FIXED-COMBINATION(S)

Normozide: labetalol/hydroCHLOROthiazide (a diuretic): 100 mg/25 mg, 200 mg/25 mg, 300 mg/25 mg.

◆CLASSIFICATION

PHARMACOTHERAPEUTIC: Alpha-, beta-adrenergic blocker. **CLINICAL:** Antihypertensive.

USES

Management of hypertension. IV for severe hypertension. **OFF-LABEL:** Management of preeclampsia, severe hypertension in pregnancy, hypertension during acute ischemic stroke, pediatric hypertension.

PRECAUTIONS

Contraindications: Hypersensitivity to labetalol. Bronchial asthma, history of obstructive airway disease, cardiogenic shock, uncompensated HF, second- or third-degree heart block (except in pts with functioning pacemaker), severe bradycardia, conditions associated with severe, prolonged hypotension. **Cautions:** Compensated HF, severe anaphylaxis to allergens, myasthenia gravis, psychiatric disease, hepatic impairment, pheochromocytoma, diabetes; concurrent use with digoxin, verapamil, or diltiaZEM; arterial obstruction, elderly. Pts with peripheral vascular disease, Raynaud's disease.

ACTION

Blocks alpha$_1$-, beta$_1$-, beta$_2$- (large doses) adrenergic receptor sites. **Therapeutic Effect:** Slows sinus heart rate; decreases peripheral vascular resistance, B/P.

PHARMACOKINETICS

Route	Onset	Peak	Duration
PO	0.5–2 hrs	2–4 hrs	8–12 hrs
IV	2–5 min	5–15 min	2–4 hrs

Incompletely absorbed from GI tract. Bioavailability: 25%. Protein binding: 50%. Metabolized in liver. Primarily excreted in urine. Not removed by hemodialysis. **Half-life:** 6–8 hrs.

⧗ LIFESPAN CONSIDERATIONS

Pregnancy/Lactation: Drug crosses placenta. Small amount distributed in breast milk. **Children:** Safety and efficacy not established. **Elderly:** Age-related peripheral vascular disease may increase susceptibility to decreased peripheral circulation. May have increased risk of orthostatic hypotension.

INTERACTIONS

DRUG: May decrease effects of beta$_2$-adrenergic agonists (e.g., **arformoterol, salmeterol), theophylline. Beta blockers (e.g., carvedilol, metoprolol), calcium channel blockers (e.g., diltiazem, verapamil), digoxin** may increase risk of bradycardia. **HERBAL: Ephedra, ginseng, yohimbe** may worsen hypertension. **Garlic** may increase antihypertensive effect. **Licorice** may cause water retention, increased serum sodium, decreased serum potassium. **FOOD:** None known. **LAB VALUES:** May increase serum antinuclear antibody titer (ANA), BUN, LDH, alkaline phosphatase, bilirubin, creatinine, potassium, triglycerides, lipoprotein, uric acid, ALT, AST.

AVAILABILITY (Rx)

Injection Solution: 5 mg/mL. **Tablets:** 100 mg, 200 mg, 300 mg.

ADMINISTRATION/HANDLING

 **IV**

◀ALERT▶ Prolonged duration of action: Monitor several hrs after administration. Excessive administration may result in prolonged hypotension and/or bradycardia.

✤ Canadian trade name   🗠 Non-Crushable Drug   🄷🄰 High Alert drug

Reconstitution • For IV infusion, dilute in D$_5$W to provide concentration of 1–2 mg/mL.

Rate of Administration • For IV push, administer at a rate of 10 mg/min. • For IV infusion, administer at rate of 2 mg/min initially. Rate is adjusted according to B/P. • Monitor B/P immediately before and q5–10min during IV administration (maximum effect occurs within 5 min).

Storage • Store at room temperature. • After dilution, IV solution is stable for 72 hrs. • Solution appears clear, colorless to light yellow. • Discard if discolored or precipitate forms.

PO
• Give without regard to food. • Tablets may be crushed.

▦ IV INCOMPATIBILITIES

Amphotericin B complex (Abelcet, AmBisome, Amphotec), ceftaroline (Teflaro), cefTRIAXone (Rocephin), furosemide (Lasix), heparin, nafcillin (Nafcil).

▦ IV COMPATIBILITIES

Amiodarone (Cordarone), calcium gluconate, dexmedetomidine (Precedex), diltiaZEM (Cardizem), DOBUTamine (Dobutrex), DOPamine (Intropin), enalapril (Vasotec), fentaNYL (Sublimaze), HYDROmorphone (Dilaudid), lidocaine, LORazepam (Ativan), magnesium sulfate, midazolam (Versed), milrinone (Primacor), morphine, nitroglycerin, norepinephrine (Levophed), potassium chloride, potassium phosphate, propofol (Diprivan).

INDICATIONS/ROUTES/DOSAGE

Hypertension
PO: ADULTS, ELDERLY: Initially, 100 mg twice daily. Adjust in increments of 100 mg twice daily q2–3days. Usual dose: 100–300 mg twice daily. May require up to 2,400 mg/day. **CHILDREN:** 1–3 mg/kg/day in 2 divided doses. **Maximum:** 10–12 mg/kg/day up to 1,200 mg/day.

Severe Hypertension, Hypertensive Crisis
IV: ADULTS: Initially, 10–20 mg (bolus over 2 min). Additional doses of 40–80 mg may be given at 10-min intervals, up to total dose of 300 mg. **CHILDREN:** 0.2–1 mg/kg/dose. **Maximum:** 40 mg/dose.
IV Infusion: ADULTS: Initially, 2 mg/min up to total dose of 300 mg. **CHILDREN:** 0.2–1 mg/kg/hr. **Maximum:** 3 mg/kg/hr or 40 mg/dose.

Dosage in Renal Impairment
No dose adjustment.

Dosage in Hepatic Impairment
Use caution.

SIDE EFFECTS

Frequent (20%–11%): Drowsiness, dizziness, excessive fatigue. **Occasional (10% or less):** Dyspnea, peripheral edema, depression, anxiety, constipation, diarrhea, nasal congestion, weakness, diminished sexual function, transient scalp tingling, insomnia, nausea, vomiting, abdominal discomfort. **Rare:** Altered taste, dry eyes, increased urination, paresthesia.

ADVERSE EFFECTS/TOXIC REACTIONS

May precipitate, aggravate HF due to decreased myocardial stimulation. Abrupt withdrawal may precipitate myocardial ischemia, producing chest pain, diaphoresis, palpitations, headache, tremor. May mask signs, symptoms of acute hypoglycemia (tachycardia, B/P changes) in diabetic pts. Rapid reduction of blood pressure may cause CVA, optic nerve infarction, ischemic changes on EKG. May cause severe orthostatic hypotension.

NURSING CONSIDERATIONS

BASELINE ASSESSMENT

Assess baseline renal function, LFT. Assess B/P, apical pulse immediately before drug administration (if pulse is 60/min or less or systolic B/P is lower than 90 mm Hg, withhold medication, contact physician). Question history of bradycardia, HF, second- or third-degree heart block, myasthenia gravis.

INTERVENTION/EVALUATION

Monitor B/P for hypotension. Assess pulse for quality, irregular rate, bradycardia.

L

Monitor EKG for cardiac arrhythmias. Assist with ambulation if dizziness occurs. Assess for evidence of HF: dyspnea (particularly on exertion or lying down), night cough, peripheral edema, distended neck veins. Monitor I&O (increase in weight, decrease in urine output may indicate HF).

PATIENT/FAMILY TEACHING

• Do not discontinue drug except upon advice of physician (abrupt discontinuation may precipitate heart failure). • Slowly go from lying to standing. • Compliance with therapy regimen is essential to control hypertension, arrhythmias. • Avoid tasks that require alertness, motor skills until response to drug is established. • Report shortness of breath, excessive fatigue, weight gain, prolonged dizziness, headache. • Do not use nasal decongestants, OTC cold preparations (stimulants) without physician approval. • Limit alcohol.

lacosamide

la-**koe**-sa-myde
(Vimpat)
Do not confuse lacosamide with zonisamide.

◆CLASSIFICATION

PHARMACOTHERAPEUTIC: Succinimide **(Schedule V). CLINICAL:** Anticonvulsant.

USES

Monotherapy or adjunctive therapy for treatment of partial-onset seizures in pts 17 yrs and older.

PRECAUTIONS

Contraindications: Hypersensitivity to lacosamide. **Cautions:** Renal/hepatic impairment, cardiac conduction problems (e.g., marked first-degree AV block, second-degree or higher AV block, sick sinus syndrome without pacemaker), myocardial ischemia, HF, pts at risk of suicide.

ACTION

Selectively enhances slow inactivation of sodium channels, stabilizing hyperexcitable neuronal membranes and inhibits neuronal firing. **Therapeutic Effect:** Reduces seizure frequency.

PHARMACOKINETICS

Completely absorbed following PO administration. Protein binding: 15%. Peak plasma concentration: 1–4 hrs after oral dosing and is reached at the end of IV infusion. Primarily excreted in urine. Steady-state levels achieved in 3 days. Removed by hemodialysis. **Half-life:** 13 hrs.

⧗ LIFESPAN CONSIDERATIONS

Pregnancy/Lactation: Use in pregnancy if benefits outweigh risk. Unknown if distributed in breast milk. **Children:** Safety and efficacy not established in pts younger than 17 yrs. **Elderly:** No age-related precautions noted.

INTERACTIONS

DRUG: Strong CYP2C9 inhibitors (e.g., fluconazole), strong CYP3A4 inhibitors (e.g., clarithromycin, ketoconazole) may increase concentration/effects. **HERBAL:** None significant. **FOOD:** None known. **LAB VALUES:** May increase serum ALT; proteinuria.

AVAILABILITY (Rx)

Injection Solution: 10 mg/mL (20 mL). **Oral Solution:** 10 mg/mL.

Tablets: 50 mg, 100 mg, 150 mg, 200 mg.

ADMINISTRATION/HANDLING

PO

• Give without regard to meals. • Do not break, crush, dissolve, or divide film-coated tablets. • Oral solution should be administered with a calibrated measuring device. • Discard any unused portion after 7 wks.

IV

• Appears as a clear, colorless solution. • Discard unused portion or if precipitate or discoloration is present. May give without further dilution. • If mixing with diluent, may be stored for 24 hrs at room temperature. Infuse over 30–60 min.

▨ IV COMPATIBILITIES

0.9% NaCl, D₅W, lactated Ringer's.

INDICATIONS/ROUTES/DOSAGE

Note: IV dose is same as oral dose. May give undiluted or mixed in compatible diluent and infused over 30–60 min.

Partial-Onset Seizures
Monotherapy
PO/IV: ADULTS, CHILDREN 17 YRS AND OLDER: Initially, 100 mg twice daily. May increase by 50 mg twice daily at wkly intervals. **Maintenance:** 150–200 mg twice daily.
Adjunctive Therapy
PO/IV: ADULTS, CHILDREN 17 YRS AND OLDER: Initially, 50 mg twice daily. May increase by 50 mg twice daily at wkly intervals. **Maintenance:** 100–200 mg twice daily. **Maximum:** 400 mg/day.

Switch from IV to PO
When switching from IV to PO form, use same equivalent daily dosage and frequency as IV administration.

Switch from PO to IV
When switching from PO to IV form, initial total daily IV dosage should be equivalent to total daily dosage and frequency of PO form and should be infused IV over 30–60 min.

Dosage in Renal Impairment
Use caution when titrating. **Mild to moderate impairment:** No dose adjustment. **Severe impairment, end-stage renal disease: Maxiumum:** 300 mg/day.

Dosage in Hepatic Impairment
Use caution when titrating. **Mild to moderate impairment: Maximum:** 300 mg/day. **Severe impairment:** Not recommended.

SIDE EFFECTS

Frequent (31%–13%): Dizziness, headache. **Occasional (11%–5%):** Nausea, double vision, vomiting, fatigue, blurred vision, ataxia, tremor, nystagmus. **Rare (4%–2%):** Vertigo, diarrhea, gait disturbances, memory impairment, depression, pruritus, injection site discomfort.

ADVERSE EFFECTS/TOXIC REACTIONS

Increased risk of suicidal ideation, behavior. Dose-dependent prolongations in PR interval noted. Leukopenia, anemia, thrombocytopenia occur rarely.

NURSING CONSIDERATIONS

BASELINE ASSESSMENT

Review history of seizure disorder (intensity, frequency, duration, level of consciousness). Initiate seizure precautions. Renal function, LFT, CBC should be performed before therapy begins and periodically during therapy. Question history of cardiac conduction disorders, depression, suicidal ideation and behavior.

INTERVENTION/EVALUATION

Observe for recurrence of seizure activity. Assess for clinical improvement (decrease in intensity/frequency of seizures). Assist with ambulation if dizziness occurs. Assess for suicidal ideation, depression, behavioral changes. Drug should be withdrawn gradually (over a minimum of 1 wk) to minimize potential for increased seizure frequency. Monitor ECG for QT prolongation.

PATIENT/FAMILY TEACHING

• Strict maintenance of drug therapy is essential for seizure control. • Avoid tasks that require alertness, motor skills until response to drug is established. • Avoid alcohol. • Report depression, suicidal ideation, unusual behavioral changes.

lactulose

lak-tyoo-lose
(Apo-Lactulose ✦, Constulose, Enulose, Generlac, Kristalose)
Do not confuse lactulose with lactose.

◆CLASSIFICATION

PHARMACOTHERAPEUTIC: Lactose derivative. **CLINICAL:** Hyperosmotic laxative, ammonia detoxicant.

USES

Prevention, treatment of portal-systemic encephalopathy (including hepatic pre-coma, coma); treatment of constipation.

PRECAUTIONS

Contraindications: Hypersensitivity to lactulose. Pts requiring a low-galactose diet. **Cautions:** Diabetes, hepatic impairment, dehydration.

ACTION

Inhibits diffusion of NH_3 into blood by converting NH_3 to NH_4^+; enhances diffusion of NH_3 from blood to gut, where it is converted to NH_4^+; produces osmotic effect in colon. **Therapeutic Effect:** Promotes increased peristalsis, bowel evacuation; decreases serum ammonia concentration.

PHARMACOKINETICS

Poorly absorbed from GI tract. Extensively metabolized in colon. Primarily excreted in feces.

☒ LIFESPAN CONSIDERATIONS

Pregnancy/Lactation: Unknown if drug crosses placenta or is distributed in breast milk. **Children:** Avoid use in pts younger than 6 yrs (usually unable to describe symptoms). **Elderly:** No age-related precautions noted.

INTERACTIONS

DRUG: None significant. **HERBAL:** None significant. **FOOD:** None known. **LAB VALUES:** May decrease serum potassium (GI loss).

AVAILABILITY (Rx)

Packets (Kristalose): 10 g, 20 g. **Solution, Oral:** 10 g/15 mL.

ADMINISTRATION/HANDLING

PO

• Store solution at room temperature. • Solution appears pale yellow to yellow, viscous liquid. Cloudiness, darkened solution does not indicate potency loss. • Drink water, juice, milk with each dose (aids stool softening, increases palatability). • Mix packets with 4 oz water.

Rectal

• Lubricate anus with petroleum jelly before enema insertion. • Insert carefully (prevents damage to rectal wall) with nozzle toward navel. • Squeeze container until entire dose expelled. • Instruct pt to retain 30–60 min in divided doses. • **Maximum:** 60 mL/day (40 g/day).

INDICATIONS/ROUTES/DOSAGE

Constipation
PO: ADULTS, ELDERLY: 15–30 mL (10–20 g)/day, up to 60 mL (40 g)/day. **CHILDREN:** 1.5–3 mL/kg/day (1–2 g/kg/day). **Maximum:** 40 g/day (60 mL/day).

Prevention of Portal-Systemic Encephalopathy
ADULTS, ELDERLY: 30–45 mL (20–30 g) 3–4 times/day. Adjust dose q1–2 days to produce 2–3 soft stools/day. **CHILDREN:** 40–90 mL/day (26.7–60 g/day) in divided doses 3–4 times/day. **INFANTS:** 2.5–10 mL/day (1.7–6.7 g/day) in 3–4 divided doses. Adjust dose q1–2 days to produce 2–3 soft stools/day.

Treatment of Portal-Systemic Encephalopathy
PO: ADULTS, ELDERLY: Initially, 30–45 mL (20–30 g) every hr to induce rapid laxation. Then, 30–45 mL 3–4 times/day. Adjust dose q1–2 days to produce 2–3 soft stools/day.

Rectal Administration (as Retention Enema)
200 g (300 mL) diluted with 700 mL water or NaCl via rectal balloon catheter. Retain 30–60 min q4–6h. (Transition to oral prior to stopping rectal administration.)

Dosage in Renal/Hepatic Impairment
No dose adjustment.

SIDE EFFECTS

Occasional: Abdominal cramping, flatulence, increased thirst, abdominal discomfort. **Rare:** Nausea, vomiting.

ADVERSE EFFECTS/TOXIC REACTIONS

Severe diarrhea may cause dehydration, electrolyte imbalance. Long-term use may result in laxative dependence, chronic constipation, loss of normal bowel function.

NURSING CONSIDERATIONS

BASELINE ASSESSMENT

Question usual stool pattern, frequency, characteristics. Conduct neurological exam in pts with elevated serum ammonia levels, symptoms of encephalopathy. Assess hydration status.

INTERVENTION/EVALUATION

Encourage adequate fluid intake. Assess bowel sounds for peristalsis. Monitor daily pattern of bowel activity, stool consistency; record time of evacuation. Assess for abdominal disturbances. Monitor serum electrolytes in pts with prolonged, frequent, excessive use of medication. Monitor encephalopathic pts for symptom improvement (alertness, orientation, ability to follow commands).

PATIENT/FAMILY TEACHING

• Evacuation occurs in 24–48 hrs of initial dose. • Institute measures to promote defecation: increase fluid intake, exercise, high-fiber diet. • Drink plenty of fluids. • If therapy was started to treat high ammonia levels, notify physician if worsening of confusion, lethargy, weakness occurs.

lamiVUDine

la-**miv**-yoo-deen
(Apo-LamiVUDine ✺, Epivir, Epivir-HBV, Heptovir ✺)

■ **BLACK BOX ALERT** ■ Serious, sometimes fatal lactic acidosis, severe hepatomegaly with steatosis (fatty liver) have occurred. Pts must be monitored for chronic hepatitis B virus infection for several months following therapy. Do not use Epivir-HBV for treatment of HIV infection.

Do not confuse Epivir with Combivir, or lamiVUDine with lamoTRIgine.

FIXED-COMBINATION(S)

Combivir: lamiVUDine/zidovudine (an antiviral): 150 mg/300 mg. **Epzicom:** lamiVUDinc/abacavir (an antiviral): 300 mg/600 mg. **Triumeq:** lamiVUDine/abacavir (antiretroviral)/dolutegravir (integrase inhibitor): 300 mg/600 mg/50 mg. **Trizivir:** lamiVUDine/zidovudine/abacavir (an antiviral): 150 mg/300 mg/300 mg.

◆CLASSIFICATION

PHARMACOTHERAPEUTIC: Nucleoside reverse transcriptase inhibitor. **CLINICAL:** Antiviral.

USES

Epivir: Treatment of HIV infection in combination with at least two other antiretroviral agents. **Epivir-HBV:** Treatment of chronic hepatitis B virus infection associated with evidence of hepatitis B viral replication and active hepatic inflammation. **OFF-LABEL:** Prophylaxis in health care workers at risk of acquiring HIV after occupational exposure to virus. Use as part of multidrug regimen.

PRECAUTIONS

Contraindications: Hypersensitivity to lamiVUDine. **Cautions:** Use in children with history of pancreatitis or risk factors for developing pancreatitis. Use in combination with interferon alfa with or without ribavirin in HIV/HBV coinfected pts; renal/hepatic impairment.

ACTION

Inhibits HIV reverse transcriptase by viral DNA chain termination. Inhibits RNA-, DNA-dependent DNA polymerase, an enzyme necessary for HIV, hepatitis B virus replication. **Therapeutic Effect:** Slows HIV replication, reduces progression of HIV infection, chronic hepatitis B virus infection.

PHARMACOKINETICS

Rapidly, completely absorbed from GI tract. Protein binding: less than 36%. Widely distributed (crosses blood-brain barrier). Primarily excreted unchanged in urine. Not removed by hemodialysis or peritoneal dialysis. **Half-life: Children:** 2 hrs. **Adults:** 5–7 hrs.

⧗ LIFESPAN CONSIDERATIONS

Pregnancy/Lactation: Drug crosses placenta. Unknown if distributed in breast milk. Breastfeeding not recommended (possibility of HIV transmission). **Children:** Safety and efficacy not established in pts younger than 3 mos. **Elderly:** Age-related renal impairment may require dosage adjustment.

INTERACTIONS

DRUG: Zalcitabine may inhibit absorption of both drugs; avoid concurrent administration. **HERBAL:** None significant. **FOOD:** None known. **LAB VALUES:** May increase Hgb, neutrophil count; serum amylase, ALT, AST, bilirubin.

AVAILABILITY (Rx)

Oral Solution: 5 mg/mL (Epivir-HBV), 10 mg/mL (Epivir). **Tablets:** 100 mg (Epivir-HBV), 150 mg (Epivir), 300 mg (Epivir).

ADMINISTRATION/HANDLING

PO
• Give without regard to meals.

INDICATIONS/ROUTES/DOSAGE

Note: Epivir tablets/oral solution contain a higher dose of lamivudine than Epivir-HBV tablets/oral solution.

HIV Infection (Epivir)
PO: ADULTS, ELDERLY: 150 mg twice daily or 300 mg once daily. **CHILDREN 4 MOS–16 YRS:** *(Oral Solution):* 4 mg/kg twice daily (up to 150 mg/dose). **INFANTS 1–3 MOS:** 4 mg/kg twice daily. **NEONATES YOUNGER THAN 30 DAYS:** 2 mg/kg twice daily. *(Tablets):* **25 KG OR MORE:** 150 mg 2 times/day or 300 mg once daily. **20–24 KG:** 75 mg in AM and 150 mg in PM or 225 mg once daily. **14–19 KG:** 75 mg 2 times/day or 150 mg once daily.

Chronic Hepatitis B (Epivir HBV)
PO: ADULTS: 100 mg/day. **CHILDREN 2–17 YRS:** 3 mg/kg/day. **Maximum:** 100 mg/day.

Dosage in Renal Impairment
Dosage and frequency are modified based on creatinine clearance.

Creatinine Clearance	Dosage HIV	Dosage Hepatitis B
30–49 mL/min	150 mg once/daily	100 mg first dose, then 50 mg once/daily
15–29 mL/min	150 mg first dose, then 100 mg once/daily	100 mg first dose, then 25 mg once/daily
5–14 mL/min	150 mg first dose, then 50 mg once/daily	35 mg first dose, then 15 mg once/daily
Less than 5 mL/min	50 mg first dose, then 25 mg once/daily	35 mg first dose, then 10 mg once/daily

Hemodialysis: Dosing post-HD recommended.

Dosage in Hepatic Impairment
No dose adjustment.

SIDE EFFECTS

Frequent (35%–10%): Headache, nausea, malaise, fatigue, nasal disturbances, diarrhea, cough, musculoskeletal pain, neuropathy, insomnia, anorexia, dizziness, fever, chills. **Occasional (9%–5%):** Depression, myalgia, abdominal cramps, dyspepsia, arthralgia.

❖ Canadian trade name   🦫 Non-Crushable Drug   🔲 High Alert drug

ADVERSE EFFECTS/TOXIC REACTIONS

Pancreatitis occurs in 13% of pediatric pts. Anemia, neutropenia, thrombocytopenia occur rarely. Lactic acidosis, severe hepatomegaly with steatosis have been reported. May cause hepatitis B virus reactivation when treatment is discontinued.

NURSING CONSIDERATIONS

BASELINE ASSESSMENT

Obtain baseline renal function test, LFT, CD4 count, viral load. Screen HIV pts for hepatitis B virus infection before initiating therapy.

INTERVENTION/EVALUATION

Monitor serum BUN, creatinine, amylase, lipase, ALT, AST, bilirubin. Assess for headache, nausea, cough. Monitor daily pattern of bowel activity, stool consistency. Modify diet or administer laxative as needed. Assess for dizziness, sleep pattern. If pancreatitis in children occurs, movement aggravates abdominal pain; sitting up, flexing at the waist may relieve the pain.

PATIENT/FAMILY TEACHING

• Continue therapy for full length of treatment. • Doses should be evenly spaced. • LamiVUDine is not a cure for HIV infection, nor does it reduce risk of transmission to others. • Avoid tasks requiring alertness, motor skills until response to drug is established. • Avoid alcohol. • Closely monitor for symptoms of pancreatitis (severe, steady abdominal pain often radiating to the back, clammy skin, hypotension; nausea/vomiting may accompany abdominal pain).

lamoTRIgine

la-**moe**-tri-jeen
(Apo-LamoTRIgine ✤, LaMICtal, LaMICtal ODT, LaMICtal XR)
■ **BLACK BOX ALERT** ■ Severe, potentially life-threatening skin rashes have been reported, including Stevens-Johnson syndrome. Risk increased with coadministration with valproic acid and rapid-dose titration.
Do not confuse LaMICtal with LamISIL or Lomotil, or lamoTRIgine with labetalol or lamiVUDine.

◆CLASSIFICATION

PHARMACOTHERAPEUTIC: Phenyltriazine. **CLINICAL:** Anticonvulsant.

USES

Immediate-Release: Adjunctive therapy in adults and children 2 yrs of age and older with generalized tonic-clonic seizures, partial seizures, and generalized seizures of Lennox-Gastaut syndrome. Conversion to monotherapy in adults treated with another enzyme-inducing antiepileptic drug (EIAED) (e.g., valproic acid, carBAMazepine, phenytoin, PHENobarbital, or primidone as the single antiepileptic drug). Long-term maintenance treatment of bipolar disorder. Treatment of pts 2 yrs and older with primary generalized tonic-clonic seizures. **Extended-release:** Adjunctive therapy for primary generalized tonic-clonic and partial-onset seizures in pts 13 yrs and older. Conversion to monotherapy in pt 13 yrs and older with partial seizures receiving treatment with a single antiepileptic drug (AED).

PRECAUTIONS

Contraindications: Hypersensitivity to lamoTRIgine. **Cautions:** Renal/hepatic impairment, pts at high risk of suicide, pts taking estrogen-containing oral contraceptives, history of adverse hematologic reaction.

ACTION

May block voltage-sensitive sodium channels, stabilizing neuronal membranes, regulating presynaptic transmitter release of excitatory amino acids. **Therapeutic Effect:** Reduces frequency of seizure activity. Delays time to occurrence of acute mood episodes (mania, depression, hypomania).

L

⌛ LIFESPAN CONSIDERATIONS

Pregnancy/Lactation: Distributed in breast milk. Breastfeeding not recommended. Increased fetal risk of oral cleft formation has been noted with use during pregnancy. **Children:** Safety and efficacy not established in pts younger than 18 yrs with bipolar disorder or in pts younger than 13 yrs with epilepsy. **Elderly:** Age-related renal impairment may require dosage adjustment.

INTERACTIONS

DRUG: CarBAMazepine, PHENobarbital, primidone, phenytoin, rifAMPin may decrease concentration. **Valproic acid** may increase concentration/effects. May decrease effects of **oral contraceptives. HERBAL:** Evening primrose may decrease seizure threshold. **FOOD:** None known. **LAB VALUES:** None significant.

AVAILABILITY (Rx)

Tablets: 25 mg, 100 mg, 150 mg, 200 mg. **Tablets (Chewable):** 5 mg, 25 mg. **Tablets (Orally Disintegrating):** 25 mg, 50 mg, 100 mg, 200 mg.

◥ Tablets (Extended-Release): 25 mg, 50 mg, 100 mg, 200 mg, 250 mg, 300 mg.

ADMINISTRATION/HANDLING

PO

• Give without regard to food. • Chewable tablets may be dispensed in water or diluted fruit juice, or swallowed whole. • Extended-release tablets must be swallowed whole; do not break, crush, dissolve, or divide. • Place orally disintegrating tablet on tongue, allow to dissolve. Pt must not break, cut, or chew. Can be swallowed without regard to food or water.

INDICATIONS/ROUTES/DOSAGE

Lennox-Gastaut, Primary Generalized Tonic-Clonic Seizures, Partial Seizures
PO: ADULTS, ELDERLY, CHILDREN OLDER THAN 12 YRS: Initially, 25 mg/day for 2 wks, then increase to 50 mg/day for 2 wks. After 4 wks, may increase by 50 mg/day at 1- to 2-wk intervals. **Maintenance:** 225–375 mg/day in 2 divided doses. **CHILDREN 2–12 YRS:** Initially, 0.3 mg/kg/day in 1–2 divided doses for 2 wks, then increase to 0.6 mg/kg/day in 1–2 divided doses for 2 wks. After 4 wks, may increase by 0.6 mg/kg/day at 1- to 2-wk intervals. **Maintenance:** 4.5–7.5 mg/kg/day in 2 divided doses. **Maximum:** 300 mg/day in 2 divided doses.

Adjusted Dosage with Antiepileptic Drugs Containing Valproic Acid
PO: ADULTS, ELDERLY, CHILDREN OLDER THAN 12 YRS: Initially, 25 mg every other day for 2 wks, then increase to 25 mg/day for 2 wks. After 4 wks, may increase by 25–50 mg/day at 1- to 2-wk intervals. **Maintenance:** 100–400 mg/day in 2 divided doses (100–200 mg/day when taking lamoTRIgine with valproic acid alone). **CHILDREN 2–12 YRS:** Initially, 0.15 mg/kg/day in 1–2 divided doses for 2 wks, then increase to 0.3 mg/kg/day in 1–2 divided doses for 2 wks. After 4 wks, may increase by 0.3 mg/kg/day at 1- to 2-wk intervals. **Maintenance:** 1–5 mg/kg/day in 2 divided doses. **Maximum:** 200 mg/day in 2 divided doses.

Adjusted Dosage with EIAED without Valproic Acid
PO: ADULTS, ELDERLY, CHILDREN OLDER THAN 12 YRS: Initially, 50 mg/day for 2 wks, then increase to 100 mg/day in 2 divided doses for 2 wks. After 4 wks, may increase by 100 mg/day at 1- to 2-wk intervals. **Maintenance:** 300–500 mg/day in 2 divided doses. **CHILDREN 2–12 YRS:** Initially, 0.6 mg/kg/day in 1–2 divided doses for 2 wks, then increase to 1.2 mg/kg/day in 1–2 divided doses for 2 wks. After 4 wks, may increase by 1.2 mg/kg/day at 1- to 2-wk intervals. **Maintenance:** 5–15 mg/kg/day in 2 divided doses. **Maximum:** 400 mg/day in 2 divided doses.

Usual Maintenance Range for Extended-Release Tablets
PT TAKING VALPROIC ACID: 200–250 mg once daily. **PT TAKING EIAED WITHOUT VALPROIC ACID:** 400–600 mg once daily. **PT NOT TAKING EIAED:** 300–400 mg once daily.

✦ Canadian trade name   **◥** Non-Crushable Drug   **▦** High Alert drug

Conversion to Monotherapy for Pts Receiving EIAEDs
PO: ADULTS, ELDERLY, CHILDREN 16 YRS AND OLDER: 500 mg/day in 2 divided doses. Titrate to desired dose while maintaining EIAED at fixed level, then withdraw EIAED by 20% each wk over a 4-wk period.

Conversion to Monotherapy for Pts Receiving Valproic Acid
PO: ADULTS, ELDERLY, CHILDREN 16 YRS AND OLDER: Titrate lamoTRIgine to 200 mg/day, maintaining valproic acid dose. Maintain lamoTRIgine dose and decrease valproic acid to 500 mg/day, no greater than 500 mg/day, then maintain 500 mg/day for 1 wk. Increase lamoTRIgine to 300 mg/day and decrease valproic acid to 250 mg/day. Maintain for 1 wk, then discontinue valproic acid and increase lamoTRIgine by 100 mg/day each wk until maintenance dose of 500 mg/day reached.

Bipolar Disorder
PO: ADULTS, ELDERLY: Initially, 25 mg/day for 2 wks, then 50 mg/day for 2 wks, then 100 mg/day for 1 wk, then 200 mg/day beginning with wk 6.

Bipolar Disorder in Pts Receiving EIAEDs
PO: ADULTS, ELDERLY: 50 mg/day for 2 wks, then 100 mg/day for 2 wks, then 200 mg/day for 1 wk, then 300 mg/day for 1 wk, then up to usual maintenance dose 400 mg/day in divided doses.

Bipolar Disorder in Pts Receiving Valproic Acid
PO: ADULTS, ELDERLY: 25 mg/day every other day for 2 wks, then 25 mg/day for 2 wks, then 50 mg/day for 1 wk, then 100 mg/day. **Usual maintenance dose with valproic acid:** 100 mg/day.

Usual Dosage for LaMICtal XR
Adjunct Therapy: Range: 200–600 mg/day.
Conversion to Monotherapy: Range: 250–500 mg/day.

Discontinuation Therapy
◀**ALERT**▶ A dosage reduction of approximately 50%/wk over at least 2 wks is recommended.

Dosage in Renal Impairment
◀**ALERT**▶ Decreased dosage may be effective in pts with significant renal impairment.

Dosage in Hepatic Impairment
Mild impairment: No dose adjustment. **Moderate to severe impairment without ascites:** Reduce dose by 25%. **Severe impairment with ascites:** Reduce dose by 50%.

SIDE EFFECTS

Frequent (38%–14%): Dizziness, headache, diplopia, ataxia, nausea, blurred vision, drowsiness, rhinitis. **Occasional (10%–5%):** Rash, pharyngitis, vomiting, cough, flu-like symptoms, diarrhea, dysmenorrhea, fever, insomnia, dyspepsia. **Rare:** Constipation, tremor, anxiety, pruritus, vaginitis, hypersensitivity reaction.

ADVERSE EFFECTS/TOXIC REACTIONS

Abrupt withdrawal may increase seizure frequency. Serious rashes, including Stevens-Johnson syndrome, have been reported. May increase risk of suicidal thoughts and behavior.

NURSING CONSIDERATIONS

BASELINE ASSESSMENT

Review history of seizure disorder (type, onset, intensity, frequency, duration, LOC), medication history (esp. other anticonvulsants), other medical conditions (e.g., renal impairment). Initiate seizure precautions. Assess baseline mood, behavior. Question history of suicidal thought and behavior.

INTERVENTION/EVALUATION

Report occurrence of rash (drug discontinuation may be necessary). Assist with ambulation if dizziness, ataxia occurs. Assess for clinical improvement (decreased intensity/frequency of seizures). Assess for visual abnormalities, headache. Monitor for suicidal ideation, depression, behavioral changes.

PATIENT/ FAMILY TEACHING

• Take medication only as prescribed; do not abruptly discontinue medication after long-term therapy. • Avoid alcohol. • Avoid tasks that require alertness, motor skills until response to drug is established. • Carry identification card/bracelet to note anticonvulsant therapy. • Strict maintenance of drug therapy is essential for seizure control. • Report any rash, fever, swelling of glands, worsening depression, suicidal ideation, unusual changes in behavior, worsening of seizure control. • May cause photosensitivity reaction; avoid exposure to sunlight, ultraviolet light.

---

lansoprazole

lan-**soe**-pra-zole
(Apo-Lansoprazole ♣, First Lansoprazole, Prevacid, Prevacid Solu-Tab, Prevacid 24HR)
Do not confuse lansoprazole with ARIPiprazole or dexlansoprazole, or Prevacid with Pravachol, PriLOSEC, or Prinivil.

FIXED-COMBINATION(S)

Prevacid NapraPac: lansoprazole/naproxen (an NSAID): 15 mg/375 mg, 15 mg/500 mg. **Prevpac:** Combination card containing amoxicillin 500 mg (4 capsules), lansoprazole 30 mg (2 capsules), clarithromycin 500 mg (2 tablets).

◆CLASSIFICATION

PHARMACOTHERAPEUTIC: Proton pump inhibitor. **CLINICAL:** Antiulcer agent.

USES

Short-term treatment (4 wks and less) of healing, symptomatic relief of active duodenal ulcer; short-term treatment (8 wks and less) for healing, symptomatic relief of erosive esophagitis. Long-term treatment of pathologic hypersecretory conditions, including Zollinger-Ellison syndrome. Short-term treatment (8 wks and less) of active benign gastric ulcer, *H. pylori*–associated duodenal ulcer (part of multidrug regimen), maintenance treatment for healed duodenal ulcer. Treatment of gastroesophageal reflux disease (GERD), NSAID-associated gastric ulcer. Reduce risk of NSAID-associated gastric ulcer in pts with history of gastric ulcer requiring NSAIDs. **OTC:** Relief of frequent heartburn (2 or more days/wk). **IV:** Short-term treatment of erosive esophagitis. **OFF-LABEL:** Stress ulcer prophylaxis in critically ill.

PRECAUTIONS

Contraindications: Hypersensitivity to lansoprazole, other proton pump inhibitors. **Cautions:** Hepatic impairment. May increase risk of hip, wrist, spine fractures; GI infections.

ACTION

Inhibits the (H^+, K^+)–ATPase enzyme system, blocking the final step in gastric acid secretion. **Therapeutic Effect:** Suppresses gastric acid secretion.

PHARMACOKINETICS

Rapid, complete absorption (food may decrease absorption) once drug has left stomach. Protein binding: 97%. Distributed primarily to gastric parietal cells. Metabolized in liver. Excreted in bile and urine. Not removed by hemodialysis. **Half-life:** 1.5 hrs (increased in hepatic impairment, elderly).

⌛ LIFESPAN CONSIDERATIONS

Pregnancy/Lactation: Unknown if distributed in breast milk. **Children:** Safety and efficacy not established. **Elderly:** No age-related precautions noted but doses greater than 30 mg not recommended.

INTERACTIONS

DRUG: May decrease concentration of **atazanavir.** May interfere with absorption of

---

ampicillin, digoxin, iron salts, keto-conazole. Sucralfate may delay absorption. May increase effect of warfarin. May decrease effect of clopidogrel. HERBAL: St. John's wort may decrease concentration/effect. FOOD: Food may decrease absorption. LAB VALUES: May increase serum LDH, alkaline phosphatase, bilirubin, cholesterol, creatinine, ALT, AST, triglycerides, uric acid; Hgb, Hct. May produce abnormal albumin/globulin ratio, electrolyte balance, platelet, RBC, WBC count.

AVAILABILITY (Rx)

Tablets, Orally Disintegrating (Prevacid Solu-Tab): 15 mg, 30 mg. Powder for Oral Suspension (First Lansoprazole): 3 mg/mL.

🖎 Capsules (Delayed-Release): (Prevacid): 15 mg, 30 mg. (Prevacid 24HR): 15 mg.

ADMINISTRATION/HANDLING

PO

• Best if taken before breakfast • Do not cut/crush delayed-release capsules. • If pt has difficulty swallowing capsules, open capsules, sprinkle granules on 1 tbsp of applesauce, give immediately. Do not crush or allow pt to chew granules.

PO (Solu-Tab)

• Place tablet on tongue; allow to dissolve, then swallow. • May give via oral syringe or nasogastric tube. • May dissolve in 4 mL (15 mg) or 10 mL (30 mg) water.

INDICATIONS/ROUTES/DOSAGE

Duodenal Ulcer

PO: ADULTS, ELDERLY: 15 mg/day, for up to 4 wks. Maintenance: 15 mg/day.

Erosive Esophagitis

PO: ADULTS, ELDERLY: 30 mg/day, for up to 8 wks. If healing does not occur within 8 wks (in 5%–10% of cases), may give for additional 8 wks. Maintenance: 15 mg/day. CHILDREN 1–11 YRS, WEIGHING GREATER THAN 30 KG: 30 mg/day for up to 12 wks; WEIGHING 30 KG OR LESS: 15 mg/day for up to 12 wks.

Gastric Ulcer

PO: ADULTS: 30 mg/day for up to 8 wks.

NSAID Gastric Ulcer

PO: ADULTS, ELDERLY: (Healing): 30 mg/day for up to 8 wks. (Prevention): 15 mg/day for up to 12 wks.

Gastroesophageal Reflux Disease (GERD)

PO: ADULTS: 15 mg/day for up to 8 wks. CHILDREN 12–17 YRS: 30 mg/day up to 8 wks. CHILDREN 1–11 YRS, WEIGHING GREATER THAN 30 KG: 30 mg/day for up to 8 wks; WEIGHING 30 KG OR LESS: 15 mg/day for up to 8 wks.

H. Pylori Infection

PO: ADULTS, ELDERLY: (triple drug therapy including amoxicillin, clarithromycin) 30 mg q12h for 10–14 days or (with amoxicillin) 30 mg 3 times/day for 14 days.

Pathologic Hypersecretory Conditions (Including Zollinger-Ellison Syndrome)

PO: ADULTS, ELDERLY: Initially, 60 mg/day. Individualize dosage according to pt needs and for as long as clinically indicated. Administer doses greater than 120 mg/day in divided doses.

Heartburn (OTC)

PO: ADULTS, ELDERLY: 15 mg once daily for 14 days. May repeat q4mos.

Dosage in Renal Impairment

No dose adjustment.

Dosage in Hepatic Impairment

Consider dose reduction in severe impairment.

SIDE EFFECTS

Occasional (3%–2%): Diarrhea, abdominal pain, rash, pruritus, altered appetite. Rare (1%): Nausea, headache.

ADVERSE EFFECTS/TOXIC REACTIONS

Bilirubinemia, eosinophilia, hyperlipidemia occur rarely. May increase risk of C. difficile infection. Chronic use may increase risk of osteoporosis, fractures.

L

NURSING CONSIDERATIONS

BASELINE ASSESSMENT

Obtain baseline lab values. Assess for epigastric/abdominal pain, evidence of GI bleeding, ecchymosis.

INTERVENTION/EVALUATION

Monitor CBC, hepatic/renal function tests. Assess for therapeutic response (relief of GI symptoms). Question if diarrhea, abdominal pain, nausea occurs. Obtain *C. difficile* PCR test in pts with persistent diarrhea, fever, abdominal pain.

PATIENT/ FAMILY TEACHING

• Do not chew, crush delayed-release capsules. • For pts who have difficulty swallowing capsules, open capsules, sprinkle granules on 1 tbsp of applesauce, swallow immediately.

lapatinib

la-**pa**-tin-ib
(Tykerb)

■ **BLACK BOX ALERT** ■ Hepatotoxicity (serum ALT or AST more than 3 times upper limit of normal [ULN] and total bilirubin more than 2 times ULN), possibly severe, has occurred. **Do not confuse lapatinib with dasatinib, erlotinib, or imatinib.**

◆CLASSIFICATION

PHARMACOTHERAPEUTIC: Tyrosine kinase inhibitor. **CLINICAL:** Antineoplastic.

USES

Combination treatment with capecitabine for the treatment of human epidermal growth receptor type 2 (HER2)–overexpressing advanced or metastatic breast cancer in pts who have received prior therapy including an anthracycline, a taxane, and trastuzumab. Combination treatment with letrozole for treatment of postmenopausal women with *HER2*-overexpressing hormone receptor–positive metastatic breast cancer for whom hormonal therapy is indicated. **OFF-LABEL:** Treatment (in combination with trastuzumab) of *HER2*-overexpressing metastatic breast cancer that progressed on prior trastuzumab-containing therapy. Treatment of *HER2*-overexpressing metastatic breast cancer with brain metastasis.

PRECAUTIONS

Contraindications: Hypersensitivity to lapatinib. **Cautions:** Left ventricular function abnormalities, prolonged QT interval or medications known to prolong QT interval, hepatic impairment. History of treatment with anthracyclines, chest wall irradiation. Avoid concurrent use with strong CYP3A4 inhibitors or inducers.

ACTION

Inhibitory action against kinases targeting intracellular components of epidermal growth factor receptor ErbB1 and a second receptor, human epidermal receptor (HER2 [ErbB2]). **Therapeutic Effect:** Inhibits tumor cell growth and metastasis.

PHARMACOKINETICS

Route	Onset	Peak	Duration
PO	30 min	4 hrs	—

Steady-state level reached within 6–7 days. Incomplete and variable oral absorption. Undergoes extensive metabolism. Protein binding: 99%. Minimally excreted in feces and plasma. **Half-life:** 24 hrs.

⧗ LIFESPAN CONSIDERATIONS

Pregnancy/Lactation: May cause fetal harm. Unknown if distributed in breast milk. **Children:** Safety and efficacy not established. **Elderly:** No age-related precautions noted.

INTERACTIONS

DRUG: QT interval–prolonging medications (e.g., amiodarone, azithromycin, ceritinib, haloperidol, moxifloxacin) may increase risk of QT interval prolongation, cardiac arrhythmias. May increase **digoxin** levels. **CYP3A4 inhibitors** (e.g., **clarithromycin, ketoconazole, ritonavir**) may increase plasma concentration. **CYP3A4 inducers** (e.g., **carBAMazepine, phenytoin, rifAMPin**) may decrease plasma concentration. **HERBAL: St. John's wort** decreases plasma concentration. **FOOD: Grapefruit products** may increase plasma concentration (potential for torsades, myelotoxicity). **LAB VALUES:** May increase serum ALT, AST, bilirubin. May decrease neutrophils, Hgb, platelets.

AVAILABILITY (Rx)

Tablets: 250 mg.

ADMINISTRATION/HANDLING

PO

• Do not break, crush, dissolve, or divide film-coated tablets. • Give at least 1 hr before or 1 hr after food. Take full dose at same time each day.

INDICATIONS/ROUTES/DOSAGE

Breast Cancer

PO: ADULTS, ELDERLY: (With capecitabine): 1,250 mg (5 tablets) once daily. **(With letrozole):** 1,500 mg once daily continuously with letrozole. Continue until disease progresses or unacceptable toxicity.

Dose Modification
Cardiac Toxicity

Discontinue with decreased left ventricular ejection fraction grade 2 or higher, or in pts with an ejection fraction that drops to lower limit of normal. May be started at a reduced dose (1,000 mg/day) at a minimum of 2 wks when ejection fraction returns to normal and pt is asymptomatic.

Pulmonary Toxicity

Discontinue with symptoms indicative of interstitial lung disease or pneumonitis grade 3 or higher.

Severe Hepatic Impairment

With capecitabine: 750 mg/day. **With letrozole:** 1,000 mg/day.

CYP3A4 Inhibitors/Inducers

Concomitant use of CYP3A4 inhibitors may require dose reduction of lapatinib (e.g., decrease to 500 mg/day with careful monitoring); CYP3A4 inducers may require dose increase of lapatinib (e.g., increase to 4,500 mg with capecitabine or 5,500 mg with letrozole).

Dosage in Renal Impairment

No dose adjustment.

Dosage in Hepatic Impairment

Mild to moderate impairment: No dose adjustment. **Severe impairment:** See dose modification.

SIDE EFFECTS

Common (65%–44%): Diarrhea, hand-foot syndrome (blistering/rash/peeling of skin on palms of hands, soles of feet), nausea. **Frequent (28%–26%):** Rash, vomiting. **Occasional (15%–10%):** Mucosal inflammation, stomatitis, extremity pain, back pain, dry skin, insomnia.

ADVERSE EFFECTS/TOXIC REACTIONS

Decreases in left ventricular ejection grade 3 or higher have been observed; 20% decrease relative to baseline is considered toxic.

NURSING CONSIDERATIONS

BASELINE ASSESSMENT

Screen for home medications that prolong QT interval. Obtain baseline EKG. Question for possibility of pregnancy. Obtain baseline CBC, serum chemistries before treatment begins and monthly thereafter.

INTERVENTION/EVALUATION

Offer antiemetics to control nausea, vomiting. Monitor daily pattern of bowel activity, stool consistency. Monitor CBC (particularly Hgb, platelets, neutrophil count), LFT. Assess hands and feet for erythema/blistering/peeling. Monitor for shortness of breath, palpitations, fatigue (decreased cardiac ejection fraction). Monitor ECG for QT prolongation. Obtain CXR if pneumonitis suspected.

PATIENT/FAMILY TEACHING

• Avoid crowds, those with known infection. • Avoid contact with those who recently received live virus vaccine. • Do not have immunizations without physician's approval (drug lowers resistance). • Promptly report fever, unusual bruising/bleeding from any site. • Ensure use of appropriate birth control measures in women. • Treatment may cause severe lung inflammation; report shortness of breath, severe cough, lung pain. • Report liver problems such as upper abdominal pain, bleeding, dark or amber-colored urine, nausea, vomiting, or yellowing of the skin or eyes.

ledipasvir/sofosbuvir

le-**dip**-as-vir/soe-**fos**-bue-vir
(Harvoni)

■ **BLACK BOX ALERT** ■ Test all pts for hepatitis B virus (HBV) infection prior to initiation. HBV reactivation was reported in HCV/HBV co-infected pts who were undergoing or had completed treatment with HCV direct-acting antivirals and were not receiving HBV antiviral therapy. HBV reactivation may cause fulminant hepatitis, hepatic failure, and death.

Do not confuse ledipasvir with daclatasvir, elbasvir, or ombitasvir, or sofosbuvir with dasabuvir.

◆CLASSIFICATION

PHARMACOTHERAPEUTIC: Combination nucleotide analog NS5A inhibitor and nucleotide analog NS5B polymerase inhibitor. **CLINICAL:** Antihepacvirus.

USES

Treatment of chronic hepatitis C virus (HCV) in adults and children 12 yrs and older or weighing at least 35 kg with genotype 1, 4, 5, or 6 infection without cirrhosis or with compensated cirrhosis; genotype 1 infection in adults with decompensated cirrhosis, in combination with ribavirin; genotype 1 or 4 infection in adults who are liver transplant recipients without cirrhosis or with compensated cirrhosis, in combination with ribavirin. Treatment in pediatric pts 12 yrs and older and weighing at least 35 kg with HCV genotype 1, 4, 5, or 6 infection without cirrhosis or with compensated cirrhosis.

PRECAUTIONS

Note: If used with ribavirin, the Contraindications and Cautions for the use of ribavirin also apply.
Contraindications: Hypersensitivity to ledipasvir, sofosbuvir. **Cautions:** Advanced hepatic disease, HIV infection, hepatitis B virus infection. Concomitant use of amiodarone (with or without beta blockers) in pts with underlying cardiac disease. Concomitant use of P-glycoprotein (P-gp) inducers not recommended.

ACTION

Ledipasvir inhibits HCV NS5A protein, essential for viral replication. Sofosbuvir is converted to its active form and inhibits NS5B RNA-dependent RNA polymerase, also essential for viral replication. **Therapeutic Effect:** Inhibits viral replication of HCV.

PHARMACOKINETICS

Widely absorbed. Ledipasvir is metabolized by oxidative processes. Sofosbuvir is metabolized in liver. Protein binding: 99.8% (ledipasvir), 61%–65% (sofosbuvir). Peak plasma concentration: 4–4.5 hrs (ledipasvir), 0.8–1 hr (sofosbuvir). Ledipasvir is excreted in feces (87%) and urine (1%). Sofosbuvir is excreted in urine (80%), feces (14%). **Half-life:** 47 hrs (ledipasvir), 0.4 hr (sofosbuvir).

L

☒ LIFESPAN CONSIDERATIONS

Pregnancy/Lactation: Unknown if ledipasvir or sofosbuvir is distributed in breast milk. When administered with ribavirin, therapy is contraindicated in pregnant women and in men whose female partners are pregnant. **Children:** Safety and efficacy not established in pts younger than 12 yrs of age or weight less than 35 kg. **Elderly:** No age-related precautions noted.

INTERACTIONS

DRUG: May enhance bradycardic effect of **amiodarone**. May increase concentration of **rosuvastatin**. Aluminum- or magnesium-containing antacids, H₂-receptor antagonists (e.g., famotidine), proton pump inhibitors (e.g., omeprazole), anticonvulsants (e.g., carBAMazepine), antimycobacterials (e.g., rifAMPin) may decrease concentration/effects. **HERBAL:** None significant. **FOOD:** None known. **LAB VALUES:** May increase serum bilirubin.

AVAILABILITY (Rx)

Tablets (Fixed-Dose Combination): 90 mg (ledipasvir)/400 mg (sofosbuvir).

ADMINISTRATION/HANDLING

PO

• Give with or without food.

INDICATIONS/ROUTES/DOSAGE

Hepatitis C Virus Infection
PO: ADULTS, ELDERLY, CHILDREN 12 YRS OF AGE AND OLDER WHO WEIGH AT LEAST 35 KG: 1 tablet (ledipasvir/sofosbuvir) once daily. See manufacturer guidelines for treatment with ribavirin.

Treatment Regimen and Duration for Adults
Genotype 1
Treatment-naïve without cirrhosis or with compensated cirrhosis (Child-Pugh A): Ledipasvir/sofosbuvir for 12 wks. Treatment for 8 wks may be considered in treatment-naïve genotype 1 pts without cirrhosis who have HCV-RNA level less than 6 million international units/mL prior to initiation. **Treatment-experienced without cirrhosis:** Ledipasvir/sofosbuvir for 12 wks. **Treatment-experienced with compensated cirrhosis (Child-Pugh A):** Ledipasvir/sofosbuvir for 24 wks. Ledipasvir/sofosbuvir plus ribavirin for 12 wks may be considered in treatment-experienced genotype 1 pts with cirrhosis who are eligible for ribavirin. **Treatment-naïve and treatment-experienced with decompensated cirrhosis (Child-Pugh B or C):** Ledipasvir/sofosbuvir plus ribavirin for 12 wks.

Genotype 1 or 4
Treatment-naïve and treatment-experienced liver transplant recipients without cirrhosis or with compensated cirrhosis (Child-Pugh A): Ledipasvir/sofosbuvir plus ribavirin for 12 wks.

Treatment Regimen and Duration for Children
Genotype 1
Treatment-naïve without cirrhosis or with compensated cirrhosis (Child-Pugh A): Ledipasvir/sofosbuvir for 12 wks. **Treatment-experienced without cirrhosis:** Ledipasvir/sofosbuvir for 12 wks. **Treatment-experienced with compensated cirrhosis (Child-Pugh A):** Ledipasvir/sofosbuvir for 24 wks.
Genotype 4, 5, or 6
Treatment-naïve and treatment-experienced without cirrhosis or with compensated cirrhosis (Child-Pugh A): Ledipasvir/sofosbuvir for 12 wks.

Dosage in Renal Impairment
Mild to moderate impairment: No dose adjustment. **Severe impairment:** Not specified; use caution.

Dosage in Hepatic Impairment
No dose adjustment.

SIDE EFFECTS

Occasional (16%–4%): Fatigue, headache, nausea, diarrhea. **Rare (3%):** Insomnia. **(Treatment with ribavirin):** **Frequent (31%–29%):** Asthenia, headache.

Occasional (18%–5%): Fatigue, myalgia, irritability, dizziness. Rare (3%): Dyspnea.

ADVERSE EFFECTS/TOXIC REACTIONS

HBV reactivation was reported in pts co-infected with HBV/HCV; may result in fulminant hepatitis, hepatic failure, death. Cardiac arrest, symptomatic bradycardia, pacemaker implantation was reported in pts taking concomitant amiodarone. Bradycardia usually occurred within hrs to days, but may occur up to 2 wks after initiation. Pts with underlying cardiac disease, advanced hepatic disease, or pts taking concomitant beta blockers are at an increased risk for bradycardia when used concomitantly with amiodarone. Psychiatric disorders including depression may occur.

NURSING CONSIDERATIONS

BASELINE ASSESSMENT

Obtain LFT, HCV-RNA level; pregnancy test in females of reproductive potential; CBC for pts treated with ribavirin. Confirm HCV genotype. Test all pts for HBV infection prior to initiation. Receive full medication history and screen for contraindications/interactions, esp. concomitant use of amiodarone. Question for history of chronic anemia, HBV infection, HIV infection, liver transplantation.

INTERVENTION/EVALUATION

Periodically monitor LFT, HCV-RNA level for treatment effectiveness. Closely monitor for exacerbation of hepatitis or HBV reactivation. If unable to discontinue amiodarone, consider inpatient cardiac monitoring for at least 48 hrs, followed by outpatient or self-monitoring of heart rate for at least 2 wks after initiation. Cardiac monitoring is also recommended in pts who discontinue amiodarone just prior to initiation. In females of reproductive potential who are taking concomitant ribavirin, reinforce birth control compliance and obtain monthly pregnancy tests. Monitor for new-onset or worsening of depression

PATIENT/FAMILY TEACHING

• Pts who take amiodarone (an antiarrhythmic) during therapy may require inpatient and outpatient cardiac monitoring (and in some cases pacemaker implantation) due to an increased risk of slow heart rate or cardiac arrest. If amiodarone therapy cannot be withheld or stopped, immediately report symptoms of slow heart rate such as chest pain, confusion, dizziness, fainting, light-headedness, memory problems, palpitations, weakness. • Treatment may be used in combination with ribavirin (inform pt of contraindications/adverse effects of ribavirin therapy). If therapy includes treatment with ribavirin, females of reproductive potential and males with female partners of reproductive potential should avoid pregnancy during treatment. • Do not breastfeed. • There is an increased risk of drug interactions with other medications. • Do not take newly prescribed medications unless approved by prescriber who originally started treatment. • Do not take herbal products. • Avoid alcohol. • Report signs of depression.

leflunomide

lee-**floo**-noe-myde
(Apo-Leflunomide ✦, Arava)

■ **BLACK BOX ALERT** ■ Do not use during pregnancy. Women of childbearing potential must be counseled regarding fetal risk, use of reliable contraceptives confirmed, possibility of pregnancy excluded. Severe hepatic injury may occur.

◆CLASSIFICATION

PHARMACOTHERAPEUTIC: Immunomodulatory agent. **CLINICAL:** Antiinflammatory, antirheumatic.

USES

Treatment of active rheumatoid arthritis (RA). Improve physical function in pts with rheumatoid arthritis. **OFF-LABEL:** Treatment of cytomegalovirus (CMV) disease. Prevention of acute/chronic rejection in recipients of solid organ transplants.

PRECAUTIONS

Contraindications: Hypersensitivity to leflunomide. Pregnancy or plans for pregnancy. Severe hepatic impairment. **Cautions:** Hepatic/renal impairment, hepatitis B or C virus infection, pts with immunodeficiency or bone marrow dysplasias, breastfeeding mothers, history of new/recurrent infections, latent TB, significant hematologic abnormalities, diabetes, concomitant use of neurotoxic medications, elderly pts.

ACTION

Inhibits pyrimidine synthesis, resulting in antiproliferative and anti-inflammatory effects. **Therapeutic Effect:** Reduces signs/symptoms of RA, retards structural damage.

PHARMACOKINETICS

Well absorbed after PO administration. Protein binding: greater than 99%. Metabolized in GI wall, liver. Excreted through renal, biliary systems. Not removed by hemodialysis. **Half-life:** 16 days.

⧖ LIFESPAN CONSIDERATIONS

Pregnancy/Lactation: Can cause fetal harm. Contraindicated in pregnancy. Unknown if distributed in breast milk. Breastfeeding not recommended. **Children:** Safety and efficacy not established in pts younger than 18 yrs. **Elderly:** No age-related precautions noted.

INTERACTIONS

DRUG: RifAMPin may increase concentration/effects. **Hepatotoxic medications (e.g., acetaminophen, ketoconazole, simvastatin)** may increase risk of side effects, hepatotoxicity. Use of **live virus vaccine** not recommended. **HERBAL: Echinacea** may decrease

effects. **FOOD:** None known. **LAB VALUES:** May increase serum ALT, AST, alkaline phosphatase, bilirubin.

AVAILABILITY (Rx)

Tablets: 10 mg, 20 mg.

ADMINISTRATION/HANDLING

PO
• Give without regard to food.

INDICATIONS/ROUTES/DOSAGE

Rheumatoid Arthritis (RA)
PO: ADULTS, ELDERLY: Initially, 100 mg/day for 3 days, then 10–20 mg/day. (Loading dose may be omitted in pts at increased risk of hepatitis or toxicity.)

Dosage in Renal Impairment
No dose adjustment.

Dosage in Hepatic Impairment
ALT 2–3 Times Upper Limit of Normal (ULN): Not recommended. **Persistent ALT Level Greater Than 3 Times ULN:** Discontinue and initiate accelerated drug elimination. Cholestyramine 8 g 3 times/day for 11 days or activated charcoal 50 g q12h for 11 days.

SIDE EFFECTS

Frequent (20%–10%): Diarrhea, respiratory tract infection, alopecia, rash, nausea.

ADVERSE EFFECTS/TOXIC REACTIONS

May cause immunosuppression. Transient thrombocytopenia, leukopenia, hepatotoxicity occur rarely. Interstitial lung disease, peripheral neuropathy.

NURSING CONSIDERATIONS

BASELINE ASSESSMENT

Obtain pregnancy test in females or reproductive potential. Question plans of breastfeeding. Obtain baseline CBC, LFT. Assess limitations in activities of daily living due to rheumatoid arthritis (RA). Obtain baseline evaluation for active TB, latent TB.

INTERVENTION/EVALUATION

Monitor tolerance to medication. Assess symptomatic relief of RA (relief of pain; improved range of motion, grip strength, mobility). Monitor LFT, CBC, signs/symptoms of severe infection or pulmonary symptoms.

PATIENT/FAMILY TEACHING

• May take without regard to food. • Improvement may take longer than 8 wks. • Avoid pregnancy.

lenalidomide

len-a-**lid**-o-myde
(Revlimid)

■ **BLACK BOX ALERT** ■ Analogue to thalidomide. High potential for significant birth defects. Hematologic toxicity (thrombocytopenia, neutropenia) occurs in 80% of pts. Greatly increases risk for DVT, pulmonary embolism in multiple myeloma pts.
Do not confuse lenalidomide with thalidomide.

◆CLASSIFICATION

PHARMACOTHERAPEUTIC: Isoxazole immunomodulator. **CLINICAL:** Immunosuppressive agent.

USES

Treatment of low- to intermediate-risk myelodysplastic syndrome (MDS) in pts with deletion 5q cytogenetic abnormality with transfusion-dependent anemia. Treatment of multiple myeloma (in combination with dexamethasone). Treatment of pts with mantle cell lymphoma that has relapsed or progressed after 2 prior therapies (one of which included bortezomib). Maintenance treatment for multiple myeloma (following autologous stem cell transplant). **OFF-LABEL:** Systemic amyloidosis, lower-risk myelodysplastic syndrome, non-Hodgkin's lymphoma. Relapsed or refractory chronic lymphocytic leukemia (CLL).

PRECAUTIONS

Contraindications: Hypersensitivity to lenalidomide. Pregnancy, women capable of becoming pregnant. **Cautions:** Renal/hepatic impairment. History of arterial thromboembolic events, hypertension, hyperlipidemia. Avoid use in pts with glucose intolerance, lactase deficiency.

ACTION

Inhibits secretion of pro-inflammatory cytokines, increases secretion of anti-inflammatory cytokines. Enhances cell-mediated immunity by stimulation of T cells. **Therapeutic Effect:** Inhibits myeloma cell growth; induces cell cycle arrest and cell death.

PHARMACOKINETICS

Well absorbed following PO administration. Protein binding: 30%. Excreted in urine. **Half-life:** 3 hrs (increased in renal impairment).

⧗ LIFESPAN CONSIDERATIONS

Pregnancy/Lactation: Contraindicated in women who are or may become pregnant, who are not using two reliable forms of contraception, or who are not abstinent. Can cause severe birth defects, fetal death. Unknown if distributed in breast milk; breastfeeding not recommended. **Children:** Safety and efficacy not established in pts younger than 18 yrs. **Elderly:** Age-related renal impairment may require caution in dosage selection. Risk of toxic reactions greater in those with renal insufficiency.

INTERACTIONS

DRUG: May increase toxic effects of **abatacept, anakinra, bisphosphonate derivatives, canakinumab, cloZAPine, leflunomide, natalizumab, nivolumab, rilonacept, tofacitinib, vedolizumab**. May increase immunosuppressive effects of **certolizumab, fingolimod, ocrelizumab**. May increase neutropenic effect of **deferiprone, cloZAPine. Denosumab, dipyrone, pimecrolimus** may increase risk of toxicity. May decrease therapeutic effect of **nivolumab. Dexamethasone,**

erythropoiesis-stimulating agents, estrogens may increase risk of thrombosis. Ocrelizumab, roflumilast, tocilizumab may increase immunosuppressive effects. May increase concentration effect of digoxin. May increase toxic effect of live vaccines; may diminish therapeutic effect of vaccines. HERBAL: Avoid echinacea (has immunostimulant properties). FOOD: None known. LAB VALUES: May decrease WBC count, Hgb, Hct platelets, troponin I, serum creatinine, sodium, T_3, T_4. May decrease serum bilirubin, glucose, potassium, magnesium.

AVAILABILITY (Rx)

Capsules: 2.5 mg, 5 mg, 10 mg, 15 mg, 25 mg.

ADMINISTRATION/HANDLING

• Store at room temperature. • Do not break, crush, dissolve, or divide capsules. • Swallow whole with water.

INDICATIONS/ROUTES/DOSAGE

Myelodysplastic Syndrome
PO: ADULTS, ELDERLY: 10 mg once daily.

Dosage Adjustments for Myelodysplastic Syndrome
Platelets:
Thrombocytopenia within 4 wks with 10 mg/day
Baseline platelets 100,000 cells/mm³ or greater: If platelets less than 50,000 cells/mm³, hold treatment. Resume at 5 mg/day when platelets return to 50,000 cells/mm³ or greater. **Baseline platelets less than 100,000 cells/mm³:** If platelets fall to 50% of baseline, hold treatment. Resume at 5 mg/day if baseline is 60,000 cells/mm³ or greater and platelets return to 50,000 cells/mm³ or greater. Resume at 5 mg/day if baseline is less than 60,000 cells/mm³ and platelets return to 30,000 cells/mm³ or greater.
Thrombocytopenia after 4 wks with 10 mg/day: If platelets less than 30,000 cells/mm³ OR less than 50,000 cells/mm³ with platelet transfusion, hold treatment.

Resume at 5 mg/day when platelets return to 30,000 cells/mm³ or greater.
Thrombocytopenia developing with 5 mg/day: If platelets less than 30,000 cells/mm³ OR less than 50,000 cells/mm³ with platelet transfusion, hold treatment. Resume at 5 mg every other day when platelets return to 30,000 cells/mm³ or greater.
Neutrophils:
Neutropenia within 4 wks with 10 mg/day
Baseline absolute neutrophil count (ANC) 1,000/mcl or greater: If ANC less than 750 cells/mm³, hold treatment. Resume at 5 mg/day when ANC 1,000 cells/mm³ or greater. **Baseline ANC less than 1,000 cells/mm³:** If ANC less than 500 cells/mm³, hold treatment. Resume at 5 mg/day when ANC 500 cells/mm³ or greater.
Neutropenia after 4 wks with 10 mg/day: If ANC less than 500 cells/mm³ for 7 days or longer or associated with fever, hold treatment. Resume at 5 mg/day when ANC 500 cells/mm³ or greater.
Neutropenia developing with 5 mg/day: If ANC less than 500 cells/mm³ for 7 days or longer or associated with fever, hold treatment. Resume at 5 mg every other day when ANC 500 cells/mm³ or greater.

Mantle Cell Lymphoma
PO: ADULTS, ELDERLY: 25 mg once daily on days 1–21 of repeated 28-day cycle. Continue until disease progression or unacceptable toxicity.

Multiple Myeloma
PO: ADULTS, ELDERLY: 25 mg/day on days 1–21 of repeated 28-day cycle (in combination with dexamethasone). Continue until disease progression or unacceptable toxicity.

Multiple Myeloma following auto-HSCT
PO: ADULTS, ELDERLY: 10 mg once daily continuously on days 1–28 of repeated 28-day cycle.

Dosage Adjustments for Multiple Myeloma
Platelets:
Thrombocytopenia: If platelets fall to less than 30,000 cells/mm³, hold treatment, monitor CBC. Resume at 15 mg/day

L

when platelets 30,000 cells/mm^3 or greater. For each subsequent fall to less than 30,000 cells/mm^3, hold treatment and resume at 5 mg/day less than previous dose when platelets return to 30,000 cells/mm^3 or greater. Do not dose to less than 5 mg/day.

Neutrophils:

Neutropenia: If neutrophils fall to less than 1,000 cells/mm^3, hold treatment, add G-CSF, follow CBC wkly. Resume at 25 mg/day when neutrophils return to 1,000 cells/mm^3 and neutropenia is the only toxicity. Resume at 15 mg/day if other toxicity is present. For each subsequent fall to less than 1,000 cells/mm^3, hold treatment and resume at 5 mg/day less than previous dose when neutrophils return to 1,000 cells/mm^3 or greater. Do not dose to less than 5 mg/day.

Dosage in Renal Impairment

	Creatinine Clearance 30–59 mL/min	Creatinine Clearance Less Than 30 mL/min (Nondialysis Dependent)	Creatinine Clearance Less Than 30 mL/min (Dialysis Dependent)
Myelodysplastic syndrome	5 mg once daily	2.5 mg once daily	2.5 mg once daily (give after dialysis)
Multiple myeloma	10 mg once daily	15 mg q48h	5 mg once daily (give after dialysis)

Dosage in Hepatic Impairment
No dose adjustment.

SIDE EFFECTS

Frequent (49%–31%): Diarrhea, pruritus, rash, fatigue. **Occasional (24%–12%):** Constipation, nausea, arthralgia, fever, back pain, peripheral edema, cough, dizziness, headache, muscle cramps, epistaxis, asthenia, dry skin, abdominal pain. **Rare (10%–5%):** Extremity pain, vomiting, generalized edema, anorexia, insomnia, night sweats, myalgia, dry mouth, ecchymosis, rigors, depression, dysgeusia, palpitations.

ADVERSE EFFECTS/TOXIC REACTIONS

Significant increased risk of deep vein thrombosis (DVT), pulmonary embolism. Thrombocytopenia occurs in 62% of pts, neutropenia in 59% of pts, and anemia in 12% of pts. Upper respiratory infection (nasopharyngitis, pneumonia, sinusitis, bronchitis, rhinitis), UTI occur occasionally. Cellulitis, peripheral neuropathy, hypertension, hypothyroidism occur in approximately 6% of pts.

NURSING CONSIDERATIONS

L

BASELINE ASSESSMENT

Obtain baseline CBC. Due to high potential for human birth defects/fetal death, female pts must avoid pregnancy 4 wks before therapy, during therapy, during dose interruptions, and 4 wks following therapy. Two reliable forms of contraception must be used even if pt has history of infertility unless it is due to hysterectomy or menopause that has occurred for at least 24 consecutive mos. Confirm two negative pregnancy tests before therapy initiation. Screen for risk of arterial, venous thrombosis. Offer emotional support.

INTERVENTION/EVALUATION

Monitor CBC, BMP, serum magnesium as appropriate. Perform pregnancy tests on women of childbearing potential: wkly during the first 4 wks, then at 4-wk intervals in pts with regular menstrual cycles or q2wks in pts with irregular menstrual cycles. Monitor for hematologic toxicity; obtain CBC wkly during first 8 wks of therapy and at least monthly thereafter. Observe for signs, symptoms of thromboembolism (shortness of breath, chest pain, extremity pain, swelling, stroke-like symptoms).

• Two reliable forms of birth control must be used at least 4 wks before, during, and for 4 wks following therapy. • A pregnancy test must be performed within 10–14 days and 24 hrs before therapy begins. • Males must always use a latex or synthetic condom during any sexual contact with females of childbearing potential even if they have undergone a successful vasectomy. • Avoid crowds; avoid those with active infection. • Treatment may cause blood clots in the arms, legs, or lungs; report arm or leg pain/swelling, difficulty breathing, chest pain.

lenvatinib

len-va-ti-nib
(Lenvima)
Do not confuse lenvatinib with dasatinib, ibrutinib, imatinib.

◆CLASSIFICATION

PHARMACOTHERAPEUTIC: Kinase inhibitor. **CLINICAL:** Antineoplastic.

USES

Treatment of locally recurrent or metastatic, progressive, radioactive iodine–refractory differentiated thyroid cancer. Treatment of advanced renal cell carcinoma (RCC) in combination with everolimus after one course of another antineoplastic.

PRECAUTIONS

Contraindications: Hypersensitivity to lenvatinib. **Cautions:** Electrolyte imbalance (hypokalemia, hypomagnesemia), hepatic/renal impairment. History of cardiac dysfunction (HF, pulmonary edema, right or left ventricular dysfunction), GI perforation/hemorrhage, hypertension, long QT interval syndrome, medications that prolong QT interval, thromboembolic events (e.g., CVA, DVT), pituitary/thyroid disease.

ACTION

Inhibits tyrosine kinase receptor activity of vascular endothelial growth factor (VEGF) receptors. Inhibits tumor angiogenesis, growth, progression. **Therapeutic Effect:** Inhibits tumor cell growth and metastasis.

PHARMACOKINETICS

Readily absorbed. Metabolized in liver. Protein binding: 98%–99%. Peak plasma concentration: 1–4 hrs. Excreted in feces (64%), urine (25%). Not removed by dialysis. **Half-life:** 28 hrs.

☒ LIFESPAN CONSIDERATIONS

Pregnancy/Lactation: Avoid pregnancy; may cause fetal harm. Female pts of reproductive potential must use effective contraception during treatment for at least 2 wks after discontinuation. Potentially distributed in breast milk. Must either discontinue drug or discontinue breastfeeding. Treatment may reduce fertility in both female and male pts. **Children:** Safety and efficacy not established. **Elderly:** No age-related precautions noted.

INTERACTIONS

DRUG: CYP3A4 inhibitors (e.g., ketoconazole, ritonavir) may increase concentration/effect. **CYP3A4 inducers (e.g., carBAMazepine, rifAMPin)** may decrease concentration/effect. **Amiodarone, ciprofloxacin, quiNIDine** may increase risk of QT interval prolongation. **Hormonal contraceptives** may increase risk of thromboembolic events. **HERBAL:** None significant. **FOOD:** None known. **LAB VALUES:** May increase serum alkaline phosphatase, ALT/AST, amylase, bilirubin, cholesterol, creatinine, lipase. May decrease serum albumin, glucose, magnesium; platelets. May increase or decrease serum calcium, potassium.

AVAILABILITY (Rx)

Capsules: 4 mg, 10 mg.

ADMINISTRATION/HANDLING

PO
• Give without regard to food. • Administer same time each day. • Do not cut, crush, divide, or open capsules.

• Should be swallowed whole. May be dissolved with 15 mL water or apple juice by first adding whole capsule to liquid; leave for 10 min, stir for 3 min, then administer. Then add 15 mL to glass, swirl, swallow additional liquid.

INDICATIONS/ROUTES/DOSAGE

Thyroid Cancer
PO: ADULTS, ELDERLY: 24 mg once daily. Continue until disease progression or unacceptable toxicity.

RCC
PO: ADULTS, ELDERLY: 18 mg once daily (in combination with everolimus). Continue until disease progression or unacceptable toxicity.

Dose Modification
Based on Common Terminology Criteria for Adverse Events (CTCAE).

Adverse Reaction	Modification	Adjusted Dose (Thyroid Cancer)
First occurrence	Interrupt until resolved to grade 0 or 1 or baseline	20 mg once daily
Second occurrence	Interrupt until resolved to grade 0 or 1 or baseline	14 mg once daily
Third occurrence	Interrupt until resolved to grade 0 or 1 or baseline	10 mg once daily

Adjusted dose for RCC is lower.

Arterial Thrombotic Event
Discontinue treatment.

Cardiac Dysfunction/Hemorrhagic Event
PO: ADULTS, ELDERLY: Interrupt treatment for grade 3 event until improved to grade 0 to 1 or baseline. Either resume at reduced dose or discontinue (depending on the severity and persistence). Discontinue for grade 4 event.

GI Perforation/Fistula Formation
Discontinue treatment.

Hypertension
PO: ADULTS, ELDERLY: Interrupt treatment for grade 3 hypertension that persists despite optimal antihypertensive therapy. Resume at reduced dose when hypertension is controlled at less than or equal to grade 2. Discontinue for life-threatening hypertension.

Proteinuria
PO: ADULTS, ELDERLY: Interrupt treatment for greater than or equal to 2 g proteinuria/24 hrs. Resume at reduced dose when proteinuria less than 2 g/24 hrs. Discontinue if nephrotic syndrome occurs.

QT Prolongation
PO: ADULTS, ELDERLY: Interrupt treatment for grade 3 or greater. Resume at reduced dose when QT prolongation resolved to grade 0 or 1 or baseline.

Renal Failure/Impairment or Hepatotoxicity
PO: ADULTS, ELDERLY: Interrupt treatment for grade 3 or 4 renal failure/impairment or hepatotoxicity until resolved to grade 0 or 1 or baseline. Either resume at reduced dose or discontinue (depending on the severity and persistence). Discontinue if hepatic failure occurs.

Reversible Posterior Leukoencephalopathy Syndrome (RPLS)
PO: ADULTS, ELDERLY: Interrupt treatment until fully resolved. Resume at reduced dose or discontinue (depending on the severity and persistence of neurologic symptoms).

Other Adverse Reactions
PO: ADULTS, ELDERLY: Reduce dose according to dose modification table. Due to limited data, there are no recommendations on resuming treatment in pts with grade 4 adverse events that resolve.

Dosage in Renal Impairment
Mild to moderate impairment: No dose adjustment. **Severe impairment:** 14 mg once daily.

Dosage in Hepatic Impairment

Mild to moderate impairment: No dose adjustment. **Severe impairment:** 14 mg once daily.

SIDE EFFECTS

Frequent (73%–29%): Hypertension, diarrhea, fatigue, asthenia, malaise, arthralgia, myalgia, decreased appetite, weight decreased, nausea, stomatitis, glossitis, mouth ulceration, mucosal inflammation, headache, vomiting, dysphonia, abdominal pain, constipation. **Occasional (25%–7%):** Oral pain, glossodynia, cough, peripheral edema, rash, dysgeusia, dry mouth, dizziness, dyspepsia, insomnia, alopecia, hypotension, dehydration, hyperkeratosis.

ADVERSE EFFECTS/TOXIC REACTIONS

Serious adverse effects may include arterial thromboembolic events (5% of pts); cardiac dysfunction (7% of pts); dental and oral infections including gingivitis, parotitis, pericoronitis, periodontitis, sialoadenitis, tooth abscess, tooth infection (10% of pts); GI perforation/fistula formation (2% of pts); hemorrhagic events (35% of pts); hepatotoxicity (4% of pts); hypertension (73% of pts); grade 3 or greater hypocalcemia (9% of pts); impairment of thyroid-stimulating hormone (57% of pts); palmar-plantar erythrodysesthesia (32% of pts); proteinuria (34% of pts); QT interval prolongation (9% of pts); renal failure (14% of pts); urinary tract infection (11% of pts). Reverse posterior leukoencephalopathy occurs rarely. The median onset of hypertension was 16 days. The most frequently reported hemorrhagic event was epistaxis. The primary risk factor for renal failure was dehydration and hypovolemia related to diarrhea and vomiting.

NURSING CONSIDERATIONS

BASELINE ASSESSMENT

Obtain baseline CBC, BMP, LFT; serum magnesium, phosphate, ionized calcium; urinalysis for proteinuria. Confirm negative pregnancy status before initiating treatment. Receive full medication history and screen for interactions. Question history of cardiac/pituitary/thyroid disease, CVA/DVT, hypertension, hepatic/renal impairment, long QT interval syndrome. Assess oral cavity for lesions, poor dentation. Ensure that B/P is controlled prior to initiation. Assess hydration status. Offer emotional support.

INTERVENTION/EVALUATION

Monitor B/P after 1 wk, then every 2 wks for the first 2 mos, then at least monthly thereafter. Monitor LFT every 2 wks for the first 2 mos, then at least monthly thereafter. Monitor for proteinuria periodically. If urine dipstick proteinuria is greater than or equal to 2+, obtain a 24-hr urine protein test. Monitor blood calcium levels at least monthly and replace as needed depending on severity, presence of EKG changes, persistence of hypocalcemia. Monitor and correct other electrolyte abnormalities as needed. Initiate medical management for nausea, vomiting, diarrhea prior to any interruption or dose reduction. Reversible posterior leukoencephalopathy syndrome should be considered in pts with altered mental status, confusion, headache, seizures, visual disturbances. Immediately report abdominal pain, GI bleeding, hemoptysis (may indicate GI perforation/fistula formation). Obtain cardiac echocardiogram, EKG if cardiac decompensation is suspected.

PATIENT/FAMILY TEACHING

• Blood levels will be monitored regularly. • Treatment may cause fetal harm. Female pts of childbearing potential should use effective contraception during treatment and up to 2 wks following discontinuation. Immediately report suspected pregnancy. • Therapy may reduce fertility in both female and male pts. • Report liver problems such as upper abdominal pain, bruising, dark or amber-colored urine, nausea, vomiting, or yellowing of the skin or eyes; heart problems such as chest tightness, dizziness, fainting, palpitations, shortness of breath; kidney problems such as dark-colored urine, decreased urine output, extremity swelling, flank pain; skin changes such as rash, skin bubbling, sloughing. • Neurologic changes including blurry vision, confusion, headache, one-sided weakness, seizures, trouble speaking may indicate high blood pressure crisis, stroke, or life-threatening brain swelling. • Report mouth ulceration, jaw pain. • Swallow capsules whole; do not chew, crush, cut, or open capsules. • Treatment may increase risk of GI bleeding, nosebleeds. • Drink plenty of fluids.

letrozole HIGH ALERT

let-roe-zole
(Apo-Letrozole ✤, <u>Femara</u>)
Do not confuse Femara with Famvir, Femhrt, or Provera, or letrozole with anastrozole.

◆CLASSIFICATION

PHARMACOTHERAPEUTIC: Aromatase inhibitor, hormone. **CLINICAL:** Antineoplastic.

USES

First-line treatment of hormone receptor–positive or hormone receptor unknown locally advanced or metastatic breast cancer. Treatment of advanced breast cancer in postmenopausal women with disease progression following antiestrogen therapy. Postsurgical treatment for postmenopausal women with hormone receptor–positive early breast cancer. Extended treatment of early breast cancer after 5 yrs of tamoxifen. **OFF-LABEL:** Treatment of ovarian (epithelial), endometrial cancer.

PRECAUTIONS

Contraindications: Hypersensitivity to letrozole, other aromatase inhibitors. Use in women who are or may become pregnant. **Cautions:** Hepatic impairment, hyperlipidemia.

ACTION

Decreases circulating estrogen by inhibiting aromatase, an enzyme that catalyzes the final step in estrogen production (inhibits conversion of androgens to estrogens). **Therapeutic Effect:** Inhibits growth of breast cancers stimulated by estrogens.

PHARMACOKINETICS

Rapidly, completely absorbed. Metabolized in liver. Primarily excreted in urine. Unknown if removed by hemodialysis. **Half-life:** Approximately 2 days.

⧗ LIFESPAN CONSIDERATIONS

Pregnancy/Lactation: Unknown if distributed in breast milk. May cause fetal harm. **Children:** Safety and efficacy not established. **Elderly:** No age-related precautions noted.

INTERACTIONS

DRUG: Tamoxifen may reduce concentration. **HERBAL:** None significant. **FOOD:** None known. **LAB VALUES:** May increase serum calcium, cholesterol, GGT, ALT, AST, bilirubin.

AVAILABILITY (Rx)

Tablets: 2.5 mg.

ADMINISTRATION/HANDLING

PO
• Give without regard to food.

INDICATIONS/ROUTES/DOSAGE

Breast Cancer (Advanced)
PO: ADULTS, ELDERLY: 2.5 mg/day. Continue until tumor progression is evident.

Breast Cancer (Early–Adjuvant Treatment)
PO: ADULTS, ELDERLY: (Postmenopausal): 2.5 mg/day for planned duration of 5 yrs. Discontinue at relapse.

Breast Cancer (Early–Extended Adjuvant Treatment)
PO: ADULTS, ELDERLY: (Postmenopausal): 2.5 mg/day for planned duration of 5 yrs (after 5 yrs of tamoxifen). Discontinue at relapse.

L

Dosage in Renal Impairment
No dose adjustment.

Dosage in Severe Hepatic Impairment
PO: **ADULTS, ELDERLY:** 2.5 mg every other day.

SIDE EFFECTS

Frequent (21%–9%): Musculoskeletal pain (back, arm, leg), nausea, headache. **Occasional (8%–5%):** Constipation, arthralgia, fatigue, vomiting, hot flashes, diarrhea, abdominal pain, cough, rash, anorexia, hypertension, peripheral edema. **Rare (4%–1%):** Asthenia, drowsiness, dyspepsia, weight gain, pruritus.

ADVERSE EFFECTS/TOXIC REACTIONS

Pleural effusion, pulmonary embolism, bone fracture, thromboembolic disorder, MI occur rarely.

NURSING CONSIDERATIONS

BASELINE ASSESSMENT

Obtain baseline CBC, chemistries, renal function, LFT. Obtain pregnancy test prior to beginning therapy. Offer emotional support.

INTERVENTION/EVALUATION

Assist with ambulation if asthenia, dizziness occurs. Assess for headache. Offer antiemetic for nausea, vomiting. Monitor CBC, thyroid function, electrolytes, renal function, LFT. Monitor for evidence of musculoskeletal pain; offer analgesics for pain relief.

PATIENT/FAMILY TEACHING

• Report if nausea, asthenia, hot flashes become unmanageable. • Discuss importance of negative pregnancy test prior to beginning therapy; discuss nonhormonal methods of birth control. • Explain possible risk to fetus if pt is or becomes pregnant before or during therapy.

leucovorin

loo-**koe**-vor-in
Do not confuse leucovorin with Leukeran.

◆CLASSIFICATION

PHARMACOTHERAPEUTIC: Folic acid antagonist. **CLINICAL:** Antidote.

USES

Antidote for folic acid antagonists (methotrexate, trimethoprim, pyrimethamine). Treatment of megaloblastic anemias when folate deficient. Palliative treatment of advanced colon cancer (with fluorouracil). IV rescue therapy after high-dose methotrexate for osteosarcoma or orally to diminish toxicity and impaired methotrexate elimination. **OFF-LABEL:** Adjunctive cofactor therapy in methanol toxicity. Prevents pyrimethamine hematologic toxicity in HIV-positive pts.

PRECAUTIONS

Contraindications: Hypersensitivity to leucovorin. Pernicious anemia, other megaloblastic anemias secondary to vitamin B_{12} deficiency. **Cautions:** Renal impairment.

ACTION

Competes with methotrexate for same transport processes into cells (limits methotrexate action on normal cells). **Therapeutic Effect:** Reverses toxic effects of folic acid antagonists. Reverses folic acid deficiency.

PHARMACOKINETICS

Readily absorbed from GI tract. Widely distributed. Metabolized in liver, intestinal mucosa. Primarily excreted in urine. **Half-life:** 15 min; metabolite, 30–35 min.

⧗ LIFESPAN CONSIDERATIONS

Pregnancy/Lactation: Unknown if drug crosses placenta or is distributed in breast milk. **Children:** May increase risk of seizures by counteracting anticonvulsant effects of **barbiturates, hydantoins. Elderly:** Age-related renal impairment may require dosage adjustment when used for rescue from effects of high-dose methotrexate therapy.

INTERACTIONS

DRUG: May decrease effects of **anticonvulsants (e.g., phenytoin).** May increase **5-fluorouracil** toxicity/effects when taken in combination. **HERBAL:** None significant. **FOOD:** None known. **LAB VALUES:** May decrease platelets, WBCs (when used in combination with 5-fluorouracil).

AVAILABILITY (Rx)

Injection, Powder for Reconstitution: 50 mg, 100 mg, 200 mg, 350 mg, 500 mg. **Injection, Solution:** 10 mg/mL. **Tablets:** 5 mg, 10 mg, 15 mg, 25 mg.

ADMINISTRATION/HANDLING

 IV

◄**ALERT**► Strict adherence to timing of 5-fluorouracil following leucovorin therapy must be maintained.
Reconstitution • Reconstitute each 50-mg vial with 5 mL Sterile Water for Injection or Bacteriostatic Water for Injection containing benzyl alcohol to provide concentration of 10 mg/mL. • Due to benzyl alcohol in 1-mg ampule and in Bacteriostatic Water for Injection, reconstitute doses greater than 10 mg/m² with Sterile Water for Injection. • Further dilute with 100–1,000 mL D₅W or 0.9% NaCl.
Rate of Administration • Do not exceed 160 mg/min if given by IV infusion (due to calcium content).
Storage • Store powdered vials for parenteral use at room temperature. • Refrigerate solution for injection vials. • Injection appears as clear, yellowish solution. • Use immediately if reconstituted with Sterile Water for Injection; stable for 7 days if reconstituted with Bacteriostatic Water for Injection.

Diluted solutions stable for 24 hrs at room temperature or 4 days refrigerated.

PO
• Scored tablets may be crushed.

▦ IV INCOMPATIBILITIES

Amphotericin B complex (Abelcet, AmBisome, Amphotec), droperidol (Inapsine), foscarnet (Foscavir).

▦ IV COMPATIBILITIES

CISplatin (Platinol AQ), cyclophosphamide (Cytoxan), DOXOrubicin (Adriamycin), etoposide (VePesid), filgrastim (Neupogen), 5-fluorouracil, gemcitabine (Gemzar), granisetron (Kytril), heparin, methotrexate, metoclopramide (Reglan), mitoMYcin (Mutamycin), piperacillin and tazobactam (Zosyn), vinBLAStine (Velban), vinCRIStine (Oncovin).

INDICATIONS/ROUTES/DOSAGE

Rescue in High-Dose Methotrexate Therapy
PO, IV, IM: ADULTS, ELDERLY, CHILDREN: 15 mg (approximately 10 mg/m²) started 24 hrs after starting methotrexate infusion; continue q6h for 10 doses, until methotrexate level is less than 0.05 micromole/L. Additional dose adjusted based on methotrexate levels.

Folic Acid Antagonist Overdose
PO: ADULTS, ELDERLY, CHILDREN: 5–15 mg/day.

Megaloblastic Anemia Secondary to Folate Deficiency
IM/IV: ADULTS, ELDERLY, CHILDREN: 1 mg or less per day.

Colon Cancer
◄**ALERT**► For rescue therapy in cancer chemotherapy, refer to specific protocols used for optimal dosage and sequence of leucovorin administration.
IV: ADULTS, ELDERLY: *(In Combination with 5-fluorouracil):* 200 mg/m² daily for 5 days. Repeat course at 4-wk intervals for 2 courses, then 4- to 5-wk intervals or 20 mg/m² daily for 5 days.

Repeat course at 4-wk intervals for 2 courses, then 4- to 5-wk intervals.

Dosage in Renal/Hepatic Impairment
No dose adjustment.

SIDE EFFECTS

Frequent: When combined with chemotherapeutic agents: diarrhea, stomatitis, nausea, vomiting, lethargy, malaise, fatigue, alopecia, anorexia. **Occasional:** Urticaria, dermatitis.

ADVERSE EFFECTS/TOXIC REACTIONS

Excessive dosage may negate chemotherapeutic effects of folic acid antagonists. Anaphylaxis occurs rarely. Diarrhea may cause rapid clinical deterioration.

NURSING CONSIDERATIONS

BASELINE ASSESSMENT

Obtain baseline CBC, LFT, renal function. Give as soon as possible, preferably within 1 hr, for treatment of accidental overdosage of folic acid antagonists.

INTERVENTION/EVALUATION

Monitor for vomiting (may need to change from oral to parenteral therapy). Observe elderly, debilitated closely due to risk for severe toxicities. Assess CBC, BMP, LFT.

PATIENT/FAMILY TEACHING

• Explain purpose of medication in treatment of cancer. • Report allergic reaction, vomiting.

---

leuprolide   HIGH ALERT

loo-proe-lide
(Eligard, Lupron ✤, <u>Lupron Depot</u>, Lupron Depot-Ped)

◆ CLASSIFICATION

PHARMACOTHERAPEUTIC: Gonadotropin-releasing hormone (GnRH) analogue. **CLINICAL:** Antineoplastic.

USES

Palliative treatment of advanced prostate carcinoma. Management of endometriosis. Treatment of anemia caused by uterine leiomyomata (fibroids). Treatment of central precocious puberty. **OFF-LABEL:** Treatment of breast cancer, infertility.

PRECAUTIONS

Contraindications: Hypersensitivity to leuprolide, GnRH, GnRH-agonist analogue. Pregnancy or women who may become pregnant, breastfeeding (Lupron Depot 3.75 mg and 11.25 mg), abnormal, undiagnosed vaginal bleeding (Lupron Depot 3.75 mg and 11.25 mg). 22.5 mg, 30 mg, 45 mg Lupron Depot contraindicated in women. **Cautions:** History of psychiatric illness, QTc prolongation or medications that prolong QTc interval, preexisting cardiac disease, chronic alcohol use, steroid therapy, seizures or medications that decrease seizures threshold.

ACTION

Inhibits gonadotropin secretion; suppresses ovarian and testicular steroidogenesis due to decreased LH/FSH levels. Decreases testosterone and estrogen. **Therapeutic Effect:** Produces pharmacologic castration, decreases growth of abnormal prostate tissue in males; causes endometrial tissue to become inactive, atrophic in females; decreases rate of pubertal development in children with central precocious puberty.

PHARMACOKINETICS

Rapidly, well absorbed after subcutaneous administration. Absorbed slowly after IM administration. Protein binding: 43%–49%. **Half-life:** 3–4 hrs.

LIFESPAN CONSIDERATIONS

Pregnancy/Lactation: **Depot:** Contraindicated in pregnancy. May cause spontaneous abortion. **Children:** Long-term safety not established. **Elderly:** No age-related precautions noted.

INTERACTIONS

DRUG: QT interval–prolonging medications (e.g., **amiodarone, azithromycin, ceritinib, haloperidol, moxifloxacin**) may increase risk of QT interval prolongation, cardiac arrhythmias. **HERBAL:** None significant. **FOOD:** None known. **LAB VALUES:** May increase serum prostatic acid phosphatase (PAP). Initially increases, then decreases serum testosterone. May increase serum ALT, AST, alkaline phosphatase, glucose, LDH, LDL, cholesterol, triglycerides. May decrease platelets, WBC.

AVAILABILITY (Rx)

Injection Depot Formulation: Eligard: 7.5 mg, 22.5 mg, 30 mg, 45 mg. **Lupron Depot-Ped:** 7.5 mg, 11.25 mg (3-month), 11.25 (monthly), 15 mg, 30 mg. **Lupron Depot:** 3.75 mg, 11.25 mg, 22.5 mg, 30 mg, 45 mg. **Injection Solution (Lupron):** 5 mg/mL.

ADMINISTRATION/HANDLING

◀ **ALERT** ▶ May be carcinogenic, mutagenic, teratogenic. Handle with extreme care during preparation/administration.

IM
Lupron Depot • Store at room temperature. • Protect from light, heat. • Do not freeze vials. • Reconstitute only with diluent provided. Follow manufacturer's instructions for mixing. • Do not use needles less than 22 gauge; use syringes provided by the manufacturer (0.5-mL low-dose insulin syringes may be used as an alternative). • Administer immediately.
Eligard • Refrigerate. • Allow to warm to room temperature before reconstitution. • Follow manufacturer's instructions for mixing. • Following reconstitution, administer within 30 min.

Subcutaneous
Lupron • Refrigerate vials. • Injection appears clear, colorless. • Discard if discolored or precipitate forms. • Administer into deltoid muscle, anterior thigh, abdomen.

INDICATIONS/ROUTES/DOSAGE

Advanced Prostatic Carcinoma
IM *(Lupron Depot):* **ADULTS, ELDERLY:** 7.5 mg q1mo, 22.5 mg q3mos, 30 mg q4mos, or 45 mg q6mos.
SQ *(Eligard):* **ADULTS, ELDERLY:** 7.5 mg every mo, 22.5 mg q3mos, 30 mg q4mos, or 45 mg q6mos.
SQ *(Lupron):* **ADULTS, ELDERLY:** 1 mg/day.

Endometriosis
IM *(Lupron Depot):* **ADULTS, ELDERLY:** 3.75 mg/mo for up to 6 mos or 11.25 mg q3mos for up to 2 doses.

Uterine Leiomyomata
IM *(with Iron [Lupron Depot]):* **ADULTS, ELDERLY:** 3.75 mg/mo for up to 3 mos or 11.25 mg as a single injection.

Precocious Puberty
IM *(Lupron Depot-Ped):* **CHILDREN GREATER THAN 37.5 KG:** 15 mg q1mo. **GREATER THAN 25 KG TO 37.5 KG:** 11.25 mg q1mo. **25 KG OR LESS:** 7.5 mg q1mo. Titrate dose upward by 3.75 mg/mo if down regulation not achieved. **LUPRON DEPOT-PED (3 MOS):** 11.25 mg or 30 mg q12wks.
SQ *(Lupron):* **CHILDREN:** Initially, 50 mcg/kg/day. Titrate upward by 10 mcg/kg/day if down regulation is not achieved.

Dosage in Renal/Hepatic Impairment
No dose adjustment.

SIDE EFFECTS

Frequent: Hot flashes (ranging from mild flushing to diaphoresis), migraines, hyperhidrosis. **Females:** Amenorrhea, spotting. **Occasional:** Arrhythmias, palpitations, blurred vision, dizziness, edema, headache, burning, pruritus, swelling at injection site, nausea, insomnia, weight gain. **Females:** Deepening voice, hirsutism, decreased libido, increased breast tenderness, vaginitis, altered mood. **Males:** Constipation, decreased testicle size, gynecomastia, impotence, decreased appetite, angina. **Rare: Males:** Thrombophlebitis.

ADVERSE EFFECTS/TOXIC REACTIONS

Occasionally, signs/symptoms of prostatic carcinoma worsen 1–2 wks after initial dosing (subsides during continued therapy). Increased bone pain and, less frequently, dysuria, hematuria, weakness, paresthesia of lower extremities may be noted. MI, pulmonary embolism occur rarely.

NURSING CONSIDERATIONS

BASELINE ASSESSMENT

Question for possibility of pregnancy before initiating therapy. Obtain serum testosterone, prostatic acid phosphates (PAP) periodically during therapy. Serum testosterone, PAP should increase during first wk of therapy. Serum testosterone then should decrease to baseline level or less within 2 wks, PAP within 4 wks. Question medical history as listed in Precautions. Offer emotional support.

INTERVENTION/EVALUATION

Monitor for arrhythmias, palpitations. Assess for peripheral edema. Assess sleep pattern. Monitor for visual difficulties. Assist with ambulation if dizziness occurs. Offer antiemetics if nausea occurs.

PATIENT/ FAMILY TEACHING

• Hot flashes tend to decrease during continued therapy. • Temporary exacerbation of signs/symptoms of disease may occur during first few wks of therapy. • Use contraceptive measures. • Report persistent, regular menstruation; pregnancy. • Avoid tasks that require alertness, motor skills until response to drug is established (potential for dizziness).

levalbuterol

lee-val-**bue**-ter-ole
(Xopenex, Xopenex HFA)
Do not confuse Xopenex with Xanax.

◆CLASSIFICATION

PHARMACOTHERAPEUTIC: Beta₂ agonist. **CLINICAL:** Bronchodilator.

USES

Treatment, prevention of bronchospasm due to reversible obstructive airway disease (e.g., asthma, bronchitis, emphysema).

PRECAUTIONS

Contraindications: History of hypersensitivity to albuterol or levalbuterol. **Cautions:** Cardiovascular disorders (cardiac arrhythmias, HF), seizures, hypertension, hyperthyroidism, diabetes, glaucoma, hypokalemia.

ACTION

Stimulates beta₂-adrenergic receptors in lungs, resulting in relaxation of bronchial smooth muscle. **Therapeutic Effect:** Relieves bronchospasm, reduces airway resistance.

PHARMACOKINETICS

Route	Onset	Peak	Duration
Inhalation	5–10 min	1.5 hrs	5–6 hrs
Nebulization	10–17 min	1.5 hrs	5–8 hrs

Half-life: 3.3–4 hrs.

⧖ LIFESPAN CONSIDERATIONS

Pregnancy/Lactation: Crosses placenta. Unknown if distributed in breast milk. **Pregnancy Category C. Children:** Safety and efficacy not established in pts younger than 12 yrs. **Elderly:** Lower initial dosages recommended.

INTERACTIONS

DRUG: Beta blockers (e.g., carvedilol, metoprolol) antagonize effects; may produce severe bronchospasm. May decrease **digoxin** concentration. **MAOIs (e.g., phenelzine, tranylcypromine), tricyclic antidepressants (e.g., amitriptyline, desipramine)** may potentiate cardiovascular effects. **Diuretics (e.g., furosemide, HCTZ)** may increase hypokalemia. **HERBAL:** None significant. **FOOD:** None known. **LAB VALUES:** May decrease serum potassium.

AVAILABILITY (Rx)

Inhalation Aerosol: 45 mcg/activation. **Solution for Nebulization:** 0.31 mg in 3-mL vials, 0.63 mg in 3-mL vials, 1.25 mg in 3-mL vials, 1.25 mg in 0.5-mL vials.

ADMINISTRATION/HANDLING

Nebulization
• No diluent necessary. • Protect from light, excessive heat. Store at room temperature. • Once foil is opened, use within 2 wks. • Use within 1 wk and protect from light after removal from pouch • Discard if solution is not colorless. • Do not mix with other medications. • Concentrated solution (1.25 mg in 0.5 mL) should be diluted with 2.5 mL 0.9% NaCl prior to use. • Give over 5–15 min.

Inhalation
• Shake well before inhalation. • Prime before initial use or if not used for more than 3 days. • Following first inhalation, wait 2 min before inhaling second dose (allows for deeper bronchial penetration). • Rinsing mouth with water immediately after inhalation prevents mouth/throat dryness.

INDICATIONS/ROUTES/DOSAGE

Treatment/Prevention of Bronchospasm
Nebulization: ADULTS, ELDERLY, CHILDREN 12 YRS AND OLDER: Initially, 0.63 mg 3 times/day 6–8 hrs apart. May increase to 1.25 mg 3 times/day with dose monitoring. **CHILDREN 5–11 YRS:** Initially, 0.31 mg 3 times/day. **Maximum:** 0.63 mg 3 times/day. **CHILDREN 4 YRS OR YOUNGER:** 0.31–1.25 mg q4–6h as needed.

Inhalation: ADULTS, ELDERLY, CHILDREN 4 YRS AND OLDER: 1–2 inhalations q4–6h.

Acute Asthma Exacerbation
Nebulization: ADULTS, ELDERLY, CHILDREN 12 YRS AND OLDER: 1.25–2.5 mg q20min for 3 doses, then 1.25–5 mg q1–4h as needed. **CHILDREN YOUNGER THAN 12 YRS:** 0.075 mg/kg (minimum dose: 1.25 mg) q20min for 3 doses, then 0.075–0.15 mg/kg q1–4h as needed.
Inhalation: ADULTS, ELDERLY, CHILDREN 12 YRS AND OLDER: 4–8 puffs q20min for up to 4 hrs, then q1–4h. **CHILDREN YOUNGER THAN 12 YRS:** 4–8 puffs q20min for 3 doses, then q1–4h.

Dosage in Renal/Hepatic Impairment
No dose adjustment.

SIDE EFFECTS

Occasional (11%–4%): Nervousness, tremor, rhinitis, flu-like illness. **Rare (less than 3%):** Tachycardia, dizziness, anxiety, viral infection, dyspepsia, dry mouth, headache, chest pain.

ADVERSE EFFECTS/TOXIC REACTIONS

Excessive sympathomimetic stimulation may produce palpitations, premature heart contraction, tachycardia, chest pain, slight increase in B/P followed by substantial decrease, chills, diaphoresis, blanching of skin. Too-frequent or excessive use may decrease bronchodilating effectiveness, lead to severe, paradoxical bronchoconstriction.

NURSING CONSIDERATIONS

BASELINE ASSESSMENT
Assess lung sounds, pulse, B/P, oxygen saturation. Note color, amount of sputum.

INTERVENTION/EVALUATION
Monitor rate, depth, rhythm, type of respiration; quality/rate of pulse, EKG, serum potassium, ABG determinations. Assess lung sounds for wheezing (bronchoconstriction). Observe for paradoxical bronchospasm.

• Increase fluid intake (decreases lung secretion viscosity). • Rinsing mouth with water immediately after inhalation may prevent mouth/throat dryness. • Avoid excessive use of caffeine derivatives (chocolate, coffee, tea, cola, cocoa). • Report if palpitations, tachycardia, chest pain, tremors, dizziness, headache occurs or shortness of breath is not relieved.

levETIRAcetam

lee-ve-tye-**ra**-se-tam
(Apo-LevETIRAcetam ✿, Keppra, Keppra XR, Spritam)
Do not confuse Keppra with Kaletra, Keflex, or Keppra XR, or levETIRAcetam with levo-FLOXacin.

◆CLASSIFICATION

PHARMACOTHERAPEUTIC: Pyrrolidine derivative. **CLINICAL:** Anticonvulsant.

USES

Adjunctive therapy in treatment of partial-onset, myoclonic, and/or primary generalized tonic-clonic seizures.

PRECAUTIONS

Contraindications: Hypersensitivity to levETIRAcetam. **Cautions:** Renal impairment, pts with depression at high risk for suicide.

ACTION

Exact mechanism unknown. May inhibit voltage-dependent calcium channels, facilitate GABA inhibitory transmission, reduce potassium current, or bind to synaptic proteins that modulate neurotransmitter release. **Therapeutic Effect:** Prevents seizure activity.

PHARMACOKINETICS

Rapidly, completely absorbed following PO administration. Protein binding: less than 10%. Metabolized primarily by enzymatic hydrolysis. Primarily excreted in urine as unchanged drug. **Half-life:** 6–8 hrs.

⧖ LIFESPAN CONSIDERATIONS

Pregnancy/Lactation: Distributed in breast milk. Breastfeeding not recommended. **Children:** Safety and efficacy not established in children 4 yrs or younger. **Elderly:** Age-related renal impairment may require dosage adjustment.

INTERACTIONS

DRUG: None significant. **HERBAL:** None significant. **FOOD:** None known. **LAB VALUES:** May decrease Hgb, Hct, RBC, WBC.

AVAILABILITY (Rx)

Injection, Solution: 100 mg/mL. **Oral Solution:** 100 mg/mL. **Tablets:** 250 mg, 500 mg, 750 mg, 1,000 mg.

🗂 **Tablets, Extended-Release:** 500 mg, 750 mg.

ADMINISTRATION/HANDLING
💉 IV

Rate of Infusion • Infuse over 15 min. **Reconstitution** • Dilute with 100 mL 0.9% NaCl or D₅W.
Storage • Store at room temperature. • Stable for 24 hrs following dilution.

▦ IV INCOMPATIBILITIES
Data not available.

▦ IV COMPATIBILITIES
DiazePAM (Valium), LORazepam (Ativan), valproate (Depacon).
PO
• Give without regard to food. • Use oral solution for pts weighing 20 kg or less. • Use tablets or oral solution for pts weighing more than 20 kg. • Oral solution should be administered with a calibrated measuring device. • Swallow extended-release and immediate-release

tablets whole; do not break, crush, dissolve, or divide.

INDICATIONS/ROUTES/DOSAGE

Partial-Onset Seizures
IV/PO: ADULTS, ELDERLY, CHILDREN 17 YRS AND OLDER: *(Immediate-Release Tablets, Oral Solution, Tablets for Oral Suspension):* Initially, 500 mg q12h. May increase by 1,000 mg/day q2wks. **Maximum:** 3,000 mg/day in 2 divided doses. *Extended-Release Tablets:* 1,000 mg once daily. May increase in increments of 1,000 mg/day q2wks. **Maximum:** 3,000 mg once daily.
IV/PO: CHILDREN 4–16 YRS: *(Oral Solution, Tablets):* 20 mg/kg/day in 2 divided doses. May increase q2wks by 10 mg/kg/dose up to 60 mg/kg/day in 2 divided doses. **Maximum:** 3,000 mg/day. *(Tablets):* **GREATER THAN 40 KG:** 500 mg twice daily. May increase q2wks by 500 mg/dose. **Maximum:** 1,500 mg twice daily. **20–40 kg:** 250 mg twice daily. May increase q2wks by 250 mg/dose. **Maximum:** 750 mg twice daily. **CHILDREN 6 MOS TO YOUNGER THAN 4 YRS:** *(Oral Solution):* 20 mg/kg/day in 2 divided doses. May increase q2wks by 10 mg/kg/dose. **Maximum:** 50 mg/kg/day in 2 divided doses. **CHILDREN 1 MO TO YOUNGER THAN 6 MOS:** *(Oral Solution):* 14 mg/kg/day in 2 divided doses. May increase q2wks by 7 mg/kg/dose. **Maximum:** 42 mg/kg/day in 2 divided doses.

Myoclonic Seizures
PO/IV: ADULTS, ELDERLY, CHILDREN 12 YRS AND OLDER: *(Immediate-Release Tablets, Oral Solution, Tablets for Oral Suspension):* Initially, 500 mg q12h. May increase by 1,000 mg/day q2wks. **Maximum:** 3,000 mg/day in 2 divided doses.

Tonic-Clonic Seizures
PO, IV: ADULTS, ELDERLY, CHILDREN 16 YRS AND OLDER: *(Immediate-Release Tablets, Oral Solution, Tablets for Oral Suspension):* Initially, 500 mg twice daily. May increase by 1,000 mg/day

q2wks up to recommended dose of 1,500 mg 2 times/day. **CHILDREN 6–15 YRS:** Initially, 10 mg/kg twice daily. May increase by 20 mg/kg/day q2wks up to recommended dose of 30 mg/kg 2 times/day.

Dosage in Renal Impairment
Dosage is modified based on creatinine clearance. **Note:** CrCl less than 50 mL/min: Not recommended with Keppra XR.

Creatinine Clearance	Dosage (Immediate-Release, IV)	Dosage (Extended-Release)
Greater than 80 mL/min:	500–1,500 mg q12h	1,000–3,000 mg q24h
50–80 mL/min:	500–1,000 mg q12h	1,000–2,000 mg q24h
30–49 mL/min:	250–750 mg q12h	500–1,500 mg q24h
Less than 30 mL/min:	250–500 mg q12h	500–1,000 mg q24h
End-stage renal disease using dialysis:	500–1,000 mg q24h; after dialysis, a 250- to 500-mg supplemental dose is recommended	NA
CRRT	250–750 mg q12h	

Dosage in Hepatic Impairment
No dose adjustment.

SIDE EFFECTS

Frequent (15%–10%): Drowsiness, asthenia, headache, infection. **Occasional (9%–3%):** Dizziness, pharyngitis, pain, depression, anxiety, vertigo, rhinitis, anorexia. **Rare (less than 3%):** Amnesia, emotional lability, cough, sinusitis, anorexia, diplopia.

ADVERSE EFFECTS/TOXIC REACTIONS

Acute psychosis, agitation, delirium, impulsivity have been reported. Sudden discontinuance increases risk of seizure activity. Serious dermatological reactions, including Stevens-Johnson syndrome and toxic epidermal necrolysis, have been reported.

L

NURSING CONSIDERATIONS

BASELINE ASSESSMENT

Review history of seizure disorder (intensity, frequency, duration, LOC). Initiate seizure precautions. Question prior hypersensitivity reaction. Obtain renal function test.

INTERVENTION/EVALUATION

Observe for recurrence of seizure activity. Assess for clinical improvement (decrease in intensity/frequency of seizures). Monitor renal function tests. Observe for suicidal ideation, depression, behavioral changes. Assist with ambulation if dizziness occurs.

PATIENT/ FAMILY TEACHING

• Drowsiness usually diminishes with continued therapy. • Avoid tasks that require alertness, motor skills until response to drug is established. • Avoid alcohol. • Do not abruptly discontinue medication (may precipitate seizures). • Strict maintenance of drug therapy is essential for seizure control. • Report mood swings, hostile behavior, suicidal ideation, unusual changes in behavior.

---

levoFLOXacin   TOP 100

lee-voe-**flox**-a-sin
(Apo-LevoFLOXacin , Iquix, Levaquin, Quixin)

■ **BLACK BOX ALERT** ■ May increase risk of tendonitis, tendon rupture. (Risk increased with concurrent corticosteroids, organ transplant, pts older than 60 yrs.) May exacerbate myasthenia gravis. **Do not confuse Levaquin with Levoxyl, Levsin/SL, or Lovenox, or levoFLOXacin with levETIRAcetam or levothyroxine.**

◆CLASSIFICATION

PHARMACOTHERAPEUTIC: Fluoroquinolone. **CLINICAL:** Antibiotic.

USES

Treatment of susceptible infections due to *S. pneumoniae, S. aureus, E. faecalis, H. influenzae, M. catarrhalis, Serratia marcescens, K. pneumoniae, E. coli, P. mirabilis, P. aeruginosa, C. pneumoniae, Legionella pneumophila, Mycoplasma pneumoniae,* including acute bacterial exacerbation of chronic bronchitis, acute bacterial sinusitis, community-acquired pneumonia, nosocomial pneumonia, complicated and uncomplicated UTI, acute pyelonephritis, complicated and uncomplicated mild to moderate skin/ skin structure infections, prostatitis. Inhalation anthrax (postexposure); plague. **Ophthalmic:** Treatment of superficial infections to conjunctiva (0.5%), cornea (1.5%). **OFF-LABEL:** Urethritis, traveler's diarrhea, diverticulitis, enterocolitis, Legionnaire's disease, peritonitis. Treatment of prosthetic joint infection.

PRECAUTIONS

Contraindications: Hypersensitivity to levoFLOXacin, other fluoroquinolones. **Cautions:** Known or suspected CNS disorders, seizure disorder, renal impairment, bradycardia, rheumatoid arthritis, elderly, hypokalemia, hypomagnesemia, myasthenia gravis, severe cerebral arteriosclerosis, prolonged QT interval, medications that potentiate QT interval prolongation, diabetes, pts at risk for tendon rupture, tendonitis (e.g., renal failure, concomitant use of corticosteroids, organ transplant recipient, rheumatoid arthritis, elderly, strenuous physical activity or exercise).

ACTION

Inhibits DNA enzyme gyrase in susceptible microorganisms, interfering with bacterial cell replication, repair. **Therapeutic Effect:** Bactericidal.

PHARMACOKINETICS

Well absorbed after PO, IV administration. Protein binding: 50%. Widely distributed. Excreted unchanged in urine. Partially removed by hemodialysis. **Half-life:** 6–8 hrs.

L

⧖ LIFESPAN CONSIDERATIONS

Pregnancy/Lactation: Distributed in breast milk. Avoid use in pregnancy. **Children:** Safety and efficacy not established in pts younger than 18 yrs. **Elderly:** Age-related renal impairment may require dosage adjustment.

INTERACTIONS

DRUG: Antacids, iron preparations, sucralfate, zinc decrease absorption. **NSAIDs** may increase risk of CNS stimulation, seizures. **Medications that prolong QT interval (e.g., amiodarone, FLUoxetine, haloperidol, sotalol, quiNIDine)** may increase risk of arrhythmias. May increase effects of **warfarin. HERBAL:** None significant. **FOOD:** None known. **LAB VALUES:** May alter serum glucose.

AVAILABILITY (Rx)

Infusion Premix: 250 mg/50 mL, 500 mg/100 mL, 750 mg/150 mL. **Injection, Solution:** 25 mg/mL. **Ophthalmic Solution:** 0.5%. **Oral Solution:** 25 mg/mL. **Tablets:** 250 mg, 500 mg, 750 mg.

ADMINISTRATION/HANDLING

 **IV**

Reconstitution • For infusion using single-dose vial, withdraw desired amount (10 mL for 250 mg, 20 mL for 500 mg). Dilute each 10 mL (250 mg) with minimum 40 mL 0.9% NaCl, D_5W, providing a concentration of 5 mg/mL.
Rate of Administration • Administer no less than 60 min for 250 mg or 500 mg; 90 min for 750 mg.
Storage • Available in single-dose 20-mL (500-mg) vials and premixed with D_5W, ready to infuse. • Diluted vials stable for 72 hrs at room temperature, 14 days if refrigerated.

PO

• Do not administer antacids (aluminum, magnesium), sucralfate, iron or multivitamin preparations with zinc within 2 hrs of administration (significantly reduces absorption). • Give tablets without regard to food. • Give oral solution 1 hr before or 2 hrs after meals.

Ophthalmic
• Place a gloved finger on lower eyelid and pull out until a pocket is formed between eye and lower lid. • Place prescribed number of drops into pocket. • Instruct pt to close eye gently (so that medication will not be squeezed out of the sac) and to apply digital pressure to lacrimal sac for 1–2 min to minimize systemic absorption.

▦ IV INCOMPATIBILITIES

Furosemide (Lasix), heparin, insulin, nitroglycerin, propofol (Diprivan).

▦ IV COMPATIBILITIES

Dexmedetomidine (Precedex), DOBUTamine (Dobutrex), DOPamine (Intropin), fentaNYL (Sublimaze), lidocaine, (Ativan), magnesium, morphine.

INDICATIONS/ROUTES/DOSAGE

Usual Dosage Range
PO, IV: ADULTS, ELDERLY: 250–500 mg q24h; 750 mg q24h for severe or complicated infections.

Bacterial Conjunctivitis
Ophthalmic: ADULTS, ELDERLY, CHILDREN 1 YR AND OLDER (QUIXIN) (0.5%): 1–2 drops q2h for 2 days while awake (up to 8 times/day), then 1–2 drops q4h while awake up to 4 times/day.

Dosage in Renal Impairment
Normal renal function dosage of 250 mg/day:

Creatinine Clearance	Dosage
20–49 mL/min	No change
10–19 mL/min	250 mg initially, then 250 mg q48h

L

Normal renal function dosage of 500 mg/day:

Creatinine Clearance	Dosage
50–80 mL/min	No change
20–49 mL/min	500 mg initially, then 250 mg q24h
10–19 mL/min	500 mg initially, then 250 mg q48h

For pts undergoing dialysis, 500 mg initially, then 250 mg q48h.

Normal renal function dosage of 750 mg/day:

Creatinine Clearance	Dosage
50–80 mL/min	No change
20–49 mL/min	Initially, 750 mg, then 750 mg q48h
10–19 mL/min	Initially, 750 mg, then 500 mg q48h
Dialysis	500 mg q48h (administer after dialysis on dialysis days)
Continuous Renal Replacement Therapy	
CVVH	500–750 mg once, then 250 mg q24h
CVVHD	500–750 mg once, then 250–500 mg q24h
CVVHDT	500–750 mg once, then 250–750 mg q24h

Dosage in Hepatic Impairment
No dose adjustment.

SIDE EFFECTS

Occasional (3%–1%): Diarrhea, nausea, abdominal pain, dizziness, drowsiness, headache. **Ophthalmic:** Local burning/discomfort, margin crusting, crystals/scales, foreign body sensation, ocular itching, altered taste. **Rare (less than 1%):** Flatulence; pain, inflammation, swelling in calves, hands, shoulder; chest pain, difficulty breathing, palpitations, edema, tendon pain. **Ophthalmic:** Corneal staining, keratitis, allergic reaction, eyelid swelling, tearing, reduced visual acuity.

ADVERSE EFFECTS/TOXIC REACTIONS

Antibiotic-associated colitis, other superinfections (abdominal cramps, severe watery diarrhea, fever) may occur. Superinfection (genital/anal pruritus, ulceration/changes in oral mucosa, moderate to severe diarrhea) may occur from altered bacterial balance in GI tract. Hypersensitivity reactions, including photosensitivity (rash, pruritus, blisters, edema, sensation of burning skin), have occurred in pts receiving fluoroquinolones. May increase risk of tendonitis, tendon rupture, peripheral neuropathy; CNS effects including agitation, anxiety, confusion, depression, dizziness, hallucinations, nightmares, paranoia, tremors, vertigo. May exacerbate muscle weakness in pts with myasthenia gravis.

NURSING CONSIDERATIONS

BASELINE ASSESSMENT

Question for hypersensitivity to levoFLOXacin, other fluoroquinolones. Question history as listed in Precautions. Receive full medication history, and screen for interactions, esp. medications that prolong QT interval. Obtain baseline EKG.

INTERVENTION/EVALUATION

Monitor serum glucose, renal function, LFT. Monitor daily pattern of bowel activity, stool consistency. Promptly report hypersensitivity reaction: skin rash, urticaria, pruritus, photosensitivity. Be alert for superinfection: fever, vomiting, diarrhea, anal/genital pruritus, oral mucosal changes (ulceration, pain, erythema). Monitor for muscle weakness, voice dystonia in pts with myasthenia gravis; pain, swelling, bruising, popping of tendons.

PATIENT/ FAMILY TEACHING

• It is essential to complete drug therapy despite symptom improvement. Early discontinuation may result in antibacterial resistance or increase risk of recurrent infection. • Report any episodes of diarrhea, esp. the first few mos after final dose. Frequent diarrhea, fever, abdominal pain, blood-streaked stool may indicate infectious diarrhea, which may be contagious to others. • Severe allergic reactions, such as hives, palpitations, rash, shortness of breath, tongue swelling, may occur. • Tendon inflammation/swelling, tendon rupture may occur; report bruising, pain, swelling in tendon areas or snapping, popping of tendons. • Immediately report nervous system problems such as anxiety, confusion, dizziness, nervousness, nightmares, thoughts of suicide, seizures, tremors, trouble sleeping. • Treatment may cause heart problems such as low heart rate, palpitations; permanent nerve damage such as burning, numbness, tingling, weakness. • Do not take aluminum- or magnesium-containing antacids, multivitamins, zinc or iron products at least 2 hrs before or 6 hrs after dose. • Drink plenty of fluids.

---

levothyroxine [TOP 100]

lee-voe-thy-**rox**-een
(Eltroxin ✦, Levoxyl, <u>Synthroid</u>, Tirosint, Unithroid)

■ **BLACK BOX ALERT** ■ Ineffective, potentially toxic for weight reduction. High doses increase risk of serious, life-threatening toxic effects, especially when used with some anorectic drugs.
Do not confuse levothyroxine with levoFLOXacin or liothyronine, or Synthroid with Symmetrel.

FIXED-COMBINATION(S)

With liothyronine, T_3 (**Thyrolar**).

◆CLASSIFICATION

PHARMACOTHERAPEUTIC: Synthetic isomer of thyroxine. **CLINICAL:** Thyroid hormone (T_4).

USES

PO: Treatment of hypothyroidism, pituitary thyroid-stimulating hormone (TSH) suppression. **IV:** Myxedema coma. **OFF-LABEL:** Management of hemodynamically unstable potential organ donors.

PRECAUTIONS

Contraindications: Hypersensitivity to levothyroxine. Acute MI, untreated subclinical or overt thyrotoxicosis, uncorrected adrenal insufficiency. **Capsule:** Inability to swallow capsules. **Cautions:** Elderly pts, angina pectoris, hypertension, other cardiovascular disease, adrenal insufficiency, myxedema, diabetes mellitus and insipidus, swallowing disorders.

ACTION

Converts to T_3, then binds to thyroid receptor proteins exerting metabolic effects through DNA and protein synthesis. **Therapeutic Effect:** Involved in normal metabolism, growth and development. Increases basal metabolic rate, enhances gluconeogenesis, stimulates protein synthesis.

PHARMACOKINETICS

Variable, incomplete absorption from GI tract. Protein binding: greater than 99%. Widely distributed. Deiodinated in peripheral tissues, minimal metabolism in liver. Eliminated by biliary excretion. **Half-life:** 6–7 days.

⧗ LIFESPAN CONSIDERATIONS

Pregnancy/Lactation: Does not cross placenta. Minimal distribution in breast milk. **Children:** No age-related precautions noted. Caution in neonates in interpreting thyroid function tests. **Elderly:** May be more sensitive to thyroid effects; individualized dosage recommended.

INTERACTIONS

DRUG: Cholestyramine, colestipol, **aluminum-** and **magnesium-containing antacids** may decrease absorption (do not administer within

L

---

668 **levothyroxine**

4 hrs). **Estrogens** may cause decrease in serum-free thyroxine. May enhance effects of **oral anticoagulants (e.g, warfarin). Sympathomimetics (e.g., norepinephrine, phenylephrine)** may increase risk of coronary insufficiency, effects of levothyroxine. May decrease effects of **insulin, oral hypoglycemic agents. HERBAL:** None significant. **FOOD:** None known. **LAB VALUES:** None known.

AVAILABILITY (Rx)

Capsules (Tirosint): 13 mcg, 25 mcg, 50 mcg, 75 mcg, 88 mcg, 100 mcg, 112 mcg, 125 mcg, 137 mcg, 150 mcg. **Injection, Powder for Reconstitution:** 100 mcg, 200 mcg, 500 mcg. **Tablets:** 25 mcg, 50 mcg, 75 mcg, 88 mcg, 100 mcg, 112 mcg, 125 mcg, 137 mcg, 150 mcg, 175 mcg, 200 mcg, 300 mcg.

ADMINISTRATION/HANDLING

◀**ALERT**▶ Do not interchange brands (known issues with bioequivalence between manufacturers).

 IV

Reconstitution • Reconstitute 200-mcg or 500-mcg vial with 5 mL 0.9% NaCl to provide concentration of 40 or 100 mcg/mL, respectively; shake until clear.

Rate of Administration • Use immediately; discard unused portions. • Give each 100 mcg or less over 1 min.

Storage • Store vials at room temperature.

PO

• Administer in the morning on an empty stomach, 30 min before food. • Administer before breakfast to prevent insomnia. • Tablets may be crushed. • Take 4 hrs apart from antacids, iron, calcium supplements.

▦ IV INCOMPATIBILITIES

Do not use or mix with other IV solutions.

INDICATIONS/ROUTES/DOSAGE

Note: Doses based on clinical response and laboratory parameters. IV dose is 50% of oral dose.

Hypothyroidism
PO: ADULTS, CHILDREN IN WHOM GROWTH AND PUBERTY ARE COMPLETE, OLDER ADULTS RECENTLY TREATED FOR HYPOTHYROIDISM OR WHO HAVE BEEN HYPOTHYROID FOR ONLY A FEW MOS: 1.6 mcg/kg/day as single daily dose. Usual maintenance: 100–125 mcg/day. **ADULTS YOUNGER THAN 50 YRS WITH CARDIAC DISEASE, OLDER THAN 50 YRS WITHOUT CARDIAC DISEASE:** Initially, 25–50 mcg/day. Adjust dose by 12.5–25 mcg/day at 6–8-wk intervals. **ADULTS (OLDER THAN 50 YRS WITH CARDIAC DISEASE):** Initially, 12.5–25 mcg/day. Adjust dose by 12.5–25 mcg/day at 6–8-wk intervals. **CHILDREN OLDER THAN 12 YRS, GROWTH AND PUBERTY INCOMPLETE:** 2–3 mcg/kg/day. **CHILDREN 6–12 YRS:** 4–5 mcg/kg/day. **CHILDREN 1–5 YRS:** 5–6 mcg/kg/day. **CHILDREN 6–12 MOS:** 6–8 mcg/kg/day. **CHILDREN 3–5 MOS:** 8–10 mcg/kg/day. **CHILDREN YOUNGER THAN 3 MOS:** 10–15 mcg/kg/day.

Myxedema Coma
IV: ADULTS, ELDERLY: Initially, 300–500 mcg, then 50–100 mcg once daily until able to tolerate PO administration.

Pituitary Thyroid-Stimulating Hormone (TSH) Suppression
PO: ADULTS, ELDERLY: Doses greater than 2 mcg/kg/day usually required to suppress TSH below 0.1 milliunits/L.

Dosage in Renal/Hepatic Impairment
No dose adjustment.

SIDE EFFECTS

Occasional: Reversible hair loss at start of therapy in children. **Rare:** Dry skin, GI intolerance, rash, urticaria, pseudotumor cerebri, severe headache in children.

underlined – top prescribed drug

ADVERSE EFFECTS/TOXIC REACTIONS

Excessive dosage produces signs/symptoms of hyperthyroidism (weight loss, palpitations, increased appetite, tremors, anxiety, tachycardia, hypertension, headache, insomnia, menstrual irregularities). Cardiac arrhythmias occur rarely. Long-term therapy may decrease bone mineral density.

NURSING CONSIDERATIONS

BASELINE ASSESSMENT

Obtain baseline TSH, T_3, T_4, weight, vital signs. Signs/symptoms of diabetes, diabetes insipidus, adrenal insufficiency, hypopituitarism may become intensified. Treat with adrenocortical steroids before thyroid therapy in coexisting hypothyroidism and hypoadrenalism.

INTERVENTION/EVALUATION

Monitor pulse for rate, rhythm (report pulse greater than 100 or marked increase). Observe for tremors, anxiety. Assess appetite, sleep pattern. **Children: (Undertreatment):** May decrease intellectual development, linear growth. **(Overtreatment):** Adversely affects brain maturation, accelerates bone age. Monitor thyroid function tests.

PATIENT/ FAMILY TEACHING

• Do not discontinue drug therapy; replacement for hypothyroidism is lifelong. • Follow-up office visits, thyroid function tests are essential. • Take medication at the same time each day, preferably in the morning. • Monitor pulse for rate, rhythm; report irregular rhythm or pulse rate over 100 beats/min. • Promptly report chest pain, weight loss, anxiety, tremors, insomnia. • Children may have reversible hair loss, increased aggressiveness during first few mos of therapy. • Full therapeutic effect may take 1–3 wks.

lidocaine

lye-doe-kane
(Lidoderm, Xylocaine)

FIXED-COMBINATION(S)

EMLA: lidocaine/prilocaine (an anesthetic): 2.5%/2.5%. **Lidosite:** lidocaine/EPINEPHrine (a sympathomimetic): 10%/0.1%. **Lidocaine with EPINEPHrine:** lidocaine/EPINEPHrine (a sympathomimetic): 2%/1:50,000, 1%/1:100,000, 1%/1:200,000, 0.5%/1:200,000. **Synéra:** lidocaine/tetracaine (an anesthetic): 70 mg/70 mg.

◆CLASSIFICATION

PHARMACOTHERAPEUTIC: Amide anesthetic. **CLINICAL:** Class 1B antiarrhythmic, anesthetic.

USES

Antiarrhythmic: Rapid control of acute ventricular arrhythmias following MI, cardiac catheterization, cardiac surgery. **Local anesthetic:** Infiltration/nerve block for dental/surgical procedures, childbirth. **Topical anesthetic:** Local skin disorders (minor burns, insect bites, prickly heat, skin manifestations of chickenpox, abrasions). Mucous membranes (local anesthesia of oral, nasal, laryngeal mucous membranes; local anesthesia of respiratory, urinary tracts; relief of discomfort of pruritus ani, hemorrhoids, pruritus vulvae). **Dermal patch:** Relief of chronic pain in postherpetic neuralgia, allodynia (painful hypersensitivity).

PRECAUTIONS

Contraindications: Hypersensitivity to lidocaine. Adams-Stokes syndrome, hypersensitivity to amide-type local anesthetics, supraventricular arrhythmias, Wolff-Parkinson-White syndrome. Severe

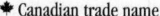

degree of SA, AV, or intraventricular heart block (except in pts with functioning pacemaker). **Cautions:** Hepatic disease, marked hypoxia, severe respiratory depression, hypovolemia, incomplete heart. History of malignant hyperthermia, shock, elderly pts, HF.

ACTION

Anesthetic: Inhibits conduction of nerve impulses. **Therapeutic Effect:** Causes temporary loss of feeling/sensation. **Antiarrhythmic:** Suppresses automaticity of conduction tissue; increases electrical stimulation threshold of ventricle, His-Purkinje system; and spontaneous depolarization of ventricle during diastole. Blocks initiation/conduction of nerve impulses by decreasing neuronal membrane's permeability to sodium ions. **Therapeutic Effect:** Inhibits ventricular arrhythmias.

PHARMACOKINETICS

Route	Onset	Peak	Duration
IV	30–90 sec	N/A	10–20 min
Local anesthetic	2.5 min	N/A	30–60 min

Completely absorbed after IV administration. Protein binding: 60%–80%. Widely distributed. Metabolized in liver. Primarily excreted in urine. Minimally removed by hemodialysis. **Half-life:** 1–2 hrs.

⏳ LIFESPAN CONSIDERATIONS

Pregnancy/Lactation: Crosses placenta. Distributed in breast milk. **Children:** No age-related precautions noted. **Elderly:** More sensitive to adverse effects. Dose, rate of infusion should be reduced. Age-related renal impairment may require dosage adjustment.

INTERACTIONS

DRUG: **Class 1 antiarrhythmics (e.g., propafenone, quinidine)** may increase cardiac effects. **HERBAL:** **St. John's wort** may decrease concentration. **FOOD:** None known. **LAB VALUES:** IM lidocaine may increase creatine kinase (CK) level. **Therapeutic serum level:** 1.5–6 mcg/mL; **toxic serum level:** greater than 6 mcg/mL.

AVAILABILITY (Rx)

Cream, Topical: 4%. **Infusion Premix:** 0.4% (4 mg/mL in 250 mL, 500 mL); 0.8% (8 mg/mL in 250 mL, 500 mL). **Injection, Solution:** 0.5% (5mg/mL), 1% (10mg/mL), 2% (20mg/mL). **Jelly, Topical:** 2%. **Solution, Topical:** 4%. **Solution, Viscous:** 2%. **Transdermal, Topical (Lidoderm):** 5%.

ADMINISTRATION/HANDLING

◀**ALERT**▶ Resuscitative equipment, drugs (including O_2) must always be readily available when administering lidocaine by any route.

 IV

◀**ALERT**▶ Use only lidocaine without preservative, clearly marked **for IV use.**
Reconstitution • For IV infusion, prepare solution by adding 2 g to 250–500 mL D_5W or 0.9% NaCl to provide concentration of 8 mg/mL or 4 mg/mL, respectively. • Commercially available preparations of 0.4% and 0.8% may be used for IV infusion. **Maximum concentration:** 4 g/250 mL (16 mg/mL). **Rate of Administration** • For IV push, use 1% (10 mg/mL) or 2% (20 mg/mL). • Administer IV push at rate of 25–50 mg/min. • Administer for IV infusion at rate of 1–4 mg/min (1–4 mL); use volume control IV set. **Storage** • Store premix solutions at room temperature.

Topical

• Not for ophthalmic use. • For skin disorders, apply directly to affected area or put on gauze or bandage, which is then applied to the skin. • For mucous membrane use, apply to desired area per manufacturer's insert. • Administer lowest dosage possible that still provides anesthesia.

Dermal Patch

Avoid exposing to external heat source. Patch should not get wet (do not wear while bathing/swimming). Patch may be cut to appropriate size.

🔳 IV INCOMPATIBILITIES

Amphotericin B complex (Abelcet, AmBisome, Amphotec).

🔳 IV COMPATIBILITIES

Amiodarone (Cordarone), calcium gluconate, dexmedetomidine (Precedex), digoxin (Lanoxin), diltiaZEM (Cardizem), DOBUTamine (Dobutrex), DOPamine (Intropin), enalapril (Vasotec), furosemide (Lasix), heparin, insulin, nitroglycerin, potassium chloride.

INDICATIONS/ROUTES/DOSAGE

Ventricular Arrhythmias
IV: ADULTS, ELDERLY: Initially, 1–1.5 mg/kg. Refractory ventricular tachycardia, fibrillation: Repeat dose at 0.5–0.75 mg/kg q10–15min after initial dose for a maximum of 3 doses. Total dose not to exceed 3 mg/kg. Follow with continuous infusion (1–4 mg/min) after return of circulation. Reappearance of arrhythmia during infusion: 0.5 mg/kg, reassess infusion. **CHILDREN, INFANTS:** Initially, 1 mg/kg (**Maximum:** 100 mg). May repeat second dose of 0.5–1 mg/kg if start of infusion longer than 15 min. **Maintenance:** 20–50 mcg/kg/min as IV infusion.

Local Anesthesia
Infiltration, Nerve Block: ADULTS: Local anesthetic dosage varies with procedure, degree of anesthesia, vascularity, duration. **Maximum dose:** 4.5 mg/kg or 300 mg. Do not repeat within 2 hrs.

Topical Local Anesthesia
Topical: ADULTS, ELDERLY: Apply to affected areas as needed.

Treatment of Localized Pain
◄**ALERT**► Transdermal patch may contain conducting metal (e.g., aluminum). Remove patch prior to MRI.

Topical *(Dermal Patch):* **ADULTS, ELDERLY:** Apply to intact skin over most painful area. **Maximum:** Up to 3 patches at a time for up to 12 hrs in a 24-hr period.

Dosage in Renal Impairment
No dose adjustment.

Dosage in Hepatic Impairment
Use caution.

SIDE EFFECTS

CNS effects generally dose-related and of short duration. **Occasional: Infiltration/Nerve Block:** Pain at injection site. **Topical:** Burning, stinging, tenderness at application site. **Rare:** Generally associated with high dose: Drowsiness, dizziness, disorientation, light-headedness, tremors, apprehension, euphoria, sensation of heat, cold, numbness; blurred or double vision, tinnitus, nausea.

ADVERSE EFFECTS/TOXIC REACTIONS

Serious adverse reactions to lidocaine are uncommon, but high dosage by any route may produce cardiovascular depression, bradycardia, hypotension, arrhythmias, heart block, cardiovascular collapse, cardiac arrest. Potential for malignant hyperthermia, CNS toxicity may occur, esp. with regional anesthesia use, progressing rapidly from mild side effects to tremors, drowsiness, seizures, vomiting, respiratory depression. Methemoglobinemia (evidenced by cyanosis) has occurred following topical application of lidocaine for teething discomfort and laryngeal anesthetic spray.

NURSING CONSIDERATIONS

BASELINE ASSESSMENT

Question for hypersensitivity to lidocaine, amide anesthetics. Obtain baseline B/P, pulse, respiratory rate, EKG, serum electrolytes.

INTERVENTION/EVALUATION

Monitor EKG, vital signs closely during and following drug administration for cardiac performance. If EKG shows arrhythmias, prolongation of PR interval or QRS complex, inform physician immediately. Assess pulse for rhythm, rate, quality. Assess B/P for evidence of hypotension. Monitor for therapeutic serum level (1.5–6 mcg/mL). For lidocaine given by all routes, monitor vital signs, LOC. Drowsiness should be considered a warning sign of high serum levels of lidocaine. **Therapeutic serum level:** 1.5–6 mcg/mL; **toxic serum level:** greater than 6 mcg/mL.

PATIENT/ FAMILY TEACHING

• **Local anesthesia:** Due to loss of feeling/sensation, protective measures may be needed until anesthetic wears off (no ambulation, including special positions for some regional anesthesia). • **Oral mucous membrane anesthesia:** Do not eat, drink, chew gum for 1 hr after application (swallowing reflex may be impaired, increasing risk of aspiration; numbness of tongue, buccal mucosa may lead to bite trauma). • **IV infusions:** Report dizziness, numbness, double vision, nausea, pain/burning, respiratory difficulty. • **Topical:** Report irritation, pain, numbness, swelling, blurred vision, tinnitus, respiratory difficulty.

---

linaclotide

lin-a-kloe-tide
(Constella ✤, Linzess)
■ **BLACK BOX ALERT** ■ Contraindicated in pediatric pts 6 yrs of age and younger. Avoid use in pediatric patients 7 yrs through 17 yrs old.

◆CLASSIFICATION

PHARMACOTHERAPEUTIC: Guanylate cyclase-C (cGMP) agonist. **CLINICAL:** Anti-constipation agent.

USES

Treatment of irritable bowel syndrome with constipation, chronic idiopathic constipation.

PRECAUTIONS

Contraindications: Hypersensitivity to linaclotide. Pediatric patients 6 yrs and younger, known or suspected mechanical GI obstruction. **Cautions:** Diarrhea.

ACTION

Binds on the luminal surface of GI epithelium. Increases cGMP, which stimulates chloride and bicarbonate into intestinal lumen. **Therapeutic Effect:** Increases intestinal fluid, accelerates transit.

PHARMACOKINETICS

Metabolized within GI tract. Minimal distribution beyond GI tissue. Minimal systemic absorption. **Half-life:** N/A.

⏳ LIFESPAN CONSIDERATIONS

Pregnancy/Lactation: Unknown if distributed in breast milk. **Children:** Avoid use in pediatric pts 7 yrs through 17 yrs. Contraindicated in pediatric pts 6 yrs and younger. **Elderly:** No age-related precautions noted.

INTERACTIONS

DRUG: None significant. **HERBAL:** None significant. **FOOD:** None known. **LAB VALUES:** None significant.

AVAILABILITY (Rx)

Capsules: 72 mcg, 145 mcg, 290 mcg.

ADMINISTRATION/HANDLING

PO
• Give on empty stomach at least 30 min prior to first meal of day. • Do not break or crush. • For pts with swallowing difficulty, capsule may be opened and sprinkled on applesauce or into 30 mL bottled water.

INDICATIONS/ROUTES/DOSAGE

Irritable Bowel Syndrome with Constipation
PO: ADULTS 18 YRS AND OLDER, ELDERLY: 290 mcg once daily.

Chronic Idiopathic Constipation
PO: ADULTS 18 YRS AND OLDER, EL-
DERLY: 72–145 mcg once daily.

Dosage in Renal/Hepatic Impairment
No dose adjustment.

SIDE EFFECTS

Frequent (16%): Diarrhea (may begin within first 2 wks of initiation of
treatment). Occasional (7%–2%): Abdominal pain, flatulence, headache,
abdominal distention. Rare (1%
and Less): Gastroesophageal reflux,
vomiting.

ADVERSE EFFECTS/TOXIC REACTIONS

Severe diarrhea was reported in 2% of
pts. Viral gastroenteritis was noted in 3%
of pts. Fecal incontinence, dehydration
was reported in 1%. Dose reduced or
suspended secondary to diarrhea, other
GI adverse reaction.

NURSING CONSIDERATIONS

BASELINE ASSESSMENT
Encourage adequate fluid intake. Assess
bowel sounds for peristalsis. Assess for
abdominal disturbances.

INTERVENTION/EVALUATION
For pts with irritable bowel syndrome,
assess for improvement in symptoms
(relief from bloating, cramping, urgency, abdominal discomfort). Monitor
daily bowel activity, stool consistency.
Monitor serum electrolytes in pts with
prolonged, frequent, or excessive use of
medication.

PATIENT/FAMILY TEACHING
• Institute measures to promote defecation: increase fluid intake, exercise,
high-fiber diet. • Report new/worsen-
ing episodes of abdominal pain, severe
diarrhea. • Do not break, crush, or
open capsule. Take whole.

linagliptin

lin-a-glip-tin
(Tradjenta)
Do not confuse linagliptin with
SAXagliptin or SITagliptin.

FIXED-COMBINATION(S)

Glyxambi: linagliptin/empagliflozin
(an antidiabetic): 5 mg/10 mg, 5
mg/25 mg. Jentadueto: linagliptin/
metFORMIN (an antidiabetic): 2.5
mg/500 mg; 2.5 mg/850 mg; 2.5
mg/1,000 mg. Jentadueto XR:
linagliptin/metFORMIN (extended-
release): 2.5 mg/1,000 mg; 5
mg/1,000 mg.

◆CLASSIFICATION

PHARMACOTHERAPEUTIC: Dipeptidyl peptidase-4 (DDP-4) inhibitor
(gliptin). CLINICAL: Antidiabetic
agent.

USES

Adjunctive treatment to diet and exercise
to improve glycemic control in pts with
type 2 diabetes alone or in combination
with other antidiabetic agents.

PRECAUTIONS

Contraindications: Hypersensitivity to
linagliptin, other DD4 inhibitors. Cautions: Concurrent use of other hypoglycemics. Not recommended for use in type
1 diabetes, diabetic ketoacidosis, history
of pancreatitis, HF.

ACTION

Slows inactivation of incretin hormones
by inhibiting DDP-4 enzyme. Therapeutic Effect: Incretin hormones increase
insulin synthesis/release from pancreas
and decrease glucagon secretion. Lowers
serum glucose levels.

PHARMACOKINETICS

Rapidly absorbed following PO administration. Peak plasma concentration: 1.5 hrs.

Extensive tissue distribution. Protein binding: 70%–99%. Minimal metabolism (90% excreted as unchanged metabolite). Excreted primarily in enterohepatic system (80%), urine (5%). **Half-life:** 12 hrs.

⧗ LIFESPAN CONSIDERATIONS

Pregnancy/Lactation: Unknown if distributed in breast milk. **Children:** Safety and efficacy not established. **Elderly:** No age-related precautions noted.

INTERACTIONS

DRUG: CYP3A4 inducers (e.g., ri-fAMPin) may decrease concentration. **Insulin, metFORMIN, SAXagliptin, SITagliptin, sulfonylureas** may increase risk of hypoglycemia. **HERBAL: Ginseng, ginger, other herbs with hypoglycemic activity** may increase risk of hypoglycemia. **FOOD:** None known. **LAB VALUES:** Decreases serum glucose. May increase serum uric acid.

AVAILABILITY (Rx)

Tablets: 5 mg.

ADMINISTRATION/HANDLING

PO
• May give without regard to food.

INDICATIONS/ROUTES/DOSAGE

Note: Dose reduction of insulin and/or insulin secretagogues may be needed.

Type 2 Diabetes Mellitus
PO: ADULTS, ELDERLY: 5 mg once daily.

Dosage in Renal/Hepatic Impairment
No dose adjustment.

SIDE EFFECTS

Occasional (5%): Nasopharyngitis. **Rare (less than 2%):** Cough, headache.

ADVERSE EFFECTS/TOXIC REACTIONS

Hypoglycemia reported in 7% of pts. Concomitant use of hypoglycemic medication may increase hypoglycemic risk. Pancreatitis, hypersensitivity reactions (angioedema, rash, urticaria, pruritus, bronchospasm) occur rarely.

NURSING CONSIDERATIONS

BASELINE ASSESSMENT

Check blood glucose, hemoglobin A1c level. Assess pt's understanding of diabetes management, routine glucose monitoring. Receive full medication history including herbal products.

INTERVENTION/EVALUATION

Monitor blood glucose, hemoglobin A1c level. Assess for hypoglycemia (diaphoresis, tremors, dizziness, anxiety, headache, tachycardia, perioral numbness, hunger, diplopia, difficulty concentrating), hyperglycemia (polyuria, polyphagia, polydipsia, nausea, vomiting, fatigue, Kussmaul breathing). Screen for glucose-altering conditions: fever, increased activity or stress, surgical procedures. Dietary consult for nutritional education.

PATIENT/FAMILY TEACHING

• Diabetes requires lifelong control. • Diet and exercise are principal parts of treatment; do not skip or delay meals. • Test blood glucose regularly. • When taking combination drug therapy or when glucose demands are altered (fever, infection, trauma, stress, heavy physical activity), have hypoglycemic treatment available (glucagon, oral dextrose). • Monitor daily calorie intake.

linezolid

lin-**ez**-oh-lid
(Apo-Linezolid ✦, <u>Zyvox</u>, Zyvoxam ✦)

Do not confuse Zyvox with Zosyn or Zovirax.

◆CLASSIFICATION

PHARMACOTHERAPEUTIC: Oxazolidinone. **CLINICAL:** Antibiotic.

USES

Treatment of susceptible infections due to aerobic and facultative, gram-positive microorganisms, including *E. faecium* (vancomycin-resistant strains only), *S. aureus* (including methicillin-resistant strains), *S. agalactiae, S. pneumoniae* (including multidrug-resistant strains), *S. pyogenes*. Treatment of pneumonia (community-acquired and hospital-acquired), skin, soft tissue infections (including diabetic foot infections), bacteremia caused by susceptible vancomycin-resistant (VRE) organisms. **OFF-LABEL:** Treatment of prosthetic joint infection. Septic arthritis.

PRECAUTIONS

Contraindications: Hypersensitivity to linezolid. Concurrent use or within 2 wks of MAOIs. **Cautions:** History of seizures, preexisting myelosuppression, medications that may cause bone marrow depression, uncontrolled hypertension, pheochromocytoma, carcinoid syndrome, untreated hyperthyroidism, diabetes, chronic infection; concurrent use of SSRIs, SNRIs, tricyclic antidepressants, triptans, buPROPion.

ACTION

Binds to bacterial ribosomal RNA sites, preventing formation of a complex essential for bacterial translation. **Therapeutic Effect:** Bacteriostatic against enterococci, staphylococci; bactericidal against streptococci.

PHARMACOKINETICS

Rapidly, extensively absorbed after PO administration. Protein binding: 31%. Metabolized in liver by oxidation. Excreted in urine. **Half-life:** 4–5.4 hrs.

⌛ LIFESPAN CONSIDERATIONS

Pregnancy/Lactation: Unknown if distributed in breast milk. **Children:** Safety and efficacy not established. **Elderly:** No age-related precautions noted.

INTERACTIONS

DRUG: CYP3A4 inducers (e.g., **carBA-Mazepine, phenytoin**) may decrease concentration/effects. **Adrenergic medications (sympathomimetics)** may increase effects. **SSRIs (e.g., escitalopram, paroxetine, sertraline), SNRIs (e.g., duloxetine, venlafaxine)** may increase risk of serotonin syndrome. **HERBAL:** Supplements containing **caffeine, tyrosine,** or **tryptophan** may precipitate hypertensive crisis. **FOOD:** Excessive amounts of **tyramine-containing foods, beverages** may cause significant hypertension. **LAB VALUES:** May decrease Hgb, neutrophils, platelets, WBC. May increase serum ALT, AST, alkaline phosphatase, amylase, bilirubin, BUN, creatinine, LDH, lipase.

AVAILABILITY (Rx)

Injection Premix: 2 mg/mL in 100-mL, 300-mL bags. **Powder for Oral Suspension:** 100 mg/5 mL. **Tablets:** 600 mg.

ADMINISTRATION/HANDLING

💧 IV

Rate of Administration • Infuse over 30–120 min. • Should be administered without further dilution.

Storage • Store at room temperature. • Protect from light. • Yellow color does not affect potency.

PO

• Give without regard to meals. • Use suspension within 21 days after reconstitution. Gently invert 3–5 times before administration. • Do not shake.

🔳 IV INCOMPATIBILITIES

Amphotericin B complex (Abelcet, AmBisome, Amphotec), co-trimoxazole (Bactrim), diazePAM (Valium), erythromycin (Erythrocin), pentamidine (Pentam IV), phenytoin (Dilantin).

🔳 IV COMPATIBILITIES

Calcium gluconate, dexmedetomidine (Precedex), heparin, magnesium, potassium chloride.

INDICATIONS/ROUTES/DOSAGE

Vancomycin-Resistant Infections (VRE)
PO, IV: ADULTS, ELDERLY, CHILDREN OLDER THAN 11 YRS: 600 mg q12h. **CHILDREN 11 YRS AND YOUNGER:** 10 mg/kg q8–12h. **Maximum:** 600 mg/dose.

Pneumonia, Complicated Skin/Skin Structure Infections
PO, IV: ADULTS, ELDERLY, CHILDREN OLDER THAN 11 YRS: 600 mg q12h. **CHILDREN 11 YRS AND YOUNGER:** 10 mg/kg q8h. **Maximum:** 600 mg/dose.

Uncomplicated Skin/Skin Structure Infections
PO: ADULTS, ELDERLY: 600 mg q12h. **CHILDREN OLDER THAN 11 YRS:** 600 mg q12h. **CHILDREN 5–11 YRS:** 10 mg/kg/dose q12h. **Maximum:** 600 mg/dose. **CHILDREN YOUNGER THAN 5 YRS:** 10 mg/kg q8h. **Maximum:** 600 mg/dose.

Usual Neonate Dosage
PO, IV: NEONATES: 10 mg/kg/dose q8–12h.

Dosage in Renal/Hepatic Impairment
No dose adjustment. Administer after HD on dialysis days.

SIDE EFFECTS

Occasional (9%–2%): Diarrhea, nausea, vomiting, insomnia, constipation, rash, dizziness, fever, headache. **Rare (less than 2%):** Altered taste, vaginal candidiasis, fungal infection, tongue discoloration.

ADVERSE EFFECTS/TOXIC REACTIONS

Thrombocytopenia, myelosuppression occur rarely. Antibiotic-associated colitis, other superinfections (abdominal cramps, severe watery diarrhea, fever) may result from altered bacterial balance in GI tract.

NURSING CONSIDERATIONS

BASELINE ASSESSMENT

Obtain appropriate culture specimens for sensitivity testing prior to therapy. Obtain baseline CBC, chemistries. Question medical history as listed in Precautions. Receive full medication history and screen for interactions.

INTERVENTION/EVALUATION

Monitor daily pattern of bowel activity, stool consistency. Mild GI effects may be tolerable, but increasing severity may indicate onset of antibiotic-associated colitis. Be alert for superinfection: fever, vomiting, diarrhea, anal/genital pruritus, oral mucosal changes (ulceration, pain, erythema). Monitor CBC, platelets, Hgb, chemistries.

PATIENT/ FAMILY TEACHING

• Continue therapy for full length of treatment. • Doses should be evenly spaced. • May cause GI upset (may take with food, milk). • Excessive amounts of tyramine-containing foods (red wine, aged cheese) may cause severe reaction (severe headache, neck stiffness, diaphoresis, palpitations). • Avoid alcohol. • Report persistent diarrhea, nausea, vomiting.

liraglutide   TOP 100

leer-a-gloo-tide
(Saxenda, Victoza)

■ **BLACK BOX ALERT** ■ Causes dose-dependent and treatment duration–dependent thyroid C-cell tumors, including medullary thyroid cancer.

FIXED-COMBINATION(S)

Xultophy: liraglutide 3.6 mg/mL and insulin degludec 100 units/mL.

◆CLASSIFICATION

PHARMACOTHERAPEUTIC: Antihyperglycemic (glucagon-like peptide-1 [GLP-1]) receptor agonist. **CLINICAL:** Antidiabetic agent.

USES

Saxenda: Adjunct to diet and increased physical activity for chronic weight management in adults with body mass index (BMI) of 30 kg/m^2 or greater, or 27 kg/m^2 or greater, with at least one co-morbid condition (e.g., hypertension, diabetes, dyslipidemia). **Victoza:** Adjunct to diet and exercise to improve glycemic control in adult pts with type 2 diabetes. Reduce risk of major cardiovascular events in adults with type 2 diabetes and established cardiovascular (CV) disease.

PRECAUTIONS

Contraindications: Hypersensitivity to liraglutide. Personal or family history of medullary thyroid carcinoma (MTC), pts with multiple endocrine neoplasia syndrome type 2 (MEN2). **(Saxenda):** Pregnancy. **Cautions:** History of pancreatitis, cholelithiasis, alcohol abuse, renal/hepatic impairment. History of angioedema to other GLP-1 receptor agonists. Do not use in type 1 diabetes or diabetic ketoacidosis. Medications requiring a narrow therapeutic index or requiring rapid GI absorption.

ACTION

Stimulates release of insulin from pancreatic beta cells, mimics enhancement of glucose-dependent insulin secretion, suppresses elevated glucagon secretion, slows gastric emptying. **Therapeutic Effect:** Improves glycemic control by increasing postmeal insulin secretion, emptying, increasing satiety.

PHARMACOKINETICS

Maximum concentration achieved in 8–12 hrs. Protein binding: 98%. Metabolized to large proteins without a specific organ as major route of elimination. **Half-life:** 13 hrs.

☒ LIFESPAN CONSIDERATIONS

Pregnancy/Lactation: Unknown if distributed in breast milk. **Children:** Safety and efficacy not established. **Elderly:** No age-related precautions noted.

INTERACTIONS

DRUG: Liraglutide has potential to alter absorption of concurrently administered **oral medications. HERBAL:** None significant. **FOOD:** None known. **LAB VALUES:** Decreases glucose serum levels (when used in combination with insulin secretagogues [e.g., sulfonylureas]).

AVAILABILITY (Rx)

Subcutaneous, Solution (Prefilled Pen): (Victoza): 18 mg/3 mL. **(Saxenda):** (Prefilled Pen) 18 mg/3 mL. Delivers doses of 0.6 mg, 1.2 mg, 1.8 mg, 2.4 mg, or 3 mg.

ADMINISTRATION/HANDLING

Subcutaneous
• Insert needle subcutaneously into upper arms, outer thigh, or abdomen, and inject solution. • Do not inject into areas of active skin disease or injury such as sunburns, skin rashes, inflammation, skin infections, or active psoriasis. • Rotate injection sites. **Storage** • Refrigerate prefilled pens. • Discard if freezing occurs. • Discard pen 30 days after initial use.

INDICATIONS/ROUTES/DOSAGE

Diabetes (Victoza) With or Without CV Disease
SQ: ADULTS, ELDERLY: Initial dose: 0.6 mg once daily for at least 1 wk. (**Note:** This dose is intended to reduce GI symptoms during initial titration; it is not effective for glycemic control.) After 1 wk, increase dose to 1.2 mg. If 1.2-mg dose does not result in acceptable glycemic control, dose can be increased to 1.8 mg.

Weight Management (Saxenda)
SQ: ADULTS, ELDERLY: Initially, 0.6 mg once daily for one week. Increase wkly by 0.6 mg/day to a target dose of 3 mg once daily. **Note:** Evaluate change in weight 16 wks after initiation. Discontinue if less than 4% of baseline weight not achieved.

Dosage in Renal/Hepatic Impairment
Use caution.

SIDE EFFECTS

Frequent (greater than 13%): Headache, nausea, diarrhea, liraglutide antibody resistance. **Occasional (13%–6%):** Diarrhea, vomiting, dizziness, nervousness, dyspepsia. **Rare (less than 6%):** Weakness, decreased appetite.

L

ADVERSE EFFECTS/TOXIC REACTIONS

Serious hypoglycemia may occur when used concurrently with insulin analogue (e.g., sulfonylurea); consider lowering dose.

NURSING CONSIDERATIONS

BASELINE ASSESSMENT

Check blood glucose concentration before administration. Discuss pt's lifestyle to determine extent of learning, emotional needs. Ensure follow-up instruction if pt/family does not thoroughly understand diabetes management or glucose testing technique. Dose is gradually increased to improve GI tolerance.

INTERVENTION/EVALUATION

Monitor blood glucose level, food intake. Assess for hypoglycemia (cool wet skin, tremors, dizziness, anxiety, headache, tachycardia, numbness in mouth, hunger, diplopia) or hyperglycemia (polyuria, polyphagia, polydipsia, nausea, vomiting, dim vision, fatigue, deep rapid breathing). Be alert to conditions that alter glucose requirements (fever, increased activity/stress, surgical procedures). Consider lowering dose of insulin analogue to reduce risk of hypoglycemia.

PATIENT/FAMILY TEACHING

• A health care provider will show you how to properly prepare and inject your medication. You must demonstrate correct preparation and injection techniques before using medication at home. • Diabetes requires lifelong control. • Prescribed diet, exercise are principal parts of treatment; do not skip/delay meals. • Continue following dietary instructions, regular exercise program, regular testing of blood glucose level. • Serious hypoglycemia may occur when used concurrently with insulin analogue (e.g., sulfonylurea). • Have source of glucose available to treat symptoms of low blood sugar.

lisdexamfetamine

lis-dex-am-**fet**-a-meen
(Vyvanse)

■ **BLACK BOX ALERT** ■ Potential for drug abuse dependency exists. Assess for abuse potential and monitor for abuse potential/dependence.
Do not confuse lisdexamfetamine with dextroamphetamine, or Vyvanse with Glucovance, Vivactil, or Vytorin.

◆CLASSIFICATION

PHARMACOTHERAPEUTIC: Amphetamine (Schedule II). **CLINICAL:** CNS stimulant.

USES

Treatment of attention-deficit/hyperactivity disorder (ADHD), moderate to severe binge eating disorder (BED).

PRECAUTIONS

Contraindications: Hypersensitivity to lisdexamfetamine, amphetamine products. Concurrent use or within 2 wks of use of MAOI. **Cautions:** Hyperthyroidism, glaucoma, agitated states, cardiovascular conditions (hypertension, recent MI, ventricular arrhythmias), elderly, psychiatric/seizures, preexisting psychosis or bipolar disorder, Tourette syndrome. Avoid use in pts with serious structural cardiac abnormalities, cardiomyopathy, arrhythmias, CAD. History of alcohol or drug abuse.

ACTION

Enhances action of DOPamine, norepinephrine by blocking reuptake from synapses, increasing levels in extraneuronal space. **Therapeutic Effect:** Improves attention span in ADHD.

PHARMACOKINETICS

Rapidly absorbed. Converted to dextroamphetamine. Excreted in urine. **Half-life:** Less than 1 hr.

⧗ LIFESPAN CONSIDERATIONS

Pregnancy/Lactation: Has potential for fetal harm. Distributed in breast milk. **Children:** Safety and efficacy not established in pts younger than 6 yrs. **Elderly:** No age-related precautions noted.

INTERACTIONS

DRUG: **MAOIs** (e.g., **phenelzine, selegiline**) may prolong/intensify effects. May decrease sedative effect of **antihistamines** (e.g., **diphenhydrAMINE**). May decrease hypotensive effects of **antihypertensives** (e.g., **amLODIPine, lisinopril, valsartan**). Effects may be decreased by **chlorproMAZINE, haloperidol, lithium, urinary acidifying agents** (**ammonium chloride, sodium acid phosphate**). May increase absorption of **PHENobarbital, phenytoin.** **Tricyclic antidepressants** (e.g., **amitriptyline, doxepin**) may increase cardiovascular effects. **HERBAL:** None significant. **FOOD:** None known. **LAB VALUES:** May increase plasma corticosteroid.

AVAILABILITY (Rx)

Capsules: 10 mg, 20 mg, 30 mg, 40 mg, 50 mg, 60 mg, 70 mg.

ADMINISTRATION/HANDLING

PO
• May be given in the morning without regard to food. • Administer capsule whole; pt must not chew. • Capsules may be opened and dissolved in water and taken immediately.

INDICATIONS/ROUTES/DOSAGE

ADHD
Note: Assess for cardiac disease and risk of abuse before initiating.
PO: **ADULTS, CHILDREN 6 YRS AND OLDER:** Initially, 30 mg once daily in the morning. May increase dosage in increments of 10 or 20 mg/day at wkly intervals until optimal response obtained. **Maximum:** 70 mg/day.

BED
PO: **ADULTS, ELDERLY:** Initially, 30 mg once daily in morning. May increase by 20 mg/day at wkly intervals to a target dose of 50–70 mg once daily. **Maximum:** 70 mg/day.

Dosage in Renal Impairment
CrCl 30 mL/min or greater: Maximum: 70 mg/day. **CrCl 15–29 mL/min:** Maximum: 50 mg/day. **CrCl less than 15 mL/min or end-stage renal disease:** Maximum: 30 mg/day.

Dosage in Hepatic Impairment
No dose adjustment.

SIDE EFFECTS

Frequent (39%): Decreased appetite. **Occasional (19%–9%):** Insomnia, upper abdominal pain, headache, irritability, vomiting, weight decrease. **Rare (6%–2%):** Nausea, dry mouth, dizziness, rash, affect change, fatigue, tic.

ADVERSE EFFECTS/TOXIC REACTIONS

Abrupt withdrawal following prolonged administration of high dosage may produce extreme fatigue (may last for wks). Prolonged administration to children with ADHD may produce a suppression of weight and/or height patterns. May produce cardiac irregularities, psychotic syndrome.

NURSING CONSIDERATIONS

BASELINE ASSESSMENT

Assess attention span, impulse control, interaction with others. Question history of cardiomyopathy, glaucoma, hypertension, hyperthyroidism, psychiatric disorder, renal impairment. Receive full medication history and screen for interactions.

INTERVENTION/EVALUATION

Monitor for CNS stimulation, increase in B/P, weight loss, pulse, sleep pattern, appetite; palpitations, cardiac arrhythmia. Observe for signs of hostility, aggression, depression.

L

PATIENT/FAMILY TEACHING

PATIENT/FAMILY TEACHING

• Take early in day. • May mask extreme fatigue. • Report pronounced dizziness, decreased appetite, dry mouth, weight loss, new or worsened psychiatric problems, palpitations, dyspnea. • Suddenly stopping treatment may cause extreme fatigue that can last for wks. Discontinuance must be done under the close supervision of health care professional.

lisinopril

lye-**sin**-o-pril
(Apo-Lisinopril ✦, Prinivil, Qbrelis, Zestril)

■ **BLACK BOX ALERT** ■ May cause fetal injury, mortality. Discontinue as soon as possible once pregnancy is detected.
Do not confuse lisinopril with fosinopril, or Prinivil with Plendil, Pravachol, Prevacid, PriLOSEC, Proventil, or Restoril, or Zestril with Desyrel, Restoril, Vistaril, Zetia, or Zostrix.
Do not confuse lisinopril's combination form Zestoretic with PriLOSEC.

FIXED-COMBINATION(S)

Prinzide/Zestoretic: lisinopril/hydroCHLOROthiazide (a diuretic): 10 mg/12.5 mg, 20 mg/12.5 mg, 20 mg/25 mg.

◆CLASSIFICATION

PHARMACOTHERAPEUTIC: ACE inhibitor. **CLINICAL:** Antihypertensive.

USES

Treatment of hypertension in adults and children 6 yrs and older. Used alone or in combination with other antihypertensives. Adjunctive therapy in management of HF. Treatment of acute MI within 24 hrs in hemodynamically stable pts to improve survival. Treatment of left ventricular dysfunction following MI.

PRECAUTIONS

Contraindications: Hypersensitivity to lisinopril, other ACE inhibitors. History of angioedema from treatment with ACE inhibitors, idiopathic or hereditary angioedema. Concomitant use with aliskiren in pts with diabetes. **Cautions:** Renal impairment, unstented unilateral/bilateral renal artery stenosis, volume depletion, ischemic heart disease, cerebrovascular disease, severe aortic stenosis, hypertrophic cardiomyopathy, HF, systolic B/P less than 100, dialysis, hyponatremia; before, during, or immediately after major surgery. Concomitant use of potassium supplements.

ACTION

Competitive inhibitor of angiotensin-converting enzyme (ACE) (prevents conversion of angiotensin I to angiotensin II, a potent vasoconstrictor; may inhibit angiotensin II at local vascular, renal sites). Decreases plasma angiotensin II, increases plasma renin activity, decreases aldosterone secretion. **Therapeutic Effect:** Reduces blood pressure.

PHARMACOKINETICS

Route	Onset	Peak	Duration
PO	1 hr	6 hrs	24 hrs

Incompletely absorbed from GI tract. Protein binding: 25%. Primarily excreted unchanged in urine. Removed by hemodialysis. **Half-life:** 12 hrs (increased in renal impairment).

⌛ LIFESPAN CONSIDERATIONS

Pregnancy/Lactation: Crosses placenta. Unknown if distributed in breast milk. **Children:** Safety and efficacy not established. **Elderly:** May be more sensitive to hypotensive effects.

INTERACTIONS

DRUG: Diuretics (e.g., **furosemide, HCTZ**) may increase hypotensive effects. May increase concentration, risk of toxicity of **lithium.** NSAIDs (e.g., **ibuprofen, ketorolac, naproxen**) may decrease effects. **Potassium-sparing diuretics (e.g., spironolactone, triamterene), potassium supplements** may cause hyperkalemia. May increase hypoglycemic effect of **oral hypoglycemic agents (e.g., glyBURIDE, metFORMIN). HERBAL:** Ephedra, ginseng, licorice, yohimbe may worsen hypertension. **Black cohosh, periwinkle** may increase antihypertensive effect. **FOOD:** None known. **LAB VALUES:** May increase serum BUN, alkaline phosphatase, bilirubin, creatinine, potassium, ALT, AST. May decrease serum sodium. May cause positive ANA titer.

AVAILABILITY (Rx)

Solution, Oral: (Qbrelis) 1 mg/mL. **Tablets:** 2.5 mg, 5 mg, 10 mg, 20 mg, 30 mg, 40 mg.

ADMINISTRATION/HANDLING

PO
• Give without regard to food. • Tablets may be crushed.

INDICATIONS/ROUTES/DOSAGE

Hypertension (Used Alone)
PO: ADULTS: Initially, 10 mg/day. May increase by 5–10 mg/day at 1- to 2-wk intervals. Range: 10–40 mg/day. **ELDERLY:** Initially, 2.5–5 mg/day. May increase by 2.5–5 mg/day at 1- to 2-wk intervals. **Maximum:** 40 mg/day. **CHILDREN 6 YRS OR OLDER:** Initially, 0.07 mg/kg once daily (up to 5 mg). Titrate at 1- to 2-wk intervals. **Maximum:** 40 mg/day.

Hypertension (in Combination with Other Antihypertensives)
◄ALERT► If possible, discontinue diuretics 48–72 hrs prior to initiating lisinopril therapy.
PO: ADULTS, ELDERLY: Initially, 2.5–5 mg/day titrated to pt's needs. Range: 10–40 mg/day.

HF
PO: ADULTS, ELDERLY: Initially, 2.5–5 mg/day. May increase by no more than 10 mg/day at intervals of at least 2 wks to a target dose of 20–40 mg once daily.

Improve Survival in Pts after MI
PO: ADULTS, ELDERLY: Initially, 5 mg, then 5 mg after 24 hrs, 10 mg after 48 hrs, then 10 mg/day for 6 wks. For pts with systolic B/P greater than 100–120 mm Hg, give 2.5 mg/day for 3 days, then 2.5–5 mg/day. Discontinue if systolic B/P less than 90 mm Hg for more than 1 hr.

Dosage in Renal Impairment
CrCl less than 30 mL/min: Not recommended in children. Titrate to pt's needs after giving the following initial dose:

Hypertension

Creatinine Clearance	Initial Dose
10–30 mL/min	5 mg
Less than 10 mL/min or Dialysis	2.5 mg

HF
CrCl less than 30 mL/min or serum creatinine greater than 3 mg/dL: Initial dose: 2.5 mg.

Acute MI
Creatinine clearance 30 mL/min or less: Initial dose: 2.5 mg.

Dosage in Hepatic Impairment
No dose adjustment.

SIDE EFFECTS

Frequent (12%–5%): Headache, dizziness, postural hypotension. **Occasional (4%–2%):** Chest discomfort, fatigue, rash, abdominal pain, nausea, diarrhea, upper respiratory infection. **Rare (1% or less):** Palpitations, tachycardia, peripheral edema, insomnia, paresthesia, confusion, constipation, dry mouth, muscle cramps.

ADVERSE EFFECTS/TOXIC REACTIONS

Excessive hypotension ("first-dose syncope") may occur in pts with HF, severe salt/volume depletion. Angioedema

---

L

(swelling of face and lips), hyperkalemia occur rarely. Agranulocytosis, neutropenia may be noted in pts with collagen vascular disease (scleroderma, systemic lupus erythematosus). Nephrotic syndrome may be noted in pts with history of renal disease.

NURSING CONSIDERATIONS

BASELINE ASSESSMENT

Obtain BMP (esp. serum BUN, creatinine, sodium, potassium; CrCl, GFR. Obtain B/P, apical pulse immediately before each dose in addition to regular monitoring (be alert to fluctuations). In pts with renal impairment, autoimmune disease, taking drugs that affect leukocytes or immune response, CBC and differential count should be performed before beginning therapy and q2wks for 3 mos, then periodically thereafter. Question history of aortic stenosis, cardiac disease, cardiomyopathy, renal impairment or stenosis.

INTERVENTION/EVALUATION

Monitor B/P, renal function tests, WBC, serum potassium. Assess for edema. Auscultate lungs for rales. Monitor I&O; weigh daily. Monitor daily pattern of bowel activity, stool consistency. Assist with ambulation if dizziness occurs. If excessive reduction in B/P occurs, place pt in supine position, feet slightly elevated.

PATIENT/ FAMILY TEACHING

• To reduce hypotensive effect, go from lying to standing slowly. • Limit alcohol intake. • Report vomiting, diarrhea, diaphoresis, swelling of face/lips/tongue, difficulty in breathing, persistent cough. • Limit salt intake. • Maintain adequate hydration. • Report decreased urinary output, dark-colored urine, swelling of the hands and feet. • Immediately report allergic reactions, esp. life-threatening swelling of the face or tongue.

lithium

lith-ee-um
(Apo-Lithium ✦, Lithobid)
■ BLACK BOX ALERT ■ Lithium toxicity is closely related to serum lithium levels and can occur at therapeutic doses. Routine determination of serum lithium levels is essential during therapy.
Do not confuse Lithobid with Levbid or Lithostat.

◆CLASSIFICATION

PHARMACOTHERAPEUTIC: Mood-stabilizing agent. **CLINICAL:** Antimanic.

USES

Management of bipolar disorder. Treatment of mania in pts with bipolar disorder. **OFF-LABEL:** Augmenting agent for depression.

PRECAUTIONS

Contraindications: Hypersensitivity to lithium. Severely debilitated pts, severe cardiovascular disease, concurrent use with diuretics, severe dehydration, severe renal disease, severe sodium depletion or dehydration. **Cautions:** Mild to moderate cardiovascular disease, thyroid disease, elderly, mild to moderate renal impairment, medications altering sodium excretion, pregnancy, pts at risk for suicide, pts with significant fluid loss, pts receiving neuromuscular blocking agents.

ACTION

Changes cation transport across cell membrane in nerve/muscle cells; influences reuptake of serotonin/norepinephrine. **Therapeutic Effect:** Stabilizes mood, reducing episodes of mania.

PHARMACOKINETICS

Rapidly, completely absorbed from GI tract. Protein binding: None. Primarily excreted unchanged in urine. Removed by hemodialysis. **Half-life:** 18–24 hrs (increased in elderly).

☒ LIFESPAN CONSIDERATIONS

Pregnancy/Lactation: Freely crosses placenta. Distributed in breast milk. **Children:** May increase bone formation or density (alter parathyroid hormone concentrations). **Elderly:** More susceptible to develop lithium-induced goiter or clinical hypothyroidism, CNS toxicity. Increased thirst, urination noted more frequently; lower dosage recommended.

INTERACTIONS

DRUG: Diuretics (e.g., furosemide), NSAIDs, metroNIDAZOLE, ACE inhibitors (e.g., enalapril, lisinopril), angiotensin II antagonists, SSRIs (e.g., escitalopram, paroxetine, sertraline), calcium channel blockers (e.g., losartan, valsartan) may increase lithium concentration, risk of toxicity. **HERBAL:** None significant. **FOOD:** None known. **LAB VALUES:** May increase serum glucose, immunoreactive parathyroid hormone, calcium. **Therapeutic serum level:** 0.6–1.2 mEq/L; **toxic serum level:** greater than 1.5 mEq/L.

AVAILABILITY (Rx)

Capsules: 150 mg, 300 mg, 600 mg. **Oral Solution:** 300 mg/5 mL. **Tablets:** 300 mg.

🐾 **Tablets (Extended-Release):** 300 mg, 450 mg.

ADMINISTRATION/HANDLING

PO
• Administer with meals, milk to decrease GI upset. • Do not break, crush, dissolve, or divide extended-release tablets.

INDICATIONS/ROUTES/DOSAGE

◀**ALERT**▶ During acute phase, a therapeutic serum lithium concentration of 0.6–1.2 mEq/L is required. For long-term control, desired level is 0.8–1 mEq/L. Monitor serum drug concentration, clinical response to determine proper dosage.

Usual Dosage
PO: ADULTS, ELDERLY, CHILDREN OLDER THAN 12 YRS: *(Immediate-Release):* 300 mg 3–4 times/day. Gradually increase based on response/tolerability. *(Extended-Release):* 450 mg twice daily. Gradually increase based on response/tolerability. Usual dose: *(Immediate-Release):* 900–1,800 mg/day in 3–4 divided doses. *(Extended-Release):* 900–1,800 mg in 2 divided doses. **CHILDREN 6–12 YRS:** *(Immediate-Release):* 15–60 mg/kg/day in 3–4 divided doses not to exceed usual adult dose.

Dosage in Renal Impairment

Creatinine Clearance	Dosage
10–50 mL/min	50%–75% normal dose
Less than 10 mL/min	25%–50% normal dose
End-stage renal disease with HD	Dose after HD

Dosage in Hepatic Impairment
No dose adjustment.

SIDE EFFECTS

◀**ALERT**▶ Side effects are dose related and seldom occur at lithium serum levels less than 1.5 mEq/L. **Occasional:** Fine hand tremor, polydipsia, polyuria, mild nausea. **Rare:** Weight gain, bradycardia, tachycardia, acne, rash, muscle twitching, peripheral cyanosis, pseudotumor cerebri (eye pain, headache, tinnitus, vision disturbances).

ADVERSE EFFECTS/TOXIC REACTIONS

Lithium serum concentration of 1.5–2.0 mEq/L may produce vomiting, diarrhea, drowsiness, confusion, incoordination, coarse hand tremor, muscle twitching,

T-wave depression on EKG. Lithium serum concentration of 2.0–2.5 mEq/L may result in ataxia, giddiness, tinnitus, blurred vision, clonic movements, severe hypotension. Acute toxicity may be characterized by seizures, oliguria, circulatory failure, coma, death.

NURSING CONSIDERATIONS

BASELINE ASSESSMENT

Question history of cardiac/thyroid disease, renal impairment. Assess hydration status. Assess mental status (e.g., mood, behavior). Serum lithium levels should be tested q3–4days during initial phase of therapy, q1–2mos thereafter, and wkly if there is no improvement of disorder or adverse effects occur.

INTERVENTION/EVALUATION

Clinical assessment of therapeutic effect, tolerance to drug effect is necessary for correct dosing-level management. Assess behavior, appearance, emotional status, response to environment, speech pattern, thought content. Monitor serum lithium concentrations, CBC with differential, urinalysis, creatinine clearance. Monitor renal, hepatic, thyroid, cardiovascular function; serum electrolytes. Assess for increased urinary output, persistent thirst. Report polyuria, prolonged vomiting, diarrhea, fever to physician (may need to temporarily reduce or discontinue dosage). Monitor for signs of lithium toxicity. Assess for therapeutic response (interest in surroundings, improvement in self-care, increased ability to concentrate, relaxed facial expression). Monitor lithium levels q3–4days at initiation of therapy (then q1–2mos). Obtain lithium levels 8–12 hrs postdose. **Therapeutic serum level:** 0.6–1.2 mEq/L; **toxic serum level:** greater than 1.5 mEq/L.

PATIENT/ FAMILY TEACHING

• Limit alcohol, caffeine intake. • Avoid tasks requiring coordination until CNS effects of drug are known.

• May cause dry mouth. • Maintain adequate salt, fluid intake (avoid dehydration). • Report vomiting, diarrhea, muscle weakness, tremors, drowsiness, ataxia. • Monitoring of serum level is necessary to determine proper dose.

lixisenatide

lix-i-sen-a-tide
(Adlyxin)
Do not confuse lixisenatide with exenatide, liraglutide.

FIXED-COMBINATION(S)

Soliqua: lixisenatide 33 mcg/mL and insulin glargine 100 units/mL.

◆CLASSIFICATION

PHARMACOTHERAPEUTIC: Antihyperglycemic (glucagon-like peptide-1 [GLP-1]) receptor agonist. **CLINICAL:** Antidiabetic agent.

USES

Adjunct to diet and exercise to improve glycemic controls in pts with type 2 diabetes mellitus.

PRECAUTIONS

Contraindications: Hypersensitivity to lixisenatide. **Cautions:** Renal impairment, severe gastroparesis, history of pancreatitis. Not recommended in pts with diabetic ketoacidosis, type 1 diabetes mellitus. Not a substitute for insulin. Medications with narrow therapeutic index or requiring rapid GI absorption.

ACTION

Increases glucose-dependent insulin secretion; decreases glucagon secretion. Slows gastric emptying. **Therapeutic Effect:** Improves glycemic control by lowering fasting glucose and postprandial blood glucose.

PHARMACOKINETICS

Widely distributed. Protein binding: not specified. Peak plasma concentration: 1–3.5 hrs. Eliminated through glomerulus filtration and proteolytic degradation. **Half-life:** 3 hrs.

☒ LIFESPAN CONSIDERATIONS

Pregnancy/Lactation: Unknown if distributed in breast milk. **Children:** Safety and efficacy not established in pts younger than 18 yrs. **Elderly:** No age-related precautions noted.

INTERACTIONS

DRUG: May increase hypoglycemic effect when added to **insulin or sulfonylureas.** May decrease the rate of absorption of **oral medications** due to delayed gastric emptying. **Oral contraceptive** should be taken 1 hr before or 11 hrs after lixisenatide. **HERBAL:** None significant. **FOOD:** None known. **LAB VALUES:** Expected to decrease serum glucose, Hgb A1c.

AVAILABILITY (Rx)

Prefilled Injector Pens: 50 mcg/mL in 3 mL (for 14 preset doses of 10 mcg/dose), 100 mcg/mL in 3 mL (for 14 preset doses of 20 mcg/dose).

ADMINISTRATION/HANDLING

Subcutaneous

Preparation • Follow instructions for preparation according to manufacturer guidelines. • Visually inspect for particulate matter or discoloration. Solution should appear clear and colorless. • Do not use if solution is cloudy or discolored or if visible particles are observed.

Administrations • Administer within 1 hr before the first meal of the day, preferably the same time each day. If a dose is missed, administer within 1 hr prior to next meal. • Insert needle subcutaneously into upper arms, outer thigh, or abdomen, and inject solution. • Do not inject into areas of active skin disease or injury such as sunburns, skin rashes, inflammation, skin infections, or active psoriasis. • Rotate injection sites.

Storage • Refrigerate unused injector pens. • Once injector pen is activated, store at room temperature for up to 14 days. • Do not freeze. • Protect from light.

INDICATIONS/ROUTES/DOSAGE

Type 2 Diabetes Mellitus
SQ: ADULTS, ELDERLY: 10 mcg once daily for 14 days. **Maintenance:** Increase to 20 mcg once daily on day 15.

Dosage in Renal Impairment
Use caution.

Dosage in Hepatic Impairment
No dose adjustment.

SIDE EFFECTS

Frequent (25%–10%): Nausea, vomiting. **Occasional (9%–1%):** Headache, diarrhea, dizziness, dyspepsia, constipation, abdominal distention, abdominal pain.

ADVERSE EFFECTS/TOXIC REACTIONS

May increase risk of acute renal failure or worsening of chronic renal impairment (esp. in pts with vomiting, dehydration). May increase risk of hypoglycemia when used with other hypoglycemic agents or insulin. Anaphylaxis reported in less than 1% of pts. Other hypersensitivity reactions including angioedema, bronchospasm, laryngeal edema occur rarely. Acute pancreatitis, hemorrhagic or necrotizing pancreatitis were reported. Immunogenicity (auto-lixisenatide antibodies) occurred in 70% of pts.

NURSING CONSIDERATIONS

BASELINE ASSESSMENT

Obtain baseline fasting glucose level, Hgb A1c; BMP. Question history of

L

renal impairment, gastroparesis, hypersensitivity reaction. Screen for use of other hypoglycemic agents or insulin. Assess pt's understanding of diabetes management, routine home glucose monitoring, medication self-administration. Assess hydration status. Obtain dietary consult for nutritional education.

INTERVENTION/EVALUATION

Monitor capillary blood glucose levels, Hgb A1c; renal function test (esp. in pts with renal impairment who report diarrhea, gastroparesis, vomiting). Assess for hypoglycemia (anxiety, confusion, diaphoresis, diplopia, dizziness, headache, hunger, perioral numbness, tachycardia, tremors), hyperglycemia (confusion, fatigue, Kussmaul breathing, nausea, polyuria, vomiting). Screen for glucose-altering conditions: fever, stress, surgical procedures, trauma. Monitor for hypersensitivity reactions; abdominal pain that radiates to the back. Encourage fluid intake. Monitor I&O.

PATIENT/FAMILY TEACHING

• Diabetes requires lifelong control. Diet and exercise are principal parts of treatment; do not skip or delay meals. • Test blood sugar regularly. • Monitor daily calorie intake. • When taking additional medications to lower blood sugar or when glucose demands are altered (fever, infection, stress trauma), have low blood sugar treatment available (glucagon, oral dextrose).
• Persistent, severe abdominal pain that radiates to the back (with or without vomiting) may indicate acute pancreatitis. • Report allergic reactions of any kind, esp. difficulty breathing, itching, rash, swelling of the face or throat. • Oral contraceptives should be taken at least 1 hr before or 11 hrs after dose. • Therapy may cause acute kidney injury or kidney failure; report decreased urine output, amber-colored urine, flank pain.

lomitapide

lom-i-**ta**-pide
(Juxtapid)
Do not confuse lomitapide with loperamide.

■ **BLACK BOX ALERT** ■ May cause hepatotoxicity. May cause hepatic steatosis (increase in hepatic fat) regardless of serum ALT, AST elevation; may be risk factor for progressive hepatic disease, including steatohepatitis and cirrhosis.

◆CLASSIFICATION

PHARMACOTHERAPEUTIC: Microsomal triglyceride transfer protein inhibitor. **CLINICAL:** Antihyperlipidemic.

USES

Treatment of homozygous familial hypercholesterolemia (HoFH) in combination with low-fat diet and other lipid-lowering therapies, including LDL-C apheresis, to reduce LDL, total cholesterol, apoprotein B, non–HDL-C.

PRECAUTIONS

Contraindications: Hypersensitivity to lomitapide. Pregnancy, breastfeeding, moderate to severe hepatic impairment, active hepatic disease including unexplained persistent elevation of serum transaminases, concomitant use of strong CYP3A4 inhibitors (e.g., ketoconazole, protease inhibitors). **Cautions:** Mild to moderate renal impairment, end-stage renal disease, mild hepatic impairment, alcohol consumption. Avoid use in pts with history of glucose-galactose malabsorption, other agents having hepatotoxic potential (e.g., acetaminophen).

ACTION

Inhibits microsomal triglyceride transfer protein in lumen of endoplasmic reticulum. Prevents assembly of apo-B-containing lipoproteins in enterocytes, hepatocytes;

inhibits synthesis of chylomicrons, very low density lipoprotein (VLDL). **Therapeutic Effect:** Decreases plasma low-density lipoprotein cholesterol (LDL-C).

PHARMACOKINETICS

Well absorbed in GI tract. Metabolized in liver. Protein binding: 99%. Peak plasma concentration: 6 hrs. Primarily excreted in feces. **Half-life:** 40 hrs.

⧖ LIFESPAN CONSIDERATIONS

Pregnancy/Lactation: Contraindicated in pregnancy. May cause fetal harm. Must use effective contraception in addition to barrier methods. Unknown if distributed in breast milk. Must either discontinue breastfeeding or discontinue therapy. **Children:** Safety and efficacy not established. **Elderly:** Increased risk for side effects, adverse reactions.

INTERACTIONS

DRUG: Acetaminophen, amiodarone, ISOtretinoin, methotrexate, tamoxifen, tetracycline may increase risk for hepatotoxicity. **Strong CYP3A4 inhibitors (e.g., ketoconazole, protease inhibitors)** contraindicated due to increased risk for myopathy, rhabdomyolysis. Moderate **CYP3A4 inhibitors (e.g., atorvastatin, oral contraceptives)** may increase concentration. May increase concentration of **warfarin.** May increase effects of **P-glycoprotein substrates (e.g., digoxin, SITagliptin). HERBAL:** None known. **FOOD: Grapefruit products** may increase absorption, toxicity. **LAB VALUES:** May increase serum alkaline phosphatase, bilirubin, ALT, AST.

AVAILABILITY (Rx)

🛡 **Capsules:** 5 mg, 10 mg, 20 mg, 30 mg, 40 mg, 60 mg.

ADMINISTRATION/HANDLING

PO
• Give with water only. • Administer without food (at least 2 hrs after evening meal). • Administer whole; do not break, crush, or open capsules.

INDICATIONS/ROUTES/DOSAGE

◀**ALERT**▶ To reduce risk for fat-soluble nutrient deficiency, recommend supplemental coadministration: vitamin E 400 international units PO daily, linolenic acid 200 mg PO daily, alpha-linolenic acid (ALA) 210 mg PO daily, eicosapentaenoic acid (EPA) 110 mg PO daily, docosahexaenoic acid (DHA) 80 mg PO daily. Because of risk for myopathy, concurrent use of simvastatin should not exceed 20–40 mg/day.

Homozygous Familial Hypercholesterolemia
PO: ADULTS, ELDERLY: Initially, 5 mg once daily for minimum of 2 wks. Gradually increase dose at 4-wk (minimum) intervals to 10 mg once daily, then 20 mg once daily, then 40 mg once daily, then 60 mg once daily based on tolerability. **Maximum:** 60 mg/day.

Dose Modification
Elevated Hepatic Enzymes
If ALT, AST is between 3–5 times upper limit of normal (ULN), reduce dose until ALT, AST less than 3 times ULN. If ALT, AST is greater than 5 times ULN, withhold dose until less than 3 times ULN, then restart at reduced dose. If hepatotoxicity occurs or bilirubin level rises greater than 2 times ULN, discontinue treatment.
End-Stage Renal Disease Receiving Dialysis, Mild Hepatic Impairment
Do not exceed 40 mg/day.
Concurrent Use of Weak CYP3A4 Inhibitors
Do not exceed 30 mg/day.
Concurrent Use of Oral Contraception
Do not exceed 40 mg/day.

Dosage in Renal Impairment
No dose adjustment. **End-stage renal disease:** Maximum: 40 mg/day.

Dosage in Hepatic Impairment
Mild impairment: Maximum: 40 mg/day. **Moderate to severe impairment:** Contraindicated.

L

SIDE EFFECTS

Frequent (79%–65%): Diarrhea, nausea. **Occasional (38%–10%):** Dyspepsia, vomiting, abdominal pain, weight loss, abdominal distention, constipation, flatulence, fatigue, back pain, gastric reflux, headache, dizziness.

ADVERSE EFFECTS/TOXIC REACTIONS

Progressive hepatic disease including steatohepatitis, cirrhosis has been reported in 6% of pts due to increased hepatic fat. May reduce absorption of fat-soluble nutrients; recommend daily supplemental replacement. Increased risk for myopathy including rhabdomyolysis (muscle pain/tenderness, weakness, dark or decreased urine output, elevated serum creatinine, CPK) when used with other antihyperlipidemics. May increase risk for supratherapeutic INR with warfarin. Infections including influenza, nasopharyngitis, gastroenteritis reported in 5% of pts. Palpitations, angina pectoris reported in 3% of pts. Increased risk for dehydration/malabsorption with galactose intolerance hereditary disorder, pancreatic disease, diarrhea.

NURSING CONSIDERATIONS

BASELINE ASSESSMENT

Obtain detailed dietary history, esp. fat consumption. Confirm negative pregnancy test before initiating treatment. Obtain baseline laboratory studies: ALT, AST, alkaline phosphatase, bilirubin, serum cholesterol, triglycerides, PT/INR (if pt is on warfarin). Confirm positive history of homozygous familial hypercholesterolemia (HoFH). Receive full medication history including vitamins, minerals, herbal products. Screen for medical history as listed in Precautions.

INTERVENTION/EVALUATION

Maintain hydration; offer fluids frequently. Monitor INR routinely (with anticoagulants). Monitor LFT with any dosage change, then every month for first year when maintenance goal reached, then every 3 mos. Obtain EKG for palpitations, shortness of breath, dizziness. Monitor for bruising, hematuria, jaundice, right upper abdominal pain, fever, lethargy, melena.

PATIENT/FAMILY TEACHING

• Avoid pregnancy. • Use appropriate contraception measures, including barrier precautions. • If pregnancy occurs, inform physician immediately. • Diarrhea may decrease effectiveness of oral contraception. • Do not breastfeed. • Maintain low-fat diet. • Report yellowing of skin, bruising, black/tarry stool, right upper quadrant pain, fever, lethargy, chest pain, palpitations. • Avoid alcohol. • Avoid grapefruit products. • Do not chew, crush, or open capsules. • Report any newly prescribed medications.

loperamide

loe-**per**-a-myde
(Apo-Loperamide ❖, Diamode, Diarr-Eze ❖, Imodium A-D, Loperacap ❖, Novo-Loperamide ❖)
Do not confuse Imodium with Indocin, or loperamide with furosemide.

FIXED-COMBINATION(S)

Imodium Advanced: loperamide/simethicone (an antiflatulent): 2 mg/125 mg.

◆CLASSIFICATION

PHARMACOTHERAPEUTIC: Antidiarrheal agent. **CLINICAL:** Antidiarrheal.

USES

Controls, provides symptomatic relief of acute nonspecific diarrhea, chronic diarrhea associated with inflammatory bowel disease; reduces volume of ileostomy discharge. **OTC:** Control symptoms of diarrhea, including traveler's diarrhea. **OFF-LABEL:** Chemotherapy-induced diarrhea, irinotecan-induced delayed diarrhea.

PRECAUTIONS

Contraindications: Hypersensitivity to loperamide. Abdominal pain without diarrhea, children younger than 2 yrs; acute dysentery, acute ulcerative colitis, bacterial enterocolitis caused by invasive organisms, including *Salmonella, Shigella, Campylobacter.* **Cautions:** Hepatic impairment, use in young children. Avoid use when inhibition of peristalsis is undesirable (e.g., potential for ileus, megacolon). Avoid use in pts with risk factors for QT prolongation.

ACTION

Directly affects intestinal wall muscles through opioid receptor. **Therapeutic Effect:** Slows intestinal motility, prolongs transit time of intestinal contents by reducing fecal volume, diminishing loss of fluid, electrolytes, increasing viscosity, bulk of stool. Increases tone of anal sphincter.

PHARMACOKINETICS

Poorly absorbed from GI tract. Protein binding: 97%. Metabolized in liver. Excreted in feces (30%), urine (less than 2%). Not removed by hemodialysis. Half-life: 7–14 hrs.

⌛ LIFESPAN CONSIDERATIONS

Pregnancy/Lactation: Unknown if drug crosses placenta or is distributed in breast milk. **Children:** Not recommended for pts younger than 2 yrs (infants younger than 3 mos more susceptible to CNS effects). **Elderly:** May mask dehydration, electrolyte depletion.

INTERACTIONS

DRUG: May increase levels/effects of **QT-prolonging agents. Ranolazine** may increase levels/effects. **HERBAL:** None

significant. **FOOD:** None known. **LAB VALUES:** None significant.

AVAILABILITY (Rx)

Capsules: 2 mg. **Liquid:** 1 mg/5 mL, 1 mg/7.5 mL. **Suspension, Oral:** 1 mg/7.5 mL. **Tablet:** 2 mg. **Tablet, Chewable:** 2 mg.

ADMINISTRATION/HANDLING

Liquid
• When administering to children, use accompanying plastic dropper to measure the liquid.

INDICATIONS/ROUTES/DOSAGE

Acute Diarrhea
PO *(Capsules):* **ADULTS, ELDERLY:** Initially, 4 mg, then 2 mg after each unformed stool. **Maximum:** 16 mg/day. **CHILDREN 9–12 YRS, WEIGHING MORE THAN 30 KG:** Initially, 2 mg 3 times/day for 24 hrs, then 0.1 mg/kg/dose after each loose stool. **Maximum:** 6 mg/day. **CHILDREN 6–8 YRS, WEIGHING 20–30 KG:** Initially, 2 mg twice daily for 24 hrs, then 0.1 mg/kg/dose after each loose stool. **Maximum:** 4 mg/day. **CHILDREN 2–5 YRS, WEIGHING 13–20 KG:** Initially, 1 mg 3 times/day for 24 hrs, then 0.1 mg/kg/dose after each loose stool. **Maximum:** 3 mg/day. **Maintenance:** 1 mg/10 kg only after loose stool but not exceeding initial dose.

Chronic Diarrhea
PO: ADULTS, ELDERLY: Initially, 4 mg, then 2 mg after each unformed stool until diarrhea is controlled. Average maintenance dose: 4–8 mg/day. **Maximum:** 16 mg/day.

Traveler's Diarrhea
PO: ADULTS, ELDERLY: Initially, 4 mg, then 2 mg after each loose bowel movement (LBM). **Maximum:** 8 mg/day. **CHILDREN 9–11 YRS:** Initially, 2 mg, then 1 mg after each LBM. **Maximum:** 6 mg/day. **CHILDREN 6–8 YRS:** Initially, 2 mg, then 1 mg after each LBM. **Maximum:** 4 mg/day.

L

✦ Canadian trade name　　　🦺 Non-Crushable Drug　　　🟥 High Alert drug

Dosage in Renal/Hepatic Impairment
No dose adjustment.

SIDE EFFECTS

Rare: Dry mouth, drowsiness, abdominal discomfort, allergic reaction (rash, pruritus).

ADVERSE EFFECTS/TOXIC REACTIONS

Toxicity results in constipation, GI irritation (nausea, vomiting), CNS depression. Activated charcoal is used to treat loperamide toxicity.

NURSING CONSIDERATIONS

BASELINE ASSESSMENT

Do not administer if GI bleeding, mechanical obstruction is suspected. Investigate cause of diarrhea (infectious vs. noninfectious). The use of antidiarrheals in the presence of *C. difficile*–associated diarrhea or other diarrhea caused by bacteria is controversial (drug may inhibit expulsion of toxic bacteria while elderly and debilitated pts are at an increased risk of mortality due to dehydration).

INTERVENTION/EVALUATION

Encourage adequate fluid intake. Assess bowel sounds for peristalsis. Monitor daily pattern of bowel activity, stool consistency. Withhold drug, notify physician promptly in event of abdominal pain, distention, fever.

PATIENT/FAMILY TEACHING

• Do not exceed prescribed dose. • May cause dry mouth. • Avoid alcohol. • Avoid tasks that require alertness, motor skills until response to drug is established. • Report diarrhea lasting more than 3 days, abdominal pain with distention, new-onset fever.

lopinavir/ritonavir

loe-**pin**-a-veer/rit-**oh**-na-veer
(<u>Kaletra</u>)
Do not confuse Kaletra with Keppra.

♦**CLASSIFICATION**

PHARMACOTHERAPEUTIC: Protease inhibitor combination. **CLINICAL:** Antiretroviral.

USES

In combination with other antiretroviral agents for treatment of HIV infection.

PRECAUTIONS

Contraindications: Hypersensitivity to lopinavir, ritonavir. Concomitant use of potent CYP3A inducers: alfuzosin, colchicine (pts with renal and/or hepatic impairment), dronedarone, elbasvir/grazoprevir, ergot derivatives (causes vasospasm, peripheral ischemia of extremities), lovastatin, lurasidone, midazolam (oral), pimozide, rifAMPin, sildenafil (for treatment of pulmonary arterial hypertension), simvastatin, St. John's wort, triazolam (increased sedation, respiratory depression); coadministration of medications highly dependent on CYP3A for clearance (increased concentrations are associated with serious adverse reactions). **Cautions:** Hepatic impairment, hepatitis B or C virus infection, cardiac disease with underlying conduction abnormalities or structural heart defects, ischemic heart disease, cardiomyopathies, congenital long QT syndrome or medications that prolong QT interval, hypokalemia, history of pancreatitis, diabetes.

ACTION

Lopinavir inhibits activity of protease, an enzyme, late in HIV replication process; ritonavir increases plasma levels of lopinavir by inhibiting CYP3A metabolism of lopinavir. **Therapeutic Effect:** Formation of immature, noninfectious viral particles.

PHARMACOKINETICS

Readily absorbed after PO administration (absorption increased when taken with food). Protein binding: 98%–99%. Metabolized in liver. Excreted primarily in feces. Not removed by hemodialysis. **Half-life:** 5–6 hrs.

⌛ LIFESPAN CONSIDERATIONS

Pregnancy/Lactation: Unknown if distributed in breast milk. Breastfeeding by HIV-infected mothers not recommended. **Children:** Safety and efficacy not established in pts younger than 6 mos. **Elderly:** Age-related renal/hepatic/cardiac impairment requires caution.

INTERACTIONS

DRUG: May increase concentration/toxicity of **amiodarone, atorvastatin, bepridil, clarithromycin, cycloSPORINE, felodipine, fluticasone, ketoconazole, lidocaine, lovastatin, midazolam, nelfinavir, niCARdipine, NIFEdipine, sildenafil, simvastatin, tacrolimus, traZODone, triazolam, warfarin.** May decrease concentration/effects of **oral contraceptives.** CYP3A4 inducers (e.g., **carBAMazepine, phenytoin, rifAMPin**) may decrease concentration/effects. May cause disulfiram-like reaction with **metroNIDAZOLE.** **HERBAL: St. John's wort** may decrease concentration/effects. **FOOD:** None known. **LAB VALUES:** May increase serum glucose, GGT, amylase, bilirubin, total cholesterol, triglycerides, uric acid, ALT, AST. May decrease platelets, serum sodium.

AVAILABILITY (Rx)

Oral Solution: 80 mg/mL lopinavir/20 mg/mL ritonavir.

🥄 **Tablets:** 100 mg lopinavir/25 mg ritonavir, 200 mg lopinavir/50 mg ritonavir.

ADMINISTRATION/HANDLING

PO
• Give tablets whole; do not break, crush, dissolve, or divide. • Does not require refrigeration. • Give tablets without regard to food. • Solution should be given with food. • Administer solution using calibrated oral syringe.

INDICATIONS/ROUTES/DOSAGE

HIV Infection
Doses based on lopinavir component.

PO: ADULTS: 800 mg once daily or 400 mg twice daily. **Pregnant Women:** 400 mg twice daily. **CHILDREN 6 MOS–18 YRS, WEIGHING GREATER THAN 40 KG:** *(Oral Solution):* 400 mg twice daily. **WEIGHING 15–40 KG:** 10 mg/kg twice daily. **WEIGHING LESS THAN 15 KG:** 12 mg/kg twice daily. **CHILDREN 14 DAYS–6 MOS:** 16 mg/kg twice daily. *(Tablets):* **WEIGHING GREATER THAN 35 KG:** 400 mg twice daily. **WEIGHING 26–35 KG:** 300 mg twice daily. **WEIGHING 15–25 KG:** 200 mg twice daily. **WEIGHING LESS THAN 15 KG:** Not recommended.

Dosage Adjustment for Combination Therapy
Efavirenz, Nelfinavir, Nevirapine: ADULTS, CHILDREN 6 MOS–18 YRS, WEIGHING GREATER THAN 45 KG: 500 mg (520-mg solution) twice daily. *(Solution):* **15–45 KG:** 11 mg/kg twice daily. **LESS THAN 15 KG:** 13 mg/kg twice daily. *(Tablet):* **31–45 KG:** 400 mg twice daily. **21–30 KG:** 300 mg twice daily. **15–20 KG:** 200 mg twice daily. **LESS THAN 15 KG:** Not recommended.

Dosage in Renal Impairment
No dose adjustment. Avoid once-daily dosing in HD pts.

Dosage in Hepatic Impairment
Use caution.

SIDE EFFECTS

Frequent (14%): Mild to moderate diarrhea. **Occasional (6%–2%):** Nausea, asthenia. Abdominal pain, headache, vomiting. **Rare (less than 2%):** Insomnia, rash.

ADVERSE EFFECTS/TOXIC REACTIONS

Anemia, leukopenia, lymphadenopathy, deep vein thrombosis (DVT), Cushing's syndrome, pancreatitis, hemorrhagic colitis occur rarely.

L

✦ Canadian trade name   🥄 Non-Crushable Drug   ⬛ High Alert drug

NURSING CONSIDERATIONS

BASELINE ASSESSMENT

Obtain baseline CBC, renal function, LFT viral load, CD4 count, cell count. Obtain baseline weight. Question medical history as listed in Precautions. Receive full medication history and screen for contraindications/interactions.

INTERVENTION/EVALUATION

Monitor electrolytes, serum glucose, cholesterol, LFT, CBC with differential, CD4 cell count, viral load. Monitor daily pattern of bowel activity, stool consistency. Assess for opportunistic infections: onset of fever, oral mucosa changes, cough, other respiratory symptoms. Check weight at least 2 times/wk. Assess for nausea, vomiting. Observe for signs/symptoms of pancreatitis (nausea, vomiting, abdominal pain).

PATIENT/FAMILY TEACHING

• Eat small, frequent meals to offset nausea, vomiting. • Lopinavir/ritonavir is not a cure for HIV infection, nor does it reduce risk of transmission to others. • Pt must continue practices to prevent HIV transmission. • Illnesses, including opportunistic infections, may still occur. • Due to high risk for drug interactions, do not take newly prescribed medication unless approved by prescriber who originally started treatment.

loratadine

lor-at-a-deen
(Alavert, Apo-Loratadine ♣, Claritin, Claritin Reditabs, Loradamed)
Do not confuse loratadine with clonidine, or Claritin with clarithromycin.

FIXED-COMBINATION(S)

Alavert Allergy and Sinus, Claritin-D: loratadine/pseudoephedrine (a sympathomimetic): 5 mg/120 mg, 10 mg/240 mg.

◆CLASSIFICATION

PHARMACOTHERAPEUTIC: H₁ antagonist, second generation. **CLINICAL:** Antihistamine.

USES

Relief of nasal, non-nasal symptoms of seasonal allergic rhinitis (hay fever). Treatment of itching due to hives (urticaria).

PRECAUTIONS

Contraindications: Hypersensitivity to loratadine. **Cautions:** Renal/hepatic impairment.

ACTION

Competes with histamine for H₁ receptor sites on effector cells. **Therapeutic Effect:** Prevents allergic responses mediated by histamine (e.g., rhinitis, urticaria, pruritus).

PHARMACOKINETICS

Route	Onset	Peak	Duration
PO	1–3 hrs	8–12 hrs	Longer than 24 hrs

Rapidly, almost completely absorbed from GI tract. Protein binding: 97%; metabolite, 73%–77%. Distributed mainly to liver, lungs, GI tract, bile. Metabolized in liver. Excreted in urine (40%) and feces (40%). Not removed by hemodialysis. **Half-life:** 8.4 hrs; metabolite, 28 hrs (increased in elderly, hepatic impairment).

⧖ LIFESPAN CONSIDERATIONS

Pregnancy/Lactation: Distributed in breast milk. **Children:** Safety and efficacy not established in pts younger than 2 yrs. **Elderly:** More sensitive to anticholinergic effects (e.g., dry mouth, nose, throat).

INTERACTIONS

DRUG: Clarithromycin, erythromycin, fluconazole, ketoconazole may increase concentration. **HERBAL: St. John's wort** may decrease concentration/effects. **FOOD: All foods** delay absorption. **LAB VALUES:** May suppress wheal, flare reactions to antigen skin testing unless drug is discontinued 4 days before testing.

AVAILABILITY (Rx)

Capsule: 5 mg. **Solution, Oral:** 5 mg/5 mL. **Syrup:** 5 mg/5 mL. **Tablets (Alavert, Claritin, Loradamed):** 10 mg. **Tablets, Chewable (Claritin):** 5 mg. **Tablets (Orally Disintegrating [Alavert]):** 5 mg, 10 mg.

ADMINISTRATION/HANDLING

PO

• May take without regard for food.

Orally Disintegrating Tablets

• Place under tongue. • Disintegration occurs within seconds, after which tablet contents may be swallowed with or without water.

INDICATIONS/ROUTES/DOSAGE

Allergic Rhinitis, Urticaria
PO: ADULTS, ELDERLY, CHILDREN 6 YRS AND OLDER: 10 mg once daily or 5 mg twice daily (Claritin Reditabs). **CHILDREN 2–5 YRS:** 5 mg once daily.

Dosage in Renal Impairment (CrCl less than 30 mL/min)
PO: ADULTS, ELDERLY, CHILDREN 6 YRS AND OLDER: 10 mg every other day. **CHILDREN 2–5 YRS:** No dose adjustment.

Dosage in Hepatic Impairment
No dose adjustment.

SIDE EFFECTS

Frequent (12%–8%): Headache, fatigue, drowsiness. **Occasional (3%):** Dry mouth, nose, throat. **Rare:** Photosensitivity.

ADVERSE EFFECTS/ TOXIC REACTIONS

None significant.

NURSING CONSIDERATIONS

BASELINE ASSESSMENT

Assess lung sounds for wheezing, skin for urticaria, other allergy symptoms.

INTERVENTION/EVALUATION

For upper respiratory allergies, increase fluids to decrease viscosity of secretions, offset thirst, replenish loss of fluids from increased diaphoresis. Monitor symptoms for therapeutic response.

PATIENT/FAMILY TEACHING

• Drink plenty of water (may cause dry mouth). • Avoid alcohol. • Avoid tasks that require alertness, motor skills until response to drug is established (may cause drowsiness). • May cause photosensitivity reactions (avoid direct exposure to sunlight).

LORazepam

lor-**az**-e-pam
(Apo-LORazepam ✦, <u>Ativan</u>, LORazepam Intensol, Novo-Lorazem ✦)
Do not confuse Ativan with Ambien or Atarax, or LORazepam with ALPRAZolam, diazePAM, Lovaza, temazepam, or Zolpidem.

◆CLASSIFICATION

PHARMACOTHERAPEUTIC: Benzodiazepine **(Schedule IV). CLINICAL:** Antianxiety, sedative-hypnotic, antiemetic, skeletal muscle relaxant, amnesiac, anticonvulsant, antitremor.

USES

PO: Management of anxiety disorders, short-term relief of symptoms of anxiety, anxiety associated with depressive

---

✦ Canadian trade name   🦅 Non-Crushable Drug   🈲 High Alert drug symptoms. Insomnia due to anxiety or transient stress. **IV:** Status epilepticus, preanesthesia for amnesia, sedation. **OFF-LABEL:** Treatment of alcohol withdrawal, psychogenic catatonia, partial complex seizures, agitation (IV administration only), antiemetic for chemotherapy; rapid tranquilization of agitated pt, status epilepticus in children.

PRECAUTIONS

Contraindications: Hypersensitivity to LORazepam, other benzodiazepines. Acute narrow-angle glaucoma, IV administration in pts with sleep apnea, severe respiratory depression (except during mechanical ventilation). **Cautions:** Neonates, renal/hepatic impairment, compromised pulmonary function, concomitant CNS depressant use, depression, history of drug dependence, alcohol abuse, or significant personality disorder, pts at risk for suicide.

ACTION

Enhances action of inhibitory neurotransmitter gamma-aminobutyric acid (GABA) in CNS, affecting memory, motor, sensory, cognitive function. **Therapeutic Effect:** Produces anxiolytic, anticonvulsant, sedative, muscle relaxant, antiemetic effects.

PHARMACOKINETICS

Route	Onset	Peak	Duration
PO	30–60 min	N/A	6–8 hrs
IV	5–20 min	N/A	6–8 hrs
IM	20–30 min	N/A	6–8 hrs

Well absorbed after PO, IM administration. Protein binding: 85%. Widely distributed. Metabolized in liver. Primarily excreted in urine. Not removed by hemodialysis. **Half-life:** 10–20 hrs.

⏳ LIFESPAN CONSIDERATIONS

Pregnancy/Lactation: May cross placenta. May be distributed in breast milk. May increase risk of fetal abnormalities if administered during first trimester of pregnancy. Chronic ingestion during pregnancy may produce fetal toxicity, withdrawal symptoms, CNS depression in neonates. **Children:** Safety and efficacy not established in pts younger than 12 yrs. **Elderly:** Use small initial doses with gradual increases to avoid ataxia, excessive sedation, or paradoxical CNS restlessness, excitement. May be more susceptible to cognitive impairment, delirium, falls, fractures.

INTERACTIONS

DRUG: Valproic acid may increase concentration/effects. **Alcohol, other CNS depressants (e.g., morphine, PHENobarbital, zolpidem)** may increase CNS depression. **HERBAL: Gotu kola, kava kava, St. John's wort, valerian** may increase CNS depression. **FOOD:** None known. **LAB VALUES:** None significant. **Therapeutic serum level:** 50–240 ng/mL; **toxic serum level:** unknown.

AVAILABILITY (Rx)

Injection Solution: 2 mg/mL, 4 mg/mL. **Oral Solution (LORazepam Intensol):** 2 mg/mL. **Tablets:** 0.5 mg, 1 mg, 2 mg.

ADMINISTRATION/HANDLING

 IV

Reconstitution • Dilute with equal volume of Sterile Water for Injection, D₅W, or 0.9% NaCl.
Rate of Administration • Give by IV push into tubing of free-flowing IV infusion (0.9% NaCl, D₅W) at a rate not to exceed 2 mg/min.
Storage • Refrigerate parenteral form. • Do not use if discolored or precipitate forms. • Avoid freezing.

IM
• Give deep IM into large muscle mass.

PO
• Give with food. • Tablets may be crushed. • Dilute oral solution in water, juice, soda, or semisolid food.

▦ IV INCOMPATIBILITIES

Aztreonam (Azactam), ondansetron (Zofran).

▦ IV COMPATIBILITIES

Bumetanide (Bumex), cefepime (Maxipime), dexmedetomidine (Precedex), diltiaZEM (Cardizem), DOBUTamine (Dobutrex), DOPamine (Intropin), heparin, labetalol (Normodyne, Trandate), milrinone (Primacor), norepinephrine (Levophed), piperacillin and tazobactam (Zosyn), potassium, propofol (Diprivan).

INDICATIONS/ROUTES/DOSAGE

Anxiety
PO: ADULTS: Initially, 2–3 mg/day in 2–3 divided doses. Usual dose: 2–6 mg/day in divided doses. Range: 1–10 mg/day. **ELDERLY:** Initially, 1–2 mg/day in divided doses. Titrate cautiously. **Maximum:** 3 mg/day in divided doses.

Insomnia Due to Anxiety
PO: ADULTS: (less than 65 yrs): 0.5–2 mg at bedtime. (65 yrs and older): 0.5–1 mg at bedtime.

Status Epilepticus
IV: ADULTS, ELDERLY, CHILDREN: 0.1 mg/kg. **Maximum:** 4 mg over 2–5 min. May repeat in 5–10 min. **NEONATES:** 0.05–0.1 mg/kg over 2–5 min. May repeat in 10–15 min.

Dosage in Renal/Hepatic Impairment
PO: No dose adjustment. **IM/IV: Mild to moderate impairment:** Use caution. Not recommended in severe impairment.

SIDE EFFECTS

Frequent (16%–7%): Drowsiness, dizziness. **Rare (less than 4%):** Weakness, ataxia, headache, hypotension, nausea, vomiting, confusion, injection site reaction.

ADVERSE EFFECTS/TOXIC REACTIONS

Abrupt or too-rapid withdrawal may result in pronounced restlessness, irritability, insomnia, hand tremor, abdominal cramping, muscle cramps, diaphoresis, vomiting, seizures. Overdose results in drowsiness, confusion, diminished reflexes, coma. **Antidote:** Flumazenil (see Appendix J for dosage).

NURSING CONSIDERATIONS

BASELINE ASSESSMENT

Offer emotional support to anxious pt. Pt must remain recumbent following parenteral administration to reduce hypotensive effect. Assess motor responses (agitation, trembling, tension), autonomic responses (cold or clammy hands, diaphoresis).

INTERVENTION/EVALUATION

Monitor B/P, respiratory rate, heart rate. For those on long-term therapy, hepatic/renal function tests, CBC should be performed periodically. Assess for paradoxical reaction, particularly during early therapy. Evaluate for therapeutic response: calm facial expression, decreased restlessness, insomnia, decrease in seizure-related symptoms. **Therapeutic serum level:** 50–240 ng/mL; **toxic serum level:** N/A.

PATIENT/ FAMILY TEACHING

• Drowsiness usually subsides during continued therapy. • Avoid tasks that require alertness, motor skills until response to drug is established. • Smoking reduces drug effectiveness. • Do not abruptly discontinue medication after long-term therapy. • Do not use alcohol, CNS depressants. • Contraception recommended for long-term therapy. • Immediately report suspected pregnancy.

losartan

loe-**sar**-tan
(Apo-Losartan ✦, Cozaar)
■ **BLACK BOX ALERT** ■ May cause fetal injury, mortality. Discontinue as soon as possible once pregnancy is detected.

L

Do not confuse Cozaar with Colace, Coreg, Hyzaar, or Zocor, or losartan with lorcaserin, valsartan.

FIXED-COMBINATION(S)

Hyzaar: losartan/hydroCHLOROthiazide (a diuretic): 50 mg/12.5 mg, 100 mg/12.5 mg, 100 mg/25 mg.

◆CLASSIFICATION

PHARMACOTHERAPEUTIC: Angiotensin II receptor antagonist. **CLINICAL:** Antihypertensive.

USES

Treatment of hypertension. Used alone or in combination with other antihypertensives. Treatment of diabetic nephropathy with an elevated creatinine and proteinuria (in pts with type 2 diabetes and history of hypertension), prevention of stroke in pts with hypertension and left ventricular hypertrophy. **OFF-LABEL:** Slow rate of progression of aortic root dilation in children with Marfan's syndrome. HF in pts intolerant of ACE inhibitors.

PRECAUTIONS

Contraindications: Hypersensitivity to losartan. Concomitant use of aliskiren in pts with diabetes. **Cautions:** Renal/hepatic impairment, unstented renal arterial stenosis, significant aortic/mitral stenosis. Concurrent use of potassium supplements. Pts with history of angioedema.

ACTION

Blocks vasoconstrictor, aldosterone-secreting effects of angiotensin II, inhibiting binding of angiotensin II to AT_1 receptors. **Therapeutic Effect:** Causes vasodilation, decreases peripheral resistance, decreases B/P.

PHARMACOKINETICS

Route	Onset	Peak	Duration
PO	N/A	6 hrs	24 hrs

Well absorbed after PO administration. Protein binding: 98%. Metabolized in liver. Excreted in urine (35%), feces (60%). Not removed by hemodialysis. **Half-life:** 2 hrs; metabolite, 6–9 hrs.

⧖ LIFESPAN CONSIDERATIONS

Pregnancy/Lactation: Has caused fetal/neonatal morbidity, mortality. Potential for adverse effects on breastfed infant. Breastfeeding not recommended. **Children:** Safety and efficacy not established. **Elderly:** May be more sensitive to hypotensive effects.

INTERACTIONS

DRUG: NSAIDs (e.g., ibuprofen, ketorolac, naproxen) may decrease effects. **Potassium-sparing diuretics (e.g., spironolactone, triamterene), potassium supplements** may increase serum potassium. **Diuretics (e.g., furosemide, HCTZ), antihypertensive medications (e.g., amLODIPine, lisinopril, valsartan)** may produce additive hypotension. May increase levels/effects of **lithium. HERBAL:** Ephedra, ginseng, licorice, yohimbe may worsen hypertension. **Black cohosh, periwinkle** may increase antihypertensive effect. **Garlic, ginger, ginseng** may increase hypoglycemic effect. **FOOD:** None known. **LAB VALUES:** May increase serum bilirubin, ALT, AST, Hgb, Hct. May decrease serum glucose.

AVAILABILITY (Rx)

Tablets: 25 mg, 50 mg, 100 mg.

ADMINISTRATION/HANDLING

PO
• May give without regard to food.

INDICATIONS/ROUTES/DOSAGE

Hypertension
PO: ADULTS, ELDERLY: Initially, 50 mg once daily. **Maximum:** May be given once or twice daily, with total daily doses ranging from 25–100 mg. **CHILDREN 6–16 YRS:** 0.7 mg/kg once daily. Adjust dose to BP response. **Maximum:** 100 mg/day.

Diabetic Nephropathy

PO: ADULTS, ELDERLY: Initially, 50 mg/day. May increase to 100 mg/day based on B/P response.

Stroke Prevention (Hypertension with Left Ventricular Hypertrophy)

PO: ADULTS, ELDERLY: 50 mg/day. **Maximum:** 100 mg/day based on BP response. Should be used in combination with a thiazide diuretic.

Renal Impairment

Not recommended if glomerular filtration rate (GFR) less than 30 mL/min.

Hepatic Impairment

PO: ADULTS, ELDERLY: Initially, 25 mg/day. May increase up to 100 mg/day.

SIDE EFFECTS

Frequent (8%): Upper respiratory tract infection. **Occasional (4%–2%):** Dizziness, diarrhea, cough. **Rare (1% or less):** Insomnia, dyspepsia, heartburn, back/leg pain, muscle cramps, myalgia, nasal congestion, sinusitis, depression.

ADVERSE EFFECTS/TOXIC REACTIONS

Overdosage may manifest as hypotension and tachycardia. Bradycardia occurs less often. Institute supportive measures.

NURSING CONSIDERATIONS

BASELINE ASSESSMENT

Obtain B/P, apical pulse immediately before each dose, in addition to regular monitoring (be alert to fluctuations). Question for possibility of pregnancy. Assess medication history (esp. diuretics).

INTERVENTION/EVALUATION

Maintain hydration (offer fluids frequently). Assess for evidence of upper respiratory infection, cough. Monitor B/P, pulse. Assist with ambulation if dizziness occurs. Monitor daily pattern of bowel activity, stool consistency.

PATIENT/FAMILY TEACHING

• Female pts of childbearing age should take measures to avoid pregnancy. • Report pregnancy as soon as possible. • Avoid tasks that require alertness, motor skills until response to drug is established (possible dizziness effect). • Report any sign of infection (sore throat, fever), chest pain. • Do not take OTC cold preparations, nasal decongestants. • Do not stop taking medication. • Limit salt intake.

lovastatin

loe-va-stat-in
(Altoprev, Apo-Lovastatin ♣, Mevacor)
Do not confuse lovastatin with atorvastatin, Leustatin, Lotensin, nystatin, pitavastatin, or pravastatin, or Mevacor with Benicar or Lipitor.

FIXED-COMBINATION(S)

Advicor: lovastatin/niacin: 20 mg/500 mg, 20 mg/750 mg, 20 mg/1,000 mg.

◆CLASSIFICATION

PHARMACOTHERAPEUTIC: HMG-CoA reductase inhibitor. **CLINICAL:** Antihyperlipidemic.

USES

Adjunct to diet to decrease elevated serum total and LDL cholesterol in primary hypercholesterolemia; primary prevention of coronary artery disease; reduction of risk of MI, unstable angina, and in coronary revascularization procedures. Slows progression of coronary atherosclerosis in pts with coronary heart disease. Adjunct to diet in adolescent pts (10–17 yrs) with heterozygous familial hypercholesterolemia having LDL greater than 189 mg/dL or LDL greater than 160 mg/dL with positive family history of premature CV disease or LDL greater than

L

160 mg/dL with presence of at least 2 other CVD risk factors.

PRECAUTIONS

Contraindications: Hypersensitivity to lovastatin. Active hepatic disease, unexplained persistent elevations of serum transaminases. Pregnancy, breastfeeding. Concomitant use of strong CYP3A4 inhibitors. **Cautions:** History of heavy/chronic alcohol use, renal impairment, hepatic disease; concomitant use of amiodarone, cycloSPORINE, fibrates, gemfibrozil, niacin, verapamil (increased risk of myopathy), elderly.

ACTION

Inhibits HMG-CoA reductase, the enzyme that catalyzes the early step in cholesterol synthesis. **Therapeutic Effect:** Decreases LDL, VLDL, triglycerides; increases HDL.

PHARMACOKINETICS

Route	Onset	Peak	Duration
PO (LDL, cholesterol reduction)	3 days	N/A	N/A

Incompletely absorbed from GI tract (increased on empty stomach). Protein binding: 95%. Hydrolyzed in liver. Primarily excreted in feces. Not removed by hemodialysis. **Half-life:** 1.1–1.7 hrs.

⏳ LIFESPAN CONSIDERATIONS

Pregnancy/Lactation: Contraindicated in pregnancy (suppression of cholesterol biosynthesis may cause fetal toxicity) and lactation. Unknown if drug is distributed in breast milk. **Children:** Safety and efficacy not established. **Elderly:** No age-related precautions noted.

INTERACTIONS

DRUG: CYP3A4 inhibitors (e.g., ketoconazole, clarithromycin) may increase concentration, risk of myopathy, rhabdomyolysis. **CycloSPORINE, fibrates, gemfibrozil, niacin, amiodarone, verapamil** may increase risk of rhabdomyolysis, acute renal failure.

HERBAL: St. John's wort may decrease concentration/effects. **FOOD:** Large quantities of **grapefruit juice** may increase risk of side effects (e.g., myalgia, weakness). **Red yeast rice** may increase concentration (2.4 mg lovastatin/600 mg rice). **LAB VALUES:** May increase serum creatine kinase (CK), transaminase.

AVAILABILITY (Rx)

Tablets: 10 mg, 20 mg, 40 mg.

📋 **Tablets (Extended-Release [Altoprev]):** 20 mg, 40 mg, 60 mg.

ADMINISTRATION/HANDLING

PO
• Immediate-release tablet given with evening meal; extended-release at bedtime. • Avoid intake of large quantities of grapefruit juice (greater than 1 quart). • Do not break, crush, dissolve, or divide extended-release tablets.

INDICATIONS/ROUTES/DOSAGE

Hypercholesterolemia
PO (Immediate-Release): ADULTS, ELDERLY: Initially, 20 mg/day. Adjust at 4-wk intervals. **Maintenance:** 10–80 mg once daily or in 2 divided doses. **Maximum:** 80 mg/day.
PO (Extended-Release): ADULTS, ELDERLY: Initially, 20–60 mg once daily at bedtime. Adjust at 4-wk intervals. **Maximum:** 60 mg once daily at bedtime.

Heterozygous Familial Hypercholesterolemia
PO (Immediate-Release): CHILDREN 10–17YRS: (LDL reduction 20% or greater): Initially, 20 mg/day; (LDL reduction less than 20%): Initially, 10 mg/day. Adjust at 4-wk intervals. Range: 10–40 mg daily.

Dosage with Concurrent Medication
Amiodarone: Maximum: 40 mg/day. **DiltiaZEM, dronedarone, verapamil: Maximum: (Immediate-Release):** 10 mg/day. **(Extended-Release):** 20 mg/day. **Lomitapide:** Consider reduction in dose.

Dosage in Renal Impairment
Use caution.

Dosage in Hepatic Impairment
No dose adjustment.

SIDE EFFECTS

Generally well tolerated. Side effects usually mild and transient. **Frequent (9%–5%):** Headache, flatulence, diarrhea, abdominal pain, abdominal cramping, rash, pruritus. **Occasional (4%–3%):** Nausea, vomiting, constipation, dyspepsia. **Rare (2%–1%):** Dizziness, heartburn, myalgia, blurred vision, eye irritation.

ADVERSE EFFECTS/ TOXIC REACTIONS

Potential for cataract development. Occasionally produces myopathy manifested as muscle pain, tenderness, weakness with elevated creatine kinase (CK). Severe myopathy may lead to rhabdomyolysis.

NURSING CONSIDERATIONS

BASELINE ASSESSMENT

Obtain dietary history. Question for possibility of pregnancy before initiating therapy. Obtain LFT, serum cholesterol, triglycerides.

INTERVENTION/EVALUATION

Monitor daily pattern of bowel activity, stool consistency. Monitor for headache, dizziness, blurred vision. Assess for rash, pruritus. Monitor serum cholesterol, triglycerides for therapeutic response. Be alert for malaise, muscle cramping/ weakness. Monitor LFT.

PATIENT/FAMILY TEACHING

• Follow special diet (important part of treatment). • Periodic lab tests are essential part of therapy. • Maintain appropriate birth control measures. • Avoid grapefruit juice, alcohol. • Report severe gastric upset, vision changes, myalgia, weakness, changes in color of urine/stool, yellowing of eyes/skin, unusual bruising.

lurasidone

loo-**ras**-i-done
(Latuda)

■ **BLACK BOX ALERT** ■ Elderly pts with dementia-related psychosis are at increased risk for mortality due to cardiovascular events, infectious diseases. Increased risk of suicidal thinking/behavior in children, adolescents, young adults.

◆CLASSIFICATION

PHARMACOTHERAPEUTIC: DOPamine, serotonin receptor antagonist. **CLINICAL:** Antipsychotic.

USES

Treatment of schizophrenia in adults and adolescents (13–17 yrs). Depression associated with bipolar I disorder as monotherapy and as adjunctive therapy with lithium or valproate.

PRECAUTIONS

Contraindications: Hypersensitivity to lurasidone. Concurrent use with strong CYP3A4 inhibitors (e.g., ketoconazole) and inducers (e.g., rifAMPin). **Cautions:** Cardiovascular disease (HF, history of MI, ischemia, conduction abnormalities), cerebrovascular disease (history of CVA in pts with dementia, seizure disorders), diabetes, Parkinson's disease, renal/hepatic impairment, pts at risk for aspiration pneumonia, pts at risk for suicide, disorders where CNS depression is a feature, pts at risk for hypotension, elderly, head trauma, alcoholism, medications that lower seizure threshold.

ACTION

Antagonizes central DOPamine type 2 and serotonin type 2 receptors. **Therapeutic Effect:** Diminishes symptoms of schizophrenia. Reduces incidence of extrapyramidal side effects.

L

PHARMACOKINETICS

Absorbed in 1–3 hrs. Steady-state concentration occurs in 7 days. Well absorbed from GI tract (unaffected by food). Protein binding: 99%. Metabolized in liver. Excreted in feces (80%), urine (9%). **Half-life:** 18 hrs.

⏳ LIFESPAN CONSIDERATIONS

Pregnancy/Lactation: Unknown if distributed in breast milk. Breastfeeding not recommended. **Children:** Safety and efficacy not established. **Elderly:** More susceptible to postural hypotension. Increased risk of cerebrovascular events (including stroke), mortality, in elderly pts with psychosis.

INTERACTIONS

DRUG: Alcohol, CNS depressants (e.g., LORazepam, morphine, zolpidem) may increase CNS depression. RifAMPin decreases concentration/effects. DiltiaZEM, ketoconazole, ritonavir may increase concentration/effects. **HERBAL:** Gotu kola, kava kava, St. John's wort, valerian may increase CNS depression. **FOOD:** Grapefruit products may increase risk of torsades, orthostatic hypotension. **LAB VALUES:** May increase prolactin levels.

AVAILABILITY (Rx)

Tablets: 20 mg, 40 mg, 60 mg, 80 mg, 120 mg.

ADMINISTRATION/HANDLING

PO
• Give with food. • Tablets may be crushed.

INDICATIONS/ROUTES/DOSAGE

Schizophrenia
PO: ADULTS, ELDERLY: Initially, 40 mg once daily with food. Increase dose based on response and tolerability. **Maximum:** 160 mg once daily with food. **Adolescents:** Initially, 40 mg once daily with food. **Maximum:** 80 mg once daily with food.

Depressive Episode Associated with Bipolar Disorder
PO: ADULTS, ELDERLY: Initially, 20 mg once daily, alone or in combination with lithium or divalproex. **Maximum:** 120 mg/day. Titration not required.

Concomitant Use of Moderate CYP3A4 Inhibitors
PO: ADULTS, ELDERLY: Initially, 20 mg/day. **Maximum:** 80 mg/day.

Moderate to Severe Renal Impairment
CrCl less than 50 mL/min: Initially, 20 mg/day. **Maximum:** 80 mg/day.

Hepatic Impairment
Mild impairment: No dose adjustment. **Moderate impairment:** Initially, 20 mg/day. **Maximum:** 80 mg/day. **Severe impairment:** Initially, 20 mg/day. **Maximum:** 40 mg/day.

SIDE EFFECTS

Frequent (15%–7%): Drowsiness, sedation, insomnia (paradoxical reaction). **Occasional (6%–3%):** Nausea, vomiting, dyspepsia, fatigue, back pain, akathisia, dizziness, agitation, anxiety. **Rare (2%–1%):** Restlessness, salivary hypersecretion, tongue spasm, torticollis, trismus.

ADVERSE EFFECTS/TOXIC REACTIONS

Extrapyramidal disorder (including cogwheel rigidity, drooling, bradykinesia, tardive dyskinesia, tremors) occurs in 5% of pts. Neuroleptic malignant syndrome (fever, muscle rigidity, irregular B/P or pulse, altered mental status, visual changes, dyspnea) occurs rarely.

NURSING CONSIDERATIONS

BASELINE ASSESSMENT

Question history as listed in Precautions. Assess behavior, appearance, emotional status, response to environment, speech pattern, thought content. Renal function, LFT should be obtained before therapy as

L

dose adjustment is required when initiating therapy.

INTERVENTION/EVALUATION

Supervise suicidal risk pt closely during early therapy (as depression lessens, energy level improves, increasing suicide potential). Monitor for potential neuroleptic malignant syndrome. Assess for therapeutic response (greater interest in surroundings, improved self-care, increased ability to concentrate, relaxed facial expression).

PATIENT/FAMILY TEACHING

• Avoid tasks that may require alertness, motor skills until response to drug is established (may cause drowsiness, dizziness). • Avoid alcohol. • Report trembling in fingers, altered gait, unusual muscle/skeletal movements, palpitations, severe dizziness, fainting, visual changes, rash, difficulty breathing. • Report suicidal ideation, unusual changes in behavior.

L

magnesium

mag-**nee**-zee-um

magnesium chloride

(Mag-Delay, Slow-Mag)

magnesium citrate

(Citroma, Citro-Mag ✤)

magnesium hydroxide

(Milk of Magnesia)

magnesium oxide

(Mag-Ox 400, Uro-Mag)

magnesium sulfate

(Epsom salt, magnesium sulfate injection)
Do not confuse magnesium sulfate with morphine sulfate.

FIXED-COMBINATION(S)

With aluminum and simethicone, an antiflatulent (**Mylanta**).

◆CLASSIFICATION

CLINICAL: Antacid, anticonvulsant, electrolyte, laxative.

USES

Magnesium chloride: Treatment/prevention of hypomagnesemia. Dietary supplement. **Magnesium citrate:** Evacuation of bowel before surgical, diagnostic procedures. Relieves occasional constipation. **Magnesium hydroxide:** Short-term treatment of constipation, symptoms of hyperacidity, laxative. **Magnesium oxide:** Relief of acid indigestion and upset stomach, short-term relief of constipation. Dietary supplement. **Magnesium sulfate:** Treatment/prevention of hypomagnesemia; prevention and treatment of seizures in severe preeclampsia or eclampsia; pediatric acute nephritis, treatment of arrhythmias due to hypomagnesemia (ventricular fibrillation, ventricular tachycardia, or torsades de pointes). **OFF-LABEL: Magnesium sulfate:** Asthma exacerbation unresponsive to conventional treatment.

PRECAUTIONS

Contraindications: Antacid: Appendicitis, symptoms of appendicitis, ileostomy, intestinal obstruction, severe renal impairment. **Laxative:** Appendicitis, HF, colostomy, hypersensitivity, ileostomy, intestinal obstruction, undiagnosed rectal bleeding. **Systemic:** Heart block, myocardial damage, IV use for pre-eclampsia/eclampsia during the 2 hrs prior to delivery. **Cautions:** Safety in children younger than 6 yrs not known. **Antacids:** Undiagnosed GI/rectal bleeding, ulcerative colitis, colostomy, diverticulitis, chronic diarrhea. **Laxative:** Diabetes, pts on low-salt diet (some products contain sugar, sodium). **Systemic:** Severe renal impairment. Myasthenia gravis or other neuromuscular diseases.

ACTION

Antacid: Acts in stomach to neutralize gastric acid. **Therapeutic Effect:** Increases pH. **Laxative:** Osmotic effect primarily in small intestine, draws water into intestinal lumen. **Therapeutic Effect:** Promotes peristalsis, bowel evacuation. **Systemic (dietary supplement replacement):** Found primarily in intracellular fluids. **Therapeutic Effect:** Essential for enzyme activity, nerve conduction, muscle contraction. Maintains and restores magnesium levels. **Anticonvulsant:** Blocks neuromuscular transmission, amount of acetylcholine released at motor end plate. **Therapeutic Effect:** Produces seizure control.

PHARMACOKINETICS

Antacid, laxative: Minimal absorption through intestine. Absorbed dose primarily excreted in urine. **Systemic:** Widely distributed. Primarily excreted in urine.

⌛ LIFESPAN CONSIDERATIONS

Pregnancy/Lactation: Antacid: Unknown if distributed in breast milk. **Parenteral:** Readily crosses placenta. Distributed in breast milk for 24 hrs after magnesium therapy is discontinued. Continuous IV infusion increases risk of magnesium toxicity in neonate. IV administration should not be used 2 hrs preceding delivery. **Children:** No age-related precautions noted. **Elderly:** Increased risk of developing magnesium deficiency (e.g., poor diet, decreased absorption, medications).

INTERACTIONS

DRUG: May decrease absorption of **quinolones** (e.g., **ciprofloxacin, levoFLOXacin), tetracycline, bisphosphonates.** May increase effects of **antihypertensives** (e.g., **amLODIPine, lisinopril). HERBAL:** None significant. **FOOD:** None known. **LAB VALUES: Antacid:** May increase gastrin production, pH. **Laxative:** May decrease serum potassium. **Systemic:** None significant.

AVAILABILITY (Rx)

MAGNESIUM CHLORIDE
Tablets (Mag-Delay, Slow-Mag): 64 mg.
MAGNESIUM CITRATE
Oral Solution (Citroma): 290 mg/5 mL.
Tablets: 100 mg.
MAGNESIUM HYDROXIDE
Suspension, Oral (Milk of Magnesia): 400 mg/5 mL, 1,200 mg/15 mL. **Tablets:** 400 mg.
MAGNESIUM OXIDE
Capsules (Uro-Mag): 140 mg. **Tablets (Mag-Ox 400):** 400 mg.
MAGNESIUM SULFATE
Infusion Solution: 10 mg/mL, 20 mg/mL, 40 mg/mL, 80 mg/mL. **Injection Solution:** 125 mg/mL, 500 mg/mL.

ADMINISTRATION/HANDLING

💉 IV

Reconstitution • Must dilute to maximum concentration of 20% for IV infusion. May give IV push, IV piggyback, or continuous infusion.

Rate of Administration • For IV push (diluted): Give no faster than 150 mg/min. For IV infusion, maximum rate of infusion is 2 g/hr.
Storage • Store at room temperature.

IM

• For adults, elderly, use 250 mg/mL (25%) or 500 mg/mL (50%) magnesium sulfate concentration. • For infants, children, do not exceed 200 mg/mL (20% diluted solution).

PO (Antacid)

• Shake suspension well before use. • Chewable tablets should be chewed thoroughly before swallowing, followed by full glass of water.

PO (Laxative)

• Drink full glass of liquid (8 oz) with each dose (prevents dehydration). • Flavor may be improved by following with fruit juice, citrus carbonated beverage. • Refrigerate citrate of magnesia (retains potency, palatability).

🔲 IV INCOMPATIBILITIES

Amphotericin B complex (Abelcet, AmBisome, Amphotec), cefepime (Maxipime), lansoprazole (Prevacid), pantoprazole (Protonix).

🔲 IV COMPATIBILITIES

Amikacin (Amikin), ceFAZolin (Ancef), ciprofloxacin (Cipro), dexmedetomidine (Precedex), DOBUTamine (Dobutrex), enalapril (Vasotec), gentamicin, heparin, HYDROmorphone (Dilaudid), insulin, linezolid (Zyvox), metoclopramide (Reglan), milrinone (Primacor), morphine, piperacillin/tazobactam (Zosyn), potassium chloride, propofol (Diprivan), tobramycin (Nebcin), vancomycin (Vancocin).

INDICATIONS/ROUTES/DOSAGE

MAGNESIUM SULFATE
Hypomagnesemia
Mild to Moderate
IV: ADULTS, ELDERLY: 1–4 g as 1 g/hr.
Maximum: 12 g/12 hrs.

Severe Deficiency
IV: ADULTS, ELDERLY: 4–8 g as 1 g/hr.
IV: CHILDREN: 25–50 mg/kg/dose over 10–20 min. **Maximum single dose:** 2 g.

Usual Dose for Neonates
IM/IV: 25–50 mg/kg/dose q8–12h for 2–3 doses.

Eclampsia/Preeclampsia
IV: ADULTS: 4–5 g infusion, then 1–2 g/hr continuous infusion. **Maximum:** 40 g/24 hrs.

MAGNESIUM CHLORIDE
Dietary Supplement
PO: ADULTS, ELDERLY: 2 tablets once daily.

Hypomagnesemia
PO: ADULTS, ELDERLY: 8–20 mEq/day.

MAGNESIUM CITRATE
Laxative
PO: ADULTS, ELDERLY, CHILDREN 12 YRS AND OLDER: 195–300 mL once or in divided doses. **6–12 YRS:** 90–210 mL once or in divided doses. **2–5 YRS:** 60–90 mL once or in divided doses.

MAGNESIUM HYDROXIDE
Antacid
PO: ADULTS, ELDERLY, CHILDREN 12 YRS AND OLDER: *(400 mg/5 mL):* 5–15 mL as needed up to 4 times/day.

Laxative
PO: ADULTS, ELDERLY, CHILDREN 12 YRS AND OLDER: *(400 mg/5 mL):* 30–60 mL at HS or in divided doses. *(Tablet):* 8 tabs/day in divided doses. **CHILDREN 6–11 YRS:** *(400 mg/5 mL):* 15–30 mL at HS. **CHILDREN 2–5 YRS:** 5–15 mL at HS.

MAGNESIUM OXIDE
Antacid/Dietary Supplement
PO: ADULTS, ELDERLY: 1–2 tablets daily.

Laxative
PO: ADULTS, ELDERLY: 2–4 tablets at bedtime or in divided doses.

Dosage in Renal Impairment
Use caution.

Dosage in Hepatic Impairment
No dose adjustment.

SIDE EFFECTS

Frequent: Antacid: Chalky taste, diarrhea, laxative effect. **Occasional: Antacid:** Nausea, vomiting, stomach cramps. **Antacid, laxative:** Prolonged use or large doses in renal impairment may cause hypermagnesemia (dizziness, palpitations, altered mental status, fatigue, weakness). **Laxative:** Cramping, diarrhea, increased thirst, flatulence. **Systemic (dietary supplement, electrolyte replacement):** Reduced respiratory rate, decreased reflexes, flushing, hypotension, decreased heart rate.

ADVERSE EFFECTS/TOXIC REACTIONS

Magnesium as antacid, laxative has no known adverse reactions. Systemic use may produce prolonged PR interval, widening of QRS interval. Magnesium toxicity may cause loss of deep tendon reflexes, heart block, respiratory paralysis, cardiac arrest. **Antidote:** 10–20 mL 10% calcium gluconate (5–10 mEq of calcium).

NURSING CONSIDERATIONS

BASELINE ASSESSMENT

Assess sensitivity to magnesium. **Antacid:** Assess GI pain (duration, location, quality, time of occurrence, relief with food, causative/exacerbative factors). **Laxative:** Assess for weight loss, nausea, vomiting, history of recent abdominal surgery. **Systemic:** Assess renal function, serum magnesium.

INTERVENTION/EVALUATION

Antacid: Assess for relief of gastric distress. Monitor renal function (esp. if dosing is long term or frequent). **Laxative:** Monitor daily pattern of bowel activity,

M

stool consistency. **Systemic:** Monitor renal function, magnesium levels, EKG for cardiac function. Test patellar reflexes before giving repeated, rapid parenteral doses (used as indication of CNS depression; suppressed reflexes may be sign of impending respiratory arrest). Patellar reflex must be present, respiratory rate should be 16/min or over before each parenteral dose. Initiate seizure precautions.

PATIENT/FAMILY TEACHING

• **Antacid:** Take at least 2 hrs apart from other medication. • Do not take longer than 2 wks unless directed by physician. • For peptic ulcer, take 1 and 3 hrs after meals and at bedtime for 4–6 wks. • Chew tablets thoroughly, followed by 8 oz of water; shake suspensions well. • Repeat dosing or large doses may have laxative effect. • **Laxative:** Drink full glass (8 oz) liquid to aid stool softening. • Use only for short term. Do not use if abdominal pain, nausea, vomiting is present. • **Systemic:** Report symptoms of hypermagnesemia (altered mental status, difficulty breathing, dizziness, fatigue, palpitations, weakness).

---

mannitol

man-it-ol
(Aridol, Osmitrol)
Do not confuse Osmitrol with esmolol.

◆CLASSIFICATION

PHARMACOTHERAPEUTIC: Polyol (sugar alcohol). **CLINICAL:** Osmotic diuretic.

USES

Reduces increased ICP due to cerebral edema, IOP due to acute glaucoma. Promotes urinary excretion of toxic substances. **OFF-LABEL:** Improves renal transplant function. Severe, traumatic brain injury.

PRECAUTIONS

Contraindications: Hypersensitivity to mannitol. Severe dehydration, active intracranial bleeding (except during craniotomy), severe pulmonary edema, congestion, severe renal disease (anuria), progressive HF. **Cautions:** Concurrent nephrotoxic agents, conditions increasing sensitivity to bronchoconstriction (e.g., recent abdominal, thoracic surgery), sepsis, preexisting renal disease, hypernatremia.

ACTION

Elevates osmotic pressure of glomerular filtrate, inhibiting tubular reabsorption of water and electrolytes, resulting in increased urine output. Reduces intracranial pressure by decreasing blood viscosity, thereby increasing cerebral blood flow/oxygen transport. **Therapeutic Effect:** Produces diuresis; reduces intraocular pressure (IOP), intracranial pressure (ICP), cerebral edema.

PHARMACOKINETICS

Route	Onset	Peak	Duration
IV (diuresis)	1–3 hrs	N/A	—
IV (reduced ICP)	15–30 min	N/A	1.5–6 hrs

Remains in extracellular fluid. Primarily excreted unchanged in urine. Removed by hemodialysis. **Half-life:** 4.7 hrs.

⧗ LIFESPAN CONSIDERATIONS

Pregnancy/Lactation: Unknown if drug crosses placenta or is distributed in breast milk. **Children:** Safety and efficacy not established in pts younger than 12 yrs. **Elderly:** Age-related renal impairment may require dosage adjustment.

INTERACTIONS

DRUG: None significant. **HERBAL: Yohimbe** may decrease effects. **FOOD:** None known. **LAB VALUES:** May decrease serum phosphate, potassium. May increase serum sodium, serum osmolality.

M

AVAILABILITY (Rx)

Injection Solution (Osmitrol): 5%, 10%, 15%, 20%, 25%.

ADMINISTRATION/HANDLING

◀**ALERT**▶ Assess IV site for patency before each dose. Pain, thrombosis noted with extravasation. In-line filter (less than 5 microns) used for concentrations over 20%.

 IV

Rate of Administration • Administer test dose for pts with oliguria. • Give IV push over 3–5 min; over 30–60 min for cerebral edema, elevated ICP. Maximum concentration: 25%. • Do not add KCl or NaCl to mannitol 20% or greater. Do not add to whole blood for transfusion.
Storage • Store at room temperature. • If crystals are noted in solution, warm bottle in hot water, shake vigorously at intervals. Cool to body temperature before administration. Do not use if crystals remain after warming procedure.

▩ IV INCOMPATIBILITIES

Cefepime (Maxipime), filgrastim (Neupogen), imipenem-cilastatin (Primaxin).

▩ IV COMPATIBILITIES

CISplatin (Platinol), furosemide (Lasix), linezolid (Zyvox), ondansetron (Zofran), propofol (Diprivan).

INDICATIONS/ROUTES/DOSAGE

Usual Dosage
Elevated Intracranial Pressure
IV: ADULTS, ELDERLY: 0.25–1 g/kg/dose. May repeat q6–8h as needed to maintain serum osmolality <300–325 mOsm/kg. **CHILDREN:** 0.25–1 g/kg/dose; repeat to maintain serum osmolality <300–320 mOsm/kg.

IOP Reduction
IV: ADULTS, ELDERLY: 1.5–2 g/kg over 30–60 min 1–1.5 hrs prior to surgery.

CHILDREN: 1–2 g/kg over 30–60 min 1–1.5 hrs prior to surgery.

Dosage in Renal Impairment
Contraindicated with severe impairment; caution with underlying renal disease.

Dosage in Hepatic Impairment
No dose adjustment.

SIDE EFFECTS

Frequent: Dry mouth, thirst. **Occasional:** Blurred vision, increased urinary frequency/volume, headache, arm pain, backache, nausea, vomiting, urticaria, dizziness, hypotension, hypertension, tachycardia, fever, angina-like chest pain.

ADVERSE EFFECTS/TOXIC REACTIONS

Fluid, electrolyte imbalance may occur due to rapid administration of large doses or inadequate urine output resulting in overexpansion of extracellular fluid. Circulatory overload may produce pulmonary edema, HF. Excessive diuresis may produce hypokalemia. Fluid loss in excess of electrolyte excretion may produce hypernatremia, hyperkalemia.

NURSING CONSIDERATIONS

BASELINE ASSESSMENT

Obtain baseline B/P, pulse. Assess skin turgor, mucous membranes, mental status, muscle strength. Obtain baseline weight, chemistry studies. Assess I&O.

INTERVENTION/EVALUATION

Monitor urinary output to ascertain therapeutic response. Monitor serum electrolytes, serum osmolarity, ICP, renal function, LFT. Assess vital signs, skin turgor, mucous membranes. Weigh daily. Monitor for signs of hypernatremia (confusion, drowsiness, thirst, dry mouth, cold/clammy skin); signs of hypokalemia (changes in muscle strength, tremors, muscle cramps, altered mental status, cardiac arrhythmias). Signs of hyperkalemia include colic, diarrhea, muscle twitching followed by weakness, paralysis, arrhythmias.

PATIENT/FAMILY TEACHING
• Expect increased urinary frequency/volume. • May cause dry mouth.

medroxyPROGES-TERone

me-**drox**-ee-proe-**jes**-ter-one
(Apo-Medroxy ✤, Depo-Provera, Depo-SubQ Provera 104, Novo-Medrone ✤, Provera)
■ **BLACK BOX ALERT** ■ Prolonged use (over 2 yrs) of contraceptive injection form may result in loss of bone mineral density. Limit long-term use (more than 2 yrs). May increase risk of dementia in postmenopausal women. Increased risk of invasive breast cancer in postmenopausal women in combination with conjugated estrogens.
Do not confuse medroxyPROGESTERone with HYDROXYprogesterone, methylPREDNISolone, or methylTESTOSTERone, or Provera with Covera, Femara, Parlodel, or Premarin.

◆CLASSIFICATION
PHARMACOTHERAPEUTIC: Hormone. **CLINICAL:** Progestin, antineoplastic, contraceptive hormone.

USES
PO: Reduction of endometrial hyperplasia in nonhysterectomized postmenopausal women (concurrently given with estrogen to women with intact uterus), treatment of secondary amenorrhea, abnormal uterine bleeding due to hormonal imbalance. **IM:** Adjunctive therapy, palliative treatment of inoperable, recurrent, metastatic endometrial carcinoma; prevention of pregnancy, endometriosis-associated pain. **OFF-LABEL:** Treatment of paraphilia/hypersexuality.

PRECAUTIONS
Contraindications: Hypersensitivity to medroxyPROGESTERone. Carcinoma of breast or other progesterone-dependent or estrogen-dependent neoplasm, history of or active thrombotic disorders (cerebral apoplexy, thrombophlebitis, thromboembolic disorders), known or suspected pregnancy, missed abortion, severe hepatic impairment, undiagnosed abnormal vaginal bleeding, cerebrovascular disease, use as pregnancy test. **Cautions:** Pts with conditions aggravated by fluid retention (asthma, seizures, migraine, cardiac/renal dysfunction), diabetes, history of mental depression, preexisting hypercholesterolemia, hypertriglyceridemia.

ACTION
Inhibits secretion of pituitary gonadotropins. **Therapeutic Effect:** Prevents follicular maturation, ovulation. Causes endometrial thinning.

PHARMACOKINETICS
Well absorbed after PO administration. Slowly absorbed after IM administration. Protein binding: 90%. Metabolized in liver. Primarily excreted in urine. **Half-life: PO:** 12–17 hrs. **IM:** 40–50 days.

⧗ LIFESPAN CONSIDERATIONS
Pregnancy/Lactation: Avoid use during pregnancy, esp. first 4 mos (congenital heart, limb reduction defects may occur). Distributed in breast milk. **Children:** Safety and efficacy not established. **Elderly:** No age-related precautions noted.

INTERACTIONS
DRUG: CYP3A inducers (e.g., carBAMazepine, phenytoin, rifAMPin) may decrease effects. **HERBAL: St. John's wort** may decrease effect of progestin contraceptive. **FOOD:** None known. **LAB VALUES:** May alter serum thyroid, LFT, PT, HDL, total cholesterol,

M

triglycerides; metapyrone test. May increase LDL.

AVAILABILITY (Rx)

Injection Suspension: 104 mg/0.65 mL prefilled syringe (Depo-SubQ Provera 104), 150 mg/mL (Depo-Provera), 400 mg/mL (Depo-Provera). **Tablets (Provera):** 2.5 mg, 5 mg, 10 mg.

ADMINISTRATION/HANDLING

IM
• Shake vial immediately before administering (ensures complete suspension). • Administer deep IM into gluteal or deltoid muscle.

SQ
• Shake vigorously prior to administration. • Inject in upper thigh or abdomen (avoid bony areas and umbilicus). • Give over 5–7 sec; do not rub injection area.

PO
• Give with food.

INDICATIONS/ROUTES/DOSAGE

Endometrial Hyperplasia
PO: ADULTS: 5–10 mg/day for 12–14 consecutive days each month starting on day 1 or 16 of cycle.

Secondary Amenorrhea
PO: ADULTS: 5–10 mg/day for 5–10 days, beginning at any time during menstrual cycle.

Abnormal Uterine Bleeding
PO: ADULTS: 5–10 mg/day for 5–10 days, beginning on calculated day 16 or day 21 of menstrual cycle.

Endometrial Carcinoma
IM: ADULTS, ELDERLY: Initially, 400–1,000 mg; repeat at 1-wk intervals.

Pregnancy Prevention
IM: *(Depo-Provera):* **ADULTS:** 150 mg q3mos (q13 wks).
SQ: *(Depo-Subq Provera 104):* **ADULTS:** 104 mg q3mos (q12–14wks).

Endometriosis-Associated Pain
SQ: *(Depo-Subq Provera 104):* **ADULTS:** 104 mg q3mos (q12–14 wks) for up to 2 yrs.

Dosage in Renal Impairment
No dose adjustment.

Dosage in Hepatic Impairment
Contraindicated with severe impairment.

SIDE EFFECTS

Frequent: Transient menstrual abnormalities (spotting, change in menstrual flow/cervical secretions, amenorrhea) at initiation of therapy. **Occasional:** Edema, weight change, breast tenderness, anxiety, insomnia, fatigue, dizziness. **Rare:** Alopecia, depression, dermatologic changes, headache, fever, nausea.

ADVERSE EFFECTS/TOXIC REACTIONS

Thrombophlebitis, pulmonary/cerebral embolism, retinal thrombosis occur rarely.

NURSING CONSIDERATIONS

BASELINE ASSESSMENT
Obtain usual menstrual history. Question for hypersensitivity to progestins, possibility of pregnancy before initiating therapy. Obtain baseline weight, serum glucose, B/P.

INTERVENTION/EVALUATION
Check weight daily; report wkly gain of 5 lb or more. Assess B/P periodically. Assess skin for rash, urticaria. Report development of chest pain, sudden shortness of breath, sudden decrease in vision, migraine headache, pain (esp. with swelling, warmth, redness) in calves, numbness of arm/leg (thrombotic disorders) immediately.

PATIENT/FAMILY TEACHING
• Report sudden loss of vision, severe headache, chest pain, coughing up of blood (hemoptysis), numbness in arm/leg, severe pain/swelling in calf, unusually

heavy vaginal bleeding, severe abdominal pain/tenderness. • Depo-Provera Contraceptive injection should be used as long-term birth control method (e.g., longer than 2 yrs) only if other birth control methods are inadequate.

megestrol HIGH ALERT

meh-**jes**-trol
(Megace, Megace ES, Megace OS ♣)

Do not confuse megestrol with mesalamine.

◆CLASSIFICATION
PHARMACOTHERAPEUTIC: Synthetic hormone. **CLINICAL:** Antineoplastic, progestin.

USES
Palliative treatment of advanced endometrial or breast carcinoma; treatment of anorexia, cachexia, unexplained significant weight loss in pts with AIDS.

PRECAUTIONS
Contraindications: Hypersensitivity to megestrol. **Suspension:** Known or suspected pregnancy. **Cautions:** History of thrombophlebitis, elderly.

ACTION
Antiestrogenic; interferes with normal estrogen cycle by decreasing release of luteinizing hormone (LH) from anterior pituitary gland by inhibiting pituitary function. May increase appetite by antagonizing metabolic effects of catabolic cytokines. **Therapeutic Effect:** Reduces tumor size. Increases appetite.

PHARMACOKINETICS
Well absorbed from GI tract. Metabolized in liver. Excreted in urine. **Half-life:** 13–105 hrs (mean 34 hrs).

☒ LIFESPAN CONSIDERATIONS
Pregnancy/Lactation: If possible, avoid use during pregnancy, esp. first 4 mos. Breastfeeding not recommended. **Children:** Safety and efficacy not established. **Elderly:** Use caution.

INTERACTIONS
DRUG: None significant. **HERBAL:** Avoid **black cohosh, dong quai** in estrogen-dependent tumors. Avoid **herbs with progestogenic properties (e.g., chaste-berry);** may increase adverse effects. **FOOD:** None known. **LAB VALUES:** May alter serum thyroid, LFT, PT, HDL, total cholesterol, triglycerides. May increase LDL.

AVAILABILITY (Rx)
Oral Suspension: 40 mg/mL (Megace), 625 mg/5 mL (Megace ES). **Tablets (Megace):** 20 mg, 40 mg.

ADMINISTRATION/HANDLING
PO
• Store tablets, oral suspension at room temperature. • Shake suspension well before use. • Oral suspension compatible with water, orange juice, apple juice. • Administer without regard to food.

INDICATIONS/ROUTES/DOSAGE
Palliative Treatment of Advanced Breast Cancer
PO: ADULTS, ELDERLY: 40 mg 4 times/day for at least 2 mos.

Palliative Treatment of Advanced Endometrial Carcinoma
PO: ADULTS, ELDERLY: 40–320 mg/day in divided doses for at least 2 mos.

Anorexia, Cachexia, Weight Loss
PO: *(Megace):* **ADULTS, ELDERLY:** 160–800 mg/day (10–20 mL/day) or (40 mg/mL suspension).

Dosage in Renal Impairment
Use caution.

M

Dosage in Hepatic Impairment
No dose adjustment.

SIDE EFFECTS

Frequent: Weight gain secondary to increased appetite. **Occasional:** Nausea, breakthrough menstrual bleeding, backache, headache, breast tenderness, carpal tunnel syndrome. **Rare:** Feeling of coldness.

ADVERSE EFFECTS/TOXIC REACTIONS

Thrombophlebitis, pulmonary embolism occur rarely.

NURSING CONSIDERATIONS

BASELINE ASSESSMENT

Question for possibility of pregnancy. Provide support to pt, family, recognizing that this drug is palliative, not curative.

INTERVENTION/EVALUATION

Monitor for tumor response. Monitor pt weight, caloric intake (appetite stimulant).

PATIENT/FAMILY TEACHING

• Contraception is imperative. • Report lower leg (calf) pain, difficulty breathing, vaginal bleeding. • May cause headache, nausea, vomiting, breast tenderness, backache.

meloxicam

mel-**ox**-i-kam
(Apo-Meloxicam ✤, Mobic, Vivlodex)
■ **BLACK BOX ALERT** ■ Increased risk of serious cardiovascular thrombotic events, including myocardial infarction, CVA. Increased risk of severe GI reactions, including ulceration, bleeding, GI perforation.

◆CLASSIFICATION

PHARMACOTHERAPEUTIC: NSAID. **CLINICAL:** Anti-inflammatory, analgesic.

USES

Relief of signs/symptoms of osteoarthritis, rheumatoid arthritis (RA). Treatment of juvenile idiopathic arthritis (JIA) in pts 2 yrs of age and older (suspension) and weighing 60 kg or more (tablets).

PRECAUTIONS

Contraindications: Hypersensitivity to meloxicam. Pts with aspirin triad (asthma, rhinitis, aspirin intolerance). History of asthma, urticaria with NSAIDs, perioperative pain in setting of CABG surgery. **Cautions:** Renal/hepatic impairment, asthma, coagulation disorders, hypertension, history of GI disease (bleeding or ulcers), concurrent use of anticoagulants, fluid retention, HF, dehydration, smoking, alcohol use, elderly, debilitated.

ACTION

Produces analgesic, antipyretic, anti-inflammatory effects by inhibiting prostaglandin synthesis. **Therapeutic Effect:** Reduces inflammatory response, intensity of pain.

PHARMACOKINETICS

Route	Onset	Peak	Duration
PO (Analgesic)	30 min	4–5 hrs	N/A

Well absorbed after PO administration. Protein binding: 99%. Metabolized in liver. Excreted equally in urine, feces. Not removed by hemodialysis. **Half-life:** 15–20 hrs.

⌛ LIFESPAN CONSIDERATIONS

Pregnancy/Lactation: Avoid use at 30 wks gestation or more (may cause premature closure of ductus arteriosus). Distributed in breast milk. **Children:** Safety and efficacy not established in children younger than 2 yrs. **Elderly:** Age-related renal impairment may require dosage adjustment. More susceptible to GI toxicity; lower dosage recommended.

INTERACTIONS

DRUG: May decrease antihypertensive effects of **ACE inhibitors (e.g., enalapril, lisinopril).** May increase risk of nephrotoxicity with **cycloSPORINE. Aspirin** may increase risk of epigastric distress (heartburn, indigestion). **Anticoagulants (e.g., heparin, warfarin), antiplatelets (e.g., aspirin, clopidogrel), NSAIDs (e.g., ibuprofen, naproxen), SNRIs (e.g., duloxetine, venlafaxine), SSRIs (e.g., escitalopram, paroxetine), thrombolytic therapy (e.g., TPA)** may increase risk of bleeding. May increase concentration, risk of toxicity of **lithium. HERBAL: Cat's claw, dong quai, evening primrose, feverfew, garlic, ginger, ginkgo, green tea, red clover** may increase antiplatelet activity, risk of bleeding. **FOOD:** None known. **LAB VALUES:** May increase serum creatinine, ALT, AST.

AVAILABILITY (Rx)

Oral Suspension: *(Mobic):* 7.5 mg/5 mL. **Tablets:** *(Mobic):* 7.5 mg, 15 mg. *(Vivlodex):* 5 mg, 10 mg.

ADMINISTRATION/HANDLING

PO

• Give with food or milk to minimize GI irritation. • Shake oral suspension gently before administering.

INDICATIONS/ROUTES/DOSAGE

Osteoarthritis, Rheumatoid Arthritis (RA)
PO: *(Mobic):* **ADULTS, ELDERLY:** Initially, 7.5 mg/day. **Maximum:** 15 mg/day (7.5 mg for pts on dialysis).

Osteoarthritis
PO: *(Vivlodex):* **ADULTS, ELDERLY:** Initially, 5 mg once daily. May increase to 10 mg once daily.

JIA
PO: *(Suspension):* **CHILDREN, 2 YRS AND OLDER:** 0.125 mg/kg once daily. **Maximum:** 7.5 mg. *(Tablets):* **CHILDREN WEIGHING 60 KG OR MORE:** 7.5 mg once daily.

Dosage in Renal Impairment
Not recommended with severe impairment.

Dosage in Hepatic Impairment
No dose adjustment.

SIDE EFFECTS

Frequent (9%–7%): Dyspepsia, headache, diarrhea, nausea. **Occasional (4%–3%):** Dizziness, insomnia, rash, pruritus, flatulence, constipation, vomiting. **Rare (less than 2%):** Drowsiness, urticaria, photosensitivity, tinnitus.

ADVERSE EFFECTS/TOXIC REACTIONS

In pts treated chronically, peptic ulcer, GI bleeding, gastritis, severe hepatic toxicity (jaundice), nephrotoxicity (hematuria, dysuria, proteinuria), severe hypersensitivity reaction (bronchospasm, angioedema) occur rarely.

NURSING CONSIDERATIONS

BASELINE ASSESSMENT

Assess onset, type, location, duration of pain/inflammation. Inspect appearance of affected joints for immobility, deformities, skin condition. Question history of GI bleeding, gastric or duodenal ulcers, hepatic/renal impairment, asthma.

INTERVENTION/EVALUATION

Monitor CBC, BMP, LFT. Assess skin for petechiae. Assess for therapeutic response: relief of pain, stiffness, swelling; increased joint mobility; reduced joint tenderness; improved grip strength. Monitor for abdominal pain, hematemesis.

PATIENT/FAMILY TEACHING

• Take with food, milk to reduce GI upset. • Report tinnitus, persistent abdominal pain/cramping, severe nausea, vomiting, difficulty breathing, unusual bruising or bleeding, rash, peripheral edema, chest pain, palpitations. • Avoid use after 30 wks gestation.

M

✦ Canadian trade name   🍶 Non-Crushable Drug   🔲 High Alert drug

melphalan

HIGH ALERT

mel-fa-lan
(Alkeran, Evomela)

■ BLACK BOX ALERT ■ Myelosuppression is common. Potentially mutagenic, leukemogenic. Hypersensitivity noted with IV administration. Must be administered by certified chemotherapy personnel. **Do not confuse Alkeran with Leukeran or Myleran, or melphalan with Mephyton or Myleran.**

◆CLASSIFICATION

PHARMACOTHERAPEUTIC: Alkylating agent. **CLINICAL:** Antineoplastic.

USES

Treatment of nonresectable epithelial ovarian carcinoma, multiple myeloma. **OFF-LABEL:** Hodgkin's lymphoma, malignant melanoma, neuroblastoma, induction regimen for bone marrow and stem cell transplantation, light chain amyloidosis, Ewing's sarcoma.

PRECAUTIONS

Contraindications: Hypersensitivity to melphalan. Resistance to prior melphalan therapy. **Cautions:** Preexisting bone marrow suppression, renal impairment, pregnancy, prior chemotherapy or irradiation.

ACTION

Inhibits protein synthesis primarily by cross-linking strands of DNA, RNA. Cell cycle–phase nonspecific. **Therapeutic Effect:** Disrupts nucleic acid function, producing tumor cell death.

PHARMACOKINETICS

Oral administration is highly variable. Incomplete intestinal absorption, variable first-pass metabolism, rapid hydrolysis may result. Protein binding: 60%–90%. Extensively metabolized in blood. Eliminated from plasma primarily by chemical hydrolysis. Partially excreted in feces; minimal elimination in urine. **Half-life: PO:** 1–1.25 hrs. **IV:** 1.5 hrs.

⧗ LIFESPAN CONSIDERATIONS

Pregnancy/Lactation: May cause fetal harm. Unknown if distributed in breast milk. **Children:** Safety and efficacy not established. **Elderly:** Age-related renal impairment may require dosage adjustment.

INTERACTIONS

DRUG: Bone marrow depressants may increase myelosuppression. **Live virus vaccines** may potentiate virus replication, increase vaccine side effects, decrease pt's antibody response to vaccine. **HERBAL: Echinacea** may decrease effects. **FOOD:** None known. **LAB VALUES:** May increase serum uric acid.

AVAILABILITY (Rx)

Injection, Powder for Reconstitution: 50 mg. **Tablets (Alkeran):** 2 mg.

ADMINISTRATION/HANDLING

 IV

Reconstitution • Reconstitute 50-mg vial with diluent supplied by manufacturer to yield 5 mg/mL solution. • Further dilute with 0.9% NaCl to final concentration not exceeding 0.45 mg/mL.
Rate of Administration • Infuse over 15–30 min at rate not to exceed 10 mg/min (total infusion should be administered within 1 hr).
Storage • Store at room temperature; protect from light. • Once reconstituted, complete administration within 60 min.

PO
• Store tablets in refrigerator; protect from light. • Give on empty stomach (1 hr before or 2 hrs after meals).

▨ IV INCOMPATIBILITIES

Amphotericin B complex (Abelcet, AmBisome, Amphotec).

M

🔲 IV COMPATIBILITIES

Acyclovir, dexamethasone (Decadron), famotidine (Pepcid), furosemide (Lasix), LORazepam (Ativan), morphine.

INDICATIONS/ROUTES/DOSAGE

Note: WBC less than 3,000 cells/mm³, platelets less than 100,000 cells/mm³: Withhold treatment until recovery.

Ovarian Carcinoma
PO: ADULTS, ELDERLY: 0.2 mg/kg/day for 5 successive days. Repeat at 4- to 5-wk intervals.

Multiple Myeloma
PO: ADULTS: Initially, 6 mg once daily for 2–3 wks, followed by up to 4 wks rest, then maintenance dose of 2 mg daily; or 0.15 mg/kg/day for 7 days with 2–6 wks rest, then maintenance dose of 0.05 mg/kg/day; or 0.25 mg/kg/day for 4 days, repeat at 4- to 6-wk intervals.
IV: ADULTS: 16 mg/m²/dose every 2 wks for 4 doses, then repeat monthly after hematologic recovery.

Dosage in Renal Impairment
IV: BUN LEVEL GREATER THAN 30 MG/DL: Decrease dosage by 50%.

Dosage in Hepatic Impairment
No dose adjustment.

SIDE EFFECTS

Frequent: Nausea, vomiting (may be severe with large dose). **Occasional:** Diarrhea, stomatitis, rash, pruritus, alopecia.

ADVERSE EFFECTS/TOXIC REACTIONS

Myelosuppression manifested as hematologic toxicity (principally leukopenia, thrombocytopenia, and, to lesser extent, anemia, pancytopenia, agranulocytosis). Leukopenia may occur as early as 5 days after drug initiation. WBC, platelet counts return to normal during 5th wk after therapy, but leukopenia, thrombocytopenia may last more than 6 wks after discontinuing drug. Hyperuricemia noted by hematuria, crystalluria, flank pain.

NURSING CONSIDERATIONS

BASELINE ASSESSMENT

Obtain CBC, then wkly thereafter. Dosage may be decreased or discontinued if WBC falls below 3,000 cells/mm³ or platelet count falls below 100,000 cells/mm³. Antiemetics may be effective in preventing/treating nausea, vomiting.

INTERVENTION/EVALUATION

Monitor CBC with differential, serum electrolytes. Monitor for stomatitis. Monitor for hematologic toxicity (fever, sore throat, signs of local infection, unusual bruising/bleeding from any site), symptoms of anemia (excessive fatigue, weakness), signs of hyperuricemia (hematuria, flank pain). Avoid IM injections, rectal temperatures, other traumas that may induce bleeding.

PATIENT/FAMILY TEACHING

• Increase fluid intake (may protect against hyperuricemia). • Maintain strict oral hygiene. • Hair loss is reversible, but new hair growth may have different color, texture. • Avoid crowds, those with infections. • Report fever, shortness of breath, cough, sore throat, bleeding, unusual bruising. • May suppress ovarian function, leading to amenorrhea.

M

---

memantine   TOP 100

me-**man**-teen
(Apo-Memantine 🍁, Ebixa 🍁, Namenda, Namenda XR)

FIXED-COMBINATION(S)

Namzaric: memantine/donepezil (a cholinesterase inhibitor): 7 mg/10 mg; 14 mg/10 mg; 21 mg/10 mg; 28 mg/10 mg.

🍁 Canadian trade name   Non-Crushable Drug   HIGH ALERT High Alert drug

◆CLASSIFICATION

PHARMACOTHERAPEUTIC: NMDA receptor antagonist. **CLINICAL:** Anti-Alzheimer's agent.

USES

Treatment of moderate to severe dementia of Alzheimer's type. **OFF-LABEL:** Treatment of mild to moderate vascular dementia.

PRECAUTIONS

Contraindications: Hypersensitivity to memantine. **Cautions:** Moderate to severe renal impairment, severe hepatic impairment, cardiovascular disease, seizure disorder, GU conditions that raise urine pH level.

ACTION

Decreases effects of glutamate, the principal excitatory neurotransmitter in the brain. Persistent CNS excitation by glutamate is thought to cause symptoms of Alzheimer's disease. **Therapeutic Effect:** May inhibit clinical deterioration in moderate to severe Alzheimer's disease.

PHARMACOKINETICS

Rapidly, completely absorbed after PO administration. Protein binding: 45%. Undergoes little metabolism; most of dose is excreted unchanged in urine. **Half-life:** 60–80 hrs.

⊠ LIFESPAN CONSIDERATIONS

Pregnancy/Lactation: Unknown if drug crosses placenta or is distributed in breast milk. **Children:** Not prescribed for this pt population. **Elderly:** No age-related precautions noted, but use is not recommended in pts with severe renal impairment (CrCl less than 9 mL/min).

INTERACTIONS

DRUG: Urine **alkalinizers (e.g., carbonic anhydrase inhibitors, sodium bicarbonate)** may decrease renal elimination. **HERBAL:** None significant. **FOOD:** None known. **LAB VALUES:** None significant.

AVAILABILITY (Rx)

Oral Solution: 2 mg/mL. **Tablets:** 5 mg, 10 mg.

🍃 Capsules (Extended-Release [Namenda XR]): 7 mg, 14 mg, 21 mg, 28 mg.

ADMINISTRATION/HANDLING

PO

• Give without regard to food. • Administer oral solution using syringe provided. Do not dilute or mix with other fluids. • Give extended-release capsules whole. Do not crush. May open capsule and sprinkle on applesauce; give immediately.

INDICATIONS/ROUTES/DOSAGE

Alzheimer's Disease

PO: ADULTS, ELDERLY *(Immediate-Release):* Initially, 5 mg once daily. May increase dosage at intervals of at least 1 wk in 5-mg increments to 10 mg/day (5 mg twice daily), then 15 mg/day (5 mg and 10 mg as separate doses), and finally 20 mg/day (10 mg twice daily). Target dose: 20 mg/day. *(Extended-Release):* Initially, 7 mg once daily. May increase at intervals of at least 7 days in increments of 7 mg. **Maximum:** 28 mg once daily. Switching from immediate-release to extended-release: Begin the day following last dose of immediate release.

10 mg twice daily: 28 mg once daily.
5 mg twice daily: 14 mg once daily.

Dosage in Renal Impairment

Creatinine Clearance	Dosage Immediate-Release	Extended-Release
30 mL/min or greater	No adjustments	No adjustments
5–29 mL/min	5 mg twice daily or 10 mg once daily	14 mg once daily

Dosage in Hepatic Impairment
Mild to moderate impairment: No dose adjustment. **Severe impairment:** Use caution.

SIDE EFFECTS

Occasional (7%–4%): Dizziness, headache, confusion, constipation, hypertension, cough. **Rare (3%–2%):** Back pain, nausea, fatigue, anxiety, peripheral edema, arthralgia, insomnia.

ADVERSE EFFECTS/TOXIC REACTIONS

None known.

NURSING CONSIDERATIONS

BASELINE ASSESSMENT

Assess cognitive, behavioral, functional deficits of pt. Assess renal function. Question history of cardiovascular disease, hepatic/renal impairment, seizure disorder.

INTERVENTION/EVALUATION

Monitor cognitive, behavioral, functional status of pt. Monitor urine pH (alterations of urine pH toward the alkaline condition may lead to accumulation of the drug with possible increase in side effects). Monitor BUN, CrCl, serum creatinine lab values.

PATIENT/FAMILY TEACHING

• Do not reduce or stop medication; do not increase dosage without physician direction. • Ensure adequate fluid intake. • If therapy is interrupted for several days, restart at lowest dose, titrate to current dose at minimum of 1-wk intervals. • Local chapter of Alzheimer's Disease Association can provide a guide to services.

meropenem

mer-oh-**pen**-em
(Merrem)
Do not confuse meropenem with doripenem, ertapenem, or imipenem.

◆CLASSIFICATION

PHARMACOTHERAPEUTIC: Carbapenem. **CLINICAL:** Antibiotic.

USES

Treatment of multidrug-resistant infections; meningitis in children 3 mos and older; intra-abdominal infections; complicated skin/skin structure infections caused by susceptible *S. aureus, S. pyogenes, S. agalactiae, S. pneumoniae, H. influenzae, N. meningitidis, M. catarrhalis, E. coli, Klebsiella, Enterobacter, Serratia, P. aeruginosa, B. fragilis.* **OFF-LABEL:** Febrile neutropenia, liver abscess, otitis external, prosthetic joint infection.

PRECAUTIONS

Contraindications: Hypersensitivity to meropenem, pts who experienced anaphylactic reactions to other beta-lactams. **Cautions:** Renal impairment, CNS disorders (particularly with history of seizures, concurrent use with valproic acid).

ACTION

Binds to penicillin-binding proteins. Inhibits bacterial cell wall synthesis. **Therapeutic Effect:** Bactericidal.

PHARMACOKINETICS

After IV administration, widely distributed into tissues and body fluids, including CSF. Protein binding: 2%. Primarily excreted unchanged in urine. Removed by hemodialysis. **Half-life:** 1 hr.

⊠ LIFESPAN CONSIDERATIONS

Pregnancy/Lactation: Unknown if distributed in breast milk. **Children:** Safety and efficacy not established in pts younger than 3 mos. **Elderly:** Age-related renal impairment may require dosage adjustment.

INTERACTIONS

DRUG: May decrease effects of **valproic acid. HERBAL:** None significant.

M

FOOD: None known. **LAB VALUES:** May increase serum BUN, alkaline phosphatase, LDH, ALT, AST, bilirubin. May decrease Hgb, Hct, WBC.

AVAILABILITY (Rx)

Injection, Powder for Reconstitution: 500 mg, 1 g.

ADMINISTRATION/HANDLING

▣ IV

Reconstitution • Reconstitute each 500 mg with 10 mL Sterile Water for Injection, 0.9% NaCl, or D_5W to provide concentration of 50 mg/mL. • Shake to dissolve until clear. • May further dilute with 0.9% NaCl or D_5W to a concentration of 1–20 mg/mL.

Rate of Administration • May give by IV push or IV intermittent infusion (piggyback). • If administering as IV intermittent infusion (piggyback), give over 15–30 min (may also give over 3 hrs); if administered by IV push, give over 3–5 min (at a concentration not greater than 50 mg/mL).

Storage • Store vials at room temperature. • After reconstitution of vials with 0.9% NaCl, stable for 2 hrs at room temperature or 18 hrs if refrigerated (with D_5W, stable for 1 hr at room temperature, 8 hrs if refrigerated). IV infusion with 0.9% NaCl stable for 4 hrs at room temperature or 24 hrs if refrigerated (with D_5W, 1 hr at room temperature or 4 hrs if refrigerated).

▦ IV INCOMPATIBILITIES

Acyclovir (Zovirax), amphotericin B (Fungizone), diazePAM (Valium), doxycycline (Vibramycin), metroNIDAZOLE (Flagyl), ondansetron (Zofran).

▦ IV COMPATIBILITIES

Dexamethasone (Decadron), DOBUTamine (Dobutrex), DOPamine (Intropin), furosemide (Lasix), heparin, magnesium, morphine.

INDICATIONS/ROUTES/DOSAGE

Usual Dosage

IV: ADULTS, ELDERLY: 1.5–6 g/day in divided doses q8h. *(Extended-Infusion):* 0.5–2 g over 3 hrs q8h. **CHILDREN, ADOLESCENTS WEIGHING MORE THAN 50 KG:** 1.5–6 g/day in divided doses q8h. **CHILDREN 3 MOS AND OLDER WEIGHING 50 KG OR LESS:** 30–120 mg/kg/day in divided doses q8h. **Maximum:** 6 g/day. **NEONATES:** 20 mg/kg/dose q8–12h.

Meningitis

IV: ADULTS, ELDERLY, CHILDREN WEIGHING 50 KG OR MORE: 2 g q8h. **CHILDREN 3 MOS AND OLDER WEIGHING LESS THAN 50 KG:** 40 mg/kg q8h. **Maximum:** 2 g/dose.

Dosage in Renal Impairment

Dosage and frequency are modified based on creatinine clearance.

Creatinine Clearance	Dosage	Interval
26–49 mL/min	Normal dose	q12h
10–25 mL/min	50% of normal dose	q12h
Less than 10 mL/min	50% of normal dose	q24h
Hemodialysis:	500 mg	q24h
Peritoneal dialysis:	Recommended dose (based on indication)	q24h

Continuous renal replacement therapy

CRRT	Dosage	Interval
Continuous venovenous hemofiltration	1 gram then 500 mg OR 1 gram	q8h OR q12h
Continuous venovenous hemodialysis/continuous venovenous hemodiafiltration	1 gram then 500 mg OR 1 gram	q6–8h OR q8–12h

Dosage in Hepatic Impairment

No dose adjustment.

SIDE EFFECTS

Frequent (5%–3%): Diarrhea, nausea, vomiting, headache, inflammation at injection site. **Occasional (2%):** Oral candidiasis, rash, pruritus. **Rare (less than 2%):** Constipation, glossitis.

ADVERSE EFFECTS/TOXIC REACTIONS

Antibiotic-associated colitis, other super-infections (abdominal cramps, severe watery diarrhea, fever) may result from altered bacterial balance in GI tract. Anaphylactic reactions have been reported. Seizures may occur in pts with CNS disorders (e.g., brain lesions, history of seizures), bacterial meningitis, renal impairment.

NURSING CONSIDERATIONS

BASELINE ASSESSMENT

Question history of hypersensitivity, allergic reaction to penicillins, cephalosporins. Inquire about history of seizures.

INTERVENTION/EVALUATION

Monitor daily pattern of bowel activity, stool consistency. Monitor for nausea, vomiting. Evaluate for inflammation at IV injection site. Assess skin for rash. Evaluate hydration status. Monitor I&O, renal function, LFT. Check mental status; be alert to tremors, possible seizures. Assess temperature, B/P twice daily, more often if necessary. Monitor serum electrolytes, esp. potassium.

PATIENT/FAMILY TEACHING

• Report persistent diarrhea, abdominal cramps, fever.

mesalamine

me-**sal**-a-meen
(Apriso, Asacol HD, Canasa, Delzicol, Lialda, Mesasal ✦, Pentasa, Rowasa, Salofalk ✦, sfRowasa)

Do not confuse Asacol with Os-Cal, Lialda with Aldara, or mesalamine with megestrol, memantine, or methenamine.

◆ CLASSIFICATION

PHARMACOTHERAPEUTIC: Salicylic acid derivative. **CLINICAL:** Anti-inflammatory agent.

USES

PO: Treatment, maintenance of remission of mild to moderate active ulcerative colitis. **Rectal:** Treatment of active mild to moderate distal ulcerative colitis, proctosigmoiditis or proctitis. **OFF-LABEL:** Crohn's disease.

PRECAUTIONS

Contraindications: Hypersensitivity to mesalamine, salicylates. **Cautions:** SulfaSALAzine, active peptic ulcer, pyloric stenosis, pericarditis, myocarditis, renal/hepatic impairment, elderly.

ACTION

Mechanism unknown. May modulate local mediators of inflammation, may inhibit tumor necrosis factor. **Therapeutic Effect:** Diminishes inflammation in colon.

PHARMACOKINETICS

Poorly absorbed from colon. Moderately absorbed from GI tract. Metabolized in liver. Unabsorbed portion excreted in feces; absorbed portion excreted in urine. Unknown if removed by hemodialysis. **Half-life:** 0.5–1.5 hrs; metabolite, 5–10 hrs.

⧖ LIFESPAN CONSIDERATIONS

Pregnancy/Lactation: Unknown if drug crosses placenta or is distributed in breast milk. **Children:** Safety and efficacy not established. **Elderly:** Age-related renal impairment may require dosage adjustment.

M

INTERACTIONS

DRUG: None known. **HERBAL:** None significant. **FOOD:** None known. **LAB VALUES:** May increase serum alkaline phosphatase, ALT, AST, bilirubin.

AVAILABILITY (Rx)

Rectal Suspension (Rowasa, sfRowasa): 4 g/60 mL. Suppositories (Canasa): 1 g.

Capsules (Controlled-Release [Pentasa]): 250 mg, 500 mg. Capsules (Delayed-Release [Delzicol]): 400 mg. Capsules (Extended-Release [Apriso]): 375 mg. Tablets (Delayed-Release): (Asacol HD): 800 mg. (Lialda): 1.2 g.

ADMINISTRATION/HANDLING

◄ALERT► Store rectal suspension, suppository, oral forms at room temperature.

PO
• Have pt swallow whole; do not break outer coating of tablet. • Give without regard to food. • **Apriso:** Do not administer with antacids. • **Lialda:** Administer once daily with meal.

Rectal
• Shake bottle well. • Instruct pt to lie on left side with lower leg extended, upper leg flexed forward. • Knee-chest position may also be used. • Insert applicator tip into rectum, pointing toward umbilicus. • Squeeze bottle steadily until contents are emptied. • Store suppositories at room temperature. Do not refrigerate.

INDICATIONS/ROUTES/DOSAGE

Treatment of Ulcerative Colitis
PO *(Capsule [Pentasa]):* ADULTS, ELDERLY: 1 g 4 times daily.
PO *(Capsule [Delzicol]):* ADULTS, ELDERLY: 800 mg 3 times daily. CHILDREN 5 YRS AND OLDER, WEIGHING 54–90 KG: 1,200 mg in morning and evening. **Maximum:** 2,400 mg/day. 33–53 KG: 1,200 mg in morning and 800 mg in evening. **Maximum:** 2,000 mg/day.

17–32 KG: 800 mg in morning and 400 mg in evening. **Maximum:** 1,200 mg/day.
PO *(Tablet [Asacol HD]):* ADULTS, ELDERLY: 1.6 g 3 times daily.
PO *(Tablet [Lialda]):* ADULTS, ELDERLY: 2.4–4.8 g once daily.

Maintenance of Remission in Ulcerative Colitis
PO *(Capsule [Pentasa]):* ADULTS, ELDERLY: 1 g 4 times daily.
PO *(Capsule [Delzicol]):* ADULTS, ELDERLY: 1.6 g/day in 2–4 divided doses.
PO *(Capsule, Extended-Release [Apriso]):* ADULTS, ELDERLY: 1.5 g once daily in the morning.
PO *(Tablet [Lialda]):* 2.4 g once daily with food.

Distal Ulcerative Colitis, Proctosigmoiditis, Proctitis
Rectal *(Retention Enema):* ADULTS, ELDERLY: 60 mL (4 g) at bedtime; retained overnight for approximately 8 hrs for 3–6 wks.
Rectal *(1 G Suppository):* ADULTS, ELDERLY: Once daily at bedtime. Continue therapy for 3–6 wks.

◄ALERT► Suppository should be retained for 1–3 hrs for maximum benefit.

Dosage of Renal/Hepatic Impairment
Use caution.

SIDE EFFECTS

Mesalamine is generally well tolerated, with only mild, transient effects. **Frequent (greater than 6%): PO:** Abdominal cramps/pain, diarrhea, dizziness, headache, nausea, vomiting, rhinitis, unusual fatigue. **Rectal:** Abdominal/stomach cramps, flatulence, headache, nausea. **Occasional (6%–2%): PO:** Hair loss, decreased appetite, back/joint pain, flatulence, acne. **Rectal:** Alopecia. **Rare (less than 2%): Rectal:** Anal irritation.

ADVERSE EFFECTS/TOXIC REACTIONS

Sulfite sensitivity may occur in susceptible pts, manifested as cramping, headache, diarrhea, fever, rash, urticaria, pruritus, wheezing. Discontinue drug immediately. Hepatitis, pancreatitis, pericarditis occur rarely with oral forms.

NURSING CONSIDERATIONS

BASELINE ASSESSMENT

Obtain BUN, serum creatinine, LFT. Assess for abdominal pain, discomfort.

INTERVENTION/EVALUATION

Encourage adequate fluid intake. Assess bowel sounds for peristalsis. Monitor daily pattern of bowel activity, stool consistency; record time of evacuation. Assess for abdominal disturbances. Assess skin for rash, urticaria. Discontinue medication if rash, fever, cramping, diarrhea occurs.

PATIENT/FAMILY TEACHING

• Report rash, fever, abdominal pain, significant diarrhea. • Avoid tasks that require alertness, motor skills until response to drug is established. • May discolor urine yellow-brown. • Suppositories stain fabrics.

---

mesna

mess-na
(Mesnex, Uromitexan ✦)

◆ CLASSIFICATION

PHARMACOTHERAPEUTIC: Cytoprotective agent. **CLINICAL:** Antineoplastic adjunct, antidote.

USES

Detoxifying agent used as protectant against hemorrhagic cystitis induced by ifosfamide. **OFF-LABEL:** Reduce incidence of cyclophosphamide-induced hemorrhagic cystitis with high-dose cyclophosphamide.

PRECAUTIONS

Contraindications: Hypersensitivity to mesna. **Cautions:** Preexisting autoimmune disorders.

ACTION

Binds with, detoxifies urotoxic metabolites of ifosfamide/cyclophosphamide. **Therapeutic Effect:** Inhibits ifosfamide/cyclophosphamide-induced hemorrhagic cystitis.

PHARMACOKINETICS

Rapidly metabolized after IV administration to mesna disulfide, which is reduced to mesna in kidneys. Protein binding: 69%–75%. Excreted in urine. **Half-life:** 24 min; metabolite: 72 min.

⧗ LIFESPAN CONSIDERATIONS

Pregnancy/Lactation: Unknown if drug crosses placenta or is distributed in breast milk. **Children:** Safety and efficacy not established. **Elderly:** Information not available.

INTERACTIONS

DRUG: None significant. **HERBAL:** None significant. **FOOD:** None known. **LAB VALUES:** May produce false-positive test result for urinary ketones.

AVAILABILITY (Rx)

Injection Solution: 100 mg/mL. **Tablets:** 400 mg.

ADMINISTRATION/HANDLING

IV

Reconstitution • Dilute with D₅W or 0.9% NaCl to concentration of 20 mg/mL. • May add to solutions containing ifosfamide or cyclophosphamide.
Rate of Administration • Administer by IV infusion over 15–30 min or by continuous infusion.
Storage • Store parenteral form at room temperature. • After dilution, in

---

✦ Canadian trade name   🦫 Non-Crushable Drug   ⬛ High Alert drug

M

0.9% NaCl or D₅W, stable for 48 hrs at room temperature (solutions of mesna and cyclophosphamide in D₅W stable for 48 hrs if refrigerated or 6 hrs at room temperature). Discard unused medication.

PO
• Administer orally in either tablet formulation or parenteral solution. • Dilute mesna solution before PO administration to decrease sulfur odor. Can be diluted (1:1 to 1:10) in carbonated cola drinks, fruit juices, milk.

▨ IV INCOMPATIBILITIES

Amphotericin B complex (Abelcet, AmBisome, Amphotec), CISplatin (Platinol).

▨ IV COMPATIBILITIES

Allopurinol (Aloprim), DOCEtaxel (Taxotere), DOXOrubicin (Adriamycin), etoposide (VePesid), gemcitabine (Gemzar), granisetron (Kytril), methotrexate, ondansetron (Zofran), PACLitaxel (Taxol), vinorelbine (Navelbine).

INDICATIONS/ROUTES/DOSAGE

Prevention of Hemorrhagic Cystitis in Pts Receiving Ifosfamide
IV: ADULTS, ELDERLY: 20% of ifosfamide dose at time of ifosfamide administration and 4 and 8 hrs after each dose of ifosfamide. **Total dose:** 60% of ifosfamide dosage.
IV/PO: 100% of ifosfamide dose, given as 20% at start time followed by 40% given orally 2 and 6 hrs after start of ifosfamide.

Dosage in Renal/Hepatic Impairment
No dose adjustment.

SIDE EFFECTS

Frequent (greater than 17%): Altered taste, soft stools. **Large doses:** Diarrhea, myalgia, headache, fatigue, nausea, hypotension, allergic reaction.

ADVERSE EFFECTS/TOXIC REACTIONS

Hematuria occurs rarely.

NURSING CONSIDERATIONS

BASELINE ASSESSMENT
◄ALERT► Each dose must be administered with ifosfamide therapy.

INTERVENTION/EVALUATION
Assess morning urine specimen for hematuria. If such occurs, dosage reduction or discontinuation may be necessary. Monitor daily pattern of bowel activity, stool consistency; record time of evacuation. Monitor B/P for hypotension.

PATIENT/FAMILY TEACHING
• Report headache, myalgia, nausea.

---

metFORMIN

met-**for**-min
(Apo-MetFORMIN ✤, Fortamet, <u>Glucophage</u>, <u>Glucophage XR</u>, Glumetza, Glycon ✤, Riomet)
■ BLACK BOX ALERT ■ Lactic acidosis occurs very rarely, but mortality rate is 50%. Risk increases with degree of renal impairment, pt's age, those with diabetes, unstable or acute HF.
Do not confuse Glucophage with Glucotrol, or metFORMIN with metroNIDAZOLE.

FIXED-COMBINATION(S)

Actoplus Met: metFORMIN/pioglitazone (an antidiabetic): 500 mg/15 mg, 850 mg/15 mg. **Avandamet:** metFORMIN/rosiglitazone (an antidiabetic): 500 mg/1 mg, 500 mg/2 mg, 500 mg/4 mg, 1,000 mg/2 mg, 1,000 mg/4 mg. **Glucovance:** metFORMIN/glyBURIDE (an antidiabetic): 250 mg/1.25 mg, 500 mg/2.5 mg, 500 mg/5 mg. **Invokamet:** metFORMIN/canagliflozin (an antidiabetic): 500 mg/50 mg, 500 mg/150 mg, 1,000 mg/50 mg, 1,000 mg/150 mg. **Janumet, Janumet XR:** metFORMIN/SITagliptin (an antidiabetic): 500 mg/50 mg, 1,000 mg/50 mg. **Jentadueto, Jentadueto**

M

XR: metFORMIN/linagliptin (an antidiabetic): 500 mg/2.5 mg; 1,000 mg/2.5 mg; 1,000 mg extended-release/2.5 mg; 1,000 mg extended-release/5 mg. **Kazano:** metFORMIN/alogliptin (an antidiabetic): 500 mg/12.5 mg; 1,000 mg/12.5 mg. **Kombiglyze XR:** metFORMIN/SAXagliptin (an antidiabetic): 500 mg/5 mg, 1,000 mg/5 mg, 1,000 mg/2.5 mg. **Metaglip:** metFORMIN/glipiZIDE (an antidiabetic): 250 mg/2.5 mg, 500 mg/2.5 mg, 500 mg/5 mg. **PrandiMet:** metFORMIN/repaglinide (an antidiabetic): 500 mg/1 mg, 500 mg/2 mg. **Synjardy:** metFORMIN/empagliflozin (an antidiabetic): 500 mg/5 mg, 1,000 mg/5 mg, 500 mg/12.5 mg, 1,000 mg/12.5 mg.

◆ CLASSIFICATION

PHARMACOTHERAPEUTIC: Biguanide antihyperglycemic. **CLINICAL:** Antidiabetic agent.

USES

Management of type 2 diabetes mellitus as monotherapy or concomitantly with oral sulfonylurea or insulin. **OFF-LABEL:** Polycystic ovarian syndrome, gestational diabetes mellitus. Prevention of type 2 diabetes.

PRECAUTIONS

◀ **ALERT** ▶ Lactic acidosis is a rare but potentially severe consequence of metFORMIN therapy. Withhold in pts with conditions that may predispose to lactic acidosis (e.g., hypoxemia, dehydration, hypoperfusion, sepsis).
Contraindications: Hypersensitivity to metFORMIN. Renal disease/dysfunction; abnormal CrCl from any cause including MI, septicemia, or shock; acute or chronic metabolic acidosis (with or without coma). **Cautions:** HF, hepatic impairment, excessive acute/chronic alcohol intake, elderly. Recommend temporary discontinuation at time of or before iodinated contrast imaging procedures in pts with CrCl of 30–60 mL/min, or with history of hepatic disease, alcoholism, HF.

ACTION

Decreases hepatic production of glucose. Decreases intestinal absorption of glucose, improves insulin sensitivity. **Therapeutic Effect:** Improves glycemic control, stabilizes/decreases body weight, improves lipid profile.

PHARMACOKINETICS

Slowly, incompletely absorbed after PO administration. Food delays, decreases extent of absorption. Protein binding: Negligible. Primarily distributed to intestinal mucosa, salivary glands. Primarily excreted unchanged in urine. Removed by hemodialysis. **Half-life:** 9–17 hrs.

⏳ LIFESPAN CONSIDERATIONS

Pregnancy/Lactation: Insulin is drug of choice during pregnancy. Distributed in breast milk in animals. **Children:** Safety and efficacy not established in children younger than 10 yrs. **Elderly:** Age-related renal impairment or peripheral vascular disease may require dosage adjustment or discontinuation.

INTERACTIONS

DRUG: **Furosemide** may increase concentration. **Cationic medications (e.g., digoxin, morphine, quiNINE, raNITIdine, vancomycin)** may increase concentration/effects. **IV contrast dye** may increase risk of metFORMIN-induced lactic acidosis, acute renal failure (discontinue metFORMIN 24–48 hrs prior to and up to 72 hrs after contrast exposure). **HERBAL:** **Garlic** may cause hypoglycemia. **FOOD:** None known. **LAB VALUES:** May alter cholesterol, LDL, triglycerides, HDL.

AVAILABILITY (Rx)

Oral Solution (Riomet): 100 mg/mL. **Tablets (Glucophage):** 500 mg, 850 mg, 1,000 mg.

🗞 **Tablets (Extended-Release):** 500 mg (Fortamet, Glucophage XR, Glumetza), 750 mg (Glucophage XR), 1,000 mg (Fortamet, Glumetza).

M

ADMINISTRATION/HANDLING

PO

• Give extended-release tablets whole. Do not break, crush, dissolve, or divide extended-release tablets. • Give with meals (to decrease GI upset). Give Fortamet with glass of water.

INDICATIONS/ROUTES/DOSAGE

◀ALERT▶ Allow 1–2 wks between dose titrations.

Diabetes Mellitus

PO *(Immediate-Release Tablets, Solution):* **ADULTS, ELDERLY:** Initially, 500 mg twice daily or 850 mg once daily. Titrate in increments of 500 mg wkly or 850 mg every other wk. May also titrate from 500 mg twice daily to 850 mg twice daily after 2 wks. **Maintenance:** 1,000–2,550 mg/day in 2–3 divided doses. **Maximum:** 2,550 mg/day. **CHILDREN 10–16 YRS:** Initially, 500 mg twice daily. **Maintenance:** Titrate in 500-mg increments wkly. **Maximum:** 2,000 mg/day.

PO *(Extended-Release Tablets [Glucophage XR]):* **ADULTS, ELDERLY:** Initially, 500 mg once daily. May increase by 500 mg at 1-wk intervals. **Maintenance:** 1,000–2,000 mg daily. **Maximum:** 2,000 mg/day.

PO *(Extended-Release Tablets [Glumetza]):* **ADULTS, ELDERLY:** Initially, 1,000 mg once daily. May increase by 500 mg at 1-wk intervals. **Maximum:** 2,000 mg/day. *[Fortamet]:* Initially, 500–1,000 mg once daily. May increase by 500 mg at 1-wk intervals. **Maximum:** 2,500 mg/day.

Dosage in Renal Impairment

Contraindicated in pts with serum creatinine greater than 1.5 mg/dL (males) or greater than 1.4 mg/dL (females). **Alternative Recommendation: CrCl 45–60 mL/min:** Continue use; monitor renal function q3–6 mos. **CrCl 30–44 mL/min:** Use caution. Consider dose reduction; monitor renal function q3mos. **CrCL less than 30 mL/min:** Discontinue use.

Dosage in Hepatic Impairment

Avoid use (risk factor for lactic acidosis).

SIDE EFFECTS

Occasional (greater than 3%): GI disturbances (diarrhea, nausea, vomiting, abdominal bloating, flatulence, anorexia) that are transient and resolve spontaneously during therapy. **Rare (3%–1%):** Unpleasant/metallic taste that resolves spontaneously during therapy.

ADVERSE EFFECTS/ TOXIC REACTIONS

Lactic acidosis occurs rarely (0.03 cases/1,000 pts) but is a serious and often fatal (50%) complication. Lactic acidosis is characterized by increase in blood lactate levels (greater than 5 mmol/L), decrease in blood pH, electrolyte disturbances. Symptoms include unexplained hyperventilation, myalgia, malaise, drowsiness. May advance to cardiovascular collapse (shock), acute HF, acute MI, prerenal azotemia.

NURSING CONSIDERATIONS

BASELINE ASSESSMENT

Verify pt has not received IV contrast dye within last 48 hrs. Obtain CBC, renal function test, fasting serum glucose, Hgb A1c.

INTERVENTION/EVALUATION

Monitor fasting serum glucose, Hgb A1c, renal function, CBC. Monitor folic acid, renal function tests for evidence of early lactic acidosis. If pt is on concurrent oral sulfonylureas, assess for hypoglycemia (cool/wet skin, tremors, dizziness, anxiety, headache, tachycardia, numbness in mouth, hunger, diplopia). Be alert to conditions that alter glucose requirements: fever, increased activity, stress, surgical procedure.

PATIENT/FAMILY TEACHING

• Discontinue metFORMIN, report immediately if evidence of lactic acidosis appears (unexplained hyperventilation, muscle aches, extreme fatigue, unusual drowsiness). • Prescribed diet is principal part of treatment; do not skip, delay meals. • Diabetes requires lifelong control. • Avoid alcohol. • Report persistent headache, nausea, vomiting, diarrhea or if skin rash, unusual bruising/bleeding, change in color of urine or stool occurs. • Do not take dose for at least 48 hrs after receiving IV contrast dye with radiologic testing.

methadone

meth-a-done
(Dolophine, Metadol ✤, Methadone Disket, Methadone Intensol, Methadose)

■ **BLACK BOX ALERT** ■ May prolong QT interval, which may cause serious arrhythmias. May cause serious, life-threatening, or fatal respiratory depression. Monitor for signs of misuse, abuse, addiction. Prolonged maternal use may cause neonatal withdrawal syndrome.

Do not confuse methadone with Mephyton, Metadate CD, Metadate ER, methylphenidate, or morphine.

◆CLASSIFICATION

PHARMACOTHERAPEUTIC: Opioid agonist **(Schedule II). CLINICAL:** Opioid analgesic. Opioid dependency management.

USES

Moderate to severe pain when a continuous around-the-clock analgesic is needed. Detoxification/maintenance treatment of opioid addiction in conjunction with social/medical services.

PRECAUTIONS

Contraindications: Hypersensitivity to methadone. Severe respiratory depression, acute or severe asthma (in absence of resuscitative equipment or unmonitored setting), hypercarbia, known or suspected paralytic ileus, concurrent use of selegiline. **Caution:** Renal/hepatic impairment, elderly/debilitated pts, risk for QT prolongation, medications that prolong QT interval, conduction abnormalities, severe volume depletion, hypokalemia, hypomagnesemia, cardiovascular disease, depression, suicidal tendencies, history of drug abuse, respiratory disease, biliary tract dysfunction, acute pancreatitis, hypothyroidism, Addison's disease, head injury, increased intracranial pressure.

ACTION

Binds with opioid receptors within CNS, causing inhibition of ascending pain pathways. **Therapeutic Effect:** Alters processes affecting analgesia, emotional response to pain; reduces withdrawal symptoms from other opioid drugs.

PHARMACOKINETICS

Route	Onset	Peak	Duration
PO	0.5–1 hr	1.5–2 hrs	6–8 hrs
IM	10–20 min	1–2 hrs	4–5 hrs
IV	N/A	15–30 min	3–4 hrs

Well absorbed after IM injection. Protein binding: 85%–90%. Metabolized in liver. Primarily excreted in urine. Not removed by hemodialysis. **Half-life:** 7–59 hrs.

⧖ LIFESPAN CONSIDERATIONS

Pregnancy/Lactation: Crosses placenta. Distributed in breast milk. Respiratory depression may occur in neonate if mother received opiates during labor. Regular use of opiates during pregnancy may produce withdrawal symptoms in neonate (irritability, excessive crying, tremors, hyperactive reflexes, fever, vomiting, diarrhea, yawning, sneezing, seizures). **Children:** Paradoxical excitement may occur. Pts younger than 2 yrs more susceptible to respiratory depressant effects. **Elderly:** More susceptible to respiratory depressant effects. Age-related renal impairment may increase risk of urinary retention.

M

M

INTERACTIONS

DRUG: Alcohol, other CNS depressants (e.g., LORazepam, morphine, zolpidem) may increase CNS effects, respiratory depression, hypotension. **CYP3A4 inducers** (e.g., carBAMazepine, PHENobarbital) may decrease concentration/effects. **CYP3A4 inhibitors** (e.g., rifAMPin, clarithromycin) may increase methadone level. **Amiodarone, erythromycin** may prolong QT interval. **MAOIs** (e.g., phenelzine, selegiline) may produce serotonin syndrome (reduce dose to ¼ of usual methadone dose). **HERBAL:** Gotu kola, kava kava, St. John's wort, valerian may increase CNS depression. **St. John's wort** may decrease concentration/effects. **FOOD:** Grapefruit products may alter concentration/effects. **LAB VALUES:** May increase serum amylase, lipase.

AVAILABILITY (Rx)

Injection Solution: 10 mg/mL. **Oral Concentrate:** 10 mg/mL. **Oral Solution:** 5 mg/5 mL, 10 mg/5 mL. **Tablets (Dispersible):** 40 mg. **Tablets:** 5 mg, 10 mg.

ADMINISTRATION/HANDLING

IM, SQ

◀**ALERT**▶ IM preferred over SQ route (SQ produces pain, local irritation, induration). • Do not use if solution appears cloudy or contains a precipitate. • Administer slowly. • Those with circulatory impairment experience higher risk of overdosage due to delayed absorption of repeated administration.

PO

• Give without regard to meals. • Oral dose for detoxification and maintenance may be given in fruit juice or water. • Dispersible tablet should not be chewed or swallowed; add to liquid, allow to dissolve before swallowing.

INDICATIONS/ROUTES/DOSAGE

Analgesia

PO: ADULTS, ELDERLY: Initially, 2.5 mg q8–12 hrs. May increase by 2.5 mg/dose or 5 mg/day q5–7 days. **CHILDREN:** 0.1 mg/kg/dose q4h for 2–3 doses then q6–12h as needed. **Maximum dose:** 10 mg. **IV, IM, SQ: ADULTS, ELDERLY:** Initially, 2.5 mg q8–12h, then titrate slowly to desired effect. **CHILDREN:** 0.1 mg/kg q4h for 2–3 doses, then q6–12h. **Maximum:** 10 mg/dose.

Dosage in Renal Impairment

CrCl less than 10 mL/min: 50–75% normal dose. Avoid in severe hepatic disease.

Dosage in Hepatic Impairment

Mild to moderate impairment: No dose adjustment. **Severe Impairment:** Avoid use.

Detoxification

PO: ADULTS, ELDERLY: Initially, dose of 20–30 mg. An additional 5–10 mg may be provided if withdrawal symptoms have not been suppressed or if symptoms reappear after 2–4 hrs. Day 1 dose not to exceed 40 mg. **Maintenance range:** Titrate to a dose that prevents withdrawal symptoms for 24 hrs, reduces craving, reduces euphoria effect of self-administered opioids, while ensuring tolerance to sedative effects of methadone. Usual range: 80–120 mg/day. Dose reduction should be in increments of less than 10% of the maintenance dose every 10–14 days. **Short-term:** Initially, titrate to 40 mg/day in 2 divided doses. Continue 40-mg dose for 2–3 days. After 2–3 days of stabilization at 40 mg, gradually decrease dose to level keeping withdrawal symptoms tolerable.

SIDE EFFECTS

Frequent: Sedation, orthostatic hypotension, diaphoresis, facial flushing, constipation, dizziness, nausea, vomiting. **Occasional:** Confusion, urinary retention, palpitations, abdominal cramps, visual changes, dry mouth, headache, decreased appetite, anxiety, insomnia. **Rare:** Allergic reaction (rash, pruritus).

ADVERSE EFFECTS/TOXIC REACTIONS

Overdose results in respiratory depression, skeletal muscle flaccidity, cold/clammy skin, cyanosis, extreme drowsiness progressing to seizures, stupor, coma. Early sign of toxicity presents as increased sedation after being on a stable dose. Cardiac toxicity manifested as QT prolongation, torsades de pointes. Tolerance to analgesic effect, physical dependence may occur with repeated use. **Antidote:** Naloxone (see Appendix J for dosage).

NURSING CONSIDERATIONS

BASELINE ASSESSMENT

Obtain baseline EKG. Assess type, location, intensity of pain. **Detoxification:** Assess pt for opioid withdrawal. Pt should be in recumbent position before drug administration by parenteral route. Obtain vital signs before giving medication. If respirations are 12/min or less (20/min or less in children), withhold medication, contact physician.

INTERVENTION/EVALUATION

Monitor vital signs 15–30 min after SQ/IM dose, 5–10 min following IV dose. Oral medication is 50% as potent as parenteral. Assess for adequate voiding. Monitor daily pattern of bowel activity, stool consistency. Assess for clinical improvement, record onset of relief of pain. Provide support to pt in detoxification program; monitor for withdrawal symptoms.

PATIENT/FAMILY TEACHING

• Methadone may produce drug dependence, has potential for being abused. • Avoid alcohol. • Do not stop taking abruptly after prolonged use. • May cause dry mouth, drowsiness. • Avoid tasks that require alertness, motor skills until response to drug is established. • Report severe drowsiness, respiratory depression.

methocarbamol

meth-oh-**kar**-ba-mal
(Robaxin, Robaxin-750)
Do not confuse Robaxin with Skelaxin.

◆ CLASSIFICATION

PHARMACOTHERAPEUTIC: Autonomic agent, carbamate derivative of guaiFENesin. **CLINICAL:** Skeletal muscle relaxant.

USES

Adjunct to rest and physical therapy for relief of discomfort associated with acute, painful musculoskeletal conditions (e.g., tetanus).

PRECAUTIONS

Contraindications: Hypersensitivity to methocarbamol. Renal impairment (injectable formulation). **Cautions:** Elderly, hepatic impairment, seizure disorders (injectable formulation).

ACTION

Skeletal muscle relaxant action may be related to its CNS depressant effects. Does not directly relax skeletal muscle, motor end plate, or nerve fiber. **Therapeutic Effect:** Relieves musculoskeletal pain.

PHARMACOKINETICS

Extensively distributed in tissues. Protein binding: 46%–50%. Converts to metabolites. Metabolized by dealkylation, hydroxylation; excreted in urine. **Half-life:** 1–2 hrs.

⧗ LIFESPAN CONSIDERATIONS

Pregnancy/Lactation: Unknown if distributed in breast milk. **Children:** Safety and efficacy not established in pts 16 yrs and younger. **Elderly:** May be more susceptible to CNS effects, anticholinergic effects. May have increased risk for falls, fractures.

M

◆ Canadian trade name   🦚 Non-Crushable Drug   🔲 High Alert drug

INTERACTIONS

DRUG: Alcohol, CNS depressants (e.g., LORazepam, morphine, zolpidem), tricyclic antidepressants (e.g., amitriptyline, doxepin) may increase sedative effects. May inhibit effect of **pyridostigmine. HERBAL: St. John's wort, valerian, kava kava, gotu kola** may increase CNS depression. **FOOD: High-fat meals** may increase absorption. **LAB VALUES:** May decrease WBC count.

AVAILABILITY (Rx)

Injection, Solution: 100 mg/mL.

 Tablets, Film-Coated: 500 mg, 750 mg.

ADMINISTRATION/HANDLING

IM/IV
(IM)
• Maximum of 5 mL can be given into each gluteal region.

(IV)
• May give undiluted at maximum rate of 3 mL/min. • May dilute with D_5W or 0.9% NaCl to concentration of 4 mg/mL. • Administer in recumbent position and remain in position for 10–15 min after IV administration.

PO
• Give without regard to food. • May crush or break tablets and mix with food or liquid.

INDICATIONS/ROUTES/DOSAGE

Muscle Spasm
PO: ADULTS, ELDERLY, CHILDREN 16 YRS AND OLDER: 1.5 g 4 times/day for 2–3 days, then 4–4.5 g/day in 3–6 divided doses.

Usual Parenteral Dose (Muscle Spasms)
IM/IV: ADULTS, ELDERLY: 1 g q8h for up to 3 days. **Maximum:** 3 g/day.

Tetanus
◄ALERT► Do not use for longer than 72 hrs.
IV: ADULTS, ELDERLY: Initially, 1–2 g by direct IV injection, then 1–2 g by IV infusion q6h until oral therapy possible.

Maximum: 24 g/day. **CHILDREN:** 15 mg/kg/dose. May repeat q6h if needed. **Maximum:** 1.8 g/m²/day.

Dosage in Renal/Hepatic Impairment
No dose adjustment. Injection contraindicated in severe renal impairment; use caution in pts with cirrhosis.

SIDE EFFECTS

Occasional: Dizziness, drowsiness, confusion, double vision, insomnia, headache, irritability, nausea, nervousness, dyspepsia, vomiting, metallic taste.

ADVERSE EFFECTS/TOXIC REACTIONS

Anaphylactic reaction (rash, pruritus, urticaria, angioneurotic edema, fever, bradycardia, hypotension, syncope) has occurred. Leukopenia, cholestatic jaundice, seizure occur rarely.

NURSING CONSIDERATIONS

BASELINE ASSESSMENT
Record onset, type, location, duration of musculoskeletal pain, inflammation. Inspect appearance of affected joints for immobility, stiffness, swelling.

INTERVENTION/EVALUATION
Assist with ambulation at all times. Evaluate for therapeutic response: relief of pain, stiffness, swelling; improved mobility; reduced joint tenderness; improved grip strength.

PATIENT/FAMILY TEACHING
• Avoid tasks that require alertness, motor skills until response to drug is established. • Avoid alcohol. • May color urine brown, black, or green. • Medication intended for short-term use (3 wks). • Report severe sedation.

---

methotrexate　　HIGH ALERT

meth-o-**trex**-ate
(Apo-Methotrexate ✤, Otrexup, Rasuvo, Trexall)

■ **BLACK BOX ALERT** ■ May cause fetal abnormalities, death. May produce potentially fatal chronic hepatotoxicity, dermatologic reactions, acute renal failure, pneumonitis, myelosuppression, malignant lymphoma, aplastic anemia, GI toxicity. Do not use for psoriasis or rheumatoid arthritis treatment in pregnant women.

Do not confuse methotrexate with metOLazone, methylPREDNISolone, or mitoXANTRONE. MTX is an error-prone abbreviation; do not use as an abbreviation.

◆CLASSIFICATION

PHARMACOTHERAPEUTIC: Antimetabolite. **CLINICAL:** Antineoplastic, antiarthritic, antipsoriatic, antirheumatic, immunosuppressant.

USES

Oncology-related: Treatment of breast, head/neck, non–small-cell lung, small-cell lung carcinomas; trophoblastic tumors, acute lymphocytic, meningeal leukemias; non-Hodgkin's lymphomas (lymphosarcoma, Burkitt's lymphoma), carcinoma of gastrointestinal tract, mycosis fungoides, osteosarcoma. **Non-oncology uses:** Psoriasis, rheumatoid arthritis (including juvenile idiopathic arthritis). **OFF-LABEL:** Treatment of acute myelocytic leukemia, bladder carcinoma, ectopic pregnancy, management of abortion, systemic lupus erythematosus, treatment of and maintenance of remission in Crohn's disease.

PRECAUTIONS

Contraindications: Hypersensitivity to methotrexate. Breastfeeding. **Additional: For pts with psoriasis or rheumatoid arthritis:** Pregnancy, hepatic disease, alcoholism, immunodeficiency syndrome, preexisting blood dyscrasias. **Cautions:** Peptic ulcer, ulcerative colitis, preexisting myelosuppression, history of chronic hepatic disease, alcohol consumption, obesity, diabetes, hyperlipidemia, use with other hepatotoxic medications, concomitant use of proton pump inhibitors. Use of NSAIDs or aspirin with lower methotrexate doses for rheumatoid arthritis.

ACTION

Competes with enzymes necessary to reduce folic acid to tetrahydrofolic acid, a component essential to DNA synthesis, repair, and cellular replication. **Therapeutic Effect:** Inhibits DNA, RNA, protein synthesis. Possesses anti-inflammatory and immunemodulating activity.

PHARMACOKINETICS

Variably absorbed from GI tract. Completely absorbed after IM administration. Protein binding: 50%–60%. Widely distributed. Metabolized in liver. Primarily excreted in urine. Removed by hemodialysis but not by peritoneal dialysis. **Half-life:** 3–10 hrs (large doses, 8–15 hrs).

⏳ LIFESPAN CONSIDERATIONS

Pregnancy/Lactation: Avoid pregnancy during methotrexate therapy and minimum 3 mos after therapy in males or at least one ovulatory cycle after therapy in females. May cause fetal death, congenital anomalies. Distributed in breast milk. Breastfeeding not recommended. **Children/Elderly:** Renal/hepatic impairment may require dosage adjustment.

INTERACTIONS

DRUG: Alcohol, hepatotoxic medications (e.g., acetaminophen, isoniazid, ketoconazole, simvastatin) may increase risk of hepatotoxicity. **Bone marrow depressants** may increase myelosuppression. **Live virus vaccines** may potentiate virus replication, increase vaccine side effects, decrease pt's antibody response to vaccine. **NSAIDs (e.g., ibuprofen, ketorolac, naproxen)** may increase risk of toxicity.

M

M

Probenecid, salicylates (e.g., aspirin) may increase concentration, risk of toxicity. **HERBAL:** Cat's claw, echinacea possess immunostimulant properties. **FOOD:** None known. **LAB VALUES:** May increase serum uric acid, AST.

AVAILABILITY (Rx)

Injection, Powder for Reconstitution: 1 g. **Injection, Autoinjector (Rasuvo):** 7.5 mg, 10 mg, 12.5 mg, 15 mg, 17.5 mg, 20 mg, 22.5 mg, 25 mg, 27.5 mg, 30 mg. **Injection Solution:** 25 mg/mL. **Injection Syringe (Otrexup):** 7.5 mg/0.4 mL, 10 mg/0.4 mL, 15 mg/0.4 mL, 20 mg/0.4 mL, 25 mg/0.4 mL. **Tablets (Trexall):** 2.5 mg, 5 mg, 7.5 mg, 10 mg, 15 mg.

ADMINISTRATION/HANDLING

◀**ALERT**▶ May be carcinogenic, mutagenic, teratogenic. Handle with extreme care during preparation/administration. Wear gloves when preparing solution. If powder or solution comes in contact with skin, wash immediately, thoroughly with soap, water. May give IM, IV, intra-arterially, intrathecally.

 IV

Reconstitution • Reconstitute powder with D_5W or 0.9% NaCl to provide concentration of 25 mg/mL or less. • For intrathecal use, dilute with preservative-free 0.9% NaCl to provide a concentration not greater than 2–4 mg/mL.
Rate of Administration • Give IV push at rate of 10 mg/min. • Give IV infusion at rate of 4–20 mg/hr (refer to specific protocol).
Storage • Store vials at room temperature. Diluted solutions stable for 24 hrs at room temperature.

▒ IV INCOMPATIBILITIES

Droperidol (Inapsine), gemcitabine (Gemzar), IDArubicin (Idamycin), midazolam (Versed), nalbuphine (Nubain).

▒ IV COMPATIBILITIES

CISplatin (Platinol AQ), cyclophosphamide (Cytoxan), DAUNOrubicin (DaunoXome), DOXOrubicin (Adriamycin), etoposide (VePesid), 5-fluorouracil, granisetron (Kytril), leucovorin, mitoMYcin (Mutamycin), ondansetron (Zofran), PAClitaxel (Taxol), vinBLAStine (Velban), vinCRIStine (Oncovin), vinorelbine (Navelbine).

INDICATIONS/ROUTES/DOSAGE

Oncology Uses
◀**ALERT**▶ Refer to individual specific protocols for optimum dosage, sequence of administration.

Head/Neck Cancer
PO, IV, IM: ADULTS, ELDERLY: 40 mg/m^2 once weekly. Continue until disease progression or unacceptable toxicity.

Breast Cancer
IV: ADULTS, ELDERLY: 40 mg/m^2 days 1 and 8 q4wks in combination with cyclophosphamide and fluorouracil.

Mycosis Fungoides
IM, PO: ADULTS, ELDERLY: 5–50 mg once weekly or 15–37.5 mg twice weekly.

Rheumatoid Arthritis (RA)
PO: ADULTS: Initially, 7.5 mg once wkly or 2.5 mg q12h for 3 doses once wkly. Adjust dose gradually to optimal response. **SQ/IM:** Initially, 7.5 mg wkly. Adjust dose gradually to optimal response. **ELDERLY:** Initially, 5–7.5 mg/wk. **Maximum:** 20 mg/wk.

Juvenile Rheumatoid Arthritis (JRA)
PO, IM, SQ: CHILDREN: Initially, 10 mg/m^2 once wkly, then 20–30 mg/m^2/wk as a single dose.

Psoriasis
PO: ADULTS, ELDERLY: Initially, 10–25 mg once wkly or 2.5–5 mg q12h for 3 doses once wkly. **IM/SQ:** 10–25 mg once wkly. Adjust dose gradually to optimal response. Titrate to lowest effective dose.

Dosage in Renal Impairment	
Creatinine Clearance	Reduce Dose to
61–80 mL/min	75% of normal
51–60 mL/min	70% of normal
10–50 mL/min	30–50% of normal
Less than 10 mL/min	Avoid use

Dosage in Hepatic Impairment
Use caution.

SIDE EFFECTS

Frequent (10%–3%): Nausea, vomiting, stomatitis, burning/erythema at psoriatic site (in pts with psoriasis). **Occasional (3%–1%):** Diarrhea, rash, dermatitis, pruritus, alopecia, dizziness, anorexia, malaise, headache, drowsiness, blurred vision.

ADVERSE EFFECTS/TOXIC REACTIONS

High potential for various severe toxicities. GI toxicity may produce gingivitis, glossitis, pharyngitis, stomatitis, enteritis, hematemesis. Hepatotoxicity more likely to occur with frequent small doses than with large intermittent doses. Pulmonary toxicity characterized by interstitial pneumonitis. Hematologic toxicity, resulting from marked myelosuppression, may manifest as leukopenia, thrombocytopenia, anemia, hemorrhage. Dermatologic toxicity may produce rash, pruritus, urticaria, pigmentation, photosensitivity, petechiae, ecchymosis, pustules. Severe nephrotoxicity produces azotemia, hematuria, renal failure.

NURSING CONSIDERATIONS

BASELINE ASSESSMENT

Rheumatoid arthritis: Assess pain, range of motion. Obtain baseline CBC, BMP, LFT, rheumatoid factor. **Psoriasis:** Assess skin lesions. Question for possibility of pregnancy in pts with psoriasis, rheumatoid arthritis (RA). Obtain all functional tests before therapy, repeat throughout therapy. Antiemetics may prevent nausea, vomiting.

INTERVENTION/EVALUATION

Monitor CBC, BMP, LFT, urinalysis, chest X-rays, serum uric acid. Monitor for hematologic toxicity (fever, sore throat, signs of local infection, unusual bruising/bleeding from any site), symptoms of anemia (excessive fatigue, weakness). Assess skin for evidence of dermatologic toxicity. Keep pt well hydrated, urine alkaline. Avoid rectal temperatures, traumas that induce bleeding. Apply 5 full min of pressure to IV sites.

PATIENT/FAMILY TEACHING

• Maintain strict oral hygiene. • Do not have immunizations without physician's approval (drug lowers resistance). • Avoid crowds, those with infection. • Avoid alcohol, aspirin. • Avoid ultraviolet sunlight exposure. • Use contraceptive measures during therapy and for 3 mos (males) or 1 ovulatory cycle (females) after therapy. • Promptly report fever, sore throat, signs of local infection, unusual bruising/bleeding from any site, diarrhea. • Hair loss is reversible, but new hair growth may have different color, texture. • Report persistent nausea/vomiting.

M

methylergonovine

meth-il-er-**goe**-noe-veen
(Methergine ✦)

◆CLASSIFICATION

PHARMACOTHERAPEUTIC: Ergot alkaloid. **CLINICAL:** Oxytocic agent, uterine stimulant.

USES

Management of uterine atony, hemorrhage and subinvolution of uterus following delivery of placenta. Control uterine hemorrhage following delivery of anterior shoulder in second stage of labor.

M

PRECAUTIONS

Contraindications: Hypersensitivity to methylergonovine. Hypertension, pregnancy, toxemia. **Cautions:** Renal/hepatic impairment, coronary artery disease, pts at risk for coronary artery disease (diabetes, obesity, smoking, hypercholesterolemia), concurrent use with CYP3A4 inhibitors (e.g., protease inhibitors), occlusive peripheral vascular disease, sepsis, second stage of labor.

ACTION

Increases tone, rate, amplitude of contraction of uterine smooth muscle. **Therapeutic Effect:** Shortens third stage of labor, reduces blood loss.

PHARMACOKINETICS

Route	Onset	Peak	Duration
PO	5–10 min	N/A	3 hrs
IV	Immediate	N/A	45 min
IM	2–5 min	N/A	3 hrs

Rapidly absorbed from GI tract after IM administration. Distributed rapidly to plasma, extracellular fluid, tissues. Metabolized in liver. Primarily excreted in urine. **Half-life:** 0.5–2 hrs.

⌛ LIFESPAN CONSIDERATIONS

Pregnancy/Lactation: Contraindicated during pregnancy. Small amounts distributed in breast milk. **Children/Elderly:** No information available.

INTERACTIONS

DRUG: **DOPamine, norepinephrine, phenylephrine, vasopressin** may increase effects. **Strong CYP3A4 inhibitors (e.g., ketoconazole, ritonavir)** may increase concentration/effect. **Beta blockers (e.g., carvedilol, labetalol, metoprolol)** may increase vasoconstrictive effect of ergot alkaloids. **Anesthetics (e.g., halothane, methoxyflurane)** may increase oxytocic effects. **HERBAL:** None significant. **FOOD:** None known. **LAB VALUES:** May decrease serum prolactin.

AVAILABILITY (Rx)

Injection Solution: 0.2　mg/mL. **Tablets:** 0.2 mg.

ADMINISTRATION/HANDLING

Note: Initial dose may be given parenterally, followed by oral regimen. IV use in life-threatening emergencies only. **Reconstitution** • Dilute with 0.9% NaCl to volume of 5 mL. **Rate of Administration** • Give over at least 1 min, carefully monitoring B/P. **Storage** • Refrigerate ampules.

▦ IV INCOMPATIBILITIES

None known.

▦ IV COMPATIBILITIES

Heparin, potassium.

INDICATIONS/ROUTES/DOSAGE

Prevention/Treatment of Postpartum, Postabortion Hemorrhage
PO: **ADULTS:** 0.2 mg 3–4 times daily. Continue for up to 7 days.
IV, IM: **ADULTS:** Initially, 0.2 mg after delivery of anterior shoulder, after delivery of placenta, or during puerperium. May repeat q2–4h as needed.

Dosage in Renal/Hepatic Impairment
Use caution.

SIDE EFFECTS

Frequent: Nausea, uterine cramping, vomiting. **Occasional:** Abdominal pain, diarrhea, dizziness, diaphoresis, tinnitus, bradycardia, chest pain. **Rare:** Allergic reaction (rash, pruritus), dyspnea, severe or sudden hypertension.

ADVERSE EFFECTS/ TOXIC REACTIONS

Severe hypertensive episodes may result in CVA, serious arrhythmias, seizures. Hypertensive effects are more frequent with pt susceptibility, rapid IV administration, concurrent use of regional anesthesia, vasoconstrictors. Peripheral ischemia may lead to gangrene.

NURSING CONSIDERATIONS

BASELINE ASSESSMENT

Determine baseline serum calcium level, B/P, pulse. Assess for any evidence of bleeding before administration.

INTERVENTION/EVALUATION

Monitor uterine tone, bleeding, B/P, pulse q15min until stable (about 1–2 hrs). Assess extremities for color, warmth, movement, pain. Report chest pain promptly. Provide support with ambulation if dizziness occurs.

PATIENT/FAMILY TEACHING

• Avoid smoking: causes increased vasoconstriction. • Report increased cramping, bleeding, foul-smelling lochia. • Report pale, cold hands/feet (possibility of diminished circulation).

---

methylnaltrexone

meth-il-nal-**trex**-own
(Relistor)
Do not confuse methylnaltrexone with naltrexone.

◆CLASSIFICATION

PHARMACOTHERAPEUTIC: Opioid receptor antagonist. **CLINICAL:** Laxative.

USES

Injection: Treatment of opioid-induced constipation in pts with advanced illness who are receiving palliative care when response to laxative therapy is insufficient. **Injection/Tablets:** Treatment of opioid-induced constipation for chronic pain unrelated to cancer.

PRECAUTIONS

Contraindications: Hypersensitivity to methylnaltrexone. Known or suspected GI obstruction. Pts at increased risk of recurrent obstruction due to potential of GI perforation. **Cautions:** Renal impairment,

history of GI tract lesions (e.g., peptic ulcer disease, GI tract malignancies).

ACTION

Blocks binding of opioids to peripheral opioid receptors within GI tract. **Therapeutic Effect:** Decreases constipating effect of opioids without reducing analgesic effect.

PHARMACOKINETICS

Absorbed rapidly. Undergoes moderate tissue distribution. Protein binding: 11%–15%. Excreted in urine (50%), feces (35%). **Half-life:** 8 hrs.

⧗ LIFESPAN CONSIDERATIONS

Pregnancy/Lactation: Unknown if distributed in breast milk (not recommended). **Children:** Safety and efficacy not established. **Elderly:** No age-related precautions noted.

INTERACTIONS

DRUG: None significant. **HERBAL:** None significant. **FOOD:** None known. **LAB VALUES:** None significant.

AVAILABILITY (Rx)

Injection, Solution: 8 mg/0.4 mL, 12 mg/0.6 mL. **Tablets:** 150 mg.

ADMINISTRATION/HANDLING

PO

• Administer with water on an empty stomach at least 30 min before first meal of day.

Subcutaneous

Preparation • Visually inspect for particulate matter or discoloration. Solution should appear colorless to pale yellow in color. Do not use if solution is cloudy, discolored, or if large particles are observed. **Administration** • Insert needle subcutaneously into upper arms, outer thigh, or abdomen, and inject solution. • Do not inject into areas of active skin disease or injury such as sunburns, skin rashes, inflammation, skin infections, or active psoriasis. • Rotate injection sites.

M

Storage • Once solution is drawn into syringe, may be stored at room temperature. • Administer within 24 hrs.

INDICATIONS/ROUTES/DOSAGE

◀ALERT▶ Usual schedule is once every other day, as needed, but no more frequently than once every 24 hrs.

Constipation (Chronic Non-Cancer Pain)
PO: ADULTS, ELDERLY: 450 mg once daily in the morning. **SQ: ADULTS, ELDERLY:** 12 mg/day. **Note:** Discontinue all laxatives prior to use.

Constipation (Advanced Illness)
SQ: ADULTS, ELDERLY WEIGHING 38 KG TO LESS THAN 62 KG: 8 mg. **ADULTS, ELDERLY WEIGHING 62–114 KG:** 12 mg. **ADULTS, ELDERLY WHOSE WEIGHT FALLS OUTSIDE THESE RANGES:** Dose at 0.15 mg/kg (round dose up to nearest 0.1 mL of volume).

Dosage in Severe Renal Impairment (CrCl Less Than 60 mL/min)
SQ: ADULTS, ELDERLY: Administer 50% of recommended dose.

Dosage in Hepatic Impairment
No dose adjustment.

SIDE EFFECTS

Frequent (29%–12%): Abdominal pain, flatulence, nausea. **Occasional (7%–5%):** Diarrhea, dizziness.

ADVERSE EFFECTS/ TOXIC REACTIONS

None known.

NURSING CONSIDERATIONS

BASELINE ASSESSMENT

Question characteristics of constipation, frequency of bowel movements. Assess bowel sounds. Question history of GI obstruction, perforation, baseline GI disease; renal impairment. Receive full medication history, including herbal products, and screen for interactions. Assess hydration status.

INTERVENTION/EVALUATION

30% of pts report defecation within 30 min after drug administration. Encourage fluid intake. Assess bowel sounds for peristalsis. Monitor daily pattern of bowel activity, stool consistency. If opioid medication is stopped, drug should be discontinued. Assess for abdominal disturbances.

PATIENT/FAMILY TEACHING

• Laxative effect usually occurs within 30 min but may take up to 24 hrs after medication administration. • Common side effects include transient abdominal pain, nausea, vomiting. • Report persistent or worsening symptoms, or if severe or persistent diarrhea occurs.

---

methylphenidate

meth-il-**fen**-i-date
(Apo-Methylphenidate ✦, Aptensio XR, Concerta, Cotempla XR, Daytrana, Metadate CD, Metadate ER, Methylin, PMS-Methylphenidate ✦, Quillichew ER, Quillivant XR, Ritalin, Ritalin LA)
■ **BLACK BOX ALERT** ■ Chronic abuse can lead to marked tolerance, psychological dependence. Abrupt withdrawal from prolonged use may lead to severe depression, psychosis.
Do not confuse Metadate ER with Metadate CD, methylphenidate with methadone, or Ritalin with Rifadin.

◆**CLASSIFICATION**

PHARMACOTHERAPEUTIC: CNS stimulant **(Schedule II). CLINICAL:** CNS stimulant.

USES

Treatment of attention-deficit hyperactivity disorder (ADHD). Management of narcolepsy. **OFF-LABEL:** Secondary mental depression (especially elderly pts, medically ill).

PRECAUTIONS

Contraindications: Hypersensitivity to methylphenidate. Use during or within 14 days following MAOI therapy; marked anxiety, tension, agitation, motor tics; family history or diagnosis of Tourette's syndrome, glaucoma. **Metadate (additional):** Severe hypertension, HF, arrhythmia, hyperthyroidism, recent MI or angina. **Cautions:** Hypertension, seizures, acute stress reaction, emotional instability, history of drug dependence, HF, recent MI, hyperthyroidism or thyrotoxicosis, known structural cardiac abnormality, bipolar disorder, cardiomyopathy, arrhythmias, alcohol abuse.

ACTION

Blocks reuptake of norepinephrine, DOPamine into presynaptic neurons. **Therapeutic Effect:** Decreases motor restlessness, fatigue. Increases motor activity, attention span, mental alertness. Produces mild euphoria.

PHARMACOKINETICS

Onset	Peak	Duration
Immediate-release	2 hrs	3–6 hrs
Sustained-release	4–7 hrs	8 hrs
Extended-release	N/A	12 hrs
Transdermal	2 hrs	N/A

Slowly, incompletely absorbed from GI tract. Protein binding: 15%. Metabolized in liver. Primarily excreted in urine. Unknown if removed by hemodialysis. **Half-life:** 2–4 hrs.

⧗ LIFESPAN CONSIDERATIONS

Pregnancy/Lactation: Unknown if drug crosses placenta or is distributed in breast milk. **Children:** May be more susceptible to developing anorexia, insomnia, stomach pain, decreased weight. Chronic use may inhibit growth. Not approved for children younger than 6 yrs. **Elderly:** No age-related precautions noted.

INTERACTIONS

DRUG: MAOIs (e.g., phenelzine, selegiline) may increase effects. **Other CNS stimulants** (e.g., caffeine, dextroamphetamine, phentermine) may have additive effect. May inhibit metabolism of **warfarin, anticonvulsants** (e.g., carBAMazepine, phenytoin), **antidepressants. HERBAL:** Ephedra may cause hypertension, arrhythmias. **Yohimbe** may increase CNS stimulation. **FOOD:** None known. **LAB VALUES:** None significant.

AVAILABILITY (Rx)

Oral Solution (Methylin): 5 mg/5 mL, 10 mg/5 mL, 10 mg/1 mL. **Tablets (Chewable [Methylin]):** 2.5 mg, 5 mg, 10 mg. **Tablets (Methylin, Ritalin):** 5 mg, 10 mg, 20 mg. **Topical Patch (Daytrana):** 10 mg/9 hrs, 15 mg/9 hrs, 20 mg/9 hrs, 30 mg/9 hrs. **Powder for Suspension, Extended-Release (Quillivant XR):** 25 mg/5 mL. **Capsules (Extended-Release [Aptensio XR]):** 10 mg, 15 mg, 20 mg, 30 mg, 40 mg, 50 mg, 60 mg. **Capsules (Extended-Release [Metadate CD]):** 10 mg, 20 mg, 30 mg, 40 mg, 50 mg, 60 mg. **Capsules (Extended-Release [Ritalin LA]):** 10 mg, 20 mg, 30 mg, 40 mg. **Tablets (Extended-Release [Concerta]):** 18 mg, 27 mg, 36 mg, 54 mg, 72 mg. **Tablets (Extended-Release [Metadate ER, Methylin ER]):** 10 mg, 20 mg. **Tablets (Extended-Release [Quillichew ER]):** 20 mg, 30 mg, 40 mg.

🦬 **Capsules (Extended-Release [Aptensio XR]):** 10 mg, 15 mg, 20 mg, 30 mg, 40 mg, 50 mg, 60 mg. **Capsules (Extended-Release [Metadate CD]):** 10 mg, 20 mg, 30 mg, 40 mg, 50 mg, 60 mg. 🦬 **Capsules (Extended-Release [Ritalin LA]):** 10 mg, 20 mg, 30 mg, 40 mg. 🦬 **Tablets (Extended-Release [Concerta]):** 18 mg, 27 mg, 36 mg, 54 mg, 72 mg. 🦬 **Tablets (Extended-Release [Metadate ER, Methylin ER]):** 10 mg, 20 mg. **Tablets, Extended Release ODT (Cotempla XR):** 8.6 mg, 17.3 mg, 25.9 mg. **Tablets Chewable (Extended-Release [Quillichew ER]):** 20 mg, 30 mg, 40 mg. 🦬 **Tablets (Sustained-Release [Ritalin SR]):** 20 mg.

ADMINISTRATION/HANDLING

◀**ALERT**▶ Sustained-release, extended-release tablets may be given in place of regular tablets once the daily dose is titrated using regular tablets and the titrated dosage corresponds to sustained-release or extended-release tablet strength.

PO

• Do not give in afternoon or evening (may cause insomnia). • Do not crush, break extended-release capsules, extended- or sustained-release tablets. • Immediate-release tablets may be crushed. • Give dose 30–45 min before meals.

• **Concerta:** Administer once daily in morning. May take without regard to food but must be taken with water, milk, or juice.
• **Methylin Chewable:** Give with at least 8 oz of water or other fluid.
• **Metadate CD, Ritalin LA:** • May be opened, sprinkled on applesauce. • Instruct pt to swallow applesauce without chewing. Do not crush or chew capsule contents.
• **Quillivant XR:** Administer in morning with or without food. Shake bottle more than 10 sec prior to administration.

Patch

• To be worn daily for 9 hrs. • Replace daily in morning. • Apply to dry, clean area of hip. • Avoid applying to waistline (clothing may cause patch to rub off). • Alternate application site daily. • Press firmly in place for 30 sec to ensure patch is in good contact with skin. • Do not cut patch.

INDICATIONS/ROUTES/DOSAGE

ADHD

PO: ADULTS: *(Immediate-Release):* 5 mg twice daily, before breakfast and lunch. May increase by 5–10 mg/day at wkly intervals. **Maximum:** 60 mg/day in 2–3 divided doses. CHILDREN 6 YRS AND OLDER: Initially, 5 mg before breakfast and lunch. May increase by 5–10 mg/day at wkly intervals. Usual dose: 20–30 mg/day in 2–3 divided doses. **Maximum:** 60 mg/day.

PO *(Concerta):* CHILDREN 6 YRS AND OLDER, ADULTS UP TO 65 YRS OF AGE: Initially, 18 mg once daily; may increase by 18 mg/day at wkly intervals. **Maximum:** 54 mg/day in children 6–12 yrs of age (up to 72 mg/day in adolescents younger than 18 yrs).

PO *(Metadate CD):* CHILDREN 6 YRS AND OLDER: Initially, 20 mg/day. May increase by 10–20 mg/day at wkly intervals. **Maximum:** 60 mg/day.

PO: *(Quillichew ER):* CHILDREN 6 YRS AND OLDER: Initially, 20 mg/day. May increase by 10 mg/15 mg or 20 mg/day at wkly intervals. **Maximum:** 60 mg/day.

PO *(Quillivant XR):* CHILDREN 6 YRS AND OLDER: Initially, 20 mg once daily in the morning. May increase in increments of 10–20 mg/day at wkly increments. **Maximum:** 60 mg/day.

PO *(Ritalin LA):* CHILDREN 6 YRS AND OLDER: Initially, 20 mg/day. May increase by 10 mg/day at wkly intervals. **Maximum:** 60 mg/day.

PO *(Metadate ER, Methylin ER):* CHILDREN 6 YRS AND OLDER: May replace regular tablets after daily dose is titrated and 8-hr dosage corresponds to sustained-release or extended-release tablet strength. **Maximum:** 60 mg/day.

PO *(Cotempla XR):* CHILDREN, 6–18 YRS: Initially, 17.3 mg once daily. May increase in weekly intervals in 8.6 to 17.3 mg increments. **Maximum:** 51.8 mg/day.

PATCH *(Daytrana):* CHILDREN 6–12 YRS, ADOLESCENTS: Initially, 10 mg daily (applied and worn for 9 hrs). Dosage is titrated to desired effect. May increase dose no more frequently than every wk.

Narcolepsy

PO: ADULTS, ELDERLY: *(Immediate-Release):* Initially, 5 mg twice daily, before breakfast and lunch. May increase by 5–10 mg/day at wkly intervals. **Maximum:** 60 mg/day in 2–3 divided doses. *(Extended Release):* May give once immediate-release is titrated. **Maximum:** 60 mg/day.

M

Dosage in Renal/Hepatic Impairment
No dose adjustment.

SIDE EFFECTS

Frequent: Anxiety, insomnia, anorexia. **Occasional:** Dizziness, drowsiness, headache, nausea, abdominal pain, fever, rash, arthralgia, vomiting. **Rare:** Blurred vision, Tourette's syndrome (uncontrolled vocal outbursts, repetitive body movements, tics), palpitations, priapism.

ADVERSE EFFECTS/ TOXIC REACTIONS

Prolonged administration to children with ADHD may delay normal weight gain pattern. Overdose may produce tachycardia, palpitations, arrhythmias, chest pain, psychotic episode, seizures, coma. Hypersensitivity reactions, blood dyscrasias occur rarely.

NURSING CONSIDERATIONS

BASELINE ASSESSMENT

ADHD: Assess attention span, impulsivity, interaction with others, distractibility. **Narcolepsy:** Observe/assess frequency of episodes. Question history of seizures.

INTERVENTION/EVALUATION

Monitor B/P, pulse, changes in ADHD symptoms. CBC with differential should be performed routinely during therapy. If paradoxical return of attention-deficit occurs, dosage should be reduced or discontinued. Monitor growth.

PATIENT/FAMILY TEACHING

• Avoid tasks that require alertness, motor skills until response to drug is established. • Sugarless gum, sips of water may relieve dry mouth. • Report any increase in seizures. • Take daily dose early in morning to avoid insomnia. • Report anxiety, palpitations, fever, vomiting, skin rash. • Report new or worsened symptoms (e.g., behavior, hostility, concentration ability). • Avoid caffeine. • Do not stop taking abruptly after prolonged use.

methylPREDNISolone

meth-il-pred-**nis**-oh-lone
(Medrol)

methylPREDNISolone acetate

(DepoMedrol)

methylPREDNISolone sodium succinate

(Solu-Medrol)
Do not confuse DepoMedrol with Solu-Medrol, Medrol with Mebaral, or methylPREDNISolone with medroxyPROGESTERone or prednisoLONE.

✦CLASSIFICATION

PHARMACOTHERAPEUTIC: Adrenal corticosteroid. **CLINICAL:** Anti-inflammatory.

USES

Anti-inflammatory or immunosuppressant in treatment of hematologic, allergic, inflammatory, autoimmune, or neoplastic disorders. **OFF-LABEL:** Acute spinal cord injury.

PRECAUTIONS

Contraindications: Hypersensitivity to methylPREDNISolone. Administration of live or attenuated virus vaccines, systemic fungal infection. **IM (additional):** Idiopathic thrombocytopenia purpura. **Cautions:** Respiratory tuberculosis, untreated systemic infections, hypertension, HF, diabetes, GI disease (e.g., peptic ulcer), myasthenia gravis, renal/hepatic impairment, seizures, cataracts, glaucoma, following acute MI, thyroid disorder, thromboembolic tendencies, cardiovascular disease, elderly pts, psychiatric conditions, pts at risk for osteoporosis.

M

ACTION

Suppresses migration of polymorpho-nuclear leukocytes, reverses increased capillary permeability. **Therapeutic Effect:** Decreases inflammation.

PHARMACOKINETICS

Route	Onset	Peak	Duration
PO	Rapid	1–2 hrs	30–36 hrs
IM	Rapid	4–8 days	1–4 wks
IV	Rapid	N/A	N/A

Well absorbed from GI tract after IM administration. Widely distributed. Metabolized in liver. Excreted in urine. Removed by hemodialysis. **Half-life:** 3.5 hrs.

⧗ LIFESPAN CONSIDERATIONS

Pregnancy/Lactation: Crosses placenta. Distributed in breast milk. May cause cleft palate (chronic use in first trimester). Breastfeeding not recommended. **Children:** Prolonged treatment or high dosages may decrease short-term growth rate, cortisol secretion. **Elderly:** No age-related precautions noted.

INTERACTIONS

DRUG: May alter effects of **warfarin.** **CYP3A inducers (e.g., phenytoin, rifAMPin)** may decrease effects. **Live virus vaccines** may decrease pt's antibody response to vaccine, increase vaccine side effects, potentiate virus replication. **HERBAL: Cat's claw, echinacea** possess immunostimulant properties. **St. John's wort** may decrease concentration. **FOOD:** None known. **LAB VALUES:** May increase serum glucose, cholesterol, lipids, amylase, sodium. May decrease serum calcium, potassium, thyroxine, hypothalamic-pituitary-adrenal (HPA) axis.

AVAILABILITY (Rx)

Injection, Powder for Reconstitution (SOLU): 40 mg, 125 mg, 500 mg, 1 g. **Injection Suspension (DEPO):** 40 mg/mL, 80 mg/mL. **Tablets (Medrol):** 2 mg, 4 mg, 8 mg, 16 mg, 32 mg. **(Medrol Dosepak):** 4 mg (21 tablets).

ADMINISTRATION/HANDLING

◄ALERT► Do **not** give methylPRED-NISolone acetate IV.

 IV

Reconstitution • For infusion, add to D_5W, 0.9% NaCl.
Rate of Administration • Give IV push over 3–15 min. • Give IV piggyback. Dose of 250 mg over 15–30 min; dose of 500–999 mg over at least 30 min; dose of 1g or greater over 1 hr.
Storage • Store vials at room temperature. Diluted solution is stable for 48 hrs at room temperature or refrigerated.

IM

• MethylPREDNISolone acetate should not be further diluted. • MethylPRED-NISolone sodium succinate should be reconstituted with Bacteriostatic Water for Injection. • Give deep IM in gluteus maximus (avoid injection into deltoid muscle).

PO

• Give with food, milk.

▦ IV INCOMPATIBILITIES

Ciprofloxacin (Cipro), diltiaZEM (Cardizem), potassium chloride, propofol (Diprivan).

▦ IV COMPATIBILITIES

Dexmedetomidine (Precedex), DOPamine (Intropin), heparin, midazolam (Versed), theophylline.

INDICATIONS/ROUTES/DOSAGE

Anti-Inflammatory, Immunosuppressive
IV: ADULTS, ELDERLY: 10–40 mg. May repeat q4–6h as needed. **CHILDREN:** 0.5–1.7 mg/kg/day or 5–25 mg/m²/day in 2–4 divided doses.

PO: ADULTS, ELDERLY: 4–48 mg/day in 1–4 divided doses. **CHILDREN:** 0.5–1.7 mg/kg/day or 5–25 mg/m²/day in 2–4 divided doses.

IM (MethylPREDNISolone Succinate): ADULTS, ELDERLY: 10–40 mg/day.

IM *(Methylprednisolone Acetate):*
ADULTS, ELDERLY: 4–120 mg single dose.
**Intra-Articular, Intralesional: ADULTS,
ELDERLY:** 4–80 mg q1–5wks.

Dosage in Renal/Hepatic Impairment
No dose adjustment.

SIDE EFFECTS

Frequent: Insomnia, heartburn, anxiety, abdominal distention, diaphoresis, acne, mood swings, increased appetite, facial flushing, GI distress, delayed wound healing, increased susceptibility to infection, diarrhea, constipation. **Occasional:** Headache, edema, tachycardia, change in skin color, frequent urination, depression. **Rare:** Psychosis, increased blood coagulability, hallucinations.

ADVERSE EFFECTS/ TOXIC REACTIONS

Long-term therapy: Hypocalcemia, hypokalemia, muscle wasting (esp. in arms, legs), osteoporosis, spontaneous fractures, amenorrhea, cataracts, glaucoma, peptic ulcer, HF. **Abrupt withdrawal after long-term therapy:** Anorexia, nausea, fever, headache, severe arthralgia, rebound inflammation, fatigue, weakness, lethargy, dizziness, orthostatic hypotension.

NURSING CONSIDERATIONS

BASELINE ASSESSMENT

Question for hypersensitivity to any of the corticosteroids, components. Obtain baselines for height, weight, B/P, serum glucose, electrolytes. Check results of initial tests (tuberculosis [TB] skin test, X-rays, EKG). Question history as listed in Precautions.

INTERVENTION/EVALUATION

Monitor I&O, daily weight; assess for edema. Monitor daily pattern of bowel activity, stool consistency. Check vital signs at least twice daily. Be alert for infection (sore throat, fever, vague symptoms). Monitor serum electrolytes, including B/P, glucose. Monitor for hypocalcemia (muscle twitching, cramps, positive Trousseau's or Chvostek's signs), hypokalemia (weakness, muscle cramps, numbness, tingling [esp. lower extremities], nausea/vomiting, irritability, EKG changes). Assess emotional status, ability to sleep. Check lab results for blood coagulability, clinical evidence of thromboembolism.

PATIENT/FAMILY TEACHING

• Take oral dose with food, milk. • Do not change dose/schedule or stop taking drug; must taper off gradually under medical supervision. • Report fever, sore throat, muscle aches, sudden weight gain or loss, edema, loss of appetite, fatigue. • Maintain strict personal hygiene; avoid exposure to disease, trauma. • Severe stress (serious infection, surgery, trauma) may require increased dosage. • Follow-up visits, lab tests are necessary. • Children must be assessed for growth retardation. • Inform dentist, other physicians of methylPREDNISolone therapy now or within past 12 mos.

metoclopramide

met-oh-**kloe**-pra-myde
(Apo-Metoclop ✦, Reglan)
■ **BLACK BOX ALERT** ■ Prolonged use may cause tardive dyskinesia.
Do not confuse metoclopramide with metOLazone or metoprolol, or Reglan with Renagel.

◆CLASSIFICATION

PHARMACOTHERAPEUTIC: DOPamine receptor antagonist. **CLINICAL:** GI emptying adjunct, peristaltic stimulant, antiemetic.

USES

ORAL: Symptomatic treatment of diabetic gastroparesis, gastroesophageal reflux.

M

IV/IM: Symptomatic treatment of diabetic gastroparesis, placement of enteral feeding tubes, prevent/treat nausea/vomiting with chemotherapy or after surgery. To stimulate gastric emptying and intestinal transit of barium when delayed emptying interferes with the radiological examination of the stomach and/or small intestine. To facilitate small bowel intubation in adults and children.

PRECAUTIONS

Contraindications: Hypersensitivity to metoclopramide. Concurrent use of medications likely to produce extrapyramidal reactions. Situations in which GI motility may be dangerous (e.g., GI hemorrhage, GI perforation/obstruction), history of seizure disorder, pheochromocytoma. **Cautions:** Renal impairment, HF, cirrhosis, hypertension, depression, Parkinson's disease, elderly.

ACTION

Stimulates motility of upper GI tract. Blocks DOPamine/serotonin receptors in chemoreceptor trigger zone. Enhances acetylcholine response in upper GI tract; increases lower esophageal sphincter tone. **Therapeutic Effect:** Accelerates intestinal transit, promotes gastric emptying. Relieves nausea, vomiting.

PHARMACOKINETICS

Route	Onset	Peak	Duration
PO	30–60 min	N/A	1–2 hrs
IV	1–3 min	N/A	1–2 hrs
IM	10–15 min	N/A	1–2 hrs

Well absorbed from GI tract. Metabolized in liver. Protein binding: 30%. Primarily excreted in urine. Not removed by hemodialysis. **Half-life:** 4–6 hrs.

⌛ LIFESPAN CONSIDERATIONS

Pregnancy/Lactation: Crosses placenta. Distributed in breast milk. **Children:** More susceptible to having dystonic reactions. **Elderly:** More likely to have parkinsonian dyskinesias after long-term therapy.

INTERACTIONS

DRUG: **Alcohol, other CNS depressants** (e.g., **LORazepam, morphine, zolpidem**) may increase CNS depressant effect. **Anticholinergics** (e.g., **scopolamine**), **opioid analgesics** (e.g., **morphine, HYDROmorphone**) may decrease effects on GI motility. **HERBAL:** None significant. **FOOD:** None known. **LAB VALUES:** May increase serum aldosterone, prolactin.

AVAILABILITY (Rx)

Injection Solution: 5 mg/mL. **Solution, Oral:** 5 mg/5 mL. **Tablets:** 5 mg, 10 mg.

 Tablets, Orally Disintegrating: 5 mg, 10 mg.

ADMINISTRATION/HANDLING

🖐 IV

Reconstitution • Dilute doses greater than 10 mg in 50 mL D_5W or 0.9% NaCl. **Rate of Administration** • Infuse over 15–30 min. • May give undiluted slow IV push at rate of 10 mg over 1–2 min. • Too-rapid IV injection may produce intense feeling of anxiety, restlessness, followed by drowsiness. **Storage** • Store vials at room temperature. • After dilution, IV infusion (piggyback) is stable for 24 hrs.

PO

• Give 30 min before meals and at bedtime. • Tablets may be crushed. • Do not cut, divide, break orally disintegrating tablets. Place on tongue, swallow with saliva.

▦ IV INCOMPATIBILITIES

Allopurinol (Aloprim), cefepime (Maxipime), furosemide (Lasix), propofol (Diprivan).

▦ IV COMPATIBILITIES

Dexamethasone, dexmedetomidine (Precedex), diltiaZEM (Cardizem), diphenhydrAMINE (Benadryl), fentaNYL (Sublimaze), heparin, HYDROmorphone (Dilaudid), morphine, potassium chloride.

INDICATIONS/ROUTES/DOSAGE

Prevention of Chemotherapy-Induced Nausea/Vomiting
IV: ADULTS, ELDERLY, CHILDREN: 1–2 mg/kg 30 min before chemotherapy; repeat q2h for 2 doses, then q3h for 3 doses.

Postop Nausea/Vomiting
IV: ADULTS, ELDERLY: 10–20 mg near end of surgery.

Gastroparesis
PO, IV: ADULTS: 10 mg 30 min before meals and at bedtime for 2–8 wks.
PO, IV: ELDERLY: Initially, 5 mg 30 min before meals and at bedtime. May increase to 10 mg.

Gastroesophageal Reflux Disease (GERD)
PO: ADULTS: 10–15 mg up to 4 times/day, or single doses up to 20 mg as needed. **ELDERLY:** Initially, 5 mg 4 times/day. May increase to 10 mg.

Facilitate Small Bowel Intubation (Single Dose)
IV: ADULTS, ELDERLY: 10 mg as a single dose. **CHILDREN 6–14 YRS:** 2.5–5 mg as a single dose. **CHILDREN YOUNGER THAN 6 YRS:** 0.1 mg/kg as a single dose.

Dosage in Renal Impairment
Dosage is modified based on creatinine clearance.

Creatinine Clearance	Dosage
Less than 40 mL/min	50% of normal dose

Dosage in Hepatic Impairment
No dose adjustment.

SIDE EFFECTS

◄ALERT► Doses of 2 mg/kg or greater, or increased length of therapy, may result in a greater incidence of side effects.
Frequent (10%): Drowsiness, restlessness, fatigue, lethargy. **Occasional (3%):** Dizziness, anxiety, headache, insomnia, breast tenderness, altered menstruation, constipation, rash, dry mouth, galactorrhea, gynecomastia. **Rare (less than 3%):** Hypotension, hypertension, tachycardia.

ADVERSE EFFECTS/TOXIC REACTIONS

Extrapyramidal reactions occur most frequently in children, young adults (18–30 yrs) receiving large doses (2 mg/kg) during chemotherapy and usually are limited to akathisia (involuntary limb movement, facial grimacing, motor restlessness). Neuroleptic malignant syndrome (diaphoresis, fever, unstable B/P, muscular rigidity) has been reported.

NURSING CONSIDERATIONS

BASELINE ASSESSMENT
Antiemetic: Assess for dehydration (poor skin turgor, dry mucous membranes, longitudinal furrows in tongue). Assess for nausea, vomiting, abdominal distention, bowel sounds.

INTERVENTION/EVALUATION
Monitor for anxiety, restlessness, extrapyramidal symptoms (EPS) during IV administration. Monitor daily pattern of bowel activity, stool consistency. Assess skin for rash. Evaluate for therapeutic response from gastroparesis (nausea, vomiting, bloating). Monitor renal function, B/P, heart rate.

PATIENT/FAMILY TEACHING
• Avoid tasks that require alertness, motor skills until response to drug is established. • Report involuntary eye, facial, limb movement (extrapyramidal reaction). • Avoid alcohol.

metOLazone

meh-**toe**-la-zone
(Zaroxolyn ✦)
Do not confuse metOLazone with metaxalone, methotrexate, metoclopramide, or metoprolol, or Zaroxolyn with Zarontin.

M

◆CLASSIFICATION

PHARMACOTHERAPEUTIC: Thiazide diuretic. **CLINICAL:** Diuretic, antihypertensive.

USES

Treatment of mild to moderate hypertension, edema due to HF, nephrotic syndrome, or impaired renal function.

PRECAUTIONS

Contraindications: Hypersensitivity to metOLazone. Anuria, hepatic coma/precoma. **Cautions:** History of hypersensitivity to sulfonamides, thiazide diuretics. Severe renal disease, severe hepatic impairment, gout, prediabetes or diabetes, elevated serum cholesterol, triglycerides.

ACTION

Blocks reabsorption of sodium, potassium, chloride at distal convoluted tubule, increasing excretion of sodium, potassium, water. **Therapeutic Effect:** Reduces B/P, promotes diuresis.

PHARMACOKINETICS

Route	Onset	Peak	Duration
PO (diuretic)	1 hr	—	24 hrs

Incompletely absorbed from GI tract. Protein binding: 95%. Primarily excreted unchanged in urine. Not removed by hemodialysis. **Half-life:** 20 hrs.

⧖ LIFESPAN CONSIDERATIONS

Pregnancy/Lactation: Crosses placenta. Small amount distributed in breast milk. Breastfeeding not recommended. **Children:** No age-related precautions noted. **Elderly:** May be more sensitive to hypotensive or electrolyte effects. Age-related renal impairment may require dosage adjustment.

INTERACTIONS

DRUG: May increase risk of **digoxin** toxicity associated with metOLazone-induced hypokalemia. May increase risk of **lithium** toxicity. **HERBAL: Ephedra, ginseng, licorice** may decrease effect. **Black cohosh, periwinkle** may enhance effect. **FOOD:** None known. **LAB VALUES:** May increase serum glucose, cholesterol, LDL, bilirubin, calcium, creatinine, uric acid, triglycerides. May decrease urinary calcium, serum magnesium, potassium, sodium.

AVAILABILITY (Rx)

Tablets: 2.5 mg, 5 mg, 10 mg.

ADMINISTRATION/HANDLING

PO
• May give with food, milk if GI upset occurs, preferably with breakfast (may prevent nocturia).

INDICATIONS/ROUTES/DOSAGE

Edema
PO: ADULTS: 2.5–10 mg/day. May increase to 20 mg/day.

Hypertension
PO: ADULTS, ELDERLY: Initially, 2.5–5 mg/day. Adjust dose to achieve maximum therapeutic effect.

Usual Pediatric Dosage (Edema, Refractory)
PO: 0.2–0.4 mg/kg/day in 1–2 divided doses.

Dosage in Renal Impairment
Mild to moderate impairment: No dose adjustment. **Severe impairment:** Use caution.

Dosage in Hepatic Impairment
No dose adjustment. Contraindicated with hepatic coma or precoma.

SIDE EFFECTS

Expected: Increased urinary frequency/volume. **Frequent (10%–9%):** Dizziness, light-headedness, headache. **Occasional (6%–4%):** Muscle cramps/spasm, drowsiness, fatigue, lethargy. **Rare (less than 2%):** Asthenia, palpitations, depression, nausea, vomiting, abdominal bloating, constipation, diarrhea, urticaria.

ADVERSE EFFECTS/ TOXIC REACTIONS

Vigorous diuresis may lead to profound water loss and electrolyte depletion, resulting in hypokalemia, hyponatremia, dehydration. Acute hypotensive episodes may occur. Hyperglycemia may occur during prolonged therapy. Pancreatitis, paresthesia, blood dyscrasias, pulmonary edema, allergic pneumonitis, dermatologic reactions occur rarely. Overdose can lead to lethargy, coma without changes in electrolytes, hydration.

NURSING CONSIDERATIONS

BASELINE ASSESSMENT

Check vital signs, esp. B/P for hypotension, before administration. Assess baseline serum electrolytes, particularly check for hypokalemia. Assess skin turgor, mucous membranes for hydration status. Assess for peripheral edema. Assess muscle strength, mental status. Note skin temperature, moisture. Obtain baseline weight. Monitor I&O.

INTERVENTION/EVALUATION

Continue to monitor B/P, vital signs, serum electrolytes, I&O, weight. Note extent of diuresis. Monitor for electrolyte disturbances (hypokalemia may result in weakness, tremors, muscle cramps, nausea, vomiting, altered mental status, tachycardia; hyponatremia may result in confusion, thirst, cold/clammy skin).

PATIENT/FAMILY TEACHING

• Expect increased urinary frequency/volume. • Slowly go from lying to standing to reduce hypotensive effect. • Avoid tasks requiring motor skills, mental alertness until response to drug is established. • Eat foods high in potassium, such as whole grains (cereals), legumes, meat, bananas, apricots, orange juice, potatoes (white, sweet), raisins.

metoprolol

me-**toe**-pro-lol
(Apo-Metoprolol ✤, Lopressor, Toprol XL)

■ **BLACK BOX ALERT** ■ Abrupt withdrawal can produce acute tachycardia, hypertension, ischemia. Drug should be gradually tapered over 1–2 wks.
Do not confuse metoprolol with atenolol, labetalol, nadolol, or stanozolol, or Toprol XL with TEGretol, TEGretol XR, or Topamax.

FIXED-COMBINATION(S)

Dutoprol: metoprolol/hydroCHLOROthiazide (a diuretic): 25 mg/12.5 mg, 50 mg/12.5 mg, 100 mg/12.5 mg. **Lopressor HCT:** metoprolol/hydrochlorothiazide (a diuretic): 50 mg/25 mg, 100 mg/25 mg, 100 mg/50 mg.

◆CLASSIFICATION

PHARMACOTHERAPEUTIC: Beta$_1$-adrenergic blocker. **CLINICAL:** Antianginal, antihypertensive, MI adjunct.

USES

Lopressor: Treatment of hemodynamically stable acute myocardial infarction (AMI) to reduce CV mortality, angina pectoris, hypertension. **Toprol XL:** Treatment of angina pectoris, to reduce mortality or hospitalizations in pts with HF already receiving ACE inhibitors, diuretics, and/or digoxin; hypertension. **OFF-LABEL:** Treatment of ventricular arrhythmias, migraine prophylaxis, essential tremor, aggressive behavior, prevent reinfarction post MI, prevent/treat atrial fibrillation/atrial flutter, hypertrophic cardiomyopathy, thyrotoxicosis.

PRECAUTIONS

Contraindications: Hypersensitivity to metoprolol. **(Immediate-Release):** MI: Severe sinus bradycardia, MI with heart

M

---

rate less than 45 beats/min or systolic B/P less than 100 mm Hg, moderate to severe HF, significant first-degree heart block, second- or third-degree heart block. *(Immediate-Release):* HTN/Angina: Sinus bradycardia, second- or third-degree heart block, cardiogenic shock, overt HF, sick sinus syndrome (except with pacemaker), severe peripheral arterial disease, pheochromocytoma. *(Extended-Release):* Severe bradycardia, second- or third-degree heart block, cardiogenic shock, decompensated HF, sick sinus syndrome (except with functioning pacemaker). **Cautions:** Arterial obstruction, bronchospastic disease, hepatic impairment, peripheral vascular disease, hyperthyroidism, diabetes mellitus, myasthenia gravis, psychiatric disease, history of severe anaphylaxis to allergens. *(Extended-Release):* Compensated HF.

ACTION

Selectively blocks beta$_1$-adrenergic receptors. **Therapeutic Effect:** Slows heart rate, decreases cardiac output, reduces B/P. Decreases myocardial ischemia severity.

PHARMACOKINETICS

Route	Onset	Peak	Duration
PO	10–15 min	1–2 hrs	N/A
PO (extended-release)	N/A	6–12 hrs	N/A
IV	Immediate	20 min	N/A

Well absorbed from GI tract. Protein binding: 12%. Widely distributed. Metabolized in liver. Primarily excreted in urine. Removed by hemodialysis. **Half-life:** 3–7 hrs.

⏳ LIFESPAN CONSIDERATIONS

Pregnancy/Lactation: Crosses placenta; distributed in breast milk. Avoid use during first trimester. May produce bradycardia, apnea, hypoglycemia, hypothermia during delivery, low-birth-weight infants. **Children:** Safety and efficacy not established. **Elderly:** Age-related peripheral vascular disease may increase susceptibility to decreased peripheral circulation.

INTERACTIONS

DRUG: Diuretics (e.g., **furosemide, HCTZ**), other antihypertensives (e.g., **amLODIPine, lisinopril, valsartan**) may increase hypotensive effect. May mask symptoms of hypoglycemia, prolong hypoglycemic effect of **insulin, oral hypoglycemics. NSAIDs** (e.g., **ibuprofen, ketorolac, naproxen**) may decrease antihypertensive effect. **Sympathomimetics** (e.g., **DOPamine, norepinephrine**), **xanthines** may mutually inhibit effects. Potent **CYP2D6 inhibitors** (e.g., **FLUoxetine, cimetidine**) may increase concentration. **Digoxin, verapamil, diltiaZEM** may increase risk of bradycardia/heart block. **HERBAL: Ephedra, ginseng, yohimbe** may worsen hypertension. **Garlic** may increase antihypertensive effect. **FOOD:** None known. **LAB VALUES:** May increase serum antinuclear antibody titer (ANA), serum BUN, lipoprotein, LDH, alkaline phosphatase, bilirubin, creatinine, potassium, uric acid, ALT, AST, triglycerides.

AVAILABILITY (Rx)

Injection Solution: 1 mg/mL. **Tablets (Immediate-Release):** 25 mg, 50 mg, 100 mg.

 Tablets (Extended-Release): 25 mg, 50 mg, 100 mg, 200 mg.

ADMINISTRATION/HANDLING

🖥 IV

Rate of Administration • May give undiluted. • Administer IV injection over 1 min. • May give by IV piggyback (in 50 mL D$_5$W or 0.9% NaCl) over 30–60 min. • Monitor EKG, B/P during administration.

Storage • Store at room temperature.

PO

• Tablets may be crushed; do not crush extended-release tablets. • Extended-release tablets may be divided in half. • Give at same time each day. • May be given with or immediately after meals (enhances absorption).

🔲 IV INCOMPATIBILITY

Amphotericin B complex (Abelcet, AmBisome, Amphotec), lidocaine, nitroglycerin.

🔲 IV COMPATIBILITIES

Amiodarone, diltiaZEM, furosemide, heparin, morphine.

INDICATIONS/ROUTES/DOSAGE

Hypertension

PO *(Immediate-Release):* **ADULTS, ELDERLY:** Initially, 50 mg twice daily. Increase at wkly (or longer) intervals. **Maintenance:** 100–450 mg/day in 2–3 divided doses. **CHILDREN:** Initially, 0.5–1 mg/kg/dose. **Maximum Initial Dose:** 25 mg. **Maximum Daily Dose:** 6 mg/kg/day or 200 mg/day, whichever is less.

PO *(Extended-Release):* **ADULTS, ELDERLY:** Initially, 25–100 mg/day as single dose. May increase at least at wkly intervals until optimum B/P attained. **Maximum:** 400 mg/day. **CHILDREN 6 YRS OR OLDER:** Initially, 1 mg/kg once daily. **Maximum:** 50 mg. May increase to 2 mg/kg/day or 200 mg/day, whichever is less.

Angina Pectoris

PO *(Immediate-Release):* **ADULTS:** Initially, 50 mg twice daily. Increase at wkly (or longer) intervals. Usual range: 50–200 mg twice daily. **Maximum:** 400 mg/day.

PO *(Extended-Release):* **ADULTS:** Initially, 100 mg/day as single dose. May increase by at least at wkly intervals until optimum clinical response achieved. **Maximum:** 400 mg/day.

HF

PO *(Extended-Release):* **ADULTS:** Initially, 12.5–25 mg/day. May double dose q2wks up to target dose of 200 mg/day.

Early Treatment of MI

IV: **ADULTS:** 5 mg q5min for up to 3 doses, followed by 25–50 mg orally q6–12h for 48–72 hrs. Transition over 2–3 days to twice daily Lopressor or once daily Toprol XL. May increase up to a maximum of 200 mg/day.

Dosage in Renal/Hepatic Impairment
No dose adjustment.

SIDE EFFECTS

Metoprolol is generally well tolerated, with transient and mild side effects. **Frequent:** Diminished sexual function, drowsiness, insomnia, unusual fatigue/weakness. **Occasional:** Anxiety, diarrhea, constipation, nausea, vomiting, nasal congestion, abdominal discomfort, dizziness, difficulty breathing, cold hands/feet. **Rare:** Altered taste, dry eyes, nightmares, paresthesia, allergic reaction (rash, pruritus).

ADVERSE EFFECTS/ TOXIC REACTIONS

Overdose may produce profound bradycardia, hypotension, bronchospasm. Abrupt withdrawal may result in diaphoresis, palpitations, headache, tremulousness, exacerbation of angina, MI, ventricular arrhythmias. May precipitate HF, MI in pts with heart disease, thyroid storm in those with thyrotoxicosis, peripheral ischemia in those with existing peripheral vascular disease. Hypoglycemia may occur in pts with previously controlled diabetes (may mask signs of hypoglycemia). **Antidote:** Glucagon (see Appendix J for dosage).

NURSING CONSIDERATIONS

BASELINE ASSESSMENT

Assess baseline renal function, LFT. Assess B/P, apical pulse immediately before drug administration (if pulse is 60/min or less or systolic B/P is less than 90 mm Hg, withhold medication, contact physician). **Antianginal:** Record onset, type (sharp, dull, squeezing), radiation, location, intensity, duration of anginal pain, precipitating factors (exertion, emotional stress).

INTERVENTION/EVALUATION

Measure B/P near end of dosing interval (determines whether B/P is controlled throughout day). Monitor B/P for hypotension, respiration for shortness of breath. Assess pulse for quality, rate, rhythm. Assess for evidence of HF: dyspnea (esp. on exertion, lying down), night cough, peripheral edema, distended neck veins. Monitor I&O (increased weight, decreased urinary output may indicate HF). Therapeutic response to hypertension noted in 1–2 wks.

PATIENT/FAMILY TEACHING

• Do not abruptly discontinue medication. • Compliance with therapy regimen is essential to control hypertension, arrhythmias. • If dose is missed, take next scheduled dose (do not double dose). • Go from lying to standing slowly. • Report excessive fatigue, dizziness. • Avoid tasks that require alertness, motor skills until response to drug is established. • Do not use nasal decongestants, OTC cold preparations (stimulants) without physician approval. • Monitor B/P, pulse before taking medication. • Restrict salt, alcohol intake.

---

metroNIDAZOLE

me-troe-nye-da-zole
(Flagyl, Metro, MetroCream, MetroGel, MetroGel-Vaginal, NidaGel ✦, Noritate, Vandazole)
Do not confuse metroNIDAZOLE with meropenem, metFORMIN, methotrexate, or miconazole.

FIXED-COMBINATION(S)

Helidac: metroNIDAZOLE/bismuth/tetracycline (an anti-infective): 250 mg/262 mg/500 mg. **Pylera:** metroNIDAZOLE/bismuth/tetracycline (an anti-infective): 125 mg/140 mg/125 mg.

◆CLASSIFICATION

PHARMACOTHERAPEUTIC: Nitroimidazole derivative. **CLINICAL:** Antibacterial, antiprotozoal.

USES

Treatment of anaerobic infections (skin/skin structure, CNS, lower respiratory tract, bone/joints, intra-abdominal, gynecologic, endocarditis, septicemia). Treatment of *H. pylori* (part of multidrug regimen); surgical prophylaxis (colorectal), trichomoniasis, amebiasis. Topical treatment of acne rosacea or inflammatory lesions. **Vaginal gel:** Treatment of bacterial vaginosis. **OFF-LABEL:** Crohn's disease, urethritis. Antibiotic-associated pseudomembranous colitis (AAPC) caused by *C. difficile*.

PRECAUTIONS

Contraindications: Hypersensitivity to metroNIDAZOLE. Pregnancy (first trimester with trichomoniasis), use of disulfiram within 2 wks, use of alcohol during therapy or within 3 days of discontinuing metroNIDAZOLE. **Cautions:** Blood dyscrasias, severe hepatic dysfunction, endstage renal disease, seizure disorder, HF, other sodium-retaining states, elderly.

ACTION

Disrupts DNA, inhibiting nucleic acid synthesis. **Therapeutic Effect:** Produces bactericidal, antiprotozoal, amebicidal, trichomonacidal effects. Produces antiinflammatory, immunosuppressive effects when applied topically.

PHARMACOKINETICS

Well absorbed from GI tract; minimally absorbed after topical application. Protein binding: less than 20%. Widely distributed; crosses blood-brain barrier. Metabolized in liver. Excreted in urine (80%), feces (15%). Removed by hemodialysis. **Half-life:** 8 hrs (increased in cirrhosis, neonates). Active metabolite prolonged in renal failure.

⧗ LIFESPAN CONSIDERATIONS

Pregnancy/Lactation: Readily crosses placenta. Distributed in breast milk. Contraindicated during first trimester in those with trichomoniasis. Topical use during pregnancy, lactation discouraged. **Children:** Safety and efficacy of topical administration not established in pts younger than 21 yrs. **Elderly:** Age-related hepatic impairment may require dosage adjustment.

INTERACTIONS

DRUG: Alcohol may cause disulfiram-type reaction (e.g., abdominal cramps, nausea, vomiting, headache, psychotic reactions). **Disulfiram** may increase risk of toxicity. May increase effects of **oral anticoagulants (e.g., warfarin).** **HERBAL:** None significant. **FOOD:** None known. **LAB VALUES:** May increase serum LDH, ALT, AST.

AVAILABILITY (Rx)

Capsules: 375 mg. **Injection (Infusion):** 500 mg/100 mL. **Suspension, Oral:** 50 mg/mL, 100 mg/mL. **Tablets (Flagyl):** 250 mg, 500 mg. **Topical Cream:** 0.75% (MetroCream), 1% (Noritate). **Topical Gel (MetroGel):** 0.75%, 1%. **Vaginal Gel (MetroGel-Vaginal, Vandazole):** 0.75%.

 Tablets (Extended-Release): 750 mg.

ADMINISTRATION/HANDLING

 IV

Rate of Administration • Infuse IV over 30–60 min. Do not give by IV bolus. **Storage** • Store at room temperature (ready-to-use infusion bags).

PO

• Give without regard to meals. Give with food to decrease GI irritation. • Extended-release tablet should be given on an empty stomach (1 hr before or 2 hrs after meals). • Do not crush extended-release tablets.

▓ IV INCOMPATIBILITIES

Amphotericin B complex (Abelcet, AmBisome, Amphotec).

▓ IV COMPATIBILITIES

Dexmedetomidine (Precedex), diltiaZEM (Cardizem), DOPamine (Intropin), heparin, HYDROmorphone (Dilaudid), LORazepam (Ativan), magnesium sulfate, midazolam (Versed), morphine.

INDICATIONS/ROUTES/DOSAGE

Amebiasis
PO: ADULTS, ELDERLY: 750 mg q8h for 5–10 days. **CHILDREN:** 35–50 mg/kg/day in divided doses q8h for 7–10 days.

Anaerobic Infections
PO, IV: ADULTS, ELDERLY: 500 mg q6–8h. **Maximum:** 4 g/day.
PO: CHILDREN, INFANTS: 30–50 mg/kg/day in divided doses q8h. **Maximum:** 2,250 mg/day.
IV: CHILDREN, INFANTS: 22.5–40 mg/kg/day in 3 divided doses. **Maximum:** 1,500 mg/day.

Intra-Abdominal Infections
IV: ADULTS, ELDERLY: 500 mg q6h. **Maximum:** 4 g/day.

Pseudomembranous Colitis
PO: ADULTS, ELDERLY: 250–500 mg 3–4 times/day. **CHILDREN:** 30 mg/kg/day in divided doses q6h for 7–10 days. **Maximum:** 2 g/day.

Bacterial Vaginosis
Intravaginal: ADULTS: 0.75% apply 1–2 times/day for 5 days. 1.3% apply once as a single dose.
◄ALERT► Centers for Disease Control and Prevention (CDC) does not recommend the use of topical agents during pregnancy.

Rosacea
Topical: ADULTS, ELDERLY: (1%): Apply to affected area once daily. **(0.75%):** Apply to affected area twice daily.

Dosage in Renal Impairment
No dose adjustment.

Dosage in Hepatic Impairment
Mild to moderate impairment: Use caution. No dose adjustment. **Severe impairment:** Reduce dose by 50% for

M

immediate-release; not recommended for extended-release.

SIDE EFFECTS

Frequent: Systemic: Anorexia, nausea, dry mouth, metallic taste. **Vaginal:** Symptomatic cervicitis/vaginitis, abdominal cramps, uterine pain. **Occasional: Systemic:** Diarrhea, constipation, vomiting, dizziness, erythematous rash, urticaria, reddish-brown urine. **Topical:** Transient erythema, mild dryness, burning, irritation, stinging, tearing when applied too close to eyes. **Vaginal:** Vaginal, perineal, vulvar itching; vulvar swelling. **Rare:** Mild, transient leukopenia; thrombophlebitis with IV therapy.

ADVERSE EFFECTS/ TOXIC REACTIONS

Oral therapy may result in furry tongue, glossitis, cystitis, dysuria, pancreatitis. Peripheral neuropathy (manifested as numbness, tingling of hands/feet) usually is reversible if treatment is stopped immediately upon appearance of neurologic symptoms. Seizures occur occasionally.

NURSING CONSIDERATIONS

BASELINE ASSESSMENT

Obtain baseline CBC, LFT. Question for history of hypersensitivity to metroNIDAZOLE, other nitroimidazole derivatives (and parabens with topical). Obtain specimens for diagnostic tests, cultures before giving first dose (therapy may begin before results are known).

INTERVENTION/EVALUATION

Monitor daily pattern of bowel activity, stool consistency. Monitor I&O, assess for urinary problems. Be alert to neurologic symptoms (dizziness, paresthesia of extremities). Assess for rash, urticaria. Monitor for onset of superinfection (ulceration/change of oral mucosa, furry tongue, vaginal discharge, genital/anal pruritus).

PATIENT/FAMILY TEACHING

• Urine may be red-brown or dark. • Avoid alcohol, alcohol-containing preparations (cough syrups, elixirs) for at least 48 hrs after last dose. • Avoid tasks that require alertness, motor skills until response to drug is established. • If taking metroNIDAZOLE for trichomoniasis, refrain from sexual intercourse until full treatment is completed. • For amebiasis, frequent stool specimen checks will be necessary. • **Topical:** Avoid contact with eyes. • May apply cosmetics after application. • MetroNIDAZOLE acts on erythema, papules, pustules but has no effect on rhinophyma (hypertrophy of nose), telangiectasia, ocular problems (conjunctivitis, keratitis, blepharitis). • Other recommendations for rosacea include avoidance of hot/spicy foods, alcohol, extremes of hot/cold temperatures, excessive sunlight.

micafungin

mye-ka-**fun**-jin
(Mycamine)

✦CLASSIFICATION

PHARMACOTHERAPEUTIC: Echinocandin antifungal. **CLINICAL:** Antifungal.

USES

Treatment of esophageal candidiasis, candidemia, candida peritonitis, abscesses, acute disseminated candidiasis, prophylaxis of *Candida* infection in pts undergoing hematopoietic stem cell transplant. **OFF-LABEL:** Treatment of infections due to *Aspergillus* spp.

PRECAUTIONS

Contraindications: Hypersensitivity to micafungin. **Cautions:** Hepatic/renal impairment, concomitant hepatotoxic medications.

ACTION

Inhibits synthesis of glucan (vital component of fungal cell formation), damaging fungal cell membrane. **Therapeutic Effect:** Decreased glucan content leads to cellular lysis.

PHARMACOKINETICS

Slowly metabolized in liver. Protein binding: greater than 99%. Primarily excreted in feces. Not removed by hemodialysis. **Half-life:** 11–21 hrs.

⌛ LIFESPAN CONSIDERATIONS

Pregnancy/Lactation: May reduce sperm count. May be embryotoxic. Unknown if distributed in breast milk. **Children:** Safety and efficacy not established. **Elderly:** No age-related precautions noted.

INTERACTIONS

DRUG: Hepatotoxic drugs (e.g., acetaminophen, ketoconazole, methotrexate, simvastatin) may increase risk of hepatic injury. May increase concentration of NIFEdipine, sirolimus, itraconazole. **HERBAL:** None significant. **FOOD:** None known. **LAB VALUES:** May increase serum creatinine, alkaline phosphatase, LDH, ALT, AST.

AVAILABILITY (Rx)

Injection, Powder for Reconstitution: 50 mg, 100 mg.

ADMINISTRATION/HANDLING

 IV

Reconstitution • Add 5 mL 0.9% NaCl (without bacteriostatic agent) to each 50-mg vial (10 mL to 100-mg vial) to yield micafungin 10 mg/mL. • Gently swirl to dissolve; do not shake. • Further dilute in 0.9% NaCl or D₅W to final concentration of 0.5–1.5 mg/mL. • Alternatively, D₅W may be used for reconstitution and dilution. • Flush existing IV line with 0.9% NaCl or D₅W before infusion.
Rate of Administration • Infuse over 60 min.

Storage • Reconstituted solution is stable for 24 hrs at room temperature. • Discard if precipitate is present.

▣ IV INCOMPATIBILITIES

Amiodarone, niCARdipine.

▣ IV COMPATIBILITIES

Bumetanide (Bumex), calcium gluconate, heparin.

INDICATIONS/ROUTES/DOSAGE

Esophageal Candidiasis
IV: ADULTS, ELDERLY: 150 mg/day for 10–30 days. **CHILDREN 4 MOS OR OLDER: (GREATER THAN 30 KG):** 2.5 mg/kg/day. (**Maximum:** 150 mg daily.) **(30 KG OR LESS):** 3 mg/kg/day.

Candida Prophylaxis in Stem Cell Pts
IV: ADULTS, ELDERLY: 50 mg/day. **CHILDREN 4 MOS OR OLDER:** 1 mg/kg/day. **Maximum:** 50 mg/day.

Candidemia, Disseminated Candidiasis, Peritonitis, Abscesses
IV: ADULTS, ELDERLY: 100 mg/day for 15 days. **CHILDREN 4 MOS OR OLDER:** 2 mg/kg/day. **Maximum:** 100 mg daily.

Dosage in Renal/Hepatic Impairment
No dose adjustment.

SIDE EFFECTS

Occasional (3%–2%): Nausea, headache, diarrhea, vomiting, fever. **Rare (1%):** Dizziness, drowsiness, pruritus, abdominal pain, dyspepsia.

ADVERSE EFFECTS/ TOXIC REACTIONS

Hypersensitivity reaction characterized by rash, pruritus, facial edema occurs rarely. Anaphylaxis, hemoglobinuria, hemolytic anemia have been reported.

NURSING CONSIDERATIONS

BASELINE ASSESSMENT

Determine baseline renal function, LFT and periodically thereafter.

M

INTERVENTION/EVALUATION

Monitor BUN, serum creatinine, CrCl, LFT. Monitor for hepatotoxicity.

PATIENT/FAMILY TEACHING

• Report liver problems such as bruising, confusion; dark amber or orange-colored urine; right upper abdominal pain; yellowing of the skin or eyes. • Report decreased urine output; dark, amber urine; swelling of the hands or feet. • Do not take OTC medications that are toxic to the liver (e.g., acetaminophen).

---

midazolam [HIGH ALERT]

mye-**da**-zoe-lam
(Apo-Midazolam ✦)

■ **BLACK BOX ALERT** ■ May cause severe respiratory depression, respiratory arrest, apnea. Initial doses in elderly should be conservative. Do not administer by rapid IV injection in neonates (may cause severe hypotension/seizures).

Do not confuse midazolam with, ALPRAZolam or LORazepam.

◆ CLASSIFICATION

PHARMACOTHERAPEUTIC: Benzodiazepine (**Schedule IV**). **CLINICAL:** Sedative, anxiolytic.

USES

Sedation, anxiolytic, amnesia before procedure or induction of anesthesia, conscious sedation before diagnostic/radiographic procedure, continuous IV sedation of intubated or mechanically ventilated pts. **OFF-LABEL:** Anxiety, status epilepticus, conscious sedation (intranasal route).

PRECAUTIONS

Contraindications: Hypersensitivity to midazolam. Acute narrow-angle glaucoma, concurrent use of potent CYP3A4 inhibitors. **Cautions:** Renal/hepatic/pulmonary impairment, impaired gag reflex, HF, treated open-angle glaucoma, obese pts, concurrent CNS depressants, alcohol dependency, elderly pts, debilitated pts.

ACTION

Enhances action of gamma-aminobutyric acid (GABA), one of the major inhibitory neurotransmitters in the brain. **Therapeutic Effect:** Produces anxiolytic, hypnotic, anticonvulsant, muscle relaxant, amnestic effects.

PHARMACOKINETICS

Route	Onset	Peak	Duration
PO	10–20 min	N/A	N/A
IV	1–5 min	5–7 min	20–30 min
IM	5–15 min	30–60 min	2–6 hrs

Well absorbed after IM administration. Protein binding: 97%. Metabolized in liver. Primarily excreted in urine. Not removed by hemodialysis. **Half-life:** 1–5 hrs.

⌧ LIFESPAN CONSIDERATIONS

Pregnancy/Lactation: Crosses placenta. Unknown if drug is distributed in breast milk. **Children:** Neonates more likely to have respiratory depression. **Elderly:** Age-related renal impairment may require dosage adjustment.

INTERACTIONS

DRUG: Alcohol, other CNS depressants (e.g., LORazepam, morphine, zolpidem) may increase CNS effects, respiratory depression, hypotensive effect. CYP3A4 inhibitors (e.g., erythromycin, ketoconazole, ritonavir) may increase concentration/sedative effect. **HERBAL:** Gotu kola, kava kava, St. John's wort, valerian may increase CNS depression. St. John's wort may decrease concentration. **FOOD:** Grapefruit products increase oral absorption, systemic availability. **LAB VALUES:** None significant.

AVAILABILITY (Rx)

Injection Solution: 1 mg/mL, 5 mg/mL.
Syrup: 2 mg/mL.

ADMINISTRATION/HANDLING

 IV

Rate of Administration • May give undiluted or as infusion. • Resuscitative equipment, O_2 must be readily available before IV administration. • Administer by slow IV injection over at least 2–5 min at concentration of 1–5 mg/mL. • Reduce IV rate in those older than 60 yrs, debilitated pts with chronic disease states, pulmonary impairment. • Too-rapid IV rate, excessive doses, or single large dose increases risk of respiratory depression/arrest.

Storage • Store vials at room temperature.

IM
• Give deep IM into large muscle mass.
Maximum concentration: 1 mg/mL.

PO
• Do not mix with grapefruit juice.

🚫 IV INCOMPATIBILITIES

Albumin, amphotericin B complex (Abelcet, AmBisome, Amphotec), ampicillin (Polycillin), ampicillin and sulbactam (Unasyn), bumetanide (Bumex), co-trimoxazole (Bactrim), dexamethasone (Decadron), fosphenytoin (Cerebyx), furosemide (Lasix), hydrocortisone (Solu-Cortef), methotrexate, nafcillin (Nafcil), sodium bicarbonate.

🚫 IV COMPATIBILITIES

Amiodarone (Cordarone), atropine, calcium gluconate, dexmedetomidine (Precedex), diltiaZEM (Cardizem), diphenhydrAMINE (Benadryl), DOBUTamine (Dobutrex), DOPamine (Intropin), etomidate (Amidate), fentaNYL (Sublimaze), glycopyrrolate (Robinul), heparin, HYDROmorphone (Dilaudid), hydrOXYzine (Vistaril), insulin, LORazepam (Ativan), milrinone (Primacor), morphine, nitroglycerin, norepinephrine (Levophed), potassium chloride, propofol (Diprivan).

INDICATIONS/ROUTES/DOSAGE

Preop Sedation
PO: CHILDREN: 0.25–0.5 mg/kg. **Maximum:** 20 mg.
IV: ADULTS, ELDERLY: 0.02–0.04 mg/kg. Usual dose: 1–2.5 mg. **CHILDREN 6–12 YRS:** 0.025–0.05 mg/kg. **Maximum:** 10 mg. **CHILDREN 6 MOS–5 YRS:** 0.05–0.1 mg/kg. **Maximum:** 6 mg.
IM: ADULTS, ELDERLY: 0.07–0.08 mg/kg 30–60 min before surgery. Usual dose: 5 mg. **CHILDREN:** 0.1–0.15 mg/kg 30–60 min before surgery. **Maximum:** 10 mg.

Continuous Sedation During Mechanical Ventilation
IV: ADULTS, ELDERLY: Initially, 0.01–0.05 mg/kg (1–5 mg in 70-kg adult). May repeat at 5- to 15-min intervals until adequate sedation achieved or continuous infusion rate of 0.02–0.1 mg/kg/hr and titrated to desired effect. **CHILDREN:** Initially, 0.05–0.2 mg/kg followed by continuous infusion of 0.06–0.12 mg/kg/hr (1–2 mcg/kg/min) titrated to desired effect. Usual range: 0.4–9.4 mcg/kg/min.

Dosage in Renal Impairment
No dose adjustment.

Dosage in Hepatic Impairment
Use caution.

SIDE EFFECTS

Frequent (10%–4%): Decreased respiratory rate, tenderness at IM or IV injection site, pain during injection, oxygen desaturation, hiccups. **Occasional (3%–2%):** Hypotension, paradoxical CNS reaction. **Rare (less than 2%):** Nausea, vomiting, headache, coughing.

ADVERSE EFFECTS/ TOXIC REACTIONS

Inadequate or excessive dosage, improper administration may result in

M

cerebral hypoxia, agitation, involuntary movements, hyperactivity, combativeness. Too-rapid IV rate, excessive doses, or single large dose increases risk of respiratory depression/arrest. Respiratory depression/apnea may produce hypoxia, cardiac arrest.

NURSING CONSIDERATIONS

BASELINE ASSESSMENT

Resuscitative equipment, oxygen must be available. Obtain vital signs before administration. Assess level of consciousness.

INTERVENTION/EVALUATION

Monitor respiratory rate, oxygen saturation continuously during parenteral administration for underventilation, apnea. Monitor vital signs, level of sedation q3–5min during recovery period. Assess level of consciousness for effectiveness.

M

midodrine

mye-doe-dreen
(Amatine ✤, Apo-Midodrine ✤)
■ **BLACK BOX ALERT** ■ Can cause marked rise in supine blood pressure; use in pts for whom orthostatic hypotension significantly impairs daily life.
Do not confuse Amatine with amantadine or protamine, or midodrine with Midrin.

◆CLASSIFICATION

PHARMACOTHERAPEUTIC: Alpha₁ agonist. **CLINICAL:** Vasopressor.

USES

Treatment of symptomatic orthostatic hypotension. **OFF-LABEL:** Vasovagal syncope, prevention of dialysis-induced hypotension.

PRECAUTIONS

Contraindications: Hypersensitivity to midodrine. Acute renal failure, persistent supine hypertension, pheochromocytoma, severe cardiac disease, thyrotoxicosis, urinary retention. **Cautions:** Renal/hepatic impairment, history of visual problems, diabetes, immobility, pts who are unable to stand. Concurrent administration with digoxin, beta blockers (e.g., metoprolol), vasoconstrictors (e.g., norepinephrine).

ACTION

Forms active metabolite desglymidodrine, an alpha₁ agonist, increasing arteriolar and venous tone. **Therapeutic Effect:** Increases standing, sitting, and supine systolic B/P in pts with orthostatic hypotension.

PHARMACOKINETICS

Route	Onset	Peak	Duration
PO	1 hr	—	2–3 hrs

Rapid absorption from GI tract following PO administration. Protein binding: Low. Undergoes enzymatic hydrolysis in systemic circulation. Excreted in urine. **Half-life:** 0.5 hr.

⧖ LIFESPAN CONSIDERATIONS

Pregnancy/Lactation: Unknown if drug crosses placenta or is distributed in breast milk. **Children:** Safety and efficacy not established. **Elderly:** Age-related renal impairment may require dosage adjustment.

INTERACTIONS

DRUG: **Digoxin** may have additive bradycardic effects. **Sodium-retaining steroids (e.g., fludrocortisone)** may increase sodium retention. **Vasoconstrictors (e.g., DOPamine, norepinephrine)** may have additive effects. **HERBAL:** None significant. **FOOD:** None known. **LAB VALUES:** None significant.

AVAILABILITY (Rx)

Tablets: 2.5 mg, 5 mg, 10 mg.

ADMINISTRATION/HANDLING

• Give without regard to food. • Last dose of day should be given 3–4 hrs before bedtime.

INDICATIONS/ROUTES/DOSAGE

Orthostatic Hypotension
PO: ADULTS, ELDERLY: 10 mg 3 times/
day (q3–4hrs). Give during the day
when pt is upright, such as upon arising, midday, and late afternoon. Do not
give later than 6 PM. **Maximum:** 30
mg/day.

Dosage in Renal Impairment
2.5 mg 3 times/day; increase gradually,
as tolerated. **Hemodialysis:** Dose after
HD unless used to prevent HD-induced
hypotension.

Dosage in Hepatic Impairment
Use caution.

SIDE EFFECTS

Frequent (20%–7%): Paresthesia, piloerection, pruritus, dysuria, supine hypertension. **Occasional (6%–1%):** Pain,
rash, chills, headache, facial flushing,
confusion, dry mouth, anxiety.

ADVERSE EFFECTS/
TOXIC REACTIONS

May cause marked increase of supine
systolic BP (supine hypertension).

NURSING CONSIDERATIONS

BASELINE ASSESSMENT

Assess sensitivity to midodrine, other
medications (esp. digoxin, sodium-
retaining vasoconstrictors). Assess
medical history, esp. for renal impairment, severe hypertension, cardiac
disease.

INTERVENTION/EVALUATION

Monitor B/P, renal, hepatic, cardiac
function.

PATIENT/FAMILY TEACHING

• Do not take last dose of the day after
evening meal or less than 4 hrs before
bedtime. • Do not give if pt will be supine. • Use caution with OTC medications that may affect B/P (e.g., cough and
cold, diet medications).

midostaurin

mye-doe-**staw**-rim
(Rydapt)
**Do not confuse midostaurin
with midodrine.**

◆CLASSIFICATION

PHARMACOTHERAPEUTIC: Tyrosine
kinase inhibitor. **CLINICAL:** Antineoplastic.

USES

Treatment of adult pts with newly diagnosed acute myeloid leukemia (AML)
who are FLT3 mutation–positive, as detected by an FDA-approved test (in combination with standard cytarabine and
daunorubicin induction and cytarabine
consolidation chemotherapy). Treatment
of adult pts with aggressive systemic mastocytosis (ASM), systemic mastocytosis
with associated hematologic neoplasm
(SM-AHN), or mast cell leukemia (MCL).

PRECAUTIONS

Contraindications: Hypersensitivity to
midostaurin. **Cautions:** Baseline anemia,
leukopenia, neutropenia, thrombocytopenia; concomitant use of strong CYP3A
inhibitors, strong CYP3A inducers; pts at
risk for hemorrhage (e.g., history of GI
bleeding, coagulation disorders, recent
trauma; concomitant use of anticoagulants, NSAIDs, antiplatelet medication).

ACTION

Inhibits multiple receptors including
FLT3 receptor signaling, and cell proliferation. **Therapeutic Effect:** Induces
apoptosis in ITD and ITD mutant expressing leukemic cells.

PHARMACOKINETICS

Widely distributed. Metabolized in liver.
Protein binding: 99.8%. Peak plasma
concentration: 1–3 hrs. Steady state
reached in 28 days. Excreted in feces
(95%), urine (5%). **Half-life:** 21 hrs.

M

◆ Canadian trade name   🐿 Non-Crushable Drug   🔲 High Alert drug

⏳ LIFESPAN CONSIDERATIONS

Pregnancy/Lactation: Avoid pregnancy; may cause fetal harm. Females of reproductive potential and males with female partners of reproductive potential should use effective contraception during treatment and for at least 4 mos after discontinuation. Unknown if distributed in breast milk. Breastfeeding not recommended. May impair fertility in both females and males. **Children:** Safety and efficacy not established. **Elderly:** No age-related precautions noted.

INTERACTIONS

DRUG: **Moderate CYP3A4 inhibitors** (e.g., **ciprofloxacin, fluconazole, verapamil**), **strong CYP3A4 inhibitors** (e.g., **erythromycin, ketoconazole, ritonavir**) may increase concentration/effect. **Strong CYP3A4 inducers** (e.g., **carBAMazepine, phenytoin, rifAMPin**) may decrease concentration/effect. **QT-prolonging agents** may enhance QT-prolonging effect. May decrease therapeutic effect of BCG. **HERBAL:** **St. John's wort** may decrease concentration/effect. **FOOD:** **Grapefruit products** may increase concentration/effect. **LAB VALUES:** May increase serum alkaline phosphatase, ALT, AST, bilirubin, creatinine, GGT, glucose, lipase, sodium, uric acid. May decrease Hgb, Hct, lymphocytes, leukocytes, neutrophils, platelets, RBCs; serum albumin, magnesium, phosphate, potassium. May increase or decrease serum calcium or sodium. May prolong aPTT.

AVAILABILITY (Rx)

 Capsules: 25 mg.

ADMINISTRATION/HANDLING

PO
• Give with food. • Administer whole; do not cut, crush, open capsules.

INDICATIONS/ROUTES/DOSAGE

Acute Myeloid Leukemia
PO: ADULTS, ELDERLY: 50 mg twice daily (at 12-hr intervals) on days 8–21 of each induction with cytarabine and daunorubicin, and on days 8–21 of each cycle of consolidation with high-dose cytarabine.

Systemic Mastocytosis, Mast Cell Leukemia
PO: ADULTS, ELDERLY: 100 mg twice daily. Continue until disease progression or unacceptable toxicity.

Dose Modification for Systemic Mastocytosis
Neutropenia
Treatment-induced ANC less than 1000 cells/mm³ in pts without MCL; treatment-induced ANC less than 500 cells/mm³ in pts with baseline ANC 500–1500 cells/mm³: Withhold treatment until ANC greater than or equal to 1000 cells/mm³, then resume at 50 mg twice daily. May increase to 100 mg twice daily if 50 mg dose is tolerated. If treatment-induced neutropenia persists for more than 21 days, permanently discontinue.

Thrombocytopenia
Platelet count less than 50,000 cells/mm³ (treatment-induced) in pts without MCL; platelet count less than 25,000 cells/mm³ (treatment-induced) in pts with baseline platelet count 25,000–75,000 cells/mm³: Withhold treatment until platelet count greater than or equal to 50,000 cells/mm³, then resume at 50 mg twice daily. May increase to 100 mg twice daily if 50-mg dose is tolerated. If treatment-induced thrombocytopenia persists for more than 21 days, permanently discontinue.

Anemia
Hgb less than 8 g/dL (treatment-induced) in pts without MCL; life-threatening anemia with baseline Hgb 8–10 g/dL (treatment-induced): Withhold treatment until Hgb greater than or equal to 8 g/dL, then resume at

50 mg twice daily. May increase to 100 mg twice daily if 50-mg dose is tolerated. If treatment-induced anemia persists for more than 21 days, permanently discontinue.

Nausea, Vomiting
CTCAE Grade 3 or 4 nausea, vomiting despite antiemetic therapy: Withhold treatment for 3 days (6 doses), then resume at 50 mg twice daily. May increase to 100 mg twice daily if 50-mg dose is tolerated.

Nonhematologic Toxicities
Any other grade toxicities: Withhold treatment until resolved to CTCAE Grade 2 or less, then resume at 50 mg twice daily. May increase to 100 mg twice daily if 50-mg dose is tolerated.

Dosage in Rena/Hepatic Impairment
Not specified; use caution.

SIDE EFFECTS

(AML) Frequent (83%–24%): Nausea, mucositis, stomatitis, laryngeal pain, vomiting, headache, petechiae, musculoskeletal pain. **Occasional (20%–7%):** Hyperglycemia, hemorrhoids, arthralgia, hyperhidrosis, insomnia, hypertension, dry skin, increased weight. **Rare (4%–3%):** Tremor, eyelid edema. **(Systemic Mastocytosis) Frequent (82%–23%):** Nausea, vomiting, diarrhea, edema, peripheral edema, fatigue, asthenia, musculoskeletal pain, back pain, extremity pain, abdominal pain, constipation, pyrexia, headache, dyspnea, bronchospasm. **Occasional (19%–6%):** Arthralgia, cough, rash, dizziness, insomnia, hypotension, dyspepsia. **Rare (5%–4%):** Vertigo, chills, mental status change.

ADVERSE EFFECTS/ TOXIC REACTIONS

Anemia, leukopenia, lymphopenia, neutropenia, thrombocytopenia are expected responses to therapy. Hypersensitivity reactions including anaphylaxis, angioedema, dyspnea, itching, flushing may occur. Infections including bronchitis, bronchopulmonary aspergillosis, colitis, cellulitis, device-related infection, erysipelas, fungal pneumonia, gastroenteritis, hepatic candidiasis, herpes zoster, nasopharyngitis, oral herpes, pneumonia, sepsis, sinusitis, splenic fungal infection, upper respiratory tract infection, urinary tract infection have occurred. Renal failure, acute kidney injury may occur. Other adverse effects including angina pectoris, cardiac failure, contusion, duodenal ulcer hemorrhage, epistaxis, gastritis, febrile neutropenia, GI bleeding, hematoma, interstitial lung disease, myocardial infarction, myocardial ischemia, pericardial effusion, pneumonitis, pulmonary congestion, pulmonary edema, thrombosis were reported. May prolong QT interval.

NURSING CONSIDERATIONS

BASELINE ASSESSMENT
Obtain ANC, CBC, BMP, LFT; serum magnesium; vital signs. Ensure electrolytes are corrected prior to initiation. In females of reproductive potential, obtain pregnancy test within 7 days of initiation. Screen for active infection. To reduce risk of nausea/vomiting, administer antiemetic before treatment. Obtain EKG in pts taking QT interval–prolonging medications. Receive full medication history and screen for interactions. Question history as listed in Precautions. Question plans of breastfeeding. Confirm compliance of effective contraception. Offer emotional support.

INTERVENTION/EVALUATION
Monitor ANC, CBC for anemia, leukopenia, neutropenia, lymphopenia, thrombocytopenia. Monitor BMP for renal insufficiency, electrolyte imbalance (esp. in pts with diarrhea, vomiting, malnutrition); LFT for transaminitis, hepatotoxicity. Diligently screen for infections, sepsis; provide appropriate antimicrobial therapy

if indicated. Obtain ABG, radiologic test if interstitial lung disease or pneumonitis suspected. Monitor for toxicities at least wkly for 4 wks, then every other wk for 8 wks, then monthly thereafter. If treatment-related toxicities occur, consider referral to specialist. Monitor for hemorrhage, melena, hematuria; hypersensitivity reactions; myocardial infarction, pulmonary disease, thrombosis. Monitor I&O.

PATIENT/FAMILY TEACHING

• Blood levels will be routinely monitored. • Treatment may depress your immune system and reduce your ability to fight infection. Report symptoms of infection such as body aches, burning with urination, chills, cough, fatigue, fever. Avoid those with active infection. • Report symptoms of kidney failure (decreased urination, amber-colored urine, flank pain, fatigue, swelling of the hands or feet); liver problems (bruising, confusion; amber, dark, orange-colored urine; right upper abdominal pain, yellowing of the skin or eyes); lung problems (severe cough, difficulty breathing, lung pain, shortness of breath). • Avoid pregnancy. Females and males of child-bearing potential should use effective contraception during treatment and for at least 4 mos after last dose. Do not breastfeed. • Treatment may impair fertility. • Avoid grapefruit products, Seville oranges, starfruit, herbal supplements. • Do not take newly prescribed medications unless approved by the prescriber who originally started treatment. • Heart attacks have occurred; immediately report chest pain, sweating, fainting, palpitations, jaw pain, pain that radiates to the left arm. • Antinausea medication will be given before treatment to reduce the risk of nausea or vomiting. • Report bleeding of any kind, esp. nosebleeds, blood in stool or urine. • Allergic reactions such as anaphylaxis, difficulty breathing, itching, flushing, rash may occur.

milnacipran

mil-**nay**-sip-ran
(Savella)

■ **BLACK BOX ALERT** ■ Increased risk of suicidal ideation and behavior in children, adolescents, and young adults 18–24 yrs with major depressive disorder, other psychiatric disorders. Not approved for use in children.

Do not confuse Savella with cevimeline or sevelamer.

◆ CLASSIFICATION

PHARMACOTHERAPEUTIC: Serotonin, norepinephrine reuptake inhibitor. **CLINICAL:** Fibromyalgia agent.

USES

Management of fibromyalgia.

PRECAUTIONS

Contraindications: Hypersensitivity to milnacipran. Concomitant use of MAOIs to treat psychiatric disorders (concurrently or within 5 days of discontinuing milnacipran or within 2 wks of discontinuing MAOI), initiation of milnacipran in pts receiving linezolid or IV methylene blue. **Cautions:** Pts with depression, pts at increased risk of suicide, other psychiatric disorders; elevated blood pressure or heart rate, seizure disorder, pts with substantial alcohol use or chronic hepatic disease, pts with history of dysuria (e.g., prostatic hypertrophy, prostatitis), controlled narrow-angle glaucoma, renal impairment, cardiovascular disease, elderly.

ACTION

Appears to inhibit serotonin and norepinephrine reuptake at CNS neuronal presynaptic membranes. **Therapeutic Effect:** Reduces chronic pain, fatigue, depression, sleep disorders associated with fibromyalgia syndrome; improves physical function.

PHARMACOKINETICS

Well absorbed following PO administration. Protein binding: 13%. Excreted unchanged in urine. Steady-state levels reached in 36–48 hrs. **Half-life:** 6–8 hrs.

⌛ LIFESPAN CONSIDERATIONS

Pregnancy/Lactation: Increased risk of fetal complications, including need for respiratory support, if given during third trimester. Unknown if distributed in breast milk. **Children:** Safety and efficacy not established in pts younger than 18 yrs. **Elderly:** Severe renal impairment requires dosage adjustment.

INTERACTIONS

DRUG: **Lithium, MAOIs (e.g., phenelzine, selegiline)** may increase risk of serotonin syndrome. **EPINEPHrine, norepinephrine** may produce paroxysmal hypertension, arrhythmias. **Intravenous digoxin** may produce tachycardia, hypotension. May inhibit antihypertensive effect of **cloNIDine.** **HERBAL:** **Gotu kola, kava kava, St. John's wort, valerian** may increase CNS depression, increase risk of serotonin syndrome. **FOOD:** None known. **LAB VALUES:** May decrease serum sodium.

AVAILABILITY (Rx)

🦋 **Tablets, Film-Coated:** 12.5 mg, 25 mg, 50 mg, 100 mg.

ADMINISTRATION/HANDLING

• Give without regard to food. • Do not break, crush, dissolve, or divide film-coated tablets.

INDICATIONS/ROUTES/DOSAGE

Fibromyalgia
PO: ADULTS, ELDERLY: Day 1: 12.5 mg once. **Days 2–3:** 25 mg/day (12.5 mg twice daily). **Days 4–7:** 50 mg/day (25 mg twice daily). **After Day 7:** 100 mg/day (50 mg twice daily thereafter). Dose may be increased to 200 mg/day (100 mg twice daily).

Dosage in Renal Impairment
Mild impairment: No dose adjustment. **Moderate impairment:** Use caution. **Severe impairment:** Reduce maintenance dose by 50% to 50 mg/day (25 mg twice daily). Based on pt response, dose may be increased to 100 mg/day (50 mg twice daily). Not recommended in end-stage renal disease.

Dosage in Hepatic Impairment
Mild to moderate impairment: No dose adjustment. **Severe impairment:** Use caution.

SIDE EFFECTS

Frequent (37%–18%): Nausea, headache. **Occasional (16%–5%):** Constipation, insomnia, hot flashes, dizziness, hyperhidrosis, palpitations, vomiting, URI. **Rare (Less Than 5%):** Dry mouth, increased B/P, anxiety, skin flushing, rash, blurred vision, abdominal pain, chest pain, chills, pruritus, paresthesia, tachycardia.

ADVERSE EFFECTS/TOXIC REACTIONS

Abrupt discontinuation may present withdrawal symptoms (dysphoria, irritability, agitation, dizziness, paresthesia, anxiety, confusion, headache, lethargy, emotional lability, tinnitus, seizures). Serotonin syndrome symptoms may include mental status changes (agitation, hallucinations), hyperreflexia, incoordination. May increase risk of bleeding events (e.g., ecchymoses, hematomas, epistaxis).

NURSING CONSIDERATIONS

BASELINE ASSESSMENT

Obtain baseline pain intensity scale, location(s) of pain, tenderness. Obtain baseline B/P, heart rate. Question for history of changes in day-to-day pain intensity.

INTERVENTION/EVALUATION

Control nausea with antiemetics. Treat complaint of headache, migraine with

M

appropriate analgesics. Monitor for increase in B/P, pulse. Question for changes in visual acuity. Assess for clinical improvement and record onset of pain control, decreased fatigue, lessening of depressive symptoms, improvement in sleep pattern. Monitor for suicidal ideation.

PATIENT/FAMILY TEACHING

• Avoid tasks that require alertness, motor skills until response to drug is established. • Do not abruptly discontinue medication. • Increase fluids, bulk to prevent constipation. • Report unusual changes in behavior, suicidal ideation; hot flushing that becomes intolerant, excessive sweating. • Caution about risk of bleeding associated with concomitant use of NSAIDs, aspirin.

---

milrinone

mil-ri-none

◆ CLASSIFICATION

PHARMACOTHERAPEUTIC: Cardiac inotropic agent. **CLINICAL:** Vasodilator.

USES

Short-term management of decompensated HF. **OFF-LABEL:** Inotropic therapy for pts unresponsive to other therapy, outpatient inotropic therapy for heart transplant candidates, palliation of symptoms in end-stage HF.

PRECAUTIONS

Contraindications: Hypersensitivity to milrinone. **Cautions:** Severe obstructive aortic or pulmonic valvular disease, history of ventricular arrhythmias, atrial fibrillation/flutter, renal impairment. Not recommended in pts with acute MI.

ACTION

Inhibits phosphodiesterase, which increases cyclic adenosine monophosphate (cAMP), potentiating delivery of calcium to myocardial contractile systems. **Therapeutic Effect:** Relaxes vascular muscle, causing vasodilation. Increases cardiac output, decreases pulmonary capillary wedge pressure, vascular resistance.

PHARMACOKINETICS

Route	Onset	Peak	Duration
IV	5–15 min	N/A	N/A

Protein binding: 70%. Metabolized in liver. Primarily excreted in urine. **Half-life:** 1.7–2.7 hrs.

⌛ LIFESPAN CONSIDERATIONS

Pregnancy/Lactation: Unknown if drug crosses placenta or is distributed in breast milk. **Children:** Safety and efficacy not established. **Elderly:** Age-related renal impairment may require dosage adjustment.

INTERACTIONS

DRUG: None significant. **HERBAL:** None significant. **FOOD:** None known. **LAB VALUES:** None significant.

AVAILABILITY (Rx)

Injection Solution (Primacor): 1 mg/mL, 10-mL vial. **Injection Solution (Premix [Primacor]):** 200 mcg/mL (100 mL, 200 mL).

ADMINISTRATION/HANDLING

IV

Reconstitution • For IV infusion, dilute 20-mg (20-mL) vial with 80 mL 0.9% NaCl or D_5W to provide concentration of 0.2 mg/mL (200 mcg/mL).
Rate of Administration • For IV injection (loading dose), administer undiluted slowly over 10 min. • Monitor for arrhythmias, hypotension during IV therapy; reduce or temporarily discontinue infusion until condition stabilizes. Infuse via infusion pump.
Storage • Diluted solutions stable for 72 hrs at room temperature.

▣ IV INCOMPATIBILITIES

Furosemide (Lasix), imipenem-cilastatin (Primaxin), procainamide (Pronestyl).

▣ IV COMPATIBILITIES

Calcium gluconate, dexamethasone (Decadron), dexmedetomidine (Precedex), digoxin (Lanoxin), diltiaZEM (Cardizem), DOBUTamine (Dobutrex), DOPamine (Intropin), heparin, HYDROmorphone (Dilaudid), lidocaine, magnesium, midazolam (Versed), morphine, nitroglycerin, potassium, propofol (Diprivan).

INDICATIONS/ROUTES/DOSAGE

Management of HF
IV: ADULTS: Initially, 50 mcg/kg over 10 min. Continue with maintenance infusion rate of 0.125–0.75 mcg/kg/min based on hemodynamic and clinical response.

Dosage in Renal Impairment

Creatinine Clearance	Dosage
50 mL/min	0.43 mcg/kg/min
40 mL/min	0.38 mcg/kg/min
30 mL/min	0.33 mcg/kg/min
20 mL/min	0.28 mcg/kg/min
10 mL/min	0.23 mcg/kg/min
5 mL/min	0.2 mcg/kg/min

Dosage in Hepatic Impairment
No dose adjustment.

SIDE EFFECTS

Occasional (3%–1%): Headache, hypotension. **Rare (less than 1%):** Angina, chest pain.

ADVERSE EFFECTS/TOXIC REACTIONS

Supraventricular/ventricular arrhythmias (12%), nonsustained ventricular tachycardia (2%), sustained ventricular tachycardia (1%) may occur. Ventricular fibrillation (0.2%) has been documented.

NURSING CONSIDERATIONS

BASELINE ASSESSMENT

Obtain baseline lab studies, esp. BN peptide. Offer emotional support (difficulty breathing may produce anxiety). Assess B/P, apical pulse rate before treatment begins and during IV therapy. Assess lung sounds; observe for edema.

INTERVENTION/EVALUATION

Monitor B/P, heart rate, cardiac output, EKG, serum potassium, renal function, signs/symptoms of HF.

---

minocycline

mye-noe-**sye**-kleen
(Apo-Minocycline ✦, Minocin, Solodyn)
Do not confuse Dynacin with Dyazide, DynaCirc, or Dynapen, or Minocin with Indocin, Mithracin, or niacin.

◆ CLASSIFICATION

PHARMACOTHERAPEUTIC: Tetracycline. **CLINICAL:** Antibiotic.

USES

Treatment of susceptible infections due to *Rickettsiae, M. pneumoniae, C. trachomatis, C. psittaci, H. ducreyi, Yersinia pestis, Francisella tularensis, Vibrio cholerae, Brucella* spp.; gram-negative organisms, including acute intestinal amebiasis, gram-negative respiratory and skin/skin structure infections. **Solodyn:** Treatment of inflammatory lesions of moderate to severe non-nodular acne. **OFF-LABEL:** Treatment of nocardiosis, community-acquired MRSA infection, rheumatoid arthritis (RA), prosthetic joint infection.

PRECAUTIONS

Contraindications: Hypersensitivity to minocycline, other tetracyclines. **Cautions:** Children younger than 8 yrs, renal impairment, hepatic impairment, sun/ultraviolet exposure (severe photosensitivity reaction). Avoid use in pregnancy.

M

ACTION

Inhibits bacterial protein synthesis by binding to ribosomes. **Therapeutic Effect:** Bacteriostatic.

PHARMACOKINETICS

Well absorbed from GI tract. Protein binding: 70%–75%. Partially excreted in feces; minimal excretion in urine. Not removed by hemodialysis. **Half-life:** 11–23 hrs.

⧖ LIFESPAN CONSIDERATIONS

Pregnancy/Lactation: Readily crosses placenta; distributed in breast milk. May inhibit fetal skeletal growth. **Children:** May cause permanent discoloration of teeth, enamel hypoplasia. Not recommended in pts younger than 8 yrs. **Elderly:** No age-related precautions noted.

INTERACTIONS

DRUG: **Aluminum-, calcium-, magnesium-containing antacids** may decrease absorption, effect. **Ergot** may increase risk of ergotism. May decrease the effects of **estrogen-containing oral contraceptives. HERBAL: Dong quai, St. John's wort** may increase risk of photosensitivity. **FOOD:** None known. **LAB VALUES:** May increase serum alkaline phosphatase, amylase, bilirubin, ALT, AST, BUN.

AVAILABILITY (Rx)

Capsules: 50 mg, 75 mg, 100 mg. **Tablets:** 50 mg, 75 mg, 100 mg.

Tablets (Extended-Release [Solodyn]): 45 mg, 55 mg, 65 mg, 80 mg, 90 mg, 105 mg, 115 mg, 135 mg.

ADMINISTRATION/HANDLING

PO

• Take without regard to food. • Give with adequate fluid (reduces risk of esophageal irritation and ulceration). • Give pellet-filled capsules, extended-release tablets whole; do not cut, crush, dissolve, or divide.

INDICATIONS/ROUTES/DOSAGE

Usual Dosage

PO: ADULTS, ELDERLY: Initially, 100–200 mg once, then 100 mg q12h or 50 mg 4 times/day. **CHILDREN OLDER THAN 8 YRS:** Initially, 4 mg/kg once, then 2 mg/kg q12h. **Maximum:** 100 mg/dose, 200 mg/day.

Acne

PO *(Solodyn):* CHILDREN 12 YRS AND OLDER, WEIGHING 126–136 KG: 135 mg once daily; **WEIGHING 111–125 KG:** 115 mg once daily; **WEIGHING 97–110 KG:** 105 mg once daily; **WEIGHING 85–96 KG:** 90 mg once daily; **WEIGHING 72–84 KG:** 80 mg once daily; **WEIGHING 60–71 KG:** 65 mg once daily; **WEIGHING 50–59 KG:** 55 mg once daily; **WEIGHING 45–49 KG:** 45 mg once daily. *(Capsule or Immediate-Release Tablet):* **ADULTS, ELDERLY:** 50–100 mg/twice daily.

Dosage in Renal/Hepatic Impairment
Use caution.

SIDE EFFECTS

Frequent: Dizziness, light-headedness, diarrhea, nausea, vomiting, abdominal cramps, possibly severe photosensitivity, drowsiness, vertigo. **Occasional:** Altered pigmentation of skin, mucous membranes, rectal/genital pruritus, stomatitis.

ADVERSE EFFECTS/ TOXIC REACTIONS

Superinfection (esp. fungal), anaphylaxis, increased ICP may occur. Bulging fontanelles occur rarely in infants.

NURSING CONSIDERATIONS

BASELINE ASSESSMENT

Question for history of allergies, esp. tetracyclines, sulfite.

INTERVENTION/EVALUATION

Assess ability to ambulate (may cause vertigo, dizziness). Monitor daily pattern

M

of bowel activity, stool consistency. Monitor renal function, LFT with long-term therapy. Assess skin for rash. Observe for signs of increased intracranial pressure (altered LOC, widened pulse pressure). Be alert for superinfection: fever, vomiting, diarrhea, anal/genital pruritus, oral mucosal changes (ulceration, pain, erythema).

PATIENT/FAMILY TEACHING

• Continue antibiotic for full length of treatment. • Space doses evenly. • Drink full glass of water with capsules or tablets. • Avoid tasks that require alertness, motor skills until response to drug is established. • Report diarrhea, rash, other new symptoms. • Protect skin from sun exposure. • Advise female pts to use additional form of birth control (may decrease effectiveness of oral contraceptives).

mirabegron

mir-a-**beg**-ron
(Myrbetriq)

◆**CLASSIFICATION**

PHARMACOTHERAPEUTIC: Beta$_3$-adrenergic agonist. **CLINICAL:** Smooth muscle relaxant.

USES

Treatment of overactive bladder with symptoms of urinary incontinence, urgency, frequency.

PRECAUTIONS

Contraindications: Hypersensitivity to mirabegron. **Cautions:** Bladder outlet obstruction, pts taking antimuscarinic medications (increases urinary retention), mild to moderate hepatic/renal impairment, history of QT-interval prolongation, medications known to prolong QT interval. Not recommended for use in pts with severe uncontrolled hypertension (SBP equal to or greater than 180 mm Hg and/or DBP equal to or greater than 110 mm Hg).

ACTION

Relaxes detrusor smooth muscle of bladder through beta$_3$ stimulation during storage phase of urinary bladder fill–void cycle. **Therapeutic Effect:** Increases bladder capacity, reduces symptoms of urinary urgency, increased voiding frequency, urge incontinence, nocturia.

PHARMACOKINETICS

Readily absorbed following PO administration; widely distributed. Protein binding: 71%. Eliminated in urine (55%), feces (35%). **Half-life:** 50 hrs.

⧗ LIFESPAN CONSIDERATIONS

Pregnancy/Lactation: Unknown if distributed in breast milk. **Children:** Safety and efficacy not established. **Elderly:** No age-related precautions noted.

INTERACTIONS

DRUG: May increase concentration of **desipramine, digoxin, metoprolol, thioridazine, flecainide, propafenone. HERBAL:** None significant. **FOOD:** None known. **LAB VALUES:** May increase GGT, LDH; temporarily increase ALT, AST.

AVAILABILITY (Rx)

🦅 **Tablets, Extended-Release:** 25 mg, 50 mg.

ADMINISTRATION/HANDLING

PO

• Give without regard to meals. • Administer with water; instruct pt to swallow whole. • Do not break, crush, dissolve, or divide film-coated tablets.

INDICATIONS/ROUTES/DOSAGE

Overactive Bladder
PO: ADULTS, ELDERLY: Initially, 25 mg once daily. Efficacy seen within 8 wks

M

---

for 25-mg dose. May increase to 50 mg once daily.

Dosage in Renal Impairment
Mild to moderate impairment: No dosage adjustment. **Severe impairment:** Do not exceed 25 mg once daily.

Dosage in Hepatic Impairment
Mild impairment: No dosage adjustment. **Moderate impairment:** Do not exceed 25 mg once daily. **Severe impairment:** Not recommended.

SIDE EFFECTS

Occasional (9%–4%): Hypertension, headache, nasopharyngitis. **Rare (2%–1%):** Constipation, arthralgia, diarrhea, tachycardia, fatigue.

ADVERSE EFFECTS/ TOXIC REACTIONS

Worsening of preexisting hypertension reported infrequently. Urinary tract infection occurred in 6% of pts, influenza in 3%, and upper respiratory infection in 1.5%.

NURSING CONSIDERATIONS

BASELINE ASSESSMENT
Check B/P; assess for hypertension. Monitor EKG. Receive full medication history, and screen for possible drug interactions. Monitor I&O (particularly in pts with history of urinary retention).

INTERVENTION/EVALUATION
Monitor ALT, AST, LDH, GGT periodically. Palpate bladder for urinary retention. Measure B/P near end of dosing interval (determines whether B/P is controlled throughout day). Periodic B/P determinations are recommended, especially in hypertensive pts. For pts taking digoxin, monitor digoxin serum level for therapeutic effect (very narrow line between therapeutic and toxic level). Assess pulse for quality, irregular rate, bradycardia. Question for evidence of headache.

PATIENT/FAMILY TEACHING
• Report urinary retention. • Do not use nasal decongestants, over-the-counter cold preparations without doctor approval. Restrict salt, alcohol intake. • Take mirabegron with water; swallow tablet whole; do not chew, crush, dissolve, or divide tablet. • May take with or without food.

mirtazapine

mir-**taz**-a-peen
(Apo-Mirtazapine ✤, Remeron, Remeron Soltab)
■ **BLACK BOX ALERT** ■ Increased risk of suicidal thinking and behavior in children, adolescents, young adults 18–24 yrs with major depressive disorder, other psychiatric disorders.
Do not confuse Remeron with Premarin, Rozerem, or Zemuron.

◆CLASSIFICATION
PHARMACOTHERAPEUTIC: Alpha-2 antagonist. **CLINICAL:** Antidepressant.

USES

Treatment of major depressive disorder (MDD).

PRECAUTIONS

Contraindications: Hypersensitivity to mirtazapine. Use of MAOIs to treat psychiatric disorders (concurrently or within 14 days of discontinuing either MAOI or mirtazapine), initiation of mirtazapine in pts receiving linezolid or IV methylene blue. **Cautions:** Renal/hepatic impairment, elderly pts, seizure disorder, suicidal ideation or behavior, alcoholism, concurrent medications that lower seizure threshold, cardiovascular disease, pts at risk for QT prolongation, medications known to prolong QT interval.

M

ACTION

Acts as antagonist at presynaptic alpha$_2$-adrenergic receptors, increasing norepinephrine, serotonin neurotransmission. Has low anticholinergic activity. **Therapeutic Effect:** Relieves depression.

PHARMACOKINETICS

Rapidly, completely absorbed after PO administration; absorption not affected by food. Protein binding: 85%. Metabolized in liver. Primarily excreted in urine. Unknown if removed by hemodialysis. **Half-life:** 20–40 hrs (longer in males [37 hrs] than females [26 hrs]).

⧗ LIFESPAN CONSIDERATIONS

Pregnancy/Lactation: Unknown if distributed in breast milk. **Children:** Safety and efficacy not established. **Elderly:** Age-related renal impairment may require dosage adjustment.

INTERACTIONS

DRUG: Alcohol, CNS depressant medications (e.g., LORazepam, morphine, zolpidem) may increase impairment of cognition, motor skills. **Serotonergic drugs (e.g., venlafaxine)** may increase risk of serotonin syndrome. **CYP3A4 inducers (e.g., carBAMazepine, phenytoin, rifAMPin)** may decrease concentration/effects. **CYP3A4 inhibitors (e.g., erythromycin, ketoconazole, ritonavir)** may increase concentration/effects. **MAOIs (e.g., phenelzine, selegiline)** may increase risk of neuroleptic malignant syndrome, hypertensive crisis, severe seizures. **HERBAL: Gotu kola, kava kava, St. John's wort, valerian** may increase CNS depression. **St. John's wort** may decrease concentration/effects, may increase risk of serotonin syndrome. **FOOD:** None known. **LAB VALUES:** May increase serum cholesterol, triglycerides, ALT.

AVAILABILITY (Rx)

Tablets: 7.5 mg, 15 mg, 30 mg, 45 mg. **Tablets (Orally Disintegrating):** 15 mg, 30 mg, 45 mg.

ADMINISTRATION/HANDLING

PO
• Give without regard to food. • May crush/break scored tablets.

Orally Disintegrating Tablets
• Give without regard to food. • Do not split tablet. • Place on tongue; dissolves without water.

INDICATIONS/ROUTES/DOSAGE

Depression
PO: ADULTS: Initially, 15 mg at bedtime. May increase by 15 mg/day q1–2wks. **Maximum:** 45 mg/day. **ELDERLY:** Initially, 7.5 mg at bedtime. May increase by 7.5–15 mg/day q1–2wks. **Maximum:** 45 mg/day.

Dosage in Renal/Hepatic Impairment
Use caution.

SIDE EFFECTS

Frequent (54%–12%): Drowsiness, dry mouth, increased appetite, constipation, weight gain. **Occasional (89%–4%):** Asthenia, dizziness, flu-like symptoms, abnormal dreams. **Rare:** Abdominal discomfort, vasodilation, paresthesia, acne, dry skin, thirst, arthralgia.

ADVERSE EFFECTS/TOXIC REACTIONS

Higher incidence of seizures than with tricyclic antidepressants (esp. in pts with no history of seizures). Overdose may produce cardiovascular effects (severe orthostatic hypotension, dizziness, tachycardia, palpitations, arrhythmias). Abrupt discontinuation from prolonged therapy may produce headache, malaise, nausea, vomiting, vivid dreams. Agranulocytosis occurs rarely.

NURSING CONSIDERATIONS

BASELINE ASSESSMENT
Assess mental status, appearance, behavior, speech pattern, level of interest, mood. Obtain baseline weight. For pts on

M

---

long-term therapy, renal function, LFT, CBC should be performed periodically.

INTERVENTION/EVALUATION

Supervise suicidal-risk pt closely during early therapy (as depression lessens, energy level improves, increasing suicide potential). Children, adolescents are at increased risk for suicidal thoughts/behavior and worsening of depression, esp. during first few mos of therapy. Assess appearance, behavior, speech pattern, level of interest, mood. Monitor for hypotension, arrhythmias.

PATIENT/FAMILY TEACHING

• Take as single bedtime dose. • Avoid alcohol, depressant/sedating medications. • Avoid tasks requiring alertness, motor skills until response to drug established. • Report worsening depression, suicidal ideation, unusual changes in behavior.

M

---

miSOPROStol

mis-oh-**pros**-tol
(Cytotec, Novo-MiSOPROStol ✦)
■ **BLACK BOX ALERT** ■ Use during pregnancy can cause abortion, premature birth, birth defects. Not recommended in women of childbearing potential unless pt is capable of complying with effective contraception.
Do not confuse Cytotec with Cytoxan, or miSOPROStol with metoprolol or miFEPRIStone.

FIXED-COMBINATION(S)

Arthrotec: miSOPROStol/diclofenac (an NSAID): 200 mcg/50 mg, 200 mcg/75 mg.

◆CLASSIFICATION

PHARMACOTHERAPEUTIC: Prostaglandin. **CLINICAL:** Antisecretory, gastric protectant.

USES

Prevention of NSAID-induced gastric ulcers and in pts at high risk for developing gastric ulcer/gastric ulcer complications. Medical termination of intrauterine pregnancy through 70 days' gestation (in conjunction with miFEPRIStone). **OFF-LABEL:** Cervical ripening, labor induction, treatment/prevention of postpartum hemorrhage, treatment of incomplete or missed abortion.

PRECAUTIONS

Contraindications: Hypersensitivity to prostaglandins; pregnancy when used to reduce NSAID-induced ulcers (produces uterine contractions). **Cautions:** Renal impairment, cardiovascular disease, elderly.

ACTION

Replaces protective prostaglandins consumed with prostaglandin-inhibiting therapies (e.g., NSAIDs). Induces uterine contractions. **Therapeutic Effect:** Reduces acid secretion from gastric parietal cells, stimulates bicarbonate production from gastric/duodenal mucosa.

PHARMACOKINETICS

Route	Onset	Peak	Duration
PO	30 min	1–1.5 hrs	3–6 hrs

Rapidly absorbed from GI tract. Protein binding: 80%–90%. Primarily excreted in urine. Unknown if removed by hemodialysis. **Half-life:** 20–40 min.

⌛ LIFESPAN CONSIDERATIONS

Pregnancy/Lactation: Unknown if distributed in breast milk. Produces uterine contractions, uterine bleeding, expulsion of products of conception (abortifacient property). **Children:** Safety and efficacy not established. **Elderly:** No age-related precautions noted.

INTERACTIONS

DRUG: Antacids may increase concentration. **HERBAL:** None significant. **FOOD:** None known. **LAB VALUES:** None significant.

AVAILABILITY (Rx)

Tablets: 100 mcg, 200 mcg.

ADMINISTRATION/HANDLING

PO

• Give with or after meals (minimizes diarrhea).

INDICATIONS/ROUTES/DOSAGE

Prevention of NSAID-Induced Gastric Ulcer

PO: ADULTS: 200 mcg 4 times/day with food (last dose at bedtime). Continue for duration of NSAID therapy. May reduce dosage to 100 mcg 4 times/day or 200 mcg 2 times/day with food. **ELDERLY:** 100–200 mcg 4 times/day with food.

Termination of Intrauterine Pregnancy

See manufacturer guidelines for miFEPRISTone.

Early Pregnancy Loss

Intravaginal: 800 mcg once; may repeat 3 or more hrs after first dose and within 7 days of no response to initial dose.

Incomplete Abortion, Postpartum Hemorrhage

PO: 600 mcg as a single dose.

Labor Induction or Cervical Ripening

Intravaginal: 25 mcg q3–6 hrs. Some pts may require 50 mcg q6 hrs. **Maximum:** 50 mcg/dose.

Dosage in Renal/Hepatic Impairment

No dose adjustment.

SIDE EFFECTS

Frequent (40%–20%): Abdominal pain, diarrhea. **Occasional (3%–2%):** Nausea, flatulence, dyspepsia, headache. **Rare (1%):** Vomiting, constipation.

ADVERSE EFFECTS/ TOXIC REACTIONS

Overdosage may produce sedation, tremor, seizures, dyspnea, palpitations, hypotension, bradycardia.

NURSING CONSIDERATIONS

BASELINE ASSESSMENT

Question for possibility of pregnancy before initiating therapy.

PATIENT/FAMILY TEACHING

• Avoid magnesium-containing antacids (minimizes potential for diarrhea).
• Women of childbearing potential must not be pregnant before or during medication therapy (may result in hospitalization, surgery, infertility, fetal death).
• Incidence of diarrhea may be lessened by taking immediately following meals.

---

mitoMYcin

mye-toe-**mye**-sin
(Mutamycin ✿)

■ **BLACK BOX ALERT** ■ Potent vesicant. Marked myelosuppression. Infiltration produces ulceration, necrosis, cellulitis, tissue sloughing. Hemolytic-uremic syndrome reported. Must be administered by certified chemotherapy personnel.

Do not confuse mitoMYcin with mithramycin or mitoXANTRONE.

◆CLASSIFICATION

PHARMACOTHERAPEUTIC: Antibiotic. **CLINICAL:** Antineoplastic.

USES

Treatment of disseminated adenocarcinoma of stomach, pancreas (in combination with other chemotherapy agents and as palliative treatment when other modalities have failed). **OFF-LABEL:** Treatment of bladder cancer, anal carcinoma; cervical, esophageal, gastric, non–small-cell lung cancer.

PRECAUTIONS

Contraindications: Hypersensitivity to mitoMYcin. Coagulation disorders, other increased bleeding tendencies,

---

M

thrombocytopenia. **Cautions:** Myelosuppression, renal (serum creatinine greater than 1.7 mg/dL)/hepatic impairment, pregnancy, prior radiation treatment.

ACTION

Alkylating agent, cross-linking with strands of DNA. **Therapeutic Effect:** Inhibits DNA, RNA synthesis.

PHARMACOKINETICS

Widely distributed. Does not cross blood-brain barrier. Metabolized in liver. Excreted in urine. **Half-life:** 50 min.

⏳ LIFESPAN CONSIDERATIONS

Pregnancy/Lactation: If possible, avoid use during pregnancy, esp. first trimester. Breastfeeding not recommended. Safety in pregnancy not established. **Children:** Safety and efficacy not established. **Elderly:** Age-related renal impairment may require dosage adjustment.

INTERACTIONS

DRUG: Bone marrow depressants may increase myelosuppression. **Live virus vaccines** may potentiate virus replication, increase vaccine side effects, decrease pt's antibody response to vaccine. **HERBAL:** Avoid **black cohosh, dong quai** in estrogen-dependent tumors. **FOOD:** None known. **LAB VALUES:** May increase serum BUN, creatinine.

AVAILABILITY (Rx)

Injection, Powder for Reconstitution: 5 mg, 20 mg, 40 mg.

ADMINISTRATION/HANDLING

◀**ALERT**▶May be carcinogenic, mutagenic, teratogenic. Handle with extreme care during preparation/administration. Give via IV push, IV infusion. Extremely irritating to vein. Injection may produce pain with induration, thrombophlebitis, paresthesia.

 IV

Reconstitution • Reconstitute with Sterile Water for Injection to provide solution containing 0.5–1 mg/mL. • Do not shake vial to dissolve. • Allow vial to stand at room temperature until complete dissolution occurs. • For IV infusion, further dilute with 50–100 mL D5W or 0.9% NaCl (concentration 20–40 mcg/mL).
Rate of Administration • Give slow IV push or by IV infusion over 15–30 min. • Extravasation may produce cellulitis, ulceration, tissue sloughing. Terminate administration immediately, inject ordered antidote. Apply ice intermittently for up to 72 hrs; keep area elevated.
Storage • Use only clear, blue-gray solutions. • Concentration of 0.5 mg/mL (reconstituted vial or syringe) is stable for 7 days at room temperature or 2 wks if refrigerated. Further diluted solution with D5W is stable for 3 hrs, 12 hrs if diluted with 0.9% NaCl at room temperature.

🚫 IV INCOMPATIBILITIES

Aztreonam (Azactam), bleomycin (Blenoxane), cefepime (Maxipime), filgrastim (Neupogen), heparin, piperacillin/tazobactam (Zosyn), sargramostim (Leukine), vinorelbine (Navelbine).

🚫 IV COMPATIBILITIES

CISplatin (Platinol AQ), cyclophosphamide (Cytoxan), DOXOrubicin (Adriamycin), 5-fluorouracil, granisetron (Kytril), leucovorin, methotrexate, ondansetron (Zofran), vinBLAStine (Velban), vinCRIStine (Oncovin).

INDICATIONS/ROUTES/DOSAGE

Refer to individual protocols.

Stomach, Pancreatic Cancer
IV: ADULTS, ELDERLY, CHILDREN: 20 mg/m² as single dose. Repeat q6–8wks.

Bladder Cancer (Non–Muscle Invasive) Intravesicular Instillation: ADULTS, ELDERLY: Low risk of recurrence: 40 mg as single dose postoperatively (retain in bladder for 1–2 hrs). High risk of recurrence: 20 mg/wk for 6 wks, then 20 mg qmo for 3 yrs (retain in bladder for 1–2 hrs).

Dose Modification for Toxicity

Leukocytes 2,000 to less than 3,000 cells/mm^3	Hold therapy until leukocytes 4,000 or more cells/mm^3; reduce dose to 70% or more in subsequent cycles
Leukocytes less than 2,000 cells/mm^3	Hold therapy until leukocytes 4,000 or more cells/mm^3; reduce dose to 50% in subsequent cycles
Platelets 25,000 to less than 75,000 cells/mm^3	Hold therapy until platelets 100,000 or more cells/mm^3; reduce dose to 70% in subsequent cycles
Platelets less than 25,000 cells/mm^3	Hold therapy until platelets 100,000 or more cells/mm^3; reduce dose to 50% in subsequent cycles

Dosage in Renal Impairment
CrCl less than 10 mL/min: Give 75% of normal dose.

Dosage in Hepatic Impairment
No dose adjustment.

SIDE EFFECTS

Frequent (greater than 10%): Fever, anorexia, nausea, vomiting. **Occasional (10%–2%):** Stomatitis, paresthesia, purple colored bands on nails, rash, alopecia, unusual fatigue. **Rare (less than 1%):** Thrombophlebitis, cellulitis with extravasation.

ADVERSE EFFECTS/ TOXIC REACTIONS

Marked myelosuppression results in hematologic toxicity manifested as leukopenia, thrombocytopenia, and, to a lesser extent, anemia (generally occurs within 2–4 wks after initial therapy). Renal toxicity may be evidenced by increased serum BUN, creatinine levels. Pulmonary toxicity manifested as dyspnea, cough, hemoptysis, pneumonia. Long-term therapy may produce hemolytic uremic syndrome, characterized by hemolytic anemia, thrombocytopenia, renal failure, hypertension.

NURSING CONSIDERATIONS

BASELINE ASSESSMENT

Obtain CBC with differential, PT, bleeding time, before and periodically during therapy. Antiemetics before and during therapy may alleviate nausea/vomiting. Offer emotional support.

INTERVENTION/EVALUATION

Monitor hematologic status, renal function studies. Assess IV site for phlebitis, extravasation. Monitor for hematologic toxicity (fever, sore throat, signs of local infection, unusual bruising/bleeding from any site), symptoms of anemia (excessive fatigue, weakness). Assess for renal toxicity (foul odor from urine, elevated serum BUN, creatinine).

PATIENT/FAMILY TEACHING

• Maintain strict oral hygiene. • Immediately report stinging, burning, pain at injection site. • Do not have immunizations without physician's approval (drug lowers resistance to infection). • Avoid contact with those who have recently received live virus vaccine. • Hair loss is reversible, but new hair growth may have different color, texture. • Report nausea/vomiting, fever, sore throat, bruising, bleeding, shortness of breath, painful urination.

M

---

modafinil

TOP 100

moe-**daf**-i-nil
(Alertec ✦, Apo-Modafinil ✦, Provigil)

◆CLASSIFICATION

PHARMACOTHERAPEUTIC: Alpha$_1$-agonist, CNS stimulant **(Schedule IV).** **CLINICAL:** Wakefulness-promoting agent, antinarcoleptic.

USES

Treatment of excessive daytime sleepiness associated with narcolepsy, shift work sleep disorder, adjunct therapy for obstructive sleep apnea/hypopnea syndrome. **OFF-LABEL:** Treatment of ADHD, multiple sclerosis–related fatigue.

PRECAUTIONS

Contraindications: Hypersensitivity to modafinil, armodafinil. **Cautions:** History of clinically significant mitral valve prolapse, left ventricular hypertrophy, renal/hepatic impairment, angina, cardiac disease, myocardial ischemia, recent MI, preexisting psychosis or bipolar disorder, Tourette's syndrome.

ACTION

Increases alpha activity, decreasing delta, theta, brain wave activity. **Therapeutic Effect:** Reduces number of sleep episodes, total daytime sleep.

PHARMACOKINETICS

Well absorbed from GI tract. Protein binding: 60%. Widely distributed. Metabolized in liver. Excreted by kidneys. Unknown if removed by hemodialysis. **Half-life:** 15 hrs.

☒ LIFESPAN CONSIDERATIONS

Pregnancy/Lactation: Unknown if excreted in breast milk. Use caution if given to pregnant women. **Children:** Safety and efficacy not established in pts younger than 16 yrs. **Elderly:** Age-related renal/hepatic impairment may require decreased dosage.

INTERACTIONS

DRUG: May decrease concentrations of **cycloSPORINE, oral contraceptives.** May increase concentrations of **tricyclic antidepressants (e.g., amitriptyline, doxepin), warfarin. Other CNS stimulants (e.g., caffeine)** may increase CNS stimulation. **HERBAL:** None significant. **FOOD:** None known. **LAB VALUES:** None significant.

AVAILABILITY (Rx)

Tablets (Provigil): 100 mg, 200 mg.

ADMINISTRATION/HANDLING

PO
• Give without regard to meals.

INDICATIONS/ROUTES/DOSAGE

Narcolepsy, Obstructive Sleep Apnea/ Hypopnea Syndrome
PO: ADULTS: 200 mg/day in the morning. **ELDERLY:** 100 mg/day in the morning.

Shift Work Sleep Disorder
PO: ADULTS: 200 mg about 1 hr prior to start of work shift.

Dosage in Renal Impairment
No dose adjustment.

Dosage in Hepatic Impairment
Mild to moderate impairment: No dose adjustment. Reduce dose 50% with severe impairment.

SIDE EFFECTS

Generally well tolerated. **Occasional (5%):** Headache, nausea, dizziness, insomnia, palpitations, diarrhea.

ADVERSE EFFECTS/ TOXIC REACTIONS

Agitation, excitation, increased B/P, insomnia may occur. Psychiatric disturbances (anxiety, hallucinations, suicidal ideation), serious allergic reactions (angioedema, Stevens-Johnson syndrome) have been noted.

M

NURSING CONSIDERATIONS

BASELINE ASSESSMENT

Obtain baseline evidence of narcolepsy or other sleep disorders, including pattern, environmental situations, length of sleep episodes. Question for sudden loss of muscle tone (cataplexy) precipitated by strong emotional responses before sleep episode. Assess frequency/severity of sleep episodes before drug therapy.

INTERVENTION/EVALUATION

Monitor sleep pattern, evidence of restlessness during sleep, length of insomnia episodes at night. Assess for dizziness, anxiety; initiate fall precautions.

PATIENT/FAMILY TEACHING

• Avoid alcohol. • Sugarless gum, sips of water may relieve dry mouth. • Do not increase dose without physician approval. • Use alternative contraceptives during therapy and 1 mo after discontinuing modafinil (reduces effectiveness of oral contraceptives).

---

mometasone

moe-**met**-a-sone
(Asmanex, Asmanex HFA, Elocon, Nasonex)

FIXED-COMBINATION(S)

Dulera: mometasone/formoterol (beta-adrenergic agonist): 100 mcg/5 mcg, 200 mcg/5 mcg.

◆CLASSIFICATION

PHARMACOTHERAPEUTIC: Adrenocorticosteroid. **CLINICAL:** Anti-inflammatory.

USES

Nasal: Treatment of nasal symptoms of seasonal/perennial allergic rhinitis in adults, children 2 yrs and older. Prophylaxis of nasal symptoms of seasonal allergic rhinitis in adults, adolescents 12 yrs and older. Treatment of nasal polyps in adults. **Inhalation:** Maintenance treatment of asthma as prophylactic therapy. **Topical:** Relief of inflammatory, pruritic manifestations of steroid-responsive dermatoses.

PRECAUTIONS

Contraindications: Hypersensitivity to mometasone, milk proteins. Primary treatment of status asthmaticus or acute bronchospasm. **Cautions:** Thyroid/hepatic/renal impairment, elderly, diabetes, cardiovascular disease, glaucoma, cataracts, myasthenia gravis, pts at risk for osteoporosis, seizures, GI disease (e.g., ulcer, colitis); following MI. Untreated systemic fungal, viral, bacterial infections.

ACTION

Inhibits release of mediators of inflammation (e.g., histamine, kinins). **Therapeutic Effect:** Improves symptoms of asthma, rhinitis.

PHARMACOKINETICS

Undetectable in plasma. Protein binding: 98%–99%. Swallowed portion undergoes extensive metabolism. Excreted in bile (74%), urine (8%). **Half-life:** 5 hrs.

⧗ LIFESPAN CONSIDERATIONS

Pregnancy/Lactation: Unknown if drug crosses placenta or is distributed in breast milk. **Children:** Prolonged treatment/high doses may decrease short-term growth rate, cortisol secretion. **Elderly:** No age-related precautions noted.

INTERACTIONS

DRUG: Ketoconazole may increase concentration (inhalation). **HERBAL:** None significant. **FOOD:** None known. **LAB VALUES:** None significant.

M

AVAILABILITY (Rx)

Cream (Elocon): 0.1%. Lotion (Elocon): 0.1%. Nasal Spray (Nasonex): 50 mcg/spray. Ointment (Elocon): 0.1%. Powder for Oral Inhaler (Asmanex): 110 mcg (delivers 100 mcg/actuation), 220 mcg (delivers 200 mcg/actuation). (Asmanex HFA): 100 mcg/actuation, 200 mcg/actuation.

ADMINISTRATION/HANDLING

Inhalation

• Do not shake or prime. • Hold twist-haler straight up with pink portion (base) on bottom, remove cap. • Exhale fully. • Firmly close lips around mouthpiece and inhale a fast, deep breath. • Hold breath for 10 sec.

Intranasal

• Instruct pt to clear nasal passages as much as possible before use. • Tilt head slightly forward. • Insert spray tip into nostril, pointing toward nasal passages, away from nasal septum. • Spray into one nostril while pt holds other nostril closed, concurrently inspires through nose to permit medication as high into nasal passages as possible.

Topical

• Apply thin layer of cream, lotion, ointment to cover affected area. Rub in gently. • Do not cover area with occlusive dressing.

INDICATIONS/ROUTES/DOSAGE

Allergic Rhinitis

Nasal Spray: ADULTS, ELDERLY, CHILDREN 12 YRS AND OLDER: 2 sprays in each nostril once daily. When used to prevent nasal rhinitis, begin 2–4 wks prior to start of pollen season. CHILDREN 2–11 YRS: 1 spray in each nostril once daily.

Asthma

Inhalation: ADULTS, ELDERLY, CHILDREN 12 YRS AND OLDER (Previous therapy with bronchodilators: (Asmanex): Initially, inhale 220 mcg (1 puff) once daily. Maximum: 440 mcg/day as single or 2 divided doses. (Previous therapy with inhaled corticosteroids): (Asmanex HFA): Initially, 100–200 mcg twice daily. Maximum: 400 mcg twice daily. (Previous therapy with oral corticosteroids): (Asmanex): 440 mcg (2 puffs) twice daily. (Asmanex HFA): 400 mcg twice daily. Reduce predniSONE no faster than 2.5 mg/day beginning after at least 1 wk of mometasone. CHILDREN 4–11 YRS: (Asmanex): 110 mcg once daily in evening.

Skin Disease

Topical: ADULTS, ELDERLY, CHILDREN 12 YRS AND OLDER: Apply cream, lotion, or ointment sparingly to affected area once daily.

Nasal Polyp

Nasal Spray: ADULTS, ELDERLY: 2 sprays (100 mcg) in each nostril twice daily. Total dose: 400 mcg.

Dosage in Renal/Hepatic Impairment

No dose adjustment.

SIDE EFFECTS

Occasional: Inhalation: Headache, allergic rhinitis, upper respiratory infection, muscle pain, fatigue. Nasal: Nasal irritation, stinging. Topical: Burning. Rare: Inhalation: Abdominal pain, dyspepsia, nausea. Nasal: Nasal/pharyngeal candidiasis. Topical: Pruritus.

ADVERSE EFFECTS/ TOXIC REACTIONS

Acute hypersensitivity reaction (urticaria, angioedema, severe bronchospasm) occurs rarely. Transfer from systemic to local steroid therapy may unmask previously suppressed bronchial asthma condition.

NURSING CONSIDERATIONS

BASELINE ASSESSMENT

Question for hypersensitivity to any corticosteroids.

INTERVENTION/EVALUATION

Teach proper use of nasal spray, oral inhaler. Instruct pt to clear nasal passages before use. Report if no improvement in symptoms or if sneezing, nasal irritation occur. Assess lung sounds for wheezing, rales.

PATIENT/FAMILY TEACHING

• Do not change dose schedule or stop taking drug; must taper off gradually under medical supervision. **Nasal:** Report if symptoms do not improve; report if sneezing, nasal irritation occur. • Clear nasal passages prior to use. **Inhalation:** Inhale rapidly, deeply; rinse mouth after inhalation. • Not indicated for acute asthma attacks. **Topical:** Do not cover affected area with bandage, dressing.

---

montelukast

mon-**tee**-loo-kast
(Apo-Montelukast ✦, Singulair)
Do not confuse Singulair with SINEquan.

◆CLASSIFICATION

PHARMACOTHERAPEUTIC: Leukotriene receptor inhibitor. **CLINICAL:** Antiasthmatic.

USES

Prophylaxis, chronic treatment of asthma. Prevention of exercise-induced bronchoconstriction. Relief of symptoms of seasonal allergic rhinitis (hay fever), perennial allergic rhinitis. **OFF-LABEL:** Urticaria.

PRECAUTIONS

Contraindications: Hypersensitivity to montelukast. **Cautions:** Systemic corticosteroid treatment reduction during montelukast therapy. Concomitant use of CYP3A4 inducers. Not for use in acute asthma attacks.

ACTION

Binds to cysteinyl leukotriene receptors, inhibiting effects of leukotrienes on bronchial smooth muscle. **Therapeutic Effect:** Decreases bronchoconstriction, vascular permeability, mucosal edema, mucus production.

PHARMACOKINETICS

Route	Onset	Peak	Duration
PO	N/A	N/A	24 hrs
PO (chewable)	N/A	N/A	24 hrs

Rapidly absorbed from GI tract. Protein binding: 99%. Extensively metabolized in liver. Excreted almost exclusively in feces. **Half-life:** 2.7–5.5 hrs (slightly longer in elderly).

⧗ LIFESPAN CONSIDERATIONS

Pregnancy/Lactation: Unknown if distributed in breast milk. Use during pregnancy only if necessary. **Children/Elderly:** No age-related precautions noted in pts older than 6 yrs or the elderly.

INTERACTIONS

DRUG: CYP3A4 inducers (e.g., carBAMazepine, PHENobarbital, rifAMPin) may decrease concentration/effects. **HERBAL: St. John's wort** may decrease concentration/effects. **FOOD:** None known. **LAB VALUES:** May increase serum ALT, AST, eosinophils.

AVAILABILITY (Rx)

Oral Granules: 4 mg per packet. **Tablets:** 10 mg. **Tablets (Chewable):** 4 mg, 5 mg.

M

ADMINISTRATION/HANDLING

PO

• May take without regard to food/ meals. When treating asthma, administer in evening. • When treating allergic rhinitis, may individualize administration times. • Granules may be given directly in mouth or mixed with carrots, rice, applesauce, ice cream, baby formula, or breast milk (do not add to any other liquid or food). • Give within 15 min of opening packet.

INDICATIONS/ROUTES/DOSAGE

Bronchial Asthma

PO: ADULTS, ELDERLY, CHILDREN 15 YRS AND OLDER: One 10-mg tablet daily, taken in the evening. **CHILDREN 6–14 YRS:** One 5-mg chewable tablet daily, taken in the evening. **CHILDREN 2–5 YRS:** One 4-mg chewable tablet daily, taken in the evening. **CHILDREN 6–23 MOS:** 4 mg (oral granules) once daily in the evening.

Seasonal Allergic Rhinitis

PO: ADULTS, ELDERLY, CHILDREN 15 YRS AND OLDER: One 10-mg tablet, taken in the evening. **CHILDREN 6–14 YRS:** One 5-mg chewable tablet, taken in the evening. **CHILDREN 2–5 YRS:** One 4-mg chewable tablet, or oral granules taken in the evening.

Perennial Allergic Rhinitis

PO: ADULTS, ELDERLY, CHILDREN 15 YRS AND OLDER: One 10-mg tablet, taken in the evening. **CHILDREN 6–14 YRS:** One 5-mg chewable tablet, taken in the evening. **CHILDREN 2–5 YRS:** One 4-mg chewable tablet or oral granules, taken in the evening. **CHILDREN 6–23 MOS:** 4 mg oral granules, taken in the evening.

Exercise-Induced Bronchoconstriction Prevention

PO: ADULTS, ELDERLY, CHILDREN 15 YRS AND OLDER: 10 mg 2 or more hrs before exercise. No additional doses within 24 hrs. **CHILDREN 6–14 YRS:** 5 mg (chew tab) 2 or more hrs prior to exercise. No additional doses within 24 hrs.

Dosage in Renal/Hepatic Impairment
No dose adjustment.

SIDE EFFECTS

ADULTS, CHILDREN 15 YRS AND OLDER: Frequent (18%): Headache. **Occasional (4%):** Influenza. **Rare (3%–2%):** Abdominal pain, cough, dyspepsia, dizziness, fatigue, dental pain. **CHILDREN 6–14 YRS: Rare (less than 2%):** Diarrhea, laryngitis, pharyngitis, nausea, otitis media, sinusitis, viral infection.

ADVERSE EFFECTS/ TOXIC REACTIONS

Suicidal ideation and behavior, depression have been noted.

NURSING CONSIDERATIONS

BASELINE ASSESSMENT

Chewable tablet contains phenylalanine (component of aspartame); parents of phenylketonuric pts should be informed. Assess lung sounds for wheezing. Assess for allergy symptoms. Question history of depression, suicidal ideation.

INTERVENTION/EVALUATION

Monitor rate, depth, rhythm, type of respirations; quality/rate of pulse. Assess lung sounds for wheezing. Monitor for change in mood, behavior.

PATIENT/FAMILY TEACHING

• Increase fluid intake (decreases lung secretion viscosity). • Take as prescribed, even during symptom-free periods as well as during exacerbations of asthma. • Do not alter/stop other asthma medications. • Drug is not for treatment of acute asthma attacks. • Report increased use or frequency of short-acting bronchodilators, changes in behavior, suicidal ideation.

morphine

mor-feen
(Duramorph, Infumorph, Kadian,
M-Eslon ✿, MS Contin, MS-IR ✿)

■ **BLACK BOX ALERT** ■ Be alert for signs of abuse, misuse, diversion. *Epidural:* Monitor for delayed sedation. *Sustained-release:* Do not crush or chew. *MS Contin:* Use only in opioid-tolerant pts requiring over 400 mg/day. *Kadian:* Use only in opioid-tolerant pts. *Duramorph:* Risk of severe and/or sustained cardiopulmonary depression.

Do not confuse morphine with HYDROmorphone, or morphine sulfate with magnesium sulfate, MS Contin with OxyCONTIN. MSO_4 and MS are error-prone abbreviations.

FIXED-COMBINATION(S)

Embeda: morphine/naloxone (an opioid antagonist): 20 mg/0.8 mg, 30 mg/1.2 mg, 50 mg/2 mg, 60 mg/2.4 mg, 80 mg/3.2 mg, 100 mg/4 mg.

◆CLASSIFICATION

PHARMACOTHERAPEUTIC: Opioid agonist **(Schedule II)**. **CLINICAL:** Opioid analgesic.

USES

Relief of moderate to severe, acute, or chronic pain; analgesia during labor, pain due to MI, dyspnea from pulmonary edema not resulting from chemical respiratory irritant. **Infumorph:** Use in devices for managing intractable chronic pain. **Extended-release:** Use only when repeated doses for extended periods of time are required around the clock.

PRECAUTIONS

Contraindications: All Formulations: Hypersensitivity to morphine. Acute or severe asthma, GI obstruction, known or suspected paralytic ileus, severe hepatic/renal impairment, severe respiratory depression. **Extended-Release:** GI obstruction, acute postoperative pain, hypercarbia. **Injection:** HF due to lung disease; arrhythmias, head injury, seizures, acute alcoholism. Labor when premature birth expected. Increased intracranial pressure. **Immediate-Release (Tablets, Oral Solution):** Hypercarbia. **Extreme Caution:** COPD, cor pulmonale, hypoxia, hypercapnia, preexisting respiratory depression, head injury, increased ICP, severe hypotension. **Cautions:** Biliary tract disease, pancreatitis, Addison's disease, cardiovascular disease, morbid obesity, adrenal insufficiency, elderly, hypothyroidism, urethral stricture, prostatic hyperplasia, debilitated pts, pts with CNS depression, toxic psychosis, seizure disorders, alcoholism.

ACTION

Binds with opioid receptors within CNS, inhibiting ascending pain pathways. **Therapeutic Effect:** Alters pain perception, emotional response to pain.

PHARMACOKINETICS

Route	Onset	Peak	Duration
Oral solution	30 min	1 hr	3–5 hrs
Tablets	30 min	1 hr	3–5 hrs
Tablets (extended-release)	N/A	3–4 hrs	8–12 hrs
IV	Rapid	0.3 hr	3–5 hrs
IM	5–30 min	0.5–1 hr	3–5 hrs
Epidural	15–60 min	1 hr	12–20 hrs
SQ	10–30 min	1.1–5 hrs	3–5 hrs
Rectal	20–60 min	0.5–1 hr	3–7 hrs

Variably absorbed from GI tract. Readily absorbed after IM, SQ administration. Protein binding: 20%–35%. Widely distributed. Metabolized in liver. Primarily excreted in urine. Removed

M

✿ Canadian trade name   🚫 Non-Crushable Drug   ▨ High Alert drug by hemodialysis. **Half-life:** 2–4 hrs (increased in hepatic disease).

⧗ LIFESPAN CONSIDERATIONS

Pregnancy/Lactation: Crosses placenta. Distributed in breast milk. May prolong labor if administered in latent phase of first stage of labor or before cervical dilation of 4–5 cm has occurred. Respiratory depression may occur in neonate if mother received opiates during labor. Regular use of opiates during pregnancy may produce withdrawal symptoms in neonate (irritability, excessive crying, tremors, hyperactive reflexes, fever, vomiting, diarrhea, yawning, sneezing, seizures). **Children:** Paradoxical excitement may occur; those younger than 2 yrs are more susceptible to respiratory depressant effects. **Elderly:** Paradoxical excitement may occur. Age-related renal impairment may increase risk of urinary retention.

INTERACTIONS

DRUG: Alcohol, other **CNS depressants** (e.g., **LORazepam, gabapentin, zolpidem**) may increase CNS effects, respiratory depression, hypotension. **MAOIs** (e.g., **phenelzine, selegiline**) may produce serotonin syndrome. (Reduce dosage to ¼ of usual morphine dose.) **HERBAL: Gotu kola, kava kava, St. John's wort, valerian** may increase CNS depression. **FOOD:** None known. **LAB VALUES:** May increase serum amylase, lipase.

AVAILABILITY (Rx)

Injection, Solution: 2 mg/mL, 4 mg/mL, 5 mg/mL, 10 mg/mL, 15 mg/mL. **Injection, Solution (Epidural, Intrathecal, IV Infusion) (Duramorph):** 0.5 mg/mL, 1 mg/mL. **Injection, Solution (Epidural or Intrathecal) (Infumorph):** 10 mg/mL, 25 mg/mL. **Injection, Solution Patient-Controlled Analgesia (PCA) Pump:** 1 mg/mL. **Solution Oral:** 10 mg/5 mL, 20 mg/5 mL. **Suppository:** 5 mg, 10 mg, 20 mg, 30 mg. **Tablets:** 15 mg, 30 mg.

 Capsules, Extended-Release: 30 mg, 45 mg, 60 mg, 75 mg, 90 mg, 120 mg. **Capsules, Sustained-Release:** 10 mg, 20 mg, 30 mg, 50 mg, 60 mg, 80 mg, 100 mg, 200 mg. **Tablets, Extended-Release:** 15 mg, 30 mg, 60 mg, 100 mg, 200 mg.

ADMINISTRATION/HANDLING

💉 IV

Reconstitution • May give undiluted. • For IV injection, may dilute in Sterile Water for Injection or 0.9% NaCl to final concentration of 1–2 mg/mL. • For continuous IV infusion, dilute to concentration of 0.1–1 mg/mL in D_5W and give through controlled infusion device.

Rate of Administration • Always administer very slowly. Rapid IV increases risk of severe adverse reactions (apnea, chest wall rigidity, peripheral circulatory collapse, cardiac arrest, anaphylactoid effects).

Storage • Store at room temperature.

IM, SQ

• Administer slowly, rotating injection sites. • Pts with circulatory impairment experience higher risk of overdosage due to delayed absorption of repeated administration.

PO

• May give without regard to food. • Mix liquid form with fruit juice to improve taste. • Do not break, crush, dissolve, or divide extended-release capsule, tablets. • **Avinza, Kadian:** May mix with applesauce immediately prior to administration.

Rectal

• If suppository is too soft, chill for 30 min in refrigerator or run cold water over foil wrapper. • Moisten suppository with cold water before inserting well into rectum.

▦ IV INCOMPATIBILITIES

Amphotericin B complex (Abelcet, AmBisome, Amphotec), cefepime (Maxipime), DOXOrubicin (Doxil), phenytoin (Dilantin).

⚕ IV COMPATIBILITIES

Amiodarone (Cordarone), atropine, bumetanide (Bumex), bupivacaine (Marcaine, Sensorcaine), dexmedetomidine (Precedex), diltiaZEM (Cardizem), diphenhydrAMINE (Benadryl), DOBUTamine (Dobutrex), DOPamine (Intropin), glycopyrrolate (Robinul), heparin, hydrOXYzine (Vistaril), lidocaine, LORazepam (Ativan), magnesium, midazolam (Versed), milrinone (Primacor), nitroglycerin, potassium, propofol (Diprivan).

INDICATIONS/ROUTES/DOSAGE
◄ **ALERT** ► Dosage should be titrated to desired effect.

Analgesia
PO *(Immediate-Release):* **ADULTS, ELDERLY:** 10–30 mg q4h as needed. *(Solution):* 10–20 mg q4h as needed. *(Tablet):* 15–30 mg q4h as needed. **CHILDREN 6 MONTHS OF AGE AND OLDER WEIGHING 50 KG OR GREATER:** 15–20 mg q3–4h as needed. **CHILDREN 6 MONTHS OF AGE AND OLDER WEIGHING LESS THAN 50 KG:** 0.2–0.5 mg/kg q3–4h as needed. **CHILDREN YOUNGER THAN 6 MONTHS:** *(Oral solution):* 0.08–0.1 mg/kg q3–4h as needed.
◄ **ALERT** ► For the AVINza dosage below, be aware that this drug is to be administered once daily only.
◄ **ALERT** ► For the Kadian dosage information below, be aware that this drug is to be administered q12h or once daily.
◄ **ALERT** ► Be aware that pediatric dosages of extended-release preparations of Kadian and AVINza have not been established.
◄ **ALERT** ► For the MS Contin dosage information below, be aware that the daily dosage is divided and given q8h or q12h.
PO *(Extended-Release [Avinza]):* **ADULTS, ELDERLY:** Dosage requirement should be established using prompt-release formulations and is based on total daily dose. AVINza is given once daily only.

PO *(Extended-Release [Kadian]):* **ADULTS, ELDERLY:** Dosage requirement should be established using prompt-release formulations and is based on total daily dose. Dose is given once daily or divided and given q12h.
PO *(Extended-Release [MS Contin]):* **ADULTS, ELDERLY:** Dosage requirement should be established using prompt-release formulations and is based on total daily dose. Daily dose is divided and given q8h or q12h.
IV: **ADULTS, ELDERLY:** 2.5–5 mg q3–4h as needed. **Note:** Repeated doses (e.g., 1–2 mg) may be given more frequently (e.g., every hr) if needed. **CHILDREN 50 KG OR GREATER:** Initially, 2–5 mg q2–4h as needed. **CHILDREN WEIGHING LESS THAN 50 KG:** Initially, 0.05 mg/kg. Range: 0.1–0.2 mg/kg q2–4h as needed. **NEONATES:** Initially, 0.05–0.1 mg/kg/dose q4–6h as needed.
IV Continuous Infusion: ADULTS, ELDERLY: 0.8–10 mg/hr. Range: Titrate up to 80 mg/hr. **CHILDREN WEIGHING 50 KG OR GREATER:** 1.5 mg/hr. **CHILDREN WEIGHING LESS THAN 50 KG:** Initially, 0.01 mg/kg/hr. Range: 0.01–0.04 mg/kg/hr (10–40 mcg/kg/hr). **NEONATES:** Initially, 0.01 mg/kg/hr (10 mcg/kg/hr). **Maximum:** 0.015–0.02 mg/kg/hr.
Note: IM injection not recommended
IM: ADULTS, ELDERLY: 5–10 mg q3–4h as needed. **CHILDREN:** 0.1–0.2 mg/kg q3–4h as needed.

Patient-Controlled Analgesia (PCA)
IV: ADULTS, ELDERLY: Usual concentration: 1 mg/mL. **Demand dose:** 1 mg (range: 0.5–2.5 mg). **Lockout interval:** 5–10 min.

Dosage in Renal Impairment

Creatinine Clearance	Dose
10–50 mL/min, CRRT	75% of normal dose
Less than 10 mL/min, HD, PD	50% of normal dose

Dosage in Hepatic Impairment
No dose adjustment.

M

SIDE EFFECTS

◄**ALERT**► Ambulatory pts, pts not in severe pain may experience nausea, vomiting more frequently than pts in supine position or who have severe pain. **Frequent:** Sedation, decreased B/P (including orthostatic hypotension), diaphoresis, facial flushing, constipation, dizziness, drowsiness, nausea, vomiting. **Occasional:** Allergic reaction (rash, pruritus), dyspnea, confusion, palpitations, tremors, urinary retention, abdominal cramps, vision changes, dry mouth, headache, decreased appetite, pain/burning at injection site. **Rare:** Paralytic ileus.

ADVERSE EFFECTS/TOXIC REACTIONS

Overdose results in respiratory depression, skeletal muscle flaccidity, cold/clammy skin, cyanosis, extreme drowsiness progressing to seizures, stupor, coma. Tolerance to analgesic effect, physical dependence may occur with repeated use. Prolonged duration of action, cumulative effect may occur in those with hepatic/renal impairment. **Antidote:** Naloxone (see Appendix J for dosage).

NURSING CONSIDERATIONS

BASELINE ASSESSMENT

Pt should be in recumbent position before drug is given by parenteral route. Assess onset, type, location, duration of pain. Obtain vital signs before giving medication. If respirations are 12/min or less (20/min or less in children), withhold medication, contact physician. Effect of medication is reduced if full pain recurs before next dose.

INTERVENTION/EVALUATION

Monitor vital signs 5–10 min after IV administration, 15–30 min after SQ, IM. Be alert for decreased respirations, B/P. Check for adequate voiding. Monitor daily pattern of bowel activity, stool consistency; avoid constipation. Initiate deep breathing, coughing exercises, particularly in those with pulmonary impairment. Assess for clinical improvement; record onset of pain relief. Consult physician if pain relief is not adequate.

PATIENT/FAMILY TEACHING

• Discomfort may occur with injection. • Change positions slowly to avoid orthostatic hypotension. • Avoid tasks that require alertness, motor skills until response to drug is established. • Avoid alcohol, CNS depressants. • Tolerance, dependence may occur with prolonged use of high doses. • Report ineffective pain control, constipation, urinary retention.

moxifloxacin

mox-i-**flox**-a-sin
(Avelox, Avelox IV, Moxeza, Vigamox)

■ **BLACK BOX ALERT** ■ May increase risk of tendonitis, tendon rupture (increased with concurrent corticosteroids, organ transplant recipients, those older than 60 yrs). May aggravate myasthenia gravis (avoid use).
Do not confuse Avelox with Avonex.

◆**CLASSIFICATION**

PHARMACOTHERAPEUTIC: Fluoroquinolone. **CLINICAL:** Antibacterial, antibiotic.

USES

Treatment of susceptible infections due to *S. pneumoniae, S. pyogenes, S. aureus, H. influenzae, M. catarrhalis, K. pneumoniae, M. pneumoniae, C. pneumoniae* including acute bacterial exacerbation of chronic bronchitis, acute bacterial sinusitis, intra-abdominal infection, community-acquired pneumonia, uncomplicated skin/skin structure infections. **Ophthalmic:** Topical treatment of bacterial conjunctivitis due to susceptible strains of bacteria.

PRECAUTIONS

Contraindications: Hypersensitivity to moxifloxacin, other quinolones. **Cautions:** Renal/hepatic impairment, bradycardia, acute myocardial ischemia, myasthenia gravis, diabetes, rheumatoid arthritis, seizures, pts with prolonged QT interval, medications known to prolong QT interval, hypokalemia, hypomagnesemia, elderly, pts with suspected CNS disorder, pts at risk for tendon rupture, tendonitis (e.g., renal failure, concomitant use of corticosteroids; solid organ transplant recipient, elderly).

ACTION

Inhibits two enzymes, topoisomerase II and IV, in susceptible microorganisms. **Therapeutic Effect:** Interferes with bacterial DNA replication. Prevents/delays emergence of resistant organisms. Bactericidal.

PHARMACOKINETICS

Well absorbed from GI tract after PO administration. Protein binding: 50%. Widely distributed throughout body with tissue concentration often exceeding plasma concentration. Metabolized in liver. Excreted in urine (20%), feces (25%) unchanged. **Half-life: PO:** 12 hrs; **IV:** 15 hrs.

LIFESPAN CONSIDERATIONS

Pregnancy/Lactation: May be distributed in breast milk. May produce teratogenic effects. **Children:** Safety and efficacy not established. **Elderly:** No age-related precautions noted.

INTERACTIONS

DRUG: Antacids, iron preparations, sucralfate may decrease absorption. **NSAIDs (e.g., ibuprofen, ketorolac, naproxen)** may increase risks of CNS stimulation/seizures. **HERBAL:** None significant. **FOOD:** None known. **LAB VALUES:** None significant.

AVAILABILITY (Rx)

Injection Infusion (Avelox IV): 400 mg (250 mL). **Ophthalmic Solution (Moxeza, Vigamox):** 0.5%. **Tablets (Avelox):** 400 mg.

ADMINISTRATION/HANDLING

 IV

Reconstitution • Available in ready-to-use containers.
Rate of Administration • Give by IV infusion only. • Avoid rapid or bolus IV infusion. • Infuse over 60 min.
Storage • Store at room temperature. • Do not refrigerate.

PO
• Give without regard to meals. • Oral moxifloxacin should be administered 4 hrs before or 8 hrs after antacids, multivitamins, iron preparations, sucralfate, didanosine chewable/buffered tablets, pediatric powder for oral solution.

Ophthalmic
• Place gloved finger on lower eyelid and pull out until a pocket is formed between eye and lower lid. • Place prescribed number of drops into pocket. • Instruct pt to close eye gently (so medication will not be squeezed out of the sac) and to apply digital pressure to lacrimal sac at inner canthus for 1 min to minimize systemic absorption.

IV INCOMPATIBILITIES

Do not add or infuse other drugs simultaneously through the same IV line. Flush line before and after use if same IV line is used with other medications.

INDICATIONS/ROUTES/DOSAGE

Usual Dose
PO, IV: ADULTS, ELDERLY: 400 mg q24h. Duration dependent on severity of infection.

Acute Bacterial Sinusitis
PO, IV: ADULTS, ELDERLY: 400 mg q24h for 10 days.

Acute Bacterial Exacerbation of Chronic Bronchitis
PO, IV: ADULTS, ELDERLY: 400 mg q24h for 5 days.

Community-Acquired Pneumonia
PO, IV: ADULTS, ELDERLY: 400 mg q24h for 7–14 days.

Intra-Abdominal Infection
PO, IV: ADULTS, ELDERLY: 400 mg q24h for 5–14 days.

Skin/Skin Structure Infection
PO, IV: ADULTS, ELDERLY: 400 mg once daily for 7–21 days.

Topical Treatment of Bacterial Conjunctivitis Due to Susceptible Strains of Bacteria
Ophthalmic: ADULTS, ELDERLY, CHILDREN 1 YR AND OLDER: (Vigamox): 1 drop 3 times/day for 7 days. **(Moxeza):** 1 drop 2 times/day for 7 days.

Dosage in Renal Impairment
No dose adjustment.

Dosage in Hepatic Impairment
Mild to moderate impairment: No dose adjustment. **Severe impairment:** Use caution.

SIDE EFFECTS

Frequent (8%–6%): Nausea, diarrhea. **Occasional: PO, IV (3%–2%):** Dizziness, headache, abdominal pain, vomiting. **Ophthalmic (6%–1%):** Conjunctival irritation, reduced visual acuity, dry eye, keratitis, eye pain, ocular itching, swelling of tissue around cornea, eye discharge, fever, cough, pharyngitis, rash, rhinitis. **Rare (1%):** Altered taste, dyspepsia, photosensitivity.

ADVERSE EFFECTS/ TOXIC REACTIONS

Pseudomembranous colitis (severe abdominal cramps/pain, severe watery diarrhea, fever) may occur. Superinfection (anal/genital pruritus, moderate to severe diarrhea, stomatitis) may occur. May increase risk of tendonitis, tendon rupture, peripheral neuropathy.

NURSING CONSIDERATIONS

BASELINE ASSESSMENT

Obtain serum BUN, creatinine; CrCl, GFR in pts with renal impairment; LFT in pts with hepatic impairment. Obtain bacterial culture and sensitivity prior to administration. Question pt's usual stool characteristics (color, frequency, consistency). Question medical history as listed in Precautions, esp. cardiac conduction disorders, CNS disorders, hypersensitivity reaction.

INTERVENTION/EVALUATION

Monitor for CNS reactions (agitation, anxiety, convulsions, depression, hallucinations, increased ICP, insomnia, nightmares, suicidal ideation and behavior), peripheral neuropathy; hypersensitivity reactions (throat and facial edema, dyspnea, urticaria, itching, hemodynamic instability); muscle weakness, voice dystonia in pts with myasthenia gravis; pain, swelling, bruising, popping of tendons. Be alert for superinfections. Obtain EKG if cardiac arrhythmia suspected or palpitations occur. Observe daily pattern of bowel activity, stool consistency (increased severity may indicate antibiotic-associated colitis). If frequent diarrhea occurs, obtain *C. difficile* toxin screen and initiate isolation precautions until test result confirmed. Antibacterial drugs that are not directed against *C. difficile* infection may need to be discontinued. Monitor I&O.

PATIENT/FAMILY TEACHING

• It is essential to complete drug therapy despite symptom improvement. Early discontinuation may result in antibacterial resistance or increase risk of recurrent infection. • Report any episodes of diarrhea, esp. during the first few mos after final dose. Frequent diarrhea, fever, abdominal pain, blood-streaked stool may indicate infectious diarrhea, which may be contagious to others. • Severe allergic reactions, such as hives, palpitations, rash, shortness of breath, swelling of tongue, may occur. • Tendon inflammation/ swelling, tendon rupture may occur; report bruising, pain, swelling in tendon areas or snapping, popping of tendons. • Immediately report nervous system problems such as anxiety, confusion, dizziness, nervousness, nightmares, thoughts of suicide, seizures, tremors, trouble sleeping. • Treatment may cause heart problems such as low heart rate, palpitations; permanent nerve damage such as burning, numbness, tingling, weakness. • Do not take aluminum- or magnesium-containing antacids, multivitamins, zinc or iron products at least 2 hrs before or 6 hrs after dose. • Drink plenty of fluids.

mupirocin

mue-peer-oh-sin
(Bactroban, Bactroban Nasal)
Do not confuse Bactroban or Bactroban Nasal with bacitracin, baclofen, or Bactrim.

◆CLASSIFICATION

PHARMACOTHERAPEUTIC: Antibacterial. **CLINICAL:** Topical antibiotic.

USES

Ointment: Topical treatment of impetigo caused by *S. aureus, S. pyogenes.* **Cream:** Treatment of traumatic skin lesions due to *S. aureus, S. pyogenes.* **Intranasal ointment:** Eradication of nasal colonization with MRSA to reduce risk of MRSA infection among high-risk pts. **OFF-LABEL:** Surgical prophylaxis to prevent wound infections (intranasal).

PRECAUTIONS

Contraindications: Hypersensitivity to mupirocin. **Cautions:** Renal impairment, burn pts.

ACTION

Inhibits bacterial protein, RNA synthesis. Less effective on DNA synthesis. **Therapeutic Effect:** Prevents bacterial growth, replication. Bacteriostatic.

PHARMACOKINETICS

Following topical administration, penetrates outer layer of skin (minimal through intact skin). Protein binding: 95%. Metabolized in liver. Excreted in urine. **Half-life:** 17–36 min.

⧗ LIFESPAN CONSIDERATIONS

Pregnancy/Lactation: Unknown if distributed in breast milk. Breastfeeding not recommended. **Children:** Safety and efficacy not established. **Elderly:** No age-related precautions noted.

INTERACTIONS

DRUG: None significant. **HERBAL:** None significant. **FOOD:** None known. **LAB VALUES:** None significant.

AVAILABILITY (Rx)

Cream, Topical (Bactroban): 2%. **Ointment, Intranasal** (1-g single-use tube) (Bactroban Nasal): 2%. **Ointment, Topical** (Bactroban): 2%.

ADMINISTRATION/HANDLING

Topical
Cream, Ointment • For topical use only. • May cover with gauze dressing. • Avoid contact with eyes.

Intranasal
• Apply ½ of the ointment from single-use tube into each nostril. • Avoid contact with eyes.

INDICATIONS/ROUTES/DOSAGE

Usual Topical Dosage
Topical Cream: ADULTS, ELDERLY, CHILDREN 3 MOS AND OLDER: Apply small amount 3 times/day for 10 days. **Topical Ointment: ADULTS, ELDERLY, CHILDREN 2 MOS AND OLDER:** Apply small amount 3 times/day for 5–14 days.

M

Usual Nasal Dosage

Intranasal: ADULTS, ELDERLY, CHILDREN 12 YRS AND OLDER: Apply small amount 2 times/day for 5–10 days.

SIDE EFFECTS

Frequent: Nasal (9%–3%): Headache, rhinitis, upper respiratory congestion, pharyngitis, altered taste. **Occasional: Nasal (2%):** Burning, stinging, cough. **Topical (2%–1%):** Pain, burning, stinging, pruritus. **Rare: Nasal (less than 1%):** Pruritus, diarrhea, dry mouth, epistaxis, nausea, rash. **Topical (less than 1%):** Rash, nausea, dry skin, contact dermatitis.

ADVERSE EFFECTS/ TOXIC REACTIONS

Superinfection may result in bacterial, fungal infections, esp. with prolonged, repeated therapy.

NURSING CONSIDERATIONS

BASELINE ASSESSMENT

Assess skin for type, extent of lesions.

INTERVENTION/EVALUATION

Monitor healing of skin lesions. In event of skin reaction, stop applications, cleanse area gently, notify physician.

PATIENT/FAMILY TEACHING

• For external use only. • Avoid contact with eyes. • Explain precautions to avoid spread of infection; teach how to apply medication. • Report skin reactions, irritation. • Report if no improvement is noted in 3–5 days.

mycophenolate

mye-koe-**fen**-o-late
(Apo-Mycophenolate ✣, CellCept, Myfortic, Novo-Mycophenolate)
■ **BLACK BOX ALERT** ■ Increased risk of congenital malformation, spontaneous abortion. Increased risk for development of lymphoma, skin malignancy. Increased susceptibility to infections. Administer under supervision of physician experienced in immunosuppressive therapy.

◆CLASSIFICATION

PHARMACOTHERAPEUTIC: Immunologic agent. **CLINICAL:** Immunosuppressant.

USES

Should be used concurrently with cycloSPORINE and corticosteroids. **Cell-Cept:** Prophylaxis of organ rejection in pts receiving allogeneic hepatic/renal/cardiac transplant. **Myfortic:** Renal transplants. **OFF-LABEL:** Treatment of hepatic transplant rejection in pts unable to tolerate tacrolimus or cycloSPORINE due to toxicity, mild heart transplant rejection, moderate to severe psoriasis, proliferative lupus nephritis, myasthenia gravis, graft-vs-host disease. Treatment of autoimmune hepatitis (refractory).

PRECAUTIONS

Contraindications: Hypersensitivity to mycophenolate, mycophenolic acid or polysorbate 80 (IV formulation). **Cautions:** Active severe GI disease, renal impairment, neutropenia, women of childbearing potential (use caution when handling).

ACTION

Suppresses immunologically mediated inflammatory response by inhibiting inosine monophosphate dehydrogenase, an enzyme that deprives lymphocytes of nucleotides necessary for DNA, RNA synthesis, thus inhibiting proliferation of T and B lymphocytes. **Therapeutic Effect:** Prevents transplant rejection.

PHARMACOKINETICS

Rapidly, extensively absorbed after PO administration (food decreases drug plasma concentration but does not affect absorption). Protein binding: 97%. Completely hydrolyzed to active metabolite mycophenolic acid. Primarily excreted in urine. Not removed by hemodialysis. **Half-life:** 17.9 hrs.

⧖ LIFESPAN CONSIDERATIONS

Pregnancy/Lactation: Unknown if drug crosses placenta or is distributed in breast milk. Breastfeeding not recommended. Increased risk of miscarriage, birth defects. Effective contraception should be used during treatment and for 6 wks after discontinuation. **Children:** Safety and efficacy not established in children younger than 3 months. **Elderly:** Age-related renal impairment may require dosage adjustment.

INTERACTIONS

DRUG: May increase concentrations of **acyclovir, ganciclovir** in pts with renal impairment. **Antacids (aluminum- and magnesium-containing), cholestyramine** may decrease absorption. **Live virus vaccines** may potentiate virus replication, increase vaccine side effects, decrease pt's antibody response to vaccine. **Other immunosuppressants (e.g., cyclophosphamide, cycloSPORINE, tacrolimus)** may increase risk of infection, lymphomas. **Probenecid** may increase concentration. **HERBAL:** Cat's claw, echinacea may decrease effects (have immunostimulant properties). **FOOD:** All foods may decrease concentration. **LAB VALUES:** May increase serum cholesterol, alkaline phosphatase, creatinine, ALT, AST. May alter serum glucose, lipids, calcium, potassium, phosphate, uric acid.

AVAILABILITY (Rx)

Capsules (CellCept): 250 mg. **Injection, Powder for Reconstitution (CellCept):** 500 mg. **Oral Suspension (CellCept):** 200 mg/mL. **Tablets (CellCept):** 500 mg.

⧖ **Tablets (Delayed-Release [Myfortic]):** 180 mg, 360 mg.

ADMINISTRATION/HANDLING

 IV

Reconstitution • Reconstitute each 500-mg vial with 14 mL D_5W. Gently agitate. • For 1-g dose, further dilute with 140 mL D_5W; for 1.5-g dose, further dilute with 210 mL D_5W, providing a concentration of 6 mg/mL.
Rate of Administration • Infuse over at least 2 hrs. • Begin infusion within 4 hrs of reconstitution.
Storage • Store at room temperature.

PO
• Give on empty stomach (1 hr before or 2 hrs after food). • Do not break, crush, or open capsules or break, crush, dissolve, or divide delayed-release tablets. Avoid inhalation of powder in capsules, direct contact of powder on skin/mucous membranes. If contact occurs, wash thoroughly, with soap, water. Rinse eyes profusely with plain water. • May store reconstituted suspension in refrigerator or at room temperature. • Suspension is stable for 60 days after reconstitution. • Suspension can be administered orally or via an NG tube (minimum size 8 French).

▦ IV INCOMPATIBILITIES

Mycophenolate is compatible only with D_5W. Do not infuse concurrently with other drugs or IV solutions.

INDICATIONS/ROUTES/DOSAGE

Prevention of Renal Transplant Rejection
PO, IV *(Cellcept):* **ADULTS, ELDERLY:** 1 g twice daily. **PO: CHILDREN 3 MONTHS AND OLDER:** *(Cellcept Suspension):* 600 mg/m²/dose twice daily. **Maximum:** 1 g twice daily.
PO *(Myfortic):* **ADULTS, ELDERLY:** 720 mg twice daily. **CHILDREN 5–16 YRS:** 400 mg/m² twice daily. **Maximum:** 720 mg twice daily.

M

Prevention of Heart Transplant Rejection
PO, IV *(Cellcept):* ADULTS, ELDERLY: 1.5 g twice daily.

Prevention of Hepatic Transplant Rejection
PO *(Cellcept):* ADULTS, ELDERLY: 1.5 g twice daily.
IV *(Cellcept):* ADULTS, ELDERLY: 1 g twice daily.

Dosage in Renal/Hepatic Impairment
No dose adjustment.

SIDE EFFECTS

Frequent (37%–20%): UTI, hypertension, peripheral edema, diarrhea, constipation, fever, headache, nausea. **Occasional (18%–10%):** Dyspepsia, dyspnea, cough, hematuria, asthenia, vomiting, edema, tremors, oral candidiasis, acne; abdominal, chest, back pain. **Rare (9%–6%):** Insomnia, respiratory tract infection, rash, dizziness.

ADVERSE EFFECTS/ TOXIC REACTIONS

Significant anemia, leukopenia, thrombocytopenia, neutropenia, leukocytosis may occur, particularly in pts undergoing renal transplant rejection. Sepsis, infection occur occasionally. GI tract hemorrhage occurs rarely. There is an increased risk of developing neoplasms. Immunosuppression results in increased susceptibility to infection.

NURSING CONSIDERATIONS

BASELINE ASSESSMENT
Women of childbearing potential should have a negative serum or urine pregnancy test within 1 wk before initiation. Assess medical history, esp. renal function, existence of active digestive system disease, drug history, esp. other immunosuppressants.

INTERVENTION/EVALUATION
CBC should be performed wkly during first mo of therapy, twice monthly during second and third mos of treatment, then monthly throughout the first yr. If rapid fall in WBC occurs, dosage should be reduced or discontinued. Assess particularly for delayed bone marrow suppression. Report any major change in assessment of pt.

PATIENT/FAMILY TEACHING
• Effective contraception should be used before, during, and for 6 wks after discontinuing therapy, even if pt has a history of infertility, other than hysterectomy. • Two forms of contraception must be used concurrently unless abstinence is absolute. • Report unusual bleeding/bruising, sore throat, mouth sores, abdominal pain, fever. • Laboratory follow-up while taking medication is important part of therapy. • Malignancies may occur.

M

nafcillin

naf-**sil**-in

◆ CLASSIFICATION

PHARMACOTHERAPEUTIC:
Penicillinase-resistant penicillin.
CLINICAL: Antibiotic.

USES

Treatment of respiratory tract, skin/skin structure infections, osteomyelitis, endocarditis, meningitis; perioperatively, esp. in cardiovascular, orthopedic procedures. Predominant treatment of infections caused by susceptible strains of staphylococci.

PRECAUTIONS

Contraindications: Hypersensitivity to nafcillin, other penicillins. **Cautions:** History of allergies, particularly cephalosporins; severe renal/hepatic impairment; asthma, pts with HF.

ACTION

Binds to bacterial membranes. **Therapeutic Effect:** Inhibits cell wall synthesis. Bactericidal.

⧗ LIFESPAN CONSIDERATIONS

Pregnancy/Lactation: Readily crosses placenta; appears in cord blood, amniotic fluid. Distributed in breast milk. May lead to rash, diarrhea, candidiasis in neonate, infant. **Children:** Immature renal function in neonate may delay renal excretion. **Elderly:** Age-related renal impairment may require dosage adjustment.

INTERACTIONS

DRUG: High doses (2 g q4h) may decrease effects of **warfarin. HERBAL:** None significant. **FOOD:** None known. **LAB VALUES:** May cause false-positive Coombs' test.

AVAILABILITY (Rx)

Injection, Powder for Reconstitution: 1 g, 2 g. **Infusion (Premix):** 1 g/50 mL, 2 g/100 mL.

ADMINISTRATION/HANDLING

◀**ALERT**▶ Space doses evenly around the clock.

🗐 IV

Reconstitution • Reconstitute each vial with 10 mL Sterile Water for Injection or 0.9% NaCl. • For intermittent IV infusion (piggyback), further dilute with 50–100 mL 0.9% NaCl or D₅W.
Rate of Administration • Infuse over 30–60 min. • Because of potential for hypersensitivity/anaphylaxis, start initial dose at few drops per min, increase slowly to ordered rate; stay with pt first 10–15 min, then check q10min. • Limit IV therapy to less than 48 hrs, if possible. Stop infusion if pt complains of pain at IV site.
Storage • Refrigerate diluted solution for up to 7 days or store at room temperature for up to 24 hrs. • Discard if precipitate forms.

IM

• Reconstitute each 500 mg with 1.7 mL Sterile Water for Injection or 0.9% NaCl to provide concentration of 250 mg/mL. • Inject IM into large muscle mass.

▦ IV INCOMPATIBILITIES

Aztreonam (Azactam), diltiaZEM (Cardizem), droperidol (Inapsine), fentaNYL, gentamicin, insulin, labetalol (Normodyne, Trandate), methylPREDNISolone (Solu-Medrol), midazolam (Versed), nalbuphine (Nubain), vancomycin (Vancocin), verapamil (Isoptin).

▦ IV COMPATIBILITIES

Acyclovir, famotidine (Pepcid), fluconazole (Diflucan), heparin, HYDROmorphone (Dilaudid), lidocaine, lipids, magnesium, morphine, potassium chloride, propofol (Diprivan).

INDICATIONS/ROUTES/DOSAGE

Usual Dosage
IV: ADULTS, ELDERLY: 0.5–2 g q4–6h. **CHILDREN: Mild to Moderate Infections:** 100–150 mg/kg/day in divided

N

doses q6h. **Maximum:** 4 g/day. **Severe Infections:** 150–200 mg/kg/day in divided doses q4–6h. **Maximum:** 12 g/day. **NEONATES:** 25 mg/kg/dose in divided doses q6–12h.

IM: **ADULTS, ELDERLY:** 500 mg q4–6h.

Dosage in Renal/Hepatic Impairment
No dose adjustment.

SIDE EFFECTS

Frequent: Mild hypersensitivity reaction (fever, rash, pruritus), GI effects (nausea, vomiting, diarrhea). **Occasional:** Hypokalemia with high IV dosages, phlebitis, thrombophlebitis (common in elderly). **Rare:** Extravasation with IV administration.

ADVERSE EFFECTS/TOXIC REACTIONS

Potentially fatal antibiotic-associated colitis, superinfections (abdominal cramps, severe watery diarrhea, fever) may result from altered bacterial balance in GI tract. Hematologic effects (esp. involving platelets, WBCs), severe hypersensitivity reactions, anaphylaxis occur rarely.

NURSING CONSIDERATIONS

BASELINE ASSESSMENT

Question for history of allergies, esp. penicillins, cephalosporins.

INTERVENTION/EVALUATION

Hold medication, promptly report rash (possible hypersensitivity), diarrhea (fever, abdominal pain, mucus/blood in stool may indicate antibiotic-associated colitis). Evaluate IV site frequently for phlebitis (heat, pain, red streaking over vein), infiltration (potential extravasation). Monitor periodic CBC, urinalysis, BMP, LFT. Be alert for superinfection: fever, vomiting, diarrhea, anal/genital pruritus, oral mucosal changes (ulceration, pain, erythema).

PATIENT/FAMILY TEACHING

• Continue antibiotic for full length of treatment. • Doses should be evenly spaced. • Discomfort may occur with IM injection. • Report IV discomfort immediately. • Report diarrhea, rash, other new symptoms.

nalbuphine

nal-bue-feen
(Nubain ✦)

◆CLASSIFICATION

PHARMACOTHERAPEUTIC: Opioid agonist, antagonist. **CLINICAL:** Opioid analgesic.

USES

Relief of moderate to severe pain, preop analgesia, obstetric analgesia, adjunct to anesthesia. **OFF-LABEL:** Opioid-induced pruritus.

PRECAUTIONS

Contraindications: Hypersensitivity to nalbuphine. **Cautions:** Hepatic/renal impairment, respiratory depression, recent MI, recent biliary tract impairment, pancreatitis, hypovolemia, head trauma, increased intracranial pressure (ICP), pregnancy, pts suspected of being opioid dependent, obesity, thyroid dysfunction, prostatic hyperplasia, urinary stricture, adrenal insufficiency, cardiovascular disease, elderly pts, debilitated pts.

ACTION

Agonist of kappa opioid receptors and partial antagonist of mu opioid receptors within CNS, inhibiting ascending pain pathways. **Therapeutic Effect:** Alters pain perception, emotional response to pain.

PHARMACOKINETICS

Route	Onset	Peak	Duration
IV	2–3 min	2–3 min	3–4 hrs
IM	Less than 15 min	30 min	3–6 hrs
SQ	Less than 15 min	N/A	3–6 hrs

Well absorbed after IM, SQ administration. Metabolized in liver. Primarily eliminated in feces by biliary secretion. **Half-life:** 3.5–5 hrs.

⌛ LIFESPAN CONSIDERATIONS

Pregnancy/Lactation: Readily crosses placenta. Distributed in breast milk. Breastfeeding not recommended. May cause fetal, neonatal adverse effects during labor/delivery (e.g., fetal bradycardia). **Children:** Paradoxical excitement may occur. Pts younger than 2 yrs more susceptible to respiratory depression. **Elderly:** More susceptible to respiratory depression. Age-related renal impairment may increase risk of urinary retention.

INTERACTIONS

DRUG: **Alcohol, other CNS depressants (e.g., LORazepam, morphine, zolpidem)** may increase CNS effects, respiratory depression, hypotension. **HERBAL:** **Gotu kola, kava kava, St. John's wort, valerian** may increase CNS depression. **FOOD:** None known. **LAB VALUES:** May increase serum amylase, lipase.

AVAILABILITY (Rx)

Injection Solution: 10 mg/mL, 20 mg/mL.

ADMINISTRATION/HANDLING

 IV

Reconstitution • May give undiluted. **Rate of Administration** • For IV push, administer each 10 mg over 3–5 min.
Storage • Store parenteral form at room temperature.

IM/Subcutaneous
• Rotate injection sites. • Administer undiluted.

💠 IV INCOMPATIBILITIES

Amphotericin B complex (Abelcet, AmBisome, Amphotec), cefepime (Maxipime), ketorolac (Toradol), nafcillin (Nafcil), piperacillin and tazobactam (Zosyn).

💠 IV COMPATIBILITIES

Dexmedetomidine (Precedex), diphenhydrAMINE (Benadryl), droperidol (Inapsine), glycopyrrolate (Robinul), hydrOXYzine (Vistaril), lidocaine, midazolam (Versed), prochlorperazine (Compazine), propofol (Diprivan).

INDICATIONS/ROUTES/DOSAGE

Analgesia
IV, IM, SQ: ADULTS, ELDERLY: 10 mg q3–6h as needed. Do not exceed maximum single dose of 20 mg or daily dose of 160 mg. **CHILDREN 1 YR AND OLDER:** 0.1–0.2 mg/kg q3–4h as needed. **Maximum:** 20 mg/dose, 160 mg/day.

Dosage in Renal/Hepatic Impairment
Use caution.

SIDE EFFECTS

Frequent (36%): Sedation. **Occasional (9%–3%):** Diaphoresis, cold/clammy skin, nausea, vomiting, dizziness, vertigo, dry mouth, headache. **Rare (less than 1%):** Restlessness, emotional lability, paresthesia, flushing, paradoxical reaction.

ADVERSE EFFECTS/TOXIC REACTIONS

Abrupt withdrawal after prolonged use may produce symptoms of narcotic withdrawal (abdominal cramping, rhinorrhea, lacrimation, anxiety, fever, piloerection [goose bumps]). Overdose results in severe respiratory depression, skeletal muscle flaccidity, cyanosis, extreme drowsiness progressing to seizures, stupor, coma. Tolerance to analgesic effect, physical dependence may occur with chronic use.

NURSING CONSIDERATIONS

BASELINE ASSESSMENT
Question medical history as listed in Precautions. Obtain vital signs before giving medication. If respirations are 12/min or less (20/min or less in children),

N

withhold medication, contact physician. Assess onset, type, location, duration of pain. Effect of medication is reduced if full pain recurs before next dose.

INTERVENTION/EVALUATION

Monitor for change in respirations, B/P, rate/quality of pulse. Monitor daily pattern of bowel activity, stool consistency. Initiate deep breathing, coughing exercises, particularly in pts with pulmonary impairment. Assess for clinical improvement, record onset of relief of pain. Consult physician if pain relief is not adequate.

PATIENT/FAMILY TEACHING

• Avoid alcohol. • Avoid tasks that require alertness, motor skills until response to drug is established. • May cause dry mouth. • May be habit forming.

---

naldemedine

nal-**dem**-e-deen
(Symproic)

♦**CLASSIFICATION**

PHARMACOTHERAPEUTIC: Opioid receptor antagonist (peripheral acting) **(Schedule II)**. **CLINICAL:** GI agent.

USES

Treatment of opioid-induced constipation (OIC) in adult pts with chronic noncancer pain, including pts with chronic pain related to prior cancer or its treatment, who do not require frequent (e.g., weekly) opioid dosage escalation.

PRECAUTIONS

Contraindications: Hypersensitivity to naldemedine. Known or suspected mechanical GI obstruction. Pts at risk of recurrent GI obstruction. **Cautions:** Severe hepatic impairment, pts with advanced illness associated with impaired structural integrity of the GI wall or conditions that may impair integrity of GI wall (e.g., Crohn's disease, diverticulitis, GI tract malignancies, intestinal adhesions, Ogilvie's syndrome, peptic ulcers, peritoneal malignancies). Concomitant use of strong CYP3A inducers, other opioid antagonists. Pts with disruption to the blood-brain barrier (may precipitate symptoms of opioid withdrawal).

ACTION

Blocks opioid binding at the peripheral mu-opioid receptors in GI tract. Inhibits the delay in GI transit times. **Therapeutic Effect:** Decreases constipating effects of opioids.

PHARMACOKINETICS

Widely distributed. Metabolized in liver. Protein binding: 93%–94%. Peak plasma concentration: 45 mins (with food: 2.5 hrs). Excreted in urine (57%), feces (35%). Not removed by dialysis. **Half-life:** 11 hrs.

⧗ LIFESPAN CONSIDERATIONS

Pregnancy/Lactation: May cross the placenta and cause fetal opiate withdrawal due to immature blood-brain barrier. Due to risk of opiate withdrawal in nursing infants, breastfeeding not recommended during treatment and for at least 3 days after discontinuation. **Children:** Safety and efficacy not established. **Elderly:** No age-related precautions noted.

INTERACTIONS

DRUG: P-gp inhibitors (e.g., amiodarone, azithromycin, carvedilol, cycloSPORINE), moderate CYP3A inhibitors (e.g., erythromycin, ciprofloxacin, diltiazem, dronedarone, fluconazole, verapamil), strong CYP3A inhibitors (e.g, ketoconazole, ritonavir) may increase concentration/effect; **Strong CYP3A inducers (e.g., carBAMazepine, phenytoin, rifAMPin)** may decrease concentration/effect. **Methylnaltrexone, opioid antagonists** may increase adverse/toxic effects. **HERBAL: St. John's wort** may decrease concentration/effect. **FOOD:** None known. **LAB VALUES:** None known.

AVAILABILITY (Rx)

Tablets: 0.2 mg.

ADMINISTRATION/HANDLING

PO
- Give with or without food.

INDICATIONS/ROUTES/DOSAGE

Opioid-Induced Constipation
PO: ADULTS, ELDERLY: 0.2 mg once daily. (Discontinue if opioid pain medication is discontinued.)

Dosage in Renal Impairment
No dose adjustment.

Dosage in Hepatic Impairment
Mild to moderate impairment: No dose adjustment. **Severe impairment:** Not recommended.

SIDE EFFECTS

Frequent (21%-12%): Abdominal pain. **Occasional (9%-3%):** Diarrhea, nausea, flatulence, vomiting, headache, hyperhidrosis.

ADVERSE EFFECTS/ TOXIC REACTIONS

Severe abdominal pain, diarrhea requiring hospitalization have occurred. GI perforation was reported in pts with baseline GI disease (Crohn's disease, diverticulitis, GI tract malignancies, peptic ulcers, Ogilvie's syndrome, peritoneal malignancies). Symptoms of opiate withdrawal including abdominal pain, anxiety, chills, diarrhea, feeling cold, flushing, hyperhidrosis, increased lacrimation, irritability, nausea were reported, esp. in pts taking methadone or with disruptions to the blood-brain barrier. May increase risk of adverse effects in pts with renal impairment.

NURSING CONSIDERATIONS

BASELINE ASSESSMENT

Discontinue all maintenance laxative therapy prior to initiation. Laxatives may be restarted if therapy has been ineffective for 3 days. Changes to analgesic dosage prior to initiation is not required. Question characteristics of constipation, frequency of bowel movements. Assess bowel sounds. Question history of GI obstruction, GI perforation, or baseline GI disease. Receive full medication history, including herbal products, and screen for interactions. Assess hydration status.

INTERVENTION/EVALUATION

Pts may be less responsive to therapy if taking opioids for less than 4 wks. Monitor for opioid withdrawal symptoms, esp. in pts taking methadone or with disruptions to blood-brain barrier. Monitor for severe, persistent, or worsening of abdominal pain; may indicate GI tract obstruction or perforation. Encourage fluid intake. Monitor daily pattern of bowel activity, stool consistency. Discontinue treatment if opioid pain medication is also discontinued. If dose is increased to 25 mg/day in pts with renal impairment, monitor for adverse effects.

PATIENT/FAMILY TEACHING

- Take with or without food. • Do not take laxatives unless approved by prescriber. • Notify prescriber if opioid pain medication is discontinued. • Immediately report severe, persistent abdominal pain; may indicate tear or blockage in GI tract. • Do not ingest grapefruit products or take herbal supplements. • Opioid withdrawal may occur in a fetus of pregnant females due to undeveloped fetal blood-brain barrier. • Do not breastfeed during treatment and for at least 3 days after last dose. • Do not take newly prescribed medication unless approved by prescriber who originally started treatment.

N

naloxegol

nal-**ox**-ee-gol
(Movantik)
Do not confuse naloxegol with naloxone.

◆CLASSIFICATION

PHARMACOTHERAPEUTIC: Mu-opioid receptor antagonist (Peripherally acting). **CLINICAL:** GI agent.

USES

Treatment of opioid-induced constipation (OIC) in adult pts with chronic non-cancer pain, including pts with chronic pain related to prior cancer or its treatment who do not require frequent (e.g., weekly) opioid dosage escalation.

PRECAUTIONS

Contraindications: Hypersensitivity to naloxegol. Known or suspected mechanical GI obstruction, pts at risk for recurrent GI obstruction. Concomitant use of strong CYP3A inhibitors. **Cautions:** Moderate to severe renal impairment, end-stage renal disease, severe hepatic impairment; pts with risk or reduction of structural wall integrity of GI tract (e.g., Crohn's disease, diverticulitis, GI tract malignancies, peptic ulcers, Ogilvie's syndrome, peritoneal metastases). Pts with disruptions to the blood-brain barrier. Concomitant use of moderate CYP3A inhibitors, P-glycoprotein (P-gp) inhibitors. Avoid concomitant use of strong CYP3A inducers, other opioid antagonists.

ACTION

Blocks opioid binding at peripheral mu-opioid receptors in GI tract. **Therapeutic Effect:** Decreases constipating effects of opioids.

PHARMACOKINETICS

Rapidly absorbed. Widely distributed. Metabolized in liver. Protein binding: 4.2%. Peak plasma concentration: less than 2 hrs. Excreted in feces (68%), urine (16%). **Half-life:** 6–11 hrs.

⌛ LIFESPAN CONSIDERATIONS

Pregnancy/Lactation: Known to cross the placenta. Use during pregnancy may induce fetal opiate withdrawal due to immature blood-brain barrier. Unknown if excreted in breast milk. Breastfeeding not recommended due to risk of opiate withdrawal in nursing infants. **Children:** Safety and efficacy not established. **Elderly:** No age-related precautions noted.

INTERACTIONS

DRUG: P-gp inhibitors (e.g., amiodarone, azithromycin, carvedilol, cycloSPORINE), moderate CYP3A inhibitors (e.g., erythromycin, ciprofloxacin, diltiazem, dronedarone, fluconazole, verapamil), strong CYP3A inhibitors (e.g., ketoconazole, ritonavir) may increase concentration/effect; may increase risk of opiate withdrawal. **Strong CYP3A inducers (e.g., carBAMazepine, phenytoin, rifAMPin)** may decrease concentration/effect. **Methylnaltrexone, opioid antagonists** may increase adverse/toxic effects. **HERBAL:** St John's wort may decrease concentration/effect. **FOOD: Grapefruit products** may increase concentration/effect. **LAB VALUES:** None known.

AVAILABILITY (Rx)

Tablets: 12.5 mg, 25 mg.

ADMINISTRATION/HANDLING

PO

• Give on empty stomach at least 1 hr prior to first meal or 2 hrs after first meal. • Swallow whole; do not chew. For pts unable to swallow tablet whole, tablets may be crushed and mixed with 120 mL water for oral administration or mixed with 60 mL for NG tube administration. After administration of crushed tablet, refill container with 120 mL (oral) or 60 mL (NG tube) of water, stir well, and give remaining contents. • Do not give with grapefruit products.

N

INDICATIONS/ROUTES/DOSAGE

Note: Discontinue all maintenance laxative therapy prior to use. May reintroduce laxatives if suboptimal response to naloxegol after 3 days.

Opioid-Induced Constipation
PO: ADULTS, ELDERLY: 25 mg once daily in AM. May reduce dose to 12.5 mg once daily if 25-mg dose is not tolerated.

Dose Modification
Concomitant use of moderate CYP3A inhibitors: 12.5 mg daily in AM. **Strong CYP3A inhibitors:** Contraindicated.

Dosage in Renal Impairment
Mild impairment: No dose adjustment. **Moderate to severe impairment (CrCl less than 60 mL/min); ESRD:** Reduce dose to 12.5 mg once daily in AM. If tolerated, may increase to 25 mg once daily in AM.

Dosage in Hepatic Impairment
Mild to moderate impairment: No dose adjustment. **Severe impairment:** Not recommended; avoid use.

SIDE EFFECTS

Frequent (21%-12%): Abdominal pain. **Occasional (9%-3%):** Diarrhea, nausea, flatulence, vomiting, headache, hyperhidrosis.

ADVERSE EFFECTS/ TOXIC REACTIONS

Severe abdominal pain, diarrhea requiring hospitalization have occurred. GI perforation was reported in pts with baseline GI disease (Crohn's disease, diverticulitis, GI tract malignancies, peptic ulcers, Ogilvie's syndrome, peritoneal malignancies). Symptoms of opiate withdrawal, including abdominal pain, anxiety, chills, diarrhea, hyperhidrosis, irritability, yawning, were reported, esp. in pts taking methadone or with disruptions to the blood-brain barrier. May increase risk of adverse effects in pts with renal impairment who have increased dose to 25 mg/day.

NURSING CONSIDERATIONS

BASELINE ASSESSMENT

Discontinue all maintenance laxative therapy prior to initiation. Laxatives may be restarted if therapy has been ineffective for 3 days. Changes to analgesic dosage prior to initiation are not required. Question characteristics of constipation, frequency of bowel movements. Assess bowel sounds. Question history of GI obstruction, perforation, baseline GI disease. Receive full medication history including herbal products and screen for interactions. Assess hydration status.

INTERVENTION/EVALUATION

Pts may be less responsive to therapy if taking opioids for less than 4 wks. Monitor for opioid withdrawal symptoms, esp. in pts taking methadone or with disruptions to blood-brain barrier. Monitor for severe, persistent, worsening of abdominal pain; may indicate GI tract obstruction, perforation. Encourage fluid intake. Monitor daily pattern of bowel activity, stool consistency. Discontinue treatment if opioid pain medication is also discontinued. If dose is increased to 25 mg/day in pts with renal impairment, monitor for increased adverse effects.

PATIENT/FAMILY TEACHING

• Take on an empty stomach in the AM at least 1 hr before or 2 hrs after morning meal. • Do not take laxatives unless approved by prescriber. • Tablets may be taken whole or crushed and mixed in water. • Notify prescriber if opioid pain medication is discontinued. • Immediately report severe, persistent abdominal pain; may indicate tear or blockage in GI tract. • Do not ingest grapefruit products or take herbal supplements. • Opioid withdrawal may occur in a fetus of pregnant females due to undeveloped fetal blood-brain barrier. • Do not breastfeed.

N

---

naloxone

nal-**ox**-own

(Evzio, Narcan, Narcan Nasal Spray)
Do not confuse naloxone with Lanoxin or naltrexone.

FIXED-COMBINATION(S)

Embeda: naloxone/morphine (an opioid agonist): 0.8 mg/20 mg, 1.2 mg/30 mg, 2 mg/50 mg, 2.4 mg/60 mg, 3.2 mg/80 mg, 4 mg/100 mg. **Suboxone (sublingual film):** naloxone/buprenorphine (an analgesic): 0.5 mg/2 mg, 1 mg/4 mg, 2 mg/8 mg, 3 mg/12 mg. **Zubsolv:** naloxone/buprenorphine: 0.36 mg/1.4 mg, 1.4 mg/5.7 mg.

◆CLASSIFICATION

PHARMACOTHERAPEUTIC: Opioid antagonist. **CLINICAL:** Antidote.

USES

Narcan: Complete or partial reversal of opioid depression including respiratory depression. Diagnosis of suspected opioid tolerance or acute opioid overdose. **Evzio, Narcan Nasal Spray:** Emergency treatment of known or suspected opioid overdose. **OFF-LABEL:** Opioid-induced pruritus.

PRECAUTIONS

Contraindications: Hypersensitivity to naloxone. **Cautions:** Cardiac/pulmonary disease. Medications with potential for adverse cardiovascular effects (e.g., hypotension, arrhythmias).

ACTION

Displaces opioids at opioid-occupied receptor sites in CNS. **Therapeutic Effect:** Reverses opioid-induced sleep/sedation, increases respiratory rate, raises B/P to normal range.

PHARMACOKINETICS

Route	Onset	Peak	Duration
IV	1–2 min	N/A	20–60 min
IM	2–5 min	N/A	20–60 min
SQ	2–5 min	N/A	20–60 min

Well absorbed after IM, SQ administration. Metabolized in liver. Primarily excreted in urine. **Half-life:** 60–100 min.

⧗ LIFESPAN CONSIDERATIONS

Pregnancy/Lactation: Unknown if drug crosses placenta or is distributed in breast milk. **Children/Elderly:** No age-related precautions noted.

INTERACTIONS

DRUG: None significant. **HERBAL:** None significant. **FOOD:** None known. **LAB VALUES:** None significant.

AVAILABILITY (Rx)

Injection, Autoinjector (Evzio): 0.4 mg/0.4 mL. **Injection Solution:** 0.4 mg/mL, 1 mg/mL. **Narcan Nasal Spray:** 4 mg/0.1 mL.

ADMINISTRATION/HANDLING

IV

Reconstitution • For IV push, may give undiluted (0.4 mg/mL or diluted with 9 mL 0.9% NaCl to concentration of 0.04 mg/mL). • For continuous IV infusion, dilute each 2 mg of naloxone with 500 mL of D₅W or 0.9% NaCl, producing solution containing 0.004 mg/mL (4 mcg/mL).
Rate of Administration • May give IV push over 30 sec.
Storage • Store parenteral form at room temperature. • Use mixture within 24 hrs; discard unused solution. • Protect from light. • Stable in D₅W or 0.9% NaCl at 4 mcg/mL for 24 hrs.

IM
• Give deep IM in large muscle mass.

▦ IV INCOMPATIBILITIES
Amphotericin B complex (Abelcet, AmBisome, Amphotec).

▨ IV COMPATIBILITIES

Heparin, ondansetron (Zofran), propofol (Diprivan).

INDICATIONS/ROUTES/DOSAGE

Note: If no response seen after a total of 10 mg, consider other causes of respiratory depression.

Opioid Overdose
IV, IM, SQ: ADULTS, ELDERLY: 0.4–2 mg q2–3min as needed. May repeat doses q20–60min. **CHILDREN 5 YRS AND OLDER, WEIGHING 20 KG OR MORE:** 2 mg/dose; if no response, may repeat q2–3min. May need to repeat doses q20–60min. **CHILDREN YOUNGER THAN 5 YRS, WEIGHING LESS THAN 20 KG:** 0.1 mg/kg (**Maximum:** 2 mg); if no response, repeat q2–3min. May need to repeat doses q20–60min. **NARCAN NASAL SPRAY: ADULTS, ELDERLY, CHILDREN:** Single spray (4 mg) into one nostril. May give q2–3min until emergency medical assistance arrives. *(Evzio):* **IM: ADULTS, ELDERLY, CHILDREN:** 0.4 mg as a single dose; may repeat q2–3min until emergency medical assistance becomes available.

Reversal of Respiratory Depression with Therapeutic Opioid Dosing
IV, IM, SQ: ADULTS, ELDERLY: Initially, 0.02–0.2 mg. Titrate to avoid profound withdrawal, seizures, arrhythmias, or severe pain. **CHILDREN:** 0.001–0.015 mg/kg. Titrate to desired effect. If administered IM or SQ, dose is to be given in divided doses.

Dosage in Renal/Hepatic Impairment
No dose adjustment.

SIDE EFFECTS

None known; little or no pharmacologic effect in absence of narcotics.

ADVERSE EFFECTS/TOXIC REACTIONS

Too-rapid reversal of narcotic-induced respiratory depression may result in agitation, nausea, vomiting, tremors, increased B/P, tachycardia, seizures.

Excessive dosage in postoperative pts may produce significant reversal of analgesia, agitation, tremors. Hypotension or hypertension, ventricular tachycardia/fibrillation, pulmonary edema may occur in pts with cardiovascular disease.

NURSING CONSIDERATIONS

BASELINE ASSESSMENT
Maintain patent airway. Obtain weight of children to calculate drug dosage.

INTERVENTION/EVALUATION
Monitor vital signs, esp. rate, depth, rhythm of respiration, during and frequently following administration. Carefully observe pt after satisfactory response (duration of opiate may exceed duration of naloxone, resulting in recurrence of respiratory depression). Assess for increased pain with reversal of opiate.

naltrexone

N

nal-**trex**-own
(Vivitrol)
Do not confuse naltrexone with naloxone.

FIXED-COMBINATION(S)

Contrave: naltrexone/bupropion (a norepinephrine-dopamine reuptake inhibitor): 8 mg/90 mg. **Troxyca ER:** naltrexone/oxyCODONE (an opioid analgesic): 1.2 mg/10 mg, 2.4 mg/20 mg, 3.6 mg/30 mg, 4.8 mg/40 mg, 7.2 mg/60 mg, 9.6 mg/80 mg.

◆CLASSIFICATION

PHARMACOTHERAPEUTIC: Opioid receptor antagonist. **CLINICAL:** Narcotic antagonist, alcohol antagonist antidote.

USES

Treatment of alcohol dependence. Blocks effects of exogenously administered opioids.

N

PRECAUTIONS

Contraindications: Hypersensitivity to naltrexone. Opioid dependence or current use of opioid analgesics, acute opioid withdrawal, failed naloxone challenge, or positive urine screen for opioids. **Cautions:** Severe hepatic impairment, pts at high risk of suicide, thrombocytopenia, depression, history of bleeding disorders, concurrent anticoagulant therapy, moderate to severe renal impairment.

ACTION

Blocks effects of endogenous opioid peptides by competitively binding at opioid receptors. **Therapeutic Effect: Alcohol deterrent:** Decreases craving, drinking days, relapse rate. **Antidote:** Blocks physical dependence of morphine, heroin, other opioids.

PHARMACOKINETICS

Route	Onset	Peak	Duration
PO	N/A	N/A	24–72 hrs
IM	N/A	2 hrs	2–4 wks

Well absorbed following PO administration. Protein binding: 21%. Metabolized in liver. Reduction in first-pass hepatic metabolism when given by intramuscular route. Excreted primarily in urine. **Half-life: PO:** 4 hrs; **IM:** 5–10 days.

⧗ LIFESPAN CONSIDERATIONS

Pregnancy/Lactation: Unknown if drug crosses placenta or is distributed in breast milk. **Children:** Safety and efficacy not established in pts younger than 18 yrs. **Elderly:** No age-related precautions noted.

INTERACTIONS

DRUG: May decrease effects of **opioid analgesics (e.g., morphine, HYDROcodone, HYDROmorphone). HERBAL:** None significant. **FOOD:** None known. **LAB VALUES:** May increase serum transaminase, ALT, AST.

AVAILABILITY (Rx)

Injection Suspension, Extended-Release Kit (Vivitrol): 380 mg/4 mL vial. **Tablets:** 50 mg.

ADMINISTRATION/HANDLING

◄**ALERT**► In pts with narcotic dependence, do not attempt treatment until pt has remained opioid free for 7–10 days. Test urine for opioids for verification. Pt should not be experiencing withdrawal symptoms.

IM

• Give in deep muscle mass of gluteal region, alternating buttocks. • Vivitrol must be suspended only in diluent supplied in kit.

Storage • Store entire diluent supplied in the kit. • All components (microspheres, diluent, preparation needle, administration needle with safety device) are required for preparation and administration. Spare administration needle is provided in case of clogging.

PO

• May take without regard to food. Administer with food or antacids or after meals to minimize adverse GI effects.

INDICATIONS/ROUTES/DOSAGE

Alcohol Dependence
PO: ADULTS, ELDERLY: 50 mg once daily. Alternative maintenance regimens may be used (e.g., 50 mg/day Monday through Friday and 100 mg on Saturday, or 100 mg every other day, or 150 mg q3days.)
IM: ADULTS, ELDERLY: (Vivitrol): 380 mg once q4wks.

Opioid Dependence
PO: ADULTS, ELDERLY: Initially, 25 mg. Observe for 1 hr. If no withdrawal signs appear, give 50 mg on day 2. Maintenance regimen is flexible, variable, and individualized. May be given as 50 mg daily, 50 mg/day Monday through Friday and 100 mg on Saturday, 100 mg every other day, or 150 mg q3days for 12 wks.
IM: ADULTS, ELDERLY: 380 mg q4wks.

Dosage in Renal Impairment
Mild impairment: No dose adjustment.
Moderate to severe impairment: Use caution.

Dosage in Hepatic Impairment
No dose adjustment. **Severe:** Use caution.

SIDE EFFECTS

Common: IM: (69%): Injection site reaction (induration, tenderness, pain, nodules, swelling, pruritus, ecchymosis). **Frequent: Alcohol Deterrent: (33%–10%):** Nausea, headache, depression. **Narcotic Addiction (10%–5%):** Insomnia, anxiety, headache, low energy, abdominal cramps, nausea, vomiting, joint/muscle pain. **Occasional: Alcohol Deterrent (4%–2%):** Dizziness, anxiety, fatigue, insomnia, vomiting, suicidal ideation. **Narcotic Addiction (5% or less):** Irritability, increased energy, dizziness, anorexia, diarrhea, constipation, rash, chills, increased thirst.

ADVERSE EFFECTS/ TOXIC REACTIONS

Signs/symptoms of opioid withdrawal include rhinorrhea, lacrimation, yawning, diaphoresis, tremor, vomiting, piloerection (goose bumps), feeling of temperature change, arthralgia, myalgia, abdominal cramps, formication (feeling of skin crawling). Accidental naltrexone overdosage produces withdrawal symptoms within 5 min of ingestion, lasts up to 48 hrs. Symptoms present as confusion, visual hallucinations, drowsiness, significant vomiting, diarrhea. Hepatotoxicity may occur with large doses.

NURSING CONSIDERATIONS

BASELINE ASSESSMENT

Treatment should not be instituted unless pt is opioid free for 7–10 days, alcohol free for 3–5 days before therapy begins. Obtain medication history (esp. opioids), other medical conditions (esp. hepatitis, other hepatic disease). If opioid dependence suspected, a naloxone challenge test should be performed (naloxone administered to verify opioid dependence and eligibility for admission to opioid treatment program).

INTERVENTION/EVALUATION

Monitor for evidence of hepatotoxicity (abdominal pain that lasts longer than a few days, white bowel movements, dark urine, jaundice). Monitor serum ALT, AST, bilirubin.

PATIENT/FAMILY TEACHING

• If heroin, other opiates are self-administered, there will be no effect. However, any attempt to overcome naltrexone's prolonged 24- to 72-hr blockade of opioid effect by taking large amounts of opioids is dangerous and may result in coma, serious injury, fatal overdose. • Naltrexone blocks effects of opioid-containing medicine (cough/ cold preparations, antidiarrheal preparations, opioid analgesics). • Report abdominal pain lasting longer than 3 days, white bowel movement, dark-colored urine, yellowing of skin or eyes.

N

naproxen

na-**prox**-en
(Aleve, Anaprox DS, Apo-Naproxen
✤, EC-Naprosyn, Naprelan, Naprosyn)

■ **BLACK BOX ALERT** ■ Increased risk of serious cardiovascular thrombotic events, including myocardial infarction, CVA. Increased risk of severe GI reactions, including ulceration, bleeding, perforation of stomach, intestines.
Do not confuse Aleve with Alesse, or Anaprox with Anaspaz or Avapro.

FIXED-COMBINATION(S)

Prevacid NapraPac: naproxen/lansoprazole (proton pump inhibitor): 375 mg/15 mg, 500 mg/15 mg.

Treximet: naproxen/SUMAtriptan (an antimigraine): 60 mg/10 mg; 500 mg/85 mg. **Vimovo:** naproxen/esomeprazole (proton pump inhibitor): 375 mg/20 mg, 500 mg/20 mg.

◆CLASSIFICATION

PHARMACOTHERAPEUTIC: NSAID.
CLINICAL: Analgesic, anti-inflammatory.

USES

Treatment of acute or long-term mild to moderate pain, primary dysmenorrhea, rheumatoid arthritis (RA), juvenile rheumatoid arthritis (JRA), osteoarthritis, ankylosing spondylitis, acute gouty arthritis, bursitis, tendonitis, fever. **OFF-LABEL:** Migraine prophylaxis.

PRECAUTIONS

Contraindications: History of asthma, urticaria; hypersensitivity to naproxen, other NSAIDs. Perioperative pain in setting of CABG surgery. **Cautions:** GI disease (bleeding, ulcers), fluid retention, renal/hepatic impairment, asthma, HF, concurrent use of anticoagulants, smoking, use of alcohol, elderly pts, debilitated pts.

ACTION

Reversibly inhibits COX-1 and COX-2 enzymes, resulting in decreased formation of prostaglandin precursors. **Therapeutic Effect:** Reduces inflammatory response, intensity of pain.

PHARMACOKINETICS

Route	Onset	Peak	Duration
PO (analgesic)	1 hr	2–4 hrs	7 hrs or less
PO (anti-inflammatory)	2 wks	2–4 wks	12 hrs

Completely absorbed from GI tract. Protein binding: 99%. Metabolized in liver. Primarily excreted in urine. Not removed by hemodialysis. **Half-life:** 13 hrs.

⧗ LIFESPAN CONSIDERATIONS

Pregnancy/Lactation: Crosses placenta. Distributed in breast milk. Avoid use during third trimester (may adversely affect fetal cardiovascular system: premature closing of ductus arteriosus). **Children:** Safety and efficacy not established in pts younger than 2 yrs. Children older than 2 yrs at increased risk for skin rash. **Elderly:** Age-related renal impairment may increase risk of hepatic/renal toxicity; reduced dosage recommended. More likely to have serious adverse effects with GI bleeding/ulceration.

INTERACTIONS

DRUG: May decrease effects of anti-hypertensives (e.g., amLODIPine, lisinopril, valsartan), diuretics (e.g., furosemide, HCTZ). Aspirin, other salicylates may increase risk of GI side effects, bleeding. **Bone marrow depressants** may increase risk of hematologic reactions. May increase risk of bleeding with heparin, oral anticoagulants (e.g., warfarin), thrombolytics (e.g., alteplase). May increase concentration, risk of toxicity of lithium. May increase risk of methotrexate toxicity. **HERBAL:** Cat's claw, dong quai, evening primrose, feverfew, garlic, ginger, ginkgo, ginseng, horse chestnut, red clover possess antiplatelet activity, may increase risk of bleeding. **FOOD:** None known. **LAB VALUES:** May prolong bleeding time. May increase serum BUN, creatinine, ALT, AST, alkaline phosphatase. May decrease Hgb, Hct, leukocytes, platelets, uric acid.

AVAILABILITY (Rx)

Capsule: 220 mg. **Oral Suspension:** 125 mg/5 mL naproxen. **Tablets:** 220 mg, 250 mg, 275 mg, 375 mg, 500 mg, 550 mg.

Tablets (Extended-Release): 375 mg, 500 mg, 750 mg.

ADMINISTRATION/HANDLING

PO

• Give controlled-release form whole. Do not break, crush, dissolve, or divide. • Best taken with food or milk (decreases GI irritation). • Shake suspension well.

INDICATIONS/ROUTES/DOSAGE

Note: Dosage expressed as naproxen base (200 mg naproxen base equivalent to 220 mg naproxen sodium).

Rheumatoid Arthritis (RA), Osteoarthritis, Ankylosing Spondylitis
PO: ADULTS, ELDERLY: *(Immediate-Release):* 500–1,000 mg/day in 2 divided doses. May increase to 1,500 mg/day for limited time. *(Extended-Release):* Initially, 750–1,000 mg once daily. May increase temporarily to 1,500 mg once daily.

Acute Gouty Arthritis
PO: ADULTS, ELDERLY: (Immediate-Release): Initially, 750 mg naproxen, then 250 mg naproxen q8h until attack subsides. *(Extended-Release):* Initially, 1,000–1,500 mg, then 1,000 mg once daily until attack subsides.

Mild to Moderate Pain, Dysmenorrhea, Bursitis, Tendonitis
PO: ADULTS, ELDERLY (Immediate-Release): Initially, 500 mg, then 500 mg q12h or 250 mg q6–8h as needed. **Maximum:** 1,250 mg on day 1, then 1,000 mg once daily. *(Extended-Release):* Initially, 1,000 mg once daily. May temporarily increase to 1,500 mg once daily, then reduce to 1,000 mg once daily.

Juvenile Idiopathic Arthritis (JIA)
PO *(Oral Suspension Recommended):* **CHILDREN OLDER THAN 2 YRS:** 10–15 mg/kg/day in 2 divided doses. **Maximum:** 1,000 mg/day.

OTC Uses (Pain, Fever)
PO: ADULTS 65 YRS AND YOUNGER, CHILDREN 12 YRS AND OLDER: Initially, 400 mg once, then 200 mg q8–12h. **ADULTS OLDER THAN 65 YRS:** 200 mg q12h. **Maximum:** 400 mg in any 8- to 12-hr period or 600 mg/day.

Dosage in Renal Impairment
Not recommended with CrCl less than 30 mL/min.

Dosage in Hepatic Impairment
Use caution.

SIDE EFFECTS

Frequent (9%–4%): Nausea, constipation, abdominal cramps/pain, heartburn, dizziness, headache, drowsiness. **Occasional (3%–1%):** Stomatitis, diarrhea, indigestion. **Rare (less than 1%):** Vomiting, confusion.

ADVERSE EFFECTS/TOXIC REACTIONS

Rare reactions with long-term use include peptic ulcer, GI bleeding, gastritis, severe hepatic reactions (cholestasis, jaundice), nephrotoxicity (dysuria, hematuria, proteinuria, nephrotic syndrome), and severe hypersensitivity reaction (fever, chills, bronchospasm).

NURSING CONSIDERATIONS

BASELINE ASSESSMENT

Assess onset, type, location, duration of pain/inflammation. Inspect appearance of affected joints for immobility, deformities, skin condition. Question history of GI bleeding, gastric or duodenal ulcers, hypertension.

INTERVENTION/EVALUATION

Assist with ambulation if dizziness occurs. Periodically monitor renal function test during chronic use. Monitor daily pattern of bowel activity, stool consistency. Evaluate for therapeutic response: relief of pain, stiffness, swelling; increased joint mobility, reduced joint tenderness, improved grip strength.

PATIENT/FAMILY TEACHING

• Avoid tasks that require alertness, motor skills until response to drug is established. • Take with food, milk. • Avoid aspirin, alcohol during therapy (increases risk of GI bleeding). • Report headache, rash, visual disturbances, weight gain, black or tarry stools, bleeding, persistent headache.

naratriptan

nar-a-**trip**-tan
(Amerge)
Do not confuse naratriptan with eletriptan or almotriptan, or Amerge with Altace or Amaryl.

◆CLASSIFICATION

PHARMACOTHERAPEUTIC: Serotonin receptor agonist. **CLINICAL:** Antimigraine.

USES

Treatment of acute migraine headache with or without aura in adults.

PRECAUTIONS

Contraindications: Hypersensitivity to naratriptan. Basilar/hemiplegic migraine, cerebrovascular disease, peripheral vascular disease, coronary artery disease, ischemic heart disease (including angina pectoris, history of MI, silent ischemia, Prinzmetal's angina), severe hepatic impairment (Child-Pugh grade C), severe renal impairment (CrCl less than 15 mL/min), uncontrolled hypertension, use within 24 hrs of ergotamine-containing preparations or another serotonin receptor agonist, 5-HT agonist (e.g., SUMAtriptan), MAOI use within 14 days. **Cautions:** Mild to moderate renal/hepatic impairment, pt profile suggesting cardiovascular risks, elderly.

ACTION

Binds selectively to serotonin receptors, producing vasoconstrictive effect on cranial blood vessels. **Therapeutic Effect:** Relieves migraine headache.

PHARMACOKINETICS

Well absorbed after PO administration. Protein binding: 28%–31%. Metabolized in liver. Eliminated primarily in urine. **Half-life:** 6 hrs (increased in hepatic/renal impairment).

⧗ LIFESPAN CONSIDERATIONS

Pregnancy/Lactation: Unknown if drug is distributed in breast milk. **Children:** Safety and efficacy not established. **Elderly:** Not recommended in the elderly.

INTERACTIONS

DRUG: Ergotamine-containing medications may produce vasospastic reaction. **SSRIs (e.g., escitalopram, paroxetine, sertraline), SNRIs (e.g., duloxetine, venlafaxine)** may produce serotonin syndrome. **HERBAL:** None significant. **FOOD:** None known. **LAB VALUES:** None significant.

AVAILABILITY (Rx)

▧ **Tablets:** 1 mg, 2.5 mg.

ADMINISTRATION/HANDLING

PO
• Give without regard to food. • Do not break, crush, dissolve, or divide tablets. Swallow whole with water.

INDICATIONS/ROUTES/DOSAGE

Acute Migraine Attack
PO: ADULTS: 1 or 2.5 mg. If headache improves but then returns, dose may be repeated after 4 hrs. **Maximum:** 5 mg/24 hrs.

Dosage in Renal/Hepatic Impairment

Hepatic Failure	Creatinine Clearance	Dosage
Mild to moderate	15–39 mL/min	Initial, 1 mg; Max: 2.5 mg/24 hrs
Severe	Less than 15 mL/min	Contraindicated

SIDE EFFECTS

Occasional (5%): Nausea. **Rare (2%):** Paresthesia, dizziness, fatigue, drowsiness, feeling of pressure in throat, neck, jaw.

ADVERSE EFFECTS/ TOXIC REACTIONS

Corneal opacities, other ocular defects may occur. Cardiac events (ischemia, coronary artery vasospasm, MI), noncardiac vasospasm-related reactions (hemorrhage, cerebrovascular accident [CVA]) occur rarely, particularly in pts with hypertension, diabetes, strong family history of coronary artery disease, obese pts, smokers, males older than 40 yrs, postmenopausal women.

NURSING CONSIDERATIONS

BASELINE ASSESSMENT

Question medical history as listed in Precautions. Question pt regarding possible precipitating symptoms, onset, location, duration of migraine.

INTERVENTION/EVALUATION

Assess for relief of migraine headache; potential for photophobia, phonophobia (sound sensitivity), nausea, vomiting.

PATIENT/FAMILY TEACHING

• Do not chew, crush, dissolve, or divide tablet; swallow whole with water. • May repeat dose after 4 hrs (maximum of 5 mg/24 hrs). • May cause dizziness, fatigue, drowsiness. • Avoid tasks that require alertness, motor skills until response to drug is established. • Report any chest pain, palpitations, tightness in throat, rash, hallucinations, anxiety, panic.

---

nateglinide HIGH ALERT

na-**te**-glye-nide
(Starlix)

◆CLASSIFICATION

PHARMACOTHERAPEUTIC: Meglitinide analogue. **CLINICAL:** Antidiabetic agent.

USES

Treatment of type 2 diabetes mellitus as an adjunct to diet and exercise.

PRECAUTIONS

Contraindications: Hypersensitivity to nateglinide. Diabetic ketoacidosis, type 1 diabetes. **Cautions:** Moderate to severe hepatic impairment, severe renal impairment, elderly pts, malnourished, adrenal/pituitary dysfunction.

ACTION

Stimulates insulin release from beta cells of pancreas by depolarizing beta cells, leading to opening of calcium channels. Resulting calcium influx induces insulin secretion. **Therapeutic Effect:** Lowers serum glucose concentration.

PHARMACOKINETICS

Route	Onset	Peak	Duration
PO	20 min	1 hr	4 hrs

Rapidly absorbed from GI tract. Protein binding: 98%. Extensive metabolism in liver. Excreted in urine (83%), feces (10%). **Half-life:** 1.5 hrs.

LIFESPAN CONSIDERATIONS

Pregnancy/Lactation: Unknown if drug crosses placenta or is distributed in breast milk. **Children:** Safety and efficacy not established. **Elderly:** Increased susceptibility to hypoglycemia.

INTERACTIONS

DRUG: Beta blockers (e.g., **carvedilol, metoprolol**) may mask symptoms of hypoglycemia. **Beta blockers (e.g., carvedilol, metoprolol), MAOIs (e.g., phenelzine, selegiline), NSAIDs (e.g., ibuprofen, ketorolac, naproxen), salicylates** may increase hypoglycemic effect. **Corticosteroids (e.g., predniSONE), sympathomimetics, thiazide diuretics (e.g., HCTZ), thyroid medications** may decrease hypoglycemic effect. **HERBAL:** Bilberry, garlic, ginger,

ginseng may increase hypoglycemic effect. **St. John's wort** may decrease concentration/effects. **FOOD:** None known. **LAB VALUES:** Decrease in serum glucose expected.

AVAILABILITY (Rx)

Tablets: 60 mg, 120 mg.

ADMINISTRATION/HANDLING

PO

• Ideally, give within 15 min of a meal, but may be given immediately before a meal to as long as 30 min before a meal.

INDICATIONS/ROUTES/DOSAGE

Diabetes Mellitus

PO: ADULTS, ELDERLY: Initial/Maintenance: 120 mg 3 times/day before meals. 60 mg 3 times/day may be given in pts close to Hgb A1c goal.

Dosage in Renal Impairment

Mild to moderate impairment: No dose adjustment. **Severe impairment:** Use caution.

Dosage in Hepatic Impairment

Mild impairment: No dose adjustment. **Moderate to severe impairment:** Use caution.

SIDE EFFECTS

Frequent (10%): Upper respiratory tract infection. **Occasional (4%–3%):** Back pain, flu-like symptoms, dizziness, arthropathy, diarrhea. **Rare (2% or less):** Bronchitis, cough.

ADVERSE EFFECTS/ TOXIC REACTIONS

Hypoglycemia occurs in less than 2% of pts.

NURSING CONSIDERATIONS

BASELINE ASSESSMENT

Check fasting serum glucose, Hgb A1c periodically to determine minimum effective dose. Discuss lifestyle to determine extent of learning, emotional needs. Ensure follow-up instruction if pt, family do not thoroughly understand diabetes

management, glucose-testing technique. At least 1 wk should elapse to assess response to drug before new dose adjustment is made.

INTERVENTION/EVALUATION

Monitor serum glucose, food intake. Assess for hypoglycemia (cool, wet skin, tremors, dizziness, anxiety, headache, tachycardia, numbness in mouth, hunger, diplopia), hyperglycemia (polyuria, polyphagia, polydipsia, nausea, vomiting, dim vision, fatigue, deep rapid breathing). Be alert to conditions that alter glucose requirements: fever, increased activity, stress, surgical procedures.

PATIENT/FAMILY TEACHING

• Diabetes requires lifelong control. • Prescribed diet, exercise are principal parts of treatment; do not skip, delay meals. • Continue to adhere to dietary instructions, regular exercise program, regular testing of serum glucose.

---

necitumumab

ne-si-**toom**-oo-mab
(Portrazza)

■ **BLACK BOX ALERT** ■
Cardiopulmonary arrest and/or sudden death reported in 3% of pts (when treated in combination with gemcitabine and cisplatin). Closely monitor serum electrolytes, esp. serum calcium, magnesium, potassium, and aggressively replace as appropriate. Hypomagnesemia occurred in 83% of pts and was severe in 20%. Monitor pts for hypomagnesemia, hypocalcemia, hypokalemia prior to each dose, during treatment, and up to 8 wks after discontinuation. Withhold treatment for CTCAE grade 3 or 4 electrolyte abnormality.
Do not confuse necitumumab with adalimumab, belimumab, daratumumab, ipilimumab, nivolumab, ofatumumab, or panitumumab.

◆CLASSIFICATION

PHARMACOTHERAPEUTIC: Epidermal growth factor receptor (EGFR) inhibitor. Monoclonal antibody. **CLINICAL:** Antineoplastic.

USES

First-line treatment (in combination with gemcitabine and CISplatin) of metastatic squamous non–small-cell lung cancer (NSCLC).

PRECAUTIONS

Contraindications: Severe hypersensitivity to necitumumab. **Cautions:** COPD, chronic arrhythmias, coronary artery disease, HF, recent MI (within 6 mos), pts at risk for electrolyte imbalance (e.g., adrenal insufficiency, alcoholism, renal failure, thyroid disorders, malnutrition, chronic diarrhea; concomitant use of medication known to cause electrolyte abnormalities); history of venous or arterial thrombosis (e.g., CVA, DVT, MI, pulmonary embolism). Not indicated for treatment of nonsquamous non–small-cell lung cancer.

ACTION

Binds to ligand-binding site of EGFR and prevents activation, expression, signaling of EGFR. **Therapeutic Effect:** Inhibits tumor cell growth and metastasis.

PHARMACOKINETICS

Widely distributed. Metabolism not specified. Elimination not specified. **Half-life:** 14 days.

⧖ LIFESPAN CONSIDERATIONS

Pregnancy/Lactation: Avoid pregnancy; may cause fetal harm. Female pts of reproductive potential should use effective contraception during treatment and for at least 3 mos after discontinuation. Unknown if distributed in breast milk. Breastfeeding not recommended during treatment and up to 3 mos after discontinuation. **Children:** Safety and efficacy not established. **Elderly:** May have increased risk of venous thromboembolism (including pulmonary embolism).

INTERACTIONS

DRUG: None known. **HERBAL:** None known. **FOOD:** None known. **LAB VALUES:** May decrease serum calcium, magnesium, potassium.

AVAILABILITY (Rx)

Injection Solution: 800 mg/50 mL (16 mg/mL).

ADMINISTRATION/HANDLING

 IV

Preparation • Visually inspect for particulate matter or discoloration. • Solution should appear clear to slightly opalescent, colorless to slightly yellow in color. Discard if solution is cloudy or particulate matter is observed. • Dilute in 250 mL 0.9% NaCl bag. • Do not use solutions containing dextrose. • Gently invert to mix. Do not shake or agitate.

Infusion Guidelines • For pts with prior grade 1 or 2 infusion reaction, premedicate with diphenhydrAMINE (or equivalent) before each subsequent infusion. • For pts with recurrent grade 1 or 2 infusion reaction (despite administration of diphenhydrAMINE), premedicate with dexamethasone (or equivalent), acetaminophen, diphenhydrAMINE (or equivalent) before each subsequent infusion. • Once infusion is complete, flush IV line with 0.9% NaCl only.

Rate of Administration • Infuse over 60 mins using infusion pump via dedicated line.

Storage • Refrigerate unused vials in original carton until time of use. • Protect from light. • May refrigerate diluted solution up to 24 hours or at room temperature up to 4 hrs.

❖ IV INCOMPATIBILITIES

Do not mix with dextrose-containing solutions. Do not infuse with other medications or electrolytes.

INDICATIONS/ROUTES/DOSAGE

Non–Small-Cell Lung Cancer
IV: ADULTS, ELDERLY: 800 mg on days 1 and 8 of each 3-wk cycle (in combination with gemcitabine and CISplatin). Continue until disease progression or unacceptable toxicity.

Dose Modification
Based on Common Terminology Criteria for Adverse Events (CTCAE).

Infusion Reactions
Any grade 1 reaction: Decrease rate by 50%. **Grade 2 reaction:** Interrupt infusion until resolved to grade 1 or 0, then resume with rate reduced by 50% for all subsequent infusions. **Grade 3 reaction:** Permanently discontinue.

Dermatological Toxicity
Grade 3 rash or acneiform rash: Withhold treatment until resolved to grade 2 or better, then reduce dose to 400 mg for at least 1 treatment cycle. If tolerated, may increase dose to 600 mg and 800 mg for subsequent cycles.
Permanent Discontinuation: Grade 3 rash or acneiform rash that does not resolve to grade 2 or better within 6 wks; worsening of skin reaction or intolerance at 400 mg dose; grade 3 skin induration or fibrosis; grade 4 dermatologic toxicity.

Electrolyte Imbalance
Withhold treatment for any grade 3 or 4 electrolyte abnormalities. Resume once abnormalities resolve to grade 2 or better.

Venous/Arterial Thrombosis
Any occurrence: Permanently discontinue.

Dosage in Renal Impairment
No dose adjustment.

Dosage in Hepatic Impairment
Mild to moderate impairment: No dose adjustment. **Severe impairment:** Not specified; use caution.

SIDE EFFECTS

Frequent (44%–29%): Rash, vomiting. **Occasional (16%–5%):** Diarrhea, dermatitis acneiform, decreased weight, stomatitis, headache, acne, pruritus, dry skin, paronychia, conjunctivitis, blurry vision, dry eye, reduced visual acuity, blepharitis, eye pain, increased lacrimation, ocular hyperemia, visual impairment, eye pruritus, skin fissures. **Rare (3%–1%):** Dysphagia, muscle spasm, oropharyngeal pain.

ADVERSE EFFECTS/TOXIC REACTIONS

All cases were reported in combination with gemcitabine and CISplatin. Pts with severe hypomagnesemia, hypokalemia, hypocalcemia are at an increased risk for cardiac arrhythmias or sudden death. Cardiopulmonary arrest and/or sudden death occurred in 3% of pts. Most cases of cardiopulmonary arrest occurred within 30 days of the last dose and involved co-morbidities including COPD, coronary artery disease, hypomagnesemia, hypertension. Hypomagnesemia reported in 83% of pts with median onset of approx. 6 wks. Severe hypomagnesemia (grade 3 or 4) reported in 20% of pts. Infusion reaction (any grade) reported in 1.5% of pts. Life-threatening venous and arterial thromboembolic events including pulmonary embolism (5% of pts), DVT (2% of pts), CVA (2% of pts), MI (1% of pts); thrombosis of mesenteric veins, pulmonary artery/vein, axillary vein, vena cava, subclavian vein; thrombophlebitis may occur. Hemoptysis reported in 10% of pts. Ocular toxicities including conjunctivitis, conjunctival hemorrhage, eye infections were reported. Severe skin toxicities occurred in 8% of pts. Immunogenicity (auto-necitumumab antibodies) occurred in 4% of pts.

NURSING CONSIDERATIONS

BASELINE ASSESSMENT

Obtain baseline BMP, serum magnesium, ionized calcium; vital signs prior to each dose. Obtain pregnancy test in female pts of reproductive potential. Receive full medication history and screen for drugs known to cause electrolyte imbalance. Assess nutritional status. Question history of CVA, DVT, pulmonary embolism, cardiac disease, recent MI; conditions known to cause electrolyte imbalance; prior hypersensitivity reaction to any drug in treatment regimen; prior infusion reaction. Offer emotional support. Conduct full dermatological exam.

INTERVENTION/EVALUATION

Diligently monitor serum electrolytes, esp. serum magnesium, potassium, calcium, ionized calcium, during therapy and up to 8 wks after discontinuation. Monitor for symptoms of hypocalcemia, hypokalemia, hypomagnesemia. Obtain EKG, vital signs if arrhythmia, chest pain, palpitations, syncope occurs. Aggressively replace electrolytes as appropriate. Pts with sudden chest pain, dyspnea, hypoxia, tachycardia should be evaluated for pulmonary embolism. Monitor for symptoms of DVT (leg or arm pain/swelling), CVA (aphasia, altered LOC, hemiplegia, vision loss, headache, homonymous hemianopsia [vision loss on the same side of both eyes]), MI (chest pain, dyspnea, syncope, diaphoresis, left arm pain, jaw pain). Monitor for hemoptysis. Assess skin for rash, hypersensitivity reaction; eyes for infection, subconjunctival hemorrhage.

PATIENT/FAMILY TEACHING

• Therapy may cause low levels of potassium, magnesium, calcium in the blood and may be life threatening. Replace electrolytes exactly as instructed. • Report symptoms of electrolyte imbalance such as fainting, fatigue, muscle cramps, palpations, paralysis, numbness or tingling, seizures, weakness. • Avoid pregnancy; treatment may cause birth defects. Female pts of childbearing potential should use effective contraception during treatment and for at least 3 mos after last dose. Do not breastfeed during therapy and for at least 3 mos after last dose. • Treatment may cause blood clots in the arms, legs, lungs, brain, heart, or abdomen. Immediately report symptoms of stroke (difficulty speaking, confusion, paralysis, vision loss), heart attack (chest pain, shortness of breath, fainting, dizziness, profuse sweating, left arm or jaw pain), lung embolism (difficulty breathing, fast heart rate, chest pain), or blood clots in the arms or legs (pain/swelling). • Report skin rashes, allergic reactions, coughing up blood; eye problems such as infection, vision impairment, collection of blood in the whites of the eyes. • Avoid sunlight, tanning beds. Wear protective clothing, high SPF sunscreen, and lip balm when outdoors.

neratinib

ne-**ra**-ti-nib
(Nerlynx)
Do not confuse neratinib with afatinib, axitinib, bosutinib, cabozantinib, dasatinib, gefitinib, imatinib, ponatinib, tofacitinib.

CLASSIFICATION

PHARMACOTHERAPEUTIC: Epidermal growth factor receptor (EGFR) inhibitor. **CLINICAL:** Antineoplastic.

USES

Extended adjuvant treatment of adult pts with early stage HER2-overexpressed/amplified breast cancer, to follow adjuvant trastuzumab-based therapy.

PRECAUTIONS

Contraindications: Hypersensitivity to neratinib. **Cautions:** Dehydration, electrolyte imbalance, hepatic impairment, irritable bowel syndrome with diarrhea. Avoid concomitant use of strong or moderate CYP3A inhibitors, CYP3A inducers; proton pump inhibitors, H_2 receptor antagonists, antacids.

ACTION

Irreversibly binds to epidermal growth factor receptor (EGFR), human epidermal growth factor receptor 2 (HER2), HER4, reducing autophosphorylation and signaling of EGFR and HER2. **Therapeutic Effect:** Exhibits antitumor activity in EGFR and/or HER2 expressing cancer cell lines.

PHARMACOKINETICS

Widely distributed. Metabolized in liver. Protein binding: 99%. Peak plasma concentration: 2–8 hrs. Excreted in feces (97%), urine (1%). **Half-life:** 7–17 hrs.

⌛ LIFESPAN CONSIDERATIONS

Pregnancy/Lactation: Avoid pregnancy; may cause fetal harm/malformations. Unknown if distributed in breast milk. Breastfeeding not recommended during treatment and for at least 1 month after last dose. Females of reproductive potential should use effective contraception during treatment and for at least 1 mo after discontinuation. **Males:** Males with female partners of reproductive potential should use effective contraception during treatment and up to 3 mos after discontinuation. **Children:** Safety and efficacy not established. **Elderly:** May have increased risk of adverse reactions/toxic effects. Use caution.

INTERACTIONS

DRUG: **Aluminum-, magnesium-, calcium-containing antacids, H_2 receptor antagonists** (e.g., **famotidine**), **proton pump inhibitors** (e.g., **omeprazole, pantoprazole**) may decrease concentration/effect. **Strong CYP3A4** inhibitors (e.g., **ketoconazole, ritonavir**), **moderate CYP3A inhibitors** (e.g., **erythromycin, ciprofloxacin, diltiazem, dronedarone, fluconazole, verapamil**) may increase concentration/effect. **CYP3A4 inducers** (e.g., **carBAMazepine, phenytoin, rifAMPin**) may decrease concentration/effect. May increase concentration of **pazopanib, topotecan.** **HERBAL:** None significant. **FOOD: Grapefruit products** may increase concentration/effect. **LAB VALUES:** May increase serum ALT, AST, bilirubin.

AVAILABILITY (Rx)

Tablets: 40 mg.

ADMINISTRATION/HANDLING

PO

• Give with food. • Administer whole; do not break, cut, crush, or divide tablets. • If a dose is missed or vomiting occurs after administration, do not give extra dose. Administer next dose at regularly scheduled time. • Take 3 hours after aluminum-, magnesium-, or calcium-containing antacids are given.

INDICATIONS/ROUTES/DOSAGE

Note: Recommend antidiarrheal prophylaxis during first 2 cycles (56 days) of therapy.

Breast Cancer
PO: ADULTS, ELDERLY: 240 mg (6 tablets) once daily for 1 yr.

Loperamide (Antidiarrheal) Prophylaxis
WKS 1–2 (DAYS 1–14): 4 mg three times/day. **WKS 3–8 (DAYS 15–56):** 4 mg twice daily. **WKS 9–52 (DAYS 57–365):** 4 mg as needed (do not exceed 16 mg/day).

Dose Reduction Schedule (Neratinib)
First dose reduction: 200 mg daily. **Second dose reduction:** 160 mg daily. **Third dose reduction:** 120 mg daily.

Dose Modification
Any CTCAE grade 3 toxicity: Withhold treatment until improved to grade 1 or 0 (or baseline), then resume at the next

reduced dose level. **Any CTCAE grade 4 toxicity:** Permanently discontinue.

Diarrhea

CTCAE grade 1 diarrhea (increase of greater than 4 stools/day over baseline); CTCAE grade 2 diarrhea (increase of 4–6 stools/day over baseline) lasting more than 5 days, CTCAE grade 3 diarrhea (increase of greater than 7 stools/day over baseline, incontinence, hospitalization, self-limiting ADLs lasting more than 2 days): Adjust antidiarrheal therapy, diet. Maintain fluid intake (approx. 2 L/day). Once improved to grade 1 or 0, start loperamide 4 mg with each administration. **Any CTCAE grade diarrhea with complications (fever, hypotension, renal failure, or grade 3 or 4 neutropenia):** Withhold treatment and adjust antidiarrheal therapy, diet. Maintain fluid intake (approx. 2 L/day). If diarrhea improves to grade 1 or 0 within 7 days, resume treatment at same dose level. If diarrhea improves to grade 1 or 0 for more than 7 days, resume treatment at the next reduced dose level. Once improved to grade 1 or 0, start loperamide 4 mg with each administration. **CTCAE grade 4 diarrhea (life-threatening event, emergent intervention indicated); recurrent grade 2 diarrhea (or higher) at 120 mg dose:** Permanently discontinue.

Hepatotoxicity

CTCAE grade 3 serum ALT elevation (greater than 5–20 times upper limit normal [ULN]) or CTCAE grade 3 serum bilirubin elevation (greater than 3–10 times ULN): Withhold treatment until improved to grade 1 or 0 and investigate cause. If serum ALT elevation improves to grade 1 or 0 within 3 wks, resume treatment at reduced dose level. **CTCAE grade 4 serum ALT elevation (greater than 20 times ULN) or CTCAE grade 4 serum bilirubin elevation (greater than 10 times ULN):** Permanently discontinue and investigate cause.

Dosage in Renal Impairment

Not specified; use caution.

Dosage in Hepatic Impairment

Mild to moderate impairment (Child-Pugh A or B): No dose adjustment. **Severe impairment (Child-Pugh C):** Reduce starting dose to 80 mg.

SIDE EFFECTS

Frequent (95%–26%): Diarrhea, nausea, abdominal pain, vomiting. **Occasional (18%–4%):** Rash (erythematous, follicular, generalized, pruritic, pustular, maculo-papular, papular, dermatitis, dermatitis acneiform, toxic skin eruption), stomatitis, mouth ulceration, oral mucosal blistering, mucosal inflammation, oropharyngeal pain, oral pain, glossodynia, glossitis, cheilitis, decreased appetite, muscle spasm, dyspepsia, nail disorder (paronychia, onychoclasis, nail discoloration, nail toxicity, abnormal nail growth, nail dystrophy), dry skin, abdominal distention, decreased weight, dehydration. **Rare (3%):** Dry mouth.

ADVERSE EFFECTS/TOXIC REACTIONS

Diarrhea reported in 95% of pts. CTCAE grade 3 diarrhea reported in 40% of pts. CTCAE grade 4 diarrhea reported in less than 1% of pts. Median time of onset of diarrhea was days to wks. Severe diarrhea, dehydration, hypotension, renal failure may occur. Hepatotoxicity reported in 5%–10% of pts.

NURSING CONSIDERATIONS

BASELINE ASSESSMENT

Obtain LFT, vital signs. Obtain BMP and screen for electrolyte imbalance. Confirm HER2-positive status. Obtain pregnancy test prior to initiation. Question current breastfeeding status. Stress the importance of antidiarrheal therapy. Question history of IBS with chronic diarrhea, hepatic impairment. Assess hydration status. Question usual bowel movement patterns, stool characteristics. Receive full medication history and screen for interactions. Offer emotional support.

N

INTERVENTION/EVALUATION

Monitor LFT monthly for the first 3 mos, then q3mos thereafter. Monitor for hepatotoxicity (abdominal pain, ascites, confusion, dark-colored urine, jaundice). Obtain BMP (note electrolytes) if severe diarrhea occurs. Ensure compliance of antidiarrheal therapy. Additional antidiarrheal medication may be needed to manage diarrhea despite treatment with loperamide. Monitor daily pattern of bowel activity, stool consistency. If treatment-related toxicities occur, consider referral to specialist. Monitor I&O. Assess skin, nails, oral mucosa for toxic reactions.

PATIENT/FAMILY TEACHING

• Treatment may cause severe diarrhea, which may lead to life-threatening dehydration or hospitalization. Take antidiarrheal medication exactly as prescribed (goal is 1–2 bowel movements/day). Report worsening of diarrhea or dehydration. • Drink plenty of fluids (at least 2 L/day if severe diarrhea occurs). • Report liver problems such as bruising; confusion; amber, dark, orange-colored urine; right upper abdominal pain; yellowing of the skin or eyes. • Treatment may cause fetal harm; avoid pregnancy. • Females of childbearing potential should use effective contraception during treatment and for at least 1 mo after last dose. Males with female partners of childbearing potential should use effective contraception during treatment and up to 3 mos after last dose. • Do not breastfeed. • Avoid grapefruit products, Seville oranges, starfruit, herbal supplements. • Acid-reducing medications may interfere with absorption; avoid use. Do not take aluminum-, magnesium-, calcium-containing antacids 3 hrs before or 3 hrs after dose. • Do not take newly prescribed medications unless approved by the prescriber who originally started treatment.

niacin
TOP 100

nye-a-sin
(Niacor, Niaspan, Slo-Niacin)
Do not confuse niacin, Niacor, or Niaspan with Minocin or Nitro-Bid.

FIXED-COMBINATION(S)

Advicor: niacin/lovastatin (HMG-CoA reductase inhibitor [statin]): 500 mg/20 mg, 750 mg/20 mg, 1,000 mg/20 mg. **Simcor:** niacin/simvastatin (HMG-CoA reductase inhibitor [statin]): 500 mg/20 mg, 500 mg/40 mg, 750 mg/20 mg, 1,000 mg/20 mg, 1,000 mg/40 mg.

◆CLASSIFICATION

PHARMACOTHERAPEUTIC: Water-soluble vitamin. **CLINICAL:** Antihyperlipidemic.

USES

Treatment of dyslipidemias, lowers risk of recurrent MI (pts with history of MI/hyperlipidemia), slow progression of CAD, treatment of hypertriglyceridemia in pts at risk for pancreatitis, dietary supplement. **OFF-LABEL:** Treatment of pellagra.

PRECAUTIONS

Contraindications: Hypersensitivity to niacin, nicotinic acid. Active peptic ulcer disease, arterial hemorrhage, significant or unexplained persistent elevations in hepatic transaminases, active hepatic disease. **Cautions:** Diabetes, gallbladder disease, unstable angina, MI, renal impairment, heavy alcohol use, concomitant use of anticoagulants, gout, history of jaundice/hepatic disease, inadequately treated hypothyroidism, elderly pts.

ACTION

Component of two coenzymes needed for tissue respiration, lipid metabolism, glycogenolysis. May inhibit release of free fatty acids from adipose tissue, increase lipoprotein lipase activity. **Therapeutic Effect:** Reduces total LDL, VLDL cholesterol levels and triglyceride levels; increases HDL cholesterol concentration.

PHARMACOKINETICS

Readily absorbed from GI tract. Widely distributed. Protein binding: 20%. Metabolized in liver. Primarily excreted in urine. **Half-life:** 45 min.

⧖ LIFESPAN CONSIDERATIONS

Pregnancy/Lactation: Not recommended for use during pregnancy/lactation. Distributed in breast milk. **Children:** No age-related precautions noted. Not recommended in pts younger than 2 yrs. **Elderly:** No age-related precautions noted.

INTERACTIONS

DRUG: Alcohol may increase risk of side effects. May increase effect of **antihypertensives (e.g., amLODIPine, lisinopril, valsartan). Lovastatin, pravastatin, simvastatin** may increase risk of acute renal failure, rhabdomyolysis. **Vasoactive drugs (e.g., calcium channel blockers, nitrates)** may increase hypotension. **HERBAL:** None significant. **FOOD:** None known. **LAB VALUES:** May increase serum uric acid, PT, amylase, bilirubin, fasting glucose, LDH, transaminase. May decrease platelets.

AVAILABILITY (OTC)

Tablets (Immediate-Release): 50 mg, 100 mg, 250 mg, 500 mg.

🥄 **Capsules (Extended-Release):** 250 mg, 500 mg. 🥄 **Tablets (Extended-Release):** 250 mg, 500 mg, 750 mg, 1,000 mg.

ADMINISTRATION/HANDLING

PO

• For pts switching from immediate-release niacin to extended-release niacin,

initiate extended-release form with low doses and titrate to therapeutic response. • Give with food. • Give aspirin 30 min before taking extended-release niacin to minimize flushing. • Do not break, crush, dissolve, or divide long-acting forms.

INDICATIONS/ROUTES/DOSAGE

Hyperlipidemia

PO *(Immediate-Release):* **ADULTS, ELDERLY:** Initially, 250 mg once daily (with evening meal). May increase dose q4–7days up to 1.5–2 g/day in 2–3 divided doses. After 2 mos may increase at 2- to 4-wk intervals to 3 g/day in 3 divided doses. **Maximum:** 6 g/day in 3 divided doses. Usual daily dose: 1.5–3 g/day.

PO *(Extended-Release):* **ADULTS, ELDERLY:** Initially, 500 mg/day at bedtime for 4 wks, then 1 g at bedtime for 4 wks. May increase by no more than 500 mg q4wks up to maximum of 2 g/day. Usual daily dose: 1–2 g/day.

Dosage for Hepatic Toxicity

Transaminases more than 3 times ULN: Discontinue therapy.

Dosage in Renal/Hepatic Impairment

No dose adjustment.

SIDE EFFECTS

Frequent: Flushing (esp. face, neck) occurring within 20 min of drug administration and lasting for 30–60 min, GI upset, pruritus. **Occasional:** Dizziness, hypotension, headache, blurred vision, burning/tingling of skin, flatulence, nausea, vomiting, diarrhea. **Rare:** Hyperglycemia, glycosuria, rash, hyperpigmentation, dry skin.

ADVERSE EFFECTS/TOXIC REACTIONS

Arrhythmias occur rarely.

NURSING CONSIDERATIONS

BASELINE ASSESSMENT

Obtain diet history, especially fat consumption. Question for history of hypersensitivity to niacin, tartrazine, aspirin. Obtain baseline serum cholesterol, triglyceride, glucose, LFT.

INTERVENTION/EVALUATION

Evaluate flushing, degree of GI discomfort. Check for headache, dizziness, blurred vision. Monitor daily pattern of bowel activity, stool consistency. Monitor LFT, serum cholesterol, triglycerides. Check serum glucose carefully in pts on insulin, oral antihyperglycemics. Assess skin for rash, dryness. Monitor serum uric acid.

PATIENT/FAMILY TEACHING

• Transient flushing of the skin, sensation of warmth, pruritus, tingling may occur. • Report dizziness (avoid sudden changes in posture). • Report nausea, vomiting, loss of appetite, yellowing of skin, dark urine, feeling of weakness. • If medically approved, take aspirin 30 min before taking extended-release niacin to minimize flushing. • Take at bedtime with low-fat snack. • Limit alcohol consumption.

---

niCARdipine

nye-**kar**-di-peen
(Cardene IV)
Do not confuse Cardene SR with Cardizem SR or codeine, or niCARdipine with NIFEdipine or niMODipine.

◆CLASSIFICATION

PHARMACOTHERAPEUTIC: Calcium channel blocker. **CLINICAL:** Antianginal, antihypertensive.

USES

PO: Immediate-release: Treatment of chronic stable (effort-associated) angina, hypertension. **Sustained-release:** Treatment of hypertension. **Parenteral:** Short-term treatment of hypertension when oral therapy not feasible or desirable. **OFF-LABEL:** Blood pressure control in acute ischemic stroke and intracranial hemorrhage.

PRECAUTIONS

Contraindications: Hypersensitivity to niCARdipine. Advanced aortic stenosis. **Cautions:** Cardiac/renal/hepatic dysfunction, HF, hypertrophic cardiomyopathy with outflow tract obstruction, aortic stenosis, coronary artery disease, portal hypertension.

ACTION

Inhibits calcium ion movement across cell membranes, depressing contraction of cardiac, vascular smooth muscle. **Therapeutic Effect:** Increases heart rate, cardiac output, myocardial oxygen delivery. Decreases systemic vascular resistance, B/P.

PHARMACOKINETICS

Route	Onset	Peak	Duration
PO	0.5–2 hrs	—	8 hrs
IV	10 min	—	8 hrs or less

Rapidly, completely absorbed from GI tract. Protein binding: 95%. Metabolized in liver. Primarily excreted in urine. Not removed by hemodialysis. **Half-life:** 2–4 hrs.

⊠ LIFESPAN CONSIDERATIONS

Pregnancy/Lactation: Unknown if distributed in breast milk. **Children:** Safety and efficacy not established. **Elderly:** Age-related renal impairment may require dosage adjustment.

INTERACTIONS

DRUG: May increase concentration of **cycloSPORINE. HERBAL: Ephedra, ginger, ginseng, yohimbe** may increase hypertension. **Licorice** may cause retention of sodium, water; may increase loss of potassium. **St. John's wort** may decrease levels. **FOOD: Grapefruit products** may alter absorption. **LAB VALUES:** None significant.

AVAILABILITY (Rx)

Capsules: 20 mg, 30 mg. **Infusion, Ready to Use:** 20 mg/200 mL, 40 mg/200 mL. **Injection Solution:** 2.5 mg/mL (10-mL vial).

 Capsules (Sustained-Release): 30 mg, 60 mg.

ADMINISTRATION/HANDLING

IV

Reconstitution • Dilute 25-mg vial with 240 mL D$_5$W, 0.45% NaCl, or 0.9% NaCl to provide concentration of 0.1 mg/mL.
Rate of Administration • Give by slow IV infusion. • Change IV site q12h if administered peripherally.
Storage • Store at room temperature. • Diluted IV solution is stable for 24 hrs at room temperature.

PO

• Give without regard to food. • Do not break, crush, or open capsules. Give whole.

⚅ IV INCOMPATIBILITIES

Ampicillin (Principen), ampicillin/sulbactam (Unasyn), cefepime (Maxipime), cefTAZidime (Fortaz), furosemide (Lasix), heparin, sodium bicarbonate.

⚅ IV COMPATIBILITIES

DiltiaZEM (Cardizem), DOBUTamine (Dobutrex), DOPamine (Intropin), EPINEPHrine, HYDROmorphone (Dilaudid), labetalol (Trandate), LORazepam (Ativan), midazolam (Versed), milrinone (Primacor), morphine, nitroglycerin, norepinephrine (Levophed), potassium chloride.

INDICATIONS/ROUTES/DOSAGE

Chronic Stable Angina
PO: ADULTS, ELDERLY: *(Immediate-Release):* Initially, 20 mg 3 times/day. Range: 20–40 mg 3 times/day (allow 3 days between dosage increases).

Hypertension
PO: ADULTS, ELDERLY: *(Immediate-Release):* Initially, 20 mg 3 times/day. Range: 20–40 mg 3 times/day (allow 3 days between dosage increases).
PO: ADULTS, ELDERLY: *(Extended-Release):* Initially, 30 mg twice daily. Range: 30–60 mg twice daily.

Acute Hypertension
IV: ADULTS, ELDERLY (GRADUAL B/P DECREASE): Initially, 5 mg/hr. May increase by 2.5 mg/hr q5–15min. **Maximum:** 15 mg/hr. After B/P goal is achieved, adjust dose to maintain desired BP.

Dosage in Renal Impairment
ADULTS, ELDERLY: (PO): Initially, give 20 mg q8h (30 mg twice daily [sustained-release capsules]), then titrate. **(IV):** No dose adjustment.

Dosage in Hepatic Impairment
ADULTS, ELDERLY: (PO): Initially, give 20 mg twice daily, then titrate. **(IV):** No dose adjustment.

SIDE EFFECTS

Frequent (10%–7%): Headache, facial flushing, peripheral edema, lightheadedness, dizziness. **Occasional (6%–3%):** Asthenia, palpitations, angina, tachycardia. **Rare (less than 2%):** Nausea, abdominal cramps, dyspepsia, dry mouth, rash.

ADVERSE EFFECTS/TOXIC REACTIONS

Overdose produces confusion, slurred speech, drowsiness, marked hypotension, bradycardia.

NURSING CONSIDERATIONS

BASELINE ASSESSMENT

Concurrent therapy with sublingual nitroglycerin may be used for relief of anginal pain. Record onset, type (sharp, dull, squeezing), radiation, location, intensity, duration of anginal pain, precipitating factors (exertion, emotional stress).

N

INTERVENTION/EVALUATION

Monitor B/P, heart rate during and following IV infusion. Assess for peripheral edema. Assess skin for facial flushing, dermatitis, rash. Question for asthenia, headache. Monitor LFT results. Assess EKG, pulse for tachycardia.

PATIENT/FAMILY TEACHING

• May take without regard to food. • Sustained-release capsule taken whole; do not break, chew, crush, or open. • Avoid alcohol, grapefruit products; limit caffeine. • Report if anginal pain not relieved or if palpitations, shortness of breath, swelling, dizziness, constipation, nausea, hypotension occurs. • Avoid tasks requiring motor skills, alertness until response to drug is established.

---

nicotine

N

nik-o-teen
(Habitrol ✿, NicoDerm ✿, Nico-Derm CQ, Nicorette, Nicorette Plus ✿, Nicotrol ✿, Nicotrol Inhaler, Nicotrol NS, Thrive)
Do not confuse NicoDerm with Nitroderm.

◆CLASSIFICATION

PHARMACOTHERAPEUTIC: Cholinergic-receptor agonist. **CLINICAL:** Smoking deterrent.

USES

Treatment to aid smoking cessation for relief of nicotine withdrawal symptoms. **OFF-LABEL: Transdermal:** Management of ulcerative colitis.

PRECAUTIONS

Contraindications: Hypersensitivity to nicotine. **Cautions:** Smoking post-MI period, severe or worsening angina, active temporomandibular joint disease (gum), pregnancy, hyperthyroidism, pheochromocytoma, insulin-dependent diabetes, severe renal impairment, eczematous dermatitis, oropharyngeal inflammation, esophagitis, peptic ulcer (delays healing in peptic ulcer disease), coronary artery disease, recent MI, serious cardiac arrhythmias, vasospastic disease, angina, hypertension, hepatic impairment, use of oral inhaler/nasal spray with bronchospastic disease.

ACTION

Binds to nicotinic-cholinergic receptors at the autonomic ganglia, in the adrenal medulla, at neuromuscular junction, and in the brain, producing both stimulating, depressant effects on peripheral, central nervous systems. **Therapeutic Effect:** Provides source of nicotine during nicotine withdrawal, reduces withdrawal symptoms.

PHARMACOKINETICS

Absorbed slowly after transdermal administration. Protein binding: 5%. Metabolized in liver. Excreted primarily in urine. **Half-life:** 4 hrs.

⧗ LIFESPAN CONSIDERATIONS

Pregnancy/Lactation: Distributed in breast milk. Use of cigarettes, nicotine gum associated with decrease in fetal breathing movements. **Children:** Not recommended in this pt population. **Elderly:** Age-related decrease in cardiac function may require dosage adjustment.

INTERACTIONS

DRUG: Smoking cessation, decreased dosage of nicotine may alter effects of **tricyclic antidepressants (e.g., amitriptyline, doxepin), theophylline. HERBAL:** None significant. **FOOD:** None known. **LAB VALUES:** None significant.

AVAILABILITY (OTC)

Chewing Gum: 2 mg, 4 mg. **Inhalation (Nicotrol Inhaler):** 10-mg cartridge. **Lozenges:** 2 mg, 4 mg. **Nasal Spray (Nicotrol NS):** 0.5 mg/spray. **Transdermal Patch:** 7 mg/24 hrs, 14 mg/24 hrs, 21 mg/24 hrs.

ADMINISTRATION/HANDLING

Gum
• Do not swallow. • Chew 1 piece when urge to smoke present. • Chew slowly and intermittently for 30 min. • Chew until distinctive nicotine taste (peppery) or slight tingling in mouth perceived, then stop; when tingling almost gone (about 1 min), repeat chewing procedure (this allows constant slow buccal absorption). • Too-rapid chewing may cause excessive release of nicotine, resulting in adverse effects similar to oversmoking (e.g., nausea, throat irritation).

Inhaler
• Insert cartridge into mouthpiece. • Puff on nicotine cartridge mouthpiece for 20 min.

Lozenge
• Do not chew or swallow. • Allow to dissolve slowly (20–30 min).

Transdermal
• Apply promptly upon removal from protective pouch (prevents evaporation, loss of nicotine). • Use only intact pouch. Do not cut patch. • Apply only once daily to hairless, clean, dry skin on upper body, outer arm. • Replace daily; rotate sites; do not use same site within 7 days; do not use same patch longer than 24 hrs. • Normal exposure to water (e.g., bathing, swimming) should not affect patch. • Wash hands with water alone after applying patch (soap may increase nicotine absorption). • Discard used patch by folding patch in half (sticky side together), placing in pouch of new patch, and throwing away in such a way as to prevent child or pet accessibility. • Patch may contain conducting metal; remove prior to MRI.

INDICATIONS/ROUTES/DOSAGE

Smoking Cessation Aid to Relieve Nicotine Withdrawal Symptoms
PO: *(Chewing Gum):* **ADULTS, ELDERLY:** 2 mg. Use 4 mg in pts who smoke first cigarette within 30 min of waking.

Chew 1 piece of gum when urge to smoke, up to 24/day. Use following schedule: wks 1–6: q1–2h (at least 9 pieces/day); wks 7–9: q2–4h; wks 10–12: q4–8h.

PO: *(Lozenge):*
◀**ALERT**▶ For pts who smoke the first cigarette within 30 min of waking, administer the 4-mg lozenge; otherwise, administer the 2-mg lozenge.
ADULTS, ELDERLY: One 4-mg or 2-mg lozenge q1–2h for the first 6 wks (use at least 9 lozenges/day first 6 wks); 1 lozenge q2–4h for wks 7–9; and 1 lozenge q4–8h for wks 10–12. **Maximum:** 1 lozenge at a time, 5 lozenges/6 hrs, 20 lozenges/day.

Transdermal: ◀**ALERT**▶ Apply 1 new patch q24h. **ADULTS, ELDERLY WHO SMOKE 10 CIGARETTES OR MORE PER DAY:** Follow the guidelines below. **Step 1:** 21 mg/day for 6 wks. **Step 2:** 14 mg/day for 2 wks. **Step 3:** 7 mg/day for 2 wks. **ADULTS, ELDERLY WHO SMOKE LESS THAN 10 CIGARETTES PER DAY:** Follow the guidelines below. **Step 1:** 14 mg/day for 6 wks. **Step 2:** 7 mg/day for 2 wks.

Nasal: ADULTS, ELDERLY: Each dose (2 sprays, 1 spray in each nostril) = 1 mg nicotine. Initially, 1–2 doses/hr. **Maximum:** 5 doses/hr (10 sprays), 40 doses/day (80 sprays). For best results, take at least 8 doses/day (16 sprays).

Inhaler *(Nicotrol):* **ADULTS, ELDERLY:** Initially, 6–16 cartridges per day. Puff on nicotine cartridge mouthpiece for about 20 min as needed. **Maximum:** 16 cartridges/day.

Dosage in Renal/Hepatic Impairment
No dose adjustment.

SIDE EFFECTS

Frequent: All forms: Hiccups, nausea. **Gum:** Mouth/throat soreness. **Transdermal:** Erythema, pruritus, burning at application site. **Occasional: All forms:** Eructation, GI upset, dry mouth, insomnia, diaphoresis, irritability. **Gum:** Hoarseness. **Inhaler:** Mouth/throat irritation, cough. **Rare: All forms:** Dizziness, myalgia, arthralgia.

ADVERSE EFFECTS/ TOXIC REACTIONS

Overdose produces palpitations, tachyarrhythmias, seizures, depression, confusion, diaphoresis, hypotension, rapid/weak pulse, dyspnea. Lethal dose for adults is 40–60 mg. Death results from respiratory paralysis.

NURSING CONSIDERATIONS

BASELINE ASSESSMENT

Screen, evaluate those with coronary heart disease (history of MI, angina pectoris), serious cardiac arrhythmias, Buerger's disease, Prinzmetal's variant angina.

INTERVENTION/EVALUATION

Monitor smoking habits, B/P, pulse, sleep pattern, skin for erythema, pruritus, burning at application site if transdermal system used.

PATIENT/FAMILY TEACHING

• Follow guidelines for proper application of transdermal system. • Chew gum slowly to avoid jaw ache, maximize benefit. • Report persistent rash, pruritus that occurs with patch. • Do not smoke while wearing patch.

NIFEdipine

nye-**fed**-i-peen
(Adalat CC, Adalat XL ✦, Afeditab CR, Apo-Nifed ✦, Nifediac CC, Nifedical XL, Procardia, Procardia XL)
Do not confuse NIFEdipine with niCARdipine or niMODipine, or Procardia XL with Cartia XT.

◆CLASSIFICATION

PHARMACOTHERAPEUTIC: Calcium channel blocker, dihydropyridine. **CLINICAL:** Antianginal, antihypertensive.

USES

Immediate-/extended-release: Treatment of angina due to coronary artery spasm (Prinzmetal's variant angina), chronic stable angina (effort-associated angina). **Extended-release:** Treatment of hypertension. **OFF-LABEL:** Treatment of Raynaud's phenomenon, pulmonary hypertension, preterm labor, prevention/treatment of high-altitude pulmonary edema.

PRECAUTIONS

Contraindications: Hypersensitivity to NIFEdipine. ST elevation myocardial infarction (STEMI). **Cautions:** Renal/hepatic impairment, obstructive coronary disease, HF, severe aortic stenosis, edema, severe left ventricular dysfunction, hypertrophic cardiomyopathy, before major surgery, bradycardia, concurrent use with beta blockers or digoxin, CYP3A4 inhibitors/inducers.

ACTION

Inhibits calcium ion movement across cell membranes, depressing contraction of cardiac, vascular smooth muscle. **Therapeutic Effect:** Increases heart rate, myocardial oxygen delivery, cardiac output. Decreases systemic vascular resistance, B/P.

PHARMACOKINETICS

Rapidly, completely absorbed from GI tract. Protein binding: 92%–98%. Metabolized in liver. Primarily excreted in urine. Not removed by hemodialysis. **Half-life:** 2–5 hrs.

⧗ LIFESPAN CONSIDERATIONS

Pregnancy/Lactation: Insignificant amount distributed in breast milk. **Children:** Safety and efficacy not established. **Elderly:** Age-related renal impairment may require dosage adjustment. Use lower initial doses and titrate to response.

INTERACTIONS

DRUG: Strong CYP3A4 inducers (e.g., rifAMPin, PHENobarbital, phenytoin, carBAMazepine) may

---

decrease concentration/effects. **CYP3A4 inhibitors (e.g., clarithromycin, ketoconazole)** may increase concentration. **Beta blockers (e.g., carvedilol, metoprolol)** may have additive effect. May increase **digoxin** concentration, risk of toxicity. **Hypokalemia-producing agents (e.g., furosemide, other diuretics)** may increase risk of arrhythmias. **HERBAL: Ephedra, garlic, ginseng, yohimbe** may increase hypertension. **Licorice** may cause retention of sodium, water; may increase loss of potassium. **St. John's wort** decreases concentration/effects. **FOOD: Grapefruit products** may increase risk for flushing, headache, tachycardia, hypotension. **LAB VALUES:** May cause positive ANA, direct Coombs' test.

AVAILABILITY (Rx)

Capsules: 10 mg, 20 mg.

Tablets, Extended-Release: 30 mg, 60 mg, 90 mg.

ADMINISTRATION/HANDLING

PO

• Do not break, crush, dissolve, or divide extended-release tablets. • Give without regard to meals (Adalat CC, Nifediac CC should be taken on an empty stomach). • Grapefruit products may alter absorption; avoid use.

Sublingual

• Capsules must be punctured, chewed, and/or squeezed to express liquid into mouth.

INDICATIONS/ROUTES/DOSAGE

Prinzmetal's Variant Angina, Chronic Stable (Effort-Associated) Angina

PO *(Immediate-Release):* **ADULTS, ELDERLY:** Initially, 10 mg 3 times/day. Increase at 7- to 14-day intervals. **Maintenance:** 10 mg 3 times/day up to 30 mg 4 times/day. **Maximum:** 180 mg/day.

PO *(Extended-Release):* **ADULTS, ELDERLY:** Initially, 30–60 mg/day. May increase at 7- to 14-day intervals. **Maximum:** 120 mg/day.

Hypertension

PO *(Extended-Release):* **ADULTS, ELDERLY:** Initially, 30–60 mg/day. May increase at 7- to 14-day intervals. **Maximum:** 90–120 mg/day. **CHILDREN 1–17 YRS:** Initially, 0.2–0.5 mg/kg/day. **Maximum:** 3 mg/kg/day or 120 mg/day.

Dosage in Renal/Hepatic Impairment
No dose adjustment.

SIDE EFFECTS

Frequent (30%–11%): Peripheral edema, headache, flushed skin, dizziness. **Occasional (12%–6%):** Nausea, shakiness, muscle cramps/pain, drowsiness, palpitations, nasal congestion, cough, dyspnea, wheezing. **Rare (5%–3%):** Hypotension, rash, pruritus, urticaria, constipation, abdominal discomfort, flatulence, sexual dysfunction.

ADVERSE EFFECTS/TOXIC REACTIONS

May precipitate HF, MI in pts with cardiac disease, peripheral ischemia. Overdose produces nausea, drowsiness, confusion, slurred speech. **Antidote:** Glucagon (see Appendix J for dosage).

NURSING CONSIDERATIONS

BASELINE ASSESSMENT

Concurrent therapy with sublingual nitroglycerin may be used for relief of anginal pain. Record onset, type (sharp, dull, squeezing), radiation, location, intensity, duration of anginal pain; precipitating factors (exertion, emotional stress). Check B/P for hypotension immediately before giving medication.

INTERVENTION/EVALUATION

Assist with ambulation if light-headedness, dizziness occurs. Assess for peripheral edema. Assess skin for flushing. Monitor LFT. Observe for signs/symptoms of HF.

PATIENT/FAMILY TEACHING

• Go from lying to standing slowly. • Report palpitations, shortness of breath, pronounced dizziness,

nausea, exacerbations of angina.
• Avoid alcohol; concomitant grapefruit product use.

niMODipine

nye-**mode**-i-peen
(Nimotop ✦, Nymalize)

■ **BLACK BOX ALERT** ■ Severe cardiovascular events, including fatalities, have resulted when capsule contents have been withdrawn by syringe and administered by IV injection rather than orally or via nasogastric tube.

Do not confuse niMODipine with niCARdipine or NIFEdipine.

◆CLASSIFICATION

PHARMACOTHERAPEUTIC: Calcium channel blocker, dihydropyridine.
CLINICAL: Cerebral vasospasm agent.

USES

Improvement of neurologic deficits due to cerebral vasospasm following subarachnoid hemorrhage from ruptured intracranial aneurysms.

PRECAUTIONS

Contraindications: Hypersensitivity to niMODipine. Concurrent use with strong CYP3A4 inhibitors (e.g., clarithromycin, voriconazole). **Cautions:** Pts with cirrhosis, baseline hypotension, bradycardia.

⏳ LIFESPAN CONSIDERATIONS

Pregnancy/Lactation: Unknown if drug crosses placenta or is distributed in breast milk. **Children:** Safety and efficacy not established. **Elderly:** Age-related renal impairment may require dosage adjustment. May experience greater hypotensive response, constipation.

ACTION

Inhibits movement of calcium ions across vascular smooth muscle cell membranes.

Exerts greatest effect on cerebral arteries. **Therapeutic Effect:** Produces favorable effect on severity of neurologic deficits due to cerebral vasospasm. May prevent cerebral vasospasm.

PHARMACOKINETICS

Rapidly absorbed from GI tract. Protein binding: 95%. Metabolized in liver. Excreted in bile (80%), urine (20%). Not removed by hemodialysis. **Half-life:** 1–2 hrs.

INTERACTIONS

DRUG: Beta blockers (e.g., **carvedilol, metoprolol**) may have additive effect, increase depression of cardiac SA/AV conduction. May increase <u>digoxin</u> concentration. **Agents inducing hypokalemia (e.g., furosemide, HCTZ, high-dose or IV insulin)** may increase risk of arrhythmias. **CYP3A4 inhibitors (e.g., erythromycin, ketoconazole, protease inhibitors)** may inhibit metabolism. **CYP3A4 inducers (e.g., rifabutin, rifAMPin)** may increase metabolism. **HERBAL:** Ephedra, garlic, ginseng, yohimbe may increase hypertension. **Licorice** may cause retention of sodium, water; may increase loss of potassium. **St. John's wort** may decrease level/effects. **FOOD:** Grapefruit products may increase concentration, risk of toxicity. **LAB VALUES:** None significant.

AVAILABILITY (Rx)

Solution, Oral (Nymalize): 60 mg/20 mL.
🖰 **Capsules:** 30 mg.

ADMINISTRATION/HANDLING
PO

• Administer 1 hr before or 2 hrs after meals. • If pt unable to swallow, place hole in both ends of capsule with 18-gauge needle to extract contents into syringe. Empty into NG tube; flush tube with 30 mL water.

N

INDICATIONS/ROUTES/DOSAGE

Subarachnoid Hemorrhage
PO: ADULTS, ELDERLY: 60 mg q4h for 21 days. Begin within 96 hrs of subarachnoid hemorrhage.

Dosage in Renal Impairment
No dose adjustment.

Dosage in Hepatic Impairment
PO: ADULTS, ELDERLY: Reduce dose to 30 mg q4h in pts with cirrhosis.

SIDE EFFECTS

Occasional (6%–2%): Hypotension, peripheral edema, diarrhea, headache. **Rare (less than 2%):** Allergic reaction (rash, urticaria), tachycardia, flushing of skin.

ADVERSE EFFECTS/TOXIC REACTIONS

Overdose produces nausea, weakness, dizziness, drowsiness, confusion, slurred speech.

NURSING CONSIDERATIONS

BASELINE ASSESSMENT

Assess level of consciousness, neurologic response, initially and throughout therapy. Monitor baseline LFT. Assess B/P, apical pulse immediately before drug administration (if pulse is 60/min or less or systolic B/P is less than 90 mm Hg, withhold medication, contact physician).

INTERVENTION/EVALUATION

Monitor CNS response, heart rate, B/P for evidence of hypotension, bradycardia. Monitor transcranial Doppler results for evidence of vasospasm.

PATIENT/FAMILY TEACHING

• Do not chew, crush, dissolve, or divide capsules. • Report palpitations, shortness of breath, swelling, constipation, nausea, dizziness. Immediately report headache, blurry vision, confusion (may indicate vasospasm).

niraparib

nye-**rap**-a-rib
(Zejula)
Do not confuse niraparib with olaparib, neratinib, or rucaparib.

◆CLASSIFICATION

PHARMACOTHERAPEUTIC: Poly(ADP-ribose) polymerase (PARP) inhibitor. **CLINICAL:** Antineoplastic.

USES

Maintenance treatment of adult pts with recurrent epithelial ovarian, fallopian tube, or primary peritoneal cancer who are in a complete or partial response to platinum-based chemotherapy.

PRECAUTIONS

Contraindications: Hypersensitivity to niraparib. **Cautions:** Baseline anemia, leukopenia, neutropenia, thrombocytopenia; history of hypertension, cardiac disease; pts at risk for hemorrhage (e.g., history of GI bleeding, coagulation disorders, recent trauma; concomitant use of anticoagulants, antiplatelet medication, NSAIDs).

ACTION

Inhibits poly(ADP-ribose) polymerase enzymatic activity, resulting in DNA damage, apoptosis, and cellular death. **Therapeutic Effect:** Induces cytotoxicity in tumor cell lines with and without BRCA deficiencies.

PHARMACOKINETICS

Well absorbed. Widely distributed. Metabolized by carboxylesterase to inactive metabolite. Protein binding: 83%. Peak plasma concentration: 3 hrs. Excreted in urine (48%), feces (39%). **Half-life:** 36 hrs.

⌛ LIFESPAN CONSIDERATIONS

Pregnancy/Lactation: Avoid pregnancy; may cause fetal harm/malformations. Unknown if distributed in breast

N

---

milk. Breastfeeding not recommended during treatment and up to 1 mo after discontinuation. Females of reproductive potential should use effective contraception during treatment and for at least 6 mos after discontinuation. May impair fertility in males. **Children:** Safety and efficacy not established. **Elderly:** No age-related precautions noted.

INTERACTIONS

DRUG: May decrease therapeutic effect of **BCG vaccine. HERBAL:** None significant. **FOOD:** None known. **LAB VALUES:** May increase serum alkaline phosphatase, ALT, AST, creatinine, GGT. May decrease ANC, Hgb, Hct, leukocytes, neutrophils, RBCs; serum potassium.

AVAILABILITY (Rx)

Capsules: 100 mg.

ADMINISTRATION/HANDLING

PO
• Give with or without food. • Administer whole; do not break, cut, crush, or open capsules. • If a dose is missed or vomiting occurs after administration, do not give extra dose. Administer next dose at regularly scheduled time. • Administration at bedtime may decrease occurrence of nausea.

INDICATIONS/ROUTES/DOSAGE

Recurrent Epithelial Ovarian, Fallopian Tube, Peritoneal Cancer
PO: ADULTS, ELDERLY: 300 mg once daily, initiated no later than 8 wks after most recent platinum-containing regimen. Continue until disease progression or unacceptable toxicity.

Dose Reduction Schedule
First dose reduction: 200 mg daily.
Second dose reduction: 100 mg daily.

Dose Modification
Note: If acute myeloid leukemia or myelodysplastic syndrome is confirmed, permanently discontinue.

Anemia, Neutropenia
ANC less than 1,000 cells/mm³, Hgb level less than 8 g/dL: Withhold treatment for maximum of 28 days until ANC improves to greater than or equal to 1,500 cells/mm³ or Hgb level improves to 9 g/dL or greater, then resume at reduced dose level. If ANC or Hgb level does not improve to an acceptable level within 28 days or if dose is already reduced to 100 mg/day, permanently discontinue.

Hematologic Toxicity Requiring Transfusion
Platelet count less than or equal to 10,000 cells/mm³: Consider transfusion, then resume at reduced dose level.

Nonhematologic Toxicity
Any nonhematologic CTCAE grade 3 or 4 toxicity when prophylactic treatment is not possible or toxicity persists despite treatment: Withhold treatment for maximum of 28 days until resolved, then resume at next lower dose level.
Any nonhematologic CTCAE grade 3 or 4 toxicity lasting more than 28 days with 100 mg/day regimen: Permanently discontinue.

Thrombocytopenia
Platelet count less than 100,000 cells/mm³: First occurrence: Withhold treatment for maximum of 28 days until improved to greater than or equal to 100,000 cells/mm³, then resume at same or reduced dose level. If platelet count is less than 75,000 cells/mm³, resume at reduced dose level. **Second occurrence:** Withhold treatment for maximum of 28 days until improved to greater than or equal to 100,000 cells/mm³, then resume at reduced dose level. If platelet count does not improve to an acceptable level within 28 days or if dose is already reduced to 100 mg/day, permanently discontinue.

Dosage in Renal Impairment
Mild to moderate impairment: No dose adjustment. **Severe impairment, ESRD:** Not specified; use caution.

Dosage in Hepatic Impairment
Mild impairment: No dose adjustment.
Moderate to severe impairment: Not specified; use caution.

SIDE EFFECTS

Frequent (74%–20%): Nausea, fatigue, asthenia, constipation, vomiting, abdominal pain/distention, insomnia, headache, decreased appetite, rash, mucositis, stomatitis, hypertension, dyspnea. **Occasional (19%–10%):** Myalgia, back pain, dizziness, dyspepsia, cough, arthralgia, anxiety, dysgeusia, dry mouth, palpitations, tachycardia, peripheral edema, decreased weight, depression.

ADVERSE EFFECTS/TOXIC REACTIONS

Anemia, neutropenia, leukopenia, thrombocytopenia are expected responses to therapy, but more severe reactions including bone marrow failure may result in life-threatening event. Fatal cases of acute myeloid leukemia, myelodysplastic syndrome reported in 1% of pts. Hypertension, hypertensive crisis reported in 9% of pts. Infections including bronchitis, conjunctivitis, nasopharyngitis (23% of pts), urinary tract infection (13% of pts) may occur. Epistaxis may occur, esp. in pts with treatment-induced thrombocytopenia.

NURSING CONSIDERATIONS

BASELINE ASSESSMENT

Obtain ANC, CBC, BMP, LFT; vital signs. Obtain pregnancy test in females of reproductive potential. Question plans of breastfeeding. Confirm compliance of effective contraception. Question history of cardiac disease, hypertension. Assess hydration status. Screen for active infection. Offer emotional support.

INTERVENTION/EVALUATION

Monitor ANC, CBC for anemia, leukopenia, neutropenia, thrombocytopenia wkly for first 4 wks, then monthly for 11 mos, then periodically thereafter. In pts with platelet count less than 10,000 cells/mm^3, consider withholding anticoagulant, antiplatelet drugs or proceed with transfusion (if applicable). Monitor for acute myeloid leukemia, myelodysplastic syndrome (bleeding or bruising easily, fatigue, frequent infections, pyrexia, hematuria, melena, weakness, weight loss, cytopenias, increased requirements for blood transfusion). Diligently screen for infections. Monitor vital signs for arrhythmia, hypertension, tachycardia. Offer antiemetic if nausea, vomiting occurs. Assess skin for rash, toxic reactions. Encourage nutritional intake.

PATIENT/FAMILY TEACHING

• Treatment may depress your immune system and reduce your ability to fight infection. Report symptoms of infection such as body aches, burning with urination, chills, cough, fatigue, fever. Avoid those with active infection. • Treatment may cause severe bone marrow depression or new-onset myeloid leukemia; report bruising, fatigue, fever, frequent infections, shortness of breath, weight loss, bleeding easily, blood in urine or stool. • Avoid pregnancy. Females and males of childbearing potential should use effective contraception during treatment and for at least 6 mos after last dose. • Do not breastfeed during treatment and for at least 1 mo after final dose. • Treatment may impair fertility in males. • Dose administration at bedtime may decrease occurrence of nausea.

nitazoxanide

nye-ta-**zox**-a-nide
(Alinia)

◆CLASSIFICATION

PHARMACOTHERAPEUTIC: Antiparasitic. **CLINICAL:** Antiprotozoal agent.

USES

Treatment of diarrhea caused by *Cryptosporidium parvum, Giardia lamblia* in children 12 mos and older, adults. **OFF-LABEL:** *C. difficile*-associated diarrhea.

PRECAUTIONS

Contraindications: Hypersensitivity to nitazoxanide. **Cautions:** Caution with use of suspension in diabetic pts (due to sucrose content), hepatic/biliary disease, renal impairment.

ACTION

Interferes with body's reaction to pyruvate: ferredoxin oxidoreductase, an enzyme essential for anaerobic energy metabolism. **Therapeutic Effect:** Produces antiprotozoal activity, reducing/terminating diarrheal episodes.

PHARMACOKINETICS

Rapidly hydrolyzed to active metabolite. Protein binding: 99%. Excreted in urine, bile, feces. **Half-life:** 2–4 hrs.

⌛ LIFESPAN CONSIDERATIONS

Pregnancy/Lactation: Unknown if distributed in breast milk. **Children:** Safety and efficacy not established in pts younger than 1 yr (suspension) and younger than 12 yrs (tablet). **Elderly:** No age-related precautions noted.

INTERACTIONS

DRUG: None significant. **HERBAL:** None significant. **FOOD:** None known. **LAB VALUES:** May increase serum creatinine, ALT.

AVAILABILITY (Rx)

Powder for Oral Suspension: 100 mg/5 mL. **Tablets:** 500 mg.

ADMINISTRATION/HANDLING

PO (Oral Suspension)
• Store unreconstituted powder at room temperature. • Reconstitute oral suspension with 48 mL water to provide concentration of 100 mg/5 mL. • Shake vigorously to suspend powder. • Reconstituted solution is stable for 7 days at room temperature. • Give with food.

PO (Tablets)
• Give with food.

INDICATIONS/ROUTES/DOSAGE

**Diarrhea Caused by *C. Parvum, G. Lamblia*
PO: ADULTS, ELDERLY, CHILDREN 12 YRS AND OLDER:** 500 mg q12h for 3 days. **CHILDREN 4–11 YRS:** 200 mg q12h for 3 days. **CHILDREN 1–3 YRS:** 100 mg q12h for 3 days.

Dosage in Renal/Hepatic Impairment
Use caution.

SIDE EFFECTS

Occasional (8%): Abdominal pain. **Rare (2%–1%):** Diarrhea, vomiting, headache.

ADVERSE EFFECTS/TOXIC REACTIONS

None known.

NURSING CONSIDERATIONS

BASELINE ASSESSMENT

Establish baseline B/P, weight, serum glucose, electrolytes. Assess for dehydration.

INTERVENTION/EVALUATION

Evaluate serum glucose in diabetics, electrolytes (therapy generally reduces abnormalities). Weigh pt daily. Encourage adequate fluid intake. Assess bowel sounds for peristalsis. Monitor daily pattern of bowel activity, stool consistency.

PATIENT/FAMILY TEACHING

• Parents of children with diabetes should be aware that the oral suspension contains 1.48 g of sucrose per 5 mL. • Therapy should provide significant improvement of diarrhea.

nitrofurantoin

nye-troe-fue-**ran**-toyn
(Apo-Nitrofurantoin ✦, Furadantin,
Macrobid, Macrodantin, Novo-
Furantoin ✦)
**Do not confuse Macrobid with
MicroK or Nitro-Bid, or nitro-
furantoin with Neurontin or
nitroglycerin.**

◆CLASSIFICATION

PHARMACOTHERAPEUTIC: Antibacterial. **CLINICAL:** Antibiotic, UTI
prophylaxis.

USES

Prevention/treatment of UTI caused
by susceptible gram-negative, gram-
positive organisms, including *E. coli*,
*S. aureus, Enterococcus, Klebsiella,
Enterobacter.*

PRECAUTIONS

Contraindications: Hypersensitivity to
nitrofurantoin. Anuria, oliguria, renal
impairment (CrCl less than 60 mL/
min), infants younger than 1 mo due
to risk of hemolytic anemia. Pregnancy
at term, during labor, or delivery, or
when onset of labor is imminent. Pts
with history of cholestatic jaundice or
hepatic impairment with previous nitrofurantoin therapy. **Cautions:** Renal
impairment, diabetes, electrolyte imbalance, anemia, vitamin B deficiency,
debilitated pts (greater risk of peripheral neuropathy), G6PD deficiency
(greater risk of hemolytic anemia),
elderly pts, prolonged therapy (may
cause pulmonary toxicity).

ACTION

Inhibits bacterial enzyme systems, interfering with metabolism and cell wall
synthesis. **Therapeutic Effect:** Bacteriostatic (bactericidal at high concentrations).

PHARMACOKINETICS

Microcrystalline form rapidly, completely absorbed; macrocrystalline form
more slowly absorbed. Food increases
absorption. Protein binding: 60%. Primarily concentrated in urine, kidneys.
Metabolized in most body tissues. Primarily excreted in urine. Removed by
hemodialysis. **Half-life:** 20–60 min.

⧗ LIFESPAN CONSIDERATIONS

Pregnancy/Lactation: Readily crosses
placenta. Distributed in breast milk. Contraindicated at term and during lactation
when infant suspected of having G6PD
deficiency. **Children:** No age-related
precautions noted in pts older than 1
mo. **Elderly:** Avoid use. More likely to
develop acute pneumonitis, peripheral
neuropathy. Age-related renal impairment may require dosage adjustment.

INTERACTIONS

**DRUG: Antacids containing magne-
sium trisilicate** may decrease absorption.
Probenecid may increase concentration,
risk of toxicity. **HERBAL:** None significant.
FOOD: None known. **LAB VALUES:** May
increase serum ALT, AST, phosphorus. May
decrease Hgb.

AVAILABILITY (Rx)

**Capsules (Macrocrystalline [Macro-
bid]):** 100 mg. **Capsules (Macrocrystalline [Macrodantin]):** 25 mg, 50 mg, 100
mg. **Oral Suspension (Microcrystalline
[Furadantin]):** 25 mg/5 mL.

ADMINISTRATION/HANDLING

PO
• Give with food, milk to enhance absorption, reduce GI upset. • May mix
suspension with water, milk, fruit juice;
shake well.

INDICATIONS/ROUTES/DOSAGE

UTI
PO: *(Furadantin,   Macrodantin):*
ADULTS, ELDERLY: 50–100 mg q6h for
7 days or at least 3 days after obtaining
sterile urine. **Maximum:** 400 mg/day.

N

✦ Canadian trade name   🐦 Non-Crushable Drug   🄷🄸🄶🄷 High Alert drug

CHILDREN, ADOLESCENTS: 5–7 mg/kg/day in divided doses q6h for 7 days or at least 3 days after obtaining sterile urine. **Maximum:** 400 mg/day.
PO: *(Macrobid):* ADULTS, ELDERLY, ADOLESCENTS: 100 mg twice daily for 7 days.

Long-Term Prevention of UTI
PO: ADULTS, ELDERLY: 50–100 mg at bedtime. CHILDREN OLDER THAN 1 MONTH: 1–2 mg/kg/day in 2 divided doses. **Maximum:** 100 mg/day.

Dosage in Renal Impairment
Contraindicated in pts with CrCl less than 60 mL/min.

Dosage in Hepatic Impairment
No dose adjustment.

SIDE EFFECTS

Frequent: Anorexia, nausea, vomiting, dark urine. **Occasional:** Abdominal pain, diarrhea, rash, pruritus, urticaria, hypertension, headache, dizziness, drowsiness. **Rare:** Photosensitivity, transient alopecia, asthmatic exacerbation in those with history of asthma.

ADVERSE EFFECTS/TOXIC REACTIONS

Superinfection, hepatotoxicity, peripheral neuropathy (may be irreversible), Stevens-Johnson syndrome, permanent pulmonary impairment, anaphylaxis occur rarely.

NURSING CONSIDERATIONS

BASELINE ASSESSMENT
Question for history of asthma. Evaluate baseline renal function, LFT. Question medical history as listed in Precautions, and screen for contraindications.

INTERVENTION/EVALUATION
Monitor CBC, BMP, LFT; I&O. Monitor daily pattern of bowel activity, stool consistency. Assess skin for rash, urticaria. Be alert for numbness/tingling, esp. of lower extremities (may signal onset of peripheral neuropathy).

Observe for signs of hepatotoxicity (fever, rash, arthralgia, hepatomegaly). Monitor respiratory status, esp. in pts with asthma.

PATIENT/FAMILY TEACHING
• Urine may become dark yellow/brown. • Take with food, milk for best results, to reduce GI upset. • Complete full course of therapy. • Avoid sun, ultraviolet light; use sunscreen, wear protective clothing. • Report cough, fever, chest pain, difficulty breathing, numbness/tingling of fingers, toes. • Rare occurrence of alopecia is transient.

nitroglycerin

nye-troe-**glis**-er-in
(Minitran, Nitro-Bid, Nitro-Dur, Nitrolingual, NitroMist, Nitrostat, Nitro-Time, Rectiv, Trinipatch ✦)
Do not confuse Nitro-Bid with Macrobid or Nicobid, Nitro-Dur with Nicoderm, nitroglycerin with nitrofurantoin or nitroprusside, or Nitrostat with Nilstat or Nystatin.

◆CLASSIFICATION

PHARMACOTHERAPEUTIC: Nitrate. **CLINICAL:** Antianginal, antihypertensive, coronary vasodilator.

USES

Treatment/prevention of angina pectoris. Extended-release, topical forms used for prophylaxis, long-term angina management. IV form used in treatment of HF, acute MI, perioperative hypertension, induction of intraoperative hypotension. **Rectiv:** Treatment of moderate to severe pain associated with chronic anal fissure. **OFF-LABEL:** Short-term management of pulmonary hypertension, esophageal spastic disorders, uterine relaxation, treatment of sympathomimetic vasopressor extravasation.

PRECAUTIONS

Contraindications: Hypersensitivity to nitroglycerin. Allergy to adhesives (transdermal); increased ICP; severe anemia; concurrent use of sildenafil, tadalafil, vardenafil (PDE5 inhibitors). **(Additional) IV:** Restrictive cardiomyopathy, pericardial tamponade, constrictive pericarditis. **Sublingual, Rectal:** Increased intracranial pressure, severe anemia. **Cautions:** Blood volume depletion, severe hypotension (systolic B/P less than 90 mm Hg), bradycardia (less than 50 beats/min), inferior wall MI and suspected right ventricular involvement.

ACTION

Dilates coronary arteries, improves collateral blood flow to ischemic areas within myocardium. IV form produces peripheral vasodilation. **Therapeutic Effect:** Decreases myocardial oxygen demand. Reduces left ventricular preload, afterload.

PHARMACOKINETICS

Route	Onset	Peak	Duration
Sublingual	1–3 min	4–8 min	30–60 min
Translingual spray	2 min	4–10 min	30–60 min
Buccal tablet	2–5 min	4–10 min	2 hrs
PO (extended-release)	20–45 min	45–120 min	4–8 hrs
Topical	15–60 min	30–120 min	2–12 hrs
Transdermal patch	40–60 min	60–180 min	18–24 hrs
IV	1–2 min	Immediate	3–5 min

Well absorbed after PO, sublingual, topical administration. Metabolized in liver, by enzymes in bloodstream. Protein binding: 60%. Excreted in urine. Not removed by hemodialysis. **Half-life:** 1–4 min.

⏳ LIFESPAN CONSIDERATIONS

Pregnancy/Lactation: Unknown if drug crosses placenta or is distributed in breast milk. **Children:** Safety and efficacy not established. **Elderly:** More susceptible to hypotensive effects. Age-related renal impairment may require dosage adjustment.

INTERACTIONS

DRUG: Alcohol, other antihypertensives (e.g., **amLODIPine, lisinopril, valsartan**), **vasodilators** may increase risk of orthostatic hypotension. Concurrent use of **sildenafil, tadalafil, vardenafil** (PDE5 inhibitors) produces significant hypotension. **HERBAL:** Ephedra, ginger, ginseng, licorice may increase hypertension. Black cohosh, goldenseal, hawthorn may cause hypotension. **FOOD:** None known. **LAB VALUES:** May increase serum methemoglobin, urine catecholamine concentrations.

AVAILABILITY (Rx)

Infusion, Pre-Mix: 25 mg/250 mL, 50 mg/500 mL, 50 mg/250 mL, 100 mg/250 mL. **Injection, Solution:** 5 mg/mL. **Ointment (Nitro-Bid):** 2%. **Ointment, Rectal (Rectiv):** 0.4%. **Translingual Spray:** 0.4 mg/spray. **Transdermal Patch:** 0.1 mg/hr, 0.2 mg/hr, 0.4 mg/hr, 0.6 mg/hr.

 Capsules, Extended-Release: 2.5 mg, 6.5 mg, 9 mg. **Tablets, Sublingual:** 0.4 mg.

ADMINISTRATION/HANDLING

◀**ALERT**▶ Cardioverter/defibrillator must not be discharged through paddle electrode overlying nitroglycerin (transdermal, ointment) application. May cause burns to pt or damage to paddle via arcing.

IV

Reconstitution • Available in ready-to-use injectable containers. • Dilute vials in D₅W or 0.9% NaCl. **Maximum concentration:** 400 mcg/mL. • Use glass bottles.

◆ Canadian trade name   🔖 Non-Crushable Drug   🔲 High Alert drug

Rate of Administration • Use micro-drop or infusion pump.

Storage • Store at room temperature. • Reconstituted solutions stable for 48 hrs at room temperature or 7 days if refrigerated.

PO

• Do not break, crush, or open extended-release capsules. • Do not shake oral aerosol canister before lingual spraying.

Sublingual

• Instruct pt to not swallow. • Dissolve under tongue. • Administer while seated. • Slight burning sensation under tongue may be lessened by placing tablet in buccal pouch. • Keep sublingual tablets in original container.

Topical

• Spread thin layer on clean, dry, hairless skin of upper arm or body (not below knee or elbow), using applicator or dose-measuring papers. Do not use fingers; do not rub/massage into skin.

Transdermal

• Apply patch on clean, dry, hairless skin of upper arm or body (not below knee or elbow). • May keep patch on when bathing/showering. • Do not cut/trim to adjust dose.

▨ IV INCOMPATIBILITIES

Alteplase (Activase), phenytoin (Dilantin).

▨ IV COMPATIBILITIES

Amiodarone (Cordarone), dexmedetomidine (Precedex), diltiaZEM (Cardizem), DOBUTamine (Dobutrex), DOPamine (Intropin), EPINEPHrine, famotidine (Pepcid), fentaNYL (Sublimaze), furosemide (Lasix), heparin, HYDROmorphone (Dilaudid), insulin, labetalol (Trandate), lidocaine, lipids, LORazepam (Ativan), midazolam (Versed), milrinone (Primacor), morphine, niCARdipine (Cardene), nitroprusside (Nipride), norepinephrine (Levophed), propofol (Diprivan).

INDICATIONS/ROUTES/DOSAGE

Angina, CAD

Translingual   Spray: ADULTS, ELDERLY: 1–2 sprays onto or under tongue q3–5min until relief is noted (no more than 3 sprays in 15-min period).

Sublingual: ADULTS, ELDERLY: One tablet (0.3–0.4 mg) under tongue. If chest pain fails to improve or worsens in 3–5 min, call 911. After the call, may take additional tablet. A third tablet may be taken 5 min after second dose (maximum of 3 tablets).

PO *(Extended-Release):* ADULTS, ELDERLY: 2.5–6.5 mg 3–4 times/day. **Maximum:** 26 mg 4 times/day.

Topical: ADULTS, ELDERLY: Initially, ½ inch upon waking and ½ inch 6 hrs later. May double dose to 1 inch and double again to 2 inches. **Maximum:** 2 doses/day including nitrate-free interval of 10–12 hrs.

Transdermal   Patch: ADULTS, ELDERLY: Initially, 0.2–0.4 mg/hr. **Maintenance:** 0.4–0.8 mg/hr. Consider patch on for 12–14 hrs, patch off for 10–12 hrs (prevents tolerance).

HF, Acute MI

IV: ADULTS, ELDERLY: Initially, 5 mcg/min via infusion pump. Increase in 5-mcg/min increments at 3- to 5-min intervals until B/P response is noted or until dosage reaches 20 mcg/min, then increase by 10–20 mcg/min q3–5min. Dosage may be further titrated according to clinical, therapeutic response up to 400 mcg/min.

Anal Fissure

RECTAL: ADULTS, ELDERLY: One inch (1.5 mg) q12h for up to 3 wks.

Dosage in Renal/Hepatic Impairment

No dose adjustment.

SIDE EFFECTS

Frequent: Headache (possibly severe; occurs mostly in early therapy, diminishes rapidly in intensity, usually disappears during continued treatment), transient flushing of face/neck, dizziness (esp. if pt is standing immobile or is in a warm environment), weakness, orthostatic hypotension. **Sublingual:** Burning, tingling sensation at oral point of dissolution. **Ointment:** Erythema, pruritus. **Occasional:** GI upset. **Transdermal:** Contact dermatitis.

ADVERSE EFFECTS/TOXIC REACTIONS

Discontinue drug if blurred vision, dry mouth occurs. Severe orthostatic hypotension may occur, manifested by syncope, pulselessness, cold/clammy skin, diaphoresis. Tolerance may occur with repeated, prolonged therapy; minor tolerance may occur with intermittent use of sublingual tablets. High doses tend to produce severe headache.

NURSING CONSIDERATIONS

BASELINE ASSESSMENT

Record onset, type (sharp, dull, squeezing), radiation, location, intensity, duration of anginal pain; precipitating factors (exertion, emotional stress). Assess B/P, apical pulse before administration and periodically following dose. Pt must have continuous EKG monitoring for IV administration. Rule out right-sided MI, if applicable (may precipitate life-threatening hypotension). Receive full medication history, and screen for interactions, esp. use of PDE5 inhibitors. Question medical history and screen for contraindications.

INTERVENTION/EVALUATION

Monitor B/P, heart rate. Assess for facial, neck flushing. Cardioverter/defibrillator must not be discharged through paddle electrode overlying nitroglycerin (transdermal, ointment) system (may cause burns to pt or damage to paddle via electrical arcing). Consider NS boluses for hypotension.

PATIENT/FAMILY TEACHING

• Go from lying to standing slowly. • Take oral form on empty stomach (however, if headache occurs during therapy, take medication with meals). • Use spray only when lying down. • Dissolve sublingual tablet under tongue; do not swallow. • Take at first sign of angina. • May take additional dose q5min if needed up to a total of 3 doses. • If not relieved within 5 min, contact physician or immediately go to emergency room. • Do not change brands. • Keep container away from heat, moisture. • Do not inhale lingual aerosol but spray onto or under tongue (avoid swallowing after spray is administered). • Expel from mouth any remaining lingual, sublingual, intrabuccal tablet after pain is completely relieved. • Place transmucosal tablets under upper lip or buccal pouch (between cheek and gum); do not chew/swallow tablet. • Avoid alcohol (intensifies hypotensive effect). If alcohol is ingested soon after taking nitroglycerin, possible acute hypotensive episode (marked drop in B/P, vertigo, diaphoresis, pallor) may occur. • Do not use within 48 hrs of sildenafil, tadalafil, vardenafil (PDE5 inhibitors); may cause acute hypotensive episode.

nivolumab

nye-**vol**-ue-mab
(Opdivo)
Do not confuse nivolumab with denosumab, adalimumab, or palivizumab.

◆CLASSIFICATION

PHARMACOTHERAPEUTIC: Monoclonal antibody. **CLINICAL:** Antineoplastic.

USES

Treatment of BRAF V600 wild-type unresectable or metastatic melanoma, as a single agent; BRAF V600 mutation-positive unresectable melanoma, as a single agent; unresectable or metastatic melanoma, in combination with ipilimumab. Treatment of metastatic non–small-cell lung cancer with progression on or after platinum-based chemotherapy. Treatment of advanced renal cell cancer in pts receiving prior antiangiogenic therapy. Treatment of classical Hodgkin lymphoma (cHL) that relapsed or progressed following autologous hematopoietic stem cell transplant (HSCT) and post-brentuximab, or 3 or more lines of systemic therapy that includes autologous HSCT. Treatment of recurrent or metastatic squamous cell carcinoma of the head and neck. Treatment of locally advanced or metastatc urothelial carcinoma with disease progression during or following platinum-containing chemotherapy; or within 12 mos of neoadjuvant or adjuvant treatment with platinum containing chemotherapy. Treatment of colorectal cancer in adults and children 12 yrs of age and older that has progressed following treatment with fluoropyrimidine, oxaliplatin and irinotecan. Treatment of hepatocellular carcinoma in pts previously treated with sorafenib.

PRECAUTIONS

Contraindications: Hypersensitivity to nivolumab. **Cautions:** Thyroid/pituitary disease, hepatic/renal impairment, interstitial lung disease, electrolyte imbalance.

ACTION

Binds PD-1 ligands to PD-1 receptor found on T cells, blocking its interaction with the ligands (PD-L1 and PD-L2). Releases PD-1 pathway–mediated inhibition of immune response (including antitumor immune response). **Therapeutic Effect:** Inhibits T-cell proliferation and cytokine production. Inhibits tumor cell growth and metastasis.

PHARMACOKINETICS

Information on metabolism and elimination is not available. Steady-state concentration reached in 12 wks. **Half-life:** 26.7 days.

⧗ LIFESPAN CONSIDERATIONS

Pregnancy/Lactation: Avoid pregnancy; may cause fetal harm. Unknown if distributed in breast milk. Females of reproductive potential should use effective contraception during treatment and up to 5 mos after discontinuation. **Children:** Safety and efficacy not established. **Elderly:** May have increased risk of endocrine/hepatic/pulmonary/optic/renal injury due to age-related diseases.

INTERACTIONS

DRUG: None known. **HERBAL:** None significant. **FOOD:** None known. **LAB VALUES: Single Therapy:** May increase serum alkaline phosphatase, ALT, AST, potassium. May decrease serum sodium. **Combo Therapy:** May increase serum alkaline phosphatase, ALT, AST, amylase, creatinine, lipase. May decrease RBC, Hct, Hgb, lymphocytes, neutrophils, platelets; serum calcium, sodium, magnesium. May increase or decrease serum calcium, potassium.

AVAILABILITY (Rx)

Injection Solution: 40 mg/4 mL, 100 mg/10 mL single-use vial.

ADMINISTRATION/HANDLING

 IV

Preparation • Visually inspect solution for particulate matter or discoloration. Solution should appear opalescent, colorless to pale yellow. Discard if solution is cloudy or contains particulate matter other than a few translucent to white proteinaceous particles. • Do not shake vial. • Withdraw required dose volume and dilute in 0.9% NaCl or 5% Dextrose injection. Final concentration will equal 1–10 mg/mL based on volume of diluent. • Mix by gentle inversion. • Do not shake. • Discard partially used or empty vials.

Rate of Administration • Infuse over 60 min using sterile, nonpyrogenic, low protein-binding, 0.2- to 1.2-micron in-line filter. • Flush IV line upon completion.

Storage • Refrigerate diluted solution up to 24 hrs or store at room temperature

N

for no more than 4 hrs (includes time of preparation and infusion). • Do not freeze.

🞙 IV INCOMPATIBILITIES

Do not infuse with other medications.

INDICATIONS/ROUTES/DOSAGE

Melanoma
IV ADULTS, ELDERLY: *(Single Agent):* 240 mg q2wks until disease progression or unacceptable toxicity. *(In combination with ipilimumab):* 1 mg/kg, followed by ipilimumab on the same day, q3wks for 4 doses. Subsequent single-agent therapy dose is 240 mg q2wks until disease progression or unacceptable toxicity.

Metastatic Non–Small-Cell Lung Cancer
IV: ADULTS, ELDERLY: 240 mg q2wks until disease progression or unacceptable toxicity.

Advanced Renal Cell Carcinoma, Urothelial Carcinoma, Hepatocellular Carcinoma
IV: ADULTS, ELDERLY: 240 mg q2wks until disease progression or unacceptable toxicity.

cHL (Recurrent or Metastatic)
IV: ADULTS, ELDERLY: 3 mg/kg q2wks until disease progression or unacceptable toxicity.

Head and Neck Carcinoma
IV: ADULTS, ELDERLY: 3 mg/kg q2wks until disease progression or unacceptable toxicity.

Dose Modification
Based on Common Terminology Criteria for Adverse Events (CTCAE).
Withhold Treatment for Any of the Following Adverse Events:
Grade 2 or 3 diarrhea or colitis; single-agent therapy–associated colitis; grade 2 pneumonitis; serum AST or ALT greater than 3–5 times upper limit of normal (ULN) or serum bilirubin 1.5–3 times ULN; grade 2 or 3 hypophysitis; grade 2 adrenal insufficiency; serum creatinine greater than 1.5–6 times ULN; grade 3 rash; first occurrence of any other grade 3 adverse reaction. When nivolumab is administered in combination with ipilimumab and nivolumab is withheld, then ipilimumab should also be withheld.
Restarting Therapy:
Resume when adverse reactions return to grade 0 or 1.
Permanently Discontinue for Any of the Following Adverse Events:
Combo-agent therapy (ipilimumab)–associated colitis; grade 3 or 4 pneumonitis; serum AST or ALT greater than 5 times ULN or serum bilirubin 3 times ULN; pts with liver metastasis who begin treatment with baseline grade 2 serum ALT or AST elevation who experience serum ALT or AST elevation greater than or equal to 50% from baseline that persists for at least 1 wk; grade 4 hypophysitis; grade 3 or 4 adrenal insufficiency; serum creatinine greater than 6 times ULN; grade 4 rash; recurrence of any other grade 3 adverse reaction; any life-threatening or grade 4 adverse reaction; requirement for predniSONE 10 mg/day or greater (or equivalent) for more than 12 wks; persistent grade 2 or 3 adverse reaction lasting longer than 12 wks.

Dosage in Renal Impairment
No dose adjustment.

Dosage in Hepatic Impairment
Mild to moderate impairment: No dose adjustment. **Severe impairment:** Not specified; use caution.

SIDE EFFECTS

Note: Percentage of side effects may vary depending on the use of single or combination therapy. **Frequent (50%–24%):** Fatigue, dyspnea, musculoskeletal pain, decreased appetite, cough, nausea, headache, constipation. **Occasional (19%–10%):** Vomiting, asthenia, diarrhea, edema, pyrexia, cough, dehydration, rash, abdominal pain, chest pain, arthralgia, decreased weight, blurred vision, pruritus, peripheral edema, generalized pain.

ADVERSE EFFECTS/ TOXIC REACTIONS

Anemia, lymphopenia, neutropenia, thrombocytopenia is an expected response to therapy. May cause severe immune-mediated events including interstitial lung disease or pneumonitis (3%–10% of pts), colitis (21%–57% of pts), hepatitis (15%–28% of pts), hypophysitis (13% of pts), renal failure or nephritis (1%–2% of pts), hyperthyroidism (1% of pts), hypothyroidism (3%–19% of pts), rash (up to 37% of pts). Other adverse events including autoimmune nephropathy, demyelination, diabetic ketoacidosis, duodenitis, erythema multiforme, exfoliative dermatitis, facial and abducens nerve paresis, gastritis, iridocyclitis, motor dysfunction, pancreatitis, psoriasis, sarcoidosis, uveitis, vasculitis, ventricular arrhythmia, vitiligo reported in less than 2% of pts. Severe infusion-related reactions reported in less than 1% of pts. Occurrence of events is dependent on use of single or combination therapy. Upper respiratory tract infections including nasopharyngitis, pharyngitis, rhinitis reported in 11% of pts. Immunogenicity (auto-nivolumab antibodies) occurred in 8.5% of pts.

NURSING CONSIDERATIONS

BASELINE ASSESSMENT

Obtain baseline CBC, BMP, ionized calcium, LFT, TSH; vital signs; urine pregnancy. Record weight in kg. Screen for history of arrhythmias, pituitary/pulmonary/thyroid disease, autoimmune disorders, diabetes, hepatic/renal impairment; allergy to predniSONE. Along with routine assessment, conduct full dermatologic exam, ophthalmologic exam/visual acuity. Receive full medication history and screen for interactions.

INTERVENTION/EVALUATION

Monitor CBC, LFT, serum electrolytes; thyroid panel if applicable. Diligently monitor for immune-mediated adverse events as listed in Adverse Effects/Toxic Reactions. Notify physician if any CTCAE toxicities occur (see Appendix M) and initiate proper treatment. Obtain chest X-ray if interstitial lung disease, pneumonitis suspected. Screen for tumor lysis syndrome in pts with high tumor burden. Monitor I&O, daily weight. If predniSONE therapy is initiated for immune-mediated events, monitor capillary blood glucose and screen for corticosteroid side effects.

PATIENT/FAMILY TEACHING

• Blood levels will be routinely monitored. • Avoid pregnancy; treatment may cause birth defects or miscarriage. Do not breastfeed. Females of childbearing potential should use effective contraception during treatment and for at least 5 mos after discontinuation. • Serious adverse reactions may affect lungs, GI tract, kidneys, or hormonal glands; anti-inflammatory medication may need to be started. • Immediately contact physician if serious or life-threatening inflammatory reactions occur in the following body systems: colon (severe abdominal pain or diarrhea); kidney (decreased or dark-colored urine, flank pain); lung (chest pain, cough, shortness of breath); liver (bruising easily, dark-colored urine, clay-colored/tarry stools, yellowing of skin or eyes); pituitary (persistent or unusual headache, dizziness, extreme weakness, fainting, vision changes); thyroid (trouble sleeping, high blood pressure, fast heart rate [overactive thyroid]), (fatigue, goiter, weight gain [underactive thyroid]).

norepinephrine

nor-ep-i-**nef**-rin
(Levophed)

■ **BLACK BOX ALERT** ■ Extravasation may produce severe tissue necrosis, sloughing. Using fine hypodermic needle, liberally infiltrate area with 10–15 mL saline solution containing 5–10 mg phentolamine. **Do not confuse Levophed with Levaquin or levoFLOXacin, or norepinephrine with EPINEPHrine.**

◆CLASSIFICATION

PHARMACOTHERAPEUTIC: Alpha, beta agonist. **CLINICAL:** Vasopressor.

USES

Severe hypotension, treatment of shock persisting after fluid volume replacement.

PRECAUTIONS

Contraindications: Hypersensitivity to norepinephrine. Hypotension related to hypovolemia (except in emergency to maintain coronary/cerebral perfusion until volume replaced), mesenteric/peripheral vascular thrombosis (unless it is lifesaving procedure). **Cautions:** Concurrent use of MAOIs.

ACTION

Stimulates beta$_1$-adrenergic receptors, alpha-adrenergic receptors, increasing contractility, heart rate and producing vasoconstriction. **Therapeutic Effect:** Increases systemic B/P, coronary blood flow.

PHARMACOKINETICS

Route	Onset	Peak	Duration
IV	Rapid	1–2 min	N/A

Localized in sympathetic tissue. Metabolized in liver. Primarily excreted in urine.

⧖ LIFESPAN CONSIDERATIONS

Pregnancy/Lactation: Readily crosses placenta. May produce fetal anoxia due to uterine contraction, constriction of uterine blood vessels. **Children/Elderly:** No age-related precautions noted.

INTERACTIONS

DRUG: MAOIs (e.g., phenelzine, selegiline), antidepressants (tricyclic) may prolong hypertension. **HERBAL:** None significant. **FOOD:** None known. **LAB VALUES:** None significant.

AVAILABILITY (Rx)

Injection Solution: 1 mg/mL.

ADMINISTRATION/HANDLING

📵 IV

Reconstitution • Add 4 mL (4 mg) to 250 mL D$_5$W (16 mcg/mL). **Maximum concentration:** 32 mL (32 mg) to 250 mL (128 mcg/mL).
Rate of Administration • Closely monitor IV infusion flow rate (use infusion pump). • Monitor B/P q2min during IV infusion until desired therapeutic response is achieved, then q5min during remaining IV infusion. • Never leave pt unattended. • Maintain B/P at 90–100 mm Hg in previously normotensive pts, and 30–40 mm Hg below preexisting B/P in previously hypertensive pts. • Reduce IV infusion gradually. Avoid abrupt withdrawal. • If using peripherally inserted catheter, it is imperative to check the IV site frequently for free flow and infused vein for blanching, hardness to vein, coldness, pallor to extremity. • If extravasation occurs, area should be infiltrated with 10–15 mL sterile saline containing 5–10 mg phentolamine (does not alter pressor effects of norepinephrine).
Storage • Do not use if solution is brown or contains precipitate. • Store at room temperature. Diluted solution stable for 24 hrs at room temperature.

🔲 IV INCOMPATIBILITIES

Pantoprazole (Protonix), regular insulin.

🔲 IV COMPATIBILITIES

Amiodarone (Cordarone), calcium gluconate, dexmedetomidine (Precedex), diltiaZEM (Cardizem), DOBUTamine (Dobutrex), DOPamine (Intropin), EPINEPHrine, esmolol (Brevibloc), fentaNYL (Sublimaze), furosemide (Lasix), haloperidol (Haldol), heparin, HYDROmorphone (Dilaudid), labetalol (Trandate), lipids, LORazepam (Ativan),

N

magnesium, midazolam (Versed), milrinone (Primacor), morphine, niCARdipine (Cardene), nitroglycerin, potassium chloride, propofol (Diprivan).

INDICATIONS/ROUTES/DOSAGE

◄ **ALERT** ► If possible, blood, fluid volume depletion should be corrected before drug is administered.

Acute Hypotension Unresponsive to Fluid Volume Replacement
IV INFUSION: ADULTS, ELDERLY: Initially, administer at 8–12 mcg/min. Adjust rate of flow to desired response. Average maintenance range: 2–4 mcg/min (varies greatly based on clinical situation). **CHILDREN:** Initially, 0.05–0.1 mcg/kg/min; titrate to desired effect. **Maximum:** 2 mcg/kg/min.

Dosage in Renal/Hepatic Impairment
No dose adjustment.

SIDE EFFECTS

Norepinephrine produces less pronounced, less frequent side effects than EPINEPHrine. **Occasional (5%–3%):** Anxiety, bradycardia, palpitations. **Rare (2%–1%):** Nausea, anginal pain, shortness of breath, fever.

ADVERSE EFFECTS/TOXIC REACTIONS

Extravasation may produce tissue necrosis, sloughing. Overdose manifested as severe hypertension with violent headache (may be first clinical sign of overdose), arrhythmias, photophobia, retrosternal or pharyngeal pain, pallor, diaphoresis, vomiting. Prolonged therapy may result in plasma volume depletion. Hypotension may recur if plasma volume is not maintained.

NURSING CONSIDERATIONS

BASELINE ASSESSMENT
Assess EKG, B/P continuously (be alert to precipitous B/P drop). Be alert to pt complaint of headache.

INTERVENTION/EVALUATION
Monitor IV flow rate diligently. Assess for extravasation characterized by blanching of skin over vein, coolness (results from local vasoconstriction); color, temperature of IV site extremity (pallor, cyanosis, mottling). Assess nailbed capillary refill. Monitor I&O; measure output hourly, report urine output less than 30 mL/hr. Once B/P parameter has been reached, IV infusion should not be restarted unless systolic B/P falls below 90 mm Hg.

nortriptyline

nor-**trip**-ti-leen
(Apo-Nortriptyline ✤, Aventyl ✤, Norventyl ✤, Pamelor)
■ **BLACK BOX ALERT** ■ Increased risk of suicidal thinking and behavior in children, adolescents, young adults 18–24 yrs with major depressive disorder, other psychiatric disorders.
Do not confuse Aventyl with Bentyl, or nortriptyline with amitriptyline, desipramine, or Norpramin.

◆CLASSIFICATION

PHARMACOTHERAPEUTIC: Tricyclic compound. **CLINICAL:** Antidepressant.

USES

Treatment of symptoms of depression. **OFF-LABEL:** Adjunctive therapy for smoking cessation, myofascial pain, postherpetic pain, orofacial pain, chronic pain, irritable bowel syndrome.

PRECAUTIONS

Contraindications: Hypersensitivity to nortriptyline. Use during acute recovery period after MI. Use of MAOI intended to treat psychiatric disorders (concurrently or within 14 days of discontinuing either nortriptyline or MAOI). Initiation of nortriptyline in pt receiving linezolid or methylene blue. **Cautions:** Prostatic hyperplasia, history of urinary retention/obstruction, narrow-angle glaucoma, diabetes, history of seizures, hyperthyroidism, cardiac/hepatic/renal disease, psychosis, increased intraocular pressure, pts at high risk for suicide, elderly pts.

ACTION

Blocks reuptake of neurotransmitters (norepinephrine, serotonin) at neuronal presynaptic membranes, increasing their availability at postsynaptic receptor sites. **Therapeutic Effect:** Relieves depression, anxiety disorders, nocturnal enuresis.

PHARMACOKINETICS

Rapidly absorbed. Widely distributed. Extensively bound to plasma proteins. Metabolized in liver. Excreted primarily in urine. **Half-life:** (Adults): 14–51 hrs. (Elderly): 23–79 hrs.

LIFESPAN CONSIDERATIONS

Pregnancy/Lactation: Crosses placenta, excreted in breast milk. **Children:** Safety and efficacy not established in children younger than 6 yrs. **Elderly:** Use caution.

INTERACTIONS

DRUG: **Alcohol, other CNS depressants (e.g., LORazepam, morphine, zolpidem)** may increase CNS effects, respiratory depression, hypotensive effects. **Cimetidine** may increase concentration, risk of toxicity. **MAOIs (e.g., phenelzine, selegiline)** may increase risk of neuroleptic malignant syndrome, seizures, hyperpyrexia, hypertensive crisis. **HERBAL:** **Gotu kola, kava kava, St. John's wort, valerian** may increase CNS depression and risk of serotonin syndrome. **FOOD:** **Grape juice, carbonated beverages** may decrease effectiveness. **Grapefruit products** may increase risk of side effects. **LAB VALUES:** May alter serum glucose, EKG readings. **Therapeutic peak serum level:** 6–10 mcg/mL; **therapeutic

trough serum level:** 0.5–2 mcg/mL. **Toxic peak serum level:** greater than 12 mcg/mL; **toxic trough serum level:** greater than 2 mcg/mL.

AVAILABILITY (Rx)

Capsules (Pamelor): 10 mg, 25 mg, 50 mg, 75 mg. **Oral Solution:** 10 mg/5 mL.

ADMINISTRATION/HANDLING

PO
• Give with food, milk if GI distress occurs. • Dilute oral solution in water, milk, or fruit juice. Give immediately. (Do not mix with grape juice/carbonated beverages.)

INDICATIONS/ROUTES/DOSAGE

◀**ALERT**▶ At least 14 days must elapse between use of MAOIs and nortriptyline. When discontinuing, gradually taper dose to minimize withdrawal symptoms.

Depression
PO: ADULTS: Initially, 25 mg 3–4 times/day up to 150 mg/day. Adjust dose based on response and tolerability. **ELDERLY:** Initially, 30–50 mg at bedtime. May increase by 25 mg every 3–7 days. **Maximum:** 150 mg/day.

Enuresis
PO: CHILDREN OLDER THAN 11 YRS: 25–35 mg/day. **8–11 YRS:** 10–20 mg/day. **6–7 YRS:** 10 mg/day.

Dosage in Renal Impairment
No dose adjustment.

Dosage in Hepatic Impairment
Use caution.

SIDE EFFECTS

Frequent: Drowsiness, fatigue, dry mouth, blurred vision, constipation, delayed micturition, orthostatic hypotension, diaphoresis, impaired concentration, increased appetite, urinary retention. **Occasional:** GI disturbances (nausea, GI distress, metallic taste), photosensitivity. **Rare:** Paradoxical reactions (agitation, restlessness, nightmares,

N

insomnia), extrapyramidal symptoms (particularly fine hand tremor).

ADVERSE EFFECTS/ TOXIC REACTIONS

High dosage may produce cardiovascular effects (severe orthostatic hypotension, dizziness, tachycardia, palpitations, arrhythmias), altered temperature regulation (hyperpyrexia, hypothermia). Abrupt discontinuation from prolonged therapy may produce headache, malaise, nausea, vomiting, vivid dreams.

NURSING CONSIDERATIONS

BASELINE ASSESSMENT

Assess for suicidal ideation/tendencies, behavior, thought content, appearance. Obtain baseline glucose, cholesterol levels. For pts on long-term therapy, hepatic/renal function tests, blood counts should be performed periodically.

INTERVENTION/EVALUATION

Supervise suicidal-risk pt closely during early therapy (as depression lessens, energy level improves, increasing suicide potential). Assess appearance, behavior, speech pattern, level of interest, mood. Monitor daily pattern of bowel activity, stool consistency. Avoid constipation with increased fluids, bulky foods. Monitor B/P, pulse for hypotension, arrhythmias, weight. Assess for urinary retention. Therapeutic peak serum level: 6–10 mcg/mL; trough serum level: 0.5–2 mcg/mL. Toxic peak serum level: greater than 12 mcg/mL; toxic trough: greater than 2 mcg/mL.

PATIENT/FAMILY TEACHING

• Slowly go from lying to standing to avoid hypotensive effect; tolerance to postural hypotension, sedative, anticholinergic effects usually develops during early therapy. • Avoid alcohol. • Avoid tasks that require alertness, motor skills until response to drug is established. • Therapeutic effect may be noted in 2 wks or longer. • Photosensitivity to sun may occur; use sunscreen, protective clothing. • Dry mouth may be relieved by sugarless gum, sips of water. • Report visual disturbances, worsening depression, suicidal ideation, unusual changes in behavior (esp. at initiation of therapy or with changes in dosage). • Do not abruptly discontinue medication.

nystatin

nye-**stat**-in
(Candistatin ✤, Nystop, Pedi-Dri)
Do not confuse nystatin with atorvastatin, fluvastatin, lovastatin, Nitrostat, pitavastatin, pravastatin, rosuvastatin, or simvastatin.

FIXED-COMBINATION(S)

Mycolog, Myco-Triacet: nystatin/triamcinolone (a steroid): 100,000 units/0.1%.

◆CLASSIFICATION

PHARMACOTHERAPEUTIC: Polyene antifungal antibiotic. **CLINICAL:** Antifungal.

USES

Treatment of cutaneous, intestinal, oral cavity, infections caused by *Candida* spp.

PRECAUTIONS

Contraindications: Hypersensitivity to nystatin. **Cautions:** None known.

ACTION

Binds to sterols in cell membrane, increasing fungal cell membrane permeability, permitting loss of potassium, other cellular components. **Therapeutic Effect:** Fungistatic.

PHARMACOKINETICS

PO: Poorly absorbed from GI tract. Eliminated unchanged in feces. **Topical:** Not absorbed systemically from intact skin.

⏳ LIFESPAN CONSIDERATIONS

Pregnancy/Lactation: Unknown if distributed in breast milk. Vaginal applicators may be contraindicated, requiring manual insertion of tablets during pregnancy. **Children:** No age-related precautions noted for suspension, topical use. Lozenges not recommended in pts younger than 5 yrs. **Elderly:** No age-related precautions noted.

INTERACTIONS

DRUG: None significant. **HERBAL:** None significant. **FOOD:** None known. **LAB VALUES:** None significant.

AVAILABILITY (Rx)

Cream: 100,000 units/g. **Ointment:** 100,000 units/g. **Oral Suspension:** 100,000 units/mL. **Tablets:** 500,000 units. **Topical Powder (Nystop, Pedi-Dri):** 100,000 units/g.

ADMINISTRATION/HANDLING

PO

• Shake suspension well before administration. • Place and hold suspension in mouth or swish throughout mouth as long as possible before swallowing. • For neonates and infants, paint into recesses of the mouth.

INDICATIONS/ROUTES/DOSAGE

Intestinal Infection

PO: ADULTS, ELDERLY: (Tablets): 500,000–1,000,000 units q8h.

Oral Candidiasis

PO: ADULTS, ELDERLY, CHILDREN: (Suspension): 400,000–600,000 units 4 times/day.

INFANTS: 200,000 units 4 times/day. **PREMATURE INFANTS:** 100,000 units 4 times/day.

Cutaneous Candidal Infections

Topical: ADULTS, ELDERLY, CHILDREN: Apply 2–3 times/day.

Dosage in Renal/Hepatic Impairment

No dose adjustment.

SIDE EFFECTS

Occasional: PO: None known. **Topical:** Skin irritation. **Vaginal:** Vaginal irritation.

ADVERSE EFFECTS/ TOXIC REACTIONS

High dosages of oral form may produce nausea, vomiting, diarrhea, GI distress.

NURSING CONSIDERATIONS

BASELINE ASSESSMENT

Confirm cultures, histologic tests were obtained for accurate diagnosis. Inspect oral mucous membranes.

INTERVENTION/EVALUATION

Assess for increased skin irritation with topical, increased vaginal discharge with vaginal application.

PATIENT/FAMILY TEACHING

• Do not miss doses; complete full length of treatment (continue vaginal use during menses). • Report nausea, vomiting, diarrhea, stomach pain. • **Vaginal:** Insert high in vagina. • Check with physician regarding douching, sexual intercourse. • **Topical:** Rub well into affected areas. • Avoid contact with eyes. • Use cream (sparingly) or powder on erythematous areas. • Keep areas clean, dry; wear light clothing for ventilation. • Separate personal items in contact with affected areas.

N

obinutuzumab

oh-bi-nue-**tooz**-ue-mab
(Gazyva)

■ **BLACK BOX ALERT** ■ Hepatitis B virus reactivation, resulting in hepatic failure, fulminant hepatitis, and death have occurred. Screen all pts for hepatitis B virus infection before initiating treatment. Progressive multifocal leukoencephalopathy (PML) including fatal PML reported.

◆CLASSIFICATION

PHARMACOTHERAPEUTIC: Monoclonal antibody. **CLINICAL:** Antineoplastic.

USES

Treatment of previously untreated chronic lymphocytic leukemia (CLL), in combination with chlorambucil. Treatment of follicular lymphoma (in combination with bendamustine) in pts who relapsed after, or are refractory to, a riTUXimab-containing regimen. Treatment of previously untreated stage II bulky, stage III, or stage IV follicular lymphoma in combination with chemotherapy and followed by obinutuzumab monotherapy.

PRECAUTIONS

Contraindications: Hypersensitivity to obinutuzumab. **Cautions:** Pts showing evidence of prior HBV infection, preexisting cardiac/pulmonary impairment; hematologic abnormalities (e.g., leukopenia, thrombocytopenia); electrolyte imbalance; avoid with active infection.

ACTION

Targets CD20 antigen expressed on surface of B lymphocytes. Mediates B-cell lysis, cellular cytotoxicity, and antibody-dependent cellular phagocytosis (macrophage ingestion). **Therapeutic Effect:** Inhibits tumor cell growth and proliferation in chronic lymphocytic leukemia.

PHARMACOKINETICS

Metabolism and elimination not specified. **Half-life:** 28 days.

⧖ LIFESPAN CONSIDERATIONS

Pregnancy/Lactation: Unknown if distributed in breast milk. Monoclonal antibodies are known to cross placenta. Effective contraception, discontinuation of breastfeeding recommended during therapy and for 18 months after discontinuation. **Children:** Safety and efficacy not established. **Elderly:** May have increased risk of adverse reactions.

INTERACTIONS

DRUG: ACE inhibitors (e.g., enalapril, lisinopril), angiotensin receptor blockers (e.g., losartan), beta blockers (e.g., metoprolol) may increase risk of hypotension. **HERBAL:** None significant. **FOOD:** None known. **LAB VALUES:** May increase serum alkaline phosphatase, ALT, AST, bilirubin, creatinine, uric acid. May decrease albumin, Hgb, Hct, lymphocytes, neutrophils, platelets; serum potassium, sodium.

AVAILABILITY (Rx)

Solution, Injection: 1,000 mg/40 mL (25 mg/mL) single-use vial.

ADMINISTRATION/HANDLING

◀**ALERT**▶ Administer via dedicated line. Do not administer IV push or bolus. Withhold hypertensive medications at least 12 hrs before and 1 hr after administration. Do not mix with dextrose-containing fluids.

 IV

Reconstitution • Visually inspect for particulate matter or discoloration. • For 100-mg dose: withdraw 40 mL solution from vial and dilute only 4 mL (100 mg) in 100 mL 0.9% NaCl for immediate administration. Dilute remaining 36 mL (900 mg) into 250 mL 0.9% NaCl at same time and refrigerate for up to 24 hrs for cycle 1: day 2. For remaining infusions (day 8 and day 15 of cycle 1 and day 1 of cycles 2–6), dilute 40 mL (1,000 mg) solution in 250 mL NaCl infusion bag. • Gently mix by inversion. • Do not shake.
Rate of Administration • Day 1 of **Cycle 1 (100 mg):** Infuse over 4 hrs

(25 mg/hr). • Do not increase infusion rate. • **Day 2 of Cycle 1 (900 mg):** Infuse at 50 mg/hr. • May increase by 50 mg/hr every 30 min to maximum rate of 400 mg/hr. • Increase rate based on tolerability.

Storage • Solution should appear clear, colorless to slightly brown. • May refrigerate diluted solution up to 24 hrs.

INDICATIONS/ROUTES/DOSAGE

Chronic Lymphocytic Leukemia (CLL)

◀ **ALERT** ▶ Premedicate with glucocorticoid, acetaminophen, and antihistamine to decrease severity of infusion reaction. Consider premedication with antihyperuricemics (allopurinol) 12–24 hrs for pts with high tumor burden or high circulating absolute lymphocyte count greater than 25×10^9/L. Recommend antimicrobial prophylaxis throughout treatment for pts with neutropenia.

IV: ADULTS/ELDERLY: Six treatment cycles of 28-day cycle. **Day 1 of Cycle 1:** 100 mg. **Day 2 of Cycle 1:** 900 mg. **Day 8 and Day 15 of Cycle 1:** 1000 mg. **Cycles 2–6:** 1000 mg on day 1 of each subsequent 28-day cycle for 5 doses. Discontinue treatment if any severe to life-threatening infusion reactions occur.

Follicular Lymphoma (Relapsed/Refractory)

IV: ADULTS, ELDERLY: Six treatment cycles of 28 days (in combination with bendamustine). **Cycle 1:** 1,000 mg on days 1, 8, 15. **Cycles 2–6:** 1,000 mg on day 1 of each subsequent 28-day cycle for 5 doses. If achieves stable disease, complete or partial response, continue obinutuzumab (as monotherapy) 1,000 mg q2mos for 2 yrs.

Follicular Lymphoma (previously untreated)

IV: ADULTS, ELDERLY: Cycle 1 (either in combination with bedamustine or with CHOP or CVP chemotherapy): 1,000 mg wkly on days 1,8 and 15. **Cycles 2–6 (in combination with bendamustine):** 1,000 mg on day 1 q28days for 5 doses. **Cycles 2–8 (in combination with CHOP):** 1,000 mg on day1 q21days for 5 doses (with CHOP), then 1,000 mg on day 1 q21 days for 2 doses (as monotherapy). **Cycles 2–8 (in combination with CVP):** 1,000 mg on day1 q21days for 7 doses. **Then as monotherapy:** 1,000 mg q2mos for up to 2 yrs beginning approximately 2 mos after last induction phase.

Dosage in Renal/Hepatic Impairment

No dose adjustment.

SIDE EFFECTS

Frequent (69%): Infusion reactions (pruritus, flushing, urticaria). **Occasional (10%):** Pyrexia, cough.

ADVERSE EFFECTS/TOXIC REACTIONS

Thrombocytopenia, neutropenia, leukopenia, lymphopenia (47%–80% of pts) are expected responses to therapy, but more severe reactions including bone marrow failure, febrile neutropenia, opportunistic infection may result in life-threatening events. Hepatitis B virus reactivation may occur. Infusion reactions including hypotension, tachycardia, dyspnea, bronchospasm, wheezing, laryngeal edema, nausea, vomiting, flushing, pyrexia may occur during infusion. Tumor lysis syndrome may present as acute renal failure, hypocalcemia, hyperuricemia, hyperphosphatemia within 12–24 hrs of infusion. Immunogenicity (autoantibodies) occurred in 13% of pts. Progressive multifocal leukoencephalopathy (PML) occurred rarely and may include weakness, paralysis, vision loss, aphasia, cognition impairment.

NURSING CONSIDERATIONS

BASELINE ASSESSMENT

Obtain baseline CBC, BMP, ionized calcium, phosphate, uric acid; vital signs. Screen for history of anemia, asthma, arrhythmias, COPD, diabetes, GI bleeding, hypertension, hepatitis B virus infection, hepatic/renal impairment, peripheral edema. Receive full medication history,

0

esp. hypertension, anticoagulant medications. Perform baseline visual acuity. Offer emotional support.

INTERVENTION/EVALUATION

Monitor CBC, serum electrolytes, LFT, vital signs. Monitor all pts for cardiovascular alterations, respiratory distress. If respiratory reactions occur, consider administration of oxygen, EPINEPHrine, albuterol treatments. Locate rapid-sequence intubation kit if respiratory compromise occurs. Monitor strict I&O, hydration status. If PML suspected, consult neurologist for proper management. Obtain EKG for palpitations, severe hypokalemia, hyponatremia.

PATIENT/FAMILY TEACHING

• Avoid pregnancy. • Report any yellowing of skin or eyes, abdominal pain, bruising, black/tarry stools, amber or bloody urine. • Fever, cough, burning with urination, body aches, chills may indicate acute infection. • Avoid use of live virus vaccines. • Avoid alcohol. • Immediately report difficult breathing, severe coughing, chest tightness, wheezing. • Paralysis, vision changes, impaired speech, altered mental status may indicate life-threatening neurologic event.

ocrelizumab

ok-re-**liz**-ue-mab
(Ocrevus)
Do not confuse ocrelizumab with certolizumab, daclizumab, efalizumab, mepolizumab, natalizumab, or omalizumab.

◆CLASSIFICATION

PHARMACOTHERAPEUTIC: Anti-CD20 monoclonal antibody. **CLINICAL:** Multiple sclerosis agent.

USES

Treatment of adult pts with relapsing or primary progressive forms of multiple sclerosis (MS).

PRECAUTIONS

Contraindications: Life-threatening infusion reaction to ocrelizumab. Active hepatitis B virus (HBV) infection confirmed by positive results for hepatitis B surface antigen (HBsAg) and anti-HBV tests. **Cautions:** History of chronic opportunistic infections (esp. bacterial, invasive fungal, mycobacterial, protozoal, viral, tuberculosis); active infection, conditions predisposing to infection (e.g., diabetes, immunocompromised pts, renal failure, open wounds); intolerance to corticosteroids; history of depression, malignancies, breast cancer. Avoid administration of live or live attenuated vaccines during treatment and after discontinuation until B-cells are no longer depleted.

ACTION

Monoclonal antibody that is directed against B cells, which express the cell surface antigen CD20 (thought to influence the course of MS through antigen presentation, autoantibody production, cytokine regulation, and formation of ectopic lymphoid aggregates in meninges). Binds to the cell surface to deplete CD20-expressing B cells. **Therapeutic Effect:** Reduces progression of MS.

PHARMACOKINETICS

Onset of action: serum CD-19+ B-cell count reduced within 14 days. Duration of action: 72 wks (Range: 27–175 wks). Antibodies are primarily cleared by catabolism. **Half-life:** 26 days.

⧗ LIFESPAN CONSIDERATIONS

Pregnancy/Lactation: May cause transient peripheral B-cell depletion and lymphocytopenia in neonates when used during pregnancy. Immunoglobulins are known to cross the placenta. Females of reproductive potential must use effective contraception during treatment and up to 6 mos after discontinuation. Unknown if distributed in breast milk; however, immunoglobulin G (IgG) is present in breast milk. Breastfeeding not recommended. **Children:** Safety and efficacy not established. **Elderly:** No age-related precautions noted.

INTERACTIONS

DRUG: May decrease effect of **BCG, vaccines** (live and attenuated). May increase adverse effects/toxicity of **belimumab, natalizumab, picrolimus, tacrolimus. HERBAL:** None significant. **FOOD:** None known. **LAB VALUES:** May decrease immunoglobulin A (IgA), immunoglobulin M (IgM), immunoglobulin G (IgG), neutrophils.

AVAILABILITY (Rx)

Injection, Solution: 300 mg/10 mL (30 mg/mL).

ADMINISTRATION/HANDLING
IV

Preparation • Visually inspect for particulate matter or discoloration. Solution should appear clear to slightly opalescent, colorless to pale brown in color. • Do not use if solution is cloudy, discolored, or if visible particles are observed. • Withdraw proper dose from vial (10 mL for 300-mg dose; 20 mL for 600-mg dose) and dilute into 0.9% NaCl bag to a final concentration of approx. 1.2 mg/mL (300-mg dose in 250 mL 0.9% NaCl; 600-mg dose in 500 mL 0.9% NaCl). • Mix by gentle inversion. • Do not shake or agitate.
Rate of Administration • **First and Second Infusion:** Start at 30 mL/hr via dedicated line using 0.2- or 0.22-micron in-line filter. If tolerated, increase rate by 30 mL/hr q30min to a maximum rate of 180 mL/hr for a duration of 2.5 hrs or longer. **Subsequent Infusions:** Start at 40 mL/hr via dedicated line using 0.2- or 0.22-micron in-line filter. If tolerated, increase rate by 40 mL/hr q30min to a maximum rate of 200 mL/hr for a duration of 3.5 hrs or longer. **Mild Infusion Reactions:** Decrease rate by 50% and continue reduced rate for at least 30 min. If tolerated, may increase infusion rate as described above. **Severe Infusion Reactions:** Interrupt infusion until symptoms resolve, then resume infusion at

50% of the initial infusion rate. **Life-threatening Infusion Reaction:** Immediately stop infusion and permanently discontinue; do not restart.
Storage • May refrigerate diluted solution up to 24 hrs or store at room temperature for up to 8 hrs (includes infusion time). • If diluted solution is refrigerated, allow to warm to room temperature before administration. • Discard solution if not administered within required time frame.

IV INCOMPATIBILITIES

Do not dilute with other IV solutions. Do not mix or infuse with other medications.

INDICATIONS/ROUTES/DOSAGE

◀**ALERT**▶ Must be administered under the direct supervision of health care professionals with access to emergency medical supplies and who are trained to manage severe infusion reactions. If a dose is missed, administer as soon as possible; do not wait until the next regularly scheduled dose. Reset administration schedule so that the next subsequent infusion is 6 mos after the most recent dose. Subsequent doses must be separated by at least 5 mos.
Premedication
• To reduce severity and frequency of infusion reaction, premedicate with methylprednisolone 100 mg (or equivalent) approx. 30 min prior to infusion and an antihistamine (e.g., diphenhydramine) approx. 30–60 min prior to infusion. • Consider an antipyretic (e.g., acetaminophen) based on previous infusion reactions.

Multiple Sclerosis
IV: ADULTS, ELDERLY: 300 mg once at wk 0 and wk 2, then 600 mg q6mos. Observe pt for at least 1 hr after completion of infusion.

Dosage in Renal/Hepatic Impairment
Mild impairment: No dose adjustment. **Moderate to severe impairment:** Not specified; use caution.

SIDE EFFECTS

Occasional (8%–5%): Back pain, cough, diarrhea, peripheral edema, extremity pain.

ADVERSE EFFECTS/ TOXIC REACTIONS

Infusion-related reactions including bronchospasm, dizziness, dyspnea, erythema, fatigue, flushing, headache, hypotension, nausea, oropharyngeal pain, nausea, pharyngeal/laryngeal edema, pruritus, pyrexia, rash, tachycardia, throat irritation, urticaria was reported in 34%–40% of pts. Serious infusion reactions requiring hospitalization occurred in less than 1% of pts. Infections including upper respiratory tract infections (40%–49% of pts), lower respiratory tract infections (10% of pts), skin infections (16% of pts), herpes infection (6% of pts) may occur. Progressive multifocal leukoencephalopathy (PML), an opportunistic viral infection of the brain caused by the JC virus, has occurred in pts treated with other anti-CD20 antibodies; may result in progressive permanent disability and death. Symptoms of PML include altered mental status, aphasia, paralysis, vision loss, weakness. HBV reactivation was reported in pts treated with other anti-CD20 antibodies; may result in fulminant hepatitis, hepatic failure, death. May increase risk of malignancies including breast cancer. Immunogenicity (auto anti-ocrelizumab antibodies) reported in 1% of pts. Depression reported in 8% of pts.

NURSING CONSIDERATIONS

BASELINE ASSESSMENT

Assess baseline symptoms of MS (e.g., bladder/bowel dysfunction, cognitive impairment, depression, dysphagia, fatigue, gait disorder, numbness/tingling, pain, seizures, spasticity, tremors, weakness). Obtain vital signs. Question history of hypersensitivity reactions, infusion-related reactions. Ensure that proper resuscitative equipment, medical supplies are readily available (e.g., albuterol, antipyretics, antihistamines, epinephrine, isotonic IV fluids, bag-valve mask, oxygen, rapid sequence intubation kit). Screen all pts for active HBV. Pts who test negative for HBsAg and positive for anti-HBcAb+ should be referred to a hepatic specialist. If applicable, immunizations should be up-to-date according to guidelines at least 6 wks prior to initiation. Question history of chronic infections, herpes infection, depression, malignancies, breast cancer. Screen for active infection. Verify use of effective contraception in females of reproductive potential.

INTERVENTION/EVALUATION

Monitor vital signs. Diligently monitor for infusion-related reactions during infusion and for at least 1 hr after completion (esp. during initial infusions). If severe or life-threatening reactions occur, immediately stop infusion and provide appropriate medical support. Due to risk of respiratory compromise, pts with bronchospasm, dyspnea, hypoxia should be given immediate supplemental oxygen, hypersensitivity medications, hemodynamic support. If laryngeal or pharyngeal edema occurs, airway protection or possible intubation may be required. Mild to moderate infusion reactions may require interruption of infusion, decrease of infusion rate, symptom management. Closely monitor for HBV reactivation, symptoms of PML, new malignancies including breast cancer, infections. Conduct neurologic assessment. Assess for symptom improvement of MS.

PATIENT/FAMILY TEACHING

• Life-threatening infusion reactions, allergic reactions may occur during infusion and up to 24 hrs after completion of infusion. Immediately report difficulty breathing, chest pain, chest tightness, chills, dizziness, fast heart rate, fever, flushing, headache, hives, itching, low blood pressure, nausea, throat pain or swelling, rash. • If applicable, vaccinations should be up-to-date at least 6 wks before starting treatment. Do not receive live vaccines. • Treatment may depress your immune system and reduce your ability to fight infection. Report symptoms of infection such as body aches, burning with urination, chills, cough, fatigue, fever. Avoid those with active infection. • Avoid pregnancy. Females of childbearing potential should use effective contraception during treatment and for at least 6 mos after last dose. Do not breastfeed. • Due to pretreatment with a corticosteroid, pts with diabetes may experience a transient rise in blood sugar levels. • PML, an opportunistic viral infection of the brain, may cause progressive, permanent disabilities and death. Report symptoms of PML such as confusion, memory loss, paralysis, trouble speaking, vision loss, seizures, weakness. • Treatment may cause reactivation of HBV, depression, new cancers including breast cancer. • Notify physician if symptoms of MS do not improve.

---

octreotide

ock-**tree**-oh-tide
(<u>SandoSTATIN</u>, <u>SandoSTATIN LAR Depot</u>)
Do not confuse SandoSTATIN with SandIMMUNE, SandoSTATIN LAR, sargramostim, or simvastatin.

◆CLASSIFICATION

PHARMACOTHERAPEUTIC: Somatostatin analogue. **CLINICAL:** Secretory inhibitory, growth hormone suppressant; antidiarrheal.

USES

Control of diarrhea and flushing in pts with metastatic carcinoid tumors, treatment of watery diarrhea associated with vasoactive intestinal peptic-secreting tumors (VIPomas), acromegaly (to reduce blood levels of growth hormone and insulin-like growth factor). **OFF-LABEL:** Control of bleeding esophageal varices, treatment of AIDS-associated secretory diarrhea, diarrhea, diarrhea associated with graft-vs-host disease, chemotherapy-induced diarrhea, insulinomas, small-bowel fistulas, Zollinger-Ellison syndrome, Cushing's syndrome, hypothalamic obesity, malignant bowel obstruction, postgastrectomy dumping syndrome, islet cell tumors, sulfonylurea-induced hypoglycemia.

PRECAUTIONS

Contraindications: Hypersensitivity to octreotide. **Cautions:** Diabetic pts with gastroparesis, renal failure, hepatic impairment, HF, concomitant medications altering heart rate or rhythm. Concurrent use of medications that prolong QT interval, elderly pts.

ACTION

Suppresses secretion of serotonin, gastrin, VIP, insulin, glucagon, secretin, pancreatic polypeptide. **Therapeutic Effect:** Prolongs intestinal transit time.

PHARMACOKINETICS

Route	Onset	Peak	Duration
SQ	N/A	N/A	Up to 12 hrs

Rapidly, completely absorbed from injection site. Protein binding: 65%. Metabolized in liver. Excreted in urine. Removed by hemodialysis. **Half-life:** 1.7–1.9 hrs.

⏳ LIFESPAN CONSIDERATIONS

Pregnancy/Lactation: Unknown if distributed in breast milk. **Children:** Safety and efficacy not established. **Elderly:** No age-related precautions noted.

INTERACTIONS

DRUG: May decrease effectiveness of cycloSPORINE. **Glucagon, growth hormone, insulin, oral antidiabetics (e.g., glipiZIDE, metFORMIN)** may alter glucose concentrations. **HERBAL:** Avoid herbs that have hypoglycemic activity **(e.g., garlic, ginger, ginseng).** **FOOD:** None known. **LAB VALUES:** May decrease serum thyroxine (T_4). May increase serum alkaline phosphatase, ALT, AST, GGT.

O

AVAILABILITY (Rx)

Injection Solution (SandoSTATIN): 50 mcg/mL, 100 mcg/mL, 200 mcg/mL, 500 mcg/mL, 1,000 mcg/mL. **Injection Suspension (SandoSTATIN LAR):** 10-mg, 20-mg, 30-mg vials.

ADMINISTRATION/HANDLING

◄**ALERT**► SandoSTATIN may be given IV, IM, SQ. SandoSTATIN LAR Depot may be given only IM. Refrigerate.

IM
• Give immediately after mixing. • Administer deep IM in large muscle mass at 4-wk intervals. • Avoid deltoid injections.

SQ
• Do not use if discolored or particulates form. • Avoid multiple injections at same site within short periods.

 IV
• Dilute in 50–100 mL 0.9% NaCl or D₅W and infuse over 15–30 min. In emergency, may give IV push over 3 min. Following dilution, stable for 96 hrs at room temperature when diluted with 0.9% NaCl (24 hrs with D₅W). Infuse over 15–30 min.

INDICATIONS/ROUTES/DOSAGE

Note: Schedule injections between meals (to decrease GI effects).

Carcinoid Tumor
IV, SQ (Sandostatin): ADULTS, ELDERLY: Initial 2 wks, 100–600 mcg/day in 2–4 divided doses. Range: 50–750 mcg.
IM (Sandostatin Lar): ADULTS, ELDERLY: Must be stabilized on SQ octreotide for at least 2 wks. 20 mg q4wks for 2 mos, then modify based on response.

Vasoactive Intestinal Peptic-Secreting Tumor (VIPoma)
IV, SQ (Sandostatin): ADULTS, ELDERLY: Initial 2 wks, 200–300 mcg/day in 2–4 divided doses. Range: 150–750 mcg.
IM (Sandostatin Lar): ADULTS, ELDERLY: Must be stabilized on SQ octreotide for at least 2 wks; 20 mg q4wks for 2 mos, then modify based on response.

Esophageal Varices
IV (Sandostatin): ADULTS, ELDERLY: Bolus of 25–100 mcg followed by IV infusion of 25–50 mcg/hr for 2–5 days.

Acromegaly
IV, SQ (Sandostatin): ADULTS, ELDERLY: Initially, 50 mcg 3 times/day. Increase as needed. Range: 300–1,500 mcg/day. Usual effective dose: 100–200 mcg 3 times/day.
IM (Sandostatin Lar): ADULTS, ELDERLY: Must be stabilized on SQ octreotide for at least 2 wks. 20 mg q4wks for 3 mos, then modify based on response. **Maximum:** 40 mg q4wks.

Dosage in Renal/Hepatic Impairment
No dose adjustment.

SIDE EFFECTS

Frequent (10%–6%; 58%–30% in Acromegaly Pts): Diarrhea, nausea, abdominal discomfort, headache, injection site pain. **Occasional (5%–1%):** Vomiting, flatulence, constipation, alopecia, facial flushing, pruritus, dizziness, fatigue, arrhythmias, ecchymosis, blurred vision. **Rare (less than 1%):** Depression, diminished libido, vertigo, palpitations, dyspnea.

ADVERSE EFFECTS/TOXIC REACTIONS

Increased risk of cholelithiasis. Prolonged high-dose therapy may produce hypothyroidism. GI bleeding, hepatitis, seizures occur rarely.

NURSING CONSIDERATIONS

BASELINE ASSESSMENT
Establish baseline B/P, weight, thyroid function, serum glucose, electrolytes.

INTERVENTION/EVALUATION
Monitor serum glucose, electrolytes, thyroid function. In acromegaly, monitor

growth hormone levels. Weigh every 2–3 days, report over 5-lb gain per wk. Monitor B/P, pulse, respirations periodically during treatment. Be alert for decreased urinary output, peripheral edema. Monitor daily pattern of bowel activity, stool consistency.

PATIENT/FAMILY TEACHING

• Therapy should provide significant improvement of severe, watery diarrhea.

---

ofatumumab

oh-fa-**tue**-mue-mab
(Arzerra)

■ **BLACK BOX ALERT** ■ Hepatitis B virus (HBV) reactivation may occur, resulting in hepatitis, hepatic failure, death. Progressive multifocal leukoencephalopathy (PML) resulting in death may occur.
Do not confuse ofatumumab with omalizumab.

◆CLASSIFICATION

PHARMACOTHERAPEUTIC: Monoclonal antibody. **CLINICAL:** Antineoplastic.

USES

Treatment of chronic lymphocytic leukemia (CLL) in pts previously untreated, relapsed, or who require extended therapy. Treatment of CLL refractory to fludarabine and alemtuzumab.

PRECAUTIONS

Contraindications: Hypersensitivity to ofatumumab. **Cautions:** Carriers of hepatitis B virus.

ACTION

Binds to CD20 molecule, the antigen on surface of B-cell lymphocytes; inhibits early-stage B-lymphocyte activation. **Therapeutic Effect:** Controls tumor growth, triggers cell death.

PHARMACOKINETICS

Eliminated through both a target-independent route and a B-cell–mediated route. Due to depletion of B cells, clearance is decreased substantially after subsequent infusions compared with first infusion. **Half-life:** 12–16 days.

⧗ LIFESPAN CONSIDERATIONS

Pregnancy/Lactation: Unknown if distributed in breast milk. **Children:** Safety and efficacy not established. **Elderly:** No age-related precautions noted.

INTERACTIONS

DRUG: Bone marrow depressants may increase myelosuppression. **Live virus vaccines** may potentiate virus replication, increase vaccine side effects, decrease pt's antibody response to vaccine. **HERBAL: Echinacea** may decrease concentration/effects. **FOOD:** None known. **LAB VALUES:** May decrease neutrophils, platelets.

AVAILABILITY (Rx)

Injection, Solution: 100 mg/5 mL, 1000 mg/50 mL.

ADMINISTRATION/HANDLING
📮 IV

◄**ALERT**► Do not give by IV push or bolus. Use in-line filter supplied with product.
Reconstitution • 300-mg dose: Withdraw and discard 15 mL from 1,000 mL 0.9% NaCl bag. • Withdraw 5 mL from each of 3 single-use 100-mg vials and add to bag. • Gently invert. • **1,000-mg dose:** Withdraw and discard 50 mL from 1,000 mL NaCl bag. Withdraw 50 mL from 1 single-use 1,000-mg vial and add to bag. • Gently invert to mix. **2,000-mg dose:** Withdraw and discard 100 mL from 1,000 mL NaCl bag. Withdraw 50 mL from 2 single-use 1,000-mg vials and add to bag. • Gently invert to mix.
Rate of Administration • Dose 1: Initiate infusion at rate of 3.6 mg/hr

0

(12 mL/hr). • **Dose 2:** Initiate infusion at rate of 24 mg/hr (12 mL/hr). • **Dose 3–12:** Initiate infusion at rate of 50 mg/hr (25 mL/hr). • If no infusion toxicity, rate of infusion may be increased every 30 min, using following table:

Interval After Start of Infusion (min)	Dose 1 (mL/hr)	Dose 2 (mL/hr)	Doses 3–12 (mL/hr)
0–30	12	12	25
31–60	25	25	50
61–90	50	50	100
91–120	100	100	200
Over 120	200	200	400

Storage • Refrigerate vials. • After dilution, solution should be used within first 12 hrs; discard preparation after 24 hrs. • Discard if discoloration is present, but solution may contain visible, translucent-to-white particulates (will be removed by in-line filter).

▨ IV COMPATIBILITIES

Prepare all doses with 0.9% NaCl. Do not mix with dextrose solutions or any other medications.

INDICATIONS/ROUTES/DOSAGE

◀**ALERT**▶ Premedicate 30 min to 2 hrs before each infusion with acetaminophen, an antihistamine, and a corticosteroid as prophylaxis for infusion reaction. Flush IV line with 0.9% NaCl before and after each dose. Interrupt infusion if infusion reaction of any severity occurs (do not resume for grade 4 reaction).

Chronic Lymphocytic Leukemia (Untreated)
IV Infusion: ADULTS, ELDERLY: Cycle 1: 300 mg, then 1,000 mg on day 8. Subsequent cycles: 1,000 mg on day 1 q28days. Continue for at least 3 cycles or a maximum of 12 cycles (in combination with chlorambucil).

Chronic Lymphocytic Leukemia (Refractory)
IV Infusion: ADULTS, ELDERLY: Recommended dosage is 12 doses given on the following schedule: 300 mg initial dose (dose 1), followed 1 wk later by 2,000 mg wkly for 7 doses (doses 2–8), followed 4 wks later by 2,000 mg every 4 wks for 4 doses (doses 9–12).

Chronic Lymphocytic Leukemia (Relapsed)
IV Infusion: ADULTS, ELDERLY: 300 mg once on day 1, then 1,000 mg on day 8, then 1,000 mg on day 1 of subsequent 28-day cycles for a maximum of 6 cycles (in combination with fludarabine and cyclophosphamide).

Extended Treatment of CLL
IV Infusion: ADULTS, ELDERLY: 300 mg once on day 1, then 1,000 mg on day 8, then 1,000 mg 7 wks later and q8wks thereafter up to a maximum of 2 yrs.

Dosage in Renal/Hepatic Impairment
No dose adjustment.

SIDE EFFECTS

Frequent (20%–14%): Fever, cough, diarrhea, fatigue, rash. **Occasional (13%–5%):** Nausea, bronchitis, peripheral edema, nasopharyngitis, urticaria, insomnia, headache, sinusitis, muscle spasm, hypertension.

ADVERSE EFFECTS/ TOXIC REACTIONS

Most common serious adverse reactions were bacterial, viral, fungal infections (including pneumonia and sepsis), septic shock, neutropenia, thrombocytopenia. Infusion reactions occur more frequently with first 2 infusions. Severe infusion reactions manifested as angioedema, bronchospasm, dyspnea, fever, chills, back pain, hypotension. Progressive multifocal leukoencephalopathy may occur. Small bowel obstruction has been noted.

NURSING CONSIDERATIONS

BASELINE ASSESSMENT
Screen pts at high risk of hepatitis B virus. Assess baseline CBC prior to therapy. Offer emotional support.

INTERVENTION/EVALUATION

Monitor renal function, electrolytes. Monitor CBC for evidence of myelosuppression during therapy, and increase frequency of monitoring in pts who develop grade 3 or 4 cytopenia. Monitor for blood dyscrasias (fever, sore throat, signs of local infection, unusual bruising/bleeding from any site), symptoms of anemia (excessive fatigue, weakness). Closely monitor for infusion reactions.

PATIENT/FAMILY TEACHING

• Do not have immunizations without physician's approval (lowers body's resistance). • Avoid contact with those who have recently received live virus vaccine. • Avoid crowds, those with infection. • Promptly report fever, sore throat, signs of infection. • Report symptoms of infusion reactions (e.g., fever, chills, breathing problems, rash); bleeding, bruising, petechiae, worsening weakness or fatigue; new neurologic symptoms (e.g., confusion, loss of balance, vision problems); symptoms of hepatitis (e.g., fatigue, yellow discoloration of skin/eyes); worsening abdominal pain, nausea.

OLANZapine

oh-**lan**-za-peen
(Apo-OLANZapine ♣, ZyPREXA, ZyPREXA Relprevv, ZyPREXA Zydis)

■ **BLACK BOX ALERT** ■ Elderly pts with dementia-related psychosis are at increased risk for mortality due to cerebrovascular events. Sedation (including coma), delirium reported following use of ZyPREXA Relprevv.

Do not confuse OLANZapine with olsalazine or QUEtiapine, or ZyPREXA with CeleXA or ZyrTEC.

FIXED-COMBINATION(S)

Symbyax: OLANZapine/FLUoxetine (an antidepressant): 6 mg/25 mg, 6 mg/50 mg, 12 mg/25 mg, 12 mg/50 mg.

◆CLASSIFICATION

PHARMACOTHERAPEUTIC: Second-generation (atypical) antipsychotic. **CLINICAL:** Antipsychotic.

USES

PO: Management of manifestations of schizophrenia. Treatment of acute mania associated with bipolar disorder as monotherapy or in combination with lithium or valproate. In combination with FLUoxetine: treatment of depressive episodes associated with bipolar I disorder and treatment of treatment-resistant bipolar depression. **IM: ZyPREXA Intramuscular:** Controls acute agitation in schizophrenia and bipolar mania. **Relprevv:** Long-acting antipsychotic for IM injection for treatment of schizophrenia. **OFF-LABEL:** Prevention of chemotherapy-induced nausea/vomiting. Acute treatment of delirium. Treatment of anorexia nervosa, Tourette's syndrome, tic disorder.

PRECAUTIONS

Contraindications: Hypersensitivity to OLANZapine. **Cautions:** Disorders in which CNS depression is prominent; cardiac disease, hemodynamic instability, prior MI, ischemic heart disease; hyperlipidemia, pts at risk for aspiration pneumonia, decreased GI motility, urinary retention, BPH, narrow-angle glaucoma, diabetes, elderly, pts at risk for suicide, Parkinson's disease, severe renal/hepatic impairment, predisposition to seizures.

ACTION

Antagonizes alpha$_1$-adrenergic, DOPamine, histamine, muscarinic, serotonin receptors. Produces anticholinergic, histaminic, CNS depressant effects. **Therapeutic Effect:** Diminishes psychotic symptoms.

PHARMACOKINETICS

Well absorbed after PO administration. Rapid absorption following IM administration. Protein binding: 93%. Widely distributed. Excreted in urine (57%), feces (30%). Not removed by dialysis. **Half-life:** 21–54 hrs.

⧗ LIFESPAN CONSIDERATIONS

Pregnancy/Lactation: Unknown if drug crosses placenta or is distributed in breast milk. **Children:** Safety and efficacy not established. **Elderly:** Use caution. Consider lower starting doses.

INTERACTIONS

DRUG: Alcohol, **CNS depressants (e.g., LORazepam, morphine, zolpidem)** may increase CNS depressant effects. **Anticholinergics** may increase anticholinergic effects. **Hepatotoxic medications (e.g., acetaminophen, simvastatin)** may increase risk of hepatotoxicity. **HERBAL:** Dong quai, St. John's wort may increase photosensitization. Gotu kola, kava kava, St. John's wort, valerian may increase CNS depression. **FOOD:** None known. **LAB VALUES:** May increase serum GGT, cholesterol, prolactin, ALT, AST.

AVAILABILITY (Rx)

Injection, Powder for Reconstitution (ZyPREXA): 10 mg. **Suspension for IM Injection (Relprevv):** 210 mg, 300 mg, 405 mg. **Tablets (ZyPREXA):** 2.5 mg, 5 mg, 7.5 mg, 10 mg, 15 mg, 20 mg. **Tablets (Orally Disintegrating [ZyPREXA Zydis]):** 5 mg, 10 mg, 15 mg, 20 mg.

ADMINISTRATION/HANDLING

PO
• Give without regard to meals.

Orally Disintegrating
• Remove by peeling back foil (do not push through foil). • Place in mouth immediately. • Tablet dissolves rapidly with saliva and may be swallowed with or without liquid.

IM (ZyPREXA Intramuscular)
• Reconstitute 10-mg vial with 2.1 mL Sterile Water for Injection to provide concentration of 5 mg/mL. • Use within

1 hr following reconstitution. • Discard unused portion.

IM (Relprevv)
• Dilute to final concentration of 150 mg/mL. • Shake vigorously to mix. • Store at room temperature for up to 24 hrs.

INDICATIONS/ROUTES/DOSAGE

Schizophrenia
PO: ADULTS, ELDERLY: Initially, 5–10 mg once daily. May increase to 10 mg/day within 5–7 days. If further adjustments are indicated, may increase by 5 mg/day at 7-day intervals. **Maintenance:** 10–20 mg/day. **Maximum:** 20 mg/day. **CHILDREN:** Initially, 2.5–5 mg/day. Titrate in 2.5- or 5-mg increments at wkly intervals. Target dose: 10 mg. **Maximum:** 20 mg/day.
IM (Long-Acting [Relprevv]): ADULTS, ESTABLISHED ON 10 MG/DAY ORALLY: 210 mg q2wks for 4 doses or 405 mg q4wks for 2 doses. **Maintenance:** 150 mg q2wks or 300 mg q4wks. **ESTABLISHED ON 15 MG/DAY ORALLY:** 300 mg q2wks for 4 doses. **Maintenance:** 210 mg q2wks or 405 mg q4wks. **ESTABLISHED ON 20 MG/DAY ORALLY:** 300 mg q2wks.

Depression Associated with Bipolar Disorder (with FLUoxetine)
PO: ADULTS, ELDERLY: Initially, 5 mg in evening. Range: 5–12.5 mg/day. **CHILDREN 10–17 yrs:** Initially, 2.5 mg once daily. Adjust dose as tolerated.

Treatment-Resistant Depression (with FLUoxetine)
PO: ADULTS, ELDERLY: Initially, 5 mg in evening. Range: 5–20 mg/day.

Bipolar Mania
PO: ADULTS, ELDERLY: (Monotherapy) Initially, 10–15 mg/day. May increase by 5 mg/day at intervals of at least 24 hrs. Range: 5–20 mg/day. **Maximum:** 20 mg/day. **(In Combination with Lithium or Valproate):** Initially, 10 mg/day. Range: 5–20 mg/day. **CHILDREN 13 YRS OF AGE AND OLDER:** Initially, 2.5–5 mg/day.

Adjust dose by 2.5–5 mg daily to target dose of 10 mg/day. Range: 2.5–20 mg/day.

Dosage for Elderly, Debilitated Pts, Pts Predisposed to Hypotensive Reactions
Initial dosage: 5 mg/day.

Control of Agitation
IM: ADULTS, ELDERLY: *(Short-Acting):* Initially, 5–10 mg. Additional doses (up to 10 mg) may be considered. However, allow at least 2 hrs (after inital dose) or 4 hrs (after second dose) to evaluate response. **Maximum:** 30 mg/day.

Dosage in Renal/Hepatic Impairment
No dose adjustment.

SIDE EFFECTS

Frequent (26%–10%): Drowsiness, agitation, insomnia, headache, nervousness, hostility, dizziness, rhinitis. **Occasional (9%–5%):** Anxiety, constipation, nonaggressive atypical behavior, dry mouth, weight gain, orthostatic hypotension, fever, arthralgia, restlessness, cough, pharyngitis, visual changes (dim vision). **Rare:** Tachycardia; back, chest, abdominal, or extremity pain; tremor.

ADVERSE EFFECTS/ TOXIC REACTIONS

Rare reactions include seizures, neuroleptic malignant syndrome, a potentially fatal syndrome characterized by hyperpyrexia, muscle rigidity, irregular pulse or B/P, tachycardia, diaphoresis, cardiac arrhythmias. Extrapyramidal symptoms (EPS), dysphagia may occur. Overdose (300 mg) produces drowsiness, slurred speech.

NURSING CONSIDERATIONS

BASELINE ASSESSMENT
Obtain baseline LFT, serum glucose, weight, lipid profile before initiating treatment. Assess behavior, appearance, emotional status, response to environment, speech pattern, thought content.

INTERVENTION/EVALUATION
Monitor B/P, serum glucose, lipids, LFT. Assess for tremors, changes in gait, abnormal muscular movements, behavior. Supervise suicidal-risk pt closely during early therapy (as depression lessens, energy level improves, increasing suicide potential). Assess for therapeutic response (interest in surroundings, improvement in self-care, increased ability to concentrate, relaxed facial expression). Assist with ambulation if dizziness occurs. Assess sleep pattern. Notify physician if extrapyramidal symptoms (EPS) occur.

PATIENT/FAMILY TEACHING
• Avoid dehydration, particularly during exercise, exposure to extreme heat, concurrent use of medication causing dry mouth, other drying effects. • Sugarless gum, sips of water may relieve dry mouth. • Report suspected pregnancy. • Take medication as prescribed; do not stop taking or increase dosage. • Slowly go from lying to standing. • Avoid alcohol. • Avoid tasks that require alertness, motor skills until response to drug is established. • Monitor diet, exercise program to prevent weight gain.

olaparib

oh-**lap**-a-rib
(Lynparza)

◆CLASSIFICATION

PHARMACOTHERAPEUTIC: Polymerase inhibitor. **CLINICAL:** Antineoplastic.

USES

Capsules/Tablets: Treatment of deleterious or suspected deleterious germline BRCA-mutated advanced ovarian cancer in pts who have been treated with three or more prior lines of chemotherapy.

Tablets only: Maintenance treatment of adults with recurrent epithelial, ovarian, fallopian tube or primary perintoneal cancer who are in complete or partial response to platinum-based chemotherapy.

PRECAUTIONS

Contraindications: Hypersensitivity to olaparib. **Cautions:** Baseline anemia, neutropenia, lymphopenia, thrombocytopenia. History of pulmonary disease. Avoid concomitant use of strong or moderate CYP3A inhibitors, strong or moderate CYP3A inducers.

ACTION

Inhibits poly (ADP-ribose) polymerase enzymes, involved in normal cellular hemostasis (e.g., DNA transcription, cell cycle regulation, and DNA repair). Disrupts cellular homeostasis, resulting in cell death. **Therapeutic Effect:** Inhibits tumor cell growth and metastasis.

PHARMACOKINETICS

Rapidly absorbed. Metabolized in liver. Protein binding: 82%. Peak plasma concentration: 1–3 hrs. Steady-state concentration: 3–4 days. Excreted in urine (44%), feces (42%). **Half-life:** 11.9 hrs.

⏳ LIFESPAN CONSIDERATIONS

Pregnancy/Lactation: Avoid pregnancy; may cause fetal harm. Females of reproductive potential should use effective contraception during treatment and for at least 6 mos after discontinuation. Unknown if distributed in breast milk. Must either discontinue drug or discontinue breastfeeding. **Children:** Safety and efficacy not established. **Elderly:** No age-related precautions noted.

INTERACTIONS

DRUG: Strong CYP3A inhibitors (e.g., clarithromycin, ketoconazole, ritonavir), moderate CYP3A inhibitors (e.g., atazanavir, ciprofloxacin) may increase concentration/effect. **Strong CYP3A inducers (e.g., carBAMazepine), moderate CYP3A inducers (e.g., nafcillin)** may decrease concentration/effect. **HERBAL: St. John's wort** may decrease concentration/effect. **FOOD: Grapefruit products, Seville oranges** may increase concentration/effect. **High-fat food** may delay absorption. **LAB VALUES:** May increase mean corpuscular volume, serum creatinine. May decrease Hct, Hgb, lymphocytes, neutrophils, RBC.

AVAILABILITY (Rx)

Capsules: 50 mg. **Tablets:** 100 mg, 150 mg.

ADMINISTRATION/HANDLING

PO

Capsules: • Give without regard to meals. • Administer capsules whole; do not break, cut, crush, or open. **Tablets:** May give with or without food. Administer tablet whole; do not break, cut, crush, or divide.

INDICATIONS/ROUTES/DOSAGE

Note: Do not substitute tablets with capsules on a mg to mg basis.

Ovarian Cancer
PO: ADULTS, ELDERLY: (Capsule) 400 mg twice daily. Continue until disease progression or unacceptable toxicity. If a dose is missed, give next dose at its scheduled time. **(Tablet)** 300 mg (2x150 mg) twice daily (100 mg tablets available for dose reduction). **Maintenance: (Tablets only)** 300 mg (2x150 mg) twice daily (100 mg tablets available for dose reduction).

Dose Modification
Dose Reduction for Adverse Reactions
PO: ADULTS, ELDERLY: Interrupt treatment until resolved. Then, decrease to 200 mg twice daily. If further dose reduction is indicated, decrease to 100 mg twice daily.
Concomitant Use of Strong CYP3A Inhibitors
PO: ADULTS, ELDERLY: 150 mg twice daily.
Concomitant Use of Moderate CYP3A Inhibitors
PO: ADULTS, ELDERLY: 200 mg twice daily.

Dosage in Renal Impairment
Mild impairment: No dose adjustment.
Moderate to severe impairment: Not specified; use caution.

Dosage in Hepatic Impairment
Not specified; use caution.

SIDE EFFECTS

Frequent (66%–21%): Fatigue, asthenia, nausea, vomiting, abdominal pain, diarrhea, dyspepsia, decreased appetite, headache, back pain, rash, myalgia, arthralgia, musculoskeletal pain, dysgeusia, cough.

ADVERSE EFFECTS/ TOXIC REACTIONS

Myelodysplastic syndrome/acute myeloid leukemia reported in 2% of pts. Pneumonitis, including fatal cases, occurred in less than 1% of pts. Respiratory tract infections including nasopharyngitis, pharyngitis, upper respiratory tract infection occurred in 43% of pts.

NURSING CONSIDERATIONS

BASELINE ASSESSMENT

Obtain baseline CBC. Do not initiate therapy until pts have recovered from hematologic toxicities caused by previous chemotherapy. Question history of pulmonary disease. Receive full medication history and screen for interactions. Offer emotional support.

INTERVENTION/EVALUATION

Monitor CBC monthly. For prolonged hematologic toxicities, interrupt treatment and monitor CBC wkly until recovery. If hematologic levels have not recovered to CTCAE grade 1 or 0 after 4 wks of treatment interruption, consider hematology consultation for further investigations such as bone marrow analysis and blood sample for cytogenetics. Monitor for myelodysplastic syndrome/acute myeloid leukemia, pneumonitis.

PATIENT/FAMILY TEACHING

• Report bleeding or bruising easily, bloody urine or stool, frequent infections, fatigue, shortness of breath, weakness, weight loss; may indicate acute bone marrow suppression or acute leukemia. • Report new or worsening respiratory symptoms such as cough, difficulty breathing, fever, wheezing; may indicate severe lung inflammation. • Do not ingest grapefruit product, Seville oranges. • Do not take herbal products. • Avoid pregnancy; treatment may cause birth defects or miscarriage. Do not breastfeed. Females of childbearing potential should use effective contraception during treatment and for at least 6 mos after stopping therapy.

olaratumab

oh-lar-**at**-ue-mab
(Lartruvo)
Do not confuse olaratumab with elotuzumab, obinutuzumab.

◆CLASSIFICATION

PHARMACOTHERAPEUTIC: Platelet-derived growth factor receptor (PDGFR) alpha blocker. Monoclonal antibody. **CLINICAL:** Antineoplastic.

USES

Treatment of adult pts with soft tissue sarcoma (STS), in combination with doxorubicin, with a histologic subtype for which an anthracycline-containing regimen is appropriate and which is not amendable to curative treatment with radiotherapy or surgery.

PRECAUTIONS

Contraindications: Hypersensitivity to olaratumab. **Cautions:** Electrolyte imbalance, pts at risk for hyperglycemia (e.g., diabetes, recent surgery, chronic use of corticosteroids).

ACTION

A human IgG-1 antibody that binds to PDGFR-alpha. Blocks receptor activation and disrupts PDGF receptor signaling. PDGF alpha receptor plays a role in cell differentiation, growth, and angiogenesis. **Therapeutic Effect:** Exhibits antitumor activity.

PHARMACOKINETICS

Widely distributed. Metabolism not specified. Excretion not specified. **Half-life:** 11 days (range: 6–24 days).

⧗ LIFESPAN CONSIDERATIONS

Pregnancy/Lactation: Avoid pregnancy; may cause fetal harm/malformations. Females of reproductive potential must use effective contraception during treatment and up to 3 mos after discontinuation. Unknown if distributed in breast milk. Breastfeeding not recommended during treatment and for at least 3 mos after discontinuation. **Children:** Safety and efficacy not established. **Elderly:** Not specified; use caution.

INTERACTIONS

DRUG: May decrease therapeutic effect of **BCG vaccine**. **HERBAL:** None significant. **FOOD:** None known. **LAB VALUES:** May increase serum alkaline phosphatase, glucose. May decrease lymphocytes, neutrophils, platelets; serum phosphate, potassium, magnesium. May prolong aPTT.

AVAILABILITY (Rx)

Injection, Solution: 190 mg/19 mL, 500 mg/50 mL.

ADMINISTRATION/HANDLING
💉 IV

Preparation • Visually inspect for particulate matter or discoloration. Solution should appear clear to slightly opalescent, colorless to slightly yellow in color. • Do not use if solution is cloudy, discolored, or if visible particles are observed. • Withdraw required dose from vial and dilute into 250 mL 0.9% NaCl bag. • Mix by gently inversion. • Do not shake or agitate. • Discard used portions from vial.

Infusion Guidelines • Do not give IV push or bolus. • Do not mix or infuse with other medications, electrolytes.

• Flush IV line with 0.9% NaCl after completion of infusion.

Rate of Administration • Infuse over 60 min via dedicated IV line.

Storage • May refrigerate diluted solution up to 24 hrs or store at room temperature for up to 4 hrs (includes infusion time). • Do not freeze. • If diluted solution is refrigerated, allow to warm to room temperature before administration. • Discard solution if not administered within required time frame.

IV INCOMPATIBILITIES

Do not dilute in dextrose-containing solutions.

INDICATIONS/ROUTES/DOSAGE

Note: Premedicate with diphenhydramine 25–50 mg IV and dexamethasone 10–20 mg IV on day 1 of cycle 1.

Soft Tissue Sarcoma
IV: ADULTS, ELDERLY: 15 mg/kg on days 1 and 8 of each 21-day cycle. Continue until disease progression or unacceptable toxicity. Administer with doxorubicin for the first 8 cycles (see manufacturer guidelines).

Dose Modification
Infusion Reaction
CTCAE grade 1 or 2 infusion reaction: Interrupt infusion until symptoms resolve, then resume infusion at 50% of the initial infusion rate. **CTCAE grade 3 or 4 infusion reaction:** Immediately stop infusion; do not restart.

Neutropenia
Neutropenic fever/infection; CTCAE grade 4 neutropenia lasting greater than 1 wk: Withhold treatment until ANC 1000 cells/mm^3 or greater, then reduce dose to 12 mg/kg. Do not increase dose for subsequent infusions.

Dosage in Renal/Hepatic Impairment
Not specified; use caution.

SIDE EFFECTS

Frequent (73%–22%): Nausea, fatigue, asthenia, musculoskeletal pain, arthralgia, back pain, bone pain, flank pain, groin pain, musculoskeletal chest pain, myalgia, muscle spasm, neck pain, extremity pain, mucositis, alopecia, vomiting, diarrhea, decreased appetite, abdominal pain, neuropathy. **Occasional (20%–11%):** Headache, anxiety, dry eyes.

ADVERSE EFFECTS/ TOXIC REACTIONS

Neutropenia, lymphopenia, thrombocytopenia are expected responses to therapy. Life-threatening infusion-related reactions including anaphylaxis, bronchospasm, cardiac arrest, chills, dyspnea, hypotension, pyrexia occurred in 14% of pts. CTCAE grade 3 or 4 infusion-related reactions occurred in 2% of pts. Immunogenicity (auto anti-olaratumab antibodies) reported in 3.5% of pts.

NURSING CONSIDERATIONS

BASELINE ASSESSMENT

Obtain ANC, CBC, BMP. Obtain pregnancy test in females of reproductive potential. Question history of hypersensitivity reactions, infusion-related reactions; diabetes. Ensure that proper resuscitative equipment, medications are readily available (e.g., albuterol, antipyretics, antihistamines, epinephrine; isotonic IV fluids; bag-valve mask, oxygen, rapid sequence intubation kit). Assess nutritional/hydration status. Offer emotional support.

INTERVENTION/EVALUATION

Monitor ANC, CBC for neutropenia, lymphopenia, thrombocytopenia; BMP for electrolyte imbalance; vital signs. Diligently monitor for infusion-related reactions. If severe or life-threatening reactions occur, immediately stop infusion and provide appropriate medical support. Due to risk of respiratory compromise, pts with bronchospasm, dyspnea, hypoxia should be given immediate supplemental oxygen, hypersensitivity medications, hemodynamic support. Mild to moderate infusion reactions may require interruption of infusion, decrease of infusion rate, symptom management. Offer antiemetic if nausea, vomiting occurs. Monitor daily pattern of bowel activity, stool consistency.

PATIENT/FAMILY TEACHING

• Life-threatening infusion reactions, allergic reactions, cardiac arrest may occur during infusion. Immediately report difficulty breathing, chest pain, chest tightness, chills, dizziness, fast heart rate, fever, flushing, headache, hives, itching, low blood pressure, nausea, throat pain or swelling, rash. • Treatment may depress your immune system and reduce your ability to fight infection. Report symptoms of infection such as body aches, burning with urination, chills, cough, fatigue, fever. Avoid those with active infection. • Females of childbearing potential should use effective contraception during treatment and for at least 3 mos after last dose. Do not breastfeed. • Generalized pain is an expected side effect. • Treatment may cause severe diarrhea. Drink plenty of fluids. • Hair loss is an expected side effect of therapy.

olmesartan TOP 100

ol-me-**sar**-tan
(Benicar, Olmetec ✦)

■ **BLACK BOX ALERT** ■ May cause fetal injury, mortality. Discontinue as soon as possible once pregnancy is detected.
Do not confuse Benicar with Mevacor.

FIXED-COMBINATION(S)

Azor: olmesartan/amLODIPine (calcium channel blocker): 20 mg/5 mg, 40 mg/5 mg, 20 mg/10 mg, 40 mg/10 mg. **Benicar HCT:** olmesartan/hydroCHLOROthiazide (a diuretic): 20 mg/12.5 mg, 40 mg/12.5 mg, 40 mg/25 mg. **Tribenzor:** olmesartan/hydroCHLOROthiazide/amLODIPine: 20 mg/12.5 mg/5 mg, 40 mg/12.5 mg/5 mg, 40 mg/25 mg/5 mg, 40 mg/12.5 mg/10 mg, 40 mg/25 mg/10 mg.

◆CLASSIFICATION

PHARMACOTHERAPEUTIC: Angiotensin II receptor antagonist. **CLINICAL:** Antihypertensive.

USES

Treatment of hypertension alone or in combination with other antihypertensives.

PRECAUTIONS

Contraindications: Hypersensitivity to olmesartan. Concomitant use with aliskiren in pts with diabetes. **Cautions:** Renal impairment, unstented unilateral or bilateral renal arterial stenosis, significant aortic/mitral stenosis. Concurrent potassium supplements; pts who are volume depleted.

ACTION

Blocks vasoconstrictor, aldosterone-secreting effects of angiotensin II by inhibiting binding of angiotensin II to AT_1 receptors in vascular smooth muscle. **Therapeutic Effect:** Causes vasodilation, decreases peripheral resistance, decreases B/P.

PHARMACOKINETICS

Moderately absorbed after PO administration. Hydrolyzed in GI tract to olmesartan. Protein binding: 99%. Excreted in urine (35%–50%), remainder in feces. Not removed by hemodialysis. **Half-life:** 13 hrs.

⧗ LIFESPAN CONSIDERATIONS

Pregnancy/Lactation: Unknown if distributed in breast milk. **Children:** Safety and efficacy not established in children younger than 6 yrs of age. **Elderly:** No age-related precautions noted.

INTERACTIONS

DRUG: NSAIDs (e.g., **ibuprofen, ketorolac, naproxen**) may decrease antihypertensive effect. **HERBAL:** Ephedra, ginseng, yohimbe may worsen hypertension. **Garlic** may increase antihypertensive effect. **FOOD:** None known.

LAB VALUES: May slightly decrease Hgb, Hct. May increase serum BUN, creatinine, bilirubin, ALT, AST.

AVAILABILITY (Rx)

Tablets: 5 mg, 20 mg, 40 mg.

ADMINISTRATION/HANDLING

PO
• Give without regard to meals.

INDICATIONS/ROUTES/DOSAGE

Hypertension
PO: ADULTS, ELDERLY: Initially, 20 mg/day. May increase to 40 mg/day after 2 wks. Lower initial dose may be necessary in pts receiving volume-depleting medications (e.g., diuretics). **CHILDREN 6–16 YRS, WEIGHING 20 TO LESS THAN 35 KG:** Initially, 10 mg once daily. Range: 10–20 mg once daily. **WEIGHING 35 KG OR GREATER:** Initially, 20 mg once daily. Range: 20–40 mg once daily. Use with caution.

SIDE EFFECTS

Occasional (3%): Dizziness. **Rare (less than 2%):** Headache, diarrhea, upper respiratory tract infection.
Dosage in Renal/Hepatic Impairment
Use caution.

ADVERSE EFFECTS/TOXIC REACTIONS

Overdosage may manifest as hypotension, tachycardia. Bradycardia occurs less often. Rare cases of rhabdomyolysis have been reported.

NURSING CONSIDERATIONS

BASELINE ASSESSMENT
Obtain B/P, apical pulse immediately before each dose in addition to regular monitoring (be alert to fluctuations). If excessive reduction in B/P occurs, place pt in supine position, feet slightly elevated. Question for possibility of pregnancy. Assess medication history (esp. diuretics).

INTERVENTION/EVALUATION
Maintain hydration. Assess for evidence of upper respiratory infection. Assist with

ambulation if dizziness occurs. Monitor serum potassium level. Assess B/P for hypertension, hypotension.

PATIENT/FAMILY TEACHING

• Maintain adequate hydration. • Avoid pregnancy. • Avoid tasks that require alertness, motor skills until response to drug is established (possible dizziness effect). • Report any signs of infection (sore throat, fever). • Therapy requires lifelong control, diet, exercise.

---

olodaterol

oh-loe-**da**-ter-ol
(Striverdi Respimat)

■ **BLACK BOX ALERT** ■ Long-acting beta$_2$-adrenergic agonists (LABA) increase risk of asthma-related deaths. Not indicated for treatment of asthma.
Do not confuse olodaterol with albuterol, indacaterol, formoterol, or salmeterol.

FIXED-COMBINATION(S)

Stiolto Respimat: olodaterol/tiotropium (bronchodilator): 2.5 mcg/2.5 mcg.

◆CLASSIFICATION

PHARMACOTHERAPEUTIC: Sympathomimetic (beta$_2$-adrenergic agonist). **CLINICAL:** Bronchodilator.

USES

Long-term, once-daily maintenance bronchodilator treatment of airflow obstruction in pts with chronic obstructive pulmonary disease (COPD), including chronic bronchitis and emphysema. Not indicated in asthma, acute deterioration of COPD.

PRECAUTIONS

Contraindications: Hypersensitivity to olodaterol. Asthma without use of long-term asthma control medication, history of hypersensitivity to sympathomimetics. **Cautions:** Diabetes, ketoacidosis, cardiovascular disorders (e.g., coronary insufficiency, arrhythmias, hypertension, hypertrophic obstructive cardiomyopathy), seizure disorder, hyperthyroidism; history of severe bronchospasm, long QT syndrome, electrolyte imbalance.

ACTION

Stimulates beta$_2$-adrenergic receptors in lungs, resulting in relaxation of bronchial smooth muscle. **Therapeutic Effect:** Relieves bronchospasm, reduces airway resistance, improves bronchodilation.

PHARMACOKINETICS

Rapidly absorbed following inhalation. Extensively distributed in tissue. Metabolized in liver. Protein binding: 60%. Peak plasma concentration: 10–20 min. Excreted in urine. **Half-life:** 45 hrs.

⧗ LIFESPAN CONSIDERATIONS

Pregnancy/Lactation: Excretion into breast milk is probable. Breastfeeding not recommended. May interfere with uterine contractility. **Children:** Safety and efficacy not established. **Elderly:** No age-related precaution noted.

INTERACTIONS

DRUG: Beta blockers (e.g., metoprolol) may decrease therapeutic effect, cause bronchospasms. **Beta$_2$-adrenergic agonists** (e.g., salmeterol) may potentiate sympathomimetic effects. **Xanthine derivatives** (e.g., theophylline), **steroids** (e.g., methylPREDNISolone), **non–potassium-sparing diuretics** (e.g., furosemide) may increase risk of hypokalemia. **Drugs that prolong QT interval** (e.g., amiodarone, azithromycin, ciprofloxacin, haloperidol), **MAOIs** (e.g., phenelzine, selegiline), and **tricyclic antidepressants** (e.g., amitriptyline, doxepin) may potentiate cardiovascular effects. **HERBAL:** Caffeine, green tea, guarana may increase sympathomimetic effects. **FOOD:** None known. **LAB VALUES:** May increase serum glucose. May decrease serum potassium.

AVAILABILITY (Rx)

Inhalation Spray (2.5 mcg/actuation): 28 metered actuations/cartridge with inhaler, 60 metered actuations/cartridge with inhaler.

ADMINISTRATION/HANDLING

Inhalation

• While taking slow, deep breath through the mouth, press and release button and continue slow inhalation as long as possible. (See manufacturer guidelines for priming instructions and further information.)

INDICATIONS/ROUTES/DOSAGE

COPD

Inhalation: ADULTS, ELDERLY: Two inhalations (2.5 mcg per inhalation for total of 5 mcg) once daily, at same time each day. **Maximum:** 5 mcg within 24-hr period.

Dosage in Renal Impairment
No dose adjustment.

Dosage in Hepatic Impairment
Mild to moderate impairment: No dose adjustment. **Severe impairment:** Use caution.

SIDE EFFECTS

Occasional (11%–4%): Nasopharyngitis, upper respiratory tract infection, bronchitis, cough, back pain. **Rare (3%–2%):** Dizziness, insomnia, dry mouth, arthralgia, urinary retention.

ADVERSE EFFECTS/ TOXIC REACTIONS

Life-threatening asthma-related events, bronchospasm, or worsening of COPD-related symptoms have been reported. Serious cardiovascular events including arrhythmias, angina pectoris, cardiac arrest, hypertension, tachycardia; flattening of T wave, prolongation of QTc interval, ST segment depression have occurred. All beta-adrenergic agonists carry risk of hyperglycemia or significant

hypokalemia. Pts with severe COPD or hypokalemia have additional increased risk of adverse effects related to hypoxia and concomitant medications.

NURSING CONSIDERATIONS

BASELINE ASSESSMENT

Obtain ABG, capillary glucose, O_2 saturation, serum potassium level, vital signs; EKG, pulmonary function test if applicable. Assess respiratory rate, depth, rhythm. Assess lung sounds for wheezing, rales. Receive full medication history and screen for drug interactions. Question history of asthma, cardiovascular disease, diabetes, long QT syndrome, seizure disorder. Teach proper inhaler priming and administration techniques.

INTERVENTION/EVALUATION

Routinely monitor capillary glucose, O_2 saturation, serum potassium level, vital signs. Auscultate lung sounds. Obtain EKG for palpitation, tachycardia; symptomatic hypokalemia. Recommend discontinuation of short-acting beta$_2$-agonists (use only for symptomatic relief of acute respiratory symptoms). Monitor for hypoglycemia.

PATIENT/FAMILY TEACHING

• Refill prescription when dose indicator on left of inhaler reaches red area of scale. • Follow manufacturer guidelines for proper use of inhaler. • Drink plenty of fluids (decreases lung secretion viscosity). • Rinse mouth with water after inhalation to decrease mouth/throat irritation. • Avoid excessive use of caffeine derivatives (chocolate, coffee, tea, cola). • Report fever, productive cough, body aches, difficulty breathing; may indicate lung infection or worsening of COPD.

olsalazine

ole-**sal**-a-zeen
(Dipentum)
Do not confuse Dipentum with Dilantin, or olsalazine with OLANZapine.

◆CLASSIFICATION

PHARMACOTHERAPEUTIC: Salicylic acid derivative. **CLINICAL:** Anti-inflammatory.

USES

Maintenance of remission of ulcerative colitis in pts intolerant of sulfaSALAzine medication.

PRECAUTIONS

Contraindications: Hypersensitivity to olsalazine. History of hypersensitivity to salicylates. **Cautions:** Renal/hepatic impairment, elderly pts, severe allergies, asthma.

ACTION

Converted to mesalamine in colon by bacterial action. Blocks local chemical mediators of inflammatory response. **Therapeutic Effect:** Reduces colonic inflammation.

PHARMACOKINETICS

Small amount absorbed. Protein binding: 99%. Metabolized by bacteria in colon. Minimal excretion in urine, feces. **Half-life:** 0.9 hr.

⧗ LIFESPAN CONSIDERATIONS

Pregnancy/Lactation: Crosses placenta; distributed in breast milk. **Children:** Safety and efficacy not established. **Elderly:** Age-related renal impairment may require dosage adjustment.

INTERACTIONS

DRUG: Heparin, warfarin may increase risk of bleeding. May increase risk of myelosuppression with **mercaptopurine, thioguanine. HERBAL:** None significant. **FOOD:** None known. **LAB VALUES:** May increase serum ALT, AST.

AVAILABILITY (Rx)

Capsules: 250 mg.

ADMINISTRATION/HANDLING

PO
• Give with food.

INDICATIONS/ROUTES/DOSAGE

Maintenance of Controlled Ulcerative Colitis
PO: ADULTS, ELDERLY: 1 g/day in 2 divided doses, preferably q12h.

Dosage in Renal/Hepatic Impairment
No dose adjustment.

SIDE EFFECTS

Frequent (10%–5%): Headache, diarrhea, abdominal pain/cramps, nausea. **Occasional (4%–2%):** Depression, fatigue, dyspepsia, upper respiratory tract infection, decreased appetite, rash, pruritus, arthralgia. **Rare (1%):** Dizziness, vomiting, stomatitis.

ADVERSE EFFECTS/ TOXIC REACTIONS

Sulfite sensitivity may occur in susceptible pts (manifested as cramping, headache, diarrhea, fever, rash, urticaria, pruritus, wheezing). Excessive diarrhea associated with extreme fatigue is rarely noted.

NURSING CONSIDERATIONS

INTERVENTION/EVALUATION

Encourage adequate fluid intake. Assess bowel sounds for peristalsis. Monitor daily pattern of bowel activity, stool consistency. Assess for abdominal disturbances. Assess skin for rash, urticaria. Medication should be discontinued if rash, fever, cramping, diarrhea occur.

PATIENT/FAMILY TEACHING

• Report if diarrhea, cramping continues or worsens or if rash, fever, pruritus occur.

omacetaxine

oh-ma-se-**tax**-een
(Synribo)

◆CLASSIFICATION

PHARMACOTHERAPEUTIC: Protein synthesis inhibitor. **CLINICAL:** Antineoplastic.

O

USES

Treatment of adult pts with chronic or accelerated phase chronic myeloid leukemia (CML) with resistance and/or intolerance to two or more tyrosine kinase inhibitors.

PRECAUTIONS

Contraindications: Hypersensitivity to omacetaxine. **Cautions:** Glucose intolerance, poorly controlled diabetes, elderly, recent GI bleeding. Avoid all use of anticoagulants, aspirin, NSAIDs; all pts with baseline platelets less than 50,000 cells/mm^3.

ACTION

Inhibits protein synthesis of Bcr-Abl tyrosine kinase, a translocation-created enzyme, created by the Philadelphia chromosome abnormality noted in chronic myeloid leukemia (CML). **Therapeutic Effect:** Inhibits tumor proliferation and growth during accelerated and chronic stages of CML.

PHARMACOKINETICS

Rapidly absorbed following SQ administration. Maximum concentration: 30 min. Protein binding: Less than 50%. Hydrolyzed via plasma esterases. **Half-life:** 6 hrs.

⌛ LIFESPAN CONSIDERATIONS

Pregnancy/Lactation: May cause fetal harm. Not recommended in nursing mothers. Unknown if distributed in breast milk. **Children:** Safety and efficacy not established. **Elderly:** Increased risk for toxicity (e.g., hematologic).

INTERACTIONS

DRUG: NSAIDs (e.g., ibuprofen, ketorolac, naproxen), anticoagulants (e.g., heparin, warfarin), antiplatelets (e.g., clopidogrel) may increase risk for bleeding. **HERBAL:** Echinacea may decrease levels/effects. **FOOD:** None known. **LAB VALUES:** May decrease platelets, Hgb, Hct, leukocytes, lymphocytes. May increase serum ALT.

AVAILABILITY (Rx)

Injection, Powder for Reconstitution: 3.5-mg vial.

ADMINISTRATION/HANDLING

◄**ALERT**► Must be administered by health care workers trained in proper chemotherapy handling and disposal procedures.

SQ
Reconstitution • Reconstitute with 1 mL 0.9% NaCl. • Gently swirl until powder is completely dissolved. • Inspect vial for particular matter or discoloration. • Reconstituted vial will provide a concentration of 3.5 mg/mL. • Avoid contact with skin.
Storage • Solution should appear clear. • May store solution at room temperature for up to 12 hrs or may refrigerate up to 24 hrs. • Discard unused solution.

INDICATIONS/ROUTES/DOSAGE

Note: If dose is missed, skip dose and resume next regularly scheduled dose.

Chronic or Accelerated Myeloid Leukemia
SQ: ADULTS, ELDERLY: Induction dose: 1.25 mg/m^2 twice daily for 14 consecutive days every 28 days, over 28-day cycle. Continue induction dose until hematologic response achieved. **Maintenance dose:** 1.25 mg/m^2 twice daily for 7 consecutive days every 28 days of a 28-day cycle. Continue until no longer achieving clinical treatment benefit.

Dosage Modification
Hematologic Toxicity: If neutrophils less than 500 cells/mm^3 or platelets less than 50,000 cells/mm^3, interrupt therapy. Restart when neutrophil count greater than or equal to 1000 cells/mm^3 or platelet count greater than or equal to 50,000 cells/mm^3 and reduce number of dosing days by 2. **Nonhematologic Toxicity:** Interrupt therapy until toxicity/adverse effects resolved. Continue indefinitely until pt no longer benefits from therapy.

Dosage in Renal/Hepatic Impairment
No dose adjustment.

SIDE EFFECTS

Chronic Phase

Frequent (45%–25%): Diarrhea, nausea, fatigue, pyrexia, asthenia. **Occasional (20%–11%):** Headache, arthralgia, cough, epistaxis, alopecia, constipation, abdominal pain, peripheral edema, vomiting, back pain, insomnia, rash.

Accelerated Phase

Occasional (19%–7%): Diarrhea, nausea, fatigue, pyrexia, asthenia, vomiting, cough, abdominal pain, chills, anorexia, headache. **Rare (7% or less):** Dyspnea, epistaxis.

ADVERSE EFFECTS/ TOXIC REACTIONS

Thrombocytopenia, neutropenia, leukopenia, lymphopenia, or myelosuppression is an expected response to therapy, but more severe reactions including bone marrow failure, febrile neutropenia may result in life-threatening events. Pts with neutropenia are at increased risk for infection. Thrombocytopenia may increase risk for intracranial hemorrhage, GI bleeding. Hyperglycemic events including hyperglycemic hyperosmolar nonketotic syndrome (HHNK) may occur. Pts with uncontrolled diabetes are at increased risk for hyperglycemic emergency.

NURSING CONSIDERATIONS

BASELINE ASSESSMENT

Obtain baseline serum chemistries, CBC, PT/INR if on anticoagulants. Question for possibility of pregnancy, current breastfeeding status. Obtain negative urine pregnancy test before initiating treatment. Obtain full medication history including herbal products, anticoagulants. Question for history of diabetes, GI bleeding. Offer emotional support.

INTERVENTION/EVALUATION

Monitor CBC wkly, then q2wks during maintenance phase. Obtain frequent blood glucose levels, especially in diabetic pts. Do not initiate therapy until negative urine pregnancy confirmed. Monitor LFT if hepatic impairment suspected. If drug exposure occurs, immediately wash affected area with soap and water. Consider isolation protocol if pt develops neutropenia.

PATIENT/FAMILY TEACHING

• Report if pregnant or planning to become pregnant. • Use barrier methods during sexual activity. • Strictly avoid pregnancy. • May cause male infertility. • Immediately report yellowing of skin or eyes, abdominal pain, bruising, black/tarry stools, dark urine, dehydration, GI bleeding, nausea, vomiting, rash. • Report fever, cough, night sweats, flu-like symptoms, skin changes. • Shortness of breath, pale skin, weakness may indicate bleeding or severe myelosuppression. • Avoid tasks that require alertness, motor skills until response to drug is established.

omalizumab

oh-ma-**liz**-ue-mab
(Xolair)

■ **BLACK BOX ALERT** ■ Anaphylaxis (severe bronchospasm, hypotension, angioedema, syncope, urticaria) has occurred after first dose and in some cases after 1 yr of regular treatment.
Do not confuse omalizumab with ofatumumab.

◆CLASSIFICATION

PHARMACOTHERAPEUTIC: Monoclonal antibody. **CLINICAL:** Anti-asthmatic.

USES

Treatment of moderate to severe persistent asthma in adults and children 6 yrs of age and older reactive to perennial allergens and with symptoms inadequately controlled with inhaled corticosteroids. Chronic idiopathic urticaria in adults and children 12 yrs and older.

PRECAUTIONS

Contraindications: Hypersensitivity to omalizumab. Do not use to treat acute bronchospasm, status asthmaticus. **Cautions:** Pts at risk for parasitic infections.

ACTION

Selectively binds to human immunoglobulin E (IgE). Inhibits binding of IgE on surface of mast cells, basophils. **Therapeutic Effect:** Prevents/reduces number of asthmatic attacks.

PHARMACOKINETICS

Absorbed slowly after SQ administration, with peak concentration in 7–8 days. Excreted primarily via hepatic degradation. **Half-life:** 26 days.

⧗ LIFESPAN CONSIDERATIONS

Pregnancy/Lactation: Because IgE is present in breast milk, omalizumab is expected to be present in breast milk. Use only if clearly needed. **Children:** Safety and efficacy not established in pts younger than 6 yrs. **Elderly:** No age-related precautions noted.

INTERACTIONS

DRUG: None significant. **HERBAL: Echinacea** may decrease effects. **FOOD:** None known. **LAB VALUES:** May increase serum IgE levels.

AVAILABILITY (RX)

Injection, Powder for Reconstitution: 150 mg/1.2 mL after reconstitution.

ADMINISTRATION/HANDLING

Subcutaneous

Reconstitution • Use only Sterile Water for Injection to prepare for SQ administration. • Medication takes 15–20 min to dissolve. • Draw 1.4 mL Sterile Water for Injection into 3-mL syringe with 1-inch, 18-gauge needle; inject contents into powdered vial. • Swirl vial for approximately 1 min (do not shake) and again swirl vial for 5–10 sec every 5 min until no gel-like particles appear in the solution. • Do not use if contents do not dissolve completely within 40 min. • Invert vial for 15 sec (allows solution to drain toward the stopper). • Using new 3-mL syringe with 1-inch 18-gauge needle, obtain required 1.2-mL dose, replace 18-gauge needle with 25-gauge needle for SQ administration.

Rate of Administration • SQ administration may take 5–10 sec to administer due to its viscosity.

Storage • Use only clear or slightly opalescent solution; solution is slightly viscous. • Refrigerate. • Reconstituted solution is stable for 8 hrs if refrigerated or within 4 hrs of reconstitution when stored at room temperature.

INDICATIONS/ROUTES/DOSAGE

◀ALERT▶ Give only under direct medical supervision. Should be administered in health care setting by health professionals. Dosage and frequency of administration are based upon total IgE levels and body weight (see table). IgE levels should be measured prior to initiating treatment and not during treatment. Pts should be observed a minimum of 2 hrs following each omalizumab treatment.

Asthma

SQ: ADULTS, ELDERLY, CHILDREN 6 YRS AND OLDER: 75–375 mg every 2 or 4 wks; dose and dosing frequency are individualized based on body weight and pretreatment IgE level (as shown in table). (Consult specific product labeling.)

Chronic Idiopathic Urticaria

SQ: ADULTS, CHILDREN 12 YRS AND OLDER: 150 mg or 300 mg q4wks. Dosing not dependent on IgE level or body weight.

Dosage in Renal/Hepatic Impairment

No dose adjustment.

4-Wk Dosing Table

Pretreatment Serum IgE Levels (units/mL)	Weight 30–60 kg	Weight 61–70 kg	Weight 71–90 kg	Weight 91–150 kg
30–100	150 mg	150 mg	150 mg	300 mg
101–200	300 mg	300 mg	300 mg	See next table
201–300	300 mg	See next table	See next table	See next table

2-Wk Dosing Table

Pretreatment Serum IgE Levels (units/mL)	Weight 30–60 kg	Weight 61–70 kg	Weight 71–90 kg	Weight 91–150 kg
101–200	See preceding table	See preceding table	See preceding table	225 mg
201–300	See preceding table	225 mg	225 mg	300 mg
301–400	225 mg	225 mg	300 mg	Do not dose
401–500	300 mg	300 mg	375 mg	Do not dose
501–600	300 mg	375 mg	Do not dose	Do not dose
601–700	375 mg	Do not dose	Do not dose	Do not dose

SIDE EFFECTS

Frequent (45%–11%): Injection site ecchymosis, redness, warmth, stinging, urticaria, viral infection, sinusitis, headache, pharyngitis. **Occasional (8%–3%):** Arthralgia, leg pain, fatigue, dizziness. **Rare (2%):** Arm pain, earache, dermatitis, pruritus.

ADVERSE EFFECTS/ TOXIC REACTIONS

Anaphylaxis, occurring within 2 hrs of first dose or subsequent doses, occurs in 0.1% of pts. Malignant neoplasms occur in 0.5% of pts.

NURSING CONSIDERATIONS

BASELINE ASSESSMENT

Obtain baseline serum total IgE level before initiation of treatment (dosage is based on pretreatment levels). Drug is not for treatment of acute exacerbations of asthma, acute bronchospasm, status asthmaticus.

INTERVENTION/EVALUATION

Monitor rate, depth, rhythm, type of respirations, quality/rate of pulse. Assess lung sounds for rhonchi, wheezing, rales. Observe lips, fingernails for cyanosis.

PATIENT/FAMILY TEACHING

• Increase fluid intake (decreases viscosity of pulmonary secretions). • Do not alter/stop other asthma medications. • Report allergic reactions (e.g., breathing difficulty, swelling of throat/tongue).

ombitasvir, paritaprevir, ritonavir, dasabuvir

om-**bit**-as-vir/**par**-i-**ta**-pre-vir/rit-**oh**-na-vir/da-**sa**-bue-vir
(Viekira Pak, Viekira XR)

Do not confuse ombitasvir with daclatasvir, or paritaprevir with boceprevir or simeprevir, or ritonavir with Retrovir, lopinavir, darunavir, or saquinavir, or dasabuvir with sofosbuvir.

◆CLASSIFICATION

PHARMACOTHERAPEUTIC: NS5A inhibitor, protease inhibitor, CYP3A inhibitor, non-nucleoside inhibitor. **CLINICAL:** Antiviral.

USES

Treatment of genotype 1 chronic hepatitis C virus (HCV) infection including those with compensated hepatic cirrhosis, with or without ribavirin.

PRECAUTIONS

Contraindications: Hypersensitivity to any component. Moderate to severe hepatic impairment; decompensated hepatic cirrhosis; contraindication or known hypersensitivity to ribavirin; concomitant use of strong CYP3A inducers, strong CYP2C8 inducers or strong CYP2C8 inhibitors; drugs highly dependent on CYP3A for clearance and for which elevated plasma concentrations are associated with serious and/or life-threatening events. Concurrent use of alfuzosin, carBAMazepine, colchicine, dronedarone, efavirenz, ergotamine, dihydroergotamine, ethinyl estradiol–containing drugs including combined oral contraceptives, gemfibrozil, lovastatin, lurasidone, midazolam (oral), phenytoin, PHENobarbital, pimozide, ranolazine, rifAMPin, sildenafil (when used for pulmonary arterial hypertension), simvastatin, St. John's wort, triazolam. **Cautions:** History of anemia, hepatitis B virus infection, HIV infection.

ACTION

Ombitasvir inhibits HCV NS5A needed for essential RNA replication and virion assembly. Paritaprevir inhibits HCV protease needed for cleavage of HCV-encoded polyproteins and viral replication. Ritonavir inhibits CYP3A clearance; increases plasma concentrations of paritaprevir. Dasabuvir inhibits HCV RNA-dependent RNA polymerase needed for replication of viral genome. **Therapeutic Effect:** Inhibits viral replication of hepatitis C virus.

PHARMACOKINETICS

Readily absorbed. Paritaprevir, ritonavir, dasabuvir metabolized in liver. Ombitasvir metabolized by amide hydrolysis. Protein binding: ombitasvir: greater than 99%, paritaprevir: 97%–99%, ritonavir: 99%, dasabuvir: 99%. Peak plasma concentration: 4–5 hrs. Steady-state concentration: 12 days. Elimination: ombitasvir: feces (92%), urine (2%); paritaprevir: feces (88%), urine (9%); ritonavir: feces (86%), urine (11%); dasabuvir: feces (94%), urine (2%). **Half-life:** Ombitasvir: 21–25 hrs; paritaprevir: 5.5 hrs; ritonavir: 4 hrs; dasabuvir: 5.5–6 hrs.

⌛ LIFESPAN CONSIDERATIONS

Pregnancy/Lactation: Avoid pregnancy; may cause fetal harm. When administered with ribavirin, therapy is contraindicated in pregnant women and in men whose female partners are pregnant. Unknown if distributed in breast milk. Concomitant use of ethinyl estradiol–containing drugs is contraindicated. Alternative contraception methods including progestin-only drugs, barrier methods, abstinence are recommended. **Children:** Safety and efficacy not established in pts younger than 18 yrs. **Elderly:** No age-related precautions noted.

INTERACTIONS

DRUG: May increase concentration/effects of **antiarrhythmics** (e.g., **amiodarone**), **antifungals** (e.g., **itraconazole**), **calcium channel blockers** (e.g., **amLODIPine, NIFEdipine**), **corticosteroids** (e.g., **fluticasone**), **immunosuppressants** (e.g., **cycloSPORINE**), **digoxin**, **HIV antiretrovirals** (e.g., **paritaprevir, rilpivirine**), **phosphodiesterase-5 inhibitors** (e.g., **sildenafil**), **sedative/hypnotics** (e.g., **temazepam**), **statins** (e.g., **atorvastatin, simvastatin**), **sirolimus, tacrolimus**. Anticonvulsants (e.g., **carBAMazepine, phenytoin**), **dexamethasone, efavirenz, omeprazole, rifAMPin** may decrease concentration/effect. **HERBAL: St. John's wort** may decrease concentration/effect. **Kava kava**

may increase risk of hepatotoxicity. **Red yeast** may increase risk of myopathy, rhabdomyolysis. **Meals** increase absorption. **FOOD: Grapefruit products, Seville oranges** may increase concentration/effect. **LAB VALUES:** May increase serum alkaline phosphatase, ALT, INR. May decrease Hct, Hgb.

AVAILABILITY (Rx)

Fixed-Dose Combination Tablets (co-packaged with dasabuvir tablets): (Viekira Pak): Ombitasvir 12.5 mg/paritaprevir 75 mg/ritonavir 50 mg; dasabuvir 250 mg. **(Viekira XR):** Ombitasvir 8.33 mg/paritaprevir 50 mg/ritonavir 33.3 mg/dasabuvir 200 mg.

ADMINISTRATION/HANDLING

PO
• Give with food. Do not cut, crush, break, or divide XR tablets.

INDICATIONS/ROUTES/DOSAGE

Hepatitis C Virus Infection
PO: ADULTS, ELDERLY: (Viekira Pak): 2 tablets of ombitasvir, paritaprevir, ritonavir once daily, plus 1 tablet of dasabuvir twice daily with or without ribavirin. **(Viekira XR):** 3 tablets once daily.

Treatment Regimen and Duration
Genotype 1a, without cirrhosis: Fixed-combination regimen with ribavirin for 12 wks. **Genotype 1a, with cirrhosis:** Fixed-combination regimen with ribavirin for 24 wks. Consider duration of 12 wks in pts with prior treatment history. **Genotype 1b, without cirrhosis:** Fixed-combination regimen for 12 wks. **Genotype 1b, with cirrhosis:** Fixed-combination regimen (with ribavirin) for 12 wks. **Recommended dose of ribavirin based on weight in kg: LESS THAN 75 KG:** 1,000 mg/day in 2 divided doses. **75 KG OR GREATER:** 1,200 mg/day in 2 divided doses. For ribavirin dose modifications, refer to prescribing information.

Dose Modification
Liver Transplant Recipients
PO: ADULTS, ELDERLY: 2 tablets of ombitasvir, paritaprevir, ritonavir once daily, plus 1 tablet of dasabuvir twice daily with ribavirin for 24 wks, irrespective of HCV genotype 1 subtype in pts with normal hepatic function and mild fibrosis.
HCV/HIV-1 Coinfection
Follow dose recommendations as listed in Treatment Regimen and Duration. Consider suppressive antiretroviral drug therapy during treatment.

Dosage in Renal Impairment
No dose adjustment.

Dosage in Hepatic Impairment
Mild impairment: No dose adjustment. **Moderate impairment:** Treatment not recommended. **Severe impairment:** Treatment contraindicated.

SIDE EFFECTS

Frequent (34%–22%): Fatigue, nausea. **Occasional (18%–14%):** Pruritus, rash, erythema, eczema, allergic dermatitis, skin exfoliation, urticaria, photosensitivity reaction, skin ulcer, insomnia, asthenia.

ADVERSE EFFECTS/ TOXIC REACTIONS

Serum ALT greater than 5 times upper limit of normal (ULN) reported in 1% of pts (usually occurred during the first 4 wks of treatment). Elevations of serum ALT were significantly higher in female pts using ethinyl estradiol–containing drugs such as contraceptive patches, combined oral contraceptives, vaginal rings. May increase risk of drug resistance in HCV/HIV-1 coinfected pts using HIV-1 protease inhibitors. Hypersensitivity reaction including angioedema may occur.

NURSING CONSIDERATIONS

BASELINE ASSESSMENT
Obtain baseline CBC, LFT, HCV-RNA level, urine pregnancy. Confirm HCV genotype.

Receive full medication history and screen for contraindications/interactions. Ethinyl estradiol–containing contraceptive drugs should be discontinued prior to initiation. Question history as listed in Precautions. To reduce risk of HIV-1 protease inhibitor drug resistance, consider suppressive antiretroviral drug therapy upon initiation.

INTERVENTION/EVALUATION

Monitor LFT periodically during the first 4 wks of treatment, then as clinically indicated thereafter. Discontinue treatment for serum ALT persistently greater than 10 times ULN; serum ALT elevation associated with increase in serum alkaline phosphatase, bilirubin, or INR; hepatic injury. Periodically monitor CBC for anemia, HCV-RNA level for treatment effectiveness. Reinforce birth control compliance. Monitor for abdominal pain, bruising, jaundice, nausea, vomiting; may indicate hepatic injury. Ethinyl estradiol–containing contraceptives may be restarted approx. 2 wks after discontinuation.

PATIENT/FAMILY TEACHING

• Treatment must be used in combination with ribavirin. • Take with meals. • Inform pt of contraindications/adverse effects of therapy. • Do not take newly prescribed medication unless approved by doctor who originally started treatment. Do not take herbal products. • Pregnancy should be avoided when combination regimen is given with ribavirin. Female pts of childbearing potential must use reliable forms of birth control such as progestin-containing contraception, barrier methods, abstinence. Immediately report suspected pregnancy. Do not breastfeed. • Report abdominal pain, bruising easily, dark-colored urine, fatigue, yellowing of the skin or eyes. • Avoid alcohol. • Report skin changes such as rash, peeling, ulcers; allergic reactions such as difficulty breathing, itching, hives, tongue swelling.

omega-3 acid-ethyl esters

TOP 100

oh-**may**-ga 3 **as**-id **eth**-il **es**-ters
(Lovaza, Epanova, Omtryg, Vascepa)
Do not confuse Lovaza with LORazepam.

◆CLASSIFICATION

PHARMACOTHERAPEUTIC: Omega-3 fatty acid. **CLINICAL:** Antihypertriglyceride agent.

USES

Adjunct to diet to reduce very high (500 mg/dL or higher) serum triglyceride levels in adult pts. Dietary supplement for pts with early risk of CAD. **OFF-LABEL:** Treatment of IgA nephropathy.

PRECAUTIONS

Contraindications: Hypersensitivity to omega-3 fatty acids. **Cautions:** Known sensitivity, allergy to fish.

ACTION

Inhibits esterification of fatty acids, prevents hepatic enzymes from catalyzing final step of triglyceride synthesis. **Therapeutic Effect:** Reduces serum triglyceride levels.

PHARMACOKINETICS

Well absorbed following PO administration. Incorporated into phospholipids. **Half-life:** N/A.

⧗ LIFESPAN CONSIDERATIONS

Pregnancy/Lactation: Unknown if distributed in breast milk. **Children:** Safety and efficacy not established in pts younger than 18 yrs. **Elderly:** No age-related precautions noted.

INTERACTIONS

DRUG: Anticoagulants (e.g., heparin, warfarin) may increase risk of bleeding. **HERBAL:** None significant. **FOOD:** None known. **LAB VALUES:** May increase serum ALT, LDL.

AVAILABILITY (Rx)

Capsules: 200 mg, 300 mg, 500 mg, 600 mg, 1000 mg, 1,200 mg.

ADMINISTRATION/HANDLING

PO
- Give without regard to meals.

INDICATIONS/ROUTES/DOSAGE

◄**ALERT►** Before initiating therapy, pt should be on standard cholesterol-lowering diet for minimum of 3–6 mos. Continue diet throughout therapy.

Usual Dosage
PO: ADULTS, ELDERLY: 4 g/day, given as a single dose (4 capsules), or 2 capsules twice daily.

Dosage in Renal/Hepatic Impairment
No dose adjustment.

SIDE EFFECTS

Occasional (5%–3%): Eructation, altered taste, dyspepsia. **Rare (2%–1%):** Rash, back pain.

ADVERSE EFFECTS/ TOXIC REACTIONS

None known.

NURSING CONSIDERATIONS

BASELINE ASSESSMENT

Assess baseline serum triglyceride level, LFT. Obtain diet history, esp. fat consumption.

INTERVENTION/EVALUATION

Monitor serum triglyceride levels for therapeutic response. Monitor serum ALT, LDL periodically during therapy. Discontinue therapy if no response after 2 mos of treatment.

PATIENT/FAMILY TEACHING

- Continue to adhere to lipid-lowering diet (important part of treatment).
- Periodic lab tests are essential part of therapy to determine drug effectiveness.

omeprazole

oh-**mep**-ra-zole
(Apo-Omeprazole ✦, Losec ✦, PriLOSEC, PriLOSEC OTC)
Do not confuse omeprazole with ARIPiprazole, pantoprazole, or esomeprazole, or PriLOSEC with Plendil, Prevacid, Prinivil, or PROzac.

FIXED-COMBINATION(S)

Yosprala: omeprazole/aspirin (a platelet aggregation inhibitor): 40 mg/81 mg, 40 mg/325 mg. **Zegerid:** omeprazole/sodium bicarbonate (an antacid): 20 mg/1,100 mg, 40 mg/ 1,100 mg. **Zegerid Powder:** 20 mg/1,680 mg, 40 mg/1,680 mg.

◆CLASSIFICATION

PHARMACOTHERAPEUTIC: Benzimidazole. **CLINICAL:** Proton pump inhibitor.

USES

Short-term treatment (4–8 wks) of erosive esophagitis (diagnosed by endoscopy), symptomatic gastroesophageal reflux disease (GERD) poorly responsive to other treatment. *H. pylori*–associated duodenal ulcer (with amoxicillin and clarithromycin). Long-term treatment of pathologic hypersecretory conditions, treatment of active duodenal ulcer or active benign gastric ulcer. Maintenance healing of erosive esophagitis. **OTC, short-term:** Treatment of frequent, uncomplicated heartburn occurring 2 or more days/wk. **OFF-LABEL:** Prevention/treatment of NSAID-induced ulcers, stress ulcer prophylaxis in critically ill pts.

PRECAUTIONS

Contraindications: Hypersensitivity to omeprazole, other proton pump inhibitors. Concomitant use with products containing rilpivirine. **Cautions:** May

0

increase risk of fractures, gastrointestinal infections. Hepatic impairment, pts of Asian descent.

ACTION

Inhibits hydrogen-potassium adenosine triphosphatase (H^+/K^+ ATP pump), an enzyme on the surface of gastric parietal cells. **Therapeutic Effect:** Increases gastric pH, reduces gastric acid production.

PHARMACOKINETICS

Route	Onset	Peak	Duration
PO	1 hr	2 hrs	72 hrs

Rapidly absorbed from GI tract. Protein binding: 95%. Primarily distributed into gastric parietal cells. Metabolized in liver. Primarily excreted in urine. Unknown if removed by hemodialysis. **Half-life:** 0.5–1 hr (increased in hepatic impairment).

⌛ LIFESPAN CONSIDERATIONS

Pregnancy/Lactation: Unknown if drug crosses placenta or is distributed in breast milk. **Children:** Safety and efficacy not established. **Elderly:** Use caution (bioavailability may be increased).

INTERACTIONS

DRUG: May decrease concentration/effects of **atazanavir, clopidogrel.** May increase concentration/effects of **diazePAM,** oral anticoagulants (e.g., **warfarin), phenytoin. HERBAL: St. John's wort** may decrease concentration/effects. **FOOD:** None known. **LAB VALUES:** May increase serum alkaline phosphatase, ALT, AST.

AVAILABILITY (Rx)

Granules for Oral Suspension: 2.5 mg/packet, 10 mg/packet. **Powder for Oral Suspension:** 2 mg/mL.

🍵 **Capsules (Delayed-Release [PriLOSEC]):** 10 mg, 20 mg, 40 mg. 🍵 **Tablets (Delayed-Release [PriLOSEC OTC]):** 20 mg.

ADMINISTRATION/HANDLING

PO

• Give before meals (breakfast preferred). • Give whole. Do not break, crush, dissolve, or divide delayed-release forms. • May open capsule, mix with applesauce, and give immediately.

PO (Suspension)

• Following reconstitution, allow to thicken (2–3 min). • Administer within 30 min.

INDICATIONS/ROUTES/DOSAGE

Active Duodenal Ulcer
PO: ADULTS, ELDERLY: 20 mg/day for 4–8 wks.

Symptomatic GERD
PO: ADULTS, ELDERLY, CHILDREN WEIGHING 20 KG OR MORE: 20 mg/day for up to 4 wks. **10–19 KG:** 10 mg/day. **5–9 KG:** 5 mg/day.

Erosive Esophagitis
PO: ADULTS, ELDERLY, CHILDREN WEIGHING 20 KG OR MORE: Treatment: 20 mg/day for 4–8 wks. **CHILDREN 1–16 YRS WEIGHING 10–19 KG:** 10 mg/day. **WEIGHING 5–9 KG:** 5 mg/day. **CHILDREN 1–11 MOS WEIGHING 10 KG OR MORE:** 10 mg/day. **WEIGHING 5–9 KG:** 5 mg/day. **WEIGHING 3–4 KG:** 2.5 mg/day. **Maintenance: ADULTS, ELDERLY, CHILDREN WEIGHING 20 KG OR MORE:** 20 mg/day for up to 12 mos (including treatment period). **ASIAN PTS, CHILDREN WEIGHING 10–19 kg:** 10 mg/day. **WEIGHING 5–9 KG:** 5 mg/day.

Pathologic Hypersecretory Conditions
Note: Doses more than 80 mg in divided doses. **PO: ADULTS, ELDERLY:** Initially, 60 mg/day up to 120 mg 3 times/day.

H. Pylori Duodenal Ulcer
PO: ADULTS, ELDERLY: 40 mg once daily (with clarithromycin) for 14 days or 20 mg twice daily (with amoxicillin and clarithromycin) for 10 days. Presence of ulcer at initiation may need 20 mg/day

(monotherapy) for 14–18 days following combination therapy.

Gastric Ulcer
PO: **ADULTS, ELDERLY:** 40 mg/day for 4–8 wks.

OTC Use (Frequent Heartburn)
PO: **ADULTS, ELDERLY:** 20 mg/day for 14 days. May repeat after 4 mos if needed.

Dosage in Renal/Hepatic Impairment
No dose adjustment.

SIDE EFFECTS

Frequent (7%): Headache. **Occasional (3%–2%):** Diarrhea, abdominal pain, nausea. **Rare (2%):** Dizziness, asthenia, vomiting, constipation, upper respiratory tract infection, back pain, rash, cough.

ADVERSE EFFECTS/ TOXIC REACTIONS

Pancreatitis, hepatotoxicity, interstitial nephritis occur rarely. May increase risk of *C. difficile* infection.

NURSING CONSIDERATIONS

INTERVENTION/EVALUATION

Evaluate for therapeutic response (relief of GI symptoms). Question if GI discomfort, nausea, diarrhea occurs.

PATIENT/FAMILY TEACHING

• Report headache, onset of black, tarry stools, diarrhea, abdominal pain. • Avoid alcohol. • Swallow capsules whole; do not chew, crush, dissolve, or divide. • Take before eating.

---

ondansetron

on-**dan**-se-tron
(Apo-Ondansetron ✦, Zofran, Zofran ODT, Zuplenz)
Do not confuse ondansetron with dolasetron, granisetron, or palonosetron, or Zofran with Zantac or Zosyn.

◆CLASSIFICATION

PHARMACOTHERAPEUTIC: Selective 5-HT$_3$ receptor antagonist. **CLINICAL:** Antinausea, antiemetic.

USES

Prevention/treatment of nausea/vomiting due to cancer chemotherapy (including high-dose CISplatin). Prevention and treatment of postop nausea, vomiting. Prevention of radiation-induced nausea, vomiting. **OFF-LABEL:** Breakthrough treatment of nausea and vomiting associated with chemotherapy, hyperemesis gravidarum.

PRECAUTIONS

Contraindications: Hypersensitivity to ondansetron, other HT$_3$ antagonists. Use of apomorphine. **Cautions:** Mild to moderate hepatic impairment, pts at risk for QT prolongation or ventricular arrhythmia (congenital long QT prolongation, medications prolonging QT interval, hypokalemia, hypomagnesemia).

ACTION

Blocks serotonin, both peripherally on vagal nerve terminals and centrally in chemoreceptor trigger zone. **Therapeutic Effect:** Prevents nausea/vomiting.

PHARMACOKINETICS

Readily absorbed from GI tract. Protein binding: 70%–76%. Metabolized in liver. Primarily excreted in urine. Unknown if removed by hemodialysis. **Half-life:** 3–6 hrs (increased in hepatic impairment).

⌛ LIFESPAN CONSIDERATIONS

Pregnancy/Lactation: Unknown if drug crosses placenta or is distributed in breast milk. **Children:** Safety and efficacy not established in children younger than 1 mo. **Elderly:** No age-related precautions noted.

INTERACTIONS

DRUG: Apomorphine may cause profound hypotension, altered LOC. **QT**

0

---

interval–prolonging medications (e.g., **amiodarone, azithromycin, ciprofloxacin, haloperidol**) may increase risk of QT interval prolongation, torsades de pointes. **HERBAL: St. John's wort** may decrease concentration. **FOOD:** None known. **LAB VALUES:** May transiently increase serum bilirubin, ALT, AST.

AVAILABILITY (Rx)

Injection Solution (Zofran): 2 mg/mL. **Oral Soluble Film (Zuplenz):** 4 mg, 8 mg. **Oral Solution (Zofran):** 4 mg/5 mL. **Tablets (Zofran):** 4 mg, 8 mg, 24 mg. **Tablets (Orally Disintegrating [Zofran ODT]):** 4 mg, 8 mg.

ADMINISTRATION/HANDLING

 IV

Reconstitution • May give undiluted. • For IV infusion, dilute with 50 mL D₅W or 0.9% NaCl before administration.
Rate of Administration • Give IV push over 2–5 min. • Give IV infusion over 15–30 min.
Storage • Store at room temperature. • Stable for 48 hrs at room temperature following dilution.

IM
• Inject undiluted into large muscle mass.

PO
• Give without regard to food.

Orally Disintegrating Tablets
• Do not remove from blister pack until needed. • Peel backing off; do not push through. • Place tablet on tongue; allow to dissolve. • Swallow with saliva.

Oral Soluble Film
• Keep film in pouch until ready to use. • Remove film strip from pouch and place on top of tongue; allow to dissolve. • Swallow after film dissolves. Do not chew or swallow film whole. • If using more than one, each should be allowed to dissolve before administering the next one.

IV INCOMPATIBILITIES

Acyclovir (Zovirax), allopurinol (Aloprim), amphotericin B (Fungizone), amphotericin B complex (Abelcet, AmBisome, Amphotec), ampicillin (Polycillin), ampicillin and sulbactam (Unasyn), cefepime (Maxipime), 5-fluorouracil, LORazepam (Ativan), meropenem (Merrem IV), methylPREDNISolone (Solu-Medrol).

IV COMPATIBILITIES

CARBOplatin (Paraplatin), CISplatin (Platinol), cyclophosphamide (Cytoxan), cytarabine (Cytosar), dacarbazine (DTIC-Dome), DAUNOrubicin (Cerubidine), dexmedetomidine (Precedex), dexamethasone (Decadron), diphenhydrAMINE (Benadryl), DOCEtaxel (Taxotere), DOPamine (Intropin), etoposide (VePesid), gemcitabine (Gemzar), heparin, HYDROmorphone (Dilaudid), ifosfamide (Ifex), magnesium, mannitol, mesna (Mesnex), methotrexate, metoclopramide (Reglan), mitoMYcin (Mutamycin), mitoXANTRONE (Novantrone), morphine, PACLitaxel (Taxol), potassium chloride, teniposide (Vumon), topotecan (Hycamtin), vinBLAStine (Velban), vinCRIStine (Oncovin), vinorelbine (Navelbine).

INDICATIONS/ROUTES/DOSAGE

Chemotherapy-Induced Nausea/Vomiting
IV: ADULTS, ELDERLY, CHILDREN 6 MOS AND OLDER: 0.15 mg/kg (**Maximum:** 16 mg/dose) 3 times/day beginning 30 min before chemotherapy, followed by subsequent doses 4 and 8 hrs after the first dose.
PO: ADULTS, ELDERLY, CHILDREN 12 YRS AND OLDER: (highly emetogenic) 24 mg 30 min before start of chemotherapy, (moderately emetogenic) 8 mg repeat dose 8 hrs after initial dose, then q12h, beginning 30 min before chemotherapy and continuing for 1–2 days after completion of chemotherapy. **CHILDREN 4–11 YRS:** 4 mg 30 min before chemotherapy, repeat 4 and 8 hrs after initial dose then q8h for 1–2 days after chemotherapy completed.

Prevention of Postop Nausea/Vomiting
IV, IM: ADULTS, ELDERLY, CHILDREN OLDER THAN 12 YRS: 4 mg as a single dose. **CHILDREN 1 MO–12 YRS WEIGHING MORE THAN 40 KG:** 4 mg as a single dose. **CHILDREN 1 MO–12 YRS WEIGHING 40 KG OR LESS:** 0.1 mg/kg as a single dose.
PO: ADULTS, ELDERLY: 16 mg 1 hr before induction of anesthesia.

Prevention of Radiation-Induced Nausea/Vomiting
PO: ADULTS, ELDERLY: (Total body irradiation): 8 mg 1–2 hrs before each fraction of radiotherapy administereded each day. (Single high-dose radiotherapy to abdomen): 8 mg 1–2 hrs before irradiation, then 8 mg q8h after first dose for 1–2 days after completion of radiotherapy. (Daily fractionated radiotherapy to abdomen): 8 mg 1–2 hrs before irradiation, then 8 mg 8 hrs after first dose for each day of radiotherapy.

Dosage in Renal Impairment
No dose adjustment.

Dosage in Hepatic Impairment
Mild to moderate impairment: No dose adjustment. **Severe impairment:** Maximum daily dose: 8 mg.

SIDE EFFECTS

Frequent (13%–5%): Anxiety, dizziness, drowsiness, headache, fatigue, constipation, diarrhea, hypoxia, urinary retention. **Occasional (4%–2%):** Abdominal pain, xerostomia, fever, feeling of cold, redness/pain at injection site, paresthesia, asthenia (loss of strength, energy). **Rare (1%):** Hypersensitivity reaction (rash, pruritus), blurred vision.

ADVERSE EFFECTS/ TOXIC REACTIONS

Hypertension, acute renal failure, GI bleeding, respiratory depression, coma, extrapyramidal effects occur rarely. QT interval prolongation, torsades de pointes may occur.

NURSING CONSIDERATIONS

BASELINE ASSESSMENT

Assess degree of nausea, vomiting. Assess for dehydration if excessive vomiting occurs (poor skin turgor, dry mucous membranes, longitudinal furrows in tongue). Provide emotional support.

INTERVENTION/EVALUATION

Monitor EKG in pts with electrolyte abnormalities (e.g., hypokalemia, hypomagnesemia), HF, bradyarrhythmias, concurrent use of other medications that may cause QT prolongation, pts receiving high doses or frequent doses. Provide supportive measures. Assess mental status. Assess bowel sounds for peristalsis. Monitor daily pattern of bowel activity, stool consistency. Record time of evacuation.

PATIENT/FAMILY TEACHING

• Relief from nausea/vomiting generally occurs shortly after drug administration. • Avoid alcohol, barbiturates. • Report persistent vomiting. • Avoid tasks that require alertness, motor skills until response to drug is established (may cause drowsiness, dizziness).

O

oritavancin

or-**it**-a-**van**-sin
(Orbactiv)
Do not confuse oritavancin with dalbavancin or telavancin.

◆CLASSIFICATION

PHARMACOTHERAPEUTIC: Lipoglycopeptide (antibacterial). **CLINICAL:** Antibiotic.

USES

Treatment of adult pts with acute bacterial skin and skin structure infections (ABSSSI) caused by susceptible strains of gram-positive microorganisms including *Staphylococcus aureus* (including methicillin-susceptible and methicillin-resistant strains), *Strepococcus agalactiae, Strepococcus dysgalactiae, Streptococcus pyogenes, Streptococcus anginosus* group *(including S. anginosus, S. intermedius, S. constellatus),* and *E. faecalis* (vancomycin-susceptible strains only).

PRECAUTIONS

Contraindications: Hypersensitivity to oritavancin. Concomitant use of IV unfractionated heparin sodium for 120 hrs (5 days) after oritavancin administration. **Cautions:** Severe hepatic impairment, history of hypersensitivity reaction to glycopeptides (e.g., vancomycin), recent *C. difficile* infection or antibiotic-associated colitis.

ACTION

Inhibits cell wall synthesis by binding to bacterial cell membrane, disrupting membrane integrity. **Therapeutic Effect:** Bactericidal.

PHARMACOKINETICS

Widely distributed. Not metabolized. Protein binding: 85%. Excreted unchanged in feces, urine. Not removed by hemodialysis. **Half-life:** 10.2 days.

⏳ LIFESPAN CONSIDERATIONS

Pregnancy/Lactation: Unknown if distributed in breast milk. **Children:** Safety and efficacy not established in pts younger than 18 yrs. **Elderly:** No age-related precautions noted.

INTERACTIONS

DRUG: Use of **heparin** within 48 hrs of dose contraindicated. May increase risk of bleeding with **warfarin. Concomitant use of other antibiotics** may increase risk of antibiotic-associated colitis. **HERBAL:** None significant. **FOOD:** None known. **LAB VALUES:** May prolong aPTT (falsely elevates aPTT for up to 120 hrs after oritavancin administration), PT/INR. May increase ALT, AST, bilirubin, uric acid. May decrease glucose.

AVAILABILITY (Rx)

Sterile Powder for Injection: 400 mg/vial.

ADMINISTRATION/HANDLING
💉 IV

◀**ALERT**▶ No preservatives or bacteriostatic agent is present in product. Aseptic technique must be used when preparing solution. Must be reconstituted with Sterile Water for Injection and subsequently diluted with 5% Dextrose in Water only.

Reconstitution • Obtain three 400-mg vials to equal required 1,200-mg dose. • Add 40 mL of Sterile Water for Injection to each vial for final concentration of 10 mg/mL per vial. • To avoid foaming, gently swirl until contents completely dissolve. • Visually inspect each vial for particulate matter or discoloration.

Dilution • Using D_5W, withdraw 120 mL from 1,000-mL bag and discard. • Withdraw 40 mL from each vial and mix into D_5W to provide a final concentration of 1.2 mg/mL.

Rate of Administration • Administer over 3 hrs.

Storage • Reconstituted solution should appear clear, colorless to pale yellow. • Infuse diluted solution within 6 hrs when stored at room temperature or 12 hrs when refrigerated. • Combined storage time and 3-hr infusion time should not exceed 6 hrs if at room temperature or 12 hrs if refrigerated.

▦ IV INCOMPATIBILITIES

Dilute using 5% Dextrose in Water only. Dilution with normal saline may cause precipitate formation. Infuse via dedicated line only. Do not piggyback through maintenance IV line.

INDICATIONS/ROUTES/DOSAGE

Acute Bacterial Skin and Skin Structure Infection
IV: ADULTS, ELDERLY: 1,200 mg as single dose.

Dosage in Renal/Hepatic Impairment
Mild to moderate impairment: No dose adjustment. **Severe impairment:** Use caution.

SIDE EFFECTS

Occasional (10%–5%): Nausea, headache, vomiting. **Rare (4%–3%):** Diarrhea, dizziness, tachycardia.

ADVERSE EFFECTS/ TOXIC REACTIONS

Serious hypersensitivity reactions including anaphylaxis, angioedema, bronchospasm, severe skin reactions, wheezing have been reported with glycopeptide antibacterial agents. *C. difficile*–associated diarrhea with severity ranging from mild diarrhea to fatal colitis has occurred. Treatment in the absence of proven or strongly suspected bacterial infection may increase risk of drug-resistant bacteria. Infusion site reactions, phlebitis, irritation, abscess, rash, pruritus have occurred. Increased incidence of osteomyelitis has been reported.

NURSING CONSIDERATIONS

BASELINE ASSESSMENT

Obtain baseline CBC (WBC), BMP, LFT, wound culture and sensitivity, vital signs. Question history of recent *C. difficile* infection, hepatic/renal impairment, hypersensitivity reaction. Assess skin wound characteristics, hydration status. Question pt's usual stool characteristics (color, frequency, consistency).

INTERVENTION/EVALUATION

Assess skin infection/wound for improvement. Monitor daily pattern of bowel activity, stool consistency; increasing severity of diarrhea may indicate antibiotic-associated colitis. If frequent diarrhea occurs, obtain *C. difficile* toxin screen and initiate isolation precautions until result confirmed. Encourage PO intake. Monitor I&O. If osteomyelitis suspected, other antimicrobial agents may be required. Screen for hypersensitivity reaction.

PATIENT/FAMILY TEACHING

• Treatment will consist of a single infusion only. • Report episodes of diarrhea, esp. the following weeks after treatment completion. Frequent diarrhea, fever, abdominal pain, blood-streaked stool may indicate *C. difficile* infection, which may be contagious to others. • Report abdominal pain, black/tarry stools, bruising, yellowing of skin or eyes; dark urine, decreased urine output; or allergic reactions including difficulty breathing, itching, hives, tongue swelling, wheezing. • Do not breastfeed. • Drink plenty of fluids. • Report symptoms of bone pain; may indicate bone infection.

orlistat

or-lye-stat
(Alli, Xenical)
Do not confuse Xenical with Xeloda.

◆CLASSIFICATION

PHARMACOTHERAPEUTIC: Gastric/pancreatic lipase inhibitor. **CLINICAL:** Obesity management agent.

USES

Management of obesity, including weight loss/maintenance, when used in conjunction with reduced-calorie diet. Reduces risk of weight regain after previous weight loss. Indicated for pts with initial BMI of 30 kg/m^2 or greater or 27 kg/m^2 or greater with other risk factors (e.g., diabetes, dyslipidemia, hypertension). **OTC:** Weight loss in overweight adults when used along with a reduced-calorie and low-fat diet.

PRECAUTIONS

Contraindications: Hypersensitivity to orlistat. Cholestasis, chronic malabsorption syndrome, pregnancy. **Cautions:** History of hyperoxaluria or calcium oxalate nephrolithiasis.

ACTION

Inhibits absorption of dietary fats by inhibiting gastric and pancreatic lipases. **Therapeutic Effect:** Resulting caloric deficit may have positive effects on weight control.

PHARMACOKINETICS

Minimal absorption after administration. Protein binding: 99%. Metabolized within GI wall. Primarily excreted in feces. Unknown if removed by hemodialysis. **Half-life:** 1–2 hrs.

⧗ LIFESPAN CONSIDERATIONS

Pregnancy/Lactation: Unknown if distributed in breast milk. Not recommended during pregnancy (contraindicated). Breastfeeding not recommended. **Children:** Safety and efficacy not established in children younger than 12 yrs. **Elderly:** No age-related precautions noted.

INTERACTIONS

DRUG: May decrease concentration/effects of **amiodarone, anticonvulsants, cycloSPORINE, levothyroxine.** May reduce absorption of **vitamin E.** May alter effect of **warfarin** by altering vitamin K level. **HERBAL:** None significant. **FOOD:** None known. **LAB VALUES:** May decrease serum glucose, cholesterol, LDL.

AVAILABILITY (Rx)

Capsules (Alli): 60 mg. **(Xenical):** 120 mg.

ADMINISTRATION/HANDLING

PO

• Multivitamin supplements containing fat-soluble vitamins should be taken once daily at least 2 hrs before or after taking orlistat. • Distribute daily fat intake over 3 main meals (GI effects may increase when taken with any 1 meal very high in fat). Administer during or up to 1 hr after each meal containing fat.

INDICATIONS/ROUTES/DOSAGE

Weight Reduction

PO: ADULTS, ELDERLY, CHILDREN 12–16 YRS: *(Xenical):* 120 mg 3 times/day. *(Alli):* 60 mg 3 times/day with each main meal containing fat (do not take if meal is occasionally missed or contains no fat).

Dosage with Other Medication

(Cyclosporine): Give 3 hrs after orlistat. *(Levothyroxine):* Give at least 4 hrs apart. Monitor thyroid function.

Dosage in Renal/Hepatic Impairment

No dose adjustment.

SIDE EFFECTS

Frequent (30%–20%): Headache, abdominal discomfort, flatulence, fecal urgency, fatty/oily stool. **Occasional (14%–5%):** Back pain, menstrual irregularity, nausea, fatigue, diarrhea, dizziness. **Rare (less than 4%):** Anxiety, rash, myalgia, dry skin, vomiting.

ADVERSE EFFECTS/ TOXIC REACTIONS

Hypersensitivity reaction occurs rarely.

NURSING CONSIDERATIONS

BASELINE ASSESSMENT

Obtain baseline laboratory tests. Obtain pt weight.

INTERVENTION/EVALUATION

Monitor serum cholesterol, LDL, glucose, changes in coagulation parameters. Monitor weight wkly.

PATIENT/FAMILY TEACHING

• Maintain nutritionally balanced, reduced-calorie diet. • Daily intake of fat, carbohydrates, protein to be distributed over 3 main meals.

oseltamivir `TOP 100`

oh-sel-**tam**-i-veer
(Tamiflu)
Do not confuse Tamiflu with Thera-flu.

◆CLASSIFICATION

PHARMACOTHERAPEUTIC: Neuraminidase inhibitor. **CLINICAL:** Antiviral.

USES

Symptomatic treatment of uncomplicated acute illness caused by influenza A or B virus in adults and children 2 wks of age and older who are symptomatic no longer than 2 days. Prevention of influenza in adults, children.

PRECAUTIONS

Contraindications: Hypersensitivity to oseltamivir. **Cautions:** Renal impairment.

ACTION

Selective inhibitor of influenza virus neuraminidase, an enzyme essential for viral replication. Acts against influenza A and B viruses. **Therapeutic Effect:** Suppresses spread of infection within respiratory system, reduces duration of clinical symptoms.

PHARMACOKINETICS

Readily absorbed after PO administration. Protein binding: 3%. Metabolized in liver. Primarily excreted in urine. **Half-life:** 6–10 hrs.

⌛ LIFESPAN CONSIDERATIONS

Pregnancy/Lactation: Unknown if distributed in breast milk. **Children:** Safety and efficacy not established in pts younger than 2 wks. **Elderly:** No age-related precautions noted.

INTERACTIONS

DRUG: Live attenuated influenza virus vaccine intranasal may interfere with effect. **HERBAL:** None significant.

FOOD: None known. **LAB VALUES:** None significant.

AVAILABILITY (Rx)

Capsules: 30 mg, 45 mg, 75 mg. **Powder for Oral Suspension:** 6 mg/mL.

ADMINISTRATION/HANDLING

PO

• Give without regard to food. • May open capsules and mix with sweetened liquid. • Oral suspension stable for 10 days (room temperature) or 17 days (refrigerated) following reconstitution.

INDICATIONS/ROUTES/DOSAGE

Treatment of Influenza

Note: Hospitalized pts may require longer treatment course. Initiate within 48 hrs of onset of symptoms. Consider duration longer than 5 days in pts with severe or complicated influenza.

PO: ADULTS, ELDERLY, CHILDREN 13 YRS AND OLDER: 75 mg twice daily for 5 days. **CHILDREN 1–12 YRS, WEIGHING MORE THAN 40 KG:** 75 mg twice daily for 5 days. **WEIGHING 24–40 KG:** 60 mg twice daily for 5 days. **WEIGHING 16–23 KG:** 45 mg twice daily for 5 days. **WEIGHING 15 KG OR LESS:** 30 mg twice daily for 5 days. **NEONATES, INFANTS AGES 2 WKS TO YOUNGER THAN 1 YR:** 3 mg/kg twice daily for 5 days.

Prevention of Influenza

Note: Initiate within 48 hrs of contact with an infected individual. Duration: 7–10 days (longer during community outbreaks). **PO: ADULTS, ELDERLY, CHILDREN 13 YRS AND OLDER:** 75 mg daily. **CHILDREN 1–12 YRS, WEIGHING MORE THAN 40 KG:** 75 mg once daily. **WEIGHING 24–40 KG:** 60 mg once daily. **WEIGHING 15–23 KG:** 45 mg once daily. **WEIGHING LESS THAN 15 KG:** 30 mg once daily. **INFANTS 9–11 mos:** 3.5 mg/kg/dose. **INFANTS 3–8 mos:** 3 mg/kg/dose.

Dosage in Renal Impairment

CrCl 31–60 mL/min: Treatment: 30 mg twice daily. Prevention: 30 mg once daily. **CrCl 11–30 mL/min:** Treatment: 30 mg once daily. Prevention: 30 mg every other

0

day. **End-stage renal disease:** Not recommended.

Dosage in Hepatic Impairment
No dose adjustment.

SIDE EFFECTS

Frequent (10%–7%): Nausea, vomiting, diarrhea. **Rare (2%–1%):** Abdominal pain, bronchitis, dizziness, headache, cough, insomnia, fatigue, vertigo.

ADVERSE EFFECTS/ TOXIC REACTIONS

Colitis, pneumonia, tympanic membrane disorder, fever occur rarely.

NURSING CONSIDERATIONS

BASELINE ASSESSMENT

Obtain baseline laboratory tests as indicated. Confirm presence of influenza A or B virus.

INTERVENTION/EVALUATION

Monitor serum glucose, renal function in pts with influenza symptoms, diabetes.

PATIENT/FAMILY TEACHING

• Begin as soon as possible from first appearance of flu symptoms (recommended within 2 days from symptom onset). • Avoid contact with those who are at high risk for influenza. • Not a substitute for flu shot.

---

osimertinib

oh-sim-**er**-ti-nib
(Tagrisso)
Do not confuse osimertinib with afatinib, dasatinib, erlotinib, ibrutinib, imatinib, olaparib, or ospemifene, or Tagrisso with Targretin or Tasigna.

◆CLASSIFICATION

PHARMACOTHERAPEUTIC: Tyrosine kinase inhibitor (TKI). **CLINICAL:** Antineoplastic.

USES

Treatment of pts with metastatic epidermal growth factor receptor (EGFR) T790M mutation-positive non–small-cell lung cancer (NSCLC), as detected by FDA-approved test, who have progressed on or after EGFR TKI therapy.

PRECAUTIONS

Contraindications: Hypersensitivity to osimertinib. **Cautions:** Baseline anemia, lymphopenia, neutropenia, thrombocytopenia; COPD, heart disease (bradycardia, cardiomyopathy, heart block, HF, recent MI), pts at risk for QTc interval prolongation or ventricular arrhythmia (congenital long QT syndrome, history for QT prolongation, medications that prolong QT interval, hypokalemia, hypomagnesemia); history of CVA, pulmonary embolism. Concomitant use of CYP3A inducers.

ACTION

Exhibits antitumor activity by irreversibly binding to mutant forms of EGFR. **Therapeutic Effect:** Inhibits tumor cell growth and metastasis.

PHARMACOKINETICS

Widely distributed. Metabolized in liver. Protein binding: Likely high. Peak plasma concentration: 3–24 hrs (median: 6 hrs). Steady state reached in 15 days. Excreted in feces (68%), urine (14%). **Half-life:** 48 hrs.

⧖ LIFESPAN CONSIDERATIONS

Pregnancy/Lactation: Avoid pregnancy; may cause fetal harm. Females of reproductive potential should use effective contraception during treatment and for at least 6 wks after discontinuation. Males with female partners of reproductive potential must use effective barrier methods during treatment and at least 4 mos after discontinuation. Unknown if distributed in breast milk. Breastfeeding not recommended during treatment and for up to 2 wks after discontinuation. May impair fertility in both females and males. **Children:** Safety and efficacy not established. **Elderly:** May have increased risk of CTCAE grade 3 or 4 adverse events. May require more frequent dose modifications.

INTERACTIONS

DRUG: QTc interval–prolonging medications (e.g., **amiodarone, FLUoxetine, haloperidol, sotalol**) may increase risk of QTc prolongation. **Strong CYP3A inducers (e.g., car-BAMazepine, phenytoin, rifAMPin)** may decrease concentration/effect. **Strong CYP3A inhibitors (e.g., clar-ithromycin, ketoconazole, ritona-vir)** may increase concentration/risk of adverse effects. **Osimertinib** may alter concentration of medications that are sensitive substrates of CYP3A, breast cancer resistance protein (BCRP), or CYP1A2 (e.g., carBAMazepine, cyclo-SPORINE, phenytoin). **HERBAL:** **St. John's wort** may decrease concentration/effect. **FOOD:** None known. **LAB VALUES:** May decrease serum sodium, magnesium; Hgb, Hct, lymphocytes, neutrophils, platelets, RBCs. May decrease diagnostic effect of *Coccidioides immitis* skin test.

AVAILABILITY (Rx)

Tablets: 40 mg, 80 mg.

ADMINISTRATION/HANDLING

PO
• Tablets are hazardous; use cytotoxic precautions during handling and disposal. Recommend single gloving when handling intact tablets; double gloving, protective gown when handling liquid preparations. • Do not divide, crush, cut, or ultrasonicate tablets. • Give without regard to food. • If a dose is missed, skip missed dose and administer the next dose on schedule. • **Pts with dysphagia:** Disperse tablet in 60 mL of water (noncarbonated) only. • Stir until dissipated into small pieces (does not completely dissolve). • Deliver orally or via gastric tube. • Rinse container with 120–240 mL of water and administer any remaining drug residue. After oral administration of residue, instruct pt to thoroughly rinse mouth with water and swallow.

INDICATIONS/ROUTES/DOSAGE

Non–Small-Cell Lung Cancer
PO: ADULTS, ELDERLY: 80 mg once daily. Continue until disease progression or unacceptable toxicity.

Dose Modification
Based on Common Terminology Criteria for Adverse Events (CTCAE).

Cardiac Toxicity
QTc interval greater than 500 msec on at least two separate ECGs: Withhold treatment until QTc interval is less than 481 msec or recovers to baseline. Once resolved, resume at 40 mg once daily.
QTc interval prolongation with symptoms of life-threatening arrhythmia: Permanently discontinue.
Asymptomatic, absolute decrease in left ventricular ejection fraction (LVEF) of 10% from baseline and below 50%: Withhold treatment for up to 4 wks. Resume treatment if improved to baseline. If not improved to baseline, permanently discontinue.

Pulmonary Toxicity
Interstitial lung disease/pneumonitis: Permanently discontinue.

Other Toxicities
Any grade 3 or higher reaction: Withhold treatment for up to 3 wks. Resume treatment at 80 mg once daily or 40 mg once daily if improved to grade 2 or lower within 3 wks. If not improved within 3 wks, permanently discontinue.
Concomitant use of strong CYP3A4 inducers: Start dose at 160 mg once daily. May decrease dose to 80 mg once daily if strong CYP3A4 inducer has been discontinued for at least 3 wks.

0

Dosage in Renal/Hepatic Impairment
Mild to moderate impairment: No dose adjustment. **Severe impairment:** Not specified; use caution.

SIDE EFFECTS

Frequent (42%–17%): Diarrhea, rash (generalized, erythematous, macular, maculopapular, papular, pustular), erythema, folliculitis, acne, dermatitis, acneiform dermatitis, dry skin, eczema, skin fissures, xerosis, nail disorders (inflammation, tenderness, discoloration, dystrophy, infection, ridging, onychoclasis, onycholysis, onychomadesis, paronychia), dry eye, blurry vision, keratitis, cataract, eye irritation, blepharitis, eye pain, increased lacrimation, vitreous floaters, nausea. **Occasional (16%–10%):** Decreased appetite, constipation, pruritus, cough, fatigue, back pain, stomatitis, headache.

ADVERSE EFFECTS/ TOXIC REACTIONS

Anemia, leukopenia, neutropenia, thrombocytopenia are expected responses to therapy. Interstitial lung disease/pneumonitis reported in 3% of pts. May cause QTc interval prolongation (up to 3% of pts); cardiac toxicities including cardiomyopathy (1% of pts), decreased LVEF (2% of pts); other adverse effects including CVA, intracranial hemorrhage; pneumonia (4% of pts); venous thromboembolism including pulmonary embolism, jugular venous thrombosis, DVT (7% of pts).

NURSING CONSIDERATIONS

BASELINE ASSESSMENT

Obtain CBC, BMP, serum magnesium; vital signs; EKG. Confirm presence of T790M mutation in tumor specimen prior to initiation. Obtain pregnancy test in females of reproductive potential. Receive full medication history and screen for interactions. Question history of CVA, DVT, pulmonary embolism, pulmonary disease, cardiac disease. Obtain baseline echocardiogram to assess LVEF. Obtain visual acuity. Screen for active infection. Offer emotional support.

INTERVENTION/EVALUATION

Monitor CBC for cytopenias; BMP, serum magnesium for electrolyte abnormalities. Pts with cough, dyspnea, fever, worsening of respiratory status should be investigated for interstitial lung disease/pneumonitis. Pts with sudden chest pain, dyspnea, hypoxia, tachycardia should be evaluated for pulmonary embolism. Monitor for symptoms of DVT (leg or arm pain/swelling); CVA, intracranial hemorrhage (aphasia, altered LOC, facial droop, headache, hemiplegia, seizures). Assess LVEF by echocardiogram q3mos during therapy or more frequently in pts suspected of HF, congestive HF. Assess for eye pain, visual changes. Monitor for skin rash/toxicities, hypersensitivity reaction. Diligently monitor for infection. Monitor daily stool pattern, consistency.

PATIENT/FAMILY TEACHING

• Blood levels, echocardiograms will be routinely monitored. • Treatment may cause life-threatening adverse effects. Report symptoms of abnormal heartbeats (dizziness, fainting, light-headedness, palpitations), heart failure (shortness of breath, fast or slow heart rate, exercise intolerance, swelling of the ankles or legs), severe lung inflammation (difficulty breathing, cough with fever, lung pain). • Avoid pregnancy; treatment may cause birth defects. Female pts of childbearing potential should use effective contraception during treatment and for at least 6 wks after last dose. Male pts with female partners of childbearing potential should use condoms, abstinence during treatment and for at least 4 mos after last dose. Do not breastfeed during therapy and for at least 2 wks after last dose. • Treatment may cause blood clots in the arms, legs, lungs, or brain. Immediately report symptoms of stroke (difficulty speaking, confusion, paralysis, vision loss), lung embolism (difficulty breathing, fast heart rate, chest pain), blood clots in the arms or legs (pain/swelling). • Do not take any newly prescribed medications unless approved by doctor who originally started treatment. • Avoid crowds, people with active infection. • Do not take herbal supplements.

oxaliplatin
HIGH ALERT

ox-**al**-i-**pla**-tin
(Eloxatin ✦)

■ **BLACK BOX ALERT** ■
Anaphylactic-like reaction may occur within minutes of administration; may be controlled with EPINEPHrine, corticosteroids, antihistamines.

Do not confuse oxaliplatin with Aloxi, CARBOplatin, or CISplatin.

◆**CLASSIFICATION**
PHARMACOTHERAPEUTIC: Platinum-containing complex. **CLINICAL:** Antineoplastic.

USES
Treatment of stage III colon cancer after complete resection of primary tumor (in combination with infusional 5-fluorouracil and leucovorin); treatment of advanced colon cancer (in combination with infusional 5-fluorouracil and leucovorin). **OFF-LABEL:** Treatment of ovarian cancer, pancreatic cancer, hepatobiliary cancer, testicular cancer, esophageal cancer, gastric cancer, non-Hodgkin's lymphoma, chronic lymphocytic leukemia.

PRECAUTIONS
Contraindications: History of allergy to oxaliplatin, other platinum compounds. **Cautions:** Previous therapy with other antineoplastic agents; radiation, renal impairment, pregnancy, immunosuppression, presence or history of peripheral neuropathy, elderly pts.

ACTION
Inhibits DNA replication by cross-linking with DNA strands. Cell cycle–phase nonspecific. **Therapeutic Effect:** Prevents cell division.

PHARMACOKINETICS
Rapidly distributed. Protein binding: 90%. Undergoes rapid, extensive nonenzymatic biotransformation. Excreted in urine. **Half-life:** 391 hrs.

⌛ LIFESPAN CONSIDERATIONS
Pregnancy/Lactation: If possible, avoid use during pregnancy, esp. first trimester. May cause fetal harm. Breastfeeding not recommended. **Children:** Safety and efficacy not established. **Elderly:** Increased incidence of diarrhea, dehydration, hypokalemia, fatigue.

INTERACTIONS
DRUG: Bone marrow depressants may increase myelosuppression, GI effects. **Live virus vaccines** may potentiate virus replication, increase vaccine side effects, decrease pt's antibody response to vaccine. **Nephrotic medications** may increase concentration. **HERBAL: Echinacea** may decrease effects. **FOOD:** None known. **LAB VALUES:** May increase serum creatinine, bilirubin, ALT, AST, INR. May prolong prothrombin time.

AVAILABILITY (Rx)
Injection, Solution: 5 mg/mL (20-mL, 40-mL vials).

ADMINISTRATION/HANDLING
◀**ALERT**▶ Wear protective gloves during handling of oxaliplatin. If solution comes in contact with skin, wash skin immediately with soap, water. Do not use aluminum needles or administration sets that may come in contact with drug; may cause degradation of platinum compounds.
◀**ALERT**▶ Pt should avoid ice, drinking cold beverages, touching cold objects during infusion and for 5 days thereafter (can exacerbate acute neuropathy).

O

IV

Reconstitution • Dilute with 250–500 mL D_5W (never dilute with sodium chloride solution or other chloride-containing solutions) to final concentration of 0.2–0.6 mg/mL.
Rate of Administration • Infuse over 2–6 hrs.
Storage • Do not freeze. • Protect from light. • Store vials at room temperature. • After dilution, solution is stable for 6 hrs at room temperature, 24 hrs if refrigerated.

🞓 IV INCOMPATIBILITIES

Do not infuse oxaliplatin with alkaline medications.

🞓 IV COMPATIBILITIES

Dexamethasone, diphenhydrAMINE (Benadryl), granisetron (Kytril), ondansetron (Zofran), palonosetron (Aloxi).

INDICATIONS/ROUTES/DOSAGE

Refer to individual protocols.
◄ **ALERT** ▶ Pretreat pt with antiemetics. Repeat courses should not be given more frequently than every 2 wks.

Advanced Colorectal Cancer
IV: **ADULTS:** 85 mg/m² q2wks until disease progression or unacceptable toxicity (in combination with fluorouracil/leucovorin).

Stage III Colon Cancer
IV: **ADULTS:** 85 mg/m² q2wks for total of 6 months (in combination with fluorouracil/leucovorin).

Dosage in Renal Impairment
CrCl less than 30 mL/min: Reduce dose to 65 mg/m².

Dosage in Hepatic Impairment
No dose adjustment.

SIDE EFFECTS

Frequent (76%–20%): Peripheral/sensory neuropathy (usually occurs in hands, feet, perioral area, throat but may present as: jaw spasm, abnormal tongue sensation, eye pain, chest pressure, difficulty walking, swallowing, writing), nausea, fatigue, diarrhea, vomiting, constipation, abdominal pain, fever, anorexia. **Occasional (14%–10%):** Stomatitis, earache, insomnia, cough, difficulty breathing, backache, edema. **Rare (7%–3%):** Dyspepsia, dizziness, rhinitis, flushing, alopecia.

ADVERSE EFFECTS/TOXIC REACTIONS

Peripheral/sensory neuropathy can occur without any prior event by drinking or holding a glass of cold liquid during IV infusion. Pulmonary fibrosis (characterized as nonproductive cough, dyspnea, crackles, radiologic pulmonary infiltrates) may warrant drug discontinuation. Hypersensitivity reaction (rash, urticaria, pruritus) occurs rarely.

NURSING CONSIDERATIONS

BASELINE ASSESSMENT

Obtain baseline renal function, WBC, platelet count. Question medical history as listed in Precautions. Offer emotional support.

INTERVENTION/EVALUATION

Monitor for decrease in WBC, platelets (myelosuppression is minimal). Monitor daily pattern of bowel activity, stool consistency. Monitor for diarrhea, GI bleeding (bright red, black tarry stool), signs of neuropathy. Pt should avoid ice or drinking, holding glass of cold liquid during IV infusion and for 5 days following completion of infusion; may precipitate/exacerbate neuropathy (occurs within hrs or 1–2 days of dosing, lasts up to 14 days). Maintain strict I&O. Assess oral mucosa for stomatitis.

PATIENT/FAMILY TEACHING

• Promptly report fever, sore throat, signs of local infection, unusual bruising/bleeding from any site, persistent diarrhea, difficulty breathing. • Do not have immunizations without physician's approval (drug lowers resistance). • Avoid contact with those who have recently taken oral polio vaccine. • Avoid cold drinks, ice, cold objects (may produce neuropathy).

OXcarbazepine

ox-kar-**baz**-e-peen
(Oxtellar XR, Trileptal)
Do not confuse OXcarbazepine with carBAMazepine, or Trileptal with TriLipix.

◆CLASSIFICATION

PHARMACOTHERAPEUTIC: Carboxamide derivative, anticonvulsant.
CLINICAL: Anticonvulsant.

USES

Trileptal: Monotherapy, adjunctive therapy in treatment of partial seizures in adults. Monotherapy in children 4 yrs and older, adjunctive therapy in children 2 yrs and older. **Oxtellar XR:** Adjunctive therapy in treatment of partial seizures in children 6–17 yrs. **OFF-LABEL:** Treatment of neuropathic pain, bipolar disorder.

PRECAUTIONS

Contraindications: Hypersensitivity to OXcarbazepine. **Cautions:** Renal impairment, sensitivity to carBAMazepine, pts at increased risk for suicide.

ACTION

Blocks sodium channels, stabilizing hyperexcited neural membranes, inhibiting repetitive neuronal firing, diminishing synaptic impulses. **Therapeutic Effect:** Prevents seizures.

PHARMACOKINETICS

Completely absorbed from GI tract. Metabolized in liver. Protein binding: 40%. Primarily excreted in urine. **Half-life:** 2 hrs; metabolite, 6–10 hrs.

⧗ LIFESPAN CONSIDERATIONS

Pregnancy/Lactation: Crosses placenta. Distributed in breast milk. **Children:** Safety and efficacy not established in children younger than 2 yrs. **Elderly:** Age-related renal impairment may require dosage adjustment.

INTERACTIONS

DRUG: Alcohol, **CNS depressants (e.g., LORazepam, morphine, zolpidem)** may have additive sedative effect. May decrease effectiveness of **felodipine, oral contraceptives, verapamil.** May increase concentration, risk of toxicity of **PHENobarbital, phenytoin.** **HERBAL:** Gotu kola, kava kava, St. John's wort, valerian may increase CNS depression. **Evening primrose** may decrease seizure threshold. **St. John's wort** may decrease concentration. **FOOD:** None known. **LAB VALUES:** May increase serum alkaline phosphatase, ALT, AST. May decrease serum sodium.

AVAILABILITY (Rx)

Oral Suspension (Trileptal): 300 mg/5 mL. **Tablets (Trileptal):** 150 mg, 300 mg, 600 mg.

Tablets, Extended-Release (Oxtellar XR): 150 mg, 300 mg, 600 mg.

ADMINISTRATION/HANDLING

PO
• Give without regard to food. Do not break, crush, dissolve, or divide extended-release tablets. Swallow whole.

INDICATIONS/ROUTES/DOSAGE

Adjunctive Treatment of Seizures
PO: ADULTS, ELDERLY: (Immediate-Release): Initially, 600 mg/day in 2 divided doses. May increase by up to 600 mg/day at wkly intervals. **Maximum:** 2,400 mg/day. **Usual maintenance dose:** 600 mg twice daily. **CHILDREN 4–16 YRS:** Initially, 8–10 mg/kg in 2 divided doses. **Maximum:** 600 mg/day. Increase dose slowly

---

◆ Canadian trade name   🌀 Non-Crushable Drug   ▦ High Alert drug

over 2 wks. **Maintenance (based on weight):** CHILDREN WEIGHING MORE THAN 39 KG: 1,800 mg/day in 2 divided doses; CHILDREN WEIGHING 29.1–39 KG: 1,200 mg/day in 2 divided doses; CHILDREN WEIGHING 20–29 KG: 900 mg/day in 2 divided doses. CHILDREN 2–3 YRS: Initially, 8–10 mg/kg/day in 2 divided doses. **Maximum:** 600 mg/day in 2 divided doses. Increase dose slowly over 2 wks up to a **maximum** of 60 mg/kg/day in 2 divided doses. *(Extended-Release):* ADULTS: Initially, 600 mg once daily. May increase by 600 mg/day at wkly intervals. Range: 1,200–2,400 mg/day. ELDERLY: Initially, 300–450 mg/day. May increase by 300–450 mg/day at wkly intervals to desired clinical response. Range: Up to 2,400 mg/day.

Conversion to Monotherapy

PO: ADULTS, ELDERLY: *(Immediate-Release):* 600 mg/day in 2 divided doses (while decreasing concomitant anticonvulsant over 3–6 wks). May increase by 600 mg/day at wkly intervals up to 2,400 mg/day. CHILDREN 4–16 YRS: Initially, 8–10 mg/kg/day in 2 divided doses with simultaneous initial reduction of dose of concomitant antiepileptic over 3–6 wks. May increase by maximum of 10 mg/kg/day at wkly intervals (see below for recommended daily dose by weight).

Initiation of Monotherapy

PO: ADULTS, ELDERLY: *(Immediate-Release):* 600 mg/day in 2 divided doses. May increase by 300 mg/day every 3 days up to 1,200 mg/day. CHILDREN 4–16 YRS: Initially, 8–10 mg/kg/day in 2 divided doses. Increase at 3-day intervals by 5 mg/kg/day to achieve maintenance dose by weight as follows:

Weight	Dosage
70+ kg	1,500–2,100 mg/day
60–69 kg	1,200–2,100 mg/day
50–59 kg	1,200–1,800 mg/day
41–49 kg	1,200–1,500 mg/day
35–40 kg	900–1,500 mg/day
25–34 kg	900–1,200 mg/day
20–24 kg	600–900 mg/day

Dosage in Renal Impairment

Mild to moderate impairment: No dose adjustment. **CrCl less than 30 mL/min:** Give 50% of normal starting dose, then titrate slowly to desired dose.

Dosage in Hepatic Impairment

Mild to moderate impairment: No dose adjustment. **Severe impairment:** Use caution with immediate-release; not recommended with extended-release.

SIDE EFFECTS

Frequent (22%–13%): Dizziness, nausea, headache. **Occasional (7%–5%):** Vomiting, diarrhea, ataxia (muscular incoordination), nervousness, dyspepsia, constipation. **Rare (4%):** Tremor, rash, back pain, epistaxis, sinusitis, diplopia.

ADVERSE EFFECTS/ TOXIC REACTIONS

Clinically significant hyponatremia may occur, manifested as leg cramping, hypotension, cold/clammy skin, increased pulse rate, headache, nausea, vomiting, diarrhea. Suicidal ideation occurs rarely.

NURSING CONSIDERATIONS

BASELINE ASSESSMENT

Review history of seizure disorder (type, onset, intensity, frequency, duration, LOC), drug history (esp. other anticonvulsants). Provide safety precautions; quiet, dark environment.

INTERVENTION/EVALUATION

Assist with ambulation if dizziness, ataxia occur. Assess for visual abnormalities, headache. Monitor serum sodium. Assess for signs of hyponatremia (nausea, malaise, headache, lethargy, confusion). Assess for clinical improvement (decrease in intensity, frequency of seizures). Monitor for worsening depression, suicidal ideation.

PATIENT/FAMILY TEACHING

• Do not abruptly stop taking medication (may increase seizure activity). • Report if rash, nausea, headache, dizziness occurs.

• May need periodic blood tests. • Avoid tasks that require alertness, motor skills until response to drug is established. • Avoid alcohol. • May decrease effectiveness of oral contraceptives.

oxybutynin

ox-i-**bue**-ti-nin
(Apo-Oxybutynin ✤, Ditropan XL, Gelnique, Oxytrol for Women)
Do not confuse oxybutynin with OxyContin.

◆CLASSIFICATION

PHARMACOTHERAPEUTIC: Anticholinergic. **CLINICAL:** Antispasmodic.

USES

Relief of symptoms (urgency, incontinence, frequency, nocturia, urge incontinence) associated with uninhibited neurogenic bladder, reflex neurogenic bladder. **Extended-Release (additional):** Treatment of symptoms associated with detrusor overactivity due to neurologic disorder (e.g., spina bifida).

PRECAUTIONS

Contraindications: Hypersensitivity to oxybutynin. Pts with or at risk for uncontrolled narrow-angle glaucoma, urinary retention, gastric retention, or conditions with severely decreased GI motility. **Cautions:** Renal/hepatic impairment, pts with bladder outflow obstruction, treated narrow-angle glaucoma, hyperthyroidism, coronary artery disease, HF, hypertension, arrhythmias, prostatic hyperplasia, myasthenia gravis, reduced GI motility, GI obstructive disorder, gastroesophageal reflux.

ACTION

Direct antispasmodic effect on smooth muscle; inhibits action of acetylcholine on smooth muscle. **Therapeutic Effect:** Increases bladder capacity, delays desire to void. Decreases urgency and frequency.

PHARMACOKINETICS

Route	Onset	Peak	Duration
PO	0.5–1 hr	3–6 hrs	6–10 hrs

Rapidly, well absorbed from GI tract. Metabolized in liver. Primarily excreted in urine. Unknown if removed by hemodialysis. **Half-life:** 1–2.3 hrs; metabolite, 7–8 hrs.

⊠ LIFESPAN CONSIDERATIONS

Pregnancy/Lactation: Unknown if drug crosses placenta or is distributed in breast milk. **Children:** No age-related precautions noted in those older than 5 yrs. **Elderly:** May be more sensitive to anticholinergic effects (e.g., dry mouth, urinary retention).

INTERACTIONS

DRUG: Medications with **anticholinergic action (e.g., antihistamines)** may increase anticholinergic effects. **Clarithromycin, erythromycin, itraconazole, ketoconazole** may alter pharmacokinetic parameters. **HERBAL:** None significant. **FOOD:** None known. **LAB VALUES:** None significant.

AVAILABILITY (Rx)

Syrup: 5 mg/5 mL. **Tablets:** 5 mg. **Topical Gel (10%) (Gelnique):** 100 mg/unit dose sachet. **(3% Gel):** 30 mg/mL. **Transdermal (Oxytrol for Women):** 3.9 mg/24 hrs.

 Tablets (Extended-Release [Ditropan XL]): 5 mg, 10 mg, 15 mg.

ADMINISTRATION/HANDLING

PO
• Give without regard to meals.
• Extended-release tablet must be swallowed whole; do not break, crush, dissolve, or divide.

Transdermal
• Apply patch to dry, intact skin on abdomen, hip, buttock. • Use new application site for each new patch; avoid reapplication

to same site within 7 days. • Normal exposure to water (e.g., bathing, swimming) should not affect patch.

Topical Gel

• *(Gelnique):* Apply contents of 1 sachet once daily to dry, intact skin on abdomen, upper arms/shoulders, or thighs. • Do not bathe/shower until 1 hr after gel is applied. • *(3% Gel):* Apply 3 mL to thigh, upper arm, or shoulder.

INDICATIONS/ROUTES/DOSAGE

Neurogenic Bladder

PO *(Immediate-Release):* **ADULTS:** 5 mg 2–3 times/day. May increase to 5 mg 4 times/day. **ELDERLY:** 2.5–5 mg 2–3 times/day. **CHILDREN OLDER THAN 5 YRS:** 5 mg twice daily. May increase to 5 mg 3 times/day.

PO *(Extended-Release):* **ADULTS, ELDERLY:** 5–10 mg/day. May increase by 5-mg increments at weekly intervals. **Maximum:** 30 mg/day. **CHILDREN 6 YRS AND OLDER:** Initially, 5–10 mg once daily. May increase in 5 mg increments at weekly intervals. **Maximum:** 20 mg/day.

Transdermal: ADULTS: 3.9 mg applied twice wkly. Apply every 3–4 days.

Topical Gel: ADULTS, ELDERLY: (10%) 100 mg once daily.

Gel 3%: Apply 3 mL (84 mg) once daily.

Dosage in Renal/Hepatic Impairment

No dose adjustment.

SIDE EFFECTS

Frequent: Constipation, dry mouth, drowsiness, decreased perspiration. **Occasional:** Decreased lacrimation/salivation, impotence, urinary hesitancy/retention, suppressed lactation, blurred vision, mydriasis, nausea/vomiting, insomnia.

ADVERSE EFFECTS/ TOXIC REACTIONS

Overdose produces CNS excitation (nervousness, restlessness, hallucinations, irritability), hypotension/hypertension, confusion, tachycardia, facial flushing, respiratory depression.

NURSING CONSIDERATIONS

BASELINE ASSESSMENT

Assess degree of dysuria, urgency, frequency, incontinence. Question medical history as listed in Precautions.

INTERVENTION/EVALUATION

Monitor for symptomatic relief. Monitor I&O; palpate bladder for urine retention. Monitor daily pattern of bowel activity, stool consistency.

PATIENT/FAMILY TEACHING

• Avoid alcohol. • May cause dry mouth (sugarless candy/gum may reduce effect). • Avoid tasks that require alertness, motor skills until response to drug is established (may cause drowsiness). • Avoid strenuous activity in warm environment.

---

oxyCODONE

ox-ee-**koe**-done
(Oxaydo, <u>OxyCONTIN</u>, OxyIR ✦, Roxicodone, Supeudol ✦, Xtampza XR)

■ **BLACK BOX ALERT** ■ **OxyContin (controlled-release):** Not intended as an "as needed" analgesic or for immediate postop pain control. Extended-release should not be crushed, broken, or chewed (otherwise leads to rapid release and absorption of potentially fatal dose). Be alert to signs of abuse, misuse, and diversion. May cause potentially life-threatening respiratory depression. Prolonged use during pregnancy can cause neonatal withdrawal syndrome. Use of CYP3A4 inhibitors may increase effects/ cause fatal respiratory depression.

Do not confuse oxyCODONE with HYDROcodone, oxybutynin, or oxyMORphone, OxyCONTIN with MS Contin or oxybutynin, or Roxicodone with Roxanol.

FIXED-COMBINATION(S)

Combunox: oxyCODONE/ibuprofen (an NSAID): 5 mg/400 mg. **Endocet:** oxyCODONE/acetaminophen (a non-narcotic analgesic): 5 mg/325 mg, 7.5 mg/325 mg, 7.5 mg/500 mg, 10 mg/325 mg, 10 mg/650 mg. **Magnacet:** oxyCODONE/acetaminophen (a non-narcotic analgesic): 2.5 mg/400 mg, 7.5 mg/400 mg, 10 mg/400 mg. **Percocet:** oxyCODONE/acetaminophen: 2.5 mg/325 mg, 5 mg/325 mg, 5 mg/500 mg, 7.5 mg/325 mg, 7.5 mg/500 mg, 10 mg/325 mg, 10 mg/650 mg. **Percocet, Roxicet, Tylox:** oxyCODONE/acetaminophen (a non-narcotic analgesic): 5 mg/500 mg. **Percodan:** oxyCODONE/aspirin (a non-narcotic analgesic): 2.25 mg/325 mg, 4.5 mg/325 mg. **Targiniq ER:** oxyCODONE/naloxone (opioid antagonist): 10 mg/5 mg, 20 mg/10 mg, 40 mg/20 mg. **Troxyca ER:** oxyCODONE/naltrexone (an opioid antagonist): 10 mg/1.2 mg, 20 mg/2.4 mg, 30 mg/3.6 mg, 40 mg/4.8 mg, 60 mg/7.2 mg, 9.6 mg/80 mg. **Xartemis XR:** oxyCODONE/acetaminophen (non-narcotic analgesic): 7.5 mg/325 mg.

◆CLASSIFICATION

PHARMACOTHERAPEUTIC: Opioid agonist **(Schedule II). CLINICAL:** Analgesic.

USES

Immediate-Release: Relief of acute or chronic, moderate to severe pain (usually in combination with nonopioid analgesics). **Extended-Release:** Around-the-clock management of moderate to severe pain when continuous analgesic is needed.

PRECAUTIONS

Contraindications: Hypersensitivity to oxyCODONE. Acute or severe bronchial asthma, hypercarbia, paralytic ileus (known or suspected), GI obstruction, significant respiratory depression. **Extreme Caution:** CNS depression, anoxia, hypercapnia, respiratory depression, seizures, acute alcoholism, shock, untreated myxedema, respiratory dysfunction. **Cautions:** Elevated ICP, hepatic/renal impairment, coma, debilitated pts, head injury, biliary tract disease, toxic psychosis, acute abdominal conditions, hypothyroidism, prostatic hypertrophy, Addison's disease, urethral stricture, COPD, history of substance abuse, elderly pts.

ACTION

Binds with opioid receptors within CNS, causing inhibition of ascending pain pathway. **Therapeutic Effect:** Alters perception of and emotional response to pain.

PHARMACOKINETICS

Route	Onset	Peak	Duration
PO (immediate-release)	10–15 min	0.5–1 hr	3–6 hrs
PO (controlled-release)	10–15 min	0.5–1 hr	Up to 12 hrs

Moderately absorbed from GI tract. Protein binding: 38%–45%. Widely distributed. Metabolized in liver. Excreted in urine. Unknown if removed by hemodialysis. **Half-life:** 2–3 hrs (5 hrs controlled-release).

⚕ LIFESPAN CONSIDERATIONS

Pregnancy/Lactation: Readily crosses placenta. Distributed in breast milk. Respiratory depression may occur in neonate if mother received opiates during labor. Regular use of opiates during pregnancy may produce withdrawal symptoms in neonate (irritability, excessive crying, tremors, hyperactive reflexes, fever, vomiting, diarrhea, yawning, sneezing, seizures). **Children:** Paradoxical excitement may occur. Pts younger than 2 yrs are more susceptible to respiratory depressant effects. **Elderly:** Age-related renal impairment may increase risk of urinary retention. May be more susceptible to respiratory depressant effects.

INTERACTIONS

DRUG: Alcohol, other CNS depressants (e.g., LORazepam, gabapentin,

zolpidem) may increase CNS effects, respiratory depression, hypotension. **CYP3A4 inhibitors (clarithromycin, ketoconazole)** may increase concentration, toxicity. **CYP3A4 inducers (carBAMazepine, rifAMPin)** may decrease concentration/effects. **MAOIs** may produce serotonin syndrome, a severe, sometimes fatal reaction (administer ¼ of usual oxyCODONE dose). **HERBAL: Gotu kola, kava kava, St. John's wort, valerian** may increase CNS depression. **FOOD: Grapefruit products** may increase potential for respiratory depression. **LAB VALUES:** May increase serum amylase, lipase.

AVAILABILITY (Rx)

◀**ALERT**▶ New formulation of controlled-release is intended to prevent medication from being cut, broken, chewed, crushed, or dissolved to reduce risk of overdose due to tampering, snorting, or injection.
Capsules: 5 mg. **Oral Concentrate:** 20 mg/mL. **Oral Solution:** 5 mg/5 mL. **Tablets:** 5 mg, 10 mg, 15 mg, 20 mg, 30 mg. **Tablets, Abuse Deterrent (Oxaydo):** 5 mg, 7.5 mg.

🔖 **Capsules (Extended-Release [Xtampza]):** 9 mg, 13.5 mg, 18 mg, 27 mg, 36 mg. **Tablets (Controlled-Release 12 Hour Abuse Deterrent [Oxy*CONTIN*]):** 10 mg, 15 mg, 20 mg, 30 mg, 40 mg, 60 mg, 80 mg.

ADMINISTRATION/HANDLING

PO
• Give without regard to meals.
• **Controlled-release:** Swallow whole; do not break, crush, dissolve, or divide.

INDICATIONS/ROUTES/DOSAGE

Note: All doses should be titrated to desired effect. Do not abruptly discontinue in physically dependent pts. **Discontinuation: (immediate-release):** Reduce dose by 25%-50% q2-4 days while monitoring for withdrawal; **(extended-release):** Gradually titrate downward.

Analgesia
PO *(Immediate-Release):* **ADULTS, ELDERLY:** Initially, 5–15 mg q4–6h as needed. Range: 5–20 mg/dose. **CHILDREN, 6–18 YRS:** 0.1–0.2 mg/kg/dose q4–6h as needed.

Opioid Naive
PO *(Controlled-Release):* **ADULTS, ELDERLY:** (Tablets) Initially, 10 mg q12h. (Capsules) Initially, 9 mg q12h.
◀**ALERT**▶ To convert from other opioids or nonopioid analgesics to oxyCODONE controlled-release, refer to OxyCONTIN package insert. Dosages are reduced in pts with severe hepatic disease.

Dosage in Renal/Hepatic Impairment
Use caution. Titrate carefully.

SIDE EFFECTS

◀**ALERT**▶ Effects are dependent on dosage amount. Ambulatory pts, pts not in severe pain may experience dizziness, nausea, vomiting, hypotension more frequently than those in supine position or having severe pain. **Frequent:** Drowsiness, dizziness, hypotension (including orthostatic hypotension), anorexia. **Occasional:** Confusion, diaphoresis, facial flushing, urinary retention, constipation, dry mouth, nausea, vomiting, headache. **Rare:** Allergic reaction, depression, paradoxical CNS hyperactivity, nervousness in children, paradoxical excitement, restlessness in elderly, debilitated pts.

ADVERSE EFFECTS/ TOXIC REACTIONS

Overdose results in respiratory depression, skeletal muscle flaccidity, cold/clammy skin, cyanosis, extreme drowsiness progressing to seizures, stupor, coma. Hepatotoxicity may occur with overdose of acetaminophen component of fixed-combination product. Tolerance to analgesic effect, physical dependence may occur with repeated use. **Antidote:** Naloxone (see Appendix J for dosage).

NURSING CONSIDERATIONS

BASELINE ASSESSMENT

Assess onset, type, location, duration of pain. Effect of medication is reduced if full pain recurs before next dose. Obtain vital signs before giving medication. If respirations are 12/min or less (20/min or less in children), withhold medication, contact physician.

INTERVENTION/EVALUATION

Palpate bladder for urinary retention. Monitor daily pattern of bowel activity, stool consistency. Initiate deep breathing, coughing exercises, esp. in pts with pulmonary impairment. Monitor pain relief, respiratory rate, mental status, B/P, LOC.

PATIENT/FAMILY TEACHING

• May cause dry mouth, drowsiness. • Avoid tasks that require alertness, motor skills until response to drug is established. • Avoid alcohol. • May be habit forming. • Do not chew, crush, dissolve, or divide controlled-release tablets. • Report severe constipation, absence of pain relief.

---

oxyMORphone

ox-ee-**mor**-fone
(Opana, Opana ER)

■ **BLACK BOX ALERT** ■ Has abuse liability. Concern about increased risk of abuse, misuse, or diversion. Prolonged use during pregnancy can cause neonatal withdrawal syndrome.
Do not confuse oxyMORphone with oxyCODONE.

◆CLASSIFICATION

PHARMACOTHERAPEUTIC: Opioid agonist **(Schedule II). CLINICAL:** Narcotic analgesic, antianxiety, preop anesthetic.

USES

Injection: Relief of moderate to severe acute pain. **PO (Immediate-release):** Relief of moderate to severe acute pain. **(Extended-release):** Relief of moderate to severe pain in pts requiring continuous treatment for extended period of time.

PRECAUTIONS

Contraindications: Hypersensitivity to oxyMORphone, morphine, acute severe bronchial asthma, severe respiratory depression, paralytic ileus (known or suspected), moderate to severe hepatic function impairment, hypercarbia. **Extreme Cautions:** Anoxia, hypercapnia, seizures, acute alcoholism, shock, untreated myxedema. **Cautions:** Hypothyroidism, prostatic hypertrophy, Addison's disease, urethral stricture, prostatic hyperplasia, toxic psychosis, renal impairment, COPD, biliary tract disease, acute pancreatitis, head injury, increased ICP, morbid obesity, mild hepatic dysfunction, history of substance abuse.

ACTION

Binds to opiate receptor sites within CNS, causing inhibition of ascending pain pathways. **Therapeutic Effect:** Reduces intensity of pain stimuli, alters pain perception, emotional response to pain.

PHARMACOKINETICS

Route	Onset	Peak	Duration
Parenteral	5–10 min	N/A	3–6 hrs

Well absorbed. Protein binding: 10%. Widely distributed. Metabolized in liver. Excreted in urine. **Half-life:** 7–9 hrs; **extended-release:** 9–11 hrs.

⊠ LIFESPAN CONSIDERATIONS

Pregnancy/Lactation: Unknown if distributed in breast milk. May prolong labor if administered in latent phase of first stage of labor or before cervical dilation of 4–5 cm has occurred.

O

Respiratory depression may occur in neonate if mother received opiates during labor. Regular use of opiates during pregnancy may produce withdrawal symptoms in the neonate (irritability, excessive crying, tremors, hyperactive reflexes, fever, vomiting, diarrhea, yawning, sneezing, seizures). **Children:** Safety and efficacy not established in those younger than 18 yrs. **Elderly:** May be more susceptible to respiratory depression, may cause paradoxical excitement. Age-related hepatic impairment, debilitation may require dosage adjustment.

INTERACTIONS

DRUG: Alcohol, other CNS depressants (e.g., LORazepam, gabapentin, zolpidem) may increase CNS effects, respiratory depression, hypotension. **Anticholinergics** may increase risk of urinary retention, severe constipation (may lead to paralytic ileus). **Propofol** increases risk of bradycardia. Decreased effect when given concurrently with **phenothiazines. HERBAL: Gotu kola, kava kava, St. John's wort, valerian** may produce CNS depressant effects. **FOOD:** None known. **LAB VALUES:** May increase serum amylase, lipase.

AVAILABILITY (Rx)

Injection: 1 mg/mL. **Tablets:** 5 mg, 10 mg. **Tablets (Extended-Release):** 5 mg, 7.5 mg, 10 mg, 15 mg, 20 mg, 30 mg, 40 mg.

ADMINISTRATION/HANDLING

IV

Rate of Administration• Administer IV push very slowly. • Rapid IV increases risk of severe adverse reactions (chest wall rigidity, apnea, peripheral circulatory collapse, anaphylactoid effects, cardiac arrest).

IM/SQ

• Inject deep IM, preferably in upper, outer quadrant of buttock. • Use short 30-gauge needle for SQ injection. • Administer slowly, rotating injection sites. • Pts with circulatory impairment experience higher risk of overdosage due to delayed absorption of repeated administration.

Storage • Store parenteral form at room temperature. Refrigerate suppository form. • Discard parenteral form if discolored or particulate forms.

PO

• Give 1 hr before or 2 hrs after meals. • Do not break, crush, dissolve, or divide extended-release tablet.

IV COMPATIBILITIES

Glycopyrrolate, hydrOXYzine, raNITIdine.

INDICATIONS/ROUTES/DOSAGE

Analgesia

IV: ADULTS 18 YRS AND OLDER, ELDERLY: Initially, 0.5 mg. Dose may be cautiously increased until satisfactory response is achieved.

◄ALERT► IM preferred over SQ route (SQ rate of absorption is less reliable).

IM/SQ: ADULTS 18 YRS AND OLDER, ELDERLY: Initially, 1–1.5 mg every 4–6 hrs as needed.

PO: ADULTS, ELDERLY: (IMMEDIATE-RELEASE): 5–10 mg q4–6h. **(EXTENDED-RELEASE):** Initially, 5 mg q12h. May increase by 5–10 mg q12h at intervals of every 3–7 days.

Dosage in Renal Impairment

Reduce initial dose with CrCl less than 50 mL/min.

Dosage in Hepatic Impairment

Reduce initial dose with mild impairment (contraindicated in moderate to severe impairment).

SIDE EFFECTS

Note: Effects are dependent on dosage amount, route of administration. Ambulatory pts, pts not in severe pain may experience dizziness, nausea, vomiting, hypotension more frequently than those in supine position or having severe pain.

Frequent (10% or higher): Drowsiness, hypotension, dizziness, nausea, vomiting, constipation, weakness. **Occasional (9%–2%):** Nervousness, headache, restlessness, malaise, confusion, anorexia, abdominal cramps, dry mouth, decreased urinary output, ureteral spasm, pain at injection site. **Rare (1% or less):** Depression, paradoxical CNS stimulation, hallucinations, rash, urticaria.

ADVERSE EFFECTS/ TOXIC REACTIONS

Overdose results in respiratory depression, skeletal muscle flaccidity, cold/clammy skin, cyanosis, extreme drowsiness progressing to convulsions, stupor, coma. Tolerance to analgesic effect, physical dependence may occur with repeated use. Prolonged duration of action, cumulative effect may occur in those with hepatic/renal impairment.

NURSING CONSIDERATIONS

BASELINE ASSESSMENT

Assess onset, type, location, duration of pain. Obtain vital signs before giving medication. If respirations are 12/min or lower, withhold medication, contact physician. Effect of medication is reduced if full pain recurs before next dose.

INTERVENTION/EVALUATION

Monitor vital signs 5–10 min after IV administration, 15–30 min after SQ, IM. Be alert for decreased respirations, B/P. To prevent pain cycles, instruct pt to request pain medication as soon as discomfort begins. Assess for clinical improvement, record onset of pain relief. Consult physician if pain relief is not adequate.

PATIENT/FAMILY TEACHING

• Discomfort may occur with injection. • Slowly go from lying to standing to avoid postural hypotension. • Avoid tasks that require alertness, motor skills until response to drug is established. • Avoid alcohol. • Tolerance/dependence may occur with prolonged use of high doses.

oxytocin

ox-ee-**toe**-sin
(Pitocin)

■ **BLACK BOX ALERT** ■ Not to be given for elective labor induction, but can be used when there is a clear medical indication for induction.
Do not confuse Pitocin with Pitressin.

◆CLASSIFICATION

PHARMACOTHERAPEUTIC: Uterine smooth muscle stimulant. **CLINICAL:** Oxytocic agent.

USES

Antepartum: Induction of labor in pts with medical indication (e.g., at or near term), to stimulate reinforcement of labor, as adjunct in managing incomplete or inevitable abortion. **Postpartum:** To produce uterine contractions during third stage of labor and to control postpartum bleeding/hemorrhage.

PRECAUTIONS

Contraindications: Hypersensitivity to oxytocin. Adequate uterine activity that fails to progress, cephalopelvic disproportion, fetal distress without imminent delivery, grand multiparity, hyperactive or hypertonic uterus, obstetric emergencies that favor surgical intervention, prematurity, unengaged fetal head, unfavorable fetal position/presentation, when vaginal delivery is contraindicated (e.g., active genital herpes infection, invasive cervical cancer, placenta previa, cord presentation). **Cautions:** Induction of labor should be for medical, not elective, reasons. Generally not recommended in fetal distress, hydramnios, partial placental previa, predisposition to uterine rupture.

ACTION

Activates receptors that trigger increase in intracellular calcium levels in uterine myofibrils; increases prostaglandin production. **Therapeutic Effect:** Stimulates uterine contractions.

PHARMACOKINETICS

Route	Onset	Peak	Duration
IV	Immediate	N/A	1 hr
IM	3–5 min	N/A	2–3 hrs

Rapidly absorbed through nasal mucous membranes. Protein binding: 30%. Distributed in extracellular fluid. Metabolized in liver, kidney. Primarily excreted in urine. **Half-life:** 1–6 min.

⌛ LIFESPAN CONSIDERATIONS

Pregnancy/Lactation: Used as indicated, not expected to present risk of fetal abnormalities. Small amounts in breast milk. Breastfeeding not recommended. **Children/Elderly:** Not used in these pt populations.

INTERACTIONS

DRUG: Caudal block anesthetics, vasopressors may increase pressor effects. **Other oxytocics** may cause cervical lacerations, uterine hypertonus, uterine rupture. **HERBAL:** None significant. **FOOD:** None known. **LAB VALUES:** None significant.

AVAILABILITY (Rx)

Injection (Pitocin): 10 units/mL. **Injection, Solution:** 30 units/500 mL.

ADMINISTRATION/HANDLING

 IV

Reconstitution • Dilute 10–40 units (1–4 mL) in 1,000 mL of 0.9% NaCl, lactated Ringer's, or D₅W to provide concentration of 10–40 milliunits/mL solution.
Rate of Administration • Give by IV infusion (use infusion device to carefully control rate of flow as ordered by physician).
Storage • Store at room temperature.

▦ IV INCOMPATIBILITIES

No known incompatibilities via Y-site administration.

▦ IV COMPATIBILITIES

Heparin, insulin (regular), multivitamins, potassium chloride, zidovudine.

INDICATIONS/ROUTES/DOSAGE

Induction or Stimulation of Labor
IV: ADULTS: 0.5–1 milliunit/min. May gradually increase in increments of 1–2 milliunits/min q30–60 minutes until desired contraction pattern is established. Rates greater than 9–10 milliunits/min are rarely required.

Abortion
IV: ADULTS: (Midterm elective abortion): 10–20 milliunits/min. **Maximum:** 30 units/12-hr dose. **(Incomplete, inevitable abortion):** 10 units as IV infusion after suction or a sharp curettage.

Control of Postpartum Bleeding
IV Infusion: ADULTS: 10–40 units in 1,000 mL IV fluid at rate sufficient to sustain uterine contractions and control uterine atony.
IM: ADULTS: 10 units (total dose) after delivery.

Dosage in Renal/Hepatic Impairment
No dose adjustment.

SIDE EFFECTS

Occasional: Tachycardia, premature ventricular contractions, hypotension, nausea, vomiting. **Rare: Nasal:** Lacrimation/tearing, nasal irritation, rhinorrhea, unexpected uterine bleeding/contractions.

ADVERSE EFFECTS/ TOXIC REACTIONS

Hypertonicity may occur with tearing of uterus, increased bleeding, abruptio placentae (i.e., placental abruption), cervical/vaginal lacerations. **Fetal:** Bradycardia, CNS/brain damage, trauma due to rapid propulsion, low Apgar score at 5 min, retinal hemorrhage occur rarely. Prolonged IV infusion of oxytocin with excessive fluid volume has caused severe water intoxication with seizures, coma, death.

NURSING CONSIDERATIONS

BASELINE ASSESSMENT

Assess baselines for vital signs, B/P, fetal heart rate. Determine frequency, duration, strength of contractions.

INTERVENTION/EVALUATION

Monitor B/P, pulse, respirations, fetal heart rate, intrauterine pressure, contractions (duration, strength, frequency) q15min. Notify physician of contractions that last longer than 1 min, occur more frequently than every 2 min, or stop. Maintain careful I&O; be alert to potential water intoxication. Check for blood loss.

PATIENT/FAMILY TEACHING

• Keep pt, family informed of labor progress.

0

PACLitaxel HIGH ALERT

pak-li-**tax**-el
(Abraxane, Apo-**PACL**itaxel ✤)

■ **BLACK BOX ALERT** ■ Myelosuppression is major dose-limiting toxicity. Must be administered by certified chemotherapy personnel. Severe hypersensitivity reactions reported.

Do not confuse PACLitaxel with DOCEtaxel, PARoxetine, or Paxil.

◆CLASSIFICATION

PHARMACOTHERAPEUTIC: Taxoid, antimitotic agent. **CLINICAL:** Antineoplastic.

USES

Conventional: Treatment of node-positive breast cancer, metastatic breast cancer after failure of combination therapy or relapse within 6 mos of adjuvant therapy; subsequent therapy for advanced ovarian cancer or as first line therapy (in combination with CISplatin). Treatment of AIDS-related Kaposi's sarcoma; non-small-cell lung cancer (NSCLC) as first line therapy (in combination with CISplatin). **Abraxane:** Treatment of breast cancer after failure of combination chemotherapy or relapse within 6 mos of adjuvant chemotherapy. First-line treatment of metastatic adenocarcinoma of pancreas. Treatment of locally advanced or metastatic NSCLC. **OFF-LABEL:** Bladder, cervical, small-cell lung, head and neck cancers. Treatment of adenocarcinoma. **Abraxane:** Recurrent/persistent ovarian, fallopian tube, primary peritoneal cancers.

PRECAUTIONS

Contraindications: Hypersensitivity to **PACL**itaxel. Hypersensitivity to drugs developed with Cremophor EL (polyoxyethylated castor oil). Treatment of solid tumors with baseline neutrophil count less than 1,500 cells/mm³; treatment of Kaposi's sarcoma with baseline neutrophil count less than 1,000 cells/mm³.

Cautions: Hepatic impairment, severe neutropenia, peripheral neuropathy.

ACTION

Increases action of tubulin dimers; stabilizes existing microtubules; inhibits their disassembly; interferes with late G_2 mitotic phase. **Therapeutic Effect:** Inhibits cellular mitosis, replication.

PHARMACOKINETICS

Does not readily cross blood-brain barrier. Protein binding: 89%–98%. Metabolized in liver. Excreted in bile/feces (71%), urine (14%). Not removed by hemodialysis. **Half-life:** 3-hr infusion: 13.1–20.2 hrs; 24-hr infusion: 15.7–52.7 hrs.

⧖ LIFESPAN CONSIDERATIONS

Pregnancy/Lactation: May cause fetal harm. Unknown if distributed in breast milk. Avoid use in pregnancy. **Children:** Safety and efficacy not established. **Elderly:** No age-related precautions noted.

INTERACTIONS

DRUG: CYP3A4, CYP2C8 inhibitors (e.g., clarithromycin, ketoconazole, ritonavir) may increase concentration/effects. **CYP3A4, CYP2C8 inducers (e.g., carBAMazepine, phenytoin, rifAMPin)** may decrease effects. **Bone marrow depressants** may increase myelosuppression. **Live virus vaccines** may potentiate virus replication, increase vaccine side effects, decrease pt's antibody response to vaccine. **HERBAL:** Avoid **black cohosh, dong quai** in estrogen-dependent tumors. **Gotu kola, kava kava, St. John's wort, valerian** may increase CNS depression. **St. John's wort** may decrease concentration. **FOOD:** None known. **LAB VALUES:** May elevate serum alkaline phosphatase, bilirubin, ALT, AST, triglycerides.

AVAILABILITY (Rx)

Injection, Powder for Reconstitution (Abraxane): 100-mg vial. **Injection Solution:** 6 mg/mL (5-mL, 16.7-mL, 25-mL, 50-mL vials).

ADMINISTRATION/HANDLING

🖥 IV

◀ALERT▶ Wear gloves during handling; if contact with skin occurs, wash hands thoroughly with soap, water. If contact with mucous membranes occurs, flush with water.

PACLitaxel
Reconstitution • Dilute with 250–1,000 mL 0.9% NaCl, D_5W to final concentration of 0.3–1.2 mg/mL.
Rate of Administration • Administer at rate per protocol (range: 1–96 hrs) through in-line filter not greater than 0.22 microns. • Monitor vital signs during infusion, esp. during first hour. • Discontinue administration if severe hypersensitivity reaction occurs.
Storage • Store unopened vials at room temperature. • Reconstituted solution is stable at room temperature for 72 hrs. • Store diluted solutions in bottles or plastic bags. Administer through polyethylene-lined administration sets (avoid plasticized PVC equipment or devices).

Abraxane (PACLitaxel—Protein Bound)
Reconstitution • Reconstitute each vial with 20 mL 0.9% NaCl to provide concentration of 5 mg/mL. • Slowly inject onto inside wall of vial; gently swirl over 2 min to avoid foaming. • Inject appropriate amount into empty PVC-type bag.
Rate of Administration • Infuse over 30 min. Do not use in-line filter.
Storage • Store unopened vials at room temperature. • Once reconstituted, use immediately but may refrigerate for up to 8 hrs.

🟦 IV INCOMPATIBILITIES

◀ALERT▶ IV compatibility: Data for Abraxane not known; avoid mixing with other medication.
Amphotericin B complex (Abelcet, AmBisome, Amphotec), DOXOrubicin liposomal (Doxil), hydrOXYzine (Vistaril), methylPREDNISolone (Solu-Medrol), mitoXANTRONE (Novantrone).

🟦 IV COMPATIBILITIES

CARBOplatin (Paraplatin), CISplatin (Platinol AQ), cyclophosphamide (Cytoxan), cytarabine (Cytosar), dacarbazine (DTIC-Dome), dexamethasone (Decadron), diphenhydrAMINE (Benadryl), DOXOrubicin (Adriamycin), etoposide (VePesid), gemcitabine (Gemzar), granisetron (Kytril), HYDROmorphone (Dilaudid), lipids, magnesium sulfate, mannitol, methotrexate, morphine, ondansetron (Zofran), potassium chloride, vinBLAStine (Velban), vinCRIStine (Oncovin).

INDICATIONS/ROUTES/DOSAGE

Note: Premedication with dexamethasone, diphenhydrAMINE, and cimetidine, famotidine, or raNITIdine recommended. Refer to individual protocols.

PACLitaxel (Conventional)
Ovarian Cancer
IV: **ADULTS, ELDERLY: (Previously Treated):** 135–175 mg/m²/dose over 3 hrs q3wks. **(Previously Untreated):** 175 mg/m² over 3 hrs q3wks (in combination with CISplatin) or 135 mg/m² over 24 hrs q3wks (in combination with CISplatin).

Breast Cancer (Adjuvant)
IV: **ADULTS, ELDERLY:** 175 mg/m² over 3 hrs for 4 cycles (give sequentially following anthracycline-containing regimen).

Breast Cancer (Metastatic/Relapsed)
IV: **ADULTS, ELDERLY:** 175 mg/m² over 3 hrs q3wks.

Non–Small-Cell Lung Cancer
IV: **ADULTS, ELDERLY:** 135 mg/m² over 24 hrs (in combination with CISplatin).

Kaposi's Sarcoma (AIDS-Related)
IV: **ADULTS, ELDERLY:** 135 mg/m²/dose over 3 hrs q3wks or 100 mg/m²/dose over 3 hrs q2wks.

Dosage in Renal Impairment
No dose adjustment.

P

Dosage in Hepatic Impairment

Transaminase Level	Bilirubin	Dose
24-HR INFUSION		
Less than 2 times ULN	1.5 mg/dL or less	135 mg/m²
2 to less than 10 times ULN	1.5 mg/dL or less	100 mg/m²
Less than 10 times ULN	1.6–7.5 mg/dL or less	50 mg/m²
3-HR INFUSION		
Less than 10 times ULN	1.25 mg/dL or less	175 mg/m²
Less than 10 times ULN	1.26–2 times ULN	135 mg/m²
Less than 10 times ULN	2.01–5 times ULN	90 mg/m²
10 times ULN or greater	Greater than 5 times ULN	Avoid use

ULN: upper limit of normal

Dose Modification

Courses of PACLitaxel should be withheld until neutrophil count is 1,500 cells/mm³ or more and platelet count is 100,000 cells/mm³ or more.

Abraxane
Breast Cancer (Metastatic)
IV Infusion: ADULTS, ELDERLY: 260 mg/m² q3wks.

Dose Modification
Severe neutropenia (ANC less than 500 cells/mm³ for 1 wk or longer); severe sensory neuropathy: Reduce dose to 220 mg/m² for subsequent courses.
Recurrence of severe neutropenia, severe neuropathy: Reduce dose to 180 mg/m² q3wks for subsequent courses.
CTCAE grade 3 sensory neuropathy: Hold until resolved to grade 2 or 1, then reduce dose for subsequent courses.
Dosage of Abraxane for serum bilirubin greater than 1.5 mg/dL: Dose unknown.

NSCLC (Locally Advanced or Metastatic)
IV: ADULTS, ELDERLY: 100 mg/m² on days 1, 8, 15 of each 21-day cycle (in combination with CARBOplatin).

Adenocarcinoma of Pancreas (Metastatic) (in combination with gemcitabine)
IV: ADULTS, ELDERLY: 125 mg/m² on days 1, 8, 15 of each 28-day cycle (in combination with gemcitabine).

Dosage in Renal Impairment
No dose adjustment.

Dosage in Hepatic Impairment

	Mild Impairment (AST Less Than 10 Times Upper Limit of Normal [ULN], Bilirubin 1.25 Times ULN or Less)	Moderate Impairment (AST Less Than 10 Times ULN, Bilirubin 1.26–2 Times ULN)	Severe Impairment	
			(AST Less Than 10 Times ULN, Bilirubin 2.01–5 Times ULN)	(AST More Than 10 Times ULN or Bilirubin > 5 Times ULN)
Breast cancer	No adjustment	Reduce dose to 200 mg/m²	Reduce dose to 130 mg/m² (may increase to 200 mg/m² in subsequent cycles)	Not recommended
NSCLC	No adjustment	Reduce dose to 75 mg/m²	Reduce dose to 50 mg/m² (may increase to 75 mg/m² in subsequent cycles)	Not recommended
Pancreatic	No adjustment	Not recommended	Not recommended	Not recommended

SIDE EFFECTS

Expected (90%–70%): Diarrhea, alopecia, nausea, vomiting. **Frequent (48%–46%):** Myalgia, arthralgia, peripheral neuropathy. **Occasional (20%–13%):** Mucositis, hypotension during infusion, pain/redness at injection site. **Rare (3%):** Bradycardia.

ADVERSE EFFECTS/TOXIC REACTIONS

Neutropenic nadir occurs at median of 11 days. Anemia, leukopenia occur commonly; thrombocytopenia occurs occasionally. Severe hypersensitivity reaction (dyspnea, severe hypotension, angioedema, generalized urticaria) occurs rarely.

NURSING CONSIDERATIONS

BASELINE ASSESSMENT

Obtain CBC (note neutrophil count), BMP, LFT prior to each course. Receive full medication history and screen for interactions. Offer emotional support.

INTERVENTION/EVALUATION

Monitor CBC, LFT, vital signs. Monitor for hematologic toxicity (fever, sore throat, signs of local infections, unusual bleeding/bruising), symptoms of anemia (excessive fatigue, weakness). Monitor daily pattern of bowel activity, stool consistency; report diarrhea. Avoid IM injections, rectal temperatures, other traumas that may induce bleeding. Hold pressure to injection sites for full 5 min.

PATIENT/FAMILY TEACHING

• Hair loss is reversible, but new hair may have different color, texture. • Do not have immunizations without physician's approval (drug lowers resistance). • Avoid crowds, persons with known infections. • Report signs of infection at once (fever, flu-like symptoms). • Report persistent nausea/vomiting. • Be alert for signs of peripheral neuropathy. • Avoid pregnancy. • Avoid tasks that may require alertness, motor skills until response to drug is established.

palbociclib

pal-boe-**sye**-klib
(Ibrance)

◆**CLASSIFICATION**

PHARMACOTHERAPEUTIC: Kinase inhibitor. **CLINICAL:** Antineoplastic.

USES

Used in combination with an aromatase inhibitor (e.g., letrozole) for treatment of postmenopausal women with estrogen receptor–positive, human epidermal growth factor receptor 2 *(HER2)*–negative advanced breast cancer as initial endocrine-based therapy for metastatic disease or in combination with fulvestrant in women with disease progression following endocrine therapy.

PRECAUTIONS

Contraindications: Hypersensitivity to palbociclib. **Cautions:** Baseline anemia, lymphopenia, neutropenia, thrombocytopenia. History of pulmonary embolism. Avoid concomitant use of strong or moderate CYP3A inhibitors, strong or moderate CYP3A inducers.

ACTION

Inhibits proliferation of tumor cells that overexpress *HER2* by blocking cellular progression from G1 into S phase of cell cycle. Promotes cellular death (apoptosis). **Therapeutic Effect:** Inhibits tumor cell growth and metastasis.

PHARMACOKINETICS

Readily absorbed. Widely distributed. Metabolized in liver. Protein binding: 85%. Peak plasma concentration: 6–12 hrs. Steady state reached in 8 days. Excreted in feces (74%), urine (18%). **Half-life:** 29 hrs.

⧗ LIFESPAN CONSIDERATIONS

Pregnancy/Lactation: Treatment is indicated for postmenopausal women.

P

However, treatment may cause fetal harm when administered during pregnancy. Females of reproductive potential should use effective contraception during treatment and up to 2 wks after discontinuation. Unknown if distributed in breast milk. Must either discontinue drug or discontinue breastfeeding. **Children:** Safety and efficacy not established. Not indicated in this population. **Elderly:** No age-related precautions noted.

INTERACTIONS

DRUG: Strong CYP3A inhibitors (e.g., clarithromycin, ketoconazole, ritonavir), moderate CYP3A inhibitors (e.g., atazanavir, ciprofloxacin) may increase concentration/effect; avoid use. **Strong CYP3A inducers (e.g., carBAMazepine, rifAMPin), moderate CYP3A inducers (e.g., nafcillin)** may decrease concentration/effect; avoid use. May increase concentration/effects of **medications with a narrow therapeutic index (e.g., cycloSPORINE, ergotamine, tacrolimus). HERBAL: St. John's wort** may decrease concentration/effect. **FOOD: Grapefruit products** may increase concentration/effect. **LAB VALUES:** May decrease Hgb, lymphocytes, neutrophils, platelets, WBC.

AVAILABILITY (Rx)

Capsules: 75 mg, 100 mg, 125 mg.

ADMINISTRATION/HANDLING

PO
• Give with food. • Administer whole; do not break, crush, cut, or open capsule. • If vomiting occurs after dosing, do not readminister dose; give dose at next scheduled time.

INDICATIONS/ROUTES/DOSAGE

Breast Cancer
PO: ADULTS, ELDERLY: 125 mg once daily for 21 days, followed by a 7-day rest period to complete a 28-day cycle. Use in combination with an aromatase inhibitor (e.g., letrozole) once daily throughout 28-day cycle or with fulvestrant 500 mg on days 1, 15, 29 and once monthly thereafter. Continue until disease progression or unacceptable toxicity.

Dose Reduction for Adverse Events

Dose Level	Dose
Recommended starting dose	125 mg/day
First dose reduction	100 mg/day
Second dose reduction	75 mg/day
Unable to tolerate 75 mg/day	Permanently discontinue

Dose Modification
Based on Common Terminology Criteria for Adverse Events (CTCAE).

Hematologic Toxicities
Grade 1 or 2: No dose adjustment. **Grade 3 (except lymphopenia unless associated with clinical events [e.g., opportunistic infection]):** No dose adjustment. Withhold treatment until recovery to less than grade 2. **Grade 3, ANC 500–1000/mm³ plus fever that is greater than or equal to 38.5°C and/or active infection:** Interrupt treatment (and initiation of the next cycle) until recovery to grade 2 or less. Resume at reduced dose upon starting.

Nonhematologic Toxicities
Grade 1 or 2: No dose adjustment. **Grade 3 or greater (if persistent despite optimal medical management):** Interrupt treatment until resolved to grade 1 or less; grade 2 or less if the event is not considered a serious medical risk. Resume at reduced dose upon starting.

Concomitant Use of Strong CYP3A Inhibitors
PO: ADULTS, ELDERLY: 75 mg once daily if unable to use alternative drug with minimal CYP3A inhibition. If CYP3A inhibitor is discontinued, increase palbociclib dose (after 3–5 half-lives of CYP3A inhibitor have elapsed) to the dose used prior to initiating strong CYP3A inhibitor.

Dosage in Renal Impairment
Mild to moderate impairment: No dose adjustment. **Severe impairment:** Not studied; use caution.

Dosage in Hepatic Impairment
Mild impairment: No dose adjustment. **Moderate to severe impairment:** Not studied; use caution.

SIDE EFFECTS

Frequent (41%–21%): Fatigue, nausea, alopecia, diarrhea. **Occasional (16%–13%):** Decreased appetite, vomiting, asthenia.

ADVERSE EFFECTS/TOXIC REACTIONS

Anemia, leukopenia, neutropenia, thrombocytopenia are expected responses to therapy. CTCAE grade 3 neutropenia reported in 57% of pts. The median onset of neutropenia was 15 days. Pulmonary embolism (5% of pts); upper respiratory tract infections including influenza, laryngitis, nasopharyngitis, pharyngitis, rhinitis, sinusitis (31% of pts); peripheral neuropathy (31% of pts); cheilitis, glossitis, glossodynia, mouth ulceration, stomatitis (25% of pts); epistaxis (11% of pts) were reported.

NURSING CONSIDERATIONS

BASELINE ASSESSMENT

Obtain baseline ANC, CBC. Confirm estrogen receptor–positive, *HER2*-negative status. Verify pregnancy status before start of each cycle. Screen for history of pulmonary embolism. Receive full medication history and screen for interactions. Assess hydration status. Screen for active infection. Offer emotional support.

INTERVENTION/EVALUATION

Monitor ANC, CBC at start of each cycle and on day 14 on the first two cycles. If any grade 3 or 4 hematologic toxicity occurs, repeat CBC 7 days after interruption of therapy and at start of next cycle. If neutropenia occurs specifically, recommend treatment interruption, dose reduction, or delay in starting treatment

for next cycle. Monitor for neurotoxicity (peripheral neuropathy), epistaxis. If chest pain, dyspnea, tachycardia occurs, provide supplemental O_2 and obtain radiologic testing to rule out pulmonary embolism.

PATIENT/FAMILY TEACHING

• Blood levels will monitored regularly. • Treatment may cause fetal harm. Women of childbearing potential should use effective contraception during treatment and up to 2 wks following discontinuation. Immediately report suspected pregnancy. Do not breastfeed. • Immediately report chest pain, difficult breathing, fast heart rate, rapid breathing; may indicate life-threatening blood clot in the lungs. • Report symptoms of bone marrow suppression or infection such as bruising easily, chills, cough, dizziness, fainting, fever, shortness of breath, weakness. • Swallow capsules whole; do not chew, crush, cut, or open capsules. • Take each dose with food. • Treatment may increase risk of infection, nosebleeds. • Drink plenty of fluids. • Do not ingest grapefruit products or herbal supplements. • Avoid crowds, those with active infection.

paliperidone

pal-ee-**per**-i-done
(Invega, Invega Sustenna, Invega Trinza)

■ **BLACK BOX ALERT** ■ Elderly pts with dementia-related psychosis are at increased risk for mortality due to cerebrovascular events.

◆CLASSIFICATION

PHARMACOTHERAPEUTIC: Benzisoxazole derivative. **CLINICAL:** Second-generation (atypical) antipsychotic.

USES

Oral: Treatment of schizophrenia. Acute treatment of schizoaffective disorder as

monotherapy or as adjunct to mood stabilizers and/or antidepressants. **Injection:** Acute and maintenance treatment of
schizophrenia. **OFF-LABEL:** Treatment of
irritability associated with autistic disorder.

PRECAUTIONS

Contraindications: Sensitivity to paliperidone, risperiDONE. **Cautions:** History of
cardiac arrhythmias, mild renal impairment
(not recommended in moderate to severe
impairment), diabetes, HF, active seizures
or predisposition to seizures, history of
seizures, cardiovascular disease, congenital
long QT syndrome, concomitant use with
other medications that prolong QT interval,
pts at risk for aspiration pneumonia. May
increase risk of stroke in pts with dementia-
related psychosis. CNS depression, concomitant use of antihypertensives, hypovolemia
or dehydration, high risk for suicide. Pts
with breast cancer, other prolactin-dependent tumors; children, adolescents.

ACTION

Exact mechanism of action is unknown, but
may antagonize DOPamine and serotonin
receptors. **Therapeutic Effect:** Suppresses behavioral response in psychosis.

PHARMACOKINETICS

Absorbed from GI tract. Metabolized in
liver. Primarily excreted in urine. **Half-
life:** 23 hrs.

⧗ LIFESPAN CONSIDERATIONS

Pregnancy/Lactation: Unknown if drug
crosses placenta or is distributed in breast
milk. **Children:** Safety and efficacy not established. **Elderly:** Potential for orthostatic
hypotension. Age-related renal impairment
may require dosage adjustment.

INTERACTIONS

DRUG: May decrease effects of **DOPamine
agonists, levodopa. Alcohol, CNS depressants (e.g., LORazepam, morphine,
zolpidem)** may increase CNS depression.
HERBAL: None significant. **FOOD:** None
known. **LAB VALUES:** May increase serum
creatine phosphatase, uric acid, triglycerides,
ALT, AST, prolactin. May decrease serum potassium, sodium, protein, glucose.

AVAILABILITY (Rx)

Injection Suspension (Invega Sustenna): 39
mg/0.25 mL, 78 mg/0.5 mL, 117 mg/0.75
mL, 156 mg/mL, 234 mg/1.5 mL. **(Invega
Trinza):** 273 mg, 410 mg, 546 mg, 819 mg.

⧗ Tablets, Extended-Release: 1.5 mg,
3 mg, 6 mg, 9 mg.

ADMINISTRATION/HANDLING

PO

• May give without regard to food.
• Do not break, crush, dissolve, or divide extended-release tablets.

IM

• Administer both initial injections (first
injection on day 1 and the second injection 1 wk later) into deltoid muscle
(helps attain therapeutic concentration
rapidly). • Maintenance doses may be
given in gluteal or deltoid muscle.

INDICATIONS/ROUTES/DOSAGE

Treatment of Schizophrenia
PO: ADULTS, ELDERLY: Initially, 6 mg once
daily in the morning. May increase dose
in increments of 3 mg/day at intervals of
more than 5 days. Range: 3–12 mg/day.
ADOLESCENTS (51 KG OR GREATER): Initially,
3 mg once daily. Range: 3–12 mg/day. **(50
KG OR LESS):** Initially, 3 mg once daily.
Range: 3–6 mg/day.
**IM: (Invega Sustenna): ADULTS, EL-
DERLY:** Initially, 234 mg on day 1 followed
by 156 mg 1 wk later (second dose may be
given 4 days before or after the wkly time
point). **Maintenance:** Following the 1-wk
initiation regimen, begin 117 mg monthly.
Range: 39–234 mg (based on response and
tolerability). Monthly maintenance dose may
be given 7 days before or after the monthly
time point. **(Invega Trinza):** 273 mg to
819 mg q3mos (based on last dose of Invega Sustenna). Three-month IM used only
after monthly IM dose established for at
least 4 mos. The last 2 mos of monthly IM
should be the same dosage strength before
starting 3-mo injections.

P

Schizoaffective Disorder
PO: ADULTS, ELDERLY: 6 mg once daily in the morning. May increase in increments of 3 mg/day at intervals of more than 4 days. **Range:** 3–12 mg/day.
IM: ADULTS, ELDERLY: Initially, 234 mg, then 156 mg 1 wk later. **Maintenance range:** 78–234 mg monthly (based on response and tolerability). May be given 7 days before or after the monthly time point.

Dosage in Renal Impairment

Creatinine Clearance	Oral Dosage	IM Dosage
50–79 mL/min	Initially, 3 mg/d Maximum: 6 mg/d	Initially, 156 mg, then 117 mg 1 wk later, then 78 mg monthly
10–49 mL/min	Initially, 1.5 mg/d Maximum: 3 mg/d	Not recommended
Less than 10 mL/min	Not recommended	Not recommended

Dosage in Hepatic Impairment
No dose adjustment.

SIDE EFFECTS

Occasional (14%–4%): Tachycardia, headache, drowsiness, akathisia, anxiety, dizziness, dyspepsia, nausea.

ADVERSE EFFECTS/TOXIC REACTIONS

Neuroleptic malignant syndrome (NMS), hyperpyrexia, muscle rigidity, change in mental status, unstable pulse or B/P, tachycardia, diaphoresis, cardiac arrhythmias, rhabdomyolysis, acute renal failure, tardive dyskinesia (protrusion of tongue, puffing of cheeks, chewing/puckering of mouth) may occur rarely. May prolong QT interval.

NURSING CONSIDERATIONS

BASELINE ASSESSMENT
Obtain baseline renal function tests. Assess behavior, appearance, emotional status, response to environment, speech pattern, thought content. Screen for comorbidities as listed in Precautions.

INTERVENTION/EVALUATION
Monitor B/P, heart rate, weight, renal function tests, EKG. Monitor for fine tongue movement (may be first sign of tardive dyskinesia). Supervise suicidal-risk pt closely during early therapy (as depression lessens, energy level improves, increasing suicide potential). Assess for therapeutic response (greater interest in surroundings, improved self-care, increased ability to concentrate, relaxed facial expression). Monitor for potential neuroleptic malignant syndrome (fever, muscle rigidity, unstable B/P or pulse, altered mental status).

PATIENT/FAMILY TEACHING
• Avoid tasks that may require alertness, motor skills until response to drug is established. • Use caution when changing position from lying or sitting to standing. • Report trembling in fingers, altered gait, unusual muscle/skeletal movements, palpitations, severe dizziness, fainting, swelling/pain in breasts, visual changes, rash, difficulty in breathing.

palonosetron

pal-oh-**noe**-se-tron
(Aloxi)
Do not confuse Aloxi with Eloxatin or oxaliplatin, or palonosetron with dolasetron, granisetron, or ondansetron.

FIXED-COMBINATION(S)

Akynzeo: palonosetron/netupitant (a substance P/neurokinin receptor antagonist): 0.5 mg/300 mg.

◆CLASSIFICATION

PHARMACOTHERAPEUTIC: 5-HT$_3$ receptor antagonist. **CLINICAL:** Antiemetic.

USES

Prevention of acute and delayed nausea/vomiting associated with initial/repeated courses of moderately or highly emetogenic chemotherapy. Prevention of postop nausea/vomiting for up to 24 hrs following surgery.

PRECAUTIONS

Contraindications: Hypersensitivity to palonosetron. **Cautions:** History of cardiovascular disease; congenital long QT syndrome, risk factors for QT prolongation (hypokalemia, hypomagnesemia), medications that prolong QT interval or reduce potassium/magnesium levels, pts at risk for ventricular arrhythmias.

ACTION

Acts centrally in chemoreceptor trigger zone, peripherally at vagal nerve terminals. **Therapeutic Effect:** Fewer episodes of nausea/vomiting associated with chemotherapy or postoperative recovery.

PHARMACOKINETICS

Protein binding: 52%. Metabolized in liver. Excreted in urine. **Half-life:** 40 hrs.

⏳ LIFESPAN CONSIDERATIONS

Pregnancy/Lactation: Unknown if distributed in breast milk. **Children:** Safety and efficacy not established. **Elderly:** No age-related precautions noted.

INTERACTIONS

DRUG: FentaNYL, lithium, MAOIs (e.g., phenelzine, selegiline), SN-RIs (e.g., DULoxetine, venlafaxine), SSRIs (e.g., citalopram, FLUoxetine, sertraline), tricyclic antidepressants (e.g., amitriptyline, doxepin) may increase risk of serotonin syndrome. **HERBAL:** None significant. **FOOD:** None known. **LAB VALUES:** May transiently increase serum bilirubin, ALT, AST.

AVAILABILITY (Rx)

Injection Solution: 0.25 mg/5 mL.

ADMINISTRATION/HANDLING

 IV

Reconstitution • Give undiluted as IV push.
Rate of Administration • Give IV push over 30 sec. Children: Infuse over 15 min. • Flush infusion line with 0.9% NaCl before and following administration.
Storage • Store at room temperature. Solution should appear colorless, clear. Discard if cloudy precipitate forms.

▦ IV COMPATIBILITIES

Famotidine (Pepcid), LORazepam (Ativan), midazolam (Versed), potassium chloride.

INDICATIONS/ROUTES/DOSAGE

Chemotherapy-Induced Nausea/Vomiting
IV: ADULTS, ELDERLY: 0.25 mg as single dose 30 min before starting chemotherapy. **CHILDREN 1 MO TO YOUNGER THAN 17 YRS:** 20 mcg/kg as single dose 30 min before starting chemotherapy. **Maximum:** 1.5 mg.

Postop Nausea/Vomiting
IV: ADULTS, ELDERLY: 0.075 mg over 10 sec immediately before induction of anesthesia.

Dosage in Renal/Hepatic Impairment
No dose adjustment.

SIDE EFFECTS

Occasional (9%–5%): Headache, constipation. **Rare (less than 1%):** Diarrhea, dizziness, fatigue, abdominal pain, insomnia.

ADVERSE EFFECTS/TOXIC REACTIONS

Overdose may produce combination of CNS stimulation, depressant effects. May prolong QT interval. 5-HT$_3$ receptor antagonists are known to potentiate serotonin syndrome, esp. in pts taking serotonergic medications.

NURSING CONSIDERATIONS

BASELINE ASSESSMENT

Obtain BMP, serum magnesium in pts at risk for hypokalemia, hypomagnesemia, QT interval prolongation. Assess for signs of dehydration due to excessive vomiting (poor skin turgor, dry mucous membranes). Question history of cardiac disease, long QT syndrome, cardiac arrhythmias. Screen for concomitant home medications that prolong QT interval, increase risk of serotonin syndrome. Provide emotional support.

INTERVENTION/EVALUATION

Monitor BMP, serum magnesium; EKG in pts suspected of arrhythmia, QT interval prolongation. Assess for symptoms of serotonin syndrome (e.g., altered mental status, tachycardia, labile B/P, diaphoresis, hyperthermia, tremor, hyperreflexia, diarrhea, seizures). Monitor for hypersensitivity reaction. Monitor pt for signs of dehydration. Assess mental status. Monitor daily pattern of bowel activity, stool consistency.

PATIENT/FAMILY TEACHING

• Relief from nausea/vomiting generally occurs shortly after drug administration. • Avoid alcohol, barbiturates. • Report persistent vomiting. • Report palpitations, light-headedness, fainting; allergic reactions of any kind.

pamidronate

pam-id-roe-nate
(Aredia✦)
Do not confuse Aredia with Adriamycin, or pamidronate with alendronate, ibandronate, or risedronate.

◆CLASSIFICATION

PHARMACOTHERAPEUTIC: Bisphosphonate. **CLINICAL:** Hypocalcemic.

USES

Treatment of moderate to severe hypercalcemia associated with malignancy (with/without bone metastases). Treatment of moderate to severe Paget's disease, osteolytic bone lesions of multiple myeloma or metastatic breast cancer. **OFF-LABEL:** Inhibits bone resorption in osteogenesis imperfecta, treatment of bone metastases of thyroid cancer, prevention of bone loss associated with androgen deprivation treatment in prostate cancer.

PRECAUTIONS

Contraindications: Hypersensitivity to pamidronate, other bisphosphonates (e.g., etidronate, tiludronate, risedronate, alendronate). **Cautions:** Renal impairment, concurrent use with other nephrotoxic medications, history of thyroid surgery. Preexisting anemia, leukopenia, thrombocytopenia.

ACTION

Inhibits bone resorption, decreases mineralization by disrupting activity of osteoclasts. **Therapeutic Effect:** Lowers serum calcium concentration.

PHARMACOKINETICS

Route	Onset	Peak	Duration
IV	24–48 hrs	3–7 days	N/A

After IV administration, rapidly absorbed by bone. Slowly excreted unchanged in urine. Unknown if removed by hemodialysis. **Half-life:** 21–35 hrs.

⧖ LIFESPAN CONSIDERATIONS

Pregnancy/Lactation: Unknown if crosses placenta. Recommend discontinuation of drug as early as possible before a planned pregnancy. Unknown if fetal harm can occur. Unknown if distributed in breast milk. **Children:** Safety and efficacy not established. **Elderly:** May become overhydrated. Careful monitoring of fluid and electrolytes indicated; recommend dilution in smaller volume.

INTERACTIONS

DRUG: **Nephrotoxic medications** (e.g., acyclovir, amphotericin B, diclofenac, gentamicin, IV contrast dye, NSAIDs, vancomycin) may increase potential for nephrotoxicity. **HERBAL:** None significant. **FOOD:** None known. **LAB VALUES:** None significant.

AVAILABILITY (Rx)

Injection, Powder for Reconstitution: 30 mg, 90 mg. **Injection Solution:** 3 mg/mL, 6 mg/mL, 9 mg/mL.

ADMINISTRATION/HANDLING

 IV

Reconstitution • Reconstitute each vial with 10 mL Sterile Water for Injection to provide concentration of 3 mg/mL or 9 mg/mL. • Allow drug to dissolve before withdrawing. • Further dilute with 250–1,000 mL sterile 0.45% or 0.9% NaCl or D_5W (1,000 mL for hypercalcemia of malignancy, 500 mL for Paget's disease, multiple myeloma, 250 mL for breast cancer).

Rate of Administration • Adequate hydration is essential in conjunction with pamidronate therapy (avoid overhydration in pts with potential for HF). • Administer as IV infusion over 2–24 hrs for treatment of hypercalcemia; over 2 hrs for breast cancer; over 4 hrs for Paget's disease or multiple myeloma.

Storage • Store parenteral form at room temperature. • Reconstituted vial is stable for 24 hrs if refrigerated; IV solution is stable for 24 hrs after dilution.

🔯 IV INCOMPATIBILITIES

Calcium-containing IV fluids.

INDICATIONS/ROUTES/DOSAGE

Hypercalcemia of Malignancy
IV Infusion: ADULTS, ELDERLY: Moderate hypercalcemia (corrected serum calcium level 12–13.5 mg/dL): 60–90 mg as a single dose over 2–24 hrs. **Severe hypercalcemia (corrected serum** calcium level greater than 13.5 mg/dL): 90 mg as a single dose over 2–24 hrs.

Paget's Disease
IV Infusion: ADULTS, ELDERLY: 30 mg/day over 4 hrs for 3 consecutive days.

Osteolytic Bone Lesion (Multiple Myeloma)
IV Infusion: ADULTS, ELDERLY: 90 mg over 4 hrs once monthly.

Osteolytic Bone Lesion (Breast Cancer)
IV Infusion: ADULTS, ELDERLY: 90 mg over 2 hrs q3–4wks.

Dosage in Renal Impairment
Not recommended.

Dosage in Hepatic Impairment
No dose adjustment.

SIDE EFFECTS

Frequent (27%–18%): Temperature elevation (at least 1°C) 24–48 hrs after administration; erythema, swelling, induration, pain at catheter site in pts receiving 90 mg; anorexia, nausea, fatigue. **Occasional (10%–1%):** Constipation, rhinitis.

ADVERSE EFFECTS/TOXIC REACTIONS

Hypophosphatemia, hypokalemia, hypomagnesemia, hypocalcemia occur more frequently with higher dosages. Anemia, hypertension, tachycardia, atrial fibrillation, drowsiness occur more frequently with 90-mg doses. GI hemorrhage occurs rarely.

NURSING CONSIDERATIONS

BASELINE ASSESSMENT

Obtain CBC, serum calcium, ionized calcium, magnesium, phosphate; renal function test level prior to therapy. Determine hydration status.

INTERVENTION/EVALUATION

Monitor serum calcium, ionized calcium, potassium, magnesium, creatinine, CBC. Provide adequate hydration; assess overhydration. Monitor I&O carefully; assess lungs for crackles, dependent body parts for edema. Monitor B/P, temperature, pulse. Assess catheter site for redness, swelling, pain. Monitor food intake, daily pattern of bowel activity, stool consistency. Be alert for potential GI hemorrhage with 90-mg dosage.

PATIENT/FAMILY TEACHING

• Report symptoms of low blood calcium levels, including confusion, muscle twitching/cramps, numbness, seizures, tingling, jaw pain. • Immediately report GI bleeding.

---

panitumumab

pan-i-**toom**-ue-mab
(Vectibix)

■ **BLACK BOX ALERT** ■ 90% of pts experience dermatologic toxicities (dermatitis acneiform, pruritus, erythema, rash, skin exfoliation, skin fissures, abscess). Severe infusion reactions (anaphylaxis, bronchospasm, fever, chills, hypotension), fatal reactions have occurred.

◆CLASSIFICATION

PHARMACOTHERAPEUTIC: Epidermal growth factor receptor (EGFR) inhibitor, monoclonal antibody. **CLINICAL:** Antineoplastic.

USES

Treatment of wild-type RAS metastatic colorectal cancer either as first-line therapy in combination with FOLFOX or as monotherapy following disease progression after prior treatment with fluoropyrimidine-, oxaliplatin-, or irinotecan-based regimens.

PRECAUTIONS

Contraindications: Hypersensitivity to panitumumab. **Cautions:** Interstitial pneumonitis, pulmonary fibrosis, pulmonary infiltrates, renal impairment, baseline electrolyte imbalance. Not indicated in pts with *RAS*-mutant metastatic colorectal cancer or for whom *RAS* mutation status is unknown.

ACTION

Binds specifically to epidermal growth factor receptor (EGFR) and competitively inhibits binding of epidermal growth factor. **Therapeutic Effect:** Inhibits tumor cell growth and metastasis.

PHARMACOKINETICS

Clearance varies by body weight, gender, tumor burden. **Half-life:** 3–10 days.

⧖ LIFESPAN CONSIDERATIONS

Pregnancy/Lactation: May cause fetal harm. May impair fertility. May decrease fetal body weight, increase risk of skeletal fetal abnormalities. Use effective contraception during and for at least 6 mos after treatment. Breastfeeding not recommended. **Children:** Safety and efficacy not established. **Elderly:** No age-related precautions noted.

INTERACTIONS

DRUG: None significant. **HERBAL:** None significant. **FOOD:** None known. **LAB VALUES:** May decrease serum magnesium, calcium.

AVAILABILITY (Rx)

Injection Solution: 20 mg/mL vial (5-mL, 20-mL vials).

ADMINISTRATION/HANDLING
🖰 IV

◀**ALERT**▶ Do not give by IV push or bolus. Use low protein-binding 0.2- or 0.22-micron in-line filter. Flush IV line before and after chemotherapy administration with 0.9% NaCl.
Reconstitution • Dilute in 100–150 mL 0.9% NaCl to provide concentration of 10 mg/mL or less. • Do not shake solution. Invert gently to mix. • Discard any unused portion.

P

Rate of Administration • Give as IV infusion over 60 min. • Infuse doses greater than 1,000 mg over 90 min.

Storage • Refrigerate vials. • After dilution, solution may be stored for up to 6 hrs at room temperature, up to 24 hrs if refrigerated. • Discard if discolored, but solution may contain visible, translucent-to-white particulates (will be removed by in-line filter).

🔲 IV INCOMPATIBILITIES

Do not mix with dextrose solutions or any other medications.

INDICATIONS/ROUTES/DOSAGE

◀ALERT▶ Stop infusion immediately in pts experiencing severe infusion reactions.

Metastatic Colorectal Cancer
IV Infusion: ADULTS, ELDERLY: 6 mg/kg given over 60 min once every 14 days. Doses greater than 1,000 mg should be infused over 90 min. Continue until disease progression or unacceptable toxicity.

Dose Modification
Infusion Reactions
Mild to moderate reactions: Reduce infusion rate by 50% for remainder of infusion. **Severe reactions:** Discontinue infusion. Depending on severity, consider permanent discontinuation.

Skin Toxicity
For all CTCAE grade 3 skin toxicities, withhold treatment for 1–2 doses until improved to better than grade 3. Then, reduce dose as follows: **First occurrence of CTCAE grade 3:** Resume at same dose. **Second occurrence of CTCAE grade 3:** Reduce dose to 80% of initial dose. **Third occurrence of CTCAE grade 3:** Reduce dose to 60% of initial dose. **Fourth occurrence of CTCAE grade 3:** Permanently discontinue.

Dosage in Renal/Hepatic Impairment
No dose adjustment.

SIDE EFFECTS

Common (65%–57%): Erythema, acneiform dermatitis, pruritus. **Frequent (26%–20%):** Fatigue, abdominal pain, skin exfoliation, paronychia (soft tissue infection around nailbed), nausea, rash, diarrhea, constipation, skin fissures. **Occasional (19%–10%):** Vomiting, acne, cough, peripheral edema, dry skin. **Rare (7%–2%):** Stomatitis, mucosal inflammation, eyelash growth, conjunctivitis, increased lacrimation.

ADVERSE EFFECTS/TOXIC REACTIONS

Pulmonary fibrosis, severe dermatologic toxicity (complicated by infectious sequelae) occur rarely. Severe infusion reactions manifested as bronchospasm, fever, chills, hypotension occur rarely. Hypomagnesemia occurs in 39% of pts. Life-threatening and/or fatal bullous fasciitis, abscess, sepsis were reported. Severe dehydration and diarrhea may increase risk of acute renal failure. Exposure to sunlight may exacerbate skin toxicities. May cause ocular toxicities including keratitis, ulcerative keratitis, corneal ulceration.

NURSING CONSIDERATIONS

BASELINE ASSESSMENT

Assess serum magnesium, calcium prior to therapy, periodically during therapy, and for 8 wks after completion of therapy. Assess *KRAS* mutational status in colorectal tumors and confirm the absence of a *RAS* mutation.

INTERVENTION/EVALUATION

Assess for skin, ocular, mucosal, pulmonary toxicity; report effects. Median time to development of skin/ocular toxicity is 14–15 days; resolution after last dosing is 84 days. Monitor serum electrolytes for hypomagnesemia, hypocalcemia. Offer antiemetic if nausea/vomiting occurs. Monitor daily pattern of bowel activity, stool consistency.

P

PATIENT/FAMILY TEACHING

• Do not have immunizations without physician's approval (drug lowers resistance). • Avoid contact with those who have recently received a live virus vaccine. • Avoid crowds, those with infection. • There is a potential risk for development of fetal abnormalities if pregnancy occurs; take measures to prevent pregnancy. • Report skin reactions, including rash, sloughing, blisters, erosions. • Report difficulty breathing, fever with cough, lung pain; may indicate life-threatening lung inflammation. • Limit sun, UV exposure. Wear protective sunscreen, hats, and clothing while outdoors.

panobinostat

pan-oh-**bin**-oh-stat
(Farydak)

■ **BLACK BOX ALERT** ■ Severe cases of diarrhea reported in 25% of pts. If diarrhea occurs, interrupt treatment, initiate antidiarrheal therapy, and then reduce or discontinue treatment. Severe and/or fatal cases of cardiac arrhythmias, cardiac ischemic events, EKG changes may occur. Electrolyte abnormalities may increase risk of arrhythmias. Obtain EKG, serum electrolytes at baseline and monitor during treatment.
Do not confuse panobinostat with febuxostat or pentostatin.

◆CLASSIFICATION

PHARMACOTHERAPEUTIC: Histone deacetylase inhibitor. **CLINICAL:** Antineoplastic.

USES

Used in combination with bortezomib and dexamethasone for treatment of pts with multiple myeloma who have received at least 2 prior regimens, including bortezomib and an immunomodulatory agent.

PRECAUTIONS

Contraindications: Hypersensitivity to panobinostat. **Cautions:** Congenital long QT syndrome, concurrent medications that prolong QT interval, electrolyte abnormalities (hypokalemia, hypomagnesemia), renal impairment. Not recommended in pts with recent MI or unstable angina, severe hepatic impairment. Concurrent use of strong CYP3A inhibitors and/or CYP3A inducers, CYP2D6 substrates not recommended. Preexisting myelosuppression. Avoid use in pts with active infection.

ACTION

Inhibits enzymatic activity of histone deacetylase. Increases acetylation of histone proteins, resulting in cell cycle arrest and/or cellular death (apoptosis). **Therapeutic Effect:** Inhibits tumor growth and metastasis. Promotes tumor cell death.

PHARMACOKINETICS

Widely distributed. Extensively metabolized. Protein binding: 90%. Peak plasma concentration: 2 hrs. Excreted in feces (44%–77%), urine (29%–51%). **Half-life:** 37 hrs.

⧗ LIFESPAN CONSIDERATIONS

Pregnancy/Lactation: Avoid pregnancy; may cause fetal harm/malformations. Females of reproductive potential should use effective contraception during treatment and up to 1 mo after discontinuation. Unknown if distributed in breast milk. **Males:** Males should use condoms during sexual activity during treatment and up to 3 mos after discontinuation. **Children:** Safety and efficacy not established. **Elderly:** May have increased risk of adverse effects (e.g., cardiac/GI/hematologic toxicities).

INTERACTIONS

DRUG: Strong **CYP3A inhibitors (e.g., clarithromycin, ketoconazole, ritonavir)** may increase concentration/effect. Strong **CYP3A inducers (e.g., carBAMazepine, rifAMPin)** may

P

decrease concentration/effect. May increase concentration/effects of **CYP2D6 substrates (e.g., metoprolol, venlafaxine)**. Medications prolonging QT interval **(e.g., amiodarone, azithromycin, ceritinib, haloperidol, moxifloxacin)** not recommended. **HERBAL: St. John's wort** may decrease concentration/effect. **FOOD: High-fat meals** may delay absorption. **Grapefruit products** may increase concentration/effect. **LAB VALUES:** May decrease Hct, Hgb, leukocytes, lymphocytes, neutrophils, platelets; serum albumin, calcium, potassium, sodium. May increase serum bilirubin, creatinine, magnesium. May increase or decrease phosphate.

AVAILABILITY (Rx)

Capsules: 10 mg, 15 mg, 20 mg.

ADMINISTRATION/HANDLING

PO

• May give without regard to food; avoid grapefruit products (dexamethasone should be given with food to decrease GI upset). • Administer capsule whole; do not break, cut, crush, or open. • If vomiting occurs after dosing, do not readminister dose; give dose at next scheduled time.

INDICATIONS/ROUTES/DOSAGE

Multiple Myeloma

PO: ADULTS, ELDERLY: 20 mg once every other day for 3 doses/wk during wk 1 and 2 of each 21-day cycle for up to 8 cycles, in combination with bortezomib and dexamethasone. Consider continuing treatment for additional 8 cycles based on tolerability. **Total duration:** Up to 16 cycles (48 wks). **Recommended dose of bortezomib:** 1.3 mg/m² as injection/day per dosing schedule. **Recommended dose of dexamethasone:** 20 mg orally/day on a full stomach per dosing schedule.

Dosing Schedule for Cycles 1–8 of 21-Day Cycle

Week 1: Panobinostat: days 1, 3, 5. Bortezomib: days 1, 4. Dexamethasone: days 1, 2, 4, 5.

Week 2: Panobinostat: days 8, 10, 12. Bortezomib: days 8, 11. Dexamethasone: days 8, 9, 11, 12.

Week 3: Rest period (all 3 drugs).

Dosing Schedule for Cycles 9–16 of 21-Day Cycle

Week 1: Panobinostat: days 1, 3, 5. Bortezomib: day 1 only. Dexamethasone: days 1, 2.

Week 2: Panobinostat: days 8, 10, 12. Bortezomib: day 8 only. Dexamethasone: days 8, 9.

Week 3: Rest period (all 3 drugs).

Dose Reduction for Adverse Events

If reduction required, reduce panobinostat in increments of 5 mg. If the reduced dose is less than 10 mg 3 times/wk, discontinue treatment. Keep same schedule (21-day cycle) when dose reduced.

Dose Modification for Clinical Toxicities

Based on Common Terminology Criteria for Adverse Events (CTCAE).

Thrombocytopenia

Grade 3: No dose adjustment. **Bortezomib:** No dose adjustment. **Grade 3 with bleeding/grade 4:** Interrupt treatment until platelet count 50,000 cells/mm³ or greater, then resume at reduced dose. **Bortezomib:** Interrupt bortezomib until platelet count 75,000 cells/mm³ or greater. If only 1 dose was held prior to resolution of platelet count, resume bortezomib at same dose. If more than 2 doses were held consecutively, resume bortezomib at reduced dose.

Neutropenia

Grade 3: No dose adjustment. **Bortezomib:** No dose adjustment. **Two or more occurrences of grade 3:** Interrupt treatment until ANC 1,000 cells/mm³ or greater, then resume at same dose. **Bortezomib:** No dose adjustment. **Grade 3 with febrile neutropenia/grade 4:** Interrupt treatment until febrile neutropenia resolves and ANC is 1,000 cells/mm³ or greater, then resume at reduced dose. **Bortezomib:** Interrupt bortezomib until febrile neutropenia resolves and ANC is 1,000 cells/mm³ or greater. If only 1 dose was held prior resolution of platelet count, resume bortezomib at same dose. If more than 2 doses were held consecutively, resume bortezomib at reduced dose.

Anemia
Grade 3: Interrupt panobinostat until Hgb greater than or equal to 10 g/dL, then resume at reduced dose. **Bortezomib:** Not specified.

Diarrhea
Grade 2: Interrupt treatment until resolved, then resume at same dose. **Bortezomib:** Consider interruption of bortezomib until resolved, then resume at same dose. **Grade 3 or hospitalization/administration of IV fluids:** Interrupt until resolved, then resume at reduced dose. **Bortezomib:** Interrupt until resolved, then resume bortezomib at reduced dose. **Grade 4:** Permanently discontinue panobinostat and bortezomib.

Nausea/Vomiting
Grade 3 or 4: Interrupt until resolved, then resume at reduced dose. **Bortezomib:** Not specified.

Other Toxicities (Other CTCAE Grades)
Any grade 2 recurrence, any other grade 3 or 4: Interrupt until resolved to grade 1 or 0, then resume at reduced dose. **Bortezomib:** Not specified. **Any other grade 3 or 4 recurrence:** Consider further dose reduction once resolved to grade 1 or 0.

Concomitant Use of Strong CYP3A Inhibitors
PO: ADULTS, ELDERLY: 10 mg per dosing schedule.

Dosage in Renal Impairment
No dose adjustment.

Dosage in Hepatic Impairment
PO: ADULTS, ELDERLY: Mild impairment: 15 mg per dosing schedule. **Moderate impairment:** 10 mg per dosing schedule. **Severe impairment:** Treatment not recommended.

SIDE EFFECTS
Frequent (60%–2%): Fatigue, asthenia, lethargy, diarrhea, nausea, peripheral edema, decreased appetite, vomiting, pyrexia. **Occasional (12%):** Decreased weight.

ADVERSE EFFECTS/TOXIC REACTIONS
Anemia, leukopenia, neutropenia, thrombocytopenia are expected responses to therapy. Diarrhea occurred in 68% of pts. Severe cases of diarrhea occurred in 25% of pts. Cardiac toxicities such as cardiac ischemic events, ST-segment depression, T-wave abnormalities were reported. Cardiac arrhythmias including atrial fibrillation, atrial flutter, bradycardia, SVT, atrial/ventricular/sinus tachycardia occurred in 12% of pts. Severe thrombocytopenia may increase risk of fatal hemorrhage. Infectious processes such as bacterial infections, invasive fungal infections, pneumonia, sepsis, viral infections were reported. Severe and/or fatal infections occurred in 31% of pts.

NURSING CONSIDERATIONS

BASELINE ASSESSMENT
Obtain CBC, BMP, LFT; serum magnesium, phosphate; EKG, vital signs. Correct electrolyte imbalances prior to each cycle. Verify platelet count is at least 100,000 cells/mm³, ANC is 1,500 cells/mm³, QTc interval is less than 450 msec on EKG prior to each cycle. Verify pregnancy status. Assess hydration status, usual stool characteristics. Question history if acute MI, unstable angina, arrhythmia. Screen for active infection.

INTERVENTION/EVALUATION
Monitor CBC, BMP; serum magnesium, phosphate wkly; LFT as indicated; vital signs. Monitor EKG periodically. If QTc interval increases to greater than 480 msec on EKG, interrupt treatment and

P

correct any electrolyte abnormalities. If QT prolongation does not resolve, permanently discontinue treatment. Initiate medical management for nausea, vomiting, diarrhea prior to any interruption or dose reduction. Consider blood transfusion in pts with severe anemia, thrombocytopenia. Diligently monitor daily pattern bowel activity, stool consistency. Start antidiarrheal therapy at first sign of loose stool/diarrhea. Obtain 2D cardiac echocardiogram, EKG if cardiac decompensation is suspected. Monitor for infection.

PATIENT/FAMILY TEACHING

• Blood levels will be monitored regularly. • Treatment may cause fetal harm. Women of childbearing potential should use effective contraception during treatment and up to 1 mo after final dose. Immediately report suspected pregnancy. Do not breastfeed. • Therapy may reduce fertility in both female and male pts. • Male pts must use condoms during sexual activity. • Report liver problems such as upper abdominal pain, bruising, dark or amber-colored urine, nausea, vomiting, or yellowing of the skin or eyes; heart problems such as chest tightness, dizziness, fainting, palpitations, shortness of breath; kidney problems such as dark-colored urine, decreased urine output, extremity swelling, flank pain; skin changes such as rash, redness. • Report mouth ulceration, jaw pain. • Swallow capsules whole; do not chew, crush, cut, or open capsules. • Treatment may increase risk of bleeding, nosebleeds. • Drink plenty of fluids. • Report the first signs of abdominal cramping, loose stool, diarrhea.

---

pantoprazole

pan-**toe**-pra-zole
(Apo-Pantoprazole ✱, Protonix)
Do not confuse pantoprazole with ARIPiprazole.

✦CLASSIFICATION

PHARMACOTHERAPEUTIC: Benzimidazole. **CLINICAL:** Proton pump inhibitor.

USES

PO: Treatment, maintenance of healing of erosive esophagitis associated with gastroesophageal reflux disease (GERD). Reduction of relapse rate of heartburn symptoms in GERD. Treatment of hypersecretory conditions including Zollinger-Ellison syndrome. **IV:** Short-term treatment of erosive esophagitis associated with GERD, treatment of hypersecretory conditions. **OFF-LABEL:** Peptic ulcer disease, active ulcer bleeding (injection), adjunct in treatment of *H. pylori*, stress ulcer prophylaxis in critically ill pts.

PRECAUTIONS

Contraindications: Hypersensitivity to pantoprazole, other proton pump inhibitors (e.g., omeprazole). **Cautions:** May increase risk of fractures, GI infections.

ACTION

Irreversibly binds to, inhibits hydrogen-potassium adenosine triphosphate, an enzyme on surface of gastric parietal cells. Inhibits hydrogen ion transport into gastric lumen. **Therapeutic Effect:** Increases gastric pH, reduces gastric acid production.

PHARMACOKINETICS

Route	Onset	Peak	Duration
PO	N/A	N/A	24 hrs

Well absorbed from GI tract. Protein binding: 98% (primarily albumin). Primarily distributed into gastric parietal cells. Metabolized in liver. Primarily excreted in urine. Not removed by hemodialysis. **Half-life:** 1 hr.

⧖ LIFESPAN CONSIDERATIONS

Pregnancy/Lactation: Unknown if drug crosses placenta or is distributed in breast milk. **Children:** Safety and efficacy not established. **Elderly:** No age-related precautions noted.

INTERACTIONS

DRUG: May increase effects of **warfarin.** May decrease effects of **atazanavir, captopril, clopidogrel, dasatinib, nelfinavir. HERBAL:** Ginger, goldenseal may decrease effect. **FOOD:** None known. **LAB VALUES:** May increase serum creatinine, cholesterol, uric acid, glucose, lipoprotein, ALT.

AVAILABILITY (Rx)

Granules for Suspension: 40 mg/packet.
Injection, Powder for Reconstitution (Protonix): 40 mg.
🍶 **Tablets (Delayed-Release [Protonix]):** 20 mg, 40 mg.

ADMINISTRATION/HANDLING
💧 IV

Reconstitution • Mix 40-mg vial with 10 mL 0.9% NaCl injection. • May be further diluted with 100 mL D_5W, 0.9% NaCl.
Rate of Administration • Infuse 10 mL solution over at least 2 min. • Infuse 100 mL solution over at least 15 min. • Flush IV line after administration.
Storage • Store undiluted vials at room temperature. • Once diluted with 10 mL 0.9% NaCl, stable for 96 hrs at room temperature; when further diluted with 100 mL, stable for 96 hrs at room temperature.

PO
• May be given without regard to food. Best given before breakfast. • Do not break, crush, dissolve, or divide tablets; give whole. • Administer oral suspension only in apple juice or applesauce. Best taken 30 min before a meal.

🔳 IV COMPATIBILITIES

DOPamine, EPINEPHrine, furosemide (Lasix), insulin (regular), potassium chloride, vasopressin.

🔳 IV INCOMPATIBILITY

DOBUTamine.

INDICATIONS/ROUTES/DOSAGE

Erosive Esophagitis
PO: ADULTS, ELDERLY: 40 mg/day for up to 8 wks. If not healed after 8 wks, may continue an additional 8 wks. **CHILDREN 5 YRS AND OLDER (WEIGHING 40 KG OR MORE):** 40 mg/day for up to 8 wks. **(WEIGHING 15–39 KG):** 20 mg/day for up to 8 wks.
IV: ADULTS, ELDERLY: 40 mg/day for 7–10 days.

Maintenance of Healing of Erosive Esophagitis
PO: ADULTS, ELDERLY: 40 mg once daily.

Hypersecretory Conditions
PO: ADULTS, ELDERLY: Initially, 40 mg twice daily. May increase to 240 mg/day.
IV: ADULTS, ELDERLY: 80 mg twice daily. May increase to 80 mg q8h.

Prevention of Re-bleeding in Peptic Ulcer Bleed (Unlabeled)
IV: ADULTS, ELDERLY: 80 mg followed by 8 mg/hr infusion for 72 hrs or 80 mg then 40 mg q12h for 72 hrs.

Dosage in Renal/Hepatic Impairment
No dose adjustment.

SIDE EFFECTS

Rare (less than 2%): Diarrhea, headache, dizziness, pruritus, rash.

ADVERSE EFFECTS/TOXIC REACTIONS

Hyperglycemia occurs rarely. May increase risk of *C.difficile*–associated diarrhea.

NURSING CONSIDERATIONS

BASELINE ASSESSMENT
Question history of GI disease, ulcers, GERD.

INTERVENTION/EVALUATION
Evaluate for therapeutic response (relief of GI symptoms). Question if GI discomfort,

P

nausea occur. Monitor for abdominal pain, diarrhea (with or without fever).

PATIENT/FAMILY TEACHING

• Report abdominal pain, diarrhea (with or without fever) that does not resolve; may indicate colon infection. • Avoid alcohol. • Swallow tablets whole; do not chew, crush, dissolve, or divide. • Best if given before breakfast. May give without regard to food.

PARoxetine

par-ox-e-teen
(Apo-PARoxetine ✦, Brisdelle, Novo-PARoxetine ✦, Paxil, Paxil CR, Pexeva)

■ **BLACK BOX ALERT** ■ Increased risk of suicidal thinking and behavior in children, adolescents, young adults 18–24 yrs with major depressive disorder, other psychiatric disorders.
Do not confuse PARoxetine with piroxicam, FLUoxetine or pyridoxine, or Paxil with Doxil, Plavix, PROzac, or Taxol.

◆CLASSIFICATION

PHARMACOTHERAPEUTIC: Selective serotonin reuptake inhibitor (SSRI). **CLINICAL:** Antidepressant, antiobsessive-compulsive, antianxiety.

USES

Treatment of major depressive disorder (MDD). Treatment of panic disorder, obsessive-compulsive disorder (OCD). Treatment of social anxiety disorder (SAD), generalized anxiety disorder (GAD), premenstrual dysphoric disorder (PMDD), post-traumatic stress disorder (PTSD). **(Brisdelle):** Treatment of moderate to severe vasomotor symptoms associated with menopause. **OFF-LABEL:** Social anxiety disorder in children, self-injurious behavior, treatment of depression and OCD in children.

PRECAUTIONS

Contraindications: Hypersensitivity to paroxetine. Concurrent use of MAOIs with or within 14 days of MAOIs intended to treat psychiatric disorders, initiation in pts treated with linezolid or methylene blue; concomitant use with thioridazine, pimozide. **(Brisdelle):** Pregnancy. **Cautions:** History of seizures, renal/hepatic impairment, pts with suicidal tendencies, elderly pts, narrow-angle glaucoma; avoid use in first trimester of pregnancy, alcohol use.

ACTION

Selectively blocks uptake of neurotransmitter serotonin at CNS neuronal presynaptic membranes, increasing its availability at postsynaptic receptor sites. **Therapeutic Effect:** Relieves depression, reduces obsessive-compulsive behavior, decreases anxiety.

PHARMACOKINETICS

Well absorbed from GI tract. Protein binding: 95%. Widely distributed. Metabolized in liver. Excreted in urine. Not removed by hemodialysis. **Half-life:** 24 hrs.

⌛ LIFESPAN CONSIDERATIONS

Pregnancy/Lactation: May impair reproductive function. Not distributed in breast milk. May increase risk of congenital malformations. **Children:** Safety and efficacy not established. **Elderly:** Age-related renal impairment may require dosage adjustment. Use caution.

INTERACTIONS

DRUG: May increase concentration, risk of toxicity of **tricyclic antidepressants (e.g., amitriptyline, doxepin). Triptans, lithium, traMADol** may increase risk of serotonin syndrome. **Aspirin, NSAIDs (e.g., ibuprofen, ketorolac, naproxen), warfarin** may increase risk of bleeding. **MAOIs (e.g., phenelzine, selegiline)** may cause confusion, agitation, severe seizures; increase risk of serotonin syndrome, hypertensive crises. **Thioridazine** may prolong QT interval. **HERBAL: Kava kava, St. John's wort, valerian** may increase CNS

---

depression, risk of serotonin syndrome. **FOOD:** None known. **LAB VALUES:** May decrease Hgb, Hct, WBC count.

AVAILABILITY (Rx)

Capsules (Brisdelle): 7.5 mg. **Oral Suspension (Paxil):** 10 mg/5 mL. **Tablets (Paxil, Pexeva):** 10 mg, 20 mg, 30 mg, 40 mg.

Tablets (Controlled-Release [Paxil CR]): 12.5 mg, 25 mg, 37.5 mg.

ADMINISTRATION/HANDLING

PO
• May give without regard to food. • Give with food, milk if GI distress occurs. • Scored tablet may be crushed. • Do not crush, break, dissolve, or divide controlled-release tablets.

INDICATIONS/ROUTES/DOSAGE

Depression
PO: *(Immediate-Release):* **ADULTS:** Initially, 20 mg/day. May increase by 10 mg/day at intervals of more than 1 wk. **Maximum:** 50 mg/day.
PO: *(Controlled-Release):* **ADULTS:** Initially, 25 mg/day. May increase by 12.5 mg/day at intervals of more than 1 wk. **Maximum:** 62.5 mg/day.

Generalized Anxiety Disorder (GAD)
PO: *(Immediate-Release):* **ADULTS:** Initially, 20 mg/day. May increase by 10 mg/day at intervals of more than 1 wk. Range: 20–50 mg/day.

Obsessive-Compulsive Disorder (OCD)
PO: *(Immediate-Release):* **ADULTS:** Initially, 20 mg/day. May increase by 10 mg/day at intervals of more than 1 wk. Range: 20–60 mg/day. Recommended dose: 40 mg/day.

Panic Disorder
PO: *(Immediate-Release):* **ADULTS:** Initially, 10–20 mg/day. May increase by 10 mg/day at intervals of more than 1 wk. Range: 10–60 mg/day.
PO *(Controlled-Release):* **ADULTS, ELDERLY:** Initially, 12.5 mg once daily. May increase by 12.5 mg/day at wkly intervals. **Maximum:** 75 mg/day.

Social Anxiety Disorder (SAD)
PO: *(Immediate-Release):* **ADULTS:** Initially, 20 mg/day. Range: 20–60 mg/day.
PO *(Controlled-Release):* **ADULTS, ELDERLY:** Initially, 12.5 mg once daily. May increase by 12.5 mg/day at wkly intervals. **Maximum:** 37.5 mg/day.

Post-Traumatic Stress Disorder (PTSD)
PO: *(Immediate-Release):* **ADULTS:** Initially, 20 mg/day. May increase by 10 mg/day at intervals of more than 1 wk. Range: 20–50 mg/day.

Premenstrual Dysphoric Disorder (PMDD)
PO: *(Controlled-Release):* **ADULTS:** Initially, 12.5 mg/day. May increase by 12.5 mg at wkly intervals. **Maximum:** 25 mg/day.

Vasomotor Symptoms
PO: **ADULTS:** *(Brisdelle):* 7.5 mg once daily at bedtime.

Usual Elderly Dosage
PO: Initially, 10 mg/day. May increase by 10 mg/day at intervals of more than 1 wk. **Maximum:** 40 mg/day.
PO *(Controlled-Release):* Initially, 12.5 mg/day. May increase by 12.5 mg/day at intervals of more than 1 wk. **Maximum:** 50 mg/day.

Dosage Renal/Hepatic Impairment
CrCl less than 30 mL/min, severe hepatic impairment. **Immediate-Release:** Initially, 10 mg/day. May increase by 10 mg/dose at wkly intervals. **Maximum:** 40 mg/day. **Extended-Release:** Initially, 12.5 mg/day. May increase by 12.5 mg/day at wkly intervals. **Maximum:** 50 mg/day. **Brisdelle:** No dosage adjustment.

SIDE EFFECTS

Frequent (26%–8%): Nausea, drowsiness, headache, dry mouth, asthenia, constipation, dizziness, insomnia, diarrhea, diaphoresis, tremor. **Occasional (6%–3%):** Decreased appetite, respiratory disturbance (e.g., increased cough), anxiety, flatulence, paresthesia, yawning, decreased libido, sexual dysfunction, abdominal discomfort. **Rare:** Palpitations, vomiting, blurred vision, altered taste, confusion.

P

✤ Canadian trade name   Non-Crushable Drug   High Alert drug

ADVERSE EFFECTS/TOXIC REACTIONS

Hyponatremia, seizures have been reported. Serotonin syndrome (agitation, confusion, diaphoresis, hallucinations, hyperreflexia) occurs rarely.

NURSING CONSIDERATIONS

BASELINE ASSESSMENT

Obtain baseline CBC, LFT, renal function test, serum sodium. Assess appearance, behavior, speech pattern, level of interest, mood.

INTERVENTION/EVALUATION

For pts on long-term therapy, CBC, LFT, renal function test should be performed periodically. Assess mental status for depression, suicidal ideation (esp. at beginning of therapy or change in dosage), anxiety, social functioning, panic attacks. Assess appearance, behavior, speech pattern, level of interest, mood.

PATIENT/FAMILY TEACHING

• May cause dry mouth. • Avoid alcohol, St. John's wort. • Therapeutic effect may be noted within 1–4 wks. • Do not abruptly discontinue medication. • Avoid tasks that require alertness, motor skills until response to drug is established. • May impair reproductive function. • Inform physician of intention for pregnancy or if pregnancy occurs. • Report worsening depression, suicidal ideation, unusual changes in behavior.

PAZOPanib

paz-**oh**-pa-nib
(Votrient)
■ **BLACK BOX ALERT** ■ Severe, fatal hepatotoxicity has been observed.

◆CLASSIFICATION

PHARMACOTHERAPEUTIC: Tyrosine kinase inhibitor. **CLINICAL:** Antineoplastic.

USES

Treatment of advanced renal cell carcinoma (RCC), advanced soft-tissue sarcoma (STS) (in pts previously treated with chemotherapy). **OFF-LABEL:** Advanced thyroid cancer.

PRECAUTIONS

Contraindications: Hypersensitivity to PAZOPanib. **Cautions:** Avoid use of strong CYP3A4 inhibitors (e.g., clarithromycin, ketoconazole) or CYP3A inducers (carBAMazepine, rifAMPin), and grapefruit products. Cautious use in pts with increased risk or history of arterial thrombotic events (e.g., angina, MI, ischemic stroke), QT prolongation, hypokalemia, hypomagnesemia, hypertension, severe hepatic impairment, history of hemoptysis, cerebral hemorrhage or significant GI hemorrhage. Concomitant use of medications that may prolong QT interval not recommended.

ACTION

Inhibits cell surface vascular endothelial growth factor receptors. **Therapeutic Effect:** Inhibits angiogenesis, blocks tumor growth.

PHARMACOKINETICS

Peak concentration occurs 2–4 hrs following oral administration. Metabolized in liver. Protein binding: greater than 99%. Excreted in feces (60%), urine (23%). **Half-life:** 31 hrs.

⊠ LIFESPAN CONSIDERATIONS

Pregnancy/Lactation: May cause fetal harm. Unknown if distributed in breast milk. **Children:** Safety and efficacy not established in pts younger than 18 yrs. **Elderly:** No age-related precautions noted.

INTERACTIONS

DRUG: **Famotidine, proton pump inhibitors** (e.g., **omeprazole, pantoprazole**) may decrease effect. **QT interval–prolonging medications** (e.g., **amiodarone, citalopram, dasatinib, haloperidol, levoFLOXacin,**

ondansetron) may prolong QT interval. **CYP3A4 inhibitors (e.g., clarithromycin, ketoconazole, ritonavir)** may increase concentration. **CYP3A4 inducers (e.g., carBAMazepine, phenytoin, rifAMPin)** may decrease concentration. **Simvastatin** may increase serum ALT. **Medications that increase gastric pH** may decrease concentration/effect. **HERBAL: St. John's wort** decreases concentration. **FOOD: Food** may increase concentration. **Grapefruit products** may increase concentration, potential for torsades de pointes, myelotoxicity. **LAB VALUES:** May decrease serum phosphorus, sodium, magnesium, glucose, WBC count. May increase serum ALT, AST.

AVAILABILITY (Rx)

Tablets: 200 mg.

ADMINISTRATION/HANDLING

PO
• Give at least 1 hr before or 2 hrs after ingestion of food. • Give tablets whole; do not break, crush, dissolve, or divide.

INDICATIONS/ROUTES/DOSAGE

Renal Cell Carcinoma, Soft-Tissue Sarcoma
PO: ADULTS, ELDERLY: 800 mg once daily. If concomitant CYP3A4 inhibitor cannot be discontinued, reduce initial dose to 400 mg/day.

Dose Adjustment for Toxicity
Prior to dose reduction, temporarily discontinue therapy if 24-hr urine protein 3 g or more (or for other toxicities). Initial dose reduction: Renal cell carcinoma: 400 mg/day. Soft tissue sarcoma: 600 mg/day. Further dose adjustment: 200 mg/day.

Dosage in Renal Impairment
No dose adjustment.

Dosage in Hepatic Impairment
Mild impairment: No dose adjustment. **Moderate impairment:** Reduce dose to 200 mg/day. **Severe impairment:** Not recommended.

SIDE EFFECTS

Frequent (52%–19%): Diarrhea, hypertension, hair color changes, nausea, fatigue, anorexia, vomiting. **Occasional (14%–10%):** Asthenia, abdominal pain, headache. **Rare (less than 10%):** Alopecia, chest pain, altered taste, dyspepsia, proteinuria, rash, decreased weight.

ADVERSE EFFECTS/TOXIC REACTIONS

Hepatotoxicity, manifested as increase in serum bilirubin, ALT, AST, has been observed and may be fatal. Hemorrhagic events (hematuria, epistaxis, hemoptysis, GI bleeding or perforation, intracranial hemorrhage) have been noted and may be fatal. Hypertension (B/P greater than 150/100 mm Hg) is common (47% of pts), usually occurring early in the first 18 wks of treatment. Hypothyroidism has been reported occasionally. Arterial thrombotic events (MI, CVA), QT prolongation, torsades de pointes have been seen rarely.

NURSING CONSIDERATIONS

BASELINE ASSESSMENT

Obtain baseline EKG, CBC, serum chemistries, LFT. Assess medical history, esp. hepatic impairment. Question history of hepatic impairment, arterial or venous thromboembolism, GI bleeding. Receive full medication history and screen for interactions.

INTERVENTION/EVALUATION

Monitor B/P, LFT periodically for elevations. Monitor CBC, serum chemistries for changes from baseline. Observe for hepatotoxicity (jaundice, dark-colored urine, unusual fatigue, right upper quadrant abdominal pain). Observe EKG for QT-interval prolongation. Monitor for evidence of bleeding, hemorrhage. Monitor daily pattern of bowel activity, stool consistency.

PATIENT/FAMILY TEACHING

• Avoid crowds, those with known infection. • Avoid contact with anyone who recently received live virus vaccine; do

P

not receive vaccinations. • Swallow tablets whole; do not chew, crush, dissolve, or divide. • No food should be taken at least 1 hr before and 2 hrs after dose is taken. • Avoid grapefruit products. • Report diarrhea, abdominal pain, yellowing of skin or sclera, discolored urine, fatigue. • Report bleeding of any kind, esp. bloody stools, nosebleeds, coughing up blood. • Treatment may increase risk of heart attack, stroke, blood clots, or heart arrhythmias.

---

pegfilgrastim

peg-fil-**gras**-tim
(<u>Neulasta</u>, Neulasta Onpro)
Do not confuse Neulasta with Lunesta, Neumega, or Neupogen.

◆CLASSIFICATION

PHARMACOTHERAPEUTIC: Colony-stimulating factor. **CLINICAL:** Hematopoietic, antineutropenic.

USES

Decreases incidence of infection (as manifested by febrile neutropenia) in cancer pts receiving myelosuppressive chemotherapy associated with febrile neutropenia. To increase survival in pts acutely exposed to myelosuppressive doses of radiation.

PRECAUTIONS

Contraindications: Hypersensitivity to pegfilgrastim, filgrastim. **Cautions:** Any malignancy with myeloid characteristics, sickle cell disease. The 6-mg fixed dose not to be used in infants, children, or adolescents weighing less than 45 kg. Do not administer within 14 days before and 24 hrs after cytotoxic chemotherapy.

ACTION

Regulates production of neutrophils within bone marrow. A glycoprotein, primarily affects neutrophil progenitor proliferation, differentiation, selected end-cell functional activation. **Therapeutic Effect:** Increases phagocytic ability, antibody-dependent destruction; decreases incidence of infection.

PHARMACOKINETICS

Readily absorbed after SQ administration. **Half-life:** 15–80 hrs.

⧗ LIFESPAN CONSIDERATIONS

Pregnancy/Lactation: Unknown if drug crosses placenta or is distributed in breast milk. **Children:** Safety and efficacy not established in children younger than 12 yrs. **Elderly:** No age-related precautions noted.

INTERACTIONS

DRUG: None significant. **HERBAL:** None significant. **FOOD:** None known. **LAB VALUES:** May increase serum LDH, alkaline phosphatase, uric acid.

AVAILABILITY (Rx)

Injection Solution: (Neulasta): 6 mg/0.6 mL syringe. **Prefilled Syringe Kit: (Neulasta Onpro):** 6 mg/0.6 mL); dose delivers over 45 min. time period about 27 hrs after application.

ADMINISTRATION/HANDLING

SQ

Storage • Store in refrigerator. Warm to room temperature prior to administering injection. • Administer to outer upper arms, abdomen (except within 2 inches of navel), front middle thigh or upper outer buttocks. Discard if left at room temperature for more than 48 hrs. • Protect from light. • Avoid freezing; but if accidentally frozen, may allow to thaw in refrigerator before administration. Discard if freezing takes place a second time. • Discard if discolored or precipitate forms.

On Body Injector (OnPro)

A health care provider must fill the injector prior to applying to pt's skin. Apply to intact, nonirritated skin on back of arms or abdomen. Delivers pegfilgrastim over

45 min. time period about 27 hrs after application. May apply on same day as chemotherapy. Keep injector at least 4 inches away from electrical equipment.

INDICATIONS/ROUTES/DOSAGE

Neutropenia (Chemotherapy-Induced)
SQ: ADULTS, ELDERLY, CHILDREN 12–17 YRS, WEIGHING MORE THAN 45 KG: Give as single 6-mg injection once per chemotherapy cycle beginning 24–72 hrs after completion of chemotherapy. ◀**ALERT**▶ Do not administer between 14 days before and 24 hrs after cytotoxic chemotherapy. Do not use in infants, children, adolescents weighing less than 45 kg.

Radiation Injury Syndrome
Note: Prefilled syringe not designed to give doses less than 6 mg. Not recommended; use caution to avoid dosing errors.
SQ: ADULTS, ELDERLY, CHILDREN WEIGHING 45 KG OR MORE: 6 mg once wkly for 2 doses. **31–44 KG:** 4 mg once wkly for 2 doses. **21–30 KG:** 2.5 mg once wkly for 2 doses. **10–20 KG:** 1.5 mg once wkly for 2 doses. **LESS THAN 10 KG:** 0.1 mg/kg once wkly for 2 doses.

Dosage in Renal/Hepatic Impairment
No dose adjustment.

SIDE EFFECTS

Frequent (72%–15%): Bone pain, nausea, fatigue, alopecia, diarrhea, vomiting, constipation, anorexia, abdominal pain, arthralgia, generalized weakness, peripheral edema, dizziness, stomatitis, mucositis, neutropenic fever.

ADVERSE EFFECTS/TOXIC REACTIONS

Allergic reactions (anaphylaxis, rash, urticaria) occur rarely. Cytopenia resulting from antibody response to growth factors occurs rarely. Splenomegaly occurs rarely. Severe sickle cell crisis reported in pts with sickle cell disease. Glomerulonephritis, capillary leak syndrome, tumor growth stimulatory effect on malignant cells, acute respiratory distress syndrome may occur.

NURSING CONSIDERATIONS

BASELINE ASSESSMENT

Obtain CBC prior to initiation and routinely thereafter. Question history of sickle cell disease, glomerulonephritis, splenic disease, hypersensitivity reaction to acrylic adhesive on body (injector uses acrylic adhesive).

INTERVENTION/EVALUATION

Monitor for allergic reactions. Assess for peripheral edema. Assess mucous membranes for evidence of stomatitis, mucositis. Assess muscle strength. Monitor daily pattern of bowel activity, stool consistency. Adult respiratory distress syndrome (ARDS) may occur in septic pts.

PATIENT/FAMILY TEACHING

• Inform pt of possible side effects, signs/symptoms of allergic reaction. • Counsel pt on importance of compliance with pegfilgrastim treatment, including regular monitoring of blood counts. • Report unusual fever or chills, severe bone pain, chest pain or palpitations.

pegloticase

peg-**loe**-ti-kase
(Krystexxa)

■ **BLACK BOX ALERT** ■ Severe infusion reactions, anaphylaxis (bronchospasm, stridor, urticaria, hypotension, dyspnea, flushing, circumoral swelling) have occurred, especially within 2 hrs of first infusion. Premedicate pt with corticosteroids, antihistamines. Should be administered in health care setting by health care providers prepared to manage infusion reactions.
Do not confuse pegloticase with Activase, cholinesterase, or pegaspargase.

◆**CLASSIFICATION**

PHARMACOTHERAPEUTIC: Uric acid enzyme. **CLINICAL:** Antigout agent.

✦ Canadian trade name　　🚫 Non-Crushable Drug　　🔲 High Alert drug

USES

Treatment of chronic gout in adult pts refractory to conventional therapy. Not recommended for treatment of asymptomatic hyperuricemia.

PRECAUTIONS

Contraindications: Hypersensitivity to pegloticase. Glucose-6-phosphate dehydrogenase (G6PD) deficiency due to hemodialysis, methemoglobinemia. **Cautions:** History of HF, elderly, debilitated.

ACTION

Decreases uric acid production by catalyzing oxidation of uric acid to allantoin, lowering serum uric acid. **Therapeutic Effect:** Lowers serum uric acid concentration.

PHARMACOKINETICS

Catalyzes oxidation of uric acid to allantoin, an inert and water-soluble purine metabolite. Readily eliminated, primarily by renal excretion. **Half-life:** 14.5 days.

⧗ LIFESPAN CONSIDERATIONS

Pregnancy/Lactation: Unknown if drug crosses placenta or is distributed in breast milk. **Children:** Safety and efficacy not established in pts younger than 18 yrs. **Elderly:** No age-related precautions noted.

INTERACTIONS

DRUG: None significant. **HERBAL:** None significant. **FOOD:** None known. **LAB VALUES:** Decreases serum uric acid (expected).

AVAILABILITY (Rx)

Injection Solution: 2-mL (8 mg/mL) single-use vials.

ADMINISTRATION/HANDLING

 IV

Reconstitution • Withdraw 1 mL from single-use vial and inject into 250 mL 0.9% NaCl or 0.45% NaCl. • Invert infusion bag a number of times to ensure thorough mixing; do not shake.
Rate of Administration • Infuse slowly over no less than 120 min.

Storage • Store in refrigerator. • Solution should appear clear; discard if particulate is present. • Allow diluted solution to reach room temperature prior to infusion. • Following dilution, solution remains stable for 4 hrs if refrigerated or at room temperature.

INDICATIONS/ROUTES/DOSAGE

◀**ALERT**▶ Give by IV infusion; do not give as IV push or IV bolus. Pt to be pretreated with corticosteroids, antihistamines to reduce risk of infusion reaction, anaphylaxis.

Gout
Note: Discontinue oral agents prior to initiating pegloticase and do not initiate during course of therapy.
IV Infusion: ADULTS, ELDERLY: 8 mg every 2 wks.

Dosage in Renal/Hepatic Impairment
No dose adjustment.

SIDE EFFECTS

Occasional (12%–9%): Nausea, ecchymosis at IV site, nasopharyngitis. **Rare (6%–5%):** Constipation, vomiting.

ADVERSE EFFECTS/TOXIC REACTIONS

Exacerbation of HF has been noted. Infusion-related reaction (urticaria, dyspnea, chest discomfort, chest pain, erythema, pruritus) occurs in 26% of pts; anaphylaxis occurs in 7% of pts. Increase in gout flares is frequently noted upon initiation of antihyperuricemic therapy due to changing serum uric acid levels.

NURSING CONSIDERATIONS

BASELINE ASSESSMENT

If gout flare occurs during treatment, prophylaxis with an NSAID or colchicine is recommended. Pts at higher risk for G6PD deficiency (e.g., pts of African or Mediterranean ancestry) should be screened for G6PD deficiency before starting therapy. Obtain serum uric acid levels prior to each infusion. If levels reach greater than 6 mg/dL, particularly when 2 consecutive levels greater than 6 mg/dL are observed, treatment should be discontinued.

INTERVENTION/EVALUATION

Monitor closely for infusion reaction during therapy and for 2 hrs post-treatment. If infusion reaction occurs during administration, infusion may be slowed, or stopped and restarted at slower rate. If severe infusion reaction occurs, discontinue infusion and institute treatment as needed. Assess for therapeutic response (reduced joint tenderness, swelling, redness, limitation of motion).

PATIENT/FAMILY TEACHING

• Educate pts on the most common signs and symptoms of infusion reaction (rash, redness of skin, difficulty breathing, flushing, chest discomfort, chest pain). • Advise pts to seek medical care immediately if they experience any symptoms of allergic reaction during or at any time after infusion.

pembrolizumab

pem-broe-**liz**-ue-mab
(Keytruda)
Do not confuse pembrolizumab with palivizumab.

◆CLASSIFICATION

PHARMACOTHERAPEUTIC: Monoclonal antibody. **CLINICAL:** Antineoplastic.

USES

Treatment of unresectable or metastatic melanoma. Treatment of metastatic head and neck squamous cell carcinoma (HN-SCC) with disease progression on or after platinum-containing chemotherapy. Treatment of metastatic non–small-cell lung (NSCL) cancer in pts with PD-L1–expressing tumors as a single agent for first line tx, with disease progression on or after platinum-containing chemotherapy;

or in combination with pemetrexed and carboplatin, as first line tx of metastatic non-squamous NSCLC. Treatment of refractory classical Hodgkin lymphoma (cHL) or relapse after 3 or more lines of therapy. Treatment of locally advanced or metastatic urothelial carcinoma not eligible for cisplatin containing chemotherapy or who have disease progression during or following platinum-containing chemotherapy; or with 12 mos of neoadjuvant or adjuvant tx with platinum containing chemotherapy. Treatment of unresectable or metastatic microsatellite instability high (MSI-H) or mismatch repair deficient solid tumors or colorectal cancer. Treatment of gastric cancer (advanced or metastatic) or gastroesophageal junction adenocarcinoma whose tumor expess PD-L1 with disease progression on or after 2 or more lines of therapy.

PRECAUTIONS

Contraindications: Hypersensitivity to pembrolizumab. **Cautions:** Thyroid disease, hepatic/renal impairment, interstitial lung disease, electrolyte imbalance, hypertriglyceridemia.

ACTION

Binds PD-1 ligands to PD-1 receptor found on T cells, blocking its interaction with the ligands (PD-L1 and PD-L2). Releases PD-1 pathway–mediated inhibition of immune response (including antitumor immune response). **Therapeutic Effect:** Inhibits T-cell proliferation and cytokine production.

PHARMACOKINETICS

Information on metabolism and elimination not available. Steady-state concentration: 18 wks. **Half-life:** 26 days.

⧗ LIFESPAN CONSIDERATIONS

Pregnancy/Lactation: Avoid pregnancy; may cause fetal harm. Unknown if distributed in breast milk. Must either discontinue drug or discontinue breastfeeding. Recommend effective contraception during treatment and up to 4 mos after discontinuation. **Children:** Safety and efficacy not established. **Elderly:** No age-related precautions noted.

INTERACTIONS

DRUG: None known. **HERBAL:** None significant. **FOOD:** None known. **LAB VALUES:** May increase serum AST, glucose, triglycerides. May decrease albumin, serum calcium, sodium.

AVAILABILITY (Rx)

Injection, Lyophilized Powder for Reconstitution: 50 mg/vial. **Injection solution:** 100 mg/4 mL.

ADMINISTRATION/HANDLING

 IV

◀ **ALERT** ▶ Use 0.2–0.5-micron in-line filter.

Reconstitution • Verify weight in kg. • Inject 2.3 mL of Sterile Water for Injection against glass wall of vial. Do not inject directly onto lyophilized powder. • Gently swirl contents until completely dissolved; do not shake. • Allow vial to stand for up to 5 min for bubbles to clear. • Visually inspect for particulate matter. • Do not use if extraneous particulate matter other than translucent to white protein-like particles observed. • Final concentration of reconstituted vial equals 25 mg/mL. • Withdraw required dose and mix into 0.9% NaCl infusion bag (diluent volume depends on dose required). • Final concentration of diluent bag should equal 1–10 mg/mL. • Allow refrigerated solution to warm to room temperature before infusing.

Rate of Administration • Infuse via dedicated line over 30 min using a 0.2–0.5-micron filter.

Storage • Reconstituted solution should appear clear to slightly opalescent, colorless to slightly yellow. • Refrigerate reconstituted or diluted solution up to 24 hrs, or at room temperature up to 4 hrs. Store time should not exceed total combined time of reconstitution, dilution, storage, and infusion.

INDICATIONS/ROUTES/DOSAGE

cHL, MSI-H Cancer:

IV: ADULTS, ELDERLY: 200 mg q3wks.
CHILDREN: 2 mg/kg (up to 200 mg) q3wks until disease progression or unacceptable toxicity.

NSCL, HNSCC, Melanoma, Urothelial Cancer, Gastric Cancer

IV: ADULTS, ELDERLY: 200 mg q3wks. Continue until disease progression or unacceptable toxicity, or in pts without disease progression for up to 24 months.

Dose Modification

Based on Common Terminology Criteria for Adverse Events (CTCAE).
Withhold treatment for any of the following adverse events: ALT or AST greater than 3–5 times upper limit of normal (ULN) or bilirubin 1.5–3 times ULN, grade 2 or 3 colitis, grade 3 hyperthyroidism, grade 2 nephritis, grade 2 pneumonitis, symptomatic hypophysitis; any grade 3 treatment-related adverse reaction. **Permanently discontinue for any of the following adverse events:** ALT or AST greater than 5 times ULN or bilirubin 3 times ULN (or pts with liver metastasis who begin treatment with grade 2 ALT, AST, if ALT or AST increases greater than or equal to 50% from baseline and lasts for at least 1 wk), grade 3 or 4 infusion-related reaction, grade 3 or 4 nephritis, grade 3 or 4 pneumonitis; inability to reduce corticosteroid dose to 10 mg/day or less (or predniSONE equivalent) after last dose; persistent grade 2 or 3 adverse reaction that does not recover to grade 0–1 within 12 wks after last dose; any severe or grade 3 treatment-related adverse reaction that reoccurs.

Dosage in Renal Impairment
No dose adjustment.

Dosage in Hepatic Impairment
Mild impairment: No dose adjustment.
Moderate to severe impairment: Not studied, use caution.

SIDE EFFECTS

Frequent (47%–20%): Fatigue, nausea, cough, pruritus, rash, decreased appetite, constipation, diarrhea, arthralgia. **Occasional (18%–11%):** Dyspnea, extremity pain, peripheral edema, vomiting, headache, chills, insomnia, myalgia, abdominal pain, back pain, pyrexia, vitiligo, dizziness, upper respiratory tract infection.

ADVERSE EFFECTS/TOXIC REACTIONS

May cause severe immune-mediated events such as pneumonitis (2.9% of pts), colitis (1% of pts), hepatitis (0.5% of pts), hypophysitis (0.5% of pts), renal failure or nephritis (0.7% of pts), hyperthyroidism (1.2% of pts), hypothyroidism (8.3% of pts). Other reported events include adrenal insufficiency, arthritis, cellulitis, exfoliative dermatitis, hemolytic anemia, myositis, myasthenic syndrome, pancreatitis, partial seizures, pneumonia, optic neuritis, rhabdomyolysis, sepsis. Immunogenicity (anti-pembrolizumab antibody formation) may occur.

NURSING CONSIDERATIONS

BASELINE ASSESSMENT

Obtain baseline CBC, BMP, ionized calcium, LFT, TSH, free T_4, vital signs, urine pregnancy. Obtain weight in kg. Screen for history of adrenal/pituitary/pulmonary/thyroid disease, autoimmune disorders, hepatic/renal impairment, allergy to predniSONE. Question plans for breastfeeding. Along with routine assessment, conduct full dermatologic exam, visual acuity.

INTERVENTION/EVALUATION

Monitor CBC, LFT, serum electrolytes; thyroid panel if applicable. Monitor for immune-mediated adverse events. Notify physician if any CTCAE toxicities occur (see Appendix M) and initiate proper treatment. Obtain chest X-ray if pneumonitis suspected. Screen for tumor lysis syndrome in pts with high tumor burden. Offer antiemetics if nausea, vomiting occurs. Monitor I&O, daily weight. If predniSONE therapy initiated, monitor capillary blood glucose and screen for corticosteroid side effects.

PATIENT/FAMILY TEACHING

• Blood levels will be routinely monitored. • Avoid pregnancy; treatment may cause birth defects or miscarriage. Do not breastfeed. • Serious adverse reactions may affect lungs, GI tract, kidneys, or hormonal glands, and predniSONE therapy may need to be started. • Immediately contact physician if serious or life-threatening inflammatory reactions occur in the following body systems: lung (chest pain, cough, shortness of breath); colon (severe abdominal pain or diarrhea); liver (bruising, clay-colored/tarry stools, yellowing of skin or eyes); pituitary (persistent or unusual headache, dizziness, extreme weakness, fainting, vision changes); kidney (decreased or dark-colored urine, flank pain); thyroid (insomnia, hypertension, tachycardia [overactive thyroid]), (fatigue, goiter, weight gain [underactive thyroid]).

PEMEtrexed

pem-e-**trex**-ed
(Alimta)
Do not confuse PEMEtrexed with methotrexate or PRALAtrexate.

◆CLASSIFICATION

PHARMACOTHERAPEUTIC: Antimetabolite. **CLINICAL:** Antineoplastic.

USES

Treatment of unresectable malignant pleural mesothelioma in combination with CISplatin. Initial treatment of locally advanced or metastatic non–squamous non–small-cell lung cancer (NSCLC) in combination with CISplatin. Single-agent maintenance treatment of NSCLC in pts whose disease has not progressed following 4 cycles of platinum-based first-line chemotherapy. **OFF-LABEL:** Treatment of bladder, cervical, ovarian, thymic malignancies; malignant pleural mesothelioma.

P

◆ Canadian trade name   Non-Crushable Drug   High Alert drug

PRECAUTIONS

Contraindications: Severe hypersensitivity to PEMEtrexed. **Cautions:** Hepatic/renal impairment, concurrent use of nephrotoxic medications, preexisting myelosuppression. Not indicated for squamous cell NSCLC.

ACTION

Disrupts folate-dependent enzymes essential for cell replication. **Therapeutic Effect:** Inhibits growth of mesothelioma cell lines.

PHARMACOKINETICS

Protein binding: 81%. Not metabolized. Excreted in urine. **Half-life:** 3.5 hrs.

⧗ LIFESPAN CONSIDERATIONS

Pregnancy/Lactation: Unknown if drug crosses placenta or is distributed in breast milk. Breastfeeding not recommended. May cause fetal harm. Not recommended during pregnancy. **Children:** Safety and efficacy not established in pts younger than 18 yrs. **Elderly:** Higher incidence of fatigue, leukopenia, neutropenia, thrombocytopenia in pts 65 yrs and older.

INTERACTIONS

DRUG: NSAIDs (e.g., ibuprofen, ketorolac, naproxen) may increase concentration/effects. **Bone marrow depressants** may increase risk of myelosuppression. **Live virus vaccines** may potentiate virus replication, increase vaccine side effects, decrease pt's antibody response to vaccine. **HERBAL: Echinacea** may decrease effects. **FOOD:** None known. **LAB VALUES:** May increase serum ALT, AST, creatinine.

AVAILABILITY (Rx)

Injection, Powder for Reconstitution: 100 mg; 500 mg.

ADMINISTRATION/HANDLING

 IV Infusion

Reconstitution • Dilute 500-mg vial with 20 mL (4.2 mL to 100-mg vial) 0.9% NaCl to provide concentration of 25 mg/mL. • Gently swirl each vial until powder is completely dissolved. • Solution appears clear and ranges in color from colorless to yellow or green-yellow. • Further dilute reconstituted solution with 100 mL 0.9% NaCl.
Rate of Administration • Infuse over 10 min.
Storage • Store at room temperature. • Diluted solution is stable for up to 24 hrs at room temperature or if refrigerated.

▩ IV INCOMPATIBILITIES

Use only 0.9% NaCl to reconstitute; flush line prior to and following infusion. Do not add any other medications to IV line.

INDICATIONS/ROUTES/DOSAGE

Refer to individual protocols.
◀ALERT▶ Pretreatment with dexamethasone (or equivalent) will reduce risk, severity of cutaneous reaction; treatment with folic acid and vitamin B_{12} beginning 1 wk before treatment and continuing for 21 days after last PEMEtrexed dose will reduce risk of side effects. Do not begin new treatment cycles unless ANC 1,500 cells/mm³ or greater, platelets 100,000 cells/mm³ or greater, and CrCl 45 mL/min or greater.

Malignant Pleural Mesothelioma
IV: ADULTS, ELDERLY: 500 mg/m² on day 1 of each 21-day cycle in combination with CISplatin.

Nonsquamous Non–Small-Cell Lung Cancer (NSCLC)
IV: ADULTS, ELDERLY: Initial treatment 500 mg/m² on day 1 of each 21-day cycle (in combination with CISplatin). **Maintenance or second-line treatment:** 500 mg/m² on day 1 of each 21-day cycle (as single agent).

Dose Modification for Toxicity
Hematologic Toxicity
Nadir ANC less than 500 cells/mm³ and platelets 50,000 cells/mm³ or more: Reduce dose to 75% of previous dose. **Nadir platelets less than 50,000 cells/mm³ without bleeding:** Reduce

P

dose to 75% of previous dose. **Nadir platelets less than 50,000 cells/mm³ with bleeding:** Reduce dose to 50% of previous dose. **Nonhematologic toxicity grade 3 or greater (excluding neurotoxicity):** Reduce dose to 75% of previous dose (excluding mucositis). **Grade 3 or 4 mucositis:** Reduce dose to 50% of previous dose.

Dosage in Renal Impairment
Not recommended with CrCl less than 45 mL/min.

Dosage in Hepatic Impairment
Grade 3 (5.1–20 times upper limit of normal) or grade 4 (greater than 20 times upper limit of normal): 75% of previous dose.

SIDE EFFECTS

Frequent (12%–10%): Fatigue, nausea, vomiting, rash, desquamation. **Occasional (8%–4%):** Stomatitis, pharyngitis, diarrhea, anorexia, hypertension, chest pain. **Rare (less than 3%):** Constipation, depression, dysphagia.

ADVERSE EFFECTS/TOXIC REACTIONS

Myelosuppression, characterized as grade 1–4 neutropenia, thrombocytopenia, anemia, was reported.

NURSING CONSIDERATIONS

BASELINE ASSESSMENT
Question for possibility of pregnancy before initiating therapy. Obtain CBC, serum chemistry tests before therapy and at regular intervals throughout therapy.

INTERVENTION/EVALUATION
Monitor Hgb, Hct, WBC, platelet count, renal/hepatic function. Monitor for hematologic toxicity (fever, sore throat, signs of local infection, unusual bruising/bleeding from any site), symptoms of anemia (excessive fatigue, weakness). Assess skin for evidence of dermatologic toxicity. Keep pt well hydrated, urine alkaline. Monitor WBC count for nadir, recovery.

PATIENT/FAMILY TEACHING
• Maintain strict oral hygiene. • Do not have immunizations without physician's approval (drug lowers resistance). • Avoid crowds, those with infection. • Use contraceptive measures during therapy. • Promptly report fever, sore throat, signs of local infection, unusual bruising/bleeding from any site. • Do not breastfeed.

penicillin G potassium

pen-i-**sil**-in G po-**tas**-ee-um
(Crystapen ♣, Pfizerpen)
Do not confuse penicillin with penicillAMINE.

◆CLASSIFICATION

PHARMACOTHERAPEUTIC: Penicillin. **CLINICAL:** Antibiotic.

USES

Treatment of susceptible infections including sepsis, meningitis, endocarditis, pneumonia. Active against gram-positive organisms (except *S. aureus*), some gram-negative organisms (e.g., *N. gonorrhoeae*), and some anaerobes and spirochetes.

PRECAUTIONS

Contraindications: Hypersensitivity to any penicillin. **Cautions:** Renal/hepatic impairment, seizure disorder, hypersensitivity to cephalosporins, pts with asthma.

ACTION

Inhibits bacterial cell wall synthesis by binding to one or more of the penicillin-binding proteins of bacteria. **Therapeutic Effect:** Bactericidal.

PHARMACOKINETICS

Protein binding: 60%. Widely distributed (poor CNS penetration). Metabolized in liver. Primarily excreted in urine. **Half-life:** 0.5–1 hr (increased in renal impairment).

⧖ LIFESPAN CONSIDERATIONS

Pregnancy/Lactation: Readily crosses placenta; distributed in breast milk. **Children:** May delay renal excretion in neonates, young infants. **Elderly:** Age-related renal impairment may require dosage adjustment.

INTERACTIONS

DRUG: Probenecid increases concentration. **HERBAL:** None significant. **FOOD:** None significant. **LAB VALUES:** May cause positive Coombs' test. May increase serum ALT, AST, alkaline phosphatase, LDH. May decrease WBC count.

AVAILABILITY (Rx)

Injection, Powder for Reconstitution: 5 million units.

ADMINISTRATION/HANDLING

 IV

Reconstitution • After reconstitution, further dilute with 50–100 mL D_5W or 0.9% NaCl for final concentration of 100,000–500,000 units/mL (50,000 units/mL for infants, neonates).
Rate of Administration • Infuse over 15–30 min.
Storage • Reconstituted solution is stable for 7 days if refrigerated.

▥ IV INCOMPATIBILITIES

DOPamine (Intropin), sodium bicarbonate.

▥ IV COMPATIBILITIES

Amiodarone (Cordarone), calcium gluconate, diltiaZEM (Cardizem), heparin, magnesium sulfate, potassium chloride.

INDICATIONS/ROUTES/DOSAGE

Usual Dosage
IV, IM: ADULTS, ELDERLY: 12–24 million units/day in divided doses q4–6h. **CHILDREN:** 100,000–300,000 units/kg/day in divided doses q4–6h. **Maximum:** 24 million units/day. **NEONATES:** 25,000–50,000 units/kg/dose q8–12h.

Dosage in Renal Impairment
Dosage interval is modified based on creatinine clearance.

Creatinine Clearance	Dosage
Greater than 50 mL/min	No dose adjustment
10–50 mL/min	75% normal dose
Less than 10 mL/min	20%–50% normal dose
Hemodialysis:	50%–100% normal dose q8–12h
Continuous renal replacement therapy	
Continuous venovenous hemofiltration:	Loading dose 4 million units, then 2 million units q4–6h
Continuous venovenous hemodialysis:	Loading dose 4 million units, then 2–3 million units q4–6h
Continuous venovenous hemodiafiltration:	Loading dose 4 million units, then 2–4 million units q4–6h

Dosage in Hepatic Impairment
No dose adjustment.

SIDE EFFECTS

Occasional: Lethargy, fever, dizziness, rash, electrolyte imbalance, diarrhea, thrombophlebitis. **Rare:** Seizures, interstitial nephritis.

ADVERSE EFFECTS/TOXIC REACTIONS

Hypersensitivity reactions ranging from rash, fever, chills to anaphylaxis occur occasionally.

NURSING CONSIDERATIONS

BASELINE ASSESSMENT

Question for history of allergies, particularly penicillins, cephalosporins.

INTERVENTION/EVALUATION

Promptly report rash (hypersensitivity), diarrhea (with fever, abdominal pain,

P

mucus, or blood in stool, may indicate antibiotic-associated colitis). Monitor I&O, urinalysis electrolytes, renal function tests for nephrotoxicity.

penicillin V potassium

pen-i-**sil**-in V po-**tas**-ee-um
(Apo-Pen-VK ✦, Novo-Pen-VK ✦, NuPen VK ✦)

◆CLASSIFICATION

PHARMACOTHERAPEUTIC: Penicillin. **CLINICAL:** Antibiotic.

USES

Treatment of infections of respiratory tract, skin/skin structure, otitis media, necrotizing ulcerative gingivitis; prophylaxis for rheumatic fever, dental procedures. **OFF-LABEL:** Prosthetic joint infection.

PRECAUTIONS

Contraindications: Hypersensitivity to any penicillin. **Cautions:** Severe renal impairment, history of allergies (particularly cephalosporins), history of seizures, asthma.

ACTION

Inhibits cell wall synthesis by binding to bacterial cell membranes. **Therapeutic Effect:** Bactericidal.

PHARMACOKINETICS

Moderately absorbed from GI tract. Protein binding: 80%. Widely distributed. Metabolized in liver. Primarily excreted in urine. **Half-life:** 1 hr (increased in renal impairment).

⧗ LIFESPAN CONSIDERATIONS

Pregnancy/Lactation: Readily crosses placenta; appears in cord blood, amniotic fluid. Distributed in breast milk in low concentrations. May lead to allergic sensitization, diarrhea, candidiasis, skin rash in infant. **Children:** Use caution in neonates and young infants (may delay renal elimination). **Elderly:** Age-related renal impairment may require dosage adjustment.

INTERACTIONS

DRUG: ACE inhibitors (e.g., enalapril, lisinopril), potassium-sparing diuretics (e.g., spironolactone), potassium supplements may increase risk of hyperkalemia. May increase **methotrexate** concentration, toxicity. **Probenecid** may increase concentration, risk of toxicity. **Tetracycline** may decrease concentration/effect. **HERBAL:** None significant. **FOOD:** None known. **LAB VALUES:** May cause positive Coombs' test. May increase serum ALT, AST, alkaline phosphatase, LDH. May decrease WBC count.

AVAILABILITY (Rx)

Powder for Oral Solution: 125 mg/5 mL, 250 mg/5 mL. **Tablets:** 250 mg, 500 mg.

ADMINISTRATION/HANDLING

PO
• Give on empty stomach 1 hr before or 2 hrs after meals (increases absorption). • After reconstitution, oral solution is stable for 14 days if refrigerated. • Space doses evenly around the clock.

INDICATIONS/ROUTES/DOSAGE

Usual Dosage
PO: ADULTS, ELDERLY, CHILDREN 12 YRS AND OLDER: 125–500 mg q6–8h. **CHILDREN YOUNGER THAN 12 YRS:** 25–75 mg/kg/day in divided doses q6–8h. **Maximum:** 2,000 mg/day.

Dosage in Renal/Hepatic Impairment
No dose adjustment.

SIDE EFFECTS

Frequent: Mild hypersensitivity reaction (chills, fever, rash), nausea, vomiting, diarrhea. **Rare:** Bleeding, allergic reaction.

P

✦ Canadian trade name   🗪 Non-Crushable Drug   🄷🄸 High Alert drug

ADVERSE EFFECTS/TOXIC REACTIONS

Severe hypersensitivity reactions, including anaphylaxis, may occur. Nephrotoxicity, antibiotic-associated colitis, other superinfections (abdominal cramps, severe watery diarrhea, fever) may result from high dosages, prolonged therapy.

NURSING CONSIDERATIONS

BASELINE ASSESSMENT

Question for history of allergies, particularly penicillins, cephalosporins.

INTERVENTION/EVALUATION

Hold medication, promptly report rash (hypersensitivity), diarrhea (with fever, abdominal pain, mucus or blood in stool may indicate antibiotic-associated colitis). Be alert for superinfection: fever, vomiting, diarrhea, anal/genital pruritus, oral mucosal change (ulceration, pain, erythema). Review Hgb levels; check for bleeding (overt/occult bleeding, ecchymosis, swelling of tissue). Monitor I&O, urinalysis, renal function tests for nephrotoxicity.

PATIENT/FAMILY TEACHING

• Continue antibiotic for full length of treatment. • Space doses evenly. • Report immediately if rash, diarrhea, bleeding, bruising, other new symptoms occur.

perampanel

per-**am**-pa-nel
(Fycompa)

■ **BLACK BOX ALERT** ■ Risk for serious neuropsychiatric events, including irritability, aggression, anger, anxiety, paranoia, euphoric mood, agitation, mental status changes. Some of these events reported as serious and life-threatening. Violent thoughts or threatening behavior were also observed. Immediately report any changes in mood or behavior that are not typical for the patient. Health care professionals should closely monitor patients during titration period when higher doses are used.

◆CLASSIFICATION

PHARMACOTHERAPEUTIC: Noncompetitive AMPA glutamate receptive antagonist. **CLINICAL:** Anticonvulsant.

USES

Treatment of partial-onset seizures with or without secondary generalized seizures. Adjunctive therapy for the treatment of primary generalized tonic-clonic seizures.

PRECAUTIONS

Contraindications: Hypersensitivity to perampanel. **Cautions:** Elderly (increased falls, dizziness, gait disturbances), severe renal/hepatic impairment, dialysis, concurrent use of CNS depressants, pts at risk for suicidal behavior.

ACTION

Noncompetitive antagonist of AMPA glutamate receptors, a primary excitatory neurotransmitter on postsynaptic neurons. **Therapeutic Effect:** Reduces frequency of seizure activity.

PHARMACOKINETICS

Rapidly, completely absorbed. Peak concentration: 0.5–2.5 hrs. Protein binding: 95%–96%. Steady-state reached in 2–3 wks. Metabolized via oxidation/glucuronidation. Excreted in feces (48%), urine (22%). **Half-life:** 105 hrs.

⧗ LIFESPAN CONSIDERATIONS

Pregnancy/Lactation: Unknown if distributed in breast milk. Use caution when breastfeeding. **Children:** Safety and efficacy not established in pts younger than 12 yrs. **Elderly:** Due to increased risk of adverse reactions in the elderly, dosing titration should proceed very slowly.

INTERACTIONS

DRUG: CYP450 inducers (e.g., carBA-Mazepine, OXcarbazepine, phenytoin) may decrease concentration/effects. May decrease effectiveness of **hormonal contraceptives containing levonorgestrel. Alcohol, other CNS depressants (e.g., LORazepam, morphine, zolpidem)** may increase CNS depression. **HERBAL:** St. John's wort, kava kava, valerian may increase CNS depression. **Evening primrose** may decrease seizure threshold. **FOOD:** None known. **LAB VALUES:** None significant.

AVAILABILITY (Rx)

🦫 **Suspension, Oral:** 0.5 mg/mL. **Tablets, Film-Coated:** 2 mg, 4 mg, 6 mg, 8 mg, 10 mg, 12 mg.

ADMINISTRATION/HANDLING

PO
• Give at bedtime. • Give tablet whole; do not break, crush, dissolve, or divide tablet. • Measure oral suspension using provided adapter and dosing syringe.

INDICATIONS/ROUTES/DOSAGE

◀**ALERT**▶ Initial starting dose should be increased when enzyme-inducing anticonvulsants are given concurrently. Individual dosing based on clinical response, tolerability. Do not use in severe hepatic/renal impairment, pts on hemodialysis.

Partial-Onset Seizures, Generalized Tonic-Clonic Seizures in Absence of an Enzyme-Inducing Anticonvulsant
PO: ADULTS, ELDERLY, CHILDREN 12 YRS AND OLDER: Initially, 2 mg once daily at bedtime. May titrate in 2-mg increments at wkly intervals (in elderly, no more frequently than every 2 wks). **Recommended maintenance dose:** (Partial Seizures): 8–12 mg/day at bedtime. (Tonic-Clonic Seizures): 8 mg/day at bedtime.

Partial-Onset Seizures, Generalized Tonic-Clonic Seizures (Concurrently Taking an Enzyme-Inducing Anticonvulsant)
PO: ADULTS, ELDERLY, CHILDREN 12 YRS AND OLDER: Initially, 4 mg once daily at bedtime. May titrate in 2-mg increments at wkly intervals (in elderly, no more frequently than

q2wks). **Recommended maintenance dose:** 8–12 mg/day at bedtime.

Dosage in Renal Impairment
CrCl less than 30 mL/min: Not recommended.

Dosage in Hepatic Impairment
PO: ADULTS, ELDERLY, CHILDREN 12 YRS AND OLDER: 2 mg once daily with wkly increase of 2 mg daily q2wks until target dose is achieved. **Mild impairment: Maximum:** 6 mg. **Moderate impairment: Maximum:** 4 mg. **Severe impairment:** Not recommended.

SIDE EFFECTS

Frequent (32%–11%): Dizziness, sleepiness, headache. **Occasional (8%–3%):** Fatigue, irritability, nausea, balance disorder, weight gain, gait disturbance, vertigo, blurred vision, vomiting, arthralgia, anxiety. **Rare (2%–1%):** Constipation, back pain, extremity pain, asthenia, oropharyngeal pain, aggression.

ADVERSE EFFECTS/TOXIC REACTIONS

Irritability, aggression, anger, anxiety, affect lability, agitation occurred rarely (2% of pts). Increased risk for seizures when anticonvulsants are withdrawn abruptly.

NURSING CONSIDERATIONS

BASELINE ASSESSMENT
Review history of seizure disorder (intensity, frequency, duration, LOC). Initiate seizure precautions. Obtain medication history (esp. use of other anticonvulsant therapy; dosage based on concurrent seizure medication). Observe clinically. Assist with ambulation until response to drug is established (32% of pts experience dizziness).

INTERVENTION/EVALUATION
Assess mental status, cognitive abilities, behavioral changes. Monitor for clinical response, tolerability to medication, dosing level during treatment and for at least 1 mo after last therapy dose. Report persistent,

severe, or worsening psychiatric symptoms or behaviors. Assess for clinical improvement (decrease in intensity, frequency of seizures).

PATIENT/FAMILY TEACHING

• Avoid alcohol (greater risk for adverse effects). • The combination of alcohol and perampanel may significantly worsen mood, increase anger. • Counsel pts, families, and caregivers of need to monitor for emergence of anger, aggression, hostility, unusual changes in mental status. • Avoid tasks that require alertness, motor skills until response to drug is established (greater risk for dizziness, sleepiness).

---

pertuzumab

per-**tue**-zue-mab
(Perjeta)

■ **BLACK BOX ALERT** ■ Can result in embryo-fetal death, birth defects. Pts must be made aware of danger to fetus, need for effective contraception. May result in cardiac failure. Assess left ventricular ejection fraction.

◆CLASSIFICATION

PHARMACOTHERAPEUTIC: *HER2* receptor antagonist. **CLINICAL:** Antineoplastic.

USES

Treatment of *HER2*-positive metastatic breast cancer in pts who have not received prior anti-*HER2* therapy or chemotherapy for metastatic disease in combination with trastuzumab and DOCEtaxel. Neoadjuvant treatment of pts with *HER2*-positive, locally advanced inflammatory, or early-stage breast cancer in combination with trastuzumab and DOCEtaxel.

PRECAUTIONS

Contraindications: Hypersensitivity to pertuzumab. **Cautions:** Conditions that may impair left ventricular function (e.g., uncontrolled hypertension, recent MI, severe cardiac arrhythmia), history of infusion-related reaction. Prior anthracycline therapy or irradiation.

ACTION

Targets human epidermal growth factor 2 (*HER2*), blocking ligand-initiated intercellular signaling, which can result in cell growth arrest and cell death. **Therapeutic Effect:** Inhibits cell growth and metastasis.

PHARMACOKINETICS

Peak plasma concentration reached after first maintenance dose. **Half-life:** 18 days.

⌛ LIFESPAN CONSIDERATIONS

Pregnancy/Lactation: May cause embryo-fetal harm. Females of reproductive potential must use effective contraception in addition to barrier methods. Unknown if distributed in breast milk. **Children:** Safety and efficacy not established. **Elderly:** No age-related precautions noted.

INTERACTIONS

DRUG: None significant. **HERBAL:** None significant. **FOOD:** None known. **LAB VALUES:** None significant.

AVAILABILITY (Rx)

Injection Solution: 420 mg/14 mL (30 mg/mL) vial.

ADMINISTRATION/HANDLING

🖐 IV

Reconstitution • Withdraw ordered volume of solution from vial. • Dilute into 250 mL 0.9% NaCl only (do not use D₅W). • Gently invert solution (do not shake).
Rate of Administration • Initial dose to be infused over 60 min. • Subsequent doses may be infused over 30–60 min.
Storage • Refrigerate vials. Store vials in outside cartons (protects from light).

• Once diluted, use immediately or refrigerate for up to 24 hrs. • Do not use if solution appears cloudy or contains particulate.

▓ IV INCOMPATIBILITIES

Do not mix with any other medications.

INDICATIONS/ROUTES/DOSAGE

◀ALERT▶ Give as an IV infusion only. Do not give by IV push or bolus. If diluted solution is not used immediately, may refrigerate for up to 24 hrs.

Breast Carcinoma
IV Infusion: ADULTS/ELDERLY: Initially, 840 mg given over 60 min, followed q3wks thereafter by 420 mg given as a 30–60 min infusion for 3–6 cycles in combination with trastuzumab and DOCEtaxel. Continue until disease progression or unacceptable toxicity.

Breast Cancer (Neoadjuvant)
IV Infusion: ADULTS, ELDERLY: 840 mg once followed by 420 mg q3wks for 3–6 cycles. May be administered as: 4 preoperative cycles of pertuzumab, trastuzumab, DOCEtaxel, then 3 postoperative cycles of 5-fluorouracil, epiRUBicin, and cyclophosphamide (FEC) **or** 3 preoperative cycles of FEC alone, then 3 preoperative cycles of pertuzumab, trastuzumab, DOCEtaxel **or** 6 cycles of pertuzumab, trastuzumab, DOCEtaxel, and CARBOplatin. **Note:** Continue trastuzumab postoperatively to complete 1 yr of treatment.

Dosage in Renal/Hepatic Impairment
No dose adjustment.

SIDE EFFECTS

Frequent (67%–21%): Diarrhea, alopecia, nausea, fatigue, rash, peripheral neuropathy, anorexia, asthenia, mucosal inflammation, vomiting, peripheral edema, myalgia, nail disorder, headache. **Occasional (19%–12%):** Stomatitis, pyrexia, dysgeusia, arthralgia, constipation, increased lacrimation, pruritus, insomnia, dizziness. **Rare**

(10%–7%): Nasopharyngitis, dry skin, paronychia.

ADVERSE EFFECTS/TOXIC REACTIONS

Neutropenia occurs in 53% of pts, anemia occurs in 23% of pts, and leukopenia occurs in 18% of pts. Upper respiratory tract infection occurs in 17% of pts. Dyspnea, febrile neutropenia occurs in 14% of pts. Pleural effusion occurs in 5% of pts, left ventricular dysfunction occurs in 4% of pts.

NURSING CONSIDERATIONS

BASELINE ASSESSMENT
Obtain baseline left ventricular ejection fraction (LVEF) before initiating therapy. Negative pregnancy test must be confirmed before initiating treatment. Obtain *HER2* testing by an FDA-approved laboratory. Assess daily serum blood chemistries, CBC.

INTERVENTION/EVALUATION
Monitor daily ANC. Monitor LVEF and withhold dosing if ordered. Assess skin, IV site for infusion-associated reactions, hypersensitivity reactions, anaphylaxis. If a significant infusion-associated reaction occurs, slow or interrupt infusion and administer appropriate medical treatment. If a reaction is noted, the most common is pyrexia. Chills, fatigue, headache, asthenia, or vomiting usually occurs during the infusion or on the same day as the infusion. Observe pt closely for 60 min after the first infusion and for 30 min after subsequent infusions. Offer antiemetics if nausea occurs.

PATIENT/FAMILY TEACHING
• Avoid pregnancy. • Use effective contraceptive measures, including condoms, during treatment and for 6 mos after treatment in women of childbearing potential. • If pregnancy occurs, inform physician immediately. • Do not breastfeed. • Alopecia is reversible, but new hair growth may have different color, texture.

P

PHENobarbital

fee-noe-**bar**-bi-tal
**Do not confuse PHENobarbital
with pentobarbital, Phenergan,
or phenytoin.**

FIXED-COMBINATION(S)

Donnatal: PHENobarbital/atropine
(an anticholinergic)/hyoscyamine (an
anticholinergic)/scopolamine (an
anticholinergic): 16.2 mg/0.0194
mg/0.1037 mg/0.0065 mg.

◆CLASSIFICATION

PHARMACOTHERAPEUTIC: Barbiturate **(Schedule IV). CLINICAL:** Anticonvulsant, hypnotic.

USES

Management of generalized tonic-clonic
(grand mal) seizures, partial seizures,
control of acute seizure episodes (status
epilepticus). **OFF-LABEL:** Treatment of
alcohol withdrawal, sedative/hypnotic
withdrawal.

PRECAUTIONS

Contraindications: Hypersensitivity to
PHENobarbital, other barbiturates, porphyria, dyspnea or airway obstruction,
use in nephritic pts (large doses), severe
hepatic impairment. Pts with history
of sedative/hypnotic addiction. Intra-
arterial or subcutaneous administration. **Cautions:** Renal/hepatic impairment, acute/chronic pain, depression,
suicidal tendencies, history of drug
abuse, elderly pts, debilitated pts, children, hemodynamically unstable pts,
hypoadrenalism, respiratory disease.

ACTION

Depresses sensory cortex, decreases
motor activity, alters cerebellar function. **Therapeutic Effect:** Induces
drowsiness, sedation, anticonvulsant
activity.

PHARMACOKINETICS

Route	Onset	Peak	Duration
PO	20–60 min	N/A	6–10 hrs
IV	5 min	30 min	4–10 hrs

Well absorbed after PO, parenteral administration. Protein binding: 20%–45%.
Rapidly and widely distributed. Metabolized in liver. Primarily excreted in
urine. Removed by hemodialysis. **Half-
life:** 53–140 hrs.

⌛ LIFESPAN CONSIDERATIONS

Pregnancy/Lactation: Readily
crosses placenta. Distributed in breast
milk. Produces respiratory depression
in neonates during labor. May cause
postpartum hemorrhage, hemorrhagic
disease in newborn. Withdrawal symptoms may appear in neonates born to
women receiving barbiturates during
last trimester of pregnancy. Lowers
serum bilirubin in neonates. **Children:** May cause paradoxical excitement. **Elderly:** May exhibit excitement,
confusion, mental depression. Use caution.

INTERACTIONS

**DRUG: Alcohol, other CNS depres-
sants (e.g., LORazepam, morphine)** may increase effects. May
decrease effects of **warfarin, oral
contraceptives. Valproic acid** may
increase concentration, risk of toxicity.
HERBAL: Evening primrose may decrease seizure threshold. **Gotu kola,
kava kava, St. John's wort, valerian** may increase CNS depression.
FOOD: None known. **LAB VALUES:** May
decrease serum bilirubin. **Therapeutic serum level:** 10–40 mcg/mL;
toxic serum level: greater than 40
mcg/mL.

AVAILABILITY (Rx)

Elixir: 20 mg/5 mL. **Oral Solution:** 20
mg/5 mL. **Injection, Solution:** 65 mg/
mL, 130 mg/mL. **Tablets:** 15 mg, 30 mg,
60 mg, 100 mg.

P

ADMINISTRATION/HANDLING

 IV

Reconstitution • May give undiluted or may dilute with NaCl.

Rate of Administration • Adequately hydrate pt before and immediately after drug therapy (decreases risk of adverse renal effects). • Do not inject IV faster than 30 mg/min for children and 60 mg/min for adults. Too-rapid IV may produce severe hypotension, marked respiratory depression. • Inadvertent intra-arterial injection may result in arterial spasm with severe pain, tissue necrosis. Extravasation in SQ tissue may produce redness, tenderness, tissue necrosis.

Storage • Store vials at room temperature.

IM

• Do not inject more than 5 mL in any one IM injection site (produces tissue irritation). • Inject deep IM into large muscle mass.

PO

• Give without regard to meals. • Tablets may be crushed. • Elixir may be mixed with water, milk, fruit juice.

IV INCOMPATIBILITIES

Amphotericin B complex (Abelcet, AmBisome, Amphotec).

IV COMPATIBILITIES

Calcium gluconate, enalapril (Vasotec), fosphenytoin (Cerebyx), propofol (Diprivan).

INDICATIONS/ROUTES/DOSAGE

Status Epilepticus
IV: ADULTS, ELDERLY, CHILDREN: 20 mg/kg. May repeat once in 10 min with a dose of 5–10 mg/kg. **CHILDREN:** 20 mg/kg (**Maximum:** 1,000 mg) over 10 min; may repeat after 15 min (**Maximum dose:** 40 mg/kg).

Seizure Control (Maintenance)
Note: Maintenance dose usually starts 12 hrs after loading dose.

PO, IV: ADULTS, ELDERLY, CHILDREN OLDER THAN 12 YRS: 1–3 mg/kg/day. **CHILDREN 5–12 YRS:** 4–6 mg/kg/day in divided doses. **CHILDREN 1–5 YRS:** 6–8 mg/kg/day in divided doses. **CHILDREN YOUNGER THAN 1 YR:** 5–8 mg/kg/day in 1–2 divided doses. **NEONATES:** 3–4 mg/kg/day given once daily.

Dosage in Renal/Hepatic Impairment
No dose adjustment.

SIDE EFFECTS

Occasional (3%–1%): Drowsiness. **Rare (less than 1%):** Confusion, paradoxical CNS reactions (hyperactivity, anxiety in children; excitement, restlessness in elderly, generally noted during first 2 wks of therapy, particularly in presence of uncontrolled pain).

ADVERSE EFFECTS/TOXIC REACTIONS

Abrupt withdrawal after prolonged therapy may produce increased dreaming, nightmares, insomnia, tremor, diaphoresis, vomiting, hallucinations, delirium, seizures, status epilepticus. Skin eruptions appear as hypersensitivity reaction. Blood dyscrasias, hepatic disease, hypocalcemia occur rarely. Overdose produces cold/clammy skin, hypothermia, severe CNS depression, cyanosis, tachycardia, Cheyne-Stokes respirations. Toxicity may result in severe renal impairment.

NURSING CONSIDERATIONS

BASELINE ASSESSMENT

Assess B/P, pulse, respirations immediately before administration. **Hypnotic:** Raise bed rails, provide environment conducive to sleep (back rub, quiet environment, low lighting). **Seizures:** Review history of seizure disorder (length, presence of auras, LOC). Observe for recurrence of seizure activity. Initiate seizure precautions.

INTERVENTION/EVALUATION

Monitor CNS status, seizure activity, hepatic/renal function, respiratory rate,

P

heart rate, B/P. Monitor for therapeutic serum level. Neurological assessments may be inaccurate until drug has properly cleared the body. **Therapeutic serum level:** 10–40 mcg/mL; **toxic serum level:** greater than 40 mcg/mL.

PATIENT/FAMILY TEACHING

• Avoid alcohol, limit caffeine. • May be habit-forming. • Do not discontinue abruptly. • May cause dizziness/drowsiness; avoid tasks that require alertness, motor skills until response to drug is established.

---

phenylephrine

fen-il-**ef**-rin

(AK-Dilate, Mydfrin, Neo-Synephrine, Sudafed PE)

■ **BLACK BOX ALERT** ■ Intravenous use should be administered by adequately trained individuals familiar with its use.

Do not confuse Mydfrin with Midrin, or Sudafed PE with Sudafed.

◆CLASSIFICATION

PHARMACOTHERAPEUTIC: Alpha-adrenergic agonist. **CLINICAL:** Nasal decongestant, mydriatic, vasopressor.

USES

Nasal decongestant: Topical application to nasal mucosa reduces nasal secretion, promoting drainage of sinus secretions. **Parenteral:** Vascular failure in shock, supraventricular tachycardia, hypotension.

PRECAUTIONS

Contraindications: Hypersensitivity to phenylephrine. **Injection:** Severe hypertension, ventricular tachycardia. **Oral:** Use within 14 days of MAOI therapy.

Cautions: Injection: Elderly, hyperthyroidism, bradycardia, partial heart block, cardiac disease, HF, cardiogenic shock, hypertension. **Oral:** Asthma, bowel obstruction, cardiac disease, ischemic heart disease, hypertension, increased intraocular pressure, elderly, prostatic hyperplasia.

ACTION

Acts on alpha-adrenergic receptors of vascular smooth muscle. Causes vasoconstriction of arterioles of nasal mucosa/conjunctiva; produces systemic arterial vasoconstriction. **Therapeutic Effect:** Decreases mucosal blood flow, relieves congestion. Increases B/P. Reduces heart rate due to decrease in cardiac output.

PHARMACOKINETICS

Route	Onset	Peak	Duration
IV	Immediate	N/A	15–20 min
IM	10–15 min	N/A	0.5–2 hrs
SQ	10–15 min	N/A	1 hr

Minimal absorption after intranasal, ophthalmic administration. Metabolized in liver, GI tract. Primarily excreted in urine. **Half-life:** 2.5 hrs.

⌛ LIFESPAN CONSIDERATIONS

Pregnancy/Lactation: Crosses placenta. Distributed in breast milk. **Children:** May exhibit increased absorption, toxicity with nasal preparation. No age-related precautions noted with systemic use. **Elderly:** More likely to experience adverse effects.

INTERACTIONS

DRUG: MAOIs (e.g., phenelzine, selegiline) may increase vasopressor effects. **Tricyclic antidepressants (e.g., amitriptyline, doxepin)** may increase cardiovascular effects. **HERBAL: Ephedra, yohimbe** may increase CNS stimulation. **FOOD:** None known. **LAB VALUES:** None significant.

AVAILABILITY (OTC)

Injection, Solution: 10 mg/mL. **Solution, Nasal Drops (Neo-Synephrine):** 0.125%, 0.25%. **Solution, Nasal Spray (Neo-Synephrine):** 0.25%, 0.5%. **Solution, Oral:** 2.5 mg/5 mL. **Tablets (Sudafed PE):** 10 mg.

ADMINISTRATION/HANDLING

 IV

Reconstitution • For IV push, dilute 1 mL of 10 mg/mL solution with 9 mL Sterile Water for Injection to provide concentration of 1 mg/mL. • For IV infusion, dilute 10–100 mg with 500 mL 0.9% NaCl or D₅W.

Rate of Administration • For IV push, give over 20–30 sec. • For IV infusion, titrate dose to maintain systolic B/P greater than 90 mm Hg.

Storage • Store vials at room temperature.

Nasal

• Instruct pt to blow nose prior to administering medication. • With head tilted back, apply drops in 1 nostril. Wait 5 min before applying drops in other nostril. • Sprays should be administered into each nostril with head erect. • Pt should sniff briskly while squeezing container, then wait 3–5 min before blowing nose gently. • Rinse tip of spray bottle.

🔲 IV INCOMPATIBILITY

Furosemide (Lasix).

🔲 IV COMPATIBILITIES

Amiodarone (Cordarone), dexmedetomidine (Precedex), DOBUTamine (Dobutrex), lidocaine, potassium chloride, propofol (Diprivan), vasopressin.

INDICATIONS/ROUTES/DOSAGE

Nasal Decongestant
◀ **ALERT** ▶ Do not use for more than 3 days.

Intranasal: ADULTS, ELDERLY, CHILDREN 12 YRS AND OLDER: 2-3 drops or 2-3 sprays of 0.25%–0.5% solution into each nostril q4h as needed. **CHILDREN 6–11 YRS:** 2-3 drops or 2-3 sprays of 0.25% solution into each nostril q4h as needed. **CHILDREN 2–5 YRS:** 1 drop of 0.125% solution (dilute 0.5% solution with 0.9% NaCl to achieve 0.125%) in each nostril. Repeat q2–4h as needed.

PO: ADULTS, ELDERLY, CHILDREN 13 YRS AND OLDER: 10 mg q4h as needed for up to 7 days. **CHILDREN 6–11 YRS:** 5 mg q4h as needed for up to 7 days. **CHILDREN 4–5 YRS:** 2.5 mg q4h as needed for up to 7 days.

Hypotension, Shock
IV Bolus: ADULTS, ELDERLY: 100–500 mcg (0.1–0.5 mg)/dose q10–15min as needed. **CHILDREN:** 5–20 mcg/kg/dose q10–15min as needed.

IV Infusion: ADULTS, ELDERLY: 100–180 mcg/min or 0.5 mcg/kg/min. Titrate to desired response. **CHILDREN:** 0.1–0.5 mcg/kg/min. Titrate to desired effect.

SIDE EFFECTS

Frequent: Nasal: Rebound nasal congestion due to overuse, esp. when used longer than 3 days. **Occasional:** Mild CNS stimulation (restlessness, nervousness, tremors, headache, insomnia, particularly in those hypersensitive to sympathomimetics, such as elderly pts). **Nasal:** Stinging, burning, drying of nasal mucosa.

ADVERSE EFFECTS/TOXIC REACTIONS

Large doses may produce tachycardia, palpitations (particularly in pts with cardiac disease), dizziness, nausea, vomiting. Overdose in pts older than 60 yrs may result in hallucinations, CNS depression, seizures. Prolonged nasal use may produce chronic swelling of nasal mucosa, rhinitis. If phenylephrine 10% ophthalmic is instilled into denuded/damaged corneal epithelium, corneal clouding may result.

P

NURSING CONSIDERATIONS

BASELINE ASSESSMENT

Obtain baseline symptomology, vital signs. Question history of hypertension, cardiac disease, asthma, recent use of MAOI therapy.

INTERVENTION/EVALUATION

Monitor B/P, heart rate. For severe hypotension or shock states, monitor central venous pressure noninvasive hemodynamic monitoring systems.

PATIENT/FAMILY TEACHING

• Discontinue drug if adverse reactions occur. • Do not use for nasal decongestion for longer than 3 days (rebound congestion). • Discontinue drug if insomnia, dizziness, weakness, tremor, palpitations occur. • **Nasal:** Stinging/burning of nasal mucosa may occur. • **Ophthalmic:** Blurring of vision with eye instillation generally subsides with continued therapy. • Discontinue medication if redness/swelling of eyelids, itching occurs.

---

phenytoin

fen-i-toyn
(Dilantin, Novo-Phenytoin ✦, Phenytek)

■ **BLACK BOX ALERT** ■ Do not exceed IV rate of 50 mg/min in adults and 1–3 mg/kg/min in pediatric pts. **Do not confuse Dilantin with Dilaudid or diltiaZEM, or phenytoin with phenelzine or fosphenytoin.**

◆CLASSIFICATION

PHARMACOTHERAPEUTIC: Hydantoin. **CLINICAL:** Anticonvulsant, antiarrhythmic.

USES

Management of generalized tonic-clonic seizures (grand mal), complex partial seizures, status epilepticus. Prevention of seizures following head trauma/neurosurgery. **OFF-LABEL:** Prevention of early post-traumatic seizures following traumatic brain injury.

PRECAUTIONS

Contraindications: Hypersensitivity to phenytoin, other hydantoins. Concurrent use of delavirdine. **IV (additional):** Second- and third-degree AV block, sinoatrial block, sinus bradycardia, Adams-Stokes syndrome. **Cautions:** Porphyria, renal/hepatic impairment, those at increased risk of suicidal behavior/thoughts, elderly/debilitated pts, low serum albumin, cardiac disease, hypothyroidism, pts of Asian descent.

ACTION

Anticonvulsant: Stabilizes neuronal membranes in motor cortex. Decreases influx of sodium during generation of nerve impulses. **Therapeutic Effect:** Decreases seizure activity.

PHARMACOKINETICS

Slowly, variably absorbed after PO administration. Protein binding: 90%–95%. Widely distributed. Metabolized in liver. Primarily excreted in urine. Not removed by hemodialysis. **Half-life:** 7–42 hrs.

⌧ LIFESPAN CONSIDERATIONS

Pregnancy/Lactation: Crosses placenta; distributed in small amount in breast milk. Fetal hydantoin syndrome (craniofacial abnormalities, nail/digital hypoplasia, prenatal growth deficiency) has been reported. Increased frequency of seizures in pregnant women due to altered absorption of metabolism of phenytoin. May increase risk of hemorrhage in neonate, maternal bleeding during delivery. **Children:** More susceptible to gingival hyperplasia, coarsening of facial features; excess body hair. **Elderly:** No age-related precautions noted but lower dosages recommended.

INTERACTIONS

DRUG: Alcohol, other CNS depressants (e.g., LORazepam, morphine, zolpidem) may increase CNS depression.

Amiodarone, cimetidine, disulfiram, FLUoxetine, isoniazid, sulfonamides may increase concentration/effects, risk of toxicity. **Calcium-containing antacids** may decrease absorption. May decrease effects of **glucocorticoids** (e.g., **dexamethasone, predniSONE**), **anticoagulants** (e.g., **heparin, warfarin**), oral contraceptives. **Lidocaine, propranolol** may increase cardiac depressant effects. **Valproic acid** may decrease metabolism, increase concentration. May increase metabolism, decrease effects of **xanthines**. **HERBAL: Evening primrose** may decrease seizure threshold. **Gotu kola, kava kava, St. John's wort, valerian** may increase CNS depression. **FOOD:** None known. **LAB VALUES:** May increase serum glucose, GGT, alkaline phosphatase. **Therapeutic serum level:** 10–20 mcg/mL; **toxic serum level:** greater than 20 mcg/mL.

AVAILABILITY (Rx)

Capsules, Extended-Release: 30 mg, 100 mg, 200 mg, 300 mg. **Injection, Solution:** 50 mg/mL. **Suspension, Oral:** 125 mg/5 mL. **Tablets, Chewable:** 50 mg.

ADMINISTRATION/HANDLING

🖢 IV

◀ **ALERT** ▶ Give by IV push or IV piggyback. IV push very painful (chemical irritation of vein due to alkalinity of solution). To minimize effect, flush vein with sterile saline solution through same IV needle and catheter after each IV push.
Reconstitution • May give undiluted or may dilute with 0.9% NaCl to a concentration of 5 mg/mL or more.
Rate of Administration • Administer 50 mg over 1 min in adults, 20 mg/min in elderly, pts with preexisting cardiovascular conditions. In neonates, administer at rate not exceeding 1–3 mg/kg/min. • Infuse diluted solutions using an in-line filter. • Severe hypotension, cardiovascular collapse occur if rate of IV injection exceeds 50 mg/min for adults. • IV toxicity characterized by CNS depression, cardiovascular collapse.
Storage • Precipitate may form if parenteral form is refrigerated (will dissolve at room temperature). • Slight yellow discoloration of parenteral form does not affect potency, but do not use if solution is cloudy or precipitate forms. Discard if not used within 4 hrs of preparation.

PO
• Give with food if GI distress occurs. • Tablets may be chewed. • Shake oral suspension well before using. • Separate administration of phenytoin with antacids or tube feeding by 2 hrs.

🔲 IV INCOMPATIBILITIES

DiltiaZEM (Cardizem), DOBUTamine (Dobutrex), enalapril (Vasotec), heparin, HYDROmorphone (Dilaudid), insulin, lidocaine, morphine, nitroglycerin, norepinephrine (Levophed), potassium chloride, propofol (Diprivan).

INDICATIONS/ROUTES/DOSAGE

Status Epilepticus
IV: ADULTS, ELDERLY, ADOLESCENTS: Loading dose: 20 mg/kg at maximum rate of 50 mg/min. May repeat in 10 min after loading dose with dose of 5–10 mg/kg. **INFANTS, CHILDREN:** Loading dose: 20 mg/kg at maximum rate of 1 mg/kg/min. May give additional dose of 5–10 mg/kg after loading dose.

Seizure Control (Maintenance)
Note: Loading dose not used in pts with history of renal/hepatic disease.
PO: ADULTS, ELDERLY: Loading Dose: 1 g divided into 3 doses given at 2-hr intervals. **Maintenance** (begins 24 hrs after loading dose): Initially 100 mg 3 times/day; adjust at no less than 7–10-day intervals. Usual dose: 100 mg 3–4 times/day up to 200 mg 3 times/day (may consider 300 mg once daily in pts established on 100 mg 3 times/day). **CHILDREN:** Initially, 5 mg/kg/day in 2–3 divided doses. Adjust dose at 7- to 10-day intervals. **Maintenance:** 4–8 mg/kg/day. **Maximum:** 300 mg/day.

P

Dosage in Renal/Hepatic Impairment
No dose adjustment.

SIDE EFFECTS

Frequent: Drowsiness, lethargy, confusion, slurred speech, irritability, gingival hyperplasia, hypersensitivity reaction (fever, rash, lymphadenopathy), constipation, dizziness, nausea. **Occasional:** Headache, hirsutism, coarsening of facial features, insomnia, muscle twitching.

ADVERSE EFFECTS/TOXIC REACTIONS

Abrupt withdrawal may precipitate status epilepticus. Blood dyscrasias, lymphadenopathy, osteomalacia (due to interference of vitamin D metabolism) may occur. Toxic phenytoin blood concentration (25 mcg/mL or more) may produce ataxia, nystagmus, diplopia. As level increases, extreme lethargy to comatose state occurs.

NURSING CONSIDERATIONS

BASELINE ASSESSMENT

Anticonvulsant: Review history of seizure disorder (intensity, frequency, duration, LOC). Initiate seizure precautions. LFT, CBC should be performed before beginning therapy and periodically during therapy. Repeat CBC 2 wks following initiation of therapy and 2 wks following administration of maintenance dose.

INTERVENTION/EVALUATION

Observe frequently for recurrence of seizure activity. Monitor ECG for cardiac arrhythmia. Assess for clinical improvement (decrease in intensity/frequency of seizures). Monitor for signs/symptoms of depression, suicidal tendencies, unusual behavior. Monitor CBC with differential, renal function, LFT, B/P (with IV use). Assist with ambulation if drowsiness, lethargy occurs. Monitor for therapeutic serum level (10–20 mcg/mL). **Therapeutic serum level:** 10–20 mcg/mL; **toxic serum level:** greater than 20 mcg/mL. **Free unbound levels: Therapeutic:** 1–2 mcg/mL; **toxic:** more than 2 mcg/mL.

PATIENT/FAMILY TEACHING

• Pain may occur with IV injection. • To prevent gingival hyperplasia (bleeding, tenderness, swelling of gums), maintain good oral hygiene, gum massage, regular dental visits. • Serum levels should be performed every mo for 1 yr after maintenance dose is established and q3mos thereafter. • Report sore throat, fever, glandular swelling, skin reaction (hematologic toxicity). • Drowsiness usually diminishes with continued therapy. • Avoid tasks that require alertness, motor skills until response to drug is established. • Do not abruptly withdraw medication after long-term use (may precipitate seizures). • Strict maintenance of drug therapy is essential for seizure control, arrhythmias. • Avoid alcohol. • Report any unusual changes in behavior.

phosphates potassium sodium

fos-fates

◆CLASSIFICATION

PHARMACOTHERAPEUTIC: Electrolyte supplement. **CLINICAL:** Mineral.

USES

Prevention and treatment of hypophosphatemia.

PRECAUTIONS

Contraindications: (K-phosphate): Hyperkalemia, hyperphosphatemia, hypocalcemia. **(Na-phosphate):** Hypocalcemia, hypernatremia, hyperphosphatemia. **Cautions:** Renal impairment, concomitant use of potassium-sparing drugs, acid-base alteration, digitalized pts, cardiac disease, metabolic alkalosis.

ACTION

Active in bone deposition, calcium metabolism, utilization of B complex vitamins. Act as buffers in maintaining acid-base balance. Exert osmotic effect in small intestine. **Therapeutic Effect:** Correct hypophosphatemia, acidify urine, prevent calcium deposits in urinary tract, promote peristalsis in GI tract.

PHARMACOKINETICS

Poorly absorbed after PO administration. PO form excreted in feces; IV form excreted in urine.

⧗ LIFESPAN CONSIDERATIONS

Pregnancy/Lactation: Use caution in pregnant women with other medical conditions (e.g., preeclampsia). **Children:** Increased risk of dehydration in pts younger than 12 yrs. **Elderly:** No age-related precautions noted.

INTERACTIONS

DRUG: ACE inhibitors (e.g., enalapril, lisinopril), NSAIDs (e.g., ibuprofen, ketorolac, naproxen), potassium-containing medications, potassium-sparing diuretics (e.g., spironolactone, triamterene), salt substitutes containing potassium phosphate may increase serum potassium. **Antacids** may decrease absorption. **Calcium-containing medications** may increase risk of calcium deposition in soft tissues, decrease phosphate absorption. **HERBAL:** None significant. **FOOD:** None known. **LAB VALUES:** None significant.

AVAILABILITY (Rx)

Injection Solution (Potassium Phosphate): 3 mmol phosphate and 4.4 mEq potassium per mL. **Injection Solution (Sodium Phosphate):** 3 mmol phosphate and 4 mEq sodium per mL.

ADMINISTRATION/HANDLING

🖐 IV

Reconstitution • Must be diluted. Soluble in all commonly used IV solutions.

Rate of Administration • Infuse over minimum of 4 hrs (usually over 6 hrs). **Maximum rate:** 0.06 mmol/kg/hr. **Storage** • Store at room temperature.

▦ IV INCOMPATIBILITY

Amiodarone, DOBUTamine (Dobutrex), pantoprazole (Protonix).

▦ IV COMPATIBILITIES

DiltiaZEM (Cardizem), enalapril (Vasotec), famotidine (Pepcid), metoclopramide (Reglan), niCARdipine (Cardene).

INDICATIONS/ROUTES/DOSAGE

Note: **(K-Phosphate):** For each mmol of phosphate, 1.5 mEq of K will be given. **(Na-Phosphate):** For each mmol of phosphate, 1.3 mEq of Na will be given.

Hypophosphatemia
Potassium/Sodium Phosphate: (Phosphate level 2.3–3 mg/dL): 0.16–0.32 mmol/kg over 4–6 hr. (Phosphate level 1.6–2.2 mg/dL): 0.32–0.64 mmol/kg over 4–6 hr. (Phosphate level <1.5 mg/dL): 0.64–1 mmol/kg over 8–12 hr.

SIDE EFFECTS

Frequent: Mild laxative effect (in first few days of therapy). **Occasional:** Diarrhea, nausea, abdominal pain, vomiting. **Rare:** Headache, dizziness, confusion, heaviness of lower extremities, fatigue, muscle cramps, paresthesia, peripheral edema, arrhythmias, weight gain, thirst.

ADVERSE EFFECTS/TOXIC REACTIONS

Hyperphosphatemia may produce extraskeletal calcification.

NURSING CONSIDERATIONS

BASELINE ASSESSMENT

Obtain BMP, serum phosphate, ionized calcium. Question history of renal impairment, cardiac disease. Receive full medication history and screen for interactions. Assess hydration status.

P

 Canadian trade name   🐄 Non-Crushable Drug   ⬛ High Alert drug

INTERVENTION/EVALUATION

Routinely monitor serum calcium, phosphorus, potassium, sodium, ALT, AST, alkaline phosphatase, bilirubin.

PATIENT/FAMILY TEACHING

• Report diarrhea, nausea, vomiting.

---

pimavanserin

pim-a-**van**-ser-in
(Nuplazid)
Do not confuse pimavanserin with eplivanserin, flibanserin, or pravastatin, or Nuplazid with Neulasta or Neupogen.

◆CLASSIFICATION

PHARMACOTHERAPEUTIC: Second-generation (atypical) antipsychotic. **CLINICAL:** Antipsychotic.

USES

Treatment of hallucinations and delusions associated with Parkinson's disease psychosis.

PRECAUTIONS

Contraindications: Hypersensitivity to pimavanserin. **Cautions:** Concomitant use of strong CYP3A4 inhibitors, strong CYP3A4 inducers. History of orthostatic hypotension, hepatic impairment. Avoid use in pts with history of cardiac arrhythmias, symptomatic bradycardia; conditions predisposing to sudden cardiac failure, torsades de pointes (congenital long QT syndrome, medications known to prolong QT interval, HF; hypokalemia, hypomagnesemia). Not approved for dementia-related psychosis unrelated to the hallucinations and delusions associated with Parkinson's disease psychosis.

ACTION

Exact mechanism unknown. Displays agonist and antagonist activity with high affinity for 5-HT$_{2A}$ receptors and low affinity to 5-HT$_{2C}$ receptors. **Therapeutic Effect:** Produces tranquilizing effect. Reduces symptoms of psychosis.

PHARMACOKINETICS

Widely distributed. Metabolized in liver. Protein binding: 95%. Peak plasma concentration: 6 hrs (range: 4–24 hrs). Excreted in feces (less than 2%), urine (less than 1%). **Half-life:** 57 hrs.

⧖ LIFESPAN CONSIDERATIONS

Pregnancy/Lactation: Unknown if distributed in breast milk. **Children:** Safety and efficacy not established. **Elderly:** No age-related precautions noted.

INTERACTIONS

DRUG: QT interval–prolonging medications (e.g., amiodarone, FLUoxetine, haloperidol, moxifloxacin, sotalol) may increase risk of QT interval prolongation. **Strong CYP3A inducers (e.g., carBAMazepine, PHENobarbital, rifAMPin)** may decrease concentration/effect. **Strong CYP3A inhibitors (e.g., clarithromycin, ketoconazole, ritonavir)** may increase concentration/effects. **HERBAL: St. John's wort** may decrease concentration/effect. **FOOD:** None known. **LAB VALUES:** None known.

AVAILABILITY (Rx)

Tablets: 17 mg.

ADMINISTRATION/HANDLING

PO
• Give without regard to food.

INDICATIONS/ROUTES/DOSAGE

Parkinson's Disease Psychosis
PO: ADULTS, ELDERLY: 34 mg (two 17-mg tablets) once daily.

Dose Modification
Concomitant use of strong CYP3A4 inhibitors: 17 mg once daily.
Concomitant use of strong CYP3A4 inducers: 34 mg once daily (dosage increase may be necessary due to reduced effectiveness).

Dosage in Renal Impairment
Mild to moderate impairment: No
dose adjustment. **Severe impairment:**
Not recommended.

Dosage in Hepatic Impairment
Not recommended.

SIDE EFFECTS

Occasional (7%–4%): Peripheral edema,
confusion, hallucinations (auditory, tac-
tile, somatic, visual), constipation. **Rare
(2%):** Gait disturbance.

ADVERSE EFFECTS/TOXIC REACTIONS

May increase risk of death in pts with
dementia-related psychosis. Drug-related
deaths were reported in 5% of pts and
were mainly cardiovascular (e.g., sudden
death, cardiac failure) or infectious (e.g.,
pneumonia) in nature. May prolong QT
interval. May increase risk for cardiac arrhythmias.

NURSING CONSIDERATIONS

BASELINE ASSESSMENT

Obtain vital signs, EKG. Assess behavior,
appearance, emotional status, response
to environment, speech pattern, thought
content. Therapy is intended only for
Parkinson's disease psychosis. Screen
pts for dementia-related psychosis. Receive full medication history and screen
for interactions. Question history of
cardiac arrhythmias, symptomatic bradycardia, HF, QT interval prolongation,
heart block.

INTERVENTION/EVALUATION

Monitor pulse rate. Obtain orthostatic vital
signs. Assess for therapeutic response
(interest in surroundings, improvement in self-care, increased ability to
concentrate, relaxed facial expressions).
Monitor for chest pain, sudden dizziness, syncope. Monitor EKG for cardiac
arrhythmias, QT interval prolongation,
torsades de pointes. Obtain serum potassium, magnesium in pts with EKG

abnormalities and replace electrolytes
as appropriate. Monitor for reduced effectiveness in pts taking concomitant
CYP3A4 inducers.

PATIENT/FAMILY TEACHING

• Do not abruptly withdraw from long-
term therapy. • Drowsiness may subside
after continued therapy. • Avoid tasks
that require alertness, motor skills until
response to drug established. • Go
slowly from lying to standing. • Avoid
alcohol. • Use caution when taking
other drugs that depress the central nervous system. • Do not take newly prescribed medications unless approved by
prescriber who originally started therapy. • Do not take herbal products.
• Therapy may cause life-threatening cardiac arrhythmias. Seek immediate medical
attention if chest pain, dizziness, fainting,
palpitations, or feelings of impending
doom occur. • Report continued hallucinations or delirium.

---

pioglitazone

pye-oh-glit-a-zone
(Actos, Apo-Pioglitazone ✦)
■ **BLACK BOX ALERT** ■ May
cause or exacerbate HF.
**Do not confuse Actos with Acti-
dose or Actonel.**

FIXED-COMBINATION(S)

Actoplus Met: pioglitazone/metFOR-
MIN (an antidiabetic): 15 mg/500 mg,
15 mg/850 mg. **Duetact:** pioglitazone/
glimepiride (an antidiabetic): 30 mg/2
mg, 30 mg/4 mg. **Oseni:** pioglitazone/
alogliptin (an antidiabetic): 15 mg/25
mg, 30 mg/25 mg, 45 mg/25 mg, 15
mg/12.5 mg, 30 mg/12.5 mg, 45 mg/
12.5 mg.

◆CLASSIFICATION

PHARMACOTHERAPEUTIC: Thiazoli-
dinedione antihyperglycemic. **CLINI-
CAL:** Antidiabetic agent.

USES

Adjunct to diet and exercise to lower serum glucose in those with type 2 diabetes. Used as monotherapy or combination therapy.

PRECAUTIONS

Contraindications: Hypersensitivity to pioglitazone. NYHA class III/IV HF (at initiation of therapy). **Cautions:** Hepatic impairment, anemia, pts with edema; avoid in pts with bladder cancer. For premenopausal, anovulatory women may result in ovulation resumption, increased risk of pregnancy. NYHA class I/II HF.

ACTION

Improves target-cell response to insulin without increasing pancreatic insulin secretion. Action dependent on presence of insulin. **Therapeutic Effect:** Lowers serum glucose concentration.

PHARMACOKINETICS

Rapidly absorbed. Protein binding: 99%. Metabolized in liver. Excreted in urine. Unknown if removed by hemodialysis. **Half-life:** 16–24 hrs.

⧗ LIFESPAN CONSIDERATIONS

Pregnancy/Lactation: Unknown if drug crosses placenta or is distributed in breast milk. Not recommended in pregnant or breastfeeding women. **Children:** Safety and efficacy not established. **Elderly:** No age-related precautions noted.

INTERACTIONS

DRUG: **CYP2C8 inhibitors (e.g., gemfibrozil)** may increase concentration/effects. **CYP2C8 inducers (e.g., rifAMPin)** may decrease concentration. **HERBAL: Garlic, ginger, ginseng** may cause hypoglycemia. **FOOD:** None known. **LAB VALUES:** May increase serum creatine kinase (CK). May decrease Hgb (by 2%–4%). May increase serum alkaline phosphatase, bilirubin, ALT. Less than 1% of pts experience ALT values 3 times the normal level.

AVAILABILITY (Rx)

Tablets: 15 mg, 30 mg, 45 mg.

ADMINISTRATION/HANDLING

PO
• Give without regard to meals.

INDICATIONS/ROUTES/DOSAGE

Diabetes
PO: ADULTS, ELDERLY: 15–30 mg once daily. **Maximum:** 45 mg once daily.

Dosage Adjustment with Strong CYP2C8 Inhibitors
Note: Not recommended in pts with symptomatic HF.
PO: ADULTS, ELDERLY: 15 mg once daily.

Dosage in Renal/Hepatic Impairment
No dose adjustment. **Note:** Hepatic injury has been associated with use. Use caution.

SIDE EFFECTS

Frequent (13%–9%): Headache, upper respiratory tract infection. **Occasional (6%–5%):** Sinusitis, myalgia, pharyngitis, aggravated diabetes, edema.

ADVERSE EFFECTS/TOXIC REACTIONS

Hepatotoxicity occurs rarely. May cause/worsen macular edema. Increased risk of HF. May increase risk of fractures. Pts with ischemic heart disease are at high risk of MI.

NURSING CONSIDERATIONS

BASELINE ASSESSMENT

Obtain baseline chemistries, esp. LFT, before initiating therapy and periodically thereafter.

INTERVENTION/EVALUATION

Monitor serum glucose, Hgb A1c, LFT. Assess for hypoglycemia (cool/wet skin, tremors, dizziness, anxiety, headache, tachycardia, numbness in mouth, hunger, diplopia), hyperglycemia (polyuria, polyphagia, polydipsia, nausea, vomiting, dim vision, fatigue, deep rapid breathing). Be alert to conditions that alter serum glucose requirements: fever, increased activity, trauma, stress, surgical procedures. Monitor for signs/symptoms of HF.

PATIENT/FAMILY TEACHING

• Be alert for signs/symptoms of hypoglycemia and take measures to manage it. • Avoid alcohol. • Report chest pain, palpitations, abdominal pain, fever, rash, hypoglycemic reactions, yellowing of skin/eyes, dark urine, light stool, nausea, vomiting. • Report any change in vision. • Report rapid weight gain, edema, difficulty breathing. • Ensure follow-up instruction if pt, family do not thoroughly understand diabetes management, glucose-testing technique.

piperacillin sodium/tazobactam sodium

pye-per-a-**sil**-in/tay-zoe-**bak**-tam (Tazocin ✚, Zosyn)
Do not confuse Zosyn with Zofran or Zyvox.

◆CLASSIFICATION

PHARMACOTHERAPEUTIC: Penicillin. **CLINICAL:** Antibiotic.

USES

Treatment of moderate to severe bacterial infections, including community-acquired/nosocomial pneumonia, intra-abdominal, pelvic, skin, and skin structure infections. Tazobactam expands piperacillin activity to include beta-lactamase–producing strains of *S. aureus, H. influenzae, Bacteroides, PsAg, Acinetobacter, Klebsiella pneumoniae, E. coli.* **OFF-LABEL:** Surgical prophylaxis, complicated intra-abdominal infections.

PRECAUTIONS

Contraindications: Hypersensitivity to piperacillin/tazobactam, any penicillin.

Cautions: History of allergies (esp. cephalosporins, beta-lactamase inhibitors), renal impairment, preexisting seizure disorder.

ACTION

Piperacillin: Inhibits cell wall synthesis by binding to bacterial cell membranes. **Therapeutic Effect:** Bactericidal. **Tazobactam:** Inactivates bacterial beta-lactamase. **Therapeutic Effect:** Protects piperacillin from enzymatic degradation, extends its spectrum of activity, prevents bacterial overgrowth.

PHARMACOKINETICS

Protein binding: 16%–30%. Widely distributed. Primarily excreted unchanged in urine. Removed by hemodialysis. **Half-life:** 0.7–1.2 hrs (increased in hepatic cirrhosis, renal impairment).

⧗ LIFESPAN CONSIDERATIONS

Pregnancy/Lactation: Readily crosses placenta; appears in cord blood, amniotic fluid. Distributed in breast milk in low concentrations. May lead to allergic sensitization, diarrhea, candidiasis, skin rash in infant. **Children:** Dosage not established for pts younger than 12 yrs. **Elderly:** Age-related renal impairment may require dosage adjustment.

INTERACTIONS

DRUG: Concurrent use of **aminoglycosides (e.g., gentamicin, tobramycin)** may cause mutual inactivation (must give at least 1 hr apart). May increase concentration, toxicity of **methotrexate. Probenecid** may increase concentration, risk of toxicity. High-dose piperacillin may increase risk of bleeding with **heparin, NSAIDs (e.g., ibuprofen, ketorolac, naproxen), platelet inhibitors (e.g., aspirin, clopidogrel), thrombolytic agents (e.g., alteplase), warfarin. HERBAL:** None significant. **FOOD:** None known. **LAB VALUES:** May increase serum sodium, alkaline phosphatase, bilirubin, LDH, ALT, AST, BUN, creatinine, PT, PTT. May decrease serum potassium. May cause positive Coombs' test.

P

AVAILABILITY (Rx)

◄ **ALERT►** Piperacillin/tazobactam is a combination product in an 8:1 ratio of piperacillin to tazobactam. **Injection Powder:** 2.25 g, 3.375 g, 4.5 g. **Premix Ready to Use:** 2.25 g (50 mL), 3.375 g (50 mL), 4.5 g (100 mL).

ADMINISTRATION/HANDLING

 IV

Reconstitution • Reconstitute each 1 g with 5 mL D_5W or 0.9% NaCl. Shake vigorously to dissolve. • Further dilute with at least 50 mL D_5W or 0.9% NaCl.
Rate of Administration • Infuse over 30 min. Expanded infusion over 3–4 hrs.
Storage • Reconstituted vial is stable for 24 hrs at room temperature or 48 hrs if refrigerated. • After further dilution, stable for 24 hrs at room temperature or 7 days if refrigerated.

▒ IV INCOMPATIBILITIES

Amphotericin B (Fungizone), amphotericin B complex (Abelcet, AmBisome, Amphotec), famotidine (Pepcid), haloperidol (Haldol), hydrOXYzine (Vistaril), vancomycin (Vancocin).

▒ IV COMPATIBILITIES

Bumetanide (Bumex), calcium gluconate, dexmedetomidine (Precedex), diphenhydrAMINE (Benadryl), DOPamine (Intropin), enalapril (Vasotec), furosemide (Lasix), granisetron (Kytril), heparin, hydrocortisone (Solu-Cortef), HYDROmorphone (Dilaudid), LORazepam (Ativan), magnesium sulfate, methylPREDNISolone (Solu-Medrol), metoclopramide (Reglan), morphine, ondansetron (Zofran), potassium chloride.

INDICATIONS/ROUTES/DOSAGE

Note: Extended Infusion: ADULTS, ELDERLY: 3.375–4.5 g over 4 hrs q8h.

Usual Dosage
IV: ADULTS, ELDERLY: 4.5 g q6–8h or 3.375 g q6h. **Maximum:** 18 g daily.

CHILDREN 10 MOS AND OLDER: 100 mg piperacillin component/kg/dose q8h. **Maximum:** 16 g/day. **CHILDREN 2–9 MOS:** 80 mg piperacillin component/kg/dose q8h. **NEONATES:** 80–100 mg piperacillin component/kg/dose q6-12.

Creatinine Clearance	Dosage
20–40 mL/min	2.25 g q6h (3.375 g q6h for nosocomial pneumonia)
Less than 20 mL/min	2.25 g q8h (2.25 g q6h for nosocomial pneumonia) Extended Infusion 3.375 g q12h

Dosage for Hemodialysis
IV: ADULTS, ELDERLY: 2.25 g q12 with additional dose of 0.75 g after each dialysis session.

Dosage for CRRT

CVVH	2.25–3.375 g q6–8h
CVVHD	2.25–3.375 g q6h
CVVHDF	3.375 g q6h

Dosage in Renal Impairment
Dosage and frequency are modified based on creatinine clearance.

Dosage in Hepatic Impairment
No dose adjustment.

SIDE EFFECTS

Frequent: Diarrhea, headache, constipation, nausea, insomnia, rash. **Occasional:** Vomiting, dyspepsia, pruritus, fever, agitation, candidiasis, dizziness, abdominal pain, edema, anxiety, dyspnea, rhinitis.

ADVERSE EFFECTS/TOXIC REACTIONS

Antibiotic-associated colitis, other superinfections (abdominal cramps, severe watery diarrhea, fever) may result from altered bacterial balance in GI tract. Overdose, more often with renal impairment, may produce seizures, neurologic reactions. Severe hypersensitivity reactions, including anaphylaxis, occur rarely.

<u>underlined</u> – top prescribed drug

NURSING CONSIDERATIONS

BASELINE ASSESSMENT

Question for history of allergies, esp. to penicillins, cephalosporins. Obtain baseline CBC with differential, BMP, LFT; urinalysis; PT, aPTT (if on anticoagulants or history of coagulopathy).

INTERVENTION/EVALUATION

Monitor daily pattern of bowel activity, stool consistency; mild GI effects may be tolerable, but increasing severity may indicate onset of antibiotic-associated colitis. Be alert for superinfection: fever, vomiting, diarrhea, anal/genital pruritus, oral mucosal changes (ulceration, pain, erythema). Monitor I&O, urinalysis. Monitor serum electrolytes, esp. potassium, renal function tests.

---

pitavastatin

pit-av-a-stat-in
(Livalo)
Do not confuse pitavastatin with atorvastatin, lovastatin, pravastatin, or simvastatin.

◆CLASSIFICATION

PHARMACOTHERAPEUTIC: HMG-CoA reductase inhibitor. **CLINICAL:** Antihyperlipidemic.

USES

Reduces elevated total cholesterol, low-density lipoproteins (LDLs), apolipoprotein B, triglycerides; increases low high-density lipoproteins (HDLs) in primary hyperlipidemia and mixed dyslipidemia. **OFF-LABEL:** Primary and secondary prevention of atherosclerotic cardiovascular disease.

PRECAUTIONS

Contraindications: Hypersensitivity to pitavastatin. Active hepatic disease, persistent or unexplained elevations of LFT; concurrent cycloSPORINE use, pregnancy,

breastfeeding. **Cautions:** History of hepatic disease, substantial alcohol consumption, moderate renal impairment. Withholding/discontinuing pitavastatin may be necessary when pt at risk for renal failure. Pts at risk for myopathy: elderly, renal impairment, inadequately treated hypothyroidism.

ACTION

Interferes with cholesterol biosynthesis by inhibiting conversion of HMG-CoA reductase to a precursor to cholesterol. **Therapeutic Effect:** Lowers total cholesterol, LDL cholesterol, apolipoprotein B (Apo B), plasma triglycerides; increases HDL cholesterol.

PHARMACOKINETICS

Poorly absorbed from GI tract. Protein binding: greater than 99%. Metabolized in liver. Primarily excreted in feces. **Half-life:** 12 hrs.

⌛ LIFESPAN CONSIDERATIONS

Pregnancy/Lactation: Contraindicated in pregnancy (suppression of cholesterol biosynthesis may cause fetal toxicity) and lactation. Unknown if drug is distributed in breast milk (risk of serious adverse reactions in nursing infants). **Children:** Safety and efficacy not established in pts younger than 18 yrs. **Elderly:** No age-related precautions noted.

INTERACTIONS:

DRUG: Increased risk of rhabdomyolysis, acute renal failure with **gemfibrozil, niacin, other fibrates.** Cyclo**SPORINE, erythromycin, rifAMPin** may increase serum pitavastatin levels. **HERBAL:** None significant. **FOOD:** None known. **LAB VALUES:** May increase serum creatine kinase (CPK), ALT, AST concentrations.

AVAILABILITY (Rx)

Tablets: 1 mg, 2 mg, 4 mg.

ADMINISTRATION/HANDLING

PO
• Give without regard to meals or time of day.

◆ Canadian trade name   🍵 Non-Crushable Drug   🄷🄸 High Alert drug

INDICATIONS/ROUTES/DOSAGE

◄**ALERT**► Before initiating therapy, pt should be on standard cholesterol-lowering diet for minimum of 3–6 mos. Continue diet throughout pitavastatin therapy.

Usual Dosage
PO: ADULTS: Initially, 2 mg/day. **Maximum:** 4 mg/day. Range: 1–4 mg/day. **Maximum dosage with erythromycin:** 1 mg/day; **with rifAMPin:** 2 mg/day.

Dosage in Renal Impairment
CrCl 30–59, 15–60 mL/min not receiving hemodialysis, or end-stage renal disease in pts on hemodialysis: Initially, 1 mg/day. **Maximum:** 2 mg/day.

Dosage in Hepatic Impairment
See contraindications.

SIDE EFFECTS

Generally well tolerated. Side effects usually mild and transient. **Rare (less than 4%):** Myalgia, constipation/diarrhea, back/extremity pain, arthralgia, headache, nasopharyngitis.

ADVERSE EFFECTS/TOXIC REACTIONS

Hypersensitivity (rash, pruritus, urticaria) occurs rarely. Myopathy, rhabdomyolysis.

NURSING CONSIDERATIONS

BASELINE ASSESSMENT

Obtain LFT, serum cholesterol, triglycerides. Question for possibility of pregnancy before initiating therapy.

INTERVENTION/EVALUATION

Monitor cholesterol and triglyceride levels; LFT. Monitor daily pattern of bowel activity, stool consistency. Check for myalgia, arthralgia, headache. Assess for rash, pruritus. Be alert for malaise, muscle cramping/weakness.

PATIENT/FAMILY TEACHING

• Follow special diet (important part of treatment). • Periodic lab tests are essential part of therapy. • Report promptly any muscle pain/weakness. • Use nonhormonal contraception.

---

plecanatide

ple-**kan**-a-tide
(Trulance)
■ **BLACK BOX ALERT** ■ Contraindicated in pts younger than 6 yrs due to risk of life-threatening dehydration and death. Safety and efficacy not established in pts younger than 18 yrs; avoid use. **Do not confuse plecanatide with exenatide, lixisenatide, pramlintide or Trulance with Truvada.**

◆CLASSIFICATION

PHARMACOTHERAPEUTIC: Guanylate cyclase-C agonist. **CLINICAL:** GI agent.

USES

Treatment of adults with chronic idiopathic constipation.

PRECAUTIONS

Contraindications: Hypersensitivity to plecanatide. Pts younger than 6 yrs of age, mechanical GI obstruction (known or suspected). **Cautions:** Dehydration. Avoid use in pts younger than 18 yrs of age.

ACTION

Binds and agonizes guanylate cyclase-C on luminal surface of intestinal epithelium, increasing cyclic guanosine monophosphate (cGMP), resulting in chloride and bicarbonate secretion into the intestinal lumen. **Therapeutic Effect:** Increases intestinal fluid and transit time.

PHARMACOKINETICS

Minimal absorption systemically; mainly confined to GI tract. Metabolized within GI tract to active metabolite. Undergoes proteolytic degradation within intestinal lumen to smaller peptides and amino acids. **Half-life:** Not specified.

⧗ LIFESPAN CONSIDERATIONS

Pregnancy/Lactation: Unknown if distributed in breast milk. **Children:** Contraindicated in pts younger than 6 yrs. Safety and efficacy not established in pts aged 6 to less than 18 yrs. Severe, possibly fatal, dehydration may occur in pediatric pts younger than 18 yrs due to increased intestinal fluid secretion; avoid use. **Elderly:** No age-related precautions noted.

INTERACTIONS

DRUG: None known. **HERBAL:** None significant. **FOOD:** None known. **LAB VALUES:** May increase serum ALT, AST.

AVAILABILITY (Rx)

Tablets: 3 mg.

ADMINISTRATION/HANDLING

PO
• Give with or without food. • If a dose is missed, skip the dose and give at next regularly scheduled time; do not double dose. • Give tablet whole; do not break, cut, or divide. • For pts with dysphagia, tablet may be crushed and mixed in applesauce, or dispersed in 30 mL of water and given orally or via NG tube. After administration of dispersed tablet, refill container with additional 30 mL of water and give remaining contents. Flush NG tube with additional 10 mL of water.

INDICATIONS/ROUTES/DOSAGE

Chronic Idiopathic Constipation
PO: ADULTS, ELDERLY: 3 mg once daily.

Dosage in Renal/Hepatic Impairment
Not specified; use caution.

SIDE EFFECTS

Occasional (5%): Diarrhea. **Rare (less than 2%):** Abdominal pain/tenderness, flatulence.

ADVERSE EFFECTS/ TOXIC REACTIONS

Severe diarrhea reported in less than 1% of pts; usually occurred within the first 3 days.

NURSING CONSIDERATIONS

BASELINE ASSESSMENT

Question characteristics of constipation, frequency of bowel movements. Assess bowel sounds. Assess hydration status.

INTERVENTION/EVALUATION

Encourage fluid intake. Monitor daily pattern of bowel activity, stool consistency. Monitor for abdominal pain, dehydration.

PATIENT/FAMILY TEACHING

• Report severe diarrhea. • Drink plenty of fluids. • Do not take laxatives unless approved by prescriber. • Tablets may be taken whole, dispersed in water, or crushed and mixed in applesauce. • Securely store tablets away from children; life-threating dehydration may occur if accidentally ingested by children younger than 6 yrs.

P

polyethylene glycol

polyethylene glycol-electrolyte solution (PEG-ES) (CoLyte, GoLYTELY)

pol-ee-**eth**-il-een-**glye**-kol
(CoLyte, GoLYTELY, Klean-Prep ✦, MiraLax, NuLytely, Peglyte ✦, TriLyte)
Do not confuse MiraLax with Mirapex.

◆CLASSIFICATION

PHARMACOTHERAPEUTIC: Osmotic/laxative. **CLINICAL:** Bowel evacuant.

✦ Canadian trade name   🗽 Non-Crushable Drug   🔴 High Alert drug

USES

Polyethylene glycol-electrolyte solution: Bowel cleansing before GI examination, colon surgery. **Polyethylene glycol:** Treatment of occasional constipation.

PRECAUTIONS

Contraindications: Hypersensitivity to polyethylene glycol. Bowel perforation, gastric retention, GI obstruction, megacolon, toxic colitis, toxic ileus. **Cautions: (Propylene glycol):** Renal impairment. **(Propylene glycol-electrolyte solution):** Ulcerative colitis, medications altering electrolytes, hyponatremia, cardiac arrhythmias, impaired gag reflex, history of seizures, elderly.

ACTION

Osmotic effect. **Therapeutic Effect:** Induces diarrhea, cleanses bowel without depleting electrolytes.

PHARMACOKINETICS

Route	Onset	Peak	Duration
PO (bowel cleansing)	1–2 hrs	N/A	N/A
PO (constipation)	2–4 days	N/A	N/A

⧗ LIFESPAN CONSIDERATIONS

Pregnancy/Lactation: Unknown if drug crosses placenta or is distributed in breast milk. **Children/Elderly:** No age-related precautions noted.

INTERACTIONS

DRUG: May decrease absorption of **oral medications** if given within 1 hr (may be flushed from GI tract). **HERBAL:** None significant. **FOOD:** None known. **LAB VALUES:** None significant.

AVAILABILITY (Rx)

Powder for Oral Solution: Propylene glycol (Miralax): 17 g/dose. **Propylene glycol-electrolyte solution (Co-Lyte, GoLYTELY):** See individual product for specific ingredients.

ADMINISTRATION/HANDLING

PO

Polyethylene Glycol-Electrolyte Solution
• Refrigerate reconstituted solutions; use within 48 hrs. • May use tap water to prepare solution. Shake vigorously for several min to ensure complete dissolution of powder. • Fasting should occur for more than 3 hrs prior to ingestion of solution (always avoid solid food less than 2 hrs prior to administration). • Only clear liquids permitted after administration. • May give via NG tube. • Rapid drinking preferred. Chilled solution is more palatable.
Polyethylene Glycol
• Add to 4- to 8-oz beverage.

INDICATIONS/ROUTES/DOSAGE

Bowel Evacuant
PO: ADULTS, ELDERLY: Before GI examination: 240 mL (8 oz) q10min until 4 L consumed or rectal effluent clear. NG tube: 20–30 mL/min until 4 L given. **CHILDREN 6 MOS AND OLDER:** 25 mL/kg/hr until rectal effluent clear. **Maximum:** 4 L.

Constipation
PO *(Miralax):* **ADULTS:** 17 g or 1 heaping tbsp/day. **CHILDREN 6 MOS AND OLDER:** 0.5–1.5 g/kg/day. **Maximum:** 17 g/day.

Dosage in Renal/Hepatic Impairment
No dose adjustment.

SIDE EFFECTS

Frequent (50%): Some degree of abdominal fullness, nausea, bloating. **Occasional (10%–1%):** Abdominal cramping, vomiting, anal irritation. **Rare (less than 1%):** Urticaria, rhinorrhea, dermatitis.

ADVERSE EFFECTS/ TOXIC REACTIONS

None known.

NURSING CONSIDERATIONS

BASELINE ASSESSMENT

Do not give oral medication within 1 hr of start of therapy (may not adequately be absorbed before GI cleansing).

INTERVENTION/EVALUATION

Assess bowel sounds for peristalsis. Monitor daily pattern of bowel activity, stool consistency. Assess for abdominal disturbances. Monitor serum electrolytes.

PATIENT/FAMILY TEACHING

• May take 2–4 days to produce a bowel movement. • Report unusual cramps, bloating, diarrhea.

pomalidomide

poe-ma-**lid**-oh-mide
(Pomalyst)

■ **BLACK BOX ALERT** ■ May cause life-threatening birth defects. Pregnancy contraindicated. Exclude pregnancy before initiating treatment. Females of reproductive potential must use two reliable forms of contraception or continuously abstain during treatment and for 4 wks after treatment. Deep vein thrombosis and pulmonary embolism may occur. Consider venous thromboembolism (VTE) prophylaxis during treatment.

◆CLASSIFICATION

PHARMACOTHERAPEUTIC: Thalidomide analogue. **CLINICAL:** Antineoplastic.

USES

Treatment of multiple myeloma in pts who have received at least two prior therapies including lenalidomide and bortezomib and who have demonstrated disease progression on or within 60 days of completion of the last therapy.

PRECAUTIONS

◀**ALERT**▶ Do not donate blood products during therapy and for 1 month after therapy discontinuation; male pts must not donate sperm.
Contraindications: Hypersensitivity to pomalidomide. Pregnancy. **Cautions:** Anemia, HF, hepatic/renal impairment, smoking, breastfeeding, or prior history of CVA, MI, DVT, PE.

ACTION

Inhibits tumor cell proliferation and induces apoptosis (cell death) of hematopoietic cells. Enhances T-cell– and natural killer (NK) cell–mediated immunity. Inhibits proinflammatory cytokines. **Therapeutic Effect:** Inhibits tumor cell growth and metastasis.

PHARMACOKINETICS

Readily absorbed following PO administration. Metabolized in liver. Protein binding: 12%–44%. Peak plasma concentration: 2–3 hrs. Excreted in urine (73%), feces (15%). **Half-life:** 8–10 hrs.

⧗ LIFESPAN CONSIDERATIONS

Pregnancy/Lactation: Pregnancy/breastfeeding contraindicated. May cause fetal harm. Unknown if distributed in breast milk. Do not breastfeed. Must verify negative pregnancy status before initiation. Must use two reliable forms of birth control (intrauterine device [IUD], tubal ligation) plus barrier methods. Avoid pregnancy for at least 4 wks after discontinuation. **Males:** Must use condoms during treatment and up to 1 mo after treatment, despite prior history of vasectomy. Do not donate sperm. **Children:** Safety and efficacy not established. **Elderly:** May have increased risk of serious adverse effects, renal failure, electrolyte imbalance.

INTERACTIONS

DRUG: CYP3A4, P-glycoprotein inhibitors (e.g., **erythromycin**, **ketoconazole**) may increase concentration/

P

effects. **CYP3A4, P-glycoprotein inducers (e.g., carBAMazepine, rifAMPin)** may decrease concentration/effects. **HERBAL:** None significant. **FOOD:** All foods may reduce absorption/concentration. **LAB VALUES:** May decrease Hgb, Hct, neutrophils, platelets, leukocytes, lymphocytes, serum calcium, potassium, sodium. May increase serum calcium, creatinine, glucose.

AVAILABILITY (Rx)

 Capsules: 1 mg, 2 mg, 3 mg, 4 mg.

ADMINISTRATION/HANDLING

PO
• Do not break, crush, or open capsule. • Give on empty stomach; must administer at least 2 hrs before or 2 hrs after meal.

INDICATIONS/ROUTES/DOSAGE

Note: Absolute neutrophil count (ANC) should be 500 cells/mm³ or greater and platelets 50,000 cells/mm³ or greater prior to starting new cycles of therapy.

Multiple Myeloma
PO: ADULTS/ELDERLY: 4 mg once daily on days 1–21 of 28-day cycle (in combination with dexamethasone). Continue until disease progression or unacceptable toxicity.

Dose Modification
Neutropenia
ANC less than 500 cells/mm³ or febrile neutropenia: Interrupt treatment until ANC is greater than 500 cells/mm³, then reduce dose to 3 mg once daily. **Any subsequent drop of ANC less than 500 cells/mm³ after prior reduction:** Interrupt treatment until ANC is greater than 500 cells/mm³, then reduce dose at 1 mg less than previous dose. Discontinue if 1-mg dose is intolerable.
Thrombocytopenia
Platelet count less than 25,000 cells/mm³: Interrupt treatment until platelet count greater than 50,000 cells/mm³, then reduce dose to 3 mg once daily.

Any subsequent platelet drop to less than 25,000 cells/mm³: Interrupt treatment until platelet count greater than 50,000 cells/mm³, then reduce dose at 1 mg less than previous dose. Discontinue if 1-mg dose is intolerable.

Dosage in Renal Impairment
Avoid use in pts with serum creatinine more than 3 mg/dL or CrCl less than 45 mL/min.

Dosage in Hepatic Impairment
Avoid use with bilirubin more than 2 mg/dL and ALT, AST more than 3 times upper limit of normal (ULN).

SIDE EFFECTS

Frequent (55%–22%): Fatigue, constipation, nausea, diarrhea, dyspnea, back pain, peripheral edema, musculoskeletal chest pain, anorexia, rash. **Occasional (20%–7%):** Dizziness, pyrexia, muscle spasms, arthralgia, pruritus, vomiting, cough, weight loss, headache, bone pain, muscular weakness, anxiety, musculoskeletal pain, peripheral neuropathy, chills, dry skin, tremor, insomnia. **Rare (6%–1%):** Hyperhidrosis, extremity pain, back pain, night sweats, constipation.

ADVERSE EFFECTS/ TOXIC REACTIONS

Myelosuppression (neutropenia, leukopenia, thrombocytopenia) is an expected outcome of therapy; may increase risk of infection such as pneumonia, upper respiratory tract infection, UTI. Neurologic events such as acute confusion, dizziness reported. Peripheral neuropathy occurred in 18% of pts. Venous thromboembolism including DVT, PE occurred in 3% of pts. Epistaxis occurred in 15% of pts. Increased risk of secondary malignancies reported. Acute renal failure reported in 16% of pts. Additional adverse events may include interstitial lung disease (ILD), neutropenic sepsis, *Pneumocystis jiroveci* pneumonia, respiratory syncytial virus infection, urinary retention, vertigo.

NURSING CONSIDERATIONS

BASELINE ASSESSMENT

Obtain vital signs, CBC with differential, serum chemistries, esp. magnesium, phosphate, ionized calcium, PT/INR, urinalysis. Confirm negative pregnancy status 10–14 days before and 24 hrs before starting treatment. Receive full medication history. Obtain baseline neurologic exam. Question history of diabetes mellitus, electrolyte imbalance, hepatic/renal impairment, pulmonary disease, thromboembolism, smoking.

INTERVENTION/EVALUATION

Monitor CBC, serum chemistries, PT/INR. Offer antiemetics for nausea, vomiting. Monitor pregnancy status every mo during treatment and for at least 4 mos after discontinuation. Obtain EKG for palpitations, chest pain, hypokalemia, hyperkalemia, hypocalcemia, bradycardia, ventricular arrhythmias. Immediately report dyspnea, chest pain, hypoxia, unilateral peripheral edema/pain (may indicate thromboembolic event). Consider sequential compression device (SCD) for immobilized pts. Perform routine neurologic assessments to screen for confusion, delirium. Monitor urine output, frequency.

PATIENT/FAMILY TEACHING

• May cause birth defects or miscarriage. Do not breastfeed. Consult with gynecologist for appropriate birth control methods. Female pts must use contraception during treatment and for at least 1 mo after treatment. Immediately report suspected pregnancy. Male pts must use condoms with spermicide during sexual activity, despite history of vasectomy. • Do not donate blood. • Swallow capsules whole; do not break, crush, or open. • Go from lying to standing slowly (prevents postural hypotension, dizziness). Avoid tasks that require alertness, motor skills until response to drug is established. • Do not smoke. • Do not eat 2 hrs before or 2 hrs after dose. • Avoid alcohol. • Report difficulty breathing, chest pain, extremity pain or swelling, dizziness, confusion.

ponatinib

poe-**na**-ti-nib
(Iclusig)

■ **BLACK BOX ALERT** ■ Arterial occlusions have occurred, including CVA, fatal MI, large arterial vessel stenosis of the brain, severe peripheral vascular disease requiring revascularization. Events may occur in pts with or without cardiovascular risks, including pts younger than 50 yrs of age. Venous thromboembolism, serious HF, or left ventricular dysfunction were reported. Hepatotoxicity, including fatal hepatic failure, may occur.

Do not confuse ponatinib with afatinib, alectinib, dasatinib, bosutinib, gefitinib, imatinib, lapatinib, lenvatinib, neratinib, or tofacitinib.

◆CLASSIFICATION

PHARMACOTHERAPEUTIC: BCR-ABL tyrosine kinase inhibitor. **CLINICAL:** Antineoplastic.

USES

Treatment of pts with chronic, accelerated, or blast phase chronic myeloid leukemia (CML) or Philadelphia chromosome (Ph+) acute lymphoblastic leukemia (ALL) for whom no other kinase inhibitor therapy is indicated. Treatment of adults with T315I-positive CML (chronic, accelerated, or blast phase) or T315I-positive ALL (Ph+ ALL). Not indicated for treatment of newly diagnosed chronic phase CML.

PRECAUTIONS

Contraindications: Hypersensitivity to ponatinib. **Cautions:** Baseline hematologic cytopenias; conditions predisposing to infection (e.g., diabetes, immunocompromised pts, open wounds), history of arterial/venous thrombosis (e.g., CVA, DVT, MI, PE), cardiac disease, cardiac conduction disorders, HF, hypertension; diabetes, electrolyte imbalance, glaucoma, hepatic impairment, hyperlipidemia, GI perforation, neuropathy (peripheral or cranial), ocular disorders, pancreatitis or alcohol abuse, history of ischemia, vascular stenosis; pts with high tumor burden; pts at risk for hemorrhage (e.g., history of intracranial/GI bleeding, coagulation disorders, recent trauma; concomitant use of anticoagulants, antiplatelets, NSAIDs).

ACTION

Inhibits viability of cells expressing native or mutant BCR-ABL tyrosine kinase, including T315I mutation, created by the Philadelphia chromosome abnormality. **Therapeutic Effect:** Inhibits tumor cell growth and metastasis.

PHARMACOKINETICS

Widely distributed. Metabolized in liver. Protein binding: greater than 99%. Peak plasma concentration: 6 hrs or less. Excreted in feces (87%), urine (5%). **Half-life:** 24 hrs (Range: 12–66 hrs).

⌛ LIFESPAN CONSIDERATIONS

Pregnancy/Lactation: Avoid pregnancy; may cause fetal harm/malformations. Unknown if distributed in breast milk. Breastfeeding not recommended during treatment and for at least 6 days after discontinuation. Females of reproductive potential and males with female partners of reproductive potential should use effective contraception during treatment and for at least 3 wks after discontinuation. May impair fertility in females. **Children:** Safety and efficacy not established. **Elderly:** May have increased risk of adverse reactions/toxic effects. Use caution.

INTERACTIONS

DRUG: **Strong CYP3A4 inhibitors (e.g., ketoconazole, ritonavir)** may increase concentration/effect. **Strong CYP3A4 inducers (e.g., carBAMazepine, phenytoin, rifAMPin)** may decrease concentration/effect. May decrease therapeutic effect of BCG vaccine. **HERBAL:** **St. John's wort** may decrease concentration/effect. **FOOD:** **Grapefruit products** may increase concentration/effect. **LAB VALUES:** May increase serum alkaline phosphatase, amylase, ALT, AST, bilirubin, creatinine, lipase, triglycerides, uric acid. May decrease Hgb, Hct, leukocytes, lymphocytes, neutrophils, platelets; serum albumin, bicarbonate, phosphate. May increase or decrease serum calcium, glucose, potassium, sodium.

AVAILABILITY (Rx)

Tablets: 15 mg, 30 mg, 45 mg.

ADMINISTRATION/HANDLING

PO
• Give with or without food. • Administer tablets whole; do not break, cut, crush, or divide.

INDICATIONS/ROUTES/DOSAGE

CML, Ph+ ALL

PO: ADULTS, ELDERLY: 45 mg once daily. Consider dose reduction in pts with chronic or accelerated phase CML who have achieved a major cytogenetic response. If an adequate response has been not achieved within 90 days, consider discontinuation.

Dose Modification
Hepatotoxicity
CTCAE grade 2 or greater serum ALT/AST elevation (greater than 3 times upper limit normal [ULN]): Withhold treatment until improved to grade 1 or 0, then resume dose based on occurrence. **Occurrence at 45-mg dose:** Resume treatment at 30-mg dose. **Occurrence**

at 30-mg dose: Resume treatment at 15-mg dose. **Occurrence at 15-mg dose:** Permanently discontinue. **Serum ALT/AST elevation greater than or equal to 3 times ULN with concurrent serum bilirubin elevation greater than 2 times ULN and serum alkaline phosphatase less than 2 times ULN:** Permanently discontinue.

Neutropenia/Thrombocytopenia

ANC less than 1000 cells/mm³; platelets less than 50,000 cells/mm³: Withhold treatment until ANC greater than or equal to 1500 cells/mm³; or platelets greater than or equal to 75,000 cells/mm³, then resume dose based on occurrence. **First occurrence:** Resume treatment at 45-mg dose. **Second occurrence:** Resume treatment at 30-mg dose. **Third occurrence:** Resume treatment at 15-mg dose.

Pancreatitis/Elevated Lipase:

Asymptomatic CTCAE grade 1 or 2 serum lipase elevation: Consider withholding treatment or reducing dose. **Asymptomatic CTCAE grade 3 or 4 serum lipase elevation (greater than 2 times ULN); asymptomatic radiologic pancreatitis (grade 2 pancreatitis):** Withhold treatment until improved to grade 1 or 0, then resume dose based on occurrence. **Occurrence at 45-mg dose:** Resume treatment at 30-mg dose. **Occurrence at 30-mg dose:** Resume treatment at 15-mg dose. **Occurrence at 15-mg dose:** Permanently discontinue. **Grade 4 pancreatitis:** Permanently discontinue.

Concomitant Use Of Strong Cyp3a4 Inhibitors

Reduce initial dose to 30 mg.

Dosage in Renal Impairment

Not specified; use caution.

Dosage in Hepatic Impairment

Mild, moderate, severe impairment (Child-Pugh A, B, or C): Reduce initial dose to 30 mg.

SIDE EFFECTS

Note: Percentages of side effects of chronic phase, accelerated phase, blast phase CML; Ph+ ALL may vary.

Frequent (69%–18%): Hypertension, abdominal pain, fatigue, asthenia, headache, dry skin, constipation, arthralgia, nausea, pyrexia, burning sensation, hyperesthesia, hypoesthesia, neuralgia, paresthesia, dysgeusia, muscular weakness, gait disturbance, areflexia, hypotonia, restless legs syndrome, myalgia, extremity pain, back pain, diarrhea, vomiting. **Occasional (17%–2%):** Dyspnea, dizziness, peripheral edema, cough, bone pain, musculoskeletal pain, mucositis, aphthous stomatitis, lip blister, mouth ulceration, mucosal eruption, oral pain, oropharyngeal pain, stomatitis, tongue ulceration, muscle spasm, conjunctival irritation, corneal abrasion/erosion, dry eye, hyperemia, eye pain, pruritus, decreased appetite, insomnia, decreased weight, generalized pain, erythema, alopecia, chills, blurry vision, tachycardia.

ADVERSE EFFECTS/ TOXIC REACTIONS

Anemia, leukopenia, lymphopenia, neutropenia, thrombocytopenia are expected responses to therapy, but more severe reactions including bone marrow failure, febrile neutropenia may be life-threatening. Fatal arterial occlusions including CVA, MI, stenosis of large arterial vessel of the brain, severe peripheral vascular disease requiring revascularization reported in 35% of pts; may occur within 2 wks of initiation (even at reduced doses of 15 mg/day). Coronary artery occlusion, MI occurred in 21% of pts. Venous thromboembolism (DVT, PE, superficial thrombophlebitis) occurred in 5–9% of pts. Life-threatening events including cardiac bradyarrhythmias (requiring pacemaker

P

implantation), complete heart block, sick sinus syndrome, atrial fibrillation with bradycardic pauses, atrial fibrillation, SVT, ventricular tachycardia; emergent hypertension (68% of pts), GI/intracranial hemorrhage (28% of pts), hepatotoxicity (54% of pts), pancreatitis (6%), HF, left ventricular dysfunction (6% of pts); infections including cellulitis, nasopharyngitis, pneumonia, sepsis, upper respiratory tract infection, UTI; ocular toxicities including blindness, conjunctival hemorrhage, cataracts, periorbital edema, ocular hyperemia, iritis, iridocyclitis, ulcerative keratinitis; peripheral edema (31% of pts), pleural effusion (2% of pts), pericardial effusion (1% of pts); peripheral neuropathy, polyneuropathy, nerve compression (20% of pts) may occur. Tumor lysis syndrome may present as acute renal failure, hypocalcemia, hyperuricemia, hyperphosphatemia. Reversible posterior leukoencephalopathy may include aphasia, cognition impairment, paralysis, vision loss, weakness. Pts with newly diagnosed CML have an increased risk of severe toxicities. Improper wound healing, GI perforation may occur.

NURSING CONSIDERATIONS

BASELINE ASSESSMENT

Obtain CBC, BMP, LFT, serum ionized calcium, phosphate, uric acid; vital signs; weight. Obtain pregnancy test in females of reproductive potential. Question plans of breastfeeding. Receive full medication history including herbal products and screen for interactions. Question history as listed in Precautions. Screen for active infection. Conduct ophthalmologic, neurologic exam. Due to increased risk of tumor lysis syndrome, assess adequate hydration prior to initiation. Consider correcting electrolyte abnormalities prior to initiation. Obtain dietary consult. Screen for risk of bleeding; active infection. Assess skin for rash, lesions. Offer emotional support.

INTERVENTION/EVALUATION

Obtain ANC, CBC for myelosuppression q2wks for 3 mos, then monthly thereafter. Monitor serum lipase monthly; BMP, LFT, serum ionized calcium, phosphate, uric acid as indicated. Monitor ECG for cardiac arrhythmias. Due to extremely high risk for arterial occlusions, be vigilant when screening for CVA (aphasia, confusion, paresthesia, hemiparesis, seizures), MI (chest pain, diaphoresis, left arm/jaw pain, increased serum troponin, ST segment elevation), vascular compromise. Be alert for serious infection, opportunistic infection, sepsis. Monitor for GI perforation, hepatotoxicity, ocular disease, pancreatitis; symptoms of thromboembolism (arm/leg pain, swelling; chest pain, dyspnea, hypoxia, tachycardia), reversible posterior leukoencephalopathy, tumor lysis syndrome; other toxicities as listed in Adverse Reactions/Toxic Effects. Monitor daily pattern of bowel activity, stool consistency. Ensure adequate hydration, nutrition. Monitor weight, I&O.

PATIENT/FAMILY TEACHING

• Treatment may cause life-threatening arterial blood clots; report symptoms of heart attack (chest pain, difficulty breathing, jaw pain, nausea, pain that radiates to the left arm, sweating), stroke (blindness, confusion, one-sided weakness, loss of consciousness, trouble speaking, seizures). • Report symptoms of DVT (swelling, pain, hot feeling in the arms or legs), lung embolism (difficulty breathing, chest pain, rapid heart rate); liver problems (abdominal pain, bruising, clay-colored stool, amber or dark-colored urine, yellowing of the skin or eyes); HF (difficulty breathing, extremity swelling, sudden loss of breath, palpitations); inflammation of the pancreas (abdominal bruising; persistent, severe abdominal pain that radiates to the back [with or without vomiting]); eye problems (blindness, blurred vision, eye inflammation or bleeding, severe eye or head pain); heart arrhythmias (chest pain, dizziness, fainting, palpitations, slow or rapid heart rate,

P

irregular heart rate); intestinal perforation (severe abdominal pain, fever, nausea). • Treatment may depress your immune system response and reduce your ability to fight infection. Report symptoms of infection such as body aches, chills, cough, fatigue, fever. Avoid those with active infection. • Treatment may cause severe bone marrow depression; report bruising, fatigue, fever, shortness of breath, weight loss, bleeding easily, bloody urine or stool. • Avoid pregnancy; may cause birth defects or miscarriage. Females and males of childbearing potential should use effective contraception during treatment and for at least 3 wks after final dose. • Do not breastfeed during treatment and for at least 6 days after final dose. • Report planned surgical/dental procedures. • Immediately report bleeding of any kind. • Do not ingest grapefruit products, herbal supplements. • Do not take newly prescribed medications unless approved by the prescriber who originally started treatment.

posaconazole

poe-sa-**kon**-a-zole
(Noxafil, Posanol ❖)
Do not confuse Noxafil with minoxidil.

◆CLASSIFICATION

PHARMACOTHERAPEUTIC: Azole derivative. **CLINICAL:** Antifungal.

USES

Prophylaxis of invasive *Aspergillus* and *Candida* infections in pts 13 yrs and older (IV for pts 18 yrs and older) who are at high risk for developing these infections due to severely immunocompromised conditions. Treatment of oropharyngeal candidiasis. **OFF-LABEL:** Salvage therapy of refractory invasive fungal infections, mucormycosis, pulmonary infections.

PRECAUTIONS

Contraindications: Hypersensitivity to posaconazole, other azole antifungals. Coadministration with pimozide, quiNIDine (may cause QT prolongation, torsades de pointes), HMG-CoA reductase inhibitors metabolized by CYP3A4 (e.g., atorvastatin, lovastatin, simvastatin), sirolimus, ergot alkaloids. **Cautions:** Renal/hepatic impairment, hypokalemia, hypomagnesemia, pts at increased risk of arrhythmias. Concomitant administration of medications that prolong QT interval, pts with long QT syndrome.

ACTION

Inhibits synthesis of ergosterol, a vital component of fungal cell wall formation. **Therapeutic Effect:** Damages fungal cell wall membrane, altering its function.

PHARMACOKINETICS

Moderately absorbed following PO administration. Absorption increased if drug is taken with food. Widely distributed. Protein binding: 98%. Not significantly metabolized. Primarily excreted in feces. **Half-life:** 20–66 hrs.

⌛ LIFESPAN CONSIDERATIONS

Pregnancy/Lactation: May cause fetal harm. Breastfeeding not recommended. **Children:** Safety and efficacy not established in pts younger than 13 yrs. **Elderly:** No age-related precautions noted.

INTERACTIONS

DRUG: May increase concentrations of **atorvastatin, cycloSPORINE, ergot alkaloids, felodipine, midazolam, phenytoin, pimozide, quiNIDine, rifabutin, simvastatin, sirolimus, tacrolimus, vinBLAStine, vinCRIStine. Cimetidine, phenytoin** may decrease concentration. **HERBAL:** None significant. **FOOD:** Concentration higher when given with **food or nutritional supplements. Grapefruit products** may decrease concentration/effects. **LAB VALUES:** May decrease WBC, RBC, Hgb,

P

Hct, platelets, serum calcium, potassium, magnesium. May increase serum glucose, bilirubin, ALT, AST, alkaline phosphatase.

AVAILABILITY (Rx)

Injection Solution: 300 mg/16.7 mL (18 mg/mL). **Oral Suspension:** 40 mg/mL.
 Tablets (Delayed-Release): 100 mg.

ADMINISTRATION/HANDLING

🗍 IV

Reconstitution • Transfer 300 mg (16.7 mL) posaconazole into 150 mL D₅W or 0.9% NaCl bag.
Rate of Administration • Infuse over 90 min via central venous line. Must be infused through in-line filter (0.22 microns) or PVD filter.
Storage • Refrigerate vials. Once diluted, use immediately. May refrigerate solution up to 24 hrs if not used immediately.

PO

• Administer with or within 20 min of full meal, liquid nutritional supplement, or acidic carbonated beverage (e.g., ginger ale) (enhances absorption). • Store oral suspension at room temperature. • Shake suspension well before use. • **Tablets:** Swallow whole; do not crush, cut, dissolve, or divide. Administer with food.

INDICATIONS/ROUTES/DOSAGE

Note: The delayed-release tablets and oral suspension are not to be used interchangeably.

Prophylaxis of Invasive *Aspergillus* and *Candida*

PO: ADULTS, ELDERLY, CHILDREN 13 YRS AND OLDER: *(Oral Suspension):* 200 mg (5 mL) 3 times/day, given with full meal or liquid nutritional supplement. *(Delayed-Release):* 300 mg twice daily on first day, then 300 mg once daily. **IV:** 300 mg twice daily on first day, then 300 mg once daily thereafter.

Oropharyngeal Candidiasis

PO: ADULTS, ELDERLY, CHILDREN 13 YRS AND OLDER: 100 mg twice daily for 1 day, then 100 mg once daily for 13 days.

Oropharyngeal Candidiasis Refractory to Fluconazole

PO: ADULTS, ELDERLY: *(Suspension):* 400 mg twice daily for 3 days, then 400 mg once daily for up to 28 days. **HIV-Infected Pts:** *(Suspension):* 400 mg twice daily on day 1, then 400 mg once daily for 7–14 days (28 days in azole refractory pts).

Dosage in Renal Impairment

PO: No dose adjustment. **IV:** Avoid use in pts with CrCl less than 50 mL/min.

Dosage in Hepatic Impairment

No dose adjustment.

SIDE EFFECTS

Common (42%–24%): Diarrhea, nausea, vomiting, headache, abdominal pain, cough. **Frequent (20%–15%):** Constipation, rigors, rash, hypertension, fatigue, insomnia, mucositis, musculoskeletal pain, edema of lower extremities, herpes simplex, anorexia. **Occasional (14%–8%):** Hypotension, epistaxis, tachycardia, pharyngitis, dizziness, pruritus, arthralgia, dyspepsia, back pain, generalized edema, weakness.

ADVERSE EFFECTS/TOXIC REACTIONS

Bacteremia occurs in 18% of pts; upper respiratory tract infection occurs in 7%. Allergic/hypersensitivity reactions, QT prolongation, hemolytic uremic syndrome, thrombotic thrombocytopenic purpura, pulmonary embolus have been reported.

NURSING CONSIDERATIONS

BASELINE ASSESSMENT

Obtain BMP, LFT, EKG. Receive full medication history and screen for interactions (esp. drugs known to prolong QT interval).

INTERVENTION/EVALUATION

Monitor LFT periodically. Monitor daily pattern of bowel activity, stool consistency. Obtain order for antiemetic if excessive vomiting occurs. Monitor B/P for hypertension, hypotension. Assess for lower extremity edema.

PATIENT/FAMILY TEACHING

• Take each dose with full meal or liquid nutritional supplement. • Report severe diarrhea, vomiting, chest pain, yellowing of skin/eyes. • Maintain strict oral hygiene.

---

potassium acetate **HIGH ALERT**

potassium bicarbonate/citrate

(Effer-K, Klor-Con EF)

potassium chloride

(Apo-K ✦, Kaon-Cl, Klor-Con, <u>Klor-Con M10</u>, <u>Klor-Con M20</u>, Micro-K)
Do not confuse Micro-K with Macrobid or Micronase.

◆CLASSIFICATION

PHARMACOTHERAPEUTIC: Electrolyte. **CLINICAL:** Potassium replenisher.

USES

Potassium acetate, potassium bicarbonate/citrate: Treatment, prevention of hypokalemia when necessary to avoid chloride or acid/base imbalance (requires bicarbonate). **Potassium chloride:** Treatment, prevention of hypokalemia.

PRECAUTIONS

Contraindications: Renal failure, hyperkalemia, conditions in which potassium retention is present. Solid oral dosage form in pts in whom there is structural, pathologic cause for delay in passage through GI tract. **Cautions:** Cardiac disease, acid-base disorders, potassium-altering disorders, digitalized pts, concomitant therapy that increases serum potassium (e.g., ACE inhibitors), renal impairment. Do not administer IV undiluted.

ACTION

Necessary for multiple cellular metabolic processes. Primary action is intracellular. **Therapeutic Effect:** Required for nerve impulse conduction, contraction of cardiac, skeletal, smooth muscle; maintains normal renal function, acid-base balance.

PHARMACOKINETICS

Well absorbed from GI tract. Enters cells by active transport from extracellular fluid. Primarily excreted in urine.

⧖ LIFESPAN CONSIDERATIONS

Pregnancy/Lactation: Unknown if drug crosses placenta or is distributed in breast milk. **Children:** No age-related precautions noted. **Elderly:** May be at increased risk for hyperkalemia. Age-related ability to excrete potassium is reduced.

INTERACTIONS

DRUG: ACE inhibitors (e.g., enalapril, lisinopril), potassium-containing medications, potassium-sparing diuretics (e.g., spironolactone, triamterene), salt substitutes may increase serum potassium concentration. **HERBAL:** None significant. **FOOD:** None known. **LAB VALUES:** None known.

AVAILABILITY (Rx)

POTASSIUM ACETATE
Injection, Solution: 2 mEq/mL.
POTASSIUM BICARBONATE AND POTASSIUM CITRATE
Tablets for Solution: (Effer-K): 10 mEq, 20 mEq, 25 mEq. **(Klor-Con EF):** 25 mEq.

✦ Canadian trade name   ▨ Non-Crushable Drug   **HIGH ALERT** High Alert drug

POTASSIUM CHLORIDE
Injection, Solution: 2 mEq/mL. **Oral Solution:** 20 mEq/15 mL, 40 mEq/15 mL. **Powder for Oral Solution:** 20 mEq/packet, 25 mEq/packet.

 Capsules, Extended-Release (Micro-K): 8 mEq, 10 mEq. **Tablets, Extended-Release:** 8 mEq, 10 mEq, 15 mEq, 20 mEq.

ADMINISTRATION/HANDLING
IV

Reconstitution • For IV infusion only, must dilute before administration, mix well, infuse slowly. • Avoid adding potassium to hanging IV.
Rate of Administration • Routinely, give at concentration of no more than 40 mEq/L, no faster than 10 mEq/hr for peripheral infusion, 40 mEq/hr for central infusion. • Check IV site closely during infusion for evidence of phlebitis (heat, pain, red streaking of skin over vein, hardness to vein), extravasation (swelling, pain, cool skin, little/no blood return).
Storage • Store at room temperature. Use admixtures within 24 hrs.

PO
• Take with or after meals, with full glass of water (decreases GI upset). • Liquids, powder, effervescent tablets: Mix, dissolve with juice, water before administering. • Do not break, crush, dissolve, or divide tablets; give whole.

IV INCOMPATIBILITIES
Amphotericin B complex (Abelcet, AmBisome, Amphotec), phenytoin (Dilantin).

IV COMPATIBILITIES
Amiodarone (Cordarone), atropine, aztreonam (Azactam), calcium gluconate, cefepime (Maxipime), ciprofloxacin (Cipro), clindamycin (Cleocin), dexamethasone (Decadron), dexmedetomidine (Precedex), digoxin (Lanoxin), diltiaZEM (Cardizem), diphenhydrAMINE (Benadryl), DOBUTamine (Dobutrex), DOPamine (Intropin), enalapril (Vasotec), famotidine (Pepcid), fluconazole (Diflucan), furosemide (Lasix), granisetron (Kytril), heparin, hydrocortisone (Solu-Cortef), insulin, lidocaine, LORazepam (Ativan), magnesium sulfate, methylPREDNISolone (Solu-Medrol), metoclopramide (Reglan), midazolam (Versed), milrinone (Primacor), morphine, norepinephrine (Levophed), ondansetron (Zofran), oxytocin (Pitocin), piperacillin and tazobactam (Zosyn), procainamide (Pronestyl), propofol (Diprivan), propranolol (Inderal).

INDICATIONS/ROUTES/DOSAGE
Treatment of Hypokalemia
Potassium Acetate
IV: ADULTS, ELDERLY: 5–10 mEq/dose (**Maximum:** 40 mEq/dose) to infuse over 2–3 hrs. **Usual Range:** 40-100 mEq/day.

Dose/rate guidelines

Serum potassium	Greater than 2.5–3.5 mEq/L	2.5 mEq/L or less
Maximum infusion rate	10 mEq/hr	40 mEq/hr
Maximum concentration	40 mEq/L	80 mEq/L
Maximum 24-hr dose	200 mEq	400 mEq

Potassium Chloride
PO: ADULTS, ELDERLY: (Mild to moderate): Initially, 10–20 mEq given 2–4 times/day. **(Severe):** Initially, 40 mEq given 3–4 times/day. (May also give 20 mEq q2–3h in conjunction with careful monitoring.) **CHILDREN:** Initially, 1–2 mEq/kg, then as needed based on lab values.
IV: ADULTS, ELDERLY: 10 mEq/hr (or less); repeat as needed based on lab values. **CHILDREN:** 0.5–1 mEq/kg/dose (**Maximum:** 40 mEq); repeat as needed based on lab values.

Dosage in Renal/Hepatic Impairment
No dose adjustment. Use caution with potassium acetate (may increase serum aluminum and/or potassium).

SIDE EFFECTS

Occasional: Nausea, vomiting, diarrhea, flatulence, abdominal discomfort with distention, phlebitis with IV administration (particularly when potassium concentration of greater than 40 mEq/L is infused). **Rare:** Rash.

ADVERSE EFFECTS/TOXIC REACTIONS

Hyperkalemia (more common in elderly, pts with renal impairment) manifested as paresthesia, feeling of heaviness in lower extremities, cold skin, grayish pallor, hypotension, confusion, irritability, flaccid paralysis, cardiac arrhythmias.

NURSING CONSIDERATIONS

BASELINE ASSESSMENT

Assess for hypokalemia (weakness, fatigue, polyuria, polydipsia). PO should be given with food or after meals with full glass of water, fruit juice (minimizes GI irritation).

INTERVENTION/EVALUATION

Monitor serum potassium (particularly in renal impairment). If GI disturbance is noted, dilute preparation further or give with meals. Be alert to decreased urinary output (may be indication of renal insufficiency). Monitor daily pattern of bowel activity, stool consistency. Assess I&O diligently during diuresis, IV site for extravasation, phlebitis. Be alert to evidence of hyperkalemia (skin pallor/coldness, complaints of paresthesia, feeling of heaviness of lower extremities).

PATIENT/FAMILY TEACHING

• Foods rich in potassium include beef, veal, ham, chicken, turkey, fish, milk, bananas, dates, prunes, raisins, avocados, watermelon, cantaloupe, apricots, molasses, beans, yams, broccoli, brussels sprouts, lentils, potatoes, spinach. • Report paresthesia, feeling of heaviness of lower extremities, tarry or bloody stools, weakness, unusual fatigue.

PRALAtrexate

pral-a-**trex**-ate
(Folotyn)
Do not confuse Folotyn with Focalin, or PRALAtrexate with methotrexate or PEMEtrexed.

◆CLASSIFICATION

PHARMACOTHERAPEUTIC: Antimetabolite. **CLINICAL:** Antineoplastic.

USES

Treatment of relapsed or refractory peripheral T-cell lymphoma (PTCL). **OFF-LABEL:** Treatment of relapsed/refractory cutaneous T-cell lymphoma.

PRECAUTIONS

Contraindications: Hypersensitivity to PRALAtrexate. **Cautions:** Moderate to severe renal impairment, hepatic impairment. Avoid use in end-stage renal disease.

ACTION

Folate analogue metabolic inhibitor that competes with enzymes necessary for tumor cell reproduction. Inhibits DNA, RNA, protein synthesis. **Therapeutic Effect:** Inhibits tumor growth.

PHARMACOKINETICS

Protein binding: 67%. Partially excreted in urine. **Half-life:** 12–18 hrs.

⌛ LIFESPAN CONSIDERATIONS

Pregnancy/Lactation: May cause fetal harm. Unknown if drug is distributed in breast milk. **Children:** Safety and efficacy not established. **Elderly:** No age-related precautions noted.

INTERACTIONS

DRUG: NSAIDs (e.g., ibuprofen, ketorolac, naproxen), probenecid, trimethoprim/sulfamethoxazole may delay clearance, increase concentration. **HERBAL:** Echinacea may decrease

P

concentration/effects.   **FOOD:** None known. **LAB VALUES:** May decrease RBC, WBC, Hgb, Hct, platelet count, serum potassium. May increase serum ALT, AST.

AVAILABILITY (Rx)

Injection Solution: 20 mg/mL.

ADMINISTRATION/HANDLING

◄ **ALERT** ► May be carcinogenic, mutagenic, teratogenic. Handle with extreme care during preparation/administration. Wear gloves when preparing solution. If powder or solution comes in contact with skin, wash immediately, thoroughly with soap, water.

◄ **ALERT** ► Pt should begin taking oral folic acid (1 mg) daily starting 10 days prior to first IV PRALAtrexate dose and continue for 30 days after last dose. Pt should also receive vitamin B_{12} (1 mg) IM injection no more than 10 wks prior to first IV PRALAtrexate dose and every 8–10 wks thereafter.

 IV

Reconstitution • Withdraw calculated dose into syringe for immediate use. • Intended for single use only. • Do not dilute.
Rate of Administration • Administer as IV push over 3–5 min into IV infusion of 0.9% NaCl.
Storage • Refrigerate vials until use, protect from light. Stable at room temperature for 72 hrs. • Discard vial if solution is discolored (solution should appear clear to yellow) or particulate matter is present.

▧ IV INCOMPATIBILITIES

Do not mix with any other medication.

INDICATIONS/ROUTES/DOSAGE

◄ **ALERT** ► Prior to any dose, mucositis should be no higher than CTCAE grade 1, platelets 100,000 cells/mm³ or greater for first dose and 50,000 cells/mm³ or greater for subsequent doses, and absolute neutrophil count (ANC) 1,000 cells/mm³ or greater.

Refractory/Relapsed Peripheral T-Cell Lymphoma
IV: **ADULTS, ELDERLY:** 30 mg/m² administered once wkly for 6 wks in 7-wk cycles. Dose may be decreased to 20 mg/m² to manage adverse reactions. Continue until disease progression or unacceptable toxicity.

Dosage in Renal Impairment
Monitor for toxicities. Avoid use in end-stage renal disease.

Dosage in Hepatic Impairment
CTCAE Grade 3: Withhold dose; decrease to 20 mg/m² when grade 2 or less. **CTCAE Grade 4:** Discontinue.

SIDE EFFECTS

Common (70%–36%): Mucositis, nausea, fatigue. **Frequent (34%–10%):** Constipation/diarrhea, pyrexia, edema, cough, epistaxis, vomiting, dyspnea, anorexia, rash, throat/abdominal/back pain, night sweats, asthenia, tachycardia, upper respiratory infection.

ADVERSE EFFECTS/TOXIC REACTIONS

Hematologic toxicity, resulting from blood dyscrasias, may manifest as thrombocytopenia (41% of pts), anemia (34% of pts), neutropenia (24% of pts), leukopenia (11% of pts). High potential for development of mucositis (70% of pts). Mucositis is less severe when folic acid, vitamin B_{12} therapy is ongoing. Sepsis, pyrexia, febrile neutropenia, dehydration have occurred. Overdosage requires general supportive care. Prompt administration of leucovorin should be considered in case of overdose, based on mechanism of action of PRALAtrexate.

NURSING CONSIDERATIONS

BASELINE ASSESSMENT

Evaluate baseline CBC with differential, renal function, LFT, serum potassium level. Question for possibility of pregnancy before initiating therapy. Assess

P

baseline vital signs, temperature. Antiemetics before and during therapy may alleviate nausea/vomiting. Initiate folic acid, vitamin B$_{12}$ administration prior to and throughout therapy.

INTERVENTION/EVALUATION

Prior to any dose: mucositis should be grade 1 or less. Platelet count 100,000 cells/mm^3 or greater for first dose (50,000 cells/mm^3 or greater for all subsequent doses). Absolute neutrophil count (ANC) 1,000 cells/mm^3 or greater. Assess for signs of mucositis (oropharyngeal ulcers, oral/throat pain, local infection). Monitor for signs of hematologic toxicity, sepsis (fever, signs of local infection, altered CBC results). Monitor hepatic/renal function. Monitor for hypokalemia (muscle cramps, weakness, EKG changes).

PATIENT/FAMILY TEACHING

• Explain importance of folic acid, vitamin B$_{12}$ therapy to reduce adverse effects. • Maintain strict oral hygiene. • Do not have immunizations without physician's approval (drug lowers body's resistance). • Avoid crowds, those with infection. • Promptly report fever, sore throat, signs of local infection, unusual bruising/bleeding from any site. • Use nonhormonal contraception. • Report persistent nausea/vomiting.

---

pramipexole

pram-i-**pex**-ole
(Apo-Pramipexole ✦, Mirapex, Mirapex ER)
Do not confuse Mirapex with Mifeprex or MiraLax.

◆CLASSIFICATION

PHARMACOTHERAPEUTIC: DOPamine receptor agonist. **CLINICAL:** Antiparkinson agent.

USES

Mirapex: Treatment of Parkinson's disease, moderate to severe primary restless legs syndrome. **Mirapex ER:** Treatment of Parkinson's disease. **OFF-LABEL: (Immediate-Release):** Depression (due to bipolar disorder), fibromyalgia.

PRECAUTIONS

Contraindications: Hypersensitivity to pramipexole. **Cautions:** History of orthostatic hypotension, pts at risk for hypotension, syncope, hallucinations, renal impairment (extended release not recommended with CrCl less than 30 mL/min), concomitant use of CNS depressants, preexisting dyskinesia, elderly pts.

ACTION

Stimulates DOPamine receptors in striatum and substantia nigra. **Therapeutic Effect:** Relieves signs/symptoms of Parkinson's disease. Improves motor function.

PHARMACOKINETICS

Rapidly, extensively absorbed after PO administration. Protein binding: 15%. Widely distributed. Steady-state concentrations achieved within 2 days. Primarily excreted in urine. Not removed by hemodialysis. **Half-life:** 8 hrs (12 hrs in pts older than 65 yrs).

⌛ LIFESPAN CONSIDERATIONS

Pregnancy/Lactation: Unknown if drug is distributed in breast milk. **Children:** Safety and efficacy not established. **Elderly:** Increased risk of hallucinations.

INTERACTIONS

DRUG: May increase plasma concentrations of **carbidopa, levodopa. HERBAL:** Gotu kola, kava kava, St. John's wort, SAMe, valerian may increase CNS depression, risk of serotonin syndrome. **FOOD:** All foods delay peak drug plasma levels by 1 hr (extent of absorption not affected). **LAB VALUES:** None significant.

P

AVAILABILITY (Rx)

Tablets: 0.125 mg, 0.25 mg, 0.5 mg, 0.75 mg, 1 mg, 1.5 mg.

Tablets (Extended-Release [Mirapex ER]): 0.375 mg, 0.75 mg, 1.5 mg, 2.25 mg, 3 mg, 3.75 mg, 4.5 mg.

ADMINISTRATION/HANDLING

PO (Mirapex)
• Give without regard to food.

PO (Mirapex ER)
• Give once daily, without regard to food. • Give whole; do not break, crush, dissolve, or divide tablets.

INDICATIONS/ROUTES/DOSAGE

Parkinson's Disease
PO: *(Immediate-Release):* **ADULTS, ELDERLY:** Initially, 0.125 mg 3 times/day. Increase no more frequently than every 5–7 days. **Maintenance:** 0.5–1.5 mg 3 times/day.
(Extended-Release): Initially, 0.375 mg once daily. May increase to 0.75 mg, then by 0.75-mg increments no more frequently than 5–7 days. **Maximum:** 4.5 mg once daily. **Note:** May switch overnight from immediate-release to extended-release at same daily dose.

Restless Legs Syndrome
PO: ADULTS, ELDERLY: *(Immediate-Release):* Initially, 0.125 mg once daily 2–3 hrs before bedtime. May increase to 0.25 mg after 4–7 days, then to 0.5 mg after 4–7 days (interval is 14 days in pts with renal impairment). **Maximum:** 0.5 mg/day.

Dosage in Renal Impairment
Dosage and frequency are modified based on creatinine clearance.

(Parkinson's Disease)
Immediate-Release

Creatinine Clearance	Initial Dosage	Maximum Dosage
30–50 mL/min	0.125 mg twice daily	0.75 mg 3 times/day
15–29 mL/min	0.125 mg once daily	1.5 mg once daily

Extended-Release
CrCl 30–50 mL/min: Initially, 0.375 mg every other day. May increase by 0.375 mg/day in 7 days or longer. **Maximum:** 2.25 mg once daily. **CrCl less than 30 mL/min:** Not recommended.

Restless Legs Syndrome
No dose adjustment.

Dosage in Hepatic Impairment
No dose adjustment.

SIDE EFFECTS

Frequent: Early Parkinson's disease (28%–10%): Nausea, asthenia, dizziness, drowsiness, insomnia, constipation. **Advanced Parkinson's disease (53%–17%):** Orthostatic hypotension, extrapyramidal reactions, insomnia, dizziness, hallucinations. **Occasional: Early Parkinson's disease (5%–2%):** Edema, malaise, confusion, amnesia, akathisia, anorexia, dysphagia, peripheral edema, vision changes, impotence. **Advanced Parkinson's disease (10%–7%):** Asthenia, drowsiness, confusion, constipation, abnormal gait, dry mouth. **Rare: Advanced Parkinson's disease (6%–2%):** General edema, malaise, angina, amnesia, tremor, urinary frequency/incontinence, dyspnea, rhinitis, vision changes. **Restless legs syndrome: Frequent (16%):** Headache, nausea. **Occasional (13%–9%):** Insomnia, fatigue. **Rare (6%–3%):** Drowsiness, constipation, diarrhea, dry mouth.

ADVERSE EFFECTS/TOXIC REACTIONS

Vascular disease, atrial fibrillation, arrhythmias, pulmonary embolism, impulsive/compulsive behavior (pathological gambling, hypersexuality, binge eating) have been reported.

NURSING CONSIDERATIONS

BASELINE ASSESSMENT

Parkinson's disease: Assess for tremor, muscle weakness and rigidity, ataxia. **Restless legs syndrome:** Assess frequency of symptoms, sleep pattern.

INTERVENTION/EVALUATION

Assess for clinical improvement. Assist with ambulation if dizziness occurs. Assess for constipation; encourage fiber, fluids, exercise.

PATIENT/FAMILY TEACHING

• Inform pt that hallucinations may occur, esp. in the elderly. • Go from lying to standing slowly. • Avoid tasks that require alertness, motor skills until response to drug is established. • If nausea occurs, take medication with food. • Avoid abrupt withdrawal. • Avoid alcohol. • Report new or increased impulsive/compulsive behaviors (e.g., gambling, sexual urges, compulsive eating or buying).

---

pramlintide   🔲 HIGH ALERT

pram-lin-tide
(SymlinPen 60, SymlinPen 120)

■ **BLACK BOX ALERT** ■ Increased risk of severe hypoglycemia; usually occurs within 3 hrs of injection. Coadministration with insulin may increase incidence.

◆CLASSIFICATION

PHARMACOTHERAPEUTIC: Amylinomimetic. **CLINICAL:** Antidiabetic agent.

USES

Adjunctive treatment in pts with type 1 or type 2 diabetes who use mealtime insulin therapy and who have failed to achieve desired glucose control despite optimal insulin therapy.

PRECAUTIONS

Contraindications: Hypersensitivity to pramlintide. Diagnosed gastroparesis, hypoglycemia unawareness. **Cautions:** Coadministration with insulin may induce severe hypoglycemia (usually within 3 hrs following administration); concurrent use of other glucose-lowering agents may increase risk of hypoglycemia. History of nausea, visual or dexterity impairment, poor compliance with insulin monitoring or current insulin therapy, pts with hemoglobin A_{1c} greater than 9%, pts with conditions or taking concurrent medications likely to impair gastric motility (e.g., anticholinergics), pts requiring medication to stimulate gastric emptying.

ACTION

Synthetic analogue of amylin. Cosecreted with insulin by pancreatic beta cells, reduces postprandial glucose increases by slowing gastric emptying time, reducing postprandial glucagon secretion, reducing caloric intake through centrally mediated appetite suppression. **Therapeutic Effect:** Improves glycemic control by reducing postprandial glucose concentrations in pts with type 1, type 2 diabetes mellitus.

PHARMACOKINETICS

	Onset	Peak	Duration
SQ	NA	20 min	3 hrs

Metabolized primarily by kidneys. Protein binding: 60%. Excreted in urine. **Half-life:** 48 min.

⧗ LIFESPAN CONSIDERATIONS

Pregnancy/Lactation: Unknown if distributed in breast milk. **Children:** Safety and efficacy not established. **Elderly:** No age-related precautions noted.

INTERACTIONS

DRUG: Anticholinergics (e.g., dicyclomine, glycopyrrolate, scopolamine) may cause additive impairment

---

of gastric motility. HERBAL: Garlic may increase hypoglycemia. FOOD: Ethanol may increase risk of hypoglycemia. LAB VALUES: None significant.

AVAILABILITY (Rx)

Injection, Solution (SymlinPen 120): Delivers fixed doses of 120 mcg. (SymlinPen 60): Delivers fixed doses of 60 mcg.

ADMINISTRATION/HANDLING

SQ

• Administer immediately before each major meal (350 or more kcal or containing 30 g or more carbohydrate). • Give in abdomen or thigh; do not give in arm (variable absorption). • Injection site should be distinct from insulin injection site. • Rotation of injection sites is essential. • Use U-100 insulin syringe for accuracy. • Always give pramlintide and insulin as separate injections.

Storage • Store unopened vials in refrigerator. • Discard if freezing occurs. • Vials that have been opened (punctured) may be stored in refrigerator or kept at room temperature for up to 30 days.

INDICATIONS/ROUTES/DOSAGE

◄ALERT► Initially, current insulin dosage in all pts with type 1, type 2 diabetes mellitus should be reduced by 50%. This includes preprandial, rapid-acting, short-acting, fixed-mixed insulins. Oral medications should be given 1 hr before or 2 hrs after pramlintide.

Type 1 Diabetes Mellitus
SQ: ADULTS, ELDERLY: Initially, 15 mcg immediately before each major meal. Titrate in 15-mcg increments every 3 days (if no significant nausea occurs) to target dose of 30–60 mcg.

Type 2 Diabetes Mellitus
SQ: ADULTS, ELDERLY: Initially, 60 mcg immediately before each major meal. After 3–7 days, increase to 120 mcg if no significant nausea occurs (if nausea occurs at 120-mcg dose, reduce to 60 mcg).

Dosage in Renal/Hepatic Impairment
No dose adjustment.

SIDE EFFECTS

TYPE 1 DIABETES MELLITUS
Frequent (48%): Nausea. Occasional (17%–11%): Anorexia, vomiting. Rare (7%–5%): Fatigue, arthralgia, allergic reaction, dizziness.
TYPE 2 DIABETES MELLITUS
Frequent (28%): Nausea. Occasional (13%–8%): Headache, anorexia, vomiting, abdominal pain. Rare (7%–5%): Fatigue, dizziness, cough, pharyngitis.

ADVERSE EFFECTS/TOXIC REACTIONS

Overdose produces severe nausea, vomiting, diarrhea, vasodilation, dizziness. No hypoglycemia was reported. Increased risk of severe hypoglycemia when given concurrently with nontitrated insulin.

NURSING CONSIDERATIONS

BASELINE ASSESSMENT
Check serum glucose concentration before administration, both before and after meals and at bedtime. Discuss lifestyle to determine extent of learning, emotional needs. Ensure follow-up instruction if pt, family does not thoroughly understand diabetes management, glucose testing technique.

INTERVENTION/EVALUATION
Risk for hypoglycemia occurs within first 3 hrs following drug administration if given concurrently with insulin. Assess for hypoglycemia (diaphoresis, tremors, dizziness, anxiety, headache, tachycardia, numbness in mouth, hunger, diplopia, difficulty concentrating). Be alert to conditions that alter glucose requirements (fever, increased activity, stress, surgical procedures).

P

PATIENT/FAMILY TEACHING

• Diabetes mellitus requires lifelong control. • Prescribed diet, exercise are principal parts of treatment; do not skip/delay meals. • Continue to adhere to dietary instructions, regular exercise program, regular testing of serum glucose. • When taking combination drug therapy, have source of glucose available to treat symptoms of low blood sugar.

---

prasugrel
TOP 100

pra-soo-grel
(Effient)

■ **BLACK BOX ALERT** ■ Serious, sometimes fatal, hemorrhage may occur.
Do not confuse Effient with Effexor, or prasugrel with praziquantel.

◆CLASSIFICATION

PHARMACOTHERAPEUTIC: Thienopyridine derivative inhibitor. **CLINICAL:** Antiplatelet agent.

USES

Reduction of thrombotic cardiovascular events (MI, CVA, stent thrombosis) in pts with acute coronary syndrome (unstable angina, non–ST-segment elevation MI, ST-segment MI) who are to be managed with percutaneous coronary intervention (PCI). **OFF-LABEL:** Initial treatment of unstable angina, STEMI in pts undergoing PCI with allergy or major GI intolerance to aspirin.

PRECAUTIONS

Contraindications: Hypersensitivity to prasugrel. Active bleeding, prior transient ischemic attack (TIA), CVA. **Cautions:** Pts who undergo coronary artery bypass graft (CABG) after receiving prasugrel, pts at risk for bleeding (age 75 yrs or older, body weight less than 60 kg, recent trauma/surgery, recent GI bleeding or active peptic ulcer disease, severe hepatic impairment).

ACTION

Inhibits binding of the enzyme adenosine phosphate (ADP) to its platelet receptor and subsequent ADP-mediated activation of a glycoprotein complex. **Therapeutic Effect:** Inhibits platelet aggregation.

PHARMACOKINETICS

Rapidly absorbed, with peak concentration occurring 30 min following administration. Metabolized in liver. Protein binding: 98%. Excreted in urine (68%), feces (27%). **Half-life:** 7 hrs.

⧗ LIFESPAN CONSIDERATIONS

Pregnancy/Lactation: Unknown if drug crosses placenta or is distributed in breast milk. **Children:** Safety and efficacy not established. **Elderly:** May have increased risk for intracranial hemorrhage; caution advised in pts 75 yrs and older.

INTERACTIONS

DRUG: Aspirin, NSAIDs (e.g., ibuprofen, ketorolac, naproxen), warfarin may increase risk of bleeding. **HERBAL: Cat's claw, dong quai, evening primrose, feverfew, garlic, ginger, ginseng, green tea, horse chestnut, red clover** may have additive platelet effects. **Ginkgo biloba** may increase risk of bleeding. **FOOD:** None known. **LAB VALUES:** May decrease Hgb, Hct, WBC, platelet count. May increase bleeding time, serum cholesterol, ALT, AST.

AVAILABILITY (Rx)

🍷 **Tablets:** 5 mg, 10 mg.

ADMINISTRATION/HANDLING

PO
• Give without regard to food. • Do not crush tablet.

INDICATIONS/ROUTES/DOSAGE

Acute Coronary Syndrome
◀ **ALERT** ▶ Consider 5 mg once daily for pts weighing less than 60 kg. Not recommended in pts 75 yrs and older.

PO: **ADULTS, ELDERLY:** Initially, 60-mg loading dose, then 10 mg once daily (in combination with aspirin) for at least 12 mos.

Dosage in Renal/Hepatic Impairment
No dose adjustment.

SIDE EFFECTS

Occasional (8%–4%): Hypertension, minor bleeding, headache, back pain, dyspnea, nausea, dizziness. **Rare (less than 4%):** Cough, hypotension, fatigue, noncardiac chest pain, bradycardia, rash, pyrexia, peripheral edema, extremity pain, diarrhea.

ADVERSE EFFECTS/TOXIC REACTIONS

Major bleeding (intracranial hemorrhage, epistaxis, GI bleeding, hemoptysis, SQ hematoma, postprocedural hemorrhage, retroperitoneal hemorrhage, retinal hemorrhage) has been reported. Severe thrombocytopenia, anemia, abnormal hepatic function, anaphylactic reaction, angioedema, atrial fibrillation occur rarely. Overdosage may require platelet transfusion to restore clotting ability.

NURSING CONSIDERATIONS

BASELINE ASSESSMENT
Obtain baseline vital signs, CBC, EKG, LFT. Question history of intracranial hemorrhage, GI bleeding, ulcers, recent surgery or trauma.

INTERVENTION/EVALUATION
Monitor vital signs for changes in B/P, pulse. Assess for signs of unusual bleeding or hemorrhage, pain. Monitor platelet count, LFT, EKG for changes from baseline.

PATIENT/FAMILY TEACHING
• It may take longer to stop minor bleeding during drug therapy. Report unusual bleeding/bruising, blood noted in stool or urine, chest/back pain, extremity pain, symptoms of stroke. • Monitor for dyspnea. • Report fever, weakness, extreme skin paleness, purple skin patches, yellowing of skin or eyes, changes in mental status. • Do not discontinue drug therapy without physician approval. • Inform physicians, dentists before undergoing any invasive procedure or surgery.

pravastatin

pra-va-sta-tin
(Apo-Pravastatin ✦, <u>Pravachol</u>)
Do not confuse pravastatin with atorvastatin, lovastatin, nystatin, pitavastatin, or simvastatin, or Pravachol with Prevacid, Prinivil, or propranolol.

FIXED-COMBINATION(S)

Pravigard: pravastatin/aspirin (anticoagulant): 20 mg/81 mg, 40 mg/81 mg, 80 mg/81 mg, 20 mg/325 mg, 40 mg/325 mg, 80 mg/325 mg.

◆CLASSIFICATION

PHARMACOTHERAPEUTIC: Hydroxymethylglutaryl CoA (HMG-CoA) reductase inhibitor. **CLINICAL:** Antihyperlipidemic.

USES

Adjunct to diet in the treatment of primary hyperlipidemias and mixed dyslipidemias to reduce total cholesterol, LDL cholesterol, apolipoprotein B, triglycerides; increase HDL cholesterol. Reduces risk of MI, revascularization, and mortality in hypercholesterolemia without clinically evident CHD. Reduces mortality risk in pts with CHD. Reduces elevated triglycerides in hypertriglyceridemia. Treatment of heterozygous familial hypercholesterolemia in pediatric pts 8–18 yrs.

PRECAUTIONS

Contraindications: Hypersensitivity to pravastatin. Active hepatic disease or unexplained, persistent elevations of LFT results. Pregnancy, breastfeeding. **Cautions:** History of hepatic disease, substantial alcohol consumption. Withholding/discontinuing pravastatin may be necessary when pt is at risk for renal failure secondary to rhabdomyolysis, elderly.

ACTION

Interferes with cholesterol biosynthesis by preventing conversion of HMG-CoA reductase to mevalonate, a precursor to cholesterol. **Therapeutic Effect:** Lowers LDL, VLDL cholesterol, plasma triglycerides; increases HDL.

PHARMACOKINETICS

Rapidly absorbed from GI tract. Protein binding: 50%. Metabolized in liver. Primarily excreted in feces via biliary system. Not removed by hemodialysis. **Half-life:** 2–3 hrs. (Half-life including all metabolites: 77 hrs.)

⌛ LIFESPAN CONSIDERATIONS

Pregnancy/Lactation: Contraindicated in pregnancy (suppression of cholesterol biosynthesis may cause fetal toxicity) and lactation. Small amount is distributed in breast milk, but there is risk of serious adverse reactions in breastfeeding infants. Breastfeeding not recommended. **Children/Elderly:** No age-related precautions noted.

INTERACTIONS

DRUG: CycloSPORINE, clarithromycin, colchicine, erythromycin, gemfibrozil, immunosuppressants, niacin increase risk of myopathy, rhabdomyolysis. **HERBAL:** St. John's wort may decrease concentration. **FOOD:** Red yeast rice contains 2.4 mg lovastatin per 600 mg rice. **LAB VALUES:** May increase serum creatine kinase (CK), transaminase.

AVAILABILITY (Rx)

Tablets: 10 mg, 20 mg, 40 mg, 80 mg.

ADMINISTRATION/HANDLING

PO
• Give without regard to meals.

INDICATIONS/ROUTES/DOSAGE

◄**ALERT►** Prior to initiating therapy, pt should be on standard cholesterol-lowering diet for 3–6 mos. Low-cholesterol diet should be continued throughout pravastatin therapy.

Hyperlipidemia, Prevention of Coronary/Cardiovascular Events
PO: ADULTS, ELDERLY: Initially, 40 mg/day. Titrate to desired response. Range: 10–80 mg/day.

Heterozygous Familial Hypercholesterolemia
PO: CHILDREN 14–18 YRS: 40 mg/day. **CHILDREN 8–13 YRS:** 20 mg/day.

Dosage with Clarithromycin
Maximum: 40 mg/day.

Dosage with CycloSPORINE
ADULTS, ELDERLY: Initially, 10 mg/day. **Maximum:** 20 mg/day.

Dosage in Renal Impairment
For adults, give 10 mg/day initially. Titrate to desired response.

Dosage in Hepatic Impairment
See contraindications.

SIDE EFFECTS

Pravastatin is generally well tolerated. Side effects are usually mild and transient. **Occasional (7%–4%):** Nausea, vomiting, diarrhea, constipation, abdominal pain, headache, rhinitis, rash, pruritus. **Rare (3%–2%):** Heartburn, myalgia, dizziness, cough, fatigue, flu-like symptoms, depression, photosensitivity.

ADVERSE EFFECTS/TOXIC REACTIONS

Potential for malignancy, cataracts. Hypersensitivity, myopathy occur rarely. Rhabdomyolysis has been reported.

P

✦ Canadian trade name   🐴 Non-Crushable Drug   🔲 High Alert drug

NURSING CONSIDERATIONS

BASELINE ASSESSMENT

Obtain dietary history, esp. fat consumption. Question for possibility of pregnancy before initiating therapy. Assess baseline serum lab results (cholesterol, triglycerides, LFT).

INTERVENTION/EVALUATION

Monitor serum cholesterol, triglyceride lab results for therapeutic response. Monitor LFT, CPK. Monitor daily pattern of bowel activity, stool consistency. Assess for headache, dizziness (provide assistance as needed). Assess for rash, pruritus. Be alert for malaise, muscle cramping/weakness; if accompanied by fever, may require discontinuation of medication.

PATIENT/FAMILY TEACHING

• Follow special diet (important part of treatment). • Periodic lab tests are essential part of therapy. • Report promptly any muscle pain/weakness, esp. if accompanied by fever, malaise. • Avoid tasks that require alertness, motor skills until response to drug is established (potential for dizziness). • Use nonhormonal contraception. • Avoid direct exposure to sunlight.

prednisoLONE

pred-**niss**-oh-lone
(Millipred, Novo-PrednisoLONE ✦, Omnipred, Orapred ODT, Pediapred, Pred Forte, Pred Mild, Prelone, Veripred)
Do not confuse Pediapred with Pediazole, prednisoLONE with predniSONE or primidone, or Prelone with PROzac.

FIXED-COMBINATION(S)

Blephamide: prednisoLONE/sulfacetamide (an anti-infective): 0.2%/10%. **Vasocidin:** prednisoLONE/sulfacetamide: 0.25%/10%.

◆CLASSIFICATION

PHARMACOTHERAPEUTIC: Adrenal corticosteroid. **CLINICAL:** Anti-inflammatory, immunosuppressant.

USES

Systemic: Endocrine, rheumatic, hematologic disorders; collagen, respiratory, neoplastic, GI diseases; allergic states; acute or chronic solid organ rejection. **Ophthalmic:** Treatment of conjunctivitis, corneal injury (from chemical/thermal burns, foreign body).

PRECAUTIONS

Contraindications: Hypersensitivity to prednisoLONE. Acute superficial herpes simplex keratitis, systemic fungal infections, varicella, live or attenuated virus vaccines. **Cautions:** Hyperthyroidism, cirrhosis, ocular herpes simplex, respiratory tuberculosis, untreated systemic infections, renal/hepatic impairment, diabetes, cataracts, glaucoma, seizure disorder, peptic ulcer disease, osteoporosis, myasthenia gravis, hypertension, HF, ulcerative colitis, thromboembolic disorders, elderly pts.

ACTION

Inhibits accumulation of inflammatory cells at inflammation sites, phagocytosis, lysosomal enzyme release/synthesis, release of mediators of inflammation. **Therapeutic Effect:** Prevents/suppresses cell-mediated immune reactions. Decreases/prevents tissue response to inflammatory process.

PHARMACOKINETICS

Protein binding: 65%–91%. Metabolized in liver. Excreted in urine. **Half-life:** 3.6 hrs.

⧗ LIFESPAN CONSIDERATIONS

Pregnancy/Lactation: Crosses placenta. Distributed in breast milk. Fetal cleft palate often occurs with chronic, first-trimester use. Breastfeeding not recommended. **Children:** Prolonged treatment or high dosages may decrease short-term growth rate, cortisol secretion. **Elderly:** May be more susceptible to developing hypertension or osteoporosis.

INTERACTIONS

DRUG: CYP3A4 inducers (e.g., carBA-Mazepine, phenytoin, rifAMPin) may decrease effects. **Live virus vaccines** increase vaccine side effects, potentiate virus replication, decrease pt's antibody response to vaccine. May increase effect of **warfarin. HERBAL:** St. John's wort may decrease concentration. **Cat's claw, echinacea** have immunostimulant properties. **Echinacea** may decrease level/effects. **FOOD:** None known. **LAB VALUES:** May increase serum glucose, lipids, sodium, uric acid. May decrease serum calcium, WBC, hypothalamic pituitary adrenal (HPA) axis function, potassium.

AVAILABILITY (Rx)

Solution, Ophthalmic: 1%. **Solution, Oral:** 15 mg/5 mL. **(Pediapred):** 5 mg/5 mL. **(Millipred):** 10 mg/5 mL. **(Veripred):** 20 mg/5 mL. **Suspension, Ophthalmic (Pred Forte):** 1%; **(Pred Mild):** 0.12%. **Syrup (Prelone):** 15 mg/5 mL. **Tablets:** 5 mg.

🐢 **Tablets, Orally Disintegrating:** 10 mg, 15 mg, 30 mg.

ADMINISTRATION/HANDLING

PO
• Give with food or fluids to decrease GI side effects.

Orally Disintegrating Tablets
• Do not break, crush, or divide tablets. • Remove from blister just prior to giving; place on tongue. • Pt may swallow whole or allow to dissolve in mouth with/without water.

Ophthalmic
• For ophthalmic solution, shake well before using. • Instill drops into conjunctival sac, as prescribed. • Avoid touching applicator tip to conjunctiva to avoid contamination.

INDICATIONS/ROUTES/DOSAGE

Usual Dosage
PO: ADULTS, ELDERLY: 5–60 mg/day in divided doses. **CHILDREN:** 0.05–2 mg/kg/day divided every 6–24 hrs.

Treatment of Conjunctivitis, Corneal Injury
Ophthalmic: ADULTS, ELDERLY, CHILDREN: 1–2 drops every hr during day and q2h during night. After response, decrease dosage to 1 drop q4h, then 1 drop 3–4 times/day.

Dosage in Renal/Hepatic Impairment
No dose adjustment.

SIDE EFFECTS

Frequent: Insomnia, heartburn, nervousness, abdominal distention, diaphoresis, acne, mood swings, increased appetite, facial flushing, delayed wound healing, increased susceptibility to infection, diarrhea, constipation. **Occasional:** Headache, edema, change in skin color, frequent urination. **Rare:** Tachycardia, allergic reaction (rash, urticaria), psychological changes, hallucinations, depression. **Ophthalmic:** Stinging/burning, posterior subcapsular cataracts.

ADVERSE EFFECTS/TOXIC REACTIONS

Long-term therapy: Hypocalcemia, hypokalemia, muscle wasting (esp. arms, legs), osteoporosis, spontaneous fractures, amenorrhea, cataracts, glaucoma, peptic ulcer, HF, immunosuppression. **Abrupt withdrawal following long-term therapy:** Anorexia, nausea, fever, headache, severe/sudden joint pain, rebound inflammation, fatigue, weakness, lethargy, dizziness, orthostatic hypotension. Sudden discontinuance may be fatal.

NURSING CONSIDERATIONS

BASELINE ASSESSMENT
Question medical history as listed in Precautions. Obtain baselines for height, weight, B/P, serum glucose, electrolytes. Check results of initial tests (tuberculosis [TB] skin test, X-rays, EKG).

P

INTERVENTION/EVALUATION

Monitor B/P, weight, serum electrolytes, glucose, results of bone mineral density test, height, weight in children. Be alert to infection (sore throat, fever, vague symptoms); assess oral cavity daily for signs of *Candida* infection. Monitor for symptoms of adrenal insufficiency, immunosuppression.

PATIENT/FAMILY TEACHING

• Report fever, sore throat, muscle aches, sudden weight gain, swelling, loss of appetite, fatigue. • Avoid alcohol, limit caffeine. • Maintain fastidious oral hygiene. • Do not abruptly discontinue without physician's approval. • Avoid exposure to chickenpox, measles. • Long-term use may significantly increase risk of serious infections.

---

predniSONE

pred-ni-sone
(Apo-PredniSONE ❋, PredniSONE Intensol, Rayos, Winpred ❋)
Do not confuse predniSONE with methylPREDNISolone, prazosin, prednisoLONE, PriLOSEC, primidone, or promethazine.

◆CLASSIFICATION

PHARMACOTHERAPEUTIC: Adrenal corticosteroid. **CLINICAL:** Antiinflammatory, immunosuppressant.

USES

Substitution therapy in deficiency states: Acute or chronic adrenal insufficiency, congenital adrenal hyperplasia, adrenal insufficiency secondary to pituitary insufficiency. **Nonendocrine disorders:** Arthritis, rheumatic carditis; allergic, collagen, intestinal tract, multiple sclerosis exacerbations; liver, ocular, renal, skin diseases; bronchial asthma, cerebral edema, malignancies. **OFF-LABEL:** Prevention of postherpetic neuralgia, relief of acute pain in pts with herpes zoster, autoimmune hepatitis.

PRECAUTIONS

Contraindications: Hypersensitivity to prednisONE. Acute superficial herpes simplex keratitis, systemic fungal infections, varicella, administration of live or attenuated virus vaccines. **Cautions:** Hyperthyroidism, cirrhosis, ocular herpes simplex, respiratory tuberculosis, untreated systemic infections, renal/hepatic impairment, following acute MI, diabetes, cataracts, glaucoma, seizures, peptic ulcer disease, osteoporosis, myasthenia gravis, hypertension, HF, ulcerative colitis, thromboembolic disorders, elderly.

ACTION

Inhibits accumulation of inflammatory cells at inflammation sites, phagocytosis, lysosomal enzyme release/synthesis, release of mediators of inflammation. **Therapeutic Effect:** Prevents/suppresses cell-mediated immune reactions. Decreases/prevents tissue response to inflammatory process.

PHARMACOKINETICS

Well absorbed from GI tract. Protein binding: 70%–90%. Widely distributed. Metabolized in liver, converted to prednisoLONE. Primarily excreted in urine. Not removed by hemodialysis. **Half-life:** 2.5–3.5 hrs.

⌛ LIFESPAN CONSIDERATIONS

Pregnancy/Lactation: Crosses placenta. Distributed in breast milk. Fetal cleft palate often occurs with chronic, first trimester use. Breastfeeding not recommended. **Children:** Prolonged treatment or high dosages may decrease short-term growth rate, cortisol secretion. **Elderly:** May be more susceptible to developing hypertension or osteoporosis.

INTERACTIONS

DRUG: CYP3A4 inducers (e.g., carBAMazepine, phenytoin, rifAMPin) may decrease effects. **Live virus vaccines** may increase vaccine side effects, potentiate virus replication, decrease pt's antibody response to vaccine. May increase effect of

---

warfarin. **HERBAL: St. John's wort** may decrease concentration. **Cat's claw, echinacea** have immunostimulant properties. **FOOD:** None known. **LAB VALUES:** May increase serum glucose, lipids, sodium, uric acid. May decrease serum calcium, potassium, WBC, hypothalamic pituitary adrenal (HPA) axis function.

AVAILABILITY (Rx)

Solution, Oral: 1 mg/mL. **Solution, Oral Concentrate (PredniSONE Intensol):** 5 mg/mL. **Tablets:** 1 mg, 2.5 mg, 5 mg, 10 mg, 20 mg, 50 mg.

🥄 **Tablet: (Delayed-Release [Rayos]):** 1 mg, 2 mg, 5 mg.

ADMINISTRATION/HANDLING
PO

• Give with food or fluids to decrease GI side effects. • Give single doses before 9 AM, multiple doses at evenly spaced intervals. • Give delayed-release tablet whole; do not break, crush, dissolve, or divide.

INDICATIONS/ROUTES/DOSAGE

Note: Dose dependent upon condition treated, pt response rather than by rigid adherence to age, weight, or body surface area.

Usual Dosage
PO: ADULTS, ELDERLY: 5–60 mg/day in divided doses. **CHILDREN:** 0.05–2 mg/kg/day in 1–4 divided doses.

Dosage in Renal/Hepatic Impairment
No dose adjustment.

SIDE EFFECTS

Frequent: Insomnia, heartburn, nervousness, abdominal distention, diaphoresis, acne, mood swings, increased appetite, facial flushing, delayed wound healing, increased susceptibility to infection, diarrhea, constipation. **Occasional:** Headache, edema, change in skin color, frequent urination. **Rare:** Tachycardia, allergic reaction (rash, urticaria), psychological changes, hallucinations, depression.

ADVERSE EFFECTS/TOXIC REACTIONS

Long-term therapy: Muscle wasting (esp. in arms, legs), osteoporosis, spontaneous fractures, amenorrhea, cataracts, glaucoma, peptic ulcer, HF. **Abrupt withdrawal following long-term therapy:** Anorexia, nausea, fever, headache, rebound inflammation, fatigue, weakness, lethargy, dizziness, orthostatic hypotension. Sudden discontinuance may be fatal.

NURSING CONSIDERATIONS

BASELINE ASSESSMENT
Question medical history as listed in Precautions. Obtain baselines for height, weight, B/P, serum glucose, electrolytes. Check results of initial tests (tuberculosis [TB] skin test, X-rays, EKG).

INTERVENTION/EVALUATION
Monitor B/P, serum electrolytes, glucose, results of bone mineral density test, height, weight in children. Be alert to infection (sore throat, fever, vague symptoms); assess oral cavity daily for signs of *Candida* infection. Monitor for symptoms of adrenal insufficiency, immunosuppression.

PATIENT/FAMILY TEACHING
• Report fever, sore throat, muscle aches, sudden weight gain, swelling, loss of appetite, or fatigue. • Avoid alcohol, minimize use of caffeine. • Maintain fastidious oral hygiene. • Do not abruptly discontinue without physician's approval. • Avoid exposure to chickenpox, measles. • Long-term use may significantly increase risk of serious infections.

pregabalin
TOP 100

pre-**gab**-a-lin
(Apo-Pregabalin ✦, Lyrica CR)
PHARMACOTHERAPEUTIC: Antinociceptive agent. **CLINICAL:** Anticonvulsant, antineuralgic, analgesic **(Schedule V).**

USES

Lyrica: Adjunctive therapy in treatment of partial-onset seizures. Management of neuropathic pain associated with diabetic peripheral neuropathy or spinal cord injury. Management of postherpetic neuralgia. Management of fibromyalgia. **Lyrica CR:** Management of neuropathic pain associated with diabetic peripheral neuropathy, postherpetic nueralgia.

PRECAUTIONS

Contraindications: Hypersensitivity to pregabalin. **Cautions:** HF, renal impairment, cardiovascular disease, diabetes, history of angioedema, pts at risk for suicide. Concurrent use of thiazolidine antidiabetics (e.g., Actos).

ACTION

Binds to calcium channel sites in CNS tissue, inhibiting excitatory neurotransmitter release. Exerts antinociceptive, anticonvulsant activity. **Therapeutic Effect:** Decreases symptoms of painful peripheral neuropathy; decreases frequency of partial seizures.

PHARMACOKINETICS

Well absorbed following PO administration. Excreted in urine unchanged. **Half-life:** 6 hrs.

⌛ LIFESPAN CONSIDERATIONS

Pregnancy/Lactation: Increased risk of fetal skeletal abnormalities. Unknown if distributed in breast milk. **Children:** Safety and efficacy not established. **Elderly:** Age-related renal impairment may require dosage adjustment.

INTERACTIONS

DRUG: Alcohol, CNS depressants (e.g., LORazepam, morphine, zolpidem) may increase sedative effect. **HERBAL:** Gotu kola, kava kava, St. John's wort, valerian may increase CNS depression. **FOOD:** None known. **LAB VALUES:** May increase CPK. May cause mild PR interval prolongation. May decrease platelet count.

AVAILABILITY (Rx)

Solution, Oral: 20 mg/mL.

📋 **Capsules (Lyrica):** 25 mg, 50 mg, 75 mg, 100 mg, 150 mg, 200 mg, 225 mg, 300 mg. **Capsules (Lyrica CR):** 82.5 mg, 165 mg, 330 mg.

ADMINISTRATION/HANDLING

• Give without regard to food. • Administer whole; do not break, crush, or open capsule. **Lyrica CR:** Give once daily in evening. Discontinue gradually over at least one wk.

INDICATIONS/ROUTES/DOSAGE

Partial-Onset Seizures
PO: ADULTS, ELDERLY: Initially, 75 mg twice daily or 50 mg 3 times/day. May increase dose based on tolerability/effect. **Maximum:** 600 mg/day.

Neuropathic Pain (Diabetes-Associated)
PO: ADULTS, ELDERLY: Initially, 50 mg 3 times/day. May be increased within 1 wk based on tolerability/effect. **Maximum:** 300 mg/day in 3 divided doses.

PO: (Lyrica CR): ADULTS, ELDERLY: Initially, 165 mg once daily. May increase to 330 mg/day within 1 wk. **Maximum:** 330 mg/day.

Postherpetic Neuralgia, Neuropathic Pain Associated with Spinal Cord Injury
PO: ADULTS, ELDERLY: Initially, 75 mg twice daily or 50 mg 3 times/day. May increase to 300 mg/day within 1 wk. May further increase to 600 mg/day after 2–4 wks. **Maximum:** 600 mg/day.

PO: (Lyrica CR): ADULTS, ELDERLY: Initially, 165 mg once daily. May increase to 330 mg/day within 1 wk. May further increase to 660 mg once daily after 2–4 wks. **Maximum:** 330 mg/day.

Fibromyalgia
PO: ADULTS, ELDERLY: Initially, 75 mg twice daily. May increase to 150 mg twice daily within 1 wk. **Maximum:** 225 mg twice daily.

Dosage in Renal Impairment

Creatinine Clearance	Daily Dosage
30–60 mL/min	75–300 mg in 2–3 divided doses
15–29 mL/min	25–150 mg in 1 or 2 doses
Less than 15 mL/min	25–75 mg once daily

Dosage for Hemodialysis

◀ **ALERT** ▶ Take supplemental dose immediately following dialysis.

Daily Dosage	Supplemental Dosage
25 mg	Single dose of 25 mg or 50 mg
25–50 mg	Single dose of 50 mg or 75 mg
75 mg	Single dose of 100 mg or 150 mg

Dosage in Hepatic Impairment
No dose adjustment.

SIDE EFFECTS

Frequent (32%–12%): Dizziness, drowsiness, ataxia, peripheral edema. **Occasional (12%–5%):** Weight gain, blurred vision, diplopia, difficulty with concentration, attention, cognition; tremor, dry mouth, headache, constipation, asthenia. **Rare (4%–2%):** Abnormal gait, confusion, incoordination, twitching, flatulence, vomiting, edema, myopathy.

ADVERSE EFFECTS/TOXIC REACTIONS

Abrupt withdrawal increases risk of seizure frequency in pts with seizure disorders; withdraw gradually over a minimum of 1 wk. May increase risk of suicidal thoughts and behavior.

NURSING CONSIDERATIONS

BASELINE ASSESSMENT

Seizure: Review history of seizure disorder (type, onset, intensity, frequency, duration, LOC). **Pain:** Assess onset, type, location, and duration of pain.

INTERVENTION/EVALUATION

Provide safety measures as needed. Assess for seizure activity. Assess for clinical improvement; record onset of relief of pain.

Assess for peripheral edema. Question for changes in visual acuity. Monitor weight.

PATIENT/FAMILY TEACHING

• Do not abruptly stop taking drug; seizure frequency may be increased. • Avoid tasks that require alterness, motor skills until response to drug is established. • Avoid alcohol. • Carry identification card, bracelet to note seizure disorder, anticonvulsant therapy.

---

primidone

prim-i-done
(Apo-Primidone ✦, Mysoline)
Do not confuse primidone with predniSONE or pyridoxine.

◆CLASSIFICATION

PHARMACOTHERAPEUTIC: Barbiturate. **CLINICAL:** Anticonvulsant.

USES

Management of partial seizures, generalized tonic-clonic (grand mal) seizures, focal seizures. **OFF-LABEL:** Treatment of essential tremor (familial tremor).

P

PRECAUTIONS

Contraindications: Hypersensitivity to primidone, PHENobarbital; porphyria. **Cautions:** Renal/hepatic impairment, pulmonary insufficiency, elderly pts, debilitated pts, children, hypoadrenalism, pts at risk for suicidal thoughts/behavior, depression, history of drug abuse.

ACTION

Decreases neuron excitability. **Therapeutic Effect:** Reduces seizure activity.

PHARMACOKINETICS

Rapidly, usually completely absorbed following PO administration. Protein binding: 99%. Metabolized in liver to PHENobarbital. Minimal excretion in urine. **Half-life:** 3–6 hrs. (PHENobarbital: 2–5 days.)

✦ Canadian trade name   🗢 Non-Crushable Drug   🔲 High Alert drug

⏳ LIFESPAN CONSIDERATIONS

Pregnancy/Lactation: Crosses placenta; distributed in breast milk. **Children, Elderly:** May produce paradoxical excitement, restlessness.

INTERACTIONS

DRUG: Alcohol, other CNS depressants (e.g., **LORazepam**, morphine, zolpidem) may increase effects. **Valproic acid** increases concentration, risk of toxicity. **HERBAL: Evening primrose** may decrease seizure threshold. **Gotu kola, kava kava, St. John's wort, valerian** may increase CNS depression. **FOOD:** None known. **LAB VALUES:** May decrease serum bilirubin. **Therapeutic serum level:** 4–12 mcg/mL; **toxic serum level:** greater than 12 mcg/mL.

AVAILABILITY (Rx)

Tablets: 50 mg, 250 mg.

ADMINISTRATION/HANDLING

PO
• Give with food to minimize GI effects.

INDICATIONS/ROUTES/DOSAGE

Seizure Control
PO: ADULTS, ELDERLY, CHILDREN 8 YRS AND OLDER: Initially, 100–125 mg/day at bedtime for days 1–3. **Days 4–6:** 100–125 mg twice daily. **Days 7–9:** 100–125 mg 3 times/day. **Usual dose:** 750–1,500 mg/day. **Maximum:** 2 g/day. **CHILDREN YOUNGER THAN 8 YRS:** Initially, 50 mg/day at bedtime for days 1–3. **Days 4–6:** 50 mg twice daily. **Days 7–9:** 100 mg twice daily. **Usual dose:** 10–25 mg/kg/day (375–750 mg) in 3–4 divided doses. **NEONATES:** 12–20 mg/kg/day in divided doses 2–4 times/day.

Dosage in Renal Impairment

Creatine Clearance	Interval
50 mL/min or greater	q12h
10–49 mL/min	q12–24h
Less than 10 mL/min	q24h
Hemodialysis (HD)	Administer dose post-HD

Dosage in Hepatic Impairment
No dose adjustment.

SIDE EFFECTS

Frequent: Ataxia, dizziness. **Occasional:** Anorexia, drowsiness, altered mental status, nausea, vomiting, paradoxical excitement. **Rare:** Rash.

ADVERSE EFFECTS/TOXIC REACTIONS

Abrupt withdrawal after prolonged therapy may produce effects ranging from markedly increased dreaming, nightmares, insomnia, tremor, diaphoresis, vomiting to hallucinations, delirium, seizures, status epilepticus. Skin eruptions may appear as hypersensitivity reaction. Blood dyscrasias, hepatic disease, hypocalcemia occur rarely. Overdose produces cold/clammy skin, hypothermia, severe CNS depression, followed by high fever, coma. May increase risk of suicidal thoughts and behavior.

NURSING CONSIDERATIONS

BASELINE ASSESSMENT

Review history of seizure disorder (intensity, frequency, duration, LOC). Observe frequently for recurrence of seizure activity. Initiate seizure precautions.

INTERVENTION/EVALUATION

Monitor for changes in behavior, depression, suicidal ideation. Monitor CBC, neurologic status (frequency, duration, severity of seizures). Monitor for **therapeutic serum level:** 4–12 mcg/mL; **toxic serum level:** more than 12 mcg/mL.

PATIENT/FAMILY TEACHING

• Do not abruptly discontinue medication after long-term use (may precipitate seizures). • Strict maintenance of drug therapy is essential for seizure control. • Avoid tasks that require alertness, motor skills until response to drug is established; drowsiness usually disappears during continued therapy. • Slowly go from lying to standing. • Avoid alcohol. • Report depression, thoughts of suicide, unusual changes in behavior.

prochlorperazine

proe-klor-**per**-a-zeen
(Apo-Prochlorperazine ✦,
Compazine, Compro)

■ **BLACK BOX ALERT** ■ Increased risk for death in elderly with dementia-related psychosis.
Do not confuse prochlorperazine with chlorproMAZINE.

◆CLASSIFICATION

PHARMACOTHERAPEUTIC: Phenothiazine. **CLINICAL:** Antiemetic, first-generation (typical) antipsychotic.

USES

Management of severe nausea/vomiting. Treatment of acute or chronic psychosis, nonpsychotic anxiety. **OFF-LABEL:** Behavioral syndromes in dementia, psychosis/agitation related to Alzheimer's dementia.

PRECAUTIONS

Contraindications: Hypersensitivity to prochlorperazine. Coma or presence of large amounts of CNS depressants (e.g., alcohol, opioids). Use in children younger than 2 yrs or weighing less than 9 kg. Postoperative nausea/vomiting following pediatric surgery. **Cautions:** History of seizures, Parkinson's disease, elderly, pts at risk for pneumonia, severe renal/hepatic impairment, decreased GI motility, urinary retention, visual problems, narrow-angle glaucoma, paralytic ileus, myasthenia gravis, cerebrovascular/cardiovascular disease.

ACTION

Acts centrally to inhibit/block DOPamine receptors in brain. **Therapeutic Effect:** Relieves nausea/vomiting.

PHARMACOKINETICS

Route	Onset*	Peak	Duration
PO	30–40 min	N/A	3–4 hrs
IM	10–20 min	N/A	4–6 hrs
Rectal	60 min	N/A	12 hrs

*As an antiemetic.

Variably absorbed after PO administration. Widely distributed. Metabolized in liver, GI mucosa. Primarily excreted in urine. Unknown if removed by hemodialysis. **Half-life:** PO: 3–5 hrs, IV: 7 hrs.

⧗ LIFESPAN CONSIDERATIONS

Pregnancy/Lactation: Crosses placenta. Distributed in breast milk. **Children:** Safety and efficacy not established in pts weighing less than 9 kg or younger than 2 yrs. **Elderly:** More susceptible to orthostatic hypotension, anticholinergic effects (e.g., dry mouth), sedation, extrapyramidal symptoms (EPS); lower dosage recommended.

INTERACTIONS

DRUG: Alcohol, other CNS depressants (e.g., **LORazepam, morphine, zolpidem**) may increase CNS, respiratory depression, hypotensive effects. **Extrapyramidal symptom (EPS)–producing medications (e.g., haloperidol metoclopramide, SSRIs)** may increase EPS. **Lithium** may decrease absorption, produce adverse neurologic effects. **MAOIs (e.g., phenelzine, selegiline), tricyclic antidepressants (e.g., amitriptyline, doxepin)** may increase anticholinergic, sedative effects. **HERBAL:** Dong quai, St. John's wort may increase photosensitization. **Gotu kola, kava kava, St. John's wort, valerian** may increase CNS depression. **FOOD:** None known. **LAB VALUES:** None significant.

AVAILABILITY (Rx)

Injection Solution: 5 mg/mL. **Suppositories (Compro):** 25 mg. **Tablets:** 5 mg, 10 mg.

ADMINISTRATION/HANDLING

🖉 IV

Rate of Administration• May give by IV push slowly. Maximum rate: 5 mg/min. **Storage •** Store at room temperature. • Protect from light. • Clear or slightly yellow solutions may be used.

P

IM
• Inject deep IM into outer quadrant of buttocks.

PO
• Should be administered with food or water.

Rectal
• Moisten suppository with cold water before inserting well into rectum.

▦ IV INCOMPATIBILITIES

Furosemide (Lasix), hydrocortisone, HYDROmorphone (Dilaudid), midazolam (Versed).

▦ IV COMPATIBILITIES

Calcium gluconate, dexmedetomidine (Precedex), diphenhydrAMINE (Benadryl), fentaNYL, heparin, metoclopramide (Reglan), morphine, potassium chloride, promethazine (Phenergan), propofol (Diprivan).

INDICATIONS/ROUTES/DOSAGE

Nausea/Vomiting
PO: ADULTS, ELDERLY: 5–10 mg 3–4 times/day. **Maximum:** 40 mg/day. **CHILDREN: GREATER THAN 39 KG:** 5–10 mg q6–8h. **Maximum:** 40 mg/day. **19–39 KG:** 2.5 mg q8h or 5 mg q12h. **Maximum:** 15 mg/day. **14–18 KG:** 2.5 mg q8–12h. **Maximum:** 10 mg/day. **9–13 KG:** 2.5 mg q12–24h. **Maximum:** 7.5 mg/day.
IV: ADULTS, ELDERLY: 2.5–10 mg. May repeat q3–4h. **Maximum:** 10 mg/dose or 40 mg/day.
IM: ADULTS, ELDERLY: 5–10 mg q3–4h. **CHILDREN:** 0.1–0.15 mg/kg/dose q8–12h. **Maximum:** 40 mg/day.
Rectal: ADULTS, ELDERLY: 25 mg twice daily.

Psychosis
PO: ADULTS, ELDERLY: 5–10 mg 3–4 times/day. **Maximum:** 150 mg/day. **CHILDREN 2–12 YRS:** 2.5 mg 2–3 times/day. **Maximum daily dose:** 25 mg for children 6–12 yrs; 20 mg for children 2–5 yrs.

IM: ADULTS, ELDERLY: 10–20 mg q4h. **CHILDREN:** 0.13 mg/kg/dose.

Nonpsychiatric Anxiety
PO: ADULTS, ELDERLY: 5 mg 3–4 times/day for up to 12 wks. **Maximum:** 20 mg/day.

Dosage in Renal/Hepatic Impairment
No dose adjustment.

SIDE EFFECTS

Frequent: Drowsiness, hypotension, dizziness, fainting (commonly occurring after first dose, occasionally after subsequent doses, rarely with oral form). **Occasional:** Dry mouth, blurred vision, lethargy, constipation, diarrhea, myalgia, nasal congestion, peripheral edema, urinary retention.

ADVERSE EFFECTS/TOXIC REACTIONS

Extrapyramidal symptoms (EPS) appear dose related and are divided into three categories: akathisia (e.g., inability to sit still, tapping of feet), parkinsonian symptoms (mask-like face, tremors, shuffling gait, hypersalivation), acute dystonias (torticollis [neck muscle spasm], opisthotonos [rigidity of back muscles], oculogyric crisis [rolling back of eyes]). Dystonic reaction may produce diaphoresis, pallor. Tardive dyskinesia (tongue protrusion, puffing of cheeks, puckering of mouth) occurs rarely and may be irreversible. Abrupt withdrawal after long-term therapy may precipitate nausea, vomiting, gastritis, dizziness, tremors. Blood dyscrasias, particularly agranulocytosis, mild leukopenia, may occur. May lower seizure threshold.

NURSING CONSIDERATIONS

BASELINE ASSESSMENT

Avoid skin contact with solution (contact dermatitis). **Antiemetic:** Assess for dehydration (poor skin turgor, dry mucous membranes, longitudinal furrows in tongue). **Antipsychotic:** Assess

---

behavior, appearance, emotional status, response to environment, speech pattern, thought content.

INTERVENTION/EVALUATION

Monitor B/P for hypotension. Assess for EPS. Monitor CBC for blood dyscrasias. Monitor for fine tongue movement (may be early sign of tardive dyskinesia). Supervise suicidal-risk pt closely during early therapy (as depression lessens, energy level improves, increasing suicide potential). Assess for therapeutic response (interest in surroundings, improvement in self-care, increased ability to concentrate, relaxed facial expression or relief of nausea, vomiting).

PATIENT/FAMILY TEACHING

• Limit caffeine. • Avoid alcohol. • Avoid tasks requiring alertness, motor skills until response to drug is established (may cause drowsiness, impairment).

promethazine

proe-meth-a-zeen
(Phenadoz, <u>Phenergan</u>, Promethegan)

■ **BLACK BOX ALERT** ■ Fatalities due to respiratory depression reported in children 2 yrs and younger. Severe tissue injury, including gangrene, may occur with intravenous injection (preferred route is deep intramuscular). Be alert for signs and symptoms of tissue injury including burning or pain at injection site, phlebitis, swelling, blistering. Risk reduced by diluting promethazine with 10–20 mL 0.9% NaCl or diluting in a minibag (piggyback); administer slowly over 10–15 min; use large veins or central venous site (no hand or wrist veins).

Do not confuse Phenergan with phenelzine, or promethazine with chlorproMAZINE or predniSONE.

FIXED-COMBINATION(S)

Phenergan with codeine: promethazine/codeine (a cough suppressant): 6.25 mg/10 mg/5 mL. **Phenergan VC:** promethazine/phenylephrine (a vasoconstrictor): 6.25 mg/5 mg/5 mL. **Phenergan VC with codeine:** promethazine/phenylephrine/codeine: 6.25 mg/5 mg/10 mg/5 mL.

◆CLASSIFICATION

PHARMACOTHERAPEUTIC: Phenothiazine.   **CLINICAL:** Antihistamine (first generation), antiemetic, sedative-hypnotic.

USES

Treatment of allergic conditions, motion sickness, nausea, vomiting. May be used as mild sedative. Adjunct to postoperative analgesia. **OFF-LABEL:** Nausea/vomiting related to pregnancy.

PRECAUTIONS

Contraindications: Hypersensitivity to promethazine, other phenothiazines. Children 2 yrs and younger (may cause fatal respiratory depression), severe CNS depression, coma, treatment of lower respiratory tract symptoms including asthma. **Cautions:** Cardiovascular/hepatic or respiratory impairment, narrow-angle glaucoma, prostatic hypertrophy, GI/GU obstruction, urinary retention, visual problems, decreased GI motility, myasthenia gravis, Parkinson's disease, elderly, bone marrow depression, asthma, peptic ulcer, history of seizures, sleep apnea, pts suspected of Reye's syndrome.

ACTION

Block postsynaptic dopaminergic receptors; competes with histamine for histamine receptors; possesses muscarinic blocking effect. **Therapeutic Effect:** Prevents allergic responses mediated by histamine (urticaria, pruritus). Prevents, relieves nausea/vomiting. Produces mild sedative effect.

P

✦ Canadian trade name   🦥 Non-Crushable Drug   🔲 High Alert drug

PHARMACOKINETICS

Route	Onset	Peak	Duration
PO	20 min	N/A	2–8 hrs
IV	3–5 min	N/A	2–8 hrs
IM	20 min	N/A	2–8 hrs
Rectal	20 min	N/A	2–8 hrs

Well absorbed from GI tract after IM administration. Protein binding: 83%. Widely distributed. Metabolized in liver. Primarily excreted in urine. Not removed by hemodialysis. **Half-life:** 9–16 hrs.

⧗ LIFESPAN CONSIDERATIONS

Pregnancy/Lactation: Readily crosses placenta. Unknown if drug is distributed in breast milk. May inhibit platelet aggregation in neonates if taken within 2 wks of birth. May produce jaundice, extrapyramidal symptoms (EPS) in neonates if taken during pregnancy. **Children:** May experience increased excitement. Not recommended for pts younger than 2 yrs. **Elderly:** More sensitive to dizziness, sedation, confusion, hypotension, hyperexcitability, anticholinergic effects (e.g., dry mouth).

INTERACTIONS

DRUG: Alcohol, CNS depressants (e.g., LORazepam, morphine, zolpidem) may increase CNS depressant effects. **Anticholinergics (e.g., dicyclomine, glycopyrrolate, scopolamine)** may increase anticholinergic effects. **MAOIs (e.g., phenelzine, selegiline)** may prolong, intensify anticholinergic, CNS depressant effects. **HERBAL: Gotu kola, kava kava, St. John's wort, valerian** may increase CNS depression. **FOOD:** None known. **LAB VALUES:** May suppress wheal/flare reactions to antigen skin testing unless discontinued 4 days before testing.

AVAILABILITY (Rx)

Injection Solution: 25 mg/mL, 50 mg/mL. **Solution, Oral:** 6.25 mg/5 mL. **Suppositories:** 12.5 mg, 25 mg, 50 mg. **Syrup:** 6.25 mg/5 mL. **Tablets:** 12.5 mg, 25 mg, 50 mg.

ADMINISTRATION/HANDLING

◄**ALERT**► IM is preferred route; avoid IV if possible. Significant tissue necrosis may occur if given subcutaneously. Inadvertent intra-arterial injection may produce significant arteriospasm, resulting in severe circulation impairment.

 IV

Reconstitution • Dilute with 10–20 mL 0.9% NaCl or prepare minibag.
Rate of Administration • Administer slowly over 10–15 min. • Use large vein or central venous site (no hand or wrist veins). • Too-rapid rate of infusion may result in transient fall in B/P, producing orthostatic hypotension, reflex tachycardia, serious tissue injury.
Storage • Store at room temperature.

IM
• Inject deep IM.

PO
• Give with food or fluids to reduce GI distress. • Scored tablets may be crushed.

Rectal
• Refrigerate suppository. • Moisten suppository with cold water before inserting well into rectum.

▨ IV INCOMPATIBILITIES

Allopurinol (Aloprim), amphotericin B complex (Abelcet, AmBisome, Amphotec), heparin, ketorolac (Toradol), nalbuphine (Nubain), piperacillin and tazobactam (Zosyn).

▨ IV COMPATIBILITIES

Dexmedetomidine (Precedex), diphenhydrAMINE (Benadryl), HYDROmorphone (Dilaudid), midazolam (Versed), morphine.

INDICATIONS/ROUTES/DOSAGE

◄**ALERT**► Contraindicated in children 2 yrs and younger.

Allergic Symptoms
PO, RECTAL: ADULTS, ELDERLY: 6.25–12.5 mg 3 times/day plus 25 mg at bedtime. **CHILDREN:** 0.125 mg/kg/dose (**Maximum:** 12.5 mg) 4 times/day plus 0.5 mg/kg/dose (**Maximum:** 25 mg) at bedtime. **IV, IM: ADULTS, ELDERLY:** 25 mg. May repeat in 2 hrs.

Motion Sickness
PO, RECTAL: ADULTS, ELDERLY: 25 mg 30–60 min before departure; may repeat in 8–12 hrs, then every morning on rising and before evening meal. **CHILDREN:** 0.5 mg/kg 30–60 min before departure; may repeat in 8–12 hrs, then every morning on rising and before evening meal. **Maximum:** 25 mg twice daily.

Prevention of Nausea/Vomiting
PO, IV, IM, Rectal: ADULTS, ELDERLY: 12.5–25 mg q4–6h as needed. **CHILDREN:** 0.25–1 mg/kg q4–6h as needed. **Maximum:** 25 mg/dose.

Sedative
PO, IV, IM, Rectal: ADULTS, ELDERLY: 25–50 mg/dose. **CHILDREN:** 12.5–25 mg/dose.

Dosage in Renal Impairment
No dose adjustment.

Dosage in Hepatic Impairment
Use caution.

SIDE EFFECTS
Frequent: Drowsiness; dry mouth, nose, throat; urinary retention; thickening of bronchial secretions. **Occasional:** Epigastric distress, flushing, visual disturbances, hearing disturbances, wheezing, paresthesia, diaphoresis, chills, disorientation, hypotension, confusion, syncope in elderly. **Rare:** Dizziness, urticaria, photosensitivity, nightmares.

ADVERSE EFFECTS/TOXIC REACTIONS
Paradoxical reaction (particularly in children) manifested as excitation, anxiety, tremor, hyperactive reflexes, seizures. Long-term therapy may produce extrapyramidal symptoms (EPS) noted as dystonia (abnormal movements), pronounced motor restlessness (most frequently in children), parkinsonism (esp. noted in elderly). Blood dyscrasias, particularly agranulocytosis, occur rarely.

NURSING CONSIDERATIONS

BASELINE ASSESSMENT
Assess allergy symptoms. Assess B/P, pulse for bradycardia, tachycardia if pt is given parenteral form. If used as antiemetic, assess for dehydration (poor skin turgor, dry mucous membranes, longitudinal furrows in tongue). Assess level of consciousness.

INTERVENTION/EVALUATION
Monitor serum electrolytes in pts with severe vomiting. Assist with ambulation if drowsiness, dizziness occurs. Monitor for relief of nausea, vomiting, allergic symptoms.

PATIENT/FAMILY TEACHING
• Drowsiness, dry mouth may be expected response to drug. • Avoid tasks that require alertness, motor skills until response to drug is established. • Sugarless gum, sips of water may relieve dry mouth. • Coffee, tea may help reduce drowsiness. • Report visual disturbances, involuntary movements, restlessness. • Avoid alcohol, other CNS depressants. • Avoid prolonged exposure to sunlight.

propafenone

proe-**paf**-e-nown
(Apo-Propafenone ✽, Rythmol SR)
■ **BLACK BOX ALERT** ■ Mortality or nonfatal cardiac arrest rate (7.7% of pts) in asymptomatic non–life-threatening ventricular arrhythmia pts with recent MI (more than 6 days but less than 2 yrs prior) reported.

✽ Canadian trade name   🍃 Non-Crushable Drug   ⬛ High Alert drug

◆CLASSIFICATION

PHARMACOTHERAPEUTIC: Class 1c antiarrhythmic. **CLINICAL:** Antiarrhythmic.

USES

Immediate-Release: Treatment of life-threatening ventricular arrhythmias (e.g., sustained ventricular tachycardias). To prolong time to recurrence of paroxysmal atrial fibrillation/flutter (PAF) or paroxysmal supraventricular tachycardia (PSVT) in pts with disabling symptoms and without structural heart disease. **Extended-Release:** Prolong the time to recurrence of atrial fibrillation/flutter or paroxysmal supraventricular tachycardia in pts with disabling symptoms without structural heart disease. **OFF-LABEL:** Treatment following cardioversion of recent-onset atrial fibrillation; supraventricular tachycardia in pts with Wolff-Parkinson-White syndrome.

PRECAUTIONS

Contraindications: Hypersensitivity to propafenone. Sinus bradycardia, bronchospastic disorders or severe obstructive pulmonary disease, cardiogenic shock, electrolyte imbalance, sinoatrial, AV, intraventricular impulse generation or conduction disorders (e.g., sick sinus syndrome, AV block) without pacemaker, uncontrolled HF, marked hypotension. **Cautions:** Renal/hepatic impairment, myasthenia gravis, concurrent use of other medications that prolong QT interval, hypokalemia, hypomagnesemia.

ACTION

Decreases fast sodium current in Purkinje/myocardial cells. Decreases excitability, automaticity; prolongs conduction velocity, refractory period. **Therapeutic Effect:** Suppresses arrhythmias.

PHARMACOKINETICS

Nearly completely absorbed following PO administration. Protein binding: 85%–97%. Metabolized in liver. Primarily excreted in feces. **Half-life:** 2–10 hrs.

⌛ LIFESPAN CONSIDERATIONS

Pregnancy/Lactation: Crosses placenta, distributed in breast milk. **Children:** Safety and efficacy not established. **Elderly:** No age-related precautions noted.

INTERACTIONS

DRUG: **Amiodarone** may affect cardiac conduction, repolarization. May increase **digoxin** concentration. May increase effects of **warfarin. CYP3A4 inhibitors (e.g., ketoconazole, erythromycin)** may increase concentration/toxicity. **HERBAL:** St. John's wort may decrease concentration/effect. **Ephedra** may worsen arrhythmias. **FOOD:** **Grapefruit products** may increase concentration. **LAB VALUES:** May cause EKG changes (e.g., QRS widening, PR interval prolongation), positive ANA titer.

AVAILABILITY (Rx)

Tablets (Rythmol): 150 mg, 225 mg, 300 mg.

Capsules (Extended-Release [Rythmol SR]): 225 mg, 325 mg, 425 mg.

ADMINISTRATION/HANDLING

PO
• May take without regard to meals. • Give whole; do not break, crush, divide, or open capsules.

INDICATIONS/ROUTES/DOSAGE

Ventricular Arrhythmias, PAT, PSVT
PO (Immediate-Release): ADULTS, ELDERLY: Initially, 150 mg q8h. May increase at 3- to 4-day intervals to 225 mg q8h, then to 300 mg q8h. **Maximum:** 900 mg/day.

Atrial Fibrillation (Prevention of Recurrence)
PO *(Immediate-Release)*: **ADULTS, ELDERLY:** Initially, 150 mg q8h. May increase at 3- to 4-day intervals to 225 mg q8h, then to 300 mg q8h. **Maximum:** 900 mg/day. *(Extended-Release)*: **ADULTS, ELDERLY:** Initially, 225 mg q12h. May increase at 5-day intervals to 325 mg q12h. **Maximum:** 425 mg q12h.

Dosage in Renal Impairment
No dose adjustment.

Dosage in Hepatic Impairment
Use caution.

SIDE EFFECTS

Frequent (13%–7%): Dizziness, nausea, vomiting, altered taste, constipation. **Occasional (6%–3%):** Headache, dyspnea, blurred vision, dyspepsia. **Rare (less than 2%):** Rash, weakness, dry mouth, diarrhea, edema, hot flashes.

ADVERSE EFFECTS/TOXIC REACTIONS

May produce, worsen arrhythmias, HF. Overdose may produce hypotension, drowsiness, bradycardia, atrioventricular conduction disturbances.

NURSING CONSIDERATIONS

BASELINE ASSESSMENT

Correct electrolyte imbalance before administering medication. Obtain baseline EKG. Screen for cardiac contraindications.

INTERVENTION/EVALUATION

Assess pulse for quality, rhythm, rate. Monitor EKG for cardiac performance or changes, particularly widening of QRS, prolongation of PR interval. Question for visual disturbances, headache, GI upset. Monitor fluid, serum electrolyte levels. Monitor daily pattern of bowel activity, stool consistency. Assess for dizziness, unsteadiness. Monitor LFT. Monitor for therapeutic serum level (0.06–1 mcg/mL).

PATIENT/FAMILY TEACHING

• Compliance with therapy regimen is essential to control arrhythmias. • Altered taste sensation may occur. • Report headache, blurred vision. • Avoid tasks that require alertness, motor skills until response to drug is established. • Report chest pain, difficulty breathing, palpitations.

propofol

proe-poe-fol
(Diprivan, Fresenius Propoven)
Do not confuse Diprivan with Diflucan or Ditropan, or propofol with fospropofol.

◆CLASSIFICATION

PHARMACOTHERAPEUTIC: Rapid-acting general anesthetic. **CLINICAL:** Sedative-hypnotic.

USES

Induction/maintenance of anesthesia. Continuous sedation in intubated and respiratory controlled adult pts in ICU. **OFF-LABEL:** Postop antiemetic, refractory status epilepticus.

PRECAUTIONS

Contraindications: Hypersensitivity to propofol, eggs, egg products, soybean or soy products. **Cautions:** Hemodynamically unstable pts, hypovolemia, severe cardiac/respiratory disease, elevated ICP, impaired cerebral circulation, preexisting pancreatitis, hyperlipidemia, history of epilepsy, seizure disorder, elderly pts, debilitated pts, pts allergic to peanuts.

ACTION

Causes CNS depression through agonist action of GABA receptors. **Therapeutic Effect:** Produces hypnosis rapidly.

P

✦ Canadian trade name   🗲 Non-Crushable Drug   🔲 High Alert drug

PHARMACOKINETICS

Route	Onset	Peak	Duration
IV	40 sec	N/A	3–10 min

Rapidly, extensively distributed. Protein binding: 97%–99%. Metabolized in liver. Primarily excreted in urine. Unknown if removed by hemodialysis. Rapid awakening can occur 10–15 min after discontinuation. **Half-life:** 3–12 hrs.

⌛ LIFESPAN CONSIDERATIONS

Pregnancy/Lactation: Unknown if drug crosses placenta. Distributed in breast milk. Not recommended for obstetrics, breastfeeding mothers. **Children:** Safety and efficacy not established. FDA-approved for use in pts 2 mos and older. **Elderly:** No age-related precautions noted; lower dosages recommended.

INTERACTIONS

DRUG: Alcohol, CNS depressants (e.g., LORazepam, morphine, zolpidem) may increase CNS, respiratory depression, hypotensive effects. **Antihypertensive medications (e.g., amLODIPine, lisinopril, valsartan)** may increase hypotensive effects. **HERBAL:** None significant. **FOOD:** None known. **LAB VALUES:** May increase serum triglycerides.

AVAILABILITY (Rx)

Injection Emulsion: 10 mg/mL.

ADMINISTRATION/HANDLING

 IV

◀**ALERT**▶ Do not give through same IV line with blood or plasma.

Reconstitution • May give undiluted, or dilute only with D₅W. • Do not dilute to concentration less than 2 mg/mL (4 mL D₅W to 1 mL propofol yields 2 mg/mL).

Rate of Administration • Too-rapid IV administration may produce marked severe hypotension, respiratory depression, irregular muscular movements. • Observe for signs of extravasation (pain, discolored skin patches, white or blue color to peripheral IV site area, delayed onset of drug action).

Storage • Store at room temperature. • Discard unused portions. • Do not use if emulsion separates. • Shake well before using.

▦ IV INCOMPATIBILITIES

Amikacin (Amikin), amphotericin B complex (Abelcet, AmBisome, Amphotec), bretylium (Bretylol), calcium chloride, ciprofloxacin (Cipro), diazePAM (Valium), digoxin (Lanoxin), DOXOrubicin (Adriamycin), gentamicin (Garamycin), methylPREDNISolone (Solu-Medrol), minocycline (Minocin), phenytoin (Dilantin), tobramycin (Nebcin), verapamil (Isoptin).

▦ IV COMPATIBILITIES

Acyclovir (Zovirax), bumetanide (Bumex), calcium gluconate, cefTAZidime (Fortaz), dexmedetomidine (Precedex), DOBUTamine (Dobutrex), DOPamine (Intropin), enalapril (Vasotec), fentaNYL, heparin, insulin, labetalol (Normodyne, Trandate), lidocaine, LORazepam (Ativan), magnesium, milrinone (Primacor), nitroglycerin, norepinephrine (Levophed), potassium chloride, vancomycin (Vancocin).

INDICATIONS/ROUTES/DOSAGE

Anesthesia

IV Infusion: ADULTS, ELDERLY: Induction, 2–2.5 mg/kg (approximately 40 mg q10sec until onset of anesthesia). **Maintenance:** Initially, 100–200 mcg/kg/min or 6–12 mg/kg/hr for 10–15 min. Usual maintenance infusion: 50–100 mcg/kg/min or 3–6 mg/kg/hr. **CHILDREN 3–16 YRS:** Induction, 2.5–3.5 mg/kg over 20–30 sec, then infusion of 125–300 mcg/kg/min or 7.5–18 mg/kg/hr.

Sedation in ICU

IV Infusion: ADULTS, ELDERLY: Initially, 5 mcg/kg/min (0.3 mg/kg/hr); increase by increments of 5–10 mcg/kg/min (0.3–0.6 mg/kg/hr) q5–10 min until desired

P

sedation level achieved. **Usual maintenance:** 5–50 mcg/kg/min (0.3–3 mg/kg/hr). Reduce dose after adequate sedation established, and adjust to response. Daily interruption with retitration (sedation vacation) recommended to minimize prolonged sedative effects.

Dosage in Renal/Hepatic Impairment
No dose adjustment.

SIDE EFFECTS

Frequent: Involuntary muscle movements, apnea (common during induction; often lasts longer than 60 sec), hypotension, nausea, vomiting, IV site burning/stinging. **Occasional:** Twitching, thrashing, headache, dizziness, bradycardia, hypertension, fever, abdominal cramps, paresthesia, coldness, cough, hiccups, facial flushing, green-tinted urine. **Rare:** Rash, dry mouth, agitation, confusion, myalgia, thrombophlebitis.

ADVERSE EFFECTS/TOXIC REACTIONS

Continuous infusion or repeated intermittent infusions of propofol may result in extreme drowsiness, respiratory depression, circulatory depression, delirium. Too-rapid IV administration may produce severe hypotension, respiratory depression, involuntary muscle movements. Pt may experience acute allergic reaction, characterized by abdominal pain, anxiety, restlessness, dyspnea, erythema, hypotension, pruritus, rhinitis, urticaria. May cause propofol infusion syndrome, a collection of metabolic disorders and organ system failures including metabolic acidosis, hyperkalemia, rhabdomyolysis, hepatomegaly; cardiac, renal failure.

NURSING CONSIDERATIONS

BASELINE ASSESSMENT

Resuscitative equipment, suction, O_2 must be available. Obtain vital signs before administration.

INTERVENTION/EVALUATION

Observe pt for signs of wakefulness, agitation. Monitor respiratory rate, B/P, heart rate, O_2 saturation, ABGs, depth of sedation, serum lipid, triglycerides (if used longer than 24 hrs). May change urine color to green. If continuous high-dose infusions do not properly induce sedation, consider additional sedatives (e.g., opioids, hypnotics, benzodiazepines) to achieve desired response.

---

propranolol HIGH ALERT

proe-**pran**-oh-lol
(Apo-Propranolol ✦, Hemangeol, <u>Inderal LA</u>, Inderal XL, InnoPran XL)
■ **BLACK BOX ALERT** ■ Severe angina exacerbation, MI, ventricular arrhythmias may occur in angina pts after abrupt discontinuation; must taper gradually over 1–2 wks. **Do not confuse Inderal LA with Adderall, Imdur, Isordil, or Toradol, or propranolol with Pravachol.**

FIXED-COMBINATION(S)

Inderide: propranolol/hydroCHLOROthiazide (a diuretic): 40 mg/25 mg, 80 mg/25 mg. **Inderide LA:** propranolol/hydroCHLOROthiazide (a diuretic): 80 mg/50 mg, 120 mg/50 mg, 160 mg/50 mg.

◆CLASSIFICATION

PHARMACOTHERAPEUTIC: Nonselective beta-adrenergic blocker. **CLINICAL:** Antihypertensive, antianginal, antiarrhythmic, antimigraine.

USES

Treatment of angina pectoris, supraventricular arrhythmias, essential tremors, hypertension, ventricular tachycardia, symptomatic treatment of obstructive hypertrophic cardiomyopathy, treatment of proliferating infantile hemangioma requiring systemic therapy, migraine headache prophylaxis, pheochromocytoma, prevention of MI. **Hemangeol:** Treatment of proliferating infantile hemangioma needing systemic therapy. **OFF-LABEL:** Treatment adjunct for anxiety, tremor due to Parkinson's disease, alcohol withdrawal, aggressive behavior, schizophrenia, antipsychotic-induced akathisia, variceal hemorrhage, acute panic.

PRECAUTIONS

Contraindications: Hypersensitivity to propranolol. Bronchial asthma, severe sinus bradycardia, cardiogenic shock, sick sinus syndrome, heart block greater than first-degree (unless pt has functional pacemaker), uncompensated HF. **Hemangeol (Additional):** Premature infants with corrected age younger than 5 wks, infants weighing less than 2 kg; asthma, history of bronchospasm, bradycardia (less than 80 beats/min), B/P less than 50/30 mm Hg, pheochromocytoma. **Cautions:** Diabetes, renal/hepatic impairment, Raynaud's disease, hyperthyroidism, myasthenia gravis, psychiatric disease, bronchospastic disease, elderly pts, history of severe anaphylaxis to allergens.

ACTION

Blocks beta₁-, beta₂-adrenergic receptors. **Therapeutic Effect:** Slows heart rate; decreases B/P, myocardial contractility, myocardial oxygen demand.

PHARMACOKINETICS

Route	Onset	Peak	Duration
PO	1–2 hrs	N/A	6 hrs

Well absorbed from GI tract. Protein binding: 93%. Widely distributed. Metabolized in liver. Primarily excreted in urine. Not removed by hemodialysis. **Half-life:** 4–6 hrs.

LIFESPAN CONSIDERATIONS

Pregnancy/Lactation: Crosses placenta. Distributed in breast milk. Avoid use during first trimester. May produce low-birth-weight infants, bradycardia, apnea, hypoglycemia, hypothermia during delivery. **Children:** No age-related precautions noted. **Elderly:** Age-related peripheral vascular disease may increase susceptibility to decreased peripheral circulation.

INTERACTIONS

DRUG: Diuretics (e.g., furosemide, HCTZ), other antihypertensives (e.g., amLODIPine, lisinopril, valsartan) may increase hypotensive effect. May mask symptoms of hypoglycemia, prolong hypoglycemic effect of **insulin, oral hypoglycemics (e.g., glipiZIDE, metFORMIN). Digoxin** may increase risk for bradycardia. **NSAIDs (e.g., ibuprofen, ketorolac, naproxen)** may decrease antihypertensive effect. **HERBAL: Ephedra, ginger, licorice, ginseng, yohimbe** may worsen hypertension. **Licorice** may increase water retention. **Garlic, periwinkle** have antihypertensive effects. **FOOD:** None known. **LAB VALUES:** May increase serum antinuclear antibody (ANA) titer, serum BUN, LDH, lipoprotein, alkaline phosphatase, potassium, uric acid, ALT, AST, triglycerides.

AVAILABILITY (Rx)

Injection Solution: 1 mg/mL. **Oral Solution:** 20 mg/5 mL, 40 mg/5 mL. **Oral Solution (Hemangeol):** 4.28 mg/mL. **Tablets:** 10 mg, 20 mg, 40 mg, 60 mg, 80 mg. **Capsules (Extended-Release [InnoPran XL]):** 80 mg, 120 mg.

 Capsules (Extended-Release [Inno-Pran XL]): 80 mg, 120 mg. **Capsules (Sustained-Release [Inderal LA]):** 60 mg, 80 mg, 120 mg, 160 mg.

ADMINISTRATION/HANDLING

IV

Reconstitution • Give undiluted for IV push. • For IV infusion, may dilute each 1 mg in 10 mL D₅W.
Rate of Administration • Do not exceed 1 mg/min injection rate. • For IV infusion, give over 30 min.

Storage • Store at room temperature. • Once diluted, stable for 24 hrs at room temperature.

PO

• May crush scored tablets. • Do not break, crush, or open extended- or sustained-release capsules. • Give immediate-release tablets on empty stomach. • Give extended-release, sustained-release without regard to food.

🔲 IV INCOMPATIBILITIES

Amphotericin B complex (Abelcet, AmBisome, Amphotec).

🔲 IV COMPATIBILITIES

Alteplase (Activase), heparin, milrinone (Primacor), potassium chloride, propofol (Diprivan).

INDICATIONS/ROUTES/DOSAGE

Hypertension
PO: ADULTS, ELDERLY: *(Immediate-Release):* Initially, 40 mg twice daily. May increase dose q3–7days. Usual dose: 120–240 mg/day in 2–3 divided doses. **Maximum:** 640 mg/day. **CHILDREN:** Initially, 1–2 mg/kg/day in 2–3 divided doses. May increase at 3- to 5-day intervals. Usual dose: 4 mg/kg/day. **Maximum:** 4 mg/kg/day up to 640 mg/day. **PO ADULTS, ELDERLY:** *(Sustained-Release): (Inderal LA):* Initially, 80 mg once daily. **Maintenance:** 120–160 mg/day. *(Extended-Release):* Initially, 80 mg at bedtime. May increase at 2- to 3-wk intervals. **Maximum:** 120 mg.

Angina
PO: ADULTS, ELDERLY: *(Immediate-Release):* 80–320 mg/day in 2–4 divided doses.
PO *(Extended-Release):* Initially, 80 mg/day. **Maximum:** 320 mg/day.

Arrhythmia
IV: ADULTS, ELDERLY: 1–3 mg. Repeat q2–5min up to total of 5 mg. **CHILDREN:** 0.01–0.15 mg/kg. **Maximum:** Infants, 1 mg; children, 3 mg.

PO: ADULTS, ELDERLY: *(Immediate-Release):* 10–30 mg q6–8h or 10–40 mg 3–4 times/day. **CHILDREN:** Initially, 0.5–1 mg/kg/day in divided doses q6–8h. May increase q3days. Usual dosage: 2–6 mg/kg/day. **Maximum:** 16 mg/kg/day or 60 mg/day.

Obstructive Hypertrophic Cardiomyopathy
PO: ADULTS, ELDERLY: *(Immediate-Release):* 20–40 mg 3–4 times/day or 80–160 mg once daily as extended-release capsule.

Adjunct to Alpha-Blocking Agents to Treat Pheochromocytoma
PO: ADULTS, ELDERLY: 30–60 mg/day in divided doses.

Migraine Headache
PO: ADULTS, ELDERLY: *(Immediate-Release):* Initially, 80 mg/day in 3–4 divided doses or 80 mg once daily. May increase by 20–40 mg/dose q3–4wks up to 160–240 mg/day in divided doses. **CHILDREN WEIGHING 35 KG OR LESS:** 10–20 mg 3 times/day. **CHILDREN WEIGHING OVER 35 KG:** 20–40 mg 3 times/day. *(Extended-Release): (Inderal LA):* **ADULTS, ELDERLY:** Initially, 80 mg daily. Effective range: 160–240 mg/day.

Reduction of Cardiovascular Mortality, Reinfarction in Pts with Previous MI
PO: ADULTS, ELDERLY: *(Immediate-Release):* Initially, 40 mg 3 times/day. Range: 180–240 mg/day in 3–4 divided doses.

Essential Tremor
PO: ADULTS, ELDERLY: Initially, 40 mg twice daily increased up to 120–320 mg/day in 3 divided doses.

Infantile Hemangioma
Note: Separate doses by at least 9 hrs during or after feeding.
PO: INFANTS 5 WKS TO 5 MOS: Initially, 0.15 mL/kg (0.6 mg/kg) twice daily. After 1 wk, increase to 0.3 mL/kg (1.1 mg/kg) twice daily. After 2 wks, increase

P

to maintenance dose of 0.4 mL/kg (1.7 mg/kg) twice daily. Maintain dose for 6 months. Readjust dose as weight increases.

Dosage in Renal/Hepatic Impairment
Use caution.

SIDE EFFECTS

Frequent: Diminished sexual function, drowsiness, difficulty sleeping, unusual fatigue/weakness. **Occasional:** Bradycardia, depression, sensation of coldness in extremities, diarrhea, constipation, anxiety, nasal congestion, nausea, vomiting. **Rare:** Altered taste, dry eyes, pruritus, paresthesia.

ADVERSE EFFECTS/TOXIC REACTIONS

Overdose may produce profound bradycardia, hypotension. Abrupt withdrawal may result in diaphoresis, palpitations, headache, tremulousness. May precipitate HF, MI in pts with cardiac disease, thyroid storm in pts with thyrotoxicosis, peripheral ischemia in pts with existing peripheral vascular disease. Hypoglycemia may occur in pts with previously controlled diabetes. **Antidote:** Glucagon (see Appendix J for dosage).

NURSING CONSIDERATIONS

BASELINE ASSESSMENT

Assess baseline renal function, LFT. Assess B/P, apical pulse immediately before administering drug (if pulse is 60/min or less or systolic B/P is less than 90 mm Hg, withhold medication, contact physician). **Angina:** Record onset, quality, radiation, location, intensity, duration of anginal pain, precipitating factors (exertion, emotional stress).

INTERVENTION/EVALUATION

Assess pulse for quality, regularity, bradycardia. Monitor EKG for cardiac arrhythmias. Assess fingers for color, numbness (Raynaud's). Assess for evidence of HF (dyspnea [particularly on exertion or lying down], night cough, peripheral edema, distended neck veins). Monitor I&O (increase in weight, decrease in urinary output may indicate HF). Assess for rash, fatigue, behavioral changes. Therapeutic response time ranges from a few days to several wks. Measure B/P near end of dosing interval (determines if B/P is controlled throughout day).

PATIENT/FAMILY TEACHING

• Do not abruptly discontinue medication. • Compliance with therapy regimen is essential to control hypertension, arrhythmia, anginal pain. • To avoid hypotensive effect, slowly go from lying to standing. • Avoid tasks that require alertness, motor skills until response to drug is established. • Report excessively slow pulse rate (less than 50 beats/min), peripheral numbness, dizziness. • Do not use nasal decongestants, OTC cold preparations (stimulants) without physician approval. • Restrict salt, alcohol intake.

propylthiouracil

proe-pil-**thye**-oh-**ure**-a-sil
(Propyl-Thyracil ✤)

■ **BLACK BOX ALERT** ■ May cause severe hepatic injury, acute hepatic failure, death.
Do not confuse propylthiouracil with Purinethol.

◆CLASSIFICATION

PHARMACOTHERAPEUTIC: Thiourea derivative.   **CLINICAL:** Antithyroid agent.

USES

Palliative treatment of hyperthyroidism; adjunct to ameliorate hyperthyroidism in preparation for surgical treatment, radioactive iodine therapy. **OFF-LABEL:** Management of thyrotoxic crises, Graves' disease, thyroid storm.

PRECAUTIONS

Contraindications: Hypersensitivity to propylthiouracil. **Cautions:** In combination with other agranulocytosis-inducing drugs.

ACTION

Blocks conversion of thyroxine to triiodothyronine in peripheral tissues. **Therapeutic Effect:** Inhibits synthesis of thyroid hormone.

PHARMACOKINETICS

Readily absorbed from GI tract. Protein binding: 80%. Metabolized in liver. Excreted in urine. **Half-life:** 1.5–5 hrs.

INTERACTIONS

DRUG: May increase concentration of **digoxin** (as pt becomes euthyroid). May increase effect of **oral anticoagulants (e.g., apixaban, warfarin).** **HERBAL:** None significant. **FOOD:** None known. **LAB VALUES:** May increase LDH, serum alkaline phosphatase, bilirubin, ALT, AST, prothrombin time.

AVAILABILITY (Rx)

Tablets: 50 mg.

ADMINISTRATION/HANDLING

PO
• Give with food.

INDICATIONS/ROUTES/DOSAGE

Hyperthyroidism
PO: ADULTS, ELDERLY: Initially, 300–400 mg/day (**ELDERLY:** 150–300 mg/day) in divided doses q8h. **Maintenance:** 100–150 mg/day in divided doses q8–12h.

Dosage in Renal/Hepatic Impairment
No dose adjustment.

SIDE EFFECTS

Frequent: Urticaria, rash, pruritus, nausea, skin pigmentation, hair loss, headache, paresthesia. **Occasional:** Drowsiness, lymphadenopathy, vertigo. **Rare:** Drug fever, lupus-like syndrome.

ADVERSE EFFECTS/TOXIC REACTIONS

Agranulocytosis (may occur as long as 4 mos after therapy), pancytopenia, fatal hepatitis have occurred.

NURSING CONSIDERATIONS

BASELINE ASSESSMENT

Obtain baseline weight, pulse. Obtain baseline T_3, T_4, TSH level, LFT.

INTERVENTION/EVALUATION

Monitor pulse, weight daily. Check for skin eruptions, pruritus, swollen lymph glands. Be alert for signs, symptoms of hepatic injury, hepatitis (nausea, vomiting, drowsiness, jaundice). Monitor hematology results for bone marrow suppression; observe for signs of infection, bleeding.

PATIENT/FAMILY TEACHING

• Space doses evenly around the clock. • Take resting pulse daily. • Report pulse rate less than 60 beats/min. • Seafood, iodine products may be restricted. • Report fever, sore throat, yellowing of skin/eyes, unusual bleeding/bruising immediately. • Report sudden or continuous weight gain, cold intolerance, depression.

pyrazinamide

peer-a-**zin**-a-mide
(Tebrazid ✦)

FIXED-COMBINATION(S)

Rifater: pyrazinamide/isoniazid/rifAMPin (an antitubercular): 300 mg/50 mg/120 mg.

◆CLASSIFICATION

PHARMACOTHERAPEUTIC: Synthetic pyrazine analogue. **CLINICAL:** Antitubercular.

P

✦ Canadian trade name   🗌 Non-Crushable Drug   🄷🄸 High Alert drug

USES

Treatment of clinical tuberculosis in conjunction with other antitubercular agents.

PRECAUTIONS

Contraindications: Hypersensitivity to pyrazinamide. Acute gout, severe hepatic dysfunction. **Cautions:** Diabetes, porphyria, renal impairment, history of gout, history of alcoholism, concurrent medication associated with hepatotoxicity.

ACTION

Exact mechanism unknown. May disrupt *Mycobacterium tuberculosis* membrane transport. **Therapeutic Effect:** Bacteriostatic or bactericidal, depending on drug concentration at infection site, susceptibility of infecting bacteria.

PHARMACOKINETICS

Well absorbed from GI tract. Protein binding: 5%–10%. Widely distributed. Metabolized in liver. Excreted in urine. **Half-life:** 9–10 hrs.

⧗ LIFESPAN CONSIDERATIONS

Pregnancy/Lactation: Unknown if drug crosses placenta or is distributed in breast milk. **Children:** Safety and efficacy not established. **Elderly:** No age-related precautions noted.

INTERACTIONS

DRUG: None significant. **HERBAL:** None significant. **FOOD:** None known. **LAB VALUES:** May increase serum ALT, AST, uric acid.

AVAILABILITY (Rx)

Tablets: 500 mg.

INDICATIONS/ROUTES/DOSAGE

Tuberculosis (in Combination With Other Antituberculars)
PO: ADULTS: Based on lean body weight. **40–55 KG:** 1,000 mg daily; **56–75 KG:** 1,500 mg daily; **76–90 KG:** 2,000 mg (**maximum dose** regardless of weight). **CHILDREN:** 30-40 mg/kg/dose once daily. **Maximum:** 2 g/day.

Dosage in Renal/Hepatic Impairment
CrCl less than 30 mL/min or receiving HD: 25–35 mg/kg/dose 3 times/wk (give after dialysis). Contraindicated in severe hepatic impairment.

SIDE EFFECTS

Frequent: Arthralgia, myalgia (usually mild, self-limited). **Rare:** Hypersensitivity reaction (rash, pruritus, urticaria), photosensitivity, gouty arthritis.

ADVERSE EFFECTS/TOXIC REACTIONS

Hepatotoxicity, gouty arthritis, thrombocytopenia, anemia occur rarely.

NURSING CONSIDERATIONS

BASELINE ASSESSMENT

Question for hypersensitivity to pyrazinamide, isoniazid, ethionamide, niacin. Ensure collection of specimens for culture, sensitivity. Obtain CBC, LFT, serum uric acid levels.

INTERVENTION/EVALUATION

Monitor LFT results; be alert for hepatic reactions: jaundice, malaise, fever, abdominal (RUQ) tenderness, anorexia, nausea, vomiting (stop drug, notify physician promptly). Check serum uric acid levels; assess for hot, painful, swollen joints, esp. big toe, ankle, knee (gout). Evaluate serum blood glucose levels, diabetic status carefully (pyrazinamide makes management difficult). Assess for rash, skin eruptions. Monitor CBC for thrombocytopenia, anemia.

PATIENT/FAMILY TEACHING

• Do not skip doses; complete full length of therapy (may be mos or yrs). • Office visits, lab tests are essential part of treatment. • Take with food to reduce GI upset. • Avoid excessive exposure to sun, ultraviolet light until photosensitivity is determined. • Report any new symptom, immediately for jaundice (yellowing sclera of eyes/skin); unusual fatigue; fever; loss of appetite; hot, painful, swollen joints.

pyridostigmine

peer-id-oh-**stig**-meen
(Mestinon, Mestinon SR ♣,
Regonol)
**Do not confuse pyridostigmine
with physostigmine, or Regonol
with Reglan or Renagel.**

◆CLASSIFICATION

PHARMACOTHERAPEUTIC: Anticholinesterase inhibitor. **CLINICAL:** Cholinergic muscle stimulant.

USES

Improvement of muscle strength in control of myasthenia gravis, reversal of effects of nondepolarizing neuromuscular
blocking agents after surgery.

PRECAUTIONS

Contraindications: Hypersensitivity to
pyridostigmine. Mechanical GI/urinary
tract obstruction. **Cautions:** Bronchial
asthma, COPD, bradycardia, seizure disorder, hyperthyroidism, cardiac arrhythmias, peptic ulcer, renal impairment.

ACTION

Prevents destruction of acetylcholine
by inhibiting the enzyme acetylcholinesterase, enhancing impulse transmission across myoneural junction.
Therapeutic Effect: Produces miosis;
increases intestinal, skeletal muscle
tone; stimulates salivary, sweat gland
secretions.

PHARMACOKINETICS

Poorly absorbed from GI tract. Metabolized in liver. Excreted primarily unchanged in urine. **Half-life:** 1–2 hrs.

⏳ LIFESPAN CONSIDERATIONS

Pregnancy/Lactation: Unknown if
drug crosses placenta or is distributed
in breast milk. **Children:** Safety and efficacy not established. **Elderly:** No age-
related precautions noted.

INTERACTIONS

DRUG: Antagonizes effects of **neuromuscular blockers (e.g., succinylcholine,
vecuronium).** Anticholinergics **(e.g.,
dicyclomine, glycopyrrolate, scopolamine)** prevent, reverse effects. **Cholinesterase inhibitors (e.g., donepezil,
tacrine)** may increase risk of toxicity.
HERBAL: None significant. **FOOD:** None
known. **LAB VALUES:** None significant.

AVAILABILITY (Rx)

Injection Solution (Regonol): 5 mg/mL.
Syrup (Mestinon): 60 mg/5 mL. **Tablets
(Mestinon):** 60 mg.

🚫 **Tablets (Extended-Release [Mestinon
Timespan]):** 180 mg.

ADMINISTRATION/HANDLING

IV, IM
• Give large parenteral doses concur-
rently with 0.6–1.2 mg atropine sulfate
IV to minimize side effects.

PO
• Give with food, milk. • Tablets may
be crushed. Do not chew, crush
extended-release tablets (may be broken). • Give larger dose at times of
increased fatigue (e.g., for those with
difficulty in chewing, 30–45 min before
meals).

▦ IV INCOMPATIBILITIES

Do not mix with any other medications.

INDICATIONS/ROUTES/DOSAGE

Note: Highly individualized dosing
ranges.

Myasthenia Gravis
PO: ADULTS, **ELDERLY:** *(Immediate-
Release):* Initially, 60 mg 3 times/day.
Dosage increased at 48-hr intervals.
Maintenance: 60 mg–1.5 g/day divided into 5–6 doses/day. (Usual dose:
600 mg/day.) **CHILDREN:** Initially, 1 mg/
kg/dose q4–6h. **Maximum:** 7 mg/
kg/24 hr divided into 5–6 doses. Usual
dose: 600 mg/day.

P

PO *(Extended-Release):* **ADULTS, ELDERLY:** 180–540 mg 1–2 times/day with at least a 6-hr interval between doses. **IV, IM:** **ADULTS, ELDERLY:** 2 mg or 1/30th of oral dose q2–3h. **CHILDREN:** 0.05–0.15 mg/kg/dose. **Maximum single dose:** 10 mg.

Dosage in Renal/Hepatic Impairment
No dose adjustment.

SIDE EFFECTS

Frequent: Miosis, increased GI/skeletal muscle tone, bradycardia, constriction of bronchi/ureters, diaphoresis, increased salivation. **Occasional:** Headache, rash, temporary decrease in diastolic B/P with mild reflex tachycardia, short periods of atrial fibrillation (in hyperthyroid pts), marked drop in B/P (in hypertensive pts).

ADVERSE EFFECTS/TOXIC REACTIONS

Overdose may produce cholinergic crisis, manifested as increasingly severe descending muscle weakness (appears first in muscles involving chewing, swallowing, followed by muscle weakness of shoulder girdle, upper extremities), respiratory muscle paralysis, followed by pelvis girdle/leg muscle paralysis. Requires withdrawal of all cholinergic drugs and immediate use of 1–4 mg atropine sulfate IV for adults, 0.01 mg/kg for infants and children younger than 12 yrs.

NURSING CONSIDERATIONS

BASELINE ASSESSMENT
Larger doses should be given at time of greatest fatigue. Assess muscle strength before testing for diagnosis of myasthenia gravis and following drug administration. Avoid large doses in pts with megacolon, reduced GI motility.

INTERVENTION/EVALUATION
Have facial tissues readily available at pt's bedside. Monitor respirations closely during myasthenia gravis testing or if dosage is increased. Assess diligently for cholinergic reaction, bradycardia in myasthenic pt in crisis. Coordinate dosage time with periods of fatigue and increased/decreased muscle strength. Monitor for therapeutic response to medication (increased muscle strength, decreased fatigue, improved chewing/swallowing functions).

PATIENT/FAMILY TEACHING
• Report nausea, vomiting, diarrhea, diaphoresis, profuse salivary secretions, palpitations, muscle weakness, severe abdominal pain, difficulty breathing.

pyridoxine (vitamin B₆)

peer-i-**dox**-een
(Pyri-500)
Do not confuse pyridoxine with PARoxetine, pralidoxime, or Pyridium.

◆CLASSIFICATION

PHARMACOTHERAPEUTIC: Water-soluble vitamin. **CLINICAL:** Vitamin deficiency supplement.

USES

Prevention/treatment of vitamin B₆ deficiency. **OFF-LABEL:** Neurological toxicities (e.g., seizure, coma) associated with isoniazid overdose. Nausea and vomiting of pregnancy.

PRECAUTIONS

Contraindications: Hypersensitivity to pyridoxine. **Cautions:** Impaired renal function, neonates.

ACTION

Coenzyme for various metabolic functions, including metabolism of proteins, carbohydrates, fats. Aids in breakdown of glycogen and in synthesis of gamma-aminobutyric acid (GABA) in CNS.

Therapeutic Effect: Prevents pyridoxine deficiency. Increases excretion of certain drugs (e.g., isoniazid) that are pyridoxine antagonists.

PHARMACOKINETICS

Readily absorbed, primarily in jejunum. Stored in liver, muscle, brain. Metabolized in liver. Primarily excreted in urine. Removed by hemodialysis. **Half-life:** 15–20 days.

⌛ LIFESPAN CONSIDERATIONS

Pregnancy/Lactation: Crosses placenta. Distributed in breast milk. High dosages in utero may produce seizures in neonates. **Children/Elderly:** No age-related precautions noted.

INTERACTIONS

DRUG: Decreases effects of **levodopa**. **HERBAL:** None significant. **FOOD:** None known. **LAB VALUES:** None significant.

AVAILABILITY (OTC)

Capsules: 250 mg. **Injection Solution:** 100 mg/mL. **Tablets:** 25 mg, 50 mg, 100 mg, 250 mg. **Tablet, Extended-Release:** 200 mg.

ADMINISTRATION/HANDLING

◄**ALERT**► Give PO unless nausea, vomiting, malabsorption occurs. Avoid IV use in cardiac pts.

IV

• Give undiluted or may be added to IV solutions and given as infusion.

PO

• Give without regard to food.

▦ IV INCOMPATIBILITIES

Do not mix with any other medications.

INDICATIONS/ROUTES/DOSAGE

Pyridoxine Deficiency
PO/IM/IV: ADULTS, ELDERLY: 10–20 mg/day for 3 wks, followed by oral therapy up to 600 mg/day.

SIDE EFFECTS

Occasional: Stinging at IM injection site. **Rare:** Headache, nausea, drowsiness, sensory neuropathy (paresthesia, unstable gait, clumsiness of hands) with high doses.

ADVERSE EFFECTS/TOXIC REACTIONS

Long-term megadoses (2–6 g for longer than 2 mos) may produce sensory neuropathy (reduced deep tendon reflexes, profound impairment of sense of position in distal limbs, gradual sensory ataxia). Toxic symptoms subside when drug is discontinued. Seizures have occurred after IV megadoses.

NURSING CONSIDERATIONS

INTERVENTION/EVALUATION

Observe for improvement of deficiency symptoms, glossitis. Evaluate for nutritional adequacy.

PATIENT/FAMILY TEACHING

• Discomfort may occur with IM injection. • Consume foods rich in pyridoxine (legumes, soybeans, eggs, sunflower seeds, hazelnuts, organ meats, tuna, shrimp, carrots, avocados, bananas, wheat germ, bran).

P

QUEtiapine   TOP 100

kwet-**eye**-a-peen
(Apo-QUEtiapine ✦, <u>SEROquel</u>,
SEROquel XR)

■ **BLACK BOX ALERT** ■ Increased risk of suicidal ideation and behavior in children, adolescents, young adults 18–24 yrs with major depressive disorder, other psychiatric disorders. Elderly with dementia-related psychosis are at increased risk for death.

Do not confuse QUEtiapine with OLANZapine, or SEROquel with SINEquan.

◆CLASSIFICATION

PHARMACOTHERAPEUTIC: Dibenzapine derivative. **CLINICAL:** Second-generation (atypical) antipsychotic.

USES

Treatment of schizophrenia. Treatment of acute manic episodes associated with bipolar disorder (alone or in combination with lithium or valproate). Maintenance treatment of bipolar disorder as an adjunct to lithium or valproic acid. Treatment of acute depressive episodes associated with bipolar disorder. Adjunctive treatment to antidepressants in major depressive disorder (MDD). **OFF-LABEL:** Delirium in critically ill pts, psychosis/agitation related to Alzheimer's dementia. Treatment of autism, treatment-resistant obsessive compulsive disorder.

PRECAUTIONS

Contraindications: Hypersensitivity to QUEtiapine. **Cautions:** Renal/hepatic impairment, preexisting abnormal lipid profile, pts at risk for aspiration pneumonia, cardiovascular disease (e.g., HF, history of MI), cerebrovascular disease, dehydration, hypovolemia, history of drug abuse/dependence, seizure disorder, hypothyroidism, pts at risk for suicide, Parkinson's disease, decreased GI motility, urinary retention, narrow-angle glaucoma, diabetes, visual problems, elderly, pts at risk for orthostatic hypotension. Avoid use in pts at risk for torsades de pointes (hypokalemia, hypomagnesemia, history of cardiac arrhythmias, congenital long QT syndrome, concurrent medications that prolong QT interval).

ACTION

Antagonizes DOPamine, serotonin, histamine, alpha$_1$-adrenergic receptors. **Therapeutic Effect:** Diminishes symptoms associated with schizophrenia/bipolar disorders.

PHARMACOKINETICS

Rapidly absorbed. Protein binding: 83%. Widely distributed in tissues; CNS concentration exceeds plasma concentration. Metabolized in liver. Primarily excreted in urine. **Half-life:** 6 hrs.

⬓ LIFESPAN CONSIDERATIONS

Pregnancy/Lactation: Unknown if drug is distributed in breast milk. Not recommended for breastfeeding mothers. **Children:** Safety and efficacy not established in children less than 10 yrs of age (bipolar mania) or less than 13 yrs of age (schizophrenia). **Elderly:** No age-related precautions noted, but lower initial and target dosages may be necessary.

INTERACTIONS

DRUG: **Medications prolonging QT interval** (e.g., **amiodarone, citalopram, dasatinib, haloperidol, levoFLOXacin, ondansetron**) may increase risk of QT prolongation. **Alcohol, other CNS depressants** (e.g., **LORazepam, morphine, zolpidem**) may increase CNS depression. May increase hypotensive effects of **antihypertensives. CYP3A4 inducers** (e.g., **phenytoin**) may increase clearance. **CYP3A4 inhibitors** (e.g., **clarithromycin, erythromycin, fluconazole, itraconazole**) may increase effects. **HERBAL:** **St. John's wort** may decrease concentration.

Gotu kola, kava kava, St. John's wort, valerian may increase CNS depression. **FOOD:** None known. **LAB VALUES:** May decrease total free thyroxine (T_4) serum levels. May increase serum cholesterol, triglycerides, ALT, AST, WBC, GGT. May produce false-positive pregnancy test result.

AVAILABILITY (Rx)

Tablets: 25 mg, 50 mg, 100 mg, 200 mg, 300 mg, 400 mg.

Tablets, Extended-Release: 50 mg, 150 mg, 200 mg, 300 mg, 400 mg.

ADMINISTRATION/HANDLING

PO
• Give immediate-release tablets without regard to food. • Do not break, crush, dissolve, or divide extended-release tablets. • Extended-release tablets should be given without regard to food or with a light meal in evening.

INDICATIONS/ROUTES/DOSAGE

Note: • When restarting pts who have been off QUEtiapine for less than 1 wk, titration is not required and maintenance dose can be reinstituted. • When restarting pts who have been off QUEtiapine for longer than 1 wk, follow initial titration schedule. • When discontinuing, gradual tapering recommended to avoid withdrawal symptoms and minimize risk of relapse.

Schizophrenia
PO: *(Immediate-Release):* **ADULTS, ELDERLY:** Initially, 25 mg twice daily, then increase in 25–50-mg increments divided 2–3 times/day on the second and third days, up to 300–400 mg/day in 2–3 divided doses by the fourth day. Further adjustments of 25–50 mg twice daily may be made at intervals of 2 days or longer. **Maintenance:** 150–750 mg/day (adults); 50–200 mg/day (elderly). *(Extended-Release):* Initially, 300 mg/day. May increase at intervals as short as 1 day up to 300 mg/day. Range: 400–800 mg/day. *(Immediate-Release):* **CHILDREN**

13 YRS AND OLDER: Initially, 25 mg twice daily on day 1, 50 mg twice daily on day 2, then increase by 100 mg/day to target dose of 400 mg twice daily on day 5. May further increase to 800 mg/day in increments of 100 mg or less daily. Range: 400–800 mg/day. **Maximum:** 800 mg. Total dose in 3 divided doses. *(Extended-Release):* Initially, 50 mg once daily on day 1, 100 mg on day 2, until 400 mg once daily is reached on day 5. Range: 400–800 mg/day. **Maximum:** 800 mg/day.

Mania in Bipolar Disorder
PO: *(Immediate-Release):* **ADULTS, ELDERLY:** Initially, 50 mg twice daily for 1 day. May increase in increments of 100 mg/day to 200 mg twice daily on day 4. May further increase in increments of 200 mg/day to 800 mg/day on day 6. Range: 400–800 mg/day. *(Extended-Release):* Initially, 300 mg on day 1 in the evening; 600 mg on day 2 and adjust between 400–800 mg/day thereafter. *(Immediate-Release):* **CHILDREN 10 YRS AND OLDER:** 25 mg twice daily on day 1, 50 mg twice daily on day 2, then increase by 100 mg/day until target dose of 400 mg/day reached on day 5. May increase up to 600 mg/day. Range: 400–600 mg/day. *(Extended-Release):* 50 mg on day 1; 100 mg on day 2; further increases of 100 mg/day until 400 mg once daily is reached on day 4; Usual range: 400–600 mg once daily.

Depression in Bipolar Disorder
PO: *(Immediate-Release):* **ADULTS, ELDERLY:** Initially, 50 mg/day on day 1, increase to 100 mg/day on day 2, then increase by 100 mg/day up to target dose of 300 mg/day. *(Extended-Release):* Initially, 50 mg on day 1 in the evening, 100 mg on day 2, 200 mg on day 3, 300 mg on day 4 and thereafter.

Adjunctive Therapy in MDD
PO: ADULTS, ELDERLY: *(Extended-Release):* Initially, 50 mg on days 1 and 2; then 150 mg on days 3 and 4; then 150–300 mg/day thereafter.

Dosage in Hepatic Impairment
(Immediate-Release): Initially, 25 mg/day. Increase by 25–50 mg/day to effective dose.
(Extended-Release): Initially, 50 mg/day, increase by 50 mg/day until effective dose.

Dosage in Renal Impairment
No dose adjustment.

SIDE EFFECTS

Frequent (19%–10%): Headache, drowsiness, dizziness. **Occasional (9%–3%):** Constipation, orthostatic hypotension, tachycardia, dry mouth, dyspepsia, rash, asthenia, abdominal pain, rhinitis. **Rare (2%):** Back pain, fever, weight gain.

ADVERSE EFFECTS/TOXIC REACTIONS

Overdose may produce heart block, hypotension, hypokalemia, tachycardia.

NURSING CONSIDERATIONS

BASELINE ASSESSMENT

Assess behavior, appearance, emotional status, response to environment, speech pattern, thought content. Obtain baseline CBC, hepatic enzyme levels before initiating treatment and periodically thereafter. Question medical history as listed in Precautions.

INTERVENTION/EVALUATION

Monitor mental status, onset of extrapyramidal symptoms. Assist with ambulation if dizziness occurs. Supervise suicidal-risk pt closely during early therapy (as psychosis, depression lessens, energy level improves, increasing suicide potential). Monitor B/P for hypotension, lipid profile, blood glucose, CBC, or worsening depression, unusual behavior. Assess pulse for tachycardia (esp. with rapid increase in dosage). Monitor daily pattern of bowel activity, stool consistency. Assess for therapeutic response (improved thought content, increased ability to concentrate, improvement in self-care). Eye exam to detect cataract formation should be obtained q6mos during treatment.

PATIENT/ FAMILY TEACHING

• Avoid exposure to extreme heat. • Drink fluids often, esp. during physical activity. • Take medication as ordered; do not stop taking or increase dosage. • Drowsiness generally subsides during continued therapy. • Avoid tasks that require alertness, motor skills until response to drug is established. • Avoid alcohol. • Slowly go from lying to standing. • Report suicidal ideation, unusual changes in behavior.

quinapril

kwin-a-pril
(Accupril, Apo-Quinapril ✦)
■ **BLACK BOX ALERT** ■ May cause fetal injury, mortality. Discontinue as soon as possible once pregnancy detected.
Do not confuse Accupril with Accolate, Accutane, Aciphex, or Monopril.

FIXED-COMBINATION(S)

Accuretic: quinapril/hydroCHLOROthiazide (a diuretic): 10 mg/12.5 mg, 20 mg/12.5 mg, 20 mg/25 mg.

◆CLASSIFICATION

PHARMACOTHERAPEUTIC: Angiotensin-converting enzyme (ACE) inhibitor. **CLINICAL:** Antihypertensive.

USES

Treatment of hypertension. Used alone or in combination with other antihypertensives. Adjunctive therapy in management of HF. **OFF-LABEL:** Treatment of pediatric hypertension.

PRECAUTIONS

Contraindications: Hypersensitivity to quinapril. History of angioedema from previous treatment with ACE inhibitors, concomitant use with aliskiren in pts with diabetes. **Cautions:** Renal impairment, hypertrophic cardiomyopathy with outflow tract obstruction, major surgery, HF, hypovolemia, unstented bilateral renal artery stenosis, hyperkalemia, concurrent potassium supplements, severe aortic stenosis, ischemic heart disease, cerebrovascular disease.

ACTION

Suppresses renin-angiotensin-aldosterone system, preventing conversion of angiotensin I to angiotensin II, a potent vasoconstrictor; may inhibit angiotensin II at local vascular renal sites. **Therapeutic Effect:** Reduces peripheral arterial resistance, B/P, pulmonary capillary wedge pressure; improves cardiac output.

PHARMACOKINETICS

Route	Onset	Peak	Duration
PO	1 hr	N/A	24 hrs

Readily absorbed from GI tract. Protein binding: 97%. Rapidly hydrolyzed to active metabolite. Primarily excreted in urine. Minimal removal by hemodialysis. **Half-life:** 1–2 hrs; metabolite, 3 hrs (increased in renal impairment).

⏳ LIFESPAN CONSIDERATIONS

Pregnancy/Lactation: Crosses placenta. Unknown if distributed in breast milk. May cause fetal, neonatal mortality or morbidity. **Children:** Safety and efficacy not established. **Elderly:** May be more sensitive to hypotensive effects.

INTERACTIONS

DRUG: Alcohol, antihypertensives (e.g., amLODIPine, lisinopril, valsartan), diuretics (e.g., furosemide, HCTZ) may increase effects. May increase concentration, risk of toxicity of lithium. NSAIDs (e.g., ibuprofen, ketorolac, naproxen) may decrease effects. **Potassium-sparing diuretics** (e.g., spironolactone, triamterene), **potassium supplements** may cause hyperkalemia. **HERBAL: Black cohosh, periwinkle** may increase antihypertensive effect. **Ginseng, yohimbe, licorice** may worsen hypertension. **FOOD:** None known. **LAB VALUES:** May increase serum BUN, alkaline phosphatase, bilirubin, creatinine, potassium, ALT, AST. May decrease serum sodium. May cause positive antinuclear antibody (ANA) titer.

AVAILABILITY (Rx)

Tablets: 5 mg, 10 mg, 20 mg, 40 mg.

ADMINISTRATION/HANDLING

PO

• Give without regard to food. • Tablets may be crushed.

INDICATIONS/ROUTES/DOSAGE

Hypertension (Monotherapy)
PO: ADULTS: Initially, 10–20 mg/day. May adjust dosage at intervals of at least 2 wks or longer. **Maintenance:** 10–40 mg once daily. **ELDERLY:** Initially, 10 mg once daily. Titrate to optimal response.

Hypertension (Combination Diuretic Therapy)
PO: ADULTS, ELDERLY: Initially, 5 mg/day titrated to pt's needs.

Adjunct to Manage HF
PO: ADULTS, ELDERLY: Initially, 5 mg twice daily. Titrate at wkly intervals to 20–40 mg/day in 2 divided doses. Target dose: 20 mg twice daily.

Dosage in Renal Impairment
Hypertension

Creatinine Clearance	Initial Dose
More than 60 mL/min	10 mg
30–60 mL/min	5 mg
10–29 mL/min	2.5 mg

HF

Creatinine Clearance	Initial Dose
Greater than 30 mL/min	5 mg
10–30 mL/min	2.5 mg

Dosage in Hepatic Impairment
No dose adjustment.

SIDE EFFECTS

Frequent (7%–5%): Headache, dizziness. **Occasional (4%–2%):** Fatigue, vomiting, nausea, hypotension, chest pain, cough, syncope. **Rare (less than 2%):** Diarrhea, cough, dyspnea, rash, palpitations, impotence, insomnia, drowsiness, malaise.

ADVERSE EFFECTS/TOXIC REACTIONS

Excessive hypotension ("first-dose syncope") may occur in pts with HF, those who are severely salt/volume depleted. Angioedema, hyperkalemia occur rarely. Agranulocytosis, neutropenia may be noted in those with collagen vascular disease (scleroderma, systemic lupus erythematosus), renal impairment. Nephrotic syndrome may be noted in those with history of renal disease.

NURSING CONSIDERATIONS

BASELINE ASSESSMENT

Obtain B/P immediately before each dose in addition to regular monitoring (be alert to fluctuations). Renal function tests should be performed before beginning therapy. In pts with prior renal disease, urine test for protein by dipstick method should be made with first urine of day before beginning therapy and periodically thereafter. In pts with renal impairment, autoimmune disease, or taking drugs that affect leukocytes or immune response, CBC, differential count should be performed before beginning therapy and q2wks for 3 mos, then periodically thereafter.

INTERVENTION/EVALUATION

Monitor B/P (if excessive reduction in B/P occurs, place pt in supine position with legs slightly elevated), renal function, serum potassium, WBC. Assist with ambulation if dizziness occurs. Question for evidence of headache. Noncola carbonated beverage, unsalted crackers, dry toast may relieve nausea.

PATIENT/ FAMILY TEACHING

• Go slowly from lying to standing. • Full therapeutic effect may take 1–2 wks. • Report any sign of infection (sore throat, fever). • Skipping doses or voluntarily discontinuing drug may produce severe rebound hypertension. • Avoid tasks that require alertness, motor skills until response to drug is established. • Avoid alcohol.

RABEprazole [TOP 100]

ra-**bep**-ra-zole
(Aciphex, Aciphex Sprinkle, Apo-RABEprazole)
Do not confuse Aciphex with Accupril or Aricept, or RABEprazole with ARIPiprazole, lansoprazole, omeprazole, or raloxifene.

◆CLASSIFICATION

PHARMACOTHERAPEUTIC: Proton pump inhibitor. **CLINICAL:** Gastric acid inhibitor.

USES

Short-term treatment (4–8 wks), maintenance of erosive or ulcerative gastroesophageal reflux disease (GERD). Treatment of daytime/nighttime heartburn, other symptoms of GERD. Short-term treatment (4 wks or less) in healing, symptomatic relief of duodenal ulcers. Long-term treatment of pathologic hypersecretory conditions, including Zollinger-Ellison syndrome. Treatment of *H. pylori* (in combination with amoxicillin and clarithromycin). Sprinkle dose form approved for treatment of GERD in children 1–11 yrs. **OFF-LABEL:** Maintenance of healing and prevention of relapse of duodenal ulcers. Treatment of NSAID-induced ulcers.

PRECAUTIONS

Contraindications: Hypersensitivity to RABE-prazole, other proton pump inhibitors (e.g., omeprazole). Concurrent use with rilpivirine-containing products. **Cautions:** Severe hepatic impairment, osteoporosis.

ACTION

Suppresses gastric acid secretion by inhibiting H⁺/K⁺–ATP pump. **Therapeutic Effect:** Increases gastric pH, reducing gastric acid production.

PHARMACOKINETICS

Rapidly absorbed from GI tract after passing through stomach relatively intact as delayed-release tablet. Protein binding: 96%. Metabolized in liver. Primarily excreted in urine. **Half-life:** 1–2 hrs (increased with hepatic impairment).

⧖ LIFESPAN CONSIDERATIONS

Pregnancy/Lactation: Unknown if drug crosses placenta or is distributed in breast milk. **Children:** Safety and efficacy not established. **Elderly:** No age-related precautions noted.

INTERACTIONS

DRUG: May increase concentration/effects of cycloSPORINE, warfarin. May decrease concentration of ketoconazole, clopidogrel, atazanavir. **HERBAL:** St. John's wort may decrease concentration/effects. **FOOD:** None known. **LAB VALUES:** May increase serum ALT, AST, thyroid-stimulating hormone (TSH).

AVAILABILITY (Rx)

🔖 **Tablets (Delayed-Release):** 20 mg. **Capsule, Sprinkle:** 5 mg, 10 mg.

ADMINISTRATION/HANDLING

PO
• May give without regard to meals; best taken after breakfast. • Do not break, crush, dissolve, or divide tablet; give whole.

Sprinkle
• May give with antacid. • Administer 30 min before a meal. • Open capsule, sprinkle on soft food. Take within 15 min of preparation. • Do not chew, crush.

INDICATIONS/ROUTES/DOSAGE

GERD (Erosive or Ulcerative)
PO: ADULTS, ELDERLY: 20 mg/day for 4–8 wks. If inadequate response, may repeat for additional 8 wks. **Maintenance:** 20 mg/day.

Short-Term Treatment of Symptomatic GERD
PO: ADULTS, ELDERLY, CHILDREN 12 YRS AND OLDER: 20 mg/day for 4 wks. If inadequate response, may repeat additional 4 wks. **CHILDREN, 1–11 YRS (15 KG OR GREATER):** 10 mg once daily for up to 12 wks. **(LESS THAN 15 KG):** 5 mg once daily

R

for up to 12 wks; may increase to 10 mg once daily.

Duodenal Ulcer
PO: **ADULTS, ELDERLY:** 20 mg/day after morning meal for 4 wks.

Pathologic Hypersecretory Conditions
PO: **ADULTS, ELDERLY:** Initially, 60 mg once daily. May increase to 60 mg twice daily.

H. Pylori **Infection**
PO: **ADULTS, ELDERLY:** 20 mg twice daily for 10–14 days (given with amoxicillin 1,000 mg and clarithromycin 500 mg).

Dosage in Renal Impairment
No dose adjustment.

Dosage in Hepatic Impairment
Mild to moderate impairment: No dose adjustment. **Severe impairment:** Use caution.

SIDE EFFECTS

Rare (Less Than 2%): Headache, nausea, dizziness, rash, diarrhea, malaise.

ADVERSE EFFECTS/TOXIC REACTIONS

Hyperglycemia, hypokalemia, hyponatremia, hyperlipemia occur rarely. May increase risk of bone fractures, *C. difficile*-associated colitis.

NURSING CONSIDERATIONS

BASELINE ASSESSMENT
Question history of GI disease, ulcers, GERD.

INTERVENTION/EVALUATION
Evaluate for therapeutic response (relief of GI symptoms). Question if GI discomfort, nausea, diarrhea, headache occurs. Assess skin for evidence of rash. Observe for evidence of dizziness; utilize appropriate safety precautions.

PATIENT/FAMILY TEACHING
• Swallow tablets whole; do not break, chew, dissolve, or divide tablets. • Report headache.

raloxifene

ra-**lox**-i-feen
(<u>Evista</u>, Apo-Raloxifene ✦)
■ **BLACK BOX ALERT** ■ Increases risk of deep vein thrombosis, pulmonary embolism. Women with coronary heart disease or pts at risk for coronary events are at increased risk for death due to stroke.
Do not confuse Evista with AVINza.

◆CLASSIFICATION

PHARMACOTHERAPEUTIC: Selective estrogen receptor modulator. **CLINICAL:** Osteoporosis preventive.

USES

Prevention/treatment of osteoporosis in postmenopausal women. Reduces risk of invasive breast cancer in postmenopausal women with osteoporosis and postmenopausal women at high risk for invasive breast cancer.

PRECAUTIONS

Contraindications: Hypersensitivity to raloxifene. Active or history of venous thromboembolic events, such as deep vein thrombosis (DVT), pulmonary embolism, retinal vein thrombosis; women who are or may become pregnant, breastfeeding. **Cautions:** Cardiovascular disease, renal/hepatic impairment, risk for venous thromboembolism, unexplained uterine bleeding, elevated triglycerides in response to oral estrogen therapy.

ACTION

Selective estrogen receptor modulator (SERM) that binds to estrogen receptors, increasing bone mineral density. Blocks estrogen effects in breast/uterus. **Therapeutic Effect:** Reduces bone resorption, increases bone mineral density, reduces incidence of fractures.

PHARMACOKINETICS

Rapidly absorbed after PO administration. Protein binding: 95%. Metabolized

R

in liver. Excreted primarily in feces. Unknown if removed by hemodialysis. **Half-life:** 27.7–32.5 hrs.

⌛ LIFESPAN CONSIDERATIONS

Pregnancy/Lactation: Unknown if distributed in breast milk. Contraindicated in pregnancy, breastfeeding. **Children:** Not used in this population. **Elderly:** No age-related precautions noted.

INTERACTIONS

DRUG: Cholestyramine reduces peak levels, extent of absorption. Do not use concurrently with **hormone replacement therapy, systemic estrogen.** May decrease effect of **warfarin** (decreases INR). **HERBAL:** None significant. **FOOD:** None known. **LAB VALUES:** May lower serum total cholesterol, LDL. May decrease platelet count, serum inorganic phosphate, albumin, calcium, protein.

AVAILABILITY (Rx)

Tablets: 60 mg.

ADMINISTRATION/HANDLING

PO
• Give without regard to meals.

INDICATIONS/ROUTES/DOSAGE

Note: Discontinue at least 72 hrs prior to and during prolonged immobilization (may increase risk for DVT/PE).

Prophylaxis/Treatment of Osteoporosis, Breast Cancer Risk Reduction
PO: ADULTS, ELDERLY: 60 mg/day.

Dosage in Renal/Hepatic Impairment
No dose adjustment.

SIDE EFFECTS

Frequent (25%–10%): Hot flashes, flu-like symptoms, arthralgia, sinusitis. **Occasional (9%–5%):** Weight gain, nausea, myalgia, pharyngitis, cough, dyspepsia, leg cramps, rash, depression. **Rare (4%–3%):** Vaginitis, UTI, peripheral edema, flatulence, vomiting, fever, migraine, diaphoresis.

ADVERSE EFFECTS/TOXIC REACTIONS

Pneumonia, gastroenteritis, chest pain, vaginal bleeding, breast pain occur rarely.

NURSING CONSIDERATIONS

BASELINE ASSESSMENT

Question history of thrombosis (CVA, DVT, PE). Question for possibility of pregnancy. Drug should be discontinued 72 hrs before and during prolonged immobilization (postop recovery, prolonged bed rest). Therapy may be resumed only after pt is fully ambulatory. Determine serum total, LDL cholesterol before therapy and routinely thereafter.

INTERVENTION/EVALUATION

Monitor serum total cholesterol, total calcium, inorganic phosphate, total protein, albumin, bone mineral density, platelet count. Diligently monitor for CVA (aphasia, blindness, confusion, paresthesia, hemiparesis, syncope), DVT (arm/leg pain, swelling), pulmonary embolism (chest pain, dyspnea, hypoxia, tachycardia).

PATIENT/FAMILY TEACHING

• Avoid prolonged restriction of movement during travel (increased risk of venous thromboembolic events). • Take supplemental calcium, vitamin D if daily dietary intake is inadequate. • Engage in regular weight-bearing exercise. • Modify, discontinue habits of cigarette smoking, alcohol consumption. • Report symptoms of DVT (swelling, pain, hot feeling in the arms or legs), lung embolism (difficulty breathing, chest pain, rapid heart rate), stroke (blindness, confusion, difficulty speaking, one-sided weakness, passing out).

raltegravir

ral-**teg**-ra-veer
(Isentress)

◆CLASSIFICATION

PHARMACOTHERAPEUTIC: Integrase inhibitor. **CLINICAL:** Antiviral.

USES

Treatment of HIV-1 infection in adults and children 4 wks and older and weighing at least 3 kg. Used in combination with at least two other antiretroviral agents. **OFF-LABEL:** Postexposure prophylaxis for occupational exposure to HIV.

PRECAUTIONS

Contraindications: Hypersensitivity to raltegravir. **Cautions:** Elderly, pts at risk for creatine kinase (CK) elevations and/or skeletal muscle abnormalities.

ACTION

Inhibits activity of HIV-1 integrase, an enzyme that incorporates viral DNA into host cell. **Therapeutic Effect:** Prevents integration and replication of viral HIV-1.

PHARMACOKINETICS

Variably absorbed following PO administration. Protein binding: 83%. Metabolized in liver. Excreted in feces (51%), urine (32%). **Half-life:** 9 hrs.

⧗ LIFESPAN CONSIDERATIONS

Pregnancy/Lactation: May cross placenta. Breastfeeding not recommended. **Children:** Safety and efficacy not established in pts younger than 4 weeks. **Elderly:** Age-related hepatic, renal, cardiac impairment requires strict monitoring.

INTERACTIONS

DRUG: Proton pump inhibitors (e.g., omeprazole, pantoprazole) may increase concentration. **Aluminum, magnesium salts, rifAMPin** may decrease levels/effect. **HERBAL: St. John's wort** may decrease concentration/effects. **FOOD:** None known. **LAB VALUES:** May increase serum glucose, bilirubin, aminotransferase, alkaline phosphatase, amylase, lipase, creatine kinase. May decrease lymphocytes, neutrophils (ANC), Hgb, platelets.

AVAILABILITY (Rx)

Packet, Oral: 100 mg. **Tablets, Chewable:** 25 mg, 100 mg.

🦰 **Tablets, Film-Coated:** 400 mg, 600 mg.

ADMINISTRATION/HANDLING

PO
• Give without regard to food. • Do not break, crush, dissolve, or divide film-coated tablets. • Chewable tablets may be chewed or taken whole. • **Oral Packet:** Mix with 5 mL water to provide a concentration of 20 mg/mL. Once mixed, measure dose with oral syringe. Give within 30 min of mixing.

INDICATIONS/ROUTES/DOSAGE

HIV Infection
PO: ADULTS, ELDERLY, CHILDREN 12 YRS AND OLDER: 400 mg twice daily. Dosage increased to 800 mg twice daily when given with rifAMPin. **CHILDREN 2–11 YRS (CHEWABLE TABLETS) 40 KG OR GREATER:** 300 mg twice daily. **28–39 KG:** 200 mg twice daily. **20–27 KG:** 150 mg twice daily. **14–19 KG:** 100 mg twice daily. **11–13 KG:** 75 mg twice daily. **CHILDREN** weighing 3–19 kg **(ORAL PACKET): 14–19 KG:** 100 mg twice daily. **11–13 KG:** 80 mg twice daily. **8–10 KG:** 60 mg twice daily. **6–7 KG:** 40 mg twice daily. **4–5 KG:** 30 mg twice daily. **3–4 KG:** 20 mg twice daily.

Dosage in Renal/Hepatic Impairment
No dose adjustment.

SIDE EFFECTS

Frequent (17%–10%): Diarrhea, nausea, headache. **Occasional (5%):** Fever. **Rare (2%–1%):** Vomiting, abdominal pain, fatigue, dizziness.

ADVERSE EFFECTS/TOXIC REACTIONS

Hypersensitivity reactions, anemia, neutropenia, MI, gastritis, hepatitis, herpes simplex, toxic nephropathy, renal failure, chronic renal failure, renal tubular necrosis occur rarely.

NURSING CONSIDERATIONS

BASELINE ASSESSMENT

Obtain baseline CBC, BMP, LFT, CD4 count, viral load prior to initiation and at periodic intervals during therapy. Offer emotional support. Obtain medication history.

INTERVENTION/EVALUATION

Closely monitor for evidence of GI discomfort. Monitor daily pattern of bowel activity, stool consistency. Monitor serum chemistry tests for marked laboratory abnormalities. Assess for opportunistic infections: onset of fever, cough, other respiratory symptoms.

PATIENT/FAMILY TEACHING

• Report fever, abdominal pain, yellowing of skin/eyes, dark urine. • Avoid tasks that require alertness, motor skills until response to drug is established. • Raltegravir is not a cure for HIV infection, nor does it reduce risk of transmission to others. • Pt may continue to experience illnesses, including opportunistic infections.

ramelteon

ra-**mel**-tee-on
(Rozerem)
**Do not confuse ramelteon with
Remeron, or Rozerem with
Razadyne or Remeron.**

◆CLASSIFICATION

PHARMACOTHERAPEUTIC: Melatonin receptor agonist. **CLINICAL:** Hypnotic.

USES

Treatment of insomnia in pts who experience difficulty with sleep onset.

PRECAUTIONS

Contraindications: Hypersensitivity to ramelteon. Concurrent fluvoxaMINE therapy, history of angioedema with previous ramelteon therapy. **Cautions:** Depression, other psychiatric conditions, alcohol consumption, other CNS depressants, moderate hepatic impairment, severe sleep apnea, COPD; concomitant strong CYP1A2 inhibitors (e.g., fluvoxaMINE).

ACTION

Selectively targets melatonin receptors thought to be involved in maintenance of circadian rhythm underlying normal sleep-wake cycle. **Therapeutic Effect:** Prevents insomnia characterized by difficulty with sleep onset.

PHARMACOKINETICS

Rapidly absorbed following PO administration. Protein binding: 82%. Substantial tissue distribution. Metabolized in liver. Excreted in urine (84%), feces (4%). **Half-life:** 2–5 hrs.

⏾ LIFESPAN CONSIDERATIONS

Pregnancy/Lactation: Unknown if distributed in breast milk. Breastfeeding not recommended. **Children:** Safety and efficacy not established. **Elderly:** Age-related hepatic impairment may require dosage adjustment.

INTERACTIONS

DRUG: Concurrent use with **alcohol** may produce additive effect. **Fluconazole, ketoconazole** may increase serum concentration/effects. **Donepezil, doxepin, fluvoxaMINE** may cause marked increase in serum level, toxicity. **RifAMPin** may decrease serum level, effects. **HERBAL: Gotu kola, kava kava, St. John's wort, valerian** may increase CNS depression. **FOOD:** Onset of action may be reduced if taken with or immediately after a **high-fat meal. LAB VALUES:** May decrease serum cortisol.

AVAILABILITY (Rx)

🍃 **Tablets, Film-Coated:** 8 mg (Rozerem).

ADMINISTRATION/HANDLING

PO
• Administer within 30 min before bedtime. • Do not give with, or immediately following, a high-fat meal. • Do not break, crush, dissolve, or divide tablet.

INDICATIONS/ROUTES/DOSAGE

Insomnia
PO: ADULTS, ELDERLY: 8 mg 30 min before bedtime.

Dosage in Renal Impairment
No dose adjustment.

R

Dosage in Hepatic Impairment
Mild to moderate impairment: No dose adjustment. **Severe impairment:** Not recommended.

SIDE EFFECTS

Frequent (7%–5%): Headache, dizziness, drowsiness (expected effect). **Occasional (4%–3%):** Fatigue, nausea, exacerbated insomnia. **Rare (2%):** Diarrhea, myalgia, depression, altered taste, arthralgia.

ADVERSE EFFECTS/TOXIC REACTIONS

May affect reproductive hormones in adults (decreased testosterone levels, increased prolactin levels), resulting in unexplained amenorrhea, galactorrhea, decreased libido, impaired fertility. Complex sleep-related behavior may occur.

NURSING CONSIDERATIONS

BASELINE ASSESSMENT

Assess B/P, pulse, respirations. Raise bed rails, provide call light. Provide environment conducive to sleep (quiet environment, low/no lighting, TV off).

INTERVENTION/EVALUATION

Assess sleep pattern of pt. Evaluate for therapeutic response: rapid induction of sleep onset, decrease in number of nocturnal awakenings.

PATIENT/FAMILY TEACHING

• Take within 30 min before going to bed; confine activities to those necessary to prepare for bed. • Avoid tasks that require alertness, motor skills until response to drug is established. • Avoid alcohol. • Do not take medication with or immediately after a high-fat meal.

---

ramipril

ram-i-pril
(Altace, Apo-Ramipril ✦)
■ **BLACK BOX ALERT** ■ May cause fetal injury, mortality. Discontinue as soon as possible once pregnancy is detected.

Do not confuse Altace with alteplase, Amaryl, or Artane, or ramipril with enalapril or Monopril.

◆CLASSIFICATION

PHARMACOTHERAPEUTIC: Angiotensin-converting enzyme (ACE) inhibitor. **CLINICAL:** Antihypertensive.

USES

Treatment of hypertension. Used alone or in combination with other antihypertensives. Treatment of HF following MI. Reduce risk of heart attack, stroke in pts at increased risk of developing major cardiovascular events. **OFF-LABEL:** HF. Delay progression of nephropathy, reduce risks of cardiovascular events in hypertensive pts with type 1 or type 2 diabetes.

PRECAUTIONS

Contraindications: Hypersensitivity to ramipril, other ACE inhibitors. History of ACE inhibitor–induced angioedema, concomitant use with aliskiren in pts with diabetes. **Cautions:** Renal impairment; elderly pts; collagen vascular disease; hyperkalemia; hypertrophic cardiomyopathy with outflow tract obstruction; unstented unilateral, bilateral renal artery stenosis; severe aortic stenosis; before, during, or immediately after major surgery; concomitant potassium supplements.

ACTION

Suppresses renin-angiotensin-aldosterone system. Blocks conversion of angiotensin I to angiotensin II, increases plasma renin activity, decreases aldosterone secretion. **Therapeutic Effect:** Reduces peripheral arterial resistance, decreasing B/P.

PHARMACOKINETICS

Route	Onset	Peak	Duration
PO	1–2 hrs	3–6 hrs	24 hrs

Well absorbed from GI tract. Protein binding: 73%. Metabolized in liver. Primarily

R

excreted in urine. Not removed by hemodialysis. **Half-life:** 5.1 hrs.

⌛ LIFESPAN CONSIDERATIONS

Pregnancy/Lactation: Crosses placenta. Distributed in breast milk. May cause fetal or neonatal mortality or morbidity. **Children:** Safety and efficacy not established. **Elderly:** May be more sensitive to hypotensive effects.

INTERACTIONS

DRUG: Alcohol, antihypertensives (e.g., amLODIPine, lisinopril, valsartan), diuretics (e.g., furosemide, HCTZ) may increase effects. May increase **lithium** concentration, risk of toxicity. **NSAIDs** may decrease effects. **Potassium-sparing diuretics (e.g., spironolactone, triamterene), potassium supplements** may cause hyperkalemia. **HERBAL: Black cohosh, periwinkle** may increase antihypertensive effect. **Ginseng, ginger, licorice, yohimbe** may worsen hypertension. **FOOD:** None known. **LAB VALUES:** May increase serum BUN, alkaline phosphatase, bilirubin, creatinine, potassium, ALT, AST. May decrease serum sodium. May cause positive antinuclear antibody (ANA) titer.

AVAILABILITY (Rx)

Capsules: 1.25 mg, 2.5 mg, 5 mg, 10 mg.

ADMINISTRATION/HANDLING

PO
• Give without regard to food. • May mix with water, apple juice/sauce.

INDICATIONS/ROUTES/DOSAGE

Hypertension (Monotherapy)
PO: ADULTS, ELDERLY: Initially, 2.5 mg/day. Titrate to desired effect. Usual dose: 5–10 mg/day.

Hypertension (in Combination with Other Antihypertensives)
PO: ADULTS, ELDERLY: Initially, 1.25 mg daily. Titrate to desired response.

HF Following MI
PO: ADULTS, ELDERLY: Initially, 1.25–2.5 mg twice daily. Continue for 1 wk, then titrate upward q3wks to target dose of 5 mg twice daily.

Risk Reduction for MI/Stroke
PO: ADULTS, ELDERLY: Initially, 2.5 mg/day for 7 days, then 5 mg/day for 21 days, then 10 mg/day as a single dose (or in divided doses in hypertensive or recent post-MI pts).

Dosage in Renal Impairment
CrCl equal to or less than 40 mL/min: 25% of normal dose.

Renal Failure and Hypertension
Initially, 1.25 mg/day titrated upward. **Maximum:** 5 mg/day.
Renal Failure and HF: Initially, 1.25 mg/day, titrated up to 2.5 mg twice daily.

Dosage in Hepatic Impairment
No dose adjustment. Discontinue for jaundice or marked elevation of hepatic enzymes.

SIDE EFFECTS

Frequent (12%–5%): Cough, headache. **Occasional (4%–2%):** Dizziness, fatigue, nausea, asthenia. **Rare (Less Than 2%):** Palpitations, insomnia, nervousness, malaise, abdominal pain, myalgia.

ADVERSE EFFECTS/TOXIC REACTIONS

Excessive hypotension ("first-dose syncope") may occur in pts with HF, severely salt or volume depleted. Angioedema, hyperkalemia occur rarely. Agranulocytosis, neutropenia may be noted in pts with collagen vascular disease (scleroderma, systemic lupus erythematosus), renal impairment. Nephrotic syndrome may be noted in those with history of renal disease. May cause angioedema of the face, neck, throat, tongue. Cholestatic jaundice, fulminant hepatic necrosis may occur.

R

✦ Canadian trade name　　🍵 Non-Crushable Drug　　▦ High Alert drug

NURSING CONSIDERATIONS

BASELINE ASSESSMENT

Obtain B/P immediately before each dose, in addition to regular monitoring (be alert to fluctuations). If excessive reduction in B/P occurs, place pt in supine position with legs elevated. Renal function tests should be performed before beginning therapy. Question history of hypersensitivity reaction, angioedema.

INTERVENTION/EVALUATION

In pts with prior renal disease, urine test for protein (by dipstick method) should be made with first urine of day before beginning therapy and periodically thereafter. In pts with renal impairment, autoimmune disease, or taking drugs that affect leukocytes or immune response, CBC, differential count should be performed before beginning therapy and q2wks for 3 mos periodically thereafter. Monitor B/P, renal function, serum potassium, WBC. Assess for cough (frequent effect). Assist with ambulation if dizziness occurs. Assess lung sounds for rales, wheezing in pts with HF. Monitor urinalysis for proteinuria. Monitor serum potassium in pts on concurrent diuretic therapy.

PATIENT/FAMILY TEACHING

• Do not discontinue medication without physician's approval. • Slowly go from lying to standing to minimize hypotensive effect. • Report palpitations, cough, chest pain. • Dizziness may occur in first few days. • Avoid tasks that require alertness, motor skills until response to drug is established. • Avoid alcohol. • Report swelling of the face, lips, or tongue.

ramucirumab

ra-mue-sir-ue-mab
(Cyramza)

■ BLACK BOX ALERT ■ May increase risk of severe, and sometimes fatal, hemorrhagic events. Permanently discontinue if severe bleeding occurs.

Do not confuse ramucirumab with ranibizumab.

◆CLASSIFICATION

PHARMACOTHERAPEUTIC: Vascular endothelial growth factor 2 antagonist. CLINICAL: Antineoplastic.

USES

As a single agent or in combination with PACLitaxel, for treatment of advanced or metastatic gastric or gastroesophageal junction adenocarcinoma with disease progression on or after prior fluoropyrimidine- or platinum-containing chemotherapy. In combination with DOCEtaxel, for treatment of metastatic non–small cell lung cancer (NSCLC) with disease progression on or after platinum-based chemotherapy. In combination with FOL-FIRI, for treatment of metastatic colorectal cancer with disease progression on or after therapy with bevacizumab, oxaliplatin, and a fluoropyrimidine.

PRECAUTIONS

Contraindications: Hypersensitivity to ramucirumab. Cautions: History of arterial/venous thromboembolism (e.g., MI, cardiac arrest, CVA, cerebral ischemia), hepatic cirrhosis, electrolyte imbalance, hypertension, GI bleeding/perforation, chronic/unhealed wounds; baseline neutropenia, thrombocytopenia.

ACTION

Binds vascular endothelial growth factor (VEGF) receptor 2 and blocks binding of VEGF ligands, VEGF-A, VEGF-C, and VEGF-D. Therapeutic Effect: Inhibits/reduces tumor vascularity and growth.

PHARMACOKINETICS

Metabolism not specified. Elimination not specified.

⌛ LIFESPAN CONSIDERATIONS

Pregnancy/Lactation: May cause fetal harm. Contraception recommended during treatment and up to 3 mos after discontinuation. Must either discontinue drug or discontinue breastfeeding. Unknown if distributed in breast milk. **Children:** Safety and efficacy not established. **Elderly:** No age-related precautions noted.

INTERACTIONS

DRUG: None known (no studies conducted). **HERBAL:** None significant. **FOOD:** None known. **LAB VALUES:** May increase urine protein. May decrease neutrophils, serum sodium.

AVAILABILITY (Rx)

Injection Solution: 100 mg/10 mL, 500 mg/50 mL.

ADMINISTRATION/HANDLING

 IV

• Do not administer IV push or bolus. • Recommend premedication with IV histamine H_1 antagonist (e.g., diphenhydramine) prior to each infusion. Pts with prior grade 1 or grade 2 infusion reaction should also be premedicated with dexamethasone (or equivalent) and acetaminophen prior to each infusion. • Thoroughly flush IV with 0.9% NaCl upon infusion completion.

Reconstitution • Calculate dose, required solution volume, and number of vials needed using weight in kg. • Vials contain either 100 mg/10 mL or 500 mL/50 mL at concentration of 10 mg/mL. • Visually inspect for particulate matter. Discard if particulate matter or discoloration observed. • Using 250 mL 0.9% NaCl bag, withdraw and discard a volume equal to the total calculated volume of solution. • Slowly add required dose to diluent bag for final volume of 250 mL. Gently invert bag to mix; do not shake.

Rate of Administration • Infuse over 60 min using 0.22-micron in-line filter via dedicated line.

Storage • Refrigerate vials in original carton until time of use. • Do not freeze. • Diluted solution may be refrigerated up to 24 hrs or stored at room temperature for up to 4 hrs. • Protect from light.

⚙ IV INCOMPATIBILITIES

Do not dilute in dextrose-containing fluids or infuse concomitantly with other electrolytes or medications.

INDICATIONS/ROUTES/DOSAGE

Gastric or Gastroesophageal Junction Cancer
IV: ADULTS, ELDERLY: 8 mg/kg every 14 days, either as a single agent or in combination with PACLitaxel. Continue until disease progression or unacceptable toxicity.

NSCLC
IV: ADULTS, ELDERLY: 10 mg/kg on day 1 of a 21-day cycle in combination with DOCEtaxel. Continue until disease progression or unacceptable toxicity.

Colorectal Cancer
IV: ADULTS, ELDERLY: 8 mg/kg q2wks, in combination with FOLFIRI (irinotecan, leucovorin, 5-fluorouracil). Continue until disease progression or unacceptable toxicity.

Dose Modification
Based on Common Terminology Criteria for Adverse Events (CTCAE).
Infusion-related reaction: Reduce infusion rate by 50% for grade 1 or grade 2 reaction. Permanently discontinue for grade 3 or grade 4 reaction.
Severe hypertension: Interrupt treatment until controlled with medical management. Permanently discontinue for severe hypertension that is not controlled with antihypertensive therapy.
Proteinuria: Interrupt treatment for urine protein level greater than or equal to 2 g/24 hrs. Restart treatment at reduced dose of 6 mg/kg every 14 days once urine protein level returns to less than 2 g/24 hrs. If level greater than or equal 2 g/24 hrs reoccurs, interrupt treatment and reduce dose to 5 mg/kg every 14 days once level returns to less

R

than 2 g/24 hrs. Permanently discontinue for urine protein level greater than 3 g/24 hrs or in the setting of nephrotic syndrome.

Wound healing complications: Interrupt treatment prior to scheduled surgery until wound is fully healed.

Arterial thromboembolic events, GI perforation, or grade 3 or grade 4 bleeding: Permanently discontinue.

Dosage in Renal Impairment
No dose adjustment.

Dosage in Hepatic Impairment
Mild to moderate impairment: No dose adjustment. **Severe impairment:** Use caution.

SIDE EFFECTS

Occasional (16%–9%): Hypertension, diarrhea, headache.
Ramucirumab plus PACLitaxel: Frequent (57%–20%): Fatigue, diarrhea, peripheral edema, hypertension, stomatitis.

ADVERSE EFFECTS/TOXIC REACTIONS

Severe, and sometimes fatal, hemorrhagic events including GI bleeding occurred in 3.4% of pts receiving single agent and in 4.3% of pts receiving combo therapy. GI perforations occurred in 0.7% of pts receiving single agent and in 1.2% of pts receiving combo therapy. Thromboembolic events including arterial thromboembolism, CVA, MI reported in 1.7% of pts. Severe hypertension occurred in 8% of pts receiving single agent and in 15% of pts receiving combo therapy despite medical management. Severe infusion-related reactions such as back pain/spasms, bronchospasm, chest pain, chills, dyspnea, flushing, hypotension, hypoxia, paresthesia, rigors/tremors, supraventricular tachycardia, wheezing occurred in 16% of pts. May cause ineffective wound healing or wound dehiscence requiring medical intervention. Reversible posterior leukoencephalopathy syndrome (RPLS) reported in less than 1% of pts. Proteinuria may indicate nephrotic

syndrome. Clinical deterioration of hepatic cirrhosis, manifested by new-onset or worsening encephalopathy, ascites, or hepatorenal syndrome, was reported in pts receiving single agent. Other adverse reactions include epistaxis, intestinal obstruction, neutropenia, severe rash, thrombocytopenia. Immunogenicity (anti-ramucirumab antibodies) occurred in 6% of pts.

NURSING CONSIDERATIONS

BASELINE ASSESSMENT

Obtain CBC, BMP, urinalysis, urine protein, vital signs. Assess skin for open wounds. Question possibility of pregnancy, current breastfeeding status. Receive full medication history including vitamins, herbal products. Question history of CVA, hepatic impairment/cirrhosis, hypertension, MI, prior hypersensitivity reaction. Offer emotional support.

INTERVENTION/EVALUATION

Monitor CBC, electrolytes, urinalysis, urine protein. Routinely assess vital signs and report hypertension. Persistent diastolic hypertension may indicate hypertensive emergency. Obtain EKG for arrhythmia, chest pain, palpitation. Consider RPLS in pts with altered mental status, confusion, headache, seizure, visual disturbances. Encourage PO intake. Screen for GI bleeding, GI perforation. Notify physician if any CTCAE toxicities occur (see Appendix M). Monitor for hypersensitivity reaction. Once infusion is completed, IV access must be flushed with NS.

PATIENT/FAMILY TEACHING

• Blood levels will be routinely monitored. • Treatment may cause severe allergic reaction or infusion-related reaction. • Avoid pregnancy; treatment may cause birth defects or miscarriage. Do not breastfeed. Contraception should be taken during treatment and up to 3 mos after discontinuation. • Neurologic changes, including altered mental status, headache, seizures, trouble speaking, may indicate high blood pressure crisis or life-threatening brain

R

swelling. • Immediately report abdominal pain, GI bleeding, vomiting blood. • Therapy may cause severe blood-clotting events such as heart attack or stroke.

raNITIdine

ra-**nit**-i-deen
(Apo-RaNITIdine ✹, Deprizine FusePaq, Zantac, Zantac-75, Zantac-150 Maximum Strength)
Do not confuse raNITIdine with amantadine or riMANTAdine, or Zantac with Xanax, Ziac, Zofran, or ZyrTEC.

◆CLASSIFICATION

PHARMACOTHERAPEUTIC: Histamine H_2-receptor antagonist. **CLINICAL:** Antiulcer.

USES

Short-term treatment of active duodenal ulcer. Prevention of duodenal ulcer recurrence. Treatment of active benign gastric ulcer, pathologic GI hypersecretory conditions, acute gastroesophageal reflux disease (GERD), including erosive esophagitis. Maintenance of healed erosive esophagitis. **OTC:** Relief of heartburn, acid indigestion, sour stomach. **OFF-LABEL:** Treatment of upper GI bleeding. Prevention of stress-induced ulcers in ICU. Anaphylaxis (adjunct therapy). Premedication to prevent taxane hypersensitivity.

PRECAUTIONS

Contraindications: Hypersensitivity to raNITIdine. **OTC:** Do not use if trouble or pain when swallowing food, vomiting with blood, or bloody or black stool is present. Do not use 150 mg with kidney disease (unless medically advised). **Cautions:** Renal/hepatic impairment, elderly pts, history of acute porphyria.

ACTION

Inhibits histamine action at histamine H_2-receptors of gastric parietal cells.

Therapeutic Effect: Inhibits gastric acid secretion. Reduces gastric volume, hydrogen ion concentration.

PHARMACOKINETICS

Rapidly absorbed from GI tract. Protein binding: 15%. Widely distributed. Metabolized in liver. Primarily excreted in urine. Not removed by hemodialysis. **Half-life: PO:** 2.5 hrs; **IV:** 2–2.5 hrs (increased with renal impairment).

🔲 LIFESPAN CONSIDERATIONS

Pregnancy/Lactation: Unknown if drug crosses placenta or is distributed in breast milk. **Children:** No age-related precautions noted. **Elderly:** Confusion more likely with hepatic/renal impairment.

INTERACTIONS

DRUG: Magnesium or aluminum antacids may decrease absorption. May decrease absorption of **atazanavir, itraconazole, ketoconazole. HERBAL:** None significant. **FOOD:** None known. **LAB VALUES:** Interferes with skin tests using allergen extracts. May increase serum ALT, AST, GGT, creatinine.

AVAILABILITY (Rx)

Capsules: 150 mg, 300 mg. **Injection Solution:** 25 mg/mL. **Syrup:** 15 mg/mL. **Tablets:** 75 mg, 150 mg, 300 mg.

ADMINISTRATION/HANDLING

 IV

**Reconstitution • For IV push, dilute each 50 mg with 20 mL 0.9% NaCl, D_5W. • For intermittent IV infusion (piggyback), dilute each 50 mg with 0.9% NaCl, D_5W to a maximum concentration of 0.5 mg/mL. • For IV infusion, dilute with 0.9% NaCl, D_5W to a maximum concentration of 2.5 mg/mL.
Rate of Administration • Administer IV push over minimum of 5 min (prevents arrhythmias, hypotension). • Infuse IV piggyback over 15–20 min. • Infuse IV infusion over 24 hrs.

Storage • IV solutions appear clear, colorless to yellow (slight darkening does not affect potency). • IV infusion (piggyback) is stable for 48 hrs at room temperature (discard if discolored or precipitate forms).

IM

• May be given undiluted. • Give deep IM into large muscle mass.

PO

• Give without regard to meals (best given with meals or at bedtime). • Do not administer within 1 hr of magnesium- or aluminum-containing antacids (decreases absorption).

▨ IV INCOMPATIBILITIES

Amphotericin B complex (Abelcet, AmBisome, Amphotec).

▨ IV COMPATIBILITIES

Dexmedetomidine (Precedex), diltiaZEM (Cardizem), DOBUTamine (Dobutrex), DOPamine (Intropin), heparin, HYDROmorphone (Dilaudid), insulin, lidocaine, LORazepam (Ativan), morphine, norepinephrine (Levophed), potassium chloride, propofol (Diprivan).

INDICATIONS/ROUTES/DOSAGE

Duodenal Ulcer

PO: ADULTS, ELDERLY: Treatment: 150 mg twice daily or 300 mg once daily. **Maintenance:** 150 mg once daily at bedtime. **CHILDREN 1 MO TO 16 YRS: Treatment:** 4–8 mg/kg/day in 2 divided doses. **Maximum:** 300 mg. **Maintenance:** 2–4 mg/kg/day once daily. **Maximum:** 150 mg/day.

Gastric Ulcer (Benign)

PO: ADULTS, ELDERLY: Treatment: 150mg 2 times/day. **Maintenance:** 150 mg once daily at bedtime. **CHILDREN 1 MO–16 YRS: Treatment:** 4–8 mg/kg/day in 2 divided doses. **Maximum:** 300 mg/day. **Maintenance:** 2–4 mg/kg/day once daily. **Maximum (healing):** 150 mg/day.

Hypersecretory Conditions

PO: ADULTS, ELDERLY: 150 mg twice daily up to 6 g/day. **IV Infusion:** 6.25 mg/hr.

GERD

PO: ADULTS, ELDERLY: 150 mg twice daily. **CHILDREN 1 MO TO 16 YRS:** 5–10 mg/kg/day in 2 divided doses. **Maximum:** 300 mg/day.

Erosive Esophagitis

PO: ADULTS, ELDERLY: Treatment: 150 mg 4 times/day. **Maintenance:** 150 mg twice daily. **CHILDREN 1 MO TO 16 YRS: Treatment:** 5–10 mg/kg/day in 2 divided doses. **Maximum:** 600 mg/day.

Prevention of Heartburn (OTC)

PO: ADULTS, ELDERLY, CHILDREN 12 YRS AND OLDER: 75–150 mg 30–60 min before eating or drinking beverages that cause heartburn. **Maximum:** 2 doses/day. Do not use more than 14 days.

Usual Parenteral Dosage

IV: ADULTS, ELDERLY: 50 mg q6–8h. **CHILDREN:** 2–4 mg/kg/day in divided doses q6–8h. **Maximum:** 50 mg/dose. **IV Infusion:** 6.25 mg/hr.

Usual Neonatal Dosage

PO: NEONATES: 2 mg/kg/dose q8h.
IV: NEONATES: Initially, 1.5 mg/kg/dose, then 1.5–2 mg/kg/day in divided doses q8h.
IV Infusion: NEONATES: Loading dose: 1.5 mg/kg, then 1–2 mg/kg/day (0.04–0.08 mg/kg/hr).

Dosage in Renal Impairment

CrCl less than 50 mL/min: Give 150 mg PO q24h or 50 mg IV q18–24h.

Dosage in Hepatic Impairment

No dose adjustment.

SIDE EFFECTS

Occasional (2%): Diarrhea. **Rare (1%):** Constipation, headache (may be severe).

ADVERSE EFFECTS/TOXIC REACTIONS

Reversible hepatitis, blood dyscrasias occur rarely.

NURSING CONSIDERATIONS

BASELINE ASSESSMENT

Obtain history of epigastric/abdominal pain.

INTERVENTION/EVALUATION

Assess mental status in elderly. Question present abdominal pain, GI distress.

PATIENT/FAMILY TEACHING

• Smoking decreases effectiveness of medication. • Do not take medicine within 1 hr of magnesium- or aluminum-containing antacids. • Transient burning/pruritus may occur with IV administration. • Report headache. • Avoid alcohol, aspirin.

---

ranolazine

ra-**noe**-la-zeen
(Ranexa)
Do not confuse Ranexa with CeleXA.

✦CLASSIFICATION

PHARMACOTHERAPEUTIC: Sodium current inhibitor. **CLINICAL:** Antianginal, anti-ischemic.

USES

Treatment of chronic angina.

PRECAUTIONS

Contraindications: Hypersensitivity to ranolazine. Hepatic cirrhosis, concurrent use of strong CYP3A inhibitors (e.g., rifAMPin, carBAMazepine) or CYP3A inducers (e.g., ketoconazole, itraconazole, fluconazole, clarithromycin, erythromycin). **Cautions:** Renal/hepatic impairment. Preexisting QT prolongation, concurrent use with medications known to prolong QT interval, pts 75 yrs of age or older, hypokalemia, hypomagnesemia.

ACTION

Inhibits inward current of sodium channel during cardiac repolarization, thereby reducing calcium influx. Decreased influx of calcium reduces ventricular tension, myocardial oxygen demand. Does not reduce heart rate, B/P. **Therapeutic Effect:** Exerts antianginal, anti-ischemic effects on cardiac tissue.

PHARMACOKINETICS

Absorption highly variable. Peak plasma concentration: 2–5 hrs. Rapidly, extensively metabolized in intestine, liver. Protein binding: 62%. Excreted in urine (75%), feces (25%). **Half-life:** 7 hrs.

⏳ LIFESPAN CONSIDERATIONS

Pregnancy/Lactation: Unknown if drug crosses placenta or is distributed in breast milk. **Children:** Safety and efficacy not established. **Elderly:** No age-related precautions noted.

INTERACTIONS

DRUG: See contraindications. **DiltiaZEM, verapamil** may increase serum concentration. May increase concentration of **cycloSPORINE, digoxin, simvastatin, sirolimus, tacrolimus. Antiarrhythmic agents, dofetilide, quiNIDine, sotalol, thioridazine, ziprasidone** may increase risk of QT prolongation. **HERBAL: St. John's wort** may decrease concentration/effects. **FOOD: Grapefruit products** may increase plasma concentration, risk of QT prolongation. **LAB VALUES:** May slightly elevate serum BUN, creatinine.

AVAILABILITY (Rx)

Tablets (Extended-Release): 500 mg, 1,000 mg.

ADMINISTRATION/HANDLING

PO
• May give without regard to food.
• Do not break, crush, dissolve, or divide extended-release tablets.

R

INDICATIONS/ROUTES/DOSAGE

Chronic Angina
PO: ADULTS, ELDERLY: Initially, 500 mg twice daily. May increase to 1,000 mg twice daily, based on clinical response. Dose should not exceed 500 mg twice daily when used concurrently with moderate CYP3A inhibitors (e.g., diltiaZEM, verapamil).

Dosage in Renal/Hepatic Impairment
No dose adjustment (discontinue if acute renal failure develops). Contraindicated in pts with cirrhosis.

SIDE EFFECTS

Occasional (6%–4%): Dizziness, headache, constipation, nausea. **Rare (2%–1%):** Peripheral edema, abdominal pain, dry mouth, vomiting, tinnitus, vertigo, palpitations.

ADVERSE EFFECTS/TOXIC REACTIONS

Overdose manifested as confusion, diplopia, dizziness, paresthesia, syncope.

NURSING CONSIDERATIONS

BASELINE ASSESSMENT

Receive full medication history and screen for contraindications. Question history of hepatic impairment, long QT syndrome. Record onset, type (sharp, dull, squeezing), radiation, location, intensity, duration of anginal pain, precipitating factors (exertion, emotional stress). Obtain baseline EKG.

INTERVENTION/EVALUATION

Assist with ambulation if dizziness occurs. Give with food if nausea occurs. Assess for relief of anginal pain. Monitor EKG, pulse for irregularities.

PATIENT/FAMILY TEACHING

• Avoid grapefruit products. • Do not chew, crush, dissolve, or divide extended-release tablets. • Avoid tasks requiring alertness, motor skills until response to drug is established.

rasagiline

ra-**sa**-ji-leen
(Azilect, Apo-Rasagiline ✦)
Do not confuse Azilect with Aricept.

◆CLASSIFICATION

PHARMACOTHERAPEUTIC: MAOI.
CLINICAL: Antiparkinson agent.

USES

Treatment of signs/symptoms of Parkinson's disease as initial monotherapy or as adjunct therapy with or without levodopa.

PRECAUTIONS

Contraindications: Hypersensitivity to rasagiline. Concurrent use with methadone, traMADol, meperidine, MAOIs within 14 days of rasagiline, cyclobenzaprine, dextromethorphan, or St. John's wort. **Cautions:** Hepatic impairment (avoid use in moderate to severe impairment); cardiovascular, cerebrovascular disease, pts with hypotension. Avoid foods high in tyramine. Do not use within 5 wks of stopping FLUoxetine; do not start tricyclic, SSRI, or SNRI within 2 wks of stopping rasagiline. History of major psychotic disorder.

ACTION

Inhibits monoamine oxidase type B, an enzyme that plays a major role in catabolism of DOPamine. Inhibition of DOPamine depletion reduces symptomatic motor deficits of Parkinson's disease. **Therapeutic Effect:** Reduces symptoms of Parkinson's disease, appears to delay disease progression.

PHARMACOKINETICS

Rapidly absorbed following PO administration. Protein binding: 88%–94%. Metabolized in liver. Excreted in urine (62%), feces (7%). **Half-life:** 1.3–3 hrs.

R

⧗ LIFESPAN CONSIDERATIONS

Pregnancy/Lactation: Unknown if distributed in breast milk. **Children:** Safety and efficacy not established. **Elderly:** No age-related precautions noted.

INTERACTIONS

DRUG: Amphetamines, other MAOIs (e.g., **phenelzine, selegiline**), **sympathomimetics** (e.g., **DOPamine, phenylephrine, pseudoephedrine**) may cause hypertensive crisis. **Anorexiants** (e.g., **dexfenfluramine, fenfluramine, sibutramine**), **CNS stimulants** (e.g., **methylphenidate**), **cyclobenzaprine, dextromethorphan, meperidine, methadone, mirtazapine, serotonin or norepinephrine reuptake inhibitors** (e.g., **citalopram, sertraline, venlafaxine**), **sibutramine, traMADol, traZODone, tricyclic antidepressants** (e.g., **amitriptyline, doxepin**), **venlafaxine** may cause serotonin syndrome. May increase risk of **atomoxetine, buPROPion** toxicity. **Ciprofloxacin, entacapone, tolcapone** may increase concentration (reduced dosage recommended). **Levodopa** may cause hypertensive/hypotensive reaction. **HERBAL: Kava kava, SAMe, St. John's wort, valerian** may increase risk of serotonin syndrome, excessive sedation. **FOOD: Caffeine, foods/ beverages containing tyramine** may result in hypertensive reaction, hypertensive crisis. **LAB VALUES:** May increase serum alkaline phosphatase, bilirubin, ALT, AST. May cause leukopenia.

AVAILABILITY (Rx)

Tablets: 0.5 mg, 1 mg.

ADMINISTRATION/HANDLING

PO
• Give without regard to food. • Avoid food, beverages containing tyramine (e.g., cheese, sour cream, yogurt, pickled herring, liver, figs, raisins, bananas, avocados, soy sauce, broad beans, yeast extracts, meat tenderizers, red wine, beer), excessive amounts of caffeine (e.g., coffee, tea).

INDICATIONS/ROUTES/DOSAGE

◀ **ALERT** ▶ When used in combination with levodopa, dosage reduction of levodopa should be considered.

Parkinson's Disease
PO: ADULTS, ELDERLY, MONOTHERAPY, ADJUNCTIVE THERAPY WITHOUT LEVODOPA: 1 mg once daily.
PO: ADULTS, ELDERLY, ADJUNCTIVE THERAPY WITH LEVODOPA: Initially, 0.5 mg once daily. If therapeutic response is not achieved, dose may be increased to 1 mg once daily. **ADJUNCTIVE THERAPY WITHOUT LEVODOPA:** 1 mg once daily.

Dose Modification
Concomitant use of CYP1A2 inhibitors, ciprofloxacin: 0.5 mg once daily.

Dosage in Hepatic Impairment
Mild impairment: 0.5 mg once daily. **Moderate to severe impairment:** Not recommended.

Dosage in Renal Impairment
No dose adjustment.

SIDE EFFECTS

Frequent (14%–12%): Headache, nausea. **Occasional (9%–5%):** Orthostatic hypotension, weight loss, dyspepsia, dry mouth, arthralgia, depression, hallucinations, constipation. **Rare (4%–2%):** Fever, vertigo, ecchymosis, rhinitis, neck pain, arthritis, paresthesia.

ADVERSE EFFECTS/TOXIC REACTIONS

Increase in dyskinesia (impaired voluntary movement), dystonia (impaired muscular tone) occurs in 18% of pts, angina occurs in 9%. Gastroenteritis, conjunctivitis occur rarely (3% of pts).

NURSING CONSIDERATIONS

BASELINE ASSESSMENT
Obtain baseline LFT, blood pressure. Receive full medication history and screen for interactions. Question history of severe hepatic impairment, cardiovascular disease.

R

INTERVENTION/EVALUATION

Give with food if nausea occurs. Monitor B/P. Instruct pt to slowly go from lying to standing to prevent orthostatic hypotension. Assess for clinical reversal of symptoms (improvement of tremor of head/hands at rest, mask-like facial expression, shuffling gait, muscular rigidity). If hallucinations or dyskinesia occurs, symptoms may be eliminated if levodopa dosage is reduced. Hallucinations generally are accompanied by confusion and, to a lesser extent, insomnia.

PATIENT/FAMILY TEACHING

• Orthostatic hypotension may occur more frequently during initial therapy. • Avoid tasks that require alertness, motor skills until response to drug is established. • Hallucinations may occur (more so in the elderly with Parkinson's disease), typically within first 2 wks of therapy. • Avoid foods that contain tyramine (cheese, sour cream, beer, wine, pickled herring, liver, figs, raisins, bananas, avocados, soy sauce, yeast extracts, yogurt, papaya, broad beans, meat tenderizers), excessive amounts of caffeine (coffee, tea, chocolate), OTC preparations for hay fever, colds, weight reduction (may produce significant rise in B/P). • Do not take any newly prescribed medications unless approved by prescriber who originally started therapy.

rasburicase

ras-**bure**-i-kase
(Elitek, Fasturtec ✦)

■ **BLACK BOX ALERT** ■ Severe hypersensitivity reactions including anaphylaxis reported. May cause severe hemolysis in pts with glucose-6-phosphate dehydrogenase (G6PD) deficiency. Screen pts at high risk for G6PD (African or Mediterranean descent) prior to therapy. Methemoglobinemia has been reported. Blood samples left at room temperature may interfere with uric acid measurements. Must collect blood samples in prechilled tubes containing heparin and immediately immerse in ice water bath. Assay plasma samples within 4 hrs of collection. Elitek enzymatically degrades uric acid in blood samples left at room temperature.

◆CLASSIFICATION

PHARMACOTHERAPEUTIC: Urate-oxidase inhibitor. **CLINICAL:** Antihyperuricemic.

USES

Initial management of uric acid levels in pts with leukemia, lymphoma, and solid tumor malignancies who are receiving chemotherapy expected to result in tumor lysis and subsequent elevation of plasma uric acid.

PRECAUTIONS

Contraindications: History of anaphylaxis or severe hypersensitivity to rasburicase. Prior drug reaction including hypersensitivity reactions, hemolysis, methemoglobinemia; G6PD deficiency. **Cautions:** Pts at high risk for G6PD deficiency (e.g., African, Mediterranean, or Southeast Asian descent).

ACTION

Catalyzes enzymatic oxidation of poorly soluble uric acid into soluble, inactive metabolites by converting uric acid into allantoin. Does not inhibit formation of uric acid. **Therapeutic Effect:** Decreases uric acid levels.

PHARMACOKINETICS

Half-life: 16–23 hrs.

⧗ LIFESPAN CONSIDERATIONS

Pregnancy/Lactation: Unknown if distributed in breast milk. Unknown if crosses placenta. May cause fetal harm. **Children/Elderly:** No age-related precautions noted.

R

INTERACTIONS

DRUG: None significant. **HERBAL:** None significant. **FOOD:** None known. **LAB VALUES:** May increase serum bilirubin, ALT. May decrease serum phosphate.

AVAILABILITY (Rx)

Injection, Powder for Reconstitution: 1.5 mg/vial, 7.5 mg/vial.

ADMINISTRATION/HANDLING

 IV

Reconstitution • Must use diluent provided in carton. • Reconstitute 1.5-mg vial with 1 mL of diluent or 7.5-mg vial with 5 mL of diluent to provide concentration of 1.5 mg/mL. • Gently swirl to mix. Do not shake. • Inspect for particulate matter or discoloration. • Inject calculated dose into appropriate volume of 0.9% NaCl to achieve a final volume of 50 mL.
Rate of Administration • Infuse over 30 min. • Do not use filter during reconstitution or infusion.
Storage • Refrigerate solution until time of use. • Discard after 24 hrs following reconstitution.

IV INCOMPATIBILITIES

Do not mix with other IV medications.

INDICATIONS/ROUTES/DOSAGE

Note: Indicated only for a single course of treatment.

Management of Hyperuricemia
IV: ADULTS, ELDERLY, CHILDREN: 0.2 mg/kg once daily up to 5 days.

Dosage in Renal/Hepatic Impairment
No dose adjustment.

SIDE EFFECTS

Frequent (50%–46%): Vomiting, fever. **Occasional (27%–13%):** Nausea, headache, abdominal pain, constipation, diarrhea, mucositis, rash.

ADVERSE EFFECTS/TOXIC REACTIONS

Hypersensitivity reactions occurred in 4.3% of pts including injection irritation, peripheral edema, urticaria, pruritus. Anaphylaxis, hemolysis, methemoglobinemia occurred in less than 1%. Pulmonary hemorrhage, respiratory failure, supraventricular arrhythmias, ischemic coronary artery disorders, sepsis, abdominal, gastrointestinal infections occurred in greater than 2% of pts. Clinical tumor lysis syndrome (TLS), manifested by hyperuricemia, hyperkalemia, hyperphosphatemia, seizure, increased serum creatinine, renal failure reported in 3% of pts. Antirasburicase antibodies reported.

NURSING CONSIDERATIONS

BASELINE ASSESSMENT

Obtain CBC, BMP, LFT, serum phosphate, uric acid level; urine pregnancy if applicable. Question for history of prior hypersensitivity reactions. Assess G6PD deficiency risk in potential candidates.

INTERVENTION/EVALUATION

Offer antiemetics to control nausea, vomiting. Monitor CBC, BMP, LFT, serum phosphate. If hypersensitivity reaction occurs, stop infusion and immediately notify physician. Screen for clinical tumor lysis syndrome, hemolysis, methemoglobinemia. Follow strict procedure when collecting uric acid levels. Obtain EKG for chest pain/tightness, hyperkalemia, dyspnea. Assess skin for rash.

PATIENT/FAMILY TEACHING

• Report any allergic reaction, bronchospasm, chest pain or tightness, cough, difficulty breathing, dizziness, fainting, rash, or itching.

---

regorafenib

re-goe-**raf**-e-nib
(Stivarga)

■ **BLACK BOX ALERT** ■ Severe, sometimes fatal, hepatotoxicity reported. Monitor hepatic function prior to and during treatment. Interrupt, reduce, or discontinue therapy if hepatotoxicity or hepatocellular necrosis occurs.

R

◆CLASSIFICATION

PHARMACOTHERAPEUTIC: Multikinase inhibitor. **CLINICAL:** Antineoplastic.

USES

Treatment of metastatic colorectal cancer in pts who have been previously treated with fluoropyrimidine/oxaliplatin/irinotecan-based chemotherapy, anti-VEGF or anti-EGFR therapy. Locally advanced, unresectable or metastatic GI stromal tumor previously treated with imatinib and SUNItinib. Treatment of hepatocellular carcinoma (HCC) previously treated with sorafenib.

PRECAUTIONS

Contraindications: Hypersensitivity to regorafenib. **Cautions:** Mild to moderate hepatic impairment (not recommended with severe hepatic impairment), hypertension (not recommended with severe or uncontrolled hypertension), recent surgical/dental procedures, chronic open wounds/ulcers, hemoptysis, concomitant warfarin therapy, cardiovascular disease, recent MI.

ACTION

Inhibits tyrosine kinase activity involved with tumor angiogenesis, oncogenesis, and maintenance of tumor microenvironment. **Therapeutic Effect:** Inhibits colorectal tumor cell growth and metastasis.

PHARMACOKINETICS

Readily absorbed following PO administration. Metabolized in liver. Protein binding: 99.5%. Peak plasma concentration: 4 hrs. Excreted in feces (71%), urine (19%). **Half-life:** 28 hrs (Range: 14–58 hrs).

⌛ LIFESPAN CONSIDERATIONS

Pregnancy/Lactation: May cause fetal harm. Not recommended in nursing mothers. Unknown if distributed in breast milk. Contraception recommended during treatment and up to 2 mos after discontinuation of therapy. **Children:** Safety and efficacy not established in pts younger than 18 yrs. **Elderly:** No age-related precautions noted.

INTERACTIONS

DRUG: Strong CYP3A4 inducers (e.g., **carBAMazepine, phenytoin**) may decrease concentration/effects. Strong **CYP3A4 inhibitors** (e.g., **clarithromycin, ketoconazole**) may increase concentration/effects. **HERBAL: St. John's wort** may decrease concentration/effects. **FOOD: Grapefruit products** may increase concentration/effects. **High-fat meal** may increase absorption/concentration. **LAB VALUES:** May decrease lymphocytes, neutrophils, platelets, serum calcium, phosphorus, potassium, sodium. May increase serum bilirubin, ALT, AST, lipase, amylase, INR, urine protein.

AVAILABILITY (Rx)

💊 **Tablets:** 40 mg.

ADMINISTRATION/HANDLING

PO
• Take at same time each day with low-fat (less than 30%) breakfast. • Give whole; do not break, crush, dissolve, or divide tablet.

INDICATIONS/ROUTES/DOSAGE

Metastatic Colorectal Cancer, GI Stromal Tumor, Hepatocellular carcinoma
PO: ADULTS/ELDERLY: 160 mg once daily for first 21 days of each 28-day cycle. Continue until disease progression or unacceptable toxicity.

Dosage Modification
Symptomatic Hypertension, Toxic Skin Reactions, Severe Side Effects (Grades 3–4)
PO: ADULTS/ELDERLY: Reduce dose to 120 mg once daily. If recovery does not occur within 7 days (despite dose reduction), interrupt treatment for minimum of 7 days and reassess. If recovery does not occur after interruption, reduce dose to 80 mg once daily; Discontinue for any of the following: intolerance of 80-mg dose; serum ALT or AST greater than 20 times upper limit of normal (ULN); serum ALT/AST greater than 3 times ULN and bilirubin

greater than 2 times ULN; recurrent serum ALT/AST greater than 5 times ULN despite dose of 120 mg; recovery failure of grade 3 or 4 side effects, toxic skin reaction.

Dosage in Renal Impairment
No dose adjustment.

Dosage in Hepatic Impairment
Mild to moderate impairment: No dose adjustment. **Severe impairment:** Not recommended.

SIDE EFFECTS

Frequent (64%–26%): Asthenia/fatigue, anorexia, diarrhea, mucositis, weight loss, hypertension, dysphonia, generalized pain, fever, rash. **Occasional (10%–5%):** Headache, alopecia, dysgeusia, musculoskeletal stiffness, dry mouth. **Rare (2% or Less):** Tremor, gastric reflux.

ADVERSE EFFECTS/ TOXIC REACTIONS

May cause GI perforation, GI fistula formation. Hemorrhaging of respiratory, GI, genitourinary tracts reported in 21% of pts. Hypertension (30% of pts) may lead to hypertensive crisis. May cause ineffective wound healing or wound dehiscence requiring medical intervention. Palmar-plantar erythrodysesthesia syndrome (PPES), a chemotherapy-induced skin condition that presents with redness, swelling, numbness, skin sloughing of hands, feet (45% of pts). Reversible posterior leukoencephalopathy syndrome (RPLS) reported in less than 1% of pts. May induce cardiac ischemia and/or MI. Severe, sometimes fatal, hepatotoxicity including hepatocellular necrosis reported in less than 1%. Various, unspecified infections reported in 31% of pts (most likely due to neutropenia).

NURSING CONSIDERATIONS

BASELINE ASSESSMENT

Obtain baseline vital signs, CBC with differential, serum magnesium, phosphate, ionized calcium, urinalysis, urine pregnancy, urine protein, LFT, amylase, lipase, PT/INR. Assess recent surgical/dental procedures. Question possibility of pregnancy, current breastfeeding status. Obtain full medication history including herbal products. Question for history of hypertension, hepatic impairment, cardiovascular disease. Assess skin for open/unhealed wounds. Offer emotional support.

INTERVENTION/EVALUATION

Monitor B/P, CBC, electrolytes, urinalysis. Monitor LFT q2wks for 2 mos, then monthly; or every wk if elevated. Persistent diastolic hypertension may indicate hypertensive emergency. Obtain EKG for palpitation, chest pain, hypokalemia, hyperkalemia, hypocalcemia, bradycardia, ventricular arrhythmias. Reverse posterior leukoencephalopathy syndrome (RPLS) should be considered in pts with seizure, headache, visual disturbances, altered mental status, malignant hypertension. Assess hydration status. Encourage PO intake. Immediately report any hemorrhaging, bloody stools, hematuria, abdominal pain, hemoptysis (may indicate GI perforation/fistula formation).

PATIENT/FAMILY TEACHING

• Blood levels will be routinely monitored. • Avoid pregnancy. Contraception should be practiced during treatment and up to 2 mos after last dose. • Report any yellowing of skin or eyes, abdominal pain, bruising, black/tarry stools, dark urine, decreased urine output, skin changes. • Report neurologic changes including confusion, seizures, vision loss, high blood pressure crisis (may indicate RPLS). • Do not take herbal products. • Notify physician before any planned surgical/dental procedures. • Do not ingest grapefruit products. • Take with low-fat food only. • Drink liquids often if diarrhea occurs (may lead to dehydration). • Immediately report bleeding of any kind. • Swallow tablet whole; do not chew, crush, dissolve, or divide.

R

---

repaglinide `HIGH ALERT`

re-**pag**-li-nide
(Apo-Repaglinide ✤, GlucoNorm ✤, Prandin)
Do not confuse Prandin with Avandia.

FIXED-COMBINATION(S)

Prandimet: repaglinide/metFORMIN (an antidiabetic): 1 mg/500 mg, 2 mg/500 mg.

◆CLASSIFICATION

PHARMACOTHERAPEUTIC: Meglitinide analogue. **CLINICAL:** Antidiabetic agent.

USES

Adjunct to diet and exercise to lower serum glucose in pts with type 2 diabetes. Used as monotherapy or in combination with metFORMIN, pioglitazone, rosiglitazone.

PRECAUTIONS

Contraindications: Hypersensitivity to repaglinide. Diabetic ketoacidosis (with or without coma), type 1 diabetes, concurrent gemfibrozil therapy. **Cautions:** Hepatic/renal impairment, elderly pts, malnourished pts, adrenal/pituitary dysfunction.

ACTION

Stimulates release of insulin from beta cells of pancreas by depolarizing beta cells, leading to opening of calcium channels. Resulting calcium influx induces insulin secretion. **Therapeutic Effect:** Lowers serum glucose concentration.

PHARMACOKINETICS

Rapidly, completely absorbed from GI tract. Protein binding: 98%. Metabolized in liver. Excreted in feces (90%), urine (8%). Unknown if removed by hemodialysis. **Half-life:** 1 hr.

⚠ LIFESPAN CONSIDERATIONS

Pregnancy/Lactation: Unknown if drug is distributed in breast milk. **Children:** Safety and efficacy not established. **Elderly:** No age-related precautions noted, but hypoglycemia may be more difficult to recognize.

INTERACTIONS

DRUG: CYP3A4 inhibitors (e.g., ketoconazole, erythromycin), CYP2C8 inhibitors (e.g., gemfibrozil) may increase concentration/toxicity. **CYP3A4 inducers (e.g., carBAMazepine, rifAMPin)** may decrease effects. **Beta blockers (e.g., carvedilol, metoprolol), NSAIDs (e.g., ibuprofen, ketorolac, naproxen)** may increase hypoglycemic effect. **HERBAL: St. John's wort** may decrease concentration. **Garlic, ginger, ginseng** may cause hypoglycemia. **FOOD: Food** decreases concentration. **LAB VALUES:** Serum alkaline phosphatase, ALT, AST may be elevated.

AVAILABILITY (Rx)

Tablets: 0.5 mg, 1 mg, 2 mg.

ADMINISTRATION/HANDLING

PO
• Ideally, give within 15 min of a meal but may be given immediately before a meal to as long as 30 min before a meal.

INDICATIONS/ROUTES/DOSAGE

Diabetes Mellitus
PO: ADULTS, ELDERLY: (Pts not previously treated or whose Hgb A1c is less than 8%): 0.5 mg before each meal. **(Pts previously treated whose Hgb A1c is greater than 8%):** 1–2 mg before each meal. May adjust dose by at least 1-wk intervals. **Range:** 0.5–4 mg 2–4 times/day. **Maximum:** 16 mg/day.

Dosage in Renal Impairment
CrCl 20–40 mL/min: Initially, 0.5 mg with meals, titrate carefully.

Dosage in Hepatic Impairment
Use caution.

R

SIDE EFFECTS

Frequent (10%–6%): Upper respiratory tract infection, headache, rhinitis, bronchitis, back pain. **Occasional (5%–3%):** Diarrhea, dyspepsia, sinusitis, nausea, arthralgia, UTI. **Rare (2%):** Constipation, vomiting, paresthesia, allergy.

ADVERSE EFFECTS/ TOXIC REACTIONS

Hypoglycemia occurs in 16% of pts. Chest pain occurs rarely.

NURSING CONSIDERATIONS

BASELINE ASSESSMENT

Check fasting serum glucose, glycosylated Hgb A1c levels periodically to determine minimum effective dose.

INTERVENTION/EVALUATION

Monitor fasting serum glucose, glycosylated Hgb A1c levels, food intake. Assess for hypoglycemia (cool/wet skin, tremors, dizziness, anxiety, headache, tachycardia, numbness in mouth, hunger, diplopia), hyperglycemia (polyuria, polyphagia, polydipsia, nausea, vomiting, dim vision, fatigue, deep or rapid breathing). Be alert to conditions that alter glucose requirements (fever, increased activity/stress, surgical procedures). Ensure follow-up instruction if pt, family do not thoroughly understand diabetes management, glucose-testing technique. At least 1 wk should elapse to assess response to drug before new dosage adjustment is made.

PATIENT/FAMILY TEACHING

• Diabetes requires lifelong control. • Prescribed diet, exercise are principal parts of treatment; do not skip, delay meals. • Continue to adhere to dietary instructions, regular exercise program, regular testing of urine or serum glucose. • When taking combination drug therapy with a sulfonylurea or insulin, have source of glucose available to treat symptoms of low blood sugar.

reslizumab

res-li-**zoo**-mab
(Cinqair)

Do not confuse reslizumab with certolizumab, daclizumab, eculizumab, efalizumab, mepolizumab, natalizumab, omalizumab, pembrolizumab, tocilizumab, or vedolizumab, or Cinqair with Cinryze, Cinolar, Cinobac, Sinemet, Singulair, or SINEquan.

◆CLASSIFICATION

PHARMACOTHERAPEUTIC: Interleukin-5 receptor antagonist. Monoclonal antibody. **CLINICAL:** Antiasthmatic.

USES

Add-on maintenance treatment of pts with severe asthma, aged 18 yrs and older, and with an eosinophil phenotype.

PRECAUTIONS

Contraindications: Hypersensitivity to reslizumab. **Cautions:** History of helminth (parasite) infection; long-term use of corticosteroids. Not indicated for treatment of other eosinophilic conditions; relief of acute bronchospasm, status asthmaticus, exercise-induced bronchospasm. History of anaphylaxis.

ACTION

Exact mechanism unknown. Inhibits signaling of interleukin-5 cytokine, reducing production and survival of eosinophils responsible for asthmatic inflammation and pathogenesis. **Therapeutic Effect:** Prevents inflammatory process. Decreases number of asthma exacerbations.

PHARMACOKINETICS

Widely distributed. Degraded into small peptides and amino acids via proteolytic enzymes. Peak plasma concentration: reached by end of infusion. Excretion not specified. **Half-life:** 24 days.

R

◆ Canadian trade name   🦺 Non-Crushable Drug   🔲 High Alert drug

⧖ LIFESPAN CONSIDERATIONS

Pregnancy/Lactation: Unknown if distributed in breast milk. However, human immunoglobulin G (IgG) is present in breast milk and is known to cross placenta. **Children:** Safety and efficacy not established in pts younger than 18 yrs. **Elderly:** No age-related precautions noted.

INTERACTIONS

DRUG: None known. **HERBAL:** None significant. **FOOD:** None known. **LAB VALUES:** May increase creatine phosphokinase (CPK).

AVAILABILITY (Rx)

Injection Solution: 100 mg/10 mL (10 mg/mL).

ADMINISTRATION/HANDLING

 IV

Preparation • Allow vial to warm to room temperature. • Visually inspect for particulate matter or discoloration. Solution should appear clear to slightly opalescent, colorless to pale yellow. • Proteinaceous particles may be present. • Air bubbles are expected and allowed. • Do not use if solution is cloudy or discolored or if foreign particles are observed. • Do not shake. • Withdraw proper dose volume from vial and dilute in 50 mL 0.9% NaCl bag. • Gently invert to mix. Do not shake (may cause foaming/precipitate formation). • Infuse via dedicated line. • After infusion is complete, flush IV line with 0.9% NaCl.
Rate of Administration • Infuse over 20–50 mins (depending on total volume of infusion), using an in-line, low protein-binding filter (pore size: 0.2 micron).
Storage • Refrigerate unused vials. • Do not freeze. • Diluted solution may be refrigerated or stored at room temperature for up to 16 hrs. • If refrigerated, allow diluted solution to warm to room temperature before use. • Protect from light.

⧖ IV INCOMPATIBILITIES

Do not mix or infuse with other medications.

INDICATIONS/ROUTES/DOSAGE

Asthma (Severe)
IV: ADULTS, ELDERLY: 3 mg/kg once q4wks.

Dosage in Renal/Hepatic Impairment
Not specified; use caution.

SIDE EFFECTS

Rare (3%–1%): Oropharyngeal pain, myalgia.

ADVERSE EFFECTS/ TOXIC REACTIONS

Life-threatening anaphylaxis reported in less than 1% of pts. Hypersensitivity reactions including bronchospasm, dyspnea, hypoxia, rash, urticaria, vomiting usually occurred during infusion or within 20 mins after completion. Less than 1% of pts reported at least one malignant neoplasm within 6 mos of initiation. Unknown if treatment will influence the immunologic response to helminth (parasite) infection. Immunogenicity (auto-reslizumab antibodies) reported in 5% of pts.

NURSING CONSIDERATIONS

BASELINE ASSESSMENT

Obtain serum CPK. Verify presence of eosinophil phenotype. Question history of hypersensitivity reaction. Therapy should be administered in a health care setting by medical professionals who are trained and prepared to readily manage anaphylaxis. Have anaphylactic medications (e.g., antihistamine, bronchodilator, corticosteroid, EPINEPHrine, H_2 receptor antagonist), intubation kit, supplemental oxygen readily available before initiation. Inhaled or systemic corticosteroids

R

should not be suddenly discontinued upon initiation. Corticosteroids that are not gradually reduced may cause withdrawal symptoms or unmask conditions that were originally suppressed with corticosteroid therapy. Pts with preexisting helminth infection should be treated prior to initiation.

INTERVENTION/EVALUATION

Obtain serum CPK in pts complaining of myalgia. Diligently observe for hypersensitivity/anaphylactic reaction during infusion and directly after completion. If anaphylaxis occurs, discontinue infusion and provide immediate resuscitation support. Early detection is vital. Assess rate, depth, rhythm of respirations, oxygen saturation for therapeutic effectiveness. Assess lungs for wheezing, rales. Obtain pulmonary function test to assess disease improvement. Interrupt or discontinue therapy if helminth infection occurs, if worsening of asthma-related symptoms occurs (esp. in pts tapering off corticosteroids). Monitor for increased use of rescue inhalers; may indicate deterioration of asthma. Monitor for primary malignancies.

PATIENT/FAMILY TEACHING

• Treatment may cause life-threatening anaphylaxis. Immediately report allergic reactions such as difficulty breathing, hives, itching, low blood pressure, rash, swelling of the face or tongue, sudden coughing, vomiting, wheezing during infusion or immediately after infusion. • Therapy not indicated for relief of acute asthma or bronchospasm. • Have a rescue inhaler readily available. • Increased use of rescue inhalers may indicate worsening of asthma. • Seek medical attention if asthma symptoms worsen or remain uncontrolled. • Do not stop corticosteroid therapy unless directed by prescriber. • Treatment may increase risk of new cancers or alter the body's immune response to parasite infections.

ribavirin

rye-ba-**vye**-rin
(Copegus, Rebetol, Ribasphere, Virazole)

■ **BLACK BOX ALERT** ■ Significant teratogenic/embryocidal effects. Hemolytic anemia is significant toxicity, usually occurring within 1–2 wks. May worsen cardiac disease and lead to fatal or nonfatal MI. Inhalation may interfere with safe and effective assisted ventilation. Monotherapy not effective for chronic hepatitis C virus infection.

Do not confuse ribavirin with riboflavin, rifAMPin, or Robaxin.

FIXED-COMBINATION(S)

With interferon alfa-2b (**Rebetron**). Individually packaged.

◆CLASSIFICATION

PHARMACOTHERAPEUTIC: Synthetic nucleoside. **CLINICAL:** Antiviral.

USES

Inhalation: Treatment of respiratory syncytial virus (RSV) infections (esp. in pts with underlying compromising conditions such as chronic lung disorders, congenital heart disease, recent transplant recipients). **Capsule/tablet/oral solution:** Treatment of chronic hepatitis C virus infection in pts with compensated hepatic disease in combination with other medications.

PRECAUTIONS

Contraindications: Hypersensitivity to ribavirin. **(Additional) Inhalation:** Women who are pregnant or may become pregnant. **Oral formulations:** Hemoglobinopathies (e.g., sickle cell anemia), men whose female partner is pregnant, women of childbearing age who are pregnant or may become pregnant. Concomitant use of didanosine. **Ribasphere, Rebetol only:** CrCl less than 50 mL/min.

R

Cautions: Inhalation: Pts requiring assisted ventilation, COPD, asthma. **PO:** Cardiac or pulmonary disease, elderly pts, history of psychiatric disorders, renal impairment, pts with sarcoidosis, pts with baseline risk of severe anemia.

ACTION

Inhibits replication of viral RNA, DNA, influenza virus RNA polymerase activity; interferes with expression of messenger RNA. **Therapeutic Effect:** Inhibits viral protein synthesis.

PHARMACOKINETICS

Readily absorbed. Peak concentrations: (Inhalation): At end of inhalation period. (Capsules): 3 hrs. (Tablets): 2 hrs. Protein binding: None. Metabolized in liver and intracellularly. Primarily excreted in urine. **Half-life:** (Inhalation): 6.5–11 hrs. (Capsules): 298 hr at steady state. (Tablets): 120–170 hrs.

⧗ LIFESPAN CONSIDERATIONS

Pregnancy/Lactation: Contraindicated in pregnancy. Females and males with females partners of reproductive potential must use 2 forms of effective contraception during treatment and for at least 6 mos after discontinuation. Unknown if excreted in breast milk. **Children/Elderly:** No age-related precautions noted.

INTERACTIONS

DRUG: Didanosine may increase risk of pancreatitis, peripheral neuropathy. May decrease effects of **didanosine. Nucleoside analogues** (e.g., **adefovir, didanosine, lamiVUDine, stavudine, zalcitabine, zidovudine**) may increase risk of lactic acidosis. **HERBAL:** None significant. **FOOD:** None known. **LAB VALUES:** None significant.

AVAILABILITY (Rx)

Capsules (Rebetol, Ribasphere): 200 mg. **Powder for Solution, Nebulization (Virazole):** 6 g. **Solution, Oral (Rebetol):** 40 mg/mL. **Tablet (Copegus):** 200 mg. **(Ribasphere):** 200 mg, 400 mg, 600 mg.

ADMINISTRATION/HANDLING

PO
• Capsules may be taken without regard to food. • Do not break, crush, or open capsules. • Use oral solution in children 5 yrs or younger, those 47 kg or less, or those unable to swallow. • Give capsules with food when combined with peginterferon alfa-2b. • Tablets should be given with food.

Inhalation
◀**ALERT**▶ May be given via nasal or oral inhalation.
• Solution appears clear, colorless; is stable for 24 hrs at room temperature. • Discard solution for nebulization after 24 hrs. • Discard if discolored or cloudy. • Add 50–100 mL Sterile Water for Injection or Inhalation to 6-g vial. • Transfer to a flask, serving as reservoir for aerosol generator. • Further dilute to final volume of 300 mL, giving solution concentration of 20 mg/mL. • Use only aerosol generator available from manufacturer of drug. • Do not give concomitantly with other drug solutions for nebulization. • Discard reservoir solution when fluid levels are low and at least q24h. • Only experienced personnel should administer drug.

INDICATIONS/ROUTES/DOSAGE

Note: Combination therapy with peginterferon alone is not recommended in HCV guidelines.

Chronic Hepatitis C Virus Infection
Rebetol, Ribasphere (Oral Capsule or Solution) (In Combination with Peginterferon alfa-2b)
PO: ADULTS, ELDERLY WEIGHING MORE THAN 105 KG: 1,400 mg daily (600 mg in morning, 800 mg in evening); **(WEIGHING 81–105 KG):** 1,200 mg daily (600 mg in morning and evening); **(WEIGHING 66–80 KG):** 1,000 mg daily (400 mg in morning, 600 mg in evening); **(WEIGHING LESS THAN 66 KG):** 800 mg daily (400 mg in morning and evening). **CHILDREN 3 YRS OR OLDER WEIGHING MORE THAN 73 KG:** 1,200 mg

R

daily (600 mg in morning and evening); **(WEIGHING 60–73 KG):** 1,000 mg daily (400 mg in morning, 600 mg in evening; **(WEIGHING 47–59 KG):** 800 mg daily (400 mg in morning and evening); **(WEIGHING LESS THAN 47 KG):** 15 mg/kg/day in 2 divided doses as oral solution.

Rebetol, Ribasphere (Oral Capsule/ Solution) (in Combination with Interferon alfa-2b)
PO: ADULTS, ELDERLY WEIGHING MORE THAN 75 KG: 1,200 mg daily (600 mg in morning and evening); **(WEIGHING 75 KG OR LESS):** 1,000 mg daily (400 mg in morning, 600 mg in evening).

Copegus, Ribasphere (Oral Tablet) (in Combination with Peginterferon alfa-2b)
PO: ADULTS, ELDERLY: Genotype 1, 4 (weighing more than 75 kg): 1,200 mg daily (600 mg in morning and evening); **(weighing 75 kg or less):** 1,000 mg daily (400 mg in morning, 600 mg in evening). Duration: 48 wks. **Genotype 2, 3:** 800 mg daily (400 mg in morning and evening). Duration: 24 wks. **CHILDREN 5 YRS AND OLDER WEIGHING 75 KG OR GREATER:** 1,200 mg daily (600 mg in morning and evening); **(WEIGHING 60–74 KG):** 1000 mg daily (400 mg in morning, 600 mg in evening); **(WEIGHING 47–59 KG):** 800 mg daily (400 mg in morning and evening); **(WEIGHING 34–46 KG):** 600 mg daily (200 mg in morning, 400 mg in evening); **(WEIGHING 23–33 KG):** 400 mg daily (200 mg in morning and evening). Duration: 24 wks for genotypes 2, 3; 48 wks for genotypes 1, 4.

Dosage in Renal Impairment
Rebetol Capsules/Oral Solution; Ribasphere Capsules
ADULTS: CrCl less than 50 mL/min: Contraindicated. **CHILDREN: Serum creatinine more than 2 mg/dL:** Discontinue treatment.
Ribasphere Tablets
ADULTS: CrCl less than 50 mL/min: Not recommended.

Copegus Tablets
CrCl 30–50 mL/min: Alternate 200 mg and 400 mg every other day. **CrCl less than 30 mL/min, end-stage renal disease:** 200 mg once daily.

Dosage in Hepatic Impairment
Contraindicated.

Severe Lower Respiratory Tract Infection Caused by Respiratory Syncytial Virus (RSV)
Inhalation: CHILDREN, INFANTS: Use with Viratek small-particle aerosol generator at concentration of 20 mg/mL (6 g reconstituted with 300 mL Sterile Water for Injection) over 12–18 hrs/day for 3–7 days.

SIDE EFFECTS

Frequent (greater than 10%): Hemolytic anemia, dizziness, headache, fatigue, fever, insomnia, irritability, depression, emotional lability, impaired concentration, alopecia, rash, pruritus, nausea, anorexia, dyspepsia, vomiting, decreased hemoglobin, hemolysis, arthralgia, musculoskeletal pain, dyspnea, sinusitis, flu-like symptoms. **Occasional (10%–1%):** Nervousness, altered taste, weakness.

ADVERSE EFFECTS/ TOXIC REACTIONS

Cardiac arrest, apnea, ventilator dependence, bacterial pneumonia, pneumonia, pneumothorax occur rarely. If treatment exceeds 7 days, anemia may occur.

NURSING CONSIDERATIONS

BASELINE ASSESSMENT
Obtain sputum specimens before giving first dose or at least during first 24 hrs of therapy. Assess respiratory status for baseline. **PO:** Obtain CBC with differential, pretreatment and monthly pregnancy test for women of childbearing age.

INTERVENTION/EVALUATION
Monitor Hgb, Hct, platelets, LFT, I&O, fluid balance carefully. Check hematology reports for anemia due to reticulocytosis when therapy exceeds 7 days. For ventilator-assisted pts, watch for "rainout"

R

---

in tubing and empty frequently; be alert to impaired ventilation/gas exchange due to drug precipitate. Assess skin for rash. Monitor B/P, respirations; assess lung sounds.

PATIENT/FAMILY TEACHING

• Report immediately any difficulty breathing, itching/swelling/redness of eyes, severe abdominal pain, bloody diarrhea, unusual bleeding/bruising. • Female pts should take measures to avoid pregnancy. • Male pts must use condoms during sexual activity.

---

ribociclib

rye-boe-**sye**-klib
(Kisqali)
Do not confuse ribociclib with palbociclib or riboflavin.

◆CLASSIFICATION

PHARMACOTHERAPEUTIC: Cyclin-dependent kinase inhibitor. **CLINICAL:** Antineoplastic.

USES

Used in combination with an aromatase inhibitor as initial endocrine-based therapy for treatment of postmenopausal women with hormone receptor–positive, human epidermal growth factor receptor 2 (HER2)-negative advanced or metastatic breast cancer.

PRECAUTIONS

Contraindications: Hypersensitivity to ribociclib. **Cautions:** Baseline hematologic cytopenias (anemia, thrombocytopenia, lymphopenia, neutropenia); electrolyte imbalance (correct abnormality prior to treatment), hepatic impairment, Avoid concomitant use of strong CYP3A inhibitors, strong CYP3A inducers, QT interval–prolonging medications. Avoid use in pts with or at risk for QTc prolongation (e.g., congenital long QT syndrome, hypokalemia, hypomagnesemia; uncontrolled,

significant cardiac disease including MI, HF, unstable angina, bradyarrhythmias).

ACTION

Blocks retinoblastoma protein phosphorylation and prevents progression through cell cycle, resulting in arrest of G_1 phase. **Therapeutic Effect:** Inhibits tumor growth.

PHARMACOKINETICS

Widely distributed. Metabolized extensively in liver via CYP3A4. Protein binding: 70%. Peak plasma concentration: 1–4 hrs. Excreted in feces (69%), urine (23%). **Half-life:** 30–55 hrs.

⧖ LIFESPAN CONSIDERATIONS

Pregnancy/Lactation: Indicated for postmenopausal women; however, may cause fetal harm/malformations when used during pregnancy. Females of reproductive potential should use effective contraception during treatment and for up to 3 wks after discontinuation. Unknown if distributed in breast milk. Breastfeeding not recommended during treatment and for up to 3 wks after discontinuation. **Children:** Safety and efficacy not established. **Elderly:** No age-related precautions noted.

INTERACTIONS

DRUG: Strong CYP3A inhibitors (e.g., clarithromycin, ketoconazole, ritonavir) may increase concentration/effect; avoid use. **Strong CYP3A inducers (e.g., carBAMazepine, phenytoin, rifAMPin)** may decrease concentration/effect; avoid use. **QT interval–prolonging medications (e.g., amiodarone, azithromycin, ceritinib, haloperidol, moxifloxacin)** may increase risk of QT interval prolongation, torsades de pointes. May increase concentration/effect of **aprepitant, bosutinib, budesonide, naloxegol, neratinib, olapanib, pimozide.** May decrease effect of **BCG vaccine.** May increase adverse effects/toxicity of **natalizumab, pimecrolimus, tacrolimus.** May decrease effect, increase toxicity of live vaccines. **HERBAL: Echinacea, St. John's wort** may decrease concentration/effect. **FOOD: Grapefruit products, pomegranate** may increase concentration/effect. **LAB VALUES:** May increase serum ALT, AST, bilirubin. May decrease ANC, Hgb, lymphocytes, leukocytes, neutrophils, platelets; serum potassium, phosphate.

AVAILABILITY (Rx)

Tablets: 200 mg. **Blister pack:** (14 tablets, 21 tablets).

ADMINISTRATION/HANDLING

PO

• Give with or without food. • Swallow whole. Do not crush, chew, or split (do not take broken or cracked tablets). If a dose is missed or vomiting occurs after administration, do not give extra dose. Administer next dose at regularly scheduled time.

INDICATIONS/ROUTES/DOSAGE

Breast Cancer
PO: ADULTS, ELDERLY: 600 mg once daily for 21 days, followed by 7 days off treatment of 28-day cycle. Use in combination with letrozole 2.5 mg once daily during 28-day cycle.
Dose Reduction for Adverse Events
Starting dose: 600 mg/day. **First dose reduction:** 400 mg/day. **Second dose reduction:** 200 mg/day. **Unable to tolerate 200 mg/day:** Permanently discontinue.

Dose Modification
Hepatotoxicity (During Treatment)
Note: Defined as hepatotoxicity without total bilirubin greater than 2 times upper limit of normal (ULN). If serum ALT, AST elevation greater than 3 times ULN with total bilirubin greater than 2 times ULN, permanently discontinue.
CTCAE grade 1 serum ALT, AST elevation (up to 3 times ULN): No dose adjustment. **CTCAE grade 2 serum ALT, AST elevation (greater than 3–5 times ULN) with baseline at less than grade 2:** Withhold treatment until recovery to less than or equal to baseline

grade, then resume at same dose level. If baseline at grade 2, do not withhold treatment. If grade 2 serum ALT, AST elevation recurs, then resume at reduced dose level. **CTCAE grade 3 serum ALT, AST elevation (greater than 5–20 times ULN):** Withhold treatment until recovery to less than or equal to baseline grade, then resume at reduced dose level. If grade 3 serum ALT, AST elevation recurs, permanently discontinue. **CTCAE grade 4 serum ALT, AST elevation (greater than 20 times ULN):** Permanently discontinue.

Hematologic
CTCAE grade 1 or 2 neutropenia (ANC 1000 cells/mm³ to less than the lower limit of normal): No dose adjustment. **CTCAE grade 3 neutropenia (ANC 500 to less than 1000 cells/mm³:** Withhold treatment until recovery to grade 2 or less, then resume at same dose level. If grade 3 neutropenia recurs, withhold treatment until recovery to grade 2 or less, then resume at reduced dose level. **CTCAE grade 3 febrile neutropenia:** Withhold treatment until recovery to grade 2 or less, then resume at reduced dose level. **Grade 4 neutropenia (ANC less than 500 cells/mm³):** Withhold treatment until recovery to grade 2 or less, then resume at reduced dose level.

QTc Interval Prolongation
QTc interval prolongation greater than 480 msec: Withhold treatment until resolved to less than 481 msec, then resume at same dose level. If QTc interval prolongation greater than 480 msec recurs, withhold treatment until resolved to less than 481 msec, then resume at reduced dose level. **QTc interval prolongation greater than 500 msec:** Withhold treatment if QTc interval prolongation greater than 500 msec on at least two separate EKGs (within same visit). If QTc interval prolongation resolves to less than 481 msec after withholding treatment, resume at

reduced dose level. **QTc interval prolongation greater than 500 msec (or greater than 60 msec from baseline) with torsades de pointes, polymorphic ventricular tachycardia, unexplained syncope, symptoms of serious arrhythmia:** Permanently discontinue.

Other Toxicities

Any other CTCAE grade 1 or 2 toxicities: No dose adjustment. **Any other CTCAE grade 3 toxicities:** Withhold treatment until resolved to grade 1 or 0, then resume at same dose level. If grade 3 toxicities recur, resume at reduced dose level. **Any other CTCAE grade 4 toxicities:** Permanently discontinue.

Concomitant Use of Strong CYP3A Inhibitors

Reduce initial dose to 400 mg once daily if strong CYP3A inhibitor cannot be discontinued. If CYP3A inhibitor is discontinued, increase ribociclib dose (after at least 5 half-lives of CYP3A inhibitor have elapsed) to the dose used prior to initiating strong CYP3A inhibitor.

Dosage in Renal Impairment
Not specified; use caution.

Dosage in Hepatic Impairment
Mild impairment: No dose adjustment. **Moderate to severe impairment:** Reduce starting dose to 400 mg once daily.

SIDE EFFECTS

Frequent (52%–17%): Nausea, fatigue, diarrhea, alopecia, vomiting, constipation, headache, back pain, decreased appetite, rash. **Occasional (14%–11%):** Pruritus, pyrexia, insomnia, dyspnea, stomatitis, peripheral edema, abdominal pain.

ADVERSE EFFECTS/ TOXIC REACTIONS

Anemia, leukopenia, lymphopenia, neutropenia, thrombocytopenia are expected responses to therapy, but more severe reactions, including febrile neutropenia, may be life threatening. CTCAE grade 3 or 4 neutropenia reported in 60% of pts. Severe hepatotoxicity reported in 10% of pts. QTc interval prolongation, infections including UTI may occur.

NURSING CONSIDERATIONS

BASELINE ASSESSMENT

Obtain ANC, CBC, BMP, LFT, serum phosphate; vital signs, weight. Obtain EKG (note QTc interval). Initiate treatment only in pts with QTc interval less than 450 msec. Obtain pregnancy test in females of reproductive potential. Question plans of breastfeeding. Question history of cardiac disease, cardiac conduction disorders, hepatic impairment. Receive full medication history including herbal products and screen for interactions. Screen for risk of bleeding, QTc interval prolongation, active infection. Obtain dietary consult. Offer emotional support.

INTERVENTION/EVALUATION

Monitor ANC, CBC for myelosuppression; LFT for hepatotoxicity q2wks for the first 2 cycles, then prior to each subsequent cycle, then as clinically indicated. Monitor BMP, serum phosphate for electrolyte imbalance; consider correcting imbalances, esp. hypokalemia, hypomagnesemia (due to increased risk of cardiac arrhythmias, torsades de pointes). Obtain repeat EKG on day 14 of the first cycle and at the beginning of the second cycle, or more frequently if QTc interval prolongation occurs. Monitor daily pattern of bowel activity, stool consistency. Assess skin for rash, lesions. Monitor weight, I&O.

PATIENT/FAMILY TEACHING

• Treatment may depress your immune system and reduce your ability to fight

R

infection. Report symptoms of infection such as body aches, burning with urination, chills, cough, fatigue, fever. Avoid those with active infection. • Report symptoms of bone marrow depression such as bruising, fatigue, fever, shortness of breath, weight loss; bleeding easily, bloody urine or stool. • Do not take newly prescribed medications unless approved by the prescriber who originally started treatment. • Report liver problems such as bruising, confusion, amber or dark-colored urine; right upper abdominal pain, yellowing of the skin or eyes; heart arrhythmias (chest pain, difficulty breathing, palpitations, passing out). • Therapy indicated for postmenopausal women; however, birth defects may occur when used during pregnancy. Females of childbearing potential should use effective contraception during treatment and for at least 3 wks after final dose. • Do not breastfeed during treatment and for up to 3 wks after final dose. • Do not ingest grapefruit products, Seville oranges, starfruit, pomegranate, herbal supplements. • Report planned surgical/dental procedures. • Immediately report bleeding of any kind.

rifabutin

rif-a-**bue**-tin
(Mycobutin)
Do not confuse rifabutin with rifAMPin.

◆CLASSIFICATION

PHARMACOTHERAPEUTIC: Rifamycin derivative. **CLINICAL:** Antimycobacterial.

USES

Prevention of disseminated *Mycobacterium avium* complex (MAC) disease in those with advanced HIV infection.

OFF-LABEL: Part of multidrug regimen for treatment of MAC. Alternative to rifAMPin as prophylaxis for latent tuberculosis infection, part of multidrug regimen for treatment of active tuberculosis infection.

PRECAUTIONS

Contraindications: Hypersensitivity to rifabutin, other rifamycins (e.g., rifAMPin). **Cautions:** Severe renal impairment. Avoid use in renal/hepatic impairment; do not give for MAC prophylaxis in pts with active TB.

ACTION

Inhibits DNA-dependent RNA polymerase. **Therapeutic Effect:** Prevents MAC disease.

PHARMACOKINETICS

Readily absorbed from GI tract. Protein binding: 85%. Widely distributed. Crosses blood-brain barrier. Extensive intracellular tissue uptake. Metabolized in liver. Excreted in urine (53%), feces (30%). Unknown if removed by hemodialysis. **Half-life:** 16–69 hrs.

⌛ LIFESPAN CONSIDERATIONS

Pregnancy/Lactation: Unknown if drug crosses placenta or is distributed in breast milk. **Children/Elderly:** No age-related precautions noted.

INTERACTIONS

DRUG: May decrease effectiveness of **oral contraceptives, clarithromycin, itraconazole.** May decrease concentration/effects of **non-nucleoside reverse transcriptase inhibitors (e.g., delavirdine, efavirenz, nevirapine), protease inhibitors (e.g., amprenavir, indinavir, ritonavir, saquinavir).** **HERBAL:** None significant. **FOOD: High-fat meals** may delay absorption. **LAB VALUES:** May increase serum alkaline phosphatase, ALT, AST.

AVAILABILITY (Rx)

Capsules: 150 mg.

R

ADMINISTRATION/HANDLING

PO
• May take with meals to reduce nausea/vomiting.

INDICATIONS/ROUTES/DOSAGE

Prevention of MAC (Advanced HIV Infection)
PO: ADULTS, ELDERLY: 300 mg once daily or 150 mg twice daily to reduce gastrointestinal upset. **CHILDREN, INFANTS:** 5 mg/kg once daily. **Maximum:** 300 mg once daily.

Dosage in Renal Impairment
CrCl less than 30 mL/min: Reduce dosage by 50%.

Dosage in Hepatic Impairment
No dose adjustment.

SIDE EFFECTS

Frequent (30%): Red-orange or red-brown discoloration of urine, feces, saliva, skin, sputum, sweat, tears. **Occasional (11%–3%):** Rash, nausea, abdominal pain, diarrhea, dyspepsia, belching, headache, altered taste, uveitis, corneal deposits. **Rare (Less Than 2%):** Anorexia, flatulence, fever, myalgia, vomiting, insomnia.

ADVERSE EFFECTS/TOXIC REACTIONS

Hepatitis, anemia, thrombocytopenia, neutropenia occur rarely. May cause uveitis, *C. difficile*–associated diarrhea.

NURSING CONSIDERATIONS

BASELINE ASSESSMENT
Obtain chest X-ray; sputum, blood cultures. Biopsy of suspicious node(s) must be done to rule out active tuberculosis. Obtain baseline CBC, serum hepatic function tests.

INTERVENTION/EVALUATION
Monitor serum LFT, platelet count, Hgb, Hct. Avoid IM injections, rectal temperatures, other traumas that may induce bleeding. Check temperature; notify physician of flu-like syndrome, rash, GI intolerance. Monitor bowel pattern, stool consistency.

PATIENT/FAMILY TEACHING
• Urine, feces, saliva, sputum, perspiration, tears, skin may be discolored brown-orange. • Soft contact lenses may be permanently discolored. • Rifabutin may decrease efficacy of oral contraceptives; nonhormonal methods should be considered. • Avoid crowds, those with infection. • Report flu-like symptoms, nausea, vomiting, dark urine, unusual bruising/bleeding from any site, any visual disturbances, diarrhea.

rifAMPin

rif-**am**-pin
(Rifadin, Rofact ✦)
Do not confuse Rifadin with Rifater or Ritalin, or rifAMPin with ribavirin, rifabutin, Rifamate, rifapentine, rifAXIMin, or Ritalin.

FIXED-COMBINATION(S)

Rifamate: rifAMPin/isoniazid (an antitubercular): 300 mg/150 mg. **Rifater:** rifAMPin/isoniazid/pyrazinamide (an antitubercular): 120 mg/50 mg/300 mg.

◆CLASSIFICATION

PHARMACOTHERAPEUTIC: Rifamycin derivative. **CLINICAL:** Antimycobacterial, antitubercular.

USES

In combination with other antitubercular agents for initial treatment, retreatment of active tuberculosis. Eliminates meningococci from nasopharynx of asymptomatic carriers. **OFF-LABEL:** Prophylaxis of *H. influenzae* type B infection, *Legionella* pneumonia, serious infections caused by *Staphylococcus* spp. (in combination with other agents). Treatment of prosthetic joint infection.

PRECAUTIONS

Contraindications: Concomitant therapy with atazanavir, darunavir, fosamprenavir, saquinavir, ritonavir, tipranavir; hypersensitivity to rifAMPin, other rifamycins. **Cautions:** Hepatic impairment, active or treated alcoholism, porphyria. Concurrent medications associated with hepatotoxicity.

ACTION

Interferes with bacterial RNA synthesis by binding to DNA-dependent RNA polymerase, preventing attachment to DNA, thereby blocking RNA transcription. **Therapeutic Effect:** Bactericidal in susceptible microorganisms.

PHARMACOKINETICS

Well absorbed from GI tract (food delays absorption). Protein binding: 80%. Widely distributed. Metabolized in liver. Primarily eliminated by biliary system. Not removed by hemodialysis. **Half-life:** 3–5 hrs (increased in hepatic impairment).

LIFESPAN CONSIDERATIONS

Pregnancy/Lactation: Crosses placenta. Distributed in breast milk. **Children/Elderly:** No age-related precautions noted.

INTERACTIONS

DRUG: Alcohol, hepatotoxic medications (e.g., acetaminophen, isoniazid, methotrexate, ketoconazole), ritonavir, saquinavir may increase risk of hepatotoxicity. May decrease effects of digoxin, disopyramide, fluconazole, methadone, mexiletine, oral anticoagulants (e.g., apixaban, warfarin), oral antidiabetics (e.g., glipiZIDE, metFORMIN), oral contraceptives, tacrolimus, tricyclic antidepressants, phenytoin, quiNIDine, tocainide, verapamil. **HERBAL:** St. John's wort

may decrease concentration. **FOOD:** Food decreases extent of absorption. **LAB VALUES:** May increase serum alkaline phosphatase, bilirubin, uric acid, ALT, AST.

AVAILABILITY (Rx)

Capsules (Rifadin): 150 mg, 300 mg. **Injection, Powder for Reconstitution:** 600 mg.

ADMINISTRATION/HANDLING

 IV

Reconstitution • Reconstitute 600-mg vial with 10 mL Sterile Water for Injection to provide concentration of 60 mg/mL. • Withdraw desired dose and further dilute with 0.9% NaCl or D₅W to concentration not to exceed 6 mg/mL.
Rate of Administration • For IV infusion only. Avoid IM, SQ administration. • Avoid extravasation (local irritation, inflammation). • Infuse over 30 min to 3 hrs.
Storage • Reconstituted vial is stable for 24 hrs. • Once reconstituted vial is further diluted, it is stable for 4 hrs in D₅W or 24 hrs in 0.9% NaCl.

PO

• Preferably give 1 hr before or 2 hrs following meals with 8 oz of water (may give with food to decrease GI upset; will delay absorption). • For pts unable to swallow capsules, contents may be mixed with applesauce, jelly. • Administer at least 1 hr before antacids, esp. those containing aluminum.

▨ IV INCOMPATIBILITY

DiltiaZEM (Cardizem).

▨ IV COMPATIBILITY

D₅W if infused within 4 hrs (risk of precipitation beyond this time period).

INDICATIONS/ROUTES/DOSAGE

Tuberculosis
Note: A four-drug regimen (ethambutol, isoniazid, pyrazinamide, rifampin) is preferred for initial, empiric treatment.

R

PO, IV: ADULTS, ELDERLY: 10 mg/kg/day. **Maximum:** 600 mg/day. **CHILDREN:** 10–20 mg/kg/day usually as a single dose. **Maximum:** 600 mg/day.

Meningococcal Carrier
PO, IV: ADULTS, ELDERLY: 600 mg twice daily for 2 days. **PO ONLY: CHILDREN 1 MO AND OLDER:** 10 mg/kg/dose q12h for 2 days. **Maximum:** 600 mg/dose. **CHILDREN YOUNGER THAN 1 MO:** 5 mg/kg/dose q12h for 2 days.

Dosage in Renal/Hepatic Impairment
No dose adjustment.

SIDE EFFECTS

Frequent: Red-orange or red-brown discoloration of urine, feces, saliva, skin, sputum, sweat, tears. **Occasional (5%–3%):** Hypersensitivity reaction (flushing, pruritus, rash). **Rare (2%–1%):** Diarrhea, dyspepsia, nausea, oral candida (sore mouth, tongue).

ADVERSE EFFECTS/ TOXIC REACTIONS

Hepatotoxicity (risk is increased when rifAMPin is taken with isoniazid), hepatitis, blood dyscrasias, Stevens-Johnson syndrome, antibiotic-associated colitis occur rarely.

NURSING CONSIDERATIONS

BASELINE ASSESSMENT
Obtain CBC, renal function test, LFT. Screen for concomitant medications known to cause hepatotoxicity. Question for hypersensitivity to rifAMPin, rifamycins. Ensure collection of diagnostic specimens.

INTERVENTION/EVALUATION
Assess IV site at least hourly during infusion; restart at another site at the first sign of irritation or inflammation. Monitor LFT, assess for hepatitis: jaundice, anorexia, nausea, vomiting, fatigue, weakness (hold rifAMPin, inform physician at once). Report hypersensitivity reactions promptly: any type of skin

eruption, pruritus, flu-like syndrome with high dosage. Monitor daily pattern of bowel activity, stool consistency (potential for antibiotic-associated colitis). Monitor CBC results for blood dyscrasias; be alert for infection (fever, sore throat), unusual bruising/bleeding, unusual fatigue/weakness.

PATIENT/FAMILY TEACHING
• Preferably take on empty stomach with 8 oz of water 1 hr before or 2 hrs after meal (with food if GI upset). • Avoid alcohol. • Do not take any other medications without consulting physician, including antacids; must take rifAMPin at least 1 hr before antacid. • Urine, feces, sputum, sweat, tears may become red-orange; soft contact lenses may be permanently stained. • Report any new symptom immediately such as yellow eyes/skin, fatigue, weakness, nausea/vomiting, sore throat, fever, flu, unusual bruising/bleeding. • If taking oral contraceptives, check with physician (reliability may be affected).

rifAXIMin

rif-**ax**-i-min
(Xifaxan, Zaxine ✦)
Do not confuse rifAXIMin with rifAMPin.

◆CLASSIFICATION

PHARMACOTHERAPEUTIC: Anti-infective. **CLINICAL:** Site-specific antibiotic.

USES

Treatment of traveler's diarrhea caused by noninvasive strains of *E. coli*. Reduction of risk for recurrence of overt hepatic encephalopathy. Treatment of irritable bowel syndrome with diarrhea (IBS-D) in adults. **OFF-LABEL:** Treatment of hepatic encephalopathy. Treatment of *C. difficile*–associated diarrhea.

PRECAUTIONS

Contraindications: Hypersensitivity to rifAXIMin, other rifamycin antibiotics. **Cautions:** Severe hepatic impairment.

ACTION

Inhibits bacterial RNA synthesis by binding to a subunit of bacterial DNA-dependent RNA polymerase. **Therapeutic Effect:** Bactericidal.

PHARMACOKINETICS

Less than 0.4% absorbed after PO administration. Primarily excreted in feces. **Half-life:** 5.85 hrs.

⧖ LIFESPAN CONSIDERATIONS

Pregnancy/Lactation: Unknown if drug is distributed in breast milk. **Children:** Safety and efficacy not established in pts younger than 12 yrs for traveler's diarrhea; younger than 18 yrs for IBS-D. **Elderly:** No age-related precautions noted.

INTERACTIONS

DRUG: None significant. **HERBAL:** None significant. **FOOD:** None known. **LAB VALUES:** None significant.

AVAILABILITY (Rx)

🗲 **Tablets:** 200 mg, 550 mg.

ADMINISTRATION/HANDLING

PO
• Give without regard to food. • Do not break, crush, dissolve, or divide film-coated tablets.

INDICATIONS/ROUTES/DOSAGE

Traveler's Diarrhea
PO: ADULTS, ELDERLY, CHILDREN 12 YRS AND OLDER: 200 mg 3 times/day for 3 days.

Hepatic Encephalopathy
PO: ADULTS, ELDERLY: 550 mg 2 times/day.

IBS-D
PO: ADULTS, ELDERLY: 550 mg 3 times/day for 14 days. May repeat up to 2 times if symptoms recur.

Dosage in Renal/Hepatic Impairment
No dose adjustment.

SIDE EFFECTS

Occasional (11%–5%): Flatulence, headache, abdominal discomfort, rectal tenesmus, defecation urgency, nausea. **Rare (4%–2%):** Constipation, fever, vomiting.

ADVERSE EFFECTS/TOXIC REACTIONS

Hypersensitivity reaction, superinfection occur rarely.

NURSING CONSIDERATIONS

BASELINE ASSESSMENT

Check baseline hydration status: skin turgor, mucous membranes for dryness, urinary status. Assess stool frequency, consistency.

INTERVENTION/EVALUATION

Encourage adequate fluid intake. Assess bowel sounds for peristalsis. Monitor daily pattern of bowel activity, stool consistency. Assess for GI disturbances, blood in stool.

PATIENT/FAMILY TEACHING

• Report if diarrhea worsens or if blood occurs in stool, fever develops within 48 hrs.

rilpivirine

ril-pi-**vir**-een
(Edurant)
Do not confuse rilpivirine with delavirdine, etravirine, or nevirapine.

FIXED-COMBINATION(S)

Complera: rilpivirine/emtricitabine (an antiretroviral)/tenofovir (TDF) (an antiretroviral): 25 mg/200 mg/300 mg. **Odefsey:** rilpivirine/emtricitabine/tenofovir (TAF): 25 mg/200 mg/25 mg.

R

◆CLASSIFICATION

PHARMACOTHERAPEUTIC: Non-nucleoside reverse transcriptase inhibitor. **CLINICAL:** Antiretroviral.

USES

Used in combination with at least two other antiretroviral agents for treatment of HIV-1 infection in treatment-naive pts with HIV-1 RNA 100,000 copies/mL or less.

PRECAUTIONS

Contraindications: Hypersensitivity to rilpivirine. Concurrent use of carBAMazepine, dexamethasone (greater than 1 dose), OXcarbazepine, PHENobarbital, phenytoin, proton pump inhibitors (see drug classification), rifabutin, rifAMPin, rifapentine, St. John's wort. **Cautions:** Severe depressive disorders, medications that increase risk of prolongation of QT interval (torsades de pointes), hypokalemia, hypomagnesemia, pts with significant transaminase elevations, hepatitis B or C virus infection. Not for treatment-experienced pts.

ACTION

Inhibits HIV-1 replication by binding to HIV-1 reverse transcriptase. **Therapeutic Effect:** Interferes with HIV replication, slowing progression of HIV infection.

PHARMACOKINETICS

Readily absorbed after PO administration. Peak concentration: 4–5 hrs. Protein binding: 99.7%. Metabolized in liver. Excreted primarily in feces. **Half-life:** 50 hrs.

⌛ LIFESPAN CONSIDERATIONS

Pregnancy/Lactation: Unknown if distributed in breast milk. HIV-infected mothers should not breastfeed infants due to risk of postnatal HIV transmission. **Children:** Safety and efficacy not established. **Elderly:** Caution due to higher risk of impaired renal/hepatic function.

INTERACTIONS

DRUG: CYP3A4 inducers (e.g., **carBA-Mazepine, PHENobarbital, phenytoin, proton pump inhibitors, rifabutin, rifAMPin**) may significantly decrease effectiveness. **Antacids, H₂-receptor antagonists (e.g., cimetidine, famotidine)** may decrease plasma concentration. **CYP3A4 inhibitors (e.g., clarithromycin, ketoconazole, verapamil)** may increase plasma concentration. **HERBAL:** St. John's wort may decrease concentration/effects. **FOOD:** Grapefruit products may increase potential for torsades de pointes. **LAB VALUES:** May increase serum creatinine, ALT, AST, bilirubin, cholesterol, triglycerides.

AVAILABILITY (Rx)

Tablets: 25 mg.

ADMINISTRATION/HANDLING

PO

• Give with a meal. Administer antacids 2 hrs before or 4 hrs after rilpivirine; H₂-receptor antagonist 12 hrs before or 4 hrs after rilpivirine.

INDICATIONS/ROUTES/DOSAGE

HIV Infection (in Combination with Other Antiretrovirals)

PO: ADULTS, ELDERLY, CHILDREN 12 YRS AND OLDER AND 35 KG OR GREATER: 25 mg once daily with a meal. With rifabutin: increase to 50 mg once daily.

Dosage in Renal/Hepatic Impairment

No dose adjustment. Use caution with severe renal impairment.

SIDE EFFECTS

Occasional (3%): Headache, insomnia, rash. **Rare (1%):** Nausea, vomiting, abdominal pain, fatigue, dizziness, abnormal dreams.

ADVERSE EFFECTS/TOXIC REACTIONS

Psychiatric disorders including depression, dysphoria, altered mood, suicidal ideation reported in 3% of pts. May

R

prolong QT interval. May develop redistribution/accumulation of body fat (lipodystrophy) or immune reconstitution syndrome.

NURSING CONSIDERATIONS

BASELINE ASSESSMENT

Obtain CBC, BMP, EKG, LFT, lipid panel, CD4 count, viral load. Receive full medication history including herbal products. Question for history of prolonged QT interval, torsades de pointes, psychiatric disorder.

INTERVENTION/EVALUATION

Closely monitor for evidence of rash. Monitor CBC, renal function, LFT.

PATIENT/FAMILY TEACHING

• Offer emotional support. • Take with food (optimizes absorption). • Report any signs of depression, thoughts of suicide, decreased urine output, abdominal pain, yellowing of skin, darkened urine, clay-colored stools, chest tightness, difficulty breathing, palpitations. • Report any newly prescribed medications. • Rilpivirine does not cure HIV infection nor reduce risk of transmission to others. • Continue to practice safe sex with barrier methods or practice abstinence.

risedronate

ris-ed-roe-nate
(Actonel, Atelvia,
Apo-Risedronate ✤)
**Do not confuse Actonel with
Actos, or risedronate with
alendronate.**

FIXED-COMBINATION(S)

Actonel with Calcium: risedronate/
calcium: 35 mg/6 × 500 mg.

◆CLASSIFICATION

PHARMACOTHERAPEUTIC: Bisphosphonate. **CLINICAL:** Calcium regulator.

USES

Actonel: Treatment of Paget's disease of bone. Treatment/prevention of osteoporosis in postmenopausal women, glucocorticoid-induced osteoporosis. Treatment of osteoporosis in men. **Atelvia:** Treatment of osteoporosis in postmenopausal women.

PRECAUTIONS

Contraindications: Hypersensitivity to risedronate, other bisphosphonates (e.g., alendronate); inability to stand or sit upright for at least 30 min; abnormalities of esophagus that delay esophageal emptying. **Cautions:** GI diseases (duodenitis, dysphagia, esophagitis, gastritis, ulcers [drug may exacerbate these conditions]), severe renal impairment (CrCl less than 30 mL/min), hypocalcemia.

ACTION

Inhibits bone resorption by action on osteoclasts or osteoclast precursors. **Therapeutic Effect:** Decreases bone resorption (indirectly increases bone mineral density). **Paget's Disease:** Inhibition of bone resorption causes a decrease (but more normal architecture) in bone formation.

PHARMACOKINETICS

Rapidly absorbed. Bioavailability decreased when administered with food. Protein binding: 24%. Not metabolized. Excreted unchanged in urine, feces. Not removed by hemodialysis. **Half-life:** 1.5 hrs (initial); 480 hrs (terminal).

⧗ LIFESPAN CONSIDERATIONS

Pregnancy/Lactation: Unknown if distributed in breast milk. **Children:** Not indicated for use in this pt population. **Elderly:** No age-related precautions noted.

INTERACTIONS

DRUG: Antacids containing aluminum, calcium, magnesium; vitamin D

✤ Canadian trade name Non-Crushable Drug ▦ High Alert drug

may decrease absorption (avoid administration within 30 min of **risedronate**). **HERBAL:** None significant. **FOOD:** None known. **LAB VALUES:** None significant.

AVAILABILITY (Rx)

Tablets: 5 mg, 30 mg, 35 mg, 150 mg. Tablets, Delayed-Release: 35 mg.

ADMINISTRATION/HANDLING

PO

Actonel: • Administer 30–60 min before any food, drink, other oral medications to avoid interference with absorption. • Give on empty stomach with full glass of plain water (not mineral water). • Pt must avoid lying down for at least 30 min after swallowing tablet (assists with delivery to stomach, reduces risk of esophageal irritation). • Give whole; do not break, crush, dissolve, or divide tablet.

Atelvia: • Take in morning immediately following breakfast with at least 4 oz water. • Remain upright for 30 min after taking dose.

INDICATIONS/ROUTES/DOSAGE

Paget's Disease
PO: *(Actonel):* **ADULTS, ELDERLY:** 30 mg/day for 2 mos. Retreatment may occur after 2-mo post-treatment observation period.

Prophylaxis, Treatment of Postmenopausal Osteoporosis
PO: *(Actonel):* **ADULTS, ELDERLY:** 5 mg/day or 35 mg once wkly or 150 mg once monthly.

Treatment of Postmenopausal Osteoporosis
PO: *(Atelvia):* **ADULTS, ELDERLY:** 35 mg once wkly.

Treatment of Male Osteoporosis
PO: *(Actonel):* **ADULTS, ELDERLY:** 35 mg once wkly.

Glucocorticoid-Induced Osteoporosis
PO: *(Actonel):* **ADULTS, ELDERLY:** 5 mg/day.

Dosage in Renal Impairment
Not recommended with CrCl less than 30 mL/min.

Dosage in Hepatic Impairment
No dose adjustment.

SIDE EFFECTS

Frequent (30%): Arthralgia. **Occasional (12%–8%):** Rash, diarrhea, constipation, nausea, abdominal pain, dyspepsia, flu-like symptoms, peripheral edema. **Rare (5%–3%):** Bone pain, sinusitis, asthenia, dry eye, tinnitus.

ADVERSE EFFECTS/TOXIC REACTIONS

Overdose produces hypocalcemia, hypophosphatemia, significant GI disturbances, osteonecrosis of jaw.

NURSING CONSIDERATIONS

BASELINE ASSESSMENT
Assess symptoms of Paget's disease (bone pain, bone deformities). Hypocalcemia, vitamin D deficiency must be corrected before therapy begins. Obtain baseline laboratory studies, esp. serum electrolytes, renal function. Verify pt is able to stand or sit upright for at least 30 min.

INTERVENTION/EVALUATION
Check serum electrolytes (esp. calcium, ionized calcium, phosphorus, alkaline phosphatase levels). Monitor I&O, BUN, creatinine in pts with renal impairment.

PATIENT/FAMILY TEACHING
• Expected benefits occur only when medication is taken with full glass (6–8 oz) of plain water first thing in the morning and at least 30 min before first food, beverage, medication of the day. Any other beverage (mineral water, orange juice, coffee) significantly reduces absorption of medication. • Do not lie down for at least 30 min after taking medication (potentiates delivery to stomach, reduces risk of esophageal irritation). • Report swallowing difficulties, pain when swallowing, chest pain, new/worsening heartburn.

R

• Consider weight-bearing exercises; modify behavioral factors (cigarette smoking, alcohol consumption). • Report jaw pain, incapacitating bone, joint, or muscle pain.

risperiDONE

ris-**per**-i-done
(Apo-RisperiDONE ♣, RisperDAL, RisperDAL Consta, RisperDAL M-Tabs, RisperiDONE M-Tab)

■ **BLACK BOX ALERT** ■ Increased risk of mortality in elderly pts with dementia-related psychosis, mainly due to pneumonia, HF.
Do not confuse RisperDAL with Restoril, or risperiDONE with rOPINIRole.

◆CLASSIFICATION

PHARMACOTHERAPEUTIC: Benzisoxazole derivative. **CLINICAL:** Second-generation (atypical) antipsychotic.

USES

(Oral): Treatment of schizophrenia, irritability/aggression associated with autistic disease in children. Treatment of acute mania associated with bipolar disorder (monotherapy in children and adults; in combination with lithium or valproate in adults). **(IM):** Management of schizophrenia, maintenance treatment of bipolar 1 disorder (monotherapy or in combination with lithium or valproate in adults). **OFF-LABEL:** Tourette's syndrome. Post-traumatic stress syndrome. Major depressive disorder.

PRECAUTIONS

Contraindications: Hypersensitivity to risperiDONE. **Cautions:** Renal/hepatic impairment, seizure disorder, cardiac disease, recent MI, breast cancer or other prolactin-dependent tumors, suicidal pts, pts at risk for aspiration pneumonia. Parkinson's disease, pts at risk for orthostatic hypotension, elderly pts, diabetes, decreased GI motility, urinary retention, BPH, xerostomia, visual problems, pts exposed to temperature extremes, preexisting myelosuppression, narrow-angle glaucoma; pts with high risk of suicide.

ACTION

May antagonize DOPamine, serotonin receptors in both CNS and periphery. **Therapeutic Effect:** Suppresses psychotic behavior.

PHARMACOKINETICS

Well absorbed from GI tract; unaffected by food. Protein binding: 90%. Metabolized in liver. Primarily excreted in urine. **Half-life:** 3–20 hrs; metabolite, 21–30 hrs (increased in elderly). **Injection:** 3–6 days.

⧗ LIFESPAN CONSIDERATIONS

Pregnancy/Lactation: Unknown if drug crosses placenta or is distributed in breast milk. Breastfeeding not recommended. **Children:** Safety and efficacy not established in children younger than 13 yrs for schizophrenia, 10 yrs for bipolar mania, and 5 yrs for autistic disorder. **Elderly:** More susceptible to postural hypotension. Age-related renal/hepatic impairment may require dosage adjustment.

INTERACTIONS

DRUG: Alcohol, other CNS depressants (e.g., LORazepam, morphine, zolpidem) may increase CNS depression. **CarBAMazepine** may decrease concentration. May decrease effects of **DOPamine** agonists, **levodopa. PARoxetine, FLUoxetine** may increase concentration, risk of extrapyramidal symptoms (EPS). **Antihypertensives** (e.g., **amLODIPine, lisinopril, valsartan**), **beta blockers** (e.g., **carvedilol, metoprolol**), **calcium channel blockers** (e.g., **diltiaZEM, verapamil**), **diuretics** (e.g., **furosemide, HCTZ**), **doxepin, pramipexole, prazosin, sildenafil** may increase

R

hypotensive effect. **HERBAL: Gotu kola, kava kava, St. John's wort, valerian** may increase CNS depression. **FOOD:** None known. **LAB VALUES:** May increase serum prolactin, glucose, AST, ALT. May cause EKG changes.

AVAILABILITY (Rx)

Injection, Powder for Reconstitution (RisperDAL Consta): 12.5 mg, 25 mg, 37.5 mg, 50 mg. **Oral Solution (RisperDAL):** 1 mg/mL. **Tablets (RisperDAL):** 0.25 mg, 0.5 mg, 1 mg, 2 mg, 3 mg, 4 mg.

Tablets (Orally Disintegrating [RisperDAL M-Tabs, RisperiDONE M-Tab]): 0.25 mg, 0.5 mg, 1 mg, 2 mg, 3 mg, 4 mg.

ADMINISTRATION/HANDLING

◀ **ALERT** ▶ Do not administer via IV route.

IM

Reconstitution • Use only diluent and needle supplied in dose pack. • Prepare suspension according to manufacturer's directions. • May be given up to 6 hrs after reconstitution, but immediate administration is recommended. • If 2 min pass between reconstitution and injection, shake upright vial vigorously back and forth to resuspend solution.

Rate of Administration • Inject IM into upper outer quadrant of gluteus maximus or into deltoid muscle in upper arm.

Storage • Store at room temperature.

PO

• Give without regard to food. • May mix oral solution with water, coffee, orange juice, low-fat milk. Do not mix with cola, tea.

Orally Disintegrating Tablet

• Remove from blister pack immediately before administration. • Using gloves, place immediately on tongue. • Tablet dissolves in seconds. • Pt may swallow with or without liquid. • Do not split or chew.

INDICATIONS/ROUTES/DOSAGE

Schizophrenia

PO: ADULTS: Initially, 1 mg twice daily. May increase gradually (1–2 mg/day at intervals of at least 24 hrs) to target dose of 6 mg/day. Range: 4–8 mg/day. **Maintenance:** Target dose of 4 mg once daily (range: 2–8 mg/day). **ELDERLY:** Initially, 0.5 mg twice daily. May increase slowly at increments of no more than 0.5 mg twice daily. Range: 2–6 mg/day. **CHILDREN 13–17 YRS:** Initially, 0.5 mg/day (as single daily dose). May increase by 0.5–1 mg/day at intervals of greater than 24 hrs to recommended dose of 3 mg/day.

IM: ADULTS, ELDERLY: Initially, 12.5–25 mg q2wks. **Maximum:** 50 mg q2wks. Dosage adjustments should not be made more frequently than every 4 wks.

Bipolar Mania

PO: ADULTS, ELDERLY: Initially, 2–3 mg as a single daily dose. May increase by 1 mg/day at 24-hr intervals. Range: 1–6 mg/day. **PO: CHILDREN 10–17 YRS:** Initially, 0.5 mg/day. May increase by 0.5 mg/day at intervals of greater than 24 hrs to recommended dose of 2.5 mg/day. **IM: ADULTS, ELDERLY:** 25 mg q2wks. **Maximum:** 50 mg q2wks. Dosage adjustments should not be made more frequently than every 4 wks.

Autism

CHILDREN 5 YRS AND OLDER WEIGHING MORE THAN 19 KG: Initially, 0.5 mg/day. May increase to 1 mg after 4 days. May further increase dose by 0.5 mg/day in greater than 2-wk intervals. Range: 0.5–3 mg/day. **CHILDREN 5 YRS AND OLDER WEIGHING 15–19 KG:** Initially, 0.25 mg/day. May increase to 0.5 mg/day after 4 days. May further increase dose by 0.25 mg/day in greater than 2-wk intervals. Range: 0.5–3 mg/day.

Dosage in Renal/Hepatic Impairment

Mild to moderate impairment: No dose adjustment. **Severe impairment:** Initial dosage for adults, elderly pts is 0.5 mg twice daily. Dosage is titrated slowly to desired effect.

SIDE EFFECTS

Frequent (26%–13%): Agitation, anxiety, insomnia, headache, constipation. **Occasional (10%–4%):** Dyspepsia, rhinitis, drowsiness, dizziness, nausea, vomiting, rash, abdominal pain, dry skin, tachycardia. **Rare (3%–2%):** Visual disturbances, fever, back pain, pharyngitis, cough, arthralgia, angina, aggressive behavior, orthostatic hypotension, breast swelling.

ADVERSE EFFECTS/TOXIC REACTIONS

Rare reactions include tardive dyskinesia (characterized by tongue protrusion, puffing of the cheeks, chewing or puckering of mouth), neuroleptic malignant syndrome (hyperpyrexia, muscle rigidity, altered mental status, irregular pulse or B/P, tachycardia, diaphoresis, cardiac arrhythmias, rhabdomyolysis, acute renal failure). Hyperglycemia, life-threatening events such as ketoacidosis and hyperosmolar coma, death have been reported.

NURSING CONSIDERATIONS

BASELINE ASSESSMENT

Renal function test, LFT should be performed before therapy begins. Assess behavior, appearance, emotional status, response to environment, speech pattern, thought content, baseline weight. Obtain fasting serum glucose, CBC.

INTERVENTION/EVALUATION

Monitor B/P, heart rate, weight, LFT, EKG. Monitor for fine tongue movement (may be first sign of tardive dyskinesia, which may be irreversible). Monitor for suicidal ideation. Assess for therapeutic response (greater interest in surroundings, improved self-care, increased ability to concentrate, relaxed facial expression). Monitor for potential neuroleptic malignant syndrome: fever, muscle rigidity, irregular B/P or pulse, altered mental status. Monitor fasting serum glucose periodically during therapy.

PATIENT/FAMILY TEACHING

• Avoid tasks that may require alertness, motor skills until response to drug is established (may cause dizziness/drowsiness). • Avoid alcohol. • Go from lying to standing slowly. • Report trembling in fingers, altered gait, unusual muscular/skeletal movements, palpitations, severe dizziness/fainting, swelling/pain in breasts, visual changes, rash, difficulty breathing.

ritonavir

rit-**oh**-na-veer
(Norvir)

■ **BLACK BOX ALERT** ■ Concurrent use with other medications (nonsedating antihistamines, sedative hypnotics, antiarrhythmics, ergot alkaloids) may result in potentially serious, life-threatening events.

Do not confuse Norvir with Norvasc, or ritonavir with Retrovir.

◆CLASSIFICATION

PHARMACOTHERAPEUTIC: Protease inhibitor. **CLINICAL:** Antiviral.

USES

Treatment of HIV infection in combination with other antiretroviral agents. May be used as "booster" for other protease inhibitors.

PRECAUTIONS

Contraindications: Hypersensitivity to ritonavir. Due to potential serious and/or life-threatening drug interactions (e.g., arrhythmias, hematologic abnormalities, seizures), the following medications should not be given concomitantly with ritonavir: alfuzosin, amiodarone, colchicine (pts with renal/hepatic impairment), dihydroergotamine, ergotamine, dronedarone, ergonovine, flecainide, lovastatin, lurasidone, methylergonovine, midazolam (oral),

R

pimozide, propafenone, quiNIDine, sildenafil (when used for pulmonary arterial hypertension), simvastatin, St. John's wort, triazolam, voriconazole (when ritonavir dose 800 mg or greater/day). **Cautions:** Hepatic impairment, cardiomyopathy, ischemic heart disease, preexisting cardiac conduction abnormalities, structural heart disease, pts with increased triglycerides, hemophilia A and B, diabetes, hepatitis B or C virus infection, medications that prolong PR interval, diabetes.

ACTION

Inhibits HIV-1 and HIV-2 proteases, rendering these enzymes incapable of processing polypeptide precursors, leading to production of noninfectious, immature HIV particles. **Therapeutic Effect:** Slows HIV replication, reducing progression of HIV infection.

PHARMACOKINETICS

Well absorbed (absorption increased with food). Protein binding: 98%–99%. Metabolized in liver. Primarily excreted in feces. Unknown if removed by hemodialysis. **Half-life:** 2.7–5 hrs.

⌛ LIFESPAN CONSIDERATIONS

Pregnancy/Lactation: Breastfeeding not recommended (possibility of HIV transmission). **Children:** No age-related precautions noted in pts older than 1 month. **Elderly:** None known.

INTERACTIONS

DRUG: See contraindications. May increase concentration of **clarithromycin, fluticasone, ketoconazole, protease inhibitors, sildenafil, statins.** May decrease concentration/effects of **methadone, phenytoin, warfarin.** **RifAMPin** may decrease concentration/effects. **HERBAL:** St. John's wort may decrease concentration/effects. **FOOD:** None known. **LAB VALUES:** May increase serum creatine kinase (CK), GGT, triglycerides, uric acid, ALT, AST, glucose. May decrease Hgb, Hct, WBC, neutrophils.

AVAILABILITY (Rx)

Capsules: 100 mg. **Oral Solution:** 80 mg/mL.

📋 **Tablets:** 100 mg.

ADMINISTRATION/HANDLING

PO
• Store capsules in refrigerator. Store tablets, oral solution at room temperature. • Protect from light. • Give without regard to meals (preferably give with food). • Give tablets whole; do not break, crush, dissolve, or divide. • May improve taste of oral solution by mixing with chocolate milk, Ensure, Advera, Boost within 1 hr of dosing.

INDICATIONS/ROUTES/DOSAGE

Note: Not recommended as primary protease inhibitor in any regimen.
Treatment of HIV Infection
PO: ADULTS, CHILDREN 12 YRS AND OLDER: 600 mg twice daily. If nausea occurs at this dosage, decrease dose to 300 mg twice daily for 1 day, then increase by 100 mg twice daily every 2–3 days to recommended dose of 600 mg twice daily. **CHILDREN 1 MO–11 YRS:** Initially, 250 mg/m²/dose twice daily. Increase by 50 mg/m²/dose q2–3days up to 350–400 mg/m²/dose. **Maximum:** 600 mg/dose twice daily.

Booster Therapy
PO: ADULTS, ELDERLY: 100–400 mg/day (usually as 100–200 mg 1–2 times/day.)

Dosage in Renal Impairment
No dose adjustment.

Dosage in Hepatic Impairment
Mild to moderate impairment: No dose adjustment. **Severe impairment:** Not recommended.

SIDE EFFECTS

Frequent: GI disturbances (abdominal pain, anorexia, diarrhea, nausea, vomiting), circumoral and peripheral paresthesia, altered taste, headache, dizziness, fatigue, asthenia. **Occasional:** Allergic reaction, flu-like symptoms, hypotension. **Rare:** Hyperglycemia.

ADVERSE EFFECTS/TOXIC REACTIONS

Hepatitis, pancreatitis occur rarely. May cause new-onset diabetes.

NURSING CONSIDERATIONS

BASELINE ASSESSMENT

Pts beginning combination therapy with ritonavir and nucleosides may promote GI tolerance by beginning ritonavir alone, then subsequently adding nucleosides before completing 2 wks of ritonavir monotherapy. Obtain baseline laboratory testing, esp. LFT, triglycerides before beginning ritonavir therapy and at periodic intervals during therapy. Offer emotional support. Obtain full medication history and screen for contraindications/interactions.

INTERVENTION/EVALUATION

Closely monitor for evidence of GI disturbances, neurologic abnormalities (particularly paresthesia). Monitor LFT, serum glucose, CD4 cell count, plasma levels of HIV RNA.

PATIENT/FAMILY TEACHING

• Continue therapy for full length of treatment. • Doses should be evenly spaced. • Ritonavir is not a cure for HIV infection, nor does it reduce risk of transmission to others. • Pts may continue to acquire illnesses associated with advanced HIV infection. • If possible, take ritonavir with food. • Taste of solution may be improved when mixed with chocolate milk, Ensure, Advera, Boost. • Report increased thirst, frequent urination, nausea, vomiting, abdominal pain.

riTUXimab

ri-**tux**-i-mab
(Rituxan)

■ **BLACK BOX ALERT** ■ Profound, occasionally fatal infusion-related reactions reported during first 30–120 min of first infusion. Tumor lysis syndrome leading to acute renal failure may occur 12–24 hrs following first dose. Severe, sometimes fatal, mucocutaneous reactions resulting in multifocal leukoencephalopathy (PML) and death reported.

Do not confuse Rituxan with Remicade, or riTUXimab with bevacizumab or inFLIXimab, brentuximab, ruxolitinib.

◆CLASSIFICATION

PHARMACOTHERAPEUTIC: Monoclonal antibody. **CLINICAL:** Disease-modifying antirheumatic drug (DMARD), antineoplastic.

USES

Treatment of CD20-positive non-Hodgkin's lymphomas (NHL): Relapsed or refractory, low-grade, or follicular B-cell NHL; follicular B-cell NHL (previously untreated); nonprogressive, low-grade B-cell NHL; diffuse large B-cell NHL, previously untreated. Treatment of CD20-positive chronic lymphocytic leukemia (CLL). Treatment of moderate to severe active rheumatoid arthritis (RA) in combination with methotrexate. Treatment of granulomatosis with polyangiitis (GPA). Treatment of microscopic polyangiitis (MPA). **OFF-LABEL:** Treatment of autoimmune hemolytic anemia, chronic immune thrombocytopenic purpura (ITP), systemic autoimmune disease (other than rheumatoid arthritis), Burkitt's lymphoma, CNS lymphoma, Hodgkin's lymphoma.

PRECAUTIONS

Contraindications: Hypersensitivity to riTUXimab, murine proteins. **Cautions:** Pts at risk for tumor lysis syndrome. Cardiac disease, elderly pts, pulmonary

R

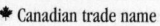 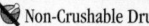

disease, renal impairment, severe active infection; history of hepatitis B virus infection.

ACTION

Binds to CD20, the antigen found on surface of B lymphocytes, B-cell non-Hodgkin's lymphoma (NHL). Activates B-cell cytotoxicity. **Therapeutic Effect:** Produces cytotoxicity, reduces tumor size. Signs/symptoms of rheumatoid arthritis are reduced; structural damage delayed.

PHARMACOKINETICS

Rapidly depletes B cells. **Half-life:** 59.8 hrs after first infusion, 174 hrs after fourth infusion.

⧖ LIFESPAN CONSIDERATIONS

Pregnancy/Lactation: Has potential to cause fetal B-cell depletion. Unknown if distributed in breast milk. Female pts of reproductive potential should use effective contraception during treatment and up to 12 mos after discontinuation. **Children:** Safety and efficacy not established. **Elderly:** Increased risk of cardiac/pulmonary adverse reactions.

INTERACTIONS

DRUG: Denosumab, tacrolimus may increase risk of adverse effects. May increase toxic effects of **abatacept, belimumab, clozapine, leflunomide, natalizumab.** Roflumilast may increase immunosuppressive effect. May increase immunosuppressive effect of **deferiprone, fingolimod, tofacitinib.** May decrease concentration/effect of **nivolumab, sipuleucel-T.** Trastuzumab may increase neutropenic effect. May decrease therapeutic effect of **vaccines;** increase risk of adverse effect of **live vaccines. HERBAL:** Echinacea may decrease therapeutic effect. **Garlic, ginger, ginseng** may increase hypoglycemic effect. **FOOD:** None known. **LAB VALUES:** May increase creatinine, LDH. May decrease Hgb, Hct, neutrophils, platelets, B-cell counts, immunoglobulin concentrations. May diminish diagnostic effect of *Coccidioides immitis* skin test.

AVAILABILITY (Rx)

Injection Solution: 10 mg/mL (10 mL, 50 mL).

ADMINISTRATION/HANDLING
💉 IV

◀**ALERT**▶ Do not give by IV push or bolus.

Reconstitution • Dilute with 0.9% NaCl or D_5W to provide final concentration of 1–4 mg/mL into infusion bag.
Rate of Administration • Initially infuse at rate of 50 mg/hr. If no hypersensitivity or infusion-related reaction, may increase infusion rate in 50 mg/hr increments q30min to maximum 400 mg/hr. • Subsequent infusion can be given at 100 mg/hr and increased by 100 mg/hr increments q30min to maximum 400 mg/hr.
Storage • Refrigerate vials. • Diluted solution is stable for 24 hrs if refrigerated or at room temperature.

🚫 IV INCOMPATIBILITIES

Do not mix with any other medications.

INDICATIONS/ROUTES/DOSAGE

Note: Refer to specific protocols.

NHL (Relapsed/Refractory, Low-Grade or Follicular CD20-Positive B-cell)
IV: ADULTS: 375 mg/m² wkly for 4 or 8 doses.

NHL (Diffuse Large B-cell)
IV: ADULTS: 375 mg/m² on day 1 of each cycle up to 8 doses.

NHL (Follicular, CD20-Positive, B-cell, Previously Untreated)
IV: ADULTS: 375 mg/m² on day 1 of each cycle up to 8 doses. **Maintenance (single agent):** 375 mg/m² q8 wks for 12 doses.

NHL (Nonprogressive, CD20-Positive, B-cell Following 6–8 Cycles of Cyclophosphamide, VinCRIStine, and PrednisoLONE [CVP Therapy])
IV: ADULTS: 375 mg/m² once wkly for 4 doses q6mos. **Maximum:** 16 doses.

R

NHL (Combination with Ibritumomab)
IV: ADULTS: 250 mg/m² day 1; repeat in 7–9 days with ibritumomab.

Rheumatoid Arthritis
IV: ADULTS: 1,000 mg every 2 wks times 2 doses in combination with methotrexate. May repeat course q24 wks (if needed, no sooner than 16 wks).

CLL
IV: ADULTS: 375 mg/m² in first cycle (on day prior to fludarabine/cyclophosphamide) and 500 mg/m² on day 1 in cycles 2–6, administered every 28 days.

GPA, MPA
IV: ADULTS: 375 mg/m² once wkly for 4 wks (in combination with methylPREDNISolone IV for 1–3 days, then daily predniSONE).

Dosage in Renal/Hepatic Impairment
No dose adjustment.

SIDE EFFECTS

Frequent (49%–10%): Fever, chills, nausea, asthenia, headache, angioedema, hypotension, rash/pruritus. **Occasional (Less Than 10%):** Myalgia, dizziness, weakness, abdominal pain, throat irritation, vomiting, neutropenia, rhinitis, bronchospasm, urticaria.

ADVERSE EFFECTS/TOXIC REACTIONS

Hypersensitivity reaction produces hypotension, bronchospasm, angioedema. Arrhythmias may occur, particularly in pts with history of preexisting cardiac conditions.

NURSING CONSIDERATIONS

BASELINE ASSESSMENT

Pretreatment with acetaminophen and diphenhydrAMINE before each infusion may prevent infusion-related effects. CBC should be obtained at regular intervals during therapy.

INTERVENTION/EVALUATION

Monitor CBC, renal function, LFT. Diligently monitor for tumor lysis syndrome in pts with high tumor burden. Monitor for an infusion-related symptoms complex consisting mainly of fever, chills, rigors that generally occurs within 30 min–2 hrs of beginning first infusion. Slowing infusion resolves symptoms.

PATIENT/FAMILY TEACHING

• Report fever, sore throat, abdominal pain, yellowing of eyes/skin, unusual bruising/bleeding.

---

rivaroxaban

rye-va-**rox**-a-ban
(Xarelto)

■ **BLACK BOX ALERT** ■ Epidural/spinal hematomas may occur in pts receiving neuraxial anesthesia or spinal puncture, resulting in long-term or permanent paralysis. Factors increasing risk of epidural/spinal hematoma include indwelling epidural catheters, concomitant drugs such as NSAIDs, platelet inhibitors, other anticoagulants; history of traumatic or repeated spinal or epidural punctures, history of spinal deformity or spinal surgery. Monitor for signs and symptoms of neurologic impairment. Consider benefits and risks before neuraxial intervention in anticoagulated pts or planned thromboprophylaxis. Increased risk of stroke may occur in pts with atrial fibrillation when discontinuing for reasons other than bleeding.
Do not confuse rivaroxaban with argatroban.

◆CLASSIFICATION

PHARMACOTHERAPEUTIC: Factor Xa inhibitor. **CLINICAL:** Anticoagulant.

USES

Prophylaxis of deep vein thrombosis (DVT) in pts undergoing knee or hip

---

replacement surgery. Prevents stroke/systemic embolism in pts with nonvalvular atrial fibrillation. Treatment of DVT/PE. Reduces risk of recurrent DVT/PE following 6 mos of treatment.

PRECAUTIONS

Contraindications: Hypersensitivity to rivaroxaban. Active major bleeding. **Cautions:** Renal/hepatic impairment, pts at increased risk of bleeding (e.g., thrombocytopenia, stroke, severe uncontrolled hypertension), elderly pts; avoid use with heparin, low molecular weight heparin (LMWH), aspirin, warfarin, NSAIDs. Pts with prosthetic heart valves or significant rheumatic heart disease.

ACTION

Selectively blocks active site of factor Xa, a key factor in the intrinsic and extrinsic pathway of blood coagulation cascade. Inhibits platelet activation and fibrin clot formation. **Therapeutic Effect:** Inhibits blood coagulation.

PHARMACOKINETICS

Rapidly absorbed after PO administration. Peak plasma concentration: 2–4 hrs. Absorption dependent on site of drug release within GI tract. Avoid administration into small intestine due to reduced absorption. Protein binding: 92%–95%. Metabolized in liver. Excreted in urine (66%), feces (28%). **Half-life:** 5–9 hrs, 11–13 hrs (elderly pts).

⧗ LIFESPAN CONSIDERATIONS

Pregnancy/Lactation: Crosses placenta. Use during pregnancy should be avoided. Unknown if excreted in breast milk. **Children:** Safety and efficacy not established. **Elderly:** May be at increased risk for bleeding due to age-related renal impairment. Use caution.

INTERACTIONS

DRUG: CYP3A4 inhibitors (e.g., **ketoconazole, clarithromycin, ritonavir**) may increase concentration, risk of bleeding. **Anticoagulants** (e.g., **heparin, warfarin**), **antiplatelets** (e.g., **aspirin, clopidogrel**), **NSAIDs** (e.g., **ibuprofen, ketorolac, naproxen**) may increase bleeding risk. **HERBAL: St. John's wort** may decrease effect. **FOOD: Grapefruit products** may increase risk of bleeding. **LAB VALUES:** May decrease platelets. May increase serum ALT, AST, bilirubin.

AVAILABILITY (Rx)

Tablets: 10 mg, 15 mg, 20 mg.

ADMINISTRATION/HANDLING

PO
• Administer doses of 15 mg or greater with food; doses of 10 mg/day may be given without regard to food. • **DVT prophylaxis (knee, hip):** Give without regard to meals. • **Nonvalvular atrial fibrillation:** Give with evening meal.

INDICATIONS/ROUTES/DOSAGE

Note: Avoid in pts with BMI greater than 40 kg/m^2 or weight greater than 120 kg due to lack of clinical data in this population.

DVT Prophylaxis, Knee Replacement
PO: ADULTS: 10 mg daily for minimum 10–14 days up to 35 days. Initiate at least 6–10 hrs after surgery once hemostasis established. **CrCl less than 30 mL/min:** Avoid use.

DVT Prophylaxis, Hip Replacement
PO: ADULTS: 10 mg daily for 10–14 days (minimum) up to 35 days. Initiate at least 6–10 hrs after surgery once hemostasis established. **CrCl less than 30 mL/min:** Avoid use.

Nonvalvular Atrial Fibrillation
PO: ADULTS: CrCl greater than 50 mL/min: 20 mg daily. **CrCl 15–50 mL/min:** 15 mg daily. **CrCl less than 15 mL/min:** Avoid use.

Treatment of DVT/PE
PO: ADULTS, ELDERLY: 15 mg twice daily for 3 wks, then 20 mg once daily.

Reduce Risk of DVT/PE (After 6 mos Treatment)
PO: ADULTS, ELDERLY: 10 mg once daily up to 6–12 mos.

Dosage in Renal Impairment
CrCl less than 30 mL/min: Avoid use in DVT/PE, postoperative thromboprophylaxis. *Nonvalvular atrial fibrillation:* **CrCl 15–50 mL/min:** 15 mg once daily with evening meal. **CrCl less than 15 mL/min:** Avoid use.

Dosage in Hepatic Impairment
Mild impairment: No dose adjustment. **Moderate to severe impairment:** Avoid use.

SIDE EFFECTS

Rare (3%–1%): Wound secretion/oozing, extremity pain, muscle spasm, syncope, pruritus.

ADVERSE EFFECTS/TOXIC REACTIONS

Increased risk of bleeding/hemorrhagic events including retroperitoneal hemorrhage, cerebral hemorrhage, subdural hematoma, epidural/spinal hematoma (esp. with epidural catheters, spinal trauma). Serious reactions including jaundice, cholestasis, cytolytic hepatitis, Stevens-Johnson syndrome, hypersensitivity reaction, anaphylaxis reported.

NURSING CONSIDERATIONS

BASELINE ASSESSMENT

Obtain CBC, serum chemistries, PT/INR, vital signs, urine pregnancy if applicable. Obtain EKG for pts with a history of atrial fibrillation. Question for history of bleeding disorders, recent surgery, spinal punctures, intracranial hemorrhage, bleeding ulcers, open wounds, anemia, renal/hepatic impairment. Receive full medication history including herbal products.

INTERVENTION/EVALUATION

Monitor CBC, serum chemistries, renal function, occult urine/stool. Be alert for complaints of abdominal/back pain,

headache, confusion, weakness, vision change (may indicate hemorrhage). Question for increased menstrual bleeding/discharge. Assess peripheral pulses; skin for ecchymosis, petechiae. Check for excessive bleeding from minor cuts, scratches. Assess urine output for hematuria. Immediately report suspected pregnancy.

PATIENT/FAMILY TEACHING

• Do not take/discontinue any medication except on advice of physician. • Avoid alcohol, aspirin, NSAIDs. • Consult physician before surgery, dental work. • Use electric razor, soft toothbrush to prevent bleeding. • Report any unusual bleeding/bruising, spinal/epidural hematomas (e.g., tingling, numbness, muscular weakness). • Report if pregnant or planning to become pregnant. • Avoid grapefruit products.

rivastigmine

riv-a-**stig**-meen
(Apo-Rivastigmine ✦, Exelon, Novo-Rivastigmine ✦)

◆CLASSIFICATION

PHARMACOTHERAPEUTIC: Acetylcholinesterase inhibitor. **CLINICAL:** Anti-Alzheimer's dementia agent.

USES

Treatment of mild to severe dementia of Alzheimer's or mild to moderate dementia of Parkinson's disease. **OFF-LABEL:** Lewy body dementia.

PRECAUTIONS

Contraindications: Hypersensitivity to rivastigmine, other carbamate derivatives (e.g., neostigmine), history of application site reactions with rivastigmine patch. **Cautions:** Peptic ulcer disease, concurrent use of NSAIDs, sick sinus syndrome, bradycardia or supraventricular conduction defects, urinary obstruction, seizure

R

disorders, asthma, COPD, pts with body weight less than 50 kg.

ACTION

Increases acetylcholine in CNS by inhibiting hydrolysis by cholinesterase. **Therapeutic Effect:** Slows progression of symptoms of Alzheimer's disease, dementia of Parkinson's disease.

PHARMACOKINETICS

Rapidly, completely absorbed. Protein binding: 40%. Widely distributed throughout body. Rapidly, extensively metabolized. Primarily excreted in urine. **Half-life:** 1.5 hrs.

⌛ LIFESPAN CONSIDERATIONS

Pregnancy/Lactation: Unknown if distributed in breast milk. **Children:** Not indicated for use in this pt population. **Elderly:** No age-related precautions noted.

INTERACTIONS

DRUG: May interfere with **anticholinergics** (e.g., **dicyclomine, glycopyrrolate, scopolamine**) effects. May have additive effect with **bethanechol.** **NSAIDs** may increase GI effects, irritation. **HERBAL:** Ginkgo biloba may increase cholinergic effects. **FOOD:** None known. **LAB VALUES:** None significant.

AVAILABILITY (Rx)

Solution, Oral: 2 mg/mL. **Transdermal Patch:** 4.6 mg/24 hrs, 9.5 mg/24 hrs, 13.3 mg/24 hrs.

 Capsules: 1.5 mg, 3 mg, 4.5 mg, 6 mg.

ADMINISTRATION/HANDLING

PO

• Give morning and evening doses with food. • Give capsule whole. • **Oral Solution:** May swallow directly from syringe or mixed with water, soda, or cold fruit juice. Stir well; use within 4 hrs of mixing.

Transdermal Patch

• May apply the day following the last oral dose. • Apply to upper or lower back, upper arm, or chest. • Avoid reapplication to same spot of skin for 14 days. • Do not apply to red, irritated, or broken skin. • Avoid eye contact. • After removal, fold patch to press adhesive together and discard.

INDICATIONS/ROUTES/DOSAGE

Alzheimer's Dementia (Mild to Moderate)
PO: ADULTS, ELDERLY: Initially, 1.5 mg twice daily. May increase at intervals of at least 2 wks to 3 mg twice daily, then 4.5 mg twice daily, and finally 6 mg twice daily. **Maximum:** 6 mg twice daily. **Transdermal:** Initially, 4.6 mg/24 hrs. May increase at intervals of at least 4 wks to 9.5 mg/24 hrs and then to 13.3 mg/24 hrs.

Alzheimer's Dementia (Severe)
Transdermal: ADULTS, ELDERLY: Initially, 4.6 mg/24 hrs. May increase at intervals of at least 4 wks to 9.5 mg/24 hrs and then to 13.3 mg/24 hrs.

Parkinson's Dementia
PO: ADULTS, ELDERLY: Initially, 1.5 mg twice daily. May increase at intervals of at least 4 wks to 3 mg twice daily, then 4.5 mg twice daily, and finally 6 mg twice daily. **Maximum:** 6 mg twice daily. **Transdermal Dosage: Note:** Initially, 4.6 mg/24 hrs. May increase after 4 wks to 9.5 mg/24 hrs and then to 13.3 mg/24 hrs.

Dosage in Renal Impairment
No dose adjustment.

Dosage in Hepatic Impairment
Oral: No dose adjustment. **Transdermal:** Maximum dose: 4.6 mg/24 hrs.

SIDE EFFECTS

Frequent (47%–17%): Nausea, vomiting, dizziness, diarrhea, headache, anorexia. **Occasional (13%–6%):** Abdominal pain, insomnia, dyspepsia (heartburn, indigestion, epigastric pain), confusion, UTI, depression. **Rare (5%–3%):** Anxiety, drowsiness, constipation, malaise, hallucinations, tremor, flatulence, rhinitis, hypertension, flu-like symptoms, weight loss, syncope.

R

ADVERSE EFFECTS/ TOXIC REACTIONS

Overdose can produce cholinergic crisis, characterized by severe nausea/vomiting, increased salivation, diaphoresis, bradycardia, hypotension, respiratory depression, seizures.

NURSING CONSIDERATIONS

BASELINE ASSESSMENT

Obtain baseline vital signs. Assess history for peptic ulcer, urinary obstruction, asthma, COPD, cardiac disease. Assess cognitive, behavioral, functional deficits.

INTERVENTION/EVALUATION

Monitor for cholinergic reaction: GI discomfort/cramping, feeling of facial warmth, excessive salivation, diaphoresis, lacrimation, pallor, urinary urgency, dizziness. Monitor for nausea, diarrhea, headache, insomnia.

PATIENT/ FAMILY TEACHING

• Take with meals (at breakfast, dinner). • Swallow capsule whole. Do not break, chew, or divide capsules. • Report nausea, vomiting, diarrhea, diaphoresis, increased salivary secretions, severe abdominal pain, dizziness.

rizatriptan

rye-za-trip-tan
(Apo-Rizatriptan ✤, Maxalt, Maxalt-MLT, Maxalt RPD ✤)

◆CLASSIFICATION

PHARMACOTHERAPEUTIC: Serotonin 5-HT$_1$ receptor agonist. **CLINICAL:** Antimigraine.

USES

Treatment of acute migraine headache with or without aura.

PRECAUTIONS

Contraindications: Hypersensitivity to rizatriptan. Basilar or hemiplegic migraine, history of stroke or transient ischemic attack; severe cardiovascular disease, coronary artery vasospasm, peripheral vascular disease, ischemic bowel disease, uncontrolled hypertension, use within 24 hrs of ergotamine-containing preparations or another serotonin receptor agonist, MAOI use within 14 days. **Cautions:** Mild to moderate renal/hepatic impairment, dialysis pts, elderly pts, pt profile suggesting cardiovascular risks (e.g., hypertension, diabetes, hypercholesterolemia).

ACTION

Binds selectively to serotonin 5-HT$_1$ receptors in cranial arteries producing vasoconstriction. **Therapeutic Effect:** Relieves migraine headache.

PHARMACOKINETICS

Well absorbed after PO administration. Protein binding: 14%. Crosses blood-brain barrier. Metabolized by liver. Excreted primarily in urine (82%), feces (12%). **Half-life:** 2–3 hrs.

⧖ LIFESPAN CONSIDERATIONS

Pregnancy/Lactation: Unknown if drug is distributed in breast milk. **Children:** Safety and efficacy not established. **Elderly:** No age-related precautions noted.

INTERACTIONS

DRUG: Ergotamine-containing medications may produce vasospastic reaction. **FLUoxetine, fluvoxaMINE, PARoxetine, sertraline** may produce hyperreflexia, incoordination, weakness. **MAOIs (e.g., phenelzine, selegiline), propranolol** may dramatically increase concentration (avoid concurrent use). **HERBAL:** None significant. **FOOD: All foods** delay peak drug concentration by 1 hr. **LAB VALUES:** None significant.

R

✤ Canadian trade name   🗣 Non-Crushable Drug   🔲 High Alert drug

AVAILABILITY (Rx)

Tablets (Maxalt): 5 mg, 10 mg. **Tablets (Orally Disintegrating [Maxalt-MLT]):** 5 mg, 10 mg.

ADMINISTRATION/HANDLING

PO

• Orally disintegrating tablet is packaged in individual aluminum pouch. • Open packet with dry hands. • Place tablet onto tongue, allow to dissolve, swallow with saliva. Administration with water is not necessary.

INDICATIONS/ROUTES/DOSAGE

Acute Migraine Headache

PO: ADULTS OLDER THAN 18 YRS, ELDERLY: 5–10 mg. If significant improvement is not attained, dose may be repeated after 2 hrs. **Maximum:** 30 mg/24 hrs. (Use 5 mg/dose in pts taking propranolol with maximum of 15 mg/24 hrs.) **CHILDREN 6–17 YRS WEIGHING 40 KG OR GREATER:** 10 mg as single dose. (Maximum 5 mg as single dose with propranolol.) **WEIGHING LESS THAN 40 KG:** 5 mg as a single dose. (Not recommended if taking propranolol.)

Dosage in Renal/Hepatic Impairment
No dose adjustment.

SIDE EFFECTS

Frequent (9%–7%): Dizziness, drowsiness, paresthesia, fatigue. **Occasional (6%–3%):** Nausea, chest pressure, dry mouth. **Rare (2%):** Headache; neck, throat, jaw pressure; photosensitivity.

ADVERSE EFFECTS/TOXIC REACTIONS

Cardiac reactions (ischemia, coronary artery vasospasm, MI), noncardiac vasospasm-related reactions (hemorrhage, CVA) occur rarely, particularly in pts with hypertension, diabetes, strong family history of coronary artery disease, obesity, smokers, males older than 40 yrs, postmenopausal women.

NURSING CONSIDERATIONS

BASELINE ASSESSMENT

Question for history of peripheral vascular disease, renal/hepatic impairment. Question pt regarding onset, location, duration of migraine, possible precipitating symptoms.

INTERVENTION/EVALUATION

Monitor for evidence of dizziness. Assess for photophobia, phonophobia (sound sensitivity, nausea, vomiting), relief of migraine headache.

PATIENT/FAMILY TEACHING

• Take single dose as soon as symptoms of an actual migraine headache appear. • Medication is intended to relieve migraine, not to prevent or reduce number of attacks. • Avoid tasks that require alertness, motor skills until response to drug is established. • Report immediately if palpitations, pain/tightness in chest/throat, pain/weakness of extremities occurs. • Do not remove orally disintegrating tablet from blister pack until just before dosing. • Use protective measures against exposure to UV light, sunlight (sunscreen, protective clothing).

roflumilast

roe-**floo**-mi-last
(Daliresp, Daxas ✦)

◆CLASSIFICATION

PHARMACOTHERAPEUTIC: Phosphodiesterase 4 (PDE4) inhibitor. **CLINICAL:** Anti-COPD agent.

USES

Adjunct to bronchodilator therapy for maintenance treatment of severe COPD associated with chronic bronchitis and history of exacerbations.

PRECAUTIONS

Contraindications: Hypersensitivity to roflumilast. Moderate to severe hepatic impairment. **Cautions:** Mild hepatic impairment, history of depression, suicidal ideation. Not indicated as bronchodilator or for relief of acute bronchospasm.

ACTION

Selectively inhibits PDE4, causing an accumulation of cyclic AMP within inflammatory/structural cells necessary in pathogenesis of COPD. Produces antiinflammatory effects. **Therapeutic Effect:** Reduces risk of exacerbation of COPD/chronic bronchitis.

PHARMACOKINETICS

Readily absorbed after PO administration. Maximum plasma concentration: 0.5–2 hrs. Protein binding: 99%. Metabolized in liver. Primarily excreted in urine (70%). **Half-life:** 17 hrs.

⌛ LIFESPAN CONSIDERATIONS

Pregnancy/Lactation: Unknown if distributed in breast milk. Not recommended for nursing mothers. **Children:** Safety and efficacy not established. **Elderly:** No age-related precautions noted.

INTERACTIONS

DRUG: CYP3A4 inducers (e.g., car-BAMazepine, phenytoin, rifAMPin) may decrease efficacy. **CYP3A4 inhibitors (e.g., erythromycin, ketoconazole)** may increase concentration. **HERBAL:** None significant. **FOOD:** None known. **LAB VALUES:** None significant.

AVAILABILITY (Rx)

Tablets: 500 mcg.

ADMINISTRATION/HANDLING

PO
• Give without regard to food.

INDICATIONS/ROUTES/DOSAGE

Adjunct in Severe COPD
PO: ADULTS, ELDERLY: 500 mcg once daily.

Dosage in Renal Impairment
No dose adjustment.

Dosage in Hepatic Impairment
Mild impairment: No dose adjustment. **Moderate to severe impairment:** Contraindicated.

SIDE EFFECTS

Occasional (10%–4%): Diarrhea, nausea, headache. **Rare (3%–2%):** Back pain, flu-like symptoms, insomnia, dizziness, decreased appetite, vomiting, abdominal pain, rhinitis, muscle spasm, tremor, dyspepsia.

ADVERSE EFFECTS/ TOXIC REACTIONS

Psychiatric events including worsening depression, suicidal ideation, anxiety reported in less than 2% of pts. Moderate to severe weight loss may result in discontinuation.

NURSING CONSIDERATIONS

BASELINE ASSESSMENT

Assess vital signs, O_2 saturation, lung sounds, body weight. Question for history of depression, anxiety, suicidal ideation, dehydration, COPD, hepatic impairment. Assess plans for breastfeeding. Obtain full medication history.

INTERVENTION/EVALUATION

Monitor vital signs, O_2 saturation, mental status, body weight. Assess for dehydration if diarrhea occurs (skin turgor, mucous membranes, decreased urine output, dizziness, dry mouth).

PATIENT/FAMILY TEACHING

• Report changes in mood or behavior, thoughts of suicide, insomnia, anxiety. • Report any weight loss. • Increase fluid intake if dehydration is suspected. • Worsening cough, fever, difficulty breathing may indicate exacerbation/infection. • Immediately report if pregnancy is suspected.

R

rolapitant

roe-**la**-pi-tant
(Varubi)
Do not confuse rolapitant with aprepitant, fosaprepitant.

◆CLASSIFICATION

PHARMACOTHERAPEUTIC: Substance P/neurokinin (P/NK) receptor antagonist. **CLINICAL:** Antinausea, antiemetic.

USES

Prevention of delayed nausea and vomiting associated with initial and repeat courses of emetogenic cancer chemotherapy, including, but not limited to, highly emetogenic chemotherapy, in combination with other antiemetic agents.

PRECAUTIONS

Contraindications: Hypersensitivity to rolapitant. Concomitant use of thioridazine. **Cautions:** Mild to moderate hepatic impairment, pts at risk for QT interval prolongation or ventricular arrhythmia (congenital long QT syndrome, medications that prolong QT interval, hypokalemia, hypomagnesemia). Not recommended in severe hepatic impairment.

ACTION

Antagonizes human substance P/NK₁ receptors. **Therapeutic Effect:** Decreases nausea and vomiting associated with chemotherapy.

PHARMACOKINETICS

Readily absorbed. Widely distributed. Metabolized in liver. Protein binding: greater than 99%. Peak plasma concentration: 4 hrs. Excreted in urine (14%), feces (73%). **Half-life:** 158 hrs.

⧗ LIFESPAN CONSIDERATIONS

Pregnancy/Lactation: Safety and efficacy not established during pregnancy. Unknown if distributed in breast milk. **Children:** Safety and efficacy not established. **Elderly:** No age-related precautions noted.

INTERACTIONS

DRUG: Thioridazine may increase risk of torsades de pointes, QT internal prolongation (contraindicated). **Strong CYP3A inducers** (e.g., **rifAMPin**) may decrease concentration/effect. May increase concentration/effect of **BCRP substrates** (e.g., **methotrexate, rosuvastatin**), **CYP2D6 substrates** (e.g., **pimozide**), **P-gp substrates** (e.g., **digoxin**). **QT interval–prolonging medications** (e.g., **amiodarone, azithromycin, ceritinib, haloperidol, moxifloxacin**) may increase risk of QT interval prolongation, cardiac arrhythmias. **HERBAL: St. John's wort** may decrease concentration/effect. **FOOD:** None significant. **LAB VALUES:** May decrease Hct, Hgb, neutrophils, RBC.

AVAILABILITY (Rx)

Emulsion, IV: 166.5 mg/92.5 ml. **Tablets:** 90 mg.

ADMINISTRATION/HANDLING

 IV

Rate of Administration • Infuse over 30 minutes. Do not dilute. • Solution is compatible with 0.9% NaCl, D5W or Lactated Ringers via Y-site.
Storage • Store at room temperature.

PO
• Administer approx. 1–2 hrs prior to chemotherapy. • Give without regard to meals. Administer prior to initiation of each chemotherapy cycle at no less than 2-wk intervals.

INDICATIONS/ROUTES/DOSAGE

Chemotherapy-Associated Nausea/Vomiting
PO: ADULTS, ELDERLY: 180 mg once on day 1 (in combination with dexamethasone and a 5-HT₃ receptor antagonist). Do not give rolapitant at intervals of less than 2 wks. **IV: ADULTS, ELDERLY:** 166.5 mg given within 2 hrs prior to initiation of chemotherapy on day 1.

Dosage in Renal Impairment
Mild to moderate impairment: No dose adjustment. **Severe impairment:** Not specified; use caution.

Dosage in Hepatic Impairment
Mild to moderate impairment: No
dose adjustment. **Severe impairment:**
Treatment not recommended.

SIDE EFFECTS

Occasional (9%–6%): Decreased appetite,
hiccups, dizziness. **Rare (4%–3%):** Abdominal pain.

ADVERSE EFFECTS/
TOXIC REACTIONS

Torsades de pointes, QT prolongation reported in pts taking thioridazine concomitantly; avoid use. Baseline electrolyte imbalance may increase risk of arrhythmias.

NURSING CONSIDERATIONS

BASELINE ASSESSMENT

Obtain CBC, BMP, serum magnesium.
Question history of arrhythmias, hepatic
impairment, congenital long QT syndrome. Receive medication history and
screen for interactions. Assess hydration
status. Obtain EKG in pts taking concomitant drugs that prolong QT interval.

INTERVENTION/EVALUATION

Periodically monitor CBC, BMP. Monitor
hydration, nutritional status, I&O. Correct electrolyte imbalances prior to each
dose. If CYP2D6 substrate medications
cannot be withheld, diligently monitor for
QT interval prolongation, ventricular arrhythmias. Assist with ambulation if dizziness occurs. Assess for anemia-related
symptoms.

PATIENT/FAMILY TEACHING

• Therapy may alter effectiveness of other
drugs. Do not take any newly prescribed
medications unless approved by doctor
who originally started treatment. • Report symptoms of arrhythmias such as
chest pain, dizziness, fainting, fatigue, palpitations, shortness of breath. • Do not
take herbal products or ingest grapefruit
products. • Report persistent nausea,
vomiting despite treatment.

romiDEPsin

roe-mi-**dep**-sin
(Istodax)
**Do not confuse romiDEPsin with
romiPLOStim.**

◆CLASSIFICATION

PHARMACOTHERAPEUTIC: Histone
deacetylase inhibitor. **CLINICAL:** Antineoplastic.

USES

Treatment of refractory cutaneous T-cell
lymphoma (CTCL) or refractory peripheral T-cell lymphoma (PTCL).

PRECAUTIONS

Contraindications: Hypersensitivity to
romiDEPsin. **Cautions:** Moderate or
severe hepatic impairment, end-stage
renal impairment, preexisting cardiac
disease, pts with QT interval prolongation, concomitant administration of
medications prolonging QT interval,
hypokalemia, hypomagnesemia. Avoid
concomitant strong CYP3A4 inhibi-
tors/inducers; caution with moderate
CYP3A4 inhibitors or P-glycoprotein
inhibitors.

ACTION

Inhibits histone deacetylase resulting in
acetyl group accumulation, which alters
chromatin structure, terminating cell
growth. **Therapeutic Effect:** Induces
cell-cycle arrest, cell death.

PHARMACOKINETICS

Extensively metabolized. Protein binding:
92%–94%. **Half-life:** 3 hrs.

⧗ LIFESPAN CONSIDERATIONS

Pregnancy/Lactation: May cause fetal
harm. Unknown if distributed in breast
milk. **Children:** Safety and efficacy not
established. **Elderly:** No age-related
precautions noted.

R

INTERACTIONS

DRUG: Coumarin-derivative anticoagulants prolong PT, INR. **Strong CYP3A4 inhibitors** (e.g., **clarithromycin, itraconazole, ritonavir**) may increase concentration. Potent **CYP3A4 inducers** (e.g., **carBAMazepine, PHENobarbital, rifabutin, rifAMPin**) may decrease concentration. **QT interval–prolonging medications** (e.g., **amiodarone, azithromycin, ceritinib, haloperidol, moxifloxacin**) may increase risk of QT interval prolongation, cardiac arrhythmias. **HERBAL:** **St. John's wort** may increase metabolism and decrease concentration. **FOOD:** **Grapefruit products** may increase concentration/effects. **LAB VALUES:** May decrease Hgb, Hct, WBC count, platelets, serum magnesium, calcium, potassium, sodium, albumin, phosphates. May increase serum glucose, ALT, AST, uric acid. May alter serum magnesium.

AVAILABILITY (Rx)

Injection, Powder for Reconstitution, 2-Vial Kit: 10 mg.

ADMINISTRATION/HANDLING

Reconstitution • Reconstitute powder with 2 mL of supplied diluent (80% propylene glycol, 20% dehydrated alcohol). • Swirl contents gently to dissolve powder. • Reconstituted solution provides 5 mg/mL. Further dilute in 500 mL 0.9% NaCl.
Rate of Administration • Infuse over 4 hrs.
Storage • Reconstituted solution is stable for at least 24 hrs at room temperature. • Solution appears clear, colorless. Discard if precipitate is present or solution is discolored.

INDICATIONS/ROUTES/DOSAGE

CTCL, PTCL
IV: ADULTS, ELDERLY: 14 mg/m^2 administered over 4 hrs on days 1, 8, and 15 of a 28-day cycle. Repeat cycles every 28 days if pt continues to benefit from and tolerates therapy.

Dose Modification
Hematologic Toxicity
Grade 3 or 4 neutropenia or thrombocytopenia: Delay treatment until ANC 1,500 cells/mm^3 or more and/or platelets 75,000 cells/mm^3 or more (or baseline), then resume at 14 mg/m^2.
Grade 4 neutropenia or thrombocytopenia requiring platelet transfusion: Delay treatment until recovered to grade 1 or 0 (or baseline), then permanently reduce dose to 10 mg/m^2.
Nonhematologic Toxicity (Excluding Alopecia)
Grade 2 or 3 toxicity: Delay treatment until recovered to grade 1 or 0 (or baseline); may restart at 14 mg/m^2.
Grade 4, recurrent grade 3 toxicity: Delay treatment until recovered to grade 1 or 0 (or baseline), then permanently reduce dose to 10 mg/m^2.
Recurrent grade 3 or 4 toxicity (with dose reduction): Permanently discontinue.

Dosage in Renal Impairment
No dose adjustment. Use caution in end-stage-renal disease.

Dosage in Hepatic Impairment
Mild impairment: No dose adjustment. **Moderate to severe impairment:** Use caution.

SIDE EFFECTS

Frequent (57%–23%): Nausea, fatigue, vomiting, anorexia. **Occasional (20%–7%):** Diarrhea, fever, distorted sense of taste, constipation, hypotension, pruritus. **Rare (4%–2%):** Dermatitis, T-wave and ST-wave changes on EKG.

ADVERSE EFFECTS/ TOXIC REACTIONS

Infection (47% of pts), including sepsis, arrhythmias, acute respiratory distress syndrome, acute renal failure. Anemia occurs in 19% of pts, thrombocytopenia in 17% of pts, neutropenia in 11% of pts.

NURSING CONSIDERATIONS

BASELINE ASSESSMENT

Provide emotional support. Baseline CBC, BMP, LFT, PT/INR, serum magnesium, ionized calcium; capillary blood glucose; EKG should be obtained prior to therapy at baseline and routinely thereafter. Inform women of childbearing potential of risk to fetus if pregnancy occurs.

INTERVENTION/EVALUATION

Calculate daily absolute neutrophil count (ANC). Closely monitor hematologic, chemistry parameters, EKG. Diligently monitor for infection. Provide antiemetics to control nausea/vomiting.

PATIENT/FAMILY TEACHING

• Diarrhea may cause dehydration, electrolyte depletion. • Do not have immunizations without physician's approval (lowers body's resistance). • Avoid contact with those who recently received live virus vaccine. • Avoid crowds, those with infection. • May reduce effectiveness of estrogen-containing contraceptives. • Report excessive nausea or vomiting, palpitations, chest pain, shortness of breath. Seek immediate medical attention if unusual bleeding occurs.

romiPLOStim

roe-mye-**ploe**-stim
(Nplate)
Do not confuse romiPLOStim with romiDEPsin.

◆CLASSIFICATION

PHARMACOTHERAPEUTIC: Recombinant fusion protein, thrombopoietin receptor agonist. **CLINICAL:** Hematologic agent.

USES

Treatment of thrombocytopenia in pts with chronic immune (idiopathic) thrombocytopenic purpura (ITP) who have had an insufficient response to corticosteroids, immunoglobulins, or splenectomy.

PRECAUTIONS

Contraindications: Hypersensitivity to romiPLOStim. **Cautions:** Myelodysplastic syndrome, hematologic malignancy, hepatic impairment, history of cerebrovascular disease, concurrent anticoagulants or antiplatelet medication.

ACTION

Binds and activates thrombopoietin (TPO) receptors on hematopoietic cells. **Therapeutic Effect:** Increases platelet production.

PHARMACOKINETICS

Concentration is dependent on dose and baseline platelet count. Peak concentration occurs in 7–50 hrs (median, 14 hrs). **Half-life:** 1–34 days (median, 3.5 days).

⧗ LIFESPAN CONSIDERATIONS

Pregnancy/Lactation: Studies suggest drug crosses placenta, is distributed in breast milk. **Children:** Safety and efficacy not established in pts younger than 18 yrs. **Elderly:** Age-related renal, hepatic, cardiac abnormalities may require dosage adjustment.

INTERACTIONS

DRUG: Anticoagulants (e.g., **apixaban, heparin, warfarin**), antiplatelets (e.g., **aspirin, clopidogrel**) may increase risk of bleeding. **HERBAL:** None significant. **FOOD:** None known. **LAB VALUES:** Increases platelet count.

AVAILABILITY (Rx)

Injection, Powder for Reconstitution: 250-mcg, 500-mcg single-use vial.

ADMINISTRATION/HANDLING

◀**ALERT**▶ Use syringe with 0.01-mL graduations for reconstitution.

R

SQ

Reconstitution • Reconstitute 0.72 mL Sterile Water for Injection to 250-mcg single-use vial for final concentration of 500 mcg/mL. • Reconstitute 1.2 mL Sterile Water for Injection to 500-mcg single-use vial for final concentration of 500 mcg/mL. • Gently swirl and invert vial to reconstitute; do not shake. • Dissolution takes less than 2 min. • Inject at abdomen, thigh, upper arm. • Do not inject at sites that are bruised, red, tender, or indurated. **Storage** • Refrigerate unreconstituted vial. • Reconstituted solution can be kept at room temperature or refrigerated for up to 24 hrs. • Protect reconstituted solution from light. • Do not use if discolored or particulate is present. • Discard unused portion.

INDICATIONS/ROUTES/DOSAGE

Thrombocytopenia
SQ: ADULTS, ELDERLY: Initially, 1 mcg/kg once wkly based on actual body weight. Adjust wkly doses by increments of 1 mcg/kg to achieve platelet count 50,000/mm^3 or greater and reduce risk of bleeding. **Maximum:** 10 mcg/kg wkly.

Dosage Adjustments

Platelet Count	Dose
Less than 50,000/mm^3	Increase by 1 mcg/kg
Greater than 200,000/mm^3 for 2 consecutive wks	Reduce by 1 mcg/kg
Greater than 400,000/mm^3	Hold dose

Dosage in Renal/Hepatic Impairment
No dose adjustment.

SIDE EFFECTS

Frequent (35%–26%): Headache, arthralgia. **Occasional (17%–6%):** Dizziness, insomnia, myalgia, extremity pain, abdominal pain, shoulder pain, paresthesia, dyspepsia.

ADVERSE EFFECTS/ TOXIC REACTIONS

Reticulin fiber deposits within the bone marrow, progressing to bone marrow fibrosis may occur. Worsening thrombocytopenia may be noted. Discontinuation of therapy may result in thrombocytopenia of greater severity than baseline, increasing risk of bleeding. Thromboembolic effects may occur. Increases risk of hematologic malignancies.

NURSING CONSIDERATIONS

BASELINE ASSESSMENT

Establish baseline CBC with differential prior to initiation, wkly during therapy and for 2 wks following discontinuation. Assess extent of RBC, WBC abnormalities. Question medical history as listed in Precautions.

INTERVENTION/EVALUATION

Monitor CBC with differential wkly during dose adjustment phase and then monthly following establishment of a stable dose.

PATIENT/FAMILY TEACHING

• Report if bruising, bleeding occur.
• Essential to receive drug therapy at scheduled times or risk of bleeding may occur.

rOPINIRole

roe-**pin**-i-role
(Requip, Requip XL)
Do not confuse rOPINIRole with RisperDAL or risperiDONE.

◆CLASSIFICATION

PHARMACOTHERAPEUTIC: DOPamine agonist. **CLINICAL:** Antiparkinson agent.

USES

Treatment of signs/symptoms of idiopathic Parkinson's disease. **Immediate-release only:** Treatment of moderate to severe primary restless legs syndrome (RLS).

PRECAUTIONS

Contraindications: Hypersensitivity to rOPINIRole. **Cautions:** History of orthostatic hypotension, cardiovascular or cerebrovascular disease, syncope, hallucinations (esp. in elderly pts), concurrent use of CNS depressants, preexisting dyskinesia, hepatic or severe renal dysfunction (end-stage renal disease [ESRD]), major psychotic disorder, elderly pts.

ACTION

Stimulates postsynaptic DOPamine receptors in caudate putamen in the brain. **Therapeutic Effect:** Relieves signs/symptoms of Parkinson's disease.

PHARMACOKINETICS

Rapidly absorbed after PO administration. Protein binding: 40%. Widely distributed. Extensively metabolized. Steady-state concentrations achieved within 2 days. Excreted in urine. Unknown if removed by hemodialysis. **Half-life:** 6 hrs.

⧗ LIFESPAN CONSIDERATIONS

Pregnancy/Lactation: Distributed in breast milk. Drug activity possible in breastfeeding infant. **Children:** Safety and efficacy not established. **Elderly:** No age-related precautions noted, but hallucinations may occur more frequently.

INTERACTIONS

DRUG: Ciprofloxacin may increase concentration. **Alcohol, CNS depressants (e.g., LORazepam, morphine, zolpidem)** may increase CNS depressant effects. **HERBAL: Gotu kola, kava kava, St. John's wort, valerian** may increase CNS depression. **FOOD: All foods** delay peak plasma levels by 1 hr but do not affect drug absorption. **LAB VALUES:** May increase serum alkaline phosphatase.

AVAILABILITY (Rx)

Tablets: 0.25 mg, 0.5 mg, 1 mg, 2 mg, 3 mg, 4 mg, 5 mg.

Tablets, Extended-Release: 2 mg, 4 mg, 6 mg, 8 mg, 12 mg.

ADMINISTRATION/HANDLING

PO
• May give without regard to meals.
• Do not break, crush, dissolve, or divide extended-release tablets.

INDICATIONS/ROUTES/DOSAGE

Parkinson's Disease
PO: (Immediate-Release): ADULTS, ELDERLY: Initially, 0.25 mg 3 times/day based on individual pt response. Dosage should be titrated with wkly increments as noted:
Week 1: 0.25 mg 3 times/day; total daily dose: 0.75 mg.
Week 2: 0.5 mg 3 times/day; total daily dose: 1.5 mg.
Week 3: 0.75 mg 3 times/day; total daily dose: 2.25 mg.
Week 4: 1 mg 3 times/day; total daily dose: 3 mg.
After week 4, may increase dose by 1.5 mg/day on wkly basis up to dose of 9 mg/day. May then further increase by 3 mg/day on wkly basis up to total dose of 24 mg/day (ESRD: 18 mg).
(Extended-Release): Initially, 2 mg once daily for 1–2 wks. May increase by 2 mg/day at 1 wk or longer interval. **Maximum:** 24 mg/day. ESRD: 18 mg.

Discontinuation Taper
Gradually taper over 7 days as follows: Decrease frequency from 3 times/day to twice daily for 4 days, then decrease from twice daily to once daily for remaining 3 days.

Restless Legs Syndrome
PO: (Immediate-Release): ADULTS, ELDERLY: 0.25 mg for days 1 and 2. May increase to 0.5 mg for days 3–7 and after 7 days to 1 mg daily. May further titrate upward in 0.5-mg increments q7days until reaching daily dose of 3 mg during week 6. Daily dose may be increased to maximum of 4 mg beginning week 7. Give all doses 1–3 hrs before bedtime. ESRD: 3 mg maximum.

R

Dosage in Renal/Hepatic Impairment
No dose adjustment. Use caution with severe renal impairment. Titrate cautiously in pts with hepatic impairment.

SIDE EFFECTS

Frequent (60%–40%): Nausea, dizziness, extreme drowsiness. **Occasional (12%–5%):** Syncope, vomiting, fatigue, viral infection, dyspepsia, diaphoresis, asthenia, orthostatic hypotension, abdominal discomfort, pharyngitis, abnormal vision, dry mouth, hypertension, hallucinations, confusion. **Rare (Less Than 4%):** Anorexia, peripheral edema, memory loss, rhinitis, sinusitis, palpitations, impotence.

ADVERSE EFFECTS/ TOXIC REACTIONS

Dyskinesia, impulsive/compulsive behavior (pathologic gambling, hypersexuality, binge eating) occur rarely.

NURSING CONSIDERATIONS

BASELINE ASSESSMENT

Parkinson's disease: Assess signs/symptoms (e.g., tremor, gait). **Restless legs syndrome:** Assess frequency of symptoms, sleep pattern.

INTERVENTION/EVALUATION

Assess for clinical improvement, clinical reversal of symptoms (improvement of tremors of head/hands at rest, masklike facial expression, shuffling gait, muscular rigidity). Assist with ambulation if dizziness occurs. Monitor B/P, daytime alertness.

PATIENT/FAMILY TEACHING

• Drowsiness, dizziness may be an initial response to drug. • Postural hypotension may occur more frequently during initial therapy. Slowly go from lying to standing. • Avoid tasks that require alertness, motor skills until response to drug is established. • If nausea occurs, take medication with food. • Hallucinations may occur, more so in the elderly than in younger pts with Parkinson's disease. • Report occurrence of falling asleep during activities of daily living, new or worsening symptoms, changes in B/P, fainting, unusual urges. • Avoid alcohol.

rosuvastatin

roe-**soo**-va-**sta**-tin
(Apo-Rosuvastatin ✱, <u>Crestor</u>)
Do not confuse rosuvastatin with atorvastatin, lovastatin, nystatin, pitavastatin, or simvastatin.

◆CLASSIFICATION

PHARMACOTHERAPEUTIC: HMG-CoA reductase inhibitor. **CLINICAL:** Antihyperlipidemic.

USES

Adjunct to diet therapy in pts with primary hyperlipidemia and mixed dyslipidemia; to decrease elevated total, LDL cholesterol, serum triglyceride levels; increases HDL. Adjunct to diet to slow progression of atherosclerosis in pts with elevated cholesterol. Treatment of primary dysbetalipoproteinemia, homozygous familial hypercholesterolemia (FH). Treatment of pts ages 10–17 yrs with heterozygous familial hypercholesterolemia (HeFH) to reduce elevated total cholesterol, LDL cholesterol, and apolipoprotein B. Primary prevention of cardiovascular disease (risk reduction of MI, stroke, arterial revascularization) without clinically evident CAD, but with multiple risk factors.

PRECAUTIONS

Contraindications: Hypersensitivity to rosuvastatin. Active hepatic disease, breastfeeding, pregnancy, unexplained, persistent elevations of hepatic enzymes. **Cautions:** Anticoagulant therapy, hepatic impairment, substantial alcohol consumption, elective major surgery, renal impairment, acute renal failure, uncontrolled hypothyroidism, elderly pts.

ACTION

Interferes with cholesterol biosynthesis by inhibiting conversion of the enzyme HMG-CoA to mevalonate, a precursor to cholesterol. **Therapeutic Effect:** Decreases LDL, VLDL, plasma triglyceride levels; increases HDL concentration.

PHARMACOKINETICS

Protein binding: 88%. Minimal hepatic metabolism. Primarily excreted in feces. **Half-life:** 19 hrs (increased in severe renal dysfunction).

⧗ LIFESPAN CONSIDERATIONS

Pregnancy/Lactation: Contraindicated in pregnancy (suppression of cholesterol biosynthesis may cause fetal toxicity), lactation. Risk of serious adverse reactions in breastfeeding infants. **Children:** Safety and efficacy not established in children younger than 7 yrs. **Elderly:** No age-related precautions noted.

INTERACTIONS

DRUG: **Aluminum- and magnesium-containing antacids** may decrease concentration/effects. Increased risk of myopathy with **cycloSPORINE, fibrate, gemfibrozil, niacin.** May increase concentrations of **estradiol, ethinyl, norgestrel.** Enhances anticoagulant effect of **warfarin. HERBAL:** None significant. **FOOD:** **Red yeast rice** contains 2.4 mg lovastatin per 600 mg rice. **LAB VALUES:** May increase serum alkaline phosphatase, bilirubin, creatinine phosphokinase, glucose, transaminases. May produce hematuria, proteinuria.

AVAILABILITY (Rx)

Tablets: 5 mg, 10 mg, 20 mg, 40 mg.

ADMINISTRATION/HANDLING

PO
• Give without regard to meals. May give at any time of day.

INDICATIONS/ROUTES/DOSAGE

Hyperlipidemia, Dyslipidemia, Atherosclerosis, Dysbetalipoproteinemia, Primary Prevention of Cardiovascular Disease
PO: ADULTS, ELDERLY: Usual starting dosage is 10 mg/day, with adjustments based on lipid levels; monitor q2–4wks until desired level is achieved. Lower starting dose of 5 mg is recommended in pts of Asian ancestry. **Maximum:** 40 mg/day. Range: 5–40 mg/day.

FH
PO: ADULTS, ELDERLY: Initially, 20 mg/day. Range: 5–40 mg/day. **Maximum:** 40 mg/day. **CHILDREN 7 YRS AND OLDER:** 20 mg once daily.

HeFH
PO: CHILDREN 10–17 YRS: Initially, 20 mg once daily. Range: 5–20 mg once daily. **8–9 YRS:** 5–10 mg once daily.

Concurrent CycloSPORINE Use
PO: ADULTS, ELDERLY: 5 mg/day maximum.

Concurrent Gemfibrozil, Atazanavir/ Ritonavir, Lopinavir/Ritonavir or Simeprevir Therapy
PO: ADULTS, ELDERLY: Initially, 5 mg/day. 10 mg/day maximum.

Dosage in Renal Impairment (CrCl Less Than 30 mL/min)
PO: ADULTS, ELDERLY: 5 mg/day; do not exceed 10 mg/day.

Dosage in Hepatic Impairment
Contraindicated in active in liver disease.

SIDE EFFECTS

Generally well tolerated. Side effects are usually mild, transient. **Occasional (9%–3%):** Pharyngitis, headache, diarrhea, dyspepsia, nausea, depression. **Rare (Less Than 3%):** Myalgia, asthenia, back pain.

R

ADVERSE EFFECTS/ TOXIC REACTIONS

Potential for ocular lens opacities. Hypersensitivity reaction, hepatitis, rhabdomyolysis occur rarely.

NURSING CONSIDERATIONS

BASELINE ASSESSMENT

Obtain dietary history, esp. fat consumption. Question for possibility of pregnancy. Assess baseline lab results: serum cholesterol, triglycerides, LFT.

INTERVENTION/EVALUATION

Monitor serum cholesterol, HDL, LDL, triglycerides for therapeutic response. Lipid levels should be monitored within 2–4 wks of initiation of therapy or change in dosage. Monitor LFT at 12 wks following initiation of therapy, at any elevation of dose, and periodically (e.g., semiannually) thereafter. Monitor CPK if myopathy is suspected. Monitor daily pattern of bowel activity, stool consistency. Assess for headache, sore throat. Be alert for myalgia, weakness.

PATIENT/FAMILY TEACHING

• Use appropriate contraceptive measures. • Periodic lab tests are essential part of therapy. • Maintain appropriate diet (important part of treatment). • Report unexplained muscle pain, tenderness, weakness, esp. if associated with fever, malaise.

rucaparib

roo-**kap**-a-rib
(Rubraca)
Do not confuse rucaparib with nertinib, niraparib, olaparib.

◆CLASSIFICATION

PHARMACOTHERAPEUTIC: Poly (ADP-ribose) polymerase (PARP) inhibitor. **CLINICAL:** Antineoplastic.

USES

Treatment of deleterious germline and/ or somatic BRCA mutation–associated (detected by FDA-approved test) advanced ovarian cancer in pts who have been treated with two or more lines of chemotherapy.

PRECAUTIONS

Contraindications: Hypersensitivity to rucaparib. **Cautions:** Baseline hematologic cytopenias (anemia, neutropenia, thrombocytopenia, lymphocytopenia).

ACTION

Inhibits poly (ADP-ribose) polymerase (PARP) enzymes (involved in DNA transcription, cell-cycle regulation, and DNA repair). By inhibiting PARP, may cause PARP DNA complexes resulting in DNA damage and cellular death. **Therapeutic Effect:** Inhibits tumor cell growth and metastasis.

PHARMACOKINETICS

Widely distributed. Metabolized in liver. Protein binding: 70%. Peak plasma concentration: 1.9 hrs. Excretion not specified. **Half-life:** 17–19 hrs.

⧗ LIFESPAN CONSIDERATIONS

Pregnancy/Lactation: Avoid pregnancy; may cause fetal harm. Females of reproductive potential should use effective contraception during treatment and up to 6 mos after discontinuation. Unknown if distributed in breast milk. Breastfeeding not recommended during treatment and for at least 2 wks after discontinuation. **Children:** Safety and efficacy not established. **Elderly:** No age-related precautions noted.

INTERACTIONS

DRUG: May decrease effect of **BCG vaccine. HERBAL:** None significant. **FOOD:** None known. **LAB VALUES:** May increase serum ALT, AST, cholesterol, creatinine. May decrease ANC, Hgb, absolute lymphocyte count, platelets.

R

AVAILABILITY (Rx)

Tablets: 200 mg, 250 mg, 300 mg.

ADMINISTRATION/HANDLING

PO

• Give with or without food. • If a dose is missed or vomiting occurs after administration, do not give extra dose. Administer next dose at regularly scheduled time.

INDICATIONS/ROUTES/DOSAGE

Note: Administer only to pts with deleterious germline and/or somatic BRCA mutation.

Ovarian Cancer

PO: ADULTS, ELDERLY: 600 mg twice daily about 12 hrs apart. Continue until disease progression or unacceptable toxicity.

Dose Reduction Schedule

Starting dose: 600 mg twice daily. **First dose reduction:** 500 mg twice daily. **Second dose reduction:** 400 mg twice daily. **Third dose reduction:** 300 mg twice daily.

Dose Modification

Adverse Events, Non-Hematologic Toxicity

Either withhold treatment or reduce dosage per dose reduction schedule.

Hematologic Toxicity

Withhold treatment until improved to CTCAE grade 1 or 0 and investigate cause. If myelodysplastic syndrome or acute myeloid leukemia confirmed, permanently discontinue.

Dosage in Renal Impairment

Mild to moderate impairment: No dose adjustment. **Severe impairment, ESRD:** Not specified; use caution.

Dosage in Hepatic Impairment

Mild impairment: No dose adjustment. **Moderate to severe impairment:** Not specified; use caution.

SIDE EFFECTS

Frequent (77%–21%): Nausea, asthenia, fatigue, vomiting, constipation, dysgeusia, decreased appetite, diarrhea, abdominal pain, dyspnea. **Occasional (17%–9%):** Dizziness, rash, pyrexia, photosensitivity reaction, pruritus.

ADVERSE EFFECTS/ TOXIC REACTIONS

Anemia, lymphopenia, neutropenia, thrombocytopenia are expected responses to therapy. Myelodysplastic syndrome/acute myeloid leukemia reported in less than 1% of pts. Infections including nasopharyngitis, pharyngitis, upper respiratory tract infection occurred in 43% of pts. Febrile neutropenia reported in less than 1% of pts. Palmarplantar erythrodysesthesia syndrome (PPES), a chemotherapy-induced skin condition, that presents with redness, swelling, numbness, skin sloughing of the hands and feet, was reported in 2% of pts.

NURSING CONSIDERATIONS

BASELINE ASSESSMENT

Obtain baseline CBC, vital signs, weight. Do not initiate therapy until pts have recovered from hematologic toxicities caused by previous chemotherapy. Obtain pregnancy test in females of reproductive potential. Question plans of breastfeeding. Question history of hepatic/renal impairment, hypercholesterolemia. Screen for risk of bleeding, active infection. Offer emotional support.

INTERVENTION/EVALUATION

Monitor CBC monthly; serum cholesterol, creatinine periodically. For prolonged hematologic toxicities caused by other chemotherapies, monitor CBC weekly until recovery. If hematologic levels have not recovered to CTCAE grade 1 or 0 after 4 wks, consider hematology consultation for further investigations including bone marrow analysis, blood sample for

R

cytogenetics. Diligently monitor for infection. Monitor for myelodysplastic syndrome, acute myeloid leukemia. Assess skin for rash, lesions, sloughing. Monitor for decreased urine output, renal dysfunction.

PATIENT/FAMILY TEACHING

• Treatment may depress your immune system response and reduce your ability to fight infection. Report symptoms of infection such as body aches, chills, cough, fatigue, fever. Avoid those with active infection. • Report bleeding or bruising easily, bloody urine or stool, frequent infections, fatigue, shortness of breath, weakness, weight loss; may indicate acute bone marrow depression or acute leukemia. • Avoid pregnancy; treatment may cause birth defects. Females of childbearing potential should use effective contraception during treatment and for at least 6 mos after last dose. • Do not breastfeed during treatment and for at least 2 wks after final dose. • Do not take herbal supplements. • Report planned surgical/dental procedures.

---

rufinamide

rue-**fin**-a-myde
(Banzel)

◆CLASSIFICATION

PHARMACOTHERAPEUTIC: Triazole derivative. **CLINICAL:** Anticonvulsant.

USES

Adjunctive therapy in treatment of seizures associated with Lennox-Gastaut syndrome in adults and children 1 yr and older.

PRECAUTIONS

Contraindications: Hypersensitivity to rufinamide. Familial short QT syndrome. **Cautions:** Other drugs that shorten QT interval, clinical depression, pts at high risk for suicide, mild to moderate hepatic impairment (not recommended in pts with severe hepatic impairment), concurrent use with hormonal contraceptives.

ACTION

Modulates activity of sodium channels. Prolongs inactive state of the sodium channel in cortical neurons, limits sustained repetitive firing of sodium-dependent action potential, inhibiting excitatory neurotransmitter release. **Therapeutic Effect:** Decreases frequency/severity of seizure activity.

PHARMACOKINETICS

Well absorbed following PO administration. Protein binding: 34%. Extensively metabolized via hydrolysis. Excreted primarily in urine. **Half-life:** 6–10 hrs.

⧖ LIFESPAN CONSIDERATIONS

Pregnancy/Lactation: May produce fetal skeletal abnormalities. May be distributed in breast milk. **Children:** Safety and efficacy not established in pts younger than 4 yrs. **Elderly:** Age-related renal, hepatic, or cardiac impairment may require initiation of therapy at low end of dosing range.

INTERACTIONS

DRUG: May increase concentration of PHENobarbital, phenytoin. May decrease concentration of carBAMazepine, lamoTRIgine. **Valproate** may increase concentration. May decrease effects of estradiol, norethindrone. **Alcohol, CNS depressants (e.g., LORazepam, morphine, zolpidem)** may increase CNS depressant effect. **HERBAL:** **Evening primrose** may decrease seizure threshold. **FOOD:** None known. **LAB VALUES:** May decrease WBC count.

AVAILABILITY (Rx)

Oral Suspension: 40 mg/mL. **Tablets, Film-Coated:** 200 mg, 400 mg.

R

ADMINISTRATION/HANDLING

PO
• Give with food. • Film-coated tablets may be cut or crushed for dosing flexibility. • Shake oral suspension well before each dose; use bottle adapter and dosing syringes provided.

INDICATIONS/ROUTES/DOSAGE

Lennox-Gastaut Seizures
PO: ADULTS, ELDERLY: Initially, 400–800 mg/day, given in 2 equally divided doses. Dose should be increased by 400–800 mg/day every 2 days. **Maximum:** 3,200 mg/day, administered in 2 equally divided doses. **CHILDREN 1 YR AND OLDER:** Treatment should be initiated at a daily dose of 10 mg/kg/day, given in 2 equally divided doses. Increase by 10-mg/kg increments every other day to a target dose of 45 mg/kg/day or 3,200 mg/day, whichever is less, administered in 2 equally divided doses.

Dosage in Renal Impairment
No dose adjustment.

Dosage in Hepatic Impairment
Mild to moderate impairment: Use caution. **Severe impairment:** Not recommended.

SIDE EFFECTS

CHILDREN: Frequent (27%–11%): Headache, dizziness, fatigue, nausea, drowsiness, diplopia. **Occasional (6%–4%):** Tremor, nystagmus, blurred vision, vomiting. **Rare (3%):** Ataxia, upper abdominal pain, anxiety, constipation, dyspepsia, back pain, gait disturbance, vertigo.
ADULTS: Frequent (17%–7%): Lethargy, vomiting, headache, fatigue, dizziness, nausea. **Occasional (5%–4%):** Influenza, nasopharyngitis, anorexia, rash, ataxia, diplopia. **Rare (3%):** Bronchitis, sinusitis, psychomotor hyperactivity, upper abdominal pain, aggression, ear infection, inattention, pruritus.

ADVERSE EFFECTS/TOXIC REACTIONS

Suicidal ideation or behavior occurs rarely, noted as early as 1 wk after initiation of therapy and persisting for at least 24 wks. Shortening of the QT interval (up to 20 msec), hypersensitivity reaction (rash, fever, urticaria) have been noted. Abrupt withdrawal may precipitate seizure, status epilepticus.

NURSING CONSIDERATIONS

BASELINE ASSESSMENT
Review history of seizure disorder (intensity, frequency, duration, level of consciousness). Obtain baseline EKG. Initiate seizure precautions.

INTERVENTION/EVALUATION
Provide safety measures as needed. Observe frequently for recurrence of seizure activity. Assess for clinical improvement (decrease in intensity, frequency of seizures). Assist with ambulation if drowsiness, lethargy occur. Question for evidence of headache.

PATIENT/FAMILY TEACHING
• Do not abruptly withdraw medication (may precipitate seizures). • Avoid tasks that require alertness, motor skills until response to drug is established. • Strict maintenance of drug therapy is essential for seizure control. • Avoid alcohol. • Female pts of childbearing age should be informed that concurrent use of rufinamide with hormonal contraceptives may render contraceptive less effective; nonhormonal forms of contraception are recommended. • Be alert for any unusual changes in mood/behavior (may increase risk of suicidal ideation/behavior).

R

ruxolitinib

rux-oh-**li**-ti-nib
(Jakafi)

◆CLASSIFICATION

PHARMACOTHERAPEUTIC: Kinase inhibitor. **CLINICAL:** Antineoplastic.

USES

Treatment of intermediate or high-risk myelofibrosis, including primary myelofibrosis, post–polycythemia vera myelofibrosis, post–essential thrombocythemia myelofibrosis. Treatment of polycythemia vera.

PRECAUTIONS

Contraindications: Hypersensitivity to ruxolitinib. **Cautions:** Pts at risk for developing bacterial, fungal, or viral infections, renal/hepatic impairment, concomitant use of strong CYP3A4 inhibitors, history of bradycardia, conduction disturbances, ischemic heart disease, HF.

ACTION

Inhibits Janus-associated kinases (JAKs) JAK1 and JAK2, which mediate the signaling of cytokines and growth factor important for hematopoiesis and immune function. **Therapeutic Effect:** Reduces symptoms of myelofibrosis, including enlarged spleen.

PHARMACOKINETICS

Rapidly absorbed after PO administration. Widely distributed. Protein binding: 97%. Metabolized in liver. Excreted in urine (74%), feces (22%). **Half-life:** 3–5 hrs.

⌛ LIFESPAN CONSIDERATIONS

Pregnancy/Lactation: Unknown if distributed in breast milk. Not recommended in nursing mothers. Must either discontinue drug or discontinue breastfeeding. **Children:** Safety and efficacy not established. **Elderly:** No age-related precautions noted.

INTERACTIONS

DRUG: Strong CYP3A4 inhibitors (e.g., clarithromycin, cycloSPORINE, HIV protease inhibitors, ketoconazole) may increase concentration/effects.

HERBAL: None known. **FOOD: Grapefruit products** may increase concentration. **LAB VALUES:** May decrease platelets, RBC, Hgb, Hct, WBC. May increase serum bilirubin, ALT, AST, cholesterol.

AVAILABILITY (Rx)

Tablets: 5 mg, 10 mg, 15 mg, 20 mg, 25 mg.

ADMINISTRATION/HANDLING

PO
• Give without regard to food.

Feeding tube
• Suspend tablet in 40 mL water and stir for 10 min. • May administer suspension within 6 hrs after tablet has dispersed. • Flush with 75 mL water after administration.

INDICATIONS/ROUTES/DOSAGE

Myelofibrosis
PO: ADULTS: 20 mg twice daily if platelets greater than 200,000 cells/mm^3, or 15 mg twice daily if platelets 100,000–200,000 cells/mm^3, or 5 mg twice daily if platelets 50,000 to less than 100,000 cells/mm^3. Dose reduction based on platelet response. **Maximum:** 25 mg twice daily.

Polycythemia Vera
PO: ADULTS, ELDERLY: Initially, 10 mg bid. Doses titrated based on safety/efficacy.

Dosage in Renal/Hepatic Impairment
Initial dose 10 mg bid.

Dosage in Renal Impairment

CrCl 15–59 mL/min	Platelets 100,000–150,000/mm^3	10 mg twice daily
CrCl 15–59 mL/min	Platelets less than 100,000/mm^3	Avoid use
End-stage renal disease (ESRD) on dialysis	Platelets 100,000–200,000/mm^3	15 mg after dialysis on days of dialysis

R

| ESRD on dialysis | Platelets greater than 200,000/mm³ | 20 mg after dialysis on days of dialysis |
| ESRD not requiring dialysis | | Avoid use |

Dosage in Hepatic Impairment

| Hepatic impairment | Platelets 100,000–150,000/mm³ | 10 mg twice daily |
| Hepatic impairment | Platelets less than 100,000/mm³ | Avoid use |

SIDE EFFECTS

Frequent (23%–14%): Bruising, dizziness, vertigo, labyrinthitis, headache. **Occasional (9%–7%):** Weight gain, flatulence.

ADVERSE EFFECTS/TOXIC REACTIONS

May cause severe thrombocytopenia (70% of pts), anemia (96% of pts), neutropenia (18% of pts), which may improve with reduced dose or by temporarily withholding regimen. Anemic pts may require blood transfusions. Increased risk of developing opportunistic bacterial, mycobacterial, fungal, viral infections including herpes zoster, urinary tract infection, urosepsis, renal infection, pyuria. Increased risk of bleeding disorders including ecchymosis, hematoma, injection site hematoma, periorbital hematoma, petechiae, purpura.

NURSING CONSIDERATIONS

BASELINE ASSESSMENT
Obtain CBC, serum chemistries, renal function, LFT, urinalysis, cholesterol level. Assess recent vaccinations status. Receive full medication history including herbal products. Question for possibility of pregnancy, renal/hepatic impairment, HIV.

INTERVENTION/EVALUATION
Monitor CBC (every 2–4 wks until doses stabilized), serum chemistries, renal function, LFT, cholesterol. Obtain urinalysis with reflex culture for suspected UTI. Routinely assess vital signs, I&O, breath sounds, gait. Monitor temperature; be alert for fever, infectious process. Avoid IM injections, rectal temperatures, other traumas that induce bleeding. Assess skin for petechiae, hematoma, purpura.

PATIENT/FAMILY TEACHING
• Report any new bruising/bleeding, bloody stools or urine, fever, chills, rash, painful urination, suspected infection, fatigue, shortness of breath. • Do not breastfeed. • Avoid grapefruit products. • Open skin lesions, blisters may signal herpes infection. • Blood work will be routinely monitored; if on dialysis, take only following dialysis.

sacubitril-valsartan

sak-**ue**-bi-tril
(Entresto)

■ **BLACK BOX ALERT** ■ May cause fetal harm, mortality. Discontinue as soon as pregnancy detected.

◆ CLASSIFICATION

PHARMACOTHERAPEUTIC: Combination of sacubitril, a neprilysin inhibitor, and valsartan, an angiotensin II receptor blocker. **CLINICAL:** Reduces risk of complications in HF.

USES

To reduce the risk of cardiovascular death and hospitalization in pts with chronic HF (NYHA class II-IV) and reduced ejection fraction.

PRECAUTIONS

Contraindications: Hypersensitivity to sacubitril or valsartan; history of angioedema related to angiotensin-converting enzyme (ACE) inhibitor or angiotensin receptor blockers (ARB); concomitant use or within 36 hrs of ACE inhibitors; concomitant use of aliskiren in pts with diabetes. **Cautions:** Baseline anemia, dehydration, hypovolemia, sodium depletion; concomitant use of potassium-sparing diuretics or potassium supplements; hepatic/renal impairment; unstented bilateral/unilateral renal artery stenosis; significant aortic/mitral stenosis. Pts with orthostatic hypotension.

ACTION

Sacubitril inhibits neprilysin, increasing peptide levels that are degraded by neprilysin (e.g., natriuretic peptides). Valsartan directly antagonizes angiotensin II receptors; blocks vasoconstrictor, aldosterone secreting effects of angiotensin II, inhibiting binding of angiotensin II to AT_1 receptors. **Therapeutic Effect:** Decreases risk of mortality in pts with chronic HF; produces vasodilation; decreases peripheral resistance; decreases B/P.

PHARMACOKINETICS

Widely distributed. Sacubitril is converted by esterases; not significantly metabolized after conversion. Valsartan is minimally metabolized in liver. Protein binding (both): 94%–97%. Peak plasma concentration: sacubitril: 30 min, valsartan: 1.5 hrs. Steady-state concentration: 3 days. Excretion: sacubitril: urine (52%–68%), feces (37%–48%); valsartan: feces (86%), urine (13%). **Half-life:** sacubitril: 1.4 hrs; valsartan: 9.9 hrs.

📋 LIFESPAN CONSIDERATIONS

Pregnancy/Lactation: Avoid pregnancy; may cause fetal harm/mortality. Unknown if distributed in breast milk. Must either discontinue drug or discontinue breastfeeding. **Children:** Safety and efficacy not established. **Elderly:** No age-related precautions noted.

INTERACTIONS

DRUG: ACE inhibitors (e.g., **enalapril, ramipril**) may increase risk of angioedema (contraindicated). **Potassium-sparing diuretics (e.g., spironolactone)** may increase risk of hyperkalemia. **NSAIDs (e.g., ibuprofen, naproxen)** may worsen renal function. May increase concentration/effect of **lithium.** **HERBAL:** Ginger, ginseng, licorice may worsen hypertension. **FOOD:** None known. **LAB VALUES:** May increase serum BUN, creatinine, potassium. May decrease Hct, Hgb.

AVAILABILITY (Rx)

Fixed-dose Combination Tablets: sacubitril/valsartan: 24 mg/26 mg, 49 mg/51 mg, 97 mg/103 mg.

ADMINISTRATION/HANDLING

PO
• Give without regard to food.

INDICATIONS/ROUTES/DOSAGE

HF
Note: Allow a 36-hr washout period when switching from or to an ACE inhibitor. After initial dose, may double dose as tolerated q2–4wks to target dose of 97 mg/103 mg.

PO: ADULTS, ELDERLY: (Previously taking high dose of ACE inhibitor [greater than 10 mg enalapril or equivalent] or ARB [greater than 160 mg valsartan or equivalent]): Initially, 49 mg/51 mg twice daily. (Previously taking low dose of ACE inhibitor [10 mg or less of enalapril or equivalent] or ARB): 24 mg/26 mg twice daily. (Not currently taking an ACE inhibitor or ARB): 24 mg/26 mg twice daily.

Dosage in Renal Impairment
PO: ADULTS, ELDERLY: Mild to moderate impairment: No dose adjustment. **Severe impairment:** Initially, 24 mg/26 mg twice daily. **Maintenance:** May double each dose every 2–4 wks up to 97 mg/103 mg twice daily based on tolerability.

Dosage in Hepatic Impairment
PO: ADULTS, ELDERLY: Mild impairment: No dose adjustment. **Moderate impairment:** Initially, 24 mg/26 mg twice daily. **Maintenance:** May double each dose every 2–4 wks up to 97 mg/103 mg twice daily based on tolerability. **Severe impairment:** Treatment not recommended.

SIDE EFFECTS

Occasional (9%): Cough, dizziness.

ADVERSE EFFECTS/ TOXIC REACTIONS

Angioedema (less than 1% of pts), hypotension (18% of pts), orthostatic hypotension (2% of pts), impairment/decrease in renal function due to inhibition of renin-angiotensin-aldosterone system (5% of pts), elevation of serum creatinine greater than 50% from baseline (1.4% of pts), renal impairment including oliguria, azotemia, acute renal failure (5% of pts), hyperkalemia (12% of pts), serum potassium elevation greater than 5.5 mEq/L (4% of pts) have occurred.

NURSING CONSIDERATIONS

BASELINE ASSESSMENT
Obtain baseline BMP; CBC in pts with baseline anemia. Obtain B/P, heart rate immediately before each dose, in addition to regular monitoring (be alert for fluctuations). Assess hydration status. Correct hydration/sodium depletion prior to initiation. Receive medication history and screen for interactions, esp. concomitant use of aliskiren, ACE inhibitors, ARBs, potassium-sparing diuretics, potassium supplements. Verify negative pregnancy status. Question history of hepatic/renal impairment, renal artery stenosis; angioedema, hypersensitivity reaction.

INTERVENTION/EVALUATION
Monitor BMP, esp. serum BUN, creatinine, potassium. Monitor for hyperkalemia, hypotension. If hypotension occurs, place pt in supine position, feet slightly elevated; consider interrupting treatment or altering dose of diuretic, antihypertensive drugs and screen for dehydration/serum sodium depletion. If pt positive for dehydration, be cautious with PO/IV administration. Overhydration may exacerbate HF. Assist with ambulation if dizziness occurs. Monitor for hypersensitivity reaction, including angioedema. If angioedema occurs, interrupt treatment and institute therapy to protect airway patency.

PATIENT/FAMILY TEACHING
• Go slowly from lying to standing. • Be cautious of fluid intake. Overhydration may lead to worsening of HF, while underhydration may lead to low blood pressure. • Report urine changes such as darkened urine, decreased output. • Immediately report allergic reactions such as difficulty breathing, itching, rash, tongue swelling; symptoms of high potassium levels such as extreme fatigue, muscle weakness,

S

palpitations; suspected pregnancy. • Do not breastfeed. • Diuretics (water pills) may increase risk of low pressure or low potassium levels.

safinamide

sa-**fin**-a-mide
(Xadago)
Do not confuse safinamide with ethionamide, niacinamide, procainamide, pyrazinamide, or Xadogo with Xanax, Xarelto, or Xalatan.

◆ CLASSIFICATION

PHARMACOTHERAPEUTIC: Monoamine oxidase type B (MAO-B) inhibitor. **CLINICAL:** Antiparkinson agent.

USES

Adjunctive treatment to levodopa/carbidopa in pts with Parkinson's disease experiencing "off" episodes. Not indicated as a monotherapy.

PRECAUTIONS

Contraindications: Hypersensitivity to safinamide. Severe hepatic impairment. Concomitant use of other MAOIs, potent inhibitors of MAOI (e.g., linezolid), amphetamine (and derivatives), cyclobenzaprine, dextromethorphan, methylphenidate, opioid medications, St. John's wort, selective serotonin-norepinephrine reuptake inhibitors (SNRIs), tricyclic or triazolopyridine antidepressants. **Cautions:** Ophthalmic disorders (e.g., any active retinopathy, history of retinal/macular degeneration, uveitis, inherited retinal conditions, history of hereditary retina disease, albinism, retinitis, pigmentosa); hypertension, psychiatric disorders (e.g., schizophrenia, bipolar disorder, psychosis); history of dyskinesia, pts with impulse control disorder; concomitant use of serotonergic drugs; moderate hepatic impairment.

ACTION

Exact mechanism in Parkinson's disease unknown. Selectively inhibits MAO-B activity. Inhibits catabolism of dopamine, increasing dopamine levels and thereby increasing dopaminergic activity in the brain. **Therapeutic Effect:** Reduces effects of Parkinson's disease.

PHARMACOKINETICS

Absorbed quickly. Widely distributed. Metabolized in liver by nonmicrosomal enzymatic activity. Protein binding: 88%. Peak plasma concentration: 2–3 hrs. Excreted primarily in urine (76%). **Half-life:** 20–26 hrs.

⧗ LIFESPAN CONSIDERATIONS

Pregnancy/Lactation: Unknown if distributed in breast milk. Breastfeeding not recommended. **Children:** Safety and efficacy not established. **Elderly:** No age-related precautions noted.

INTERACTIONS

DRUG: Amphetamine (or derivatives), cyclobenzaprine, methylphenidate, isoniazid, IV methylene blue opioids (e.g., fentanyl, tramadol), linezolid, other MAOIs (e.g., phenelzine, selegiline), SNRIs (e.g., duloxetine, venlafaxine), tricyclic antidepressants (e.g., amitriptyline) may increase risk of serotonin syndrome, hypertensive crisis; use contraindicated. **Dextromethorphan** may increase risk of psychosis, abnormal behavior. **HERBAL: St. John's wort** may increase risk of serotonin syndrome. **FOOD:** Foods/beverages that are high in tyramine (e.g., aged cheese, pickled herring, red wine) may cause release of norepinephrine, resulting in hypertension. **LAB VALUES:** May increase serum ALT, AST.

AVAILABILITY (Rx)

Tablets: 50 mg, 100 mg.

ADMINISTRATION/HANDLING

PO
• Give with or without food at the same time every day. • If a dose is missed or

S

vomiting occurs after administration, do not give extra dose. Administer next dose at regularly scheduled time.

INDICATIONS/ROUTES/DOSAGE

Parkinson's Disease

PO: ADULTS, ELDERLY: 50 mg once daily. If response is inadequate, may increase to 100 mg once daily after 2 wks of treatment. (When discontinuing from 100 mg/day, decrease to 50 mg/day for 1 wk before discontinuing therapy to avoid risk of withdrawal-emergent hyperpyrexia and confusion.)

Dosage in Renal Impairment
Not specified; use caution.

Dosage in Hepatic Impairment
Mild impairment: No dose adjustment. **Moderate impairment:** Do not exceed maximum dose of 50 mg/day. **Severe impairment:** Treatment contraindicated. If hepatic impairment progresses from moderate to severe impairment, permanently discontinue.

SIDE EFFECTS

Frequent (21%): Dyskinesia. **Occasional (3%):** Nausea. **Rare (2% or less):** Orthostatic hypotension, anxiety, cough, dyspepsia.

ADVERSE EFFECTS/ TOXIC REACTIONS

Hypertension, worsening of hypertension, hypertensive crisis was reported. Life-threatening serotonin syndrome may include mental status changes (agitation, hallucinations, delirium, coma), autonomic instability (tachycardia, labile blood pressure, dizziness, sweating, flushing, hyperthermia), neuromuscular symptoms (tremor, rigidity, myoclonus [localized muscle twitching], hyperactive reflexes, incoordination). May cause sudden onset of sleep (without warning) during normal daily activities or while driving, which may result in accidents, injury. Impulsive or compulsive behaviors including gambling, sexual urges, binge eating, intense urge to spend money have occurred. Neuroleptic malignant

syndrome (hyperpyrexia, muscle rigidity, altered mental status, autonomic instability [irregular pulse or blood pressure, tachycardia, diaphoresis, and cardiac arrhythmia], elevated creatinine, phosphokinase, myoglobinuria [rhabdomyolysis], acute renal failure) may be associated with rapid dose reduction, withdrawal, changes that increase central dopaminergic tone. Hypersensitivity reactions (including angioedema), retinal degeneration, loss of photoreceptors, major psychotic episodes (psychosis, hallucinations), dyskinesia, falls were reported.

NURSING CONSIDERATIONS

BASELINE ASSESSMENT

Obtain B/P. Assess symptoms of Parkinson's disease (e.g., muscular rigidity, pen rolling motion, gait disturbance, tremors), emotional state. Receive full medication history and screen for contraindications/ interactions. Question history of ocular disease (personal or family history), dyskinesia, compulsive/impulsive behavior, psychosis, falls. Due to risk of suddenly falling asleep, discuss avoidance of driving vehicles, operating machinery. Conduct baseline ophthalmologic exam, visual acuity. Initiate fall precautions.

INTERVENTION/EVALUATION

Periodically monitor B/P. Assess for clinical improvement, reversal of symptoms (improvement of hand, head tremor at rest, mask-like facial expression, muscular rigidity). Monitor for dyskinesia (difficulty with movement), psychosis/ hallucinations; symptoms of serotonin syndrome, neuroleptic malignant syndrome. Question for episodes of sudden-onset sleep, accidents, falls, impulsivity. Assess for new-onset ocular/retinal disorders. Monitor for hypersensitivity reactions. Assist with ambulation.

PATIENT/FAMILY TEACHING

• Therapy may cause sudden sleep without drowsiness or warning, which may cause accidents and injury. Avoid tasks that require alertness, motor skills until response to drug is established. Driving, operating machinery is extremely risky. • Report symptoms of overproduction of serotonin including confusion, excessive talking, hallucinations, headache, hyperactivity, insomnia, racing thoughts, seizure activity, tremors; sexual dysfunction, fever. • Rapid dose reduction or withdrawal may cause neuroleptic malignant syndrome (confusion, high fever, muscle rigidity, high or irregular B/P, heart arrhythmias), a life-threatening condition that can be confused with symptoms of severe infection. • Report vision changes; impulsive binge eating, gambling, sexual urges, inability to stop spending money; swelling of the face, tongue, throat. • Due to high risk of drug interactions, do not take newly prescribed medication, herbal supplements unless approved by prescriber who originally started treatment. • Avoid foods high in tyramine (aged, cured, fermented, pickled, smoked food).

salmeterol

sal-**met**-er-all
(Serevent Diskhaler Disk ✤, Serevent Diskus)

■ **BLACK BOX ALERT** ■ Long-acting beta₂-adrenergic agonists may increase risk of asthma-related deaths and asthma-related hospitalizations in pediatric and adolescent pts. Use only as adjuvant therapy.

Do not confuse salmeterol with Solu-Medrol, or Serevent with Atrovent, Combivent, Serentil, or Sinemet.

FIXED-COMBINATION(S)

Advair Diskus: salmeterol/fluticasone (a corticosteroid): 50 mcg/100 mcg, 50 mcg/250 mcg, 50 mcg/500 mcg. **Advair HFA:** salmeterol/fluticasone (a corticosteroid): 21 mcg/45 mcg, 21 mcg/115 mcg, 21 mcg/230 mcg.

◆CLASSIFICATION

PHARMACOTHERAPEUTIC: Beta₂-adrenergic agonist (long-acting). **CLINICAL:** Bronchodilator.

USES

Prevention of exercise-induced bronchospasm, bronchospasm; maintenance treatment of asthma and prevention of bronchospasm in pts with reversible obstructive airway disease, including those with symptoms of nocturnal asthma. Long-term maintenance treatment of bronchospasm associated with COPD (including emphysema and chronic bronchitis).

PRECAUTIONS

Contraindications: Hypersensitivity to salmeterol. Treatment of status asthmaticus, acute episodes of asthma or COPD. Use as monotherapy in treatment of asthma without concomitant long-term asthma control medication (e.g., inhaled corticosteroids). **Cautions:** Not for acute symptoms; may cause paradoxical bronchospasm, severe asthma. Cardiovascular disorders (coronary insufficiency, arrhythmias, hypertension), seizure disorders, diabetes, hyperthyroidism, hepatic impairment, hypokalemia.

ACTION

Stimulates beta₂-adrenergic receptors in lungs, resulting in relaxation of bronchial smooth muscle. **Therapeutic Effect:** Relieves bronchospasm, reducing airway resistance.

PHARMACOKINETICS

Route	Onset	Peak	Duration
Inhalation (asthma)	30–45 min	2–4 hrs	12 hrs
Inhalation (COPD)	2 hrs	3.25–4.75 hrs	12 hrs

Low systemic absorption; acts primarily in lungs. Protein binding: 95%. Metabolized in liver. Excreted in urine (25%), feces (60%). **Half-life:** 5.5 hrs.

⌛ LIFESPAN CONSIDERATIONS

Pregnancy/Lactation: Unknown if distributed in breast milk. **Children:** No age-related precautions in pts older than 4 yrs. **Elderly:** Lower dosages may be needed (may be more susceptible to tachycardia, tremors).

INTERACTIONS

DRUG: Beta blockers (e.g., carvedilol, metoprolol) may reduce effect; may produce bronchospasm. **CYP3A4 inhibitors (e.g., ketoconazole, protease inhibitors)** may increase concentration, risk of QT prolongation. **MAOIs (e.g., phenelzine, selegiline), tricyclic antidepressants (e.g., amitriptyline, doxepin)** may increase concentration/effects (wait 14 days after stopping MAOIs, tricyclic antidepressants before starting salmeterol). **HERBAL:** None significant. **FOOD:** None known. **LAB VALUES:** May decrease serum potassium. May increase serum glucose.

AVAILABILITY (Rx)

Powder for Oral Inhalation: 50 mcg/inhalation.

ADMINISTRATION/HANDLING

Inhalation
• Do not shake or prime. Before inhaling the dose, breath out fully (do not exhale into Diskus device). Activate and use only in level horizontal position. • Inhale quickly and deeply through Diskus. • Hold breath as long as possible before exhaling slowly. • Do not use a spacer or wash mouthpiece.

INDICATIONS/ROUTES/DOSAGE

Maintenance and Prevention Therapy for Asthma, Bronchospasm
Inhalation: *(Diskus):* ADULTS, ELDERLY, CHILDREN 4 YRS AND OLDER: 1 inhalation (50 mcg) q12h (used in combination with inhaled corticosteroids not as monotherapy).

Prevention of Exercise-Induced Bronchospasm
Inhalation: *(Diskus):* ADULTS, ELDERLY, CHILDREN 4 YRS AND OLDER: 1 inhalation at least 30 min before exercise. Additional doses should not be given for 12 hrs. Do not administer if already giving salmeterol twice daily.

Maintenance Therapy for COPD
Inhalation: *(Diskus):* ADULTS, ELDERLY: 1 inhalation (50 mcg) q12h.

Dosage in Renal/Hepatic Impairment
No dose adjustment.

SIDE EFFECTS

Frequent (28%): Headache. **Occasional (7%–3%):** Cough, tremor, dizziness, vertigo, throat dryness/irritation, pharyngitis. **Rare (Less Than 3%):** Palpitations, tachycardia, nausea, heartburn, GI distress, diarrhea.

ADVERSE EFFECTS/ TOXIC REACTIONS

May prolong QT interval (can precipitate ventricular arrhythmias). Hypokalemia, hyperglycemia may occur.

NURSING CONSIDERATIONS

BASELINE ASSESSMENT

Question history of cardiac disease, hepatic impairment, seizure disorder. Screen for concomitant medications known to prolong QT interval. Assess lung sounds, vital signs.

INTERVENTION/EVALUATION

Monitor rate, depth, rhythm, type of respiration; quality/rate of pulse, B/P. Assess lungs for wheezing, rales, rhonchi. Periodically evaluate serum potassium levels.

PATIENT/FAMILY TEACHING

• Not for relief of acute episodes. • Keep canister at room temperature (cold decreases effects). • Do not stop medication or exceed recommended dosage. • Report chest pain, dizziness. • Wait at least 1 full min before second

S

---

inhalation. • Administer dose 30–60 min before exercise when used to prevent exercise-induced bronchospasm. • Avoid excessive use of caffeine derivatives (coffee, tea, colas, chocolate).

sargramostim

sar-**gra**-moe-stim
(Leukine)
Do not confuse Leukine with leucovorin or Leukeran.

◆CLASSIFICATION

PHARMACOTHERAPEUTIC: Colony-stimulating factor. **CLINICAL:** Hematopoietic agent.

USES

Acute Myelogenous Leukemia (AML: following induction chemotherapy): Shortens time to neutrophil recovery; reduces incidence of severe infections. **Bone Marrow Transplant (allogeneic or autologous):** For graft failure, engraftment delay. **Myeloid reconstitution** following allogeneic or autologous bone marrow transplant. **Peripheral stem cell transplant (allogeneic or autologous):** Mobilizes hematopoietic progenitor cells. **OFF-LABEL:** Primary prophylaxis of neutropenia; treatment of radiation-induced myelosuppression.

PRECAUTIONS

Contraindications: Hypersensitivity to sargramostim. Concurrent (24 hrs preceding or following) myelosuppressive chemotherapy or radiation, pts with excessive leukemic myeloid blasts in bone marrow or peripheral blood (greater than 10%), known hypersensitivity to yeast-derived products. **Cautions:** Preexisting HF, fluid retention, cardiovascular disease, pulmonary disease (hypoxia, pulmonary infiltrates), renal/hepatic impairment.

ACTION

Stimulates proliferation/differentiation and functional activity of eosinophils, monocytes, neutrophils, and macrophages. **Therapeutic Effect:** Assists bone marrow in making new WBCs, increases their chemotactic, antifungal, antiparasitic activity. Increases cytoneoplastic cells, activates neutrophils to inhibit tumor cell growth.

PHARMACOKINETICS

Route	Onset	Peak	Duration
IV (increase WBCs)	7–14 days	N/A	1 wk

Detected in serum within 5 min after SQ administration. **Peak serum levels:** 1–3 hrs. **Half-life: IV:** 1 hr; **SQ:** 3 hrs.

☒ LIFESPAN CONSIDERATIONS

Pregnancy/Lactation: Unknown if drug crosses placenta or is distributed in breast milk. **Children:** Safety and efficacy not established. **Elderly:** No age-related precautions noted.

INTERACTIONS

DRUG: None significant. **HERBAL:** None significant. **FOOD:** None known. **LAB VALUES:** May increase serum ALT, AST, bilirubin, creatinine. May decrease serum albumin.

AVAILABILITY (Rx)

Injection, Powder for Reconstitution: 250 mcg.

ADMINISTRATION/HANDLING

Subcutaneous
May be given without further dilution.

 IV

Reconstitution • To 250-mcg vial, add 1 mL Sterile Water for Injection (preservative free) or Bacteriostatic Water for Injection. Direct diluent to side of vial, gently swirl contents to avoid foaming; do not shake or vigorously agitate. • After reconstitution, further dilute in 25–50 mL 0.9% NaCl to a concentration of 10 mcg/mL or

S

greater. If final concentration less than 10 mcg/mL, 1 mg of human albumin per 1 mL of 0.9% NaCl should be added to provide a final albumin concentration of 0.1% (e.g., 1 mL 5% albumin per 50 mL 0.9% NaCl).

◄**ALERT**► Albumin is added before addition of sargramostim (prevents drug adsorption to components of drug delivery system).

Rate of Administration • Give each single dose over 30 min, 2 hr, 6 hr, or continuous infusion.

Storage • Refrigerate powder, reconstituted solution, diluted solution for injection. • Do not shake. • Reconstituted solutions are clear, colorless. • Use within 6 hrs; discard unused portions. • Use 1 dose per vial; do not reenter vial.

🔲 IV INCOMPATIBILITIES

Amphotericin B complex (Abelcet, AmBisome, Amphotec), ondansetron (Zofran).

🔲 IV COMPATIBILITIES

Dexamethasone (Decadron), diphenhydrAMINE (Benadryl), famotidine (Pepcid), granisetron (Kytril), heparin, metoclopramide (Reglan), promethazine (Phenergan).

INDICATIONS/ROUTES/DOSAGE

Neutrophil Recovery Following Chemotherapy in AML

IV Infusion: ADULTS 55 YRS OR OLDER: 250 mcg/m²/day (as 4-hr infusion) starting approximately 4 days following completion of induction chemotherapy (if day 10 bone marrow is hypoplastic with less than 5% blasts). Continue until ANC is greater than 1,500 cells/mm³ for 3 consecutive days or a maximum of 42 days. If WBC greater than 50,000 cells/mm³ and/or ANC greater that 20,000 cells/mm³, interrupt treatment or reduce dose by 50%.

Myeloid Recovery Following Bone Marrow Transplant (BMT)

IV Infusion: ADULTS, ELDERLY: Usual parenteral dosage: 250 mcg/m²/day (as 2-hr infusion). Begin 2–4 hrs after autologous bone marrow infusion and not less than 24 hrs after last dose of chemotherapy or last radiation treatment, when post marrow infusion ANC is less than 500/mm³. Continue until ANC greater than 1,500 cells/mm³ for 3 consecutive days. If WBC greater than 50,000/mm³ and/or ANC greater that 20,000/mm³, interrupt treatment or reduce dose by 50%. Discontinue if blast cells appear or underlying disease progresses.

Bone Marrow Transplant Failure, Engraftment Delay

IV Infusion: ADULTS, ELDERLY: 250 mcg/m²/day for 14 days. Infuse over 2 hrs. May repeat after 7 days off therapy if engraftment has not occurred. A third course with 500 mcg/m²/day for 14 days may be tried if engraftment still has not occurred.

Stem Cell Transplant, Mobilization

IV, SQ: ADULTS: 250 mcg/m²/day IV (as 24-hr infusion) or SQ once daily. Continue same dose throughout peripheral blood progenitor cell collection. If WBC greater than 50,000 cells/mm³, reduce dose by 50%.

Stem Cell Transplant, Post-transplant

IV, SQ: ADULTS, ELDERLY: 250 mcg/m²/day IV (as 24-hr infusion) or SQ once daily beginning immediately following infusion of progenitor cells. Continue until ANC greater than 1,500 cells/mm³ for 3 consecutive days.

Dosage in Renal/Hepatic Impairment

No dose adjustment.

SIDE EFFECTS

Frequent: GI disturbances (nausea, diarrhea, vomiting, stomatitis, anorexia, abdominal pain), arthralgia or myalgia, headache, malaise, rash, pruritus. **Occasional:** Peripheral edema, weight gain, dyspnea, asthenia, fever, leukocytosis, capillary leak syndrome (fluid retention, irritation at local injection site, peripheral edema). **Rare:** Tachycardia, arrhythmias, thrombophlebitis.

S

ADVERSE EFFECTS/ TOXIC REACTIONS

Pleural/pericardial effusion occurs rarely after infusion.

NURSING CONSIDERATIONS

BASELINE ASSESSMENT

Obtain CBC, BMP, LFT, vital signs. Question history of cardiac/pulmonary disease, renal/hepatic impairment.

INTERVENTION/EVALUATION

Monitor CBC with differential, serum renal/hepatic function, pulmonary function, vital signs, weight. Monitor for supraventricular arrhythmias during administration (particularly in pts with history of cardiac arrhythmias). Assess closely for dyspnea during and immediately following infusion (particularly in pts with history of lung disease). If dyspnea occurs during infusion, cut infusion rate by half. If dyspnea continues, stop infusion immediately. If neutrophil count exceeds 20,000 cells/mm^3 or platelet count exceeds 500,000/mm^3, stop infusion or reduce dose by half, based on clinical condition of pt. Blood counts return to normal or baseline 3–7 days after discontinuation of therapy.

PATIENT/FAMILY TEACHING

• Report difficulty breathing, esp. during or immediately after infusion. • May increase risk of cardiac arrhythmias; report dizziness, fainting, palpitations. • Treatment may cause edema, fluid collection in the lungs or around the heart.

sarilumab

sar-**il**-ue-mab
(Kevzara)

■ **BLACK BOX ALERT** ■ Tuberculosis (TB), invasive fungal infections, other opportunistic infections leading to hospitalization and death were reported. Avoid use in pts with active infection. Withhold treatment until serious infection is controlled. Test for TB prior to and during treatment, regardless of initial result; if positive, start treatment for TB prior to initiation.

Do not confuse sarilumab with adalimumab, avelumab, belimumab, brodalumab, dupilumab, ipilimumab, nivolumab, or panitumumab.

◆CLASSIFICATION

PHARMACOTHERAPEUTIC: Interleukin-6 receptor antagonist. Monoclonal antibody. **CLINICAL:** Antirheumatic, disease modifying.

USES

May use as monotherapy or in combination with non-biologic DMARDs (do not use in combination with biologic DMARDs). Treatment of adults with moderately to severely active rheumatoid arthritis who have had an inadequate response or intolerance to one or more DMARDs.

PRECAUTIONS

Contraindications: Hypersensitivity to sarilumab. **Cautions:** Hyperlipidemia, hypertriglyceridemia, active hepatic disease or hepatic impairment; recent travel or residence in endemic TB or mycosis areas; history of chronic opportunistic infections (esp. bacterial, invasive fungal, mycobacterial, protozoal, viral, TB); conditions predisposing to infection (e.g., diabetes, immunocompromised pts, renal failure, open wounds); history of HIV, herpes zoster, hepatitis B virus (HBV) infection, malignancies; baseline neutropenia, thrombocytopenia; pts at risk for GI perforation (Crohn's disease, diverticulitis, GI tract malignancies, peptic ulcers, peritoneal malignancies). Not recommended in pts with active infection, concomitant use of biological DMARDs; baseline ANC less than 2000 cells/mm^3, platelet count less than 150,000 cells/mm^3, serum ALT, AST above 1.5 times upper limit of normal (ULN).

ACTION

Binds to interleukin-6 (IL-6) receptor, inhibiting signaling of IL-6, a cytokine involved in inflammatory and immune responses. **Therapeutic Effect:** Reduces inflammation of RA.

PHARMACOKINETICS

Widely distributed. Peak plasma concentration: 2–4 days. Excretion (200 mg dose): linear, non-saturable proteolytic pathway. (150 mg dose): Non-linear, saturable target medicated pathway. **Half-life:** Concentration dependent: 200 mg q2wks (up to 10 days); 150 mg q2wks (up to 8 days).

⌛ LIFESPAN CONSIDERATIONS

Pregnancy/Lactation: Crosses the placental barrier, esp. during the third trimester. Unknown if distributed in breast milk; however, maternal immunoglobulin G (IgG) is present in breast milk. **Children:** Safety and efficacy not established. **Elderly:** Use caution (increased incidence of infections).

INTERACTIONS

DRUG: May decrease concentration/effect of **atorvastatin, oral contraceptives.** May decrease therapeutic effect of **BCG vaccines;** increase risk of adverse effects/toxic reactions of **live vaccines, belimumab, natalizumab, pimecrolimus, tacrolimus. HERBAL: Echinacea** may decrease effect. **FOOD:** None known. **LAB VALUES:** May increase serum ALT, AST, cholesterol, LDL, HDL, triglycerides. May decrease leukocytes, neutrophils, platelets.

AVAILABILITY (Rx)

Injection, Solution: 150 mg/1.14 mL, 200 mg/1.14 mL.

ADMINISTRATION/HANDLING

Subcutaneous

Preparation • Remove prefilled syringe from refrigerator and allow solution to warm to room temperature (approx. 30 min) with needle cap intact. • Visually inspect for particulate matter or discoloration. Solution should appear clear, colorless to slightly yellow in color. Do not use if solution is cloudy, discolored, or visible particles are observed.

Administration • Insert needle subcutaneously into upper arms, outer thigh, or abdomen and inject solution. • Do not inject into areas of active skin disease or injury such as sunburns, skin rashes, inflammation, skin infections, or active psoriasis. • Do not administer IV or intramuscularly. • Rotate injection sites.

Storage • Refrigerate in original carton until time of use. • Protect from light. • May store at room temperature for up to 14 days. Once warmed to room temperature, do not place back into refrigerator. • Do not freeze or expose to heating sources. • Do not shake.

INDICATIONS/ROUTES/DOSAGE

Note: Do not initiate if ANC is less than 2,000 cells/mm^3; platelets less than 150,000 cells/mm^3; or serum ALT or AST greater than 1.5 times ULN.

Rheumatoid Arthritis

SQ: ADULTS, ELDERLY: 200 mg once q2wks.

Dose Modification

Neutropenia

ANC greater than 1000 cells/mm^3: No dose adjustment. **ANC 500–1000 cells/mm^3:** Withhold treatment until ANC greater than 1000 cells/mm^3, then resume at 150 mg once q2wks. May increase to 200 mg once q2wks as clinically indicated. **ANC less than 500 cells/mm^3:** Permanently discontinue.

Hepatotoxicity

Serum ALT elevation up to 3 times ULN: Consider modifying dose of concomitant DMARDs. **Serum ALT elevation greater than 3–5 times ULN:** Withhold treatment until serum ALT less than 3 times ULN, then resume at 150 mg once q2wks. May increase to

S

200 mg once q2wks as clinically indicated. **Serum ALT elevation greater than 5 times ULN:** Permanently discontinue.

Serious Infection

Withhold treatment until serious infection is controlled, then resume as clinically indicated.

Thrombocytopenia

Platelet count 50,000–100,000 cells/ mm³: Withhold treatment until platelet count greater than 100,000 cells/mm³, then resume at 150 mg once q2wks. May increase to 200 mg once q2wks as clinically indicated. **Platelet count less than 50,000 cells/mm³:** Permanently discontinue if confirmed by repeat testing.

Dosage in Renal Impairment

Mild to moderate impairment: No dose adjustment. **Severe impairment:** Not specified; use caution.

Dosage in Hepatic Impairment

Not specified; use caution.

SIDE EFFECTS

Rare (4%–2%): Injection site reactions (pain, erythema, pruritus).

ADVERSE EFFECTS/ TOXIC REACTIONS

Serious, sometimes fatal, infections including aspergillosis, candidiasis, cellulitis, Cryptococcus, histoplasmosis, pneumonia, sepsis, tuberculosis; bacterial, mycobacterial, invasive fungal, opportunistic, viral infections were reported. Nasopharyngitis, upper respiratory tract infections, urinary tract infections occurred in 2–4% of pts. Neutropenia may increase risk of serious infection. GI perforation may occur, esp. in pts with history of diverticulitis or concomitant use of NSAIDs, corticosteroids. May increase risk for new malignancies. Hypersensitivity reactions including rash, urticaria reported in less than 1% of pts. May increase risk of HBV reactivation, which may result in fulminant hepatitis, hepatic failure, death. Immunogenicity (auto-sarilumab antibodies) was reported.

NURSING CONSIDERATIONS

BASELINE ASSESSMENT

Obtain CBC (note neutrophil, platelet count), LFT, lipid panel. Assess onset, location, duration of pain, inflammation. Inspect appearance of affected joints for immobility, deformities. Pts should be evaluated for active tuberculosis and tested for latent infection prior to initiation and periodically during therapy. Induration of 5 mm or greater with tuberculin skin testing should be considered a positive test result when assessing if treatment for latent tuberculosis is necessary. Question history of chronic infections, opportunistic infections, herpes infection. Screen for active infection. Assess skin for open wounds. Question history of active hepatic disease, GI perforation, malignancies, HIV, HBV, hypersensitivity reactions. Receive full medication history and screen for interactions. Assess pt's willingness to self-inject medication.

INTERVENTION/EVALUATION

Assess for therapeutic response: relief of pain, stiffness, swelling; increased joint mobility; reduced joint tenderness; improved grip strength. Monitor neutrophil count, platelet count, LFT 4–6 wks after initiation, then q3mos thereafter. Monitor lipid panel 4–6 wks after initiation, then q6mos thereafter. Monitor for symptoms of tuberculosis, including those who tested negative for latent tuberculosis infection prior to initiating therapy. Interrupt or discontinue treatment if serious infection, opportunistic infection, or sepsis occurs and initiate appropriate antimicrobial therapy. Closely monitor for HBV reactivation.

PATIENT/FAMILY TEACHING

• Treatment may depress your immune system and reduce your ability to fight infection. Report symptoms of infection such as body aches, burning with urination, chills, cough, fatigue, fever. Avoid those with active infection. • Do not receive live vaccines. • Expect frequent tuberculosis

S

screening. Report travel plans to possible endemic areas. • A health care provider will show you how to properly prepare and inject medication. You must demonstrate correct preparation and injection techniques before using medication at home. • Report allergic reactions such as itching, hives, rash. • Immediately report severe or persistent abdominal pain, bloody stool, fever; may indicate tear in GI tract. • Treatment may cause reactivation of HBV, new cancers. • Therapy may decrease platelet count, which may increase risk of bleeding. • Report liver problems such as bruising, confusion, amber or dark-colored urine; right upper abdominal pain; yellowing of the skin or eyes.

sAXagliptin

sax-a-**glip**-tin
(Onglyza)
Do not confuse SAXagliptin with SITagliptin or SUMAtriptan.

FIXED-COMBINATION(S)

Kombiglyze XR: SAXagliptin/metFORMIN (an antidiabetic): 2.5 mg/1,000 mg, 5 mg/500 mg, 5 mg/1,000 mg.

◆CLASSIFICATION

PHARMACOTHERAPEUTIC: DDP-4 inhibitor (gliptins). **CLINICAL:** Antidiabetic agent.

USES

Adjunctive treatment to diet and exercise to improve glycemic control in pts with type 2 diabetes as monotherapy or in combination with other antidiabetic agents.

PRECAUTIONS

Contraindications: Hypersensitivity to SAXagliptin. Type 1 diabetes, ketoacidosis. **Cautions:** Concurrent use of other glucose-lowering agents may increase risk of hypoglycemia, moderate to severe

renal impairment, end-stage renal disease requiring hemodialysis, concurrent use of strong CYP3A4 inhibitors (e.g., clarithromycin).

ACTION

Slows the inactivation of incretin hormones by inhibiting DDP-4 enzyme. Incretin hormones increase insulin synthesis/release from pancreas and decrease glucagon secretion. **Therapeutic Effect:** Regulates glucose homeostasis.

PHARMACOKINETICS

Route	Onset	Peak	Duration
Oral	—	—	24 hrs

Rapidly absorbed following PO administration. Extensively metabolized. Excreted by both renal and hepatic pathways. **Half-life:** 2.5 hrs; metabolite, 3.1 hrs.

⧖ LIFESPAN CONSIDERATIONS

Pregnancy/Lactation: Unknown if distributed in breast milk. **Children:** Safety and efficacy not established. **Elderly:** Age-related renal impairment may require dosage adjustment.

INTERACTIONS

DRUG: CYP3A4 inhibitors (e.g., clarithromycin, ketoconazole) may increase concentration. CYP3A4 inducers (e.g., carBAMazepine, phenytoin, rifampin) may decrease concentration. **HERBAL:** Herbal supplements that have hypoglycemic effects increase risk of hypoglycemia. **FOOD:** Grapefruit products may increase concentration. **LAB VALUES:** May slightly decrease WBCs, lymphocytes. May increase serum creatinine.

AVAILABILITY (Rx)

Tablets, Film-Coated: 2.5 mg, 5 mg.

ADMINISTRATION/HANDLING

PO
• May give without regard to food. • Do not break, crush, dissolve, or divide film-coated tablets.

INDICATIONS/ROUTES/DOSAGE

Type 2 Diabetes

PO: ADULTS OVER 18 YRS, ELDERLY: 2.5 or 5 mg once daily. **Concurrent Strong CYP3A4 Inhibitors (e.g., ketoconazole):** 2.5 mg once daily. **Hemodialysis:** Give dose after dialysis.

Dosage in Renal Impairment

Mild impairment: No dose adjustment. **Moderate to severe impairment: CrCl less than 50 mL/min:** 2.5 mg once daily.

Dosage in Hepatic Impairment

No dose adjustment.

SIDE EFFECTS

Occasional (7%): Headache. **Rare (3%–1%):** Peripheral edema, sinusitis, abdominal pain, gastroenteritis, vomiting, rash.

ADVERSE EFFECTS/TOXIC REACTIONS

Lymphopenia, rash occur rarely. Upper respiratory tract infection, urinary tract infection occur in approximately 7% of pts.

NURSING CONSIDERATIONS

BASELINE ASSESSMENT

Check serum blood glucose before administration. Discuss lifestyle to determine extent of learning, emotional needs. Ensure follow-up instruction if pt or family does not thoroughly understand diabetes management or glucose-testing technique.

INTERVENTION/EVALUATION

Assess for hypoglycemia (diaphoresis, tremors, dizziness, anxiety, headache, tachycardia, perioral numbness, hunger, diplopia, difficulty concentrating), hyperglycemia (polyuria, polyphagia, polydipsia, nausea, vomiting, dim vision, fatigue, deep, rapid breathing). Be alert to conditions that alter glucose requirements (fever, increased activity or stress, surgical procedures).

PATIENT/FAMILY TEACHING

• Diabetes requires lifelong control. Prescribed diet and exercise are principal parts of treatment; do not skip or delay meals. • Continue to adhere to dietary instructions, regular exercise program, regular testing of blood glucose. • When taking combination drug therapy or when glucose demands are altered (fever, infection, trauma, stress, heavy physical activity), have a source of glucose available to treat symptoms of hypoglycemia.

scopolamine

skoe-**pol**-a-meen
(Trans-Derm Scop, Transderm-V)

FIXED-COMBINATION(S)

Donnatal: scopolamine/atropine (anticholinergic)/hyoscyamine (anticholinergic)/PHENobarbital (sedative): 0.0065 mg/0.0194 mg/0.1037 mg/16.2 mg.

◆CLASSIFICATION

PHARMACOTHERAPEUTIC: Anticholinergic. **CLINICAL:** Antinausea, antiemetic.

USES

Prevention of motion sickness, postop nausea/vomiting. **OFF-LABEL:** Breakthrough treatment of nausea/vomiting associated with chemotherapy.

PRECAUTIONS

Contraindications: Hypersensitivity to scopolamine. Narrow-angle glaucoma. **Cautions:** Hepatic/renal impairment, cardiac disease (hypertension, HF), seizure disorder, psychoses, coronary artery disease, prostatic hyperplasia, urinary retention, reflux esophagitis, ulcerative colitis, hyperthyroidism, GI obstruction, hiatal hernia, elderly pts.

ACTION

Competitively inhibits action of acetylcholine at muscarinic receptors. Reduces excitability of labyrinthine receptors, depressing conduction in vestibular cerebellar pathway. **Therapeutic Effect:** Prevents motion-induced nausea/vomiting.

⧖ LIFESPAN CONSIDERATIONS

Pregnancy/Lactation: Crosses placenta; unknown if distributed in breast milk. **Children:** May be more susceptible to adverse effects. **Elderly:** Dizziness, hallucinations, confusion may require dosage adjustment. Use caution.

INTERACTIONS

DRUG: Anticholinergics (e.g., dicyclomine, glycopyrrolate), antihistamines (e.g., diphenhydraMINE), tricyclic antidepressants (e.g., amitriptyline, doxepin) may increase anticholinergic effects. **CNS depressants (e.g., LORazepam, morphine, zolpidem)** may increase CNS depression. **HERBAL:** None significant. **FOOD: Grapefruit products** may increase concentration/effects. **LAB VALUES:** May interfere with gastric secretion test.

AVAILABILITY (Rx)

Transdermal System (Trans-Derm Scop): 1.5 mg.

ADMINISTRATION/HANDLING

Transdermal
• Apply patch to hairless area behind one ear. • If dislodged or on for more than 72 hrs, replace with fresh patch. • Do not cut/trim. • Limit contact with water.

INDICATIONS/ROUTES/DOSAGE

Prevention of Motion Sickness

Transdermal: ADULTS: One system at least 4 hrs prior to exposure (best if 12 hrs before) and q72h as needed.

Postop Nausea/Vomiting

Transdermal: ADULTS, ELDERLY: 1 system no sooner than 1 hr before surgery and removed 24 hrs after surgery.

Dosage in Renal/Hepatic Impairment
No dose adjustment.

SIDE EFFECTS

Frequent (Greater Than 15%): Dry mouth, drowsiness, blurred vision. **Rare (5%–1%):** Dizziness, restlessness, hallucinations, confusion, difficulty urinating, rash.

ADVERSE EFFECTS/ TOXIC REACTIONS

None known.

NURSING CONSIDERATIONS

BASELINE ASSESSMENT

Assess for use of other CNS depressants, drugs with anticholinergic action, history of narrow-angle glaucoma. Question medical history as listed in Precautions.

INTERVENTION/EVALUATION

Monitor for dehydration. Observe for improvement of symptoms.

PATIENT/FAMILY TEACHING

• Avoid tasks requiring alertness, motor skills until response to drug is established (may cause drowsiness, disorientation, confusion). • Use only 1 patch at a time; do not cut. • Wash hands after administration.

secukinumab

sek-ue-**kin**-ue-mab
(Cosentyx, Cosentyx Sensor Pen)
Do not confuse secukinumab with canakinumab, ranibizumab, trastuzumab, ustekinumab

◆CLASSIFICATION

PHARMACOTHERAPEUTIC: Human interleukin-17A antagonist. **CLINICAL:** Antipsoriasis agent.

USES

Treatment of moderate to severe plaque psoriasis in adult pts who are candidates for systemic therapy or phototherapy,

S

active psoriatic arthritis (PsA), active ankylosing spondylitis (AS).

PRECAUTIONS

Contraindications: Hypersensitivity to secukinumab. **Cautions:** Elderly pts, active Crohn's disease, HIV infection, concomitant immunosuppressants, conditions predisposing to infections (e.g., diabetes, renal failure, immunocompromised pts, open wounds), hypersensitivity to latex (injector pen/prefilled syringe), preexisting or recent-onset CNS demyelinating disorders (e.g., multiple sclerosis, polyneuropathy), pts with chronic or recurrent infection or who have been exposed to tuberculosis, hematologic cytopenias. Administration of live vaccines not recommended.

ACTION

Binds to and inhibits interaction of interleukin-17A receptor, a cytokine that is involved in inflammatory and immune response. May reduce epidermal neutrophils in psoriatic plaques. **Therapeutic Effect:** Alters biologic immune response; reduces inflammation.

PHARMACOKINETICS

Widely distributed. Degraded into small peptides and amino acids via catabolic pathway. Peak plasma concentration: 6 days. Steady state reached in 24 wks. Excretion not defined. **Half-life:** 22–31 days.

⧗ LIFESPAN CONSIDERATIONS

Pregnancy/Lactation: Unknown if distributed in breast milk. **Children:** Safety and efficacy not established. **Elderly:** No age-related precautions noted.

INTERACTIONS

DRUG: May decrease efficacy/immune response of **live vaccines;** may increase risk of toxic effects of **live vaccines. HERBAL:** None significant. **FOOD:** None known. **LAB VALUES:** May significant.

AVAILABILITY (Rx)

Injector Pen: 150 mg/mL solution. **Prefilled Syringe:** 150 mg/mL solution.

ADMINISTRATION/HANDLING

Subcutaneous

Injector Pen/Prefilled Syringe
• Follow instructions for preparation according to manufacturer guidelines. **Administration** • Insert needle subcutaneously into upper arms, outer thigh, or abdomen and inject solution. • Do not inject into areas of active skin disease or injury such as sunburns, skin rashes, inflammation, skin infections, or active psoriasis. • Rotate injection sites.
Storage • Refrigerate until time of use. • Allow injector pen/prefilled syringe/vial to warm to room temperature before use (15–30 min). Do not freeze.

INDICATIONS/ROUTES/DOSAGE

Plaque Psoriasis
SQ: ADULTS, ELDERLY: 300 mg every wk for 5 wks, then 300 mg q4wks. Each 300-mg dose is given as 2 separate injections of 150 mg each.

PsA, AS
Note: With coexistent plaque psoriasis, use dose for plaque psoriasis.
SQ: ADULTS, ELDERLY: Initially, 150 mg at wks 0, 1, 2, 3, and 4, then q4wks or 150 mg q4wks. For PsA, may consider dose of 300 mg.

Dosage in Renal/Hepatic Impairment
Not studied; use caution.

SIDE EFFECTS:

Rare (4%-1%): Diarrhea, urticaria, rhinorrhea.

ADVERSE EFFECTS/ TOXIC REACTIONS

May increase risk of infection including tuberculosis. Infection processes including nasopharyngitis (11% of pts), upper respiratory tract infection (2.5% of pts), mucocutaneous infection with candida (1.2% of pts), rhinitis, pharyngitis, oral herpes (1% of pts) have occurred. May cause exacerbation of Crohn's disease. Hypersensitivity reactions including anaphylaxis were reported. Immunogenicity (auto-secukinumab antibodies) occurred in less than 1% of pts.

NURSING CONSIDERATIONS

BASELINE ASSESSMENT

Obtain baseline vital signs. Pts should be evaluated for active tuberculosis and tested for latent infection prior to initiating treatment and periodically during therapy. Induration of 5 mm or greater with tuberculin skin testing should be considered a positive test result when assessing if treatment for latent tuberculosis is necessary. Antifungal therapy should be considered for those who reside or travel to regions where mycoses are endemic. Do not initiate therapy during active infection. Question history of active Crohn's disease, hepatitis B or C virus infection, HIV infection, demyelinating disorders, cardiovascular disease; concomitant use of immunosuppressive agents.

INTERVENTION/EVALUATION

Monitor for symptoms of tuberculosis, including those who tested negative for latent tuberculosis infection prior to initiating therapy. Interrupt or discontinue treatment if serious infection, opportunistic infection, or sepsis occurs, and initiate appropriate antimicrobial therapy. Monitor skin for disease improvement. Monitor for hypersensitivity reaction.

PATIENT/FAMILY TEACHING

• Treatment may lower your immune system response and reduce your ability to fight infection. • Report symptoms of infection such as body aches, chills, cough, fatigue, fever. • Do not receive live vaccines. • Expect frequent tuberculosis screening. • Report travel plans to possible endemic areas. • Avoid

those with active infection. • Injector pen/prefilled syringe should not be used by pts with latex allergy. • Immediately report itching, hive, rash, swelling of the face or tongue; may indicate allergic reaction. • Treatment may cause worsening of Crohn's disease.

selegiline

se-**le**-ji-leen
(Apo-Selegiline 🍁, Eldepryl, Emsam, Zelapar)
Do not confuse Eldepryl with Elavil or enalapril, selegiline with Salagen, sertraline, or Stelazine, or Zelapar with Zaleplon, Zemplar, or ZyPREXA.

◆CLASSIFICATION

PHARMACOTHERAPEUTIC: MAOI. **CLINICAL:** Antiparkinson agent, antidepressant.

USES

Oral: Adjunct to levodopa/carbidopa in treatment of Parkinson's disease. **Transdermal:** Treatment of major depressive disorder (MDD). **OFF-LABEL:** Treatment of ADHD, early Parkinson's disease.

PRECAUTIONS

Contraindications: Hypersensitivity to selegiline. Concurrent use of meperidine. **Orally disintegrating tablet (additional):** Concurrent use of cyclobenzaprine, dextromethorphan, methadone, St. John's wort, tramadol, oral selegiline, other MAOIs within 14 days of selegiline. **Transdermal (additional):** Pheochromocytoma; concurrent use of bupropion, SSRIs (e.g., fluoxetine), SNRIs (e.g., duloxetine), tricyclic antidepressants, buspirone, tramadol, methadone, dextromethorphan, St. John's wort, mirtazapine, cyclobenzaprine, oral selegiline, other MAOIs, carBAMazepine, oxcarbazepine, sympathomimetics (e.g., amphetamines, cold

S

products containing vasoconstrictors). Elective surgery requiring general anesthesia, local anesthesia containing sympathomimetics; foods high in tyramine content. **Cautions:** Renal/hepatic impairment, depression, elderly pts, major psychiatric disorder; pts at high risk of suicide; pts at high risk of hypotension (cerebrovascular disease, cardiovascular disease, hypovolemia).

ACTION

Irreversibly inhibits activity of monoamine oxidase type B (enzyme that breaks down DOPamine), thereby increasing dopaminergic action. **Therapeutic Effect:** Relieves signs/symptoms of Parkinson's disease (tremor, akinesia, posture/equilibrium disorders, rigidity). Improves mood with MDD.

PHARMACOKINETICS

Route	Onset	Peak	Duration
PO	1 hr	—	24–72 hrs

Rapidly absorbed from GI tract. Crosses blood-brain barrier. Protein binding: 90%. Metabolized in liver. Primarily excreted in urine. **Half-life: PO:** 10 hrs. **Transdermal:** 18–25 hrs.

⧗ LIFESPAN CONSIDERATIONS

Pregnancy/Lactation: Unknown if drug crosses placenta or is distributed in breast milk. **Children:** Safety and efficacy not established. **Elderly:** No age-related precautions noted.

INTERACTIONS

DRUG: FLUoxetine, fluvoxaMINE, PARoxetine, sertraline, venlafaxine may cause mania, serotonin syndrome (altered mental status, restlessness, diaphoresis, diarrhea, fever). **Meperidine** may cause serotonin syndrome reaction (e.g., excitation, diaphoresis, rigidity, hypertension/hypotension, coma, death). **Tricyclic antidepressants (e.g., amitriptyline, doxepin)** may cause diaphoresis, hypertension, syncope, altered mental status, hyperpyrexia, seizures, tremors (wait 14 days between stopping selegiline and starting tricyclic antidepressants). **HERBAL: Kava kava, SAMe, St. John's wort, valerian** may increase risk of serotonin syndrome, excessive sedation. **FOOD: Tyramine-rich foods** may produce hypertensive reactions. **LAB VALUES:** None significant.

AVAILABILITY (Rx)

Capsules: 5 mg. **Tablets:** 5 mg. **Tablets (Orally Disintegrating [Zelapar]):** 1.25 mg. **Transdermal (Emsam):** 6 mg/24 hrs, 9 mg/24 hrs, 12 mg/24 hrs.

ADMINISTRATION/HANDLING

PO
• Give without regard to meals. • Avoid tyramine-containing foods, large quantities of caffeine-containing beverages.

PO (Orally Disintegrating Tablets)
• Give in morning before breakfast and without liquid. • Peel off backing with dry hands (do not push tablets through foil). • Immediately place on top of tongue, allow to disintegrate. • Avoid food, liquids for 5 min before and after taking selegiline.

Transdermal
• Apply to dry, intact skin on upper torso or thigh, outer surface of upper arm. • Avoid exposure to external heat source. • Normal exposure to water unlikely to affect adhesion. • If patch becomes loose, press back into place. If patch falls of again, apply a new patch; follow same dose schedule. • Rotate application sites.

INDICATIONS/ROUTES/DOSAGE

Adjunctive Treatment of Parkinson's Disease
PO: ADULTS: *(Eldepryl):* 10 mg/day in divided doses, such as 5 mg at breakfast and lunch, given concomitantly with each dose of carbidopa and levodopa. **ELDERLY:** Initially, 5 mg in the morning. May increase up to 10 mg/day. **ADULTS,**

S

ELDERLY: *(Zelapar):* Initially, 1.25 mg daily for at least 6 wks. May increase to maximum of 2.5 mg/day.

Major Depressive Disorder
Transdermal: ADULTS: Initially, 6 mg/24 hrs. May increase in 3 mg/24 hrs increments at minimum of 2 wks. **Maximum:** 12 mg/24 hrs. **ELDERLY:** 6 mg/24 hrs **(maximum)**.

Dosage in Renal/Hepatic Impairment
Orally disintegrating tablet: Not recommended in severe impairment.
Oral: Use caution.
Transdermal: No dose adjustment.

SIDE EFFECTS

Frequent (10%–4%): Nausea, dizziness, light-headedness, syncope, abdominal discomfort. **Occasional (3%–2%):** Confusion, hallucinations, dry mouth, vivid dreams, dyskinesia. **Rare (1%):** Headache, myalgia, anxiety, diarrhea, insomnia.

ADVERSE EFFECTS/ TOXIC REACTIONS

Symptoms of overdose may vary from CNS depression (sedation, apnea, cardiovascular collapse, death) to severe paradoxical reactions (hallucinations, tremor, seizures). Impaired motor coordination, (loss of balance, blepharospasm, facial grimaces, feeling of heaviness in lower extremities), depression, nightmares, delusions, overstimulation, sleep disturbance, anger, hallucinations, confusion may occur.

NURSING CONSIDERATIONS

BASELINE ASSESSMENT

Receive full medication history and screen for contraindications/interactions. Question medical history as listed in Precautions. Assess current state of mental health.

INTERVENTION/EVALUATION

Be alert to neurologic effects (headache, lethargy, mental confusion, agitation).

Monitor for evidence of dyskinesia (difficulty with movement). Assess for clinical reversal of symptoms (improvement of tremors of head/hands at rest, mask-like facial expression, shuffling gait, muscular rigidity). Monitor for unusual behavior, worsening depression, suicidal ideation, especially at initiation of therapy or with changes in dosage.

PATIENT/FAMILY TEACHING

• Tolerance to dizziness, light-headedness develops during therapy. • To reduce hypotensive effect, slowly go from lying to standing. • Avoid tasks that require alertness, motor skills until response to drug is established. • Dry mouth, drowsiness, dizziness may be an expected response to drug. • Avoid alcohol. • Report worsening depression, unusual behavior, thoughts of suicide. • Avoid tyramine-rich foods. • Do not take newly prescribed medications unless approved by prescriber who originally started treatment. • Do not take herbal supplements.

sertraline

ser-tra-leen
(Apo-Sertraline ✦, PMS-Sertraline ✦, Zoloft)
■ **BLACK BOX ALERT** ■ Increased risk of suicidal ideation and behavior in children, adolescents, young adults 18–24 yrs with major depressive disorder, other psychiatric disorders.
Do not confuse sertraline with selegiline, Serentil, or Serevent, or Zoloft with Zocor.

◆CLASSIFICATION

PHARMACOTHERAPEUTIC: Selective serotonin reuptake inhibitor.
CLINICAL: Antidepressant, anxiolytic, obsessive-compulsive disorder adjunct.

S

USES

Treatment of major depressive disorders, panic disorder, obsessive-compulsive disorder (OCD), post-traumatic stress disorder (PTSD), premenstrual dysphoric disorder (PMDD), social anxiety disorder. **OFF-LABEL:** Eating disorders, bulimia nervosa, generalized anxiety disorder (GAD).

PRECAUTIONS

Contraindications: Hypersensitivity to sertraline. MAOI use within 14 days (concurrently or within 14 days of stopping an MAOI or sertraline). Concurrent use of oral concentrate (contains alcohol) with disulfiram. Concurrent use with pimozide; initiation in pts treated with linezolid or methylene blue. **Cautions:** Seizure disorder, hepatic impairment, pts at risk for uric acid nephropathy, elderly pts, pts in third trimester of pregnancy, pts at high risk for suicide, family history of bipolar disorder or mania, pts with risk factors for QT prolongation (e.g., hypokalemia, hypomagnesemia), alcoholism. Pts in whom weight loss is undesirable.

ACTION

Blocks reuptake of the neurotransmitter serotonin at CNS neuronal presynaptic membranes, increasing availability at postsynaptic receptor sites. **Therapeutic Effect:** Relieves depression, reduces obsessive-compulsive behavior, decreases anxiety.

PHARMACOKINETICS

Incompletely, slowly absorbed from GI tract; food increases absorption. Protein binding: 98%. Widely distributed. Metabolized in liver. Excreted in urine (45%), feces (45%). Not removed by hemodialysis. **Half-life:** 26 hrs.

⏳ LIFESPAN CONSIDERATIONS

Pregnancy/Lactation: Unknown if drug crosses placenta or is distributed in breast milk. **Children:** Children and adolescents are at increased risk for suicidal ideation and behavior or worsening of depression, esp. during the first few mos of therapy. **Elderly:** No age-related precautions noted, but lower initial dosages recommended.

INTERACTIONS

DRUG: Anticoagulants (e.g., heparin, rivaroxaban, warfarin), antiplatelets (e.g., aspirin, clopidogrel), NSAIDs (e.g., ibuprofen, ketorolac, naproxen), thrombolytics (e.g., alteplase) may increase risk of bleeding. May increase concentration, risk of toxicity of **highly protein-bound medications (e.g., digoxin, warfarin).** MAOIs (e.g., phenelzine, selegiline) may cause neuroleptic malignant syndrome, serotonin syndrome. Concomitant use of other **serotonergic drugs (e.g., buspirone, carBAMazepine, fentanyl, linezolid, SNRIs [e.g., duloxetine, venlafaxine], triptans [e.g., sumatriptan])** may cause serotonin syndrome. May increase concentration, toxicity of **tricyclic antidepressants (e.g., amitriptyline, doxepin).** **HERBAL:** Gotu kola, kava kava, St. John's wort, valerian may increase CNS depression. **St. John's wort** may increase risk of serotonin syndrome. **FOOD:** None known. **LAB VALUES:** May increase total serum cholesterol, triglycerides, ALT, AST. May decrease serum uric acid.

AVAILABILITY (Rx)

Oral Concentrate: 20 mg/mL. **Tablets:** 25 mg, 50 mg, 100 mg.

ADMINISTRATION/HANDLING

PO

• Give with food, milk if GI distress occurs. • Oral concentrate must be diluted before administration. Mix with 4 oz water, ginger ale, lemon/lime soda, or orange juice *only.* Give immediately after mixing.

---

underlined – top prescribed drug

INDICATIONS/ROUTES/DOSAGE

Depression

PO: ADULTS: Initially, 50 mg/day. May increase by 50 mg/day at 7-day intervals up to 200 mg/day. **ELDERLY:** Initially, 25 mg/day. May increase by 25–50 mg/day at 7-day intervals up to 200 mg/day.

Obsessive-Compulsive Disorder (OCD)

PO: ADULTS, CHILDREN 13–17 YRS: Initially, 50 mg/day with morning or evening meal. May increase by 50 mg/day at 7-day intervals up to 200 mg/day. **ELDERLY, CHILDREN 6–12 YRS:** Initially, 25 mg/day. May increase by 25–50 mg/day at 7-day intervals. **Maximum:** 200 mg/day.

Panic Disorder, Post-Traumatic Stress Disorder (PTSD), Social Anxiety Disorder (SAD)

PO: ADULTS, ELDERLY: Initially, 25 mg/day. May increase by 50 mg/day at 7-day intervals. Range: 50–200 mg/day. **Maximum:** 200 mg/day.

Premenstrual Dysphoric Disorder (PMDD)

PO: ADULTS: Initially, 50 mg/day either daily throughout menstrual cycle or limited to luteal phase of menstrual cycle. May increase up to 150 mg/day per menstrual cycle in 50-mg increments when dosing throughout menstrual cycle or 100 mg/day when dosing during luteal phase only.

Dosage in Renal Impairment

No dose adjustment.

Dosage in Hepatic Impairment

Use caution.

SIDE EFFECTS

Frequent (26%–12%): Headache, nausea, diarrhea, insomnia, drowsiness, dizziness, fatigue, rash, dry mouth. **Occasional (6%–4%):** Anxiety, nervousness, agitation, tremor, dyspepsia, diaphoresis, vomiting, constipation, sexual dysfunction, visual disturbances, altered taste. **Rare (Less Than 3%):** Flatulence, urinary frequency, paresthesia, hot flashes, chills.

ADVERSE EFFECTS/ TOXIC REACTIONS

Serotonin syndrome (seizures, arrhythmias, high fever), neuroleptic malignant syndrome (muscle rigidity, cognitive changes), suicidal ideation have occurred.

NURSING CONSIDERATIONS

BASELINE ASSESSMENT

Assess appearance, behavior, speech patterns, level of interest, mood. For pts on long-term therapy, CBC, renal function, LFT should be performed periodically.

INTERVENTION/EVALUATION

Assess mental status for depression, suicidal ideation (esp. at beginning of therapy or change in dosage), anxiety, social function, panic attack. Monitor daily pattern of bowel activity, stool consistency. Assist with ambulation if dizziness occurs.

PATIENT/FAMILY TEACHING

• Dry mouth may be relieved by sugarless gum, sips of water. • Report headache, fatigue, tremor, sexual dysfunction. • Avoid tasks that require alertness, motor skills until response to drug is established (may cause dizziness, drowsiness). • Take with food if nausea occurs. • Inform physician if pregnancy occurs. • Avoid alcohol. • Do not take OTC medications without consulting physician. • Report worsening of depression, suicidal ideation.

sevelamer

se-**vel**-a-mer
(Renagel, Renvela)
Do not confuse Renagel with Reglan, Regonol, or Renvela, or sevelamer with Savella.

◆CLASSIFICATION

PHARMACOTHERAPEUTIC: Polymeric phosphate binder. **CLINICAL:** Electrolyte modifier, antihyperphosphatemia agent.

USES

Reduction of serum phosphorus in pts with chronic renal disease on hemodialysis.

PRECAUTIONS

Contraindications: Hypersensitivity to sevelamer. Bowel obstruction. **Cautions:** Dysphagia, severe GI tract motility disorders, major GI tract surgery.

ACTION

Binds with dietary phosphorus in GI tract, allowing phosphorus to be eliminated through normal digestive process, decreasing serum phosphorus level. **Therapeutic Effect:** Decreases incidence of hypercalcemic episodes in pts receiving calcium acetate treatment.

PHARMACOKINETICS

Not absorbed systemically. Unknown if removed by hemodialysis.

⧖ LIFESPAN CONSIDERATIONS

Pregnancy/Lactation: Not distributed in breast milk. **Children:** Safety and efficacy not established. **Elderly:** No age-related precautions noted.

INTERACTIONS

DRUG: May decrease concentration/effect of **fluoroquinolones (e.g., levo-FLOXacin)**. **HERBAL:** None significant. **FOOD:** May cause reduced absorption of **vitamins D, E, K, folic acid**. **LAB VALUES:** Expected to decrease serum phosphate.

AVAILABILITY (Rx)

Powder for Oral Suspension (Renvela): 0.8 g/pack, 2.4 g/pack.

🔖 **Tablets (Renagel):** 400 mg, 800 mg. **(Renvela):** 800 mg.

ADMINISTRATION/HANDLING

PO

• Give with meals. • Space other medication by at least 1 hr before or 3 hrs after sevelamer. • Give tablets whole; do not break, crush, dissolve, or divide. • **Oral Suspension:** Mix 0.8 g with 30 mL water (2.4 g with 60 mL water). Stir vigorously to suspend (does not dissolve) just prior to drinking.

INDICATIONS/ROUTES/DOSAGE

Hyperphosphatemia

PO: ADULTS, ELDERLY: 800–1,600 mg with each meal, depending on severity of hyperphosphatemia (5.5–7.4 mg/dL: 800 mg 3 times/day; 7.5–8.9 mg/dL: 1,200–1,600 mg 3 times/day; 9 mg/dL or greater: 1,600 mg 3 times/day). **Maintenance:** Based on serum phosphorus concentrations. Goal range: 3.5–5.5 mg/dL.

Serum Phosphorus

Concentration	Dosage
Greater than 5.5 mg/dL	Increase by 400–800 mg per meal at 2-wk intervals
3.5–5.5 mg/dL	Maintain current dosage
Less than 3.5 mg/dL	Decrease by 400–800 mg per meal

Dosage in Renal/Hepatic Impairment
No dose adjustment.

SIDE EFFECTS

Frequent (20%–11%): Infection, pain, hypotension, diarrhea, dyspepsia, nausea, vomiting. **Occasional (10%–1%):** Headache, constipation, hypertension, increased cough.

ADVERSE EFFECTS/ TOXIC REACTIONS

Thrombosis occurs rarely.

NURSING CONSIDERATIONS

BASELINE ASSESSMENT

Obtain baseline chemistries, esp serum calcium, phosphate; assess for bowel obstruction.

S

INTERVENTION/EVALUATION

Monitor serum phosphate, bicarbonate, chloride, calcium.

PATIENT/FAMILY TEACHING

• Take with meals, swallow tablets whole; do not chew, crush, dissolve, or divide tablets. • Report persistent headache, nausea, vomiting, diarrhea, hypotension.

simeprevir

sim-e-pre-veer
(Galexos, Olysio)

■ **BLACK BOX ALERT** ■ Test all pts for hepatitis B virus (HBV) infection prior to initiation. HBV reactivation was reported in HBV/HBC coinfected pts who were undergoing or had completed treatment with HCV direct-acting antivirals and were not receiving HBV antiviral therapy. HBV reactivation may cause fulminant hepatitis, hepatic failure, and death.

Do not confuse simeprevir with sofosbuvir.

◆CLASSIFICATION

PHARMACOTHERAPEUTIC: Protease inhibitor. **CLINICAL:** Antiviral.

USES

Treatment of genotypes 1 and 4 chronic hepatitis C virus infection, in combination with other antihepaciviral therapy, in adults without cirrhosis or with compensated cirrhosis.

PRECAUTIONS

Contraindications: Hypersensitivity to simeprevir. Pregnancy, male partners of pregnant women, breastfeeding, any contraindications to other antihepacivirals used in combination for treatment of chronic hepatitis C. **Cautions:** Pts of East Asian ancestry, sulfa allergy, or history of HIV, sun exposure, severe hepatic impairment. Latent or current HBV. Do not use as monotherapy. Combination with ribavirin is contraindicated with pregnancy. Avoid use in combination with peginterferon and ribavirin with decompensated cirrhosis.

ACTION

Inhibits hepatitis C virus (HCV) protease needed for cleavage of HCV-encoded polyproteins by binding to active serine protease sites. **Therapeutic Effect:** Inhibits viral replication of hepatitis C virus.

PHARMACOKINETICS

Well absorbed after PO administration. Metabolized in liver. Protein binding: 99.9%. Peak plasma concentration: 4–6 hrs. Excreted primarily in feces via biliary route (91%). **Half-life:** 10–13 hrs.

⌛ LIFESPAN CONSIDERATIONS

Pregnancy/Lactation: Strictly avoid pregnancy. May cause birth defects or fetal demise. Women of childbearing age must use two different forms of reliable of birth control during treatment and for at least 6 mos after discontinuation. Do not initiate therapy until negative pregnancy test confirmed. Unknown if distributed in breast milk. Breastfeeding contraindicated. **Children:** Safety and efficacy not established. **Elderly:** No age-related precautions noted. **Race:** Pts of East Asian ancestry may have increased risk of adverse reactions due to increased drug exposure/sensitivity.

INTERACTIONS

DRUG: May increase concentration/effects of **antiarrhythmics (e.g., amiodarone, quiNIDine), calcium channel blockers (e.g., felodipine, NIFEdipine), cycloSPORINE, digoxin, sedative/hypnotics (e.g., midazolam, triazolam), statins (e.g., atorvastatin, simvastatin), sildenafil, vardenafil.** May decrease

S

concentration/effects of **sirolimus, tacrolimus. CYP3A4 inducers (e.g., carBAMazepine, rifAMPin)** may decrease concentration/effects. **CYP3A4 inhibitors (e.g., itraconazole, fluconazole, clarithromycin, ritonavir)** may increase concentration/effects. **HERBAL: St. John's wort** may decrease concentration/effects. **Milk thistle** *(Silybum marianum)* may increase concentration/effects. **FOOD:** None known. **LAB VALUES:** May increase serum alkaline phosphatase, bilirubin.

AVAILABILITY (Rx)

🟦 **Capsules:** 150 mg.

ADMINISTRATION/HANDLING

PO
• Administer with food. • Administer capsule whole; do not break, crush, or open.

INDICATIONS/ROUTES/DOSAGE

◀ **ALERT** ▶ Must use in combination with other antihepacivirals. Not recommended as monotherapy. Dose reduction of simeprevir not recommended. Combination therapy with peginterferon/ribavirin not recommended in HCV treatment guidelines.

Chronic Hepatitis C Infection (with Peginterferon Alfa and Ribavirin)
PO: ADULTS/ELDERLY: 150 mg daily with food for 12 wks (with peginterferon alfa and ribavirin).
Treatment Naïve, Prior Relapsers (Including Cirrhosis): Extend peginterferon alfa and ribavirin therapy for additional 12 wks after completing 12-wk triple therapy (24 wks total).
Prior Nonresponders (Including Cirrhosis): Extend peginterferon alfa and ribavirin therapy for additional 36 wks after completing 12-wk triple therapy (48 wks total).

Chronic Hepatitis C Infection (with Sofosbuvir)
PO: ADULTS, ELDERLY: (Treatment naïve or treatment experienced without

cirrhosis): 150 mg daily with food for 12 wks. **(Treatment naïve or treatment experienced with cirrhosis):** 150 mg daily with food for 24 wks.

Treatment Futility
If HCV RNA viral load greater than or equal to 25 IU/mL at wk 4, discontinue simeprevir, peginterferon alfa, and ribavirin. If HCV RNA viral load greater than or equal to 25 IU/mL at wk 12 or 24, discontinue peginterferon alfa and ribavirin (simeprevir already completed at wk 12). Discontinue therapy if serious adverse effects occur.

Dosage in Renal Impairment
No dose adjustment.

Dosage in Hepatic Impairment
Not recommended in moderate to severe impairment.

SIDE EFFECTS

Frequent (28%–22%): Rash, pruritus, nausea. **Occasional (16%–12%):** Myalgia, dyspnea.

ADVERSE EFFECTS/ TOXIC REACTIONS

Increased risk of thromboembolic events associated with peginterferon alfa. Dermatologic events/photosensitivity including generalized rash, erythema, eczema, maculopapular rash, dermatitis, skin exfoliation, rash erythematosus, urticaria, allergic dermatitis, cutaneous vasculitis, skin eruption, photodermatosis, sunburn reported. Mild to moderate dyspnea reported in 12% of pts. Pts of East Asian ancestry may have increased risk of photosensitivity.

NURSING CONSIDERATIONS

BASELINE ASSESSMENT
Obtain baseline vital signs, CBC, HCV-RNA level, complete metabolic panel, liver function test. Confirm hepatitis C genotype. Receive full history of home

S

medications including herbal products. Screen for contraindications to peginterferon alfa and ribavirin. Confirm negative pregnancy test before initiating treatment. Question history of anemia, HIV, hepatitis B, liver transplantation, pulmonary disease, renal impairment. Conduct dermatologic exam, noting baseline skin characteristics, moles, lesions.

INTERVENTION/EVALUATION

Assess vital signs routinely. Monitor CBC, HCV-RNA levels, electrolytes accordingly. Obtain urine pregnancy every mo and for 6 mos after discontinuation in female pts of childbearing age. Reinforce birth control compliance. Monitor for intrauterine device failures if applicable. Monitor international normalized ratio (INR) level if on warfarin. Monitor for bruising, dyspnea, hematuria, DVT, pulmonary embolism. Encourage nutritional intake and assess for anorexia, weight loss.

PATIENT/FAMILY TEACHING

• Treatment must be used in combination with peginterferon, ribavirin. Inform pts of side effects/contraindications of triple-medication regimen. Periodic lab tests are an essential part of therapy. • Report any newly prescribed medications. • Do not take herbal products. • Women of childbearing age must use two different forms of reliable birth control during treatment and for at least 6 mos after treatment. Do not breastfeed. • Notify physician if female partner becomes pregnant. • Report difficulty breathing, weakness, dizziness, weight loss. • Avoid alcohol. • Take with meals. Do not use tanning beds. Limit sun exposure; use protective UV measures. Immediately report any changes to skin including rash, skin peeling, ulcers, or new moles/lesions.

simvastatin

sim-va-sta-tin
(Apo-Simvastatin ✸, Zocor)
Do not confuse simvastatin with atorvastatin, lovastatin, nystatin, pitavastatin, or pravastatin, or Zocor with Cozaar, Lipitor, Zoloft, or ZyrTEC.

FIXED-COMBINATION(S)

Juvisync: simvastatin/SITagliptin (an antidiabetic agent): 10 mg/100 mg, 20 mg/100 mg, 40 mg/100 mg. **Simcor:** simvastatin/niacin (an antilipemic agent): 20 mg/500 mg, 40 mg/500 mg, 20 mg/750 mg, 20 mg/1,000 mg, 40 mg/1,000 mg. **Vytorin:** simvastatin/ezetimibe (a cholesterol absorption inhibitor): 10 mg/10 mg, 20 mg/10 mg, 40 mg/10 mg, 80 mg/10 mg.

◆CLASSIFICATION

PHARMACOTHERAPEUTIC: Hydroxymethylglutaryl-CoA (HMG-CoA) reductase inhibitor. **CLINICAL:** Antihyperlipidemic.

USES

Secondary prevention of cardiovascular events in pts with hypercholesterolemia and coronary heart disease (CHD) or at high risk for CHD. Treatment of hyperlipidemias to reduce elevations in total serum cholesterol, LDL-C, apolipoprotein B, triglycerides, VLDL-C and increase HDL-C. Treatment of homozygous familial hypercholesterolemia. Treatment of heterozygous familial hypercholesterolemia in adolescents (10–17 yrs, females more than 1 yr postmenarche).

PRECAUTIONS

Contraindications: Hypersensitivity to simvastatin. Active hepatic disease or unexplained, persistent elevations of hepatic function test results, pregnancy, breastfeeding, concurrent use of strong CYP3A4 inhibitors (e.g., clarithromycin,

S

---

cycloSPORINE, gemfibrozil). **Cautions:** History of hepatic disease, diabetes, severe renal impairment, substantial alcohol consumption. Withholding or discontinuing simvastatin may be necessary when pt is at risk for renal failure secondary to rhabdomyolysis. Concomitant use of other medications associated with myopathy.

ACTION

Interferes with cholesterol biosynthesis by inhibiting conversion of the enzyme HMG-CoA to mevalonate. **Therapeutic Effect:** Decreases LDL, cholesterol, VLDL, triglyceride levels; increase in HDL concentration.

PHARMACOKINETICS

Well absorbed from GI tract. Protein binding: 95%. Metabolized in liver. Excreted in feces (60%), urine (13%). Unknown if removed by hemodialysis.

Route	Onset	Peak	Duration
PO (to reduce cholesterol)	3 days	14 days	N/A

⌛ LIFESPAN CONSIDERATIONS

Pregnancy/Lactation: Contraindicated in pregnancy (suppression of cholesterol biosynthesis may cause fetal toxicity), lactation. Risk of serious adverse reactions in breastfeeding infants. **Children:** Safety and efficacy not established in children less than 10 yrs of age or in premenarchal girls. **Elderly:** No age-related precautions noted.

INTERACTIONS

DRUG: CycloSPORINE, CYP3A4 inhibitors (e.g., ketoconazole, erythromycin), amiodarone, calcium channel blockers (e.g., diltiaZEM, verapamil), colchicine, fibrates, gemfibrozil, niacin, ranolazine may increase risk of acute renal failure, rhabdomyolysis. **HERBAL:** St. John's wort may decrease concentration. **FOOD: Grapefruit products** may increase concentration, toxicity. **Red yeast rice** contains 2.4 mg **lovastatin** per 600 mg rice. **LAB VALUES:** May increase serum creatine kinase (CK), transaminase.

AVAILABILITY (Rx)

Tablets: 5 mg, 10 mg, 20 mg, 40 mg, 80 mg.

ADMINISTRATION/HANDLING

PO
• Give without regard to meals.
• Administer in evening for maximum efficacy.

INDICATIONS/ROUTES/DOSAGE

Note: Limit 80-mg dose to pts taking simvastatin longer than 12 mos without evidence of myopathy.

Prevention of Cardiovascular Events
PO: ADULTS, ELDERLY: 10–20 mg once daily. Range: 5–40 mg/day.

Hyperlipidemias
PO: ADULTS, ELDERLY: Initially, 10–20 mg once daily. (Pts with CHD or CHD risk equivalents): Initially, 40 mg/day. Range: 5–40 mg/day.

Homozygous Familial Hypercholesterolemia
PO: ADULTS, ELDERLY: 40 mg once daily in evening.

Heterozygous Familial Hypercholesterolemia
PO: CHILDREN 10–17 YRS: 10 mg once daily in evening. Range: 10–40 mg/day.

Dosing Adjustment with Medications
CycloSPORINE, gemfibrozil: Do not exceed 10 mg/day. **Amiodarone, amLODIPine, ranolazine:** Do not exceed 20 mg/day. **DiltiaZEM, dronedarone, verapamil:** Do not exceed 10 mg/day. **Lomitapide:** Reduce simvastatin dose by 50% when initiating lomitapide. Do not exceed 20 mg/day.

Dosage in Renal Impairment
CrCl less than 30 mL/min: Initially, 5 mg/day.

Dosage in Hepatic Impairment
Contraindicated with active hepatic disease.

SIDE EFFECTS

Generally well tolerated. Side effects are usually mild and transient. **Occasional (3%–2%):** Headache, abdominal pain/cramps, constipation, upper respiratory tract infection. **Rare (Less Than 2%):** Diarrhea, flatulence, asthenia, nausea/vomiting, depression.

ADVERSE EFFECTS/ TOXIC REACTIONS

Potential for ocular lens opacities. Hypersensitivity reaction, hepatitis occur rarely. Myopathy (muscle pain, tenderness, weakness with elevated serum creatine kinase [CK], sometimes taking the form of rhabdomyolysis) has occurred.

NURSING CONSIDERATIONS

BASELINE ASSESSMENT

Obtain dietary history, esp. fat consumption. Question for possibility of pregnancy before initiating therapy. Question for history of hypersensitivity to simvastatin. Assess baseline lab results: serum cholesterol, LDL, VLDL, HDL, triglycerides, LFT.

INTERVENTION/EVALUATION

Monitor serum cholesterol, triglyceride lab results for therapeutic response. Monitor LFT. Monitor daily pattern of bowel activity, stool consistency. Assess for headache, myopathy.

PATIENT/FAMILY TEACHING

• Use appropriate contraceptive measures. • Periodic lab tests are essential part of therapy. • Maintain appropriate diet. Avoid grapefruit products. • Report unexplained muscle pain, tenderness, weakness.

sirolimus

sir-**oh**-li-mus
(Rapamune)

■ **BLACK BOX ALERT** ■ Increased susceptibility to infection and potential for development of lymphoma. Not recommended for liver or lung transplant pts. Use only by physicians experienced in immunosuppressive therapy and management of transplant pts.
Do not confuse Rapamune with Rapaflo, or sirolimus with everolimus, pimecrolimus, tacrolimus, or temsirolimus.

◆CLASSIFICATION

PHARMACOTHERAPEUTIC: mTOR kinase inhibitor. **CLINICAL:** Immunosuppressant.

USES

Prophylaxis of organ rejection in pts receiving renal transplant (in combination with cycloSPORINE and corticosteroids). Treatment of lymphangioleiomyomatosis. **OFF-LABEL:** Prophylaxis of organ rejection in heart transplant recipients. Prevention of acute graft-vs-host disease in allogeneic stem cell transplantation. Treatment of refractory acute or chronic graft-vs-host disease. Rescue agent for acute and chronic organ rejection.

PRECAUTIONS

Contraindications: Hypersensitivity to sirolimus. **Cautions:** Cardiovascular disease (HF, hypertension); pulmonary disease, hepatic impairment, renal impairment, hyperlipidemia, perioperative period due to increased chance of surgical complications from impaired wound and tissue healing. Concurrent use with medications that may alter renal function.

ACTION

Inhibits T-lymphocyte activation and proliferation in response to antigenic and cytokine stimulation, and inhibits antibody production. **Therapeutic Effect:** Inhibits acute rejection of allografts and prolongs graft survival.

S

PHARMACOKINETICS

Rapidly absorbed from GI tract. Protein binding: 92%. Extensively metabolized in liver. Primarily excreted in feces (91%). **Half-life:** 57–63 hrs.

⌛ LIFESPAN CONSIDERATIONS

Pregnancy/Lactation: Unknown if drug crosses placenta or is distributed in breast milk. **Children:** Safety and efficacy not established in pts younger than 13 yrs. **Elderly:** No age-related precautions noted.

INTERACTIONS

DRUG: CYP3A4 inducers (e.g., carBAMazepine, rifabutin, rifAMPin) may decrease concentration/effects. **CYP3A4 inhibitors (e.g., clarithromycin, erythromycin, itraconazole, verapamil)** may increase concentration, toxicity. May increase concentration/effects of **cycloSPORINE** (take sirolimus 4 hrs after cycloSPORINE for renal transplant). **HERBAL: St. John's wort** may decrease concentration. **Cat's claw, echinacea** possess immunostimulant properties. **Garlic, ginger, ginseng** may increase hypoglycemia. **FOOD: Grapefruit products** may increase risk of myelotoxicity, nephrotoxicity. **LAB VALUES:** May increase serum ALT, AST, alkaline phosphatase, LDH, BUN, creatine phosphate, cholesterol, triglycerides, creatinine. May alter WBC, serum glucose, calcium. May decrease Hgb, Hct.

AVAILABILITY (Rx)

Oral Solution: 1 mg/mL.

🔖 **Tablets:** 0.5 mg, 1 mg, 2 mg.

ADMINISTRATION/HANDLING

• Doses should be taken 4 hrs after cycloSPORINE. • Take consistently with or without food. • Do not break, crush, dissolve, or divide tablets. • Mix oral solution with only water or orange juice, stir vigorously, drink immediately.

INDICATIONS/ROUTES/DOSAGE

◀ **ALERT** ▶ Tablets and oral solution are not bioequivalent. (However, clinical equivalence shown at 2 mg dose.)

Prevention of Organ Transplant Rejection (Low to Moderate Risk)
PO: ADULTS, CHILDREN 13 YRS AND OLDER WEIGHING MORE THAN 40 KG: Loading dose: 6 mg on day 1. **Maintenance:** 2 mg/day. **ADULTS, CHILDREN 13 YRS AND OLDER WEIGHING LESS THAN 40 KG:** Loading dose: 3 mg/m^2 on day 1. **Maintenance:** 1 mg/m^2/day.

Prevention of Organ Transplant Rejection (High Risk)
PO: ADULTS: Loading dose: Up to 15 mg on day 1. **Maintenance:** 5 mg/day. Obtain trough between 5–7 days. Continue therapy for 1 yr following transplantation. Further adjustments based on clinical status.

Lymphangioleiomyomatosis
PO: ADULTS, ELDERLY: Initially, 2 mg/day with dosage adjustment to maintain concentration between 5–15 ng/mL.

Dosage in Renal Impairment
No dose adjustment.

Dosage in Hepatic Impairment
Loading dose: No change. **Maintenance dose: Mild to moderate impairment:** Reduce dose by 33%. **Severe impairment:** Reduce dose by 50%.

SIDE EFFECTS

Occasional: Hypercholesterolemia, hyperlipidemia, hypertension, rash. **High doses (5 mg/day):** Anemia, arthralgia, diarrhea, hypokalemia, peripheral edema, thrombocytopenia.

ADVERSE EFFECTS/ TOXIC REACTIONS

Hepatotoxicity occurs rarely. Skin carcinoma (including basal cell, squamous cell, melanoma) has been observed.

NURSING CONSIDERATIONS

BASELINE ASSESSMENT

Obtain LFT. Assess for pregnancy, lactation. Question for medication usage (esp. cycloSPORINE, diltiaZEM, ketoconazole, rifAMPin). Determine if pt has chickenpox, herpes zoster, malignancy, infection.

INTERVENTION/EVALUATION

Monitor serum renal function, LFT periodically. Monitor serum cholesterol, triglycerides, platelets; Hgb.

PATIENT/FAMILY TEACHING

• Avoid those with colds, other infections. • Avoid grapefruit products. • Avoid exposure to sunlight, artificial light sources. • Strict monitoring is essential in identifying, preventing symptoms of organ rejection. • Do not chew, crush, dissolve, or divide tablets.

SITagliptin

sit-a-**glip**-tin
(Januvia)
Do not confuse Januvia with Enjuvia, Jantoven, or Janumet, or SITagliptin with SAXagliptin or SUMAtriptan.

FIXED-COMBINATION(S)

Janumet, Janumet XR: SITagliptin/metFORMIN (an antidiabetic): 50 mg/500 mg, 50 mg/1,000 mg. **Juvisync:** SITagliptin/simvastatin (an antilipidemic agent): 100 mg/10 mg, 100 mg/20 mg, 100 mg/40 mg.

◆CLASSIFICATION

PHARMACOTHERAPEUTIC: DPP-4 inhibitors (gliptins). **CLINICAL:** Antidiabetic agent.

USES

Adjunctive treatment to diet, exercise to improve glycemic control in pts with type 2 diabetes as monotherapy or in combination with other antidiabetic agents.

PRECAUTIONS

Contraindications: Hypersensitivity to SITagliptin. **Cautions:** Type I diabetes, diabetic ketoacidosis, renal impairment, end-stage renal disease, history of pancreatitis, angioedema with other DPP-4 inhibitors. Concurrent use of other glucose-lowering agents may increase risk of hypoglycemia.

ACTION

Inhibits DPP-4 enzyme, causing prolonged active incretin levels. Incretin regulates glucose homeostasis. **Therapeutic Effect:** Regulates glucose homeostasis. Increases synthesis and release of insulin from pancreatic cells; lowers glucagon secretion from pancreas, decreases hepatic glucose production.

PHARMACOKINETICS

Route	Onset	Peak	Duration
PO	N/A	1–4 hrs	24 hrs

Rapidly absorbed. Protein binding: 38%. Excreted in urine (87%), feces (13%). **Half-life:** 12 hrs.

⧗ LIFESPAN CONSIDERATIONS

Pregnancy/Lactation: Unknown if distributed in breast milk. **Children:** Safety and efficacy not established. **Elderly:** No age-related precautions noted.

INTERACTIONS

DRUG: None known. **HERBAL:** None significant. **FOOD:** None known. **LAB VALUES:** May slightly increase WBCs, particularly neutrophil count. May increase serum creatinine.

AVAILABILITY (Rx)

🗳 **Tablets (Film-Coated):** 25 mg, 50 mg, 100 mg.

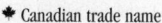
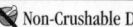

ADMINISTRATION/HANDLING

PO
• May give without regard to food.
• Do not break, crush, dissolve, or divide film-coated tablets.

INDICATIONS/ROUTES/DOSAGE

Type 2 Diabetes
PO: ADULTS OVER 18 YRS, ELDERLY: 100 mg once daily.

Dosage in Renal Impairment
Moderate impairment: (CrCl equal to or greater than 30 mL/min to less than 50 mL/min): 50 mg once daily. **Severe impairment:** (CrCl less than 30 mL/min or dialysis pt): 25 mg once daily.

Dosage in Hepatic Impairment
No dose adjustment.

SIDE EFFECTS

Occasional (5% and greater): Headache, nasopharyngitis. **Rare (3%–1%):** Diarrhea, abdominal pain, nausea.

ADVERSE EFFECTS/ TOXIC REACTIONS

Hypersensitivity reactions including angioedema, Stevens-Johnson syndrome reported. Acute pancreatitis occurs rarely.

NURSING CONSIDERATIONS

BASELINE ASSESSMENT
Check serum glucose concentration before administration. Assess renal function. Discuss lifestyle to determine extent of learning, emotional needs. Ensure follow-up instruction if pt, family do not thoroughly understand diabetes management, glucose-testing technique.

INTERVENTION/EVALUATION
Monitor serum glucose, Hgb A1c, BUN, creatinine. Assess for hypoglycemia (diaphoresis, tremor, dizziness, anxiety, headache, tachycardia, perioral numbness, hunger, diplopia, difficulty concentrating), hyperglycemia (polyuria, polyphagia, polydipsia, nausea, vomiting, dim vision, fatigue, deep, rapid breathing). Be alert to conditions that alter glucose requirements (fever, increased activity, stress, trauma, surgical procedures).

PATIENT/FAMILY TEACHING
• Diabetes requires lifelong control.
• Prescribed diet, exercise are principal part of treatment; do not skip, delay meals. • Continue to adhere to dietary instructions, regular exercise program, regular testing of serum glucose. • When taking combination drug therapy or when glucose demands are altered (fever, infection, trauma, stress, heavy physical activity), have source of glucose available to treat symptoms of hypoglycemia. • Report nausea, vomiting, anorexia, severe abdominal pain, pancreatitis.

---

sodium bicarbonate

soe-dee-um bye-**kar**-boe-nate

◆CLASSIFICATION

PHARMACOTHERAPEUTIC: Alkalinizing agent. **CLINICAL:** Antacid electrolyte, urinary/systemic alkalinizer.

USES

Management of metabolic acidosis, gastric hyperacidity. Alkalinization agent for urine; hyperkalemia treatment; management of overdose of tricyclic antidepressants and aspirin. **OFF-LABEL:** Prevention of contrast-induced nephropathy.

PRECAUTIONS

Contraindications: Hypersensitivity to sodium bicarbonate. Hypernatremia, alkalosis, unknown abdominal pain, hypocalcemia, severe pulmonary edema. **Cautions:** HF, edematous states, renal insufficiency, cirrhosis.

ACTION

Dissociates to provide bicarbonate ion. **Therapeutic Effect:** Neutralizes

---

hydrogen ion concentration, raises blood, urinary pH.

PHARMACOKINETICS

Route	Onset	Peak	Duration
PO	15 min	N/A	1–3 hrs
IV	Immediate	N/A	8–10 min

Well absorbed following PO administration, sodium bicarbonate dissociates to sodium and bicarbonate ions. With increased hydrogen ion concentrations, bicarbonate ions combine with hydrogen ions to form carbonic acid, which then dissociates to CO_2, which is excreted by the lungs. Plasma concentration regulated by kidney (ability to form, excrete bicarbonate).

⧗ LIFESPAN CONSIDERATIONS

Pregnancy/Lactation: May produce hypernatremia, increase tendon reflexes in neonate or fetus whose mother is administered chronically high doses. May be distributed in breast milk. **Children:** No age-related precautions noted. Do not use as antacid in pts younger than 6 yrs. **Elderly:** Age-related renal impairment may require dosage adjustment.

INTERACTIONS

DRUG: May increase concentration, toxicity of **quiNIDine, quiNINE.** May decrease effects of **lithium. HERBAL:** None significant. **FOOD: Milk, other dairy products** may result in milk-alkali syndrome. **LAB VALUES:** May increase serum, urinary pH.

AVAILABILITY (Rx)

Injection Solution (Rx): 0.5 mEq/mL (4.2%), 1 mEq/mL (8.4%). **Tablets (OTC):** 325 mg, 650 mg.

ADMINISTRATION/HANDLING

◻ IV

◀ALERT▶ For direct IV administration in neonates or infants, use 0.5 mEq/mL concentration.

Reconstitution • May give undiluted. **Rate of Administration** • For IV push, give up to 1 mEq/kg over 1–3 min for cardiac arrest. • For IV infusion, do not exceed rate of infusion of 1 mEq/kg/hr. • For children younger than 2 yrs, premature infants, neonates, administer by slow infusion, up to 10 mEq/min.
Storage • Store at room temperature.

PO
• Give 1–3 hrs after meals.

▦ IV INCOMPATIBILITIES

Amiodarone (Cordarone), ascorbic acid, calcium chloride, diltiaZEM (Cardizem), DOBUTamine (Dobutrex), DOPamine (Intropin), HYDRO-morphone (Dilaudid), magnesium sulfate, midazolam (Versed), norepinephrine (Levophed), ondansetron (Zofran).

▦ IV COMPATIBILITIES

Dexmedetomidine (Precedex), furosemide (Lasix), heparin, insulin, lidocaine, mannitol, milrinone (Primacor), morphine, phenylephrine (Neo-Synephrine), potassium chloride, propofol (Diprivan), vancomycin (Vancocin).

INDICATIONS/ROUTES/DOSAGE

◀ALERT▶ May give by IV push, IV infusion, or orally. Dose individualized based on severity of acidosis, laboratory values, pt age, weight, clinical conditions. Do not fully correct bicarbonate deficit during the first 24 hrs (may cause metabolic alkalosis).

Cardiac Arrest
◀ALERT▶ Routine use not recommended.

IV: ADULTS, ELDERLY: Initially, 1 mEq/kg. May repeat with 0.5 mEq/kg in 10 min one time during continued cardiopulmonary arrest. Use in postresuscitation phase is based on arterial blood pH, partial pressure of carbon dioxide in arterial blood ($PaCO_2$), base deficit

S

calculation. **CHILDREN, INFANTS:** Initially, 0.5–1 mEq/kg. Repeat in 10 min one time, or as indicated by pt's acid-base status.

Metabolic Acidosis (Mild to Moderate)
IV: ADULTS, ELDERLY, CHILDREN: 2–5 mEq/kg over 4–8 hrs. May repeat based on acid-base status.

Prevention of Contrast-Induced Nephropathy
IV Infusion: ADULTS, ELDERLY: 154 mEq/L sodium bicarbonate in D₅W solution: 3 mL/kg/hr 1 hr immediately before contrast injection, then 1 mL/kg/hr during contrast exposure and for 6 hrs after procedure.

Metabolic Acidosis (Associated with Chronic Renal Failure)
PO: ADULTS, ELDERLY: Initially, 15.4–23.1 mEq/day in divided doses. Titrate to normal serum bicarbonate level of 23–29 mEq/L.

Renal Tubular Acidosis (Distal)
PO: ADULTS, ELDERLY: 0.5–2 mEq/kg/day in 4–6 divided doses. **CHILDREN:** 2–3 mEq/kg/day in divided doses.

Renal Tubular Acidosis (Proximal)
PO: ADULTS, ELDERLY, CHILDREN: 5–10 mEq/kg/day in divided doses. Maintenance dose to maintain serum bicarbonate in normal range.

Urine Alkalinization
PO: ADULTS, ELDERLY: Initially, 4 g, then 1–2 g q4h. **Maximum:** 16 g/day (8 g/day in adults older than 60 yrs). **CHILDREN:** 1–10 mEq/kg/day in divided doses q4–6h.

Antacid
PO: ADULTS, ELDERLY: 300 mg–2 g 1–4 times/day.

Hyperkalemia
IV: ADULTS, ELDERLY: 50 mEq over 5 min.

SIDE EFFECTS

Frequent: Abdominal distention, flatulence, belching.

ADVERSE EFFECTS/ TOXIC REACTIONS

Excessive, chronic use may produce metabolic alkalosis (irritability, twitching, paresthesia, cyanosis, slow or shallow respirations, headache, thirst, nausea). Fluid overload results in headache, weakness, blurred vision, behavioral changes, incoordination, muscle twitching, elevated B/P, bradycardia, tachypnea, wheezing, coughing, distended neck veins. Extravasation may occur at the IV site, resulting in tissue necrosis, ulceration.

NURSING CONSIDERATIONS

BASELINE ASSESSMENT
Assess for signs and symptoms of acidosis, alkalosis. Do not give PO medication within 1 hr of antacids.

INTERVENTION/EVALUATION
Monitor serum, urinary pH, CO_2 level, serum electrolytes, plasma bicarbonate levels. Watch for signs of metabolic alkalosis, fluid overload. Assess for clinical improvement of metabolic acidosis (relief from hyperventilation, weakness, disorientation). Monitor daily pattern of bowel activity, stool consistency. Monitor serum phosphate, calcium, uric acid levels. Assess for relief of gastric distress.

sodium chloride

so-dee-um **klor**-ide
(Muro 128, Nasal Moist, Ocean, SalineX)

◆CLASSIFICATION
PHARMACOTHERAPEUTIC: Salt. **CLINICAL:** Electrolyte, isotonic volume expander, ophthalmic adjunct, bronchodilator.

S

USES

Parenteral: Source of hydration; prevention/treatment of sodium, chloride deficiencies (hypertonic for severe deficiencies). Prevention of muscle cramps, heat prostration occurring with excessive perspiration. **Nasal:** Restores moisture, relieves dry, inflamed nasal membranes. **Ophthalmic:** Therapy in reduction of corneal edema, diagnostic aid in ophthalmoscopic exam.

PRECAUTIONS

Contraindications: Hypersensitivity to sodium chloride. Fluid retention, hypernatremia, hypertonic uterus. **Cautions:** HF, renal impairment, cirrhosis, hypertension, edema. Do not use sodium chloride preserved with benzyl alcohol in neonates.

ACTION

Sodium is a major cation of extracellular fluid. **Therapeutic Effect:** Controls water distribution, fluid and electrolyte balance, osmotic pressure of body fluids; maintains acid-base balance.

PHARMACOKINETICS

Well absorbed from GI tract. Widely distributed. Primarily excreted in urine and, to a lesser degree, in sweat, tears, saliva.

LIFESPAN CONSIDERATIONS

Pregnancy/Lactation: No precautions noted. **Children/Elderly:** No age-related precautions noted.

INTERACTIONS

DRUG: May decrease effect of **lithium**. **HERBAL:** None significant. **FOOD:** None known. **LAB VALUES:** None significant.

AVAILABILITY (Rx)

Injection (Concentrate) (Rx): 23.4% (4 mEq/mL). **Injection Solution (Rx):** 0.45%, 0.9%, 3%. **Irrigation (Rx):** 0.45%, 0.9%. **Nasal Gel (Nasal Moist) (OTC):** 0.65%. **Nasal Solution (OTC):** 0.4% (SalineX), 0.65% (Nasal Moist, Ocean). **Ophthalmic Ointment (OTC** [Muro 128]): 5%. **Ophthalmic Solution (OTC** [Muro 128]): 2%, 5%.

 Tablets (OTC): 1 g.

ADMINISTRATION/HANDLING

IV

• Hypertonic solutions (3% or 5%) are administered via large vein; avoid infiltration; do not exceed 100 mL/hr. • Vials containing 2.5–4 mEq/mL (concentrated NaCl) must be diluted with D_5W or $D_{10}W$ before administration.

PO

• Do not crush/break enteric-coated or extended-release tablets. • Administer with full glass of water.

Nasal

• Instruct pt to begin inhaling slowly just before releasing medication into nose. • Instruct pt to inhale slowly, then release air gently through mouth. • Continue technique for 20–30 sec.

Ophthalmic

• Place gloved finger on lower eyelid and pull out until pocket is formed between eye and lower lid. • Place prescribed number of drops (or ¼–½ inch of ointment) into pocket. • Instruct pt to close eye gently for 1–2 min so that medication will not be squeezed out of sac. • When lower lid is released, have pt keep eye open without blinking for at least 30 sec for solution; for ointment have pt close eye, roll eyeball around to distribute medication. • When using drops, apply gentle finger pressure to lacrimal sac at inner canthus for 1 min to minimize systemic absorption.

INDICATIONS/ROUTES/DOSAGE

◄ALERT► Dosage based on age, weight, clinical condition; fluid, electrolyte, acid-base balance status.

Usual Parenteral Dosage
IV: ADULTS, ELDERLY, CHILDREN: Determined by laboratory determinations

S

(mEq). Dosage varies widely based on clinical conditions.

Usual Oral Dosage
PO: ADULTS, ELDERLY: 1–2 g 3 times/day.

Usual Nasal Dosage
Intranasal: ADULTS, ELDERLY, CHILDREN: 2–3 sprays as needed.

Usual Ophthalmic Dosage
Ophthalmic Solution: ADULTS, ELDERLY: Apply 1–2 drops q3–4h.
Ophthalmic Ointment: ADULTS, ELDERLY: Apply once daily or as directed.

SIDE EFFECTS

Frequent: Facial flushing. Occasional: Fever; irritation, phlebitis, extravasation at injection site. Ophthalmic: Temporary burning, irritation.

ADVERSE EFFECTS/ TOXIC REACTIONS

Too-rapid administration may produce peripheral edema, HF, pulmonary edema. Excessive dosage may produce hypokalemia, hypervolemia, hypernatremia.

NURSING CONSIDERATIONS

BASELINE ASSESSMENT

Obtain baseline serum electrolyte studies. Assess fluid balance (I&O, daily weight, lung sounds, edema).

INTERVENTION/EVALUATION

Monitor fluid balance (I&O, daily weight, lung sounds, edema), IV site for extravasation. Monitor serum electrolytes, acid-base balance, B/P. Hypernatremia associated with edema, weight gain, elevated B/P; hyponatremia associated with muscle cramps, nausea, vomiting, dry mucous membranes.

PATIENT/FAMILY TEACHING

• Temporary burning, irritation may occur upon instillation of eye medication. • Discontinue eye medication and report if severe pain, headache, rapid change in vision (peripheral, direct), sudden appearance of floating spots, acute redness of eyes, pain on exposure to light, double vision occurs.

sodium polystyrene sulfonate

so-dee-um pol-ee-**stye**-reen
(Kayexalate, Kionex, PMS-Sodium Polystyrene Sulfonate ✿, SPS)
Do not confuse Kayexalate with Kaopectate.

◆CLASSIFICATION

PHARMACOTHERAPEUTIC: Cation exchange resin. CLINICAL: Antihyperkalemic.

USES

Treatment of hyperkalemia.

PRECAUTIONS

Contraindications: Hypersensitivity to sodium polystyrene sulfonate. Hypokalemia, neonates with reduced GI motility, intestinal obstruction/perforation. Oral administration in neonates. Cautions: Severe HF, hypertension, edema. Use in premature or low-birth-weight infants, use in children when administering rectally. Avoid use in pts at risk for constipation/impaction.

ACTION

Releases sodium ions in exchange primarily for potassium ions across intestinal wall. **Therapeutic Effect:** Moves potassium from blood into intestine to be expelled from the body.

PHARMACOKINETICS

Onset: 2–24 hrs. Eliminated only in feces.

⧗ LIFESPAN CONSIDERATIONS

Pregnancy/Lactation: Unknown if drug crosses placenta or is distributed in breast

S

milk. **Children:** Safety and efficacy not established. Contraindicated in neonates. **Elderly:** Increased risk for fecal impaction.

INTERACTIONS

DRUG: Cation-donating antacids, laxatives (e.g., **magnesium hydroxide**) may decrease effect; may cause systemic alkalosis in pts with renal impairment. **HERBAL:** None significant. **FOOD:** None known. **LAB VALUES:** May decrease serum calcium, magnesium, potassium. May increase serum sodium.

AVAILABILITY (Rx)

Powder for Suspension (Kayexalate, Kionex): 15 g/4 level tsp (480 g). **Suspension (SPS):** 15 g/60 mL.

ADMINISTRATION/HANDLING

PO
• Shake suspension well prior to administration. • Do not mix with orange juice. • Chilling suspension will increase palatability.

Rectal
• After initial cleansing enema, insert large rubber tube into rectum well into sigmoid colon; tape in place. • Introduce suspension (with 100 mL aqueous vehicle) via gravity. • Flush with 50–100 mL fluid and clamp. • Pt must retain for several hrs if possible. • Irrigate colon with non–sodium-containing solution to remove resin.

INDICATIONS/ROUTES/DOSAGE

Hyperkalemia
PO: ADULTS, ELDERLY: 60 mL (15 g) 1–4 times/day. **CHILDREN:** 1 g/kg/dose q6h.
Rectal: ADULTS, ELDERLY: 30–50 g as needed q6h. **CHILDREN:** 1 g/kg/dose q2–6h.

Dosage in Renal/Hepatic Impairment
No dose adjustment.

SIDE EFFECTS

Frequent: High dosage: Anorexia, nausea, vomiting, constipation. **High dosage in elderly:** Fecal impaction (severe stomach pain with nausea/vomiting).

Occasional: Diarrhea, sodium retention (decreased urination, peripheral edema, increased weight).

ADVERSE EFFECTS/TOXIC REACTIONS

Potassium deficiency may occur. Early signs of hypokalemia include confusion, delayed thought processes, extreme weakness, irritability, EKG changes (often associated with prolonged QT interval; widening, flattening, or inversion of T wave; prominent U waves). Hypocalcemia, manifested by abdominal/muscle cramps, occurs occasionally. Arrhythmias, severe muscle weakness may be noted.

NURSING CONSIDERATIONS

BASELINE ASSESSMENT
Does not rapidly correct severe hyperkalemia (may take hrs to days). Consider other measures in medical emergency (IV calcium, IV sodium bicarbonate/glucose/insulin, dialysis).

INTERVENTION/EVALUATION
Monitor serum potassium levels frequently. Assess pt's clinical condition, EKG (valuable in determining when treatment should be discontinued). Also monitor serum magnesium, calcium levels. Monitor daily pattern of bowel activity, stool consistency (fecal impaction may occur in pts on high dosages, particularly in elderly).

S

sofosbuvir/ velpatasvir/ voxilaprevir

soe-**fos**-bue-vir/vel-**pat**-as-vir/vox-i-la-pre-vir
(Vosevi)

■■ **BLACK BOX ALERT** ■ Test all pts for hepatitis B virus (HBV) infection prior to initiation. HBV reactivation was reported in HBV/HBC co-infected pts who were undergoing or had completed treatment with HCV direct-acting antivirals and were not receiving HBV antiviral therapy. HBV reactivation may cause fulminant hepatitis, hepatic failure, and death. **Do not confuse sofosbuvir with boceprevir, dasabuvir, fosamprenavir, or simeprevir; or velpatasvir with daclatasvir, grazoprevir, or paritaprevir; or voxilaprevir with boceprevir, grazoprevir, or paritaprevir.**

◆CLASSIFICATION

PHARMACOTHERAPEUTIC: NS5A inhibitor, polymerase inhibitor, NS3/4A inhibitor, NS5B RNA polymerase inhibitor. **CLINICAL:** Antihepaciviral.

USES

Treatment of adults with chronic hepatitis C virus (HCV) infection without cirrhosis or with compensated cirrhosis who have genotype 1, 2, 3, 4, 5, or 6 infection and have previously been treated with an HCV regimen containing an NS5A inhibitor or who have genotype 1a or 3 infection and have previously been treated with an HCV regimen containing sofosbuvir without an NS5A inhibitor.

PRECAUTIONS

Contraindications: Hypersensitivity to sofosbuvir, velpatasvir, voxilaprevir. Concomitant use of rifAMPin. **Cautions:** Moderate to severe hepatic impairment, HIV infection. Concomitant use of amiodarone, beta blockers. Pts with underlying cardiac disease and/or advanced liver disease may increase risk of bradycardia. Concomitant use of P-glycoprotein inducers, moderate or strong CYP2C8 inducers, moderate or strong CYP3A4 inducers not recommended.

ACTION

Sofosbuvir inhibits the HCV NS5B RNA-dependent RNA polymerase, velpatasvir inhibits the HCV NS5A protein, voxilaprevir inhibits the NS3/4A protease, necessary for proteolytic cleavage of HCV-encoded polyprotein. **Therapeutic Effect:** Inhibits viral replication of hepatitis C virus.

PHARMACOKINETICS

Widely distributed. Metabolized in liver. Protein binding: sofosbuvir: 61%–65%; velpatasvir: greater than 99.5%; voxilaprevir: greater than 99%. Peak plasma concentration: sofosbuvir: 2 hrs; velpatasvir: 4 hrs; voxilaprevir: 4 hrs. Excreted in sofosbuvir: urine (80%), feces (14%); velpatasvir: feces (94%), urine (0.4%); voxilaprevir: primarily in feces. **Half-life:** sofosbuvir: 0.5 hrs; velpatasvir: 17 hrs; voxilaprevir: 33 hrs.

⧖ LIFESPAN CONSIDERATIONS

Pregnancy/Lactation: Unknown if distributed in breast milk. **Children:** Safety and efficacy not established. **Elderly:** No age-related precautions noted.

INTERACTIONS

DRUG: Amiodarone may increase risk of symptomatic bradycardia. **Aluminum- or magnesium-containing antacids, H₂-receptor antagonists (e.g., famotidine), proton pump inhibitors (e.g., omeprazole)** may decrease concentration/effect of velpatasvir. **Anticonvulsants (e.g., carBAMazepine, phenytoin), antimycobacterials (e.g., rifabutin, rifAMPin), tipranavir/ritonavir** may decrease concentration/effects. **Moderate or potent inducers of CYP2B6, CYP2C8, CYP3A4, P-glycoprotein (e.g., carBAMazepine, phenytoin, oxcarbazepine)** may decrease concentration/effect. May increase concentration/effect of **rosuvastatin, digoxin**. **HERBAL: St. John's wort** may significantly decrease concentration/effect. **FOOD:** None known. **LAB VALUES:** May increase serum bilirubin, creatine kinase, lipase.

AVAILABILITY (Rx)

Tablets (fixed-dose combination): 400 mg (sofosbuvir)/100 mg velpatasvir/100 mg (voxilaprevir).

ADMINISTRATION/HANDLING

PO
• Give with food.

INDICATIONS/ROUTES/DOSAGE

Hepatitis C Virus Infection
PO: ADULTS, ELDERLY: 1 tablet (sofosbuvir/velpatasvir/voxilaprevir) once daily for 12 wks.
Dosage in Renal Impairment
Mild to moderate impairment: No dose adjustment. **Severe impairment, ESRD:** Not recommended due to higher exposure of sofosbuvir.
Dosage in Hepatic Impairment
Mild impairment: No dose adjustment. **Moderate to severe impairment:** Not recommended due to higher exposure of voxilaprevir.

SIDE EFFECTS

Frequent (21%–13%): Headache, fatigue, diarrhea, nausea. **Occasional (6%–1%):** Asthenia, insomnia, rash.

ADVERSE EFFECTS/ TOXIC REACTIONS

HBV reactivation was reported in pts co-infected with HBV/HVC; may result in fulminant hepatitis, hepatic failure, death. Cardiac arrest, symptomatic bradycardia, pacemaker implantation were reported in pts taking concomitant amiodarone. Bradycardia usually occurred within hrs to days, but may occur up 2 wks after initiation. Pts with underlying cardiac disease, advanced hepatic disease, or pts taking concomitant beta blockers are at an increased risk for bradycardia when used concomitantly with amiodarone. Psychiatric disorders including depression may occur. Angioedema, blistering skin rashes may occur.

NURSING CONSIDERATIONS

BASELINE ASSESSMENT

Obtain renal function test, LFT, HCV-RNA level; serum lipase, CPK; pregnancy test in females of reproductive potential. Confirm hepatitis C virus genotype. Question history of renal impairment, hepatic disease unrelated to HCV infection; HIV infection; concomitant use of antiretroviral therapy. Receive full medication history and screen for interactions (esp. concomitant use of amiodarone).

INTERVENTION/EVALUATION

Monitor serum lipase, CK. Periodically monitor HCV-RNA level for treatment effectiveness. If unable to discontinue amiodarone, recommend inpatient cardiac monitoring for at least 48 hrs, followed by outpatient or self-monitoring of HR for at least 2 wks after initiation. Cardiac monitoring is also recommended in pts who discontinue amiodarone just prior to initiation. Encourage nutritional intake. Monitor for new-onset or worsening of depression.

PATIENT/FAMILY TEACHING

• Pts who take amiodarone (an antiarrhythmic) during therapy may require inpatient and outpatient cardiac monitoring (and in some cases, pacemaker implantation) due to an increased risk of slow heart rate or cardiac arrest. If amiodarone therapy cannot be withheld or stopped, immediately report symptoms of slow heart rate such as chest pain, confusion, dizziness, fainting, light-headedness, memory problems, palpitations, weakness. • There is a high risk of drug interactions with other medications. Do not take newly prescribed medications unless approved by prescriber who originally started treatment. • Do not take herbal products. • Avoid alcohol. • Report signs of depression.

solifenacin

sol-i-**fen**-a-sin
(VESIcare)

◆CLASSIFICATION

PHARMACOTHERAPEUTIC: Anticholinergic agent, muscarinic receptor antagonist. **CLINICAL:** Urinary antispasmodic.

USES

Treatment of overactive bladder with symptoms of urinary frequency, urgency, or urge incontinence.

PRECAUTIONS

Contraindications: Hypersensitivity to solifenacin. Gastric retention, uncontrolled narrow-angle glaucoma, urinary retention. **Cautions:** Bladder outflow obstruction, GI obstructive disorders, decreased GI motility, controlled narrow-angle glaucoma, renal/hepatic impairment, congenital or acquired QT prolongation, concurrent medications that prolong QT interval, hypokalemia, hypomagnesemia, hot weather and/or exercise.

ACTION

Inhibits muscarinic receptors. **Therapeutic Effect:** Decreases urinary bladder contractions, increases residual urine volume, decreases detrusor muscle pressure.

PHARMACOKINETICS

Well absorbed. Protein binding: 98%. Metabolized in liver. Excreted in urine (69%), feces (23%). **Half-life:** 40–68 hrs.

⌛ LIFESPAN CONSIDERATIONS

Pregnancy/Lactation: Unknown if drug crosses placenta or is distributed in breast milk. **Children:** Safety and efficacy not established. **Elderly:** No age-related precautions noted.

INTERACTIONS

DRUG: CYP3A4 inhibitors (e.g., **ketoconazole, erythromycin, azole antifungals, clarithromycin**) may increase concentration/effects. **HERBAL:** St. John's wort may decrease concentration/effects. **FOOD:** Grapefruit products may increase effects. **LAB VALUES:** None known.

AVAILABILITY (Rx)

Tablets: 5 mg, 10 mg.

ADMINISTRATION/HANDLING

PO
• Give without regard to food. Swallow tablets whole, with liquids.

INDICATIONS/ROUTES/DOSAGE

Overactive Bladder
PO: **ADULTS, ELDERLY:** 5 mg/day; if tolerated, may increase to 10 mg/day.

Dosage with CYP3A4 Inhibitors
Maximum: 5 mg/day.

Dosage in Renal/Hepatic Impairment
Severe renal impairment: (CrCl less than 30 mL/min) or moderate hepatic impairment: Maximum dosage is 5 mg/day. Not recommended in severe hepatic impairment.

SIDE EFFECTS

Frequent (28%–13%): Dry mouth, constipation. **Occasional (5%–3%):** Blurred vision, UTI, dyspepsia, nausea. **Rare (2%–1%):** Dizziness, dry eyes, fatigue, depression, edema, hypertension, epigastric pain, vomiting, urinary retention.

ADVERSE EFFECTS/ TOXIC REACTIONS

Angioneurotic edema, GI obstruction occur rarely. Overdose can result in severe anticholinergic effects.

NURSING CONSIDERATIONS

BASELINE ASSESSMENT

Assess symptoms of overactive bladder before beginning the drug. Question medical history as listed in Precautions. Screen for concomitant medications known to prolong QT interval. Obtain baseline EKG.

INTERVENTION/EVALUATION

Monitor I&O, anticholinergic effects, creatinine clearance. Assess for decrease in symptoms. Obtain bladder scan if urinary retention is suspected.

PATIENT/FAMILY TEACHING

• Avoid tasks requiring alertness, motor skills until response to drug is established. • Anticholinergic side effects include constipation, urinary retention, blurred vision, heat prostration in hot environment. • Use caution during exercise, exposure to heat.

S

somatropin

soe-ma-**troe**-pin
(Genotropin, Genotropin Miniquick, Humatrope, Norditropin, Nutropin, Nutropin AQ, Omnitrope, Saizen, Serostim, Zomacton, Zorbtive)
Do not confuse somatropin with SUMAtriptan.

◆CLASSIFICATION

PHARMACOTHERAPEUTIC: Polypeptide hormone. **CLINICAL:** Growth hormone.

USES

Adults: Growth deficiency due to pituitary disease, hypothalamic disease, surgery, radiation, or trauma; AIDS-related wasting or cachexia. **Zorbtive:** Short bowel syndrome. **Children:** Long-term treatment of growth failure due to lack of or inadequate endogenous growth hormone secretion; chronic renal insufficiency; short stature associated with Turner's syndrome, Noonan's syndrome, or homeobox gene deficiency; idiopathic short stature. **OFF-LABEL:** Treatment of pediatric HIV pts with wasting/cachexia; HIV adipose redistribution syndrome.

PRECAUTIONS

Contraindications: Hypersensitivity to growth hormone. Pts with Prader-Willi syndrome with growth hormone deficiency who are severely obese or have severe respiratory impairment, Prader-Willi syndrome without growth hormone deficiency, children with closed epiphyses, acute critical illness due to complications after open heart or abdominal surgery, multiple accidental trauma, acute respiratory failure, active neoplasia, diabetic retinopathy. Active malignancy, progression of active growing intracranial lesion or tumor. **Cautions:** Diabetes, elderly pts.

ACTION

Stimulates cartilaginous growth areas of long bones; increases number, size of skeletal muscle cells; influences size of organs; increases RBC mass by stimulating erythropoietin. Influences metabolism of carbohydrates (decreases insulin sensitivity), fats (mobilizes fatty acids), minerals (retains phosphorus, sodium, potassium by promotion of cell growth), proteins (increases protein synthesis). **Therapeutic Effect:** Stimulates growth.

PHARMACOKINETICS

Well absorbed after SQ, IM administration. Localized primarily in kidneys, liver. **Half-life: IV:** 20–30 min; **SQ, IM:** 3–5 hrs.

⧗ LIFESPAN CONSIDERATIONS

Pregnancy/Lactation: Unknown if drug is distributed in breast milk. **Children/Elderly:** No age-related precautions noted.

INTERACTIONS

DRUG: Corticosteroids (e.g., hydrocortisone, predniSONE) may inhibit growth response. **Oral estrogens** may decrease response to somatropin. **HERBAL:** None significant. **FOOD:** None known. **LAB VALUES:** May increase serum alkaline phosphatase, inorganic phosphorus, parathyroid hormone. May decrease glucose tolerance. May slightly decrease thyroid function.

AVAILABILITY (Rx)

Injection, Powder for Reconstitution (Genotropin): 5 mg, 12 mg. **(Genotropin Miniquick):** 0.2 mg, 0.4 mg, 0.6 mg, 0.8 mg, 1 mg, 1.2 mg, 1.4 mg, 1.6 mg, 1.8 mg, 2 mg. **(Omnitrope):** 5.8 mg. **(Saizen):** 5 mg, 8.8 mg. **(Serostim):** 4 mg, 5 mg, 6 mg. **(Zomacton):** 5 mg, 10 mg. **(Zorbtive):** 8.8 mg. **Injection Solution: (Norditropin):** 5 mg/1.5 mL, 10 mg/1.5 mL, 15 mg/1.5 mL. **(Nutropin AQ):** 10 mg/mL, 5 mg/mL, 2.5 mg/mL. **(Omnitrope):** 5 mg/1.5 mL, 10 mg/1.5 mL.

S

(Norditropin FlexPro Pen): 5 mg/1.5 mL, 10 mg/1.5 mL, 30 mg/3 mL.

ADMINISTRATION/HANDLING

◀ALERT▶ **Neonate:** Benzyl alcohol as a preservative has been associated with fatal toxicity (gasping syndrome) in premature infants. Reconstitute with Sterile Water for Injection only. Use only 1 dose per vial. Discard unused portion.

Reconstitution

Genotropin, Genotropin Miniquick: Reconstitute with diluent provided.

Humatrope: Reconstitute with 1.5–5 mL diluent provided, swirl gently, do not shake.

Humatrope Cartridge: Dilute with solution provided with cartridge only.

Nutropin: Reconstitute each 5 mg with 1.5–5 mL diluent, swirl gently, do not shake.

Omnitrope: Reconstitute with diluents provided, swirl gently, do not shake.

Saizen: 5 mg: Reconstitute with 1–3 mL diluent provided, swirl gently, do not shake. 8.8 mg: Reconstitute with 2–3 mL diluent provided, swirl gently, do not shake.

Serostim: Reconstitute with Sterile Water for Injection.

Zorbtive: Reconstitute with 1–2 mL Bacteriostatic Water for Injection.

Storage

Long-term storage: Refrigerate all products except Zorbtive. Once reconstituted, Humatrop, Nutropin, Saigen, Zorbtive stable for 14 days, Genotropin for 21 days, Humatrope Cartridge for 28 days. **Genotropin Miniquick:** Refrigerate, use within 24 hrs.

INDICATIONS/ROUTES/DOSAGE

Growth Hormone Deficiency

SQ: *(Genotropin, Omnitrope):* **ADULTS:** 0.04 mg/kg wkly divided in 6–7 equal doses/wk. May increase at 4- to 8-wk intervals to maximum of 0.08 mg/kg/wk. **CHILDREN:** 0.16–0.24 mg/kg wkly divided into equal daily doses.

SQ: *(Humatrope):* **ADULTS:** 0.006 mg/kg once daily. May increase to maximum of 0.0125 mg/kg/day. **CHILDREN:** 0.18–0.3 mg/kg wkly divided into alternate-day doses or 6 doses/wk.

SQ: *(Norditropin):* **ADULTS:** 0.004 mg/kg/day. May increase after 6 wks up to 0.016 mg/kg/day. **CHILDREN:** 0.024–0.036 mg/kg/dose 6–7 days/wk.

SQ: *(Nutropin, Nutropin AQ):* **ADULTS:** 0.006 mg/kg once daily. May increase to maximum of 0.025 mg/kg/day (younger than 35 yrs) or 0.0125/kg/day (35 yrs and older). **CHILDREN:** 0.3–0.7 mg/kg wkly divided into equal daily doses.

SQ: *(Saizen):* **ADULTS:** 0.005 mg/kg/day. May increase up to 0.01 mg/kg/day after 4 wks. **CHILDREN:** 0.18 mg/kg/wk divided into equal daily doses or 0.06 mg/kg 3 times/wk or as 0.03 mg/kg administered 6 days/wk.

Chronic Renal Insufficiency

SQ: *(Nutropin, Nutropin AQ):* **CHILDREN:** 0.35 mg/kg wkly divided into equal daily doses. Continue until the time of renal transplantation.

Turner's Syndrome

SQ: *(Humatrope, Nutropin, Nutropin AQ):* **CHILDREN:** 0.375 mg/kg wkly divided into equal doses 3–7 times/wk. *(Genotropin, Omnitrope):* 0.33 mg/kg wkly divided into 6–7 doses. *(Norditropin):* Up to 0.067 mg/kg/day.

AIDS-Related Wasting

SQ: *(Serostim):* **ADULTS WEIGHING MORE THAN 55 KG:** 6 mg once daily at bedtime. **ADULTS WEIGHING 45–55 KG:** 5 mg once daily at bedtime. **ADULTS WEIGHING 35–44 KG:** 4 mg once daily at bedtime. **ADULTS WEIGHING LESS THAN 35 KG:** 0.1 mg/kg once daily at bedtime.

Short Bowel Syndrome

SQ: *(Zorbtive):* **ADULTS:** 0.1 mg/kg/day. **Maximum:** 8 mg/day.

Dosage in Renal/Hepatic Impairment

No dose adjustment.

SIDE EFFECTS

Frequent: Otitis media, other ear disorders (with Turner's syndrome). **Occasional:** Carpal tunnel syndrome, gynecomastia, myalgia, peripheral edema, fatigue, asthenia. **Rare:** Rash, pruritus, visual changes, headache, nausea, vomiting, injection site pain/swelling, abdominal pain, hip/knee pain.

ADVERSE EFFECTS/ TOXIC REACTIONS

Pancreatitis occurs rarely.

NURSING CONSIDERATIONS

BASELINE ASSESSMENT

Obtain baseline lab chemistries, thyroid function, serum glucose level. Obtain full medical history (drug has multiple contraindications).

INTERVENTION/EVALUATION

Monitor bone growth, growth rate in relation to pt's age. Monitor serum calcium, glucose, phosphorus levels; renal, parathyroid, thyroid function. Observe for decreased muscle wasting in AIDS pts.

PATIENT/FAMILY TEACHING

• Follow correct procedure to reconstitute drug for administration and for safe handling/disposal of needles. • Regular follow-up with physician is important part of therapy. • Report development of severe headache, visual changes, pain in hip/knee, limping.

sonidegib

soe-ni-**deg**-ib
(Odomzo)

■ **BLACK BOX ALERT** ■ May cause embryo-fetal death/severe malformations when given during pregnancy. Verify pregnancy status before initiation. Female patients of reproductive potential must use effective contraception during treatment and for at least 20 mos after discontinuation. Due to the potential risk of exposure through semen, male patients must use condoms during sexual activity (even after a vasectomy) during treatment and for at least 8 mos after discontinuation.

Do not confuse sonidegib with vismodegib.

◆CLASSIFICATION

PHARMACOTHERAPEUTIC: Hedgehog pathway inhibitor. **CLINICAL:** Antineoplastic.

USES

Treatment of adult pts with locally advanced basal cell carcinoma that has recurred following surgery or radiation therapy, or those who are not candidates for surgery or radiation.

PRECAUTIONS

Contraindications: Hypersensitivity to sonidegib. **Cautions:** Renal/hepatic impairment. Avoid concomitant use of strong or moderate CYP3A inhibitors, strong or moderate CYP3A inducers.

ACTION

Inhibits cell migration, proliferation, survival of tumor cells. Binds to and inhibits Smoothened, a transmembrane protein involved in Hedgehog signal transduction. **Therapeutic Effect:** Inhibits tumor cell growth and metastasis.

PHARMACOKINETICS

Poorly absorbed after PO administration (less than 10%). Metabolized in liver. Protein binding: greater than 97%. Peak plasma concentration: 2–4 hrs. Steady state reached in 4 mos. Excreted in feces (70%), urine (30%). **Half-life:** 28 days.

⏳ LIFESPAN CONSIDERATIONS

Pregnancy/Lactation: May cause fetal death/malformations. Unknown if distributed in breast milk. Must either discontinue drug or discontinue breastfeeding. Female patients of reproductive potential must use effective contraception during treatment and up to 20 mos after discontinuation. May compromise female fertility. **Males:** Male patients must use condoms during sexual activity (even after a vasectomy)

S

during treatment and up to 8 mos after discontinuation. **Children:** Safety and efficacy not established. **Elderly:** May have increased risk of severe musculoskeletal adverse events (e.g., muscle spasms, myopathy).

INTERACTIONS
DRUG: Strong CYP3A inhibitors (e.g., clarithromycin, ketoconazole), moderate CYP3A inhibitors (e.g., atazanavir, fluconazole) may increase concentration/effect. **Strong CYP3A inducers (e.g., carBAMazepine, phenytoin, rifAMPin)** may decrease concentration/effect. **Statins (e.g., simvastatin)** may increase risk of rhabdomyolysis. **HERBAL: St. John's wort** may decrease concentration/effect. **FOOD: High-fat meals** may increase absorption/concentration. **LAB VALUES:** May increase serum ALT/AST, amylase, creatinine, CK, glucose, lipase. May decrease Hct, Hgb, lymphocytes.

AVAILABILITY (Rx)
Capsules: 200 mg.

ADMINISTRATION/HANDLING
PO
• Give on an empty stomach at least 1 hr before or 2 hrs after a meal.

INDICATIONS/ROUTES/DOSAGE
Basal Cell Carcinoma
PO: ADULTS, ELDERLY: 200 mg once daily. Continue until disease progression or unacceptable toxicity.

Dose Modification
Interrupt therapy for severe or intolerable musculoskeletal adverse reactions; first occurrence of serum CK level 2.5–10 times upper limit of normal (ULN); recurrent serum CK level 2.5–5 times ULN. Once resolved, resume at 200 mg once daily.

Discontinuation
Permanently discontinue treatment for serum CK level greater than 2.5 times

ULN with worsening renal function; serum CK level greater than 10 times ULN; recurrent serum CK level greater than 5 times ULN; recurrent severe or intolerable musculoskeletal adverse reactions.

Renal Impairment
No dose adjustment.

Hepatic Impairment
Mild impairment: No dose adjustment. **Moderate to severe impairment:** Not studied; use caution.

SIDE EFFECTS
Frequent (54%–23%): Muscle spasm, alopecia, dysgeusia, fatigue, nausea, diarrhea, musculoskeletal pain, decreased appetite. **Occasional (19%–10%):** Myalgia, abdominal pain, headache, generalized pain, vomiting, pruritus.

ADVERSE EFFECTS/ TOXIC REACTIONS
Musculoskeletal events occurred in 68% of pts. Common Terminology Criteria for Adverse Events (CTCAE) grade 3 or 4 musculoskeletal events (9% of pts) may require administration of muscle relaxants, analgesics/narcotics, magnesium supplementation, IV hydration. Serum CK level elevations usually occur before musculoskeletal pain or spasms. Increased serum CK levels reported in 61% of pts. The median onset of serum CK elevation was approx. 12 wks. May increase risk of rhabdomyolysis. Amenorrhea lasting longer than 18 mos has occurred.

NURSING CONSIDERATIONS
BASELINE ASSESSMENT
Obtain baseline capillary blood glucose, CBC, LFT, serum CK level, renal function test. Verify negative pregnancy status before initiation. Question current breastfeeding status. Receive medication history and screen for interactions. Assess hydration status. Offer emotional support.

INTERVENTION/EVALUATION

Monitor renal function, serum CK levels periodically and with any musculoskeletal adverse events. If musculoskeletal adverse reactions occur with serum CK levels greater than 2.5 times ULN, obtain serum CK level at least wkly until resolution. Offer antiemetics for nausea/vomiting. Monitor urine color, output. Serum CK level elevation or worsening of renal function may indicate rhabdomyolysis. Monitor pregnancy status during therapy.

PATIENT/FAMILY TEACHING

• Treatment may cause severe muscle damage, which may cause kidney damage. • Report dark-colored urine or decreased urine output despite hydration. • Immediately report musculoskeletal symptoms such as muscle pain/spasms/tenderness/weakness. • Do not donate blood or blood products during treatment and up to 20 mos after discontinuation. • Males must use condoms during sexual activity during treatment and up to 8 mos following discontinuation. • Treatment may cause birth defects or miscarriage. • Immediately report suspected pregnancy. • Hair loss is an expected side effect. • Swallow capsules whole; do not chew, crush, cut or open. • Take on empty stomach at least 1 hr before or 2 hrs after a meal.

SORAfenib

soe-**raf**-e-nib
(NexAVAR)
Do not confuse NexAVAR with NexIUM, or SORAfenib with imatinib or SUNItinib.

◆**CLASSIFICATION**

PHARMACOTHERAPEUTIC: Multikinase inhibitor. **CLINICAL:** Antineoplastic.

USES

Treatment of advanced renal cell carcinoma, unresectable hepatocellular carcinoma, locally recurrent or metastatic progressive differentiated thyroid carcinoma refractory to radioactive iodine treatment. **OFF-LABEL:** Recurrent or metastatic angiosarcoma, resistant gastrointestinal stromal tumor.

PRECAUTIONS

Contraindications: Hypersensitivity to SORAfenib. Use in combination with CARBOplatin and PACLitaxel in pts with squamous cell lung cancer. **Cautions:** Underlying or poorly controlled hypertension, pts with congenital long QT syndrome, medications that prolong QT interval, electrolyte imbalance (hypokalemia, hypomagnesemia), unstable coronary artery disease, recent MI, HF, concurrent use with strong CYP3A4 inducers.

ACTION

Decreases tumor cell proliferation by interacting with multiple intracellular, cell surface kinases. **Therapeutic Effect:** Inhibits tumor growth and metastasis

PHARMACOKINETICS

Metabolized in liver. Protein binding: 99.5%. Excreted mainly in feces, with lesser amount excreted in urine. **Half-life:** 25–48 hrs.

⌛ LIFESPAN CONSIDERATIONS

Pregnancy/Lactation: May cause fetal harm. Adequate contraception should be used during therapy and for at least 2 wks after therapy completion. Unknown if distributed in breast milk. Breastfeeding not recommended. **Children:** Safety and efficacy not established. **Elderly:** No age-related precautions noted.

INTERACTIONS

DRUG: Strong CYP3A4 inducers (e.g., **carBAMazepine, PHENobarbital, rifAMPin**) may decrease concentration. **QT interval–prolonging   medications**

S

(e.g., **amiodarone, azithromycin, ceritinib, haloperidol, moxifloxacin**) may increase risk of QT interval prolongation, cardiac arrhythmias. **HERBAL: St. John's wort** may decrease concentration. **FOOD: High-fat meals** decrease effectiveness. **LAB VALUES:** May increase serum lipase, amylase, bilirubin, alkaline phosphatase, transaminases. May decrease serum phosphorus, lymphocytes, WBCs, Hgb, Hct.

AVAILABILITY (Rx)

Tablets: 200 mg (NexAVAR).

ADMINISTRATION/HANDLING

PO
• Give 1 hr before or 2 hrs after eating (high-fat meal reduces effectiveness).
• Swallow tablet whole; do not break, crush, dissolve, or divide tablet.

INDICATIONS/ROUTES/DOSAGE

Renal Cell Carcinoma, Hepatocellular Carcinoma, Thyroid Carcinoma
PO: ADULTS, ELDERLY: 400 mg (2 tablets) twice daily without food. Continue until disease progression or unacceptable toxicity.

Dosage in Renal Impairment

Creatinine Clearance	Dosage
40–59 mL/min	400 mg twice daily
20–39 mL/min	200 mg twice daily
Hemodialysis	200 mg once daily

Dosage in Hepatic Impairment
Bilirubin greater than 1 to 1.5 times upper limit of normal (ULN) and/or AST greater than ULN: 400 mg twice daily. **Bilirubin greater than 1.5 to 3 times ULN and any AST:** 200 mg twice daily. **Albumin less than 2.5 g/dL (any bilirubin/AST):** 200 mg once daily.

SIDE EFFECTS

Frequent (43%–16%): Diarrhea, rash, fatigue, exfoliative dermatitis, alopecia, nausea, pruritus, hypertension, anorexia, vomiting. **Occasional (15%–10%):** Constipation, minor bleeding, dyspnea, sensory neuropathy, cough, abdominal pain, dry skin, weight loss, joint pain, headache. **Rare (9%–1%):** Acne, flushing, stomatitis, mucositis, dyspepsia, arthralgia, myalgia, hoarseness.

ADVERSE EFFECTS/ TOXIC REACTIONS

Anemia, neutropenia, thrombocytopenia, leukopenia occur in less than 10% of pts. Pancreatitis, gastritis, erectile dysfunction occur occasionally. Hemorrhage, cardiac ischemia/infarction, hypertensive crisis occur rarely.

NURSING CONSIDERATIONS

BASELINE ASSESSMENT
Monitor B/P wkly during first 6 wks of therapy and routinely thereafter. CBC, serum chemistries including electrolytes, renal function, LFT, chest X-ray should be performed before therapy begins and routinely thereafter.

INTERVENTION/EVALUATION
Determine serum amylase, lipase, phosphate concentrations frequently during therapy. Monitor CBC for evidence of myelosuppression. Monitor for blood dyscrasias (fever, sore throat, signs of local infection, unusual bruising/bleeding from any site), symptoms of anemia (excessive fatigue, weakness). Monitor for signs of neuropathy (gait disturbances, fine motor control difficulties, numbness).

PATIENT/FAMILY TEACHING
• Report any episode of chest pain.
• Do not have immunizations without physician's approval (drug lowers resistance). Avoid contact with those who have recently taken live virus vaccine.
• Promptly report fever, sore throat, signs of local infection, unusual bruising/bleeding from any site. • Swallow whole; do not chew, crush, dissolve, or divide tablet. • Avoid administration after high-fat meals.

S

sotalol

soe-ta-lol

(Apo-Sotalol , Betapace, Betapace AF, Novo-Sotalol ♣, Sorine, Sotylize)

■ **BLACK BOX ALERT** ■ Initiation, titration to occur in a hospital setting with continuous EKG to monitor potential onset of life-threatening arrhythmias. Betapace should not be substituted for Betapace AF.

Do not confuse Betapace with Betapace AF, or sotalol with Stadol or Sudafed.

◆CLASSIFICATION

PHARMACOTHERAPEUTIC: Nonselective beta-adrenergic blocking agent. **CLINICAL:** Antiarrhythmic.

USES

Betapace, Betapace AF, Sorine, Sotylize: Treatment of documented, life-threatening ventricular arrhythmias. **Betapace, Betapace AF, Sotylize:** Maintain normal sinus rhythm in pts with symptomatic atrial fibrillation/flutter. **OFF-LABEL:** Fetal tachycardia, treatment of atrial fibrillation with hypertrophic cardiomyopathy.

PRECAUTIONS

Contraindications: Hypersensitivity to sotalol. Cardiogenic shock, congenital or acquired long QT syndrome, second- or third-degree heart block (unless functioning pacemaker is present), sinus bradycardia, uncontrolled HF, bronchial asthma or related bronchospastic conditions. **Betapace, Betapace AF, Sotylize (additional):** Baseline QT interval greater than 450 msec, bronchospastic conditions, CrCl less than 40 mL/min, serum potassium less than 4 mEq/L, sick sinus syndrome. **Cautions:** Pts with history of ventricular tachycardia, ventricular fibrillation, cardiomegaly, compensated HF, diabetes mellitus, QT interval prolongation, concurrent medications that prolong QT interval, hypokalemia, hypomagnesemia, renal impairment, within first 2 wks post MI, peripheral vascular disease, Raynaud's syndrome, myasthenia gravis, psychiatric disease, bronchospastic disease. Concurrent use of digoxin, verapamil, diltiaZEM, history of severe anaphylaxis to allergens.

ACTION

Prolongs cardiac action potential, effective refractory period, QT interval. Decreases heart rate, AV node conduction; increases AV node refractoriness. **Therapeutic Effect:** Produces antiarrhythmic activity.

PHARMACOKINETICS

Route	Onset	Peak	Duration
PO	1–2 hrs	2.5–4 hrs	8–16 hrs

Well absorbed from GI tract. Protein binding: None. Widely distributed. Primarily excreted unchanged in urine. Removed by hemodialysis. **Half-life:** 12 hrs (increased in elderly, renal impairment).

⊠ LIFESPAN CONSIDERATIONS

Pregnancy/Lactation: Crosses placenta. Distributed in breast milk. **Children:** Safety and efficacy not established. **Elderly:** Age-related peripheral vascular disease may increase susceptibility to decreased peripheral circulation. Age-related renal impairment may require dosage adjustment.

INTERACTIONS

DRUG: Calcium channel blockers (e.g., dilTIAZem, verapamil) may increase effect on AV conduction, B/P. May mask symptoms of hypoglycemia, prolong hypoglycemic effects of **insulin, oral hypoglycemics (e.g., glipizide, metformin). QT prolonging medications (e.g., amiodarone, ciprofloxacin, haloperidol, ketoconazole, ondansetron)** may increase risk of prolonged QT interval. **HERBAL: Ephedra** may worsen arrhythmias. **FOOD: None** known. **LAB VALUES:** May increase serum BUN, glucose, alkaline phosphatase,

S

LDH, lipoprotein, ALT, AST, triglycerides, potassium, uric acid.

AVAILABILITY (Rx)

Solution, Intravenous: 150 mg/10 mL. **Solution, Oral (Sotylize):** 5 mg/mL. **Tablets:** 80 mg (Betapace, Betapace AF, Sorine), 120 mg (Betapace, Betapace AF, Sorine), 160 mg (Betapace, Betapace AF, Sorine), 240 mg (Sorine).

ADMINISTRATION/HANDLING

PO
• Give without regard to food. • Give at same time each day.

INDICATIONS/ROUTES/DOSAGE

Ventricular Arrhythmias
PO: ADULTS, ELDERLY: Initially, 80 mg twice daily. May increase in 80-mg increments at 3-day intervals. Range: 160–320 mg/day in 2–3 divided doses. **Maximum:** 640 mg/day in life-threatening refractory arrhythmias.
IV: Initially, 75 mg infused over 5 hrs twice daily. Range: 75–150 mg twice daily. **Maximum:** 300 mg twice daily.

Atrial Fibrillation, Atrial Flutter
PO: ADULTS, ELDERLY: Initially, 80 mg twice daily. May increase to 120–160 mg twice daily.
IV: Initially, 75 mg infused over 5 hrs twice daily. Usual dose: 112.5 mg twice daily. **Maximum:** 150 mg twice daily.

Usual Dosage for Children
PO: Initially, 90 mg/m^2/day in 3 divided doses. May incrementally increase up to a maximum of 180 mg/m^2/day. **Maximum:** 320 mg/day.

Dosage in Renal Impairment
Dosage interval is modified based on creatinine clearance.

BETAPACE, SORINE

Creatinine Clearance	Dosage
Greater than 60 mL/min	12 hrs
40–60 mL/min	24 hrs
Less than 40 mL/min	Contraindicated

BETAPACE AF

Creatinine Clearance	Dosage
Greater than 60 mL/min	12 hrs
40-60 mL/min	24 hrs
Less than 40 mL/min	Contraindicated

Dosage in Hepatic Impairment
No dose adjustment.

SIDE EFFECTS

Frequent: Diminished sexual function, drowsiness, insomnia, asthenia. **Occasional:** Depression, cold hands/feet, diarrhea, constipation, anxiety, nasal congestion, nausea, vomiting. **Rare:** Altered taste, dry eyes, pruritus, paresthesia of fingers, toes, scalp.

ADVERSE EFFECTS/ TOXIC REACTIONS

Bradycardia, HF, hypotension, bronchospasm, hypoglycemia, prolonged QT interval, torsades de pointes, ventricular tachycardia, premature ventricular complexes may occur.

NURSING CONSIDERATIONS

BASELINE ASSESSMENT

Pt must be on continuous cardiac monitoring upon initiation of therapy. Do not administer without consulting physician if pulse is 60 beats/min or less. Assess creatinine clearance before dosing. Question medical history as listed in Precautions.

INTERVENTION/EVALUATION

Diligently monitor for arrhythmias. Assess B/P for hypotension, pulse for bradycardia. Assess for HF: dyspnea, peripheral edema, jugular vein distention, increased weight, rales in lungs, decreased urinary output.

PATIENT/FAMILY TEACHING

• Do not discontinue, change dose without physician approval. • Avoid tasks requiring alertness, motor skills until response to drug is established (may cause drowsiness). • Periodic lab tests, EKGs are essential part of therapy. • Report rapid heartbeat, chest pain, swelling of ankles/legs, difficulty breathing.

spironolactone

spir-**on**-oh-**lak**-tone
(Aldactone, CaroSpir)

■ **BLACK BOX ALERT** ■ Has been shown to produce tumors in chronic toxicity studies.
Do not confuse Aldactone with Aldactazide.

FIXED-COMBINATION(S)

Aldactazide: spironolactone/hydro-CHLOROthiazide (a thiazide diuretic): 25 mg/25 mg, 50 mg/50 mg.

◆CLASSIFICATION

PHARMACOTHERAPEUTIC: Aldosterone antagonist. **CLINICAL:** Potassium-sparing diuretic, antihypertensive, antihypokalemic.

USES

Management of edema associated with excessive aldosterone excretion or with HF that is unresponsive to other therapies; hypertension; hypokalemia, nephrotic syndrome, severe HF; primary hyperaldosteronism. Cirrhosis of liver accompanied by edema or ascites. **OFF-LABEL:** Treatment of edema, hypertension in children, female acne, female hirsutism. Ascites due to cirrhosis.

PRECAUTIONS

Contraindications: Hypersensitivity to spironolactone. Acute renal insufficiency, significant impairment of renal excretory function, anuria, hyperkalemia, Addison's disease, concomitant use with eplerenone. **Cautions:** Dehydration, hyponatremia, concurrent use of supplemental potassium, elderly pts, mild renal impairment, declining renal function, ACE inhibitors or angiotensin receptor blockers.

ACTION

Interferes with sodium reabsorption by competitively inhibiting action of aldosterone in distal tubule, promoting sodium and water excretion, increasing potassium retention. **Therapeutic Effect:** Produces diuresis, lowers B/P.

PHARMACOKINETICS

Well absorbed from GI tract (absorption increased with food). Protein binding: 91%–98%. Metabolized in liver to active metabolite. Primarily excreted in urine. Unknown if removed by hemodialysis. **Half-life:** 78–84 min.

⊠ LIFESPAN CONSIDERATIONS

Pregnancy/Lactation: Active metabolite excreted in breast milk. Breastfeeding not recommended. **Children:** No age-related precautions noted. **Elderly:** May be more susceptible to developing hyperkalemia. Age-related renal impairment may require dosage adjustment.

INTERACTIONS

DRUG: ACE inhibitors (e.g., captopril, lisinopril), angiotensin receptor blockers (e.g., valsartan), potassium-containing medications, potassium supplements may increase risk of hyperkalemia. May increase half-life of **digoxin. NSAIDs (e.g., ibuprofen, ketorolac, naproxen)** may decrease antihypertensive effect. **HERBAL:** Avoid **natural licorice** (possesses mineralocorticoid activity). **FOOD: Food** increases absorption. **LAB VALUES:** May increase urinary calcium excretion, serum BUN, glucose, creatinine, magnesium, potassium, uric acid. May decrease serum sodium.

AVAILABILITY (Rx)

Suspension, Oral: 25 mg/5 ml. **Tablets:** 25 mg, 50 mg, 100 mg.

ADMINISTRATION/HANDLING

PO
• Take with food to reduce GI irritation and increase absorption. **Suspension:**

S

◆ Canadian trade name   🦃 Non-Crushable Drug   ▨ High Alert drug

• Shake well. • May give with or without food (give consistently with respect to food).

INDICATIONS/ROUTES/DOSAGE

Edema
PO: ADULTS, ELDERLY: 25–200 mg/day as single dose or in 2 divided doses. **CHILDREN:** 1–3.3 mg/kg/day in divided doses q12–24h. **Maximum:** 100 mg. **NEONATES:** 1–3 mg/kg/day in divided doses q12–24h.

Hypertension
PO: ADULTS, ELDERLY: 25–50 mg/day in 1–2 doses/day. **Maximum:** 100 mg. **CHILDREN:** 1–3.3 mg/kg/day in divided doses q12–24h. **Maximum:** 100 mg.

Hypokalemia
PO: ADULTS, ELDERLY: 25–100 mg/day as single dose or in 2 divided doses.

Primary Aldosteronism
PO: ADULTS, ELDERLY: 400 mg/day for 4 days up to 3–4 wks, then maintenance dose of 100–400 mg/day as single dose or in 2 divided doses.

HF
PO: ADULTS, ELDERLY: 12.5–25 mg/day adjusted based on pt response, evidence of hyperkalemia. **Maximum:** 50 mg.

Dosage in Renal Impairment
CrCl 50 mL/min or greater: Initially, 12.5–25 mg once daily. **Maintenance:** 25 mg once or twice daily. **CrCl 30–49 mL/min:** Initially, 12.5 mg once daily or every other day. **Maintenance:** 12.5–25 mg once daily. **CrCl less than 30 mL/min:** Not recommended.

Dosage in Hepatic Impairment
No dose adjustment.

SIDE EFFECTS

Frequent: Hyperkalemia (in pts with renal insufficiency, those taking potassium supplements), dehydration, hyponatremia, lethargy. **Occasional:** Nausea, vomiting, anorexia, abdominal cramps, diarrhea, headache, ataxia, drowsiness, confusion, fever. **Male:** Gynecomastia, impotence, decreased libido. **Female:** Menstrual irregularities (amenorrhea, postmenopausal bleeding), breast tenderness. **Rare:** Rash, urticaria, hirsutism.

ADVERSE EFFECTS/ TOXIC REACTIONS

Severe hyperkalemia may produce arrhythmias, bradycardia, EKG changes (tented T waves, widening QRS complex, ST segment depression). May proceed to cardiac standstill, ventricular fibrillation. Cirrhosis pts at risk for hepatic decompensation if dehydration, hyponatremia occurs. Pts with primary aldosteronism may experience rapid weight loss, severe fatigue during high-dose therapy.

NURSING CONSIDERATIONS

BASELINE ASSESSMENT
Weigh pt; initiate strict I&O. Evaluate hydration status by assessing mucous membranes, skin turgor. Obtain baseline serum electrolytes, renal/hepatic function, urinalysis. Assess for edema; note location, extent. Check baseline vital signs, note pulse rate/regularity.

INTERVENTION/EVALUATION
Monitor serum electrolyte values, esp. for increased potassium, BUN, creatinine. Monitor B/P. Monitor for hyponatremia: mental confusion, thirst, cold/clammy skin, drowsiness, dry mouth. Monitor for hyperkalemia: colic, diarrhea, muscle twitching followed by weakness/paralysis, arrhythmias. Obtain daily weight. Note changes in edema, skin turgor.

PATIENT/FAMILY TEACHING
• Expect increase in volume, frequency of urination. • Therapeutic effect takes several days to begin and can last for several days when drug is discontinued. This may not apply if pt is on a potassium-losing drug concomitantly (diet, use of supplements should be established by physician). • Report irregular or slow pulse, symptoms of electrolyte imbalance (see previous Intervention/Evaluation).

• Avoid foods high in potassium, such as whole grains (cereals), legumes, meat, bananas, apricots, orange juice, potatoes (white, sweet), raisins. • Avoid alcohol. • Avoid tasks that require alertness, motor skills until response to drug is established (may cause drowsiness).

sulfamethoxazole-trimethoprim

sul-fa-meth-**ox**-a-zole-trye-**meth**-oh-prim
(Apo-Sulfatrim ✤, Bactrim, Bactrim DS, Sulfatrim)
Do not confuse Bactrim with bacitracin or Bactroban.

FIXED-COMBINATION(S)

Bactrim, Septra: sulfamethoxazole/trimethoprim: 5:1 ratio remains constant in all dosage forms (e.g., 400 mg/80 mg).

◆CLASSIFICATION

PHARMACOTHERAPEUTIC: Sulfonamide/folate antagonist. **CLINICAL:** Antibiotic.

USES

Treatment of susceptible infections due to *S. pneumoniae, H. influenzae, E. coli, Klebsiella* spp., *Enterobacter* spp., *M. morganii, P. mirabilis, P. vulgaris, S. flexneri, Pneumocystis jiroveci,* including acute or complicated and recurrent or chronic UTI, *Pneumocystis jiroveci* pneumonia (PCP), shigellosis, enteritis, otitis media, chronic bronchitis, traveler's diarrhea. Prophylaxis of PCP. **OFF-LABEL:** Chronic prostatitis, prophylaxis for UTI, MRSA infections, prosthetic joint infection.

PRECAUTIONS

Contraindications: Hypersensitivity to any sulfa medication, trimethoprim. History of drug-induced immune thrombocytopenia

with sulfonamides or trimethoprim, infants younger than 4 wks, megaloblastic anemia due to folate deficiency, severe hepatic/renal impairment. **Cautions:** Pts with G6PD deficiency, impaired renal/hepatic function, porphyria, pts with allergies or asthma, elderly pts, alcoholism, thyroid dysfunction, concurrent anticonvulsant therapy.

ACTION

Blocks bacterial folic acid synthesis and growth. **Therapeutic Effect:** Bactericidal in susceptible microorganisms.

PHARMACOKINETICS

Rapidly, well absorbed from GI tract. Protein binding: 45%–60%. Widely distributed. Metabolized in liver. Excreted in urine. Minimally removed by hemodialysis. **Half-life:** sulfamethoxazole, 6–12 hrs; trimethoprim, 6–17 hrs (increased in renal impairment).

⧖ LIFESPAN CONSIDERATIONS

Pregnancy/Lactation: Contraindicated during pregnancy at term and during lactation. Readily crosses placenta. Distributed in breast milk. May produce kernicterus in newborn. **Children:** Contraindicated in pts younger than 2 mos; may increase risk of kernicterus in newborn. **Elderly:** Increased risk for severe skin reaction, myelosuppression, decreased platelet count.

INTERACTIONS

DRUG: May increase/prolong effects, increase adverse effects of **phenytoin, digoxin, oral hypoglycemics (e.g., glipiZIDE, metFORMIN), warfarin.** May increase effects of **methotrexate. HERBAL: Dong quai, St. John's wort** may increase photosensitization reaction. **FOOD:** None known. **LAB VALUES:** May increase serum BUN, creatinine, ALT, AST, bilirubin.

AVAILABILITY (Rx)

◄ALERT► All dosage forms have same 5:1 ratio of sulfamethoxazole (SMZ) to trimethoprim (TMP).

S

Injection Solution: SMZ 80 mg and TMP 16 mg per mL. Oral Suspension: SMZ 200 mg and TMP 40 mg per 5 mL. Tablets (Bactrim): SMZ 400 mg and TMP 80 mg. Tablets (Double Strength [Bactrim DS, Septra DS]): SMZ 800 mg and TMP 160 mg.

ADMINISTRATION/HANDLING

IV

Reconstitution • For IV infusion (piggyback), dilute each 5 mL with 75–125 mL D_5W. • Do not mix with other drugs or solutions.

Rate of Administration • Infuse over 60–90 min. Must avoid bolus or rapid infusion. • Do not give IM. • Ensure adequate hydration.

Storage • IV infusion (piggyback) stable for 2 hrs (5 mL/75 mL D_5W), 4 hrs (5 mL/100 mL D_5W), 6 hrs (5 mL/125 mL D_5W). • Discard if cloudy or precipitate forms.

PO

• Store tablets, suspension at room temperature. • Administer without regard to meals. • Give with at least 8 oz water.

🔲 IV INCOMPATIBILITIES

Fluconazole (Diflucan), foscarnet (Foscavir), midazolam (Versed), vinorelbine (Navelbine).

🔲 IV COMPATIBILITIES

Dexmedetomidine (Precedex), diltiaZEM (Cardizem), heparin, HYDROmorphone (Dilaudid), LORazepam (Ativan), magnesium sulfate, morphine, niCARdipine (Cardene).

INDICATIONS/ROUTES/DOSAGE

Usual Adult/Elderly Dosage Range
PO: 1–2 double-strength tablets q12–24h. **IV:** 8–20 mg/kg/day as trimethoprim in divided doses q6–12h.

Usual Dosage Range, Children Older Than 4 wks Mild to Moderate Infection
PO: CHILDREN: 8 mg/kg/day as trimethoprim in divided doses q12h.

Severe Infections
PO: CHILDREN: 15–20 mg/kg/day as trimethoprim in divided doses q6h.
IV: CHILDREN: 8–12 mg/kg/day as trimethoprim in divided doses q6–12h.

Dosage in Renal Impairment

Creatinine Clearance	Dosage
15–30 mL/min	50% of usual dosage
Less than 15 mL/min	Not recommended
HD	2.5–10 mg/kg trimethoprim q24h (or 5–20 mg/kg 3 times/wk) (give after HD)
CRRT	2.5–7.5 mg/kg trimethoprim q12h

Dosage in Hepatic Impairment
No dose adjustment.

SIDE EFFECTS

Frequent: Anorexia, nausea, vomiting, rash (generally 7–14 days after therapy begins), urticaria. **Occasional:** Diarrhea, abdominal pain, pain/irritation at IV infusion site. **Rare:** Headache, vertigo, insomnia, seizures, hallucinations, depression.

ADVERSE EFFECTS/TOXIC REACTIONS

Rash, fever, sore throat, pallor, purpura, cough, shortness of breath may be early signs of serious adverse effects. Fatalities are rare but have occurred in sulfonamide therapy following Stevens-Johnson syndrome, toxic epidermal necrolysis, fulminant hepatic necrosis, agranulocytosis, aplastic anemia, other blood dyscrasias. Myelosuppression, decreased platelet count, severe dermatologic reactions may occur, esp. in the elderly.

NURSING CONSIDERATIONS

BASELINE ASSESSMENT

Obtain history for hypersensitivity to trimethoprim or any sulfonamide, sulfite sensitivity, bronchial asthma. Determine serum renal, hepatic, hematologic baselines.

S

INTERVENTION/EVALUATION

Monitor daily pattern of bowel activity, stool consistency. Assess skin for rash, pallor, purpura. Check IV site, flow rate. Monitor renal, hepatic, hematology function. Assess I&O. Check for CNS symptoms (headache, vertigo, insomnia, hallucinations). Monitor vital signs at least twice daily. Monitor for cough, shortness of breath. Assess for overt bleeding, ecchymosis, edema.

PATIENT/FAMILY TEACHING

• Continue medication for full length of therapy. • Space doses evenly around the clock. • Take oral doses with 8 oz water and drink several extra glasses of water daily. • Report immediately any new symptoms, esp. rash, other skin changes, bleeding/bruising, fever, sore throat, diarrhea. • Avoid prolonged exposure to UV, direct sunlight.

---

sulfaSALAzine

sul-fa-sal-a-zeen
(Apo-SulfaSALAzine ✦, Azulfidine, Azulfidine EN-tabs, Salazopyrin ✦, Salazopyrin EN-Tabs ✦)
Do not confuse Azulfidine with Augmentin or azaTHIOprine, or sulfaSALAzine with sulfADIAZINE or sulfiSOXAZOLE.

◆CLASSIFICATION

PHARMACOTHERAPEUTIC: 5-Aminosalicylic acid derivative. **CLINICAL:** Anti-inflammatory.

USES

Treatment of mild to moderate ulcerative colitis, adjunctive therapy in severe ulcerative colitis, rheumatoid arthritis (RA), juvenile rheumatoid arthritis. **OFF-LABEL:** Treatment of ankylosing spondylitis, Crohn's disease, psoriasis, psoriatic arthritis.

PRECAUTIONS

Contraindications: Hypersensitivity to sulfaSALAzine, sulfa, salicylates; porphyria; GI or GU obstruction. **Cautions:** Severe allergies, bronchial asthma, impaired hepatic/renal function, G6PD deficiency, blood dyscrasias, history of recurring or chronic infections.

ACTION

Modulates local mediators of inflammatory response. **Therapeutic Effect:** Decreases inflammatory response, interferes with GI secretion. Effect appears topical rather than systemic.

PHARMACOKINETICS

Poorly absorbed from GI tract. Cleaved, absorbed in colon by intestinal bacteria, forming sulfapyridine and mesalamine (5-ASA). Widely distributed. Metabolized via colonic intestinal flora. Primarily excreted in urine. **Half-life:** 5.7–10 hrs.

☒ LIFESPAN CONSIDERATIONS

Pregnancy/Lactation: May produce infertility, oligospermia in men while taking medication. Readily crosses placenta; if given near term, may produce jaundice, hemolytic anemia, kernicterus in newborn. Distributed in breast milk. Pt should not breastfeed premature infant or those with hyperbilirubinemia or G6PD deficiency. **Children:** No age-related precautions noted in pts older than 2 yrs. **Elderly:** No age-related precautions noted.

INTERACTIONS

DRUG: Hepatotoxic medications (e.g., **acetaminophen, isoniazid, ketoconazole, simvastatin, SSRIs**) may increase risk of hepatotoxicity. **HERBAL: Dong quai, St. John's wort** may increase photosensitization. **FOOD:** Impairs folate absorption. **LAB VALUES:** None significant.

S

AVAILABILITY (Rx)

Tablets (Azulfidine): 500 mg.

🔖 **Tablets (Delayed-Release [Azulfidine EN-tabs]):** 500 mg.

ADMINISTRATION/HANDLING

PO

• Space doses evenly (intervals not to exceed 8 hrs). • Administer after meals or with food. • Swallow enteric-coated tablets whole; do not break, crush, dissolve, or divide. • Give with 8 oz of water; encourage several glasses of water between meals.

INDICATIONS/ROUTES/DOSAGE

Ulcerative Colitis

PO: ADULTS, ELDERLY: Initially, 3-4 g/day in divided doses q8h. May initiate at 1-2 g/day to reduce GI intolerance. **Maximum:** 6 g/day. **Maintenance:** 2 g/day in divided doses at intervals less than or equal to q8h. **CHILDREN 6 YRS AND OLDER:** Initially, 40–60 mg/kg/day in 3–6 divided doses. **Maximum (initial dose):** 4 g/day. **Maintenance:** 30 mg/kg/day in 4 divided doses at intervals less than or equal to q8h. **Maximum (maintenance dose):** 2 g/day.

Rheumatoid Arthritis (RA)

PO: *(Delayed-Release Tablets):* **ADULTS, ELDERLY:** Initially, 0.5–1 g/day for 1 wk. Increase by 0.5 g/wk, up to 2 g/day in 2 divided doses. **Maximum:** 3 g/day (if response to 2 g/day is inadequate after 12 wks of treatment).

Juvenile Rheumatoid Arthritis (JRA)

PO: *(Delayed-Release Tablets):* **CHILDREN:** Initially, 10 mg/kg/day. May increase by 10 mg/kg/day at wkly intervals. Range: 30–50 mg/kg/day. **Maximum:** 2 g/day.

Dosage in Renal/Hepatic Impairment

Use caution.

SIDE EFFECTS

Frequent (33%): Anorexia, nausea, vomiting, headache, oligospermia (generally reversed by withdrawal of drug). **Occasional (3%):** Hypersensitivity reaction (rash, urticaria, pruritus, fever, anemia). **Rare (Less Than 1%):** Tinnitus, hypoglycemia, diuresis, photosensitivity.

ADVERSE EFFECTS/TOXIC REACTIONS

Anaphylaxis, Stevens-Johnson syndrome, hematologic toxicity (leukopenia, agranulocytosis), hepatotoxicity, nephrotoxicity occur rarely.

NURSING CONSIDERATIONS

BASELINE ASSESSMENT

Question for hypersensitivity to medications. Check initial urinalysis, CBC, serum renal function, LFT.

INTERVENTION/EVALUATION

Monitor I&O, urinalysis, renal function tests; ensure adequate hydration (minimum output 1,500 mL/24 hrs) to prevent nephrotoxicity. Assess skin for rash (discontinue drug, notify physician at first sign). Monitor daily pattern of bowel activity, stool consistency. (Dosage increase may be needed if diarrhea continues, recurs.) Monitor CBC closely; assess for and report immediately any hematologic effects (bleeding, ecchymoses, fever, pharyngitis, pallor, weakness, purpura). Monitor LFT; observe for jaundice.

PATIENT/FAMILY TEACHING

• May cause orange-yellow discoloration of urine, skin. • Space doses evenly around the clock. • Take after or with food with 8 oz of water; drink several glasses of water between meals. • Swallow enteric-coated tablets whole; do not chew, crush, dissolve, or divide tablets. • Continue for full length of treatment; may be necessary to take drug even after symptoms relieved. • Routinely monitor blood levels. • Inform dentist, surgeon of sulfaSALAzine therapy. • Avoid exposure to sun, ultraviolet light until photosensitivity determined (may last for mos after last dose).

S

SUMAtriptan

soo-ma-**trip**-tan
(Apo-SUMAtriptan ✦, Imitrex,
Onzetra, Sumavel DosePro, Xsail,
Zembrace SymTouch)
**Do not confuse SUMAtriptan
with SAXagliptin, SITagliptin,
somatropin, or ZOLMitriptan.**

FIXED-COMBINATION(S)

Treximet: SUMAtriptan/naproxen (an
NSAID): 85 mg/500 mg, 10 mg/60 mg.

◆CLASSIFICATION

PHARMACOTHERAPEUTIC: Seroto-
nin 5-HT$_1$ receptor agonist. **CLINICAL:**
Antimigraine.

USES

PO, SQ, Intranasal, Transdermal:
Acute treatment of migraine headache
with or without aura. **SQ:** Treatment of
cluster headaches.

PRECAUTIONS

Contraindications: Hypersensitivity to
SUMAtriptan. Management of hemiplegic or basilar migraine, peripheral
vascular disease, CVA, ischemic heart
disease (including angina pectoris, history of MI, silent ischemia, Prinzmetal's
angina), severe hepatic impairment,
transient ischemic attack, uncontrolled
hypertension, MAOI use within 14
days, use within 24 hrs of ergotamine
preparations or another 5-HT$_1$ agonist. **Cautions:** Mild to moderate hepatic impairment, history of seizure disorder, controlled hypertension, elderly
pts.

ACTION

Binds selectively to serotonin 5-HT$_1$ receptors in cranial arteries, producing
vasoconstrictive effect on cranial blood
vessels. **Therapeutic Effect:** Relieves
migraine headache.

PHARMACOKINETICS

Route	Onset	Peak	Duration
Nasal	15 min	N/A	24–48 hrs
PO	30 min	2 hrs	24–48 hrs
SQ	10 min	1 hr	24–48 hrs

Rapidly absorbed after SQ administration. Absorption after PO administration is incomplete; significant amounts
undergo hepatic metabolism, resulting
in low bioavailability (about 14%).
Protein binding: 10%–21%. Widely
distributed. Undergoes first-pass metabolism in liver. Excreted in urine.
Half-life: 2 hrs.

⧗ LIFESPAN CONSIDERATIONS

Pregnancy/Lactation: Unknown if distributed in breast milk. **Children:** Safety
and efficacy not established. **Elderly:**
No age-related precautions noted.

INTERACTIONS

**DRUG: Ergotamine-containing medi-
cations** may produce vasospastic reaction.
MAOIs (e.g., phenelzine, selegiline)
may increase concentration, half-life. **SS-
RIs (e.g., escitalopram, paroxetine,
sertraline)** and **SNRIs (e.g., duloxetine, venlafaxine)** may increase risk
of serotonin syndrome. **HERBAL:** None
significant. **FOOD:** None known. **LAB
VALUES:** None significant.

AVAILABILITY (Rx)

Injection, Prefilled Autoinjector: 4 mg/0.5
mL, 6 mg/0.5 mL. **(Zembrace Sym-
Touch):** 3-mg prefilled syringe. **Injection
Solution (Imitrex):** 4 mg/0.5 mL, 6 mg/0.5
mL. **(Sumavel DosePro):** 4 mg/0.5 mL, 6
mg/0.5 mL. **Nasal Powder (Onzetra, Xsail):
Capsules:** 11 mg (to be used with Xsail
breath powdered nasal device). **Nasal
Spray (Imitrex Nasal):** 5 mg/actuation, 20
mg/actuation. **Tablets (Imitrex):** 25 mg,
50 mg, 100 mg.

ADMINISTRATION/HANDLING

SQ
• Follow manufacturer's instructions for
autoinjection device use. • Administer

S

needleless (Sumavel DosePro) only to abdomen or thigh.

PO
• Swallow tablets whole. Do not break, crush, dissolve, or divide. • Take with full glass of water.

Nasal
• Unit contains only one spray—do not test before use. • Instruct pt to gently blow nose to clear nasal passages. • With head upright, close one nostril with index finger, breathe out gently through mouth. • Have pt insert nozzle into open nostril about ½ inch, close mouth and, while taking a breath through nose, release spray dosage by firmly pressing plunger. • Instruct pt to remove nozzle from nose and gently breathe in through nose and out through mouth for 10–20 sec; do not breathe in deeply.

INDICATIONS/ROUTES/DOSAGE

Acute Migraine Headache
PO: ADULTS, ELDERLY: 25–100 mg. Dose may be repeated after at least 2 hrs. **Maximum:** 100 mg/single dose; 200 mg/24 hrs.
SQ: ADULTS, ELDERLY: Up to 6 mg. **Maximum:** Up to two 6-mg injections/24 hrs (separated by at least 1 hr). **(Zembrace SymTouch):** 3-mg single dose. **Maximum:** 12 mg/24 hrs. Separate dose by at least 1 hr.
Intranasal: ADULTS, ELDERLY: (Spray): 5–20 mg; may repeat in 2 hrs. **Maximum:** 40 mg/24 hrs. **(Nasal Powder):** 11 mg in each nostril. **Maximum:** 44 mg/24 hrs separated by at least 2 hrs.

Dosage in Renal Impairment
No dose adjustment.

Dosage in Hepatic Impairment
Mild to moderate impairment: Maximum PO dose: 50 mg. **Severe impairment:** Contraindicated.

SIDE EFFECTS

Frequent: PO (10%–5%): Tingling, nasal discomfort. **SQ (greater than 10%):** Injection site reactions, tingling, warm/hot sensation, dizziness, vertigo. **Nasal (greater than 10%):** Altered taste, nausea, vomiting. **Occasional: PO (5%–1%):** Flushing, asthenia, visual disturbances. **SQ (10%–2%):** Burning sensation, numbness, chest discomfort, drowsiness, asthenia. **Nasal (5%–1%):** Nasopharyngeal discomfort, dizziness. **Rare: PO (less than 1%):** Agitation, eye irritation, dysuria. **SQ (less than 2%):** Anxiety, fatigue, diaphoresis, muscle cramps, myalgia. **Nasal (less than 1%):** Burning sensation.

ADVERSE EFFECTS/TOXIC REACTIONS

Excessive dosage may produce tremors, redness of extremities, reduced respirations, cyanosis, seizures, paralysis. Serious arrhythmias occur rarely, esp. in pts with hypertension, obesity, smokers, diabetes, strong family history of coronary artery disease. Serotonin syndrome may occur (agitation, confusion, hallucinations, hyperreflexia, myoclonus, shivering, tachycardia).

NURSING CONSIDERATIONS

BASELINE ASSESSMENT
Receive full medical history, medication history and screen for contraindications. Obtain pregnancy test in female pts of reproductive potential. Question regarding onset, location, duration of migraine, possible precipitating symptoms.

INTERVENTION/EVALUATION
Evaluate for relief of migraine headache and resulting photophobia, phonophobia (sound sensitivity), nausea, vomiting.

PATIENT/FAMILY TEACHING
• Follow proper technique for loading of autoinjector, injection technique, discarding of syringe. • Do not use more than 2 injections during any 24-hr period and allow at least 1 hr between injections. • Report immediately if wheezing, palpitations, skin rash, facial swelling, pain/tightness in chest/throat occur.

SUNItinib

soo-**nit**-in-ib
(Sutent)

■ **BLACK BOX ALERT** ■ Hepato-toxicity may be severe and/or result in fatal liver failure.

Do not confuse SUNItinib with imatinib or SORAfenib.

◆CLASSIFICATION

PHARMACOTHERAPEUTIC: Tyrosine kinase inhibitor, vascular endothelial growth factor. **CLINICAL:** Antineoplastic.

USES

Treatment of GI stromal tumor after disease progression while on or demonstrating intolerance to imatinib. Treatment of advanced renal cell carcinoma. Adjuvant treatment of adults at high risk of recurrent RCC following nephrectomy. Treatment of pancreatic neuroendocrine tumor (PNET). **OFF-LABEL:** Non-GI stromal tumor, soft tissue sarcomas, advanced thyroid cancer.

PRECAUTIONS

Contraindications: Hypersensitivity to SUNItinib. **Cautions:** Cardiac dysfunction, bradycardia, electrolyte imbalance, bleeding tendencies, hypertension, history of prolonged QT interval, medications that prolong QT interval, hypokalemia, hypomagnesemia, concurrent use of strong CYP3A4 inducers or inhibitors, HF, renal/hepatic impairment, pregnancy.

ACTION

Inhibitory action against multiple kinases, growth factor receptors, stem cell factor receptors, colony-stimulating factor receptors, glial cell-line neurotrophic factor receptors. **Therapeutic Effect:** Prevents tumor cell growth, produces tumor regression, inhibits metastasis.

PHARMACOKINETICS

Metabolized in liver. Protein binding: 95%. Excreted in feces (61%), urine (16%). **Half-life:** 40–60 hrs.

⧖ LIFESPAN CONSIDERATIONS

Pregnancy/Lactation: Has potential for embryotoxic, teratogenic effects. Breastfeeding not recommended. **Children:** Safety and efficacy not established. **Elderly:** No age-related precautions noted.

INTERACTIONS

DRUG: Strong CYP3A4 inhibitors (e.g., **clarithromycin**, **itraconazole**, **ketoconazole**, **voriconazole**) may increase concentration, toxicity. **Strong CYP3A4 inducers** (e.g., **carBAMazepine**, PHENobarbital, **phenytoin**, **rifAMPin**) may decrease concentration/effects. **QT interval–prolonging medications** (e.g., **amiodarone**, **azithromycin**, **ceritinib**, **haloperidol**, **moxifloxacin**) may increase risk of QT interval prolongation, cardiac arrhythmias. **HERBAL:** St. John's wort may decrease concentration. **FOOD:** Grapefruit products may increase concentration, potential for torsades de pointes, myelotoxicity. **LAB VALUES:** May increase serum alkaline phosphatase, bilirubin, amylase, lipase, creatinine, ALT, AST. May alter serum potassium, sodium, uric acid. May produce thrombocytopenia, neutropenia. May decrease serum phosphate, thyroid function levels.

AVAILABILITY (Rx)

Capsules: 12.5 mg, 25 mg, 37.5 mg, 50 mg.

ADMINISTRATION/HANDLING

PO
• Give without regard to food. Avoid grapefruit products.

INDICATIONS/ROUTES/DOSAGE

GI Stromal Tumor, Renal Cell Carcinoma, RCC (Adjuvant Treatment)
PO: ADULTS, ELDERLY: 50 mg once daily for 4 wks, followed by 2 wks off in 6-wk cycle.

S

Pancreatic Neuroendocrine Tumor
PO: ADULTS, ELDERLY: 37.5 mg once daily continuously without a scheduled off-treatment period.

Dose Modification
PO: ADULTS, ELDERLY: Dosage increase or reduction in 12.5-mg increments is recommended based on safety and tolerability.

Dosage in Renal Impairment
No initial dose adjustment; subsequent adjustment may be needed.

Dosage in Hepatic Impairment
No dose adjustment initially; grade 3 or 4 hepatotoxicity during treatment: withhold/discontinue if hepatotoxicity does not resolve.

SIDE EFFECTS

Stromal tumor: Common (42%–30%): Fatigue, diarrhea, anorexia, abdominal pain, nausea, hyperpigmentation. **Frequent (29%–18%):** Mucositis/stomatitis, vomiting, asthenia, altered taste, constipation, fever. **Occasional (15%–8%):** Hypertension, rash, myalgia, headache, arthralgia, back pain, dyspnea, cough. **Renal carcinoma: Common (74%–43%):** Fatigue, diarrhea, nausea, mucositis/stomatitis, dyspepsia, altered taste. **Frequent (38%–20%):** Rash, vomiting, constipation, hyperpigmentation, anorexia, arthralgia, dyspnea, hypertension, headache, abdominal pain. **Occasional (18%–11%):** Limb pain, peripheral/periorbital edema, dry skin, hair color change, myalgia, cough, back pain, dizziness, fever, tongue pain, flatulence, alopecia, dehydration.

ADVERSE EFFECTS/TOXIC REACTIONS

Palmar-plantar erythrodysesthesia syndrome (PPES) occurs occasionally (14%), manifested as blistering/rash/peeling of skin on palms of hands, soles of feet. Bleeding, decrease in left ventricular ejection fraction, deep vein thrombosis (DVT), pancreatitis, neutropenia, seizures occur rarely.

NURSING CONSIDERATIONS

BASELINE ASSESSMENT

Question possibility of pregnancy. Obtain baseline CBC, BMP, LFT before beginning therapy and prior to each treatment. Obtain baseline EKG, thyroid function tests. Question medical history as listed in Precautions.

INTERVENTION/EVALUATION

Assess eye area, lower extremities for early evidence of fluid retention. Offer antiemetics to control nausea, vomiting. Monitor daily pattern of bowel activity, stool consistency. Monitor CBC for evidence of neutropenia, thrombocytopenia; assess LFT for hepatotoxicity. Monitor for PPES. Monitor B/P.

PATIENT/FAMILY TEACHING

• Avoid crowds, those with known infection. • Avoid contact with anyone who recently received live virus vaccine. • Do not have immunizations without physician's approval (drug lowers resistance). • Avoid pregnancy; use effective contraceptive measures. • Promptly report fever, unusual bruising/bleeding from any site.

suvorexant

soo-voe-**rex**-ant
(Belsomra)

◆CLASSIFICATION

PHARMACOTHERAPEUTIC: Orexin receptor antagonist. **CLINICAL:** Sedative-hypnotic.

USES

Treatment of insomnia, characterized by difficulties with sleep onset and/or sleep maintenance.

PRECAUTIONS

Contraindications: Hypersensitivity to suvorexant. History of narcolepsy. **Cautions:** History of COPD, depression, debilitation, drug dependency, obstructive sleep apnea, respiratory disease, pts at high risk of suicide; concomitant use of CNS depressants, strong CYP3A4 inhibitors/inducers. Concomitant use of other insomnia medications not recommended.

ACTION

Suppresses wake drive of the orexin neuropeptide signaling system, the central promoter of wakefulness. Blocks binding of orexin neuropeptides orexin A and orexin B to receptors of OX1R and OX2R. **Therapeutic Effect:** Induces sleep with fewer nighttime awakenings; improves sleep pattern.

PHARMACOKINETICS

Rapidly absorbed. Metabolized in liver. Protein binding: greater than 99%. Peak plasma concentration: 2 hrs. Excreted in feces (66%), urine (23%). **Half-life:** 12 hrs.

⧗ LIFESPAN CONSIDERATIONS

Pregnancy/Lactation: Unknown if distributed in breast milk. **Children:** Safety and efficacy not established. **Elderly:** No age-related precautions noted.

INTERACTIONS

DRUG: **Alcohol, CNS depressants** (e.g., **LORazepam, morphine, zolpidem**) may increase CNS depression. **Moderate CYP3A4 inhibitors** (e.g., **ciprofloxacin, diltiaZEM**), **strong CYP3A4 inhibitors** (e.g., **ketoconazole, clarithromycin**) may increase concentration/ effect, CNS depression. **CYP3A4 inducers** (e.g., **rifAMPin, phenytoin**) may decrease concentration/effect. May increase concentration/effect of **digoxin.** **HERBAL:** **Gotu kola, kava kava, valerian** may increase CNS depression. **St. John's wort** may decrease concentration/effect. **FOOD:** **Meals** may decrease absorption/ effect. **Grapefruit products** may increase concentration/effect. **LAB VALUES:** May increase serum cholesterol.

AVAILABILITY (Rx)

Tablets: 5 mg, 10 mg, 15 mg, 20 mg.

ADMINISTRATION/HANDLING

PO
• Administer no more than once per night, within 30 min of bedtime. • Do not administer unless 7 hrs or greater is dedicated for sleep. • For faster sleep onset, do not give with or immediately after meal.

INDICATIONS/ROUTES/DOSAGE

Insomnia
PO: **ADULTS, ELDERLY:** 10 mg once at bedtime. May increase to 20 mg at bedtime.

Dose Modification
Concomitant use with other CNS depressants, moderate CYP3A4 inhibitors: Decrease starting dose to 5 mg once at bedtime. May increase to 10 mg once at bedtime. **Concomitant use of strong CYP3A4 inhibitors:** Not recommended. **Daytime somnolence:** Decrease dose or discontinue if daytime somnolence.

Dosage in Renal Impairment
No dose adjustment.

Dosage in Hepatic Impairment
Mild to moderate impairment: No dose adjustment. **Severe impairment:** Not recommended.

SIDE EFFECTS

Occasional (7%): Headache, somnolence. **Rare (3%–2%):** Dizziness, diarrhea, dry mouth, upper respiratory tract infection, abnormal dreams, cough.

ADVERSE EFFECTS/TOXIC REACTIONS

Obese pts and female pts may have increased exposure-related effects compared to nonobese pts and male pts, respectively. May impair daytime wakefulness even when taken as prescribed. Impairment can occur in the absence of symptoms and may not be reliably detected by ordinary clinical exam. CNS

S

depression may persist for up to several days. May increase risk of falling asleep while driving. Abnormal thinking and behavioral changes such as amnesia, anxiety, lowered sexual inhibition, hallucinations, "sleep driving," preparing and eating meals, making phone calls have been reported. May increase risk of suicidal ideation, worsening of depression. Sleep paralysis (inability to move or speak for up to several min during sleep-wake transitions) and hypnagogic/hypnopompic hallucinations (including vivid and disturbing perceptions) may occur.

NURSING CONSIDERATIONS

BASELINE ASSESSMENT

Assess sleep pattern, ability to fall asleep. Provide environment conductive to restful sleep. Initiate fall precautions. Raise bed rails, provide call light. Receive full medication history, including herbal products, and screen for medication interactions. Question history of comorbidities, esp. mental health disorders, substance abuse.

INTERVENTION/EVALUATION

Monitor sleep pattern. Evaluate for therapeutic response: decrease in number of nocturnal awakenings, increase in length of sleep. Diligently monitor for daytime somnolence and CNS depressant effects regardless of compliance. Worsening of insomnia, emergence of new cognitive or behavioral abnormalities, or treatment failure after 7–10 days may indicate underlying psychiatric disorder.

PATIENT/FAMILY TEACHING

• Report nighttime episodes of sleep-driving, preparing food, making phone calls, or having sex while not fully awake. • Do not abruptly discontinue medication after long-term use. • Avoid tasks that require alertness, motor skills until drug response established. • Treatment may cause next-day impairment, drowsiness, or falling asleep while driving despite taking medication as prescribed (esp. pts taking higher doses). • Do not ingest alcohol or grapefruit products. • Do not take drug unless a full night can be dedicated to sleep. • Immediately report worsening of depression or thoughts of suicide.

S

tacrolimus

ta-**kroe**-li-mus
(Advagraf ✹, Astagraf XL, Envarsus
XR, <u>Prograf</u>, Protopic)

■ **BLACK BOX ALERT** ■ Increased
susceptibility to infection and
potential for development of
lymphoma. Extended-release associated with increased mortality in
female liver transplant recipients.
Topical form associated with rare
cases of malignancy. Topical form
should be used only for short-term
and intermittent treatment. Use in
children younger than 2 yrs of age
not recommended. Use only 0.03%
ointment for children 2–15 yrs of
age. Administer under supervision
of physician experienced in immunosuppressive therapy.
**Do not confuse Protopic with
Protonix, or tacrolimus with
everolimus, pimecrolimus,
sirolimus, or temsirolimus.**

◆CLASSIFICATION

PHARMACOTHERAPEUTIC: Immunologic agent. **CLINICAL:** Immunosuppressant.

USES

PO, Injection: Prevention of organ rejection in pts receiving allogeneic liver, kidney,
heart transplant. Should be used concurrently with adrenal corticosteroids. In
heart and kidney transplant pts, should be
used in conjunction with azaTHIOprine or
mycophenolate. **Topical:** Moderate to severe atopic dermatitis in immunocompetent pts. **OFF-LABEL:** Prevention of organ
rejection in lung, small bowel recipients;
prevention and treatment of graft-vs-host
disease in allogeneic hematopoietic stem
cell transplantation.

PRECAUTIONS

Contraindications: Hypersensitivity to tacrolimus. **Cautions:** Hypersensitivity to
HCO-60 polyoxyl 60 hydrogenated castor
oil (used in solution for injection).
Renal/hepatic impairment, concurrent

use with other nephrotoxic drugs (e.g.,
cycloSPORINE), concurrent use of strong
CYP3A4 inhibitors or inducers. Avoid use
of potassium-sparing diuretics, ACE inhibitors, potassium-based salt substitutes. Pts at risk for pure red cell aplasia
(e.g., concurrent use of mycophenolate);
pts at risk for QT prolongation, hypokalemia, hypomagnesemia. **Topical:** Exposure to sunlight.

ACTION

Inhibits T-lymphocyte activation by binding to intracellular proteins, forming a
complex, inhibiting phosphatase activity.
Therapeutic Effect: Suppresses immunologically mediated inflammatory response; prevents organ transplant rejection.

PHARMACOKINETICS

Variably absorbed after PO administration (food reduces absorption). Protein
binding: 99%. Metabolized in liver. Primarily excreted in feces. Not removed by
hemodialysis. **Half-life:** 21–61 hrs.

⧖ LIFESPAN CONSIDERATIONS

Pregnancy/Lactation: Crosses placenta. Hyperkalemia, renal dysfunction
noted in neonates. Distributed in breast
milk. Breastfeeding not recommended.
Children: May require higher dosages
(decreased bioavailability, increased
clearance). May make post-transplant
lymphoproliferative disorder more common, esp. in pts younger than 3 yrs.
Elderly: Age-related renal impairment
may require dosage adjustment.

INTERACTIONS

**DRUG: Aluminium-containing antac-
ids** may increase concentration. **Strong
CYP3A4 inhibitors (e.g., clarithromycin, ketoconazole, ritonavir),
calcium channel blockers (e.g.,
diltiazem, verapamil)** may increase
concentration/effects. **Strong CYP3A4
inducers (e.g., carBAMazepine,
phenytoin, rifAMPin)** may decrease
concentration/effects. May increase
concentration of **cycloSPORINE.** May

T

decrease therapeutic effects of **live vaccines. HERBAL:** Echinacea, St. John's wort may decrease concentration/effects. **FOOD:** Food decreases rate/extent of absorption. **Grapefruit products** may increase concentration, toxicity (potential for nephrotoxicity). **LAB VALUES:** May increase serum glucose, BUN, creatinine, potassium, triglycerides, cholesterol, bilirubin, amylase, ALT, AST. May decrease serum magnesium, Hgb, Hct, platelets. May alter leukocytes.

AVAILABILITY (Rx)

Capsules (Prograf): 0.5 mg, 1 mg, 5 mg. **Injection Solution (Prograf):** 5 mg/mL. **Ointment (Protopic):** 0.03%, 0.1%.

 Capsule, Extended-Release (Astagraf XL): 0.5 mg, 1 mg, 5 mg. **Tablet, Extended-Release (Envarsus XR):** 0.75 mg, 1 mg, 4 mg.

ADMINISTRATION/HANDLING

IV

Reconstitution • Dilute with appropriate amount (250–1,000 mL, depending on desired dose) 0.9% NaCl or D₅W to provide concentration between 0.004 and 0.02 mg/mL.

Rate of Administration • Give as continuous IV infusion. • Continuously monitor pt for anaphylaxis for at least 30 min after start of infusion. • Stop infusion immediately at first sign of hypersensitivity reaction.

Storage • Store diluted infusion solution in glass or polyethylene containers and discard after 24 hrs. • Do not store in PVC container (decreased stability, potential for extraction).

PO

• Avoid grapefruit products. • **Immediate-Release:** Administer without regard to food. Be consistent with timing of administration.

• **Extended-Release.** Administer at least 1 hr before or 2 hrs after a meal. Do not crush, cut, dissolve, or divide; swallow whole.

Topical

• For external use only. • Do not cover with occlusive dressing. • Rub gently, completely onto clean, dry skin.

🖼 IV INCOMPATIBILITY

Acyclovir.

🖼 IV COMPATIBILITIES

Calcium gluconate, dexamethasone (Decadron), diphenhydrAMINE (Benadryl), DOBUTamine (Dobutrex), DOPamine (Intropin), furosemide (Lasix), heparin, HYDROmorphone (Dilaudid), insulin, leucovorin, LORazepam (Ativan), morphine, nitroglycerin, potassium chloride.

INDICATIONS/ROUTES/DOSAGE

Note: Give initial postoperative dose no sooner than 6 hrs after liver or heart transplant and within 24 hrs of kidney transplant.

Prevention of Liver Transplant Rejection
PO: ADULTS, ELDERLY: *(Immediate-Release):* 0.1–0.15 mg/kg/day in 2 divided doses 12 hrs apart. Titrate to target trough concentration. **CHILDREN:** 0.15–0.2 mg/kg/day in 2 divided doses 12 hrs apart. Titrate to target trough concentration.
IV: ADULTS, ELDERLY, CHILDREN: 0.03–0.05 mg/kg/day as continuous infusion.

Prevention of Kidney Transplant Rejection
PO: ADULTS, ELDERLY: *(Immediate-Release):* 0.2 mg/kg/day (in combination with azaTHIOprine) in 2 divided doses 12 hrs apart or 0.1 mg/kg/day (in combination with mycophenolate). Titrate to target trough concentration. ***(Extended-Release): (With Basiliximab Induction):*** (Prior to or within 48 hrs of transplant completion): 0.15–0.2 mg/kg once daily (in combination with corticosteroids and mycophenolate). Titrate to target trough concentration. ***(Without Basiliximab Induction):*** Preoperative dose: 0.1 mg/kg (administer within 12 hrs prior to reperfusion). Postoperative dosing: 0.2 mg/kg once daily

(in combination with corticosteroids and mycophenolate). Give at least 4 hrs after preoperative dose and within 12 hrs of reperfusion. Titrate to target trough concentration.

IV: ADULTS, ELDERLY: 0.03–0.05 mg/kg/day as continuous infusion.

Prevention of Heart Transplant Rejection
Note: Recommend in combination with azaTHIOprine or mycophenolate.
PO: ADULTS, ELDERLY: Initially, 0.075 mg/kg/day in 2 divided doses 12 hrs apart. Titrate to target trough concentration.
IV: ADULTS, ELDERLY: 0.01 mg/kg/day as continuous infusion.

Atopic Dermatitis
Topical: ADULTS, ELDERLY, CHILDREN 15 YRS AND OLDER: Apply 0.03% or 0.1% ointment to affected area twice daily. **CHILDREN 2–15 YRS:** Use 0.03% ointment. Continue treatment for 1 wk after symptoms have resolved. If no improvement within 6 wks, re-examine to confirm diagnosis.

SIDE EFFECTS

Frequent (Greater Than 30%): Headache, tremor, insomnia, paresthesia, diarrhea, nausea, constipation, vomiting, abdominal pain, hypertension. **Occasional (29%–10%):** Rash, pruritus, anorexia, asthenia, peripheral edema, photosensitivity.

ADVERSE EFFECTS/TOXIC REACTIONS

Nephrotoxicity (elevated serum creatinine, decreased urinary output), neurotoxicity (tremor, headache, altered mental status), pleural effusion occur commonly. Thrombocytopenia, leukocytosis, anemia, atelectasis, sepsis, infection occur occasionally.

NURSING CONSIDERATIONS

BASELINE ASSESSMENT
Assess medical history, esp. renal function; medication history, use of other immunosuppressants. Have aqueous solution of EPINEPHrine 1:1,000, O_2 available at bedside before beginning IV infusion. Assess pt continuously for first 30 min following start of infusion and at frequent intervals thereafter.

INTERVENTION/EVALUATION
Closely monitor pts with renal impairment. Monitor lab values, esp. serum creatinine, serum potassium, CBC with differential, LFT. Monitor I&O closely. CBC should be performed wkly during first mo of therapy, twice monthly during second and third mos of treatment, then monthly throughout the first yr. Report any major change in pt assessment.

PATIENT/FAMILY TEACHING
• Avoid crowds, those with infection. • Report decreased urination, chest pain, headache, dizziness, respiratory infection, rash, unusual bleeding/bruising. • Avoid exposure to sun, artificial light (may cause photosensitivity reaction). • Do not take within 2 hrs of taking antacids. Do not take with grapefruit products.

---

tamoxifen ■ HIGH ALERT

ta-**mox**-fen
(Apo-Tamox ❖, Nolvadex-D ❖, Soltamox)

■ **BLACK BOX ALERT** ■ Serious, possibly life-threatening CVA, pulmonary emboli, uterine malignancy (endometrial adenocarcinoma, uterine sarcoma) have occurred.
Do not confuse tamoxifen with pentoxifylline, tamsulosin, or temazepam.

◆CLASSIFICATION

PHARMACOTHERAPEUTIC: Selective estrogen receptor modulator (SERM). **CLINICAL:** Antineoplastic.

USES

Adjunct treatment in advanced breast cancer after primary treatment with surgery and radiation, reduction of risk of breast cancer in women at high risk, reduction of risk of invasive breast cancer in women with ductal carcinoma *in situ* (DCIS), metastatic breast cancer in women and men. **OFF-LABEL:** Ovarian cancer (advanced and/or recurrent), treatment of endometrial cancer; risk reduction of breast cancer in women with Paget's disease of the breast.

PRECAUTIONS

Contraindications: Hypersensitivity to tamoxifen. Concomitant warfarin therapy when used in treatment of breast cancer in high-risk women, history of deep vein thrombosis (DVT) or pulmonary embolism (in high-risk women for breast cancer and in women with DCIS). **Cautions:** Thrombocytopenia, pregnancy, history of thromboembolic events, hyperlipidemia, concomitant strong CYP2D6 inhibitors and/or moderate CYP2D6 inhibitors.

ACTION

Competes with estradiol for estrogen-receptor binding sites in breast, uterus, vaginal cells. **Therapeutic Effect:** Inhibits DNA synthesis, estrogen response. Slows tumor growth.

PHARMACOKINETICS

Well absorbed from GI tract. Metabolized in liver. Primarily excreted in feces. **Half-life:** 7 days.

⧖ LIFESPAN CONSIDERATIONS

Pregnancy/Lactation: If possible, avoid use during pregnancy, esp. first trimester. May cause fetal harm. Unknown if distributed in breast milk. Breastfeeding not recommended. Nonhormonal contraceptives recommended during therapy and for at least 2 mos after discontinuation. **Children:** Safe and effective in girls 2–10 yrs with McCune-Albright syndrome, precocious puberty. **Elderly:** No age-related precautions noted.

INTERACTIONS

DRUG: May increase effect of **warfarin.** May decrease effect of **anastrozole. Cytotoxic agents** may increase risk of thromboembolic events. **Moderate/strong CYP2D6 inhibitors (e.g., FLUoxetine, sertraline)** may decrease efficacy and increase risk of breast cancer. **HERBAL:** Avoid **black cohosh, dong quai** in estrogen-dependent tumors. **St. John's wort** may decrease concentration/effects. **FOOD:** None known. **LAB VALUES:** May increase serum cholesterol, calcium, triglycerides, AST, ALT.

AVAILABILITY (Rx)

Solution, Oral (Soltamox): 10 mg/5 mL. **Tablets:** 10 mg, 20 mg.

ADMINISTRATION/HANDLING

PO
• Give without regard to food. • Use supplied dosing cup for oral solution.

INDICATIONS/ROUTES/DOSAGE

Metastatic Breast Cancer
(Males and Females)
PO: **ADULTS, ELDERLY:** 20–40 mg/day. Give doses greater than 20 mg/day in 2 divided doses.

Breast Cancer Treatment
PO: **ADJUVANT THERAPY (FEMALES), PRE-MENOPAUSAL WOMEN:** 20 mg once daily for 5 yrs.
POSTMENOPAUSAL WOMEN: Duration of 2–3 yrs, followed by an aromatase inhibitor to complete 5 yrs.

Ductal Carcinoma *in Situ* (DCIS)
PO: **ADULTS, ELDERLY:** 20 mg once daily for 5 yrs.

Breast Cancer Risk Reduction
PO: **ADULTS, ELDERLY:** 20 mg once daily for 5 yrs.

Dosage in Renal/Hepatic Impairment
No dose adjustment.

SIDE EFFECTS

Frequent: Women (greater than 10%): Hot flashes, nausea, vomiting. **Occasional: Women (9%–1%):** Changes in menstruation, genital itching, vaginal discharge, endometrial hyperplasia, polyps. **Men:** Impotence, decreased libido. **Men and women:** Headache, nausea, vomiting, rash, bone pain, confusion, weakness, drowsiness.

ADVERSE EFFECTS/TOXIC REACTIONS

Retinopathy, corneal opacity, decreased visual acuity noted in pts receiving extremely high dosages (240–320 mg/day) for longer than 17 mos.

NURSING CONSIDERATIONS

BASELINE ASSESSMENT

Obtain estrogen receptor assay prior to therapy. Obtain baseline breast and gynecologic exams, mammogram results. CBC, serum calcium levels should be checked before and periodically during therapy.

INTERVENTION/EVALUATION

Be alert to increased bone pain; ensure adequate pain relief. Monitor I&O, weight. Observe for edema, esp. of dependent areas, signs and symptoms of DVT. Assess for hypercalcemia (increased urinary volume, excessive thirst, nausea, vomiting, constipation, hypotonicity of muscles, deep bone/flank pain, renal stones).

PATIENT/FAMILY TEACHING

• Report vaginal bleeding/discharge/itching, leg cramps, weight gain, shortness of breath, weakness. • May initially experience increase in bone, tumor pain (appears to indicate good tumor response). • Report persistent nausea, vomiting. • Nonhormonal contraceptives are recommended during treatment.

tamsulosin

tam-**soo**-loe-sin
(Flomax, Apo-Tamsulosin ✦)
Do not confuse Flomax with Flonase, Flovent, Foltx, Fosamax, or Volmax, or tamsulosin with tamoxifen or terazosin.

FIXED-COMBINATION(S)

Jalyn: tamsulosin/dutasteride (an androgen hormone inhibitor): 0.4 mg/0.5 mg.

◆CLASSIFICATION

PHARMACOTHERAPEUTIC: Alpha₁-adrenergic blocker. **CLINICAL:** Benign prostatic hyperplasia agent.

USES

Treatment of symptoms of benign prostatic hyperplasia (BPH). **OFF-LABEL:** Treatment of bladder outlet obstruction or dysfunction. To facilitate expulsion of ureteral stones (distal).

PRECAUTIONS

Contraindications: Hypersensitivity to tamsulosin. **Cautions:** Concurrent use of phosphodiesterase (PDE5) inhibitors (e.g., sildenafil, tadalafil, vardenafil), pts with orthostatic hypotension.

ACTION

Antagonist of alpha receptors in prostate. **Therapeutic Effect:** Relaxes smooth muscle in bladder neck and prostate; improves urinary flow, symptoms of prostatic hyperplasia.

PHARMACOKINETICS

Well absorbed, widely distributed. Protein binding: 94%–99%. Metabolized in liver. Primarily excreted in urine. Unknown if removed by hemodialysis. **Half-life:** 9–13 hrs.

T

✦ Canadian trade name   🦺 Non-Crushable Drug   🔲 High Alert drug

⧗ LIFESPAN CONSIDERATIONS

Pregnancy/Lactation: Not indicated for use in women. **Children:** Not indicated in this pt population. **Elderly:** No age-related precautions noted.

INTERACTIONS

DRUG: **Other alpha-adrenergic blocking agents** (e.g., **doxazosin, prazosin, terazosin**) may increase alpha-blockade effects. **Sildenafil, tadalafil, vardenafil** may cause symptomatic hypotension. **CYP3A4 inhibitors** (e.g., **clarithromycin, ketoconazole, ritonavir**) may increase concentration. **HERBAL:** Avoid **saw palmetto** (limited experience with this combination). **Black cohosh, periwinkle** may increase hypotensive effect. **St. John's wort** may decrease concentration/effects. **FOOD: Grapefruit products** may increase risk for orthostatic hypotension. **LAB VALUES:** None known.

AVAILABILITY (Rx)

 Capsules: 0.4 mg.

ADMINISTRATION/HANDLING

PO
• Give at same time each day, 30 min after the same meal. • Do not break, crush, or open capsule.

INDICATIONS/ROUTES/DOSAGE

Benign Prostatic Hyperplasia (BPH)
PO: ADULTS: 0.4 mg once daily, approximately 30 min after same meal each day. May increase dosage to 0.8 mg if inadequate response in 2–4 wks.

Dosage in Renal/Hepatic Impairment
No dose adjustment.

SIDE EFFECTS

Frequent (9%–7%): Dizziness, drowsiness. **Occasional (5%–3%):** Headache, anxiety, insomnia, orthostatic hypotension. **Rare (Less Than 2%):** Nasal congestion, pharyngitis, rhinitis, nausea, vertigo, impotence.

ADVERSE EFFECTS/TOXIC REACTIONS

First-dose syncope (hypotension with sudden loss of consciousness) may occur within 30–90 min after initial dose. May be preceded by tachycardia (pulse rate of 120–160 beats/min).

NURSING CONSIDERATIONS

BASELINE ASSESSMENT

Assess history of prostatic hyperplasia (difficulty initiating urine stream, dribbling, sense of urgency, leaking). Question for sensitivity to tamsulosin, or use of other alpha-adrenergic blocking agents. Obtain vital signs.

INTERVENTION/EVALUATION

Assist with ambulation if dizziness occurs. Monitor renal function, I&O, weight changes, peripheral edema, B/P. Monitor for first-dose syncope.

PATIENT/FAMILY TEACHING

• Take at same time each day, 30 min after the same meal. • Go from lying to standing slowly. • Avoid tasks that require alertness, motor skills until response to drug is established. • Do not break, crush, open capsule. • Avoid grapefruit products.

tapentadol

ta-**pen**-ta-dol
(Nucynta, Nucynta ER, Nucynta IR ✦)
Do not confuse tapentadol with traMADol.

◆CLASSIFICATION

PHARMACOTHERAPEUTIC: Centrally acting synthetic analgesic (Schedule II). **CLINICAL:** Analgesic.

USES

Nucynta: Relief of moderate to severe acute pain in adults 18 yrs and older.

Nucynta ER: Management of moderate to severe chronic or neuropathic pain associated with diabetic peripheral neuropathy when around-the-clock analgesic is needed for extended period.

PRECAUTIONS

Contraindications: Hypersensitivity to tapentadol. Severe respiratory depression, acute or severe bronchial asthma, hypercapnia in uncontrolled settings, known or suspected paralytic ileus, concurrent use or ingestion within 14 days of MAOI use. **Cautions:** Respiratory disease or respiratory compromise (e.g., hypoxia, hypercapnia, or decreased respiratory reserve), asthma, COPD, severe obesity, sleep apnea syndrome, CNS depression, pts with head injury, intracranial lesions, pancreatic or biliary disease, renal or hepatic impairment, seizure disorder, conditions that increase risk of seizures, pts at risk for hypotension, adrenal insufficiency, concurrent use with serotonergic agents, elderly pts, debilitated or cachetic pts. History of substance abuse.

ACTION

Binds to mu-opioid receptors in the central nervous system, causing inhibition of ascending pain pathways; increases norepinephrine by inhibiting its reabsorption into nerve cells. **Therapeutic Effect:** Produces analgesia. Reduces level of pain perception.

PHARMACOKINETICS

Metabolized in liver. Primarily excreted in the urine. Widely distributed. Protein binding: 20%. **Half-life:** 4 hrs.

⧗ LIFESPAN CONSIDERATIONS

Pregnancy/Lactation: Unknown if drug crosses placenta or is distributed in breast milk. **Children:** Not recommended for use in this pt population. **Elderly:** Age-related renal impairment may increase risk of side effects.

INTERACTIONS

DRUG: Alcohol, CNS depressants (e.g., **LORazepam, morphine, zolpidem**) may increase CNS depression, respiratory depression. **MAOIs** (e.g., **phenelzine, selegiline**), **SSRIs** (e.g., **FLUoxetine**), **tricyclic antidepressants** (e.g., **amitriptyline**), **triptans** (e.g., **SUMAtriptan**) may increase risk of serotonin syndrome. **HERBAL: Kava kava, St. John's wort, valerian** may increase CNS depression. **St. John's wort** may increase risk for serotonin syndrome. **FOOD:** None known. **LAB VALUES:** None significant.

AVAILABILITY (Rx)

Tablets: 50 mg, 75 mg, 100 mg.

🐾 **Tablets, Extended-Release:** 50 mg, 100 mg, 150 mg, 200 mg, 250 mg.

ADMINISTRATION/HANDLING

PO
• Give without regard to food. • Tablets may be crushed. • Give extended-release tablets whole; do not break, crush, dissolve, or divide.

INDICATIONS/ROUTES/DOSAGE

Note: Not recommended in severe renal or hepatic impairment.

Pain Control
PO: ADULTS, ELDERLY: Nucynta: 50–100 mg q4–6h as needed. **Maximum:** 600 mg/day (700 mg on day 1). **Nucynta ER:** Initially, 50 mg twice daily (12 hrs apart). May increase by 50 mg twice daily q3days to effective dose. Range: 100–250 mg twice daily. **Maximum:** 500 mg/day.

Conversion to Extended-Release
Oral Opioids: Discontinue all other opioids when extended-release tapentadol is initiated. Begin with a dose that is 50% of estimated tapentadol needed with immediate-release rescue medications as a supplement.

Immediate-Release tapentadol: Use same total daily dose but divide into 2 equal doses given twice daily. Maximum dose: 500 mg daily.

Dosage in Renal Impairment
CrCl 30 mL/min or greater: No adjustment. **CrCl less than 30 mL/min:** Not recommended.

Dosage in Hepatic Impairment
Immediate-release: Moderate impairment: 50 mg q8h. **Maximum:** 3 doses/24 hrs. **Extended-release:** Initially, 50 mg/day. **Maximum:** 100 mg/day.

SIDE EFFECTS

Frequent (Greater Than 10%): Nausea, dizziness, vomiting, sleepiness, headache.

ADVERSE EFFECTS/TOXIC REACTIONS

Respiratory depression, serotonin syndrome have been reported.

NURSING CONSIDERATIONS

BASELINE ASSESSMENT

Assess onset, type, location, and duration of pain. Obtain vital signs before giving medication. If respirations are 12/min or lower, withhold medication, contact physician. Question medical history as listed in Precautions.

INTERVENTION/EVALUATION

Be alert for decreased respirations or B/P. Initiate deep breathing and coughing exercises, particularly in pts with impaired pulmonary function. Assess for clinical improvement and record onset of pain relief.

PATIENT/FAMILY TEACHING

• Avoid tasks that require alertness, motor skills until response to drug is established. • Avoid alcohol, CNS depressants. • Report nausea, vomiting, shortness of breath, difficulty breathing.

tedizolid

ted-eye-**zoe**-lid
(Sivextro)
Do not confuse tedizolid with linezolid.

◆CLASSIFICATION

PHARMACOTHERAPEUTIC: Oxazolidinone-class antibacterial. **CLINICAL:** Antibiotic.

USES

Treatment of adult pts with acute bacterial skin and skin structure infections (ABSSSI) caused by susceptible strains of gram-positive microorganisms including *Staphylococcus aureus* (including methicillin-susceptible and methicillin-resistant strains), *S. agalactiae*, *S. anginosus* group (including *S. anginosus*, *S. intermedius*, *S. constellatus*), *S. pyogenes*, and *E. faecalis*.

PRECAUTIONS

Contraindications: Hypersensitivity to tedizolid. **Cautions:** History of *C. difficile* infection or antibiotic-associated colitis, myelosuppression, neutropenia, peripheral/optic neuropathy.

ACTION

Inhibits cellular protein synthesis by binding to 50S subunit of bacterial ribosome. **Therapeutic Effect:** Antibiotic.

PHARMACOKINETICS

Readily absorbed following PO administration. Protein binding: 70%–90%. Peak plasma concentration: PO: 3 hrs; IV: end of infusion. Excreted in feces (82%), urine (18%). Minimally removed by hemodialysis. **Half-life:** 12 hrs.

⧖ LIFESPAN CONSIDERATIONS

Pregnancy/Lactation: Unknown if distributed in breast milk. **Children:** Safety and efficacy not established in pts younger than 18 yrs. **Elderly:** No age-related precautions noted.

INTERACTIONS

DRUG: None significant. **HERBAL:** None significant. **FOOD:** None known. **LAB VALUES:** May decrease Hgb, platelets, neutrophils. May increase serum ALT, AST.

AVAILABILITY (Rx)

Lyophilized Powder for Injection: 200 mg/vial. **Tablets:** 200 mg.

ADMINISTRATION/HANDLING

 IV

• Vials contain no preservatives or bacteriostatic agents. • Must reconstitute with Sterile Water for Injection and subsequently dilute with 0.9% NaCl only. • Do not inject as IV push or bolus.
Reconstitution • Reconstitute vial with 4 mL of Sterile Water for Injection. • To avoid foaming, alternate between gentle swirling and inversion until powder is completely dissolved. If foaming occurs, let vial stand until foam dispersed. • Visually inspect for particulate matter or discoloration. Do not use if particulate matter is observed. • Withdraw 4 mL of solution with vial in upright position; do not invert vial during draw-up. • Further dilute in 250 mL 0.9% NaCl. • Gently invert bag to mix; do not shake.
Rate of Administration • Infuse over 1 hr via dedicated line.
Storage • Reconstituted solution should appear clear, colorless to yellow. • Administer within 24 hrs of reconstitution. • May refrigerate or store solution at room temperature up to 24 hrs.

PO
• Give without regard to meal.

IV INCOMPATIBILITIES

Any solutions containing divalent cations (e.g., Ca^{2+}, Mg^{2+}), lactated Ringer's injection. Do not infuse with other medications.

INDICATIONS/ROUTES/DOSAGE

Acute Bacterial Skin and Skin Structure Infection
PO/IV: ADULTS, ELDERLY: 200 mg once daily for 6 days.

Dosage in Renal/Hepatic Impairment
No dose adjustment.

SIDE EFFECTS

Occasional (8%–3%): Nausea, headache, diarrhea, vomiting. **Rare (2%):** Dizziness, dermatitis, insomnia.

ADVERSE EFFECTS/TOXIC REACTIONS

Safety and efficacy in pts with neutropenia not established. Antibacterial activity may be reduced in the absence of granulocytes. *C. difficile*–associated diarrhea with severity ranging from mild diarrhea to fatal colitis has been reported for up to 2 mos following administration. Treatment in the absence of proven or strongly suspected bacterial infection may increase risk of drug-resistant bacteria. Infusion/hypersensitivity reactions (pruritus, urticaria, flushing, hypertension, palpitations, tachycardia), optic disorders (asthenopia, blurry vision, neuropathy, visual impairment, vitreous floaters), neurologic disorders (hypoesthesia, paresthesia, peripheral neuropathy, cranial nerve VII paralysis), infections (oral candidiasis, vulvovaginal mycotic infection) occur rarely.

NURSING CONSIDERATIONS

BASELINE ASSESSMENT

Obtain baseline CBC (note WBC, bands), wound culture/sensitivity, vital signs. Question history of recent *C. difficile* infection, hypersensitivity reaction. Assess skin wound characteristics; hydration status. Question pt's usual stool characteristics (color, frequency, consistency).

INTERVENTION/EVALUATION

Monitor skin infection/wound for improvement. Monitor daily pattern of

T

bowel activity, stool consistency; increasing severity may indicate antibiotic-associated colitis. If frequent diarrhea occurs, obtain *C. difficile* toxin screen and initiate isolation precautions until result confirmed. Encourage PO intake. Monitor I&O. Monitor for infusion-related/hypersensitivity reaction.

PATIENT/FAMILY TEACHING

• It is essential to complete drug therapy despite symptom improvement. Early discontinuation may result in antibacterial resistance or an increased risk of recurrent infection. • Report episodes of diarrhea, esp. following wks after treatment completion. Frequent abdominal pain, blood-streaked stool, diarrhea, fever, may indicate infectious diarrhea, which may be contagious. • Drink plenty of fluids.

---

teduglutide

te-due-**gloo**-tide
(Gattex)
Do not confuse teduglutide with liraglutide or albiglutide, or Gattex with Gas-X.

◆CLASSIFICATION

PHARMACOTHERAPEUTIC: Human glucagon-like peptide-2. **CLINICAL:** Short bowel syndrome (short gut syndrome, short gut) agent.

USES

Treatment of adults with short bowel syndrome (SBS) who are dependent on parenteral support.

PRECAUTIONS

Contraindications: Hypersensitivity to teduglutide. **Cautions:** Cardiovascular disease, HF, pts at increased risk for malignancy, biliary tract (gallbladder, pancreatic) disease, hypervolemia, stenosis, renal impairment.

ACTION

Analogue of naturally occurring peptide secreted by L cells of distal intestine, known to increase intestinal, portal blood flow, and inhibit gastric secretion. **Therapeutic Effect:** Improves intestinal absorption.

PHARMACOKINETICS

Degrades into small peptides, amino acids via catabolic pathway. Primarily excreted in urine. Bioavailability: 86–89% following SQ injection. Peak plasma concentration: 3–5 hrs. **Half-life:** 1.3–2 hrs.

⧗ LIFESPAN CONSIDERATIONS

Pregnancy/Lactation: Unknown if distributed in breast milk. **Children:** Safety and efficacy not established. **Elderly:** No age-related precautions noted.

INTERACTIONS

DRUG: May increase absorption of any **concomitant oral medication.** **HERBAL:** None significant. **FOOD:** None known. **LAB VALUES:** None significant.

AVAILABILITY (Rx)

Injection, Powder for Reconstitution: 5 mg (delivers maximum of 0.38 mL containing 3.8 mg teduglutide).

ADMINISTRATION/HANDLING

Subcutaneous
Reconstitution • If diluent syringe (contains 0.5 mL Sterile Water for Injection) has a white snap-off cap, snap or twist off white cap. • If diluent syringe has a gray screw top, unscrew top counterclockwise. • Push prefilled syringe into vial containing teduglutide. • After all diluent has gone into vial, remove syringe, needle and discard. • Allow vial to sit for 30 sec. • Gently roll vial for 15 sec (do not shake) and let stand for 2 min. • Withdraw prescribed dose, discard remaining fluid.

Administration • Insert needle subcutaneously into upper arms, outer thigh, or abdomen, and inject solution. • Do not inject into areas of active skin disease or injury such as sunburns, skin rashes, inflammation, skin infections, or active psoriasis. • Do not administer IV or intramuscularly. • Rotate injection sites.

Storage • Store kit in refrigerator. • Reconstituted solution should appear as a clear, colorless to light straw-colored liquid. • Discard if particulate is present. • Drug should be completely dissolved before solution is withdrawn from vial.

INDICATIONS/ROUTES/DOSAGE

Short Bowel Syndrome
SQ: ADULTS/ELDERLY: 0.05 mg/kg once daily.

Dosage in Moderate to Severe Renal Impairment
SQ: ADULTS/ELDERLY: CrCl less than 50 mL/min: 50% dose reduction.

Dosage in Hepatic Impairment
No dose adjustment.

SIDE EFFECTS

Frequent (30%–22%): Abdominal pain, nausea, injection site reactions. **Occasional (18%–14%):** Headache, abdominal distention, vomiting. **Rare (9%):** Flatulence, hypersensitivity, appetite disorders, sleep disturbances.

ADVERSE EFFECTS/TOXIC REACTIONS

Upper respiratory tract infection occurs in 12% of pts. Fluid overload (hypervolemia) reported in 7% of pts. Potential for hypovolemia is increased in pts with cardiovascular disease, HF. Therapy increases risk for acceleration for neoplastic growth. Cholecystitis, cholangitis, cholelithiasis, pancreatitis have been reported.

NURSING CONSIDERATIONS

BASELINE ASSESSMENT

Obtain baseline serum chemistries, LFT, lipase, amylase. Colonoscopy (or alternate imaging) with removal of polyps should be completed within 5 mos prior to initiating treatment.

INTERVENTION/EVALUATION

Follow-up colonoscopy (or alternate imaging) is recommended at the end of 1 year. If no polyp is found, subsequent colonoscopies should be done no less frequently than every 5 yrs. If a polyp is found, adherence to current polyp follow-up guidelines is recommended. Discovery of intestinal obstruction, intestinal malignancy necessitates discontinuation of treatment. Subsequent laboratory assessments, LFT are recommended every 6 mos. If clinically meaningful elevation is seen, further diagnostic workup is recommended as clinically indicated.

PATIENT/FAMILY TEACHING

• Teach proper use and administration of medication. • Be aware of need for any new supplies. • Instruct pt in preparation of medication, and observe correct administration technique. • Report yellowing of skin or eyes, dark urine, changes in stool color or consistency, severe abdominal pain, nausea, vomiting, sudden weight gain, swelling, or difficulty breathing.

telavancin

tel-a-**van**-sin
(Vibativ)

■ **BLACK BOX ALERT** ■ Pts with preexisting renal impairment (CrCl less than 50 mL/min) who are treated for hospital-acquired pneumonia may have increased mortality risk when compared to vancomycin. May cause new or worsening renal impairment. May cause fetal harm (low birth weight, limb malformations). Women of childbearing potential should have pregnancy test before treatment; avoid use during pregnancy unless benefit to pt outweighs fetal risk.

Do not confuse telavancin with dalbavancin or oritavancin; or Vibativ with Vibra-Tabs or vigabatrin.

◆CLASSIFICATION

PHARMACOTHERAPEUTIC: Lipo-glycopeptide antibacterial. **CLINICAL:** Antibiotic.

USES

Treatment of complicated skin, soft tissue infections (cSSSI) caused by gram-positive microorganisms, including methicillin-susceptible or methicillin-resistant *S. aureus*, vancomycin-susceptible *Enterococcus*. Treatment of hospital-acquired and ventilator-associated bacterial pneumonia (HABP/VABP) caused by susceptible isolates of *S. aureus*.

PRECAUTIONS

Contraindications: Prior hypersensitivity reactions to telavancin. Concomitant use of IV unfractionated heparin. **Cautions:** Renal impairment (CrCl 50 mL/min or less), concurrent therapy with other nephrotoxic medications (e.g., NSAIDs, ACE inhibitors, aminoglycosides). Avoid use in pts with history of congenital QT syndrome, known prolongation of QT interval, uncompensated HF, severe left ventricular hypertrophy, or receiving treatment with other drugs known to prolong QT interval, hypokalemia, hypomagnesemia, known vancomycin hypersensitivity.

ACTION

Inhibits bacterial cell wall synthesis by blocking polymerization and cross-linking of peptidoglycan. Disrupts membrane potential and changes cell wall permeability. **Therapeutic Effect:** Bactericidal. Antibiotic.

PHARMACOKINETICS

Not metabolized in liver; pathway unspecified. Protein binding: 90%. Primarily excreted unchanged in urine. Not removed by hemodialysis. **Half-life:** 8–9 hrs.

⏳ LIFESPAN CONSIDERATIONS

Pregnancy/Lactation: May cause fetal harm at regular dosage. Unknown if distributed in breast milk. **Children:** Safety and efficacy not established. **Elderly:** Age-related renal impairment may increase risk of nephrotoxicity; dosage adjustment recommended.

INTERACTIONS

DRUG: Telavancin may increase levels/effects of **dronedarone, nilotinib, pimozide, quiNINE, tetrabenazine, thioridazine, ziprasidone.** QT interval–prolonging medications (e.g., **amiodarone, azithromycin, ceritinib, haloperidol, moxifloxacin**) may increase risk of QT interval prolongation, cardiac arrhythmias. **HERBAL:** None significant. **FOOD:** None known. **LAB VALUES:** May alter serum potassium. May increase serum bilirubin, ALT, AST, BUN, creatinine; PT, aPTT, INR. May decrease Hgb, Hct, WBC count.

AVAILABILITY (Rx)

Injection, Powder for Reconstitution: 250 mg, 750 mg.

ADMINISTRATION/HANDLING
💉 IV

◀**ALERT**▶ Give by intermittent IV infusion (piggyback). Do not give by IV push (may result in hypotension).

Reconstitution • Reconstitute with 45 mL Sterile Water for Injection, D_5W, or 0.9% NaCl to provide concentration of 15 mg/mL (total volume approximately 50 mL). • Prior to administration, further dilute with D_5W or 0.9% NaCl to final concentration of 0.6–8 mg/mL. • Do not shake.

Rate of Administration • Infuse over at least 60 min. Flush line with D₅W or 0.9% NaCl before and after administration.

Storage • Discard if particulate is present. • Following reconstitution, drug is stable for 4 hrs at room temperature or 72 hrs if refrigerated in vial or infusion bag.

▧ IV INCOMPATIBILITIES

Amphotericin, colistimethate, levoFLOXacin (Levaquin), micafungin (Mycomine).

▧ IV COMPATIBILITIES

Azithromycin, caspofungin, cefepime, cefTAZidime, cefTRIAXone, ciprofloxacin, doripenem, doxycycline, gentamicin, ertapenem, fluconazole, meropenem, tobramycin, pantoprazole, piperacillin-tazobactam, tigecycline.

INDICATIONS/ROUTES/DOSAGE

Usual Parenteral Dosage
IV Infusion: ADULTS, ELDERLY: 10 mg/kg once every 24 hrs for 7–14 days (cSSSI); 14–21 days (HABP/VABP). Duration based on severity, infection site, and clinical progress of pt.

Dosage in Renal Impairment

Creatinine Clearance	Dosage
50 mL/min or greater	10 mg/kg every 24 hrs
30–49 mL/min	7.5 mg/kg every 24 hrs
10–29 mL/min	10 mg/kg every 48 hrs
Less than 10 mL/min	No dose adjustment (not studied)

Dosage in Hepatic Impairment
No dose adjustment (unless concomitant renal impairment).

SIDE EFFECTS

Frequent (33%–27%): Altered taste, nausea. **Occasional (14%–6%):** Vomiting, foamy urine, diarrhea, dizziness, pruritus. **Rare (4%–2%):** Rigors, rash, infusion site pain, anorexia, infusion site erythema.

ADVERSE EFFECTS/TOXIC REACTIONS

Nephrotoxicity (acute kidney injury, acute tubular necrosis, renal failure), diarrhea due to *C. difficile* may occur. "Red-man syndrome" (characterized by erythema on face, neck, upper torso), tachycardia, hypotension, myalgia, angioedema may occur from too-rapid rate of infusion. May cause QT interval prolongation.

NURSING CONSIDERATIONS

BASELINE ASSESSMENT

Obtain pregnancy test prior to treatment. Obtain baseline serum BUN, creatinine, creatinine clearance prior to initiating therapy, every 48–72 hrs, and after treatment is completed. Obtain culture and sensitivity tests before giving first dose (therapy may begin before results are known). Question history of renal impairment, long QT interval syndrome, HF.

INTERVENTION/EVALUATION

Monitor renal function tests, I&O. Assess skin for rash. Avoid rapid infusion ("red-man syndrome"). Monitor daily pattern of bowel activity, stool consistency. Obtain *C. difficile* PCR test if diarrhea occurs. Monitor ECG for QT interval prolongation, cardiac arrhythmias.

PATIENT/FAMILY TEACHING

• Use effective contraception during treatment. • Report rash, signs/symptoms of nephrotoxicity, diarrhea. • Blood levels will be monitored routinely. • Report chest pain, irregular heart rhythm, palpitations, passing out.

T

---

telmisartan

tel-mi-**sar**-tan
(Micardis ♣, Apo-Telmisartan ♣)
■ **BLACK BOX ALERT** ■ May cause fetal injury, mortality. Discontinue as soon as possible once pregnancy is detected.

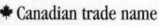 ♣ Canadian trade name   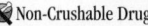 Non-Crushable Drug   ⊞ᴴᴵᴳᴴ High Alert drug

FIXED-COMBINATION(S)

Micardis HCT: telmisartan/hydro-CHLOROthiazide (a diuretic): 40 mg/12.5 mg, 80 mg/12.5 mg. **Twynsta:** telmisartan/amLODIPine (a calcium channel blocker): 40 mg/5 mg, 40 mg/10 mg, 80 mg/5 mg, 80 mg/10 mg.

♦CLASSIFICATION

PHARMACOTHERAPEUTIC: Angiotensin II receptor antagonist. **CLINICAL:** Antihypertensive.

USES

Treatment of hypertension alone or in combination with other antihypertensives. Reduces cardiovascular risk in pts 55 yrs of age and older unable to take ACE inhibitors and at high risk of major cardiovascular event (e.g., MI, stroke).

PRECAUTIONS

Contraindications: Hypersensitivity to telmisartan. Concurrent use with aliskiren in pts with diabetes. **Cautions:** Hypovolemia, hyperkalemia, hepatic/renal impairment, renal artery stenosis (unilateral, bilateral), biliary obstructive disease, significant aortic/mitral stenosis. Concurrent use with ramipril not recommended. Avoid potassium supplements.

ACTION

Blocks vasoconstrictor and aldosterone-secreting effects of angiotensin II, inhibiting binding of angiotensin II to AT_1 receptors. **Therapeutic Effect:** Causes vasodilation, decreases peripheral resistance, decreases B/P.

PHARMACOKINETICS

Route	Onset	Peak	Duration
PO (reduce B/P)	1–2 hrs	—	24 hrs

Rapidly, completely absorbed. Protein binding: greater than 99%. Metabolized in liver. Excreted in feces. Unknown if removed by hemodialysis. **Half-life:** 24 hrs.

⌛ LIFESPAN CONSIDERATIONS

Pregnancy/Lactation: May cause fetal harm. Unknown if drug is distributed in breast milk. **Children:** Safety and efficacy not established. **Elderly:** No age-related precautions noted.

INTERACTIONS

DRUG: NSAIDs (e.g., **ibuprofen, ketorolac, naproxen**) may decrease antihypertensive effect. May increase **digoxin** concentration, risk of toxicity. **HERBAL: Ephedra, ginger, licorice, ginseng, yohimbe** may worsen hypertension. **Black cohosh, periwinkle** may increase antihypertensive effect. **FOOD:** None known. **LAB VALUES:** May increase serum BUN, creatinine, uric acid, cholesterol. May decrease Hgb, Hct.

AVAILABILITY (Rx)

Tablets: 20 mg, 40 mg, 80 mg.

ADMINISTRATION/HANDLING

PO
• Give without regard to meals.

INDICATIONS/ROUTES/DOSAGE

Hypertension
PO: ADULTS, ELDERLY: Initially, 40 mg once daily. Usual range: 40–80 mg/day.

Cardiovascular Risk Reduction
PO: ADULTS, ELDERLY: 80 mg once daily.

Dosage in Renal Impairment
No dose adjustment.

Dosage in Hepatic Impairment
Use with caution.

SIDE EFFECTS

Occasional (7%–3%): Upper respiratory tract infection, sinusitis, back/leg pain, diarrhea. **Rare (1%):** Dizziness, headache, fatigue, nausea, heartburn, myalgia, cough, peripheral edema.

T

ADVERSE EFFECTS/TOXIC REACTIONS

Overdosage may manifest as hypotension, tachycardia; bradycardia occurs less often.

NURSING CONSIDERATIONS

BASELINE ASSESSMENT

Obtain B/P, apical pulse immediately before each dose, in addition to regular monitoring (be alert to fluctuations). If excessive reduction in B/P occurs, place pt in supine position, feet slightly elevated. Assess medication history (esp. diuretics). Question for history of hepatic/renal impairment, renal artery stenosis. Obtain serum BUN, creatinine, Hgb, Hct, vital signs (particularly B/P, pulse rate).

INTERVENTION/EVALUATION

Monitor B/P, pulse, serum electrolytes, renal function. Monitor for hypotension when initiating therapy.

PATIENT/FAMILY TEACHING

• Avoid tasks that require alertness, motor skills until response to drug is established (possible dizziness effect). • Maintain proper hydration. • Avoid pregnancy. • Immediately report suspected pregnancy. • Report any sign of infection (sore throat, fever). • Avoid excessive exertion during hot weather (risk of dehydration, hypotension).

telotristat ethyl

tel-**oh**-tri-state **eth**-il
(Xermelo)
Do not confuse telotristat with Triostat, or Xermelo with Xarelto.

◆CLASSIFICATION

PHARMACOTHERAPEUTIC: Tryptophan hydroxylase inhibitor. **CLINICAL:** GI agent.

USES

Treatment of carcinoid syndrome diarrhea in combination with somatostatin analog (SSA) therapy in adults with symptoms inadequately controlled by SSA therapy.

PRECAUTIONS

Contraindications: Hypersensitivity to telotristat, telotristat ethyl. **Cautions:** Pts with advanced carcinoid tumors may be at risk for altered structural integrity of the GI wall. Conditions that may impair integrity of GI wall (e.g., Crohn's disease, diverticulitis, GI tract malignancies, intestinal adhesions, Ogilvie's syndrome, peptic ulcers, peritoneal malignancies).

ACTION

Inhibits enzyme tryptophan hydroxylase (TPH). TPH converts tryptophan to 5-hydroxytryptophan, and then to serotonin, reducing overproduction and biosynthesis of peripheral serotonin. **Therapeutic Effect:** Reduces frequency of carcinoid syndrome diarrhea.

PHARMACOKINETICS

Does not cross blood-brain barrier Undergoes hydrolysis via carboxylesterases to active metabolite telotristat. Protein binding: greater than 99%. Peak plasma concentration: 1-3 hrs (telotristat). Excreted in feces (93%), urine (less than 1%). **Half-life:** 5 hrs (telotristat).

⌛ LIFESPAN CONSIDERATIONS

Pregnancy/Lactation: Unknown if crosses placenta or distributed in breastmilk. May increase risk of constipation in nursing infants. **Children:** Safety and efficacy not established. **Elderly:** No age-related precautions noted.

INTERACTIONS

DRUG: Octreotide may decrease concentration/effect (gived short acting octreotide at least 30 min after telotristat ethyl). **HERBAL:** None significant. **FOOD:** High-fat meals increases drug exposure. **LAB VALUES:** May increase alkaline phosphatase, ALT, AST, GGT.

T

AVAILABILITY (Rx)

Tablets: 250 mg.

ADMINISTRATION/HANDLING

PO

• Give with food. • If applicable, give short-acting octreotide at least 30 mins after telotristat ethyl. • If a dose is missed, do not give extra dose. Administer next dose at regularly scheduled time.

INDICATIONS/ROUTES/DOSAGE

Carcinoid Syndrome Diarrhea
PO: ADULTS, ELDERLY: 250 mg 3 times/day.

Dosage in Renal Impairment
Creatinine clearance greater that 20 mL/min: No dose adjustment. **ESRD requiring hemodialysis:** Not studied; use caution.

Dosage in Hepatic Impairment
Mild impairment: No dose adjustment. **Moderate to severe impairment:** Not studied; use caution.

SIDE EFFECTS

Occasional (13%–5%): Nausea, headache, peripheral edema, flatulence, decreased appetite, pyrexia, abdominal pain, abdominal distension, constipation.

ADVERSE EFFECTS/TOXIC REACTIONS

Severe constipation resulting in GI perforation, bowel obstruction may occur. Depression reported in 9% of pts.

NURSING CONSIDERATIONS

BASELINE ASSESSMENT

Question characteristics of diarrhea, frequency of bowel movements. Assess bowel sounds. Question history of GI obstruction, GI perforation, baseline GI disease. Assess hydration status.

INTERVENTION/EVALUATION

Assess bowel sounds. Monitor for severe, persistent, or worsening of abdominal pain. Discontinue if severe constipation, severe abdominal pain, GI perforation, bowel obstruction occurs. Monitor daily pattern of bowel activity, stool consistency.

PATIENT/FAMILY TEACHING

• Take with food. • Immediately report severe, persistent abdominal pain; abdominal distension, fever, nausea, vomiting; may indicate tear or blockage in GI tract. • Report severe constipation. • Do not breastfeed. • If therapy includes somatostatin, take somatostatin at least 30 mins after dose.

---

temozolomide

tem-oh-**zoe**-loe-myde
(Temodal ✦, <u>Temodar</u>)
Do not confuse Temodar with Tambocor.

◆CLASSIFICATION

PHARMACOTHERAPEUTIC: Imidazotetrazine derivative, alkylating agent. **CLINICAL:** Antineoplastic.

USES

Treatment of adults with refractory anaplastic astrocytoma, newly diagnosed glioblastoma multiforme (concomitantly with radiotherapy, then as maintenance therapy). **OFF-LABEL:** Malignant glioma, metastatic melanoma, metastatic CNS lesions, cutaneous T-cell lymphomas, advanced neuroendocrine tumors, soft tissue sarcoma, pediatric neuroblastoma. Ewing's sarcoma (recurrent or progressive).

PRECAUTIONS

Contraindications: Hypersensitivity to temozolomide, dacarbazine. **Cautions:** Severe renal/hepatic impairment, pregnancy.

ACTION

Produces cytotoxic effect through alkylation of DNA, causing DNA double strand breaks

---

and apoptosis. **Therapeutic Effect:** Inhibits DNA replication, causing cell death.

PHARMACOKINETICS

Rapidly, completely absorbed after PO administration. Protein binding: 15%. Peak plasma concentration: 1 hr. Penetrates blood-brain barrier. Excreted in urine (38%), feces (19%). **Half-life:** 1.6–1.8 hrs.

LIFESPAN CONSIDERATIONS

Pregnancy/Lactation: May cause fetal harm. May produce malformation of external organs, soft tissue, skeleton. If possible, avoid use during pregnancy. Unknown if drug is distributed in breast milk. **Children:** Safety and efficacy not established. **Elderly:** Pts older than 70 yrs may experience higher risk of developing grade 4 neutropenia, grade 4 thrombocytopenia.

INTERACTIONS

DRUG: Medications causing blood dyscrasias (altering blood cell counts) may increase leukopenic, thrombocytopenic effects. **Valproic acid** may decrease oral clearance. **Bone marrow depressants** may increase myelosuppression. **Live virus vaccines** may potentiate virus replication, increase vaccine side effects, decrease pt's antibody response to vaccine. **HERBAL: Echinacea** may decrease effects. **FOOD:** All foods decrease rate, extent of drug absorption. **LAB VALUES:** May decrease Hgb, neutrophils, platelets, WBC count, lymphocytes.

AVAILABILITY (Rx)

Capsules: 5 mg, 20 mg, 100 mg, 140 mg, 180 mg, 250 mg. **Injection, Powder for Reconstitution:** 100 mg.

ADMINISTRATION/HANDLING

IV

• Reconstitute each 100-mg vial with 41 mL Sterile Water for Injection to provide concentration of 2.5 mg/mL. • Swirl gently; do not shake. • Do NOT further dilute. • Infuse over 90 min. • Stable for 14 hrs (includes infusion time).

PO

• Food reduces rate, extent of absorption; increases risk of nausea, vomiting. • For best results, administer at bedtime. • Give capsule whole with glass of water. Do not break, open, or crush capsules.

INDICATIONS/ROUTES/DOSAGE

Anaplastic Astrocytoma (Refractory)

IV Infusion, PO: ADULTS, ELDERLY: Initially, 150 mg/m²/day for 5 consecutive days of 28-day treatment cycle. Subsequent doses of 100–200 mg/m²/day based on platelet count, absolute neutrophil count (ANC) during previous cycle. **Maintenance:** 200 mg/m²/day for 5 days q4wks if ANC greater than 1,500 cells/mm³ and platelets more than 100,000 cells/mm³. Continue until disease progression is observed. Minimum: 100 mg/m²/day for 5 days q4wks.

Glioblastoma Multiforme

Note: *Pneumocystis carinii* pneumonia (PCP) prophylaxis required during concomitant phase and continue in pts who develop lymphocytopenia until recovery to grade 1 or less. **IV Infusion, PO: ADULTS, ELDERLY:** 75 mg/m² daily for 42 days (with focal radiotherapy) if ANC 1,500 cells/mm³ or greater, platelet count 100,000 cells/mm³ or greater, and nonhematologic toxicity grade 1 or less. **Maintenance: (begin 4 wks after concomitant phase): (Cycle 1):** 150 mg/m² once daily for 5 days followed by 23 days without treatment. **(Cycles 2–6):** May increase to 200 mg/m² once daily for 5 days followed by 23 days without treatment if ANC greater than 1,500 cells/mm³, platelets greater than 100,000 cells/mm³, and nonhematologic toxicity with previous cycle is grade 2 or less (exclude alopecia, nausea, vomiting).

Dosage in Renal/Hepatic Impairment

No dose adjustment. Use caution in severe hepatic impairment.

SIDE EFFECTS

Frequent (53%–33%): Nausea, vomiting, headache, fatigue, constipation, seizure. **Occasional (16%–10%):** Diarrhea, asthenia, fever, dizziness, peripheral edema, incoordination, insomnia. **Rare (9%–5%):** Paresthesia, drowsiness, anorexia, urinary incontinence, anxiety, pharyngitis, cough.

ADVERSE EFFECTS/TOXIC REACTIONS

Myelosuppression is characterized by neutropenia and thrombocytopenia, with elderly pts and women showing higher incidence of developing severe myelosuppression. Usually occurs within first few cycles; is not cumulative. Nadir occurs in approximately 26–28 days, with recovery within 14 days of nadir. May increase occurrence of *Pneumocystis carinii* pneumonia, myelodysplastic syndrome including myeloid leukemia, or secondary malignancies.

NURSING CONSIDERATIONS

BASELINE ASSESSMENT

Obtain baseline CBC. Before dosing, ANC must be greater than 1,500 cells/mm³ and platelet count greater than 100,000 cells/mm³. Potential for nausea, vomiting (readily controlled with antiemetic therapy). Offer emotional support.

INTERVENTION/EVALUATION

Obtain CBC on day 22 (21 days after first dose) or within 48 hrs of that day, and wkly, until ANC is greater than 1,500 cells/mm³ and platelet count is greater than 100,000 cells/mm³. Monitor for hematologic toxicity (fever, sore throat, signs of local infection, unusual bruising/bleeding from any site), symptoms of anemia (excessive fatigue, weakness).

PATIENT/FAMILY TEACHING

• To reduce nausea/vomiting, take on an empty stomach at bedtime. • Promptly report fever, sore throat, signs of local infection, unusual bruising/bleeding from any site, or difficulty breathing. • Avoid crowds, those with infection. • Do not have immunizations without physician's approval. • Avoid pregnancy.

temsirolimus

tem-sir-**oh**-li-mus
(Torisel)
Do not confuse temsirolimus with everolimus, sirolimus, or tacrolimus.

◆CLASSIFICATION

PHARMACOTHERAPEUTIC: Kinase inhibitor. **CLINICAL:** Antineoplastic.

USES

Treatment of advanced renal cell carcinoma.

PRECAUTIONS

Contraindications: Hypersensitivity to temsirolimus. Moderate-severe hepatic impairment; serum bilirubin greater than 1.5 times upper limit of normal (ULN). **Cautions:** Hypersensitivity to sirolimus, mild hepatic impairment, diabetes, hyperlipidemia. Concurrent use with other medication that may cause angioedema (e.g., ACE inhibitors).

ACTION

Prevents activation of mTOR (mammalian target of rapamycin), preventing tumor cell division. **Therapeutic Effect:** Inhibits tumor cell growth, produces tumor regression.

PHARMACOKINETICS

Metabolized in liver. Excreted primarily in feces. **Half-life:** 17 hrs.

⌛ LIFESPAN CONSIDERATIONS

Pregnancy/Lactation: May cause fetal harm. Unknown if distributed in breast milk. **Children:** Safety and efficacy not established. **Elderly:** No age-related precautions noted.

INTERACTIONS

DRUG: CYP3A4 inhibitors (e.g., clarithromycin, ketoconazole, ritonavir) may increase concentration. **CYP3A4 inducers** (e.g., **carBAMazepine, phenytoin, rifAMPin**) may decrease concentration. **FOOD: Grapefruit products** may increase plasma concentration. **HERBAL: St. John's wort** may decrease plasma concentration. **Flaxseed, garlic, ginger, ginkgo biloba, ginseng, omega-3** may increase risk of bleeding. **LAB VALUES:** May increase serum bilirubin, alkaline phosphatase, AST, creatinine, glucose, cholesterol, triglycerides. May decrease WBCs, neutrophils, Hgb, platelets, serum phosphorus, potassium.

AVAILABILITY (Rx)

Injection Solution Kit: 25 mg/mL supplied with 1.8-mL diluent vial.

ADMINISTRATION/HANDLING

 IV

Reconstitution • Inject 1.8 mL of diluent into vial. • The vial contains an overfill of 0.2 mL (30 mg/1.2 mL). • Due to the overfill, the drug concentration of resulting solution will be 10 mg/mL. • A total volume of 3 mL will be obtained, including the overfill. • Mix well by inverting the vial. Allow sufficient time for air bubbles to subside. • Mixture must be injected rapidly into 250 mL 0.9% NaCl. • Invert bag to mix; avoid excessive shaking (may cause foaming).
Rate of Administration • Administer through an in-line filter not greater than 5 microns; infuse over 30–60 min. • Final diluted infusion solution should be completed within 6 hrs from the time drug solution and diluent mixture is added to the 250 mL 0.9% NaCl.
Storage • Refrigerate kit. • Reconstituted solution appears clear to slightly turbid, colorless to yellow, and free from visible particulates. • The 10 mg/mL drug solution/diluent mixture is stable for up to 24 hrs at room temperature. • Solutions diluted for infusion (in 250 mL 0.9% NaCl) must be infused within 6 hrs of preparation.

🚫 IV INCOMPATIBILITIES

Both acids and bases degrade solution; combinations of temsirolimus with agents capable of modifying solution pH should be avoided.

INDICATIONS/ROUTES/DOSAGE

◄ALERT► Pretreat with IV diphenhydrAMINE 25–50 mg, 30 min before infusion.

Renal Cancer
IV: ADULTS/ELDERLY: 25 mg once wkly. Treatment should continue until disease progresses or unacceptable toxicity occurs.

Dose Modification
Concomitant CYP3A4 inhibitors: Consider dose of 12.5 mg/wk. **Concomitant CYP3A4 inducers:** Consider dose of 50 mg/wk.

Dosage in Renal Impairment
No dose adjustment.

Dosage in Hepatic Impairment
Mild impairment: Reduce dose to 15 mg/wk. **Moderate to severe impairment:** Contraindicated.

SIDE EFFECTS

Common (51%–32%): Asthenia, rash, mucositis, nausea, edema (facial edema, peripheral edema), anorexia. **Frequent (28%–20%):** Generalized pain, dyspnea, diarrhea, cough, fever, abdominal pain, constipation, back pain, impaired taste. **Occasional (19%–8%):** Weight loss, vomiting, pruritus, chest pain, headache, nail disorder, insomnia, nosebleed, dry skin, acne, chills, myalgia.

ADVERSE EFFECTS/TOXIC REACTIONS

UTI occurs in 15% of pts, hypersensitivity reaction in 9%, pneumonia in 8%, upper respiratory tract infection, hypertension, conjunctivitis in 7%.

T

NURSING CONSIDERATIONS

BASELINE ASSESSMENT

Question possibility of pregnancy. Obtain baseline CBC, serum chemistries, renal function, LFT routinely thereafter. Offer emotional support.

INTERVENTION/EVALUATION

Offer antiemetics to control nausea, vomiting. Monitor daily pattern of bowel frequency, stool consistency. Assess skin for evidence of rash, edema. Monitor CBC, particularly Hgb, platelets, neutrophil count; LFT, renal function tests. Monitor for shortness of breath, fatigue, hypertension. Assess oropharynx for stomatitis, mucositis.

PATIENT/FAMILY TEACHING

• Avoid crowds, those with known infection. • Avoid contact with anyone who recently received live virus vaccine. • Do not have immunizations without physician's approval (drug lowers body resistance). • Promptly report fever, unusual bruising/bleeding from any site.

---

tenecteplase **HIGH ALERT**

ten-**eck**-te-plase
(TNKase)
Do not confuse TNKase with tPA.

◆CLASSIFICATION

PHARMACOTHERAPEUTIC: Tissue plasminogen activator. **CLINICAL:** Thrombolytic.

USES

Management of ST-elevation myocardial infarction (STEMI) for lysis of thrombi to restore perfusion and reduce mortality.

PRECAUTIONS

Contraindications: Hypersensitivity to tenecteplase. Active internal bleeding, cerebral aneurysm, AV malformation, bleeding diathesis, history of CVA, intracranial or intraspinal surgery or trauma within past 2 mos, intracranial neoplasm, severe uncontrolled hypertension. **Cautions:** Recent major surgery, GI or genitourinary (GU) bleeding, trauma, acute pericarditis, subacute bacterial endocarditis, pregnancy, severe hepatic impairment, hemorrhagic ophthalmic conditions, concurrent use of anticoagulants, elderly pts, cerebrovascular disease, hemostatic defects.

ACTION

Produced by recombinant DNA that binds to fibrin and converts plasminogen to plasmin. Initiates fibrinolysis by degrading fibrin clots, fibrinogen, other plasma proteins. **Therapeutic Effect:** Exerts thrombolytic action (dissolves clots).

PHARMACOKINETICS

Extensively distributed to tissues. Completely eliminated by hepatic metabolism. **Half-life:** 90–130 min.

⧖ LIFESPAN CONSIDERATIONS

Pregnancy/Lactation: Unknown if distributed in breast milk. **Children:** Safety and efficacy not established. **Elderly:** May have increased risk of intracranial hemorrhage, stroke, major bleeding; caution advised.

INTERACTIONS

DRUG: Anticoagulants (e.g., **heparin, warfarin**), **aspirin, dipyridamole, glycoprotein IIb/IIIa inhibitors** increase risk of bleeding. **HERBAL: Cat's claw, dong quai, evening primrose, feverfew, garlic, ginkgo biloba, ginseng, red clover** may increase risk of bleeding. **FOOD:** None known. **LAB VALUES:** Decreases plasminogen, fibrinogen levels during infusion, decreasing clotting time (confirms presence of lysis). May decrease Hgb, Hct.

AVAILABILITY (Rx)

Injection, Powder for Reconstitution: 50 mg.

ADMINISTRATION/HANDLING

 IV

Reconstitution • Add 10 mL Sterile Water for Injection without preservative

---

to vial to provide concentration of 5 mg/mL. • Gently swirl until dissolved. Do not shake. • If foaming occurs, leave vial undisturbed for several min.

Rate of Administration • Administer as IV push over 5 sec.

Storage • Store at room temperature. • If possible, use immediately, but may refrigerate up to 8 hrs after reconstitution. • Appears as colorless to pale yellow solution. • Do not use if discolored or contains particulates. • Discard after 8 hrs.

⚅ IV INCOMPATIBILITIES

Do not mix with dextrose-containing solutions or any other medications.

INDICATIONS/ROUTES/DOSAGE

◀ **ALERT** ▶ Give as single IV bolus over 5 sec. Precipitate may occur when given in IV line containing dextrose. Flush line with saline before and after administration.

Acute MI
IV: ADULTS: Dosage is based on pt's weight. Treatment should be initiated as soon as possible after onset of symptoms.

Weight (kg)	(mg)	(mL)
90 or more	50	10
80–less than 90	45	9
70–less than 80	40	8
60–less than 70	35	7
Less than 60	30	6

Dosage in Renal/Hepatic Impairment
No dose adjustment.

SIDE EFFECTS

Frequent: Bleeding (minor, 21.8%; major, 4.7%).

ADVERSE EFFECTS/TOXIC REACTIONS

Internal bleeding, including intracranial, retroperitoneal, GI, GU, respiratory sites, may occur. Lysis of coronary thrombi may produce atrial or ventricular arrhythmias, stroke.

NURSING CONSIDERATIONS

BASELINE ASSESSMENT

Obtain baseline B/P, apical pulse. Record weight. Evaluate 12-lead EKG, cardiac enzymes, serum electrolytes. Assess Hgb, Hct, platelet count, thrombin time, aPTT, PT, fibrinogen level before therapy is instituted. Type and hold blood. Screen for contraindications (e.g., history of CVA, bleeding of any kind, uncontrolled hypertension).

INTERVENTION/EVALUATION

Monitor continuous EKG for arrhythmias, B/P, pulse, respirations q15min until stable, then hourly or per protocol. Check peripheral pulses, heart and lung sounds. Monitor for chest pain relief; notify physician of continuation/recurrence (note location, type, intensity). Assess for overt or occult blood in any body substance. Monitor aPTT per protocol. Maintain B/P. Avoid any trauma that might increase risk of bleeding (e.g., injections, shaving). Assess neurologic status with vital signs.

---

tenofovir

ten-**oh**-foe-veer
(Vemlidy, Viread)

■ **BLACK BOX ALERT** ■ Lactic acidosis, severe hepatomegaly with steatosis (fatty liver), including fatalities, have occurred.

FIXED-COMBINATION(S)

Atripla: tenofovir (TDF)/efavirenz/emtricitabine (antiretroviral agents): 300 mg/600 mg/200 mg. **Complera:** tenofovir (TDF)/emtricitabine/rilpivirine (antiretroviral agents): 300 mg/200 mg/25 mg. **Descovy:** tenofovir (TAF)/emtricitabine: 25 mg/200 mg. **Genvoya:** tenofovir (TAF)/elvitegravir/cobicistat/emtricitabine: 10 mg/150 mg/150 mg/200 mg. **Odefsey:** tenofovir (TAF)/emtricitabine/rilpivirine: 25 mg/200 mg/25 mg. **Stribild:** tenofovir (TDF)/elvitegravir (an integrase inhibitor)/cobicistat (a pharmacokinetic enhancer)/emtricitabine (a nucleoside

T

reverse transcriptase inhibitor): 300 mg/150 mg/150 mg/200 mg. **Truvada:** tenofovir (TDF)/emtricitabine (an antiretroviral agent): 300 mg/200 mg.

◆CLASSIFICATION

PHARMACOTHERAPEUTIC: Nucleotide analogue (reverse transcriptase inhibitor). **CLINICAL:** Antiretroviral.

USES

Viread: Treatment of HIV-1 infection in combination with at least two other antiretroviral agents. Treatment of chronic hepatitis B virus infection in pts with hepatic disease. **Vemlidy:** Treatment of chronic hepatitis B virus infection in adults with compensated hepatic disease.

PRECAUTIONS

Contraindications: Hypersensitivity to tenofovir. **Cautions:** Hepatic/renal impairment, pts at risk for hepatic disease (e.g., obesity), concurrent nephrotoxic medications, pts with low body weight, risk factors or prior history of pancreatitis, elderly pts. Pts with history of fractures or with risk factors for bone loss, osteoporosis.

ACTION

Inhibits HIV reverse transcriptase by interfering with HIV viral RNA–dependent DNA polymerase. Inhibits replication of hepatitis B virus (HBV) by inhibiting HBV polymerase. **Therapeutic Effect:** Slows HIV replication, reduces HIV RNA levels (viral load). Inhibits HBV replication.

PHARMACOKINETICS

Bioavailability in fasted pts is approximately 25%. High-fat meals increase bioavailability. Protein binding: 0.7%–7.2%. Excreted in urine. Removed by hemodialysis. **Half-life:** 17 hrs.

⧗ LIFESPAN CONSIDERATIONS

Pregnancy/Lactation: Crosses placenta and is distributed in breast milk. Complete avoidance of breastfeeding by HIV-infected women is recommended to decrease potential transmission of HIV. **Children:** Safety and efficacy not established in children younger than 2 yrs. **Elderly:** No age-related precautions noted.

INTERACTIONS

DRUG: May increase **didanosine** concentration. May decrease concentrations of **atazanavir, indinavir, lamiVUDine, lopinavir, ritonavir. HERBAL:** None significant. **FOOD: High-fat food** increases bioavailability. **LAB VALUES:** May increase serum ALT, AST, creatinine, phosphate, protein; urinary glucose. May decrease neutrophils.

AVAILABILITY (Rx)

Tablets: *(Vemlidy):* 25 mg. *(Viread):* 150 mg, 200 mg, 250 mg, 300 mg. **Oral Powder:** 40 mg per 1 g of oral powder.

ADMINISTRATION/HANDLING

PO
• (Vemlidy) Give with food. (Viread) May be given without regard to meals. • Give oral powder with soft food. Do not mix in liquid; use only the supplied dosing scoop to measure powder.

INDICATIONS/ROUTES/DOSAGE

Hepatitis B
PO: *(Vemlidy):* ADULTS, ELDERLY: 25 mg once daily with food. *(Viread):* ADULTS, ELDERLY, CHILDREN 12 YRS AND OLDER: 300 mg once daily.

HIV (in Combination with Other Antiretroviral Agents)
PO: *(Viread):* ADULTS, ELDERLY, CHILDREN 12 YRS AND OLDER (WEIGHT 35 KG OR GREATER): 300 mg once daily. CHILDREN 2 YRS AND OLDER (WEIGHT LESS THAN 35 KG): 8 mg/kg/dose once daily. **Maximum:** 300 mg/day.

Dosage in Renal Impairment

Creatinine Clearance	Dosage
30–49 mL/min	300 mg q48h
10–29 mL/min	300 mg q72–96h
Hemodialysis	300 mg q7days or after approximately 12 hrs of dialysis

Dosage in Hepatic Impairment
No dose adjustment.

SIDE EFFECTS

Occasional: GI disturbances (diarrhea, flatulence, nausea, vomiting).

ADVERSE EFFECTS/TOXIC REACTIONS

Lactic acidosis, hepatomegaly with steatosis (excess fat in liver) occur rarely; may be severe.

NURSING CONSIDERATIONS

BASELINE ASSESSMENT

Obtain baseline laboratory testing, esp. serum renal function, triglycerides, LFT and at periodic intervals during therapy.

INTERVENTION/EVALUATION

Closely monitor for evidence of GI discomfort. Monitor daily pattern of bowel activity, stool consistency. Monitor CBC, reticulocyte count, serum renal function, LFT, CD4 cell count, HIV, RNA plasma levels, bone density.

PATIENT/FAMILY TEACHING

• Continue therapy for full length of treatment. • Tenofovir is not a cure for HIV infection, nor does it reduce risk of transmission to others. • Take with a high-fat meal (increases absorption). • Report persistent abdominal pain, nausea, vomiting.

terbutaline

ter-**bue**-ta-leen
(Bricanyl ✤)

■ **BLACK BOX ALERT** ■ Should not be used for prolonged tocolysis (longer than 48–72 hrs).
Do not confuse terbutaline with terbinafine.

◆CLASSIFICATION

PHARMACOTHERAPEUTIC: Beta₂-adrenergic agonist. **CLINICAL:** Bronchodilator, premature labor inhibitor.

USES

Symptomatic relief of reversible bronchospasm due to bronchial asthma, bronchitis, emphysema. **OFF-LABEL:** Delays premature labor in pregnancies between 20 and 34 wks.

PRECAUTIONS

Contraindications: Hypersensitivity to terbutaline. Cardiac arrhythmias associated with tachycardia, tachycardia caused by digoxin toxicity.**(Additional)Injection:** Prolonged prevention or management of preterm labor. **Oral:** Prevention or treatment of preterm labor. **Cautions:** Cardiac impairment, diabetes, glaucoma, hypertension, hyperthyroidism, history of seizures.

ACTION

Stimulates beta₂-adrenergic receptors, resulting in relaxation of uterine, bronchial smooth muscle. **Therapeutic Effect:** Inhibits uterine contractions. Relieves bronchospasm, reduces airway resistance.

PHARMACOKINETICS

Partially absorbed in GI tract following PO administration. Protein binding: 14%–25%. Metabolized in liver. Excreted in urine (30%–50%), feces (unspecified). **Half-life:** 11–16 hrs.

⌛ LIFESPAN CONSIDERATIONS

Pregnancy/Lactation: Crosses placenta; distributed in breast milk. **Children:** Safety and efficacy not established in pts younger than 6 yrs. **Elderly:** Increased risk of tremors, tachycardia due to sympathomimetic sensitivity.

INTERACTIONS

DRUG: May decrease effects of **beta blockers (e.g., labetolol, metoprolol). Digoxin, sympathomimetics (e.g., dopamine, norepinephrine)** may increase risk of arrhythmias. **MAOIs (e.g., phenelzine, selegiline)** may increase risk of hypertensive crisis. **Tricyclic antidepressants (e.g., amitriptyline, nortriptyline)** may increase cardiovascular effects. **HERBAL: Ephedra, yohimbe** may cause

T

CNS stimulation. **FOOD:** None known. **LAB VALUES:** May decrease serum potassium. May increase serum glucose.

AVAILABILITY (Rx)

Injection Solution: 1 mg/mL. **Tablets:** 2.5 mg, 5 mg.

ADMINISTRATION/HANDLING

 IV

• May administer undiluted, direct IV over 5–10 min or continuous infusion diluted in D$_5$W or 0.9% NaCl.

SQ

• Do not use if solution appears discolored. • Inject subcutaneously into lateral deltoid region.

PO

• Give without regard to food (give with food if GI upset occurs). • Tablets may be crushed.

INDICATIONS/ROUTES/DOSAGE

Bronchospasm
PO: ADULTS, ELDERLY, CHILDREN 15 YRS AND OLDER: Initially, 5 mg 3 times/day. **Maintenance:** 2.5–5 mg 3 times/day q6h while awake. **Maximum:** 15 mg/day. **CHILDREN 12–14 YRS:** 2.5 mg 3 times/day. **Maximum:** 7.5 mg/day. **CHILDREN YOUNGER THAN 12 YRS:** Initially, 0.05 mg/kg/dose q8h. May increase up to 0.15 mg/kg/dose. **Maximum:** 5 mg/24 hr.
SQ: ADULTS, CHILDREN 12 YRS AND OLDER: Initially, 0.25 mg. Repeat in 15–30 min for 3 doses. Total dose of 0.75 mg should not be exceeded. **CHILDREN YOUNGER THAN 12 YRS:** 0.01 mg/kg/dose q15–20min for 3 doses. May repeat q2–6h as needed.

Preterm Labor
◀ **ALERT** ▶ IV form should be used with caution in pregnancy; do not administer for longer than 48–72 hrs.
IV: ADULTS: Acute: 2.5–10 mcg/min. May increase gradually q15–20min up to 17.5–30 mcg/min. **SQ:** 0.25 mg q20min–3 hrs.

Dosage in Renal/Hepatic Impairment
No dose adjustment.

SIDE EFFECTS

Frequent (38%–23%): Tremor, anxiety. **Occasional (11%–10%):** Drowsiness, headache, nausea, heartburn, dizziness. **Rare (3%–1%):** Flushing, asthenia, oropharyngeal dryness, irritation (with inhalation therapy).

ADVERSE EFFECTS/TOXIC REACTIONS

Too-frequent or excessive use may lead to decreased drug effectiveness and/or severe, paradoxical bronchoconstriction. Excessive sympathomimetic stimulation may cause palpitations, extrasystoles, tachycardia, chest pain, slight increase in B/P followed by a substantial decrease, chills, diaphoresis, skin blanching.

NURSING CONSIDERATIONS

BASELINE ASSESSMENT

Bronchospasm: Offer emotional support (high incidence of anxiety due to difficulty in breathing, sympathomimetic response to drug). **Preterm labor:** Assess baseline maternal pulse, B/P, frequency and duration of contractions, fetal heart rate. Question history of cardiac arrhythmias, narrow-angle glaucoma, hypertension, seizures.

INTERVENTION/EVALUATION

Bronchospasm: Monitor rate, depth, rhythm, type of respiration; quality, rate of pulse. Assess lung sounds for rhonchi, wheezing, rales. Monitor ABGs. Observe lips, fingernails for cyanosis. Observe for clavicular retractions, hand tremor. Evaluate for clinical improvement (quieter, slower respirations, relaxed facial expression, cessation of clavicular retractions). **Preterm labor:** Monitor for frequency, duration, strength of contractions. Diligently monitor maternal and fetal heart rate.

PATIENT/FAMILY TEACHING
* Report persistent palpitations, chest pain, muscle tremor, dizziness, headache, flushing, breathing difficulties. * May cause nervousness, anxiety, shakiness. * Avoid excessive use of caffeine derivatives (chocolate, coffee, tea, cola, cocoa).

---

teriflunomide

ter-i-**floo**-noe-myde
(Aubagio)
Do not confuse teriflunomide with leflunomide.

■ **BLACK BOX ALERT** ■ May result in major birth defects. Pregnancy must be excluded before initiating therapy and must be avoided during treatment or prior to completion of an accelerated elimination procedure. Severe hepatic injury may occur. Do not initiate with acute/chronic liver disease or serum ALT greater than 2 times upper limit of normal.

◆CLASSIFICATION

PHARMACOTHERAPEUTIC: Pyrimidine synthesis inhibitor, immunomodulatory agent. **CLINICAL:** Multiple sclerosis agent.

USES

Treatment of relapsing forms of multiple sclerosis.

PRECAUTIONS

Contraindications: Hypersensitivity to teriflunomide. Pregnant women or women of childbearing potential who are not using reliable contraception, severe hepatic impairment, concurrent use of leflunomide. **Cautions:** Concomitant neurotoxic medications, diabetes, pulmonary disease, severe immunodeficiency or bone marrow dysplasia, history of significant hematologic abnormalities, uncontrolled infection, history of new/recurrent infections, pts older than 60 yrs.

ACTION

Inhibits pyrimidine synthesis, exhibiting anti-inflammatory and antiproliferative properties. **Therapeutic Effect:** May slow progression of multiple sclerosis.

PHARMACOKINETICS

Well absorbed following PO administration. Peak concentration: 1–4 hrs. Protein binding: greater than 99%. Metabolized by hydrolysis. Excreted in urine (23%), feces (38%). **Half-life:** 18–19 days.

⧖ LIFESPAN CONSIDERATIONS

Pregnancy/Lactation: May produce embryo-fetal toxicity. Pregnancy contraindicated. Avoid breastfeeding. Detected in human semen. **Children:** Safety and efficacy not established in pts younger than 18 yrs. **Elderly:** No age-related precautions noted.

INTERACTIONS

DRUG: May increase concentration/effects of **CYP2C8 substrates (e.g., repaglinide, PACLitaxel, pioglitazone, or rosiglitazone), oral contraceptives.** May decrease concentration/effects of **warfarin, CYP1A2 substrates (e.g., DULoxetine, tiZANidine). HERBAL:** None significant. **FOOD:** None known. **LAB VALUES:** May increase serum potassium, ALT, AST, alkaline phosphatase, bilirubin. May decrease WBCs, neutrophil count.

AVAILABILITY (Rx)

Tablets: 7 mg, 14 mg.

ADMINISTRATION/HANDLING

PO
* Give without regard to food.

INDICATIONS/ROUTES/DOSAGE

Multiple Sclerosis
PO: ADULTS, ELDERLY: 7 mg or 14 mg once daily.

Adjustment of Toxicity
ALT elevation greater than 3 times ULN: Discontinue teriflunomide and initiate drug elimination procedures: cholestyramine

T

---

8 g q8h for 11 days (if not tolerated, may decrease to 4 g q8h) or activated charcoal 50 g q12h for 11 days. **Note:** The 11 days do not need to be consecutive unless plasma concentration needs to be lowered rapidly.

Dosage in Renal Impairment
No dose adjustment.

Dosage in Hepatic Impairment
Mild to moderate impairment: No dose adjustment. **Severe impairment:** Contraindicated.

SIDE EFFECTS

Frequent (19%–6%): Headache, diarrhea, nausea, alopecia, paresthesia, upper abdominal pain. **Occasional (4%–3%):** Hypertension, oral herpes, anxiety, hypertension, toothache, musculoskeletal pain. **Rare (2%–1%):** Seasonal allergy, sciatica, burning sensation, carpal tunnel syndrome, blurred vision, acne, pruritus, myalgia, abdominal distention, conjunctivitis.

ADVERSE EFFECTS/TOXIC REACTIONS

Influenza occurs in 12% of pts, upper respiratory infection with sinusitis, bronchitis in 9%. Cystitis, sinusitis, viral gastroenteritis may occur. Neutropenia, leukopenia occur rarely.

NURSING CONSIDERATIONS

BASELINE ASSESSMENT

Because of high potential for birth defects/fetal death, female pts must avoid pregnancy. Obtain baseline PPD for latent TB. Obtain CBC, hepatic function test results prior to treatment and monthly for 6 mos thereafter. Obtain baseline pregnancy test. Assess baseline symptoms of MS (e.g., bladder/bowel dysfunction, cognitive impairment, depression, dysphagia, fatigue, gait disorder, numbness/tingling, pain, seizures, spasticity, tremors, weakness).

INTERVENTION/EVALUATION

Monitor for signs/symptoms of infection. Treatment should not be initiated if pt has active infection; discontinuation of treatment must be considered. If drug-induced hepatic impairment, peripheral neuropathy, severe skin reaction occur, discontinue medication, begin accelerated elimination procedure (cholestyramine or charcoal for 11 days). Monitor for symptom improvement of MS.

PATIENT/FAMILY TEACHING

• Women of childbearing potential must be counseled regarding fetal risk, use of reliable contraceptives confirmed, possibility of pregnancy excluded. • May take without regard to food. • Report symptoms of infection such as body aches, chills, cough, fatigue, fever.

teriparatide

ter-i-**par**-a-tide
(Forteo)
■ **BLACK BOX ALERT** ■ Increased risk of osteosarcoma; risk dependent on dose and duration.

◆CLASSIFICATION

PHARMACOTHERAPEUTIC: Parathyroid hormone. **CLINICAL:** Osteoporosis agent.

USES

Treatment of postmenopausal women with osteoporosis who are at increased risk for fractures. Treatment of men with primary or hypogonadal osteoporosis who are at high risk for fractures. High-risk pts include those with a history of osteoporotic fractures, who have failed previous osteoporosis therapy, or were intolerant of previous osteoporosis therapy. Treatment of glucocorticoid-induced osteoporosis in men and women.

PRECAUTIONS

Contraindications: Hypersensitivity to teriparatide. **Cautions:** Conditions that increase risk of osteosarcoma (e.g., Paget's disease, unexplained elevations of alkaline phosphatase level, children or young adults with open epiphyses, prior skeletal radiation therapy, implant therapy), hypercalcemia, hypercalcemic disorders (e.g., hyperparathyroidism), bone metastases, history of skeletal malignancies, metabolic bone diseases other than osteoporosis, cardiac disease, renal/hepatic impairment, pts at risk for orthostasis, active or recent urolithiasis.

ACTION

Stimulates osteoblast function. Increases calcium absorption from GI tract/renal tubular reabsorption. **Therapeutic Effect:** Increases bone mineral density, bone mass/strength, reduces osteoporosis-related fractures.

PHARMACOKINETICS

Extensively absorbed following SQ injection. Metabolized in liver. Excreted in urine. **Half-life:** 1 hr.

⌛ LIFESPAN CONSIDERATIONS

Pregnancy/Lactation: Unknown if drug crosses placenta or is distributed in breast milk. **Children:** Safety and efficacy not established. **Elderly:** No age-related precautions noted.

INTERACTIONS

DRUG: None significant. **HERBAL:** None significant. **FOOD:** None known. **LAB VALUES:** May increase serum calcium (transient), uric acid.

AVAILABILITY (Rx)

Injection Solution: 600 mcg/2.4 mL (injector pen containing 28 daily doses of 20 mcg).

ADMINISTRATION/HANDLING

Subcutaneous

• Refrigerate, but minimize time out of refrigerator. Do not freeze; discard if frozen. • Administer into thigh, abdominal wall.

INDICATIONS/ROUTES/DOSAGE

Osteoporosis

SQ: ADULTS, ELDERLY: 20 mcg once daily into thigh, abdominal wall.

Dosage in Renal/Hepatic Impairment
No dose adjustment.

SIDE EFFECTS

Occasional: Leg cramps, nausea, dizziness, headache, orthostatic hypotension, tachycardia.

ADVERSE EFFECTS/TOXIC REACTIONS

Angina pectoris has been reported.

NURSING CONSIDERATIONS

BASELINE ASSESSMENT

Obtain urinary, serum calcium, ionized calcium levels, serum parathyroid hormone levels, bone mineral density.

INTERVENTION/EVALUATION

Monitor bone mineral density, urinary/serum calcium levels, serum parathyroid hormone levels. Observe for symptoms of hypercalcemia. Monitor B/P for hypotension, pulse for tachycardia. Question medical history as listed in Precautions.

PATIENT/FAMILY TEACHING

• Go from lying to standing slowly.
• Report persistent symptoms of hypercalcemia (nausea, vomiting, constipation, lethargy, asthenia).

---

testosterone

tes-**tos**-te-rone
(Andriol ✹, Androderm, <u>AndroGel Pump</u>, Aveed, Axiron, Depo-Testosterone, EC-Rx Testosterone, FIRST-Testosterone, FIRST-Testosterone MC, Fortesta, Natesto, Striant, Testim, Testopel, Vogelxo Pump)

■ **BLACK BOX ALERT** ■ Virilization in children and women may occur following secondary exposure to testosterone gel. Aveed: Serious pulmonary oil microembolism reaction and anaphylaxis reported during or immediately after administration. **Do not confuse testosterone with testolactone.**

◆CLASSIFICATION

PHARMACOTHERAPEUTIC: Androgen. **CLINICAL:** Sex hormone.

USES

Androgen replacement therapy in treatment of delayed male puberty, male hypogonadism (congenital or acquired), inoperable female breast cancer pts who are 1–5 yrs postmenopausal.

PRECAUTIONS

Contraindications: Hypersensitivity to testosterone. Breastfeeding, pregnant or who may become pregnant, prostate (known or suspected) or breast cancer in males. **Depo-Testosterone (additional):** Severe cardiac/hepatic/renal disease. **Cautions:** Renal/hepatic/cardiac dysfunction, pts with history of MI or CAD; conditions influenced by edema (e.g., seizure disorder, migraines).

ACTION

Promotes growth, development of male sex organs, maintains secondary sex characteristics in androgen-deficient males. **Therapeutic Effect:** Relieves androgen deficiency.

PHARMACOKINETICS

Well absorbed after IM administration. Protein binding: 98%. Metabolized in liver. Primarily excreted in urine. Unknown if removed by hemodialysis. **Half-life:** 10–100 min.

⧗ LIFESPAN CONSIDERATIONS

Pregnancy/Lactation: Contraindicated in pregnant women, women who may become pregnant, or during lactation. **Children:** Safety and efficacy not established; use with caution. **Elderly:** May increase risk of hyperplasia, stimulate growth of occult prostate carcinoma.

INTERACTIONS

DRUG: May decrease serum glucose, requiring **insulin** adjustments. **HERBAL:** **St. John's wort** may decrease concentration/effects. **FOOD:** None known. **LAB VALUES:** May increase Hgb, Hct, LDL, serum alkaline phosphatase, bilirubin, calcium, potassium, sodium, AST. May decrease HDL.

AVAILABILITY (Rx)

Cream (First Testosterone, MC): 2%. **Cream, Transdermal (EC-Rx Testosterone):** 0.2%, 0.4%, 10%, 20%. **Ointment (First Testosterone):** 2% **Gel, Topical (AndroGel, Testim):** 1%, 1.62%. **(Vogelxo):** 50-mg packet or tube, 12.5 mg/actuation metered dose pump. **(Fortesta):** 10 mg/actuation. **Injection (Cypionate [Depo-Testosterone]):** 100 mg/mL, 200 mg/mL. **(Enanthate [Delatestryl]):** 200 mg/mL. **(Aveed [undecanoate]):** 750 mg/3 mL. **Mucoadhesive, for Buccal Application (Striant):** 30 mg. **Nasal Gel (Natesto):** 5.5 mg/actuation. **Pellet, for Subcutaneous Implantation:** 12.5 mg, 25 mg, 37.5 mg, 50 mg, 75 mg. **Solution (Metered Dose Pump [Axiron]):** 30 mg/activation. **Transdermal System (Androderm):** 2 mg/day or 4 mg/day.

ADMINISTRATION/HANDLING

IM

• Give deep in gluteal muscle. • Do not give IV. • Warming or shaking redissolves crystals that may form in long-acting preparations. • Wet needle of syringe may cause solution to become cloudy; this does not affect potency.

Buccal

(Striant): • Apply to gum area (above incisor tooth). • Hold firmly in place for 30 sec to ensure adhesion. Instruct pt to not chew or swallow. • Not affected by food, toothbrushing, gum, chewing, alcoholic beverages. • Remove before placing new system.

Transdermal

(Androderm): • Apply to clean, dry area on skin on back, abdomen, upper arms, thighs. • Do not use tape to secure. Avoid bathing, swimming for at least 3 hrs after each application. • Do not apply to bony prominences (e.g., shoulder) or oily, damaged, irritated skin. Do not apply to scrotum. • Rotate application site with 7-day interval to same site.

Transdermal Gel
(AndroGel, Testim, Vogelxo): • Apply (morning preferred) to clean, dry, intact skin of shoulder, upper arms. (AndroGel 1% may also be applied to abdomen.) • Upon opening packet(s), squeeze entire contents into palm of hand, immediately apply to application site. • Allow to dry. • Do not apply to genitals.
(Fortesta): • Apply to skin of front and inner thighs.

Topical Solution
(Axiron): • Apply using applicator to axilla at same time each morning. • Avoid washing site for 2 hrs after application.

INDICATIONS/ROUTES/DOSAGE

Male Hypogonadism
IM: ADULTS: 50–400 mg q2–4wks or 75–100 mg/wk or 150–200 mg q2wks. **(Aveed):** 750 mg at initiation, 4 wks and q10 wks thereafter. **ADOLESCENTS:** Initiation of pubertal growth: 25–75 mg q3–4wks, gradually titrate q6–9mos to 100–150 mg. Duration: 3–4yrs. **Maintenance Virilizing Dose:** 200–250 mg q3–4wks. May convert to other testosterone replacement dosages once expected adult height and adequate virilization achieved.
SQ: (Pellets): ADULTS: 150–450 mg q3–6mos.
Topical Gel: (Fortesta): 40 mg once daily in morning. Range: 10–70 mg. **(Vogelxo):** 50 mg once daily (one tube or one packet or 4 pump actuations).
Topical Solution: (Axiron): ADULTS, ELDERLY: 60 mg once daily (1 pump activation of 30 mg to each axilla). Range: 30–120 mg.
Transdermal Patch: (Androderm): ADULTS, ELDERLY: Start therapy with 4 mg/day patch applied at night. Apply patch to abdomen, back, thighs, upper arms. Dose adjustment based on testosterone levels.

TransdermalGel: **(AndroGel):ADULTS, ELDERLY: (AndroGel 1%):** Initial dose of 5 g delivers 50 mg testosterone and is applied once daily to abdomen, shoulders, upper arms. May increase to 7.5 g, then to 10 g, if necessary. **(AndroGel 1.62%):** Initial dose of 40.5 mg applied once daily in the morning to shoulder and upper arms. May increase to 81 mg. Further adjustments based on testosterone levels.
Transdermal Gel: (Testim): ADULTS, ELDERLY: Initial dose of 5 g delivers 50 mg testosterone and is applied once daily to the shoulders, upper arms. May increase to 10 g (100 mg testosterone).
Buccal: (Striant): ADULTS, ELDERLY: 30 mg q12h.
Nasal Gel: (Natesto): ADULTS ELDERLY: 11 mg (2 actuations, 1 per each nostril) 3 times/day.

Delayed Male Puberty
IM: (Cypionate or enanthate): ADOLESCENTS: 50–200 mg q2–4wks for limited duration.
SQ: (Pellets): ADULTS: 150–450 mg q3–6mos.

Breast Carcinoma
IM: (Testosterone Cypionate, Testosterone Ethanate): ADULTS: 200–400 mg q2–4wks.

Dosage in Renal/Hepatic Impairment
Use caution.

SIDE EFFECTS

Frequent: Gynecomastia, acne. **Females:** Hirsutism, amenorrhea, other menstrual irregularities; deepening of voice; clitoral enlargement (may not be reversible when drug is discontinued). **Occasional:** Edema, nausea, insomnia, oligospermia, priapism, male-pattern baldness, bladder irritability, hypercalcemia (in immobilized pts, those with breast cancer), hypercholesterolemia, inflammation/pain at IM injection site. **Transdermal:** Pruritus, erythema, skin irritation. **Rare:** Polycythemia (with high dosage), hypersensitivity.

T

ADVERSE EFFECTS/TOXIC REACTIONS

Peliosis hepatitis (presence of blood-filled cysts in parenchyma of liver), hepatic neoplasms, hepatocellular carcinoma have been associated with prolonged high-dose therapy. Anaphylactic reactions occur rarely. Venous thromboembolism (e.g., DVT, PE) reported.

NURSING CONSIDERATIONS

BASELINE ASSESSMENT

Establish baseline weight, B/P, Hgb, Hct. Check LFT, electrolytes, cholesterol. Wrist X-rays may be ordered to determine bone maturation in children. Question history of hepatic/renal impairment, seizure disorder, thromboembolism (CVA, MI, pulmonary embolism).

INTERVENTION/EVALUATION

Weigh daily, report wkly gain of more than 5 lb; evaluate for edema. Monitor I&O. Monitor B/P. Assess serum electrolytes, cholesterol, Hgb, Hct (periodically for high dosage), LFT, radiologic exam of wrist, hand (when using in prepubertal children). With breast cancer or immobility, check for hypercalcemia (lethargy, muscle weakness, confusion, irritability). Ensure adequate intake of protein, calories. Assess for virilization. Monitor sleep patterns. Monitor for CVA (aphasia, confusion, paresthesia, hemiparesis, seizures), MI (chest pain, diaphoresis, left arm/jaw pain, increased serum troponin, ST segment elevation), pulmonary embolism (chest pain, dyspnea, hypoxia, tachycardia).

PATIENT/FAMILY TEACHING

• Regular visits to physician and monitoring tests are necessary. • Do not take any other medication without consulting physician. • Maintain diet high in protein, calories. • Food may be better tolerated in small, frequent feedings. • Weigh daily; report 5 lb/wk gain. • Report nausea, vomiting, acne, pedal edema. • **Females:** Promptly report menstrual irregularities, hoarseness, deepening of voice. • **Males:** Report frequent erections, difficulty urinating, gynecomastia. • Treatment may cause arterial or venous blood clots; report symptoms of heart attack (chest pain, difficulty breathing, jaw pain, nausea, pain that radiates to the left arm, sweating), stroke (blindness, confusion, one-sided weakness, loss of consciousness, trouble speaking, seizures); DVT (swelling, pain, hot feeling in the arms or legs), lung embolism (difficulty breathing, chest pain, rapid heart rate).

tiaGABine

tye-**a**-ga-been
(Gabitril)
Do not confuse tiaGABine with tiZANidine.

◆CLASSIFICATION

PHARMACOTHERAPEUTIC: Selective GABA reuptake inhibitor. **CLINICAL:** Anticonvulsant.

USES

Adjunctive therapy for treatment of partial seizures in adults and children 12 yrs or older.

PRECAUTIONS

Contraindications: Hypersensitivity to tiaGABine. **Cautions:** Hepatic impairment. Pts at risk for suicidal behavior/thoughts.

ACTION

Enhances activity of gamma-aminobutyric acid (GABA), the major inhibitory neurotransmitter in the CNS. **Therapeutic Effect:** Inhibits seizure activity.

PHARMACOKINETICS

Rapidly absorbed from GI tract. Protein binding: 96%. Metabolized in liver. Primarily excreted in feces. **Half-life:** 2–5 hrs.

☒ LIFESPAN CONSIDERATIONS

Pregnancy/Lactation: May produce teratogenic effects. Distributed in breast milk. **Children:** Safety and efficacy not established in pts younger than 12 yrs. **Elderly:** Age-related hepatic impairment may require dosage adjustment.

INTERACTIONS

DRUG: CarBAMazepine, PHENobarbital, phenytoin may increase clearance. May alter effects of **valproic acid. HERBAL: Evening primrose** may decrease seizure threshold. **St. John's wort** may decrease concentration. **Gotu kola, kava kava, St. John's wort, valerian** may increase CNS depression. **FOOD:** None known. **LAB VALUES:** None significant.

AVAILABILITY (Rx)

Tablets: 2 mg, 4 mg, 12 mg, 16 mg.

ADMINISTRATION/HANDLING

• Give with food.

INDICATIONS/ROUTES/DOSAGE

Note: Pts not taking enzyme-inducing antiepileptic drugs (AEDs): Lower doses required and slower titration may be needed.

Partial Seizures
PO: ADULTS, ELDERLY: (Pts receiving enzyme-inducing AED regimens): Initially, 4 mg once daily. May increase by 4–8 mg/day at wkly intervals. **Maintenance:** 32–56 mg/day in 2–4 divided doses. **CHILDREN 12–18 YRS:** Initially, 4 mg once daily for 1 wk. May increase by 4 mg in 2 divided doses for 1 wk, then may increase by 4–8 mg at wkly intervals thereafter. **Maximum:** 32 mg/day in 2–4 divided doses.

Dosage in Renal Impairment
No dose adjustment.

Dosage in Hepatic Impairment
Use caution.

SIDE EFFECTS

Frequent (34%–20%): Dizziness, asthenia (loss of strength, energy), drowsiness, nervousness, confusion, headache, infection, tremor. **Occasional:** Nausea, diarrhea, abdominal pain, impaired concentration.

ADVERSE EFFECTS/TOXIC REACTIONS

Overdose characterized by agitation, confusion, hostility, weakness. Full recovery occurs within 24 hrs of discontinuation. Depression, suicidal ideation.

NURSING CONSIDERATIONS

BASELINE ASSESSMENT
Review history of seizure disorder (intensity, frequency, duration, level of consciousness). Observe frequently for recurrence of seizure activity. Initiate seizure precautions.

INTERVENTION/EVALUATION
For pts on long-term therapy, serum hepatic/renal function tests, CBC should be performed periodically. Assist with ambulation if dizziness occurs. Assess for clinical improvement (decrease in intensity, frequency of seizures). Monitor for depression, unusual behavior, suicidal ideation or thoughts.

PATIENT/FAMILY TEACHING
• Go from lying to standing slowly. • Avoid tasks that require alertness, motor skills until response to drug is established. • Avoid alcohol. • Report worsening seizure activity, thoughts of suicide, increased depression.

ticagrelor

tye-**ka**-grel-or
(Brilinta)

■ **BLACK BOX ALERT** ■ May cause significant, sometimes fatal bleeding. Do not use with active bleeding or history of intracranial bleeding. Do not initiate in pts planning urgent coronary artery bypass graft (CABG) surgery. Discontinue at least 5 days prior to any surgery. Suspect bleeding in any pt who is hypotensive and has had recent

---

percutaneous coronary intervention (PCI), CABG, or other surgical procedures. If possible, manage bleeding without discontinuing therapy to decrease risk of cardiovascular events. Aspirin maintenance doses greater than 100 mg/day may reduce effectiveness and should be strictly avoided.

◆CLASSIFICATION

PHARMACOTHERAPEUTIC: $P2Y_{12}$ platelet aggregation inhibitor. **CLINICAL:** Antiplatelet.

USES

Reduce rate of cardiovascular death, MI, stroke in pts with acute coronary syndrome (ACS) or history of MI. Reduce rate of stent thrombosis in pts who have been stented for treatment of ACS.

PRECAUTIONS

Contraindications: Hypersensitivity to ticagrelor. History of intracranial hemorrhage, active pathologic bleeding, severe hepatic impairment. **Cautions:** Moderate hepatic impairment, renal impairment, history of hyperuricemia or gouty arthritis. Pts at increased risk of bradycardia, concurrent use of strong CYP3A4 inhibitors or inducers, elderly pts. (Recommend holding dose 5 days before planned surgery if applicable.) Pts with risk factors for bleeding (e.g., trauma, peptic ulcer disease).

ACTION

Reversibly inhibits platelet $P2Y_{12}$ ADP receptor to prevent signal transduction and platelet activation. **Therapeutic Effect:** Reduces platelet aggregation.

PHARMACOKINETICS

Readily absorbed after PO administration. Protein binding: 99%. Metabolized in liver. Primarily excreted in feces (58%), urine (26%). **Half-life:** 7–9 hrs.

⧖ LIFESPAN CONSIDERATIONS

Pregnancy/Lactation: Unknown if distributed in breast milk. Must either discontinue breastfeeding or discontinue drug therapy. **Children:** Safety and efficacy not established. **Elderly:** No age-related precautions noted.

INTERACTIONS

DRUG: Aspirin greater than 100 mg/day may decrease effectiveness. **CYP3A4 inhibitors** (e.g., **clarithromycin, ketoconazole, ritonavir**) may increase concentration/effects. **CYP3A4 inducers** (e.g., **carBAMazepine, phenytoin, rifAMPin**) may decrease concentration/effects. **Anticoagulants** (e.g., **warfarin**), **antiplatelets** (e.g., **aspirin, clopidogrel**), **NSAIDs** (e.g., **ibuprofen, ketorolac, naproxen**) may increase risk of bleeding. May increase concentration of **digoxin, simvastatin, lovastatin. HERBAL: St. John's wort** may decrease effectiveness. **Fenugreek, feverfew, flaxseed, garlic, ginger, ginkgo biloba, ginseng, omega-3, red clover** with anticoagulant/antiplatelet activity may increase risk of bleeding. **FOOD: Grapefruit products** may increase potential for bleeding. **LAB VALUES:** May increase serum uric acid, creatinine.

AVAILABILITY (Rx)

Tablets: 60 mg, 90 mg.

ADMINISTRATION/HANDLING

PO
• Give without regard to meals. • May be crushed, mixed with water, and drunk immediately (refill glass with water, stir and drink contents).

INDICATIONS/ROUTES/DOSAGE

Acute Coronary Syndrome
PO: ADULTS: Initially, 180 mg once, then 90 mg twice daily. Give with aspirin 325 mg once (loading dose), then maintain with aspirin 75–100 mg daily. Continue for up to 12 mos, then decrease dose to 60 mg twice daily.

---

underlined – top prescribed drug

Dosage in Renal Impairment
No dose adjustment.

Dosage in Hepatic Impairment
Mild impairment: No dose adjustment.
Moderate impairment: Use caution.
Severe impairment: Avoid use.

SIDE EFFECTS

Occasional (13%–7%): Dyspnea, headache. **Rare (5%–3%):** Cough, dizziness, nausea, diarrhea, back pain, fatigue.

ADVERSE EFFECTS/TOXIC REACTIONS

Life-threatening events including intracranial bleeding, epistaxis, intrapericardial bleeding with cardiac tamponade, hypovolemic shock requiring vasopressive support or blood transfusion reported. Pts with history of sick sinus syndrome, second- or third-degree AV block, bradycardic syncope have increased risk of bradycardia. May induce episodes of atrial fibrillation, hypotension, hypertension. Gynecomastia reported in less than 1% of men.

NURSING CONSIDERATIONS

BASELINE ASSESSMENT

Obtain CBC, serum chemistries, renal function, LFT. Question for history of bleeding, stomach ulcers, colon polyps, head trauma, cardiac arrhythmias, unstable angina, recent MI, hepatic impairment, hypertension, stroke. Receive full medication history including herbal products. Question for history of COPD, chronic bronchitis, emphysema, asthma, exertional dyspnea.

INTERVENTION/EVALUATION

Routinely screen for bleeding. Assess skin for bruising, hematoma. Monitor renal function, uric acid, digoxin levels if applicable. Report hematuria, epistaxis, coffee-ground emesis, black/tarry stools. Monitor EKG for chest pain, shortness of breath, syncope.

PATIENT/FAMILY TEACHING

• It may take longer to stop bleeding during therapy. • Do not vigorously blow nose. • Use soft toothbrush, electric razor to decrease risk of bleeding. • Immediately report bloody stool, urine, or nosebleeds. • Report all newly prescribed medications. • Inform physician of any planned dental procedures or surgeries.

tigecycline

tye-gee-**sye**-kleen
(Tygacil)

■ **BLACK BOX ALERT** ■ An increase in all-cause mortality observed in Phase 3 and 4 clinical trials. Use is reserved when alternate treatment are not appropriate.

◆CLASSIFICATION

PHARMACOTHERAPEUTIC: Glycylcycline. **CLINICAL:** Antibiotic.

USES

Treatment of susceptible infections due to *E. coli, E. faecalis, S. aureus, S. agalactiae, S. anginosus* group (includes *S. anginosus, S. intermedius, S. constellatus*), *S. pyogenes, B. fragilis, Citrobacter freundii, E. cloacae, K. oxytoca, K. pneumoniae, B. thetaiotaomicron, B. uniformis, B. vulgatus, C. perfringens, Peptostreptococcus micros* including complicated skin/skin structure infections, complicated intra-abdominal infections, community-acquired bacterial pneumonia.

PRECAUTIONS

Contraindications: Hypersensitivity to tigecycline. **Cautions:** Hypersensitivity to tetracyclines, pregnancy, hepatic impairment, monotherapy for pts with intestinal perforation. Do not use for diabetic foot infections, healthcare (hospital)-acquired pneumonia, or ventilator-associated pneumonia.

ACTION

Inhibits protein synthesis by binding to ribosomal receptor sites of bacterial cell wall. **Therapeutic Effect:** Bacteriostatic effect.

T

PHARMACOKINETICS

Extensive tissue distribution, minimally metabolized. Excreted by biliary/fecal route (59%), urine (33%). Protein binding: 71%–89%. **Half-life:** Single dose: 27 hrs; following multiple doses: 42 hrs.

⏳ LIFESPAN CONSIDERATIONS

Pregnancy/Lactation: May cause fetal harm. May be distributed in breast milk. Permanent discoloration of the teeth (brown-gray) may occur if used during tooth development. **Children:** Safety and efficacy not established in pts younger than 8 yrs. Use is reserved for when no effective alternative is available. **Elderly:** No age-related precautions noted.

INTERACTIONS

DRUG: May decrease effects of **oral contraceptives.** May increase concentration of **warfarin,** increase bleeding time. **HERBAL:** None significant. **FOOD:** None known. **LAB VALUES:** May increase serum alkaline phosphatase, amylase, BUN, bilirubin, glucose, LDH, ALT, AST. May decrease Hgb, WBCs, thrombocytes, serum potassium, protein.

AVAILABILITY (Rx)

Injection, Powder for Reconstitution (Tygacil): 50-mg vial.

ADMINISTRATION/HANDLING

 IV

Reconstitution • Add 5.3 mL 0.9% NaCl or D₅W to each 50-mg vial. • Swirl gently to dissolve. • Resulting solution is 10 mg/mL. • Immediately withdraw 5 mL reconstituted solution and add to 100 mL 0.9% NaCl or D₅W bag for infusion (final concentration should not exceed 1 mg/mL).
Rate of Administration • Administer over 30–60 min every 12 hrs. • May be given through a dedicated line or piggyback. If same line is used for sequential infusion of several different drugs, line should be flushed before and after infusion of tigecycline with either 0.9% NaCl or D₅W.

Storage • Reconstituted solution is stable for up to 6 hrs at room temperature or up to 24 hrs if refrigerated. • Reconstituted solution appears yellow to red-orange. • Discard if solution is discolored (green, black) or precipitate forms.

▦ IV INCOMPATIBILITIES

Amphotericin B, methylPREDNISolone, voriconazole.

▦ IV COMPATIBILITIES

Amikacin, azithromycin, aztreonam, cefepime, cefTAZidime, ciprofloxacin, doripenem, ertapenem, fluconazole, gentamicin, linezolid, piperacillin-tazobactam, potassium chloride, telavancin, tobramycin, vancomycin.

INDICATIONS/ROUTES/DOSAGE

Systemic Infections
IV: ADULTS OVER 18 YRS, ELDERLY: Initially, 100 mg, followed by 50 mg every 12 hrs for 5–14 days. **CHILDREN 12 YRS AND OLDER:** 50 mg q12h. **CHILDREN 8–11 YRS:** 1.2 mg/kg q12h. **Maximum dose:** 50 mg.

Dosage in Renal Impairment
No dose adjustment.

Dosage in Hepatic Impairment
No dose adjustment in mild to moderate impairment.

Dosage in Severe Hepatic Impairment
IV: ADULTS OVER 18 YRS, ELDERLY: Initially, 100 mg, followed by 25 mg every 12 hrs.

SIDE EFFECTS

Frequent (29%–13%): Nausea, vomiting, diarrhea. **Occasional (7%–4%):** Headache, hypertension, dizziness, increased cough, delayed healing. **Rare (3%–2%):** Peripheral edema, pruritus, constipation, dyspepsia, asthenia (loss of strength, energy), hypotension, phlebitis, insomnia, rash, diaphoresis.

ADVERSE EFFECTS/TOXIC REACTIONS

Dyspnea, abscess, pseudomembranous colitis (abdominal cramps, severe watery diarrhea, fever) ranging from mild to life-threatening may result from altered bacterial balance in GI tract.

NURSING CONSIDERATIONS

BASELINE ASSESSMENT

Obtain baseline CBC, hepatic function test. Question for history of allergies, esp. tetracyclines, before therapy.

INTERVENTION/EVALUATION

Monitor daily pattern of bowel activity, stool consistency. Be alert for superinfection: fever, anal/genital pruritus, oral mucosal changes (ulceration, pain, erythema). Nausea, vomiting may be controlled by antiemetics.

PATIENT/FAMILY TEACHING

• Report diarrhea, rash, mouth soreness, other new symptoms.

---

tiotropium TOP 100

tye-oh-**trope**-ee-yum
(Spiriva HandiHaler, Spiriva Respimat)
Do not confuse Spiriva with Inspra, or tiotropium with ipratropium.

FIXED-COMBINATION(S)

Stiolto Respimat: tiotropium/olodaterol (a bronchodilator): 2.5 mcg/2.5 mcg.

◆CLASSIFICATION

PHARMACOTHERAPEUTIC: Anticholinergic. **CLINICAL:** Bronchodilator.

USES

Long-term maintenance treatment of bronchospasm associated with COPD, including chronic bronchitis, emphysema, and for reducing COPD exacerbations. Maintenance treatment of asthma in pts 6 yrs and older.

PRECAUTIONS

Contraindications: Hypersensitivity to tiotropium. History of hypersensitivity to ipratropium. **Cautions:** Narrow-angle glaucoma, prostatic hypertrophy, bladder neck obstruction, moderate to severe renal impairment, history of hypersensitivity to atropine, myasthenia gravis.

ACTION

Competitively and reversibly inhibits action of acetylcholine at muscarinic receptors in bronchial smooth muscle. **Therapeutic Effect:** Relieves bronchospasm.

PHARMACOKINETICS

Binds extensively to tissue. Protein binding: 72%. Metabolized by oxidation. Excreted in urine. **Half-life:** 5–6 days.

LIFESPAN CONSIDERATIONS

Pregnancy/Lactation: Unknown if distributed in breast milk. **Children:** Safety and efficacy not established. **Elderly:** Higher frequency of dry mouth, constipation, UTI noted with increasing age.

INTERACTIONS

DRUG: Concurrent administration with **anticholinergics (e.g., ipratropium)** may increase adverse effects. **HERBAL:** None significant. **FOOD:** None known. **LAB VALUES:** None significant.

AVAILABILITY (Rx)

Inhalation Spray (Spiriva Respimat): 1.25 mcg/actuation, 2.5 mcg/actuation.
Powder for Inhalation (Spiriva): 18 mcg/capsule (in blister packs).

ADMINISTRATION/HANDLING

Inhalation (Spiriva)

• Open dustcap of HandiHaler by pulling it upward, then open mouthpiece. • Place capsule in center chamber and firmly close mouthpiece until a click is heard, leaving the dustcap open. • Hold HandiHaler device with mouthpiece upward, press piercing button completely in once, and release. • Instruct pt to breathe out completely before breathing

T

---

in slowly and deeply but at rate sufficient to hear the capsule vibrate. • Have pt hold breath as long as it is comfortable until exhaling slowly. • Instruct pt to repeat once again to ensure full dose is received.

Spiriva Respimat • Refer to manufacturer's pt instructions.

Storage • Store at room temperature. Do not expose capsules to extreme temperature, moisture. • Do not place capsules in HandiHaler device. • Use immediately once foil is peeled back or removed.

INDICATIONS/ROUTES/DOSAGE

COPD (Maintenance Treatment, Reduction of COPD Exacerbations)
Inhalation: *(Spiriva):* **ADULTS, ELDERLY:** 18 mcg (1 capsule)/day via HandiHaler inhalation device. **(Spiriva Respimat):** 2 inhalations (2.5 mg/inhalation) once daily.

Asthma
Inhalation: *(Spiriva Respimat):* **ADULTS, ELDERLY, CHILDREN 6 YRS AND OLDER:** 2 inhalations of 1.25 mcg once daily. Maximum benefit may take up to 4–8 wks.

Dosage in Renal Impairment
CrCl 60 mL/min or less: Use caution in moderate to severe impairment.

Dosage in Hepatic Impairment
No dose adjustment.

SIDE EFFECTS

Frequent (16%–6%): Dry mouth, sinusitis, pharyngitis, dyspepsia, UTI, rhinitis. **Occasional (5%–4%):** Abdominal pain, peripheral edema, constipation, epistaxis, vomiting, myalgia, rash, oral candidiasis.

ADVERSE EFFECTS/TOXIC REACTIONS

Angina pectoris, depression, flu-like symptoms, glaucoma, increased intra-ocular pressure occur rarely.

NURSING CONSIDERATIONS

BASELINE ASSESSMENT
Question history of glaucoma, bladder outlet obstruction, renal impairment, myasthenia gravis. Auscultate lung sounds.

INTERVENTION/EVALUATION
Monitor rate, depth, rhythm, type of respiration; quality, rate of pulse. Assess lung sounds for rhonchi, wheezing, rales. Monitor ABGs. Observe for clavicular retractions, hand tremor. Evaluate for clinical improvement (quieter, slower respirations, relaxed facial expression, cessation of clavicular retractions).

PATIENT/FAMILY TEACHING
• Increase fluid intake (decreases lung secretion viscosity). • Do not use more than 1 capsule for inhalation in a 24h period. • Rinsing mouth with water immediately after inhalation may prevent mouth/throat dryness, thrush. • Avoid excessive use of caffeine derivatives (chocolate, coffee, tea, cola, cocoa). • Report eye pain/discomfort, blurred vision, visual halos.

tipiracil/trifluridine

trye-**flure**-i-deen/tye-**pir**-a-sil (Lonsurf)
Do not confuse trifluridine with floxuridine, or tipiracil with tipifarnib or Pipracil.

◆CLASSIFICATION

PHARMACOTHERAPEUTIC: Nucleoside metabolic inhibitor/thymidine phosphorylase inhibitor. **CLINICAL:** Antineoplastic.

USES

Treatment of pts with metastatic colorectal cancer who have been previously treated with fluoropyrimidine-, oxaliplatin-, and irinotecan-based chemotherapy, an anti–vascular endothelial growth factor (VEGF) biological therapy, and if RAS wild-type, an anti–epidermal growth factor (EGFR) therapy.

PRECAUTIONS

Contraindications: Hypersensitivity to trifluridine or tipiracil. **Cautions:** Baseline anemia, leukopenia, neutropenia, thrombocytopenia; active infection, pts at increased risk of infection (e.g., diabetes, indwelling catheters), pts with high tumor burden, history of pulmonary embolism; pregnancy, moderate to severe hepatic impairment.

ACTION

Trifluridine interferes with DNA synthesis and cell proliferation of cancer cells. Tipiracil increases exposure of trifluridine by inhibiting metabolism via thymidine phosphorylase. **Therapeutic Effect:** Inhibits tumor cell growth and metastasis.

PHARMACOKINETICS

Rapidly absorbed. Metabolized by thymidine phosphorylase (not metabolized in liver). Protein binding: trifluridine: 96%; tipiracil: 8%. Peak plasma concentration: 2 hrs. Excreted primarily in urine (50%). **Half-life:** trifluridine: 1.4 hrs (2.1 hrs at steady state); tipiracil: 2.1 hrs (2.4 hrs at steady state).

⏳ LIFESPAN CONSIDERATIONS

Pregnancy/Lactation: Avoid pregnancy; may cause fetal harm. Female pts of reproductive potential must use effective contraception during treatment. Unknown if distributed in breast milk. Breastfeeding not recommended. **Males:** Due to risk of potential exposure, male pts must use condoms during sexual activity during treatment and up to 3 mos after discontinuation. **Children:** Safety and efficacy not established. **Elderly:** May have increased risk of neutropenia, thrombocytopenia.

INTERACTIONS

DRUG: Not specified (no formal studies conducted). **HERBAL:** None significant. **FOOD:** None known. **LAB**

VALUES: Expected to decrease Hct, Hgb, platelets, neutrophils, RBC, WBC.

AVAILABILITY (Rx)

Fixed-Dose Combination Tablets: trifluridine/tipiracil: 15 mg/6.14 mg, 20 mg/8.19 mg.

ADMINISTRATION/HANDLING

PO
• Give within 1 hr of completion of morning and evening meals. Do not give on empty stomach.

INDICATIONS/ROUTES/DOSAGE

Note: Do not initiate the cycle until ANC is 1,500 cells/mm^3 or greater; febrile neutropenia is resolved; platelet count is 75,000 cells/mm^3 or greater; grade 3 or 4 nonhematologic toxicity is resolved to grade 1 or 0.

Colorectal Cancer
PO: ADULTS, ELDERLY: (Dose based on trifluridine component) 35 mg/m^2 (rounded to nearest 5-mg increment) twice daily on days 1–5 and days 8–12 of 28-day cycle. Continue until disease progression or unacceptable toxicity. **Maximum:** 80 mg/dose (based on trifluridine component).

Dose Modification
Based on Common Terminology Criteria for Adverse Events (CTCAE).

Hematologic/Nonhematologic Toxicity
Interrupt treatment for ANC less than 500 cells/mm^3; febrile neutropenia; platelet count less than 50,000 cells/mm^3; grade 3 or 4 nonhematologic toxicity. Do not restart until ANC is 1,500 cells/mm^3 or greater; febrile neutropenia is resolved; platelet count is 75,000 cells/mm^3 or greater; grade 3 or 4 nonhematologic toxicity is resolved to grade 1 or 0 (except grade 3 nausea and/or vomiting controlled by antiemetic therapy; grade 3 diarrhea responsive to antidiarrheal medication). Once resolved, resume at decreased incremental dose of 5 mg/m^2 from previous dose. A maximum of

T

3 dose reductions is allowed to dosage minimum of 20 mg/m² twice daily. Do not increase dose after it has been reduced.

Dosage in Renal Impairment

Mild to moderate impairment: No dose adjustment. **Severe impairment:** Not studied; use caution.

Dosage in Hepatic Impairment

Mild impairment: No dose adjustment. **Moderate to severe impairment:** Not studied; use caution.

SIDE EFFECTS

Frequent (52%–19%): Asthenia, fatigue, nausea, diarrhea, decreased appetite, vomiting, abdominal pain, pyrexia. **Occasional (8%–7%):** Stomatitis, dysgeusia, alopecia.

ADVERSE EFFECTS/TOXIC REACTIONS

Severe and/or life-threatening myelosuppression including anemia (77% of pts), grade 3 anemia (18% of pts), neutropenia (67% of pts), grade 3 or 4 neutropenia (27% and 11% of pts), thrombocytopenia (42% of pts), grade 3 or 4 thrombocytopenia (5% and 1% of pts), febrile neutropenia (3.8% of pts) may occur. Infectious processes including nasopharyngitis, urinary tract infection reported in 2%–4% of pts. Pulmonary embolism occurred in 2% of pts. Interstitial lung disease occurs rarely.

NURSING CONSIDERATIONS

BASELINE ASSESSMENT

Obtain baseline CBC and screen for anemia, neutropenia, thrombocytopenia. Obtain vital signs. Verify pregnancy status before start of each cycle. Screen for active infection, history of pulmonary embolism. Assess hydration status. Question pt's usual stool characteristics (color, frequency, consistency).

INTERVENTION/EVALUATION

Follow proper handling and disposal procedures for cytotoxic drugs. Monitor ANC, CBC on day 15 of each cycle. If any grade 3 or 4 hematologic toxicity occurs, repeat ANC, CBC more frequently. If chest pain, dyspnea, tachycardia occurs, provide supplemental O_2 and obtain radiologic testing to rule out pulmonary embolism. Diligently monitor for infection. Monitor daily stool pattern, consistency. Encourage PO intake. Monitor for bleeding if thrombocytopenia occurs.

PATIENT/FAMILY TEACHING

• Blood levels will be monitored regularly. • Treatment may cause fetal harm. Female pts of childbearing potential should use effective contraception during treatment. Immediately report suspected pregnancy. Do not breastfeed. • Male pts must use condoms during sexual activity. • Immediately report chest pain, difficult breathing, fast heart rate, rapid breathing; may indicate life-threatening blood clot in the lungs. • Report symptoms of bone marrow suppression or infection such as bruising easily, chills, cough, dizziness, fainting, fever, shortness of breath, weakness, or burning with urination. • Avoid crowds, those with active infection. • Take within 1 hr of breakfast and evening meal. • Drink plenty of fluids. • Report diarrhea, nausea, vomiting that is not controlled by antinausea, antidiarrheal medication. • Report bleeding of any kind.

tipranavir

tye-**pran**-a-veer
(Aptivus)

■ **BLACK BOX ALERT** ■ May cause hepatitis (including fatalities), hepatic dysfunction. Pts with HBV or HCV at greater risk. Intracranial hemorrhage has occurred (in combination with ritonavir).

◆CLASSIFICATION

PHARMACOTHERAPEUTIC: Protease inhibitor. **CLINICAL:** Antiretroviral.

USES

Treatment of HIV infection in combination with ritonavir and other antiretroviral agents (limited to highly treatment experienced or multi–protease inhibitor resistant pts).

PRECAUTIONS

Contraindications: Hypersensitivity to tipranavir. Moderate to severe hepatic impairment, medications dependent on CYP3A for clearance, concurrent use of tipranavir/ritonavir with strong CYP3A inducers: alfuzosin, amiodarone, bepridil, dihydroergotamine, ergonovine, ergotamine, flecainide, lovastatin, lurasidone, methylergonovine, midazolam (oral), pimozide, propafenone, quiNIDine, rifAMPin, sildenafil (pulmonary arterial hypertension), simvastatin, St. John's wort, triazolam. **Cautions:** Hemophilia, known sulfonamide allergy, mild hepatic impairment, pts at increased risk for bleeding from trauma, surgery, concurrent antiplatelet/anticoagulant therapy. Pts coinfected with HBV or HCV.

ACTION

Binds to HIV-1 protease activity sites. Inhibits cleavage of viral protein precursors into functional proteins necessary for infectious HIV. **Therapeutic Effect:** Prevents formation of mature infectious viral cells.

PHARMACOKINETICS

Incompletely absorbed following PO administration. Protein binding: 98%–99%. Metabolized in liver. Excreted in feces (82%), urine (4%). **Half-life:** 6 hrs.

⏳ LIFESPAN CONSIDERATIONS

Pregnancy/Lactation: Unknown if drug crosses placenta or is distributed in breast milk. **Children:** Safety and efficacy not established in children younger than 2 yrs. **Elderly:** Age-related hepatic impairment may require dosage adjustment.

INTERACTIONS

DRUG: May interfere with metabolism of **amiodarone, bepridil, ergotamine, midazolam, oral contraceptives.** **CarBAMazepine, PHENobarbital, phenytoin, rifAMPin** may decrease concentration. May increase concentration of **colchicine, HMG-CoA reductase inhibitors (e.g., simvastatin), fluoxetine, PARoxetine, sertraline. HMG-CoA reductase inhibitors** may increase risk of myopathy including rhabdomyolysis. **HERBAL: St. John's wort** may lead to loss of virologic response, potential resistance to tipranavir. **FOOD: High-fat meals** may increase bioavailability. **LAB VALUES:** May increase serum cholesterol, triglycerides, amylase, ALT, AST. May decrease WBC count.

AVAILABILITY (Rx)

Capsules: 250 mg. **Oral Solution:** 100 mg/mL.

ADMINISTRATION/HANDLING

PO

• May take without regard to food. When taken with ritonavir tablets, must be taken with meals. • Store unopened bottles of capsules in refrigerator. • Do not freeze/refrigerate oral solution. • Once bottle is opened, capsules may be stored at room temperature for 60 days. Use oral solution within 60 days after opening.

INDICATIONS/ROUTES/DOSAGE

Note: Must be taken with ritonavir.

HIV Infection

PO: ADULTS, ELDERLY: 500 mg administered with 200 mg of ritonavir twice daily. **CHILDREN 2–18 YRS:** 14 mg/kg with 6 mg/kg ritonavir twice daily. **Maximum:** 500 mg with 200 mg ritonavir twice daily.

Dosage in Renal Impairment
No dose adjustment.

Dosage in Hepatic Impairment
Mild impairment: Use caution. **Moderate to severe impairment:** Contraindicated.

T

SIDE EFFECTS

Frequent   (11%): Diarrhea. **Occasional (7%–2%):** Nausea, fever, fatigue, headache, depression, vomiting, abdominal pain, weakness, rash. **Rare (Less Than 2%):** Abdominal distention, anorexia, flatulence, dizziness, insomnia, myalgia.

ADVERSE EFFECTS/TOXIC REACTIONS

Bronchitis occurs in 3% of pts. Anemia, neutropenia, thrombocytopenia, diabetes mellitus, hepatic failure, hepatitis, peripheral neuropathy, pancreatitis occur rarely.

NURSING CONSIDERATIONS

BASELINE ASSESSMENT

Obtain baseline LFT before beginning therapy and at periodic intervals during therapy. Offer emotional support. Obtain full medication history and screen for interactions. Review medical history for HBV or HCV.

INTERVENTION/EVALUATION

Closely monitor for evidence of GI discomfort. Monitor daily pattern of bowel activity, stool consistency. Assess skin for evidence of rash. Monitor serum chemistry tests for marked laboratory abnormalities, particularly hepatic profile, CD4 cell count, HIV RNA plasma levels. Assess for opportunistic infections (onset of fever, oral mucosa changes, cough, other respiratory symptoms).

PATIENT/FAMILY TEACHING

• Eat small, frequent meals to offset nausea, vomiting. • Continue therapy for full length of treatment. • Doses should be evenly spaced. • Tipranavir is not a cure for HIV infection, nor does it reduce risk of transmission to others. • Pt may continue to experience illnesses, including opportunistic infections. • Diarrhea can be controlled with OTC medication.

tiZANidine

tye-**zan**-i-deen
(Apo-TiZANidine ✿, Zanaflex)
Do not confuse tiZANidine with tiaGABine.

◆CLASSIFICATION

PHARMACOTHERAPEUTIC: Alpha₂-adrenergic agonist. **CLINICAL:** Antispastic.

USES

Acute and intermittent management of muscle spasticity (spasms, stiffness, rigidity), spasticity associated with multiple sclerosis or spinal cord injury.

PRECAUTIONS

Contraindications: Hypersensitivity to tiZANidine. Concurrent use with strong CYP1A2 inhibitors. **Cautions:** Renal/hepatic disease, pts at risk for severe hypotensive effects, cardiac disease, psychiatric disorders, elderly pts.

ACTION

Increases presynaptic inhibition of spinal motor neurons mediated by alpha₂-adrenergic agonists, reducing facilitation to postsynaptic motor neurons. **Therapeutic Effect:** Reduces muscle spasticity.

PHARMACOKINETICS

Metabolized in liver. Primarily excreted in urine. **Half-life:** 2 hrs.

INTERACTIONS

DRUG: Alcohol, other CNS depressants (e.g,. **LORazepam, morphine, zolpidem**) may increase CNS depressant effects. **Antiarrhythmics (e.g., amiodarone, sotalol), cimetidine, oral contraceptives, acyclovir** may increase risk of bradycardia, hypotension, or CNS depression. **Strong CYP1A2 inhibitors (e.g., ciprofloxacin, fluvoxaMINE)** may increase concentration/adverse effects (contraindicated). **HERBAL:** Gotu kola, kava kava, St. John's wort, valerian may increase CNS depression. Black cohosh, hawthorn, periwinkle may increase hypotensive effect. FOOD: None known. LAB VALUES: May increase serum alkaline phosphatase, ALT, AST.

AVAILABILITY (Rx)

Capsules: 2 mg, 4 mg, 6 mg. Tablets: 2 mg, 4 mg.

ADMINISTRATION/HANDLING

PO

• Capsules may be opened and sprinkled on food. • May give without regard to food. • Administration should be consistent and not switched between giving with or without food.

INDICATIONS/ROUTES/DOSAGE

Muscle spasticity

PO: ADULTS, ELDERLY: Initially, 2 mg up to 3 times/day at 6- to 8-hr intervals as needed. Can be gradually increased in 2- to 4-mg increments with a minimum of 1–4 days between dosage increases. Maximum: 36 mg/24 hrs in divided doses. Discontinuation of Therapy: Gradually taper dose by 2–4 mg daily.

Dosage in Renal Impairment

May require dose reduction/less frequent dosing. CrCl less than 25 mL/min: Reduce dose by 50%. If higher doses needed, increase dose instead of frequency.

Dosage in Hepatic Impairment

Avoid use if possible. If used, monitor for adverse effects (e.g., hypotension).

SIDE EFFECTS

Frequent (49%–41%): Dry mouth, drowsiness, asthenia. Occasional (16%–4%): Dizziness, UTI, constipation. Rare (3%): Nervousness, amblyopia, pharyngitis, rhinitis, vomiting, urinary frequency.

ADVERSE EFFECTS/TOXIC REACTIONS

Hypotension may be associated with bradycardia, orthostatic hypotension, and, rarely, syncope. Risk of hypotension increases as dosage increases; hypotension is noted within 1 hr after administration. May cause visual hallucinations.

NURSING CONSIDERATIONS

BASELINE ASSESSMENT

Record onset, type, location, duration of muscular spasm. Check for immobility, stiffness, swelling. Obtain LFT.

INTERVENTION/EVALUATION

Assist with ambulation at all times. For those on long-term therapy, serum hepatic/renal function tests should be performed periodically. Evaluate for therapeutic response (decreased intensity of skeletal muscle pain/tenderness, improved mobility, decrease in spasticity). Go from lying to standing slowly.

PATIENT/FAMILY TEACHING

• Avoid tasks that require alertness, motor skills until response to drug is established. • Avoid sudden changes in posture. • May cause hypotension, sedation, impaired coordination. • Avoid alcohol.

tobramycin

toe-bra-mye-sin
(TOBI, Tobrex)

■ BLACK BOX ALERT ■ May cause neurotoxicity, nephrotoxicity, ototoxicity. Ototoxicity usually is irreversible. Increased risk of neuromuscular blockade, including respiratory paralysis, particularly when given after anesthesia or muscle relaxants. May cause fetal harm.

Do not confuse tobramycin with vancomycin, or Tobrex with TobraDex.

FIXED-COMBINATION(S)

TobraDex: tobramycin/dexamethasone (a steroid): 0.3%/0.1% per mL or per g. Zylet: tobramycin/loteprednol: 0.3%/0.5%.

◆CLASSIFICATION

PHARMACOTHERAPEUTIC: Aminoglycoside. **CLINICAL:** Antibiotic.

USES

Treatment of susceptible infections due to *P. aeruginosa,* other gram-negative organisms including skin/skin structure, bone, joint, respiratory tract infections; postop, burn, intra-abdominal infections; complicated UTI; septicemia; meningitis. **Ophthalmic:** Superficial eye infections: blepharitis, conjunctivitis, keratitis, corneal ulcers. **Inhalation:** Bronchopulmonary infections *(Pseudomonas aeruginosa)* in pts with cystic fibrosis.

PRECAUTIONS

Contraindications: Hypersensitivity to tobramycin, other aminoglycosides (crosssensitivity) and their components. **Cautions:** Renal impairment, preexisting auditory or vestibular impairment, conditions that depress neuromuscular transmission, Parkinson's disease, myasthenia gravis, hypocalcemia, pregnancy, elderly pts.

ACTION

Irreversibly binds to protein on bacterial ribosomes. **Therapeutic Effect:** Interferes with protein synthesis of susceptible microorganisms.

PHARMACOKINETICS

Rapid, complete absorption after IM administration. Protein binding: less than 30%. Widely distributed (does not cross blood-brain barrier; low concentrations in CSF). Excreted unchanged in urine. Removed by hemodialysis. **Half-life:** 2–4 hrs (increased in renal impairment, neonates; decreased in cystic fibrosis, febrile or burn pts).

⏳ LIFESPAN CONSIDERATIONS

Pregnancy/Lactation: Drug readily crosses placenta; distributed in breast milk. May cause fetal nephrotoxicity. Ophthalmic form should not be used in breastfeeding mothers and only when specifically indicated in pregnancy.

Children: Immature renal function in neonates, premature infants may increase risk of toxicity. **Elderly:** Age-related renal impairment may increase risk of toxicity; dosage adjustment recommended.

INTERACTIONS

DRUG: Nephrotoxic medications (e.g., NSAIDs, IV contrast, lisinopril, furosemide), ototoxic medications (e.g., bumetanide, furosemide) may increase risk of nephrotoxicity, ototoxicity. **Neuromuscular blockers (e.g., cisatracurium, vecuronium)** may increase neuromuscular blockade. **HERBAL:** None significant. **FOOD:** None known. **LAB VALUES:** May increase serum BUN, bilirubin, creatinine, alkaline phosphatase, LDH, ALT, AST. May decrease serum calcium, magnesium, potassium, sodium. Therapeutic peak serum level: 5–20 mcg/mL; therapeutic trough serum level: 0.5–2 mcg/mL. Toxic peak serum level: greater than 20 mcg/mL; toxic trough serum level: greater than 2 mcg/mL.

AVAILABILITY (Rx)

Infusion, Premix: 60 mg/50 mL, 80 mg/100 mL. **Inhalation Powder (TOBI Podhaler):** 28 mg in a capsule. **Injection, Powder for Reconstitution:** 1.2 g. **Injection, Solution:** 10 mg/mL, 40 mg/mL. **Ointment, Ophthalmic (Tobrex):** 0.3%. **Solution, Nebulization (TOBI):** 60 mg/mL. **Solution, Ophthalmic (Tobrex):** 0.3%.

ADMINISTRATION/HANDLING

◀**ALERT**▶ Coordinate peak and trough lab draws with administration times.

 IV

Reconstitution • Dilute with 50–100 mL D₅W or 0.9% NaCl. Amount of diluent for infants, children depends on individual need.

Rate of Administration • Infuse over 30–60 min.

Storage • Store vials at room temperature. • Solutions may be discolored by light or air (does not affect potency). • Reconstituted solution stable for 24 hrs at room temperature or 96 hrs if refrigerated.

IM

• To minimize discomfort, give deep IM slowly. • Less painful if injected into gluteus maximus rather than lateral aspect of thigh.

Inhalation

• Refrigerate. • May store at room temperature up to 28 days after removing from refrigerator. • Do not use if cloudy or contains particulates. • **Podhaler:** Pt must not swallow capsules. • Doses should be as close as possible to 12 hrs apart and not less than 6 hrs apart. • Use Podhaler device supplied.

Ophthalmic

• Place gloved finger on lower eyelid, pull out until pocket is formed between eye and lower lid. • Place correct number of drops (¼–½ inch ointment) into pocket. • **Solution:** Apply digital pressure to lacrimal sac for 1–2 min (minimizes drainage into nose/throat, reducing risk of systemic effects). • **Ointment:** Instruct pt to close eye for 1–2 min, rolling eyeball (increases contact area of drug to eye). • Remove excess solution/ointment around eye.

▧ IV INCOMPATIBILITIES

Amphotericin B complex (Abelcet, AmBisome, Amphotec), heparin, indomethacin (Indocin), piperacillin-tazobactam (Zosyn), propofol (Diprivan), sargramostim (Leukine, Prokine).

▧ IV COMPATIBILITIES

Amiodarone (Cordarone), calcium gluconate, cefepime, ceftaroline, cefTAZidime, dexmedetomidine (Precedex), diltiaZEM (Cardizem), furosemide (Lasix), HYDROmorphone (Dilaudid), insulin, linezolid (Zyvox), magnesium sulfate, midazolam (Versed), morphine, niCARdipine (Cardene), tigecycline (Tygacil).

INDICATIONS/ROUTES/DOSAGE

◀**ALERT**▶ Space parenteral doses evenly around the clock. Dosage based on ideal body weight. Peak, trough levels determined periodically to maintain desired serum concentrations (minimizes risk of toxicity). Recommended peak level: 4–10 mcg/mL; trough level: 0.5–2 mcg/mL.

Usual Parenteral Dosage

IV: ADULTS, ELDERLY, 3–7.5 mg/kg/day in 3 divided doses. Once-daily dosing: 4–7 mg/kg every 24 hrs. **CHILDREN 5 YRS AND OLDER:** 2–2.5 mg/kg/dose q8h. **CHILDREN YOUNGER THAN 5 YRS:** 2.5 mg/kg/dose q8h. **NEONATES LESS THAN 1 KG (14 DAYS OR YOUNGER):** 5 mg/kg/dose q48h; **(15–28 DAYS):** 5 mg/kg/dose q36h. **1–2 KG (7 DAYS OR YOUNGER):** 5 mg/kg/dose q48h; **(8–28 DAYS):** 5 mg/kg/dose q36h. **GREATER THAN 2 KG (7 DAYS OR YOUNGER):** 4 mg/kg q24h; **(8–28 DAYS):** 4–5 mg/kg q12–24hrs.

Usual Ophthalmic Dosage

Ophthalmic Ointment: ADULTS, ELDERLY, CHILDREN 2 MOS AND OLDER: Apply ½ inch to conjunctiva q8–12h (q3–4h for severe infections).

Ophthalmic Solution: ADULTS, ELDERLY, CHILDREN 2 MOS AND OLDER: 1–2 drops in affected eye q4h (2 drops/hr for severe infections).

Usual Inhalation Dosage (Cystic Fibrosis)

Inhalation High Dose: ADULTS, CHILDREN 6 YRS AND OLDER: 300 mg q12h 28 days on, 28 days off. **Tobi Podhaler:** Four 28-mg capsules twice daily for 28 days followed by 28 days off.

Dosage in Renal Impairment

Dosage and frequency modified based on degree of renal impairment, serum drug concentration. After loading dose of 1–2 mg/kg, maintenance dose and frequency are based on serum creatinine levels, creatinine clearance.

Creatinine Clearance	Dosing Interval
41–60 mL/min	q12h
21–40 mL/min	q24h
10–20 mL/min	q48h
Less than 10 mL/min	q72h
Hemodialysis	Loading dose 2–3 mg/kg then 1–2 mg/kg q48–72h

Creatinine Clearance	Dosing Interval
Continuous renal replacement therapy	Loading dose 2–3 mg/kg then 1–2.5 mg/kg q24–48h

Dosage in Hepatic Impairment
No dose adjustment.

SIDE EFFECTS

Occasional: IM: Pain, induration. **IV:** Phlebitis, thrombophlebitis. **Topical:** Hypersensitivity reaction (fever, pruritus, rash, urticaria). **Ophthalmic:** Tearing, itching, redness, eyelid swelling. **Rare:** Hypotension, nausea, vomiting.

ADVERSE EFFECTS/TOXIC REACTIONS

Nephrotoxicity (acute kidney injury, acute tubular necrosis, renal failure) may be reversible if drug is stopped at first sign of symptoms. Irreversible ototoxicity (dizziness, ringing/roaring in ears, hearing loss), neurotoxicity (headache, dizziness, lethargy, tremor, visual disturbances) occur occasionally. Risk increases with higher dosages or prolonged therapy or if solution is applied directly to mucosa. Superinfections, particularly fungal infections, may result from bacterial imbalance with any administration route. Anaphylaxis may occur.

NURSING CONSIDERATIONS

BASELINE ASSESSMENT

Dehydration must be treated before beginning parenteral therapy. Question for history of allergies, esp. aminoglycosides, sulfite (and parabens for topical, ophthalmic routes). Establish baseline hearing acuity. Obtain baseline lab tests, esp. renal function.

INTERVENTION/EVALUATION

Monitor I&O (maintain hydration), urinalysis, renal function. Monitor results of peak/trough blood tests. **Therapeutic serum level:** peak: 5–20 mcg/mL; trough: 0.5–2 mcg/mL. **Toxic serum level:** peak: greater than 20 mcg/mL; trough: greater than 2 mcg/mL. Be alert

to ototoxic, neurotoxic symptoms. Evaluate IV site for phlebitis (heat, pain, red streaking over vein). Assess for rash. Be alert for superinfection, particularly anal/genital pruritus, changes of oral mucosa, diarrhea. When treating pts with neuromuscular disorders, assess respiratory response carefully. **Ophthalmic:** Assess for redness, swelling, itching, tearing.

PATIENT/FAMILY TEACHING

• Report any hearing, visual, balance, urinary problems, even after therapy is completed. • **Ophthalmic:** Blurred vision, tearing may occur briefly after application. • Report persistent tearing, redness, irritation.

tocilizumab

toe-si-**liz**-oo-mab
(Actemra)

■ **BLACK BOX ALERT** ■ Tuberculosis, serious invasive fungal infections, other opportunistic infections have occurred. Test for tuberculosis prior to and during treatment, regardless of initial result. Consider treatment of latent TB prior to initiation.

◆CLASSIFICATION

PHARMACOTHERAPEUTIC: Interleukin (IL)-6 receptor inhibitor. **CLINICAL:** Antirheumatic arthritis agent.

USES

Treatment of moderate to severe rheumatoid arthritis in adults who had inadequate response to disease-modifying antirheumatic drugs (DMARDs). Treatment of active systemic juvenile idiopathic arthritis (SJIA) in pts 2 yrs of age and older. Treatment of active polyarticular juvenile idiopathic arthritis (PJIA) in pts 2 yrs and older. Treatment of adults and children 2 yrs of age and older with chimeric antigen receptor (CAR) T cell-induced severe or life-threatening cytokine release syndrome. Treatment of giant cell arteritis in adults.

PRECAUTIONS

Contraindications: Hypersensitivity to tocilizumab. **Cautions:** Platelet count 100,000 cells/mm³ or less, ANC less than 2,000 cells/mm³, ALT, AST greater than 1.5 times upper limit of normal (ULN) prior to treatment. Do not administer to pts with active infection. Preexisting or recent-onset CNS demyelinating disorders, including multiple sclerosis; pts with chronic or recurrent infection or who have been exposed to tuberculosis; hematologic cytopenia, hepatic impairment, elderly pts, pts at increased risk of GI perforation. Avoid live vaccinations.

ACTION

Binds to IL-6 receptors, inhibiting signals of proinflammatory cytokines. **Therapeutic Effect:** Inhibits/slows structural joint damage, improves physical function.

PHARMACOKINETICS

Distributed in steady state of plasma and tissue compartments. Undergoes biphasic elimination from circulation. **Half-life:** 11–13 days.

⧖ LIFESPAN CONSIDERATIONS

Pregnancy/Lactation: Unknown if distributed in breast milk. **Children:** Safety and efficacy not established in conditions other than SJIA. **Elderly:** Cautious use due to increased risk of serious infections, malignancy.

INTERACTIONS

DRUG: Anakinra, abatacept, corticosteroids, methotrexate may increase risk of infection. **Live vaccines** not recommended. May decrease effects of **lovastatin, simvastatin, oral contraceptives, phenytoin, warfarin. HERBAL: Echinacea** may alter levels/effects. **FOOD:** None known. **LAB VALUES:** May increase serum ALT, AST, lipids. May decrease platelets, neutrophils.

AVAILABILITY (Rx)

Injection Solution: 20 mg/mL (80 mg/4 mL, 200 mg/10 mL, 400 mg/20 mL). **Syringe for Subcutaneous Administration:** 162 mg/0.9 mL. (Intended only for adults with RA.)

ADMINISTRATION/HANDLING

 ◀**ALERT**▶ Do not infuse IV push or bolus.

▣ IV

Reconstitution • Dilute in 100 mL 0.9% NaCl (50 mL 0.9% NaCl for SJIA pts weighing less than 30 kg). • Prior to mixing, withdraw and discard volume of NaCl equal to volume of patient-dosed solution. • Invert bag to avoid foaming. • Inject solution and dilute for mixture that equals 50 mL or 100 mL in NaCl bag.

Rate of Administration • Infuse over 1 hr.

Storage • Refrigerate vials; do not freeze. • Diluted solutions may be stored for 24 hrs at room temperature or refrigerated. • Protect from light until time of use. • Solution appears colorless. Discard solution if it appears cloudy, discolored, or contains particulate.

INDICATIONS/ROUTES/DOSAGE

Note: Do not infuse concomitantly in same IV line with other drugs. Do not begin if ANC less than 2,000 cells/mm³, platelets less than 100,000 cells/mm³, or ALT or AST more than 1.5 times ULN.

Moderate to Severely Active Rheumatoid Arthritis
IV Infusion: ADULTS, ELDERLY: 4 mg/kg every 4 wks initially. May increase to 8 mg/kg every 4 wks. **Maximum:** 800 mg per dose. **SQ: ADULTS, ELDERLY (100 KG OR GREATER):** 162 mg/wk. **(LESS THAN 100 KG):** 162 mg every other wk. May increase to every wk based on clinical response.

Cytokine Release Syndrome
IV: ADULTS, CHILDREN greater than 30 kg: 8 mg/kg. Pts less than 30 kg: 12 mg/kg. If no clinical improvement, 3 additional doses may be given with an interval of at least 8 hrs.

Giant Cell Arteritis
SQ: ADULTS, ELDERLY: 162 mg once every wk (in combination with tapering course

T

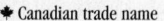 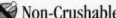

of glucocorticoid). May be given alone following discontinuation of glucocorticoid.

Dosage Modification

Hepatic enzyme levels greater than ULN.

Lab Value	Recommendation
1–3 times ULN	Dose modify concomitant DMARDs or reduce dose to 4 mg/kg until ALT, AST normalized
Greater than 3–5 times ULN	Interrupt treatment until ALT, AST less than 3 times ULN, then follow guidelines for 1–3 times ULN
Greater than 5 times ULN	Discontinue treatment

SJIA

IV: CHILDREN MORE THAN 30 KG: 8 mg/kg q2wks. **CHILDREN 30 KG OR LESS:** 12 mg/kg q2wks.

PJIA

IV: CHILDREN MORE THAN 30 KG: 8 mg/kg q4wks. **CHILDREN 30 KG OR LESS:** 10 mg/kg q4wks.

Dosage in Renal Impairment

Mild impairment: No dose adjustment. **Moderate to severe impairment:** Use caution (not studied).

Dosage in Hepatic Impairment

Not recommended.

SIDE EFFECTS

Occasional (8%–6%): Upper respiratory tract infection, nasopharyngitis, headache, hypertension. **Rare (5%–3%):** Infusion reaction, dizziness, bronchitis, rash, oral ulceration.

ADVERSE EFFECTS/TOXIC REACTIONS

Up to 48% of pts experience elevated ALT, AST. Neutropenia, thrombocytopenia occur in 4% of pts. Serious infections, including sepsis, pneumonia, tuberculosis, invasive fungal infections, hepatitis B, have occurred. Anaphylactic reaction, rash, pruritus, urticaria, bronchospasm, swelling, dyspnea occur in less than 0.2% of pts; hypersensitivity reactions (hypertension, headaches, flushing) occur more frequently. Increased risk of lymphoma, melanoma. New onset or exacerbation of CNS demyelinating disorders, including multiple sclerosis. Risk of gastric perforation with concomitant use of NSAIDs, corticosteroids.

NURSING CONSIDERATIONS

BASELINE ASSESSMENT

Evaluate pt for active tuberculosis and test for latent infection prior to initiating treatment and periodically during therapy. Induration of 5 mm or greater with tuberculin skin testing should be considered a positive test result when assessing for latent tuberculosis. Antifungal therapy should be considered for pts who reside or travel to regions where mycoses are endemic. Do not initiate therapy during an active infection. Viral reactivation can occur in cases of herpes zoster, HIV. Assess baseline lab results (hepatic enzymes, cholesterol, triglycerides, platelets, neutrophils) q4–8wks during treatment. Pts should report history of diverticulitis, weakened immune system, HIV, hepatic disease, GI bleeding, hemoptysis, diarrhea, weight loss, cancer, prior cancer treatment, use of NSAIDs, glucocorticosteroids.

INTERVENTION/EVALUATION

Monitor hepatitis B carriers during and several months following therapy. If reactivation occurs, consider interrupting treatment. Monitor pts for signs/symptoms of tuberculosis regardless of baseline PPD. Discontinue treatment if pt develops acute infection, opportunistic infection, or sepsis and initiate appropriate antimicrobial therapy. Monitor warfarin, theophylline, cycloSPORINE levels for therapeutic ranges. Modify, interrupt, or discontinue treatment if ALT, AST is 1–5 times ULN.

PATIENT/FAMILY TEACHING

• Inform pt that therapy may lower immune system response. • Detail any concomitant immunosuppressive therapy, methotrexate. • Report any history of HIV, fungal infections, hepatitis B, multiple sclerosis, hemoptysis, tuberculosis, or close relatives with active tuberculosis. • Report any travel plans to possible endemic areas. • Report signs/symptoms of stomach pain to evaluate risk of gastric perforation or history of taking NSAIDs, corticosteroids, methotrexate. • Pt will need blood levels drawn q4–8wks during treatment along with routine tuberculosis screening. • Seek immediate medical attention if adverse reaction occurs. • Do not receive live vaccines during therapy. • Notify physician if pregnant or planning on becoming pregnant. • During treatment, report any signs of liver problems, such as stomach pains, yellowing of skin/eyes, dark-amber urine, clay-colored or bloody stools, fatigue, reduced appetite, coffee-ground emesis. • Pt must adhere to strict dosing schedule. • Decreased platelet count may lead to risk of bleeding.

tofacitinib

toe-fa-**sye**-ti-nib
(Xeljanz, Xeljanz XR)
Do not confuse tofacitinib with tipifarnib or Xeljanz with Xeloda.
■ **BLACK BOX ALERT** ■
Increased risk for developing bacterial, viral, invasive fungal, other opportunistic infections including tuberculosis, cryptococcosis, pneumocystosis that may lead to hospitalization or death; infections often occurred in combination with other immunosuppressants (methotrexate, corticosteroids). Closely monitor for development of infection. Test for latent tuberculosis prior to treatment and during treatment, regardless of initial result. Treatment for latent TB should be initiated before use. Malignancies including lymphoma, nonmelanoma skin cancer reported. Increased rate of Epstein-Barr virus–associated post-transplant lymphoproliferative disorder observed in renal transplant pts who are treated with tofacitinib and other immunosuppressive therapy drugs.

◆CLASSIFICATION

PHARMACOTHERAPEUTIC: Janus kinase (JAK) inhibitor. **CLINICAL:** Antirheumatic agent.

USES

Treatment of adult pts with moderate to severe active rheumatoid arthritis with previous inadequate response or intolerance to methotrexate. May be used as monotherapy or in combination with methotrexate or other nonbiologic disease-modifying antirheumatic drugs (DMARDs). Do not use in combination with other biologic DMARDs or with potent immunosuppressants (e.g., azaTHIOprine, cycloSPORINE).

PRECAUTIONS

Contraindications: Hypersensitivity to tofacitinib. **Cautions:** Pts exposed to TB, history of serious opportunistic infections, conditions that predispose to infections (e.g., diabetes), pts at risk for GI perforation (e.g., diverticulitis), pts who resided or traveled in areas where TB is endemic, moderate to severe renal impairment, elderly pts, hepatic impairment, history of anemia, hyperlipidemia, hepatitis, Asian ancestry, pts with history of interstitial lung disease, heart rate less than 60 bpm, conduction abnormalities, ischemic heart disease, HF.

ACTION

Inhibits JAK enzymes, which are involved in stimulating hematopoiesis and immune cell functioning. **Therapeutic Effect:** Reduces inflammation, tenderness, swelling of joints; slows or prevents progressive joint destruction in rheumatoid arthritis (RA).

PHARMACOKINETICS

Rapidly absorbed following PO administration. Protein binding: 40%. Peak concentration: 30–60 min. Metabolized in liver. Excreted primarily in urine. **Half-life:** 3 hrs.

⌛ LIFESPAN CONSIDERATIONS

Pregnancy/Lactation: Not recommended in nursing mothers. Must either

T

discontinue drug or discontinue breast-feeding. Unknown if distributed in breast milk. **Children:** Safety and efficacy not established. **Elderly:** Increased risk for serious infections, malignancy.

INTERACTIONS

DRUG: May alter effects of **live virus vaccines. Immunosuppressants (e.g., azaTHIOprine, cycloSPORINE)** may increase risk for added immunosuppression, infection. **CYP3A4 inhibitors (e.g., ketoconazole), CYP2C19 inhibitors (e.g., fluconazole)** may increase concentration/effects. **CYP3A4 inducers (e.g., rifAMPin, phenytoin)** may decrease concentration/effects. **HERBAL: St. John's wort** may decrease concentration/effect. **FOOD:** None known. **LAB VALUES:** May increase ALT, AST, bilirubin, lipids, creatinine. May decrease Hgb, neutrophils, lymphocytes.

AVAILABILITY (Rx)

Tablets, Film-Coated: (Xeljanz): 5 mg. (Xeljanz XR): 11 mg.

ADMINISTRATION/HANDLING

PO
• Give without regard to food. • Do not cut, split, crush, or chew XR tablet.

INDICATIONS/ROUTES/DOSAGE

◀**ALERT**▶ Do not initiate treatment in pts with baseline active infection (systemic/localized), severe hepatic impairment, lymphocytes less than 500 cells/mm^3, ANC less than 1,000 cells/mm^3, Hgb less than 9 g/dL.

Moderate to Severe Rheumatoid Arthritis
PO: ADULTS/ELDERLY: (Xeljanz): 5 mg twice daily. (**Xeljanz XR**): 11 mg once daily.

Dose Modification
Reduce to 5 mg once daily for any of the following: moderate to severe renal impairment, moderate hepatic impairment, concurrent use of potent CYP3A4 inhibitors, concurrent use of one or more moderate CYP3A4 or potent CYP2C19 inhibitors.

Lymphopenia
Interrupt treatment until lymphocytes greater than or equal to 500 cells/mm^3. Discontinue if lymphocytes less than 500 cells/mm^3 after repeat testing.

Neutropenia
Interrupt treatment until neutrophils greater than 1,000 cells/mm^3. Discontinue if neutrophils less than 500 cells/mm^3 after repeat testing.

Anemia
Interrupt treatment until Hgb greater than or equal to 9 g/dL or baseline Hgb decreases less than or equal to 2 g/dL after repeat testing.

Hepatotoxicity
Interrupt treatment until diagnosis of drug-induced hepatic injury has been excluded.

Dosage in Renal Impairment
Mild impairment: No dose adjustment. **Moderate to severe impairment:** 5 mg once daily.

Dosage in Hepatic Impairment
Mild impairment: No dose adjustment. **Moderate impairment:** 5 mg once daily. **Severe impairment:** Not recommended.

SIDE EFFECTS

Rare (4%–2%): Upper respiratory tract infection, diarrhea, nasopharyngitis, headache, hypertension.

ADVERSE EFFECTS/TOXIC REACTIONS

Neutropenia, lymphopenia may increase risk for infection. Serious infections may include aspergillosis, BK virus, cellulitis, coccidioidomycosis, cryptococcus, cytomegalovirus, esophageal candidiasis, histoplasmosis, invasive fungal infections, listeriosis, pneumocystosis, pneumonia, tuberculosis, UTI, sepsis. Increased risk for various malignancies. May induce viral reactivation of hepatitis B or C virus infection, herpes zoster, HIV. Epstein-Barr virus–associated post-transplant lymphoproliferative disorder reported in 2% of pts with renal transplant. Increased risk for GI perforation.

NURSING CONSIDERATIONS

BASELINE ASSESSMENT

Obtain vital signs, CBC, BMP, LFT, lipid panel, urine pregnancy test results. Evaluate for active tuberculosis (TB) and test for latent infection prior to and during treatment. Induration of 5 mm or greater with purified protein derivative (PPD) is considered positive result when assessing for latent TB. Question possibility of pregnancy or breastfeeding. Screen for history/co-morbidities. Obtain full medication history including vitamins, herbal products.

INTERVENTION/EVALUATION

Obtain CBC every 4–8 wks, then every 3 mos, lipid panel 4–8 wks after initiation; hepatic function panel if hepatic impairment suspected. Monitor for TB regardless of baseline PPD. Consider discontinuation if pt develops acute infection, opportunistic infection, sepsis; initiate appropriate antimicrobial therapy. Immediately report any hemorrhaging, melena, abdominal pain, hemoptysis (may indicate GI perforation).

PATIENT/FAMILY TEACHING

• Routinely monitor blood levels. • Therapy will lower immune system response. • Do not receive live virus vaccines. • Other immunosuppressant drugs may increase risk for infection. • Expect routine TB screening. • Fever, cough, burning with urination, body aches, chills, skin changes may indicate infection. • Report history of HIV, recent infections, hepatitis B or C, TB or close relatives who have active TB. • Report any travel plans to possible endemic areas. • Notify physician if pregnant or planning pregnancy. • Do not breastfeed. • Immediately report bleeding of any kind. • Yellowing of skin or eyes, right upper quadrant abdominal pain, bruising, clay-colored stool, dark urine may indicate liver problem. • Avoid grapefruit products.

tolterodine

tol-**ter**-oh-deen
(Detrol, Detrol LA, Unidet ✦)
Do not confuse Detrol with Ditropan, or tolterodine with fesoterodine.

◆CLASSIFICATION

PHARMACOTHERAPEUTIC: Muscarinic receptor antagonist. **CLINICAL:** Antispasmodic.

USES

Treatment of overactive bladder in pts with symptoms of urinary frequency, urgency, or urge incontinence.

PRECAUTIONS

Contraindications: Hypersensitivity to tolterodine or fesoterodine. Gastric retention, uncontrolled narrow-angle glaucoma, urinary retention. **Cautions:** Renal impairment, clinically significant bladder outflow obstruction (risk of urinary retention), GI obstructive disorders (e.g., pyloric stenosis [risk of gastric retention]), treated narrow-angle glaucoma, myasthenia gravis, prolonged QT interval (congenital/medications), hypokalemia, hypomagnesemia), hepatic impairment, elderly.

ACTION

Antagonist of muscarinic receptors mediating urinary bladder contraction. Increases residual urine volume, reduces detrusor muscle pressure. **Therapeutic Effect:** Decreases urinary frequency, urgency.

PHARMACOKINETICS

Immediate-release form rapidly, well absorbed after PO administration. Protein binding: 96%. Metabolized in liver. Primarily excreted in urine. Unknown if removed by hemodialysis. **Half-life:** Immediate-release: 2–10 hrs. Extended-release: 7–18 hrs.

T

⧖ LIFESPAN CONSIDERATIONS

Pregnancy/Lactation: Unknown if drug is distributed in breast milk. Breastfeeding not recommended. **Children:** Safety and efficacy not established. **Elderly:** No age-related precautions noted.

INTERACTIONS

DRUG: CYP3A4 inhibitors (e.g., clarithromycin, ketoconazole, ritonavir) may increase concentration. **FLUoxetine** may inhibit drug metabolism. **HERBAL: St. John's wort** may decrease concentration/effects. **FOOD:** None known. **LAB VALUES:** None known.

AVAILABILITY (Rx)

Tablets (Detrol): 1 mg, 2 mg.

🍷 **Capsules (Extended-Release [Detrol LA]):** 2 mg, 4 mg.

ADMINISTRATION/HANDLING

PO
• May give without regard to food.
• Give extended-release capsules whole; do not break, crush, or open.

INDICATIONS/ROUTES/DOSAGE

Overactive Bladder
PO: ADULTS, ELDERLY (IMMEDIATE-RELEASE): 1–2 mg twice daily **(WITH CYP3A4 INHIBITORS):** 1 mg twice daily. **(EXTENDED-RELEASE):** 2–4 mg once daily. **(WITH CYP3A4 INHIBITORS):** 2 mg once daily.

Dosage in Renal/Hepatic Impairment
Mild to moderate impairment: (IM-MEDIATE-RELEASE): 1 mg twice daily. Use caution. (EXTENDED-RELEASE): 2 mg once daily. Use caution. **Severe impairment:** Not recommended.

SIDE EFFECTS

Frequent (40%): Dry mouth. **Occasional (11%–4%):** Headache, dizziness, fatigue, constipation, dyspepsia, upper respiratory tract infection, UTI, dry eyes, abnormal vision (accommodation problems), nausea, diarrhea. **Rare (3%):** Drowsiness, chest/back pain, arthralgia, rash, weight gain, dry skin.

ADVERSE EFFECTS/TOXIC REACTIONS

Overdose can result in severe anticholinergic effects, including abdominal cramps, facial warmth, excessive salivation/lacrimation, diaphoresis, pallor, urinary urgency, blurred vision, prolonged QT interval.

NURSING CONSIDERATIONS

BASELINE ASSESSMENT

Assess degree of overactive bladder (urinary urgency, frequency, incontinence). Question history as listed in Precautions.

INTERVENTION/EVALUATION

Assist with ambulation if dizziness occurs. Question for visual changes. Monitor incontinence, postvoid residuals.

PATIENT/FAMILY TEACHING

• May cause blurred vision, dry eyes/mouth, constipation. • Report any confusion, altered mental status. • Avoid tasks that require alertness, motor skills until response to drug is established.

topiramate

toe-**peer**-a-mate
(Apo-Topiramate ✦, Qudexy XR, <u>Topamax</u>, Topamax Sprinkle, Trokendi XR)
Do not confuse Topamax or topiramate with TEGretol, TEGretol XR, or Toprol XL.

◆CLASSIFICATION

PHARMACOTHERAPEUTIC: Carbonic anhydrase inhibitor. **CLINICAL:** Anticonvulsant.

USES

Monotherapy for treatment of partial-onset or primary generalized tonic-clonic seizures in pts 2 yrs and older (immediate-release, Qudexy XR) or 6 yrs and older (Trokendi XR). Adjunctive therapy for partial-onset, primary generalized tonic-clonic seizures or seizures associated with

Lennox-Gastaut syndrome in pts 2 yrs and older (immediate-release, Qudexy XR) or 6 yrs and older (Trokendi XR). Prevention of migraine headache. **OFF-LABEL:** Neuropathic pain, diabetic neuropathy, prophylaxis of cluster headaches, infantile spasms.

PRECAUTIONS

Contraindications: Hypersensitivity to topiramate. (Extended-Release): Recent alcohol use (within 6 hrs prior to or after); pts with metabolic acidosis who are taking metFORMIN. **Cautions:** Hepatic/renal impairment, elderly pts, pts who are at high risk for suicide, respiratory impairment, pts with congenital metabolism dysfunction or decreased mitochondrial activity. During strenuous exercise, exposure to high environmental temperature, concomitant use of medications with anticholinergic activity.

ACTION

Blocks neuronal sodium channels, enhances GABA activity; antagonizes glutamate receptors and weakly inhibits carbonic anhydrase. **Therapeutic Effect:** Decreases seizure activity.

PHARMACOKINETICS

Rapidly absorbed after PO administration. Protein binding: 15%–41%. Metabolized in liver. Primarily excreted unchanged in urine. Removed by hemodialysis. **Half-life:** 21 hrs.

⌛ LIFESPAN CONSIDERATIONS

Pregnancy/Lactation: Unknown if distributed in breast milk. **Children:** No age-related precautions noted in pts older than 2 yrs. **Elderly:** Age-related renal impairment may require dosage adjustment.

INTERACTIONS

DRUG: Alcohol, other CNS depressants (e.g., **LORazepam, morphine, zolpidem**) may increase CNS depression. **CarBAMazepine, phenytoin, valproic acid** may decrease concentration/effects. **Carbonic anhydrase**

inhibitors may increase risk of kidney stone formation and severity of metabolic acidosis. May decrease effectiveness of **oral contraceptives. HERBAL: Evening primrose** may decrease seizure threshold. **FOOD:** None known. **LAB VALUES:** May reduce serum bicarbonate, increase ALT, AST.

AVAILABILITY (Rx)

Capsules (Sprinkle): 15 mg, 25 mg. **Tablets:** (Topamax, Topiragen) 25 mg, 50 mg, 100 mg, 200 mg.

◥ **Tablets:** (Topamax, Topiragen) 25 mg, 50 mg, 100 mg, 200 mg. **Capsules, Extended-Release (Trokendi XR):** 25 mg, 50 mg, 100 mg, 200 mg. **Qudexy XR:** 25 mg, 50 mg, 100 mg, 150 mg, 200 mg.

ADMINISTRATION/HANDLING

PO
• Do not break, crush, dissolve, or divide tablets (bitter taste). • Give without regard to meals. • Sprinkle capsules may either be swallowed whole or contents sprinkled on teaspoonful of soft food and swallowed immediately; do not chew. • **Trokendi XR:** Give whole. Do not sprinkle on food, chew, or crush. **Qudexy XR:** Swallow whole; may open and sprinkle on spoonful of soft food.

INDICATIONS/ROUTES/DOSAGE

Note: Do not abruptly discontinue; taper gradually to prevent rebound effects.

Adjunctive Treatment of Partial-Onset Seizures, Lennox-Gastaut Syndrome (LGS), Tonic-Clonic Seizures
PO: ADULTS, ELDERLY, CHILDREN 17 YRS AND OLDER: *(Immediate-Release):* Initially, 25 mg once or twice daily for 1 wk. May increase by 25–50 mg/day at wkly intervals. Usual maintenance dose: 100–200 mg twice daily (partial-onset) or 200 mg 2 times/day (primary tonic-clonic). **Maximum:** 400 mg/day. **CHILDREN 2–16 YRS:** Initially, 1–3 mg/kg/day to maximum of 25 mg at night for 1 wk. May increase by 1–3 mg/kg/day at wkly intervals given in 2 divided doses. **Maintenance:** 5–9

T

◆ Canadian trade name   ◥ Non-Crushable Drug   〓 High Alert drug mg/kg/day in 2 divided doses. **ADULTS, ELDERLY:** *(Extended-Release):* Initially, 25–50 mg/day. Increase by 25–50 mg/day at wkly intervals, up to 400 mg/day. **CHILDREN 2 YRS AND OLDER:** Initially, 25 mg (based on range of 1–3 mg/kg) once daily at bedtime for 1 wk. Increase dose by 1–3 mg/kg at 1–2 wk intervals up to 5–9 mg/kg once daily.

Monotherapy with Partial-Onset, Tonic-Clonic Seizures
PO: ADULTS, ELDERLY, CHILDREN 10 YRS AND OLDER: *(Immediate-Release):* Initially, 25 mg twice daily. May increase at wkly intervals up to 400 mg/day according to the following schedule: Wk 1, 25 mg twice daily. Wk 2, 50 mg twice daily. Wk 3, 75 mg twice daily. Wk 4, 100 mg twice daily. Wk 5, 150 mg twice daily. Wk 6, 200 mg twice daily. **CHILDREN 2–9 YRS:** Initially, 25 mg/day. Then 25 mg 2 times/day wk 2; then increase by 25–50 mg/day at wkly intervals up to minimum dose. (See table below.) **ADULTS, ELDERLY, CHILDREN 10 YRS OR OLDER:**

Wgt.	Minimum	Maximum
11 kg or less	150 mg/day in 2 divided doses	250 mg/day in 2 divided doses
12–22 kg	200 mg/day in 2 divided doses	300 mg/day in 2 divided doses
23–31 kg	200 mg/day in 2 divided doses	350 mg/day in 2 divided doses
32–38 kg	250 mg/day in 2 divided doses	350 mg/day in 2 divided doses
39 or greater	250 mg/day in 2 divided doses	400 mg/day in 2 divided doses

(Extended-Release): **(Qudexy XR, Trokendi XR):** Initially, 50 mg once daily. Increase by 50 mg/day at wkly intervals for first 4 wks, then by 100 mg/day for wks 5 and 6, up to 400 mg/day. **CHILDREN 2–9 YRS: (Qudexy XR): 6–9 YRS: (Trokendi XR):** Initially, 25 mg once daily in evening. May increase to 50 mg once daily in wk 2, then 25–50 mg/day at wkly intervals over 5–7 wks up to **minimum daily dose (32 KG OR MORE):** 250 mg; **(12–31 KG):** 200 mg; **(11 KG OR LESS):** 150 mg.

Maximum daily dose: (38 KG OR MORE): 400 mg; **(23–38 KG):** 350 mg; **(12–22 KG):** 300 mg; **(11 KG OR LESS):** 250 mg.

Migraine Prevention
PO: ADULTS, ELDERLY, CHILDREN 12 YRS AND OLDER: *(Immediate-Release):* Initially, 25 mg/day. May increase by 25 mg/day at 7-day intervals up to a total daily dose of 100 mg/day in 2 divided doses. *Extended-Release:* **(Qudexy XR):** Initially, 25 mg once daily at bedtime. May increase wkly by 25 mg increments up to 100 mg once daily.

Dosage in Renal Impairment
Reduce drug dosage by 50% and titrate more slowly in pts who have CrCl less than 70 mL/min.

Dosage in Hepatic Impairment
Use caution.

SIDE EFFECTS

Frequent (30%–10%): Drowsiness, dizziness, ataxia, nervousness, nystagmus, diplopia, paresthesia, nausea, tremor. **Occasional (9%–3%):** Confusion, breast pain, dysmenorrhea, dyspepsia, depression, asthenia, pharyngitis, weight loss, anorexia, rash, musculoskeletal pain, abdominal pain, difficulty with coordination, sinusitis, agitation, flu-like symptoms. **Rare (3%–2%):** Mood disturbances (e.g., irritability, depression), dry mouth, aggressive behavior, impaired heat regulation.

ADVERSE EFFECTS/TOXIC REACTIONS

Psychomotor slowing, impaired concentration, language problems (esp. word-finding difficulties), memory disturbances occur occasionally. Metabolic acidosis, suicidal ideation occur rarely.

NURSING CONSIDERATIONS

BASELINE ASSESSMENT

Seizures: Review history of seizure disorder (intensity, frequency, duration, level of consciousness). Initiate seizure precautions. Provide quiet, dark environment. Question for sensitivity to topiramate, pregnancy, use of other anticonvulsant medication (esp. carBAMazepine, valproic acid, phenytoin). **Migraine:** Assess pain location, duration, intensity. Assess renal function.

INTERVENTION/EVALUATION

Observe frequently for recurrence of seizure activity. Assess for clinical improvement (decrease in intensity/frequency of seizures). Monitor renal function tests, LFT. Assist with ambulation if dizziness occurs.

PATIENT/FAMILY TEACHING

• Avoid tasks that require alertness, motor skills until response to drug is established (may cause dizziness, drowsiness, impaired concentration). • Drowsiness usually diminishes with continued therapy. • Avoid use of alcohol, other CNS depressants. • Do not abruptly discontinue drug (may precipitate seizures). • Strict maintenance of drug therapy is essential for seizure control. • Do not chew, crush, dissolve, or divide tablets (bitter taste). • Maintain adequate fluid intake (decreases risk of renal stone formation). • Report blurred vision, eye pain. • Report suicidal ideation, depression, unusual behavior. • Use caution with activities that may increase core temperature (exposure to extreme heat, dehydration). • Instruct pt to use alternative/additional means of contraception (topiramate decreases effectiveness of oral contraceptives).

---

topotecan $\boxed{\text{HIGH ALERT}}$

toe-poe-**tee**-kan
(Hycamtin)

■ **BLACK BOX ALERT** ■ Must be administered by personnel trained in administration/handling of chemotherapeutic agents. Potent immunosuppressant; severe neutropenia (absolute neutrophil count [ANC] less than 500 cells/mm³) occurs in 60% of pts. Do not administer with baseline neutrophils less than 1,500 cells/mm³ and platelets less than 100,000 cells/mm³.

Do not confuse Hycamtin with Hycomine, Mycamine, or topotecan with irinotecan.

◆CLASSIFICATION

PHARMACOTHERAPEUTIC: DNA topoisomerase inhibitor. **CLINICAL:** Antineoplastic.

USES

Treatment of metastatic ovarian cancer, relapsed or refractory small cell lung cancer, recurrent or resistant cervical cancer (in combination with CISplatin). **OFF-LABEL:** Treatment of central nervous system lesions/lymphoma, Ewing's sarcoma, rhabdomyosarcoma, neuroblastoma, acute myeloid leukemia.

PRECAUTIONS

Contraindications: Hypersensitivity to topotecan. Baseline neutrophil count less than 1,500 cells/mm³ and platelet count less than 100,000 cells/mm³, severe myelosuppression. **Cautions:** Mild myelosuppression, renal impairment, breastfeeding, pregnancy, elderly pts. Pts at risk for developing interstitial lung disease (e.g., lung cancer, pulmonary fibrosis).

ACTION

Interacts with topoisomerase I, an enzyme that relieves torsional strain in DNA by inducing reversible single-strand breaks. Prevents religation of DNA strand, resulting in damage to double-strand DNA, cell death. **Therapeutic Effect:** Produces cytotoxic effect.

PHARMACOKINETICS

Hydrolyzed to active form after IV administration. Protein binding: 35%. Excreted in urine. **Half-life:** 2–3 hrs (increased in renal impairment).

⧖ LIFESPAN CONSIDERATIONS

Pregnancy/Lactation: May cause fetal harm. Avoid pregnancy; breastfeeding not recommended. **Children:** Safety and efficacy not established. **Elderly:**

T

Age-related renal impairment may require dosage adjustment.

INTERACTIONS

DRUG: Live virus vaccines may potentiate virus replication, increase vaccine side effects, decrease pt's antibody response to vaccine. **Other bone marrow depressants** may increase risk of myelosuppression. **HERBAL:** Echinacea may decrease effectiveness. **FOOD:** None known. **LAB VALUES:** May increase serum bilirubin, ALT, AST, alkaline phosphatase. May decrease RBC, leukocyte, neutrophil, platelet counts, Hgb, Hct.

AVAILABILITY (Rx)

Injection, Powder for Reconstitution: 4 mg (single-dose vial). **Injection, Solution:** 1 mg/mL (4 mL).

 Capsule: 0.25 mg, 1 mg.

ADMINISTRATION/HANDLING

◀ALERT▶ Because topotecan may be carcinogenic, mutagenic, teratogenic, handle drug with extreme care during preparation/administration.

PO
• May take with or without food.
• Swallow whole; do not break, crush, dissolve, or divide capsule. • Do not give replacement dose if vomiting occurs.

 IV

Reconstitution • Reconstitute each 4-mg vial (lyophilized powder) with 4 mL Sterile Water for Injection. • Further dilute with 50–100 mL 0.9% NaCl or D₅W. **Rate of Administration** • Administer as IV infusion over 30 min. • Extravasation associated with only mild local reactions (erythema, ecchymosis). **Storage** • Store vials (lyophilized powder) at room temperature; refrigerate diluted solution. Diluted solution for infusion stable for 24 hrs at room temperature.

▥ IV INCOMPATIBILITIES

Dexamethasone (Decadron), 5-fluorouracil, mitoMYcin (Mutamycin).

▥ IV COMPATIBILITIES

CARBOplatin (Paraplatin), CISplatin (Platinol AQ), cyclophosphamide (Cytoxan), DOXOrubicin (Adriamycin), etoposide (VePesid), gemcitabine (Gemzar), granisetron (Kytril), ondansetron (Zofran), PACLitaxel (Taxol), palonosetron (Aloxi), vinCRIStine (Oncovin).

INDICATIONS/ROUTES/DOSAGE

◀ALERT▶ Do not give topotecan if baseline neutrophil count is less than 1,500 cells/mm³ and platelet count is less than 100,000 cells/mm³. For retreatment, neutrophils should be greater than 1,000 cells/mm³, platelets greater than 100,000 cells/mm³, and Hgb 9 g/dL or greater.

Ovarian Carcinoma, Small Cell Lung Cancer
IV: ADULTS, ELDERLY: 1.5 mg/m²/day over 30 min for 5 consecutive days, beginning on day 1 of 21-day course. Minimum of 4 courses recommended. If severe neutropenia (neutrophil count less than 1,500 cells/mm³) occurs during treatment, reduce dose for subsequent courses by 0.25 mg/m² or administer filgrastim (G-CSF) no sooner than 24 hrs after last dose of topotecan.
PO *(Small Cell Lung Cancer):* **ADULTS, ELDERLY:** 2.3 mg/m²/day for 5 days; repeat q21days (dose rounded to nearest 0.25 mg). **For severe neutropenia or prolonged neutropenia, platelets less than 25,000 cells/mm³, recovery from grade 3 or 4 diarrhea:** Reduce dose by 0.4 mg/m²/day for subsequent cycles.

Cervical Cancer
IV: ADULTS, ELDERLY: 0.75 mg/m²/day for 3 days (followed by CISplatin 50 mg/m² on day 1 only). Repeat q21days (baseline neutrophil count greater than 1,500 cells/mm³ and platelet count greater than 100,000 cells/mm³). For severe febrile neutropenia (neutrophils less than 1,000 cells/mm³ with temperature of 38°C) or platelet count less than 25,000 cells/mm³: Reduce dose to 0.6 mg/m²/day for

subsequent cycles. If necessary, further decrease dose to 0.45 mg/m²/day.

Dosage in Renal Impairment
IV: No dosage adjustment is necessary in pts with mild renal impairment (CrCl 40–60 mL/min). For moderate renal impairment (CrCl 20–39 mL/min), give 0.75 mg/m².
PO: CrCl 30–49 mL/min: 1.5 mg/m²/day. May increase by 0.4 mg/m²/day following first cycle if no GI/hematologic toxicities occur. **CrCl less than 30 mL/min:** Decrease dose to 0.6 mg/m²/day. May increase by 0.4 mg/m²/day following first cycle if no GI/hematologic toxicities occur.

Dosage in Hepatic Impairment
No dose adjustment.

SIDE EFFECTS

Frequent (77%–21%): Nausea, vomiting, diarrhea, total alopecia, headache, dyspnea. **Occasional (9%–3%):** Paresthesia, constipation, abdominal pain. **Rare:** Anorexia, malaise, arthralgia, asthenia, myalgia.

ADVERSE EFFECTS/TOXIC REACTIONS

Severe neutropenia (absolute neutrophil count [ANC] less than 500 cells/mm³) occurs in 60% of pts (develops at median of 11 days after day 1 of initial therapy). Thrombocytopenia occurs in 26% of pts. Severe anemia (RBC count less than 8 g/dL) occurs in 40% of pts (develops at median of 15 days after day 1 of initial therapy). Severe diarrhea may occur.

NURSING CONSIDERATIONS

BASELINE ASSESSMENT

Offer emotional support. Assess CBC with differential before each dose. Myelosuppression may precipitate life-threatening hemorrhage, infection, anemia. If platelet count drops, minimize trauma to pt (e.g., IM injections, pt positioning). Premedicate with antiemetics on day of treatment, starting at least 30 min before administration.

INTERVENTION/EVALUATION

Assess for bleeding, signs of infection, anemia. Monitor hydration status, I&O, serum electrolytes (severe diarrhea, vomiting are common side effects). Monitor CBC for evidence of myelosuppression. Monitor renal function, LFT. Assess response to medication; provide interventions (e.g., small, frequent meals; antiemetics for nausea/vomiting). Question for complaints of headache. Assess breathing pattern for evidence of dyspnea.

PATIENT/FAMILY TEACHING

• Hair loss is reversible but new hair may have different color, texture. • Diarrhea may cause dehydration, electrolyte depletion. • Antiemetic and antidiarrheal medications may reduce side effects. • Notify physician if diarrhea, vomiting, persistent fever, bruising/bleeding, yellowing of eyes/skin occur. • Do not have immunizations without physician's approval (drug lowers resistance). • Avoid contact with those who have recently received live virus vaccine.

---

torsemide

tore-se-myde
(Demadex)
Do not confuse torsemide with furosemide.

◆CLASSIFICATION

PHARMACOTHERAPEUTIC: Loop diuretic. **CLINICAL:** Antihypertensive, diuretic.

USES

Treatment of hypertension either alone or in combination with other antihypertensives. (Not recommended for initial treatment of hypertension.) Edema associated with HF, hepatic/renal impairment.

PRECAUTIONS

Contraindications: Hypersensitivity to torsemide or any sulfonylurea. Anuria,

---

other sulfonylureas. **Cautions:** Pts with cirrhosis, hypotension, hypokalemia.

ACTION

Enhances excretion of sodium, chloride, potassium, water at ascending limb of loop of Henle. Reduces plasma, extracellular fluid volume. **Therapeutic Effect:** Produces diuresis, relieves edema; lowers B/P.

PHARMACOKINETICS

Route	Onset	Peak	Duration
PO, IV (diuresis)	30–60 min	1–2 hrs	6–8 hrs

Rapidly, well absorbed from GI tract. Protein binding: 97%–99%. Metabolized in liver. Primarily excreted in urine. Not removed by hemodialysis. **Half-life:** 2–4 hrs.

⧖ LIFESPAN CONSIDERATIONS

Pregnancy/Lactation: Unknown if drug is distributed in breast milk. **Children:** Safety and efficacy not established. **Elderly:** No age-related precautions noted.

INTERACTIONS

DRUG: NSAIDs (e.g., ibuprofen, ketorolac, naproxen), aspirin may increase risk of renal impairment. May increase risk of **digoxin** toxicity associated with torsemide-induced hypokalemia. May increase risk of **lithium** toxicity. **Other hypokalemia-causing medications (e.g., HCTZ)** may increase risk of hypokalemia. **HERBAL: Ephedra, ginseng, yohimbe, licorice** may worsen hypertension. **Black cohosh** may increase antihypertensive effect. **FOOD:** None known. **LAB VALUES:** May increase serum BUN, creatinine, uric acid. May decrease serum calcium, chloride, magnesium, potassium, sodium.

AVAILABILITY (Rx)

Injection Solution: 10 mg/mL. **Tablets:** 5 mg, 10 mg, 20 mg, 100 mg.

ADMINISTRATION/HANDLING

 IV

Rate of Administration

◀**ALERT**▶ Flush IV line with 0.9% NaCl before and following administration.
• May give undiluted as IV push over minimum of 2 min.
Storage • Store at room temperature.

PO

• Give without regard to food. Give with food to avoid GI upset, preferably with breakfast (prevents nocturia).

▦ IV COMPATIBILITY

Milrinone (Primacor).

INDICATIONS/ROUTES/DOSAGE

Hypertension

PO: ADULTS, ELDERLY: Initially, 2.5–5 mg/day. May increase to 10 mg/day if no response in 4–6 wks. If still not effective, add additional antihypertensive. Range: 5–10 mg/day.

Edema Associated with HF

PO, IV: ADULTS, ELDERLY: Initially, 10–20 mg/day. May increase by approximately doubling dose until desired therapeutic effect is attained. **Maximum dose:** PO: 200 mg; IV: 100–200 mg.

Edema Associated with Chronic Renal Failure

PO, IV: ADULTS, ELDERLY: Initially, 20 mg/day. May increase by approximately doubling dose until desired therapeutic effect is attained. **Maximum dose:** 200 mg/day.

Hepatic Cirrhosis

PO: ADULTS, ELDERLY: Initially, 5–10 mg/day given with aldosterone antagonist or potassium-sparing diuretic. May increase by approximately doubling dose until desired therapeutic effect is attained. **Maximum single dose:** 40 mg.

Dosage in Renal/Hepatic Impairment

No dose adjustment.

T

SIDE EFFECTS

Frequent (10%–4%): Headache, dizziness, rhinitis. **Occasional (3%–1%):** Asthenia, insomnia, nervousness, diarrhea, constipation, nausea, dyspepsia, edema, EKG changes, pharyngitis, cough, arthralgia, myalgia. **Rare (Less Than 1%):** Syncope, hypotension, arrhythmias.

ADVERSE EFFECTS/TOXIC REACTIONS

Ototoxicity may occur with too-rapid IV administration or with high doses; must be given slowly. Overdose produces acute, profound water loss, volume/electrolyte depletion, dehydration, decreased blood volume, circulatory collapse.

NURSING CONSIDERATIONS

BASELINE ASSESSMENT

Obtain serum electrolyte levels, esp. potassium. Obtain baseline weight; check for edema. Assess lungs for crackles, signs of HF. Obtain B/P.

INTERVENTION/EVALUATION

Monitor B/P, serum electrolytes (esp. potassium), I&O, weight. Notify physician of any hearing abnormality. Note extent of diuresis. Assess lungs for rales. Check for signs of edema, particularly of dependent areas. Although less potassium is lost with torsemide than with furosemide, assess for signs of hypokalemia (change of muscle strength, tremor, muscle cramps, altered mental status, cardiac arrhythmias).

PATIENT/FAMILY TEACHING

• Take medication in morning to prevent nocturia. • Expect increased urinary volume, frequency. • Report palpitations, muscle weakness, cramps, nausea, dizziness. • Do not take other medications (including OTC drugs) without consulting physician. • Eat foods high in potassium such as whole grains (cereals), legumes, meat, bananas, apricots, orange juice, potatoes (white, sweet), raisins.

trabectedin

tra-**bek**-te-din
(Yondelis)

◆CLASSIFICATION

PHARMACOTHERAPEUTIC: Alkylating agent. **CLINICAL:** Antineoplastic.

USES

Treatment of unresectable or metastatic soft tissue sarcoma (liposarcoma or leiomyosarcoma) in pts who have received a prior anthracycline-containing regimen.

PRECAUTIONS

Contraindications: Hypersensitivity reaction, anaphylactic reaction to trabectedin. **Cautions:** Baseline anemia, neutropenia, thrombocytopenia; chronic liver disease, cirrhosis, hepatic impairment, hepatitis; renal impairment; history of DVT, pulmonary embolism; recent MI, cardiomyopathy, HF. Concomitant use of strong CYP3A inducers, strong CYP3A inhibitors not recommended.

ACTION

Binds to guanine residues in the minor groove of DNA, leading to cell cycle disruption and cellular death. **Therapeutic Effect:** Inhibits tumor cell growth and metastasis.

PHARMACOKINETICS

Widely distributed. Metabolized in liver. Protein binding: 97%. Excreted in feces (58%), urine (6%). Hemodialysis not expected to enhance elimination. **Half-life:** 175 hrs.

⌛ LIFESPAN CONSIDERATIONS

Pregnancy/Lactation: Avoid pregnancy; may cause fetal harm/malformations. Female pts of reproductive potential should use effective contraception during treatment and up to 2 mos after discontinuation. Breastfeeding not recommended. **Males:** Male pts with female partners of reproductive potential should use

T

barrier methods, abstinence during treatment and up to 5 mos after discontinuation. May impair fertility in both females and males. **Children:** Safety and efficacy not established. **Elderly:** Safety and efficacy not established.

INTERACTIONS

DRUG: **Strong CYP3A inducers** (e.g., **carBAMazepine, PHENobarbital, rifAMPin)** may decrease concentration/effect. **Strong CYP3A inhibitors** (e.g., **clarithromycin, ketoconazole, ritonavir)** may increase concentration/effects. **HERBAL:** **St. John's wort** may decrease concentration/effect. **FOOD:** **Grapefruit products** may increase concentration/effect. **LAB VALUES:** May decrease Hgb, Hct, platelets, neutrophils, RBCs; serum albumin, phosphate. May increase serum alkaline phosphatase, ALT, AST, bilirubin, CPK, creatinine. May reduce diagnostic effect of *Coccidioides immitis* skin test.

AVAILABILITY (Rx)

Powder for Reconstitution: 1 mg.

ADMINISTRATION/HANDLING

 IV

Reconstitution • Contents are hazardous; use cytotoxic precautions during handling and disposal. • Reconstitute with 20 mL Sterile Water for Injection for final concentration of 0.05 mg/mL. • Shake until fully dissolved. • Visually inspect solution for particulate matter or discoloration. Solution should appear clear, colorless to pale brownish-yellow in color. Discard if solution is discolored or particles are observed. • Dilute in 500 mL 0.9% NaCl or D_5W bag. • See manufacturer guidelines for materials/containers that are compatible with diluted solution.

Infusion Guidelines • Premedicate with dexamethasone 20 mg IV (or appropriate corticosteroid) 30 min prior to each infusion. • Infuse diluted solution immediately after reconstitution. • Use an in-line, 0.2-micron polyethersulfone filter. • Infuse via dedicated central venous line using an infusion pump.

Rate of Administration • Infuse over 24 hrs.

Storage • Refrigerate unused vials. • Diluted solution must be administered within 30 hrs of reconstitution.

🔳 IV INCOMPATIBILITIES

Do not mix or infuse with other medications.

INDICATIONS/ROUTES/DOSAGE

Liposarcoma, Leiomyosarcoma
IV: **ADULTS, ELDERLY:** 1.5 mg/m^2 once q3wks until disease progression or unacceptable toxicity.

Dosage in Renal Impairment
CrCl greater than or equal to 30 mL/min: No dose adjustment.
CrCl greater less than 30 mL/min or end-stage renal disease: Not specified; use caution.

Dosage in Hepatic Impairment
Mild impairment: No dose adjustment. **Moderate impairment:** 0.9 mg/m^2 once q3wks. **Severe impairment:** Not recommended.

Dose Reduction for Normal Hepatic Function or Mild Hepatic Impairment
Initial dose: 1.5 mg/m^2 once q3wks. **First dose reduction:** 1.2 mg/m^2 once q3wks. **Second dose reduction:** 1 mg/m^2 once q3wks.

Dose Reduction for Moderate Hepatic Impairment
Initial dose: 0.9 mg/m^2 once q3wks. **First dose reduction:** 0.6 mg/m^2 once q3wks. **Second dose reduction:** 0.3 mg/m^2 once q3wks.

Dose Modification
Hepatotoxicity
Serum ALT/AST greater than 2.5 times upper limit of normal (ULN): Delay next dose for up to 3 wks.

Serum alkaline phosphatase greater than 2.5 times ULN; serum ALT/AST greater than 5 times ULN; total serum bilirubin greater than ULN: Delay next dose for up to 3 wks, then resume at reduced dose level.

Hematologic Toxicity

Absolute neutrophil count (ANC) less than 1,500 cells/mm³: Delay next dose for up to 3 wks.

ANC less than 1,000 cells/mm³ with fever or infection; ANC less than 500 cells/mm³ lasting more than 5 days: Delay next dose for up to 3 wks, then resume at reduced dose level.

Platelet count less than 100,000 cells/mm³: Delay next dose for up to 3 wks.

Platelet count less than 25,000 cells/mm³: Delay next dose for up to 3 wks, then resume at reduced dose level.

Nonhematologic Toxicity

CPK greater than 2.5 times ULN: Delay next dose for up to 3 wks.

CPK greater than 5 times ULN: Delay next dose for up to 3 wks, then resume at reduced dose level.

Decreased LVEF less than lower limit of normal or clinical evidence of cardiomyopathy: Delay next dose for up to 3 wks.

Decreased LVEF with an absolute decrease of 10% or more from baseline and less than lower limit of normal, or clinical evidence of cardiomyopathy: Delay next dose for up to 3 wks, then resume at reduced dose level.

Any other grade 3 or 4 reaction: Delay next dose for up to 3 wks, then resume at reduced dose level.

Permanent Discontinuation

Permanently discontinue for persistent adverse effects requiring a delay of treatment for more than 3 wks; continued adverse effects after reducing dose to 1 mg/m² in pts with normal hepatic function, or 0.3 mg/m² in pts with preexisting moderate hepatic impairment; severe hepatic dysfunction with bilirubin 2 times ULN, and ALT/AST 3 times ULN, and alkaline phosphatase less than 2 times ULN in prior treatment cycle in pts with baseline normal hepatic function; exacerbation of hepatic dysfunction in pts with preexisting moderate hepatic impairment.

SIDE EFFECTS

Frequent (75%–25%): Nausea, fatigue, asthenia, malaise, vomiting, decreased appetite, constipation, diarrhea, peripheral edema, dyspnea, headache. **Occasional (15%–11%):** Insomnia, arthralgia, myalgia, paresthesia.

ADVERSE EFFECTS/TOXIC REACTIONS

Anemia, neutropenia, thrombocytopenia are expected responses to therapy. Life-threatening, sometimes fatal, neutropenic sepsis (3% of pts) may occur. Grade 3 or 4 neutropenia (43% of pts), febrile neutropenia (5% of pts) were reported. Fatal rhabdomyolysis, muscular toxicity may result in renal failure. CPK elevation occurred in 32% of pts; grade 3 or 4 CPK elevation occurred in 6% of pts. Hepatotoxicity, including hepatic failure, may occur. LFT elevation occurred in 70%–90% of pts. Cardiomyopathy including decreased ejection fraction, diastolic dysfunction, HF, right ventricular dysfunction reported in 6% of pts; grade 3 or 4 cardiomyopathy reported in 4% of pts. Drug extravasation may result in tissue necrosis requiring debridement. Other adverse effects may include phlebitis (15% of pts), pulmonary embolism (less than 10% of pts), hypersensitivity reaction.

NURSING CONSIDERATIONS

BASELINE ASSESSMENT

Obtain ANC, CBC, CPK, BMP, LFT; vital signs prior to each dose and periodically thereafter. Obtain baseline echocardiogram to assess LVEF. Verify placement of central venous line. Receive full medication history. Assess nutritional status. Question history of DVT, pulmonary embolism, cardiac disease, recent MI; renal/hepatic impairment; prior hypersensitivity reaction. Screen for active infection. Offer emotional support.

INTERVENTION/EVALUATION

Monitor ANC, CBC for anemia, neutropenia, thrombocytopenia; CPK, serum creatinine for rhabdomyolysis, renal failure; LFT for hepatotoxicity; BMP for electrolyte imbalance (esp. in pts with diarrhea, vomiting, malnutrition); vital signs. Assess LVEF by echocardiogram at 2- to 3-mo intervals (or more frequently in pts with cardiomyopathy). Diligently screen for infections, sepsis. Monitor for DVT (leg or arm pain/swelling), rhabdomyolysis (decreased urinary output, amber-colored urine, fatigue, muscle pain/weakness), pulmonary embolism (sudden chest pain, dyspnea, hypoxia, tachycardia), HF (dyspnea, fatigue, palpitations, edema, exercise intolerance); hypersensitivity reaction; side effects of dexamethasone (e.g., hyperglycemia, weight loss, decreased appetite). Monitor I&O. Monitor daily pattern of bowel activity, stool consistency.

PATIENT/FAMILY TEACHING

• Treatment may depress your immune system and reduce your ability to fight infection. Report symptoms of infection such as body aches, chills, cough, fatigue, fever. Avoid those with active infection. • Blood levels, echocardiograms will be routinely monitored. • Life-threatening events, such as heart failure (shortness of breath, fast or slow heart rate, exercise intolerance, swelling of the ankles or legs), liver injury or failure (abdominal pain, easy bruising, clay-colored stools, dark-amber urine, fatigue, loss of appetite, yellowing of skin or eyes), muscle toxicity (muscle pain/weakness, kidney failure), blood clots in lungs (difficulty breathing, fast heart rate, chest pain), may occur. • Avoid pregnancy. Female pts of childbearing potential should use effective contraception during treatment and for at least 2 mos after last dose. Do not breastfeed. Male pts with female partners of reproductive potential should use condoms during sexual activity

for at least 5 mos after last dose. • Treatment may impair fertility. • Avoid grapefruit products, herbal supplements. • Do not receive live vaccines.

---

traMADol

tram-a-dol
(Apo-TraMADol ✦, ConZip, Synapryn FusePaq, Ultram)
Do not confuse traMADol with tapentadol, Toradol, or Trandate, or Ultram with Ultracet.

FIXED-COMBINATION(S)

Ultracet: traMADol/acetaminophen (a non-narcotic analgesic): 37.5 mg/325 mg.

◆CLASSIFICATION

PHARMACOTHERAPEUTIC: Centrally acting synthetic opioid. **CLINICAL:** Analgesic.

USES

Immediate-Release: Management of moderate to moderately severe pain. **Extended-Release:** Around-the-clock management of moderate to moderately severe pain for extended period.

PRECAUTIONS

Contraindications: Hypersensitivity to traMADol, opioids. **(Additional) Immediate-Release, Extended-Release:** Acute alcohol intoxication, concurrent use of centrally acting analgesics, hypnotics, opioids, psychotropic drugs, hypersensitivity to opioids. **(Additional) ConZip:** Severe/acute bronchial asthma, hypercapnia, significant respiratory depression. **Caution:** CNS depression, anoxia, advanced hepatic cirrhosis, respiratory depression, elevated ICP, history of seizures or risk for seizures, hepatic/renal impairment, treatment of acute abdominal conditions, opioid-dependent pts, head injury, myxedema, hypothyroidism, hypoadrenalism, pregnancy. Avoid use in pts who are

T

suicidal or addiction prone, emotionally disturbed, depressed, heavy alcohol users, elderly pts, debilitated pts.

ACTION

Binds to mu-opioid receptors, inhibits reuptake of norepinephrine, serotonin, inhibiting ascending and descending pain pathways. **Therapeutic Effect:** Reduces pain.

PHARMACOKINETICS

Route	Onset	Peak	Duration
PO	Less than 1 hr	2–3 hrs	9 hrs

Rapidly, almost completely absorbed after PO administration. Protein binding: 20%. Metabolized in liver (reduced in pts with advanced cirrhosis). Primarily excreted in urine. Minimally removed by hemodialysis. **Half-life:** 6–7 hrs (increased in renal/hepatic failure).

☒ LIFESPAN CONSIDERATIONS

Pregnancy/Lactation: Crosses placenta. Distributed in breast milk. **Children:** Safety and efficacy not established in children 16 yrs or less. **Elderly:** Age-related renal impairment may require dosage adjustment.

INTERACTIONS

DRUG: Alcohol, other CNS depressants (e.g., LORazepam, morphine, zolpidem) may increase CNS depression. CarBAMazepine decreases concentration/effects. CYP2D6 inhibitors (e.g., PARoxetine), CYP3A4 inhibitors (e.g., clarithromycin, ketoconazole, ritonavir), triptans, selective serotonin reuptake inhibitors (SSRIs), tricyclic antidepressants (e.g., amitriptyline, doxepin) may increase risk of seizures, risk of serotonin syndrome. **HERBAL:** Gotu kola, kava kava, St. John's wort, valerian may increase CNS depression. St. John's wort may increase risk of serotonin syndrome. **FOOD:** None known. **LAB VALUES:** May increase serum creatinine, ALT, AST. May decrease Hgb. May cause proteinuria.

AVAILABILITY (Rx)

Tablets (Immediate-Release) (Ultram): 50 mg. **Capsules (Variable-Release) (ConZip):** 100 mg (25 mg immediate/75 mg extended), 200 mg (50 mg immediate/150 mg extended), 300 mg (50 mg immediate/250 mg extended). **Suspension, Oral (Synapryn FusePaq):** 10 mg/mL.

🐄 **Tablets (Extended-Release) (Ultram ER):** 100 mg, 200 mg, 300 mg.

ADMINISTRATION/HANDLING

PO

• Give without regard to meals but consistently with or without meals. • Extended-Release: Swallow whole; do not break, crush, dissolve, or divide.

INDICATIONS/ROUTES/DOSAGE

Moderate to Moderately Severe Pain
PO *(Immediate-Release):* ADULTS, ELDERLY, CHILDREN 17 YRS AND OLDER: 50–100 mg q4–6h. **Maximum:** 400 mg/day for pts 75 yrs and younger; 300 mg/day for pts older than 75 yrs.

PO *(Extended-Release):* ADULTS, ELDERLY, CHILDREN 18 YRS AND OLDER: Initially, 100 mg once daily. Titrate q5days. **Maximum:** 300 mg once daily.

Dosage in Renal Impairment
Immediate-Release: For pts with CrCl less than 30 mL/min, increase dosing interval to q12h. **Maximum:** 200 mg/day. Do not use extended-release.

Dosage in Hepatic Impairment
Immediate-Release: Cirrhosis: Dosage is decreased to 50 mg q12h. Do not use extended-release with severe hepatic impairment.

SIDE EFFECTS

Frequent (25%–15%): Dizziness, vertigo, nausea, constipation, headache, drowsiness. **Occasional (10%–5%):** Vomiting, pruritus, CNS stimulation (e.g., nervousness, anxiety, agitation, tremor, euphoria, mood swings, hallucinations), asthenia, diaphoresis, dyspepsia, dry mouth, diarrhea. **Rare (less than 5%):** Malaise, vasodilation, anorexia, flatulence, rash,

T

---

blurred vision, urinary retention/frequency, menopausal symptoms.

ADVERSE EFFECTS/TOXIC REACTIONS

Seizures reported in pts receiving traMA-Dol within recommended dosage range. May have prolonged duration of action, cumulative effect in pts with hepatic/renal impairment, serotonin syndrome (agitation, hallucinations, tachycardia, hyperreflexia). May cause suicidal ideation and behavior.

NURSING CONSIDERATIONS

BASELINE ASSESSMENT

Assess onset, type, location, duration of pain. Assess drug history, esp. carBAMazepine, analgesics, CNS depressants, MAOIs. Review past medical history, esp. epilepsy, seizures. Assess renal function, LFT.

INTERVENTION/EVALUATION

Monitor pulse, B/P, renal/hepatic function. Assist with ambulation if dizziness, vertigo occurs. Dry crackers, cola may relieve nausea. Palpate bladder for urinary retention. Monitor daily pattern of bowel activity, stool consistency. Sips of water may relieve dry mouth. Assess for clinical improvement, record onset of relief of pain.

PATIENT/FAMILY TEACHING

• May cause dependence. • Avoid alcohol, OTC medications (analgesics, sedatives). • May cause drowsiness, dizziness, blurred vision. • Avoid tasks requiring alertness, motor skills until response to drug is established. • Report severe constipation, difficulty breathing, excessive sedation, seizures, muscle weakness, tremors, chest pain, palpitations.

trametinib

tra-**me**-ti-nib
(Mekinist)
Do not confuse trametinib with imatinib or tipifarnib.

◆CLASSIFICATION

PHARMACOTHERAPEUTIC: Kinase inhibitor. **CLINICAL:** Antineoplastic.

USES

Used as a single agent or in combination with dabrafenib for treatment of unresectable or metastatic melanoma with BRAF V600E or V600L mutations, as detected by FDA-approved test. Single-agent regimen is not indicated in pts who have received prior BRAF-inhibitor therapy.

PRECAUTIONS

Contraindications: Hypersensitivity to trametinib. **Cautions:** Cardiac/pulmonary impairment, preexisting diabetes or diabetes.

ACTION

Inhibits mitogen-activated extracellular kinase (MEK). **Therapeutic Effect:** Inhibits tumor cell growth, causing apoptosis.

PHARMACOKINETICS

Rapidly absorbed after PO administration. Protein binding: 97.4%. Peak plasma concentration: 1.5 hrs. Metabolized in liver. Excreted in feces (80%), urine (20%). **Half-life:** 3.9–4.8 days.

⧗ LIFESPAN CONSIDERATIONS

Pregnancy/Lactation: Avoid pregnancy. May cause fetal harm. Must use effective nonhormonal contraception during treatment and for at least 4 wks after discontinuation (intrauterine device, barrier methods). Unknown if distributed in breast milk. Must either discontinue breastfeeding or discontinue treatment. **Children:** Safety and efficacy not established. **Elderly:** May have increased risk of adverse effects, skin lesions, primary malignancies. **Males:** May decrease sperm count.

INTERACTIONS

DRUG: May decrease levels/effect of **ARIPiprazole, ibrutinib, SAXagliptin, simeprevir. HERBAL:** None known. **FOOD:** High-fat meals may decrease absorption/effect. **LAB VALUES: SINGLE**

REGIMEN: May increase serum alkaline phosphatase, ALT, AST. May decrease serum albumin; Hgb, Hct. **COMBINATION REGIMEN:** May increase serum alkaline phosphatase, ALT, AST, bilirubin, calcium, creatinine, glucose, GGT, potassium. May decrease Hgb, Hct, leukocytes, lymphocytes, neutrophils, platelets; serum albumin, calcium, magnesium, phosphorus, potassium, sodium.

AVAILABILITY (Rx)

Tablets: 0.5 mg, 2 mg.

ADMINISTRATION/HANDLING

PO

• Administer at least 1 hr before or 2 hrs after meal.

INDICATIONS/ROUTES/DOSAGE

Melanoma

PO: ADULTS/ELDERLY: 2 mg once daily (either as a single agent or in combination with dabrafenib). Continue until disease progression or unacceptable toxicity.

Dose Reduction Schedule

Trametinib Regimen: FIRST DOSE REDUCTION: 1.5 mg once daily. **SECOND DOSE REDUCTION:** 1 mg once daily. Discontinue if unable to tolerate 1-mg dose.
Dabrafenib Combination Regimen: FIRST DOSE REDUCTION: 100 mg twice daily. **SECOND DOSE REDUCTION:** 75 mg twice daily.
THIRD DOSE REDUCTION: 50 mg twice daily. Discontinue if unable to tolerate 50-mg dose.

Dose Modification

Based on Common Terminology Criteria for Adverse Events (CTCAE) grading 1–4.
Cardiac: ASYMPTOMATIC DECREASE IN LEFT VENTRICULAR EJECTION FRACTION (LVEF) GREATER THAN 10% FROM BASELINE: Withhold trametinib up to 4 wks. If LVEF improved, resume at lower dose level. Discontinue if not improved. Do not modify dabrafenib dose. **SYMPTOMATIC HF OR DECREASE IN LVEF GREATER THAN 20% FROM BASELINE:** Discontinue

trametinib. Withhold dabrafenib until improved, then resume at lower dose level.
CUTANEOUS EVENTS: INTOLERABLE GRADE 2 SKIN TOXICITY OR GRADE 3–4 TOXICITY: Withhold both regimens for up to 3 wks. If improved, resume both at lower dose level. Discontinue both regimens if not improved. **FEBRILE EVENTS: FEVER OF 101.3°F–104°F:** Do not modify trametinib dose. Withhold dabrafenib until fever resolved, then resume at either same dose or lower dose level.
FEVER GREATER THAN 104°F OR FEVER COMPLICATED BY DEHYDRATION, HYPOTENSION, RENAL FAILURE: Withhold trametinib until resolved, then resume at either same dose or lower dose level. Withhold dabrafenib until resolved, then resume at either lower dose level or discontinue.
New Primary Malignancies: CUTANEOUS: No changes required for either regimen. **NONCUTANEOUS:** Do not change trametinib dose. Discontinue dabrafenib in pts who develop RAS mutation-positive malignancies.
Nonspecific Adverse Reactions: INTOLERABLE GRADE 2 OR ANY GRADE 3: Withhold both regimens until resolved to grade 0–1, then resume at lower dose level. Discontinue both regimens if not improved.
FIRST OCCURRENCE OF ANY GRADE 4 REACTIONS: Withhold both regimens until resolved to grade 0–1, then resume at lower dose level or discontinue.
Ocular Toxicities: GRADE 2–3 RETINAL PIGMENT EPITHELIAL DETACHMENTS: Withhold trametinib up to 3 wks. If improved to grade 0–1, resume at lower dose level. Discontinue if not improved. Do not modify dabrafenib. **RETINAL VEIN OCCLUSION:** Discontinue trametinib. Do not modify dabrafenib. **UVEITIS OR IRITIS:** Do not modify trametinib. Withhold dabrafenib for up to 6 wks. If improved to grade 0–1, then resume at same dose level. Discontinue if not improved.
Pulmonary: INTERSTITIAL LUNG DISEASE: Discontinue trametinib. Do not modify dabrafenib.

T

Venous Thromboembolism (Uncomplicated DVT or PE): Withhold trametinib for up to 3 wks. If improved to grade 0–1, then resume at lower dose level. Discontinue if not improved. Do not modify dabrafenib. **LIFE-THREATENING PE:** Discontinue both regimens.

Dosage in Renal/Hepatic Impairment
No dose adjustment.

SIDE EFFECTS

Single Regimen:
Frequent (57%–32%): Rash, diarrhea, lymphedema, peripheral edema. **Occasional (19%–10%):** Dermatitis acneiform, hypertension, stomatitis, mouth ulceration, mucosal ulceration, abdominal pain, dry skin, pruritus, paronychia, folliculitis, cellulitis, dizziness, dysgeusia, blurred vision, dry eye.
Combination Regimen:
Frequent (71%–40%): Pyrexia, chills, fatigue, rash, nausea, vomiting. **Occasional (36%–11%):** Diarrhea, abdominal pain, peripheral edema, headache, cough, arthralgia, night sweats, myalgia, constipation, decreased appetite, back pain, dry skin, insomnia, dermatitis acneiform, dizziness, muscle spasm, extremity pain, actinic keratosis, erythema, oral/throat pain, urinary tract infection, pruritus, dry mouth, dehydration.

ADVERSE EFFECTS/TOXIC REACTIONS

Primary malignancies including basal or squamous cell carcinoma, keratoacanthoma, pancreatic adenocarcinoma, glioblastoma (brain cancer) reported. DVT, PE reported in 9% of pts. May increase cell proliferation of wild-type BRAF melanoma or new malignant melanomas. Serious, sometimes fatal intracranial or gastric bleeding occurred in 5% of pts. Other hemorrhagic events may include conjunctival/gingival/rectal/hemorrhoidal/vaginal bleeding, epistaxis (nosebleed), melena (bloody stools). Cardiomyopathy, HF, decreased LVEF reported in 7%–9% of pts. Ocular toxicities such as retinal

vein occlusion, retinal detachment, vision loss, glaucoma, uveitis, iritis reported. Cough, dyspnea, hypoxia, pleural effusion, infiltrates may indicate interstitial lung disease. Serious febrile reactions may lead to renal failure, severe dehydration, hypotension, rigors. Skin toxicities including palmar-plantar erythrodysesthesia syndrome (PPES), papilloma have occurred. Hyperglycemia reported in 2%–5% of pts. Other effects may include hypertension, rhabdomyolysis. May prolong QT interval of cardiac cycle.

NURSING CONSIDERATIONS

BASELINE ASSESSMENT
Obtain baseline CBC, serum metabolic panel (with LFT), magnesium, phosphate, ionized calcium, capillary glucose level, vital signs. Obtain BRAF V600E mutation history, negative pregnancy status, ophthalmologic exam with visual acuity, echocardiogram, EKG before initiating treatment. Assess skin for moles, lesions, papillomas. Question current breastfeeding status. Receive full medication history including herbal products. Question any history as listed in PRECAUTIONS. Offer emotional support.

INTERVENTION/EVALUATION
Offer emotional support. Monitor CBC, serum electrolytes, capillary blood glucose, stool characteristics routinely. Monitor for signs of hyperglycemia (thirst, polyuria, confusion, dehydration). Assess skin for new lesions, toxicities every 2 mos during treatment and at least 6 mos after discontinuation. Obtain LVEF by echocardiogram 1 mo after initiation, then every 2–3 mos; ophthalmologic exam with any vision changes. Immediately report any altered mental status, bleeding events, vision changes, eye pain/swelling/infection, fever, urinary changes. Screen for bleeding of any kind. If dyspnea or leg swelling occurs, contact physician and initiate appropriate medical therapy (may require oxygen therapy, EKG, or radiologic test to rule out DVT, PE, or ILD).

PATIENT/FAMILY TEACHING

• Blood work, cardiac function tests, eye exams will be performed routinely. • Treatment may lead to heart failure, vision changes, lung complications, difficulty breathing, fever, skin toxicities (such as severe rash, peeling), high blood pressure, severe diarrhea. • Report bloody stools/urine, heavy menstruation, or nosebleeds. • Do not breastfeed. • Avoid pregnancy; nonhormonal contraception should be used during treatment and up to 4 wks after treatment. • Take medication at least 1 hr before or at least 2 hrs after meal (food reduces absorption). • Report any increased urination, thirst, confusion (may indicate high blood sugar); chest pain, eye pain, fever, leg swelling, new skin moles or lesions, vision changes. • Minimize sunlight exposure. • Males may experience a decreased sperm count. • Report any newly prescribed medications.

---

trastuzumab

tras-**too**-zoo-mab
(Herceptin)

■ **BLACK BOX ALERT** ■
Anaphylactic reaction, infusion reaction, acute respiratory distress syndrome have been associated with fatalities. Reduction in left ventricular ejection fraction, severe heart failure may result in thrombus formation, stroke, cardiac death. Exposure during pregnancy may result in pulmonary hypoplasia, skeletal malformations, neonatal death.
Do not confuse trastuzumab with ado-trastuzumab.

♦CLASSIFICATION

PHARMACOTHERAPEUTIC: HER2 receptor antagonist. Monoclonal antibody. **CLINICAL:** Antineoplastic.

USES

Treatment of HER2-overexpressing breast cancer (adjuvant), metastatic breast cancer,

metastatic gastric or gastroesophageal junction adenocarcinoma (in pts without prior treatment). **OFF-LABEL:** Treatment of HER2-positive metastatic breast cancer in pts who have not received prior anti-HER2 therapy or in pts whose cancer has progressed on prior trastuzumab therapy (in combination with lapatinib).

PRECAUTIONS

Contraindications: Hypersensitivity to trastuzumab. **Cautions:** Preexisting cardiac disease or dysfunction, preexisting pulmonary disease or extensive pulmonary tumor involvement, pregnancy.

ACTION

Binds to HER2 protein, overexpressed in 25%–30% of primary breast cancers, inhibiting proliferation of tumor cells. **Therapeutic Effect:** Inhibits growth of tumor cells, mediates antibody-dependent cellular cytotoxicity.

PHARMACOKINETICS

Half-life: 11–23 days.

⌛ LIFESPAN CONSIDERATIONS

Pregnancy/Lactation: Women should use effective contraception during treatment and for at least 7 mos after discontinuation. Unknown if distributed in breast milk. Breastfeeding not recommended. **Children:** Safety and efficacy not established. **Elderly:** Age-related cardiac dysfunction may require dosage adjustment.

INTERACTIONS

DRUG: None significant. **HERBAL:** None significant. **FOOD:** None known. **LAB VALUES:** None significant.

AVAILABILITY (Rx)

Injection, Powder for Reconstitution: 440 mg.

ADMINISTRATION/HANDLING
IV

Reconstitution • Reconstitute with 20 mL Bacteriostatic Water for Injection to yield concentration of 21 mg/mL.

♦ Canadian trade name   Non-Crushable Drug   High Alert drug

• Add calculated dose to 250 mL 0.9% NaCl (do not use D_5W). • Gently mix contents in bag.
Rate of Administration • Do not give IV push or bolus. • Give loading dose (4 mg/kg) over 90 min. Give maintenance infusion (2 mg/kg) over 30 min.
Storage • Refrigerate. • Reconstituted solution appears colorless to pale yellow. • Reconstituted solution in vial is stable for 28 days if refrigerated after reconstitution with Bacteriostatic Water for Injection (if using Sterile Water for Injection without preservative, use immediately; discard unused portions). • Solution diluted in 250 mL 0.9% NaCl stable for 24 hrs if refrigerated.

⬛ IV INCOMPATIBILITIES

Do not mix with D_5W or any other medications.

INDICATIONS/ROUTES/DOSAGE

Breast Cancer (Adjuvant)
IV: ADULTS, ELDERLY: (With concurrent PACLitaxel or DOCEtaxel): Initially, 4 mg/kg as 90-min infusion, then 2 mg/kg wkly as 30-min infusion for 12 wks followed 1 wk later (when concurrent chemotherapy completed) by 6 mg/kg infusion over 30–90 min q3wks for total therapy duration of 52 wks. **(With DOCEtaxel/CARBOplatin):** Initially, 4 mg/kg as 90-min infusion, then 2 mg/kg wkly as 30-min infusion for a total of 18 wks, followed 1 wk later (when concurrent chemotherapy completed) by 6 mg/kg infused over 30–90 min q3wks for total therapy duration of 52 wks. **(Following multimodality chemotherapy):** Initially, 8 mg/kg over 90 min, then 6 mg/kg over 30–90 min q3wks for total of 52 wks.

Breast Cancer (Metastatic)
IV: ADULTS, ELDERLY: (Either as single agent or in combination with PACLitaxel): Initially, 4 mg/kg as 90-min infusion, then 2 mg/kg as 30-min infusion wkly until disease progression.

Gastric Cancer
IV: ADULTS, ELDERLY: (In combination with CISplatin and either capecitabine or fluorouracil for 6 cycles, then as monotherapy): Initially, 8 mg/kg over 90 min, then 6 mg/kg over 30–90 min q3wks until disease progression.

Dosage Adjustment in Cardiotoxicity
Left ventricular ejection fraction (LVEF) 16% or greater decrease from baseline WNL (within normal limits) or LVEF below normal limits and 10% or greater decrease from baseline: Hold treatment for 4 wks. Repeat LVEF q4wks. Resume therapy if LVEF returns to normal limits in 4–8 wks and remains at 15% or less decrease from baseline.

Dosage in Renal/Hepatic Impairment
No dose adjustment.

SIDE EFFECTS

Frequent (Greater Than 20%): Pain, asthenia, fever, chills, headache, abdominal pain, back pain, infection, nausea, diarrhea, vomiting, cough, dyspnea. **Occasional (15%–5%):** Tachycardia, HF, flu-like symptoms, anorexia, edema, bone pain, arthralgia, insomnia, dizziness, paresthesia, depression, rhinitis, pharyngitis, sinusitis. **Rare (Less Than 5%):** Allergic reaction, anemia, leukopenia, neuropathy, herpes simplex.

ADVERSE EFFECTS/TOXIC REACTIONS

Cardiomyopathy, ventricular dysfunction, HF occur rarely. Pancytopenia may occur.

NURSING CONSIDERATIONS

BASELINE ASSESSMENT

Evaluate left ventricular function. Obtain baseline echocardiogram, EKG, multigated acquisition (MUGA) scan. Obtain CBC at baseline and at regular intervals during therapy.

INTERVENTION/EVALUATION

Frequently monitor for deteriorating cardiac function. Assist with ambulation if asthenia occurs. Monitor for fever, chills, abdominal pain, back pain. Offer antiemetics if nausea, vomiting occur. Monitor daily pattern of bowel activity, stool consistency.

PATIENT/FAMILY TEACHING
• Do not have immunizations without physician's approval (lowers resistance). • Avoid contact with those who have recently taken oral polio vaccine. • Avoid crowds, those with infection.

traZODone

traz-o-done
(Apo-TraZODone ✦,
Novo-TraZODone ✦, Oleptro)
■ **BLACK BOX ALERT** ■ Increased risk of suicidal ideation and behavior in children, adolescents, young adults 18–24 yrs with major depressive disorder, other psychiatric disorders.
Do not confuse traZODone with traMADol or ziprasidone.

◆**CLASSIFICATION**
PHARMACOTHERAPEUTIC: Serotonin reuptake inhibitor. **CLINICAL:** Antidepressant.

USES
Treatment of major depressive disorder (MDD). **OFF-LABEL:** Insomnia.

PRECAUTIONS
Contraindications: Hypersensitivity to traZODone. Use of MAOIs (concurrently or within 14 days of discontinuing traZODone or MAOI); initiation in pt receiving linezolid or IV methylene blue. **Cautions:** Cardiac disease, arrhythmias, cerebrovascular disease, hepatic/renal impairment, pts at high risk of suicide. Conditions predisposing to priapism (e.g., sickle cell anemia); concurrent use of antihypertensives; history of seizure disorder or conditions predisposing to seizures (e.g., alcoholism); elderly pts.

ACTION
Blocks reuptake of serotonin at neuronal presynaptic membranes, increasing its availability at postsynaptic receptor sites. **Therapeutic Effect:** Relieves depression.

PHARMACOKINETICS
Well absorbed from GI tract. Protein binding: 85%–95%. Metabolized in liver. Primarily excreted in urine. Unknown if removed by hemodialysis. **Half-life:** 5–9 hrs (increased in elderly).

⧗ LIFESPAN CONSIDERATIONS
Pregnancy/Lactation: Drug crosses placenta; minimally distributed in breast milk. **Children:** Safety and efficacy not established in pts younger than 6 yrs. **Elderly:** More likely to experience sedative, hypotensive effects; lower dosage recommended.

INTERACTIONS
DRUG: CYP3A4 inhibitors (e.g., ritonavir, ketoconazole) increase concentration/effects. May increase concentration of **digoxin, phenytoin. HERBAL: Gotu kola, kava kava, St. John's wort, valerian** may increase CNS depression and serotonin syndrome. **FOOD:** None known. **LAB VALUES:** May decrease WBC, neutrophil counts.

AVAILABILITY (Rx)
Tablets: 50 mg, 100 mg, 150 mg, 300 mg.
🗲 **Tablets:** (Extended-Release [Oleptro]): 150 mg, 300 mg.

ADMINISTRATION/HANDLING
PO
• *(Immediate-Release):* Give shortly after snack, meal (reduces risk of dizziness). • Tablets may be crushed.
• *(Extended-Release):* Give whole or break in half along score line but do not crush or chew. Take on empty stomach.

INDICATIONS/ROUTES/DOSAGE

◀**ALERT**▶ Therapeutic effect may take up to 6 wks to occur.

Depression

PO: ADULTS: *(Immediate-Release):* Initially, 150 mg/day in 3 equally divided doses. Increase by 50 mg/day at 3- to 4-day intervals until therapeutic response is achieved. **Maximum:** 600 mg/day (inpatients); 400 mg/day (outpatients). **ELDERLY:** Initially, 25–50 mg at bedtime. May increase by 25–50 mg every 3–7 days. Range: 75–150 mg/day. *Tablets (Extended-Release):* **ADULTS, ELDERLY:** Initially, 150 mg once daily. May increase by 75 mg q3days. **Maximum:** 375 mg/day. **ADOLESCENTS 13–18 YRS:** *(Immediate-Release):* Initially, 25–50 mg/day. May increase to 100–150 mg/day in divided doses. **CHILDREN 6–12 YRS:** *(Immediate-Release):* Initially, 1.5–2 mg/kg/day in divided doses. May increase gradually q3–4 days to 6 mg/kg/day in 3 divided doses.

Dosage in Renal/Hepatic Impairment
Use caution.

SIDE EFFECTS

Frequent (9%–3%): Drowsiness, dry mouth, light-headedness, dizziness, headache, blurred vision, nausea, vomiting. **Occasional (3%–1%):** Nervousness, fatigue, constipation, myalgia/arthralgia, mild hypotension. **Rare:** Photosensitivity reaction.

ADVERSE EFFECTS/TOXIC REACTIONS

Priapism, altered libido, retrograde ejaculation, impotence occur rarely. Appears to be less cardiotoxic than other antidepressants, although arrhythmias may occur in pts with preexisting cardiac disease.

NURSING CONSIDERATIONS

BASELINE ASSESSMENT

Assess mental status, mood, behavior. For pts on long-term therapy, serum hepatic/renal function tests, blood counts should be performed periodically. Elderly pts are more likely to experience sedative, hypotensive effects. Question history as listed in PRECAUTIONS.

INTERVENTION/EVALUATION

Monitor for suicidal ideation (esp. at beginning of therapy or dosage change). Assess appearance, behavior, speech pattern, level of interest, mood. Monitor WBC, neutrophil count, hepatic enzymes. Assist with ambulation if dizziness, light-headedness occurs.

PATIENT/FAMILY TEACHING

• Immediately discontinue medication, consult physician if priapism occurs. • **Immediate-Release:** May take after meal, snack. • **Extended-Release:** Take on empty stomach. • May take at bedtime if drowsiness occurs. • Change positions slowly to avoid hypotensive effect. • Avoid tasks that require alertness, motor skills until response to drug is established. • Tolerance to sedative, anticholinergic effects usually develops during early therapy. • Photosensitivity to sun may occur. • Dry mouth may be relieved by sugarless gum, sips of water. • Report visual disturbances, worsening depression, suicidal ideation, unusual changes in behavior. • Do not abruptly discontinue medication. • Avoid alcohol.

tretinoin **HIGH ALERT**

tret-i-noyn
(Atralin, Avita, Refissa, Rejuva-A , Renova, Retin-A, Retin-A Micro, Tretin X, Vesanoid ❋)

■ **BLACK BOX ALERT** ■ High risk for teratogenicity; major fetal abnormalities, spontaneous abortions. Pts with acute promyelocytic leukemia (APL) are at severe risk for reactions (fever, dyspnea, acute respiratory distress syndrome [pulmonary infiltrates, pleural effusions, pericardial effusions]), edema, hepatic, renal, and/or multiorgan failure; 40% develop leukocytosis. **Do not confuse tretinoin with ISOtretinoin, phenytoin, or triamcinolone.**

FIXED-COMBINATION(S)

With octyl methoxycinnamate and oxybenzone, moisturizers, and SPF-12, a sunscreen **(Retin-A Regimen Kit)**.

◆CLASSIFICATION

PHARMACOTHERAPEUTIC: Retinoid. **CLINICAL:** Antiacne, transdermal, antineoplastic.

USES

Topical: Treatment of acne vulgaris, photodamaged skin. **PO:** Induction of remission in pts with acute promyelocytic leukemia (APL). **OFF-LABEL (PO):** Maintenance therapy in APL, combination therapy (arsenic trioxide) for remission induction in APL. **Topical:** Some skin cancers.

PRECAUTIONS

Contraindications: Hypersensitivity to tretinoin. Sensitivity to parabens (used as preservative in gelatin capsule). **Extreme Caution: Topical:** Eczema, sun exposure. **Cautions: Topical:** Those with considerable sun exposure in their occupations, hypersensitivity to sun. **PO:** Elevated serum cholesterol/triglycerides, concurrent use of antifibrinolytic agents.

ACTION

Antiacne: Decreases cohesiveness of follicular epithelial cells. Increases turnover of follicular epithelial cells. **Therapeutic Effect:** Causes expulsion of blackheads. Bacterial skin counts are not altered. **Transdermal:** Exerts effects on growth/differentiation of epithelial cells. **Therapeutic Effect:** Alleviates fine wrinkles, hyperpigmentation. **Antineoplastic:** Induces maturation, decreases proliferation of acute promyelocytic leukemia (APL) cells. **Therapeutic Effect:** Repopulation of bone marrow and peripheral blood with normal hematopoietic cells.

PHARMACOKINETICS

Topical: Minimally absorbed. **PO:** Well absorbed following PO administration. Protein binding: greater than 95%. Metabolized in liver. Primarily excreted in urine. **Half-life:** 0.5–2 hrs.

⌛ LIFESPAN CONSIDERATIONS

Pregnancy/Lactation: Topical: Use during pregnancy only if clearly necessary. Unknown if distributed in breast milk. **PO:** Teratogenic, embryotoxic effect. **Children/Elderly:** Safety and efficacy not established.

INTERACTIONS

DRUG: TOPICAL: Retinoids (e.g., acitretin, oral tretinoin) may increase drying, irritative effects. **PO: Tetracyclines** may increase risk of pseudotumor cerebri, intracranial hypertension. **Aminocaproic acid** may increase risk of thrombotic complications. **CYP3A4 inducers (e.g., PHENobarbital, rifAMPin)** may decrease concentration/effects. **CYP3A4 inhibitors (e.g., clarithromycin, ketoconazole, ritonavir)** may increase concentration, risk of toxicity. **HERBAL: St. John's wort** may decrease concentration/effects. **Dong quai, St. John's wort** may increase photosensitization. **Vitamin A** supplementation may increase vitamin A toxicity. **FOOD:** None known. **LAB VALUES: PO:** Leukocytosis occurs commonly (40%). May elevate serum hepatic function tests, cholesterol, triglycerides.

AVAILABILITY (Rx)

Cream: 0.02% (Renova), 0.025% (Avita, Retin-A, Tretin X), 0.05% (Refissa, Retin-A, Tretin X), 0.1% (Retin-A). **Gel:** 0.01% (Retin-A, Tretin X), 0.025% (Avita, Retin-A, Tretin X), 0.04% (Retin-A Micro), 0.1% (Retin-A Micro).

🦘 **Capsules: (Vesanoid):** 10 mg.

ADMINISTRATION/HANDLING

PO
• Do not crush/break capsule. • Administer with a meal.

Topical

• Thoroughly cleanse area before applying tretinoin. • Lightly cover only affected area. Liquid may be applied with fingertip, gauze, cotton; do not rub onto unaffected skin. • Keep medication away from eyes, mouth, angles of nose, mucous membranes. • Wash hands immediately after application.

INDICATIONS/ROUTES/DOSAGE

Acne

Topical: ADULTS, CHILDREN 12 YRS AND OLDER: Apply once daily at bedtime or in the evening.

Remission Induction in Acute Promyelocytic Leukemia (APL)

PO: ADULTS, ELDERLY, CHILDREN: 45 mg/ m^2/day given as 2 evenly divided doses until complete remission is documented. Discontinue therapy 30 days after complete remission or after 90 days of treatment, whichever comes first.

Remission Maintenance in APL

PO: ADULTS, ELDERLY: 45 mg/m^2/day in 2 divided doses for 15 days q3mos for 2 yrs. **CHILDREN:** 25 mg/m^2/day in 2 divided doses for 15 days q3mos for 2 yrs.

Dosage in Renal/Hepatic Impairment
No dose adjustment.

SIDE EFFECTS

Topical: Temporary change in pigmentation, photosensitivity. Local inflammatory reactions (peeling, dry skin, stinging, erythema, pruritus) are to be expected and are reversible with discontinuation of tretinoin. **Frequent: PO (87%–54%):** Headache, fever, dry skin/oral mucosa, bone pain, nausea, vomiting, rash. **Occasional: PO (26%–6%):** Mucositis, earache or feeling of fullness in ears, flushing, pruritus, diaphoresis, visual disturbances, hypotension/hypertension, dizziness, anxiety, insomnia, alopecia, skin changes. **Rare (Less Than 6%):** Altered visual acuity, temporary hearing loss.

ADVERSE EFFECTS/TOXIC REACTIONS

PO: Retinoic acid syndrome (fever, dyspnea, weight gain, abnormal chest auscultatory findings [pulmonary infiltrates, pleural/pericardial effusions], episodic hypotension) occurs commonly (25%), as does leukocytosis (40%). Syndrome generally occurs during first month of therapy (sometimes after first dose). High-dose steroids (dexamethasone 10 mg IV) at first suspicion of syndrome reduce morbidity, mortality. Pseudotumor cerebri may be noted, esp. in children (headache, nausea, vomiting, visual disturbances). **Topical:** Possible tumorigenic potential when combined with ultraviolet radiation.

NURSING CONSIDERATIONS

BASELINE ASSESSMENT

PO: Inform women of childbearing potential of risk to fetus if pregnancy occurs. Instruct on need for use of 2 reliable forms of contraceptives concurrently during therapy and for 1 mo after discontinuation of therapy, even in infertile women. Pregnancy test should be obtained within 1 wk prior to institution of therapy. Obtain initial serum LFT, cholesterol, triglyceride levels.

INTERVENTION/EVALUATION

PO: Monitor LFT, hematologic, coagulation profiles, cholesterol, triglycerides. Monitor for signs/symptoms of pseudotumor cerebri in children.

PATIENT/FAMILY TEACHING

• **Topical:** Avoid exposure to sunlight, tanning beds; use sunscreens, protective clothing. • Protect affected areas from wind, cold. • If skin is already sunburned, do not use drug until fully healed. • Keep tretinoin away from eyes, mouth, angles of nose, mucous membranes. • Do not use medicated, drying, abrasive soaps; wash face no more than 2–3 times/day with gentle soap. • Avoid use of preparations containing alcohol,

T

menthol, spice, lime (e.g., shaving lotions, astringents, perfume). • Mild redness, peeling are expected; decrease frequency or discontinue medication if excessive reaction occurs. • Nonmedicated cosmetics may be used; however, cosmetics must be removed before tretinoin application. • Improvement noted during first 24 wks of therapy. • **Antiacne:** Therapeutic results noted in 2–3 wks; optimal results in 6 wks. • **Oral:** Avoid tasks requiring motor skills, alertness until response to drug is established. • Avoid alcohol. • Avoid exposure to sunlight, tanning beds. • Report persistent vomiting, diarrhea, unusual bleeding/bruising, acute abdominal pain, vision changes, or if pregnancy is suspected.

trospium

tro-spee-um
(Trosec ✦)

◆CLASSIFICATION

PHARMACOTHERAPEUTIC: Anticholinergic. **CLINICAL:** Antispasmotic.

USES

Treatment of overactive bladder with symptoms of urge urinary incontinence, urgency, urinary frequency.

PRECAUTIONS

Contraindications: Hypersensitivity to trospium. Gastric retention, uncontrolled narrow-angle glaucoma, urinary retention. **Cautions:** Decreased GI motility, renal/hepatic impairment, obstructive GI disorders, ulcerative colitis, intestinal atony, myasthenia gravis, controlled narrow-angle glaucoma, bladder flow obstruction, Alzheimer's disease, hot weather/exercise, elderly pts.

ACTION

Antagonizes effect of acetylcholine on muscarinic receptors, producing parasympatholytic action. **Therapeutic Effect:** Reduces smooth muscle tone in bladder.

PHARMACOKINETICS

Minimally absorbed after PO administration. Protein binding: 50%–85%. Distributed in plasma. Excreted in feces (82%), urine (6%). **Half-life:** 20 hrs.

⌛ LIFESPAN CONSIDERATIONS

Pregnancy/Lactation: Unknown if drug crosses placenta or is distributed in breast milk. **Children:** Safety and efficacy not established. **Elderly:** Higher incidence of dry mouth, constipation, dyspepsia, UTI, urinary retention in pts 75 yrs and older.

INTERACTIONS

DRUG: Other anticholinergic agents increase severity, frequency of side effects, may alter absorption of other drugs due to anticholinergic effects on GI motility. **Morphine, procainamide, tenofovir, vancomycin** may increase concentration. **HERBAL:** None significant. **FOOD: High-fat meals** may reduce absorption. **LAB VALUES:** None significant.

AVAILABILITY (Rx)

Tablets: 20 mg. Capsules, Extended-Release: 60 mg.

ADMINISTRATION/HANDLING

PO
• Store at room temperature. • Give at least 1 hr before meals or on an empty stomach. • Do not break, crush, dissolve, or divide tablets or extended-release capsules; swallow whole. • Administer tablets at bedtime, capsules in morning with full glass of water, 1 hr before eating.

INDICATIONS/ROUTES/DOSAGE

Overactive Bladder
PO: ADULTS: *(Immediate-Release):* 20 mg twice daily. **ELDERLY 75 YRS AND OLDER:** 20 mg once daily at bedtime. *(Extended-Release):* 60 mg once daily.

Dosage in Renal Impairment
For pts with CrCl less than 30 mL/min, immediate-release dosage reduced to

20 mg once daily at bedtime. Extended-release not recommended.

Dosage in Hepatic Impairment
Mild impairment: No dose adjustment.
Moderate to severe impairment: Use with caution.

SIDE EFFECTS

Frequent (20%): Dry mouth. **Occasional (10%–4%):** Constipation, headache. **Rare (Less Than 2%):** Fatigue, upper abdominal pain, dyspepsia (heartburn, indigestion, epigastric pain), flatulence, dry eyes, urinary retention.

ADVERSE EFFECTS/TOXIC REACTIONS

Overdose may result in severe anticholinergic effects, characterized by nervousness, restlessness, nausea, vomiting, confusion, diaphoresis, facial flushing, hypertension, hypotension, respiratory depression, irritability, lacrimation. Supraventricular tachycardia and hallucinations occur rarely.

NURSING CONSIDERATIONS

BASELINE ASSESSMENT
Assess for presence of dysuria, urinary urgency, frequency, incontinence.

INTERVENTION/EVALUATION
Monitor for symptomatic relief. Monitor I&O; palpate bladder for retention. Monitor daily pattern of bowel activity, stool consistency. Dry mouth may be relieved by sips of tepid water.

PATIENT/FAMILY TEACHING
• Report nausea, vomiting, diaphoresis, increased salivary secretions, palpitations, severe abdominal pain. • Swallow tablets, extended-release capsules whole. • Give 1 hr before meals.

T

umeclidinium

ue-**mek**-li-**din**-ee-um
(Incruse Ellipta)
Do not confuse umeclidinium with aclidinium or clidinium.

FIXED-COMBINATION(S)

Anoro Ellipta: umeclidinium/vilanterol (bronchodilator): 62.5 mcg/25 mcg. **Trelegy Ellipta:** umeclidium/fluticasone (corticosteroid)/vilantrol (bronchodilator): 62.5 mcg/100 mcg/25 mcg.

◆CLASSIFICATION

PHARMACOTHERAPEUTIC: Anticholinergic. **CLINICAL:** Bronchodilator.

USES

Long-term, once-daily maintenance treatment of airflow obstruction in pts with COPD including chronic bronchitis and/or emphysema.

PRECAUTIONS

Contraindications: Hypersensitivity to umeclidinium. Severe hypersensitivity to milk proteins or any drug components. **Cautions:** Bladder neck obstruction, myasthenia gravis, narrow-angle glaucoma, prostatic hypertrophy, urinary retention. Not recommended in pts with acutely deteriorating COPD requiring emergent relief of acute symptoms.

ACTION

Inhibits muscarinic M_3 receptor in lungs, resulting in relaxation of bronchial smooth muscle. **Therapeutic Effect:** Relieves bronchospasm, reduces airway resistance, improves bronchodilation.

PHARMACOKINETICS

Rapidly absorbed following inhalation. Primarily metabolized by enzyme cytochrome P4502D6. Protein binding: 89%. Peak concentration: 5–15 min. Steady state reached within 14 days. **Half-life:** 11 hrs.

⧖ LIFESPAN CONSIDERATIONS

Pregnancy/Lactation: Unknown if distributed in breast milk. Must either discontinue drug or discontinue breastfeeding. **Children:** Not indicated in this pt population. **Elderly:** No age-related precautions noted.

INTERACTIONS

DRUG: Anticholinergics (e.g., atropine, dicyclomine, glycopyrrolate, scopolamine), medications with anticholinergic properties (e.g., diphenhydrAMINE) may increase effects/risk of toxicity. **HERBAL:** None significant. **FOOD:** None known. **LAB VALUES:** None known.

AVAILABILITY (Rx)

Inhalation Powder: 62.5 mcg/capsule (in blister packs containing 7 or 30 doses).

ADMINISTRATION/HANDLING

Inhalation
Administration • Follow instructions for preparation according to manufacturer guidelines. • Do not shake or prime. Prior to inhaling dose, exhale fully (do not exhale into inhaler). Close lips tightly around inhaler and inhale (rapidly, steadily, and deeply). Do not breathe through nose or block air vent with fingers. • Remove mouthpiece and hold breath for 3–4 sec, then breathe out slowly and gently. Do not close container until medication has been inhaled. • Close lid cover.
Storage • Store at room temperature up to 6 wks after opening tray. • Do not refrigerate or freeze. • Protect from sunlight and moisture. • Discard after counter reaches 0. • Do not reuse inhaler.

INDICATIONS/ROUTES/DOSAGE

COPD
Inhalation: ADULTS, ELDERLY: One inhalation (62.5 mcg) once daily, at same time each day. **Maximum:** 1 inhalation/24 hrs.

U

Dose Modification

Deterioration of COPD: Discontinue treatment. Institute short-acting bronchodilators and supportive pulmonary therapy.

Dosage in Renal Impairment

No dose adjustment.

Dosage in Hepatic Impairment

Mild to moderate impairment: No dose adjustment. **Severe impairment:** Use caution.

SIDE EFFECTS

Occasional (8%–5%): Nasopharyngitis, upper respiratory tract infection. **Rare (3%–1%):** Cough, arthralgia, viral respiratory tract infection, pharyngitis, myalgia, abdominal pain, toothache, tachycardia.

ADVERSE EFFECTS/TOXIC REACTIONS

Life-threatening asthma-related events, bronchospasm, worsening of COPD-related symptoms have been reported. Hypersensitivity reactions may occur (esp. in pts with undiagnosed severe milk protein allergy or allergy to products containing lactose). Worsening of narrow-angle glaucoma (eye pain, blurry vision, visual halos, colored images in association with red eyes from conjunctival congestion and corneal edema) may occur. May cause worsening of urinary retention, esp. in pts with prostatic hypertrophy or bladder neck obstruction.

NURSING CONSIDERATIONS

BASELINE ASSESSMENT

Obtain baseline O_2 saturation, vital signs; pulmonary function test, if applicable. Assess respiratory rate, depth, rhythm. Assess lung sounds for wheezing, rales. Screen for concomitant use of anticholinergic medications. Question history of asthma, BPH, bladder neck obstruction, glaucoma. Teach proper inhaler priming and administration techniques. Conduct ophthalmologic exam in pts with narrow-angle glaucoma.

INTERVENTION/EVALUATION

Routinely monitor O_2 saturation, vital signs. Auscultate lung sounds and monitor for symptom improvement. Recommend discontinuation of short-acting beta$_2$-agonists while on long-term therapy. Monitor for COPD deterioration, narrow-angle glaucoma, urinary retention/obstruction. Monitor for increased use of rescue inhaler; may indicate worsening of respiratory status.

PATIENT/FAMILY TEACHING

• Report fever, productive cough, body aches, paradoxical bronchospasm, difficulty breathing; may indicate lung infection, worsening of COPD. • Therapy not intended for acute COPD symptom relief, and extra doses are not advised. • Report symptoms of acute narrow-angle glaucoma, urinary retention, bladder distention. • Refill prescription when counter on left of inhaler reaches red area of scale. • Follow manufacturer guidelines for proper use of inhaler. • Drink plenty of fluids (decreases lung secretion viscosity). • Rinse mouth with water after inhalation to decrease mouth/throat irritation.

ustekinumab

yoo-ste-**kin**-ue-mab
(Stelara)
Do not confuse Stelara with Aldara, or ustekinumab with inFLIXimab or riTUXimab.

◆ CLASSIFICATION

PHARMACOTHERAPEUTIC: Interleukin-12, interleukin-23 inhibitor, monoclonal antibody. **CLINICAL:** Antipsoriasis agent.

USES

Treatment of adults, adolescents 12 yrs or older with moderate to severe plaque psoriasis who are candidates for systemic therapy or phototherapy. Treatment of adults with active psoriatic arthritis alone or in combination with methotrexate.

Treatment of adults with moderate to severe active Crohn's disease.

PRECAUTIONS

Contraindications: Hypersensitivity to ustekinumab. **Cautions:** History of chronic infection, recurrent infection, active tuberculosis, prior malignancy, renal/hepatic impairment. Avoid use of live vaccines.

ACTION

Strongly binds with cellular components involved in responses to inflammation and immune system, thereby decreasing likelihood of aggravating psoriatic eruptions. **Therapeutic Effect:** Significantly slows growth, migration of circulating total lymphocytes (predominant in psoriatic lesions).

PHARMACOKINETICS

Following subcutaneous injections, clearance is affected by body weight, is not affected by gender or race. Degraded into small peptides and amino acids via catabolic pathways. Steady state reached in 28 wks. **Half-life:** 10–126 days.

⏳ LIFESPAN CONSIDERATIONS

Pregnancy/Lactation: Unknown if distributed in breast milk. **Children:** Not indicated for use in this pt population. **Elderly:** Age-related increased incidence of infection requires cautious use.

INTERACTIONS

DRUG: Immunosuppressive agents (e.g., **abatacept, cyclosporine, fingolimod, methotrexate, sirolimus**) increase risk of infection. **Abciximab, trastuzumab** may increase concentration/effects. May decrease therapeutic effects of **vaccines,** increase risk of adverse effects of **live vaccines. HERBAL: Echinacea** may decrease concentration/effects. **FOOD:** None known. **LAB VALUES:** May increase lymphocyte count.

AVAILABILITY (Rx)

Injection Solution (Prefilled Syringes): 45 mg/0.5 ml, 90 mg/ml.

ADMINISTRATION/HANDLING

 IV

Infuse over at least 1 hr. Use with in-line protein-binding filter (0.2 microns).

Subcutaneous

• Do not inject into areas where skin is tender, bruised, erythematous, indurated. • Avoid areas where psoriasis is present. • Administer into thigh, abdomen, buttocks, upper arm. • Refrigerate unopened vial. • Solution appears colorless to light yellow. Discard if solution contains more than a few small translucent or white particles or is cloudy.

INDICATIONS/ROUTES/DOSAGE

Plaque Psoriasis

SQ: ADULTS, ELDERLY WEIGHING 100 KG OR LESS: Initially, 45 mg, then 45 mg 4 wks later, followed by 45 mg every 12 wks. **WEIGHING MORE THAN 100 KG:** Initially, 90 mg, then 90 mg 4 wks later, followed by 90 mg every 12 wks. **Note:** 45 mg also efficacious; however, 90 mg is recommended due to greater efficacy. **CHILDREN 12 YRS AND OLDER: (GREATER THAN 100 KG):** Initially, 90 mg, repeat in 4 wks, then q12 wks. **(61–100 KG):** Initially, 45 mg, repeat in 4 wks, then q12 wks. **(60 KG OR LESS):** Initially, 0.75 mg/kg, repeat in 4 wks, then q12 wks.

Psoriatic Arthritis

SQ: ADULTS, ELDERLY: Initially, 45 mg repeated in 4 wks followed by 45 mg q12wks. **PTS WITH COEXISTENT MODERATE TO SEVERE PLAQUE PSORIASIS WEIGHING MORE THAN 100 KG:** Initially, 90 mg repeated in 4 wks, then 90 mg q12wks.

Crohn's Disease

IV INFUSION: ADULTS, ELDERLY: Initially, (as a single dose) 520 mg (greater than 85 kg); 390 mg (56–85 kg); 260 mg (up to 54 kg). **SQ (Maintenance):** 90 mg q8wks beginning 8 wks following the IV induction dose.

Dosage in Renal/Hepatic Impairment

No dose adjustment.

U

✦ Canadian trade name    Non-Crushable Drug   🔲 High Alert drug

SIDE EFFECTS

Occasional (8%–4%): Nasopharyngitis, upper respiratory tract infection, headache. **Rare (3%–1%):** Fatigue, diarrhea, back pain, dizziness, pruritus, injection site erythema, myalgia, depression.

ADVERSE EFFECTS/TOXIC REACTIONS

Worsening of psoriasis, thrombocytopenia, malignancies, serious infections (cellulitis, diverticulitis, gastroenteritis, pneumonia, osteomyelitis, UTI, postoperative wound infection) has been noted. Reversible posterior leukoencephalopathy syndrome (headache, seizures, confusion, visual disturbances) occurs rarely.

NURSING CONSIDERATIONS

BASELINE ASSESSMENT

Pts should not receive live vaccines during treatment, 1 yr prior to initiating treatment, or 1 yr following discontinuation of treatment. Inform pt of duration of treatment and required monitoring procedures. Assess skin prior to therapy; document extent and location of psoriasis lesions. Test pt for tuberculosis infection prior to initiating treatment.

INTERVENTION/EVALUATION

Closely monitor for signs/symptoms of active tuberculosis during and after treatment. Assess skin throughout therapy for evidence of improvement of psoriasis lesions. Monitor for worsening of lesions.

PATIENT/FAMILY TEACHING

• If appropriate, pt may self-inject after proper training in preparation and injection technique. • Report any signs of infection. • If new diagnosis of malignancy occurs, inform physician of current treatment with ustekinumab.

valACYclovir

val-a-**sye**-kloe-veer
(Apo-ValACYclovir ♣, <u>Valtrex</u>)
Do not confuse valACYclovir with acyclovir or valGANciclovir, or Valtrex with Valcyte.

◆CLASSIFICATION

PHARMACOTHERAPEUTIC: Nucleoside analogue DNA polymerase inhibitor. **CLINICAL:** Antiviral.

USES

Treatment of herpes zoster (shingles) in immunocompetent pts. Treatment of initial and recurrent genital herpes in immunocompetent adults. Prevention of recurrent genital herpes and reduction of transmission of genital herpes in immunocompetent pts. Suppression of genital herpes in HIV-infected pts. Treatment of cold sores, chickenpox in immunocompetent children. **OFF-LABEL:** Prophylaxis and treatment of cancer-related HSV, VZV.

PRECAUTIONS

Contraindications: Hypersensitivity to acyclovir, valACYclovir. **Cautions:** Renal impairment, concurrent use of nephrotoxic agents, elderly pts.

ACTION

Converted to acyclovir by intestinal/hepatic metabolism. Competes for viral DNA polymerase; inhibits incorporation into viral DNA. **Therapeutic Effect:** Inhibits DNA synthesis and viral replication.

PHARMACOKINETICS

Rapidly absorbed after PO administration. Protein binding: 13%–18%. Rapidly converted by hydrolysis to active compound acyclovir. Widely distributed to tissues, body fluids (including CSF). Primarily excreted in urine. Removed by hemodialysis. **Half-life:** (acyclovir) 2.5–3.3 hrs (increased in renal impairment).

⌛ LIFESPAN CONSIDERATIONS

Pregnancy/Lactation: May cross placenta. May be distributed in breast milk. **Children:** Safety and efficacy not established in children younger than 2 yrs (chickenpox); younger than 12 yrs (cold sores). **Elderly:** Age-related renal impairment may require dosage adjustment.

INTERACTIONS

DRUG: Nephrotoxic medications (e.g., **lisinopril, gentamicin, IV contrast media**) may increase risk of nephrotoxicity, renal impairment. **HERBAL:** None significant. **FOOD:** None known. **LAB VALUES:** None significant.

AVAILABILITY (Rx)

Tablets: 500 mg, 1,000 mg.

ADMINISTRATION/HANDLING

PO
• Give without regard to meals. • If GI upset occurs, give with meals.

INDICATIONS/ROUTES/DOSAGE

Herpes Zoster (Shingles)
PO: ADULTS, ELDERLY: 1 g 3 times/day for 7 days.

Herpes Simplex (Cold Sores)
PO: ADULTS, ELDERLY: 2 g twice daily for 1 day (separate by 12 hrs).

Initial Episode of Genital Herpes
PO: ADULTS, ELDERLY: 1 g twice daily for 10 days.

Recurrent Episodes of Genital Herpes
PO: ADULTS, ELDERLY: 500 mg twice daily for 3 days.

Suppressive Therapy of Genital Herpes
PO: ADULTS, ELDERLY: (HIV infected): 500 mg twice daily. **(Immunocompetent):** 1 g once daily (500 mg once daily in pts with 9 or fewer recurrences/yr).

Chickenpox
PO: CHILDREN 2–17 YRS: 20 mg/kg/dose 3 times/day for 5 days. **Maximum:** 1 g 3 times/day.

V

Dosage in Renal Impairment
Dosage and frequency are modified based on creatinine clearance. **HD:** Give dose postdialysis.

Cold Sores/Herpes Zoster

Creatinine Clearance	Herpes Zoster	Cold Sores
30–49 mL/min	1 g q12h	1 g q12h × 2 doses
10–29 mL/min	1 g q24h	500 mg q12h × 2 doses
Less than 10 mL/min	500 mg q24h	500 mg as single dose

Genital Herpes

Creatinine Clearance	Initial Episode	Recurrent Episode	Suppressive Therapy
10–29 mL/min	1 g q24h	500 mg q24h	500 mg q24–48h
Less than 10 mL/min	500 mg q24h	500 mg q24h	500 mg q24–48h

Dosage in Hepatic Impairment
No dose adjustment.

SIDE EFFECTS
Frequent: Herpes zoster (17%–10%): Nausea, headache. **Genital herpes (17%):** Headache. **Occasional: Herpes zoster (7%–3%):** Vomiting, diarrhea, constipation (50 yrs and older), asthenia, dizziness (50 yrs and older). **Genital herpes (8%–3%):** Nausea, diarrhea, dizziness. **Rare: Herpes zoster (3%–1%):** Abdominal pain, anorexia. **Genital herpes (3%–1%):** Asthenia, abdominal pain.

ADVERSE EFFECTS/TOXIC REACTIONS
Neutropenia, thrombocytopenia, renal failure occur rarely.

NURSING CONSIDERATIONS
BASELINE ASSESSMENT
Question for history of allergies, particularly to valACYclovir, acyclovir. Tissue cultures for herpes zoster, herpes simplex should be obtained before giving first dose (therapy may proceed before results are known). Assess medical history, esp. HIV infection, bone marrow or renal transplantation, renal/hepatic impairment. Assess characteristics, frequency of lesions.

INTERVENTION/EVALUATION
Monitor CBC, LFT, renal function, urinalysis. Evaluate cutaneous lesions. Provide analgesics, comfort measures for herpes zoster (esp. exhausting to elderly). Encourage fluids. Keep pt's fingernails short, hands clean.

PATIENT/FAMILY TEACHING
• Drink adequate fluids. • Do not touch lesions with fingers to avoid spreading infection to new site. • **Genital herpes:** Continue therapy for full length of treatment. • Space doses evenly. • Avoid sexual intercourse during duration of lesions to prevent infecting partner. • ValACYclovir does not cure herpes. • Report if lesions recur or do not improve. • Pap smears should be done at least annually due to increased risk of cervical cancer in women with genital herpes. • Initiate treatment at first sign of recurrent episode of genital herpes or herpes zoster (early treatment within first 24–48 hrs is imperative for therapeutic results).

valbenazine

val-**ben**-a-zeen
(Ingrezza)
Do not confuse with carBAMazepine, deutetrabenazine, or tetrabenazine.

◆CLASSIFICATION
PHARMACOTHERAPEUTIC: Pharmacotherapeutic classification. **CLINICAL:** Monoamine uptake regulator.

USES

Treatment of adults with tardive dyskinesia.

PRECAUTIONS

Contraindications: Hypersensitivity to valbenazine. **Cautions:** Pts at risk for falls, severe osteoporosis; concomitant use with strong CYP2D6 inhibitors, strong CYP3A4 inhibitors or in a poor CYP2D6 metabolizer, QTc interval–prolonging medications. Pts with congenital QT syndrome, arrhythmias associated with prolonged QT interval. Pts with depression or suicidal ideation, moderate to severe hepatic impairment. Avoid use in severe renal impairment.

ACTION

Exact mechanism of action for dyskinesia unknown. Thought to be mediated by reversible inhibition of VMAT2, a transporter that regulates uptake of monoamine from the cytoplasm to the synaptic vesicle for storage and release. **Therapeutic Effect:** Reduces abnormal involuntary movements; improves motor function.

PHARMACOKINETICS

Widely distributed. High-fat meals decrease absorption. Metabolized by hydrolysis to active metabolite. Protein binding: greater than 99%. Peak plasma concentration: 30–60 min (metabolite: 4–8 hrs). Excreted in urine (60%), feces (30%). **Half-life:** 15–22 hrs.

⌛ LIFESPAN CONSIDERATIONS

Pregnancy/Lactation: Unknown if distributed in breast milk. Breastfeeding not recommended during treatment and for at least 5 days after discontinuation. **Children:** Safety and efficacy not established. **Elderly:** No age-related precautions noted.

INTERACTIONS

DRUG: Deutetrabanzine, tetrabenzine may enhance adverse/toxic effects. **Strong CYP3A4 inhibitors** (e.g., **clarithromycin, ketoconazole, ritonavir**), strong CYP2D6 inhibitors (e.g., **fluoxetine, PARoxetine, quinidine**) may increase concentration/effect. **Strong CYP3A4 inducers** (e.g., **carBAMazepine, phenytoin, rifAMPin**) may decrease concentration/effect. May increase concentration/adverse effects of **MAOIs** (e.g., **phenelzine, selegiline**). **QT interval–prolonging medications** (e.g., **amiodarone, azithromycin, ceritinib, haloperidol, moxifloxacin, sotalol**) may increase risk of QTc interval prolongation, torsades de pointes, sudden cardiac death. **HERBAL:** St. John's wort may decrease concentration/effects. **FOOD:** None known. **LAB VALUES:** May increase alkaline phosphatase, bilirubin, prolactin, glucose.

AVAILABILITY (Rx)

Capsules: 40 mg, 80 mg.

ADMINISTRATION/HANDLING

PO
• Give with or without food.

INDICATIONS/ROUTES/DOSAGE

Tardive Dyskinesia
PO: ADULTS, ELDERLY: 40 mg once daily. May increase to 80 mg once daily if tolerated after 7 days.
Dose Modification
CYP2D2 poor metabolizers: Consider reducing dose based on tolerability.
Dosage in Renal Impairment
Mild to moderate: No dose adjustment. **Severe:** Not recommended.
Dosage in Hepatic Impairment
Mild impairment: No dose adjustment. **Moderate to severe impairment:** 40 mg once daily.

SIDE EFFECTS

Occasional (13%–3%): Somnolence, fatigue, sedation, dry mouth, constipation, attention disturbance, blurry vision, urinary retention, gait disturbance, dizziness, balance disorder, vomiting. **Rare (2%):** musculoskeletal disorders, arthralgia.

V

ADVERSE EFFECTS/TOXIC REACTIONS

May increase risk of falls, injury. Elevated serum alkaline phosphatase, bilirubin may indicate risk of cholestasis. May cause QTc prolongation in pts who are CYP2D6 poor metabolizers or taking concomitant CYP2D6 inhibitors, which may increase the risk of torsades de pointes, sudden cardiac death. VMAT2 inhibitors are associated with elevated serum prolactin levels, which may cause low estrogen levels, thereby increasing risk of amenorrhea, galactorrhea, gynecomastia, osteoporosis.

NURSING CONSIDERATIONS

BASELINE ASSESSMENT

Obtain baseline LFTs, EKG (pts at risk for QT prolongation). Assess for depression or suicidal ideation. Assess baseline of abnormal involuntary movements. Receive full medication history and screen for interactions. Initiate fall precautions. Offer emotional support.

INTERVENTION/EVALUATION

Assess for clinical improvement, reversal of symptoms (lip smacking, puckering, tongue protrusion or chewing, jaw movement, rapid blinking of the eye; slow, deliberate movements; rapid jerking motion that interrupts normal coordinated movement). Assist with ambulation.

PATIENT/FAMILY TEACHING

• Therapy is not a cure, but it may help with abnormal involuntary movements associated with disease. • Do not take newly prescribed medications unless approved by prescriber that originally started treatment. • Report fainting, chest pain, palpitations, irregular heart rhythm. • Avoid tasks that require alertness, motor skills until response to drug is established. • Do not breastfeed during treatment and for at least 5 days after final dose.

valGANciclovir

val-gan-**sye**-kloe-veer
(Apo-ValGANciclovir ✦, Valcyte)
■ **BLACK BOX ALERT** ■ May adversely affect spermatogenesis, fertility. Risk for granulocytopenia, anemia, thrombocytopenia.
Do not confuse Valcyte with Valium or Valtrex, or valGANciclovir with valACYclovir.

◆CLASSIFICATION

PHARMACOTHERAPEUTIC: Synthetic nucleoside. **CLINICAL:** Antiviral.

USES

Adults: Treatment of cytomegalovirus (CMV) retinitis in AIDS. Prevention of CMV disease in high-risk renal, cardiac, renal-pancreas transplant pts. **Children:** Prevention of CMV disease in high-risk renal (4 mos to 16 yrs) and cardiac transplant pts (1 mo to 16 yrs).

PRECAUTIONS

Contraindications: Hypersensitivity to valGANciclovir, ganciclovir. **Cautions:** Use extreme caution in children due to long-term carcinogenicity, reproductive toxicity. Renal impairment, concurrent nephrotoxic medications, preexisting bone marrow suppression or cytopenias, history of cytopenic reactions to other drugs, elderly pts(at greater risk for renal impairment).

ACTION

Inhibits binding of deoxyguanosine triphosphate to DNA polymerase. **Therapeutic Effect:** Inhibits viral DNA synthesis.

PHARMACOKINETICS

Well absorbed, rapidly converted to ganciclovir by intestinal mucosal cells and hepatocytes. Widely distributed including CSF, ocular tissue. Slowly metabolized intracellularly. Primarily excreted in urine. Removed by hemodialysis. **Half-life:** Ganciclovir: 4 hrs (increased in renal impairment).

⧖ LIFESPAN CONSIDERATIONS

Pregnancy/Lactation: Avoid pregnancy; may cause fetal harm/malformations. Female pts of reproductive potential should use effective contraception during treatment. Avoid breastfeeding; may be resumed no sooner than 72 hrs after last dose. May impair fertility in both females and males. **Children:** Safety and efficacy not established in pts younger than 1 month. **Elderly:** Age-related renal impairment may require dosage adjustment.

INTERACTIONS

DRUG: Bone marrow depressants may increase myelosuppression. May increase risk of toxicity of **didanosine, mycophenolate. Probenecid** may decrease renal clearance, increase concentration. **Zidovudine (AZT)** may increase risk of hematologic toxicity. **HERBAL:** None significant. **FOOD: All foods** maximize drug bioavailability. **LAB VALUES:** May decrease creatinine clearance, platelet count, neutrophils, Hgb, Hct. May increase serum creatinine.

AVAILABILITY (Rx)

Powder for Oral Solution: 50 mg/mL (100 mL).

🍸 **Tablets:** 450 mg.

ADMINISTRATION/HANDLING

PO
• Take with meals. • Do not break, crush, dissolve, or divide tablets; give whole (potential carcinogen). • Avoid contact with skin. • Wash skin with soap, water if contact occurs. • Store oral suspension in refrigerator. Discard after 49 days.

INDICATIONS/ROUTES/DOSAGE

Note: Do not use if absolute neutrophil count (ANC) less than 500 cells/mm³,

platelets less than 25,000 cells/mm³, or Hgb less than 8 g/dL.

Cytomegalovirus (CMV) Retinitis
PO: ADULTS: Initially, 900 mg (two 450-mg tablets) twice daily for 21 days. **Maintenance:** 900 mg once daily.

Prevention of CMV After Transplant
PO: ADULTS, ELDERLY: 900 mg once daily beginning within 10 days of transplant and continuing until 100 days (heart, kidney, or pancreas transplant) or 200 days (kidney transplant) post-transplant. **CHILDREN 1 MO–16 YRS:** Once daily based on body surface area (BSA) and CrCl using formula: (Dose = $7 \times$ BSA $\times$ CrCl). **Maximum:** 900 mg/day.

Dosage in Renal Impairment
Dosage and frequency are modified based on creatinine clearance.

Creatinine Clearance	Induction Dosage	Maintenance Dosage
60 mL/min or higher	900 mg twice daily	900 mg once daily
40–59 mL/ min	450 mg twice daily	450 mg once daily
25–39 mL/ min	450 mg once daily	450 mg every 2 days
10–24 mL/ min	450 mg every 2 days	450 mg twice wkly

Dosage in Hepatic Impairment
No dose adjustment.

SIDE EFFECTS

Frequent (16%–9%): Diarrhea, neutropenia, headache. **Occasional (8%–3%):** Nausea. **Rare (Less Than 3%):** Insomnia, paresthesia, vomiting, abdominal pain, fever.

ADVERSE EFFECTS/TOXIC REACTIONS

Hematologic toxicity, including severe neutropenia (most common), anemia, thrombocytopenia, leukopenia, aplastic anemia, pancytopenia, bone marrow suppression may occur. Retinal detachment occurs rarely. Overdose may result in renal toxicity. May decrease sperm production, fertility.

V

NURSING CONSIDERATIONS

BASELINE ASSESSMENT

Obtain baseline CBC, serum chemistries, renal function, urinalysis; pregnancy test. Receive full medication history.

INTERVENTION/EVALUATION

Monitor I&O, ensure adequate hydration (minimum 1,500 mL/24 hrs). Diligently evaluate CBC for decreased WBCs, Hgb, Hct, platelets; changes in urinary characteristics, consistency. Question pt regarding vision, therapeutic improvement, complications.

PATIENT/FAMILY TEACHING

• ValGANciclovir provides suppression, not cure, of CMV retinitis. • Frequent blood tests are necessary during therapy because of toxic nature of drug. • Ophthalmologic exam q4–6wks during treatment is advised. • Report any new symptom promptly. • May temporarily or permanently inhibit sperm production in men, suppress fertility in women. • Barrier contraception should be used during and for 90 days after therapy (mutagenic potential). • Swallow whole; do not chew, crush, dissolve, or divide. • Avoid handling broken/crushed tablets, oral solution. • Report fever, chills, unusual bleeding/bruising, urinary changes.

---

valproic acid

val-**pro**-ick **as**-id
(Apo-Divalproex ✿, Depacon, Depakene, <u>Depakote</u>, <u>Depakote ER</u>, Depakote Sprinkle, Novo-Divalproex ✿, Stavzor)

■ **BLACK BOX ALERT** ■ Embryo, fetal neural tube defects (spina bifida) have occurred. Life-threatening pancreatitis, complete hepatic failure have occurred.

Do not confuse Depakene with Depakote.

◆**CLASSIFICATION**

PHARMACOTHERAPEUTIC: Histone deacetylase inhibitor. **CLINICAL:** Anticonvulsant, antimanic, antimigraine.

USES

Monotherapy/adjunctive therapy of complex partial seizures, simple and complex absence seizures. Adjunctive therapy of multiple seizures including absence seizures. **Additional uses for Depakote, Depakote ER, Stavzor:** Treatment of manic episodes with bipolar disorder, prophylaxis of migraine headaches. **OFF-LABEL:** Refractory status epilepticus, diabetic neuropathy. Mood stabilizer for behaviors in dementia.

PRECAUTIONS

Contraindications: Hypersensitivity to valproic acid. Active hepatic disease, urea cycle disorders, known mitochondrial disorders; migraine prevention in pregnant women. **Cautions:** Children younger than 2 yrs. Pts at risk for hepatotoxicity. History of hepatic impairment, bleeding abnormalities, pts at high risk for suicide, elderly pts.

ACTION

Directly increases concentration of inhibitory neurotransmitter gamma-aminobutyric acid (GABA). **Therapeutic Effect:** Decreases seizure activity, stabilizes mood, prevents migraine headache.

PHARMACOKINETICS

Well absorbed from GI tract. Protein binding: 80%–90%. Metabolized in liver. Primarily excreted in urine. Not removed by hemodialysis. **Half-life:** 9–16 hrs (may be increased in hepatic impairment, elderly pts, children younger than 18 mos).

⌛ LIFESPAN CONSIDERATIONS

Pregnancy/Lactation: Drug crosses placenta; is distributed in breast milk.

V

Children: Increased risk of hepatotoxicity in pts younger than 2 yrs. **Elderly:** No age-related precautions, but lower dosages recommended.

INTERACTIONS

DRUG: Carbapenems (e.g., meropenem), CYP3A4 inducers (e.g., carBAMazepine, phenytoin, rifAMPin) may decrease concentration/effects. May alter effect of **warfarin.** May increase concentration of **lamoTRIgine. Topiramate** may increase risk of elevated serum ammonia levels. **HERBAL: Evening primrose** may decrease seizure threshold. **FOOD:** None known. **LAB VALUES:** May increase serum LDH, bilirubin, ALT, AST. **Therapeutic serum level:** 50–100 mcg/mL; **toxic serum level:** greater than 100 mcg/mL.

AVAILABILITY (Rx)

Capsules (Depakene): 250 mg. **Capsules, Sprinkle (Depakote Sprinkle):** 125 mg. **Injection, Solution (Depacon):** 100 mg/mL. **Syrup (Depakene):** 250 mg/5 mL.

 Tablets, Delayed-Release (Depakote): 125 mg, 250 mg, 500 mg. **Tablets, Extended-Release (Depakote ER):** 250 mg, 500 mg.

ADMINISTRATION/HANDLING

💧 IV

Reconstitution • Dilute each single dose with at least 50 mL D₅W, 0.9% NaCl, or lactated Ringer's.
Rate of Administration • Infuse over 60 min at rate of 20 mg/min or less. • Alternatively, single doses of up to 45 mg/kg given over 5–10 min (1.5–6 mg/kg/min).
Storage • Store vials at room temperature. • Diluted solutions stable for 24 hrs. • Discard unused portion.

PO
• May give without regard to food. Do not mix oral solution with carbonated beverages (may cause mouth/throat irritation). • May sprinkle capsule (Depakote Sprinkle) contents on applesauce and give immediately (do not chew sprinkle beads). • Give delayed-release/extended-release tablets whole. Do not crush, break, open delayed-release capsule (Stavzor). • Regular-release and delayed-release formulations usually given in 2–4 divided doses/day. Extended-release formulation (Depakote ER) usually given once daily.

🔲 IV INCOMPATIBILITIES

None known.

🔲 IV COMPATIBILITIES

Cefepime, cefTAZidime.

INDICATIONS/ROUTES/DOSAGE

Seizures
PO: ADULTS, ELDERLY, CHILDREN 10 YRS AND OLDER: Initially, 10–15 mg/kg/day in 1–3 divided doses. May increase by 5–10 mg/kg/day at wkly intervals up to 60 mg/kg/day. **Usual adult dosage:** 1,000–2,500 mg/day.
IV: ADULTS, ELDERLY, CHILDREN: Same frequency as oral dose.

Manic Episodes
PO: *(Depakote):* ADULTS, ELDERLY: Initially, 750 mg/day in divided doses. **Maximum:** 60 mg/kg/day.
PO: *(Extended-Release [Depakote ER]):* Initially, 25 mg/kg/day once daily. **Maximum:** 60 mg/kg/day. **(Delayed-Release [Stavzor]):** Initially, 750 mg/day in divided dose. Titrate to lowest therapeutic dose. **Maximum:** 60 mg/kg/day.

Prevention of Migraine Headaches
PO: *(Extended-Release [Depakote ER]):* ADULTS, ELDERLY: Initially, 500 mg/day for 7 days. May increase up to 1,000 mg/day.
PO: *(Delayed-Release [Depakote]):* ADULTS, ELDERLY, CHILDREN 16 YRS AND OLDER: Initially, 250 mg twice daily. May increase up to 1,000 mg/day.
ADULTS, ELDERLY, CHILDREN 12 YRS AND OLDER: *(Stavzor):* 250 mg twice daily. May increase to 1,000 mg/day.

V

Dosage in Renal Impairment
No dose adjustment.

Dosage in Hepatic Impairment
Mild to moderate impairment: Not recommended. **Severe impairment:** Contraindicated.

SIDE EFFECTS

Frequent: Epilepsy: Abdominal pain, irregular menses, diarrhea, transient alopecia, indigestion, nausea, vomiting, tremors, fluctuations in body weight. **Mania (22%–19%):** Nausea, drowsiness. **Occasional: Epilepsy:** Constipation, dizziness, drowsiness, headache, skin rash, unusual excitement, restlessness. **Mania (12%–6%):** Asthenia, abdominal pain, dyspepsia, rash. **Rare: Epilepsy:** Mood changes, diplopia, nystagmus, spots before eyes, unusual bleeding/bruising.

ADVERSE EFFECTS/TOXIC REACTIONS

Hepatotoxicity may occur, particularly in first 6 mos of therapy. May be preceded by loss of seizure control, malaise, weakness, lethargy, anorexia, vomiting rather than abnormal LFT results. Blood dyscrasias may occur.

NURSING CONSIDERATIONS

BASELINE ASSESSMENT

Anticonvulsant: Review history of seizure disorder (intensity, frequency, duration, level of consciousness). Initiate safety measures, quiet dark environment. CBC should be performed before and 2 wks after therapy begins, then 2 wks following maintenance dose. Obtain baseline LFT. **Antimanic:** Assess behavior, appearance, emotional status, response to environment, speech pattern, thought content. **Antimigraine:** Question pt regarding onset, location, duration of migraine, possible precipitating symptoms.

INTERVENTION/EVALUATION

Monitor CBC, LFT, serum ammonia. **Anticonvulsant:** Observe frequently for recurrence of seizure activity. Assess skin for ecchymoses, petechiae. Monitor for clinical improvement (decrease in intensity/frequency of seizures). **Antimanic:** Question for suicidal ideation. Assess for therapeutic response (interest in surroundings, increased ability to concentrate, relaxed facial expression). **Antimigraine:** Evaluate for relief of migraine headache and resulting photophobia, phonophobia, nausea, vomiting. **Therapeutic serum level:** 50–100 mcg/mL; **toxic serum level:** greater than 100 mcg/mL.

PATIENT/ FAMILY TEACHING

• Do not abruptly discontinue medication after long-term use (may precipitate seizures). • Strict maintenance of drug therapy is essential for seizure control. • Avoid tasks that require alertness, motor skills until response to drug is established. • Drowsiness usually disappears during continued therapy. • Avoid alcohol. • Report liver problems such as nausea, vomiting, lethargy, altered mental status, weakness, loss of appetite, abdominal pain, yellowing of skin, unusual bruising/bleeding. • Report if seizure control worsens, suicidal ideation (depression, unusual changes in behavior, suicidal thoughts) occurs.

valsartan

val-**sar**-tan
(Apo-Valsartan ✽, Diovan)
■ **BLACK BOX ALERT** ■ May cause fetal injury, mortality. Discontinue as soon as possible once pregnancy is detected.
Do not confuse Diovan with Zyban, or valsartan with losartan or Valstar.

FIXED-COMBINATION(S)

Diovan HCT: valsartan/hydroCHLOROthiazide (a diuretic): 80 mg/12.5

mg, 160 mg/12.5 mg, 160 mg/25 mg, 320 mg/12.5 mg, 320 mg/25 mg. **Byvalson:** valsartan/nebivolol (a beta blocker): 80 mg/5 mg. **Exforge:** valsartan/amLODIPine (a calcium channel blocker): 160 mg/5 mg, 160 mg/10 mg, 320 mg/5 mg, 320 mg/10 mg. **Exforge HCT:** valsartan/amLODIPine (a calcium channel blocker)/hydroCHLOROthiazide (a diuretic): 160 mg/5 mg/12.5 mg, 160 mg/5 mg/25 mg, 160 mg/10 mg/12.5 mg, 160 mg/10 mg/25 mg, 320 mg/10 mg/25 mg. **Valturna:** valsartan/aliskiren (a direct renin inhibitor): 160 mg/150 mg, 320 mg/300 mg.

◆CLASSIFICATION

PHARMACOTHERAPEUTIC: Angiotensin II receptor antagonist. **CLINICAL:** Antihypertensive.

USES

Treatment of hypertension alone or in combination with other antihypertensives. Treatment of HF (NYHA Class II–IV). Reduce mortality in high-risk pts (left ventricular failure/dysfunction) following MI.

PRECAUTIONS

Contraindications: Hypersensitivity to valsartan. Concomitant use with aliskiren in pts with diabetes. **Cautions:** Concurrent use of potassium-sparing diuretics or potassium supplements, mild to severe hepatic impairment, unstented bilateral/unilateral renal artery stenosis, renal impairment, significant aortic/mitral stenosis, elderly pts.

ACTION

Directly antagonizes angiotensin II receptors. Blocks vasoconstrictor, aldosterone-secreting effects of angiotensin II, inhibiting binding of angiotensin II to AT_1 receptors. **Therapeutic Effect:** Produces vasodilation, decreases peripheral resistance, decreases B/P.

PHARMACOKINETICS

Poorly absorbed after PO administration. Food decreases peak plasma concentration. Protein binding: 95%. Metabolized in liver. Excreted in feces (83%), urine (13%). Unknown if removed by hemodialysis. **Half-life:** 6 hrs.

⌛ LIFESPAN CONSIDERATIONS

Pregnancy/Lactation: May cause fetal harm. Unknown if distributed in breast milk. **Children:** Safety and efficacy not established. **Elderly:** No age-related precautions noted.

INTERACTIONS

DRUG: NSAIDs (e.g., ibuprofen, ketorolac, naproxen) may decrease antihypertensive effects. **Potassium-sparing drugs (e.g., spironolactone, triamterene), potassium supplements** may increase serum potassium. **Diuretics (e.g., furosemide, HCTZ)** may produce additive hypotensive effects. **HERBAL: Ginger, ginseng, licorice** may worsen hypertension. **Black cohosh, periwinkle** may increase antihypertensive effects. **FOOD:** None known. **LAB VALUES:** May increase serum bilirubin, ALT, AST, BUN, creatinine, potassium. May decrease Hgb, Hct, WBC.

AVAILABILITY (Rx)

Tablets: 40 mg, 80 mg, 160 mg, 320 mg.

ADMINISTRATION/HANDLING

PO
• Give without regard to meals.

INDICATIONS/ROUTES/DOSAGE

Hypertension
PO: ADULTS, ELDERLY: Initially, 80–160 mg/day in pts who are not volume depleted. **Maximum:** 320 mg/day. **CHILDREN 6–16 YRS:** Initially, 1.3 mg/kg once daily (**Maximum:** 40 mg). May increase up to 2.7 mg/kg once daily (**Maximum:** 160 mg/day).

HF
PO: ADULTS, ELDERLY: Initially, 20–40 mg twice daily. May increase up to 160 mg twice daily. **Maximum:** 320 mg/day.

V

Post-MI, Left Ventricular Dysfunction

PO: ADULTS, ELDERLY: May initiate 12 hrs or longer following MI. Initially, 20 mg twice daily. May increase within 7 days to 40 mg twice daily. May further increase up to target dose of 160 mg twice daily.

Dosage in Renal Impairment

CrCl greater than 30 mL/min: No dose adjustment. **CrCl 30 mL/min or less: ADULTS:** Safety/efficacy not established. **CHILDREN 6–16 YRS:** Not recommended.

Dosage in Hepatic Impairment

No dose adjustment.

SIDE EFFECTS

Rare (2%–1%): Insomnia, fatigue, heartburn, abdominal pain, dizziness, headache, diarrhea, nausea, vomiting, arthralgia, edema.

ADVERSE EFFECTS/TOXIC REACTIONS

Overdosage may manifest as hypotension, tachycardia. Bradycardia occurs less often. Viral infection, upper respiratory tract infection (cough, pharyngitis, sinusitis, rhinitis) occur rarely.

NURSING CONSIDERATIONS

BASELINE ASSESSMENT

Obtain CBC, BMP, LFT. Obtain B/P, apical pulse immediately before each dose, in addition to regular monitoring (be alert to fluctuations). If excessive reduction in B/P occurs, place pt in supine position, feet slightly elevated. Question for possibility of pregnancy. Assess medication history (esp. diuretic). Question for history of hepatic/renal impairment, renal artery stenosis, history of severe HF.

INTERVENTION/EVALUATION

Maintain hydration (offer fluids frequently). Assess for evidence of upper respiratory infection. Monitor serum electrolytes, renal function, LFT, Hgb, Hct, urinalysis, B/P, pulse. Observe for symptoms of hypotension.

PATIENT/ FAMILY TEACHING

• Females of childbearing potential must use effective contraception during treatment. • Inform physician as soon as possible if pregnancy occurs. • Report any sign of infection (sore throat, fever). • Do not stop taking medication. • Report swelling of extremities, chest pain, palpitations; decreased urine output, amber-colored urine, fatigue, yellowing of the skin or eyes.

vancomycin

van-koe-**mye**-sin

(Vancocin)

Do not confuse vancomycin with clindamycin, gentamicin, tobramycin, or Vibramycin.

◆CLASSIFICATION

PHARMACOTHERAPEUTIC: Tricyclic glycopeptide antibiotic. **CLINICAL:** Antibiotic.

USES

Systemic: Treatment of infections caused by staphylococcal, streptococcal spp. bacteria. **PO:** Treatment of *C. difficile*–associated diarrhea and treatment of enterocolitis caused by *S. aureus* (including MRSA). **OFF-LABEL:** Treatment of infections caused by gram-positive organisms in pts with serious allergies to beta-lactam antibiotics; treatment of beta-lactam–resistant gram-positive infections. Surgical prophylaxis, treatment of prosthetic joint infection.

PRECAUTIONS

Contraindications: Hypersensitivity to vancomycin. **Cautions:** Renal impairment; concurrent therapy with other ototoxic, nephrotoxic medications, elderly pts, dehydration.

ACTION

Binds to bacterial cell walls, altering cell membrane permeability, inhibiting RNA synthesis. **Therapeutic Effect:** Bactericidal.

PHARMACOKINETICS

PO: Poorly absorbed from GI tract. Primarily excreted in feces. **Parenteral:** Widely distributed (except CSF). Protein binding: 10%–50%. Primarily excreted unchanged in urine. Not removed by hemodialysis. **Half-life:** 4–11 hrs (increased in renal impairment).

⊠ LIFESPAN CONSIDERATIONS

Pregnancy/Lactation: Drug crosses placenta, distributed in breast milk following IV administration. **Children:** Close monitoring of serum levels recommended in premature neonates, young infants. **Elderly:** Age-related renal impairment may increase risk of ototoxicity, nephrotoxicity; dosage adjustment recommended.

INTERACTIONS

DRUG: Aminoglycosides (e.g., gentamicin, tobramycin), amphotericin B, CISplatin may increase risk of ototoxicity, nephrotoxicity of parenteral vancomycin. **HERBAL:** None significant. **FOOD:** None known. **LAB VALUES:** May increase BUN. **Therapeutic peak serum level:** (Not routinely obtained) 20–40 mcg/mL; **therapeutic trough serum level:** 10–20 mcg/mL. **Toxic peak serum level:** greater than 40 mcg/mL; **toxic trough serum level:** greater than 20 mcg/mL.

AVAILABILITY (Rx)

Capsules (Vancocin): 125 mg, 250 mg. **Infusion (Premix [Vancocin HCl]):** 500 mg/100 mL, 750 mg/150 mL, 1 g/200 mL. **Injection, Powder for Reconstitution (Vancocin HCl):** 500 mg, 750 mg, 1 g. **Solution, Oral:** 25 mg/mL, 50 mg/mL. **Suspension, Oral:** 50 mg/mL.

ADMINISTRATION/HANDLING

 IV

◀ **ALERT** ▶ Give by intermittent IV infusion (piggyback) or continuous IV infusion. Do not give IV push (may result in exaggerated hypotension or "red man" syndrome).

Reconstitution • For intermittent IV infusion (piggyback), reconstitute each 500-mg vial with 10 mL Sterile Water for Injection (20 mL for 1-g vial) to provide concentration of 50 mg/mL. • Further dilute with D₅W or 0.9% NaCl to final concentration not to exceed 5 mg/mL.

Rate of Administration • Administer over 60 min or longer (30 min for each 500 mg recommended). • Monitor B/P closely during IV infusion.

Storage • Reconstituted vials are stable for 14 days at room temperature or if refrigerated. • Diluted solutions are stable for 14 days if refrigerated or 7 days at room temperature. • Discard if precipitate forms.

PO

• May give with food. • Powder for injection may be reconstituted and diluted for oral administration.

▦ IV INCOMPATIBILITIES

Albumin, amphotericin B complex (Abelcet, AmBisome, Amphotec), aztreonam (Azactam), ceFAZolin (Ancef), cefotaxime (Claforan), cefOXitin (Mefoxin), cefTAZidime (Fortaz), cefTRIAXone (Rocephin), cefuroxime (Zinacef), foscarnet (Foscavir), heparin, nafcillin (Nafcil), piperacillin and tazobactam (Zosyn).

▦ IV COMPATIBILITIES

Amiodarone (Cordarone), calcium gluconate, dexmedetomidine (Precedex), diltiaZEM (Cardizem), HYDROmorphone (Dilaudid), insulin, LORazepam (Ativan), magnesium sulfate, midazolam (Versed), morphine, niCARdipine (Cardene), potassium chloride, propofol (Diprivan).

V

INDICATIONS/ROUTES/DOSAGE

Note: A loading dose of 25–30 mg/kg may be used to rapidly achieve target concentration for complicated infections in seriously ill pts.

Usual Parenteral Dosage

IV: ADULTS, ELDERLY: 15–20 mg/kg/dose q8–12h. Dosage requires adjustment in renal impairment. **CHILDREN OLDER THAN 1 MO:** 10–15 mg/kg/dose q6h. **Maximum:** 2,000 mg/dose. **NEONATES:** 15 mg/kg q24h up to 10–15 mg/kg/dose q6–24h.

Staphylococcal Enterocolitis, Antibiotic-Associated Pseudomembranous Colitis Caused by *Clostridium Difficile*

PO: ADULTS, ELDERLY: 125–500 mg 4 times/day for 7–10 days. **CHILDREN:** 40 mg/kg/day in 3–4 divided doses for 7–10 days. **Maximum:** 2 g/day.

Dosage in Renal Impairment

After loading dose, subsequent dosages and frequency are modified based on creatinine clearance, severity of infection, and serum concentration of drug.

Dosage in Hepatic Impairment

No dose adjustment.

SIDE EFFECTS

Frequent: PO: Bitter/unpleasant taste, nausea, vomiting, mouth irritation (with oral solution). **Rare: Parenteral:** Phlebitis, thrombophlebitis, pain at peripheral IV site, dizziness, vertigo, tinnitus, chills, fever, rash, necrosis with extravasation. **PO:** Rash.

ADVERSE EFFECTS/TOXIC REACTIONS

Nephrotoxicity (acute kidney injury, acute tubular necrosis, renal failure), ototoxicity (temporary or permanent hearing loss) may occur. Too-rapid infusion may cause "red man syndrome," a common adverse reaction characterized by pruritus, urticaria, erythema, angioedema, tachycardia, hypotension, myalgia, maculopapular rash (usually appears on face, neck, upper torso). Cardiovascular toxicity (cardiac depression, arrest) occurs rarely. Onset usually occurs within 30 min of start of infusion, resolves within hrs following infusion. May result from too-rapid rate of infusion.

NURSING CONSIDERATIONS

BASELINE ASSESSMENT

Avoid other ototoxic, nephrotoxic medications if possible. Obtain culture, sensitivity test before giving first dose (therapy may begin before results are known). Consider placement of central venous line/PICC line.

INTERVENTION/EVALUATION

Monitor serum renal function tests, I&O. Assess skin for rash. Check hearing acuity, balance. Monitor B/P carefully during infusion. Monitor for "red man" syndrome. Evaluate IV site for phlebitis (heat, pain, red streaking over vein). Obtain vancomycin peak/trough level as ordered by physician or pharmacist. **Therapeutic serum level: peak:** 20–40 mcg/mL; **trough:** 10–20 mcg/mL. **Toxic serum level: peak:** greater than 40 mcg/mL; **trough:** greater than 20 mcg/mL.

PATIENT/ FAMILY TEACHING

• Continue therapy for full length of treatment. • Doses should be evenly spaced. • Report ringing in ears, hearing loss, changes in urinary frequency or consistency. • Lab tests are important part of total therapy.

vandetanib

van-**det**-a-nib
(Caprelsa)

■ **BLACK BOX ALERT** ■ Can prolong QT interval (torsades de pointes and sudden cardiac death reported). Do not use in pts with hypokalemia, hypocalcemia, hypomagnesemia, congenital long

QT syndrome. Electrolyte imbalances must be corrected prior to initiating therapy. If medication that prolongs QT interval is needed, more frequent EKG monitoring is recommended. EKGs should be obtained during wks 2–4 and wks 8–12 after starting therapy and 3 mos thereafter. Any dose reduction or interruption related to QT prolongation greater than 2 wks must have frequent EKG monitoring as noted above. Only certified prescribers and pharmacies with a restricted distribution program are able to prescribe and dispense.

◆CLASSIFICATION

PHARMACOTHERAPEUTIC: Tyrosine kinase inhibitor. **CLINICAL:** Antineoplastic.

USES

Treatment of symptomatic or progressive medullary thyroid cancer in pts with unresectable locally advanced or metastatic disease.

PRECAUTIONS

Contraindications: Hypersensitivity to vandetanib. Congenital long QT syndrome. **Cautions:** Pregnancy, concurrent medications that prolong QT interval, hypokalemia, hypomagnesemia, hypothyroidism, cerebrovascular disease, moderate to severe renal/hepatic impairment, hypertension, uncompensated HF, history of torsades de pointes.

ACTION

Inhibits tyrosine kinases including epidermal growth factor (EGF) and vascular endothelial growth factor (VEGF). Inhibits cell migration, proliferation, survival, and angiogenesis (new blood vessel formation). **Therapeutic Effect:** Inhibits thyroid tumor cell growth and metastasis.

PHARMACOKINETICS

Slowly absorbed following PO administration. Peak concentration: 4–10 hrs. Metabolized in liver. Protein binding: 90%. Excreted in feces (44%), urine (25%). **Half-life:** 19 days.

⌛ LIFESPAN CONSIDERATIONS

Pregnancy/Lactation: May cause fetal harm. Avoid pregnancy. Must use effective contraception during treatment and for at least 4 mos after treatment. Unknown if distributed in breast milk. **Children:** Safety and efficacy not established. **Elderly:** No age-related precautions noted.

INTERACTIONS

DRUG: Medications prolonging QT interval (e.g., amiodarone, azithromycin, ciprofloxacin, clarithromycin, erythromycin, haloperidol) may increase risk of QT prolongation. **CYP3A4 inducers** (e.g., carBAMazepine, OXcarbazepine, phenytoin, rifAMPin) may decrease concentration/effects. **HERBAL:** St. John's wort may decrease concentration/effect. **FOOD:** Grapefruit products may increase risk of torsades de pointes, myelotoxicity. **LAB VALUES:** May decrease WBC, Hgb, neutrophils. May increase serum bilirubin, ALT, AST, creatinine; urine protein. May alter serum calcium, glucose, magnesium, potassium.

AVAILABILITY (Rx)

Tablets: 100 mg, 300 mg.

ADMINISTRATION/HANDLING

PO

• Give without regard to food. • Do not crush. • May disperse in 2 oz of noncarbonated water and stir for 10 min until tablet is evenly dispersed (will not completely dissolve). Administer dispersion immediately. Rinse residue in glass with 4 oz water and administer. Can be given via feeding tube. • Direct contact of crushed tablets with skin or mucous membranes should be strictly avoided. If contact occurs, wash thoroughly.

Storage • Contact pharmacy to properly discard out-of-date tablets.

V

♦ Canadian trade name　　　🦖 Non-Crushable Drug　　　🔲 High Alert drug

INDICATIONS/ROUTES/DOSAGE

Thyroid Cancer
PO: ADULTS, ELDERLY: 300 mg once daily. Continue until disease progression or unacceptable toxicity.

Dosage Adjustment for QT Prolongation or Toxicity
Interrupt therapy until resolved or improved, then restart at 100–200 mg once daily.

Dosage in Renal Impairment
CrCl less than 50 mL/min: 200 mg once daily. Closely monitor QT interval.

Dosage in Hepatic Impairment
Mild impairment: No dose adjustment. **Moderate to severe impairment:** Not recommended.

SIDE EFFECTS

Frequent (57%–21%): Diarrhea/colitis, rash, dermatitis acneiform/acne, nausea, headache, fatigue, anorexia, abdominal pain. **Occasional (15%–10%):** Dry skin, vomiting, asthenia, photosensitivity, insomnia, nasopharyngitis, dyspepsia, cough, pruritus, weight decrease, depression.

ADVERSE EFFECTS/TOXIC REACTIONS

Prolonged QT interval resulting in torsades de pointes, ventricular arrhythmias, sudden cardiac death have been reported. Frequent diarrhea may result in electrolyte imbalances. Severe skin reactions, including Stevens-Johnson syndrome, have been reported. Interstitial lung disease (ILD) or pneumonitis reported (may result in respiratory-related death). Consider ILD in pts with hypoxia, pleural effusion, cough, dyspnea. Ischemic cerebrovascular events have been reported. Life-threatening events including hypertensive crisis, reversible posterior leukoencephalopathy syndrome (RPLS) have been noted. Adverse reactions resulting in death included respiratory failure/arrest, aspiration pneumonia, cardiac failure, sepsis, GI bleeding.

NURSING CONSIDERATIONS

BASELINE ASSESSMENT
Obtain CBC with differential, serum chemistries, magnesium, ionized calcium, TSH, UA, EKG, vital signs. Obtain negative urine pregnancy before therapy. Question for history of congenital long QT syndrome, HF, arrhythmias, hepatic/renal impairment, seizures, CVA, hemorrhagic events, HTN. Obtain full medication history including contraception. Perform full head-to-toe exam including visual acuity, thorough skin assessment.

INTERVENTION/EVALUATION
Monitor blood levels including electrolytes esp. during episodes of diarrhea. Obtain EKG during wks 2–4, wks 8–12, then every 3 mos thereafter. Obtain EKG for palpitations, chest pain, hypokalemia, hyperkalemia, hypocalcemia, bradycardia, ventricular arrhythmias, syncope. Report any respiratory changes including dyspnea, cough (may indicate ILD). Reversible posterior leukoencephalopathy syndrome should be considered in pts with seizures, headache, visual disturbances, confusion, altered mental status. Ophthalmologic exams including slit lamp recommended in pts with visual disturbances.

PATIENT/FAMILY TEACHING
• Blood levels, EKGs will be routinely monitored. • Strictly avoid pregnancy. Contraception should be taken during treatment and 4 mos after discontinuation. • Changes in mental status, seizures, headache, blurry vision, trouble speaking, one-sided weakness may indicate stroke, high blood pressure crisis, or life-threatening brain swelling. Immediately report any newly prescribed medications. • Do not take herbal products. • Limit exposure to sunlight. • Report any yellowing of skin or eyes, abdominal pain, bruising, black/tarry stools, dark urine, decreased urine output, skin changes. • Report palpitations, chest pain, shortness of breath, dizziness, fainting (may indicate arrhythmia).

V

---

varenicline

var-**en**-i-kleen
(Champix ✦, Chantix)
■ **BLACK BOX ALERT** ■ Risk of psychiatric symptoms and suicidal behavior. Agitation, hostility, depressed mood have been reported.

◆CLASSIFICATION

PHARMACOTHERAPEUTIC: Selective partial nicotine agonist. **CLINICAL:** Smoking deterrent.

USES

Aid to smoking-cessation treatment.

PRECAUTIONS

Contraindications: Hypersensitivity to varenicline. **Cautions:** Renal impairment, history of suicidal ideation or preexisting psychiatric illness, bipolar disorder, depression, schizophrenia. History of seizures or factors that lower seizure threshold.

ACTION

Prevents nicotine stimulation of mesolimbic system associated with nicotine addiction. **Therapeutic Effect:** Decreases desire to smoke.

PHARMACOKINETICS

Completely absorbed following PO administration. Absorption unaffected by food, time-of-day dosing. Peak plasma concentration: 3–4 hrs. Steady state reached within 4 days. Protein binding: 20%. Minimal metabolism. Removed by hemodialysis. Primarily excreted unchanged in urine. **Half-life:** 24 hrs.

⏳ LIFESPAN CONSIDERATIONS

Pregnancy/Lactation: Unknown if distributed in breast milk. **Children:** Not recommended. **Elderly:** Age-related renal impairment may require dosage adjustment.

INTERACTIONS

DRUG: Cimetidine may increase effect. May increase concentration/effect of **nicotine. HERBAL:** None significant. **FOOD:** None known. **LAB VALUES:** None significant.

AVAILABILITY (Rx)

🔖 **Tablets (Film-Coated):** 0.5 mg, 1 mg.

ADMINISTRATION/HANDLING

• Give after meal and with full glass of water. • Do not break, crush, dissolve, or divide film-coated tablets.

INDICATIONS/ROUTES/DOSAGE

◄**ALERT**► Therapy should start 1 wk before stopping smoking.

Smoking Deterrent
PO: ADULTS, ELDERLY: Days 1–3: 0.5 mg once daily. **Days 4–7:** 0.5 mg twice daily. **Day 8–end of treatment:** 1 mg twice daily. Therapy should last for total of 12 wks. Pts who have successfully stopped smoking at the end of 12 wks should continue with an additional 12 wks of treatment to increase likelihood of long-term abstinence.

Dosage in Renal Impairment
CrCl less than 30 mL/min: 0.5 mg once daily. **Maximum:** 0.5 mg twice daily. **End-stage renal disease, undergoing hemodialysis: Maximum:** 0.5 mg once daily.

Dosage in Hepatic Impairment
No dose adjustment.

SIDE EFFECTS

Frequent (30%–13%): Nausea, insomnia, headache, abnormal dreams. **Occasional (8%–5%):** Constipation, abdominal discomfort, fatigue, dry mouth, flatulence, altered taste, dyspepsia, vomiting, anxiety, depression, irritability. **Rare (3%–1%):** Drowsiness, rash, increased appetite, lethargy, nightmares, gastroesophageal reflux disease, rhinorrhea, agitation, mood swings.

V

✦ Canadian trade name   🔖 Non-Crushable Drug   🔲 High Alert drug

ADVERSE EFFECTS/TOXIC REACTIONS

Abrupt withdrawal may cause irritability, sleep disturbances in 3% of pts. Hypertension, angina pectoris, arrhythmia, bradycardia, coronary artery disease, gingivitis, anemia, lymphadenopathy occur rarely. May cause bizarre behavior, suicidal ideation.

NURSING CONSIDERATIONS

BASELINE ASSESSMENT

Screen, evaluate for coronary heart disease (history of MI, angina pectoris), cardiac arrhythmias, suicidal ideation. Assess smoking pack/yr history.

INTERVENTION/EVALUATION

Discontinue use if cardiovascular symptoms occur or worsen. Monitor for psychiatric symptoms (changes in behavior, mood, level of interest, appearance). Assess for cravings, noncompliance with cessation.

PATIENT/FAMILY TEACHING

• Initiate treatment 1 wk before quit-smoking date. • Take with food and with full glass of water. • With twice-daily dosing, take 1 tablet in morning, 1 in evening. • Report persistent nausea, insomnia. • Report change in behavior, mood, level of interest, appearance.

vasopressin

vay-soe-**pres**-in
(Pressyn ✦, Pressyn AR ✦, Vasostrict)
Do not confuse Pitressin with Pitocin.

◆CLASSIFICATION

PHARMACOTHERAPEUTIC: Posterior pituitary hormone. **CLINICAL:** Vasopressor, antidiuretic.

USES

Prevention/control of polydipsia, polyuria, dehydration in pts with neurogenic diabetes insipidus or differential diagnosis of diabetes insipidus. **Vasoconstriction:** To increase blood pressure in adults with vasodilatory shock who remain hypotensive despite fluids and catecholamines. **OFF-LABEL:** Adjunct in treatment of acute massive GI hemorrhage or esophageal varices.

PRECAUTIONS

Contraindications: Hypersensitivity to vasopressin. **Cautions:** Seizure disorder, migraine, asthma, vascular disease, renal/cardiac disease, goiter (with cardiac complications), arteriosclerosis, nephritis, elderly pts.

ACTION

Increases reabsorption of water by renal tubules. Directly stimulates smooth muscle in GI tract. **Therapeutic Effect:** Causes peristalsis, vasoconstriction. Decreases urine output.

PHARMACOKINETICS

Route	Onset	Peak	Duration
IV	N/A	N/A	0.5–1 hr
IM, SQ	1–2 hrs	N/A	2–8 hrs

Distributed throughout extracellular fluid. Metabolized in liver, kidney. Primarily excreted in urine. **Half-life:** 10–20 min.

⧗ LIFESPAN CONSIDERATIONS

Pregnancy/Lactation: Caution in giving to breastfeeding women. **Children/Elderly:** Caution due to risk of water intoxication/hyponatremia.

INTERACTIONS

DRUG: Alcohol, demeclocycline, lithium, norepinephrine may decrease antidiuretic effect. **CarBAMazepine, chlorproPAMIDE, clofibrate** may increase antidiuretic effect. **HERBAL:** None significant. **FOOD:** None known. **LAB VALUES:** None significant.

AVAILABILITY (Rx)

Injection Solution: 20 units/mL.

ADMINISTRATION/HANDLING

 IV

Reconstitution • Dilute with D_5W or 0.9% NaCl to concentration of 0.1–1 unit/mL (usual concentration: 100 units/500 mL D_5W).
Rate of Administration • Give as IV infusion.
Storage • Store at room temperature.

IM, SQ
• Give with 1–2 glasses of water to reduce side effects.

▦ IV INCOMPATIBILITIES

Furosemide (Lasix), phenytoin (Dilantin).

▦ IV COMPATIBILITIES

Amiodarone, argatroban, diltiaZEM (Cardizem), DOBUTamine (Dobutrex), DOPamine (Intropin), heparin, insulin, milrinone (Primacor), nitroglycerin, norepinephrine (Levophed), pantoprazole (Protonix), phenylephrine (Neo-Synephrine).

INDICATIONS/ROUTES/DOSAGE

Diabetes Insipidus
NOTE: May be administered intranasally by nasal spray or on cotton pledgets; dosage is individualized.
IM, SQ: ADULTS, ELDERLY: 5–10 units 2–4 times/day. **CHILDREN:** 2.5–10 units, 2–4 times/day.

Vasodilatory Shock
IV Infusion: ADULTS, ELDERLY: Initially, 0.01 units/min. Titrate by 0.005 units/min at 10–15-min intervals. **Maximum:** 0.07 units/min.

Dosage in Renal/Hepatic Impairment
No dose adjustment.

SIDE EFFECTS

Frequent: Pain at injection site (with vasopressin tannate). **Occasional:** Abdominal cramps, nausea, vomiting, diarrhea, dizziness, diaphoresis, pale skin, circumoral pallor, tremors, headache, eructation, flatulence. **Rare:** Chest pain, confusion, allergic reaction (rash, urticaria, pruritus, wheezing, difficulty breathing, facial/peripheral edema), sterile abscess (with vasopressin tannate).

ADVERSE EFFECTS/TOXIC REACTIONS

Anaphylaxis, MI, water intoxication have occurred. Elderly, very young are at higher risk for water intoxication.

NURSING CONSIDERATIONS

BASELINE ASSESSMENT
Establish baselines for weight, B/P, pulse, serum electrolytes, Hgb, Hct, urine specific gravity.

INTERVENTION/EVALUATION
Monitor I&O closely, restrict intake as necessary to prevent water intoxication. Weigh daily if indicated. Check B/P, pulse frequently. Monitor serum electrolytes, Hgb, Hct, urine specific gravity. Evaluate injection site for erythema, pain, abscess. Report side effects to physician for dose reduction. Be alert for early signs of water intoxication (drowsiness, listlessness, headache, seizures). Observe for evidence of GI bleeding. Withhold medication, report immediately any chest pain, allergic symptoms.

PATIENT/FAMILY TEACHING
• Promptly report headache, chest pain, shortness of breath, other symptoms.
• Stress importance of I&O. • Avoid alcohol. • Report confusion, seizure activity.

V

vedolizumab

ve-doe-**liz**-ue-mab
(Entyvio)
Do not confuse vedolizumab with certolizumab, eculizumab, natalizumab, omalizumab, tocilizumab.

✦ Canadian trade name   🦫 Non-Crushable Drug   🔲 High Alert drug

◆CLASSIFICATION

PHARMACOTHERAPEUTIC: Selective adhesion molecule inhibitor. Monoclonal antibody. **CLINICAL:** GI agent.

USES

Treatment of adult pts with moderately to severely active ulcerative colitis (UC) who have had an inadequate response with, lost response to, or were intolerant to a tumor necrosis factor (TNF) blocker or immunomodulator; or had an inadequate response with, were intolerant to, or demonstrated dependence on corticosteroids. Treatment of adult pts with moderately to severely active Crohn's disease (CD) who have had an inadequate response with, lost response to, or were intolerant to a TNF blocker or immunomodulator; or had an inadequate response with, were intolerant to, or demonstrated dependence on corticosteroids.

PRECAUTIONS

Contraindications: Hypersensitivity to vedolizumab. **Cautions:** Hepatic impairment, immunocompromised pts, live vaccine administration. Active infections (not recommended during active infection), conditions predisposing to infections (e.g., diabetes, renal failure, open wounds, indwelling catheters). Preexisting or recent-onset CNS demyelinating disorders including multiple sclerosis.

ACTION

Binds to T-lymphocyte integrin receptors and blocks the interaction with mucosal addressin cell adhesion molecule-1 (MAdCAM-1). Inhibits migration and homing of memory T-lymphocytes into inflamed GI tissue. **Therapeutic Effect:** Reduces chronic inflammation of colon.

PHARMACOKINETICS

Metabolism not specified. Excretion not specified. **Half-life:** 25 days.

⧗ LIFESPAN CONSIDERATIONS

Pregnancy/Lactation: Unknown if distributed in breast milk. Use caution when administering to nursing women. **Children:** Safety and efficacy not established. **Elderly:** No age-related precautions noted.

INTERACTIONS

DRUG: Natalizumab may increase risk of progressive multifocal leukoencephalopathy (PML). **Other TNF blockers (e.g., inFLIXimab)** may increase risk of infection. **HERBAL:** None significant. **FOOD:** None known. **LAB VALUES:** May increase serum ALT, AST, bilirubin.

AVAILABILITY (Rx)

Lyophilized Powder for Injection: 300 mg.

ADMINISTRATION/HANDLING
💧 IV

• Do not administer IV push or bolus. • Reconstitute with Sterile Water for Injection and subsequently dilute with 0.9% NaCl only. • After infusion completed, flush IV line with 30 mL of 0.9% NaCl.

Reconstitution • Remove flip cap and swab with alcohol. • Reconstitute vial with 4.8 mL Sterile Water for Injection. Direct stream toward glass wall to avoid excessive foaming. • Gently swirl contents for at least 15 sec until completely dissolved. • Do not shake or invert vial. • Allow solution to sit at room temperature for up to 20 min to allow remaining foam to settle and powder to dissolve. If not fully dissolved after 20 min, allow additional 10 min for dissolution. Do not use if product is not dissolved within 30 min. • Visually inspect for particulate matter and discoloration. Do not use if discolored or if particle matter is observed. • Prior to withdrawing solution, invert vial 3 times to ensure mixing. • Withdraw 5 mL and further dilute in 250 mL 0.9% NaCl bag. • Infuse immediately.

V

Rate of Administration • Infuse over 30 min.

Storage • Reconstituted solution should appear clear to opalescent, colorless to light brownish yellow and free of particles. • May refrigerate diluted solution for up to 4 hrs.

INDICATIONS/ROUTES/DOSAGE

Ulcerative Colitis and Crohn's Disease
IV: ADULTS, ELDERLY: 300 mg once at wk 0, wk 2, and wk 6, then every 8 wks thereafter. Discontinue in pts who do not show evidence of therapeutic benefit by wk 14.

Dosage in Renal Impairment
Use caution.

Dosage in Hepatic Impairment
Use caution. Discontinue for jaundice or signs/symptoms of hepatic injury.

SIDE EFFECTS

Occasional (13%–4%): Nasopharyngitis, headache, arthralgia, nausea, pyrexia, upper respiratory tract infection, fatigue, cough, bronchitis, influenza, back pain. **Rare (3%):** Rash, pruritus, sinusitis, oropharyngeal pain, extremity pain.

ADVERSE EFFECTS/TOXIC REACTIONS

Infusion-related reactions, including anaphylaxis, characterized by bronchospasm, dyspnea, flushing, hypotension, laryngeal edema, nausea, pyrexia, tachycardia, wheezing, vomiting, reported in less than 1% of pts. May increase risk of severe infections such as anal abscess, cytomegaloviral colitis, giardiasis, *Listeria* meningitis, *Salmonella* sepsis, TB, UTI, which may lead to fatal sepsis. PML (weakness, paralysis, vision loss, aphasia, cognition impairment) has occurred rarely; however, immunocompromised pts are at increased risk for development. Drug-induced hepatotoxicity with serum ALT, AST greater than 3 times upper limit of normal reported in less than 2% of pts. Malignancies including B-cell lymphoma,

breast cancer, colon cancer, lung cancer of primary neuroendocrine carcinoma, lung neoplasm, malignant hepatic neoplasm, melanoma, renal cancer, squamous cell carcinoma, transitional cell carcinoma occur rarely. Immunogenicity (anti-vedolizumab antibodies) occurred in 4%–13% of pts.

NURSING CONSIDERATIONS

BASELINE ASSESSMENT
Obtain CBC, LFT. Prior to initiating treatment, all pts should be up to date with all immunizations according to proper guidelines. Continuously screen for active infection. Evaluate for active TB and test for latent infection prior to and during treatment. Induration of 5 mm or greater with tuberculin skin test should be considered a positive result when assessing for latent TB. Antifungal therapy should be considered for those who reside in or travel to regions where mycoses are endemic. Have supplemental oxygen, anaphylaxis kit readily available. Conduct full neurologic exam. Question history of malignancies.

INTERVENTION/EVALUATION
Routinely monitor LFT. Withhold treatment if acute infection, opportunistic infection, sepsis occurs and initiate appropriate antimicrobial therapy. Monitor for hypersensitivity reaction. Infusion-related reactions generally occur within 2 hrs after infusion. Consider administration of antihistamine, antipyretic, and/or corticosteroid if mild to moderate hypersensitivity reaction occurs. If anaphylaxis occurs, provide immediate resuscitation support. Monitor for new onset or worsening of neurologic symptoms, esp. in pts with CNS disorders; may indicate PML.

PATIENT/FAMILY TEACHING
• Blood levels, TB screening will be routinely monitored. • Therapy may lower immune system response. Report travel plans to possible endemic areas. • Do not receive live vaccines unless approved by your doctor.

V

• Report history of fungal infections, multiple sclerosis, TB or close relatives who have active TB. • Infusion may cause severe allergic reactions such as face/tongue swelling, hives, itching, low blood pressure, trouble breathing, or, in some cases, anaphylaxis. • Do not breastfeed. • Abdominal pain, bruising, clay-colored stools, dark-amber urine, fatigue, loss of appetite, yellowing of skin or eyes may indicate liver problem. • Paralysis, vision changes, impaired speech, altered mental status may indicate life-threatening neurologic event called progressive multifocal leukoencephalopathy (PML).

vemurafenib

vem-ue-**raf**-e-nib
(Zelboraf)

◆**CLASSIFICATION**

PHARMACOTHERAPEUTIC: BRAF kinase inhibitor. **CLINICAL:** Antineoplastic.

USES

Treatment of unresectable or metastatic melanoma with a BRAF V600E mutation as detected by FDA-approved test. Treatment of Erdheim-Chester disease (ECD) in pts with a BRAF V600E mutation.

PRECAUTIONS

Contraindications: Hypersensitivity to vemurafenib. **Cautions:** Avoid sun exposure. Prior radiation therapy. Prolonged QT syndrome, concurrent use of medications that prolong QT interval, hepatic impairment, uncorrected electrolyte imbalance (hypokalemia, hypomagnesemia), elderly pts.

ACTION

Inhibits kinase activity of certain mutated forms of BRAF. **Therapeutic Effect:** Blocks tumor cell proliferation in melanoma with the mutation.

PHARMACOKINETICS

Readily absorbed after PO administration. Protein binding: 99%. Minimally metabolized in liver. Primarily excreted in feces (94%). **Half-life:** 57 hrs. Range: 30–120 hrs.

⧗ LIFESPAN CONSIDERATIONS

Pregnancy/Lactation: Avoid pregnancy. May cause fetal harm. Must use effective contraception during treatment and for at least 2 mos after discontinuation. Unknown if distributed in breast milk. Must either discontinue breastfeeding or discontinue therapy. **Children:** Safety and efficacy not established. **Elderly:** May have increased risk of adverse reactions, side effects.

INTERACTIONS

DRUG: Antiarrhythmics (e.g., amiodarone, procainamide, quiNIDine, sotalol), azithromycin, barbiturates, ciprofloxacin, dexamethasone, fluconazole, haloperidol, phenothiazines, phenytoins, traZODone, tricyclic antidepressants, vardenafil, voriconazole may prolong QT interval. **CYP3A4 inhibitors** (e.g., clarithromycin, ketoconazole, rifAMPin) may alter concentration. May increase bleeding effect with **warfarin**. **HERBAL:** None significant. **FOOD:** None known. **LAB VALUES:** May increase serum alkaline phosphatase, ALT, AST, gammaglutamyl transferase (GGT), bilirubin.

AVAILABILITY (Rx)

▧ Film-Coated Tablets: 240 mg.

ADMINISTRATION/HANDLING

PO
• Give in morning and evening approximately 12 hrs apart. • Give without regard to food. • Do not break, crush, dissolve, or divide tablets; swallow whole. • Give with full glass of water.

INDICATIONS/ROUTES/DOSAGE

Note: Management of adverse drug reactions may require dose reduction, treatment interruption, or discontinuation.

V

ECD, Melanoma
PO: ADULTS, ELDERLY: 960 mg twice daily (in morning and evening about 12 hrs apart). Continue until disease progression or unacceptable toxicity.

Dosage Modification
Based on Common Terminology Criteria for Adverse Events (CTCAE). **Grade 1 or grade 2 (tolerable):** No dose adjustment. **Grade 2 (intolerable) or grade 3:** *First incident:* Interrupt treatment until toxicity returns to grade 0 or 1, then resume at 720 mg twice daily. *Second incident:* Interrupt treatment, then resume at 480 mg twice daily. *Third incident:* Discontinue. **Grade 4:** *First incident:* Interrupt treatment, then resume at 480 mg twice daily. *Second incident:* Discontinue.

Dosage in Renal/Hepatic Impairment
Mild to moderate impairment: No dose adjustment.
Severe impairment: Use with caution.

SIDE EFFECTS

Frequent (53%–33%): Arthralgia, alopecia, fatigue, rash, nausea. **Occasional (28%–11%):** Diarrhea, hyperkeratosis, headache, pruritus, pyrexia, dry skin, extremity pain, anorexia, vomiting, peripheral edema, erythema, dysgeusia, myalgia, constipation, asthenia. **Rare (8%–5%):** Maculopapular rash, actinic keratosis, musculoskeletal pain, back pain, cough, papular rash.

ADVERSE EFFECTS/TOXIC REACTIONS

Cutaneous squamous cell carcinoma (cuSCC) and keratoacanthomas reported in 24% of pts. Pts at increased risk of cuSCC include elderly pts, pts with prior skin cancer, chronic sun exposure. Hypersensitivity reactions including erythema, hypotension, anaphylaxis reported. Mild to severe photosensitivity was reported. Serious dermatologic reactions include Stevens-Johnson syndrome, toxic epidermal necrolysis. Ophthalmologic reactions including uveitis reported. Increased LFT may lead to discontinuation.

NURSING CONSIDERATIONS

BASELINE ASSESSMENT
Confirm presence of BRAF V600E mutation. Review history for previous radiation therapy. Obtain serum chemistries, renal function test, serum magnesium, ionized calcium, EKG, PT/INR if taking warfarin. Assess skin for moles, lesions, papilloma, and perform full dermatologic exam. Obtain baseline ophthalmologic exam, visual acuity. Assess medication history for QT-prolonging drugs. Obtain negative urine pregnancy before initiating treatment. Offer emotional support.

INTERVENTION/EVALUATION
Monitor EKG 15 days after initiation, then monthly for first 3 mos, then q3mos thereafter. Routinely assess skin and for 6 mos after discontinuation. Immediately report any new skin lesions. Obtain EKG for palpitations, chest pain, hypokalemia, hyperkalemia, hypocalcemia, bradycardia, ventricular arrhythmias, syncope. Monitor PT/INR while pt is on warfarin. Pruritus, difficulty breathing, erythema, hypotension may indicate anaphylaxis.

PATIENT/FAMILY TEACHING
• Blood levels, EKG, eye examinations are routinely ordered. • Strictly avoid pregnancy. Contraception should be used during treatment and for 2 mos after last dose. • Avoid sunlight exposure. • Report any skin changes, including new warts, sores, reddish bumps that bleed or do not heal, change in mole size or color. • Report yellowing of skin or eyes, abdominal pain, bruising, black/tarry stools, dark urine, decreased urine output, skin changes. • Report palpitations, chest pain, shortness of breath, dizziness, fainting (may indicate arrhythmia).

venetoclax

ven-**et**-oh-klax
(Venclexta)

V

Do not confuse venetoclax or
Venclexta with Venelex.

◆CLASSIFICATION

PHARMACOTHERAPEUTIC: B-cell
lymphoma-2 inhibitor. Antiapoptotic
protein. **CLINICAL:** Antineoplastic.

USES

Treatment of pts with chronic lymphocytic leukemia (CLL) with 17p deletion,
as detected by an FDA-approved test, who
have received at least one prior therapy.

PRECAUTIONS

Contraindications: Hypersensitivity to
venetoclax. Concomitant use of strong
CYP3A inhibitors at initiation and during
ramp-up phase. **Cautions:** Baseline anemia, leukopenia, neutropenia, thrombocytopenia; concomitant use of moderate
CYP3A inhibitors, P-gp inhibitors; active
infection or pts at increased risk of infection (diabetes, kidney failure, indwelling
catheters, open wounds), hepatic/renal
impairment, electrolyte imbalance; history of gout; pts at high risk for tumor
lysis syndrome (high tumor burden).

ACTION

Binds to and inhibits B-cell lymphoma-2
protein and displaces proapoptotic proteins, restoring process of apoptosis.
Therapeutic Effect: Inhibits tumor cell
growth and metastasis.

PHARMACOKINETICS

Widely distributed. Metabolized in liver.
Protein binding: highly bound (unspecified). Peak plasma concentration: 5–8
hrs. Excreted in feces (greater than
99%). **Half-life:** 26 hrs.

⧗ LIFESPAN CONSIDERATIONS

Pregnancy/Lactation: Avoid pregnancy; may cause fetal harm/malforma-
tions. Female and male pts of reproductive
potential should use effective contraception during treatment and for at least 30
days after discontinuation. Unknown if
distributed in breast milk. Breastfeeding
not recommended. May impair fertility
in males. **Children:** Safety and efficacy
not established. **Elderly:** No age-related
precautions noted.

INTERACTIONS

DRUG: Strong CYP3A inhibitors
(e.g., **clarithromycin, ketoconazole, ritonavir**) may significantly
increase concentration/effect; use
contraindicated. **Moderate CYP3A
inhibitors** (e.g., **erythromycin,
ciprofloxacin, diltiaZEM, dronedarone, fluconazole, verapamil**),
P-gp inhibitors (e.g., **amiodarone,
azithromycin, captopril, carvedilol,
cycloSPORINE, felodipine, ranolazine, ticagrelor**) may increase
concentration/effect; consider alternative therapy. **Strong CYP3A inducers**
(e.g., **carBAMazepine, phenytoin,
rifAMPin**) may decrease concentra-
tion/effect. **HERBAL: St. John's wort**
may decrease concentration/effect.
**FOOD: Grapefruit products, Seville
oranges, starfruit** may increase con-
centration/effect. Low-fat meals, high-fat
meals increase exposure/concentration.
LAB VALUES: May decrease Hgb, Hct,
neutrophils, platelets, RBCs; serum calcium, potassium. Tumor lysis syndrome
may result in elevated serum phosphate,
potassium, uric acid.

AVAILABILITY (Rx)

Tablets: 10 mg, 50 mg, 100 mg.

ADMINISTRATION/HANDLING

PO
• Give with food and water at same
time each day. • Administer tablets
whole; do not cut, crush, or divide. • If a dose is missed by no more
than 8 hrs, administer as soon as possible. If dose is missed by more than 8
hrs or if vomiting occurs after dosing,
skip dose and administer the next dose
on schedule.

V

INDICATIONS/ROUTES/DOSAGE

CLL

PO: ADULTS, ELDERLY: Week 1: 20 mg once daily for 7 days. **Week 2:** 50 mg once daily for 7 days. **Week 3:** 100 mg once daily for 7 days. **Week 4:** 200 mg once daily for 7 days. **Week 5 and beyond:** 400 mg once daily. Continue until disease progression or unacceptable toxicity.

Dose Modification

Based on Common Terminology Criteria for Adverse Events (CTCAE). For pts with dose interruption greater than 1 wk during 5-wk ramp-up phase or greater than 2 wks at 400 mg daily dose, reassess risk of tumor lysis syndrome to determine if reinitiation with a reduced dose is needed. Consider discontinuation in pts who require reduced dosage of less than 100 mg for more than 2 wks.

Dose Reduction Schedule

Note: During ramp-up phase, continue reduced dose for 1 wk before increasing dose.
Dose interruption at 400 mg: Resume at 300 mg.
Dose interruption at 300 mg: Resume at 200 mg.
Dose interruption at 200 mg: Resume at 100 mg.
Dose interruption at 100 mg: Resume at 50 mg.
Dose interruption at 50 mg: Resume at 20 mg.
Dose interruption at 20 mg: Resume at 10 mg.

Tumor Lysis Syndrome

Any occurrence of blood chemistry abnormalities: Withhold next dose, then resume at same dose if resolved within 24–48 hrs of last dose. If not resolved within 48 hrs, resume at reduced dose.
Any event of tumor lysis syndrome: Resume at reduced dose once resolved.

Grade 3 or 4 Nonhematologic Toxicity

First occurrence: Withhold treatment until resolved to grade 1 or baseline, then resume at same dose.

Second and subsequent occurrences: Withhold treatment until resolved, then follow dose reduction schedule (or reduce dose at prescriber's discretion).

Hematologic Toxicity

First occurrence of grade 3 or 4 neutropenia with infection or fever; grade 4 hematologic toxicity (except lymphopenia): Withhold treatment until resolved to grade 1 or baseline, then resume at same dose.
Second and subsequent occurrences: Withhold treatment until resolved, then follow dose reduction schedule (or reduce dose at prescriber's discretion).

Concomitant Use CYP3A Inhibitors, P-gp Inhibitors

Strong CYP3A inhibitors: Avoid inhibitor or reduce venetoclax dose by at least 75%.
Moderate CYP3A inhibitors or P-gp Inhibitors: Avoid inhibitor or reduce venetoclax dose by at least 50%.

Dosage in Renal/Hepatic Impairment

Mild to moderate impairment: No dose adjustment.
Severe impairment: Not specified; use caution.

SIDE EFFECTS

Frequent (35%–14%): Diarrhea, nausea, fatigue, pyrexia, vomiting, headache, constipation. **Occasional (13%–10%):** Cough, peripheral edema, back pain.

ADVERSE EFFECTS/TOXIC REACTIONS

Anemia, neutropenia, thrombocytopenia are expected responses to therapy. Grade 3 or 4 neutropenia reported in 41% of pts. Pts with high tumor burden, renal impairment, concomitant use of strong or moderate CYP3A inhibitors, P-gp inhibitors may experience life-threatening tumor lysis syndrome, which mainly occurs during the 5-wk ramp-up phase and as early as 6–8 hrs after dose (hospitalization may be necessary). Tumor lysis syndrome may cause renal failure requiring emergent dialysis. Other reactions may include upper respiratory tract infection, pneumonia, autoimmune hemolytic anemia.

NURSING CONSIDERATIONS

BASELINE ASSESSMENT

Obtain ANC, CBC, BMP, renal function test; serum phosphate, calcium; vital signs prior to initiation and periodically thereafter. Obtain pregnancy test in female pts of reproductive potential. Question history of hepatic/renal impairment, gout. Assess all pts for high risk of tumor lysis syndrome and provide adequate hydration and antihyperuricemics (according to manufacturer guidelines) prior to first dose. Conduct tumor burden assessments including blood chemistries, radiologic testing (e.g., CT scan). Correct electrolyte imbalances prior to initiation. Receive full medication history (esp. CYP3A inhibitors, P-gp inhibitors, drugs with narrow therapeutic index). Screen for active infection. Offer emotional support.

INTERVENTION/EVALUATION

Monitor ANC, CBC for anemia, leukopenia, neutropenia, thrombocytopenia. Diligently monitor for tumor lysis syndrome (acute renal failure, electrolyte imbalance, cardiac arrhythmias, seizures). Monitor for infection and provide appropriate antimicrobial therapy if indicated. To reduce risk of neutropenia-associated infection, consider administration of granulocyte-colony stimulating factor (e.g., filgrastim). Monitor for toxicities if discontinuation of CYP3A inhibitors, P-gp inhibitors is unavoidable. Monitor I&O. Assess hydration status.

PATIENT/FAMILY TEACHING

• Treatment may depress your immune system and reduce your ability to fight infection. Report symptoms of infection such as body aches, chills, cough, fatigue, fever. Avoid those with active infection. • Therapy may cause tumor lysis syndrome (a condition caused by the rapid breakdown of cancer cells), which can cause kidney failure and may lead to death. Report decreased urination, amber-colored urine, confusion, difficulty breathing, fatigue, fever, muscle or joint pain, palpitations, seizures, vomiting. • Drink at least 6–8 glasses of water every day. • Avoid pregnancy. Female and male pts of childbearing potential should use effective contraception during treatment and for at least 30 days after last dose. Do not breastfeed. • Treatment may impair fertility. • Avoid grapefruit products, Seville oranges, starfruit, herbal supplements. • Do not take newly prescribed medications unless approved by prescriber who originally started therapy. • Do not receive live vaccines.

venlafaxine

ven-la-**fax**-een
(Apo-Venlafaxine XR* Effexor XR)

■ **BLACK BOX ALERT** ■ Increased risk of suicidal ideation and behavior in children, adolescents, young adults 18–24 yrs with major depressive disorder, other psychiatric disorders.

◆ CLASSIFICATION

PHARMACOTHERAPEUTIC: Serotonin-norepinephrine reuptake inhibitor (SNRI). **CLINICAL:** Antidepressant.

USES

Treatment of depression. Treatment of generalized anxiety disorder (GAD), social anxiety disorder (SAD). Treatment of panic disorder, with or without agoraphobia. **OFF-LABEL:** Treatment of attention-deficit hyperactivity disorder (ADHD), obsessive-compulsive disorder (OCD), hot flashes, diabetic neuropathy, post-traumatic stress disorder (PTSD).

PRECAUTIONS

Contraindications: Hypersensitivity to venlafaxine. Use of MAOIs intended to treat psychiatric disorders concurrently or within 14 days of discontinuing MAOI. Initiation of MAOI to treat psychiatric disorder within 7 days of discontinuing venlafaxine, initiation in pts receiving linezolid or IV methylene blue. **Cautions:** Seizure disorder, renal/hepatic impairment, pts at high risk for suicide, recent MI, mania, volume-depleted pts, narrow-angle glaucoma, HF, hyperthyroidism, abnormal platelet function, elderly pts.

ACTION

Potentiates CNS neurotransmitter activity by inhibiting reuptake of serotonin, norepinephrine, and, to lesser degree, DOPamine. **Therapeutic Effect:** Relieves depression.

PHARMACOKINETICS

Well absorbed from GI tract. Protein binding: 25%–30%. Metabolized in liver. Primarily excreted in urine. Not removed by hemodialysis. **Half-life:** 3–7 hrs; metabolite, 9–13 hrs (increased in hepatic/renal impairment).

⌛ LIFESPAN CONSIDERATIONS

Pregnancy/Lactation: Unknown if distributed in breast milk. **Children:** Children, adolescents are at increased risk for suicidal ideation and behavior, worsening depression, esp. during first few mos of therapy. **Elderly:** Use caution.

INTERACTIONS

DRUG: **CYP3A4 inhibitors (e.g., clarithromycin, ketoconazole)** may increase concentration/effects. **MAOIs (e.g., phenelzine, selegiline)** may cause neuroleptic malignant syndrome, autonomic instability (including rapid fluctuations of vital signs), extreme agitation, hyperthermia, altered mental status, myoclonus, rigidity, coma. **Triptans (e.g., almotriptan, SUMAtriptan),** **selegiline, SSRIs, traZODone, tricyclic antidepressants (e.g., amitripyline, doxepin)** may increase risk of serotonin syndrome. May increase risk of bleeding with **NSAIDs (e.g., ibuprofen, ketorolac, naproxen), aspirin, warfarin.** **HERBAL: Gotu kola, kava kava, St. John's wort, valerian** may increase CNS depression. **St. John's wort** may increase risk of serotonin syndrome. **FOOD: Grapefruit products** may increase concentration/effect. **LAB VALUES:** May increase serum cholesterol CPK, LDH, prolactin, GGT.

AVAILABILITY (Rx)

Tablets: 25 mg, 37.5 mg, 50 mg, 75 mg, 100 mg.
Capsules (Extended-Release [Effexor XR]): 37.5 mg, 75 mg, 150 mg.
🎗 **Capsules (Extended-Release [Effexor XR]):** 37.5 mg, 75 mg, 150 mg. **Tablets (Extended-Release):** 37.5 mg, 75 mg, 150 mg, 225 mg.

ADMINISTRATION/HANDLING

PO
• Give with food. • Scored tablet may be crushed. • Do not break, crush, dissolve, or divide extended-release tablets. • May open capsule, sprinkle on applesauce. Give immediately without chewing and follow with full glass of water.

INDICATIONS/ROUTES/DOSAGE

Depression
PO: *(Immediate-Release):* **ADULTS, ELDERLY:** Initially, 37.5–75 mg/day in 2–3 divided doses with food. May increase up to 75 mg/day at intervals of 4 days or longer. Usual dose: 75–225 mg/day. **Maximum:** 375 mg/day in 3 divided doses.
PO: *(Extended-Release):* **ADULTS, ELDERLY:** Initially, 37.5–75 mg/day as single dose with food. May increase by 75 mg/day at intervals of 4 days or longer. Usual dose: 75–225 mg once daily. **Maximum:** 225 mg/day.

V

Generalized Anxiety Disorder (GAD)
PO: *(Extended-Release):* **ADULTS, ELDERLY:** Initially, 37.5–75 mg/day. May increase by 75 mg/day at 4-day intervals up to 225 mg/day.

Panic Disorder
PO: *(Extended-Release):* **ADULTS, ELDERLY:** Initially, 37.5 mg/day. May increase to 75 mg after 7 days followed by increases of 75 mg/day at 7-day intervals up to 225 mg/day.

Social Anxiety Disorder (SAD)
PO: *(Extended-Release):* **ADULTS, ELDERLY:** 75 mg once daily.

Dosage in Renal/Hepatic Impairment
Consider decreasing venlafaxine dosage by 50% in pts with moderate hepatic impairment, 25% in pts with mild to moderate renal impairment, 50% in pts on dialysis (withhold dose until completion of dialysis). When discontinuing therapy, taper dosage slowly over 2 wks.

SIDE EFFECTS

Frequent (greater than 20%): Nausea, drowsiness, headache, dry mouth. **Occasional (20%–10%):** Dizziness, insomnia, constipation, diaphoresis, nervousness, asthenia, ejaculatory disturbance, anorexia. **Rare (less than 10%):** Anxiety, blurred vision, diarrhea, vomiting, tremor, abnormal dreams, impotence.

ADVERSE EFFECTS/TOXIC REACTIONS

Sustained increase in diastolic B/P of 10–15 mm Hg occurs occasionally. Serotonin syndrome (agitation, confusion, hallucinations, hyperreflexia), neuroleptic malignant syndrome (muscular rigidity, fever, cognitive changes), suicidal ideation have occurred.

NURSING CONSIDERATIONS

BASELINE ASSESSMENT
Obtain initial weight, B/P. Assess appearance, behavior, speech pattern, level of interest, mood. Assess risk of suicide.

INTERVENTION/EVALUATION
Monitor signs/symptoms of depression, B/P, weight. Assess sleep pattern for evidence of insomnia. Check during waking hours for drowsiness, dizziness, anxiety; provide assistance as necessary. Assess appearance, behavior, speech pattern, level of interest, mood for therapeutic response. Monitor for suicidal ideation (esp. at initiation of therapy or changes in dosage).

PATIENT/ FAMILY TEACHING
• Take with food to minimize GI distress. • Do not increase, decrease, suddenly stop medication. • Avoid tasks that require alertness, motor skills until response to drug is established. • Report if breastfeeding, pregnant, or planning to become pregnant. • Avoid alcohol. • Report worsening depression, suicidal ideation, unusual changes in behavior.

verapamil

ver-**ap**-a-mil
(Apo-Verap ✦, Calan, Calan SR, Isoptin SR, Novo-Veramil SR ✦, Verelan, Verelan PM)
Do not confuse Calan with Covera-HS or Verelan with Voltaren.

FIXED-COMBINATION(S)

Tarka: verapamil/trandolapril (an ACE inhibitor): 240 mg/1 mg, 180 mg/2 mg, 240 mg/2 mg, 240 mg/4 mg.

◆CLASSIFICATION

PHARMACOTHERAPEUTIC: Calcium channel blocker (non-dihydropyridine). **CLINICAL:** Antihypertensive, antianginal, antiarrhythmic (class IV), hypertrophic cardiomyopathy therapy adjunct.

USES

Parenteral: Management of supraventricular tachyarrhythmias (SVT), temporary control of rapid ventricular rate in atrial flutter/fibrillation. **PO:** Treatment of hypertension, angina pectoris, supraventricular tachyarrhythmias (SVT), atrial fibrillation/flutter (rate control).

PRECAUTIONS

Contraindications: Hypersensitivity to verapamil. Atrial fibrillation/flutter in presence of accessory bypass tract (e.g., Wolff-Parkinson-White, Lown-Ganong-Levine syndromes), severe left ventricular dysfunction, cardiogenic shock, second- or third-degree heart block (except with pacemaker), hypotension (SBP less than 90 mm Hg), sick sinus syndrome (except with pacemaker). **IV (additional):** Current use of IV beta-blocking agents, ventricular tachycardia. **Cautions:** Renal/hepatic impairment, concomitant use of beta blockers and/or digoxin, myasthenia gravis, elderly pts, hypertrophic cardiomyopathy. Avoid use in HF.

ACTION

Inhibits calcium ion entry across cardiac, vascular smooth-muscle cell membranes, dilating coronary arteries, peripheral arteries, arterioles. **Therapeutic Effect:** Decreases heart rate, myocardial contractility; slows SA, AV conduction. Decreases total peripheral vascular resistance by vasodilation.

PHARMACOKINETICS

Well absorbed from GI tract. Protein binding: 90% (60% in neonates). Metabolized in liver. Primarily excreted in urine. Not removed by hemodialysis. **Half-life: (single dose):** 2–8 hrs, **(multiple doses):** 4.5–12 hrs.

⧖ LIFESPAN CONSIDERATIONS

Pregnancy/Lactation: Drug crosses placenta; distributed in breast milk. Breastfeeding not recommended. **Children:** No age-related precautions noted. **Elderly:** Age-related renal impairment may require dosage adjustment.

INTERACTIONS

DRUG: Beta blockers (e.g., carvedilol, metoprolol) may have additive negative effects on heart rate, AV conduction, or contractility. **Statins (e.g., simvastatin)** may increase risk of myopathy, rhabdomyolysis. May increase concentration of **cycloSPORINE, carBAMazepine.** May increase **digoxin** concentration. **CYP3A4 inducers (e.g., carBAMazepine, phenytoin, rifAMPin)** may decrease concentration/effects. **HERBAL:** St. John's wort may decrease concentration/effects. **Ephedra, ginseng, ginger, licorice, yohimbe, black cohosh, periwinkle** may worsen hypertension. **FOOD: Grapefruit products** may increase concentration. **LAB VALUES:** EKG may show prolonged PR interval. **Therapeutic serum level:** 0.08–0.3 mcg/mL; **toxic serum level:** N/A.

AVAILABILITY (Rx)

Injection Solution: 2.5 mg/mL. **Tablets:** 40 mg, 80 mg, 120 mg.

 Capsules (Extended-Release): 100 mg, 120 mg, 180 mg, 200 mg, 240 mg, 300 mg, 360 mg.

 Capsules (Extended-Release): 100 mg, 120 mg, 180 mg, 200 mg, 240 mg, 300 mg, 360 mg. **Tablets (Extended-Release):** 120 mg, 180 mg, 240 mg.

ADMINISTRATION/HANDLING

🖥 IV

Reconstitution • May give undiluted.
Rate of Administration
• Administer IV push over 2 min for adults, children; give over 3 min for elderly. • Continuous EKG monitoring during IV injection is required for children, recommended for adults. • Monitor EKG for rapid ventricular rate, extreme bradycardia, heart block, asystole, prolongation of PR interval. Notify physician of any significant changes. • Monitor B/P q5–10min. • Pt should remain recumbent for at least 1 hr after IV administration.

V

Storage • Store vials at room temperature.

PO
• Do not give with grapefruit products.
• Do not crush or cut extended-release tablets, capsules. Give extended-release tablets with food. • Sustained-release capsules may be opened and sprinkled on applesauce, then swallowed immediately (do not chew).

▧ IV INCOMPATIBILITIES

Albumin, amphotericin B complex (Abelcet, AmBisome, Amphotec), nafcillin (Nafcil), propofol (Diprivan), sodium bicarbonate.

▧ IV COMPATIBILITIES

Amiodarone (Cordarone), calcium chloride, calcium gluconate, dexamethasone (Decadron), digoxin (Lanoxin), DOBUTamine (Dobutrex), DOPamine (Intropin), furosemide (Lasix), heparin, HYDROmorphone (Dilaudid), lidocaine, magnesium sulfate, metoclopramide (Reglan), milrinone (Primacor), morphine, multivitamins, nitroglycerin, norepinephrine (Levophed), potassium chloride, potassium phosphate, procainamide (Pronestyl), propranolol (Inderal).

INDICATIONS/ROUTES/DOSAGE

Supraventricular Tachyarrhythmias (SVT)
IV: ADULTS, ELDERLY: Initially, 2.5–5 mg over 2 min. May give 5–10 mg 15–30 min after initial dose. **Maximum total dose:** 20–30 mg. **CHILDREN 1–15 YRS:** 0.1–0.3 mg/kg over 2 min. **Maximum initial dose:** 5 mg. May repeat in 30 min. **Maximum second dose:** 10 mg.

Angina, Unstable Angina, Chronic Stable Angina
PO: *(Immediate-Release):* **ADULTS:** Initially, 80–120 mg 3 times/day. For elderly pts, those with hepatic dysfunction, initially 40 mg 3 times/day. Titrate to optimal dose. **Maintenance:** 240–480 mg/day in 3–4 divided doses. Usual range: 80–160 mg 3 times/day.

Atrial Fibrillation (rate control)
IV: ADULTS, ELDERLY: Initially, 0.075–0.15 mg/kg (usual: 5–10 mg) over 2 min. May repeat with 10 mg after 15–30 min. **PO:** *(Immediate-Release):* 240–480 mg/day in 3–4 divided doses.

Hypertension
PO: *(Immediate-Release):* **ADULTS, ELDERLY:** Initially, 40–80 mg 3 times/day. Range: 240–480 mg/day in divided doses.
PO: *(Extended-Release [Calan SR]):* **ADULTS, ELDERLY:** Initially, 120–180 mg once daily. May increase at wkly intervals to 240 mg once daily, then 180 mg twice daily. **Maximum:** 240 mg twice daily.
PO: *(Extended-Release [Verelan]):* **ADULTS, ELDERLY:** Initially, 120–240 mg once daily. May increase dose at wkly intervals to 240 mg/day, then 360 mg/day, then 480 mg/day maximum.
PO: *(Extended-Release [Verelan PM]):* **ADULTS, ELDERLY:** Initially, 100–200 mg once daily at bedtime. May increase dose at wkly intervals to 300 mg once daily, then 400 mg once daily maximum.

Chronic Atrial Fibrillation (Rate Control), SVT
PO: *(Immediate-Release):* **ADULTS, ELDERLY:** 240–480 mg/day in 3–4 divided doses. Usual range: 120–360 mg/day.

Dosage for Renal Impairment
CrCl less than 10 mL/min: Dose reduction (50%–75%) of normal dose recommended.

Dosage in Hepatic Impairment
Dose reduction (20%–50%) of normal dose recommended.

SIDE EFFECTS

Frequent (7%): Constipation. **Occasional (4%–2%):** Dizziness, light-headedness, headache, asthenia, nausea, peripheral edema, hypotension. **Rare (less than 1%):** Bradycardia, dermatitis, rash.

ADVERSE EFFECTS/TOXIC REACTIONS

Rapid ventricular rate in atrial flutter/fibrillation, marked hypotension, extreme bradycardia, HF, asystole, second- or third-degree AV block occur rarely.

NURSING CONSIDERATIONS

BASELINE ASSESSMENT

Obtain baseline EKG. Record onset, type (sharp, dull, squeezing), radiation, location, intensity, duration of anginal pain, precipitating factors (exertion, emotional stress). Check B/P for hypotension, pulse for bradycardia immediately before giving medication.

INTERVENTION/EVALUATION

Assess pulse for quality, rate, rhythm. Monitor B/P. Monitor EKG for cardiac changes, particularly prolongation of PR interval. Notify physician of any significant EKG interval changes. Assist with ambulation if dizziness occurs. Assess for peripheral edema. For those taking oral form, monitor daily pattern of bowel activity, stool consistency. **Therapeutic serum level:** 0.08–0.3 mcg/mL; **toxic serum level:** N/A.

PATIENT/FAMILY TEACHING

• Do not abruptly discontinue medication. • Compliance with therapy regimen is essential to control anginal pain. • Go from lying to standing slowly. • Avoid tasks that require alertness, motor skills until response to drug is established. • Limit caffeine. • Avoid or limit alcohol. • Report continued, persistent angina pain, irregular heartbeats, shortness of breath, swelling, dizziness, constipation, nausea, hypotension. • Avoid grapefruit products.

vilazodone

vil-**az**-oh-done
(Viibryd)

■ **BLACK BOX ALERT** ■ Increased risk of suicidal ideation and behavior in children, adolescents, and young adults 18–24 yrs of age with major depressive disorder, other psychiatric disorders.

◆CLASSIFICATION

PHARMACOTHERAPEUTIC: Selective serotonin reuptake inhibitor. **CLINICAL:** Antidepressant.

USES

Treatment of major depressive disorder.

PRECAUTIONS

Contraindications: Hypersensitivity to vilazodone. Use of MAOIs intended to treat psychiatric disorders (with or within 14 days of stopping vilazodone or MAOI), starting vilazodone in pts receiving linezolid or methylene blue. **Cautions:** Seizure disorder, pts at risk for suicide, hepatic impairment, elderly pts.

ACTION

Enhances serotonergic activity in CNS by selectively inhibiting reuptake of serotonin. **Therapeutic Effect:** Relieves depression.

PHARMACOKINETICS

Readily absorbed from GI tract. Peak concentration: 4–5 hrs. Widely distributed. Protein binding: 96%–99%. Metabolized in liver. **Half-life:** 25 hrs.

⊠ LIFESPAN CONSIDERATIONS

Pregnancy/Lactation: Unknown if drug crosses placenta or is excreted in breast milk. **Children:** Safety and efficacy not established. **Elderly:** No age-related precautions noted.

INTERACTIONS

DRUG: Aspirin, NSAIDs (e.g., ibuprofen, ketorolac, naproxen), warfarin may increase risk of bleeding. Strong CYP3A4 inhibitors (e.g., ketoconazole, nefazodone, ritonavir)

V

may increase concentration. **Almotriptan, busPIRone, eletriptan, naratriptan, SNRIs (e.g., venlafaxine), SSRIs (e.g., sertraline), SUMAtriptan, traMADol, tryptophan** may increase risk of serotonin syndrome. **HERBAL: St. John's wort** may increase risk of serotonin syndrome. **FOOD:** None known. **LAB VALUES:** None significant.

AVAILABILITY (Rx)

Tablets: 10 mg, 20 mg, 40 mg.

ADMINISTRATION/HANDLING

PO
• Give with food (administration without food can result in inadequate drug concentration, may diminish effectiveness).

INDICATIONS/ROUTES/DOSAGE

Depression
PO: ADULTS, ELDERLY: Initially, 10 mg once daily for 7 days, followed by 20 mg once daily. May increase to 40 mg once daily after a minimum of 7 days. **Note:** When discontinuing treatment, reduce dose gradually. From 40 mg/day: taper to 20 mg/day for 4 days, then 10 mg/day for 3 days. From 20 mg/day: taper to 10 mg/day for 7 days.

Concomitant Moderate/Strong CYP3A4 Inhibitors
PO: ADULTS, ELDERLY: 20 mg/day.

Concomitant Strong CYP3A4 Inducers
May increase dose to 80 mg/day when used concomitantly for more than 14 days.

Dosage in Renal/Hepatic Impairment
No dose adjustment.

SIDE EFFECTS

Frequent (28%–23%): Diarrhea, nausea. **Occasional (9%–3%):** Dizziness, dry mouth, insomnia, vomiting, decreased libido, abnormal dreams, fatigue, sweating. **Rare (2%):** Dyspepsia, flatulence, paresthesia, restlessness, arthralgia, abnormal orgasm, delayed ejaculation, increased appetite, palpitations, tremor.

ADVERSE EFFECTS/TOXIC REACTIONS

Serotonin syndrome (agitation, confusion, hallucinations, hyperreflexia), neuroleptic malignant syndrome (fever, muscular rigidity, cognitive changes).

NURSING CONSIDERATIONS

BASELINE ASSESSMENT
Assess behavior, appearance, emotional status, response to environment, speech pattern, thought content, risk of suicide.

INTERVENTION/EVALUATION
Monitor B/P, heart rate, weight. Monitor for suicidal ideation (esp. at initiation of therapy or changes in dosage). Assess for therapeutic response (greater interest in surroundings, improved self-care, increased ability to concentrate, relaxed facial expression).

PATIENT/FAMILY TEACHING
• Avoid tasks that may require alertness, motor skills until response to drug is established (may cause dizziness). • Slowly go from lying to standing. • Take with food. • Do not suddenly stop taking medication; withdraw gradually. • Report suicidal ideation, signs of mania/hypomania. Avoid alcohol.

---

vinBLAStine

vin-**blas**-teen

■ **BLACK BOX ALERT** ■ Must be administered by personnel trained in administration/handling of chemotherapeutic agents. For IV use only. Fatal if given intrathecally (ascending paralysis, death). Vesicant; avoid extravasation. **Do not confuse vinBLAStine with vinCRIStine or vinorelbine.**

◆ CLASSIFICATION

PHARMACOTHERAPEUTIC: Vinca alkaloid. **CLINICAL:** Antineoplastic.

USES

Treatment of Hodgkin's lymphoma, lymphocytic lymphoma, histiocytic lymphoma, advanced stage of mycosis fungoides, advanced testicular carcinoma, Kaposi's sarcoma, Letterer-Siwe disease, breast carcinoma, choriocarcinoma. **OFF-LABEL:** Treatment of bladder, ovarian cancer; non–small-cell lung cancer; soft tissue sarcoma, melanoma.

PRECAUTIONS

Contraindications: Hypersensitivity to vinBLAStine. Bacterial infection, significant granulocytopenia (unless as a result of condition being treated). **Cautions:** Hepatic impairment, severe leukopenia, neurotoxicity, recent exposure to radiation therapy, chemotherapy, ischemic heart disease, preexisting pulmonary disease.

ACTION

Binds to tubulin, inhibiting microtubule formation; may interfere with nucleic acid, protein synthesis. **Therapeutic Effect:** Inhibits cell division by disrupting mitotic spindle.

PHARMACOKINETICS

Does not cross blood-brain barrier. Protein binding: 99%. Metabolized in liver. Primarily excreted in feces. **Half-life:** 24.8 hrs.

🔀 LIFESPAN CONSIDERATIONS

Pregnancy/Lactation: If possible, avoid use during pregnancy, esp. during first trimester. Breastfeeding not recommended. Aspermia has been reported in males. **Children/Elderly:** No age-related precautions noted.

INTERACTIONS

DRUG: May decrease concentration/anticonvulsant effects of **phenytoin**. **CYP3A4 inhibitors (e.g., erythromycin, ketoconazole)** may increase level/toxicity. **Bone marrow depressants** may increase myelosuppression. **Live virus vaccines** may potentiate virus replication, increase vaccine side effects, decrease pt's antibody response to vaccine. **HERBAL: St. John's wort** may decrease concentration. Avoid **black cohosh, dong quai** in estrogen-dependent tumors. **FOOD:** None known. **LAB VALUES:** May increase serum uric acid.

AVAILABILITY (Rx)

Injection, Powder for Reconstitution: 10 mg. **Injection Solution:** 1 mg/mL.

ADMINISTRATION/HANDLING

◄**ALERT**► May be carcinogenic, mutagenic, teratogenic. Handle with extreme care during preparation and administration. Give by IV injection. Leakage from IV site into surrounding tissue may produce extreme irritation. Avoid eye contact with solution (severe eye irritation, possible corneal ulceration may result). If eye contact occurs, immediately irrigate eye with water.

IV

Note: In order to prevent inadvertent intrathecal administration, dispense as a piggyback. (not a syringe).
Reconstitution • Reconstitute 10-mg vial with 10 mL 0.9% NaCl to provide concentration of 1 mg/mL. Using 1 mg/ml solution, further dilute in 25–50 mL D₅W or 0.9% NaCl.
Rate of Administration • Infuse over 5–15 min. Prolonged administration time and/or increased volume may increase risk of vein irritation and extravasation.
Storage • Refrigerate unopened vials. • Solution appears clear, colorless. • Following dilution, solution is stable for up to 21 days if protected from light (consult manufacturer prescribing information). • Discard if solution is discolored or precipitate forms.

🔳 IV INCOMPATIBILITY

Furosemide (Lasix).

⚙ IV COMPATIBILITIES

Allopurinol (Aloprim), CISplatin (Platinol AQ), cyclophosphamide (Cytoxan), DOXOrubicin (Adriamycin), etoposide (VePesid), 5-fluorouracil, gemcitabine (Gemzar), granisetron (Kytril), heparin, leucovorin, methotrexate, ondansetron (Zofran), PACLitaxel (Taxol), vinorelbine (Navelbine).

INDICATIONS/ROUTES/DOSAGE

◀**ALERT**▶ Dosage individualized based on clinical response, tolerance to adverse effects. When used in combination therapy, consult specific protocols for optimum dosage, sequence of drug administration.

Usual Dosage

IV: ADULTS, ELDERLY: Initially, 3.7 mg/m^2 (adjust dose q7days based on WBC response) up to 5.5 mg/m^2 (second wk), 7.4 mg/m^2 (third wk), 9.25 mg/m^2 (fourth wk), and 11.1 mg/m^2 (fifth wk). **Maximum:** 18.5 mg/m^2. **CHILDREN:** 3–6 mg/m^2 q7–14days. **Maximum:** 12.5 mg/m^2/wk.

Dosage in Renal Impairment

No dose adjustment.

Dosage in Hepatic Impairment

Direct serum bilirubin concentration 1.5–3 mg/dL: Reduce dose by 50%. **Greater than 3 mg/dL:** Avoid use.

SIDE EFFECTS

Frequent: Nausea, vomiting, alopecia. **Occasional:** Constipation, diarrhea, rectal bleeding, headache, paresthesia (occur 4–6 hrs after administration, persist for 2–10 hrs), malaise, asthenia, dizziness, pain at tumor site, jaw/face pain, depression, dry mouth. **Rare:** Dermatitis, stomatitis, phototoxicity, hyperuricemia.

ADVERSE EFFECTS/TOXIC REACTIONS

Hematologic toxicity manifested most commonly as leukopenia, less frequently as anemia. WBC reaches its nadir 4–10 days after initial therapy, recovers within 7–14 days (high dosage may require 21-day recovery period). Thrombocytopenia is usually mild and transient, with recovery occurring in a few days. Hepatic insufficiency may increase risk of toxicity. Acute shortness of breath, bronchospasm may occur, particularly when administered concurrently with mitoMYcin.

NURSING CONSIDERATIONS

BASELINE ASSESSMENT

Nausea, vomiting easily controlled by antiemetics. Discontinue therapy if WBC, platelet counts fall abruptly (unless drug is clearly destroying tumor cells in bone marrow). Obtain CBC wkly or before each dosing. Offer emotional support.

INTERVENTION/EVALUATION

If neutrophils fall below 2,000 cells/mm^3, assess diligently for signs of infection. Assess for stomatitis; maintain strict oral hygiene. Monitor for hematologic toxicity: infection (fever, sore throat, signs of local infection), unusual bruising/bleeding from any site, symptoms of anemia (excessive fatigue, weakness). Monitor daily pattern of bowel activity, stool consistency. Avoid constipation. Extravasation may result in cellulitis, phlebitis. Large amount of extravasation may result in tissue sloughing. If extravasation occurs, give local injection of hyaluronidase, apply warm compresses.

PATIENT/FAMILY TEACHING

• Immediately report any pain/burning at injection site during administration. • Pain at tumor site may occur during or shortly after injection. • Do not have immunizations without physician approval (drug lowers resistance). • Avoid crowds, those with infection. • Promptly report fever, sore throat, signs of local infection, unusual bruising/bleeding from any site. • Hair loss is reversible, but new hair growth may have different color, texture. • Report persistent nausea/vomiting. • Avoid constipation by increasing fluids, bulk in diet, exercise as tolerated.

V

vinCRIStine

vin-**cris**-teen
(Marqibo, Vincasar PFS)

■ **BLACK BOX ALERT** ■ Must be administered by personnel trained in administration/handling of chemotherapeutic agents. For IV use only. Fatal if given intrathecally (ascending paralysis, death). Vesicant; avoid extravasation. Marqibo and Vincasar are not interchangeable. **Do not confuse vinCRIStine with vinBLAStine.**

◆CLASSIFICATION

PHARMACOTHERAPEUTIC: Vinca alkaloid. **CLINICAL:** Antineoplastic.

USES

Vincasar: Treatment of acute lymphocytic leukemia (ALL), Hodgkin's lymphoma, advanced non-Hodgkin's lymphomas, neuroblastoma, rhabdomyosarcoma, Wilms tumor. **Marqibo:** Relapsed Philadelphia chromosome negative (Ph⁻) ALL in adults whose disease has progressed after 2 or more antileukemic therapies. **OFF-LABEL: Vincasar:** Treatment of multiple myeloma, chronic lymphocytic leukemia (CLL), brain tumors, small cell lung cancer, ovarian germ cell tumors, Ewing's sarcoma, gestational trophoblastic tumors, retinoblastoma.

PRECAUTIONS

Contraindications: Hypersensitivity to vinCRIStine. Demyelinating form of Charcot-Marie-Tooth syndrome. Intrathecal administration. **Caution:** Hepatic impairment, pts receiving radiation therapy through ports (including liver), neurotoxicity, preexisting neuromuscular disease, hepatobiliary dysfunction, elderly.

ACTION

Binds to tubulin, inhibiting microtubule formation; may interfere with nucleic acid/protein synthesis. **Therapeutic Effect:** Inhibits cell division by disrupting mitotic spindle.

PHARMACOKINETICS

Does not cross blood-brain barrier. Protein binding: 75%. Metabolized in liver. Primarily excreted in feces by biliary system. **Half-life:** 24 hrs. Marqibo: 45 hrs.

⧗ LIFESPAN CONSIDERATIONS

Pregnancy/Lactation: If possible, avoid use during pregnancy, esp. first trimester. May cause fetal harm. Breastfeeding not recommended. **Children:** No age-related precautions noted. **Elderly:** More susceptible to neurotoxic effects.

INTERACTIONS

DRUG: May decrease concentration/anticonvulsant effects of **phenytoin. Itraconazole** may increase severity of neuromuscular side effects. **Live virus vaccines** may potentiate virus replication, increase vaccine side effects, decrease pt's antibody response to vaccine. **HERBAL: St. John's wort, echinacea** may decrease concentration. **FOOD:** None known. **LAB VALUES:** May increase serum uric acid.

AVAILABILITY (Rx)

Injection Solution (Vincasar): 1 mg/mL. **Injection Suspension (Marqibo):** 5 mg/31 mL.

ADMINISTRATION/HANDLING

Note: In order to prevent inadvertent intrathecal administration, dispense as a piggyback. (not a syringe).

 IV

◀**ALERT▶** May be carcinogenic, mutagenic, teratogenic. Handle with extreme care during preparation and administration. Use extreme caution in calculating, administering vinCRIStine. Overdose may result in serious or fatal outcome.

Vincasar
Reconstitution • Dilute in 25–50 mL D₅W or 0.9% NaCl.

V

 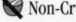

Rate of Administration • Administer as 5–10 min infusion (preferred). • Do not inject into extremity with impaired, potentially impaired circulation caused by compression or invading neoplasm, phlebitis, varicosity.

Storage • Refrigerate unopened vials. • Solution appears clear, colorless. • Discard if solution is discolored or precipitate forms. • Diluted solutions are stable for 7 days refrigerated or 2 days at room temperature.

Marqibo
Note:
• Calculate dose of vinCRIStine and remove volume equal to volume of intended solution from 100 mL 0.9% NaCl or D$_5$W infusion bag. Inject vinCRIStine into infusion bag (total volume: 100 mL).

Rate of Administration • Administer over 60 min.

Storage • Solution must be administered within 12 hrs of preparation.

▨ IV INCOMPATIBILITIES

Furosemide (Lasix), IDArubicin (Idamycin).

▨ IV COMPATIBILITIES

Allopurinol (Aloprim), CISplatin (Platinol AQ), cyclophosphamide (Cytoxan), cytarabine (Ara-C, Cytosar), DOXOrubicin (Adriamycin), etoposide (VePesid), 5-fluorouracil, gemcitabine (Gemzar), granisetron (Kytril), leucovorin, methotrexate, ondansetron (Zofran), PACLitaxel (Taxol), vinorelbine (Navelbine).

INDICATIONS/ROUTES/DOSAGE

Usual Dosage (Vincasar)
IV: ADULTS, ELDERLY: 1.4 mg/m^2, frequency may vary based on protocol. **CHILDREN WEIGHING MORE THAN 10 KG:** 1.5–2 mg/m^2, frequency may vary based on protocol. **CHILDREN WEIGHING LESS THAN 10 KG:** 0.05 mg/kg once wkly. **Maximum:** 2 mg.

Dosage in Renal Impairment
No dose adjustment.

Dosage in Hepatic Impairment

Bilirubin	Dosage
Bilirubin greater than 3 mg/dL	50% of normal

All (Marqibo)
IV: ADULTS, ELDERLY: 2.25 mg/m^2 q7days. Infuse over 1 hr.

Dosage in Renal/Hepatic Impairment (Marqibo)
No dose adjustment.

SIDE EFFECTS

Expected: Peripheral neuropathy (occurs in nearly every pt; first clinical sign is depression of Achilles tendon reflex). **Frequent:** Peripheral paresthesia, alopecia, constipation/obstipation (upper colon impaction with empty rectum), abdominal cramps, headache, jaw pain, hoarseness, diplopia, ptosis/drooping of eyelid, urinary tract disturbances. **Occasional:** Nausea, vomiting, diarrhea, abdominal distention, stomatitis, fever. **Rare:** Mild leukopenia, mild anemia, thrombocytopenia.

ADVERSE EFFECTS/TOXIC REACTIONS

Acute dyspnea, bronchospasm may occur, esp. when administered concurrently with mitoMYcin. Prolonged or high-dose therapy may produce foot/wrist drop, difficulty walking, slapping gait, ataxia, muscle wasting. Acute uric acid nephropathy may occur.

NURSING CONSIDERATIONS

BASELINE ASSESSMENT
Obtain baseline CBC, LFT. Offer emotional support. Question history of hepatic impairment, neuromuscular disease.

INTERVENTION/EVALUATION
Monitor serum uric acid levels, renal/hepatic function studies, CBC. Assess Achilles tendon reflex. Monitor daily pattern of bowel activity, stool consistency.

Monitor for ptosis, diplopia, blurred vision. Question pt regarding urinary changes. Extravasation produces stinging, burning, edema at injection site. Terminate injection immediately, locally inject hyaluronidase, apply heat (disperses drug, minimizes discomfort, cellulitis).

PATIENT/FAMILY TEACHING

• Immediately report any pain/burning at injection site during administration. • Hair loss is reversible, but new hair growth may have different color/texture. • Report persistent nausea/vomiting. • Report signs of peripheral neuropathy (burning/numbness of bottom of feet, palms of hands). • Report fever, sore throat, unusual bleeding/bruising, shortness of breath.

---

vinorelbine

vin-oh-**rel**-been
(Navelbine)

■ **BLACK BOX ALERT** ■ Must be administered by personnel trained in administration/handling of chemotherapeutic agents. For IV use only. Fatal if given intrathecally (ascending paralysis, death). Extravasation produces thrombophlebitis, local tissue necrosis. May produce severe granulocytopenia. Granulocyte counts should be 1,000 cells/mm³ or greater prior to initiation.

Do not confuse vinorelbine with vinBLAStine or vinCRIStine.

◆CLASSIFICATION

PHARMACOTHERAPEUTIC: Vinca alkaloid. **CLINICAL:** Antineoplastic.

USES

Single agent or in combination with CISplatin for treatment of unresectable, advanced, non–small-cell lung cancer (NSCLC). **OFF-LABEL:** Treatment of metastatic breast cancer, cervical carcinoma, ovarian carcinoma, malignant pleural mesothelioma, soft tissue sarcoma, small-cell lung cancer.

PRECAUTIONS

Contraindications: Hypersensitivity to vinorelbine. Granulocyte count before treatment of less than 1,000 cells/mm³. **Cautions:** Compromised marrow reserve due to prior chemotherapy/radiation therapy; hepatic impairment, neurotoxicity, neuropathy, pulmonary impairment.

ACTION

Binds to tubulin, inhibiting microtubule formation; may interfere with nucleic acid protein synthesis. **Therapeutic Effect:** Prevents cellular division by disrupting formation of mitotic spindle.

PHARMACOKINETICS

Widely distributed after IV administration. Protein binding: 80%–90%. Metabolized in liver. Primarily excreted in feces by biliary system. **Half-life:** 28–43 hrs.

⧗ LIFESPAN CONSIDERATIONS

Pregnancy/Lactation: If possible, avoid use during pregnancy, esp. during first trimester. May cause fetal harm. Unknown if distributed in breast milk. Breastfeeding not recommended. **Children:** Safety and efficacy not established. **Elderly:** No age-related precautions noted.

INTERACTIONS

DRUG: Bone marrow depressants may increase risk of myelosuppression. **CISplatin** significantly increases risk of granulocytopenia. **Live virus vaccines** may potentiate virus replication, increase vaccine side effects, decrease pt's antibody response to vaccine. **MitoMYcin** may produce an acute pulmonary reaction. **PACLitaxel** may increase neuropathy. **CYP3A4 inhibitors (e.g., erythromycin, ketoconazole)** may increase concentration/

V

 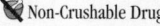

effects. **HERBAL: St. John's wort** may decrease concentration. **FOOD:** None known. **LAB VALUES:** May increase serum bilirubin, alkaline phosphatase, ALT, AST.

AVAILABILITY (Rx)

Injection Solution: 10 mg/mL (1-mL, 5-mL vials).

ADMINISTRATION/HANDLING

 IV

◄ **ALERT** ► IV needle, catheter must be correctly positioned before administration. Leakage into surrounding tissue produces extreme irritation, local tissue necrosis, thrombophlebitis. Handle drug with extreme care during administration; wear protective clothing per protocol. If solution comes in contact with skin/mucosa, immediately wash thoroughly with soap, water.

Reconstitution • Must be diluted and administered via syringe or IV bag.

SYRINGE DILUTION

• Dilute calculated vinorelbine dose with D₅W or 0.9% NaCl to concentration of 1.5–3 mg/mL.

IV BAG DILUTION

• Dilute calculated vinorelbine dose with D₅W, 0.45% or 0.9% NaCl, 5% dextrose and 0.45% NaCl, Ringer's or lactated Ringer's to concentration of 0.5–2 mg/mL.

Rate of Administration • Administer diluted vinorelbine over 6–10 min into side port of free-flowing IV closest to IV bag followed by flushing with 75–125 mL of one of the solutions. • If extravasation occurs, stop injection immediately; give remaining portion of dose into another vein.

Storage • Refrigerate unopened vials. • Protect from light. • Unopened vials are stable at room temperature for 72 hrs. • Do not administer if particulate has formed. • Diluted vinorelbine may be used for up to 24 hrs under normal room light when stored in polypropylene syringes or polyvinyl chloride bags at room temperature.

▨ IV INCOMPATIBILITIES

Acyclovir (Zovirax), allopurinol (Aloprim), amphotericin B (Fungizone), amphotericin B complex (Abelcet, AmBisome, Amphotec), ampicillin (Omnipen), ceFAZolin (Ancef), cefTRIAXone (Rocephin), cefuroxime (Zinacef), 5-fluorouracil (5-FU), furosemide (Lasix), ganciclovir (Cytovene), methylPREDNISolone (Solu-Medrol), sodium bicarbonate.

▨ IV COMPATIBILITIES

Calcium gluconate, CARBOplatin (Paraplatin), CISplatin (Platinol AQ), cyclophosphamide (Cytoxan), cytarabine (ARA-C, Cytosar), dacarbazine (DTIC), DAUNOrubicin (Cerubidine), dexamethasone (Decadron), diphenhydrAMINE (Benadryl), DOXOrubicin (Adriamycin), etoposide (VePesid), gemcitabine (Gemzar), granisetron (Kytril), HYDROmorphone (Dilaudid), IDArubicin (Idamycin), methotrexate, morphine, ondansetron (Zofran), vinBLAStine (Velban), vinCRIStine (Oncovin).

INDICATIONS/ROUTES/DOSAGE

◄ **ALERT** ► Dosage adjustments should be based on granulocyte count obtained on the day of treatment, as follows:

Granulocyte Count (cells/mm³) on Day of Treatment	Dosage
1,500 or higher	100% of starting dose
1,000–1,499	50% of starting dose
Less than 1,000	Do not administer

NSCLC Monotherapy
IV Injection: ADULTS, ELDERLY: 30 mg/m² administered wkly over 6–10 min.

NSCLC Combination Therapy with CISplatin
IV Injection: ADULTS, ELDERLY: 25–30 mg/m² every wk.

Dosage in Renal Impairment
No dose adjustment. **HD:** Decrease dose to 20 mg/m²/wk given post-HD or on non-HD days.

Dosage in Hepatic Impairment	
Bilirubin	**Dosage**
2 mg/dL or less	100% of dose
2.1–3 mg/dL	50% of dose
Greater than 3 mg/dL	25% of dose

SIDE EFFECTS

Frequent (35%–12%): Asthenia, nausea, constipation, erythema, pain, vein discoloration at injection site, fatigue, peripheral neuropathy manifested as paresthesia, hyperesthesia, diarrhea, alopecia. **Occasional (10%–5%):** Phlebitis, dyspnea, loss of deep tendon reflexes. **Rare:** Chest pain, jaw pain, myalgia, arthralgia, rash.

ADVERSE EFFECTS/TOXIC REACTIONS

Bone marrow depression is manifested mainly as granulocytopenia (may be severe). Other hematologic toxicities (neutropenia, thrombocytopenia, leukopenia, anemia) increase risk of infection, bleeding. Acute shortness of breath, severe bronchospasm occur infrequently, particularly in pts with preexisting pulmonary dysfunction. Hepatic toxicity may occur.

NURSING CONSIDERATIONS

BASELINE ASSESSMENT

Review medication history. Obtain CBC prior to each dose. Granulocyte count should be at least 1,000 cells/mm³ before vinorelbine administration. Granulocyte nadirs occur 7–10 days following dosing. Do not give hematologic growth factors within 24 hrs before administration of chemotherapy or earlier than 24 hrs following cytotoxic chemotherapy. Advise women of childbearing potential to avoid pregnancy during drug therapy. Offer emotional support.

INTERVENTION/EVALUATION

Diligently monitor injection site for swelling, redness, pain. Frequently monitor for myelosuppression during and following therapy (infection [fever, sore throat, signs of local infection], unusual bleeding/bruising, anemia [excessive fatigue, weakness]). Monitor pts developing severe granulocytopenia for evidence of infection, fever. Crackers, dry toast, sips of cola may help relieve nausea. Monitor daily pattern of bowel activity, stool consistency. Question for tingling, burning, numbness of hands/feet (peripheral neuropathy). Pt complaint of "walking on glass" is sign of hyperesthesia.

PATIENT/FAMILY TEACHING

• Immediately report redness, swelling, pain at injection site. • Avoid crowds, those with infection. • Do not have immunizations without physician's approval. • Promptly report fever, signs of infection, unusual bruising/bleeding from any site, difficulty breathing. • Avoid pregnancy. • Hair loss is reversible, but new hair growth may have different color, texture.

vismodegib

vis-moe-**deg**-ib
(Erivedge)

■ **BLACK BOX ALERT** ■ May result in embryo-fetal death or severe birth defects including missing digits, midline defects, irreversible malformations due to embryotoxic and teratogenic properties. Verify pregnancy status prior to initiation. Advise use of effective contraception in female pts. Advise male pts of potential exposure risk through seminal fluid.

◆CLASSIFICATION

PHARMACOTHERAPEUTIC: Hedgehog pathway inhibitor. **CLINICAL:** Antineoplastic.

USES

Treatment of adult pts with metastatic basal cell carcinoma, locally advanced basal cell carcinoma with recurrence after surgery, or pts who are not candidates for surgery or radiation.

V

PRECAUTIONS

◀ **ALERT** ▶ Do not donate blood products for at least 7 mos after discontinuation.

Contraindications: Hypersensitivity to vismodegib. **Cautions:** Hepatic/renal impairment. History of significant cardiac disease.

ACTION

An inhibitor of Hedgehog pathway, binding to and inhibiting smoothened, a transmembrane protein involved in Hedgehog signal transduction. **Therapeutic Effect:** Inhibits tumor cell growth and metastasis of basal cell carcinoma.

PHARMACOKINETICS

Metabolized in liver. Protein binding: 99%. Excreted in feces (82%), urine (4%). **Half-life:** 4 days (daily dosing), 12 days (single dose).

⌛ LIFESPAN CONSIDERATIONS

Pregnancy/Lactation: May cause fetal harm. Not recommended in nursing mothers. Must either discontinue drug or discontinue breastfeeding. Unknown if distributed in breast milk. Contraception recommended prior to first dose, during treatment and up to 24 mos after discontinuation. During treatment (including interruption) and for 3 mos after treatment, male pts should not donate sperm and should use condoms with spermicide if partner is of childbearing potential. **Children:** Safety and efficacy not established. **Elderly:** Safety and efficacy not established.

INTERACTIONS

DRUG: P-glycoprotein inhibitors (e.g., **clarithromycin, erythromycin**) may increase concentration/effects. **Antacids, H$_2$ blockers** (e.g., **famotidine**), **proton pump inhibitors** (e.g., **pantoprazole**) may decrease concentration/effect. **HERBAL:** None significant. **FOOD:** None known. **LAB VALUES:** May decrease potassium, sodium, GFR. May increase serum BUN, creatinine.

AVAILABILITY (Rx)

🏷 **Capsules:** 150 mg.

ADMINISTRATION/HANDLING

PO
• Give without regard to food. • Give whole. Do not break, crush, or open capsule.

INDICATIONS/ROUTES/DOSAGE

Advanced or Metastatic Basal Cell Carcinoma
PO: ADULTS/ELDERLY: 150 mg once daily. Continue until disease progression or unacceptable toxicity.

Dosage in Renal/Hepatic Impairment
No dose adjustment.

SIDE EFFECTS

Frequent (71%–40%): Muscle spasm, alopecia, dysgeusia, weight loss, fatigue. **Occasional (30%–11%):** Nausea, amenorrhea, diarrhea, anorexia, constipation, vomiting, arthralgia, loss of taste.

ADVERSE EFFECTS/TOXIC REACTIONS

May cause spontaneous abortion, fetal demise, birth defects. Azotemia (renal impairment) reported in 2% of pts.

NURSING CONSIDERATIONS

BASELINE ASSESSMENT

Obtain negative pregnancy test (urine/serum) before initiation, BMP. Question current breastfeeding status. Assess skin, moles for other possible malignancies. Offer emotional support.

INTERVENTION/EVALUATION

Obtain STAT human chorionic gonadotropin (HCG) level if pregnancy suspected, BMP if electrolyte imbalance or renal impairment suspected. Encourage fluid intake if diarrhea occurs. Offer antiemetics for nausea/vomiting. Report oliguria, dark or concentrated urine.

PATIENT/FAMILY TEACHING
• Avoid pregnancy. • May cause birth defects or miscarriage. • Do not breastfeed. • Male pts must use condoms with spermicide during sexual activity, despite history of vasectomy. • Female pts must use contraception for at least 7 mos after stopping treatment. • Immediately report suspected pregnancy. • Do not donate blood for at least 7 mos after stopping treatment. • Swallow capsules whole; do not break, crush, or open. • Hair loss is an expected side effect. • Strictly monitor menstrual cycle. • Report dark-colored urine or decreased urine output despite hydration.

vitamin D (vitamin D analogues)

calcitriol

kal-si-**trye**-ole
(Calcijex ✦, Rocaltrol, Vectical)

doxercalciferol

dox-er-kal-**sif**-e-role
(Hectorol)

ergocalciferol

er-goe-kal-**sif**-e-role
(Drisdol)

paricalcitol

par-i-**kal**-si-tol
(Zemplar)

◆CLASSIFICATION

PHARMACOTHERAPEUTIC: Fat-soluble vitamin. **CLINICAL:** Vitamin D analogue.

USES

Calcitriol: Manage hypocalcemia in pts on chronic renal dialysis, secondary hypoparathyroidism in chronic kidney disease (CKD), manage hypocalcemia in hypoparathyroidism. **(Topical):** Treatment of mild to moderate plaque psoriasis. **Doxercalciferol:** Treatment of secondary hyperparathyroidism in CKD. **Ergocalciferol:** Treatment of refractory rickets, hypophosphatemia, hypoparathyroidism, dietary supplement. **Paricalcitol: (Intravenous):** Treatment/prevention of secondary hyperparathyroidism associated with stage 5 CKD. **(PO):** Treatment/prevention of secondary hyperparathyroidism associated with stage 3 and 4 CKD and stage 5 CKD pts on hemodialysis or peritoneal dialysis. **OFF-LABEL: Calcitriol:** Vitamin D–dependent rickets. **Ergocalciferol:** Prevention/treatment of vitamin D deficiency in pts with CKD, osteoporosis prevention.

PRECAUTIONS

Contraindications: Hypersensitivity to cholecalciferol, ergocalciferol. Vitamin D toxicity, hypercalcemia. **Cautions:** Pts with malabsorption syndrome. Concurrent use with digoxin.

ACTION

Calcitriol: Stimulates calcium transport in intestines, resorption in bones, and tubular reabsorption in kidney; suppresses parathyroid hormone (PTH) secretion/synthesis. **Doxercalciferol:** Regulates blood calcium levels, stimulates bone growth, suppresses PTH secretion/synthesis. **Ergocalciferol:** Promotes active absorption of calcium and phosphorus, increasing serum levels to allow bone mineralization; mobilizes calcium and phosphate from bone, increases reabsorption of calcium and phosphate by renal tubules. **Paricalcitol:** Suppresses PTH secretion/synthesis. **Therapeutic Effect:** Essential for absorption, utilization of calcium, phosphate, control of PTH levels.

V

PHARMACOKINETICS

Calcitriol: Rapidly absorbed. Protein binding: 99.9%. Metabolized to active metabolite (ergocalciferol). Excreted in feces (49%), urine (16%). **Half-life:** 5–8 hrs. **Doxercalciferol:** Metabolized in liver. **Half-life:** 32–37 hrs. **Ergocalciferol:** Metabolized in liver. **Paricalcitol:** Readily absorbed. Protein binding: 99.8%. Metabolized in liver. Primarily excreted in feces. **Half-life:** 5–7 hrs.

⌛ LIFESPAN CONSIDERATIONS

Pregnancy/Lactation: Unknown if drug crosses placenta. Infant risk cannot be excluded. **Children/Elderly:** No age-related precautions noted.

INTERACTIONS

DRUG: Magnesium-containing antacids may increase risk of hypermagnesemia. **Calcium-containing products, concurrent vitamin D (or derivatives)** may increase risk of hypercalcemia. May increase **digoxin** toxicity due to hypercalcemia (may cause arrhythmias). **HERBAL:** None significant. **FOOD:** None known. **LAB VALUES:** May increase serum cholesterol, calcium, magnesium, phosphate, ALT, AST, BUN, creatinine.

AVAILABILITY (Rx)

Calcitriol
Capsules, Softgel (Rocaltrol): 0.25 mcg, 0.5 mcg. Injection Solution: 1 mcg/mL. Oral Solution (Rocaltrol): 1 mcg/mL.

Doxercalciferol
Capsules, Softgel (Hectorol): 0.5 mcg, 1 mcg, 2.5 mcg. Injection Solution (Hectorol): 2 mcg/mL.

Ergocalciferol
Capsules (Drisdol): 50,000 units (1.25 mg). Liquid, Oral (Drisdol): 8,000 units/mL (200 mcg/mL). Tablets: 400 units.

Paricalcitol
Capsules, Gelatin (Zemplar): 1 mcg, 2 mcg, 4 mcg. Injection Solution (Zemplar): 2 mcg/mL.

ADMINISTRATION/HANDLING

Calcitriol
PO
• May take without regard to food.

 IV
• May give as IV bolus at end of dialysis.

Doxercalciferol
PO
• May take without regard to food.

 IV
• May give as IV bolus via catheter at end of dialysis.

Ergocalciferol
PO
• May take without regard to food.

Paricalcitol
PO
• May take without regard to food. • For 3 times/wk dosing, give no more frequently than every other day.

 IV
• Give bolus anytime during dialysis. • Do not give more frequently than every other day.

INDICATIONS/ROUTES/DOSAGE

Calcitriol
Hypocalcemia on Chronic Renal Dialysis
PO: ADULTS, ELDERLY: (ROCALTROL): Initially, 0.25 mcg/day or every other day. May increase by 0.25 mcg/day at 4- to 8-wk intervals. Range: 0.5–1 mcg/day.
IV: ADULTS, ELDERLY: 1–2 mcg 3 times/wk. Adjust dose at 2- to 4-wk intervals. Range: 0.5–4 mcg 3 times/wk.

Hypocalcemia in Hypoparathyroidism
PO: ADULTS, CHILDREN 6 YRS AND OLDER: (ROCALTROL): Initially, 0.25 mcg/day. May increase at 2- to 4-wk intervals. Range: 0.5–2 mcg/day. **CHILDREN 1–5 YRS:** 0.25–0.75 mcg once daily. **CHILDREN YOUNGER THAN 1 YR:** 0.04–0.08 mcg/kg once daily. **NEONATES:** 1 mcg once daily first 5 days of life.

V

Secondary Hyperparathyroidism Associated with Moderate to Severe CKD Not on Dialysis

PO: ADULTS, ELDERLY, CHILDREN 3 YRS AND OLDER: (ROCALTROL): Initially, 0.25 mcg/day. May increase to 0.5 mcg/day. **CHILDREN YOUNGER THAN 3 YRS:** Initially, 0.01–0.015 mcg/kg/day.

Doxercalciferol
Secondary Hyperparathyroidism (Dialysis)

PO: ADULTS, ELDERLY: Initial dose (intact parathyroid hormone [iPTH] greater than 400 pg/mL): 10 mcg 3 times/wk at dialysis. Dose titrated to lower iPTH to 150–300 pg/mL, with dosage adjustments made at 8-wk intervals. **Maximum:** 20 mcg 3 times/wk.

IV: ADULTS, ELDERLY: Initial dose (iPTH greater than 400 pg/mL): 4 mcg 3 times/wk after dialysis, given as bolus dose. Dose titrated to lower iPTH to 150–300 pg/mL, with dosage adjustments made at 8-wk intervals. **Maximum:** 18 mcg/wk.

Secondary Hyperparathyroidism (Predialysis)

PO: ADULTS, ELDERLY: Initially, 1 mcg/day. Titrate dose to lower iPTH to 35–70 pg/mL for stage 3 CKD and 70–110 pg/mL for stage 4 CKD. **Maximum:** 3.5 mcg/day.

Ergocalciferol
Dietary Supplement

PO: ADULTS, ELDERLY, CHILDREN: 10 mcg (400 units)/day. **NEONATES:** 10–20 mcg (400–800 units)/day.

Hypoparathyroidism

PO: ADULTS, ELDERLY: 625 mcg–5 mg (25,000–200,000 units)/day (with calcium supplements). **CHILDREN:** 1.25–5 mg (50,000–200,000 units)/day (with calcium supplements).

Nutritional Rickets, Osteomalacia

PO: ADULTS, ELDERLY, CHILDREN: 25–125 mcg (1,000–5,000 units)/day for 8–12 wks. **ADULTS, ELDERLY (WITH MALABSORPTION SYNDROME):** 250–7,500 mcg (10,000–300,000 units)/day. **CHILDREN (WITH MALABSORPTION SYNDROME):** 250–625 mcg (10,000–25,000 units)/day.

Vitamin D–Dependent Rickets

PO: ADULTS, ELDERLY: 250 mcg–1.5 mg (10,000–60,000 units)/day. **CHILDREN:** 75–125 mcg (3,000–5,000 units)/day. **Maximum:** 1,500 mcg (60,000 units)/day.

Vitamin D–Resistant Rickets

PO: ADULTS, ELDERLY, CHILDREN: 300 mcg–12.5 mg (12,000–500,000 units)/day.

Hypophosphatemia

PO: ADULTS, ELDERLY: 250–1,500 mcg (10,000–60,000 units)/day with phosphate supplements. **CHILDREN:** 1,000–2,000 mcg (40,000–80,000 units)/day with phosphate supplements.

Plaque Psoriasis

Topical: ADULTS, ELDERLY: Apply to affected area twice daily.

Paricalcitol
Secondary Hyperparathyroidism in Stage 5 CKD

IV: ADULTS, ELDERLY, CHILDREN 5 YRS AND OLDER: Initially, 0.04–0.1 mcg/kg given as bolus dose no more frequently than every other day at any time during dialysis. May increase by 2–4 mcg every 2–4 wks. Dose is based on serum iPTH levels.

Secondary Hyperparathyroidism in Stages 3 and 4 CKD

Note: Initial dose based on baseline serum iPTH levels. Dose adjusted q2wks based on iPTH levels relative to baseline.
PO: ADULTS, ELDERLY: (iPTH 500 PG/ML OR LESS): 1 mcg/day or 2 mcg 3 times/wk. **(iPTH GREATER THAN 500 PG/ML):** 2 mcg/day or 4 mcg 3 times/wk.

Dosage in Renal/Hepatic Impairment
No dose adjustment.

SIDE EFFECTS

Frequencies not defined. **Calcitriol:** Cardiac arrhythmias, headache, pruritus, hypercalcemia, polydipsia, abdominal pain, metallic taste, nausea, vomiting, myalgia, soft tissue calcification. **Doxercalciferol:** Edema, pruritus, nausea, vomiting, headache, dizziness, dyspnea, malaise, hypercalcemia. **Ergocalciferol:** Hypercalcemia, hypervitaminosis D, decreased renal function, soft tissue calcification, bone demineralization, nausea, constipation, weight loss. **Paricalcitol:** Edema, nausea, vomiting, hypercalcemia.

ADVERSE EFFECTS/TOXIC REACTIONS

Early signs of overdose manifested as weakness, headache, drowsiness, nausea, vomiting, dry mouth, constipation, muscle/bone pain, metallic taste. Later signs of overdose evidenced by polyuria, polydipsia, anorexia, weight loss, nocturia, photophobia, rhinorrhea, pruritus, disorientation, hallucinations, hyperthermia, hypertension, cardiac dysrhythmias.

NURSING CONSIDERATIONS

BASELINE ASSESSMENT

Obtain baseline serum calcium, ionized calcium, phosphorus, alkaline phosphatase, creatinine, PTH.

INTERVENTION/EVALUATION

Monitor serum, urinary calcium levels, serum phosphate, magnesium, BUN, creatine, alkaline phosphatase determinations (therapeutic calcium level: 9–10 mg/dL), PTH measurements. Estimate daily dietary calcium intake. Encourage adequate fluid intake. Monitor for signs/symptoms of vitamin D intoxication.

PATIENT/FAMILY TEACHING

• Adequate calcium intake should be maintained. • Dietary phosphorus may need to be restricted (foods high in phosphorus include beans, dairy products, nuts, peas, whole-grain products). • Oral formulations may cause hypersensitivity reactions. Avoid excessive doses. • Report signs/symptoms of hypercalcemia (headache, weakness, drowsiness, nausea, dry mouth, constipation, metallic taste, muscle or bone pain). • Maintain adequate hydration. • Avoid changes in diet or supplemental calcium intake (unless directed by health care professional). • Avoid magnesium-containing antacids in pts with renal failure.

---

vorapaxar

vor-a-**pax**-ar
(Zontivity)

■ **BLACK BOX ALERT** ■ Avoid use in pts with history of CVA, intracranial hemorrhage (ICH), TIA or with active pathologic bleeding. Antiplatelet agents increase risk of bleeding, including ICH and fatal bleeding.

◆CLASSIFICATION

PHARMACOTHERAPEUTIC: Protease-activated receptor-1 antagonist. **CLINICAL:** Antiplatelet.

USES

To reduce thrombotic cardiovascular events in pts with history of MI or peripheral artery disease (PAD). Reduces rate of a combined endpoint of cardiovascular death, CVA, MI, and urgent coronary revascularization.

PRECAUTIONS

Contraindications: Hypersensitivity to vorapaxar. History of stroke, intracranial hemorrhage, transient ischemic attack; active bleeding. **Cautions:** Hepatic impairment, pts at increased risk of bleeding (anticoagulant use, elderly, low body weight, trauma) or with history of bleeding disorders.

V

ACTION

Inhibits thrombin-induced and thrombin receptor agonist peptide (TRAP)–induced platelet aggregation. **Therapeutic Effect:** Inhibits platelet aggregation, reduces incidence of thrombus.

PHARMACOKINETICS

Readily absorbed. Widely distributed. Metabolized in liver. Protein binding: greater than 99%. Peak plasma concentration: 1 hr. Steady state reached in 21 days. Excreted in feces (58%), urine (25%). **Half-life:** 5–13 days.

⌛ LIFESPAN CONSIDERATIONS

Pregnancy/Lactation: Unknown if distributed in breast milk. **Children:** Safety and efficacy not established. **Elderly:** May have increased risk of bleeding.

INTERACTIONS

DRUG: Aspirin, anticoagulants (e.g., warfarin), fibrinolytics (e.g., tissue plasminogen activator), NSAIDs (e.g., ibuprofen, ketorolac, naproxen), serotonin norepinephrine reuptake inhibitors (e.g., DULoxetine), SSRIs (e.g., PARoxetine) may increase risk of bleeding. **Strong CYP3A4 inducers (e.g., rifAMPin)** may decrease concentration/effects; **CYP3A4 inhibitors (e.g., clarithromycin, ketoconazole)** may increase concentration/effects. **HERBAL: St. John's wort** may decrease concentration/effects. **FOOD:** None known. **LAB VALUES:** May decrease Hbg, Hct; serum iron.

AVAILABILITY (Rx)

Tablets: 2.08 mg.

ADMINISTRATION/HANDLING

PO
• Give without regard to meals.

INDICATIONS/ROUTES/DOSAGE

Reduction of Thrombotic Cardiovascular Events (Pts with PAD, MI)
PO: ADULTS, ELDERLY: 2.08 mg once daily (in combination with aspirin and/or clopidogrel).

Dosage in Renal Impairment
No dose adjustment.

Dosage in Hepatic Impairment
Mild to moderate impairment: No dose adjustment.
Severe impairment: Not recommended.

SIDE EFFECTS

Rare (2%): Depression, rash, skin eruptions, exanthemas.

ADVERSE EFFECTS/TOXIC REACTIONS

Hemorrhagic events (25% of pts) including fatal bleeding (less than 1%), GI bleeding (4%), ICH (less than 1%) have been reported. Vorapaxar increases risk of moderate to severe bleeding by 55%.

NURSING CONSIDERATIONS

BASELINE ASSESSMENT

Obtain baseline CBC, PFA level. Question history of CVA, intracranial hemorrhage (ICH), transient ischemic attack (TIA) (therapy contraindicated); anemia, bleeding ulcers, GI/genitourinary (GU) bleeding, recent surgery, spinal punctures, open wounds; hepatic impairment. Receive full medication history including herbal products.

INTERVENTION/EVALUATION

Monitor CBC. Question for increased menstrual bleeding/discharge. Monitor for confusion, headache, hemiparesis, vision change (may indicate ICH); hematuria, GI bleeding. Assess peripheral pulses; skin for ecchymosis, petechiae. Check for excessive bleeding from minor cuts, scratches, skin tears. Consider transfusion of platelets or RBCs if severe bleeding occurs.

PATIENT/FAMILY TEACHING

• It may take longer to stop bleeding. • Bruising may occur more easily. • Report unexpected, prolonged, excessive bleeding of any kind, or blood

V

❦ Canadian trade name   🍃 Non-Crushable Drug   🄷🄸🄶🄷 High Alert drug in sputum, stool, urine, or vomitus. • Avoid alcohol, over-the-counter anti-inflammatories such as aspirin, ibuprofen, or naproxen. • Consult doctor before any planned surgery, dental work. • Use electric razor, soft toothbrush to prevent bleeding. • Report confusion, headache, one-sided weakness, trouble speaking, or vision problems; may indicate life-threatening bleeding of brain.

voriconazole

vor-i-**kon**-a-zole
(Vfend, Apo-Voriconazole ✦)
Do not confuse voriconazole with fluconazole.

◆CLASSIFICATION

PHARMACOTHERAPEUTIC: Triazole derivative. **CLINICAL:** Antifungal.

USES

Treatment of invasive aspergillosis, esophageal candidiasis. Treatment of serious fungal infections caused by *Scedosporium apiospermum, Fusarium* spp. Treatment of candidemia in non-neutropenic pts. Treatment of disseminated *Candida* infections of skin and viscera. **OFF-LABEL:** Empiric treatment of fungal meningitis or osteoarticular infections, coccidioidomycosis in HIV pts, fungal endophthalmitis, infection prophylaxis of graft-vs-host disease or pts with allogeneic hematopoietic stem cell transplant.

PRECAUTIONS

Contraindications: Hypersensitivity to voriconazole. Concurrent administration of barbiturates (long acting), carBAMazepine, efavirenz (400 mg/day or greater), ergot alkaloids, pimozide, quiNIDine (may cause prolonged QT interval, torsades de pointes), rifabutin, rifAMPin, ritonavir (800 mg/day or

greater), sirolimus, St. John's wort. **Cautions:** Severe renal/hepatic impairment, hypersensitivity to other azole antifungal agents. Pts at risk for acute pancreatitis, pts with fructose intolerance, glucose-galactose malabsorption; concomitant nephrotoxic medications; hypokalemia, hypomagnesemia, hypocalcemia. May prolong QT interval; use caution in pts with history of QT syndrome, concomitant medications that prolong QT interval, electrolyte imbalance.

ACTION

Interferes with fungal cytochrome activity, decreasing ergosterol synthesis, inhibiting fungal cell membrane formation. **Therapeutic Effect:** Damages fungal cell wall membrane.

PHARMACOKINETICS

Rapidly, completely absorbed after PO administration. Widely distributed. Protein binding: 58%. Metabolized in liver. Primarily excreted as metabolite in urine. **Half-life:** Variable, dose dependent.

⚖ LIFESPAN CONSIDERATIONS

Pregnancy/Lactation: May cause fetal harm. **Children:** Safety and efficacy not established in pts younger than 12 yrs. **Elderly:** No age-related precautions noted.

INTERACTIONS

DRUG: May increase concentration, risk of toxicity of **ALPRAZolam, calcium channel blockers (e.g., dilTIAZem, verapamil), cycloSPORINE, efavirenz, ergot alkaloids, HMG-CoA reductase inhibitors (e.g., lovastatin), methadone, midazolam, protease inhibitors (e.g., amprenavir, saquinavir), rifabutin, sirolimus, tacrolimus, triazolam, warfarin. CarBAMazepine, rifabutin, rifAMPin, ritonavir** may decrease concentration/effect. **QT interval–prolonging medications (e.g., amiodarone,**

V

azithromycin, ceritinib, haloperidol, moxifloxacin) may increase risk of QT interval prolongation, cardiac arrhythmias. **HERBAL: St. John's wort** may significantly decrease concentration. **FOOD: Grapefruit products** may increase concentration. **LAB VALUES:** May increase serum alkaline phosphatase, ALT, AST, bilirubin, creatinine. May decrease potassium.

AVAILABILITY (Rx)

Injection, Powder for Reconstitution: 200 mg. **Powder for Oral Suspension:** 200 mg/5 mL. **Tablets:** 50 mg, 200 mg.

ADMINISTRATION/HANDLING

 IV

Reconstitution • Reconstitute 200-mg vial with 19 mL Sterile Water for Injection to provide concentration of 10 mg/mL. Further dilute with 0.9% NaCl or D5W to provide concentration of 0.5–5 mg/mL.
Rate of Administration • Infuse over 1–2 hrs at a rate not to exceed 3 mg/kg/hr. • Do not infuse concomitantly into same line with other drug infusions. • Do not infuse concomitantly even in separate lines with concentrated electrolyte solutions or blood products.
Storage • Store powder for injection at room temperature. • Use reconstituted solution immediately. • Do not use after 24 hrs when refrigerated.

PO

• Give 1 hr before or 1 hr after a meal. • Do not mix oral suspension with any other medication or flavoring agent. • Shake suspension for about 10 sec before use.

▓ IV INCOMPATIBILITY

Tigecycline (Tygacil).

▓ IV COMPATIBILITIES

Anidulafungin, caspofungin, ceftaroline, doripenem.

INDICATIONS/ROUTES/DOSAGE

Invasive Aspergillosis
IV: ADULTS, ELDERLY, CHILDREN 12 YRS AND OLDER: Initially, 6 mg/kg q12h for 2 doses, then 4 mg/kg q12h, then oral maintenance dose. **(LESS THAN 40 KG):** 100 mg q12h (**Maximum:** 300 mg/day). **(40 KG OR GREATER):** 200 mg q12h (**Maximum:** 400 mg/day). **CHILDREN 3–11 YRS OF AGE: (HIV exposed):** Initially, 9 mg/kg (**Maximum:** 400 mg) q12h for 2 doses, then 8 mg/kg (**Maximum:** 200 mg) q12h. **(Non–HIV exposed):** 8 mg/kg/dose q12h.
PO: (HIV exposed): Initially, 9 mg/kg (**Maximum:** 400 mg) q12h for 2 doses, then 7 mg/kg (**Maximum:** 200 mg) q12h. **(Non–HIV exposed):** 9 mg/kg/dose q12h.

Candidemia, Other Deep Tissue Candida Infections
IV: ADULTS, ELDERLY, CHILDREN 12 YRS AND OLDER: Initially, 6 mg/kg q12h for 2 doses, then 3–4 mg/kg q12h, then oral maintenance dose. **LESS THAN 40 KG:** 100 mg q12h (**Maximum:** 300 mg/day). **40 KG OR GREATER:** 200 mg q12h (**Maximum:** 600 mg/day).

Esophageal Candidiasis
PO: ADULTS, ELDERLY WEIGHING 40 KG OR MORE: 200 mg q12h for minimum of 14 days, then at least 7 days following resolution of symptoms. **Maximum:** 600 mg/day. **ADULTS, ELDERLY WEIGHING LESS THAN 40 KG:** 100 mg q12h for minimum of 14 days, then at least 7 days following resolution of symptoms. **Maximum:** 300 mg/day.

Dosage in Pts Receiving Phenytoin
IV: Increase maintenance dose to 5 mg/kg q12h.
PO: Increase 200 mg q12h to 400 mg q12h (pts weighing 40 kg or more) or 100 mg q12h to 200 mg q12h (pts weighing less than 40 kg).

V

Dosage in Pts Receiving Efavirenz
Increase dose to 400 mg q12h and reduce efavirenz to 300 mg/day.

Dosage in Renal Impairment
No dose adjustment. IV dosing not recommended in pts with CrCl 50 mL/min or less.

Dosage in Hepatic Impairment
Mild to moderate impairment: Reduce maintenance dose by 50%.
Severe impairment: Use only if benefits outweigh risks. Monitor closely for toxicity.

SIDE EFFECTS

Frequent (20%–6%): Abnormal vision, fever, nausea, rash, vomiting. **Occasional (5%–2%):** Headache, chills, hallucinations, photophobia, tachycardia, hypertension.

ADVERSE EFFECTS/TOXIC REACTIONS

Hepatotoxicity (jaundice, hepatitis, hepatic failure), acute renal failure have occurred in severely ill pts.

NURSING CONSIDERATIONS

BASELINE ASSESSMENT
Obtain baseline serum hepatic/renal function tests; EKG. Correct electrolyte deficiencies prior to initiating treatment. Receive full medication history and screen for interactions. Question medical history as listed in Precautions.

INTERVENTION/EVALUATION
Monitor serum renal function, LFT. Monitor visual function (visual acuity, visual field, color perception) for drug therapy lasting longer than 28 days.

PATIENT/FAMILY TEACHING
• Take at least 1 hr before or 1 hr after a meal. • Avoid grapefruit products. • Avoid driving at night. • Report visual changes (blurred vision, photophobia, yellowing of skin/eyes). • Avoid performing hazardous tasks if changes in vision occur. • Avoid direct sunlight. • Women of childbearing potential should use effective contraception.

vorinostat

vor-**in**-o-stat
(Zolinza)
Do not confuse vorinostat with Votrient.

◆CLASSIFICATION

PHARMACOTHERAPEUTIC: Histone deacetylase inhibitor. **CLINICAL:** Antineoplastic.

USES

Treatment of cutaneous manifestations in pts with cutaneous T-cell lymphoma (CTCL) with progressive, persistent, or recurrent disease, on or following two systemic therapies.

PRECAUTIONS

Contraindications: Hypersensitivity to vorinostat. **Cautions:** History of deep vein thrombosis (DVT), diabetes mellitus, hepatic impairment, preexisting hypokalemia, hypomagnesemia, pts with history of QT prolongation or medications that prolong QT interval. Use caution during perioperative period in pts requiring bowel surgery.

ACTION

Inhibits activity of histone deacetylase enzymes that catalyze removal of acetyl groups of proteins, causing accumulation of acetylated histones. **Therapeutic Effect:** Terminates cell growth, causes apoptosis.

PHARMACOKINETICS

Protein binding: 71%. Metabolized to inactive metabolites. Excreted in urine. **Half-life:** 2 hrs.

⧖ LIFESPAN CONSIDERATIONS

Pregnancy/Lactation: May cause fetal harm. Unknown if distributed in breast milk. **Children:** Safety and efficacy not established. **Elderly:** No age-related precautions noted.

INTERACTIONS

DRUG: May increase effect of **warfarin**. **Valproic acid** increases risk of GI bleeding, thrombocytopenia. **QT interval–prolonging medications (e.g., amiodarone, azithromycin, ceritinib, haloperidol, moxifloxacin)** may increase risk of QT interval prolongation, cardiac arrhythmias. **HERBAL:** None significant. **FOOD:** None known. **LAB VALUES:** May decrease serum calcium, potassium, sodium, phosphate, platelet count. May increase serum glucose, creatinine; urine protein.

AVAILABILITY (Rx)

🗩 **Capsules:** 100 mg.

ADMINISTRATION/HANDLING

PO
• Do not break, crush, dissolve, or divide capsules. • Give with food. • Maintain adequate hydration during treatment.

INDICATIONS/ROUTES/DOSAGE

Cutaneous T-Cell Lymphoma (CTCL)
PO: ADULTS, ELDERLY: 400 mg once daily with food. Continue until disease progression or unacceptable toxicity.

Dose Modification
Intolerance or Toxicity: Reduce dose to 300 mg once daily.
Unable to tolerate daily dose: May further reduce to 300 mg once daily for 5 consecutive days per wk (5 out of 7 days).

Dosage in Renal Impairment
Use caution.

Dosage in Hepatic Impairment
Mild to moderate impairment: 300 mg once daily.
Severe impairment: 100–200 mg once daily.

SIDE EFFECTS

Frequent (50%–24%): Fatigue, diarrhea, nausea, altered taste, anorexia. **Occasional (21%–11%):** Weight decrease, muscle spasms, alopecia, dry mouth, chills, vomiting, constipation, dizziness, peripheral edema, headache, pruritus, cough, fever.

ADVERSE EFFECTS/TOXIC REACTIONS

Thrombocytopenia occurs in 25% of pts, anemia in 15%. Pulmonary embolism occurs in 4% of pts. Deep vein thrombosis (DVT) occurs rarely.

NURSING CONSIDERATIONS

BASELINE ASSESSMENT

Obtain baseline EKG. Baseline PT, INR, CBC, serum chemistry tests, esp. serum potassium, calcium, magnesium, glucose, creatinine should be obtained prior to therapy and every 2 wks during first 2 mos of therapy and monthly thereafter. Inform women of childbearing potential of risk to fetus if pregnancy occurs.

INTERVENTION/EVALUATION

Monitor CBC, serum electrolytes; PT/INR q2wks for 2 mos, then monthly. Monitor signs/symptoms of DVT. Encourage fluid intake, approximately 2 L/day input. Assess for evidence of dehydration. Provide antiemetics to control nausea/vomiting. Monitor daily pattern of bowel activity, stool consistency.

PATIENT/FAMILY TEACHING

• Drink at least 2 L/day of fluids to prevent dehydration. • Report persistent vomiting, diarrhea. • Report shortness of breath, pain in any extremity.

V

vortioxetine

vor-tye-ox-e-teen
(Trintellix)

Do not confuse vortioxetine with FLUoxetine, PARoxetine, or venlafaxine.

■ **BLACK BOX ALERT** ■ Antidepressants have an increased risk of suicidal ideation and behavior in children, adolescents, and young adults. Monitor closely for worsening or emergence of suicidal thoughts and behaviors.

◆CLASSIFICATION

PHARMACOTHERAPEUTIC: Selective serotonin reuptake inhibitor (SSRI). **CLINICAL:** Antidepressant.

USES

Treatment of major depressive disorder.

PRECAUTIONS

Contraindications: Hypersensitivity to vortioxetine. Use of monoamine oxidase inhibitors (MAOIs). Do not use MAOIs within 21 days of stopping vortioxetine; do not use vortioxetine within 14 days of stopping an MAOI. **Cautions:** History of angioedema, dehydration, hyponatremia, pts at risk for bleeding, hepatic impairment, seizure disorder, elderly pts, pts at high risk of suicide, family history of bipolar disorder, mania, hypomania.

ACTION

Blocks reuptake of neurotransmitter serotonin at CNS presynaptic membranes, increasing availability at postsynaptic receptor sites. **Therapeutic Effect:** Relieves depression.

PHARMACOKINETICS

Readily absorbed following PO administration. Metabolized in liver, primarily through oxidation. Protein binding: 98%. Peak plasma concentration: 7–11 hrs. Steady state reached within 2 wks. Excreted in urine (59%), feces (26%). **Half-life:** 66 hrs.

⌛ LIFESPAN CONSIDERATIONS

Pregnancy/Lactation: May cause fetal harm when administered in third trimester. Unknown if distributed in breast milk. Exposed neonates are at increased risk of apnea, cyanosis, prolonged hospitalization, pulmonary hypertension, seizures, serotonin syndrome. **Children:** Safety and efficacy not established in pediatric population. **Elderly:** May have increased risk of dehydration, hyponatremia.

INTERACTIONS

DRUG: Strong CYP inducers (e.g., carBAMazepine, phenytoin, riFAMPin) may decrease concentration/effects. **Strong CYP2D6 inhibitors (e.g., buPROPion, FLUoxetine, PARoxetine)** may increase concentration/effect. **MAOIs** contraindicated; may cause malignant hyperthermia, hypertensive crisis, hyperreflexia, seizures, serotonin syndrome. **Serotonergic drugs (e.g., busPIRone, fentaNYL, linezolid, traMADol, tricyclic antidepressants, triptans)** may increase risk of serotonin syndrome. **Anticoagulants, antiplatelets, NSAIDs** may increase risk of bleeding. **Diuretics** may increase risk of hyponatremia. **HERBAL: St. John's wort** may increase risk of serotonin syndrome. **FOOD:** None known. **LAB VALUES:** May decrease serum sodium.

AVAILABILITY (Rx)

Tablets: 5 mg, 10 mg, 20 mg.

ADMINISTRATION/HANDLING

PO
• Give without regard to meals. May administer with milk or food if GI upset occurs.

V

INDICATIONS/ROUTES/DOSAGE

Major Depressive Disorder
PO: ADULTS/ELDERLY: Initially, 10 mg once daily. May increase to 20 mg as tolerated. **Maintenance:** 5–20 mg once daily.

Dose Modification
Concomitant Use of Strong CYP2D6 Inhibitors: Reduce dose by half of intended therapy. **Maximum:** 10 mg once daily. **Concomitant Use of Strong CYP Inducers:** If coadministered for more than 14 days, consider increasing vortioxetine dose. **Maximum:** Do not exceed more than 3 times original dose. **CYP2D6 poor metabolizers: Maximum:** 10 mg once daily.
Discontinuation: Gradually taper dose to minimize incidence of withdrawal symptoms and to allow detection of re-emerging symptoms.

Dosage in Renal Impairment
No dose adjustment.

Dosage in Hepatic Impairment
Mild to moderate impairment: No dose adjustment. **Severe impairment:** Not recommended.

SIDE EFFECTS

Frequent (32%–22%): Nausea, sexual dysfunction. **Occasional (10%–3%):** Diarrhea, dizziness, dry mouth, constipation, vomiting, flatulence, abnormal dreams, pruritus.

ADVERSE EFFECTS/TOXIC REACTIONS

Life-threatening serotonin syndrome may include mental status changes (agitation, hallucinations, delirium, coma), autonomic instability (tachycardia, labile blood pressure, dizziness, sweating, flushing, hyperthermia), neuromuscular symptoms (tremor, rigidity, myoclonus [localized muscle twitching], hyperactive reflexes, incoordination), seizures, GI symptoms (nausea, vomiting, diarrhea). May increase risk of bleeding events such as ecchymosis, hematoma, epistaxis (nosebleed), petechiae. Mania/hypomania may indicate baseline bipolar disorder. Syndrome of inappropriate antidiuretic hormone (SIADH), also known as water intoxication or dilutional hyponatremia, may induce seizures, coma, or death. Angioedema, dyspnea, rash may indicate allergic reaction. May increase risk of suicidal ideation and behavior once treatment is therapeutic. May alter sexual drive, ease of arousal, ease of reaching orgasm, or cause erectile dysfunction in men or decreased lubrication in women.

NURSING CONSIDERATIONS

BASELINE ASSESSMENT
Obtain baseline electrolytes. Note serum sodium level. Assess appearance, behavior, speech pattern, level of interest, mood. Screen for history of bipolar disorder, bleeding events, SIADH, prior allergic reactions to drug class. Receive full medication history including herbal products.

INTERVENTION/EVALUATION
Monitor serum sodium levels. Screen for signs of SIADH (confusion, seizures). Offer emotional support. Assess mental status for depression, suicidal ideation (esp. during first few mo of therapy or with dosage change), anxiety, social function. Monitor daily pattern of bowel activity, stool consistency. Assist with ambulation if dizziness occurs. Monitor pt for symptoms of serotonin syndrome, mania/hypomania. Offer antiemetic for nausea, vomiting. Monitor for allergic reactions.

PATIENT/FAMILY TEACHING
• Dry mouth may be relieved with sugarless gum, sips of water. • Report neurologic changes: confusion, excessive

V

talking, hallucinations, headache, hyperactivity, insomnia, racing thoughts, seizure-like activity, tremors; sexual dysfunction; fever; or any type of allergic reaction • Avoid tasks that require alertness, motor skills until response to drug is established (may cause dizziness, drowsiness). • Take with food if nausea occurs. • Report pregnancy. • Avoid alcohol. • Do not take OTC medications such as aspirin or ibuprofen without consulting physician. • Immediately report thoughts of suicide, self-destructive behavior, or violence. • Sexual dysfunction such as inability to reach orgasm, difficulty maintaining an erection, or lack of sexual drive may occur. • Do not suddenly stop treatment. Dose must be gradually reduced over time.

V

warfarin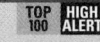

war-far-in
(Apo-Warfarin ♣, Coumadin,
Jantoven, Novo-Warfarin ♣)

■ **BLACK BOX ALERT** ■ May
cause major or fatal bleeding. Risk
factors include history of GI bleeding, hypertension, cerebrovascular
disease, heart disease, malignancy,
trauma, anemia, renal insufficiency,
age 65 yrs and older, high anticoagulation factor (INR greater than 4).
Consider cardiac/hepatic function,
age, nutritional status, concurrent
medications, risk of bleeding when
dosing warfarin. Genetic variations
have been identified as factors associated with dosage and bleeding
risk. Genotyping tests are available.
**Do not confuse Coumadin with
Kemadrin, or Jantoven with
Janumet or Januvia.**

◆CLASSIFICATION

PHARMACOTHERAPEUTIC: Vitamin
K antagonist. **CLINICAL:** Anticoagulant.

USES

Prophylaxis, treatment of thromboembolic disorders and embolic complications arising from atrial fibrillation or
valve replacement. Risk reduction of
systemic embolism following MI (e.g., recurrent MI, stroke). **OFF-LABEL:** Adjunct
treatment in transient ischemic attacks.

PRECAUTIONS

Contraindications: Hypersensitivity to warfarin. Hemorrhagic tendencies (e.g.,
cerebral aneurysms, bleeding from GI
tract), recent or potential surgery of
eye or CNS, neurosurgical procedures,
open wounds, severe uncontrolled or
malignant hypertension, spinal puncture procedures, uncontrolled bleeding, ulcers, unreliable or noncompliant
pts, unsupervised pts, blood dyscrasias,
pericarditis or pericardial effusion, pregnancy (except in women with mechanical

heart valves at high risk for thromboembolism), bacterial endocarditis, threat-
ened abortion. Major regional lumbar
block anesthesia or traumatic surgery,
eclampsia/preeclampsia. **Cautions:** Active tuberculosis, acute infection, diabetes, heparin-induced thrombocytopenia
and deep vein thrombosis, pts at risk for
hemorrhage, moderate to severe renal
impairment, moderate to severe hypertension, thyroid disease, polycythemia
vera, vasculitis, open wound, menstruat-
ing and postpartum women, indwelling
catheters, trauma, prolonged dietary deficiencies, disruption of GI normal flora,
history of peptic ulcer disease, protein C
deficiency, elderly.

ACTION

Interferes with hepatic synthesis of vitamin K–dependent clotting factors, resulting in depletion of coagulation factors II,
VII, IX, X. **Therapeutic Effect:** Prevents
further extension of formed existing clot;
prevents new clot formation, secondary
thromboembolic complications.

PHARMACOKINETICS

Route	Onset	Peak	Duration
PO	1.5–3 days	5–7 days	2–5 days

Well absorbed from GI tract. Protein
binding: 99%. Metabolized in liver. Primarily excreted in urine. Not removed by
hemodialysis. **Half-life:** 20–60 hrs.

⧗ LIFESPAN CONSIDERATIONS

Pregnancy/Lactation: Contraindicated in pregnancy (fetal, neonatal hemorrhage, intrauterine death). Crosses
placenta; is not distributed in breast milk.
Children: More susceptible to effect.
Elderly: Increased risk of hemorrhage;
lower dosage recommended.

INTERACTIONS

DRUG: Amiodarone, azole antifungals, cimetidine, disulfiram,
fluvoxaMINE sulfamethoxazole-tri-
methoprim, levothyroxine, metro-
NIDAZOLE, NSAIDs (e.g., ibuprofen,

W

ketorolac, naproxen), omeprazole, platelet aggregation inhibitors (e.g., clopidogrel), salicylates (e.g., aspirin), thrombolytic agents (e.g., alteplase), thyroid hormones may increase effect. Griseofulvin, CYP3A inducers (e.g., carBAMazepine, phenytoin, rifAMPin), vitamin K may decrease effects. Alcohol may enhance anticoagulant effect. HERBAL: Cat's claw, dong quai, evening primrose, feverfew, garlic, ginger, ginkgo biloba, ginseng possess antiplatelet activity, may increase risk of bleeding. Ginseng, St. John's wort may decrease effect. FOOD: Foods rich in vitamin K (e.g., spinach, brussels sprouts, meat) may decrease effect. Cranberry juice may increase effect. LAB VALUES: None known.

AVAILABILITY (Rx)

Tablets (Coumadin, Jantoven): 1 mg, 2 mg, 2.5 mg, 3 mg, 4 mg, 5 mg, 6 mg, 7.5 mg, 10 mg.

ADMINISTRATION/HANDLING

PO
• Give without regard to food. Give with food if GI upset occurs. • Give at same time each day.

INDICATIONS/ROUTES/DOSAGE

◄ALERT► Initial dosing must be individualized.

Anticoagulant
PO: ADULTS, ELDERLY: Initially, 2–5 mg/ daily for 2 days OR 5–10 mg daily for 1–2 days, adjusting the dose based on INR results. Usual maintenance dose: 2–10 mg/day, but may vary outside these guidelines. CHILDREN: Initially, 0.2 mg/ kg/day. Maximum: 10 mg. Maintenance: Adjust based on INR.

Dosage in Renal/Hepatic Impairment
No dose adjustment. Closely monitor INR.

SIDE EFFECTS

Occasional: GI distress (nausea, anorexia, abdominal cramps, diarrhea).

Rare: Hypersensitivity reaction (dermatitis, urticaria), esp. in those sensitive to aspirin.

ADVERSE EFFECTS/TOXIC REACTIONS

Bleeding complications ranging from local ecchymoses to major hemorrhage (intracranial hemorrhage, GI/GU/nasal/ oral/rectal bleeding) may occur. Hepatotoxicity, blood dyscrasias, necrosis, vasculitis, local thrombosis occur rarely. Antidote: Vitamin K. Amount based on INR, significance of bleeding. Range: 2.5–10 mg given orally or slow IV infusion (see Appendix J for dosage).

NURSING CONSIDERATIONS

BASELINE ASSESSMENT
Cross-check dose with co-worker. Obtain CBC, PT/INR before administration and daily following therapy initiation. When stabilized, follow with INR determination q4–6wks. Obtain genotyping prior to initiating therapy if available. Screen for major active bleeding. Question recent history of bleeding, recent trauma, surgical procedures, epidural anesthesia.

INTERVENTION/EVALUATION
Monitor INR diligently. Assess CBC for anemia; urine/stool for occult blood. Be alert to complaints of abdominal/ back pain, severe headache, confusion, seizures, hemiparesis, aphasia (may be sign of hemorrhage). Decrease in B/P, increase in pulse rate may be sign of hemorrhage. Question for increase in amount of menstrual discharge. Assess peripheral pulses; skin for ecchymoses, petechiae. Check for excessive bleeding from minor cuts, scratches. Assess gums for erythema, gingival bleeding.

PATIENT/FAMILY TEACHING
• Take medication at same time each day. • Blood levels will be monitored routinely. • Do not take, discontinue any other medication except on advice of physician. • Avoid alcohol, aspirin, drastic

---

W

dietary changes. • Consult with physician before surgery, dental work. • Urine may become red-orange. • Falls, subtle injuries, esp. head or abdominal trauma, can be life-threatening. • Report bleeding, bruising, red or brown urine, black stools. • Use electric razor, soft toothbrush to prevent bleeding. • Report coffee-ground vomitus, blood-tinged mucus from cough. • Do not use any OTC medication without physician approval (may interfere with platelet aggregation). • Seek immediate medical attention for stroke-like symptoms (confusion, difficulty speaking, headache, one-sided weakness); bloody stool or urine.

W

zafirlukast

za-**fir**-loo-kast
(Accolate)
Do not confuse Accolate with Accupril, Accutane, or Aclovate.

◆CLASSIFICATION

PHARMACOTHERAPEUTIC: Leukotriene receptor antagonist. **CLINICAL:** Antiasthma.

USES

Prophylaxis, chronic treatment of bronchial asthma in adults and children 5 yrs and older. **OFF-LABEL:** Chronic urticaria.

PRECAUTIONS

Contraindications: Hypersensitivity to zafirlukast. Hepatic impairment. **Cautions:** Elderly pts. Not approved for acute asthma attacks, status asthmaticus.

ACTION

Competitive antagonist of leukotriene receptor. Leukotriene production and receptor occupation are associated with pathophysiology of asthma. **Therapeutic Effect:** Reduces airway edema, smooth muscle constriction; alters cellular activity associated with inflammatory process. Reduces signs/symptoms of asthma.

PHARMACOKINETICS

Rapidly absorbed after PO administration (food reduces absorption). Protein binding: 99%. Metabolized in liver. Primarily excreted in feces. Unknown if removed by hemodialysis. **Half-life:** 10 hrs.

⧗ LIFESPAN CONSIDERATIONS

Pregnancy/Lactation: Drug is distributed in breast milk. Do not administer to breastfeeding women. **Children:** Safety and efficacy not established in pts younger than 5 yrs. **Elderly:** No age-related precautions noted.

INTERACTIONS

DRUG: Erythromycin, theophylline may decrease concentration/effect. **Aspirin** may increase concentration/effects. May increase effects of **warfarin** (increases INR). **HERBAL:** None significant. **FOOD: Food** decreases bioavailability by 40%. **LAB VALUES:** None significant.

AVAILABILITY (Rx)

Tablets: 10 mg, 20 mg.

ADMINISTRATION/HANDLING

PO
• Give 1 hr before or 2 hrs after meals.

INDICATIONS/ROUTES/DOSAGE

Bronchial Asthma
PO: ADULTS, ELDERLY, CHILDREN 12 YRS AND OLDER: 20 mg twice daily. **CHILDREN 5–11 YRS:** 10 mg twice daily.

Dosage in Renal Impairment
No dose adjustment.

Dosage in Hepatic Impairment
Contraindicated.

SIDE EFFECTS

Frequent (13%): Headache. **Occasional (3%):** Nausea, diarrhea. **Rare (Less Than 3%):** Generalized pain, asthenia, myalgia, fever, dyspepsia, vomiting, dizziness.

ADVERSE EFFECTS/ TOXIC REACTIONS

Concurrent administration of inhaled corticosteroids increases risk of upper respiratory tract infection.

NURSING CONSIDERATIONS

BASELINE ASSESSMENT

Obtain medication history. Assess LFT. Auscultate lung sounds.

INTERVENTION/EVALUATION

Monitor rate, depth, rhythm, type of respiration; quality, rate of pulse. Assess lung sounds for rhonchi, wheezing, rales. Monitor LFT.

Z

PATIENT/FAMILY TEACHING

• Increase fluid intake (decreases lung secretion viscosity). • Take as prescribed, even during symptom-free periods. • Do not use for acute asthma episodes. • Do not alter, stop other asthma medications. • Do not breastfeed. • Report nausea, jaundice, abdominal pain, flu-like symptoms, worsening of asthma.

zanamivir

zan-**am**-i-veer
(Relenza Diskhaler)

◆CLASSIFICATION

PHARMACOTHERAPEUTIC: Neuraminidase inhibitor. **CLINICAL:** Antiviral, anti-influenza.

USES

Treatment of uncomplicated acute illness due to influenza virus A and B in adults, children 7 yrs and older who have been symptomatic for less than 2 days. Prevention of influenza A and B in adults and children 5 yrs and older.

PRECAUTIONS

Contraindications: Hypersensitivity to zanamivir. **Cautions:** Not recommended in respiratory disease (e.g., COPD, asthma), renal/hepatic impairment.

ACTION

Inhibits influenza virus enzyme neuraminidase, essential for viral replication. **Therapeutic Effect:** Prevents viral release from infected cells.

PHARMACOKINETICS

Systemically absorbed, approximately 4%–17%. Protein binding: less than 10%. Not metabolized. Excreted unchanged in urine. **Half-life:** 2.5–5.1 hrs.

⧗ LIFESPAN CONSIDERATIONS

Pregnancy/Lactation: Unknown if drug crosses placenta or is distributed in breast milk. **Children:** Safety and efficacy not established in pts younger than 7 yrs (treatment) or younger than 5 yrs (prevention). **Elderly:** No age-related precautions noted.

INTERACTIONS

DRUG: May decrease levels/effect of **influenza virus vaccine. HERBAL:** None significant. **FOOD:** None known. **LAB VALUES:** None significant.

AVAILABILITY (Rx)

Powder for Inhalation: 5 mg/blister.

ADMINISTRATION/HANDLING

Inhalation

• Instruct pt to use Diskhaler device provided, exhale completely; then, holding mouthpiece 1 inch away from lips, inhale and hold breath as long as possible before exhaling. • Rinse mouth with water immediately after inhalation (prevents mouth/throat dryness). • Store at room temperature.

INDICATIONS/ROUTES/DOSAGE

Treatment of Influenza Virus
Inhalation: ADULTS, ELDERLY, CHILDREN 7 YRS AND OLDER: 2 inhalations (one 5-mg blister per inhalation for total dose of 10 mg) twice daily (approximately 12 hrs apart) for 5 days.

Prevention of Influenza Virus
Inhalation: ADULTS, ELDERLY, CHILDREN 5 YRS AND OLDER: 2 inhalations (10 mg) once daily for duration of exposure period (10 days for household exposure, 28 days for community exposure).

Dosage in Renal/Hepatic Impairment
No dose adjustment.

SIDE EFFECTS

Occasional (3%–2%): Diarrhea, sinusitis, nausea, bronchitis, cough, dizziness,

---

♣ Canadian trade name   🗟 Non-Crushable Drug   [HIGH ALERT] High Alert drug

Z

headache. **Rare (Less Than 1.5%):** Malaise, fatigue, fever, abdominal pain, myalgia, arthralgia, urticaria.

ADVERSE EFFECTS/ TOXIC REACTIONS

May produce neutropenia. Bronchospasm may occur in those with history of COPD, bronchial asthma. Neuropsychiatric events (e.g., confusion, seizures, hallucinations) have been reported.

NURSING CONSIDERATIONS

BASELINE ASSESSMENT

Pts requiring an inhaled bronchodilator at same time as zanamivir should use the bronchodilator before zanamivir administration.

INTERVENTION/EVALUATION

Provide assistance if dizziness occurs. Monitor daily pattern of bowel activity, stool consistency.

PATIENT/FAMILY TEACHING

• Follow manufacturer guidelines for use of delivery device. • Avoid contact with those who are at high risk for influenza. • Continue treatment for full 5-day course. • Doses should be evenly spaced. • In pts with respiratory disease, an inhaled bronchodilator should be readily available.

zidovudine

zye-**doe**-vue-deen
(Apo-Zidovudine ✱, Novo-AZT ✱, Retrovir)
■ **BLACK BOX ALERT** ■ Neutropenia, severe anemia may occur. Lactic acidosis, severe hepatomegaly with steatosis (fatty liver), including fatalities, have occurred. Symptomatic myopathy, myositis associated with prolonged use.
Do not confuse Retrovir with acyclovir or ritonavir.

FIXED-COMBINATION(S)

Combivir: zidovudine/lamiVUDine (an antiviral): 300 mg/150 mg. **Trizivir:** zidovudine/lamiVUDine/abacavir (an antiviral): 300 mg/150 mg/ 300 mg.

◆CLASSIFICATION

PHARMACOTHERAPEUTIC: Nucleoside reverse transcriptase inhibitors. **CLINICAL:** Antiretroviral.

USES

Treatment of HIV infection in combination with at least two other antiretroviral agents. Prevention of maternal/fetal HIV transmission. **OFF-LABEL:** Prophylaxis in health care workers at risk for acquiring HIV after occupational exposure (part of multidrug regimen).

PRECAUTIONS

Contraindications: Potentially life-threatening allergic reactions to zidovudine or its components. **Cautions:** Bone marrow compromise, renal/hepatic dysfunction. Combination with interferon with or without ribavirin in HIV/hepatitis C virus (HCV) co-infection.

ACTION

Interferes with viral RNA-dependent DNA polymerase, an enzyme necessary for viral HIV replication. **Therapeutic Effect:** Slows HIV replication, reducing progression of HIV infection.

PHARMACOKINETICS

Rapidly, completely absorbed from GI tract. Protein binding: 25%–38%. Metabolized in liver. Crosses blood-brain barrier and is widely distributed, including to CSF. Primarily excreted in urine. Minimal removal by hemodialysis. **Half-life:** 0.5–3 hrs (increased in renal impairment).

⊠ LIFESPAN CONSIDERATIONS

Pregnancy/Lactation: Unknown if drug crosses placenta or is distributed

Z

in breast milk. Unknown if fetal harm or effects on fertility can occur. **Children:** No age-related precautions noted. **Elderly:** Information not available.

INTERACTIONS

DRUG: Bone marrow depressants, ganciclovir may increase myelosuppression. May be antagonistic with **DOXOrubicin.** Hematologic toxicities may occur with **interferon alfa. HERBAL:** None significant. **FOOD:** None known. **LAB VALUES:** May increase mean corpuscular volume (MCV).

AVAILABILITY (Rx)

Capsules (Retrovir): 100 mg. **Injection Solution (Retrovir):** 10 mg/mL. **Syrup (Retrovir):** 50 mg/5 mL. **Tablets:** 300 mg.

ADMINISTRATION/HANDLING

 **IV**

Reconstitution • Must dilute before administration. • Remove calculated dose from vial and add to D₅W to provide concentration no greater than 4 mg/mL.

Rate of Administration • Infuse over 1 hr. May infuse over 30 min in neonates.

Storage • After dilution, IV solution is stable for 24 hrs at room temperature; 48 hrs if refrigerated. • Use within 8 hrs if stored at room temperature or 24 hrs if refrigerated to minimize potential for microbial-contaminated solution. • Do not use if solution is discolored or precipitate forms.

PO

• Keep capsules in cool, dry place. Protect from light. • May administer without regard to food. • Space doses evenly around the clock. • Pt should maintain an upright position when given medication to prevent esophageal ulceration.

IV INCOMPATIBILITIES

None known.

IV COMPATIBILITIES

Dexamethasone (Decadron), DOBUTamine (Dobutrex), DOPamine (Intropin), heparin, LORazepam (Ativan), morphine, potassium chloride.

INDICATIONS/ROUTES/DOSAGE

HIV Infection

PO: ADULTS, ELDERLY: 300 mg q12h. **CHILDREN 4 WKS TO 18 YRS WEIGHING 30 KG OR MORE:** 300 mg q12h. **WEIGHING 9–29 KG:** 9 mg/kg q12h. **WEIGHING 4–8 KG:** 12 mg/kg q12h. **PREMATURE NEONATES, GA 35 WKS OR GREATER:** 4 mg/kg q12h, increase to 12 mg/kg q12h after 4 wks of age. **GA 30–34 WKS:** 2 mg/kg q12h for 2 wks, then 3 mg/kg q12h, then 12 mg/kg q12h after 6–8 wks. **GA LESS THAN 30 WKS:** 2 mg/kg q12h, then 3 mg/kg q12h at 4 wks of age, then 12 mg/kg q12h after 8–10 wks of age.

IV: ADULTS, ELDERLY, CHILDREN OLDER THAN 12 YRS: 1 mg/kg/dose q4h around the clock. **CHILDREN 12 YRS AND YOUNGER, FULL-TERM NEONATES:** 3 mg/kg/dose q12h. **PREMATURE NEONATES:** 1.5–2.3 mg/kg/dose q12h based on gestation at birth.

Prevention of Maternal/Fetal HIV Transmission

Note: Zidovudine should be given IV near delivery regardless of antepartum regimen or mode of delivery in women with HIV RNA level greater than 1,000 copies/mL (or unknown status). Other antiretrovirals should be continued orally. Zidovudine IV is not required in pts receiving HIV therapy with HIV RNA level less than 1,000 copies/mL near delivery.

IV (During Labor and Delivery): 2 mg/kg loading dose, then IV infusion of 1 mg/kg/hr until delivery. For scheduled cesarean section, begin IV zidovudine 3 hrs before surgery. **NEONATAL:** Begin 6–12 hrs after birth and continue for first 6 wks of life. Use IV route only until oral therapy can be administered.

PO: FULL-TERM INFANTS: 4 mg/kg/dose q12h (IV: 3 mg/kg/dose q12h). **INFANTS**

Z

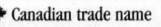

30–34 WKS' GESTATION: 2 mg/kg/dose q12h; increase to 3 mg/kg/dose at 2 wks of age (IV: 1.5 mg/kg/dose q12h; increase to 2.3 mg/kg/dose q12h at 2 wks of age). **INFANTS LESS THAN 30 WKS' GESTATION:** 2 mg/kg/dose q12h; increase to 3 mg/kg/dose at 4 wks of age (IV: 1.5 mg/kg/dose q12h; increase to 2.3 mg/kg/dose q12h at 4 wks of age).

Dosage in Renal Impairment
ADULTS, ELDERLY: CrCl less than 15 mL/min, including hemodialysis or peritoneal dialysis: PO: 100 mg q8h or 300 mg once daily. **IV:** 1 mg/kg q6–8hr. **INFANTS OLDER THAN 6 WKS, CHILDREN, ADOLESCENTS: GFR 10 mL/min/1.73m² or greater:** No adjustment. **GFR less than 10 mL/min/1.73m²:** Administer 50% of dose q8h.

Dosage in Hepatic Impairment
No dose adjustment.

SIDE EFFECTS

Expected (46%–42%): Nausea, headache. **Frequent (20%–16%):** Abdominal pain, asthenia, rash, fever, acne. **Occasional (12%–8%):** Diarrhea, anorexia, malaise, myalgia, drowsiness. **Rare (6%–5%):** Dizziness, paresthesia, vomiting, insomnia, dyspnea, altered taste.

ADVERSE EFFECTS/ TOXIC REACTIONS

Anemia (occurring most commonly after 4–6 wks of therapy), granulocytopenia are particularly significant in pts with pretherapy low baselines. Neurotoxicity (ataxia, fatigue, lethargy, nystagmus, seizures) may occur.

NURSING CONSIDERATIONS

BASELINE ASSESSMENT

Avoid drugs that are nephrotoxic, cytotoxic, myelosuppressive; may increase risk of toxicity. Obtain specimens for viral diagnostic tests before starting therapy (therapy may begin before results are obtained). Check hematology reports for accurate baseline.

INTERVENTION/EVALUATION

Monitor CBC, reticulocyte count, CD4 cell count, HIV RNA plasma levels. Check for bleeding. Assess for headache, dizziness. Monitor daily pattern of bowel activity, stool consistency. Evaluate skin for acne, rash. Be alert to development of opportunistic infections (fever, chills, cough, myalgia). Monitor I&O, serum renal function, LFT. Check for insomnia.

PATIENT/FAMILY TEACHING

• Doses should be evenly spaced around the clock. • Zidovudine is not a cure for HIV infection, nor does it reduce risk of transmission to others. Acts to reduce symptoms and slows or arrests progress of disease. • Do not take any medications without physician's approval. • Bleeding from gums, nose, rectum may occur and should be reported to physician immediately. • Blood counts are essential because of bleeding potential. • Dental work should be done before therapy or after blood counts return to normal (often wks after therapy has stopped). • Inform physician if muscle weakness, difficulty breathing, headache, inability to sleep, unusual bleeding, rash, signs of infection occur.

ziprasidone

zi-**pras**-i-done
(Geodon, Zeldox ✤)
■ **BLACK BOX ALERT** ■ Increased risk of mortality in elderly pts with dementia-related psychosis, mainly due to pneumonia, HF.
Do not confuse ziprasidone with traZODone.

◆CLASSIFICATION

PHARMACOTHERAPEUTIC: Second-generation (atypical) antipsychotic. **CLINICAL:** Antipsychotic.

Z

USES

Treatment of schizophrenia, acute agitation in pts with schizophrenia. Treatment of acute mania or mixed episodes associated with bipolar disorder with or without psychosis. Maintenance treatment of bipolar disorder as adjunct to lithium or valproic acid. **OFF-LABEL:** Major depressive disorder (adjunct to antidepressants).

PRECAUTIONS

Contraindications: Hypersensitivity to ziprasidone. Conditions associated with risk of prolonged QT interval, congenital long QT syndrome, concurrent use of other QT-prolongation medications (e.g., amiodarone, moxifloxacin, tacrolimus, thioridazine). Uncompensated HF. Recent MI. **Cautions:** Pts with bradycardia, hypokalemia, hypomagnesemia may be at greater risk for torsades de pointes. History of MI or unstable heart disease, seizures, cardiac arrhythmias, disorders in which CNS depression is a feature; pts at risk for aspiration pneumonia, hypotension, suicide; elderly, diabetes, hepatic impairment, Parkinson's disease, pts with breast cancer or other prolactin-dependent tumors.

ACTION

Exact mechanism unknown. Antagonizes alpha-adrenergic, DOPamine, histamine, serotonin receptors; inhibits reuptake of serotonin, norepinephrine. **Therapeutic Effect:** Diminishes symptoms of schizophrenia, depression.

PHARMACOKINETICS

Well absorbed after PO administration. Food increases bioavailability. Protein binding: 99%. Metabolized in liver. Excreted in feces. Not removed by hemodialysis. **Half-life: PO:** 7 hrs; **IM:** 2–5 hrs.

☒ LIFESPAN CONSIDERATIONS

Pregnancy/Lactation: Unknown if drug crosses placenta or is distributed in breast milk. **Children:** Safety and efficacy not established. **Elderly:** No age-related precautions noted. Use caution.

INTERACTIONS

DRUG: Alcohol, other CNS depressants (e.g., LORazepam, morphine, zolpidem) may increase CNS depression. **CarBAMazepine** may decrease concentration. **Ketoconazole** may increase concentration. **QT interval–prolonging medications (e.g., amiodarone, azithromycin, ceritinib, haloperidol, moxifloxacin)** may increase risk of QT interval prolongation, cardiac arrhythmias. **HERBAL: Gotu kola, kava kava, St. John's wort, valerian** may increase CNS depression. **St. John's wort** may decrease concentration. **FOOD: All foods** enhance bioavailability. **LAB VALUES:** May prolong QT interval. May increase serum glucose, prolactin levels.

AVAILABILITY (Rx)

Capsules: 20 mg, 40 mg, 60 mg, 80 mg. **Injection, Powder for Reconstitution:** 20 mg.

ADMINISTRATION/HANDLING

IM

• Store vials at room temperature; protect from light. • Reconstitute each vial with 1.2 mL Sterile Water for Injection to provide concentration of 20 mg/mL. • Reconstituted solution stable for 24 hrs at room temperature or 7 days if refrigerated.

PO

• Give with food containing at least 500 calories (increases bioavailability).

INDICATIONS/ROUTES/DOSAGE

◀**ALERT**▶ Dosage greater than 80 mg twice daily is not recommended in most pts. **To discontinue therapy:** Gradually discontinue to avoid withdrawal symptoms, minimize risk of relapses.

Schizophrenia

PO: ADULTS, ELDERLY: Initially, 20 mg twice daily with food. Titrate at intervals

Z

of no less than 2 days based on response and tolerability. **Maintenance:** 40–100 mg twice daily.

Acute Agitation (Schizophrenia)
IM: ADULTS, ELDERLY: 10 mg q2h or 20 mg q4h. **Maximum:** 40 mg/day. Switch to oral therapy as soon as possible.

Bipolar Disorder (acute and maintenance as adjunct to lithium or valproate)
PO: ADULTS, ELDERLY (Acute): Initially, 40 mg twice daily. May increase to 60–80 mg twice daily on second day of treatment. **Maintenance:** 40–80 mg twice daily.

Dosage in Renal Impairment
Oral: No dose adjustment. **IM:** Use caution.

Dosage in Hepatic Impairment
Use caution.

SIDE EFFECTS

Frequent (30%–16%): Headache, drowsiness, dizziness. **Occasional:** Rash, orthostatic hypotension, weight gain, restlessness, constipation, dyspepsia. **Rare:** Hyperglycemia, priapism.

ADVERSE EFFECTS/ TOXIC REACTIONS

Prolongation of QT interval (as seen on EKG) may produce torsades de pointes, a form of ventricular tachycardia. Pts with bradycardia, hypokalemia, hypomagnesemia are at increased risk.

NURSING CONSIDERATIONS

BASELINE ASSESSMENT
Assess pt's behavior, appearance, emotional status, response to environment, speech pattern, thought content. EKG should be obtained to assess for QT prolongation before instituting medication. Blood chemistry for serum magnesium, potassium should be obtained before beginning therapy and routinely thereafter.

INTERVENTION/EVALUATION
Assess for therapeutic response (greater interest in surroundings, improved self-care, increased ability to concentrate, relaxed facial expression). Monitor weight.

PATIENT/FAMILY TEACHING
• Avoid tasks that require alertness, motor skills until response to drug is established. • Avoid alcohol. • Report chest pain, shortness of breathing, irregular heartbeats, fainting, palpitations.

ziv-aflibercept

ziv-a-**flib**-er-sept
(Zaltrap)
Do not confuse ziv-aflibercept with abatacept, Aricept, or etanercept.

■ **BLACK BOX ALERT** ■ Severe, and sometimes fatal, hemorrhagic events including GI hemorrhage were reported in pts receiving concomitant FOLFIRI therapy. Do not initiate in pts with severe hemorrhage. Fatal GI perforation may occur. Discontinue treatment in pts with impaired wound healing. Withhold treatment for at least 4 wks prior to elective surgery. Do not resume treatment for at least 4 wks after major surgery until wound is fully healed.

◆CLASSIFICATION

PHARMACOTHERAPEUTIC: Vascular endothelial growth factor (VEGF) inhibitor. **CLINICAL:** Antineoplastic.

USES

Treatment of metastatic colorectal cancer (mCRC) (in combination with 5-fluorouracil, leucovorin, irinotecan [FOLFIRI]) in pts resistant to or has progressed following an oxaliplatin-containing regimen.

PRECAUTIONS

Contraindications: Hypersensitivity to ziv-aflibercept. **Cautions:** Baseline hematologic cytopenias, (neutropenia, leukopenia, thrombocytopenia), conditions predisposing to infection (e.g., diabetes, renal failure, immunocompromised pts, open wounds), pts at risk for bleeding (e.g., history of intracranial/GI/GU bleeding, coagulation disorders, recent trauma; concomitant use of anticoagulants, antiplatelet medication, NSAIDS), hypertension, elderly pts, history of arterial/venous thrombosis (e.g., CVA, DVT, MI, pulmonary embolism), GI perforation or hemorrhage.

ACTION

A recombinant fusion protein, comprising portions of binding domains of vascular endothelial growth factor (VEGF) receptors. Acts as a decoy receptor that prevents VEGF receptor binding/activation. **Therapeutic Effect:** Produces anti-angiogenesis/tumor regression.

PHARMACOKINETICS

Half-life: 6 days. (Range: 4–7 days).

⏳ LIFESPAN CONSIDERATIONS

Pregnancy/Lactation: Avoid pregnancy; may cause fetal harm. Females of reproductive potential and males should use effective contraception during therapy and for at least 3 mos after discontinuation. Unknown if distributed in breast milk. **Children:** Safety and efficacy not established. **Elderly:** May have increased risk of side effects, esp. diarrhea, dehydration, dizziness, weakness, weight loss.

INTERACTIONS

DRUG: May decrease therapeutic effect of **BCG (intravesical)**. **Anticoagulants (e.g., heparin, warfarin), antiplatelets (e.g., aspirin, clopidogrel), NSAIDS (e.g., diclofenac, ibuprofen, naproxen), thrombolytic therapy (e.g., tPA)** may increase risk of bleeding in pts with treatment-induced thrombocytopenia. **HERBAL:** None significant.

FOOD: None known. **LAB VALUES:** May increase serum ALT, AST, serum creatinine; urine protein. May decrease leukocytes, neutrophils, platelets.

AVAILABILITY (Rx)

Injection, Solution: 100 mg/4 mL (25mg/mL), 200 mg/8mL (25 mg/mL).

ADMINISTRATION/HANDLING

 IV

Preparation • Visually inspect for particulate matter or discoloration. Solution should appear clear, colorless to pale yellow in color. Discard if solution is cloudy, discolored, or if visible particles are observed. • Withdraw proper dose from vial and dilute in 0.9% NaCl or D_5W to a final concentration of 0.6–8 mg/mL. Use polyvinyl chloride (PVC) infusion bags containing bis (2-ethylhexyl) phthalate (DEHP) or polyolefin. • Mix by gentle inversion. • Do not shake or agitate. • Discard unused portions.

Rate of Administration • Infuse over 60 min via dedicated IV line using an in-line 0.2-micron polyethersulfone filter and an infusion set made of one of the following: polypropylene, polyethylene-lined PVC, polyurethane, DEHP-free PVC-containing trioctyl-trimellitate (TOTM), PVC containing DEHP. • Do not use in-line filters made of polyvinylidene fluoride (PVDF) or nylon. • Do not administer as IV push or bolus.

Storage • Refrigerate unused vials. • Do not shake. • Protect from light. • May refrigerate diluted solution for up to 24 hrs or at controlled room temperature for up to 8 hrs.

IV INCOMPATIBILITIES

Do not infuse with other medications or solutions.

INDICATIONS/ROUTES/DOSAGE

Note: Delay treatment until ANC 1,500/mm³ or greater.

Metastatic Colorectal Cancer
IV: ADULTS, ELDERLY: 4 mg/kg q2wks (in combination with 5-fluorouracil,

leucovorin, and irinotecan). Continue until disease progression or unacceptable toxicity.

Dose Modification
Hypertension (Treatment-Induced)
Severe hypertension, recurrent hypertension: Withhold treatment until hypertension is controlled, then permanently reduce to 2 mg/kg q2wks.

Proteinuria
Urine protein greater than or equal to 2 g/24 hrs: Withhold treatment until urine protein less than 2 g/24 hrs, then resume at previous dose. **Recurrent urine protein greater than 2 g/24 hrs:** Withhold treatment until urine protein less than 2 g/24hrs, then resume with a permanent reduction to 2 mg/kg q2wks.

Permanent Discontinuation
Permanently discontinue if severe hemorrhage, GI perforation, impaired wound healing, fistula formation, hypertensive crisis, arterial thromboembolism, nephrotic syndrome, thrombotic microangiopathy, reversible posterior leukoencephalopathy occurs.

Dosage in Renal/Hepatic Impairment
No dose adjustment.

SIDE EFFECTS

Frequent (57%–24%): Diarrhea, fatigue, stomatitis, abdominal pain, decreased appetite. **Occasional (13%–9%):** Asthenia, dyspnea, headache. **Rare (3%–2%):** Skin hyperpigmentation, dystonia, oropharyngeal pain, dehydration, rhinorrhea, hemorrhoids, proctalgia.

ADVERSE EFFECTS/ TOXIC REACTIONS

Leukopenia, neutropenia, thrombocytopenia are expected responses to therapy, but more severe reactions including bone marrow depression, febrile neutropenia may be life-threatening. Severe, sometimes fatal, hemorrhagic events including intracranial/GI/GU/nasal/postprocedural hemorrhage may occur. GI perforations

occurred in less than 1% of pts. May cause impaired wound healing or wound dehiscence requiring medical intervention, GI or non-GI fistula formation, severe hypertension, severe proteinuria, nephrotic syndrome, severe diarrhea, dehydration. Arterial thromboembolism including CVA, MI, TIA reported in up to 3% of pts. Reversible posterior leukoencephalopathy syndrome (RPLS) may present as aphasia, altered mental status, paralysis, vision loss, weakness. UTI reported in 6% of pts. Palmar-plantar erythrodysesthesia syndrome (PPES), a chemotherapy-induced skin condition that presents with redness, swelling, numbness, skin sloughing of the hands and feet, reported in 4% of pts. Immunogenicity (auto-ziv-afilbercept antibodies) occurred in up to 3% of pts.

NURSING CONSIDERATIONS

BASELINE ASSESSMENT

Obtain CBC, BUN, serum creatinine, LFT; urine protein; vital signs. Obtain pregnancy test in females of reproductive potential. Question for recent surgeries, dental procedures. Question history of thromboembolism (CVA, DVT, MI, pulmonary embolism), hypertension, hemorrhagic events. Screen for active infection. Screen for home medications that may increase risk of hemorrhage. Conduct dermatologic exam; assess for open wounds, lesions, surgical incisions. Obtain dietary consult. Assess hydration status. Offer emotional support.

INTERVENTION/EVALUATION

Monitor ANC, CBC for myelosuppression prior to each cycle; renal function test, LFT, urine protein periodically. Monitor B/P at least q2wks. Persistent diastolic hypertension may indicate hypertensive crisis. If urine dipstick proteinuria is greater than or equal to 2+, obtain 24-hr urine protein test. Withhold treatment for at least 4 wks prior to elective surgery or for at least 4 wks after major surgery and until wound is fully healed. Due to high risk for arterial occlusions, be vigilant when screening for CVA (aphasia, confusion, paresthesia, hemiparesis, seizures), MI (chest pain, diaphoresis, left arm/jaw pain, increased serum troponin, ST segment elevation). RPLS should be considered in pts with altered mental status, confusion, headache, seizures, visual disturbances. Report abdominal pain, fever, hemoptysis, melena (may indicate GI perforation/fistula formation). Monitor skin for impaired wound healing, new skin lesions, rash, sloughing. Monitor for decreased urine output, renal dysfunction, nephrotic syndrome. Encourage fluid intake. Monitor daily pattern of bowel activity, stool consistency.

PATIENT/FAMILY TEACHING

• Life-threatening blood clots of the arteries and veins have occurred; report symptoms of heart attack (chest pain, difficulty breathing, jaw pain, nausea, pain that radiates to the left arm, sweating), stroke (blindness, confusion, one-sided weakness, loss of consciousness, trouble speaking, seizures), DVT (swelling, pain, hot feeling in the arms or legs), lung embolism (difficulty breathing, chest pain, rapid heart rate). Report liver problems (abdominal pain, bruising, clay-colored stool, amber or dark-colored urine, yellowing of the skin or eyes); skin changes (sloughing, rash, poor healing of wounds). • Life-threatening bleeding may occur; report bloody stool or urine, rectal bleeding, nosebleeds, vomiting up blood. • Treatment may depress your immune system response and reduce your ability to fight infection. Report symptoms of infection such as body aches, chills, cough, fatigue, fever. Avoid those with active infection. • Avoid pregnancy; treatment may cause birth defects. Females and males of childbearing potential should use effective contraception during treatment and for at least 3 mos after last dose. • Nervous system changes, including altered mental status, seizures, headache, blurry vision, high blood pressure, trouble speaking,

one-sided weakness, may indicate stroke, high blood pressure crisis, life-threatening brain dysfunction/swelling. • Notify physician before any planned surgeries/dental procedures. • Severe diarrhea may lead to dehydration; drink plenty of fluids.

zoledronic acid

zoe-le-**dron**-ik **as**-id
(Aclasta ✦, Reclast, <u>Zometa</u>)
Do not confuse Zometa with Zofran or Zoladex.

◆CLASSIFICATION

PHARMACOTHERAPEUTIC: Bisphosphonate. **CLINICAL:** Calcium regulator, bone resorption inhibitor.

USES

Zometa: Treatment of hypercalcemia of malignancy, bone metastases from solid tumors. Treatment of multiple myeloma osteolytic lesions. **Reclast:** Treatment and prevention of postmenopausal osteoporosis, glucocorticoid-induced osteoporosis, treatment of Paget's disease. Treatment of osteoporosis in men to increase bone mass. **OFF-LABEL:** Prevention of bone loss associated with aromatase inhibitor therapy in postmenopausal women with breast cancer or androgen deprivation therapy in men with prostate cancer. Post–renal transplant bone loss.

PRECAUTIONS

Contraindications: Hypersensitivity to zoledronic acid, other bisphosphonates (e.g., alendronate, risedronate). **Reclast Only:** CrCl less than 35 mL/min, acute renal impairment, hypocalcemia. **Cautions:** Elderly. **(Oncology Indications):** History of aspirin-sensitive asthma, mild to moderate renal impairment. **(Non-Oncology Indications):** Pts with disturbances of calcium and mineral metabolism (e.g., hypoparathyroidism, malabsorption syndrome).

Z

✦ Canadian trade name   🔖 Non-Crushable Drug   🔲 High Alert drug

ACTION

Inhibits bone resorption by action on osteoclasts. Inhibits osteoclast activity/skeletal calcium release induced by tumors; inhibits osteoclast-mediated resorption. **Therapeutic Effect: (Tumor):** Increases urinary calcium, phosphorus excretion; decreases serum calcium, phosphorus levels. **(Osteoporosis):** Reduces bone turnover.

⌛ LIFESPAN CONSIDERATIONS

Pregnancy/Lactation: Unknown if drug crosses placenta or is distributed in breast milk. Recommend discontinuation of therapy as early as possible prior to a planned pregnancy. **Children:** Safety and efficacy not established. **Elderly:** Age-related renal impairment may require dosage adjustment.

INTERACTIONS

DRUG: Loop diuretics (e.g., furosemide) may increase risk for hypocalcemia. **Nephrotoxic drugs (e.g., IV contrast dye, furosemide, lisinopril, rifAMPin)** may increase risk for nephrotoxicity. **HERBAL:** None significant. **FOOD:** None known. **LAB VALUES:** May decrease serum magnesium, calcium, phosphate.

AVAILABILITY (Rx)

Injection Solution: 4 mg/5 mL vial, 4 mg/100 mL single-use ready-to-use bottle. 5 mg diluted in 100 mL ready-to-infuse solution.

ADMINISTRATION/HANDLING

◀**ALERT**▶ Pt should be adequately rehydrated before administration of zoledronic acid.

IV (Zometa)

Reconstitution • Further dilute Zometa with 100 mL 0.9% NaCl or D₅W.
Rate of Administration • Adequate hydration is essential in conjunction with zoledronic acid. • Administer as IV infusion over not less than 15 min (increases risk of deterioration in renal function).

Storage • Store intact vials at room temperature. • Infusion of solution must be completed within 24 hrs.

IV (Reclast)

• Administer as IV infusion over not less than 15 min. • Follow infusion with a 10-mL 0.9% NaCl flush of IV line.

▨ IV INCOMPATIBILITIES

Do not mix with other medications.

INDICATIONS/ROUTES/DOSAGE

Hypercalcemia Malignancy (Zometa)
IV Infusion: ADULTS, ELDERLY: 4 mg IV infusion given over no less than 15 min. Retreatment may be considered, but at least 7 days should elapse to allow for full response to initial dose.

Multiple Myeloma, Osteolytic Lesions, Bone Metastases from Solid Tumors (Zometa)
IV: ADULTS, ELDERLY: 4 mg q3–4wks.

Paget's Disease (Reclast)
IV: ADULTS, ELDERLY: 5 mg as a single dose. Data about retreatment not available (seldom required within 5 yrs).

Osteoporosis Treatment (Reclast)
IV: ADULTS, ELDERLY: 5 mg once yearly. Consider discontinuing after 3–5 yrs in pts with low risk of fractures.

Treatment/Prevention of Glucocorticoid-Induced Osteoporosis (Reclast)
IV: ADULTS, ELDERLY: 5 mg once yearly.

Prevention of Postmenopausal Osteoporosis (Reclast)
IV: ADULTS, ELDERLY: 5 mg once q2yrs.

Dosage in Renal Impairment
(Reclast): CrCl less than 35 mL/min: Contraindicated.
(Zometa): (Multiple Myeloma, Metastatic Bone Lesions of Solid Tumors)

Creatinine Clearance	Dosage
50–60 mL/min	3.5 mg
40–49 mL/min	3.3 mg
30–39 mL/min	3 mg
Less than 30 mL/min	Not recommended

Z

(Zometa): (Hypercalcemia of Malignancy)
Mild to moderate impairment: No adjustment. **Severe impairment: (SCr greater than 4.5 mg/dL):** Use caution only after considering risk versus benefit.

Dosage in Hepatic Impairment
No dose adjustment.

SIDE EFFECTS

Frequent (44%–26%): Fever, nausea, vomiting, constipation. **Occasional (15%–10%):** Hypotension, anxiety, insomnia, flu-like symptoms (fever, chills, bone pain, myalgia, arthralgia). **Rare:** Conjunctivitis.

ADVERSE EFFECTS/ TOXIC REACTIONS

Renal toxicity may occur if IV infusion is administered in less than 15 min.

NURSING CONSIDERATIONS

BASELINE ASSESSMENT

Prior to initiation, obtain dental exam for pts at risk for osteonecrosis. Establish baseline serum electrolytes, renal function test.

INTERVENTION/EVALUATION

Monitor serum renal function, CBC. Assess vertebral bone mass (document stabilization, improvement). Monitor serum calcium, phosphate, magnesium, creatinine levels. Assess for fever. Monitor food intake, daily pattern of bowel activity, stool consistency. Check I&O, serum BUN, creatinine in pts with renal impairment.

ZOLMitriptan

zole-mi-**trip**-tan
(<u>Zomig</u>, Zomig Rapimelt ,
Zomig-ZMT)
Do not confuse ZOLMitriptan with almotriptan, rizatriptan or sumatriptan.

◆CLASSIFICATION

PHARMACOTHERAPEUTIC: Serotonin 5-HT$_1$ receptor agonist. **CLINICAL:** Antimigraine.

USES

Oral: Treatment of acute migraine attack with or without aura in adults. **Nasal:** Treatment of acute migraine with or without aura in adults and children 12 yrs and older. **OFF-LABEL:** Short-term prevention of menstrual migraines.

PRECAUTIONS

Contraindications: Hypersensitivity to ZOLMitriptan. Arrhythmias associated with conduction disorders (e.g., Wolff-Parkinson-White syndrome), basilar or hemiplegic migraine, coronary artery disease, ischemic heart disease (including angina pectoris, history of MI, silent ischemia, Prinzmetal's angina), uncontrolled hypertension, use within 24 hrs of ergotamine-containing preparations or another serotonin receptor agonist, MAOI used within 14 days. **Additional for nasal spray:** Cerebrovascular syndromes (e.g., stroke), peripheral vascular disease. **Cautions:** Hepatic impairment, pt profile suggesting cardiovascular risks (e.g., hypertension, hypercholesterolemia, smoker, obesity, diabetes), elderly.

ACTION

Binds selectively to serotonin receptors, producing vasoconstrictive effect on cranial blood vessels. **Therapeutic Effect:** Relieves migraine headache.

PHARMACOKINETICS

Well absorbed after PO administration. Protein binding: 25%. Metabolized in liver. Excreted in urine (60%), feces (30%). **Half-life:** 2.8–3.7 hrs.

⧗ LIFESPAN CONSIDERATIONS

Pregnancy/Lactation: Unknown if drug is distributed in breast milk. **Children:** Safety and efficacy not established

Z

---

in pts younger than 12 yrs. **Elderly:** No age-related precautions noted.

INTERACTIONS

DRUG: Ergotamine-containing medications may produce vasospastic reaction. **FLUoxetine, fluvoxaMINE, PARoxetine, sertraline** may produce hyperreflexia, incoordination, weakness. **MAOIs (e.g., phenelzine, selegiline)** may dramatically increase concentration. **HERBAL:** None significant. **FOOD:** None known. **LAB VALUES:** None significant.

AVAILABILITY (Rx)

Nasal Spray (Zomig): 2.5 mg, 5 mg.
Tablets: 2.5 mg, 5 mg.

🖝 **Tablets (Orally Disintegrating [Zomig-ZMT]):** 2.5 mg, 5 mg.

ADMINISTRATION/HANDLING

PO
• Give without regard to food. Tablets may be broken.

Orally Disintegrating Tablet (ODT)
• Give whole; do not break, crush, cut. • Place on pt's tongue; allow to dissolve. • Not necessary to administer with liquid.

Nasal
• Instruct pt to clear nasal passages as much as possible before use. • With head upright, pt should close one nostril with index finger, breathe out gently through mouth. • Instruct pt to insert nozzle into open nostril about ½ inch, close mouth, and while taking a breath through nose, release spray dosage by firmly pressing plunger. • Have pt remove nozzle from nose, gently breathe in through nose and out through mouth for 15–20 sec. Tell pt to avoid breathing in deeply.

INDICATIONS/ROUTES/DOSAGE

Acute Migraine Attack
PO: ADULTS, ELDERLY, CHILDREN OLDER THAN 18 YRS: Initially, 1.25–2.5 mg (**maximum:** 5 mg). If headache returns, may repeat dose after 2 hrs. **Maximum:** 10 mg/24 hrs.

Orally Disintegrating Tablet: ADULTS, ELDERLY: Initially, 2.5 mg (**maximum:** 5 mg) at onset of migraine headache. If headache returns, may repeat dose after 2 hrs. **Maximum:** 10 mg/24 hrs.

Intranasal: ADULTS, ELDERLY, CHILDREN 12 YRS AND OLDER: Initially, 2.5 mg (**maximum:** 5 mg). If headache returns, may repeat dose after 2 hrs. **Maximum:** 10 mg/24 hrs.

Dosage in Renal Impairment
No dose adjustment.

Dosage in Hepatic Impairment
Nasal/ODT: Mild impairment: No dose adjustment. **Moderate to severe impairment:** Not recommended. **Tablet: Mild:** No dose adjustment. **Moderate to severe impairment:** Initially, 1.25 mg. (**Maximum daily dose:** 5 mg in severe impairment.)

SIDE EFFECTS

Frequent (8%–6%): PO: Dizziness, paresthesia, neck/throat/jaw pressure, drowsiness. **Nasal:** Altered taste, paresthesia. **Occasional (5%–3%): PO:** Warm/hot sensation, asthenia, chest pressure. **Nasal:** Nausea, drowsiness, nasal discomfort, dizziness, asthenia, dry mouth. **Rare (2%–1%):** Diaphoresis, myalgia.

ADVERSE EFFECTS/ TOXIC REACTIONS

Cardiac events (ischemia, coronary artery vasospasm, MI), noncardiac vasospasm-related reactions (hemorrhage, stroke) occur rarely, particularly in pts with hypertension, diabetes, strong family history of coronary artery disease; pts who are obese; smokers; males older than 40 yrs; postmenopausal women.

NURSING CONSIDERATIONS

BASELINE ASSESSMENT
Question for history of peripheral vascular disease, coronary artery disease,

Z

renal/hepatic impairment, MAOI use. Question pt regarding onset, location, duration of migraine, possible precipitating factors.

INTERVENTION/EVALUATION

Monitor for evidence of dizziness. Monitor B/P, esp. in pts with hepatic impairment. Assess for relief of migraine headache, migraine potential for photophobia, phonophobia (sound sensitivity, light sensitivity, nausea, vomiting).

PATIENT/FAMILY TEACHING

• Take single dose as soon as symptoms of actual migraine attack appear. • Medication is intended to relieve migraine, not to prevent or reduce number of attacks. • Lie down in dark, quiet room for additional benefit after taking medication. • Avoid tasks that require alertness, motor skills until response to drug is established. • Report chest pain; palpitations; tightness in throat; edema of face, lips, eyes; rash; easy bruising; blood in urine or stool; pain or numbness in arms or legs.

zolpidem

zole-**pi**-dem
(Ambien, Ambien CR, Edluar, Intermezzo, Sublinox ♣, Zolpimist)
Do not confuse Ambien with ativan, or zolpidem with zaleplon.

◆CLASSIFICATION

PHARMACOTHERAPEUTIC: Hypnotic, miscellaneous (Schedule IV). **CLINICAL:** Sedative-hypnotic.

USES

Ambien, Edluar, Zolpimist: Short-term treatment of insomnia (with difficulty of sleep onset). **Ambien CR:** Treatment of insomnia (with difficulty of sleep onset and/or sleep maintenance).

Intermezzo: Treatment of insomnia characterized by middle-of-the-night awakening followed by difficulty returning to sleep in pts with 4 or more hrs of sleep time remaining.

PRECAUTIONS

Contraindications: Hypersensitivity to zolpidem. **Cautions:** Hepatic impairment, pts with depression, history of drug dependence, sleep apnea, COPD, respiratory disease, myasthenia gravis, debilitated pts, elderly.

ACTION

Enhances action of inhibitory neurotransmitter gamma-aminobutyric acid (GABA). **Therapeutic Effect:** Induces sleep with fewer nightly awakenings, improves sleep quality.

PHARMACOKINETICS

Route	Onset	Peak	Duration
PO	30 min	N/A	6–8 hrs

Rapidly absorbed from GI tract. Protein binding: 92%. Metabolized in liver; excreted in urine. Not removed by hemodialysis. **Half-life:** 1.4–4.5 hrs (increased in hepatic impairment).

⧗ LIFESPAN CONSIDERATIONS

Pregnancy/Lactation: Drug crosses placenta and is distributed in breast milk. **Children:** Safety and efficacy not established. **Elderly:** More likely to experience falls or confusion; decreased initial doses recommended. Age-related hepatic impairment may require dosage adjustment.

INTERACTIONS

DRUG: Alcohol, other CNS depressants (e.g., gabapentin, LORazepam, morphine) may increase CNS depression. **HERBAL: Gotu kola, kava kava, valerian** may increase CNS depression. **St. John's wort** may decrease concentration/effect. **FOOD:** None known. **LAB VALUES:** None significant.

Z

AVAILABILITY (Rx)

Oral Solution (Zolpimist): 5 mg/actuation. **Tablets:** 5 mg, 10 mg. **Tablets (Sublingual [Edluar]):** 5 mg, 10 mg. **(Intermezzo):** 1.75 mg, 3.5 mg.

Tablets (Extended-Release): 6.25 mg, 12.5 mg.

ADMINISTRATION/HANDLING

PO
• For faster sleep onset, do not give with or immediately after a meal. • Do not break, crush, dissolve, or divide Ambien CR tablets; give whole. • Edluar sublingual tablets to be placed under tongue and allowed to disintegrate. Do not swallow or administer with water. • Spray Zolpimist directly into mouth over tongue.

INDICATIONS/ROUTES/DOSAGE

Note: Dosage adjustment is recommended for female pts.

Insomnia
PO, Spray, Sublingual: *(Edluar, Zolpimist):* **ADULTS:** (males) 10 mg, (females) 5 mg immediately before bedtime. **ELDERLY, DEBILITATED:** 5 mg immediately before bedtime.
(Intermezzo): **ADULTS, ELDERLY:** (males) 3.5 mg, (females) 1.75 mg, taken once in middle of night with 4 or more hrs of expected sleep yet to come.
PO: *(Extended-Release):* **ADULTS:** (males) 6.25–12.5 mg, (females) 6.25 mg immediately before bedtime. **ELDERLY, DEBILITATED:** 6.25 mg immediately before bedtime.

Dosage in Renal Impairment
No dose adjustment; use caution.

Dosage in Hepatic Impairment
Mild to moderate impairment: *(Immediate-Release Tablet, Spray, Sublingual Tablet):* 5 mg. *(Extended-Release Tablet):* 6.25 mg. *(Intermezzo):* 1.75 mg. **Severe impairment:** Avoid use.

SIDE EFFECTS

Occasional (7%): Headache, change in appetite. **Rare (less than 2%):** Dizziness, nausea, diarrhea, muscle pain, sleepwalking.

ADVERSE EFFECTS/ TOXIC REACTIONS

Overdose may produce severe ataxia (clumsiness, unsteadiness), bradycardia, diplopia, severe drowsiness, nausea, vomiting, difficulty breathing, unconsciousness. Abrupt withdrawal following long-term use may produce weakness, facial flushing, diaphoresis, vomiting, tremor. Drug tolerance/dependence may occur with prolonged use of high dosages. May cause amnesic events that include cooking, sleepwalking, sexual activity, driving.

NURSING CONSIDERATIONS

BASELINE ASSESSMENT

Assess B/P, pulse, respirations, mental status, sleep patterns. Raise bed rails, provide call light. Provide environment conducive to sleep (back rub, quiet environment, low lighting). Do not give unless a full night of sleep is planned.

INTERVENTION/EVALUATION

Monitor sleep pattern of pt. Evaluate for therapeutic response to insomnia: decrease in number of nocturnal awakenings, increase in length of sleep. Monitor daytime alertness, respiratory rate, behavior profile.

PATIENT/FAMILY TEACHING

• Do not abruptly discontinue medication after long-term use. • Avoid alcohol and tasks that require alertness, motor skills until response to drug is established. • Tolerance, dependence may occur with prolonged use of high dosages. • Do not break, chew, crush, dissolve, or divide Ambien CR tablets; swallow whole. • Therapy may need to be discontinued if cooking, driving, sleepwalking occurs without recollection. • Do not take unless a full 8 hrs of sleep is planned.

Z

---

zonisamide

zoe-**nis**-a-mide
(Zonegran)
Do not confuse Zonegran with SINEquan, or zonisamide with lacosamide.

◆CLASSIFICATION

PHARMACOTHERAPEUTIC: Anticonvulsant, miscellaneous. **CLINICAL:** Anticonvulsant.

USES

Adjunctive therapy in treatment of partial seizures in adults, children older than 16 yrs with epilepsy. **OFF-LABEL:** Bipolar disorder.

PRECAUTIONS

Contraindications: Hypersensitivity to zonisamide. Allergy to sulfonamides. **Cautions:** Renal/hepatic impairment, pts at high risk for suicide or metabolic acidosis (e.g., severe respiratory disease).

ACTION

Exact mechanism unknown. May stabilize neuronal membranes, suppress neuronal hypersynchronization by blocking sodium, calcium channels. **Therapeutic Effect:** Reduces seizure activity.

PHARMACOKINETICS

Well absorbed after PO administration. Metabolized in liver. Extensively bound to RBCs. Protein binding: 40%. Primarily excreted in urine. **Half-life:** 63 hrs (plasma), 105 hrs (RBCs).

⧖ LIFESPAN CONSIDERATIONS

Pregnancy/Lactation: Crosses placenta. Unknown if distributed in breast milk. **Children:** Safety and efficacy not established in pts younger than 16 yrs. **Elderly:** No age-related precautions noted, but lower dosages recommended.

INTERACTIONS

DRUG: Alcohol, other CNS depressants (e.g., LORazepam, morphine, zolpidem) may increase sedative effect. **CYP3A4 inducers** (e.g., carBAMazepine, PHENobarbital, phenytoin, valproic acid) may increase metabolism, decrease effect. **HERBAL:** None significant. **FOOD:** None known. **LAB VALUES:** May increase serum BUN, creatinine.

AVAILABILITY (Rx)

🖐 **Capsules:** 25 mg, 50 mg, 100 mg.

ADMINISTRATION/HANDLING

PO
• May give with or without food. • Do not crush, break capsules. Give capsules whole. • Do not give to pts allergic to sulfonamides.

INDICATIONS/ROUTES/DOSAGE

Note: Do not use if CrCl is less than 50 mL/min.

Partial Seizures
PO: ADULTS, ELDERLY, CHILDREN OLDER THAN 16 YRS: Initially, 100 mg/day. May increase to 200 mg/day after 2 wks. Further increases to 300 mg/day and 400 mg/day can be made with minimum of 2 wks between adjustments. Range: 100–600 mg/day.

Dosage in Renal Impairment
Not recommended with CrCl less than 50 mL/min.

Dosage in Hepatic Impairment
Use with caution.

SIDE EFFECTS

Frequent (17%–9%): Drowsiness, dizziness, anorexia, headache, agitation, irritability, nausea. **Occasional (8%–5%):** Fatigue, ataxia, confusion, depression, impaired memory/concentration, insomnia, abdominal pain, diplopia, diarrhea, speech difficulty. **Rare (4%–3%):** Paresthesia, nystagmus, anxiety, rash, dyspepsia, weight loss.

Z

ADVERSE EFFECTS/ TOXIC REACTIONS

Overdose characterized by bradycardia, hypotension, respiratory depression, coma. Leukopenia, anemia, thrombocytopenia occur rarely.

NURSING CONSIDERATIONS

BASELINE ASSESSMENT

Review history of seizure disorder (intensity, frequency, duration, level of consciousness). Initiate seizure precautions. CBC, LFT should be performed before therapy begins and periodically during therapy.

INTERVENTION/EVALUATION

Observe frequently for recurrence of seizure activity. Assess for clinical improvement (decrease in intensity, frequency of seizures). Assist with ambulation if dizziness occurs.

PATIENT/FAMILY TEACHING

• Strict maintenance of drug therapy is essential for seizure control. • Avoid tasks that require alertness, motor skills until response to drug is established. • Avoid alcohol. • Report if rash, back/ abdominal pain, blood in urine, fever, sore throat, ulcers in mouth, easy bruising occur. • Report worsening depression, unusual behavior, suicidal ideation.

Z

CALCULATION OF DOSES

Frequently, dosages ordered do not correspond exactly to what is available and must be calculated.

RATIO/PROPORTION:

A pt is to receive 65 mg of a medication. It is available as 80 mg/2 mL. What volume (mL) needs to be administered to the patient?

STEP 1: Set up ratio.

$$\frac{80 \text{ mg}}{2 \text{ mL}} = \frac{65 \text{ mg}}{x \ (\text{mL})}$$

STEP 2: Cross multiply and divide each side by the number with x to determine volume to be administered.

$$80 \text{ mg} \times (x) \text{ mL} = 65 \text{ mg} \times 2 \text{ mL}$$
$$80 \, x = 130$$
$$x = \frac{130}{80} = 1.625 \text{ mL}$$

CALCULATIONS IN MICROGRAMS PER KILOGRAM PER MINUTE (mcg/kg/min):

A 63-year-old pt (weight 165 lb) is to receive medication A at a rate of 8 mcg/kg/min. Given a solution containing medication A in a concentration of 500 mg/250 mL, at what rate (mL/hr) would you infuse this medication?

STEP 1: Convert to same units. In this problem, the dose is expressed in mcg/kg; therefore, convert weight to kg (2.2 lb = 1 kg) and drug concentration to mcg/mL (1 mg = 1,000 mcg).

$$165 \text{ lb divided by } 2.2 = 75 \text{ kg}$$

$$\frac{500 \text{ mg}}{250 \text{ mL}} = \frac{2 \text{ mg}}{\text{mL}} = \frac{2,000 \text{ mcg}}{\text{mL}}$$

STEP 2: Number of mcg/hr.

$$(75 \text{ kg}) \times 8 \text{ mcg/kg/min} = 600 \text{ mcg/min or } 36,000 \text{ mcg/hr}$$

STEP 3: Number of mL/hr.

$$36,000 \text{ mcg/hr divided by } 2,000 \text{ mcg/mL} = 18 \text{ mL/hr}$$

CONTROLLED DRUGS (UNITED STATES)

Schedule I: Medications having no legal medical use. These substances may be used for research purposes with proper registration (e.g., heroin, LSD).

Schedule II: Medications having a legitimate medical use but are characterized by a very high abuse potential and/or potential for severe physical and psychic dependency. Emergency telephone orders for limited quantities of these drugs are authorized, but the prescriber must provide a written, signed prescription order (e.g., morphine, amphetamines, hydrocodone, oxycodone).

Schedule III: Medications having significant abuse potential (less than Schedule II). Telephone orders are permitted (e.g., codeine in combination with other substances such as butalbital).

Schedule IV: Medications having a low abuse potential. Telephone orders are permitted (e.g., benzodiazepines, tramadol, zolpidem).

Schedule V: Medications having the lowest abuse potential of the controlled substances. Some Schedule V products may be available without a prescription (e.g., certain cough preparations containing limited amounts of an opiate).

WOUND CARE

A wound is any process that disrupts the normal structure and function of tissues. Wounds can be closed (e.g., bruise, sprain) or open (e.g., abrasion, surgical wound). The most common chronic wounds are nonhealing surgical wounds, pressure ulcers, diabetic foot ulcers, and venous ulcers.

TYPES OF OPEN WOUNDS

Superficial	Damage only to the epithelium; heals rapidly via regeneration of epithelial cells.
Partial thickness	Involves the dermal layer and is associated with blood vessel damage.
Full thickness	Involves subcutaneous fat and deeper layers (e.g., muscle, bone).
	Requires the longest time to heal.
	Connective tissue needs to regenerate; contraction occurs during the healing process.

WOUND HEALING

Wound healing is a complex process resulting in restored cell structure and tissue layers after an injury. When skin is damaged, it begins to heal from the bottom layer up and from the outside inward. Wound healing involves cellular, physiologic, biochemical, and molecular processes. They are interdependent and overlapping. An acute wound usually heals within several wks, whereas chronic wounds take 6 wks or longer to heal. Additionally, other factors can delay the healing process. These include trauma/edema, infection, necrosis, lack of oxygen delivery to the tissues, advanced age, obesity, chronic diseases (e.g., diabetes, anemia), vascular insufficiency, immobility, pressure necrosis, and immunodeficiency.

Wound healing can be divided into three phases: inflammation, proliferation, and maturation.

Inflammation	Occurs within seconds of the injury and can last up to 3 days.
	Associated with redness, heat, swelling, and pain.
	Immediate vasoconstriction of damaged blood vessels and coagulation limiting blood loss occurs.
	Following vasoconstriction, histamine and other chemical mediators are released from damaged cells, causing vasodilation and release of growth factors essential for wound healing (e.g., increased capillary permeability and release of exudate).
Proliferation	Granulation tissue composed of macrophages, fibroblasts, immature collagen, blood vessels, and ground substance is formed.
	Fibroblasts stimulate production of collagen and elastin, increasing the strength of the wound and stimulating growth of new blood vessels.
	As granulation fills the wound site, the edges of the wound pull together, decreasing the surface of the wound.

	Epithelialization then occurs: Epithelial cells migrate from the wound edge, covering the wound and resulting in scar formation.
	This phase usually lasts 2 to 3 wks.
Maturation	Collagen fibers cross link and reorganize, increasing the strength of scar. This process can take anywhere from 3 wks to 2 yrs.

WOUND DRESSINGS

Dressings play a major role in wound management. They protect the wound, keeping it moist, and thus promote healing (only diabetic, dry, gangrenous toes require a moisture-free environment for effective healing).

Hydrocolloid, hydrogel, film, and foam dressing can handle large amounts of exudate and promote auto-debridement. Alginate and collagen-based dressings promote granulation of tissue. Silver and iodine dressings are used to avoid infections, which may delay wound healing.

WOUND CARE PRODUCTS

Description	General Uses	Comments
Alginate dressings: Spun fibers of brown seaweed that act as ion exchange mechanisms to absorb serous fluid or exudate, forming a gel-like covering that conforms to the shape of the wound. Facilitate autolytic debridement and maintain a moist wound environment. **Products:** Algicell, Carra Sorb. Available as ropes, pads.	Abrasions/ lacerations/skin tears Arterial/venous ulcers Deep and tunneling wounds Diabetic ulcers Pressure ulcers Second-degree burns Odorous wounds Contaminated and infected wounds	Good for moderately to heavily exudative wounds and hemorrhagic wounds Can be left in place until soaked with exudate Requires a secondary dressing (e.g., transparent film, foam, hydrocolloids) Do not moisten prior to use Nonadhesive, nonocclusive Contraindicated in third-degree burns; not recommended for dry or minimally exudative wounds
Collagenase ointment: Sterile enzymatic de-briding ointment that possesses the ability to digest collagen in necrotic tissue. **Products:** Santyl.	Debriding chronic dermal ulcers and severely burned areas	Can be used for infected wounds Gauze is used as a secondary dressing Discontinue when granulation tissue is present Optimal pH for enzymatic action is 6-8 Avoid acidic agents for cleansing; avoid detergents and agents containing heavy metal (e.g., mercury or silver), which may adversely affect enzymatic activity

Description	General Uses	Comments
Trypsin, castor oil, Peru balsam: Trypsin is a mild debriding agent that helps shed damaged skin cells. **Castor oil** acts as a lubricant to protect tissue. **Peru balsam** increases blood flow to a wound area, reduces wound odor. **Products:** Granulex, Xenaderm. Available as gel, ointment, spray.	Promotes healing/ treatment of decubitus ulcers, varicose ulcer, and dehiscent wounds	Can be used for infected wounds Avoid concurrent use of silver-containing products (may reduce efficacy) Promotes healing and relieves pain caused by bed sores and other skin ulcers
Hydrophilic polyurethane foam: Also called open cell foam dressings. Sheets of foamed solutions of polymers containing variably sized open cells that can hold wound exudate away from wound bed. Maintains moist wound environment. **Products:** Curafoam, Lyofoam. Available as sheets in a wide variety of formulations.	Moderate to heavy exudative wounds with or without a clean granular wound bed Diabetic ulcers, pressure ulcers, venous stasis ulcers Draining surgical incisions Superficial burns Tube and drain sites	Contraindicated for use in third-degree burns Not recommended for wounds with little to no exudate or when tunneling is present Good for cavitating wounds Highly absorbent, semiocclusive dressing Usual dressing change is up to 3 times/wk Can be worn during bathing
Hydrocolloids: Formulations of elastomeric, adhesive, and gelling agents; the most common absorbent ingredient is carboxymethylcellulose. Most hydrocolloids are backed with a semiocclusive film layer. The wound side of the dressing is adhesive, adhering to a moist surface as well as to dry skin but not to the moist wound bed. As wound fluid is absorbed, the hydrocolloid forms a viscous gel in the wound bed, enhancing a moist wound environment. **Products:** Hydrocol, Tegasorb. Available as dressings, granules, patches, paste.	Minimal to moderate exudate in partial and full thickness wounds Cuts and abrasions First- and second-degree burns Pressure ulcers Stasis ulcers	Not for wounds producing heavy exudate, infected wounds, dry escharcovered wounds May provide pain relief Good for chronic wounds that are epithelializing Can be left in place for up to 7 days Contraindicated for third-degree burns Can shower while wearing

Continued

Description	General Uses	Comments
Hydrogels: Glycerin- or water-based dressings designed to hydrate the wound. May absorb small amounts of exudate. **Products:** Curacel, Duo Derm, Intra Site. Available as gel, sheets, gauze.	Partial and full thickness wounds Dry to minimal exudate Cuts and abrasions First- and second-degree burns Pressure ulcers Stasis ulcers	Not for wounds producing moderate to heavy exudate Not for infected wounds May provide pain relief Good for wounds that are debriding Good for keeping a dry wound moist Can be left in place for 1-3 days
Iodine compounds: Cadexomer iodine: Iodine is complexed with a polymeric cadexomer starch vehicle, forming a topical gel or paste. The cadexomer moiety absorbs exudate and debris and releases iodine for antimicrobial activity. **Products:** Iodosorb, Iodoflex. Available as gel, dressing, ointment, powder.	Chronic nonhealing, exuding wounds including pressure or leg ulcers and exuding, infected wounds	Requires use of a secondary dressing Contraindicated in pts with iodine sensitivity, Hashimoto's thyroiditis, nontoxic nodular goiter, children Dressing to be changed when it turns white, indicating that the iodine has been depleted Do not use on dry necrotic tissue
Silver compounds Silver sulfadiazine cream: Silver possesses bactericidal properties. Has been shown to reduce bacterial density, vascular margination, migration of inflammatory cells. Enhances rate of re-epithelialization. **Products:** Silvadene, SSD, Thermazene.	Prevent infection in second- and third-degree burns Prevent or treat infection in chronic wounds	May have cytotoxic effects that could delay wound healing Allergic reactions may occur Use should be limited to a 2- to 4-wk period Bacteria may become resistant with prolonged use Avoid use with collagenase- or trypsin-containing debriding agents
Transparent film dressings: Polyurethane sheets coated on one side with an adhesive that is inactivated by moisture and will not adhere to a moist surface such as the wound bed. Have no absorbent capacity and are impermeable to fluids and bacteria but are semipermeable to oxygen and water vapor. **Products:** Bioclusive, CarraFilm, Tegaderm HP. Available in a variety of sizes and features.	Prophylaxis on high-risk intact skin Superficial wounds with minimal or no exudate Wounds on elbows, heels, or flat surfaces; covering of blisters; and retention of primary dressing	Prevents wound desiccation and contamination by bacteria Contraindicated in third-degree burns Promotes autolysis of necrotic tissue in the wound; maintains moist environment Avoid in arterial ulcers and infected wounds requiring frequent monitoring Do not use as primary dressing on wounds with depth or tunneling May provide pain relief Usually changed up to 3 times/wk

Description	General Uses	Comments
Becaplermin gel: Recombinant formulation of platelet-derived growth factor that promotes cell mitogenesis and proliferation of cells involved in wound repair. Enhances formation of granulation tissue. **Products:** Regranex.	Diabetic foot ulcers that extend into subcutaneous tissue or beyond and have an adequate blood supply	Usually applied daily Adequate blood supply and absence of necrotic tissue are needed for efficacy Repeated use (3 or more tubes) may increase risk of cancer-related death Use cautiously in pts with known malignancy

DRUGS OF ABUSE

Substance	Brand/ Street Names	Administered	Effects of Intoxication	Potential Health Consequences
Amphetamine	Adderall, Dexedrine; bennies, black beauties, hearts, speed, truck drivers, uppers	Injection, smoked, snorted	Increased heart rate, blood pressure, body temperature, metabolism; increased energy, mental alertness; tremors; reduced appetite; irritability; anxiety; panic; violent behavior; psychosis	Weight loss, insomnia, cardiac or cardiovascular complications, stroke, seizures, addiction, tremor, irritability
Barbiturates	Nembutal, Seconal, Phenobarbital; barbs, reds, phennies, yellows, yellow jackets	Injection, oral	Reduction of pain and anxiety; feeling of well-being; lowered inhibitions; slowed pulse/ breathing; lowered blood pressure; poor concentration; sedation, drowsiness	Confusion, fatigue; impaired coordination, memory, judgment; respiratory depression or arrest; addiction; depression; unusual excitement; fever; irritability; slurred speech; dizziness
Benzodiazepines	Ativan, Librium, Valium, Xanax; candy, downers, tranks, Xannies, Xannie bars	Oral	Reduction of pain and anxiety; feeling of well-being; lowered inhibitions; slowed pulse/breathing; lowered blood pressure; poor concentration; sedation, drowsiness	Confusion, fatigue; impaired coordination, memory, judgment; respiratory depression or arrest; addiction; dizziness

Substance	Brand/ Street Names	Administered	Effects of Intoxication	Potential Health Consequences
Bupropion	*Wellbutrin;* poor man's cocaine	Oral	Increased heart rate, B/P, and temperature; mental alertness; feel euphoric, exhilarated, energetic	Seizures, tachycardia, arrhythmias, loss of consciousness
Cocaine	Blow, bump, candy, coke, crack, rock, snow, toot	Injection, smoked, snorted	Increased heart rate, blood pressure, body temperature, metabolism; increased energy, mental alertness; tremors; reduced appetite; irritability; anxiety; panic; violent behavior; psychosis	Weight loss, insomnia, cardiac or cardiovascular complications, stroke, seizures, addiction, nasal damage from snorting, rapid or irregular heartbeat, headaches, malnutrition
Codeine	*Fiorinal with codeine, Tylenol with codeine;* Captain Cody, schoolboy, loads, pancakes and syrup	Injection, oral	Pain relief, euphoria, drowsiness	Respiratory depression and arrest, nausea, confusion, constipation, sedation, unconsciousness, coma, tolerance, addiction
Dextromethorphan	Found in some cough and cold medications; poor man's PCP, velvet, Robo, Triple C	Oral	Impaired motor function, feeling of being separated from one's body and environment; euphoria; slurred speech; confusion; dizziness; distorted visual perceptions	

Continued

Substance	Brand/ Street Names	Administered	Effects of Intoxication	Potential Health Consequences
Flunitraze-pam	*Rohypnol;* for- get-me pill, Mexican Valium, roofies, roofinol, rope, rophies	Oral, snorted	Sedation, muscle relaxation, confusion, memory loss, dizziness, impaired coordination, reduced pain/anxiety, feeling of well-being	Addiction; confusion, fatigue, memory loss, respiratory depression
Gabapentin	*Neurontin, Lyrica, Lycia; gabbie*	Oral	Self-treatment of alcohol, cocaine, or opioid craving; euphoria, relaxation	Diarrhea, double vision, drowsiness, lethargic, slurred speech
GHB	Georgia home boy, grievous bodily harm, liquid ecstasy, goop, liquid X	Oral	Drowsiness, nausea, headache, disorientation, loss of coordination, memory loss	Unconsciousness, seizures, coma, confusion, nausea, vomiting, headache
Heroin	Smack, brown sugar, dope, junk, white horse, China white	Injection, smoked, snorted	Euphoria, drowsiness, impaired coordination, dizziness, confusion, nausea, sedation, feeling of heaviness in the body, slowed breathing	Constipation, confusion, sedation, respiratory depression, coma, addiction
Hydroco-done	*Vicodin, Lortab;* vike, watson-387	Oral	Pain relief, euphoria, drowsiness	Respiratory depression and arrest, nausea, confusion, constipation, sedation, unconsciousness, coma, tolerance, addiction

Substance	Brand/Street Names	Administered	Effects of Intoxication	Potential Health Consequences
Inhalants	Solvents (paint thinner, glues), nitrites (laughing gas, snappers, poppers)	Inhaled through nose or mouth	Stimulation, loss of inhibition, headache, nausea or vomiting, slurred speech, loss of motor coordination, wheezing	Cramps, muscle weakness, depression, memory impairment, damage to cardiovascular and nervous systems, unconsciousness, sudden death
Ketamine	*Ketalar;* cat Valium, Special K, kit kat, vitamin K	Injection, snorted, smoked	Increased heart rate and blood pressure, impaired motor function, feelings of being separated from one's body and environment; at high doses: delirium, depression, respiratory depression or arrest; death	Memory loss, numbness, nausea/vomiting, anxiety, tremors, respiratory depression
Loperamide	*Imodium;* poor man's methadone	Oral	Reducing symptoms of opioid withdrawal	CNS depression, intestinal blockage
LSD	Acid, cubes, microdot, yellow sunshine, blotter, bloomers	Oral, absorbed through mouth tissues	Altered states of perception and feeling; hallucinations; nausea; increased body temperature, heart rate, blood pressure; loss of appetite; sweating; sleeplessness; numbness; dizziness; weakness; tremors; impulsive behavior; rapid shifts in emotion	Flashbacks, hallucinogen persisting perception disorder

Continued

Substance	Brand/ Street Names	Administered	Effects of Intoxication	Potential Health Consequences
Marijuana	Blunt, ganja, grass, joint, Mary Jane, pot, reefer, sinsemilla, skunk, weed	Oral, smoked	Euphoria, relaxation, slowed reaction time, impaired balance and coordination, increased heart rate and appetite, impaired learning and memory, anxiety, panic attacks, psychosis	Cough, impaired memory and learning, anxiety, panic attacks, frequent respiratory infections, possible mental health decline, addiction
MDMA	Ecstasy, Adam, clarity, Eve, lover's speed, peace, Molly	Injection, oral, snorted	Mild hallucinogenic effects, increased tactile sensitivity, empathic feelings, lowered inhibition, anxiety, chills, sweating, teeth clenching, muscle cramping	Reduced appetite, irregular heartbeat, heart failure, impaired memory, hyperthermia, addiction
Mescaline	Buttons, cactus, peyote	Oral, smoked	Altered states of perception and feeling; hallucinations; nausea; increased body temperature, heart rate, blood pressure; loss of appetite; sweating; sleeplessness; numbness; dizziness; weakness; tremors; impulsive behavior; rapid shifts in emotion	Loss of appetite, nausea, weakness, chronic mental disorders

Substance	Brand/ Street Names	Administered	Effects of Intoxication	Potential Health Consequences
Metham-phetamine	*Desoxyn*; meth, ice, crank, crystal, go fast, speed	Oral, injection, smoked, snorted	Increased heart rate, blood pressure, body temperature, metabolism; increased energy, mental alertness; tremors; reduced appetite; irritability; anxiety; panic; violent behavior; psychosis	Weight loss, insomnia, cardiac or cardiovascular complications, stroke, seizures, addiction, severe dental problems, behavior/memory loss, impaired memory and learning, tolerance, addiction
Methylphe-nidate	*Ritalin*; JIF, MPH, Skippy, smart drug, vitamin R	Injection, oral, snorted	Increase or decrease in blood pressure; psychotic episodes	Digestive problems, loss of appetite, weight loss, reduced appetite, rapid irregular heartbeat, heart failure, seizures, stroke
Morphine	*Roxanol, Dura-morph*; M, Miss Emma, monkey, white stuff	Injection, oral, smoked	Pain relief, euphoria, drowsiness	Respiratory depression and arrest, nausea, confusion, constipation, sedation, unconsciousness, coma, tolerance, addiction
Oxycodone	*OxyContin, Percodan*; oxy-cotton, oxycet, hillbilly heroin, killers, OCs	Injection, oral	Pain relief, euphoria, drowsiness	Respiratory depression and arrest, nausea, confusion, constipation, sedation, unconsciousness, coma, tolerance, addiction

Continued

Substance	Brand/ Street Names	Administered	Effects of Intoxication	Potential Health Consequences
PCP	*Phencyclidine;* angel dust, boat, hog, love boat, peace pill	Injection, oral, smoked	Impaired motor function, feelings of being separated from one's body and environment, analgesia, psychosis, aggression, violence, slurred speech, loss of coordination, hallucinations	Memory loss, loss of appetite, panic, aggression, violence
Psilocybin	Magic mushrooms, purple passion, shrooms	Oral	Altered states of perception and feeling, hallucinations, nausea, nervousness, paranoia, panic	Chronic mental disorders
Quetiapine	*Seroquel;* baby heroin, Suzie-Q, Q-ball	Oral	Reduced anxiety, sedation	Arrhythmias, coma, death (with overdose)

EQUIANALGESIC DOSING

Guidelines for equianalgesic dosing of commonly used analgesics are presented in the following table. The dosages are approximate to 10 mg of morphine intramuscularly. These guidelines are for the management of acute pain in the opioid-naïve pt. Dosages may vary for the opioid-tolerant pt and for the management of chronic pain. Dosing adjustments for renal or hepatic insufficiency may also be necessary. Clinical response is the criterion that must be applied for each pt with titration to desired response.

Name	Equianalgesic Oral Dose	Equianalgesic Parenteral Dose (IV, IM, SQ)
Codeine	200 mg	100–130 mg
Fentanyl	Not available	0.1 mg (100 mcg)
Hydrocodone	30–45 mg	Not available
Hydromorphone (Dilaudid)	7.5–8 mg	1.5–2 mg
Hydromorphone (Dilaudid) (Controlled-Release)	7.5 mg	N/A
Meperidine (Demerol)	300 mg	75 mg
Methadone (Dolophine)	10–20 mg	10 mg
Morphine	30 mg	10 mg
Oxycodone (OxyContin)	20–30 mg	Not available
Oxymorphone	10 mg	1 mg
Oxymorphone (Extended-Release)	10 mg	N/A

HERBALS: COMMON NATURAL MEDICINES

The use of herbal therapies is increasing in the United States. Because of the rise in the use of herbal therapy, the following is presented to provide some basic information on some of the more popular herbs. Please note this is not an all-inclusive list, which is beyond the scope of this handbook.

Name	Uses	Comments
Aloe vera	Orally: osteoarthritis, inflammatory bowel diseases (e.g., ulcerative colitis), fever, itching, inflammation. Topically: burns, wound healing, psoriasis, sunburn, frostbite, cold sores.	Well tolerated. Orally can cause abdominal pain, cramps; topically can cause burning, itching, contact dermatitis. May lower blood glucose levels and have additive effects with antidiabetic medications.
Bilberry	Orally: improve visual acuity (e.g., night vision, cataracts), atherosclerosis, chronic fatigue syndrome, venous insufficiency, varicose veins, hemorrhoids. Topically: mild inflammation of mouth and throat mucous membranes.	Can inhibit platelet aggregation, increase risk of bleeding when combined with antiplatelet or anticoagulant medications (e.g., aspirin, clopidogrel, enoxaparin, warfarin). May lower blood glucose.
Bitter orange	Orally: appetite stimulant, dyspepsia. Topically: inflammation of the eyelid, conjunctiva, retina.	May cause hypertension, cardiovascular toxicity. May increase concentration/effects of midazolam; concurrent use with MAOIs may increase blood pressure (avoid use); combination with caffeine can increase blood pressure, heart rate.
Black cohosh	Orally: symptoms of menopause, premenstrual syndrome (PMS), dysmenorrhea, dyspepsia, inducing labor in pregnant women, anxiety, fever, cough, cardiovascular disease, cognitive function, infertility, osteoarthritis, osteoporosis, rheumatoid arthritis. Topically: acne, mole, and wart removal; improve skin appearance.	Can cause GI upset, rash, headache, dizziness, increased weight, cramping, breast tenderness, vaginal spotting/bleeding. May decrease effects of cisplatin; may increase risk of hepatic damage with hepatotoxic medications.

Name	Uses	Comments
Capsicum (cayenne pepper)	Orally: dyspepsia, flatulence, diarrhea, cramps, toothache, hyperlipidemia. Topically: pain of shingles, osteoarthritis, rheumatoid arthritis, postherpetic neuralgia, diabetic neuralgia, trigeminal neuralgia.	Orally can cause upper abdominal discomfort (e.g., gas, bloating, nausea, diarrhea, belching); topically can cause burning, stinging, erythema. May increase effects/adverse effects of antiplatelet medications.
Chamomile	Prepared as a tea and used as a mild sedative, relaxant, and sleeping aid; used for indigestion, itching, and inflammation.	Large amounts may cause vomiting.
Chastberry	Orally: menstrual irregularities (e.g., dysmenorrhea, amenorrhea, metrorrhagia).	Can cause GI upset, headache, diarrhea, nausea, itching, urticaria, rash, insomnia, increased weight, irregular menstrual bleeding. Can interfere with efficacy of oral contraceptives, hormone replacement therapy.
Clove (clove oil)	Orally: dyspepsia, expectorant, diarrhea, halitosis, flatulence, nausea, vomiting. Topically: toothache, mouth and throat inflammation.	Topically can cause tissue irritation, allergic dermatitis.
Co-enzyme Q-10	Heart failure, angina, diabetes, hypertension.	Can cause GI side effects (e.g., nausea, vomiting, diarrhea, appetite suppression, heartburn, epigastric discomfort). Can decrease blood pressure and have an additive effect with antihypertensive medications; may reduce anticoagulant effects of warfarin.
Cranberry	Prevention/treatment of urinary tract infections, neurogenic bladder, urinary deodorizer in incontinence, kidney stones, prevention of urinary catheter blockage.	Usually well tolerated. Large amounts can cause GI upset, diarrhea, nausea, vomiting. Greater than 1,000 mL daily can increase risk of uric acid, kidney stone formation.
DHEA	Slow or reverse aging, weight loss, metabolic syndrome, increase immune and cognitive function.	At high dose can cause acne, hirsutism, hair loss, voice deepening, insulin resistance, altered menstrual pattern. May interfere with antiestrogen effects of anastrozole, letrozole, or other aromatase inhibitors; may overcome estrogen receptor antagonist activity of tamoxifen in estrogen receptor positive cancer cells.

Continued

Name	Uses	Comments
Dong quai	Dysmenorrhea, premenstrual syndrome, menopausal symptoms.	May cause photosensitivity and photodermatitis. May increase effect/risk of bleeding with antiplatelet and anticoagulant medications (e.g., aspirin, warfarin).
Echinacea	Treat/prevent common cold, influenza, other upper respiratory tract infections.	Usually well tolerated. Can cause GI effects (e.g., nausea, abdominal pain, diarrhea, vomiting). Stimulates immune function—may exacerbate autoimmune diseases (e.g., multiple sclerosis, rheumatoid arthritis, systemic lupus erythematosus).
Eucalyptus	Orally: infections, fever, dyspepsia, expectorant for coughs. Topically: inflammation of respiratory tract mucous membranes, rheumatoid arthritis, nasal stuffiness.	Orally: GI effects (e.g., nausea, vomiting, diarrhea). Topically (prolonged exposure/large amounts): agitation, drowsiness, muscle weakness, ataxia.
Evening primrose oil	Premenstrual syndrome (PMS), endometriosis, symptoms of menopause (e.g., hot flashes).	May increase risk of bruising/bleeding with antiplatelet/anticoagulant medications (e.g., aspirin, clopidogrel, enoxaparin, warfarin).
Feverfew	Orally: fever, headaches, prevention of migraines, menstrual irregularities. Topically: toothaches, antiseptic.	Orally: GI effects (e.g., heartburn, nausea, diarrhea, constipation, abdominal pain, bloating, flatulence). Topically: contact dermatitis. May have additive effects, increase risk of bleeding with antiplatelet medications.
Fish oil	Hyperlipidemia, hypertriglyceridemia, hypertension, stroke, depression, rheumatoid arthritis, osteoporosis, psoriasis, Crohn's disease.	Can cause a fishy aftertaste, halitosis, heartburn, dyspepsia, nausea, loose stools, rash. May have additive effect with antihypertensive medication.
Garlic	Hypertension, hyperlipidemia, age-related vascular changes, atherosclerosis, chronic fatigue syndrome, menstrual disorders, coronary heart disease, peripheral arterial disease.	Dose-related effects including breath/body odor, mouth and GI burning/irritation, heartburn, flatulence, nausea, vomiting, diarrhea. May increase effects of antiplatelets (e.g., aspirin, clopidogrel, enoxaparin), anticoagulants (e.g., warfarin); may decrease effects of oral contraceptives, cyclosporine, protease inhibitors, and non-nucleoside reverse transcriptase inhibitors (NNRTIs).

Name	Uses	Comments
Ginger	Motion sickness, morning sickness, dyspepsia, rheumatoid arthritis, osteoarthritis, loss of appetite, migraine headache, diarrhea, flatulence, irritable bowel syndrome, dysmenorrhea.	Usually well tolerated. At high doses of 5 g/day may cause abdominal discomfort, heartburn, diarrhea, irritant effect in mouth and throat. May increase risk of bleeding with antiplatelet medications and anticoagulants (e.g., aspirin, clopidogrel, enoxaparin, warfarin).
Ginkgo	Dementia (including Alzheimer's), vascular dementia, mixed dementia.	Mild GI upset, headache, dizziness, constipation, palpitations, allergic skin reactions. Large doses can cause diarrhea, nausea, vomiting, weakness. Decreases platelet aggregation; may increase risk of bleeding with antiplatelet and anticoagulants (e.g., aspirin, clopidogrel, enoxaparin, warfarin).
Ginseng	Increases resistance to environmental stress, improves well-being, boosts energy, diuretic.	May cause insomnia, vaginal bleeding, headache, hypertension, hypotension, decreased appetite, edema. May decrease effectiveness of warfarin.
Glucosamine	Osteoarthritis, glaucoma, temporomandibular joint arthritis.	May cause mild GI effects (e.g., nausea, heartburn, diarrhea, constipation). May increase risk of bleeding with anticoagulants (e.g., warfarin).
Gotu kola	Reduce fatigue, anxiety, depression, improve memory and intelligence.	May cause GI upset, nausea, drowsiness. May cause additive sedative effects/side effects with CNS depressants (e.g., clonazepam, lorazepam, zolpidem).
Grapefruit	Hyperlipidemia, atherosclerosis, weight loss and obesity.	May increase concentrations/effects of benzodiazepines, calcium channel blockers, carbamazepine, carvedilol, clomipramine, cyclosporine, estrogens, lovastatin, simvastatin, atorvastatin.
Green tea	Improves cognitive performance and mental alertness.	Can cause nausea, vomiting, abdominal bloating, dyspepsia, flatulence, diarrhea. Higher doses can cause dizziness, insomnia, fatigue, agitation. May increase effects of amphetamines, caffeine.

Continued

Name	Uses	Comments
Hawthorn	Congestive HF, coronary heart disease, angina, arrhythmias.	Generally well tolerated. Can cause vertigo, dizziness, nausea, GI complaints, fatigue, sweating, rash.
Kava kava	Anxiety disorders, stress, attention-deficit hyperactivity disorder (ADHD), insomnia, restlessness.	GI upset, headache, dizziness, drowsiness, enlarged pupils and disturbances of oculomotor equilibrium and accommodation, dry mouth, allergic skin reactions. May increase drowsiness, motor reflex depression with alcohol, benzodiazepines, other CNS depressants.
L-carnitine	Treatment of primary L-carnitine deficiency, acute myocardial infarction, supplement to total parenteral nutrition, L-carnitine deficiency in those requiring hemodialysis.	Can cause nausea, vomiting, abdominal cramps, heartburn, gastritis, diarrhea, body odor, seizures.
Licorice	Gastric and duodenal ulcers, sore throat, bronchitis, dyspepsia, cough, osteoarthritis, chronic gastritis, menopausal symptoms, osteoporosis, bacterial/viral infections.	Excessive ingestion can cause pseudohyperaldosteronism with sodium and water retention, hypokalemia, alkalosis. May lead to hypertension, edema, arrhythmias. May reduce effect of antihypertensive medication therapy, warfarin.
Melatonin	Jet lag, insomnia, shift-work disorder.	Can cause daytime drowsiness, headache, dizziness. May increase effect of antiplatelets, anticoagulants (e.g., aspirin, clopidogrel, enoxaparin, warfarin). May cause additive sedation with CNS depressants (e.g., alcohol, benzodiazepines).
Milk thistle	Liver disorders, chronic inflammatory liver disease, hepatic cirrhosis, chronic hepatitis.	Usually well tolerated. Can cause nausea, diarrhea, dyspepsia, flatulence, abdominal bloating, anorexia.
Nettle	Urinary disorders associated with benign prostatic hyperplasia (e.g., nocturia, frequency, dysuria, urinary retention).	Generally well tolerated. May cause GI complaints, sweating, allergic skin reactions. May decrease effects of warfarin.
Peppermint	Common cold, cough, inflammation of mouth and pharynx, sinusitis, fever, cramps of upper GI tract, dyspepsia, flatulence, irritable bowel syndrome (IBS), fever, tension headache.	Can cause heartburn, nausea, vomiting, allergic reactions including flushing and headache. May increase concentration/effects of cyclosporine.

Name	Uses	Comments
Red yeast	Maintain desirable cholesterol levels in healthy people; reduce cholesterol in hyperlipidemia; indigestion; diarrhea; improve blood circulation.	Can cause abdominal discomfort, heartburn, flatulence, dizziness. May increase cyclosporine concentration.
SAMe	Depression, anxiety, heart disease, fibromyalgia, osteoarthritis, tendonitis, dementia, Alzheimer's disease, Parkinson's disease.	Higher doses can cause flatulence, nausea, vomiting, diarrhea, constipation, headache, mild insomnia, anorexia, sweating, dizziness, nervousness. May have additive adverse effects with MAOIs including hypertension, hyperthermia, agitation, confusion, coma. May have additive serotonergic effects and serotonin syndromelike effects (e.g., agitation, tremors, tachycardia, diarrhea, hyperreflexia, shivering, diaphoresis) with antidepressants.
Saw palmetto	Symptoms of benign prostatic hyperplasia (BPH).	Can cause dizziness, headache, GI complaints (e.g., nausea, vomiting, constipation, diarrhea). May increase effect of antiplatelets, anticoagulants (e.g., aspirin, clopidogrel, enoxaparin, warfarin). May interfere with contraceptives.
St. John's wort	Depression, anxiety, heart palpitations; mood disturbances associated with menopause, ADHD, obsessive-compulsive disorder (OCD), seasonal affective disorder (SAD), premenstrual syndrome (PMS), social phobia.	Usually well tolerated. Can cause insomnia, vivid dreams, restlessness, agitation, irritability, GI discomfort, diarrhea, fatigue, dry mouth, dizziness, headache. May decrease effect of alprazolam, amitriptyline, oral contraceptives, cyclosporine, imatinib, irinotecan, NNRTIs, phenytoin, protease inhibitors, tacrolimus, warfarin. May cause additive serotonergic effects with antidepressants, paroxetine, sertraline, tramadol.
Turmeric	Osteoarthritis, rheumatoid arthritis, dyspepsia, abdominal pain, Crohn's disease, ulcerative colitis, diarrhea, flatulence, loss of appetite, hepatitis, *H. pylori*, peptic ulcers, irritable bowel syndrome.	Usually well tolerated. Can cause dyspepsia, diarrhea, distention, GERD, nausea, vomiting. May increase risk of bleeding with antiplatelets/anticoagulants. May increase risk of hypoglycemia with antidiabetic drugs.

Continued

Name	Uses	Comments
Valerian	Insomnia, anxiety-associated restlessness, sleeping disorders.	Can cause headache, excitability, insomnia, gastric discomfort, dry mouth, vivid dreams, morning drowsiness. May have additive sedative effects with alcohol, benzodiazepines, other CNS depressants.
Yohimbe	Aphrodisiac, impotence, exhaustion, angina, hypertension, diabetic neuropathy, postural hypotension.	Can cause excitation, tremors, insomnia, anxiety, hypertension, tachycardia, dizziness, irritability, headache, fluid retention, rash, nausea, vomiting. High doses can cause respiratory depression. May have additive effects with MAOIs. Tyramine-containing foods increase risk of hypertensive crisis.

LIFESPAN, CULTURAL ASPECTS, AND PHARMACOGENOMICS OF DRUG THERAPY

LIFESPAN

Drug therapy is unique to pts of different ages. Age-specific competencies involve understanding the development and health needs of the various age groups. Pregnant pts, children, and elderly people represent different age groups with important considerations during drug therapy.

CHILDREN

In pediatric drug therapy, drug administration is guided by the age of the child, weight, level of growth and development, and height. The dosage ordered is to be given either by kilogram of body weight or by square meter of body surface area, which is based on the height and weight of the child. Many dosages based on these calculations must be individualized based on pediatric response.

If the oral route of administration is used, often syrup or chewable tablets are given. Additionally, sometimes medication is added to liquid or mixed with foods. Remember to never force a child to take oral medications because choking or emotional trauma may ensue.

If an intramuscular injection is ordered, the vastus lateralis muscle in the midlateral thigh is used because the gluteus maximus is not developed until walking occurs and the deltoid muscle is too small. For intravenous medications, administer very slowly in children. If given too quickly, high serum drug levels will occur with the potential for toxicity.

PREGNANCY

Women of childbearing years should be asked about the possibility of pregnancy before any drug therapy is initiated. Advise a woman who is either planning a pregnancy or believes she may be pregnant to inform her physician immediately. During pregnancy, medications given to the mother pass to the fetus via the placenta. Teratogenic (fetal abnormalities) effects may occur. Breastfeeding while the mother is taking certain medications may not be recommended due to the potential for adverse effects on the newborn.

The choice of drug ordered for pregnant women is based on the stage of pregnancy because the fetal organs develop during the first trimester. Cautious use of drugs in women of reproductive age who are sexually active and who are not using contraceptives is essential to prevent the potential for teratogenic or embryotoxic effects.

ELDERLY

Elderly people are more likely to experience an adverse drug reaction owing to physiologic changes (e.g., visual, hearing, mobility changes, chronic diseases) and cognitive changes (short-term memory loss or alteration in the thought process) that may lead to multiple medication dosing. In chronic disease states such as hypertension, glaucoma, asthma, or arthritis, the daily ingestion of multiple medications increases the potential for adverse reactions and toxic effects.

Decreased renal or hepatic function may lower the metabolism of medications in the liver and reduce excretion of medications, thus prolonging the half-life of the drug and the potential for toxicity. Dosages in elderly people should initially be smaller than for the general adult population and then slowly titrated based on pt response and therapeutic effect of the medication.

CULTURE

The term *ethnopharmacology* was first used to describe the study of medicinal plants used by indigenous cultures. More recently, it is being used as a reference to the action and effects of drugs in people from diverse racial, ethnic, and cultural backgrounds. Although there are insufficient data from investigations involving people from diverse backgrounds that would provide reliable information on ethnic-specific responses to all medications, there is growing evidence that modifications in dosages are needed for some members of racial and ethnic groups. There are wide variations in the perception of side effects by pts from diverse cultural backgrounds. These differences may be related to metabolic differences that result in higher or lower levels of the drug, individual differences in the amount of body fat, or cultural differences in the way individuals perceive the meaning of side effects and toxicity. Nurses and other health care providers need to be aware that variations can occur with side effects, adverse reactions, and toxicity so that pts from diverse cultural backgrounds can be monitored.

Some cultural differences in response to medications include the following:

African Americans: Generally, African Americans are less responsive to beta blockers (e.g., propranolol [Inderal]) and angiotensin-converting enzyme (ACE) inhibitors (e.g., enalapril [Vasotec]).

Asian Americans: On average, Asian Americans have a lower percentage of body fat, so dosage adjustments must be made for fat-soluble vitamins and other drugs (e.g., vitamin K used to reverse the anticoagulant effect of warfarin).

Hispanic Americans: Hispanic Americans may require lower dosages and may experience a higher incidence of side effects with tricyclic antidepressants (e.g., amitriptyline).

Native Americans: Alaskan Eskimos may suffer prolonged muscle paralysis with the use of succinylcholine when administered during surgery.

There has been a desire to exert more responsibility over one's health and, as a result, a resurgence of self-care practices. These practices are often influenced by folk remedies and the use of medicinal plants. In the United States, there are several major ethnic population subgroups (white, black, Hispanic, Asian, and Native Americans). Each of these ethnic groups has a wide range of practices that influence beliefs and interventions related to health and illness. At any given time, in any group, treatment may consist of the use of traditional herbal therapy, a combination of ritual and prayer with medicinal plants, customary dietary and environmental practices, or the use of Western medical practices.

AFRICAN AMERICANS

Many African Americans carry the traditional health beliefs of their African heritage. Health denotes harmony with nature of the body, mind, and spirit, whereas illness is seen as disharmony that results from natural causes or divine punishment. Common practices to the art of healing include treatments with herbals and rituals known empirically to restore health. Specific forms of healing include using home remedies, obtaining medical advice from a physician, and seeking spiritual healing.

Examples of healing practices include the use of hot baths and warm compresses for rheumatism, the use of herbal teas for respiratory illnesses, and the use of kitchen condiments in folk remedies. Lemon, vinegar, honey, saltpeter, alum, salt, baking soda, and Epsom salt are common kitchen ingredients used. Goldenrod, peppermint, sassafras, parsley, yarrow, and rabbit tobacco are a few of the herbals used.

HISPANIC AMERICANS

The use of folk healers, medicinal herbs, magic, and religious rituals and ceremonies are included in the rich and varied customs of Hispanic Americans. This ethnic group believes that God is responsible for allowing health or illness to occur. Wellness may be viewed as good luck, a reward for good behavior, or a blessing from God. Praying, using herbals and spices, wearing religious objects such as medals, and maintaining a balance in diet and physical activity are methods considered appropriate in preventing evil or poor health.

Hispanic ethnopharmacology is more complementary to Western medical practices. After the illness is identified, appropriate treatment may consist of home remedies (e.g., use of vegetables and herbs), use of over-the-counter patent medicines, and use of physician-prescribed medications.

ASIAN AMERICANS

For Asian Americans, harmony with nature is essential for physical and spiritual well-being. Universal balance depends on harmony among the elemental forces: fire, water, wood, earth, and metal. Regulating these universal elements are two forces that maintain physical and spiritual harmony in the body: the *yin* and the *yang*. Practices shared by most Asian cultures include meditation, special nutritional programs, herbology, and martial arts.

Therapeutic options available to traditional Chinese physicians include prescribing herbs, meditation, exercise, nutritional changes, and acupuncture.

NATIVE AMERICANS

The theme of total harmony with nature is fundamental to traditional Native American beliefs about health. It is dependent on maintaining a state of equilibrium among the physical body, the mind, and the environment. Health practices reflect this holistic approach. The method of healing is determined traditionally by the medicine man, who diagnoses the ailment and recommends the appropriate intervention.

Treatment may include heat, herbs, sweat baths, massage, exercise, diet changes, and other interventions performed in a curing ceremony.

EUROPEAN AMERICANS

Europeans often use home treatments as the front-line interventions. Traditional remedies practiced are based on the magical or empirically validated experience of ancestors. These cures are often practiced in combination with religious rituals or spiritual ceremonies.

Household products, herbal teas, and patent medicines are familiar preparations used in home treatments (e.g., saltwater gargle for sore throat).

PHARMACOGENOMICS

Traditionally, medications are prescribed using a "one size fits all" philosophy. In general, the genetic makeup is similar in all humans, regardless of race or sex. However, people inherit variations in their genes, which can affect the way a person responds to a medication. A genetic variation may make a medication stay in the body longer, causing serious side effects, or a variation may make the medication less potent.

For example, two people taking the same cancer medication may have very different responses. One may have severe, life-threatening side effects, whereas the second may have few, if any, side effects. The drug may shrink a tumor in one person but not in another.

Pharmacogenomics examines how a person's genetic makeup affects response to medications. Although widespread application still lies in the future, pharmacogenomics has the potential to personalize medical therapies. Physicians eventually will be able to prescribe medications based on an individual's genotype, thereby maximizing effectiveness and minimizing side effects.

PHARMACOGENOMICS

Pharmacogenomics is an expanding field that explores the effect of inter-individual genetic differences on pharmacokinetics, pharmacodynamics, drug efficiency, and safety of drug treatments. Pharmacogenomic biomarkers (proteins) can provide predictive tools for improving drug response and reducing adverse drug reactions. These biomarkers mainly originate from genes encoding drug-metabolizing enzymes, drug transporters, drugs targets, and human leukocyte antigens. Currently, more than 100 drugs contain pharmacogenomic information in the package labeling. The goal is to develop personalized genetic-based strategies that will optimize therapeutic outcomes.

Personalized treatments are especially warranted when prescribing medications with a narrow therapeutic index or when toxicity can be life threatening. Antineoplastics, anticoagulants, and anti-HIV therapies are often administered at maximum tolerated doses. This approach can result in toxicity and/or produce a poor response to therapy. Severe adverse drug reactions are one of the most common reasons for hospital admissions. Genetic testing for drug responses is expected to decrease hospitalizations by as much as 30%.

Carbamazepine (Tegretol) has been linked to dose-dependent side effects and life-threatening adverse effects. It is metabolized by enzymes encoded by the CYP3A4 gene to its active metabolite. An association has been found between the HLA-B*1502 allele and risk of Stevens-Johnson syndrome/toxic epidermal necrolysis, particularly in Asians. Before initiating carbamazepine treatment in high-risk patients, genetic testing for the HLA-B*1502 allele is recommended by the Food and Drug Administration (FDA).

Tumor cells carry the same genetic polymorphisms of normal cells. However, malignant cells are genetically unstable and can produce genetic changes that can alter disposition of active drug at the tumor site. Genetic analysis of tumors can help predict therapeutic benefit (or lack thereof) of targeted biologics such as **trastuzumab (Herceptin)** for ERBB2 *(HER2)*-amplified breast cancers or **erlotinib (Tarceva)** for epidermal growth factor receptor (EGFR)-overexpressing lung cancers.

Genetic mutations in tumors can also predict resistance to treatment, as noted in colorectal cancers, where activating mutations in *KRAS* are known to be a predictive marker for resistance to the EGFR-specific monoclonal antibodies **cetuximab (Erbitux)** and **panitumumab (Vectibix).**

By utilizing the information provided by pharmacogenomic testing, drug therapy is changing to a more individualized approach. Anticipated benefits of pharmacogenomics include creation of better vaccines, safer medications targeted to specific diseases, and more appropriate dosing of medications at the onset of therapy. Ultimately, we may see a decrease in health care costs due to more efficient clinical trials, reduced adverse drug reactions, and less time needed to find effective therapy for patients.

Appendix H

NORMAL LABORATORY VALUES

HEMATOLOGY/COAGULATION

Test	Normal Range
Activated partial thromboplastin time (aPTT)	25–35 sec
Erythrocyte count (RBC count)	M: 4.5–5.5 million cells/mm^3 F: 4.0–4.9 million cells/mm^3
Hematocrit (HCT, Hct)	M: 41%–50% F: 36%–44%
Hemoglobin (Hb, Hgb)	M: 13.5–16.5 g/dL F: 12.0–15.0 g/dL
Leukocyte count (WBC count)	4.5–10.0 thousand cells/mm^3
Leukocyte differential count	
Basophils	0%–0.75%
Eosinophils	1%–3%
Lymphocytes	25%–33%
Monocytes	3%–7%
Neutrophils—bands	3%–5%
Neutrophils—segmented	54%–62%
Mean corpuscular hemoglobin (MCH)	26–34 pg/cell
Mean corpuscular hemoglobin concentration (MCHC)	31%–37% Hb/cell
Mean corpuscular volume (MCV)	80–100 fL
Partial thromboplastin time (PTT)	60–85 sec
Platelet count (thrombocyte count)	100–450 thousand/mm^3
Prothrombin time (PT)	11–13.5 sec
RBC count (see Erythrocyte count)	

CLINICAL CHEMISTRY (SERUM PLASMA, URINE)

Test	Normal Range
Alanine aminotransferase (ALT)	8–36 units/L 8–78 units/L (children 0–2 mos)
Albumin	3.2–5 g/dL
Alkaline phosphatase	33–131 (adults 25–60 yrs) 51–153 (adults older than 60 yrs)
Amylase	30–110 units/L
Aspartate aminotransferase (AST)	5–35 units/L
Bilirubin (direct)	0–0.3 mg/dL
Bilirubin (total)	0.1–1.2 mg/dL
BUN	7–20 mg/dL

1273

Test	Normal Range
Calcium, ionized	2.24–2.46 mEq/L
Calcium (total)	8.6–10.3 mg/dL
Carbon dioxide (CO_2) total	23–30 mEq/L
Chloride	95–108 mEq/L
Cholesterol (total) 　HDL cholesterol 　LDL cholesterol	Less than 200 mg/dL 40–60 mg/dL Less than 160 mg/dL
Creatinine	0.5–1.4 mg/dL
Creatinine clearance	M: 80–125 mL/min/1.73 m^2 F: 75–115 mL/min/1.73 m^2
Creatine kinase (CK) isoenzymes 　CK-BB 　CK-MB (cardiac) 　CK-MM (muscle)	0% 0%–3.9% 96%–100%
Creatine phosphokinase (CPK)	8–150 units/L
Ferritin	13–300 ng/mL
Glucose (preprandial)	Less than 115 mg/dL
Glucose (fasting)	60–110 mg/dL
Glucose (nonfasting, 2 hrs postprandial)	Less than 120 mg/dL
Hemoglobin A1c	Less than 8
Iron	66–150 mcg/dL
Iron-binding capacity, total (TIBC)	250–420 mcg/dL
Lactate dehydrogenase (LDH)	56–194 units/L
Lipase	23–208 units/L
Magnesium	1.6–2.5 mg/dL
Osmolality	289–308 mOsm/kg
Oxygen saturation	90–95 (arterial) 40–70 (venous)
pH	7.35–7.45 (arterial) 7.32–7.42 (venous)
Phosphorus, inorganic	2.8–4.2 mg/dL
Potassium	3.5–5.2 mEq/L
Protein (total)	6.5–7.9 g/dL
Sodium	134–149 mEq/L
Thyroid-stimulating hormone (TSH)	0.7–6.4 milliunits/L (adults 20 yrs or younger) 0.4–4.2 milliunits/L (adults 21–54 yrs) 0.5–8.9 milliunits/L (adults 55–87 yrs)
Transferrin	Greater than 200 mg/dL
Triglycerides (TG)	45–155 mg/dL
Urea nitrogen	7–20 mg/dL
Uric acid	M: 2–8 mg/dL F: 2–7.5 mg/dL

CYTOCHROME P450 (CYP) ENZYMES

Most drugs are eliminated from the body, at least in part, by being changed chemically to a less lipid-soluble product (i.e., metabolized) and thus more likely to be excreted from the body via the kidney or bile. Drugs may go through two different metabolic processes: phase 1 and phase 2 metabolism.

In phase 1 metabolism, hepatic microsomal enzymes found in the endothelium of liver cells metabolize drugs via hydrolysis and oxidation and reduction reactions. These chemical reactions make the drug more water soluble. In phase 2 metabolism, large water-soluble substances (e.g., glucuronic acid, sulfate) are attached to the drug, forming inactive, or significantly less active, water-soluble metabolites. Phase 2 processes include glucuronidation, sulfation, conjugation, acetylation, and methylation.

Virtually any of the phase 1 and phase 2 enzymes can be inhibited, and some of these enzymes can be induced by drugs. Inhibiting the activity of metabolic enzymes results in increased concentrations of the drug (substrate), whereas inducing metabolic enzymes results in decreased concentrations of the drug (substrate).

The term "cytochrome P450" (CYP enzymes) refers to a family of more than 100 enzymes in the human body that modulate various physiologic functions. First identified in the 1950s, the CYP enzyme system contains two large subgroups: steroidogenic and xenobiotic enzymes. Only the xenobiotic group is involved in the metabolism of drugs. The xenobiotic group includes four major enzyme families: CYP1, CYP2, CYP3, and CYP4. The primary role of these families is the metabolism of drugs. These families are further subdivided into subfamilies designated by a capital letter and given a specific enzyme number (1, 2, 3, etc.) according to the similarity in amino acid sequence it shares with other enzymes (e.g., CYP1A2).

The key CYP450 enzymes include CYP1A2, CYP2C9, CYP2C19, CYP2D6, and CYP3A4 and may be responsible for metabolism of 75% of all drugs, with the CYP3A subfamily responsible for nearly half of this activity.

The CYP enzymes are found in the endoplasmic reticulum of cells in a variety of human tissue but are primarily concentrated in the liver and intestine. CYP enzymes can be both inhibited and induced, leading to increased or decreased serum concentration of the drug (along with its effects).

The following tables of CYP substrates, inhibitors, and inducers provide a perspective on drugs that are affected by, or affect, cytochrome P450 (CYP) enzymes. **CYP substrate** includes drugs reported to be metabolized, at least in part, by one or more CYP enzymes. **CYP inhibitor** includes drugs reported to inhibit one or more CYP enzymes. **CYP inducer** contains drugs reported to induce one or more CYP enzymes.

P450 ENZYMES: SUBSTRATES, INHIBITORS, INDUCERS
CYP1A2 ENZYME

CYP1A2 SUBSTRATES	CYP1A2 INHIBITORS	CPY1A2 INDUCERS
Caffeine	Cimetidine (Tagamet)	Barbiturates
Clozapine (Clozaril)	Ciprofloxacin (Cipro)	Carbamazepine (Tegretol)
Mirtazapine (Remeron)	Fluvoxamine	Rifampin (Rifadin)
Olanzapine (Zyprexa)	Zileuton (Zyflo)	Smoking
Ramelteon (Rozerem)		
Ropinirole (Requip)		
Tizanidine (Zanaflex)		

- CYP1A2 enzyme is increasingly involved in drug interactions.
- More potent inhibitors include cimetidine, ciprofloxacin, and fluvoxamine.
- Smoking is the most important inducer, but rifampin and barbiturates also can increase enzyme activity.
- Example of reaction: Tizanidine plasma concentrations increased more than 30-fold when the inhibitor fluvoxamine was given concurrently.

CYP2C9 ENZYME

CYP2C9 SUBSTRATES	CYP2C9 INHIBITORS	CYP2C9 INDUCERS
Candesartan (Atacand)	Amiodarone (Cordarone)	Barbiturates
Celecoxib (Celebrex)	Clopidogrel (Plavix)	Carbamazepine (Tegretol)
Diclofenac (Voltaren)	Fluconazole (Diflucan)	Rifampin (Rifadin)
Glipizide (Glucotrol)	Metronidazole (Flagyl)	St. John's wort
Glyburide (DiaBeta)	Sulfamethoxazole	
Ibuprofen (Advil, Motrin)	Valproic acid (Depakote)	
Irbesartan (Avapro)		
Meloxicam (Mobic)		
Warfarin (Coumadin)		

- More potent inhibitors include amiodarone, metronidazole, and sulfamethoxazole.
- All of the inducers can substantially increase enzyme activity.
- Both warfarin and oral hypoglycemics are of serious concern with regard to drug interactions. Substrates warranting attention include warfarin and oral hypoglycemics.

CYP2C19 ENZYME

CYP2C19 SUBSTRATES	CYP2C19 INHIBITORS	CYP2C19 INDUCERS
Citalopram (Celexa)	Cimetidine (Tagamet)	Barbiturates
Diazepam (Valium)	Clopidogrel (Plavix)	Carbamazepine (Tegretol)
Escitalopram (Lexapro)	Esomeprazole (Nexium)	Rifampin (Rifadin)
Omeprazole (Prilosec)	Fluconazole (Diflucan)	St. John's wort
Pantoprazole (Protonix)	Fluvoxamine	
Sertraline (Zoloft)	Modafinil (Provigil)	

- Inhibition by itself does not frequently cause adverse effects compared with other CYP enzymes because many of the substrates do not have serious toxicity.
- Inhibition or induction of the enzyme nonetheless may result in an adverse drug interaction.
- Racial background is important in the likelihood of being deficient in this enzyme (e.g., 3%–5% of Caucasians and 12%–23% of Asians are poor metabolizers of this enzyme).

CYP2D6 ENZYME

CYP2D6 SUBSTRATES	CYP2D6 INHIBITORS	CYP2D6 INDUCERS
Amitriptyline (Elavil)	Amiodarone (Cordarone)	See comment below
Atomoxetine (Strattera)	Bupropion (Wellbutrin)	
Duloxetine (Cymbalta)	Fluoxetine (Prozac)	
Fluoxetine (Prozac)	Paroxetine (Paxil)	
Metoclopramide (Reglan)		
Metoprolol (Lopressor)		
Paroxetine (Paxil)		
Risperidone (Risperdal)		
Tamoxifen (Nolvadex)		
Tolterodine (Detrol)		
Tramadol (Ultram)		
Venlafaxine (Effexor)		

- Potent inhibitors include fluoxetine and paroxetine.
- Evidence suggests that this enzyme is not very susceptible to enzyme induction.
- Genetics, rather than drug therapy, accounts for most ultra-rapid metabolizers (e.g., Greeks, Portuguese, Saudis, and Ethiopians have high enzyme activity).

CYP3A4 ENZYME

CYP3A4 SUBSTRATES	CYP3A4 INHIBITORS	CYP3A4 INDUCERS
Alfuzosin (Uroxatral)	Amiodarone (Cordarone)	Carbamazepine (Tegretol)
Alprazolam (Xanax)	Clarithromycin (Biaxin)	Efavirenz (Sustiva)
Budesonide (Entocort EC)	Diltiazem (Cardizem)	Phenobarbital
Carbamazepine (Tegretol)	Erythromycin (Ery-Tab)	Rifampin (Rifadin)
Cyclosporine (Neoral)	Fluconazole (Diflucan)	St. John's wort
Fluticasone (Flovent)	Fluoxetine (Prozac)	
Lovastatin (Mevacor)	Itraconazole (Sporanox)	
Repaglinide (Prandin)	Ketoconazole (Nizoral)	
Sildenafil (Viagra)	Verapamil (Calan, Isoptin)	
Simvastatin (Zocor)		
Tadalafil (Cialis)		

- This enzyme metabolizes about half of all medications on the market.
- Drug toxicity of CYP3A4 substrates due to inhibition of CYP3A4 is relatively common.
- This enzyme is very sensitive to induction, tending to lower plasma concentrations of substrates, resulting in reduced efficacy of the substrate.
- Most potent inhibitors include clarithromycin, itraconazole, and ketoconazole.
- Rifampin is a potent inducer and may reduce serum concentrations of substrates by as much as 90%.

ANTIDOTE/REVERSAL AGENTS

Agent	Antidote/ Reversal Agents	Dosage
Acetaminophen	Acetylcysteine (Acetadote, Mucomyst)	PO: ADULTS, CHILDREN: Loading dose: 140 mg/kg, then 70 mg/kg q4h for a total of 18 doses. Total dose delivered: 1,330 mg/kg. IV: ADULTS, CHILDREN: Loading dose: 150 mg/kg over 60 min, then 50 mg/kg over 4 hrs, then 100 mg/kg over 16 hrs. Total dose delivered: 300 mg/kg.
Anticholinergic agents (e.g., atropine)	Physostigmine	IM/IV/SQ: ADULTS: Initially, 0.5–2 mg, then repeat q20min until response occurs or adverse effects occur. Repeat 1–4 mg q30–60min as life-threatening symptoms recur. IV: CHILDREN (Reserve for life-threatening situation only): 0.01–0.03 mg/kg/dose. May repeat after 15–20 min to maximum total dose of 2 mg, or until response occurs or adverse cholinergic effects occur.
Apixaban (Eliquis)	Kcentra Prothrombin Complex concentrate (Factors II, VII, IX, X, Protein C, Protein S)	Dose based on pre-dose INR, expressed in units of factor IX activity. (Give with Vitamin K) **INR 2 to <4:** 25 units/kg. **Maximum:** 2,500 units. **INR 4–6:** 35 units/kg. **Maximum:** 3,500 units. **INR >6:** 50 units/kg. **Maximum:** 5,000 units.
Arsenic	Dimercaprol (BAL in oil)	Mild Poisoning IM: ADULTS, CHILDREN: 2.5 mg/kg/dose q6h for 2 days, then q12h for 1 day, then once daily for 10 days. Severe Poisoning IM: ADULTS, CHILDREN: 3 mg/kg/dose q4h for 2 days, then q6h for 1 day, then q12h for 10 days.
Benzodiaze- pines (e.g., midazolam)	Flumazenil (Romazicon)	IV: ADULTS: 0.2 mg over 30 sec. May give 0.3-mg dose after 30 sec if desired LOC not obtained. Additional doses of 0.5 mg can be given over 30 sec at 1-min intervals up to cumulative dose of 3 mg. CHILDREN: 0.01 mg/kg (**maximum: 0.2 mg**) with repeat doses of 0.01 mg/kg (**maximum: 0.2 mg**) given every minute to maximum total cumulative dose of 1 mg.
Beta blockers (e.g., propranolol)	Glucagon	IV: ADULTS: 5–10 mg over 1 min, followed by infusion of 1–10 mg/hr.
Calcium channel blockers (e.g., verapamil)	Glucagon	IV: ADULTS: 5–10 mg over 1 min, followed by infusion of 1–10 mg/hr.

Continued

1279

Agent	Antidote/ Reversal Agents	Dosage
Carbamate pesticides	Atropine	IV: ADULTS: Initially, 1–5 mg doubled q5min until signs of muscarinic excess abate. IV INFUSION: ADULTS: 0.5–1 mg/hr. IM: ADULTS (Mild symptoms): 2 mg. If severe symptoms develop after first dose, 2 additional doses should be repeated in 10 min. (Severe symptoms): Immediately administer three 2-mg doses. IV: CHILDREN: 0.02–0.05 mg/kg q10-20min until atropine effect observed, then q1–4h for at least 24 hrs. IM: 0.5–2 mg/dose based on weight (0.5 mg: 15–40 lb, 1 mg: 41–90 lb, 2 mg: greater than 90 lb). (Mild symptoms): 1 injection. (Severe symptoms): 2 additional injections given in rapid succession 10 min after receiving first injection.
Dabigatran (Pradaxa)	Idarucizumab (Praxbind)	IV: 5 g (give as 2 separate 2.5 g doses no more than 15 minutes apart).
Digoxin (Lanoxin)	Digoxin immune FAB (Digibind)	**ADULTS** Unknown amount of ingestion: 800 mg IV infusion if acute ingestion, 240 mg IV infusion if chronic ingestion. **Dosing for Ingestion of Single Large Dose** Dose (in no. of vials) = (Total digitalis body load in mg)/(0.5 mg of digitalis bound per vial). Total digitalis body load in mg = (No. of tablets/capsules ingested) × (mg strength of tablet/capsule) × (bioavailability of tablet/capsule). Digoxin tablets and elixir are 80% bioavailable. Digoxin capsules and injection are 100% bioavailable. **Dosing Based on Serum Level** Digoxin: Dose (in no. of vials) = (Serum digoxin level in ng/mL) × (weight in kg)/(100). Digitoxin: Dose (in no. of vials) = (Serum digitoxin level in ng/mL) × (weight in kg)/(1,000). **CHILDREN** **Dosing for Ingestion of Single Large Dose** Dose (in no. of vials) = (Total digitalis body load in mg)/(0.5 mg of digitalis bound per vial). Total digitalis body load in mg = (No. of tablets/capsules ingested) × (mg strength of tablet/capsule) × (bioavailability of tablet/capsule). Digoxin tablets and elixir are 80% bioavailable. Digoxin capsules and injection are 100% bioavailable. WEIGHING 20 kg or less: Dilution of reconstituted vial to 1 mg/mL may be desirable for doses of 3 mg or less. Dose (in no. of mg) = Dose (in no. of vials) × 38 mg/vial. Dose (in no. of vials) = (Serum digoxin level in ng/mL) × (weight in kg)/(100).

Agent	Antidote/ Reversal Agents	Dosage
Edoxaban (Savaysa)	see apixaban (Eliquis)	see apixaban (Eliquis)
Ethylene glycol	Fomepizole (Antizol)	IV: ADULTS, CHILDREN: Loading dose 15 mg/kg, then 10 mg/kg q12h for 4 doses, then 15 mg/kg q12h thereafter until ethylene glycol levels reduced to less than 20 mg/dL and patient is asymptomatic with normal pH.
Extravasation vasoconstrictive agents (e.g., dopamine)	Phentolamine (Regitine)	ADULTS, CHILDREN: Infiltrate area with small amount of solution made by diluting 5–10 mg in 10 mL 0.9% NaCl within 12 hrs of extravasation. In general, do not exceed 0.1–0.2 mg/kg (5 mg total).
Heparin	Protamine	IV: ADULTS, CHILDREN: Dosage is determined by most recent dosage of heparin or low molecular weight heparin (LWH): 1 mg protamine neutralizes 90–115 units of heparin and 1 mg (100 units) of LWH. **Maximum:** 50 mg.
Iron	Deferoxamine (Desferal)	Acute IM: ADULTS: Initially, 1,000 mg, then 500 mg q4h for 2 doses. Additional doses of 0.5 g q4–12h. **Maximum:** 6 g/24 hrs. CHILDREN 3 YRS AND OLDER: 90 mg/kg/ dose q8h (not to exceed 1 g/dose). **Maximum:** 6 g/24 hrs. IV: ADULTS, CHILDREN: 15 mg/kg/hr. **Maximum:** 6 g/24 hrs. Chronic IM: ADULTS: 500–1,000 mg/day. IV: ADULTS, CHILDREN: 15 mg/kg/hr. **Maximum:** 12 g/24 hrs.
Isoniazid	Pyridoxine (vitamin B$_6$)	IV: ADULTS, CHILDREN: Total dose of pyridoxine equal to amount of isoniazid ingested as first dose 1–4 g IV, then 1 g IM q30min until total dose completed. If not known, give 5 g at rate of 1 g/min. May repeat q5–10min.
Lead	Calcium EDTA	Symptomatic Treat for 3–5 days; give in conjunction with dimercaprol. IM: ADULTS, CHILDREN: 167 mg/m^2 q4h. IV: ADULTS, CHILDREN: 1 g/m2 as 8- to 24-hr infusion or divided q12h. Lead Encephalopathy Treat for 5 days; give concurrently with dimercaprol. IM: ADULTS, CHILDREN: 250 mg/m^2 q4h. IV: ADULTS, CHILDREN: 50 mg/kg/day as 24-hr continuous infusion.

Continued

Agent	Antidote/Reversal Agents	Dosage
Lead	Dimercaprol (BAL in oil)	**Mild** IM: ADULTS, CHILDREN: Loading dose 4 mg/kg, then 3 mg/kg/dose q4h for 2–7 days. Begin calcium EDTA with second dose. **Severe and Lead Encephalopathy** IM: ADULTS, CHILDREN: 4 mg/kg/dose q4h for 3–5 days. Begin calcium EDTA with second dose.
Lead	Succimer (Chemet)	PO: ADULTS, CHILDREN: 10 mg/kg/dose q8h for 5 days, then q12h for 14 days. **Maximum:** 500 mg/dose. Note: For children younger than 5 yrs, dose based on mg/m^2.
Methanol	Fomepizole (Antizol)	IV: ADULTS, CHILDREN: Loading dose 15 mg/kg, then 10 mg/kg q12h for 4 doses, then 15 mg/kg q12h thereafter until ethylene glycol levels reduced to less than 20 mg/dL and patient is asymptomatic with normal pH.
Opioids (e.g., morphine)	Naloxone (Narcan)	IV/IM/SQ: ADULTS: 0.4–2 mg/dose. May repeat every 2–3 min as needed. Therapy may need to be reassessed if no response is seen after cumulative dose of 10 mg. CHILDREN (5 YRS OR OLDER or WEIGHING 20 KG OR GREATER): 2 mg/dose IV/IM/SQ. May repeat every 2–3 min as needed. Therapy may need to be reassessed if no response is seen after cumulative dose of 10 mg. CHILDREN (WEIGHING LESS THAN 20 KG): 0.1 mg/kg/dose. May repeat every 2–3 min as needed.
Organophosphate pesticides	Atropine	IV: ADULTS: Initially, 1–5 mg doubled q5min until signs of muscarinic excess abate. IV INFUSION: ADULTS: 0.5–1 mg/hr. IM: ADULTS (Mild symptoms): 2 mg. If severe symptoms develop after first dose, 2 additional doses should be repeated in 10 min. (Severe symptoms): Immediately administer three 2-mg doses. IV: CHILDREN: 0.02–0.05 mg/kg q10–20min until atropine effect observed, then q1–4h for at least 24 hrs. IM: 0.5–2 mg/dose based on weight (0.5 mg: 15–40 lb, 1 mg: 41–90 lb, 2 mg: greater than 90 lb). (Mild symptoms): 1 injection. (Severe symptoms): 2 additional injections given in rapid succession 10 min after receiving first injection.

Agent	Antidote/Reversal Agents	Dosage
Organophosphate pesticides	Pralidoxime (Protopam)	IM/IV: ADULTS: 1–2 g. Repeat in 1–2 hrs if muscle weakness has not been relieved, then at 10- to 12-hr intervals if cholinergic signs recur. CHILDREN: 20–50 mg/kg/dose. Repeat in 1–2 hrs if muscle weakness is not relieved, then at 10- to 12-hr intervals if cholinergic signs recur.
Rivaroxaban (Xarelto)	See apixaban (Eliquis)	see apixaban (Eliquis)
Warfarin (Coumadin)	Phytonadi- one (vitamin K)	PO/IV/SQ: ADULTS: 2.5–10 mg/dose. May repeat in 12–48 hrs if given PO, 6–8 hrs if given by IV or SQ route. CHILDREN: 0.5–5 mg depending on need for further anticoagulation, severity of bleeding.

PREVENTING MEDICATION ERRORS AND IMPROVING MEDICATION SAFETY

Medication safety is a high priority for the health care professional. Prevention of medication errors and improved safety for the pt are important, esp. in today's health care environment when today's pt is older and sometimes sicker and the drug therapy regimen can be more sophisticated and complex.

A medication error is defined by the National Coordinating Council for Medication Error Reporting and Prevention (NCC MERP) as "any preventable event that may cause or lead to inappropriate medication use or pt harm while the medication is in the control of the health care professional, pt, or consumer."

Most medication errors occur as a result of multiple, compounding events as opposed to a single act by a single individual.

Use of the wrong medication, strength, or dose; confusion over sound-alike or look-alike drugs; administration of medications by the wrong route; miscalculations (esp. when used in pediatric pts or when administering medications intravenously); and errors in prescribing and transcription all can contribute to compromising the safety of the pt. The potential for adverse events and medication errors is definitely a reality and is potentially tragic and costly in both human and economic terms.

Health care professionals must take the initiative to create and implement procedures to prevent medication errors from occurring and implement methods to reduce medication errors. The first priority in preventing medication errors is to establish a multidisciplinary team to improve medication use. The goal for this team would be to assess medication safety and implement changes that would make it difficult or impossible for mistakes to occur. Some important criteria in making improved medication safety successful include the following:

* Promote a nonpunitive approach to reducing medication errors.
* Increase the detection and the reporting of medication errors, near misses, and potentially hazardous situations that may result in medication errors.
* Determine root causes of medication errors.
* Educate about the causes of medication errors and ways to prevent these errors.
* Make recommendations to allow organization-wide, system-based changes to prevent medication errors.
* Learn from errors that occur in other organizations and take measures to prevent similar errors.

Some common causes and ways to prevent medication errors and improve safety include the following:

Handwriting: Poor handwriting can make it difficult to distinguish between two medications with similar names. Also, many drug names sound similar, esp. when the names are spoken over the telephone, poorly enunciated, or mispronounced.

* Take time to write legibly.
* Keep phone or verbal orders to a minimum to prevent misinterpretation.

- Repeat back orders taken over the telephone.
- When ordering a new or rarely used medication, print the name.
- Always specify the drug strength, even if only one strength exists.
- Express dosages for oral liquids only in metric weights or volumes (e.g., mg or mL), not by teaspoon or tablespoon.
- Print generic and brand names of look-alike or sound-alike medications.

Zeros and decimal points: Hastily written orders can present problems even if the name of the medication is clear.

- Never leave a decimal point "naked." Place a zero before a decimal point when the number is less than a whole unit (e.g., use 0.25 mg or 250 mcg, **not** .25 mg).
- Never have a trailing zero following a decimal point (e.g., use 2 mg, **not** 2.0 mg).

Abbreviations: Errors can occur because of a failure to standardize abbreviations. Establishing a list of abbreviations that should never be used is recommended.

- Never abbreviate unit as "U"; spell out "unit."
- Do not abbreviate "once daily" as OD or QD or "every other day" as QOD; spell it out.
- Do not use D/C, as this may be misinterpreted as either discharge or discontinue.
- Do not abbreviate drug names; spell out the generic and/or brand names.

Ambiguous or incomplete orders: These types of orders can cause confusion or misinterpretation of the writer's intention. Examples include situations when the route of administration, dose, or dosage form has not been specified.

- Do not use slash marks—they may be read as the number one (1).
- When reviewing an unusual order, verify the order with the person writing the order to prevent any misunderstanding.
- Read over orders after writing.
- Encourage that the drug's indication for use be provided on medication orders.
- Provide complete medication orders—do not use "resume preop" or "continue previous meds."
- Provide the age and, when appropriate, the weight of the pt.

High-alert medications: Medications in this category have an increased risk of causing significant pt harm when used in error. Mistakes with these medications may or may not be more common but may be more devastating to the pt if an error occurs. A list of high-alert medications can be obtained from the Institute for Safe Medication Practices (ISMP) at www.ismp.org.

Technology available today that can be used to address and help solve potential medication problems or errors includes the following:

- Electronic prescribing systems—This refers to computerized prescriber order entry systems. Within these systems is the capability to incorporate medication safety alerts (e.g., maximum dose alerts, allergy screening). Additionally, these systems should be integrated or interfaced with pharmacy and laboratory systems to provide drug-drug and drug-disease interactions alerts and include clinical order screening capability.
- Bar codes—These systems are designed to use bar-code scanning devices to validate identity of pts, verify medications administered, document administration, and provide safety alerts.

- "Smart" infusion pumps—These pumps allow users to enter drug infusion protocols into a drug library along with predefined dosage limits. If a dosage is outside the limits established, an alarm is sounded and drug delivery is halted, informing the clinician that the dose is outside the recommended range.
- Automated dispensing systems; point-of-use dispensing system—These systems should be integrated with information systems, esp. pharmacy systems.
- Pharmacy order entry system—This should be fully integrated with an electronic prescribing system with the capability of producing medication safety alerts. Additionally, the system should generate a computerized medication administration record (MAR), which would be used by the nursing staff while administering medications.

Medication reconciliation: Medication errors generally occur at transition points in the pt's care (admission, transfer from one level of care to another [e.g., critical care to general care area], and discharge). Incomplete documentation can account for up to 60% of potential medication errors. Therefore, it becomes necessary to accurately and completely reconcile medication across the continuum of care. This includes the name, dosage, frequency, and route of medication administration.

Medication reconciliation programs are a process of identifying the most accurate list of all medications a pt is taking and using this list to provide correct medications anywhere within the health care system. The focus is on not only compiling a list but using the list to reduce medication errors and provide quality pt care.

Additional Strategies to Reduce Medication Errors

The ISMP, FDA, and other agencies have identified high-risk areas associated with medication errors. They include the following:

At-risk population: At-risk populations primarily include pediatric and geriatric pts. For both, this risk is due to altered pharmacokinetic parameters with little published information regarding medication use in these groups. Additionally, in the pediatric population, the risk is due to the need for calculating doses based on age and weight, lack of available dosage forms, and concentrations for smaller children.

In a USP report, more than one-third of medication errors reaching the pt occurred in pts 65 yrs of age and older. Almost 40% of people 60 yrs and older take at least five medications. More than 50% of fatal hospital medication errors involve seniors. In the senior population, age-related physiologic changes (e.g., decreased renal function, reduced muscle mass) increase the risk for adverse events.

Avoid abbreviations and nomenclature: The confusion caused by abbreviations has prompted the ISMP to develop a list of abbreviations that should be avoided (see back cover of handbook).

Recognize prescription look-alike and sound-alike medications: The ISMP has developed an extensive list of confused drug names (see www.jointcommission.org). See individual monographs for **DO NOT CONFUSE** information.

Focus on high alert medications: High alert medications are medications that bear a heightened risk of causing significant pt harm if incorrectly used. High alert medications in the handbook have a colored background for the entire monograph.

Look for duplicate therapies and interactions: Drug interactions and duplicate therapies can increase risk of adverse reactions. Refer to individual monographs for significant interaction information (drug, herbal, food).

Report errors to improve process: This action plays an important role in preventing further errors. The intent is to identify system failures that can be altered to prevent further errors.

PARENTERAL FLUID ADMINISTRATION

Replacing fluids in the body is based on body fluid needs. Water comprises approximately 60% of the adult body. Approximately 40% is intracellular fluid and 20% is extracellular fluid, of which 15% is interstitial (tissues) and 5% is intravascular. The walls separating these compartments are porous, allowing water to move freely between them. Small particles such as sodium and chloride can pass through the walls, but larger molecules such as proteins and starches usually are unable to pass through the walls.

Hydrostatic and osmotic pressures are forces that move water and regulate the body's water. Intravenous fluid manipulates these two pressures. Hydrostatic pressure reflects the weight and volume of water. The greater the volume, the higher the blood pressure.

Effects of Osmotic Pressure: *Osmosis* is the diffusion of water across a semipermeable membrane from an area of high concentration to an area of low concentration (water moves into the compartment of higher concentration of particles, or solute). This is similar to the action of a sponge soaking up water. This pull is referred to as *osmotic pressure*. It is the number of particles in each compartment that keeps water where it is supposed to be. By administering fluids with more (or fewer) particles than blood plasma, fluid is pulled into the compartment where it is needed the most.

How do we know where the water is needed? To assess water balance, measure the *osmolality* of blood plasma (number of particles [osmoles] in a kilogram of fluid). *Osmolarity* is the number of particles in a liter of fluid. Normal serum osmolality is approximately 300 milliosmoles (mOsm) per liter.

Crystalloids are made of substances that form crystals (e.g., sodium chloride) and are small, so easy movement between compartments is possible. Crystalloids are categorized by their tonicity (a synonym for osmolality). An isotonic solution has the same number of particles (osmolality) as plasma and will not promote a shift of fluids into or out of cells. Examples of isotonic crystalloid solutions are 0.9% sodium chloride and lactated Ringer's solution. Dextrose 5% in water is another isotonic crystalloid. However, it is quickly metabolized, and the fluid quickly becomes hypotonic. Hypotonic solutions (e.g., D5W, 0.45% sodium chloride) are a good source of free water, causing a shift out of the vascular bed and into cells by way of osmosis. Hypotonic solutions are given to correct cellular dehydration and hypernatremia. Hypertonic solutions have more particles than body water and pull water back into the circulation, which can shrink cells.

SODIUM CHLORIDE
USES

- Extracellular fluid replacement when chloride loss is greater than or equal to sodium loss
- Treatment of metabolic alkalosis in the presence of fluid loss; chloride ions cause a compensatory decrease of bicarbonate ions
- Sodium depletion, extracellular fluid volume deficit with sodium deficit
- Initiation and termination of blood transfusion, preventing hemolysis of RBCs (occurs with dextrose in water solutions)

SIDE EFFECTS/ABNORMALITIES

- Hypernatremia
- **Acidosis:** 0.9% sodium chloride contains one-third more chloride ions than is present in extracellular fluid; excess chloride ions cause loss of bicarbonate, resulting in acidosis
- **Hypokalemia:** Increased potassium excretion at the same time extracellular fluid is increasing, which further decreases potassium concentration in extracellular fluid
- Circulatory overload

DEXTROSE (GLUCOSE)

EFFECTS

- Provides calories for essential energy
- Improves hepatic function because it is converted into glycogen
- Spares body protein, preventing unnecessary breakdown of protein tissue
- Prevents ketosis
- Stored in the liver as glycogen, causing a shift of potassium from extracellular to intracellular fluid compartment

USES

- Dehydration
- Hyponatremia
- Hyperkalemia
- Vehicle of drug delivery and nutrition

Note: Once infused, dextrose is rapidly metabolized to water and carbon dioxide, becoming hypotonic rather than isotonic.

SIDE EFFECTS/ABNORMALITIES

- Dehydration: Osmotic diuresis occurs if dextrose is given faster than the pt's ability to metabolize it
- Hypokalemia (see Effects)
- Hyperinsulinism due to rapid infusion of hypertonic solution
- Water intoxication due to an imbalance based on increase in extracellular fluid volume from water alone

SELECTED PARENTERAL FLUIDS

Solution	Comments
Dextrose 5% in water (D_5W)	Supplies approximately 170 cal/L and free water to aid in renal excretion of solutes Avoid excessive volumes in pts with increased antidiuretic hormone activity or to replace fluids in hypovolemic pts
0.9% Sodium chloride (0.9% NaCl)	Isotonic fluid commonly used to expand extracellular fluid in presence of hypovolemia Can be used to treat mild metabolic alkalosis

Continued

Solution	Comments
0.45% Sodium chloride (0.45% NaCl)	Hypotonic solution that provides sodium, chloride, and free water; sodium and chloride allow kidneys to select and retain needed amounts Free water is desirable as aid to kidneys in elimination of solutes
3% Sodium chloride	Used only to treat severe hyponatremia
Lactated Ringer's solution	Isotonic solution that contains sodium, potassium, calcium, and chloride in approximately the same concentrations as found in plasma Used to treat hypovolemia, burns, and fluid loss as bile or diarrhea

COMMON TERMINOLOGY CRITERIA FOR ADVERSE EVENTS (CTCAE)

The Common Terminology Criteria for Adverse Events (CTCAE) is descriptive terminology used for reporting an adverse event (AE) in a concise and standardized manner. It is supported by the U.S. Department of Health and Human Services, National Institutes of Health, and National Cancer Institute. An AE term is a unique representation of a specific event that can be used for medical documentation and scientific analyses. Along with cancer medications, other drugs may use the CTCAE system for dose and treatment modifications.

CTCAE terms are grouped by system organ classes, such as *Blood/Lymphatic, GI, Nervous, Renal,* and *Respiratory* disorders. Within each system organ class, AEs are listed and accompanied by a brief description. A grading scale is then provided for each AE term, and each grade refers to a specific severity.

The CTCAE grading scale displays grades 1–5 with particular descriptions and/or recommendations. The severity for each AE is based on the following generalized guidelines: **Grade 1**: Asymptomatic or mild symptoms; clinical or diagnostic observations only; intervention not indicated. **Grade 2**: Moderate; minimal, local, or noninvasive intervention indicated; limiting age-appropriate instrumental activity of daily living (ADL). **Grade 3**: Severe or medically significant but not immediately life threatening; hospitalization or prolonged hospitalization indicated; disabling; limiting self-care ADL. **Grade 4**: Life-threatening consequences; urgent intervention indicated. **Grade 5**: Death related to AE.

CTCAE EXAMPLES

Adverse Event	Grade				
	1	2	3	4	5
Blood/ Lymphatic **Anemia**	Hgb < lower limit of normal– 10 g/dL	Hgb 8–10 g/dL	Hgb <8 g/dL; transfusion indicated	Life-threatening consequences Urgent intervention indicated	Death
Gastrointestinal **Diarrhea**	Increase of <4 stools/ day over baseline Mild ostomy output	Increase of 4–6 stools/day over baseline Moderate ostomy output	Increase of 7 stools/day over baseline Severe ostomy output Hospitalization required	Life-threatening consequences Urgent intervention indicated	Death
General **Fever**	38–39°C (100.4– 102.2°F)	>39–40°C (102.3– 104°F)	> 40°C (>104° F) for less than 24 hrs	> 40°C (>104°F) for more than 24 hrs	Death

Adverse Event	Grade				
	1	2	3	4	5
Infections **UTI**	N/A	Localized; local intervention indicated (topical, antifungal, antiviral)	IV antibiotic, antifungal, antiviral intervention indicated. Radiologic or surgical intervention indicated	Life-threatening consequences Urgent intervention indicated	Death
Investigations **Lipase increased**	>ULN–1.5 times ULN	> 1.5–2 times ULN	>2–5 times ULN	> 5 times ULN	N/A
Metabolism/ Nutrition **Hyperkalemia**	> ULN–5.5 mmol/L	> 5.5–6 mmol/L	> 6–7 mmol/L	> 7 mmol/L; life-threatening consequences	Death

ULN, Upper limit of normal.

---

bold – generic drug name   regular type – trade name

---

bold – generic drug name   regular type – trade name

---

bold page # – main drug entry

bold – generic drug name   regular type – trade name

bold page # – main drug entry

---

bold – generic drug name